INCONTINENCE

EDITORS

PAUL ABRAMS - LINDA CARDOZO - SAAD KHOURY -
ALAN WEIN

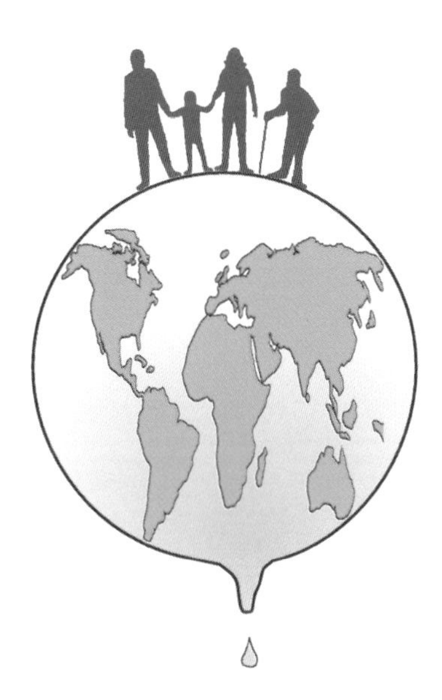

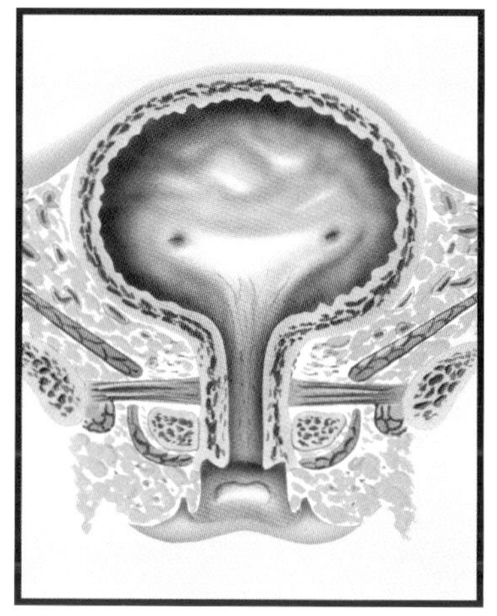

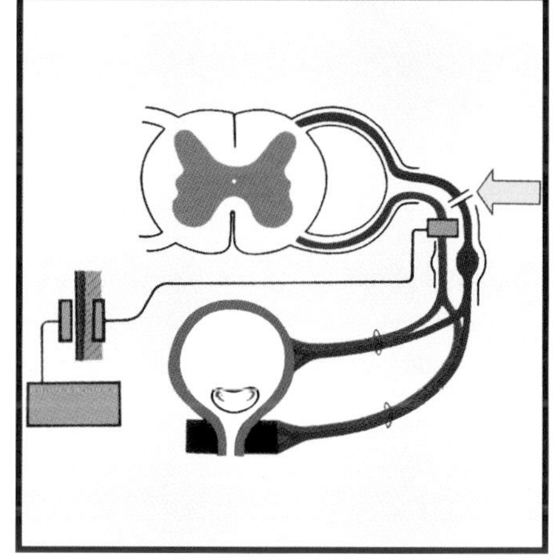

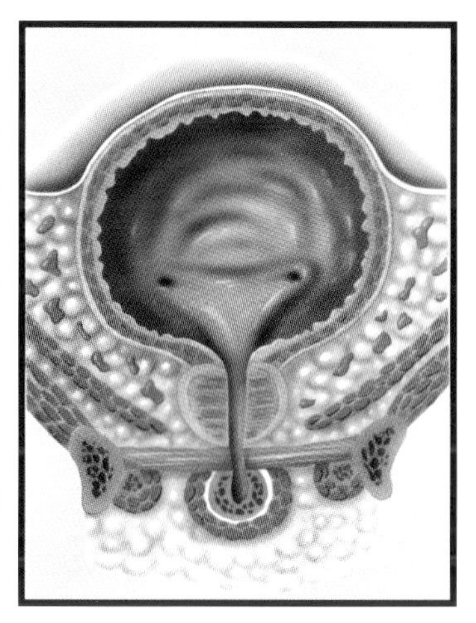

2nd International Consultation on Incontinence Paris, July 1-3, 2001

2nd Edition 2002

Aknowledgement

We would like to thank :

• The Bristol Urological Institute and

• The Urology Department at La Pitié Hospital in Paris and its chairman
Professor F. Richard

for kindly providing logistic assistance for the editing of this book.

We would also like to thank all the contributors for their enthusiastic support and help.

Distributor : Plymbridge Distributors Ltd
Estover Road, Plymouth PL6 7PY, United Kingdom
Customer Services : Tel. : +44 1752 202301 - Fax: +44 1752 202333
E-mail : cservs@plymbridge.com

ISBN 1 898452 55 5

FOREWORD

The First International Consultation on Incontinence held in 1998 highlighted the plight of some 200 million sufferers from urinary incontinence worldwide. Urinary incontinence represents a particular and severe problem in certain developing areas of the world, where labour and birth injuries lead to catastrophic leakage. Untreated vesico-vaginal fistula, particularly in sub Saharan Africa, affects millions of women causing ostracizism from society. Because of the enormity of this particular problem, the second consultation had a specific committee to highlight the subject, to advance the understanding of the causes of birth injury, to lead to improved treatment for the many untreated women, and most importantly, to begin preventative programmes.

There were three new committees in the 2nd ICI: Pelvic Organ Prolapse, Faecal Incontinence and Incontinence in the Developing World, (mentioned above). The first consultation stressed the importance of a multidisciplinary approach to continence care, and the new committees on pelvic organ prolapse and faecal incontinence recognize that, particularly in women, urinary incontinence coexists with prolapse and faecal incontinence in many instances. This is also true, to a more limited extent, in men with coexisting faecal incontinence. The task of these two committees was very considerable and they had to outline the basic science, and investigation and management techniques within a single chapter.

The report of these two chapters will lay the foundation for a broadening of the multidisciplinary approach to pelvic disorders. Already there are various models of a new ways of working with close collaboration between urologists, gynaecologists and coloproctologists, working within a multidisciplinary team with nurses and physiotherapists. From the research and investigation point of view, we were very dependent on our colleagues from other disciplines such as the basic sciences, epidemiology, social science and engineering.

The 2nd World Health Organisation sponsored consultation on incontinence was held in Paris in July 2001. The structure of the consultation followed the successful formula developed by the ICUD (the International Consultation on Urological Diseases which is recognized as a WHO, Non Governmental Organization) and used for the 1st ICI held in Monaco in 1998 and published the following year. Once again an international faculty of almost 200 individuals from a wide range of professions and specialities were grouped into a series of subcommittees, each with a specific area of responsibility.

The spectrum of subcommittees spanned from Basic Science through to Assessment and Investigation to Therapy. These committees were further divided into specific patient groups for children, women, men, neurological patients and the frail elderly. Subcommittee members were selected according to their academic reputation giving due recognition to the need to provide balance between specialities and geographical regions. A chairperson was selected for each subcommittee and was responsible for the drafting of that committees' chapter. Many committees met at least once before the consultation in Paris, to progress their report.

Each chairperson presented his or her committees' main discussions and recommendations in Paris, their chapter was then modified accordingly, in the light of the consultation.

This book details the evidence reviewed by each committee. Each chapter uses a modification of the Oxford System for evaluating evidence and providing recommendations. The system used during the consultation utilized a simplified system with five levels of evidence (1 to 5) and four grades of recommendation (A to D). This system worked well for the treatment committees but there is, as yet, no system that can be used to evaluate the evidence from the basic science and investigation committees. Nevertheless, the consultation feels that continued efforts to specify the evidence base for the recommendations are of vital importance.

The book's final chapter is the Recommendations of the International Scientific Committee which includes all subcommittee chairs together with the members of the Steering Committee. This chapter has been expanded to include algorithms for the treatment of faecal incontinence and pelvic organ prolapse. Furthermore, the 1998 algorithms have been extensively reconfigured in the light of new evidence and in order to facilitate their use. The algorithms from 1998 were published in the journal "Lancet" and it is the intention of the 2nd ICI to publish the new algorithms in an equally prestigious journal.

The consultation hopes that its' work will begin to help those millions who suffer incontinence and in particular, its' social consequences. We must all work to break down the social taboos that prevent many sufferers from obtaining help for their problem. We must also increase our efforts to prevent incontinence and in particular, the catastrophic birth related fistulae that afflict so many women in the developing world.

Paul Abrams and the Scientific Committee

Some of the members of the international committees
Paris - July 1-3, 2002

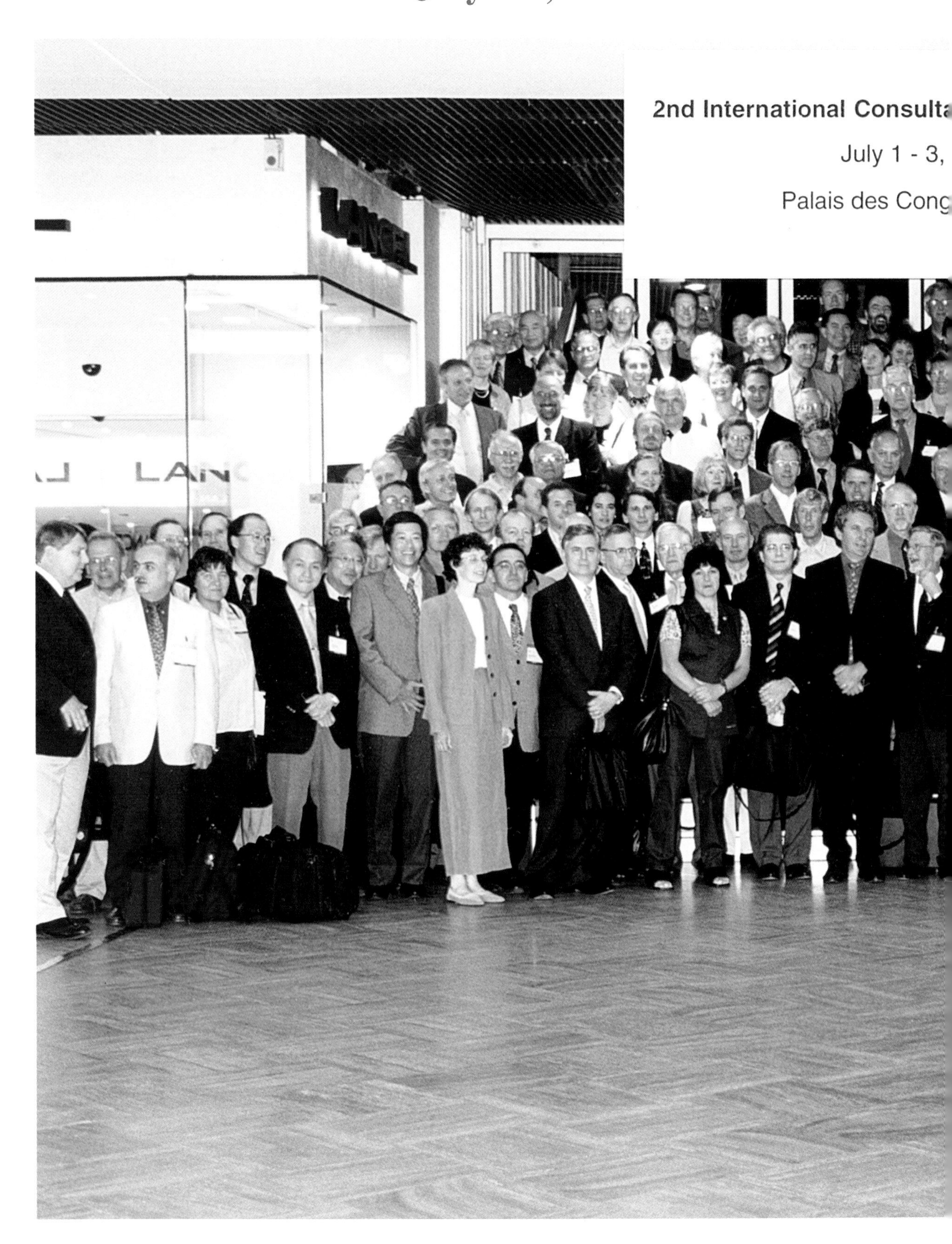

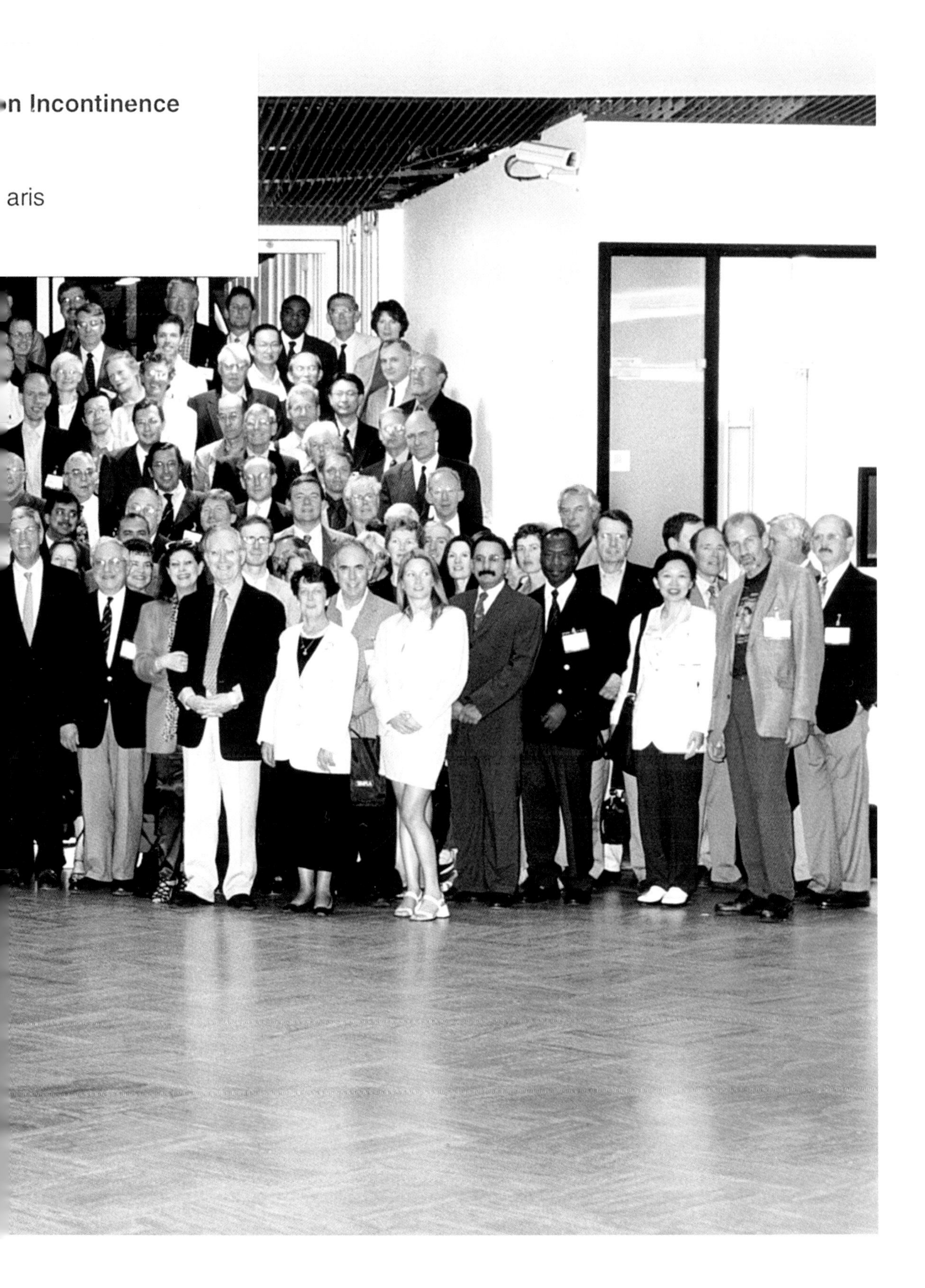
n Incontinence
aris

Editors

P. Abrams, *U.K.*

L. Cardozo, *U.K*

S. Khoury, *France*

A. Wein *USA*

Members of the Committees

(Alphabetical order - Chairmen in bold print)

08c	ANDERSEN	Jens T.	Denmark
9	***ANDERSSON***	***K-Erik***	***Sweden***
9	APPELL	Rodney	USA
12	ARROWSMITH	Steven	USA
08c	***ARTIBANI***	***Walter***	***Italy***
9	AWAD	Said	Canada
6	BADIA	Xavier	Spain
11c	BARRETT	David	USA
7	BATISTA	Jose	Spain
7	BAUER	Stuart	USA
08b	BENSON	Tom	USA
10d	BENVENUTI	Francesco	Italy
14	BITKER	M-Olivier	France
16	BLAIVAS	Jerry	USA
2	BLOK	Bertil	The Netherlands
11a	BLOOM	David	USA
10c	***BO***	***Kari***	***Norway***
4	BOITEUX	Jean Paul	France
10c	BOURCIER	Alain	France
10a	BOWER	Wendy	Australia
2	BRADING	Alison	U.K
12	BRIGGS	Nimi	Nigeria
5	***BRUBAKER***	***Linda***	***USA***
11b	BRUSCHINI	Humero	Brazil
5	BUMP	Richard	USA
3	BURGIO	Kathryn	USA
15	BUTLER	Ursula	U.K.
11c	CASTRO	David	Spain
10e	CHANCELLOR	Michael	USA
9	CHAPPLE	Chirstopher	U.K
10e	CHARTIER-KASTLER	E.	France
15	CHRISTIANSEN	John	Denmark
6	CORCOS	Jacques	Canada
11d	COSTA	Pierre	France
10d	COTTENDEN	Alan	U.K
7	CRAGGS	Mike	U.K
1	CREED	Kate	Australia
11c	DANESHGARI	Firouz	USA
2	DE GROAT	William	USA
1	DELANCEY	John	USA
1	DELMAS	Vincent	France
13	DENIS	Louis	Belgium
3	DIOKNO	Ananias	USA
1	DIXON	John	U.K.
08c	DJURHUUS	Jens C.	Denmark
11c	DMOCHOWSKI	Roger	USA
6	***DONOVAN***	***Jenny***	***UK***
9	DRUTZ	Harold	Canada
10c	DUBEAU	Catherine	USA
9	FINKBEINER	Alex	USA
11a	FISCH	Margit	Germany
10d	FONDA	David	Australia
9	FOURCROY	Jean	USA
08b	FOWLER	Clare	U.K.
08c	GAJEWSKI	Jerzy	Canada
13	GARTLEY	Cheryl	USA
11c	GHONIEM	Gamal M.	USA
1	GOSLING	John	USA
6	GOTOH	Momokazu	Japan
7	GRIFFITHS	Derek	USA
11d	GRISE	Philippe	France
13	GRUENWALD	Ilan	Israel
9	HAAB	Francois	France
11b	HANUS	Tomas	Czech Republic
15	HARARI	Danielle	U.K.
10c	HAY-SMITH	Jean	New Zealand
16	HERRERA	Hector	USA
11b	***HERSCHORN***	***Sender***	***Canada***
3	HERZOG	A.Regula	USA
7	HILTON	Paul	UK
3	HJALMAS	Kjell	Sweden
7	***HOMMA***	***Yukio***	***Japan***
14	HU	Teh- Wei	USA
13	HUAT CHYE	Peter Lim	Singapore
3	***HUNSKAR***	***Steinar***	***Norway***
08a	HURT	Glenn	USA

10e	IGAWA	Yashuhiko	Japan
5	JACQUETIN	Bernard	France
11c	JARVIS	Gerry	U.K
16	JONAS	Udo	Germany
2	KAKIZAKI	Hidehiro	Japan
6	KELLEHER	Con	U.K.
10d	KIRSCHNER-HERMANNS	R.	Germany
4	KOELBL	Heinz	Germany
10b	KONDO	Atsuo	Japan
10e	KOVINDHA	Apichana	Thailand
7	KRAMER	Guus	Germany
16	KUSEK	John	USA
1	LANDON	David	U.K
3	LAPITAN	Mela	Philippines
12	LASSEY	Anyetei	Ghana
08a	LAYCOCK	Jo	U.K
2	LEVIN	Robert	USA
7	LOSE	Gunnar	Denmark
11b	LOW	Anthony	Australia
6	LUKACS	Bertrand	France
4	MACARAK	Edward	USA
10e	MADERSBACHER	Helmut	Austria
16	MATTIASSON	Anders	Sweden
3	MCGROTHER	Catherine	U.K.
5	MESSELINK	Bert	The Netherlands
5	MILANI	Rodolfo	Italy
13	MILLARD	Richard	Australia
10d	MILLER	Karen	USA
11a	MITCHELL	Michael	USA
14	MOORE	Kate	Australia
2	***MORRISON***	***John***	***Arab Emirates***
4	MOSTWIN	Jacek	USA
11d	MUNDY	Anthony	U.K.
6	NAUGHTON	Michelle	USA
15	NELSON	Richard	USA
13	***NEWMAN***	***Diane***	***USA***
10a	NIJMAN	Rien	The Netherlands
11c	NITTI	Victor	USA
10b	NORDLING	Jorgen	Denmark
1	NORTON	Peggy	USA
15	***NORTON***	***Christine***	***U.K.***
16	NYBERG	Leroy	USA
10c	NYGAARD	Ingrid	USA
08c	OSTERGARD	Donald	USA
14	OUSLANDER	Joseph	USA
10d	PALMER	Mary	USA
08a	PALMTAG	Hans	Germany
11c	PARAISO	M.Fidela	USA
16	***PAYNE***	***Christopher***	***USA***
15	PEMBERTON	John	USA
11d	PERKASH	Inder	USA
16	PETERS	Tim	U.K.
4	PETRI	Eckhard	Germany
08c	RAZ	Shlomo	USA
10d	RESNICK	Neil	USA
12	RIENHARDT	Gunther	South Africa
13	ROBERTS	Richard	USA
7	ROSIER	Peter	The Netherlands
15	ROVNER	Eric	USA
11b	RUUD BOSCH	JLH	The Netherlands
3	SANDVIK	Hogne	Norway
4	SCHAFER	Werner	Germany
11b	SCHICK	Erik	Canada
5	SCHUESSLER	Bernhard	Switzerland
6	SHAW	Chris	U.K
08a	SHULL	Bob	USA
10b	SIROKY	Mike	USA
11c	SMITH	Anthony	U.K.
11a	SNYDER	Howard	USA
15	STANTON	Stuart	U.K.
10c	STASKIN	David	USA
2	***STEERS***	***William***	***USA***
11d	STOEHRER	Manfred	Germany
11d	STONE	Anthony	USA
16	STOTHERS	Mary-Ann	Canada
14	SUBAK	Leslee	USA
15	SULTAN	Abdul	U.K.
10b	TAMMELA	Teuvo	Finland
2	THOR	Karl B.	USA
10b	TONG LONG LIN	Alex	China
08c	TUBARO	Andrea	Italy
11d	VALE	Paulo	Portugal
10a	VAN GOOL	Jan	The Netherlands
16	VAN KERREBROECK	P.	The Netherlands
14	VERSI	Eboo	USA
08b	VODUSEK	David	Slovenia
14	WAGNER	Todd	USA
12	***WALL***	***Lewis***	***USA***
16	WEBER	Ann	USA
5	WEIDNER	Alison	USA
13	WILLIAMS	Kate	UK
10c	***WILSON***	***Don***	***New Zealand***
11a	WOODHOUSE	Christopher	U.K.
10c	WYMAN	Jean	USA
10e	WYNDAELE	Jacques	Belgium
4	YAMAGUCHI	Osamu	Japan
08b	YANG	Claire	USA
08a	YANG	Yong	China
5	ZIMMERN	Philippe	USA
14	ZINNER	Norman	USA
08a	ZUBIETA	Ricardo	Chile

MEMBERS OF THE COMMITTEES *(by Committee)*

1. ANATOMY, CELLULAR AND GROSS

CREED	Kate	Australia
DELANCEY	John	USA
DELMAS	Vincent	France
DIXON	John	U.K.
GOSLING	John	USA
LANDON	David	U.K
NORTON	Peggy	USA

2. BASIC NEUROPHYSIOLOGY AND NEUROPHARMACOLOGY

BLOK	Bertil	The Netherlands
BRADING	Alison	U.K
DE GROAT	William	USA
KAKIZAKI	Hidehiro	Japan
LEVIN	Robert	USA
MORRISON	***John***	***Arab Emirates***
STEERS	***William***	***USA***
THOR	Karl B.	USA

3. EPIDEMIOLOGY

BURGIO	Kathryn	USA
DIOKNO	Ananias	USA
HERZOG	A.Regula	USA
HJALMAS	Kjell	Sweden
HUNSKAR	***Steinar***	***Norway***
LAPITAN	Mela	Philippines
MCGROTHER	Catherine	U.K.
SANDVIK	Hogne	Norway

4. PATHOPHYSIOLOGY

BOITEUX	Jean Paul	France
KOELBL	Heinz	Germany
MACARAK	Edward	USA
MOSTWIN	Jacek	USA
PETRI	Eckhard	Germany
SCHAFER	Werner	Germany
YAMAGUCHI	Osamu	Japan

5. INCONTINENCE RELATED TO PELVIC FLOOR FUNCTION

BRUBAKER	***Linda***	***USA***
BUMP	Richard	USA
JACQUETIN	Bernard	France
MESSELINK		The Netherlands
MILANI	Rodolfo	Italy
SCHUESSLER	Bernhard	Switzerland
WEIDNER	Alison	USA
ZIMMERN	Philippe	USA

6. SYMPTOM AND QUALITY OF LIFE ASSESSMENT

BADIA	Xavier	Spain
CORCOS	Jacques	Canada
DONOVAN	***Jenny***	***U.K***
GOTOH	Momokazu	Japan
KELLEHER	Con	U.K.
LUKACS	Bertrand	France
NAUGHTON	Michelle	USA
SHAW	Chris	U.K

7. URODYNAMICS

BATISTA	Jose	Spain
BAUER	Stuart	USA
CRAGGS	Mike	U.K
GRIFFITHS	Derek	USA
HILTON	Paul	U.K
HOMMA	***Yukio***	***Japan***
KRAMER	Guus	Germany
LOSE	Gunnar	Denmark
ROSIER	Peter	The Netherlands

8. OTHER INVESTIGATIONS

A. PHYSICAL EXAMINATION

HURT	Glenn	USA
LAYCOCK	Jo	U.K
PALMTAG	Hans	Germany
SHULL	Bob	USA
YANG	Yong	China
ZUBIETA	Ricardo	Chile

B. NEUROPHYSIOLOGY

BENSON	Tom	USA
FOWLER	Clare	U.K.
VODUSEK	David	Slovenia
YANG	Claire	USA

C. IMAGING AND OTHER INVESTIGATINGS

ANDERSEN	Jens Thorup	Denmark
ARTIBANI	***Walter***	***Italy***
DJURHUUS	Jens C.	Denmark
GAJEWSKI	Jerzy	Canada
OSTERGARD	Donald	USA
RAZ	Shlomo	USA
TUBARO	Andrea	Italy

9. PHARMACOLOGIC TREATMENT

ANDERSSON	***Karl-Erik***	***Sweden***
APPELL	Rodney	USA
AWAD	Said	Canada
CHAPPLE	Christopher	U.K
DRUTZ	Harold	Canada
FINKBEINER	Alex	USA
FOURCROY	Jean	USA
HAAB	Francois	France

10. CONSERVATIVE TREATMENT

A. CHILDREN

BOWER	Wendy	Australia
NIJMAN	Rien	The Netherlands
NYGAARD	Ingrid	USA
VAN GOOL	Jan	The Netherlands

B. MEN

KONDO	Atsuo	Japan
NORDLING	Jorgen	Denmark

SIROKY	Mike	USA
TAMMELA	Teuvo	Finland
TONG LONG LIN	Alex	China

C. WOMEN

BO	***Kari***	***Norway***
BOURCIER	Alain	France
HAY-SMITH	Jean	New Zealand
NYGAARD	Ingrid	USA
STASKIN	David	USA
WILSON	***Don***	***New Zealand***
WYMAN	Jean	USA

D. ELDERLY

BENVENUTI	Francesco	Italy
COTTENDEN	Alan	U.K
DUBEAU	Catherine	USA
FONDA	David	Australia
KIRSCHNER-HERMANNS	Ruth	Germany
MILLER	Karen	USA
PALMER	Mary	USA
RESNICK	Neil	USA

E. NEUROPATHIC

CHANCELLOR	Michael	USA
CHARTIER-KASTLER	Emmanuel	France
IGAWA	Yashuhiko	Japan
KOVINDHA	Apichana	Thailand
MADERSBACHER	Helmut	Austria
WYNDAELE	Jean Jacques	Belgium

11. SURGICAL TREATMENT

A. CHILDREN

WOODHOUSE	Christopher	U.K.
BLOOM	David	USA
FISCH	Margit	Germany
MITCHELL	Michael	USA
SNYDER	Howard	USA

B. MEN

RUUD BOSCH	JLH	The Netherlands
HANUS	Tomas	Czech
LOW	Anthony	Australia
SCHICK	Erik	Canada
BRUSCHINI	Humero	Brazil
HERSCHORN	***Sender***	***Canada***

C. WOMEN

COSTA	Pierre	France
DANESHGARI	Firouz	USA
JARVIS	Gerry	U.K
DMOCHOWSKI	Roger	USA
GHONIEM	Gamal M.	USA
NITTI	Victor	USA
PARAISO	Marie Fidela	USA
SMITH	Anthony	U.K.

D. NEUROPATHIC

VALE	Paulo	Portugal
BARRETT	David	USA
MUNDY	Anthony	U.K.
CASTRO	David	Spain
GRISE	Philippe	France
PERKASH	Inder	USA
STOEHRER	Manfred	Germany
STONE	Anthony	USA

12. INCONTINENCE IN THE DEVELOPING WORLD

ARROWSMITH	Steven	USA
BRIGGS	Nimi	Nigeria
LASSEY	Anyetei	Ghana
RIENHARDT	Gunther	South Africa
WALL	***Lewis***	***USA***

13. PROMOTION, ORGANISATION AND EDUCATION IN CONTINENCE CARE

DENIS	Louis	Belgium
GARTLEY	Cheryl	USA
GRUENWALD	Ilan	Israel
HUAT CHYE	Peter	Singapore
MILLARD	Richard	Australia
NEWMAN	***Diane***	***USA***
ROBERTS	Richard G.	USA
WILLIAMS	Kate	U.K

14. ECONOMICS OF INCONTINENCE

BITKER	Marc-Olivier	France
HU	Teh- Wei	USA
MOORE	Kate	Australia
OUSLANDER	Joseph	USA
SUBAK	Leslee	USA
VERSI	Eboo	USA
WAGNER	Todd	USA
ZINNER	Norman	USA

15. ASSESSMENT AND MANAGEMENT OF FAECAL INCONTINENCE

BUTLER	Ursula	U.K.
CHRISTIANSEN	John	Denmark
HARARI	Danielle	U.K.
NELSON	Richard	USA
NORTON	***Christine***	***U.K.***
PEMBERTON	John	USA
ROVNER	Eric	USA
STANTON	Stuart	U.K.
SULTAN	Abdul	U.K

6. RESEARCH AND OUTCOMES

BLAIVAS	Jerry	USA
HERRERA	Hector	USA
JONAS	Udo	Germany
KUSEK	John	USA
MATTIASSON	Anders	Sweden
NYBERG	Leroy	USA
PAYNE	***Christopher***	***USA***
PETERS	Tim	U.K.
STOTHERS	Mary-Ann	Canada
VAN KERREBROECK	Philip	The Netherlands
WEBER	Ann	USA

Levels of Evidence and Grades of Recommendation

The International Consultation on Urological Diseases (ICUD) is a non-governmental organisation registered with the World Health Organisation (WHO). The ICUD in consultation with WHO advises on the structure of consensus consultations. In the last ten years Consultations have been organised on BPH, Prostate Cancer, Urinary Stone Disease, Nosocomial Infections, Erectile Dysfunction and Incontinence. These consultations have looked at published evidence and produced recommendations at four levels; highly recommended, recommended, optional and not recommended. This method has been useful but the ICUD believes that there should be more explicit statements of the levels of evidence that generate the subsequent grades of recommendations. The ICUD would be delighted if other bodies, such as journals, were to take up the proposed system.

The AHCPR have used specified evidence levels to justify recommendations for the investigation and treatment of a variety of conditions. The Oxford Centre for Evidence Based Medicine have produced a widely accepted adaptation of the work of AHCPR and this has been recently updated. (June 5th 2001 http:// cebm. jr2. ox.ac.uk/)

The ICUD has examined the Oxford guidelines and discussed with the Oxford group, their applicability to the Consultations organised by ICUD. It is highly desirable that the recommendations made by the Consultation follows an accepted grading system backed up by explicit levels of evidence.

The ICUD proposes that future consultations should use a somewhat modified version of the Oxford system which can be directly 'mapped' onto the Oxford system.

A. Therapeutic Interventions

All interventions should be judged by the body of evidence for their efficacy, tolerability and cost effectiveness. It is accepted that at present little data exists on cost effectiveness for most interventions.

Levels of Evidence

Firstly, it should be stated that any level of evidence may be positive (the therapy works) or negative (the therapy doesn't work).

Level 1 evidence (incorporates Oxford 1a, 1b, 1c) usually involves one or more randomised controlled trials or 'all or none' studies in which no treatment is not an option, for example in vesicovaginal fistula.

Level 2 evidence includes good quality prospective 'cohort studies' (and incorporates Oxford 1a, 1b and 1c). These may include a single group when individuals who develop the condition are matched from within the original cohort group. There can be parallel cohorts where those with the condition in the first group are matched by those in the second group.

Level 3 evidence includes good quality retrospective 'case-control studies' where a group of patients who have a condition are matched (for age, sex etc) by control individuals from a general population. (incorporates Oxford 3a and 3b)

Level 4 evidence includes good quality 'case series' where a group of patients all with the same condition/disease/therapeutic intervention, are described, without matching control.

Level 5 evidence includes expert opinion were the opinion is based not on evidence but on 'first principles' (e.g. physiological or anatomical) or bench research. The Delphi process can be used to give 'expert opinion' greater authority. In the Delphi process a series of questions are posed to a panel; the answers are collected into a series of 'options'; the options are serially ranked; if a 75% agreement is reached then a Delphi consensus statement can be made.

Where there is disparity of evidence, for example if there were three well conducted RCT's showing that Drug A was superior to placebo, but one RCT showing no difference, then there has to be an individual judgement as to the level of evidence selected and the rationale explained.

Grades of Recommendation

The ICUD will use the four grades from the Oxford system. As with levels of evidence the grades of evidence may apply either positively (do the procedure) or negatively (don't do the procedure).

Grade A recommendation usually depends on consistent level 1 evidence and often means that the recommendation is effectively mandatory and placed within a clinical care pathway. However, there will be occasions where excellent evidence (level 1) does not lead to a Grade A recommendation, for example, if the therapy is prohibitively expensive, dangerous or unethical.

A grade A recommendation can follow from Level 2 evidence, for example, rectus sheath sling for stress incontinence has never been the subject of RCT's against another procedure such as colposuspension for the same condition.

Grade B recommendation usually depends on consistent level 2 and or 3 studies, or 'majority evidence' from RCT's.

Grade C recommendation usually depends on level 4 studies or 'majority evidence' from level 2/3 studies or Dephi processed expert opinion.

Grade D recommendation is given when the evidence is inconsistent/inconclusive or non-existent for studies that may vary in type from RCT's to case series, or for expert opinion delivered without any analytical process, such as by Dephi.

B. Assessment and Investigation

From initial discussions with the Oxford group it is clear that application of levels of evidence/grades of recommendation to investigate is much more complex than for interventions. The ICUD recommend, that, as a minimum, any test should be subjected to three questions:

does the test have good technical performance, for example, do three aliguots of the same urine sample give the same result when subjected to 'stix' testing?

Does the test have good diagnostic performance, for example, are abdominal leak point pressure measurements significantly different in women with and without urodynamic stress incontinence?

Does the test have clinical relevance that is, does the test alter clinical management, does the test predict outcome?

Where possible the ICUD system (modified from the Oxford system) should be used for assessment or investigation techniques.

C. Basic Science and Epidemiology

The proposed ICUD system does not easily fit into these areas of science. Further research needs to be carried out, in order to develop explicit levels of evidence that can lead to recommendations as to the soundness of data in these important aspects of medicine.

Conclusion

The ICUD believes that it's consultation should follow the ICUD system of levels of evidence and grades of recommendation, were possible. This system can be mapped directly to the Oxford system.

There are aspects to the ICUD system which require further research, particularly to include cost effectiveness, and also factors such as patient preference, for which no evidence exists.

P. Abrams and the Committee

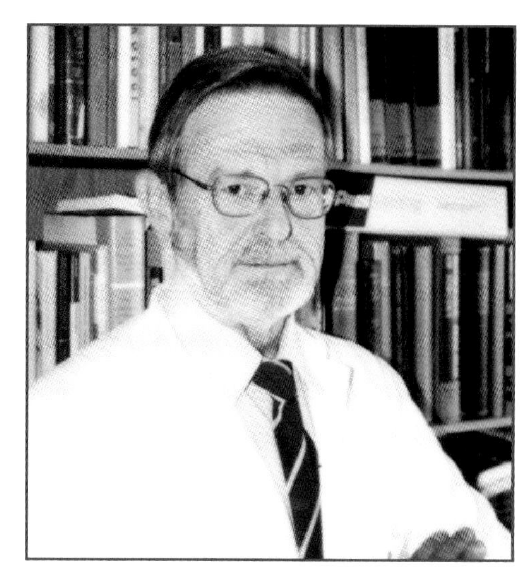

Professor Tage Hald

Honorary President of the 2nd International Consultation on Incontinence

Tage Hald: a pioneering surgeon, great teacher and true European.

I first met Tage Hald in 1975 in the Railway Hotel, a magnificent and majestic Victorian monument to the great days of the railway, in Glasgow during the 6th International Continence Society annual meeting. That encounter summed up Professor Hald's qualities beautifully: he held court to a mixed group of young and older colleagues, showering us with urological wisdom, amusing stories and great hospitality, in equal measures (single malt whisky, I hazily recollect). Then and subsequently, he gave freely of his time to the most junior of us: a sure sign of a great teacher.

Tage Hald is a "country boy" having been born in Jutland, an area that he's now returned to in order to grow his own forest. Even before his medical graduation, he had an international reputation! He had represented Denmark as a freestyle swimmer. He had also spent a good deal of time studying languages to a high level. Indeed his appointment as the Chairman of the Standardisation Committee of the International Continence Society owed much to the fact that he spoke, and certainly wrote, better grammatical English than most native English speakers! After graduation from the University of Copenhagen, he spent a year as a research fellow at New York State University and in 1969 was awarded a Doctorate in Medical Science for his thesis on "Neruogenic Dysfunction of the Urinary Bladder". His collaborations with the late lamented Bill Bradley, an American Neurologist, were recognized worldwide as of the highest quality and culminated in their book on Neurourology. As Chairman of urology, and from 1985 Professor of Surgery, at the University of Copenhagen, he developed a department of exceptional quality and with his collegues put Scandinavian urology in general and Danish urology in particular, 'on the map'.

His early interest in neurourology brought him into the field of incontinence and urodynamics at it's infancy in the late 60's. His knowledge and authority led to he and his co-workers having considerable influence during this important development phase of this new field of investigation and treatment. In urodynamics, he worked with a small Danish company to build urodynamic equipment of the highest quality, now a world leader in this field. He recognized the fact that a new method of investigation needed to be accompanied by an agreed set of definitions and terminology. As the first chairman of the ICS Standardisation Committee he provided the foundations on which a new method of investigation could develop quickly and become accepted worldwide within a relatively short time. He supervised the publication of the first standardization reports and remained chairman until his protégé Jens Thorup Andersen succeeded him in 1986.

Tage Hald has been honoured many times in his own country and abroad. He has been President of both the Danish Urological Association (1978-1982) and the Danish Surgical Society (1988-1990). His eloquence as a speaker, and his dexterity as a surgeon meant numerous visiting professorships worldwide, awards, and honorary memberships of surgical and scientific societies.

In recent years he took a particular interest in the effects of ageing on the lower urinary tract and chaired a committee on that topic in the successive WHO consultations on "BPH". With the ageing population this topic will assume increasing importance and it is typical of Tage Hald that he had the foresight to appreciate it's significance more than 10 years ago.

It is most appropriate that he is now honoured as the President of the 2nd International Consultation on Incontinence.

Paul Abrams
Chairman of the 2nd ICI, 2001.

CONTENTS

Incontinence

2nd International Consultation on Incontinence Paris, July 1-3, 2001

2nd Edition 2002

ORDER FORM

Order from : **Plymbridge Distributors Ltd**
Estover Road, Plymouth PL6 7PY, United Kingdom
Customer Services : Tel. : +44 1752 202301 - Fax: +44 1752 202333
E-mail: cservs@plymbridge.com

ISBN	Author/Title (MRn°)	Quantity	Unit Price	total
1 898452 55 5	- Book "INCONTINENCE" 2nd Edition 2002		£ 100	
	- CD Rom "INCONTINENCE 2nd Edition 2002		£ 70	
	- BOOK + CD Rom		£ 120	

Mailing costs

	BOOK or Book + CD Rom	CD Rom alone
U.K	£ 5	£ 1.50
Europe	£ 14	£ 2

Sub total ________

Shipping ________

Total Enclosed ________

USA - BOOK or Book+ CD Rom
Surface £ 12 ❑ - Air £ 22 ❑ - DHL £26 ❑

USA - CD Rom alone
Surface £ 2 ❑ - Air £ 4 ❑ - DHL £ 13 ❑

REST OF THE WORLD
BOOKor Book + CD Rom £ 27 AIR ❑
CD Rom alone £ 4 AIR ❑

______ ***Cheque enclosed*** : Cheque must be drawn ***in sterling*** on a UK clearing Bank

______ ***Charge to*** : ❑ Visa ❑ MasterCard ❑ American Express

Card Number : ______________________ Exp Date : ____________

Name on the Card : ______________________ Issue Number: ____________

Signature : ____________________

Name : ____

Address (in full) : ____

____

____

Telephone N°: ____________________ Fax N°: ____________________

________________________________ Please print your name and

________________________________ address in **CAPITAL LETTERS**

INCONTINENCE

EDITORS

PAUL ABRAMS - LINDA CARDOZO - SAAD KHOURY -
ALAN WEIN

Committee 1

Gross Anatomy and Cell Biology of the Lower Urinary Tract

Chairmen

J. DeLancey (USA),

J. Gosling (USA)

Members

K. Creed (Austriala),

J. Dixon (U.K.),

V. Delmas (France),

D.Landon (U.K.),

P. Norton (USA)

.

CONTENTS

Gross Anatomy and Cell Biology of the Lower Urinary Tract

J. DeLancey, J. Gosling,

K. Creed, J. Dixon, V. Delmas, D. Landon, P. Norton

SUMMARY

The structure and relationships of the male and female lower urinary tract have been considered with particular emphasis placed on those morphological components believed to be of importance in the maintenance of urinary continence. The autonomic innervation of the detrusor has been reviewed and the location of the vesical plexus and its constituent neurons has been noted. The location of this plexus close to the bladder neck renders the innervation of the detrusor vulnerable during surgical procedures in this region. The motor innervation of detrusor smooth muscle is considered to be mainly cholinergic in type and sympathetic influences are believed to act on autonomic neurons rather than directly on bladder smooth muscle. Encapsulated sensory nerve terminals are occasionally observed in the adventitia of the urinary bladder although most presumptive sensory nerves are thought to reside in the submucosa. The structure and innervation of the male bladder neck has been described and this region serves to prevent reflux of seminal fluid at the time of ejaculation. In both sexes the role of the bladder neck in maintaining urinary continence remains uncertain. The location and innervation of striated muscle within the wall of the urethra (rhabdosphincter, external urethral sphincter) in both sexes has been described. In the female this muscle forms an omega shaped sphincter which is thickest in the middle one third of the urethra and consists mainly of small diameter, slow twitch fibres. In the male, both large and small diameter fast and slow twitch fibres form the sphincter which lies at, and below, the apex of the prostate. In both sexes the sphincter is anatomically separate from the medial fibres forming the pelvic diaphragm. The structure and innervation of the levator ani have been described particularly with respect to the effects of parturition on the pelvic floor musculature. Finally the relevance of fascial thickenings in maintaining support for pelvic viscera has been considered. Whilst thickenings of the endopelvic fascia have been described macroscopically, their relative importance by comparison with the active muscle tone exerted by the pelvic floor remains to be determined. The anatomy of the anal sphincter mechanism has also been considered.

The upright posture of human beings means that gravitational forces and abdominal pressure generated by the striated muscle activity associated with normal posture both combine to exert continuous force on the outflow tract, and thus a continuous occlusive force has to be generated to maintain continence. This is achieved via both dynamic forces in the smooth and striated muscles of the urethral wall, and passive forces in the vascular filling of the lamina propria and the apposition of its surfaces. The dynamic occlusion forces need to be increased to prevent leakage with sudden rises in intrabdominal pressure, and decreased in synchrony with the elevation of the bladder pressure in micturition. Again a complex neuronal network is apparent in the urethral walls, with sensory fibres and several classes of motor nerve.

Throughout this report we have attempted to indicate those aspects of lower urinary tract morphology which require further investigation in order to clarify their role and relative significance in the prevention of urinary incontinence.

I. MACROSCOPIC ANATOMY OF THE URINARY BLADDER

In both sexes, the urinary bladder lies in the anterior (ventral) part of the pelvic cavity. The proportion of the cavity that it occupies is dependent upon the volume of fluid contained within the vesical lumen. The full bladder is approximately spherical in shape, becoming more tetrahedral in form as emptying occurs. It is in the contracted state that the anatomical relationships of the urinary bladder are best considered. In the following account, the relations of the urinary bladder will be described separately for each sex.

1. External features

Although the urinary bladder is highly variable in shape it is convenient, if not strictly accurate, to consider the viscus as a tetrahedron, possessing an anterior, an inferior (caudal) and two posterolateral (dorsolateral) angles. The anterior angle is directed forwards and upwards and is attached to the urachus, a fibrous cord ascending in the extraperitoneal tissues of the abdominal wall as far as the umbilicus. The urachus is the embryological remnant of the allantois and occasionally remains patent throughout life. This condition may be unrecognized clinically until the bladder neck or urethra becomes obstructed, whereupon urine is discharged from the umbilicus. The two posterolateral angles are those regions in which the ureters pierce the bladder wall; the inferior angle corresponds to the bladder neck and associated internal urethral meatus. The distal 1-2 cm of each ureter is surrounded by an incomplete collar of detrusor smooth muscle which forms a sheath (of Waldeyer) separated from the ureteric muscle coat by a connective tissue sleeve. The ureters pierce the posterior aspect of the bladder (fig. 1) and run obliquely through its wall for a distance of 1.5-2.0 cm before terminating at the ureteric orifices. This arrangement is believed to assist in the prevention of ureteric reflux since the intramural ureters are thought to be occluded during increases in bladder pressure.

As a tetrahedron, the urinary bladder also possesses four surfaces which are readily discernible in the contracted organ. The two inferolateral surfaces conform to the pelvic walls and floor to which they become more closely related as bladder distension increases. The posterior surface, or base, of the bladder is small and varies in size to only a minor degree as the organ fills and empties. This surface extends between the entrances of the ureters into the bladder wall and the posterior aspect of the bladder neck. The superior surface (fundus) varies the most in shape and area, expanding upwards and forwards as the organ fills.

2. Internal features

When viewed from within, the mucosa lining the wall of the bladder presents three distinct apertures, namely, the ureteric orifices and the internal urethral meatus (fig. 2). These lie relatively close to one another and delimit the trigonal region of the bladder. The two lateral orifices appear slit-like and are formed by the internal openings of the ureters. Frequently, these two orifices are connected by a prominent ridge known as the interureteric bar. Extending inferomedially from the ureteric orifices, a pair of ridges corresponding to the lateral edges of the trigone extend as far as the internal urethral meatus. The latter lies in the midline and forms a circular aperture on the luminal aspect of the bladder neck region. With the exception of the trigone, the bladder mucosa is comparatively rugose in the undistended organ but becomes smoother as filling proceeds. The trigone is characterized by a relatively flattened appearance with a smooth urothelial covering and retains its appearance and size irrespective of the degree of distension of the bladder.

3. Relations of the female urinary bladder

In the female, the inferolateral surfaces of the bladder are closely applied to the fascia which covers the pelvic walls and floor (fig. 3). The lateral pelvic walls are formed by the obturator internus muscles, covered on their medial aspects by the obturator fasicae. The latter give attachment to the levator ani muscles which, together with the coccygeus, form the pelvic floor. The levator muscles are covered on their superior aspects by a further layer of fascia (the pelvic fascia).

Several nerves and blood vessels course in the fascia adjacent to the inferolateral surface of the bladder. The nerves include the obturator nerve and part of the pelvic plexus of autonomic nerves (the vesical plexus). The arteries related to these surfaces of the bladder are the superior vesical arteries (which continue anteriorly as the obliterated umbilical arteries), the obturator arteries and the inferior vesical and vaginal arteries. The obturator veins are discrete vessels which accompany the obturator arteries; the vesical veins form a network of venous channels, the vesical venous plexus, which lies adjacent to the bladder's inferolateral surface. The posterior relations are the cervix of the uterus and the vagina (fig. 4). The extravaginal portion of the cervix lies against the superior part of the base of the bladder while the anterior vaginal wall is in contact with most of the remaining areas of the bladder base. The superior relations of the female bladder are somewhat variable because the size, position and presence of the uterus are subject to alteration. The non-gravid uterus commonly inclines forwards

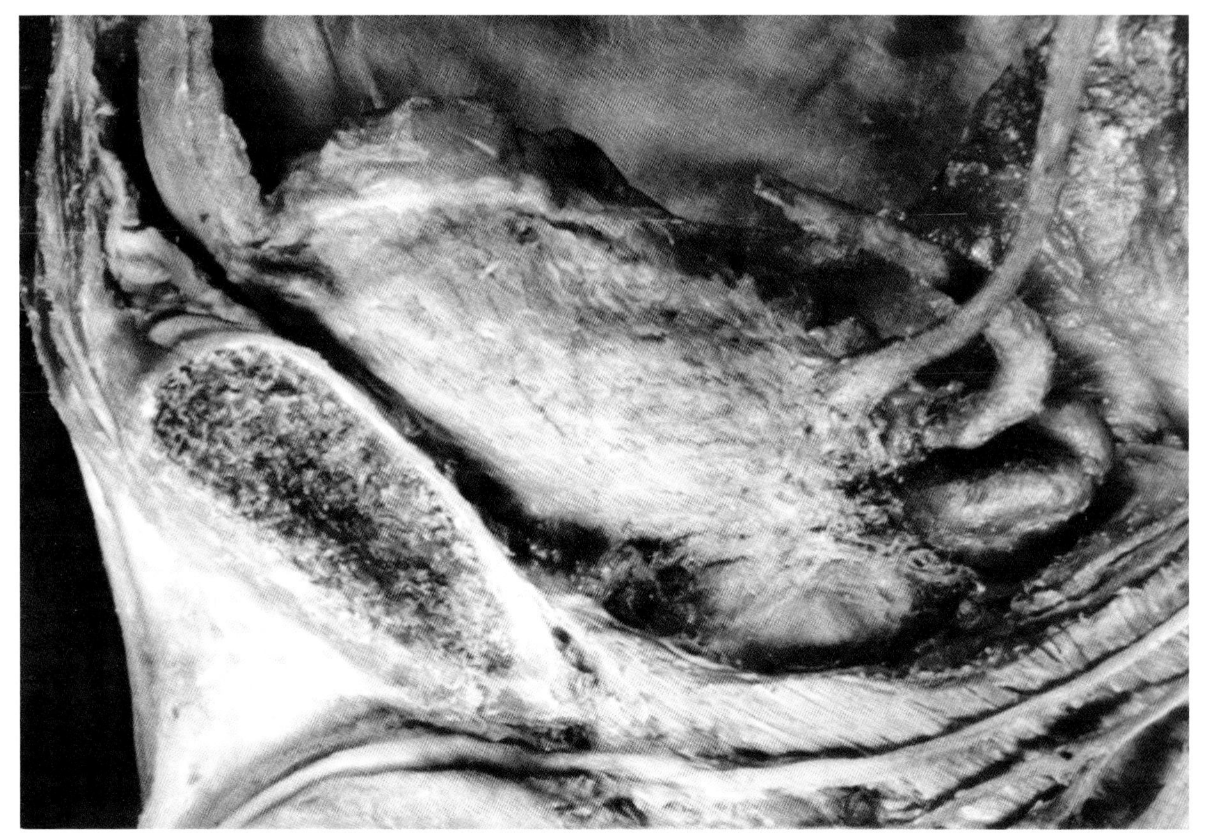

Figure 1 : Lateral view of the male bladder after removal of the left pelvic wall. The left ureter enters the posterior surface of the bladder and is crossed by the terminal portion of the ductus deferens.

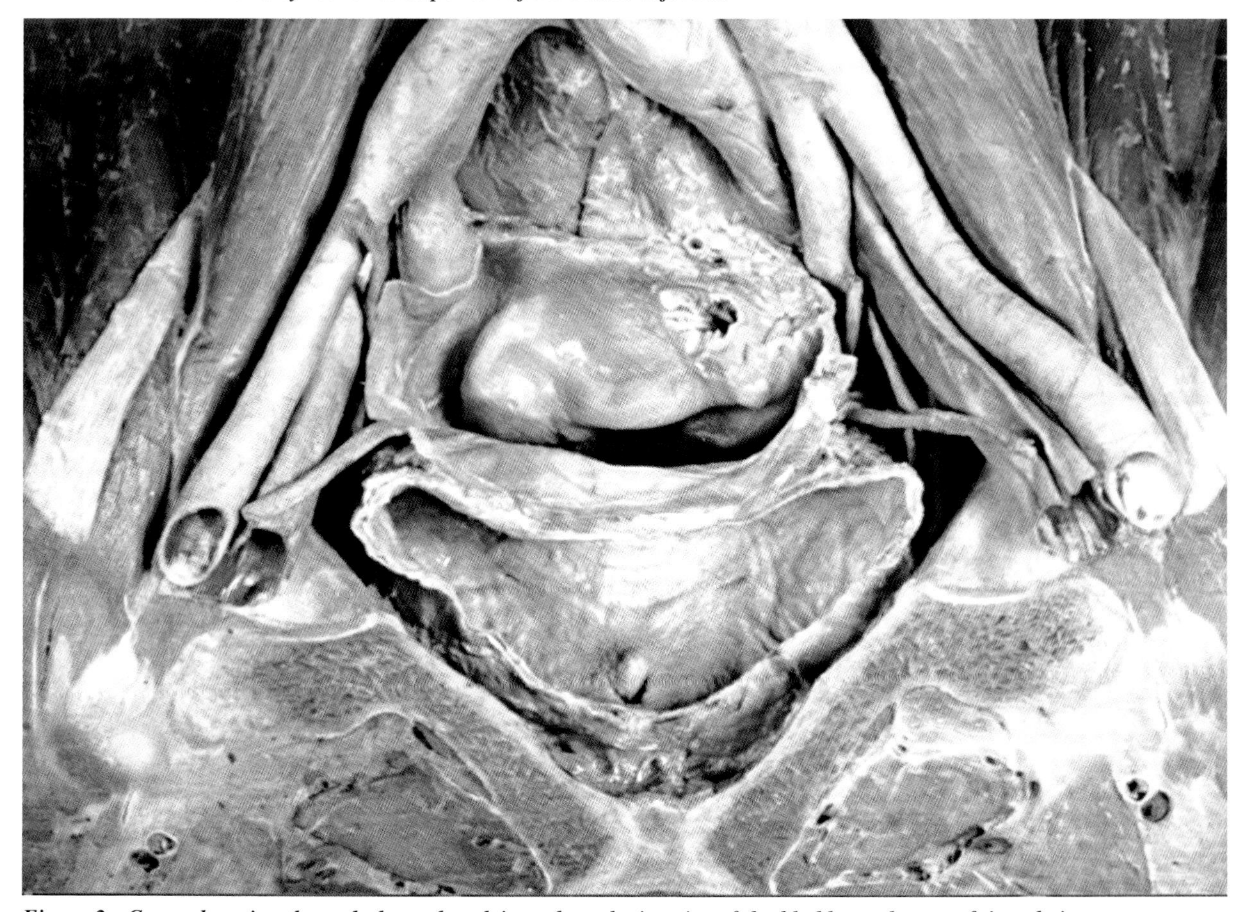

Figure 2 : Coronal section through the male pelvis to show the interior of the bladder and some of its relations.

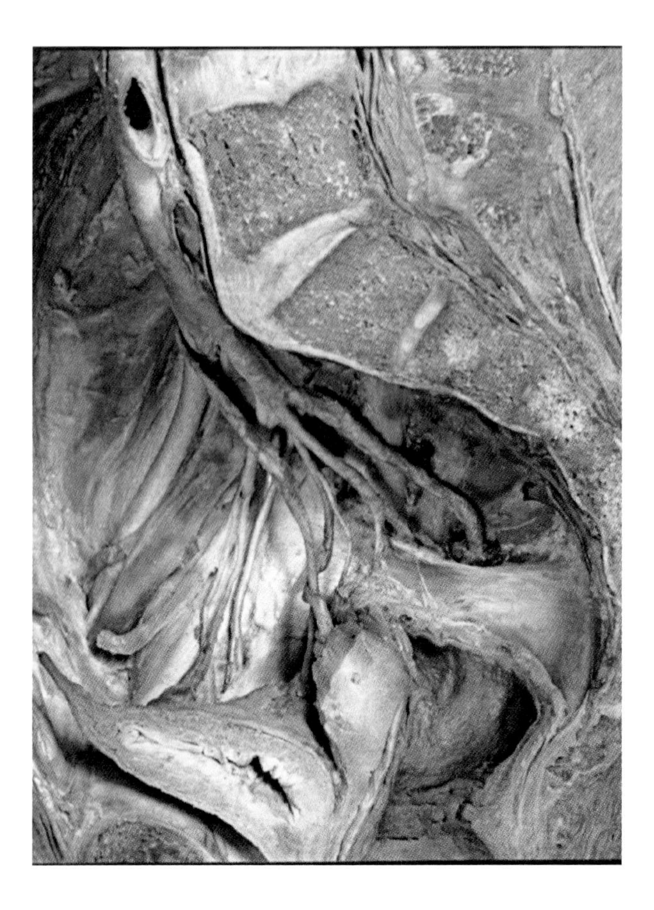

Figure 3 : Female pelvis dissected to show some of the structures which relate to the infrolateral aspect of the bladder.

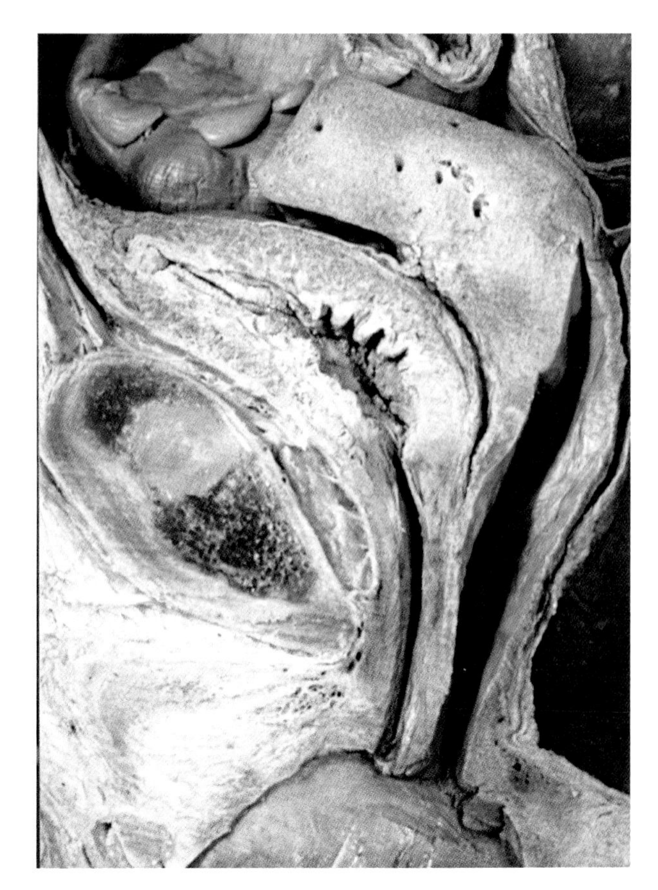

Figure 4 : Median sagittal section through the female pelvis to show the bladder and some of its relations.

and upwards and lies on the posterior part of the superior surface of the bladder (fig. 5). The remainder of the superior surface of the bladder is related to coils of intestine. However, a normal variant may occur whereby the body of the uterus is retroverted and directed towards the rectum and sacrum, thereby leaving the entire superior surface of the bladder in contact with intestines.

Between the bladder and the pubic bones lies adipose tissue, the terminations of the arcus tendineus fascia pelvis to the pubic bones, and numerous veins (see below). Vesical filling results in direct contact between the bladder and the anterior abdominal wall above the pubic symphysis. The peritoneum from the anterior abdominal wall continues onto the superior surface of the bladder (fig. 6) but extends posteriorly only as far as the isthmus of the uterus onto which it is reflected to form the uterovesical pouch.

4. Relations of the male urinary bladder

The inferolateral surfaces of the bladder are related to fascia and to the walls and floor of the pelvis (fig. 7) as described in the female. The base or posterior surface of the bladder is related to the seminal vesicles, the ampullae of the ducti deferentes, the rectum and the rectovesical pouch of peritoneum. The seminal vesicles and ampullae are applied to the lateral parts of the bladder base. These structures are partly covered by peritoneum which continues for a short distance from the superior surface of the bladder onto its base. This peritoneum caps the ampullae of the ducti deferentes and the seminal vesicles before being reflected at the rectovesical pouch onto the anterior surface of the rectum. When the rectum is distended its ampulla lies in close contact with the base of the bladder. However, when the rectum or bladder, or both, are relatively empty, coils of intestine frequently intervene and occupy the rectovesical pouch.

The prostate gland, surrounded by the prostatic venous plexus, lies inferior to the bladder neck (fig. 8). Between the bladder and the pubic bones lies the retropubic space containing adipose tissue and the puboprostatic and pubovesical ligaments. As bladder filling occurs the organ comes to occupy more of the retropubic space; further filling results in the superior surface of the bladder extending above the pubis, thereby displacing the peritoneum from the anterior abdominal wall. Thus, the anterior aspect of the distended bladder is in direct contact with the abdominal wall without the intervention of peritoneum. The whole of the superior surface of the bladder and the median portion of its base are covered by peritoneum and are related to intestines consisting of ileum, sigmoid colon and rectum.

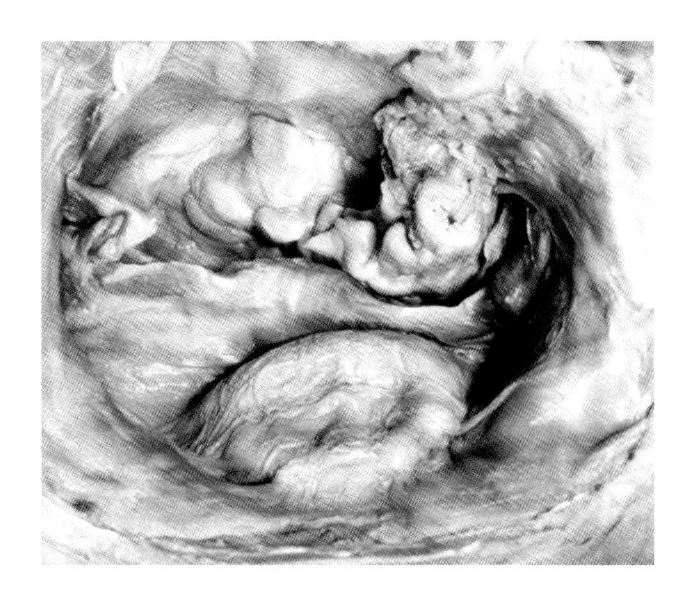

Figure 5 : Superior view of peritoneum and organs within the female pelvis. The small intestine and most of the sigmoid colon have been removed.

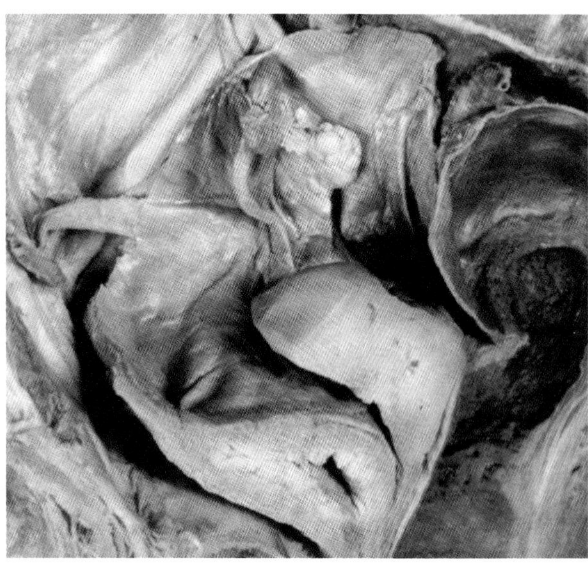

Figure 6 : The superior surface of the bladder is covered by peritoneum. In this dissection the fat which occupied the retropubic space has been removed.

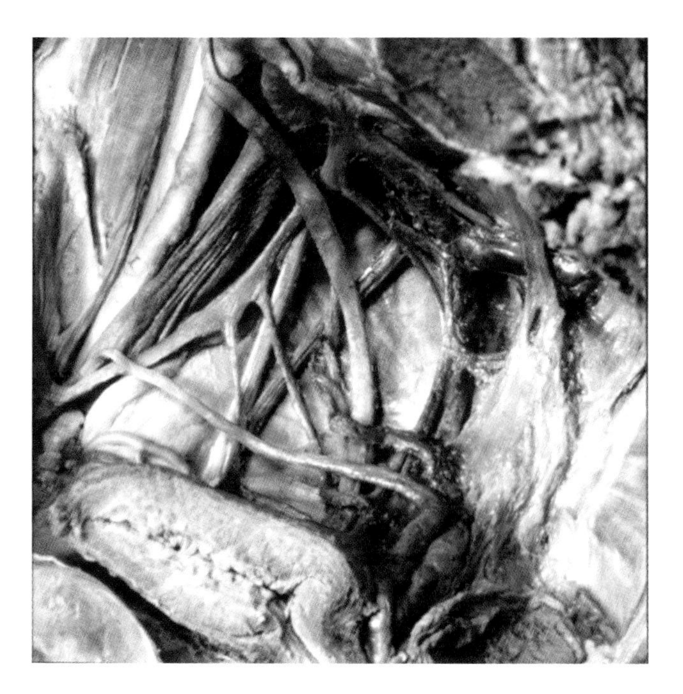

Figure 7 : Some of the structures which relate to the infrolateral and posterior surfaces of the male bladder. The pelvic plexus forms a flat sheet which extends upto the seminal vesicle and ductus deferens.

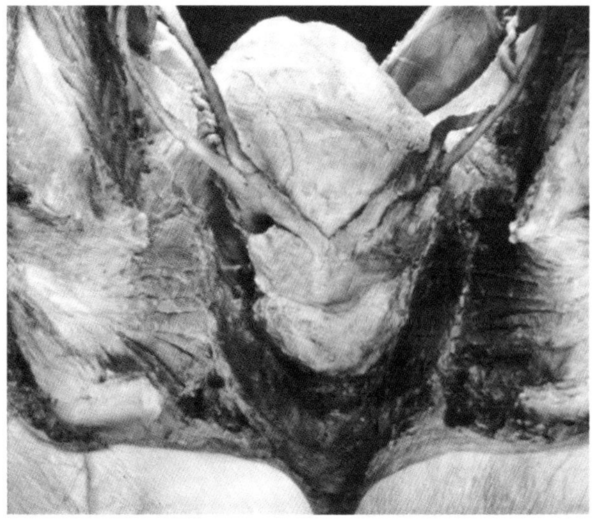

Figure 8 : Removal of the rectum and the posterior wall of the pelvis exposes the bladder, ducti deferentes, seminal vesicles and prostate.

II. EXTRINSIC INNERVATION OF THE LOWER URINARY TRACT

Efferent sympathetic and parasympathetic fibres are conveyed to the bladder and urethra via the hypogastric and pelvic splanchnic nerves, respectively. These nerves as well as the pudendal nerves convey afferent (sensory) fibres to the spinal cord. The sympathetic fibres are derived from the lower two thoracic and upper two lumbar segments of the spinal cord. The parasympathetic fibres arise from the second to the fourth sacral segments of the spinal cord (the nervi erigentes or pelvic splanchnic nerves). The hypogastric and pelvic splanchnic nerves from each side unite to form the right or left pelvic plexus, which lies lateral to the rectum, internal genital organs, and bladder (fig. 9). That part of each pelvic plexus specifically related to the urinary bladder is referred to as the vesical plexus of autonomic nerves and contains both sympathetic and parasympathetic ganglion cells and nerve fibres together with occasional small intensely fluorescent (SIF) cells [1].

Afferent impulses arising from sensory nerve endings in the wall of the bladder and urethra pass to the spinal cord via the pudendal, pelvic splanchnic, and hypogastric nerves. The pudendal nerve transmits sensation mainly from the urethral mucosa (in addition to that from the skin of the genital area and the anal canal) and also transmits proprioceptive impulses from the striated muscle of the pelvic floor. The afferent pathway of the micturition reflex is carried in the pelvic splanchnic nerves, together with those afferents concerned with bladder mucosal pain and lower ureteric pain. The part played by the hypogastric nerves in relaying sensation from the lower urinary tract is not well defined. A detailed consideration of bladder afferent nerves is provided later in this report.

III. THE BLADDER WALL

1. SMOOTH MUSCLE

a) Cellular morphology

The individual smooth muscle cells in the bladder wall are typical smooth muscle cells – they are long spindle shaped cells with a central nucleus, and when fully relaxed are several hundred microns long, and five to six microns in diameter at their widest, where the nucleus is. As shown in figures 10 and 11, the cytoplasm is packed with the normal myofilaments, and the membranes contain regularly spaced dense bands, with membrane vesicles (caveoli) between them. There are also scattered dense bodies in the cytoplasm. Mitochondria and fairly sparse elements of sarcoplasmic reticulum (mostly near the nucleus) are also present. The smooth muscle cells are arranged in muscle bundles (fig. 12). These range extensively in size. In human detrusor the muscle bundles are large, often a few mm in diameter, and composed of several smaller sub-bundles [2]. The bundles are not clearly arranged in distinct layers, but run in all directions in the detrusor. Amongst the smooth muscle cells can be found cells having long dendritic processes extending parallel to the smooth muscle fibres, which contain vimentin, an intermediate filament expressed by cells of mesenchymal origin (fig. 13) [3].

Within the main bundles the smooth muscle cells may exist in groups of small functional units, or fascicles [4]. Intermediate junctions are seen, where adjacent cells have dense bands similarly aligned on their membranes, the gaps between the cells being quite narrow and filled with dense basement membrane. In the trigone the bundles are smaller and clearly differentiated into two layers [5]. The orientation and interaction between the smooth muscle cells in the bladder are important, since this will determine how the bladder wall behaves and what effect activity in the cells will have on its shape and intraluminal pressure.

b) Contractile machinery

As far as is known, the contractile system in the bladder smooth muscle is similar to other smooth muscles, in that shortening occurs by interaction between thin and thick filaments. The thin actin filaments are anchored at the membranes on the dense bands, or in the cytoplasm on the dense bodies, and interact with the thick filaments through cross bridges formed by the heads of myosin molecules. Relatively few papers have been published which have specifically studied the contractile machinery in detrusor smooth muscle (but see below). From studies on other smooth muscles, it is clear that a spectrum exists from those specialised for producing phasic activity (such as the ureter) and those specialized for maintaining continuous tone (such as some vascular smooth muscles). In both cases the contractile system is a myosin-activated system. Cross bridge cycling is initiated when the ATPase activity of the myosin heads is switched on (fig. 14). This is achieved by phosphorylation of one of two light chains on the cross bridge, through a specific enzyme, myosin light chain kinase, which is activated by a rise in the intracellular calcium [Ca^{2+}], with a half-maximal concentration at about 1μM. Tonically active smooth muscle may generate force with low expenditure of metabolic energy, through activation of a 'latch state' in the cross bridges, in which dephosphorylation of attached cross bridges occurs, allowing maintenance of force without energy expenditure. Information about

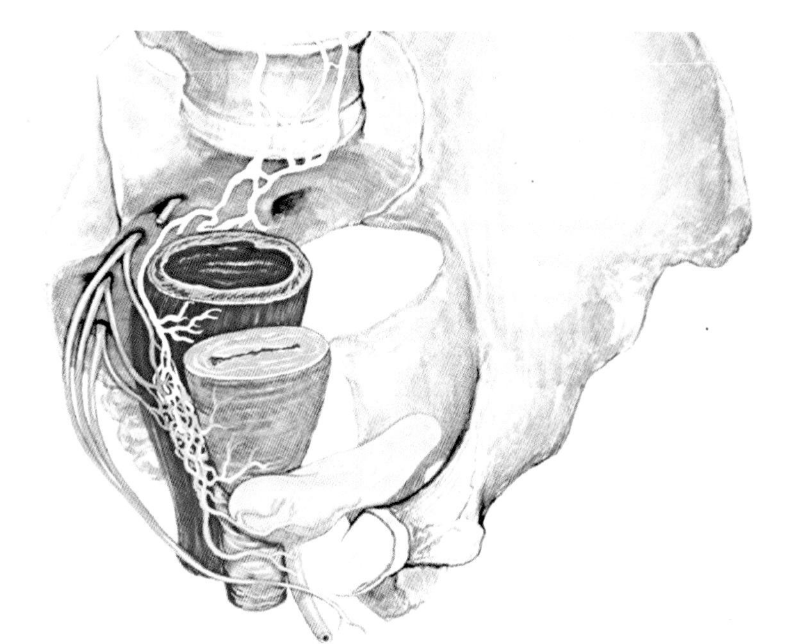

Figure 9 : A diagram illustrating the autonomic nerves which form the pelvic plexus in the female.

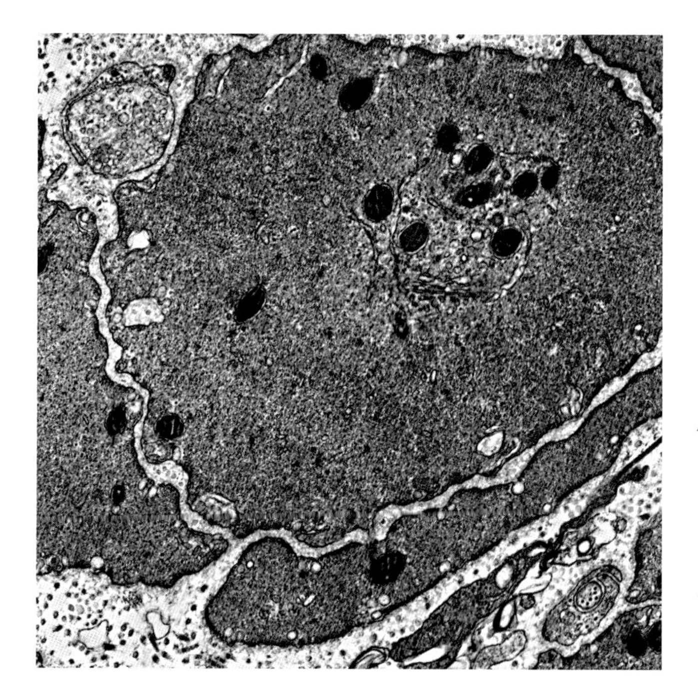

Figure 10 : Transverse section of a muscle bundle in the bladder of a rat. In the centre a large muscle cell profile shows mitochondria, Golgi apparatus, sarcoplasmic reticulum, caveolae and other surface invaginations; most of the profile is occupied by myofilaments and dense bodies. To the top left is an axon packed with vesicles and only partly covered by a Schwann cell; the exposed axolemma lies very close to the surface of the muscle cell. To the bottom right a small axonal profile, which is the intervaricose portion of a terminal axon, displays only 6 microtubules and a vesicle and is fully wrapped by a Schwann cell. Source: Giorgio Gabella, unpublished.

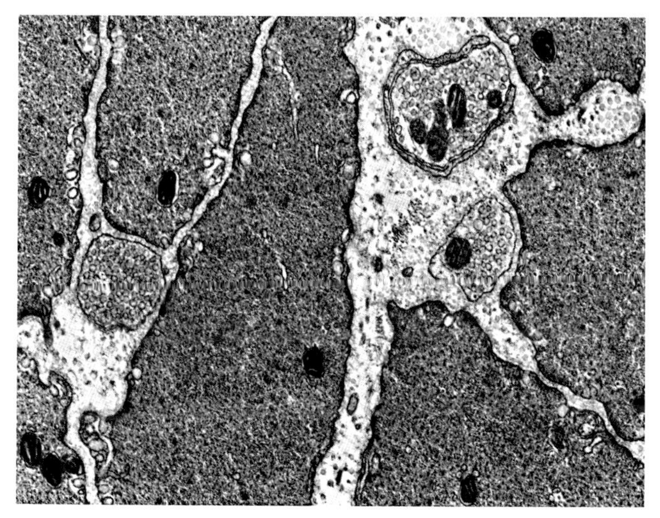

Figure 11 : Transmission electron micrograph of a muscle bundle of the rat bladder showing partial profiles of muscle cells and three axons packed with vesicles; two of the axons are near to their end and are devoid of Schwann cell wrapping while lying very close to the surface of 1-3 muscle cells. The third axonal profile is wrapped by a Schwann cell except for a small region (a window) where the axolemma is directly exposed to the extracellular space and faces at close distance the surface of a muscle cells. All three axons are regarded as forming a neuro-muscular junction. Source: Giorgio Gabella, unpublished.

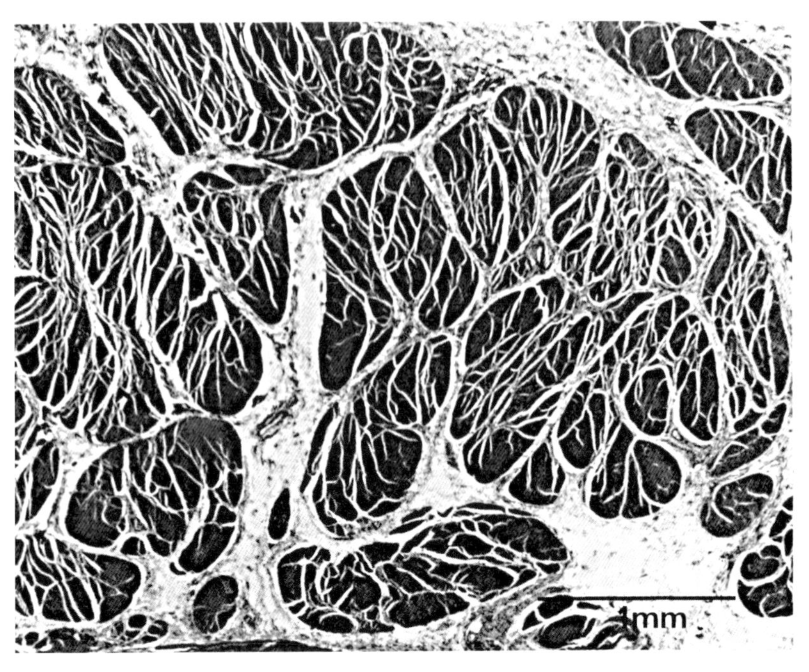

Figure 12 : Low magnification cross section of muscle bundles from normal human detrusor. Note that the muscle cells are arranged into small bundles or fasicles that are grouped together into larger bundles divided from each other by connective tissue containing collagen.

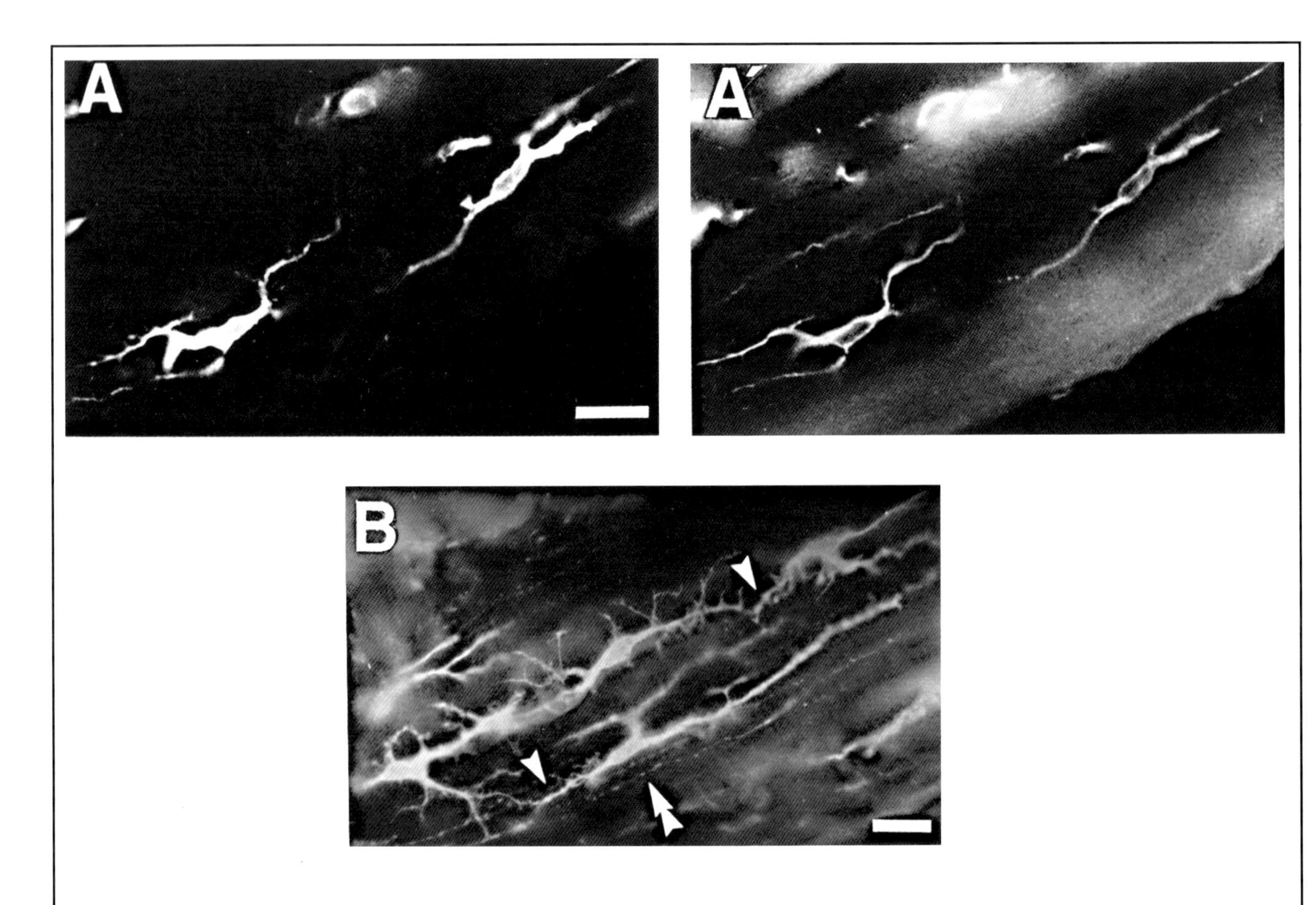

Figure 13 : Interstitial cells in the guinea-pig bladder. In A and B the cells show immunofluorescence to cGMP after exposure to sodium nitroprusside. In A', the cells shown in A have also been labeled with a fluorescent antibody to vimentin. These interstitial cells have long dendritic processes that run in parallel to the smooth muscle cells. Scale bars 25 µm. From Smet et al., 1996 [3]

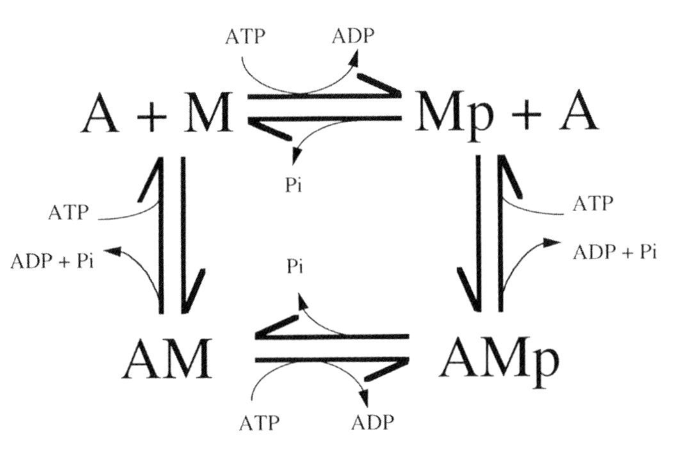

Figure 14 : Activation of contractile machinery. Normal rapid cross bridge cycling on the right of the figure occurs between phosphorylated myosin heads (Mp) and actin (A), and involves the breakdown of one ATP molecule for each cycle. Cycling is switched on by phosphorylation of the regulatory light chains of the myosin head, catalyzed by the enzyme Myosin Light Chain Kinase (MLCK). Intracellular free calcium binds to calmodulin, which then activates MLCK. Dephosphorylation of the myosin heads (M) is achieved by phosphatases. Dephosphorylation of the attached cross bridges (AM) is thought to alter the kinetics of detachment, resulting in a «latch» bridge shown on the left of the figure, which detaches from the thin filament more slowly than in the phosphorylated state.

smooth muscle contraction and the differences between this and striated muscle can be found in the following references [6-12].

Contractions of detrusor smooth muscle are more phasic in nature than seen in many other smooth muscles: during continuous excitation they show a transient phasic contraction which declines to a much smaller tonic component [13,14] that may be important for ensuring bladder emptying, but which tends towards the resting state. Changes in the contractile proteins occur in developing bladders, and during bladder hypertrophy, and several studies have mapped these changes [15-20]. Alterations in the intracellular environment may also affect contractility by altering myofibril Ca^{2+}- sensitivity [21].

c) Muscle mechanics

The great compliance of the detrusor in normal bladders, and the possibility that changes in compliance occur in various forms of dysfunction, have stimulated considerable research into the mechanical properties of the detrusor. Detrusor smooth muscle exhibits gross muscle mechanical properties common to other smooth muscle. Thus it is possible to construct length-tension and force-velocity curves (figs. 15 & 16), although their interpretation is considerably more problematic than for striated muscles. The force-velocity relationship is variable, for example the maximum shortening velocity declines during the contraction and the velocity of shortening at any load is dependent on the previous contractile history of the muscle. These mechanical phenomena are believed to be dependent on the rate of cross-bridge cycling under these different conditions. An additional problem has been to correlate the contractile behaviour of the whole bladder to that occurring in the individual muscle cells of the detrusor mass. This has been attempted by correlating the in vivo and in vitro properties of the bladder and detrusor strip preparations as well as comparing the mechanical properties of multicellular detrusor preparations and isolated smooth muscle cells [22-24].

The detrusor shows some special mechanical features. As might be expected, the length-tension relationship is relatively broad, allowing tension to be developed over a large range of resting muscle lengths [25]. The tissue shows visco-elasticity, and the visco-elastic properties of the detrusor will influence the eventual translation of muscle tension into changes in bladder wall tension. The muscle is also known to exhibit significant stress-relaxation, whereby a rapid stretch of detrusor is followed by a partial visco-elastic relaxation of stress [26, 27]. The rate of stress-relaxation is a function of the initial rate of stretch. The evaluation of those factors, whether passive or active, which determine the rate and extent of stress relaxation is important, since they will affect the measurements of bladder wall compliance [28-30].

d) Contractile characteristics of smooth muscle strips in vitro

Isolated detrusor strips show spontaneous mechanical activity to a variable extent. It is more frequently seen in bladders from small mammals, [31] but can also be seen in strips from human detrusor, particularly if a strip is left unstimulated. Spontaneous contractions normally start from a baseline of zero tension, and are brief phasic contractions of variable height, but much smaller than the maximal force the strip can generate. Spontaneous fused tetanic contractions such as those commonly seen in smooth muscles from the gastro-intestinal tract and uterus, are almost never seen in normal bladders, although they are commonly seen in strips from unstable bladders (fig. 17). Evoked contractions often show two components, a rapid phasic contraction which with continuous activation relaxes into a smaller tonic response, which is also not well maintained.

e) Membrane electrical properties

Early work from detrusor of small mammals has shown that the smooth muscle of the detrusor is able to support a regenerative action potential from a resting potential of -50 to -60 mV [32-34]. Similar action potentials can be recorded from strips of human detrusor muscle. The action potentials may have after hyperpolarizations (fig. 18) and several different K channels, such as

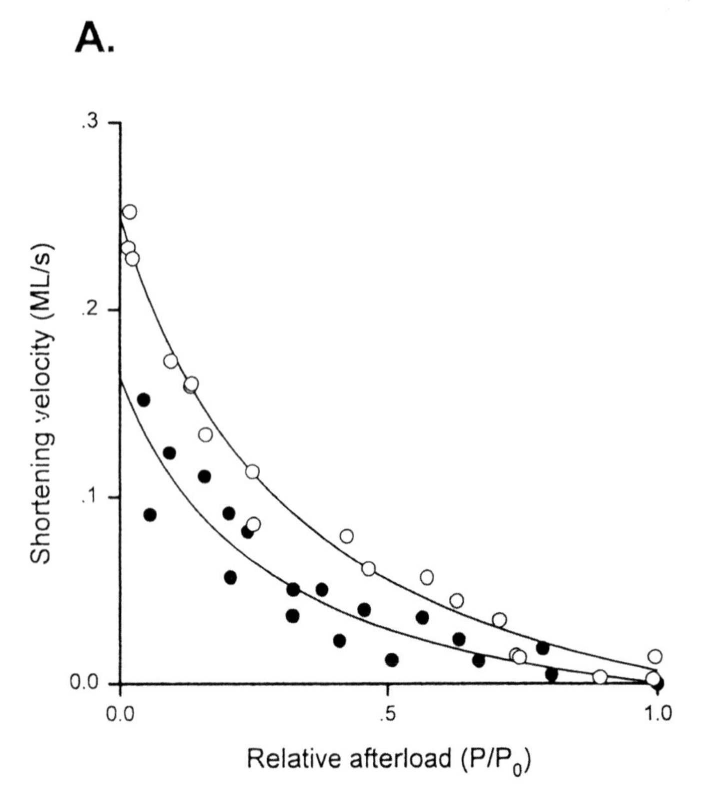

Figure 15 : Force velocity relationship of smooth muscle strips dissected from normal (open circles) and hypertrophic (filled circles) rat bladders. The shortening velocity, in muscle lengths (ML) per second, is plotted against the relative afterload (P/Po). The lines are fits to the Hill equation (v = b(1-P/Po)/(P/Po + a/Po)) where Po is isometric force and a and b are constants. From Sjuve et al, 1996 [20].

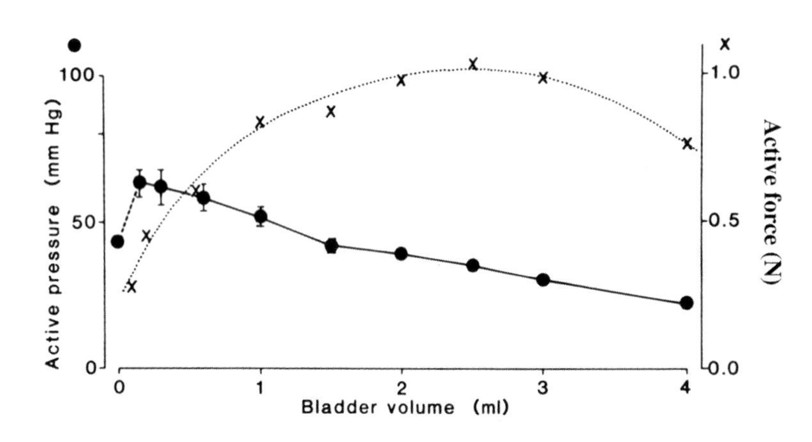

Figure 16 : Relationship between bladder volume (and hence muscle length) active pressure (in response to supra-maximal stimulation of the pelvic nerves) and active force generated in the longitudinally oriented musculature of the guinea-pig bladder. Note how the active force remains nearly constant and maximal over a wide range of volumes, and hence cell lengths. From Uvelius & Gabella, 1980 [2].

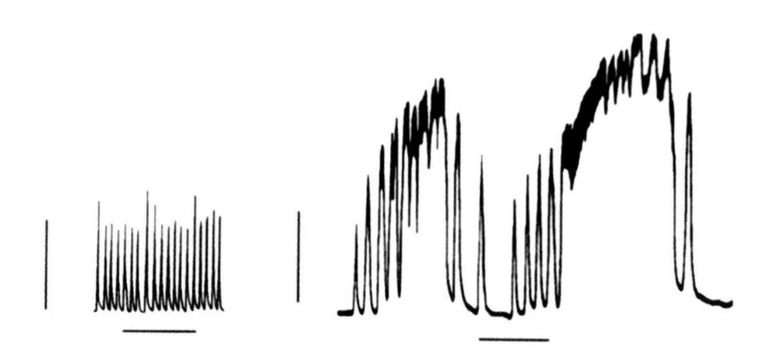

Figure 17 : Spontaneous mechanical activity recorded from strips of pig detrusor. On the right is typical activity in a strip from a normal bladder. Note the contractions vary in height, but relax to the baseline and show no fused tetanus. On the left is an example of spontaneous activity from a strip dissected from an unstable bladder (instability induced by partial urethral obstruction). Note the spontaneous fused tetanic contractions. Vertical lines represent force (0.5 gms wt), and horizontal lines time (1 min).

delayed rectifier and transient outward channels and both large and small Ca^{2+}-activated K^+ channels, appear to be involved in determining their shape [35-38]. The upstroke is supported by Ca^{2+} influx through L-type Ca^{2+} channels. In addition a potassium (K^+) channel opened by reduced intracellular ATP has been demonstrated, [39,40] which on activation is profoundly inhibitory to the spontaneous activity [41]. Several other conductances have been demonstrated in detrusor smooth muscle which include a non-specific cation channel linked to the P2X receptor [42] and stretch-activated cation channels [43]. In human detrusor, electrical properties have been studied in isolated myocytes, and similar properties are seen to those in smaller mammals [44].

f) Propagation of electrical responses

The lack of fused tetanic contractions in normal detrusor smooth muscle strips suggests that the electrical coupling between the cells may be relatively poorly developed, and this is supported by the absence of gap junctions between the cells [45], and by measurements of tissue impedance, [46,47] which suggest that detrusor is less well coupled electrically than other smooth muscles. In the guinea-pig detrusor, records of the effect of current injection into one cell on neighbouring cells (within 40 μm) showed only about 25% of the cells to be coupled electrically (fig. 19) [32, 48]. Poor coupling could be a feature of normal detrusor to prevent synchronous activation of the smooth muscle cells during bladder filling. Some degree of coupling within a muscle bundle clearly does exist, since it is possible to measure the length constant of a bundle [48] but in the absence of morphologically demonstrable gap junctions there is little evidence as to what allows the coupling to occur. Such propagation requires the presence of either low-resistance gap junctions or mechanoreceptive cell-to-cell junctions (the intermediate junctions or stretch activated channels could play a role here). It has been suggested that a change in the properties of the cell coupling may underlie the generation of the unsuppressible detrusor contractions occurring in unstable bladders, although the evidence is at present conflicting [49, 50].

Some interesting observations have been made on the changing properties of the detrusor as it develops in rats from the new-born to adulthood. In the newborn detrusor spontaneous activity is absent, although low doses of excitatory agonists induce high amplitude phasic contractions that are almost maximal in amplitude. This type of activity then appears spontaneously during early post-natal development and as development continues, the adult pattern of low-amplitude phasic contractions develops. The implication of these findings is that the poor coupling between muscle cells observed in the adult detrusor may be preceded by a phase of good coupling. This phase co-incides with the somatovesical

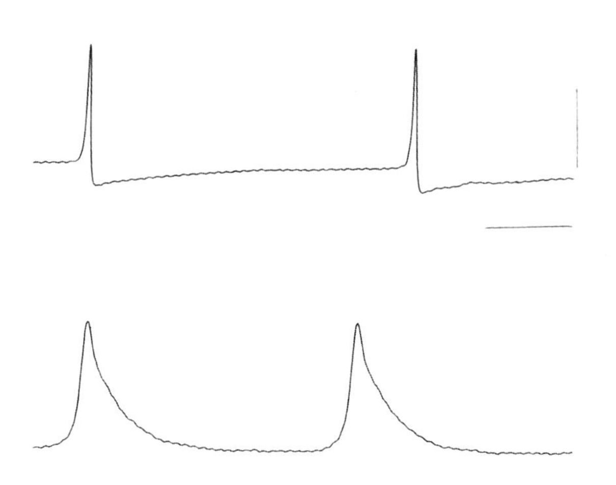

Figure 18 : Action potentials recorded with a microelectrode from smooth muscle cells of guinea-pig detrusor. The top records are in normal conditions. Note the relatively rapid repolarization and pronounced after-hyperpolarization, both of which involve K channels. The bottom records are after application of 5 mM procaine, which has little effect on the upstroke, since this is caused by current flowing through calcium channels, but markedly prolongs the repolarization and abolished the after hyperpolarization. Procaine blocks K channels non-specifically. Horizontal bar 0.2 sec, vertical bar 50 mV.

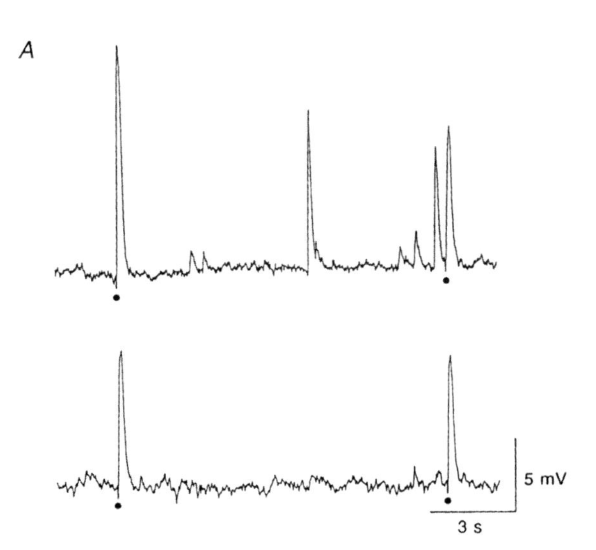

Figure 19 : A. Excitatory junction potentials (EJPs) recorded with microelectrodes from two cells in guinea-pig bladder separated by a distance of 40 μm in the axial direction. Nifedipine (10 μM) present throughout to block action potentials. Transmural stimulation (at the dots) evoked EJPs simultaneously in both cells, because of the dense innervation. However spontaneous EJPs arising in the upper cell were not recorded in the lower cell, implying poor coupling between them. From Bramich, N. & Brading, A.F. J. Physiol (Lond) 492, 185, 1996.

reflex micturition that is seen in newborn rats, activated by the mother licking the perineal area. At this age the dense excitatory innervation has not fully developed, and good coupling may be necessary to ensure bladder emptying [51-54].

g) Neuronal control of contractile behaviour

Normal bladder function requires co-ordinated detrusor relaxation and urethral sphincter contraction during the filling phase of the micturition cycle and the converse during micturition itself. Although to some extent the properties of the smooth muscles themselves help towards this end during the filling phase, control of the smooth muscle activity is achieved through the autonomic nervous system by the effects of excitatory and inhibitory transmitters, integration of which is brought about by the activity in sensory nerves and control centres in the spinal cord, pons, and forebrain [55].

1) Structural aspects: In most species, including humans, ganglia are present in the bladder wall, although the rat detrusor does not contain them. Most of these are presumably ganglia in parasympathetic pathway's and will supply the smooth muscle, although there is good evidence that the ganglia are heterogeneous [56, 57] and could be involved in local reflexes. Histochemical studies have shown that numerous guinea-pig intramural neurones stain with quinacrine, which labels ATP, providing support for the dual purinergic, cholinergic nature of the innervation (see below) [58]. Immunohistochemical studies [56] have looked at the distribution of peptides in the intramural ganglia of human detrusor. These contain immunoreactivity to vasoactive intestinal peptide, nitric oxide synthase, neuropeptide Y, and galanin, but are heterogeneous with regard to their content of these antigens, with the proportion of immunopositive cells ranging from 58-84%. Occasional neurones with immunoreactivity to the catecholamine-synthesising enzyme, tyrosine hydroxylase, are also observed. No cell somata, however, appear immunoreactive for enkephalin, substance P, calcitonin gene-related peptide or somatostatin.

The only detailed electron-microscopic study of the innervation of the detrusor using serial sectioning has been carried out in the rat [59]. This study has shown a uniform dense innervation with the penetrating nerves branching repeatedly into long varicose fibres largely encased in a Schwann cell sheath. The terminal varicosities become devoid of the Schwann cell sheath and lie close to the muscle cells forming a neuro-muscular junction with a gap normally of 30-50 nm (see fig. 11). The naked varicosities are packed with small agranular vesicles and a lesser number of dense-cored vesicles, although some large electron-lucent vesicles are occasionally seen. The density of the innervation is such that each smooth muscle cell receives at least one junction, and some may receive two. This study shows no evidence of separate purinergic and cholinergic nerves, although functionally purinergic innervation is important in the rat.

2) Functional studies: Detrusor strips demonstrate phasic contractions to selective stimulation of their intrinsic nerves [60, 31] Selective stimulation can be achieved using short pulses (0.05 msec), and the selectivity confirmed by demonstrating that the contractions are blocked by tetrodotoxin. If the pulse width of the stimuli is increased, direct activation of the smooth muscle cells can occur, which is tetrodotoxin resistant. Most mammalian bladder strips contract to single stimuli of their intrinsic nerves. Maximum contractions with tetanic trains of 5 sec train length usually occur at frequencies of about 40 Hz (fig. 20). If trains are prolonged, a biphasic contraction with a rapid transient phase declining to a smaller more prolonged slow phase can be seen in most non-human bladders (fig. 21) [14]. The slow phase is abolished by atropine and enhanced in the presence of cholinesterase inhibitors, suggesting that the excitatory transmitter is acetylcholine, but the rapid phasic response shows considerable atropine resistance, and can be abolished by desensitisation of the P2x-purinoceptors with α, β-methylene ATP, suggesting that ATP is normally a co-transmitter with acetylcholine [34, 61, 62]. In contrast, detrusor strips from normal human bladders produce little response to single stimuli and require repetitive activation of the intrinsic nerves to induce a response, and the response can be completely abolished by atropine [31], suggesting that the response is purely cholinergic (fig. 22). Evidence suggests that the detrusor possesses both M2 and M3 cholinoreceptors [63-65]. Although M2 receptors predominate in receptor binding studies, it is the M3 receptor that is thought to mediate contraction.

Although purinergic innervation does not appear to be important in the normal human bladder, it seems probable that ATP is released with acetylcholine, and this innervation may become important in unstable bladders. The detrusors of mammalian bladders possess excitatory P2x receptors, [42, 66] inhibitory P2y receptors [67] and possibly other types of purinoceptor (fig. 23) [68-70]. Excitatory effects on the detrusor may also be mediated by local release of tachykinins (substance P, neurokinin A) and other peptides from sensory nerves in the bladder wall. These have been shown to produce diverse biological effects, such as smooth muscle contraction, facilitation of neurotransmitter release from nerves, vasodilatation, and increased plasma permeability [71-74]. The actions of the tachykinins are mediated by activation of three distinct receptor subtypes termed NK1, NK2, and NK3 [75].

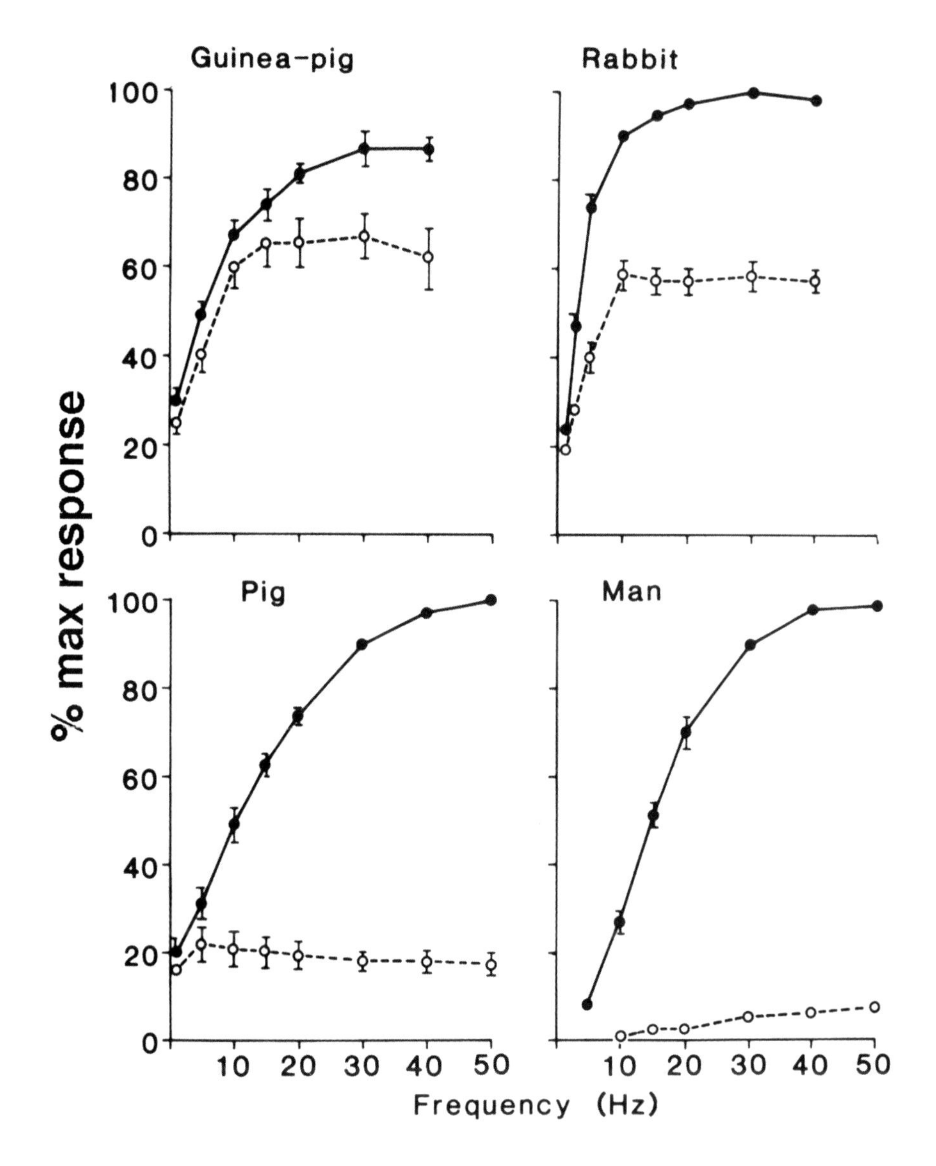

Figure 20 : Responses of detrusor strips from varies species to electrical field stimulation of the intrinsic nerves, using 5 sec trains at different frequencies. The solid points are controls, and the open circles and dotted lines the response in the presence of muscarinic receptor blockade (atropine 5.10-7 - 10-6M). Note that in the guinea-pig, rabbit and pig, the tissues respond to stimuli at 1 Hz, with atropine resistant contractions. The size of the atropine resistant component at higher frequencies is species dependent, being large in the guinea-pig, and virtually absent in the human.

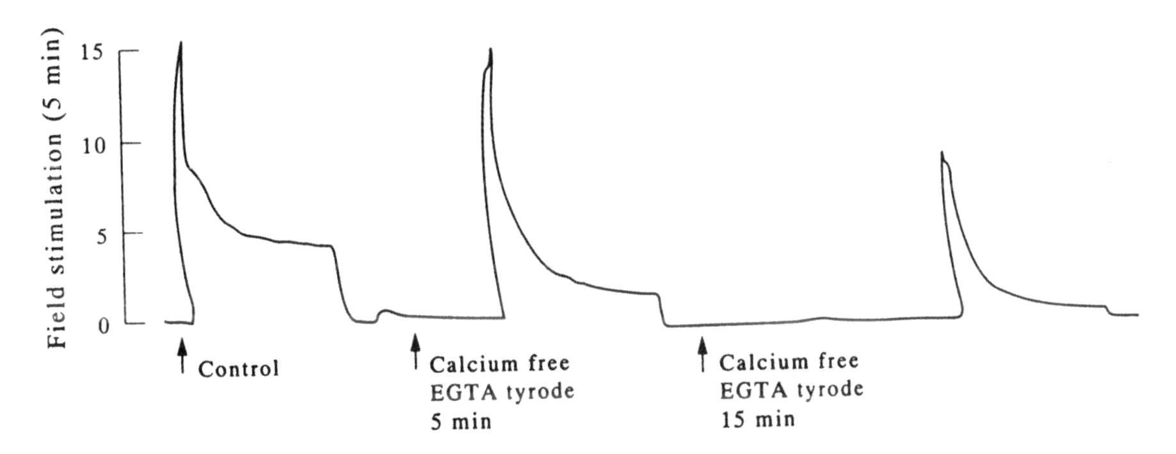

Figure 21 : Responses of rabbit bladder smooth muscle to 5 min trains of electrical field stimulation (32 Hz, 80 V). Note transient peak followed by decline to a prolonged plateau. The peak component was initially less susceptible to calcium free solution than the plateau. From Zhao et al. 1993 [14].

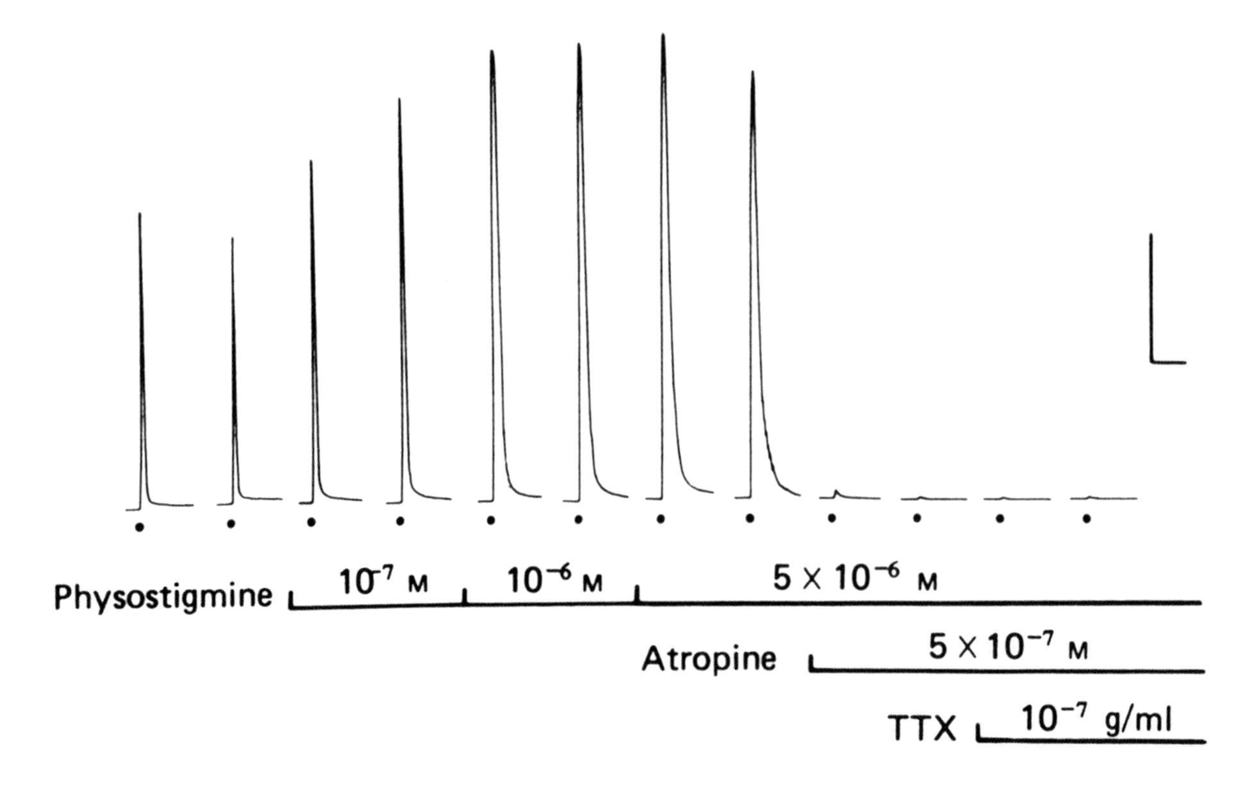

Figure 22 : Responses of a strip of human detrusor to stimulation of its intrinsic nerves for 5 sec at 20 Hz. Note the size of the response is progressively enhanced as the cholinesterase is inhibited with physostigmine, and that the contractions are virtually abolished by 5.10-7M atropine. Horizontal bar represents 2 min, and vertical bar 2 gm wt.

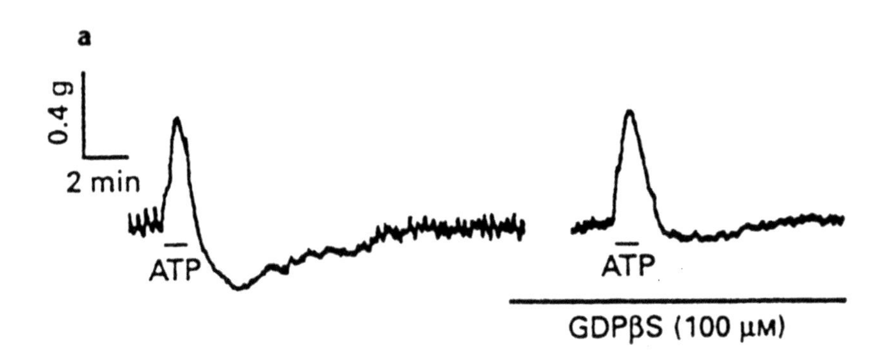

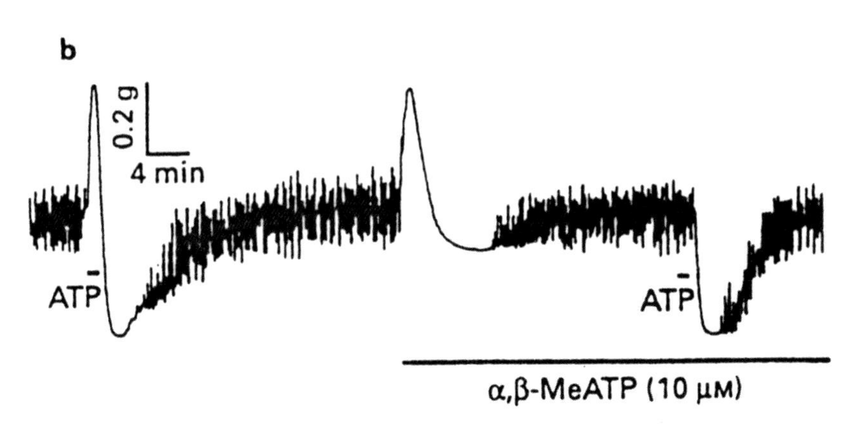

Figure 23 : Responses of marmoset detrusor strip to ATP (1 mn, 60 sec application).

(a) Stimulation with ATP in the absence and presence of the G-protein inactivator, GDPβS which abolishes P2y mediated effects. Note that the relaxant phase is abolished, leaving a pure contractile response.

(b) Stimulation with ATP in the absence and presence of P2x receptor desensitization with, α, β-Me ATP. Desensitaization of the P2x receptors abolishes the contractile response, and leaves a pure relaxant response. From McMurray et al. 1998. [67].

There is normally no rise in bladder pressure during the filling phase until the bladder is near its full capacity, hence it has been suggested that activation of inhibitory nerves may be involved in keeping the smooth muscles quiescent. However morphological studies show a dense but uniform acetylcholinesterase positive innervation of the detrusor, and there is little evidence for direct innervation by adrenergic nerves [76, 77] Electron microscope studies confirm the dense but uniform innervation by nerves that contain predominantly the small clear vesicles that are characteristic of cholinergic nerves (see fig. 11) [59]. The response of the detrusor to catecholamines varies between species, and depends on which area of the detrusor is being investigated. An α-receptor-mediated contraction of the trigone and bladder neck regions is commonly seen (fig. 24) and β-receptor mediated relaxant responses can also be found, and both β2 and β3 may be present (figures 25 & 26) [78, 79].

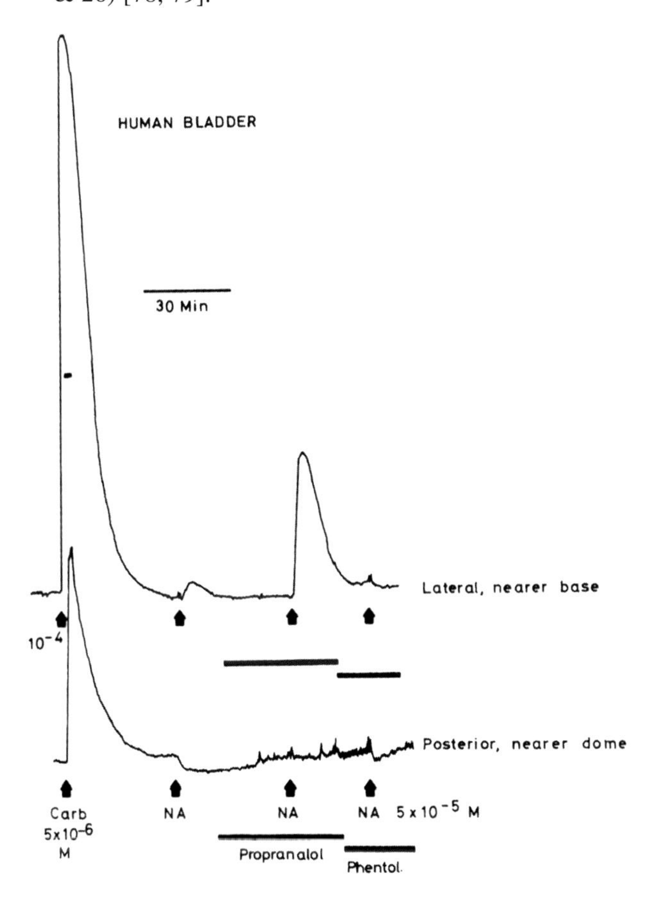

Figure 24 : Responses of strips of smooth muscle from the human bladder, taken from the base (above) or the dome (below). Both strips respond to carbachol, but the response to noradrenaline varies. The basal strip contracts weakly, but the response is enhanced by blocking β-adrenoceptors with propranalol, and abolished by blocking the α-adrenoceptors with phentolamine. In contrast, the strip from the dome relaxes to noradrenaline , but the response is mediated by β-adrenoceptors since it is abolished by propranalol and unaffected by phentolamine.

Although the evidence for anything other than a postganglionic parasympathetic input to the detrusor is poor, there is, however, evidence that inhibitory pathways to the bladder do exist, although it seems likely that these terminate at the level of the intramural ganglia. In the rabbit, many sympathetic fibres terminate on vesical parasympathetic ganglia and inhibit neurotransmission via α 2-adrenoceptors [80]. In the human bladder several types of presynaptic input onto intramural ganglia have been demonstrated [55]. It has also been shown that GABA inhibits bladder function in humans and other mammals through specific receptors both in the central nervous system and in the periphery [81-83].

In both humans and guinea pigs, varicose nitric oxide synthase-immunoreactive nerve terminals provided a moderate innervation to the detrusor muscle of the bladder body [3]. However, the smooth muscle cells do not react to stimulation with sodium nitroprusside either by relaxing or by expressing cGMP-immunoreactivity (the normal pathway for NO-mediated smooth muscle relaxation), although numerous interstitial cells throughout the bladder body demonstrated an intense induction of cGMP-immunoreactivity by sodium nitroprusside (see fig. 13). The function of these cells, and of the nitrergic nerves in the detrusor is unknown.

h) Excitation-contraction and receptor-effector coupling

The trigger for contraction in all smooth muscles is a rise in intracellular free calcium concentration. Calcium may either enter down its electrochemical gradient from the extracellular medium, or be released from intracellular calcium stores. Excitation-contraction coupling describes the link between changes in the membrane potential and tension development, and receptor-effector coupling the pathways between receptor activation and alterations in contractile activity. The involvement of calcium entry through the membrane and store release vary markedly in different smooth muscles. The patterns in bladder and urethra are clearly different, although currently the details in both tissues arc poorly undcrstood.

The detrusor produces calcium-based action potentials, and it seems likely that the spontaneous contractile activity of strips is triggered by these. However, the frequency of spontaneous action potentials recorded with microelectrodes in single cells within a strip are usually higher than the frequency of the phasic contractions recorded from strips [84,85] This, and the lack of fused tetanic contractions which normally are seen in other smooth muscles with high frequency action potentials, suggests that the action potentials may not be well syn-

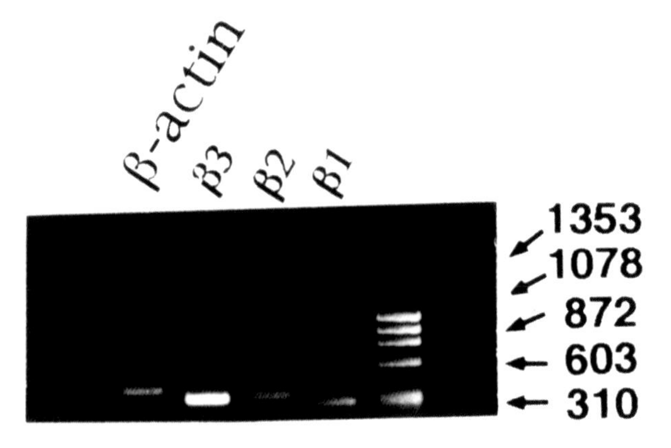

Figure 25 : Demonstration of the presence of β1, β2 and β3-adrenoceptors in human detrusor. Total RNA was extracted from the detrusor, and amplification of the mRNA for β1, β2 and β3-adrenoceptors was carried out using the reverse transcription / polymerase chain reaction (RT/PCR). The figure shows the results of agarose gel electrophoresis and size fractionation of the products. From right to left, the first lane is a negative control (PCR product using primers specific for β3-adrenoceptors without RT), the next lane shows the presence of β-actin, a smooth muscle marker, the next three lanes show the presence of the three β-adrenoceptors and the last lane is a size marker.

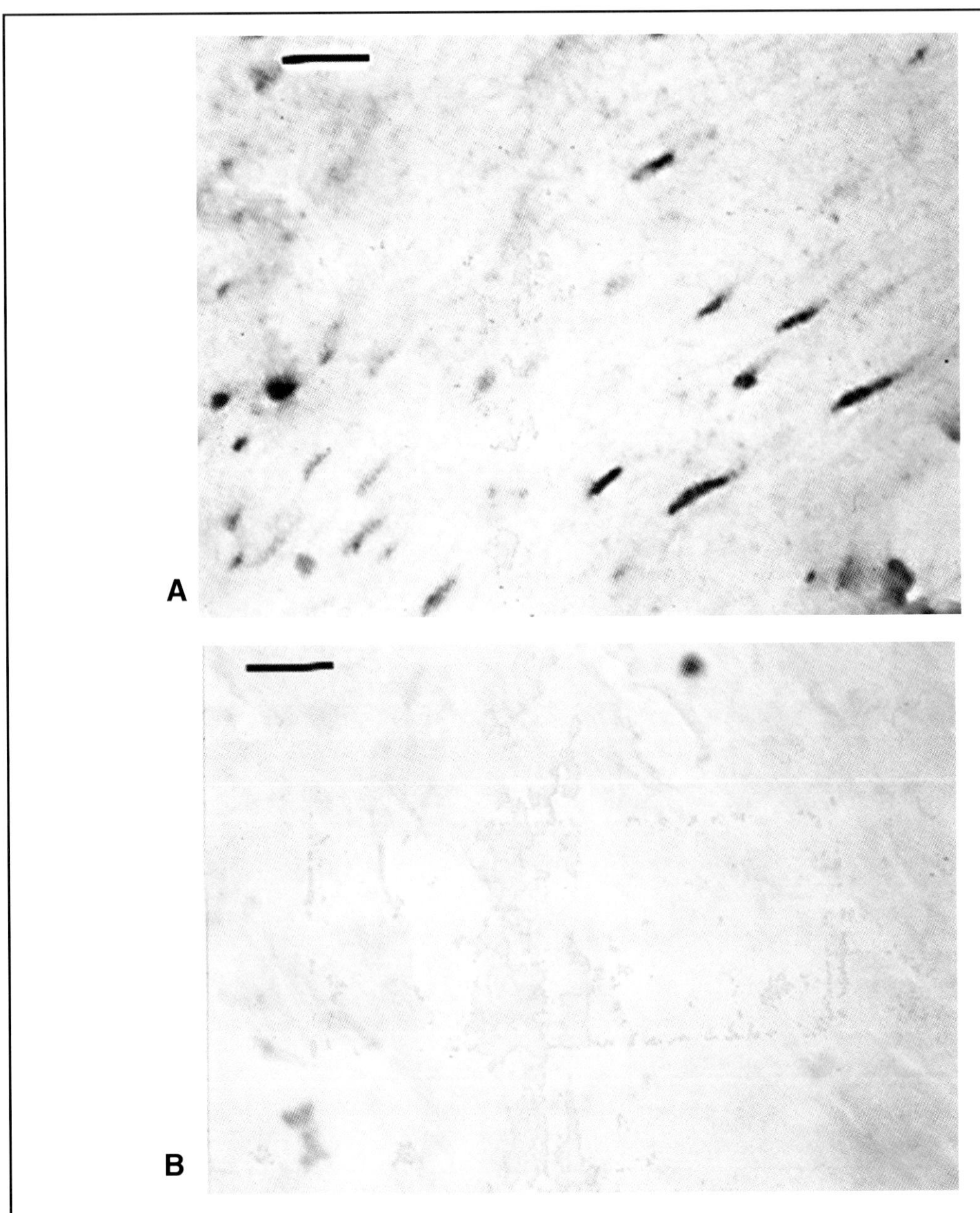

Figure 26 : In situ hybndization of β3-adrenoceptors from human detrusor. (a) Blue stain indicates positive hybridization of a digoxtgenin-11-d-UTP labelled antisense oligonucleotide probe, suggesting the expression of β3-adrenoceptor mRNA. (b) Negative control, using a digoxtgenin-11-d-UTP labelled sense oligonucleotide probe. Bars denote 400 μM.

chronized in detrusor strips. The spontaneous phasic contractions are usually much smaller than the maximal contraction that can be evoked by nerve stimulation, and thus it appears that Ca^{2+} entering in the spikes does not elevate the free calcium levels sufficiently to cause much activation of the contractile machinery. In other smooth muscles, calcium entering in the spikes has been shown to activate release of calcium from internal stores by a calcium-activated calcium release channel. Evidence that such channels exist in the detrusor has been provided from studies on the effects of caffeine, a drug known to sensitise these channels and cause Ca^{2+} release from stores (fig. 27) [86, 87]. However the response to caffeine is transient and much smaller than seen in other smooth muscles. The sarcoplasmic reticulum also acts as a powerful Ca^{2+} accumulating organelle to terminate the contraction, via active transport using a magnesium (Mg^{2+})-dependent ATPase [88].

The role of excitation contraction coupling in the response of the detrusor to transmitters is less clear. In detrusor muscle from non-human mammals, intrinsic nerve stimulation generates excitatory junction potentials and triggers synchronous action potentials in detrusor smooth muscle [46 48]. The junction potentials are mediated by activation of P2x purinoceptors, which open non-selective cation channels, depolarising the membrane, and activating L-type Ca^{2+} channels. The contractile response can be abolished by L-type Ca channel blockers, implicating Ca^{2+} entry and possibly Ca^{2+}-induced Ca^{2+} release from internal stores in the contractile response. This mechanism does not seem to be apparent in normal human detrusor, but is sometimes seen in unstable detrusor [89, 90].

It is unclear what the role of electrophysiological changes are in the contractile response to acetylcholine. Activation of muscarinic receptors produces little change in the membrane potential, [84, 85] but spike frequency is increased at concentrations able to elicit large contractions. Whole cell patch clamp studies show that acetylcholine causes an outward K^+ current, presumably mediated through calcium activated K^+ channels. M3 receptors are thought to act through increased polyphosphoinositide hydrolysis, inositol triphosphate (IP3) production (fig. 28) and release of intracellular calcium stores [63, 91, 92]. The rise in intracellular Ca^{2+} will initiate contraction and may open Ca^{2+}-activated K^+ channels. This pathway also generates diacylglycerol in the membrane, which can activate protein kinase C which may be involved in generating the tonic element of the response through modulation of Ca^{2+} and K^+ channels (fig. 29) [13,14]. M2 receptors mediate inhibition of adenylate cyclase, with the reduction of cAMP levels. Since elevated cAMP levels mediate smooth muscle relaxation, the role of the M2 receptors could be to render the smooth muscle more easily excited [93].

With reference to the release of calcium through activation of IP3 receptors, it is interesting that the response to muscarinic receptor activation can be blocked by L-type calcium channel blockers [94]. It is currently believed that Ca^{2+} influx through Ca^{2+}-channels aids in filling intracellular stores and that open K^+-channels keep the membrane potential sufficiently negative to prevent too large a Ca^{2+} influx through this route [39, 95].

i) The role of the smooth muscle in the bladder wall

The role of the detrusor smooth muscle is to maintain the integrity of the bladder without generating significant intravesical pressure during filling, and to contract synchronously during micturition to elevate the intravesical pressure sufficiently and for long enough to empty the bladder. There is also smooth muscle in the trigone. This has different properties and innervation to the detrusor, [5] and may play a role in preventing reflux up the ureters during micturition. Changes in the properties of the detrusor could clearly result in major alterations in the behaviour of the bladder, and might result in significant dysfunction. Indeed such changes have been clearly demonstrated in patients and animals with unstable bladders, and there is currently argument as to whether such changes are a cause of unstable contractions or the result of other factors which may underlie instability. Those interested in pursuing this are referred to the proceedings of the consensus conference on the overactive bladder [95, 96].

2. Stroma

The bladder stroma could be defined as the bladder wall minus the smooth muscle and the urothelium. The main constituents are collagen and elastin in a matrix composed of proteoglycans. The main cells are fibroblasts. The passive mechanical properties of the bladder wall depends on the viscoelastic properties of the stroma and of the relaxed detrusor muscle (e.g. [97, 98]). Collagen and elastin are generally thought to be intimately related to bladder compliance.

a) Bladder wall collagen

Microanatomical organisation: The amount of collagen in the bladder wall is considerable; more than a third of the bladder dry weight is collagen [99, 100] A detailed morphological analysis of the collagen distribution in the human bladder [101] found differences in the collagen arrangement in the mucosal, muscular and serosal layers. The mucosal layer could be divided into 3 portions (fig. 30). Just under the urothelium there was a superficial portion interwoven densely by thin collagen fibrils running in all directions, forming a felt-like structure. Deeper to this there was a thicker intermedia-

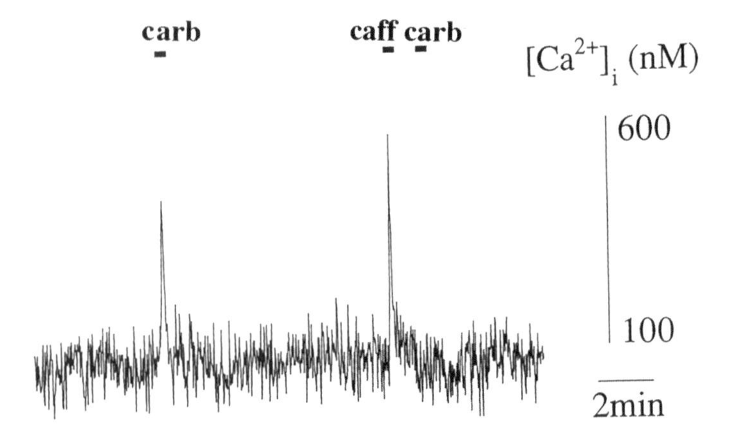

Figure 27 : Intracellular calcium transients in a smooth muscle cell from guinea-pig detrusor. Carbachol (10-4 M) causes a transient elevation of intracellular calcium as does caffeine (10 mM). Caffeine appears to empty the intracellular stores completely, since carbachol applied immediately after caffeine no longer elicits a calcium transient.

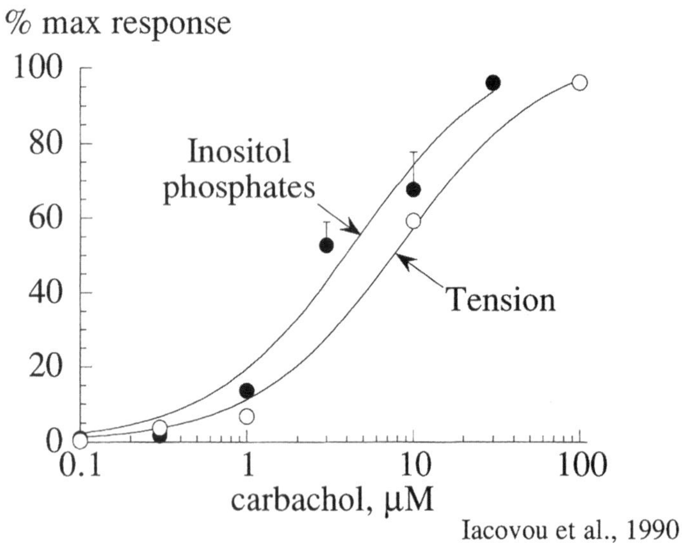

Figure 28 : The effects of carbachol on intracellular inositol phosphates and tension in guinea-pig detrusor. Adapted from Iacovou et al., 1990 [91].

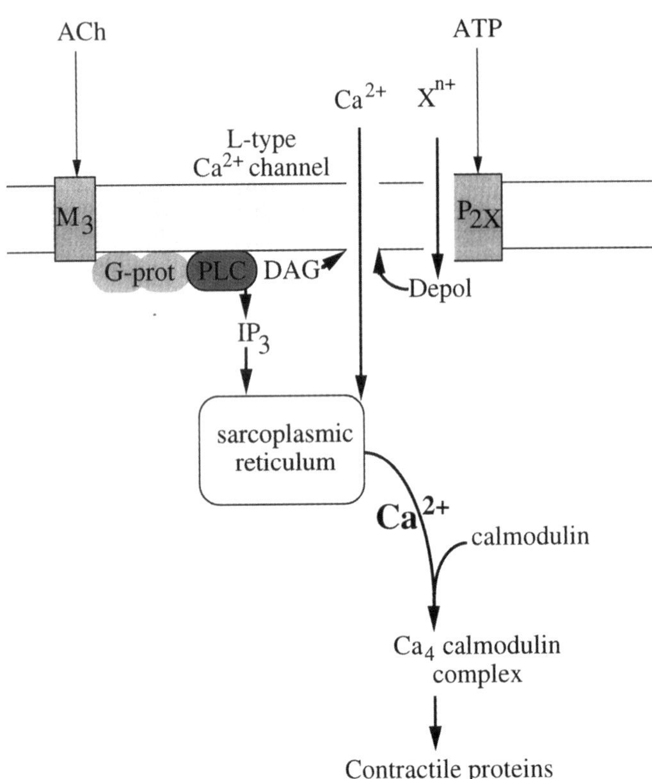

Figure 29 : Diagram of pathways involved in the response of detrusor to acetylcholine (ACh) and ATP. ACh interacts with M_3-muscarinic receptors and activates phospholipase C (PLC) through a G-protein, leading to the production of inositol tris phosphate (IP_3) and diacylglycerol (DAG). IP3 elicits release of calcium from the sarcoplasmic reticulum through IP_3-receptors, and DAG may modulate voltage sensitive calcium channels in the plasma membrane. ATP acting through P_{2x} purinoceptors opens non-selective cation channels in the membrane, leading to depolarization which opens voltage sensitive calcium channels. Both lead to entry of calcium. This triggers release of further calcium from the stores through ryanodine receptors. The rise in intracellular free calcium concentration triggers contraction, and may also open various calcium-activated channels in the membrane (such as calcium activated K channels), which can modulate the response.

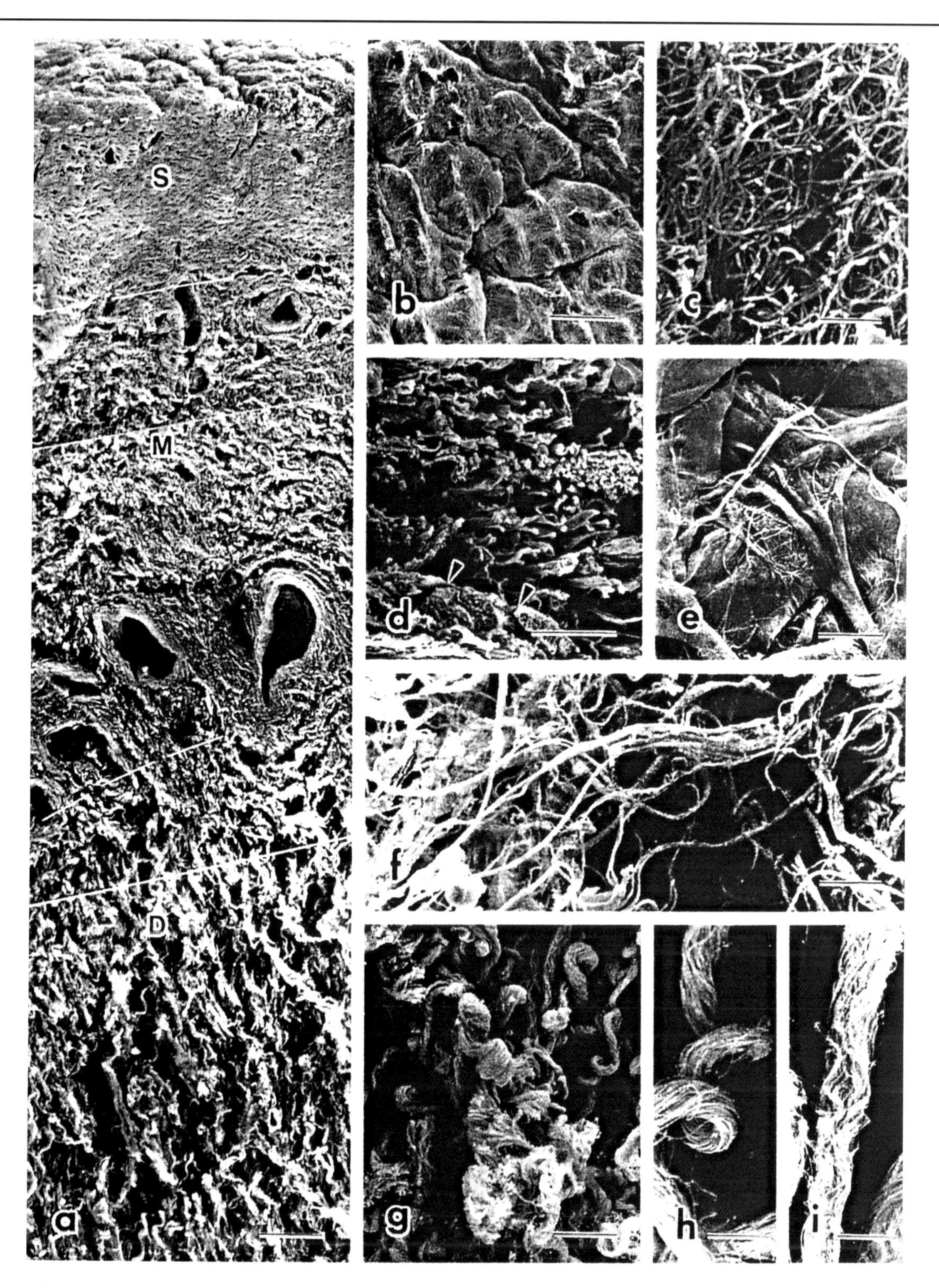

Figure 30 : Collagen and elastin components of the mucosal layer of the urinary bladder of a 54-year-old male.(a) Low power view of the cut face of the mucosal layer. Bar 100 μM. The dotted line shows the innermost surface. Superficial (S), middle (M) and deep (D) portions are distinguishable according to the arrangement and density of the collagen fibrils. Numerous small holes for capillaries and nerves are seen in the superficial portion, and canals for larger vessels in the middle and deep portions. (b) and (c) lower and higher magnification of collagen fibres forming the innermost surface of the superficial portion just under the epithelium. Bars 20 μM and 2 μM. (d) stacks of collagen bundles in the middle portion running between the smooth muscle cells, the sheaths of which are indicated by arrowheads. Bar 50 μM. (e) flat tape-like collagen bundles arranged in two dimensions ruin parallel to the mucosal coat. Bar 5 μM. (f) loose network of elastin fibres in the middle portion. Bar 20 μM. (g) and (h) lower and higher magnification of loose network of curled collagen bundles in the deep portion from unstretched bladder. Bars 20 μM and 5 μM. (i) straight collagen bundle from deep part of stretched bladder. Bar 5 μM. From Murakumo et al., 1995 [101].

te portion with parallel bundles of thick collagen fibrils. A discontinuous muscularis mucosa separated this layer from the deep portion of the mucosa. This portion was the thickest, and contained a loose network of thick twisted strands of thin collagen bundles. These strands were strongly curled in the empty bladder, but straightened as the bladder was filled. The muscular layer consists mainly of muscle bundles, running in various directions. A rich amount of collagen fibres is found between the bundles. The collagen fibres are arranged in thick bundles often running transversely to the bundle they surround. Within the muscle bundles winding collagen fibrils form thin lace-like sheaths surrounding the individual smooth muscle cells. Outside the muscular layer there is a loose sub-serosal network of collagen bundles.

No such detailed morphological analysis exists for bladders from other species, but in the rat most of the collagen fibrils are found in the mucosa and between the muscle bundles [100]. Fibroblasts, which are common outside the muscle bundles are rarely seen within.

Relative amount of interstitial tissue: Most of the bladder wall collagen is found in the connective tissue outside the muscle bundles. Changes in relation between the amount of muscle and non-muscle tissue in the bladder wall would therefore influence collagen concentration. In the rat infravesical obstruction or bladder denervation induce hypertrophy of the detrusor smooth muscle and the collagen concentration decreases [100, 102].

In man, the proportion of connective tissue relative to muscle in the bladder is lower in childhood than in the fetus [103]. Ageing is associated with a relative decrease in smooth muscle in both males and females [104]. Despite this, the collagen concentration in the adult male is not influenced by age [99]. This could perhaps be related to the decreased packing density of submucosal collagen during ageing [105].

Collagen subtypes: Today a considerable number of collagen types are known. In the bladder types I, III and IV are the most important ones (see e.g.[106]). Types I and III form fibrils with a typical banding. There seems to be a correlation between the ratio of type III-to-type I collagen content and bladder compliance. In the foetal bovine bladder the increase in compliance during the second and third trimester is paralleled by a decreased ratio of type III:I collagen [107]. The adult bovine bladder has, on the other hand, a decreased compliance and an increased type III:I ratio. Also, the type III:I ratio is increased in low compliant dysfunctional human bladders [108] compared with age-matched controls. The increased amount of collagen type III is mainly between the cells in the smooth muscle bundles [109].

b) Bladder wall elastin

Elastic fibres are amorphous structures composed of elastin and a microfibrillar component located mainly around the periphery of the amorphous component [110]. In the mature fibre, the amorphous component composes about 90%. The microfibrils contain a number of proteins; possibly the most important ones are the glycoproteins fibrillin and microfibril associated glycoproteins (MAGP).

Elastin fibres are sparse in the bladder, compared to collagen [101] but are found in all layers (see fig. 30). Anti-elastin immunohistochemistry [110] has shown that the elastin in the mucosa-submucosa appears to be arranged in fibres parallel to the urothelial lining. Elastin was also found between and in the smooth muscle bundles, although the organisation was less regular.

The elastin fibres can also be stained by antibodies against fibrillin and MAGP. These however, also cause an intense staining of the urothelium, suggesting the presence of microfibrillar protein in the absence of amorphous elastin. Most of these microfibrillar proteins seem to be localised together with collagen type IV in the basement membrane, [111] but the staining pattern also suggests that there is some fibrillin between the urothelial cells.

Elastin can be demonstrated histologically in increasing amounts from 20 weeks gestation in the human bladder [112]. The amount of elastin seems to have increased in the obstructed foetal bladder showing that the turnover of elastin can be influenced by pathophysiological conditions.

c) Bladder proteoglycans

The non-fibrillar matrix in the stroma is largely composed of a gel of proteoglycans and water. Proteoglycans are glycoproteins with glycosaminoglycans covalently attached. The arrangement of the proteoglycans in the matrix creates a compartment of tissue water which has a viscous behaviour when subjected to deformation. The resistance to tissue deformation is further increased because the proteoglycans in the bladder wall are compressed as compared to their state in solution. The non-fibrillar matrix has not attracted the same interest in recent research as the fibrils embedded in the matrix, and consequently, the number of reports are limited.

The different proteoglycans do not have similar distribution in the bladder wall. Heparin sulphate is localised to the basement membrane under the urothelium [113]. The mucosa contains the highest amount of chondroitin sulphate proteoglycan (CSPG) in the bladder, [114] while the submucosa is the richest site of decorin and hyaluronan, a glycosaminoglycan. Hyaluronan is most concentrated along the transition between the mucosa and the submucosa. The uneven distribution of the proteoglycans would be expected to give different biomechanical properties to the different layers of the stroma; e.g. decorin, which is less hydrated than CSPG, would decrease submucosal compliance. Hyaluronan, which creates a more hydrated matrix than the other molecules, could create a loose matrix for movement of the mucosa over the submucosa during changes of bladder filling [114].

Pathophysiological processes can influence the proteoglycan distribution. In trabeculated bladders the high hyaluronan concentration has moved from the transition between mucosa and submucosa to the deep submucosa [114]. Apparently, the influence of possible changes in the non-fibrillar matrix has to be taken into account when explaining changes in bladder compliance secondary to neurogenic lesions or obstruction.

d) The role of the stroma

In the past there has been an intense interest in bladder and urethral muscle. The stroma has, however, more or less been considered as a passive low metabolic tissue filling out the space between muscle bundles, vessels and nerves. In recent years the important role of the stroma in the adaptation of the bladder to pathophysiological conditions has been more appreciated. Collagen and elastin have been found to modify and better adapt to e.g. increased functional demands, but changes can also lead to decreased compliance. The cells in the stroma include myofibroblasts which under certain conditions can differentiate into new smooth muscle cells. In arteries, disruption of elastin in the stroma [115] can stimulate proliferation of smooth muscle. Although no such mechanisms are yet known in the bladder, it is possible that there could be a more intimate relation between changes in the composition of the stroma and muscle function and growth than is appreciated at present.

3. Blood vessels

a) Structure and properties

The bladder vasculature is a multi-layer vascular plexus with morphological as well as functional implications. The vascular anatomy of the urinary bladder is not fully known, however the presence of an extramural as well as intramural and submucosal plexus has been shown [116]. The muscularis and submucosa contain relatively few vessels, and the arteries and veins run predominantly in the connective tissue between the muscle bundles, with mainly capillaries penetrating between the smooth muscle fascicles (fig. 31). In thick sections of the bladder the tortuous course of the blood vessels is clearly apparent (fig. 32). In contrast, the underside of the epithelium is scored by numerous grooves which are occupied by a dense network of blood capillaries. These vascular grooves allow a large number of capillaries to run at a distance of only a few microns from the epithelium (fig. 33) [117]. These capillaries are partially fenestrated, with the fenestrated areas being predominantly located on the aspect of the capillary facing the urothelial basal lamina (fig.34). Fenestrated capillaries are a regular feature of many organs and tissues; they have been shown to be more permeable to both water and solutes than the more usual non-fenestrated capillaries in terms of both uptake (e.g. endocrine glands and the intestinal epithelium) and leakage (e.g. renal glomerulus and spinal and autonomic ganglia), and fenestrations are also transiently expressed in some developing tissues (e.g. dental pulp), and during regeneration following damage (e.g. peripheral nerve and striated muscle). The presence of fenestrae in the endothelial cells of the sub-urothelial capillary plexus may indicate that it has a role in the uptake of substances with an endocrine function, e.g. ATP, secreted by the urothelium, to be transported to more remote sites of action, e.g. the detrusor, autonomic ganglia and the CNS.

Because of the large increase in surface area of the bladder wall during filling, the blood vessels will need to be able to lengthen considerably, and to maintain a good blood flow, mechanisms may have to be present to ensure that the overall resistance of the vessels as they lengthen does not increase sufficiently to reduce the effective perfusion of the tissue. Several techniques have been used in order to study blood flow in the intact urinary bladder. However, almost no studies have been carried out on conscious subjects and most studies have been performed in various animal models [118]. Radioactive microspheres and radio-labelled tracer washout have been used to study the blood flow in rabbit, pig and dog bladders [119, 120]. Recently laser Doppler probes placed in the bladder wall have been used to evaluate blood flow in the human bladder [121, 122] and pig bladder [123] and in vivo models for the study of the rat urinary bladder micro-circulation have also been developed to allow the evaluation of the microcirculatory response to vasoactive agents [124].

The effect of bladder filling on the blood flow has been investigated by several groups, with variable results. The majority of reports have shown that the blood flow is reduced by the distension during bladder filling [122, 118]. In patients with a low compliant bladder there is a marked increase in the intravesical pressure and a more pronounced decrease in bladder blood flow as compared with normal controls [121]. The principal determinant of blood flow in the bladder wall seems to be the pressure within its lumen (see figs.35, 36). During normal filling the blood flow is able to adapt to the large increase in surface area until the pressure

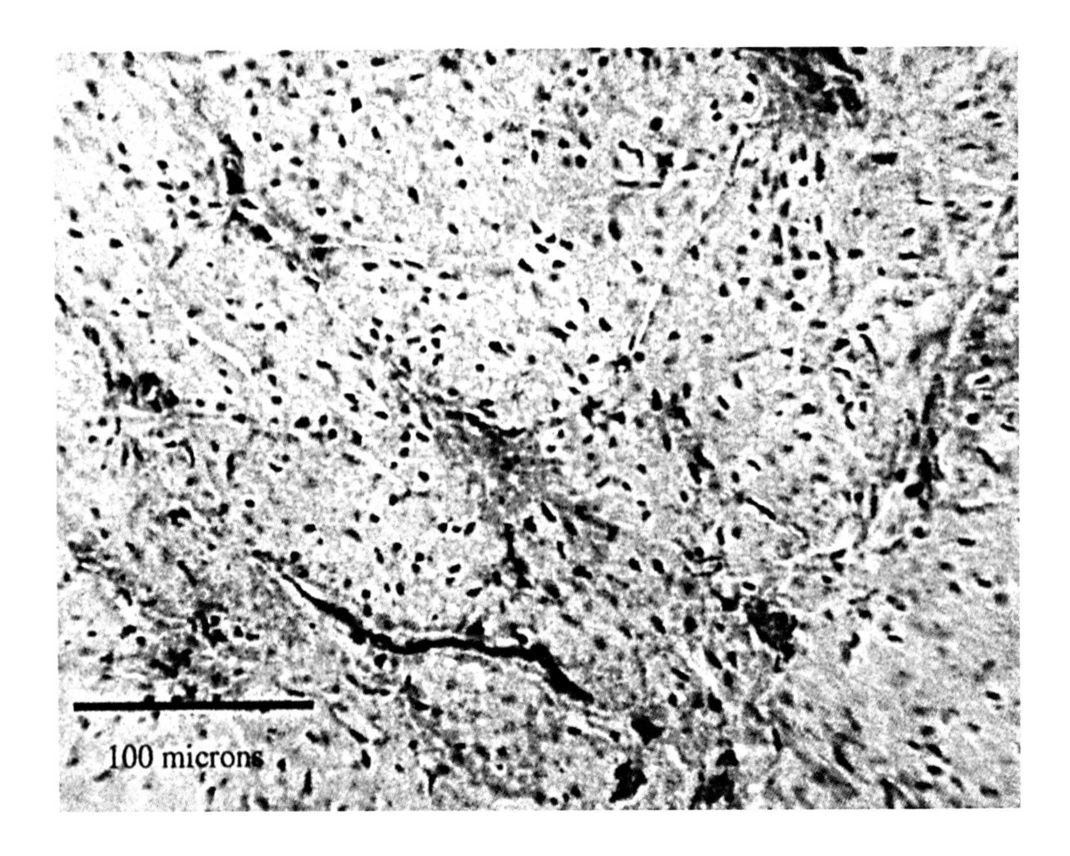

Figure 31 : Section of pig detrusor through smooth muscle bundles, stained to reveal endothelial cells. Note that capillaries run between the smooth muscle bundles, but do not penetrate into them.

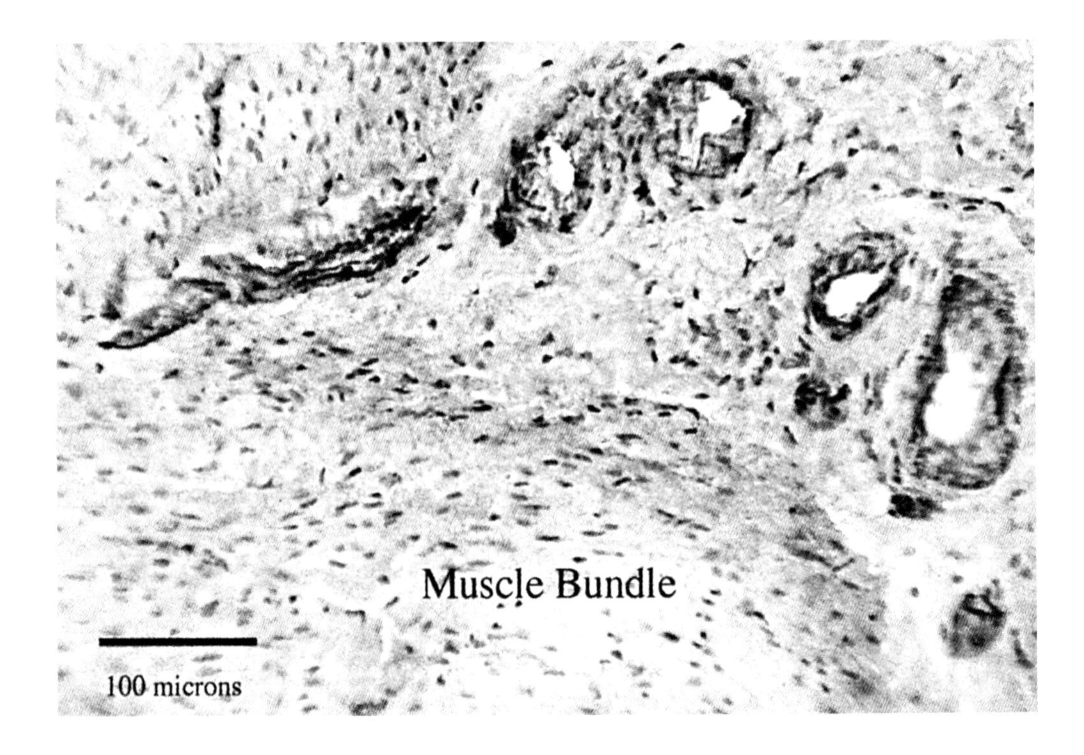

Figure 32 : Tortuous course of small artery in the pig bladder wall.

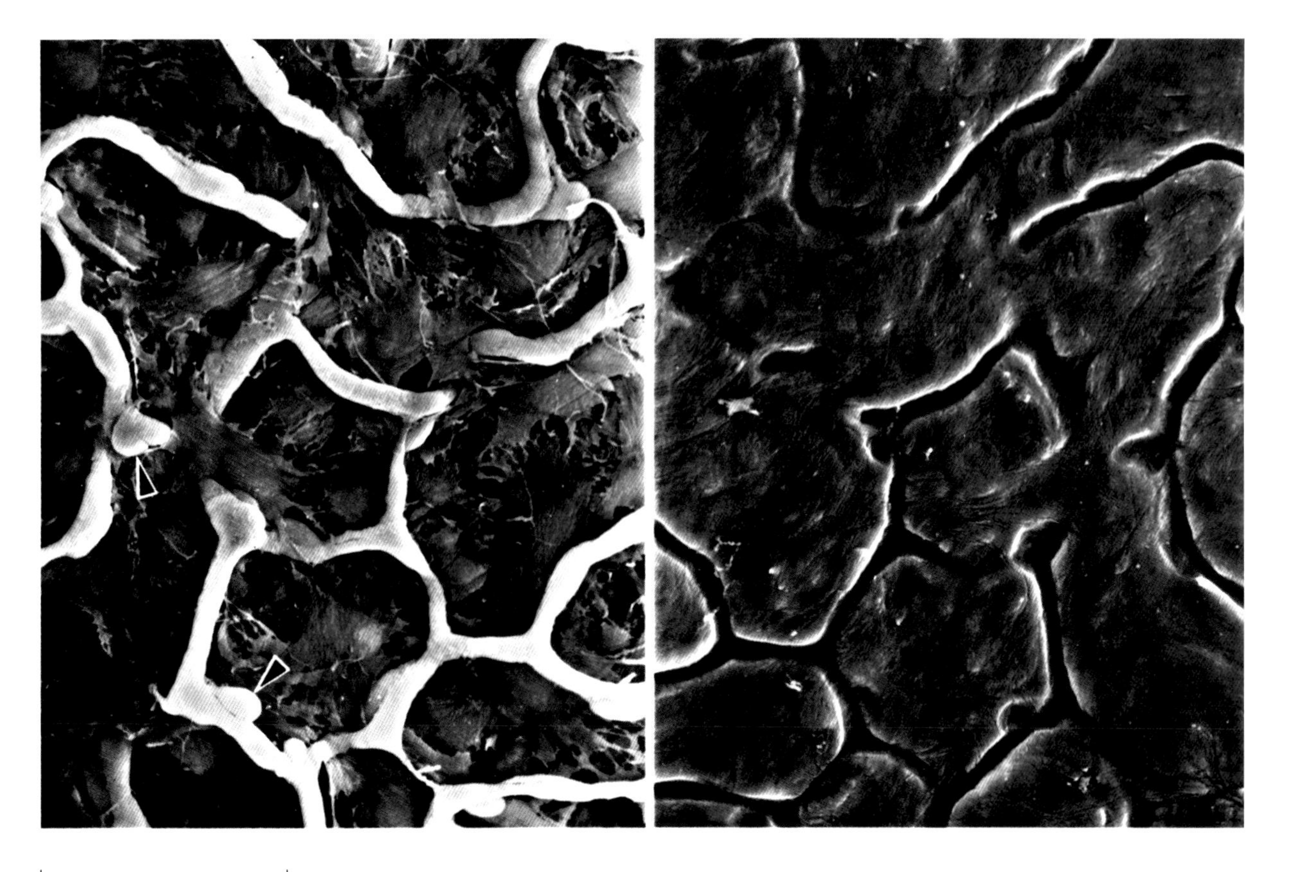

Figure 33 : Scanning electron micrographs of a rat bladder mucosa; two complementary pairs show the interface between the lamina propria (left side) and the underside of the epithelium (right side). The capillaries form a network lying on a sheet of mucosal fibroblasts, and they correspond to the grooves seen on the underside of the epithelium. In the bottom pair of micrographs an axons with varicosities is visible. The arrowheads point to pericytes lying on the interstitial surface of the capillaries. (from Inoue and Gabella, 1992 [117]).

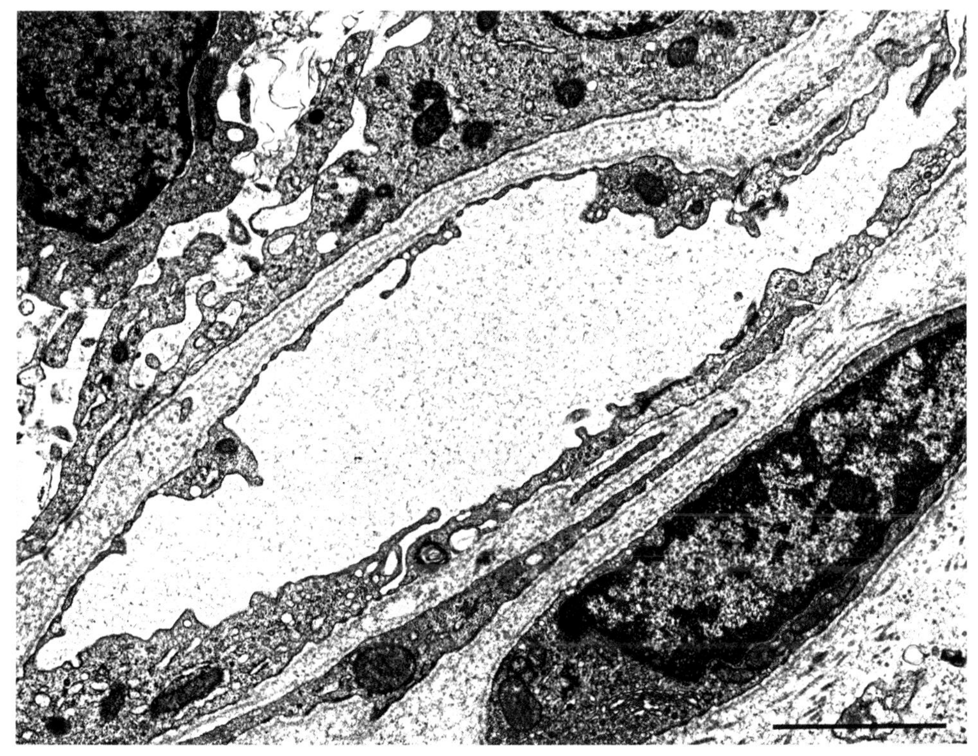

Figure 34 : An example of an element of the suburothelial capillary plexus showing the fenestrated endothelial wall facing the deep surface of the urothelium. Scale = 2 µm.

Urodynamic recording and blood flow in normal pig (compliant bladder)

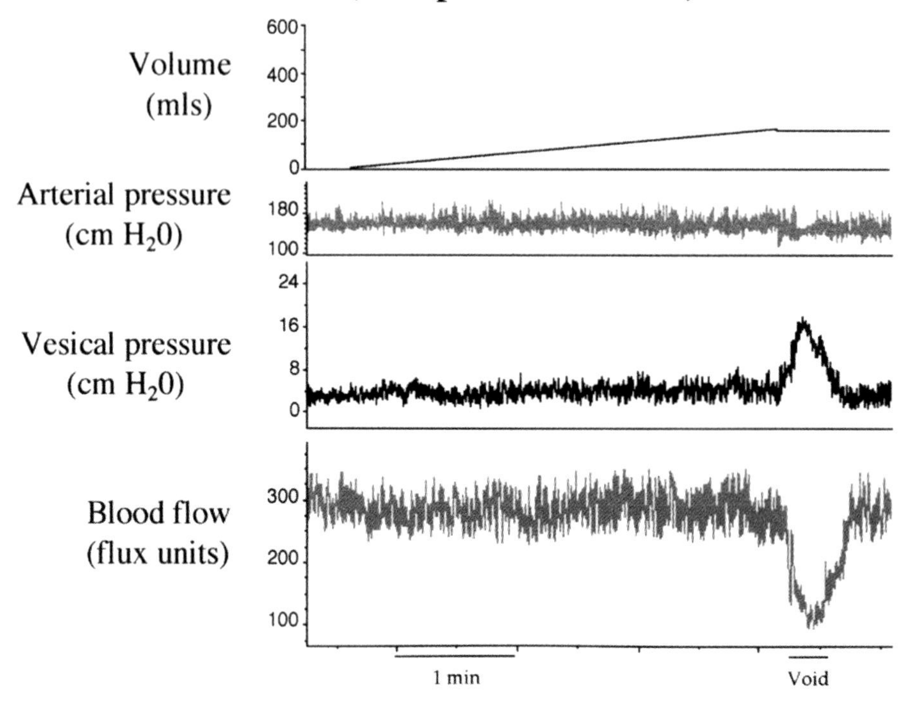

Figure 35 : Cystometrogram, blood pressure and blood flow in the bladder wall during the micturition cycle in a female pig with a normally compliant bladder. Note little pressure rise in detrusor during filling, and no fall in blood flow until the voiding contraction raises the detrusor pressure.

Urodynamic recording and blood flow in normal pig (non-compliant bladder)

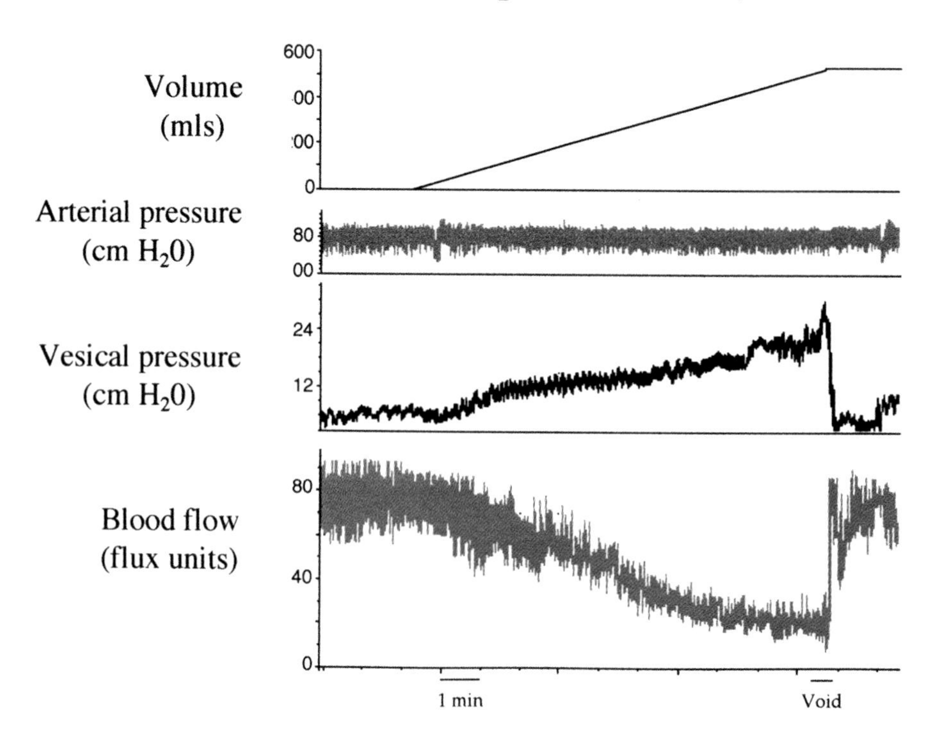

Figure 36 : Cystometrogram, blood pressure and blood flow in the bladder wall during the micturition cycle in a female pig with a poorly compliant bladder. In this case the blood pressure in the bladder wall falls as the detrusor pressure rises.

increases in the bladder (see [118]). In the cat vasodilatation has been observed [125] during filling which suggests that local factors are involved in ensuring good perfusion of the bladder during the vascular rearrangement necessary with the increased surface area. Locally produced prostaglandins were implicated. The reflex cardiovascular responses to bladder distension in patients with spinal lesions [126] also suggest that neuronal pathways exist as well as local factors which could mediate control of blood vessels during filling. Bladder vasodilatation in response to pelvic nerve stimulation in the cat has been seen, [127] and pudendal nerve stimulation leads to an increased blood flow in the sphincteric regions of the dog urinary tract [128].

Histochemical and immunohistochemical studies have demonstrated the presence of catecholamine-containing, acetylcholinesterase-positive, vasoactive intestinal polypeptide-, substance P-, [Met] enkephalin- and gastrin-immunoreactive nerves on the adventitial-medial border of blood vessels in the pig urinary tract [129].

b) Roles of the blood vessels

The urinary bladder requires a rich blood supply to maintain its functions, the storage and release of urine. The blood flow is important for tissue oxygenation and for the transport of nutrients and humoral factors as well as for the removal of metabolites. When the detrusor is deprived of oxygen and a metabolic substrate, as would occur in ischaemia, its contractile ability rapidly declines [130,131] and a rigor contraction develops [132]. It has been suggested that ischaemia and reperfusion might lead to damage to intramural neurones and result in the patchy denervation and altered smooth muscle function seen in bladders of people with detrusor instability [50].

The subepithelial capillary plexus may be associated with maintenance of the barrier function of the urothelium, [133] reducing any exposure of the detrusor smooth muscle to substances diffusing from the urine, It may also play a role in epithelial transport function and be necessary for urothelial metabolism.

4. UROTHELIUM

In the urinary tract, epithelia have continuously decreasing permeability from the extremely permeable kidney glomerular membrane down to the transitional epithelium of the ureter and bladder. The mammalian kidney produces urine which may vary considerably in ionic composition and tonicity, and one would expect that an important function of the bladder urothelium will be to prevent equilibration of the urine with the body fluids. The urinary epithelium is specialized, the cells form a continuous layer (fig. 37) and are joined with tight junctions. They have specialized cell-surface proteins, and ion pumps plus proteoglycans and glycoproteins, all of which function together to maintain the impermeability of the membrane [134-139]. These same mechanisms also present an active defence against bacterial colonisation.

The urothelium, once categorized as "transitional" in type, is a stratified epithelium consisting of a minimum of two layers of cells; a superficial layer of capping or umbrella cells, and a basal layer separated from the submucosa/lamina propria by a continuous extracellular basal lamina. In histological preparations these two layers usually appear to be separated by one or more layers of "intermediate" cells. Evidence of epithelial cell division is rarely seen but can occur in superficial and deeper layers.

The superficial cells have large nuclei with prominent nucleoli and dispersed chromatin, are often multinucleate and are linked to their neighbours at their luminal aspect by tight junctions, zonulae adhaerentes and small desmosomes. They are highly pleomorphic, varying from flattened squamous to narrowly columnar in response to the degree of distention of the bladder lumen. Their cytoplasm contains dispersed small mitochondria, golgi complexes and rough endoplasmic reticulum, with varying numbers of large complex lysosomes. In the normal bladder their cell membranes are polarized, with the majority on their external surface in contact with the urine having a characteristic asymmetric trilaminar structure. They possess an irregular and angular profile due to their content of a family of particulate transmembrane proteins, the uroplakins, which stiffen the membrane to produce an assembly of semi-ridgid plaques. The immediately underlying cytoplasm contains numerous elliptical vesicles having the same trilaminar membrane structure and which can on occasions be seen to make direct contact with the surface membrane [fig. 37]. It has been claimed that these vesicles may contribute addition uroplakin-containing membrane to the cell surface when this is stretched by distention of the bladder wall. The lateral and basal surfaces of the umbrella cells lack the uroplakin component, are covered with fine folds and microvilli, and are linked to their lateral and deeper neighbouring cells by occasional small desmosomes (fig. 38, 39).

In many human bladder biopsies, however, surface cells with the usual angular, uroplakin-containing surface membranes are replaced, wholly or in part, by others lacking both these features and the sub-surface vacuoles, and having a flat surface mambrane bearing numerous well formed and regularly ordered microvilli covered by a conspicuous glycocalyx coat, and which also tend to contain larger and more numerous mitochondria (figs. 40, 41, 42). This change may represent a functional adaptation of the superficial cells to chan-

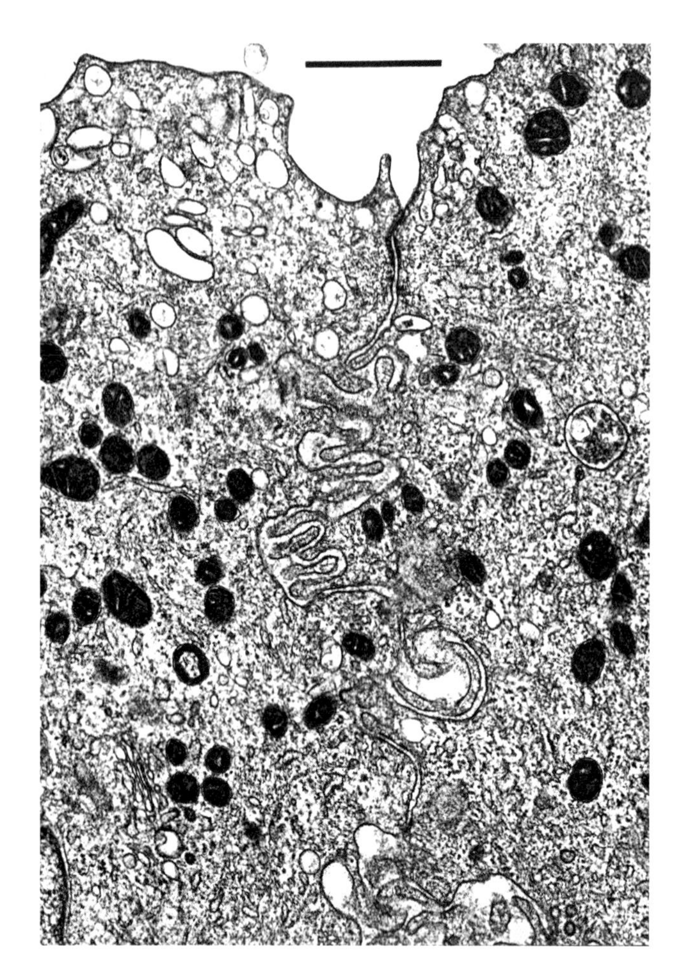

Figure 37 : The interface between two superficial cells. Scale = 1 μm

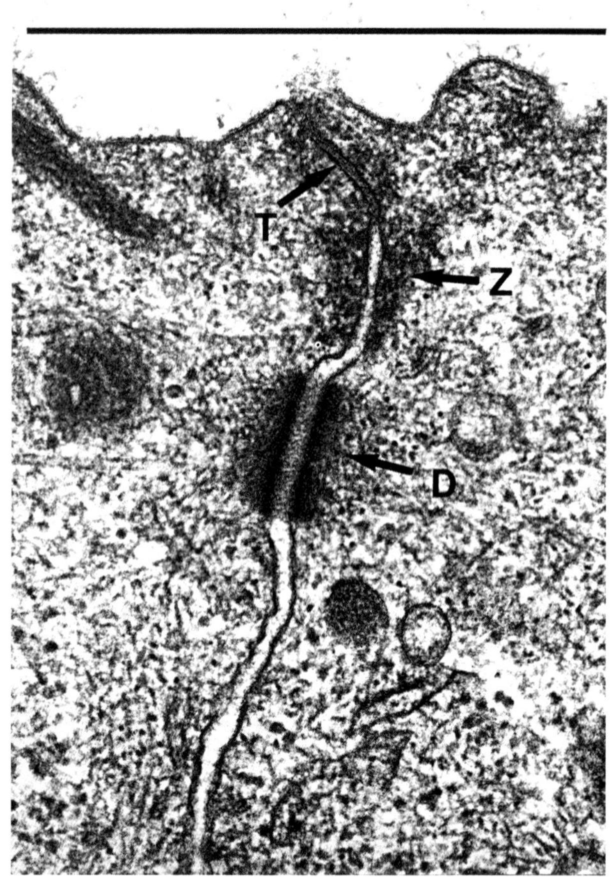

Figure 38 : Fine structure of the intercellular attachments at the luminal surface of two superficial cells; the tight junction (T), the zonula adhaerens (z) and a desmosome (D). Scale = 1 μm.

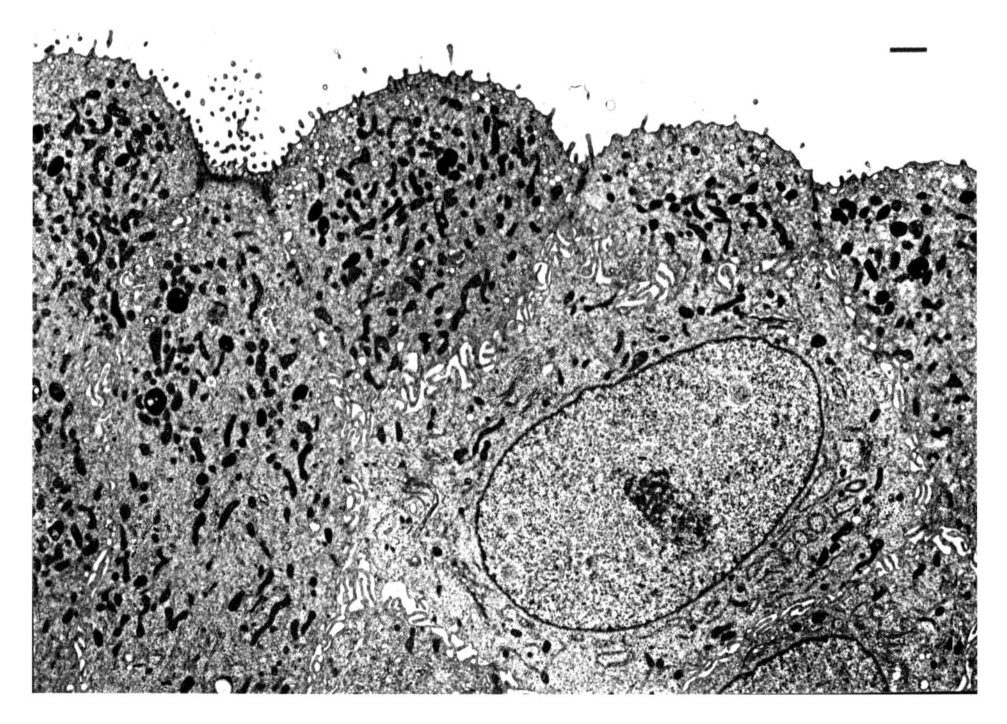

Figure 39 : An example of urothelial surface cells lacking the usual angular surface profile and bearing numerous micro-villi. Scale = 1 μm.

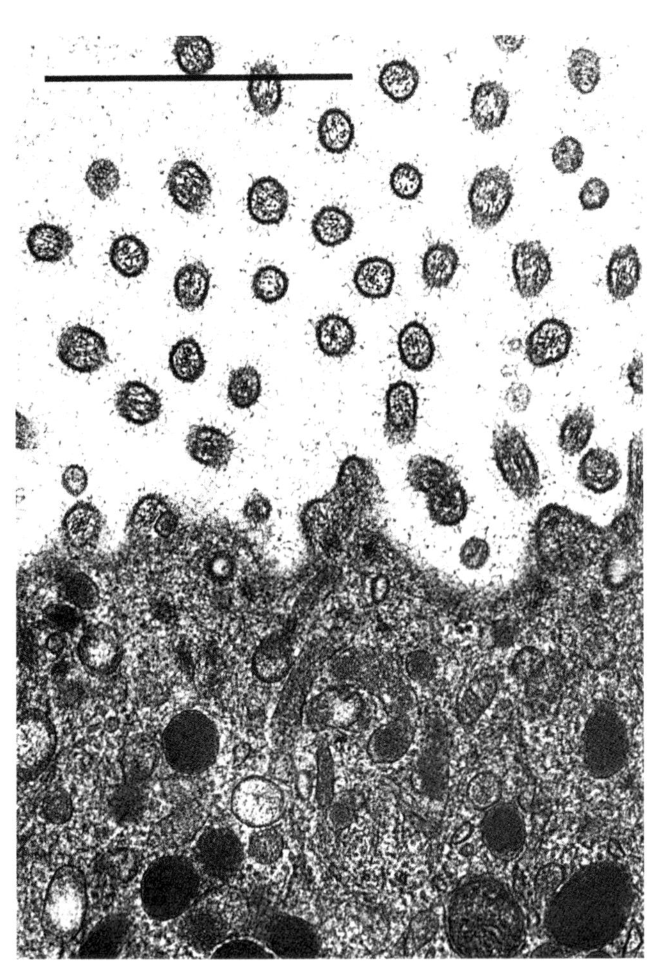

Figure 40 : A detailed view of the microvilli on the surface of such a cell. Scale = 1μm.

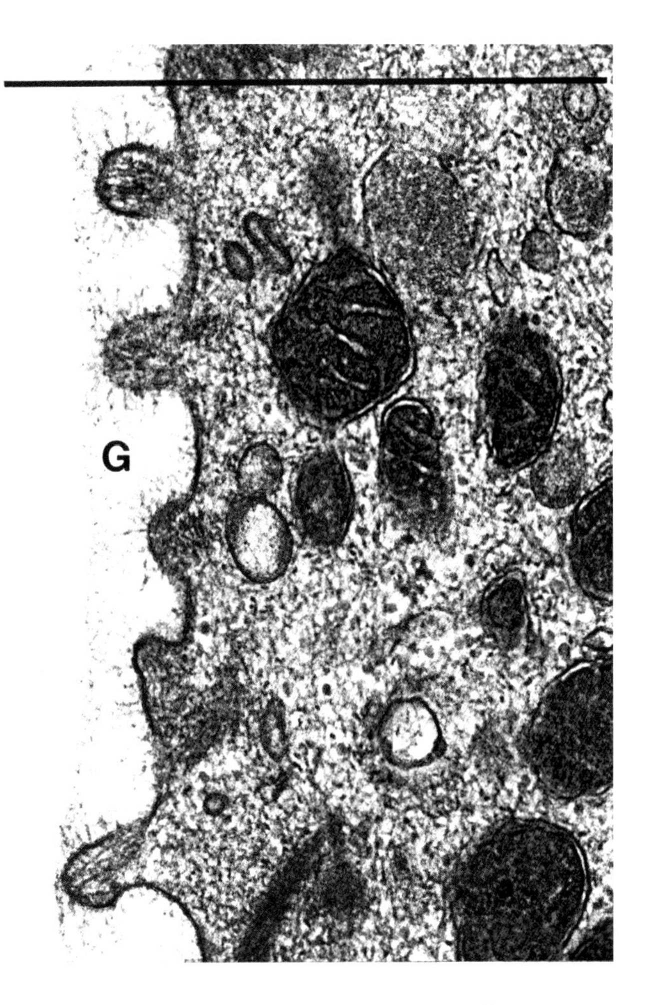

Figure 41 : The surface glycocalyx on a microvillous urothelial surface cell. Scale = 1μ.

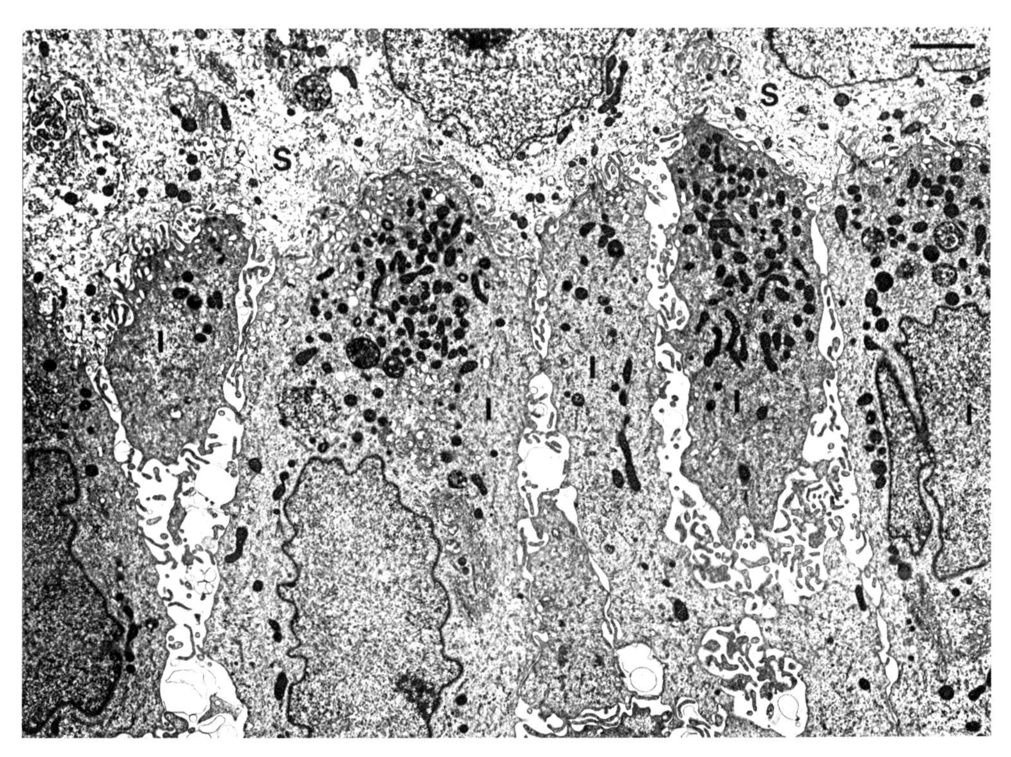

Figure 42 : A row of intermediate urothelial cells (I) showing their relationship to the deep surface of the superficial cell (S), and the differences between these in respect of their cytoplasmic density and organelle content. Scale = 2μ.

ge in their local environment, or their replacement by the insertion of deeper cells into the surface layer.

The deepest cells of the urothelium have basal processes which are closely adherent to the underlying basal lamina, with occasional hemidesmosomal attachments thereto, and abut those of their neighbours but without showing any specialized points of contact. Their cell bodies are generally columnar, having numerous folds and villi on their lateral and apical surfaces, and are adherent one to another only by means of scattered small desmosomes; they are thus well adapted to adjust their shape to the degree of stretch applied to the urothelium. Their nuclei are characteristically ellipsoid and indented, and are distinguishable from those of the umbrella cells by possession of a prominent rim of heterochromatin; their cytoplasm is polarized in that the majority of the cell organelles, including mitochondria, golgi complexes, rough endoplasmic reticulum and lysosomes are concentrated on the luminal aspect of the nucleus (fig. 43). The intermediate cells have similar cytological characteristics to the basal cells and can only be identified by their lack of contact with the basal lamina, a feature that is difficult to establish with certainty in tissue sections through such an irregularly convoluted structure.

In biopsy specimens of human bladder wall the intercellular space between the three classes of urothelial cells varies greatly in its extent, both between and within individual specimens, reflecting the degree of stretch of the membrane and other factors, such as the presence of underlying inflammation of the lamina propria; the only constraints on the relationships and separation of the urothelial cells being their apparently randomly scattered desmosomal contacts and the attachment of the basal cells to the urothelial basal lamina. This intercellular space appears to be freely accessible to leucocytes, mast cells and macrophages which can penetrate the basal lamina and migrate between the urothelial cells up to the level of the zonulae adhaerentes linking the margins of the umbrella cells. Hence the urothelial cells of all layers are open to continuous immunological surveillance.

Although structural features, i.e. the presence of tight junctions between adjacent apical cells, support the concept of an impermeable membrane, physiological experiments suggest otherwise. Although apical epithelial cells in the bladder are impermeable to water they actively transport sodium [140-142]. Sulphated polysaccharides, especially glycosaminoglycans, covering apical cells (fig. 41) act as an epithelial barrier to small molecules. Disruption of this polysaccharide layer increases permeability to urea and has been linked to inflammatory or hypersensitivity disorders of the bladder, such as interstitial cystitis [135].

A consensus has not been reached concerning the physiological role of active transmembrane transport mechanisms in the bladder. One function may be in epithelial cell volume regulation during changes accompanying distension [140]. Another role may be to actively maintain urine hypertonicity. A subepithelial vascular network could function as a countercurrent exchanger to maintain a hyperosmotic urine [143]. In addition, the microvasculature of the bladder can change with disease. Following obstruction, luminal diameters of intramural vessels increase and become more sensitive to alpha-adrenergic agonists [144]. Epithelial permeability could provide a mechanism for exposing smooth muscle to intravesical contents, thereby altering bladder contractility [143]. Investigators have demonstrated that intravesical installations of anti-neoplastic drugs, anticholinergic agents [145] and calcium channel antagonists, [146] influence detrusor function and access systemic circulation.

It is well recognised that the composition of the urine may have a marked effect on the volumes of urine voided. This could come about through penetration of small molecules through the urothelium having a direct sensitising effect on the dense meshwork of subepithelial sensory nerves, [147] or by production of substances by the urothelium that have this effect. ATP has recently been shown to be produced by epithelial cells in response to increased hydrostatic pressure changes in rabbit bladder, [142] and proposed to modulate sensory nerve activity. In the human urothelium iNOS activity has also been found after various treatments (e.g. cytokines or treatment with BCG) [148,149]. Recently it was found that patients with bladder inflammation showed a 30-60 fold increase in bladder NO levels [150]. Patients with interstitial cystitis or cystitis due to irradiation, BCG treatment or infection all showed a marked increase in the production of bladder NO. It is unclear whether the increased NO formation seen during inflammation has a role in the urgency symptoms found during such conditions. It is however likely that increased bladder NO levels can be used to distinguish between urgency caused by inflammation as compared to the urgency due to impaired function in the sensory afferent innervation. Thus, measurement of NO may be used to monitor inflammation in the urinary bladder.

5. Intrinsic innervation of the urinary bladder

a) Motor innervation

The urinary bladder is profusely supplied with autonomic nerve fibres, which form a dense plexus among the detrusor smooth muscle cells. The majority of these nerves contain acetylcholinesterase (fig. 44), and while

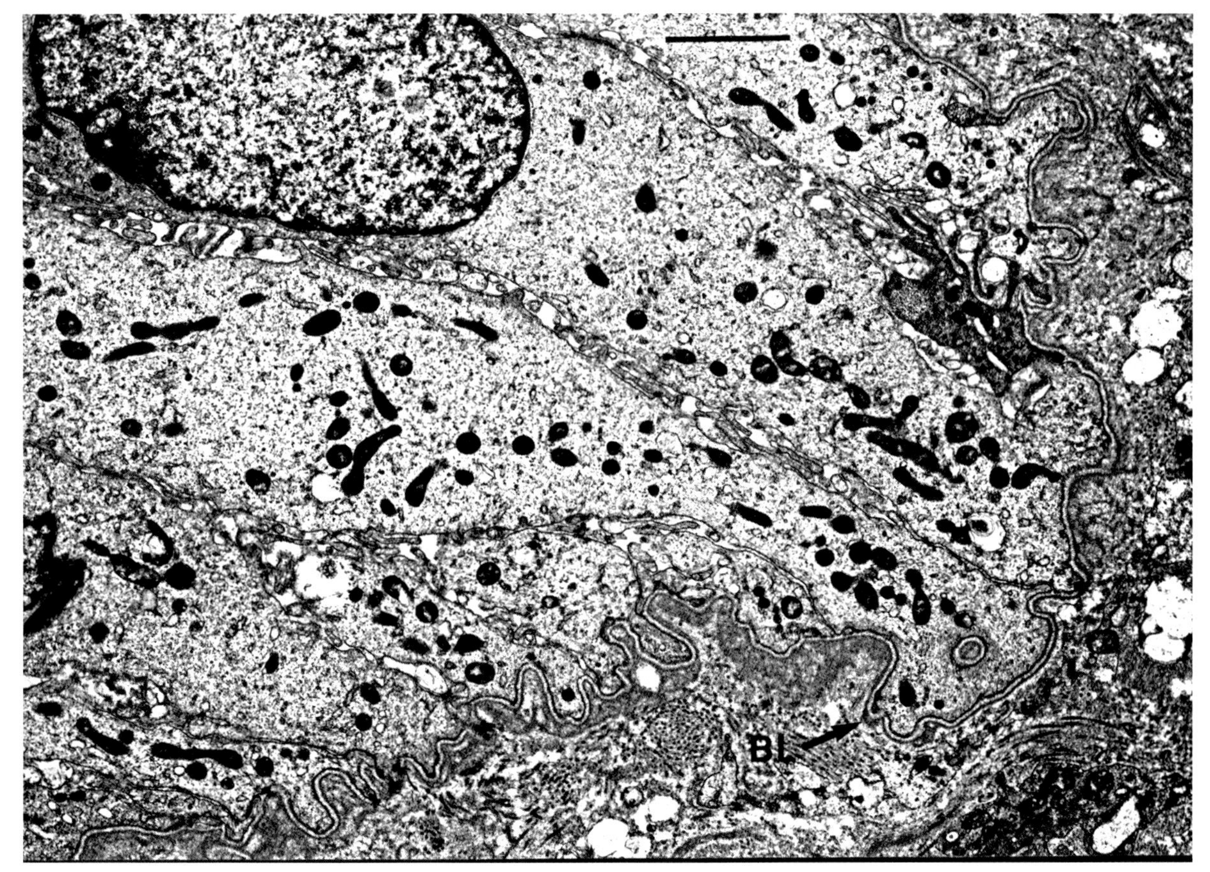

Figure 43 : The basal processes of several basal urothelial cells showing their contact with the basal lamina (BL) and underlying lamina propria. Scale = 2μ.

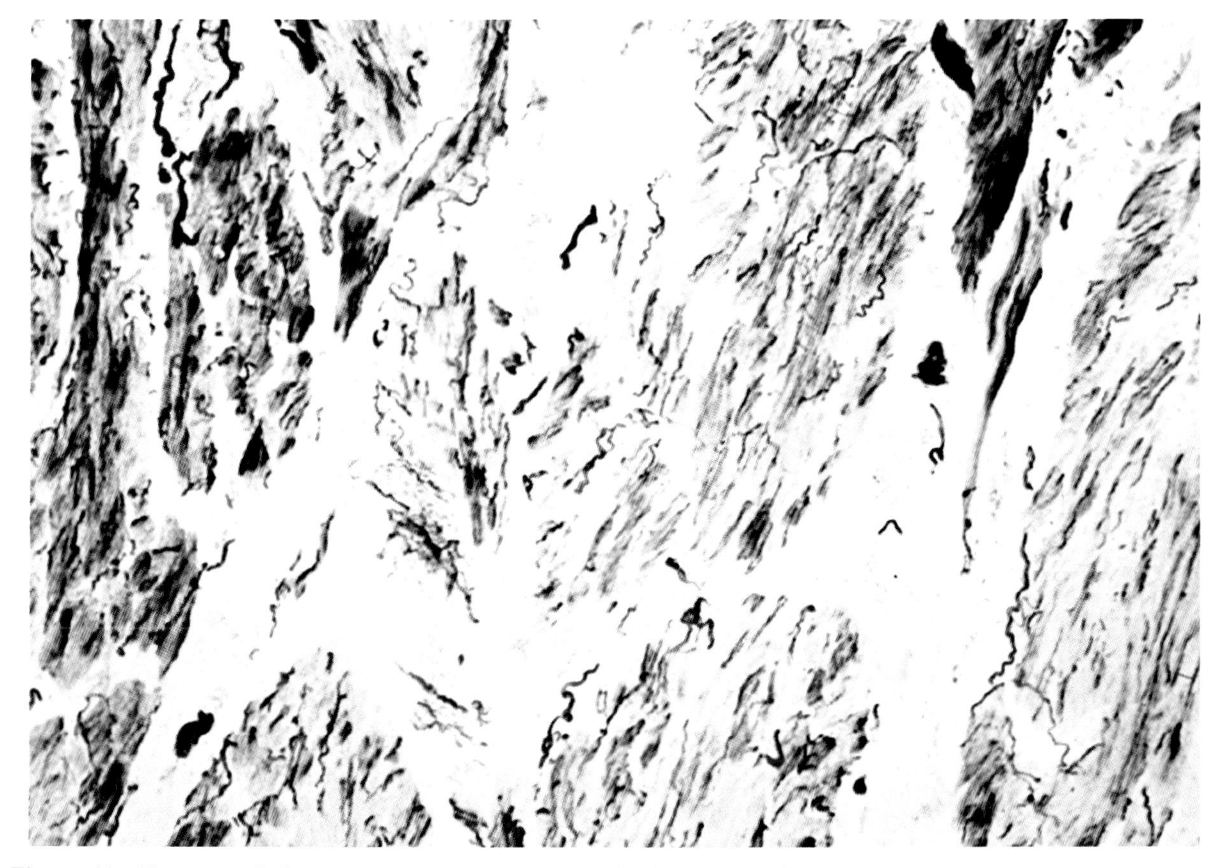

Figure 44 : Numerous cholinesterase positive nerves supply the detrusor muscle. X100

they occur in profusion throughout the muscle coat of the bladder, some muscle bundles appear to be more richly innervated than others. The majority of the autonomic nerves innervating the detrusor muscle are considered to be excitatory cholinergic in type [151], and contraction of the normal human detrusor is mediated almost exclusively through muscarinic receptor stimulation by released acetylcholine. Both nitric oxide synthase (NOS) and neuropeptide Y (NPY) are co-localised in some of these cholinergic nerves [3, 56]. The human detrusor possesses an exceedingly sparse supply of sympathetic noradrenergic nerves [152-158]. Although nerves of this type generally accompany the vasculature to the bladder (fig. 45), they rarely extend among the smooth muscle cells of the detrusor. In addition, there is evidence for the occurrence of a nonadrenergic noncholinergic transmission in the human lower urinary tract, but so far the presence of such a transmitter, either excitatory or inhibitory, has not been definitely established. As indicated above, several neuropeptides, including vasoactive intestinal peptide (VIP) and NPY, have been demonstrated in a percentage of nerves within the detrusor muscle [56, 158, 159]. However, the precise function of these peptides as neurotransmitters and/or neuromodulators remains to be defined.

b) Sensory innervation

The urinary bladder is supplied by afferent nerves travelling via the pelvic splanchnic and hypogastric nerves [160]. The cell bodies reside in dorsal root ganglia in the lumbosacral region, and no local afferent neurons are known to exist within the bladder itself [160]. A smaller group of sensory nerves extends to the striated urethral sphincter muscle via the pudendal nerve. The sensory nerves supplying the bladder are either thin myelinated A delta or unmyelinated fibres, and terminate as free nerve endings [160, 161]. A population of afferent nerves function as slowly adapting tension receptors, which respond to physiological distension in a graded manner. The same nerves also respond to bladder contraction, indicating that tension, rather than stretch, is the effective stimulus. In addition, the bladder is supplied by polymodal nociceptors. These fibres are typically unmyelinated and respond to stimuli associated with tissue damage, such as inflammatory mediators and ischaemia. The nocioeptors also respond to cold, but not to stretch within physiological parameters [160, 162].

In the human bladder, presumptive sensory nerves containing calcitonin gene-related peptide (CGRP) are rare, comprising less than 5% of the total bladder innervation, and are restricted in their distribution [56, 159]. CGRP nerves are typically found in the subepithelium, around blood vessels, and surrounding intramural ganglion cells [56, 159]. The fibres occasionally penetrate into the epithelium, particularly in the urethra. Unlike the situation in animals, CGRP fibres only very rarely project to the detrusor muscle in the human bladder [56, 159].

The projections of presumptive sensory fibres in the human bladder are consistent with their assumed role as tension receptors. In addition, the fibres may act as touch receptors if the walls of the bladder or urethra coapt, or as chemoreceptors of urine content. It has also been suggested that chemicals released by the bladder as a result of stretch, such as prostaglandins [163], nitric oxide, or ATP [164], may influence sensory transmission. The presence of presumptive sensory nerve terminals around local ganglion cells indicates that sensory collaterals may influence ganglionic neurotransmission [56]. Such transmission may become more prominent when the bladder functions abnormally [165]. Two neurochemically distinct subpopulations of presumptive sensory fibres have been identified in the human. One class contains CGRP and tachykinins such as substance P (SP) and neurokinin A, and the other class, representing 75% of the total afferent fibres, contains CGRP only [159]. Since these nerves account for such a small proportion of the total bladder innervation, it is possible that other populations of sensory nerves exist in human bladder which cannot be detected with these neurochemical markers. Electron microscope (EM) studies have identified SP-containing nerves in human bladder as being unmyelinated [166]. Myelinated nerves have also been detected in human bladder deep lamina propria by EM, and these fibres do not contain SP [166]. It is likely that these nerves are sensory, since the postganglionic parasympathetic and sympathetic nerves are unmyelinated. A detailed confocal/EM study examining the distribution and neurochemistry of myelinated nerves in human bladder would yield much valuable information.

Pacinian corpuscles have been identified in the subserosal region of the human bladder [167]. These specialised sensory endings are extremely rare, and appear to be associated with noradrenergic fibres [168]. Pacinian corpuscles act as rapidly adapting pressure receptors – it is therefore unlikely that such fibres can transmit information related to slow bladder distension. The subserosal location of the receptors reinforces this argument. Pacinian corpuscles are most likely to be activated by rapid changes in bladder or abdominal pressure, as occurs during coughing or physical exertion. Such information may be used in "guarding reflexes" to close the striated urethral sphincter.

The sensory nerves that supply the bladder exhibit a remarkable plasticity. Collateral sprouting, and the formation of new and sometimes aberrant connections can occur as a result of spinal injury, inflammation [169],

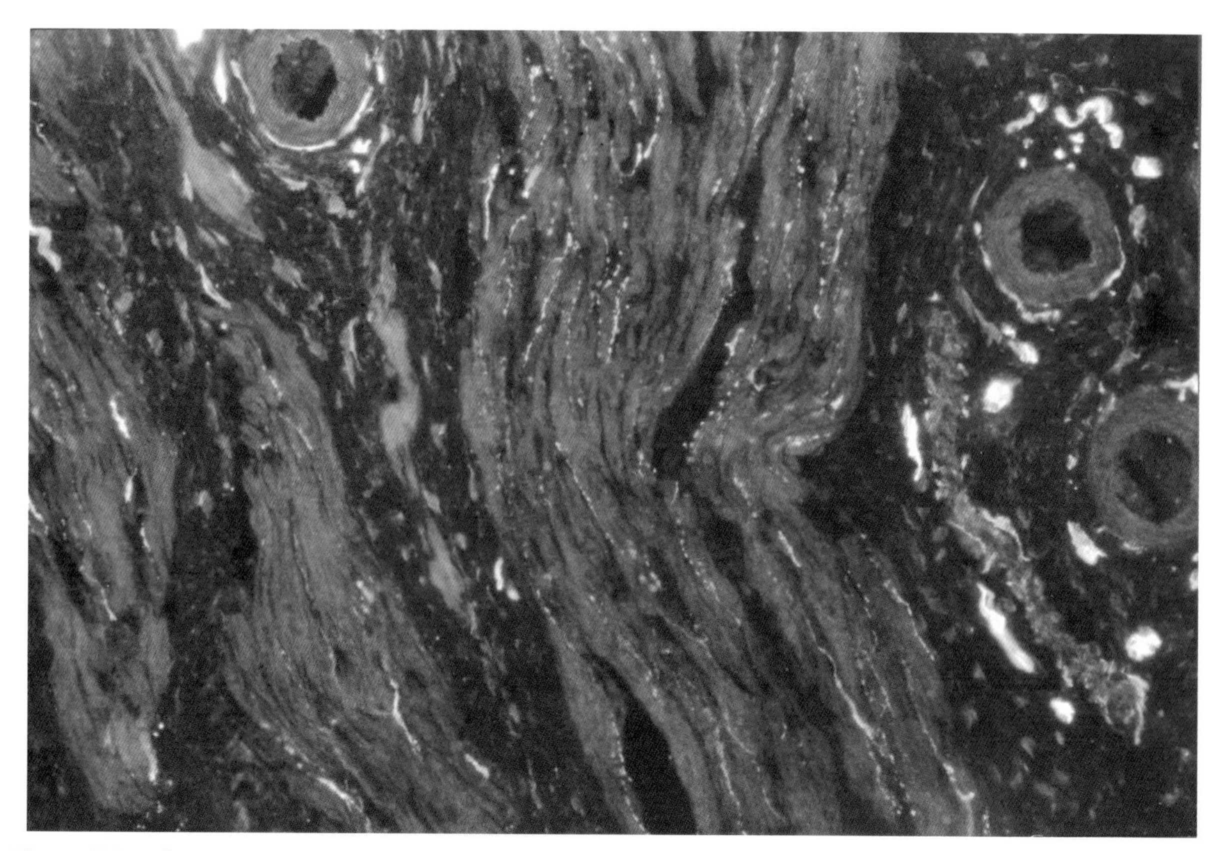

Figure 45 A : The general nerve marker protein gene product 9.5 demonstrates the rich detrusor and perivascular innervation. X200

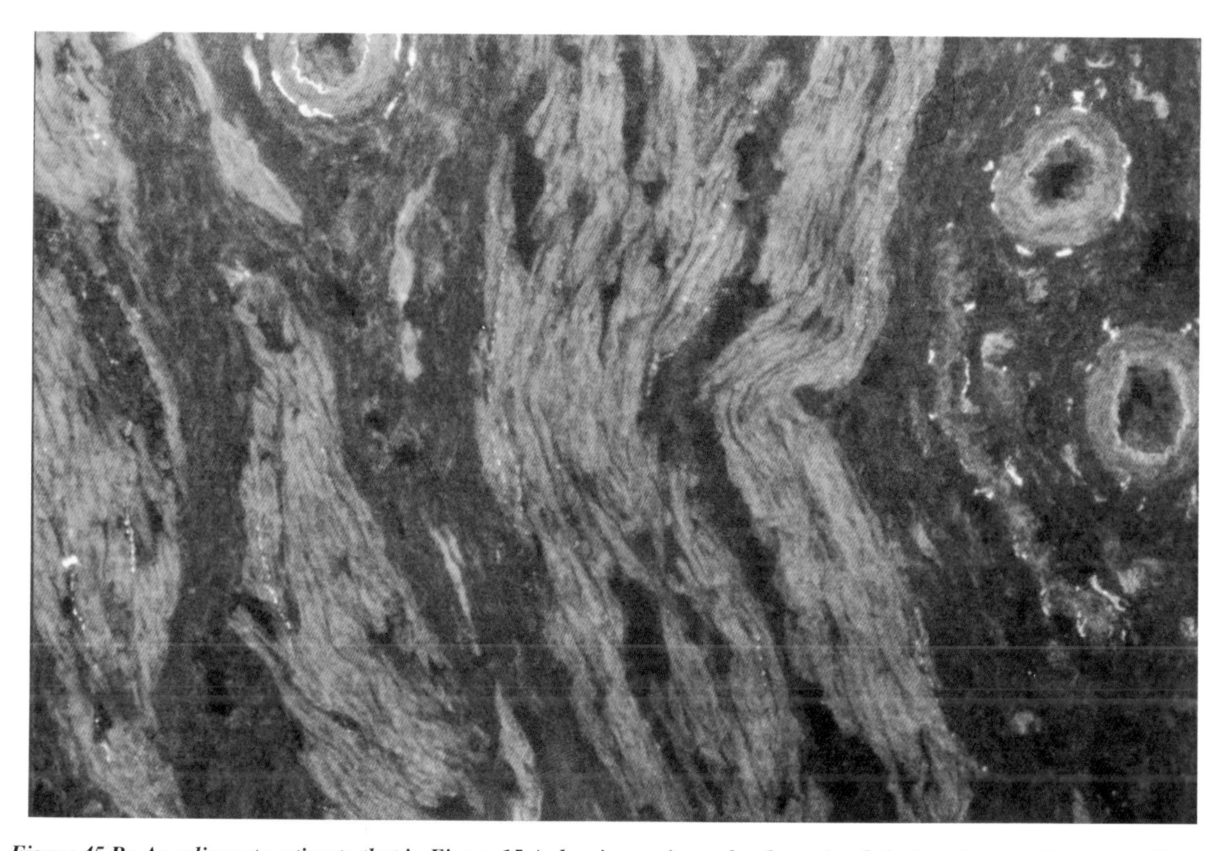

Figure 45 B : An adjacent section to that in Figure 15.A showing perivascular dopamine β- hydroxylase positive nerves. Few such nerves are present in the detrusor muscle bundles. X200

nerve injury [170] or bladder hypertrophy [171] in animals. This may occur at both the level of the spinal cord and within the periphery [171]. Recently it has been shown that the density of SP-containing presumptive sensory nerves is elevated in women suffering from bladder pain [173]. Similarly, the innervation of the bladder subepithelium by nerves containing SP and CGRP is increased in women with idiopathic detrusor instability [159]. This increase is relatively selective, and does not involve other populations of nerves. The role of sensory neuron plasticity in bladder malfunction, and the involvement of neuronal growth factors [170, 174] in this process clearly needs further investigation.

Although it has been assumed that the subepithelial plexus of nerves in human bladder is composed of sensory nerves, the evidence is as yet lacking. Many nerves in this region supply the rich vascular bed of the subepithelium, and need not, therefore, be afferent. While CGRP and SP have proved useful as markers, a definitive neurochemical marker for human afferent nerves is required. The finding that capsaicin-senitive sensory nerves express a vanilloid receptor [175] should aid in the future identification of sensory fibres in humans. Similarly, the trkA NGF receptor is expressed by many visceral sensory neurons [176], and may be useful in detecting putative sensory fibres. Myelin-specific antibodies, and the detection of myelinated fibres in the bladder by EM will also prove useful [166]. If the neurochemistry of myelinated fibres can be unravelled, it will go a long way towards establishing a marker for bladder sensory nerves. This work will form a solid foundation for examining the role of sensory nerve plasticity in the development of incontinence. Such research needs the development of a robust and reproducible test for assessing and quantifying lower urinary tract sensation [162, 177].

c) Autonomic ganglia

Small clusters of autonomic ganglion cells occur throughout all regions of the human bladder wall, being especially numerous in the adventitia of the bladder base. These intramural ganglia together with those which populate the vesical plexus consist of different types of neurons on the basis of their histochemistry and immunochemistry [56]. One type contains noradrenaline and corresponds to the short noradrenergic neuron described in association with the genital tract of other species [178]. In addition to presumptive cholinergic (excitatory) preganglonic nerves, some ganglion cells receive noradrenergic (possibly inhibitory) input [56, 179] (fig. 46). Recent studies, however, have demonstrated that the types of neuron associated with the lower urinary tract are much more complex than was previously believed [56].

d) Paraganglia

In addition to autonomic ganglia, numerous paraganglia [180] have been demonstrated in association with the human urinary bladder, being especially obvious in late fetal and early postnatal life. These paraganglia are located among the ramifications of the pelvic plexus, and the constituent cells receive a direct autonomic innervation. Many of the paraganglia that are present during fetal and early postnatal life contain specialized encapsulated sensory corpuscles (fig. 47) resembling small pacinian corpuscles [181, 182]. The functional significance of this developmental association remains obscure, as does the subsequent fate of these corpuscular nerve endings. However, occasional isolated corpuscles have been observed in the adventitia of the bladder in older children. The paraganglion cells are rich in catecholamines [183] and as a consequence contain large amounts of dopamine β-hydroxylase (DBH). However, the functional significance of the paraganglia and their relationship to developing autonomic ganglia remains to be determined.

IV. BLADDER NECK

The smooth muscle of this region is histologically, histochemically and pharmacologically distinct from that which comprises the detrusor proper, hence, the bladder neck should be considered as a separate functional unit. The arrangement of smooth muscle in this region is quite different in males and females and consequently each sex will be described separately.

1. Female bladder neck

The female bladder neck consists of morphologically distinct smooth muscle, since the large diameter muscle bundles characteristic of the detrusor are replaced in the region of the bladder neck by those of small diameter (fig. 48). The majority of muscle bundles in the female bladder neck extend obliquely or longitudinally into the urethral wall. There is no anatomical smooth muscle sphincter at the bladder neck, and it remains to be determined whether this region plays a significant part in the maintenance of female urinary continence.

In contrast with the rich sympathetic innervation in the male, the smooth muscle of the female bladder neck possesses fewer noradrenergic nerves, but is well supplied with presumptive cholinergic fibres [152]. The role played by this type of nerve in the functional control of the bladder neck remains uncertain. In strips of bladder neck taken from female dogs stimulation invariably produces a large relaxation this is blocked by nitric oxide inhibitors to reveal a small tonic contraction (Creed and Van der Werf, personal communication).

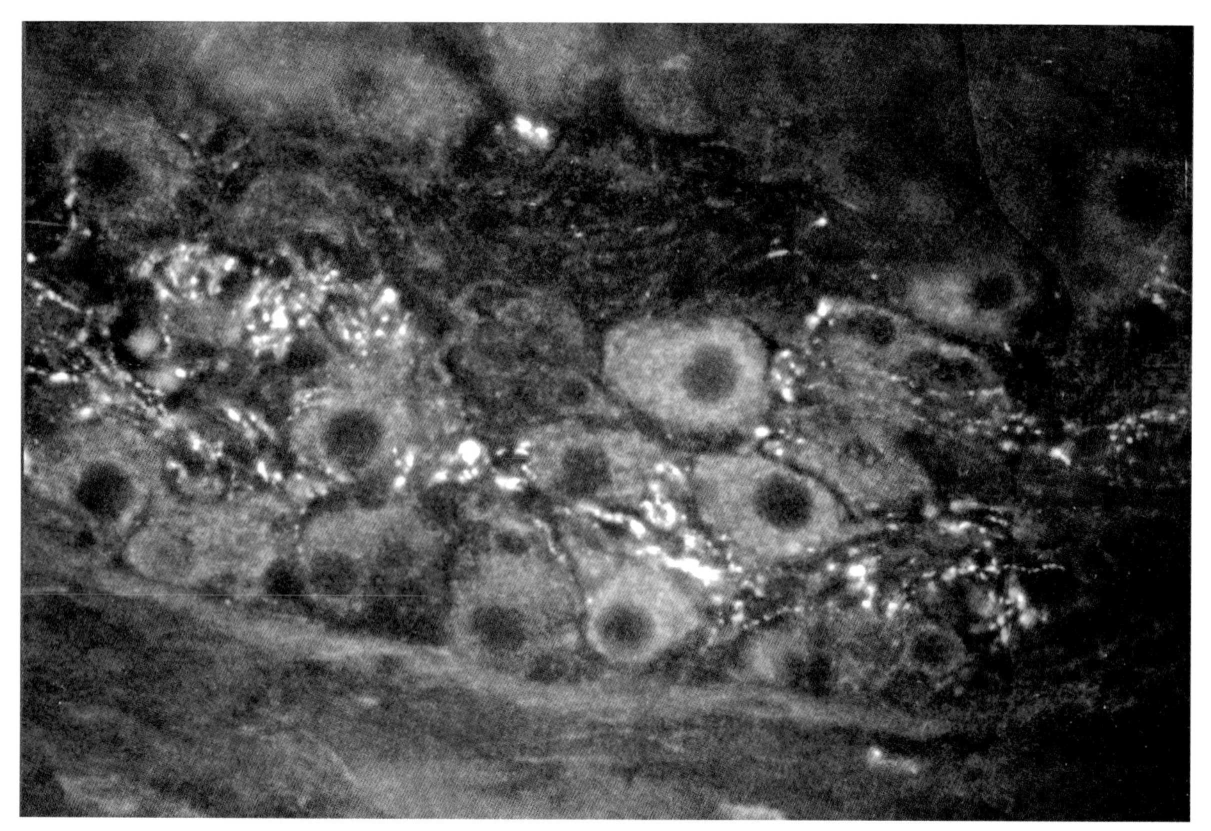

Figure 46 : Numerous dopamine β- hydroxylase-immunoreactive nerve fibres and terminals seen in close association with non-reactive (presumptive cholinergic) neurons in the vesicle plexus. X400

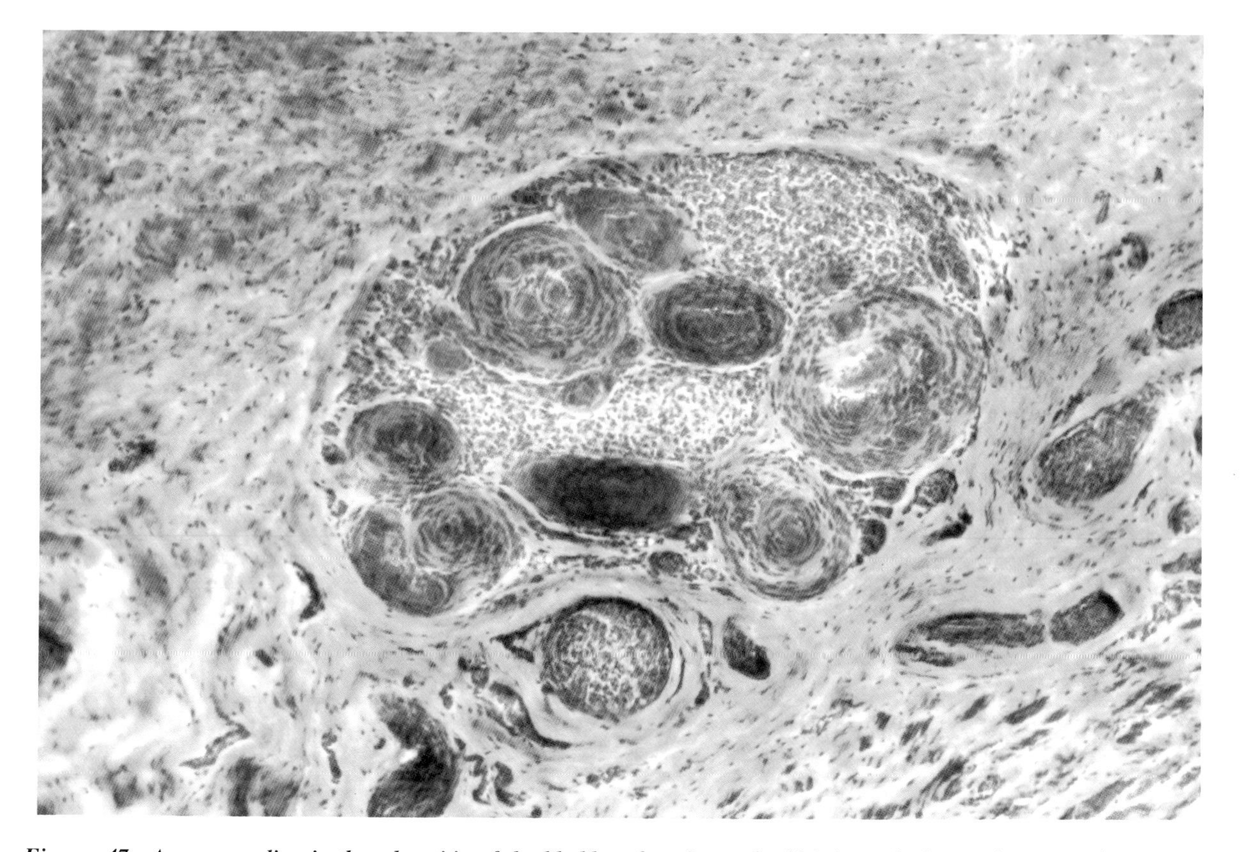

Figure 47 : A paraganglion in the adventitia of the bladder of an 8 month old infant which contains several sensory corpuscles. Massons trichrome. X200

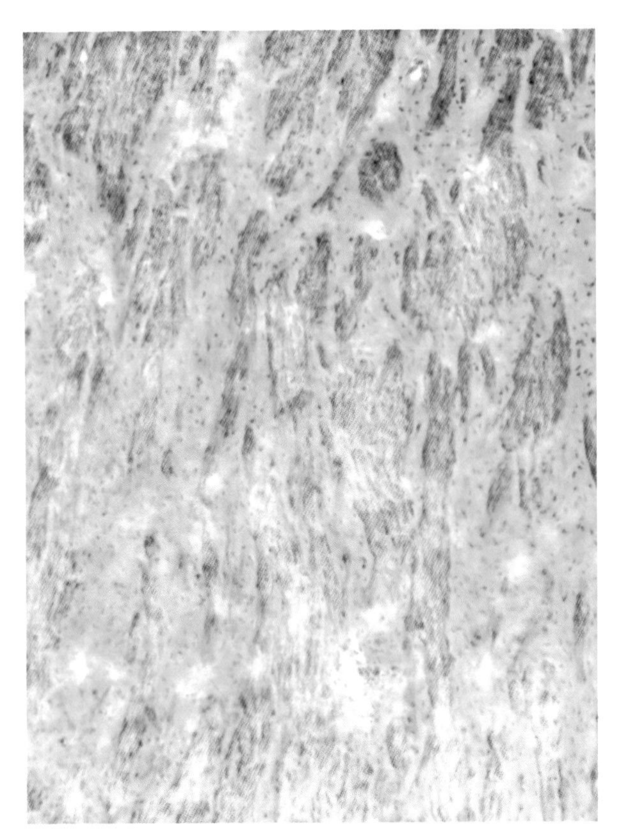

Figure 48 : Small diameter muscle bundles in the female bladder neck. Massons trichrome. X200

2. Male bladder neck

At the male bladder neck, the smooth muscle cells form a complete circular collar which extends distally to surround the proximal portion of the urethra. Because of the location and orientation of its constituent fibres, the terms internal, proximal or preprostatic urethral sphincter have been used as alternatives for this particular component of urinary tract smooth muscle. Distally, bladder neck muscle merges with, and become indistinguishable from, the musculature in the stroma and capsule of the prostate gland.

In the male, bladder neck smooth muscle is supplied with cholinergic (parasympathetic) nerves and also possesses a rich noradrenergic (sympathetic) innervation [153]. A similar distribution of autonomic nerves occurs in the smooth muscle of the prostate gland, seminal vesicles and ducti deferentes. On stimulation the sympathetic nerves cause contraction of smooth muscle in the wall of the genital tract resulting in seminal emission. Concomitant sympathetic stimulation of bladder neck muscle causes sphincteric closure of the region, thereby preventing reflux of ejaculate into the bladder [184].

Although this genital function of the male bladder neck is well established it is not known whether the smooth muscle of this region normally plays an active role in maintaining urinary continence. Recently, NOS positive nerve fibres have been described amongst the smooth muscle of the region [185]. Furthermore precontracted smooth muscle strips produce a relaxation response to nerve stimulation which is blocked by NO inhibitors. However the precise role of this type of nerve in the functional control of the bladder neck and urethra has yet to be established.

V. THE FEMALE URETHRA

The female urethra (fig. 49) is a fibromuscular tube 3-4 cm long and begins at the internal urethral meatus of the bladder. Embedded in the anterior wall of the vagina it inclines downwards and forwards through a gap in the pelvic floor and terminates in the vestibule at the external meatus between the clitoris and the vaginal opening.

The female urethra is comprised of different regions along its length and can be understood by dividing the length of the urethral lumen into fifths, each 20 % of the total length [186]. In the first quintile, the lumen of the urethra is surrounded by the vesical neck (0 – 20%). Next the sphincter urethrae and smooth muscle encircly the lumen from 20 – 60%. The arch shaped compressor urethrae and urethrovaginal sphincter are found from 60%-80% while the distal component includes only fibrous tissue and no significant contractile elements.

The striated urogenital sphincter muscle [187] has two components as this division implies (fig. 49). The urethral sphincter (rhabdosphincter) is circular in orientation and forms the outermost layer of the muscular wall. It is often deficient in the portion adjacent to the vagina, but can form a complete circle, especially in the young. The more distal portion that lies adjacent to the perineal membrane is comprised of two arch shaped straps of muscle. The compressor urethrae arises laterally near the ischiopubic rami while the urethrovaginal sphincter closely follow thc wall of thc vagina. Interestingly these muscles seem to be preserved with advancing age while the more proximal sphincter deteriorates, indicating the separate nature of these two elements.

The striated sphincter can be contracted to increase urethra closure during times of urgent need and micturition occurs when bladder pressure is higher than urethral pressure and is typically produced by contraction of the detrusor muscle of the bladder wall accompanied by relaxation of the intramural striated and smooth sphincters.

The wall of the female urethra comprises an outer muscle coat and an inner epithelial membrane which

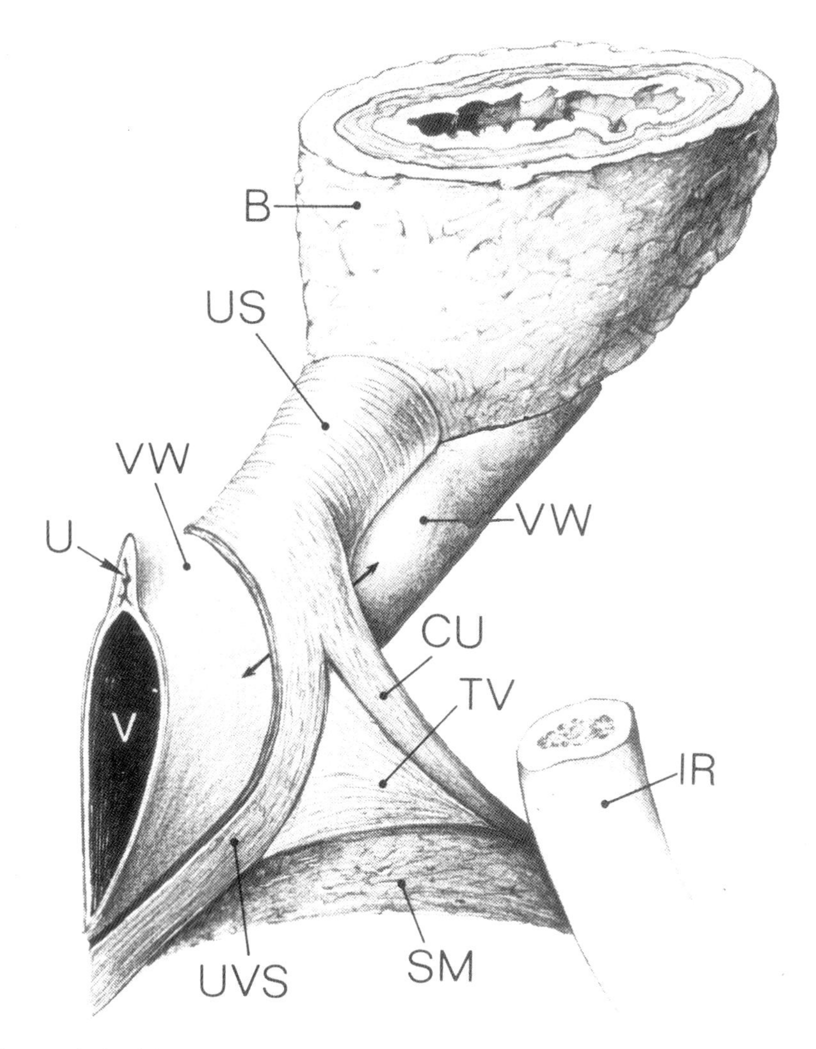

Figure 49 : Striated urogenital sphincter muscle showing its urethral sphincter (US), compressor urethrae (CU) and urethrovaginal sphincter (UVS). Also shown, B, bladder; IR, ischiopubic ramus; SM, smooth muscle; TV transverse vaginal muscle; U, urethra; V, vagina; VW, vaginal wall. After Oelrich

lines the lumen and is continuous with the epithelium of the bladder. The muscle coat consists of the previously described outer sleeve of striated muscle (striated urogenital sphincter or rhabdosphincter) together with an inner coat of smooth muscle fibres.

The striated muscle cells are of the slow twitch (type I) variety (fig. 50, 51) and are relatively small with diameters of 15-20 μm on average [188]. These fibres exert tone upon the urethral lumen over prolonged periods, especially in relation to the middle third of its length. Periurethral striated muscle of the levator ani aids urethral closure during events which require rapid, albeit short-lived, increases in urethral resistance.

The smooth muscle coat extends throughout the length of the urethra and consists of slender muscle bundles, the majority of which are orientated obliquely or longitudinally and are associated with a considerable quantity of connective tissue. Of these layers, circular and longitudinal, the latter is by far the more prominent (189). The few circularly arranged muscle cells occur in the outer aspect of the smooth muscle layer and intermingle with the striated muscle forming the inner part of the striated sphincter. Proximally the urethral smooth muscle extends as far as the bladder neck. When traced distally, urethral smooth muscle bundles terminate in the subcutaneous tissue surrounding the external urethral meatus. The smooth muscle of the female urethra is associated with relatively few noradrenergic nerves but receives an extensive presumptive cholinergic parasympathetic nerve supply [152] identical in appearance to that which supplies the detrusor. From a functional point of view it seems unlikely that competence of the female bladder neck and proximal urethra is solely the result of smooth muscle activity in the absence of an anatomical sphincter. The innervation and longitudinal orientation of most of the muscle fibres suggest that urethral smooth muscle in the female is active during micturition, serving to shorten and widen the urethral lumen.

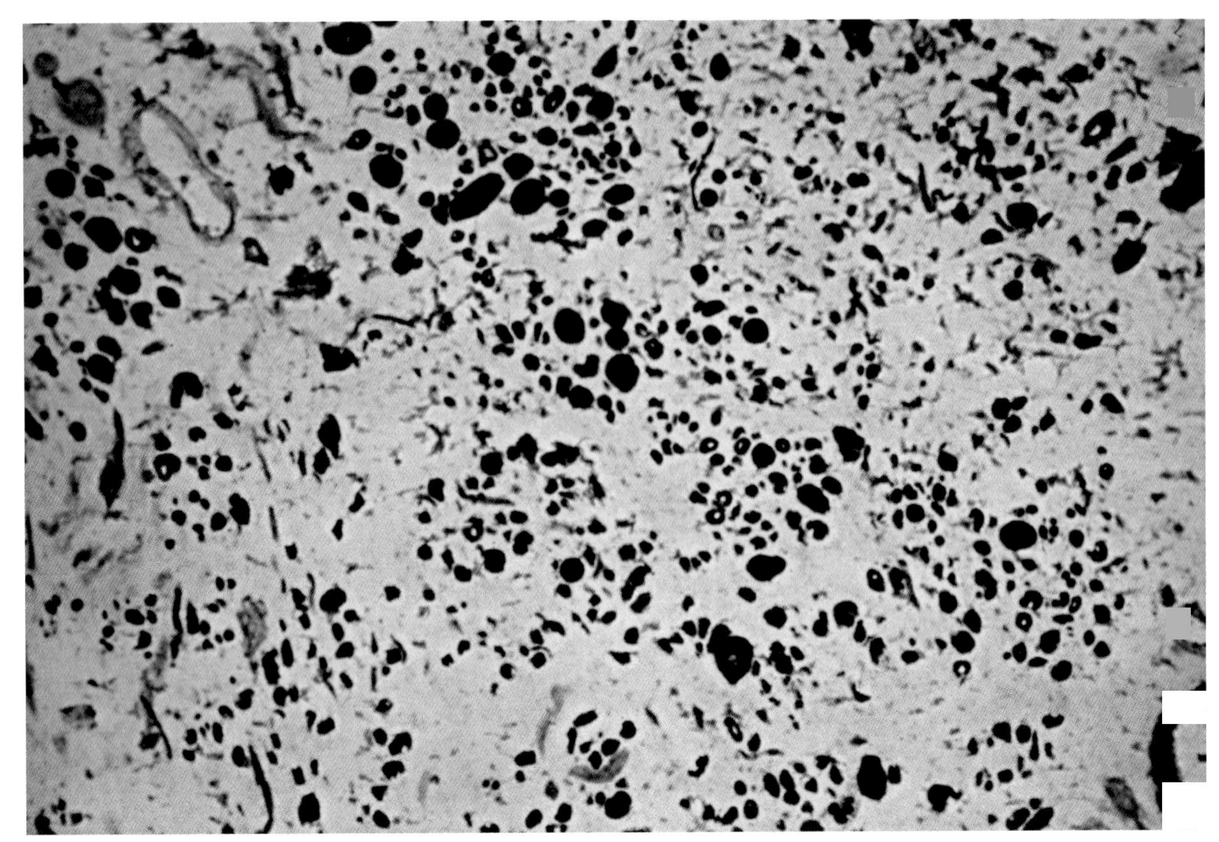

Figure 50 : Female intramural urethral striated muscle showing darkly stained slow twitch (type I) fibres. X150

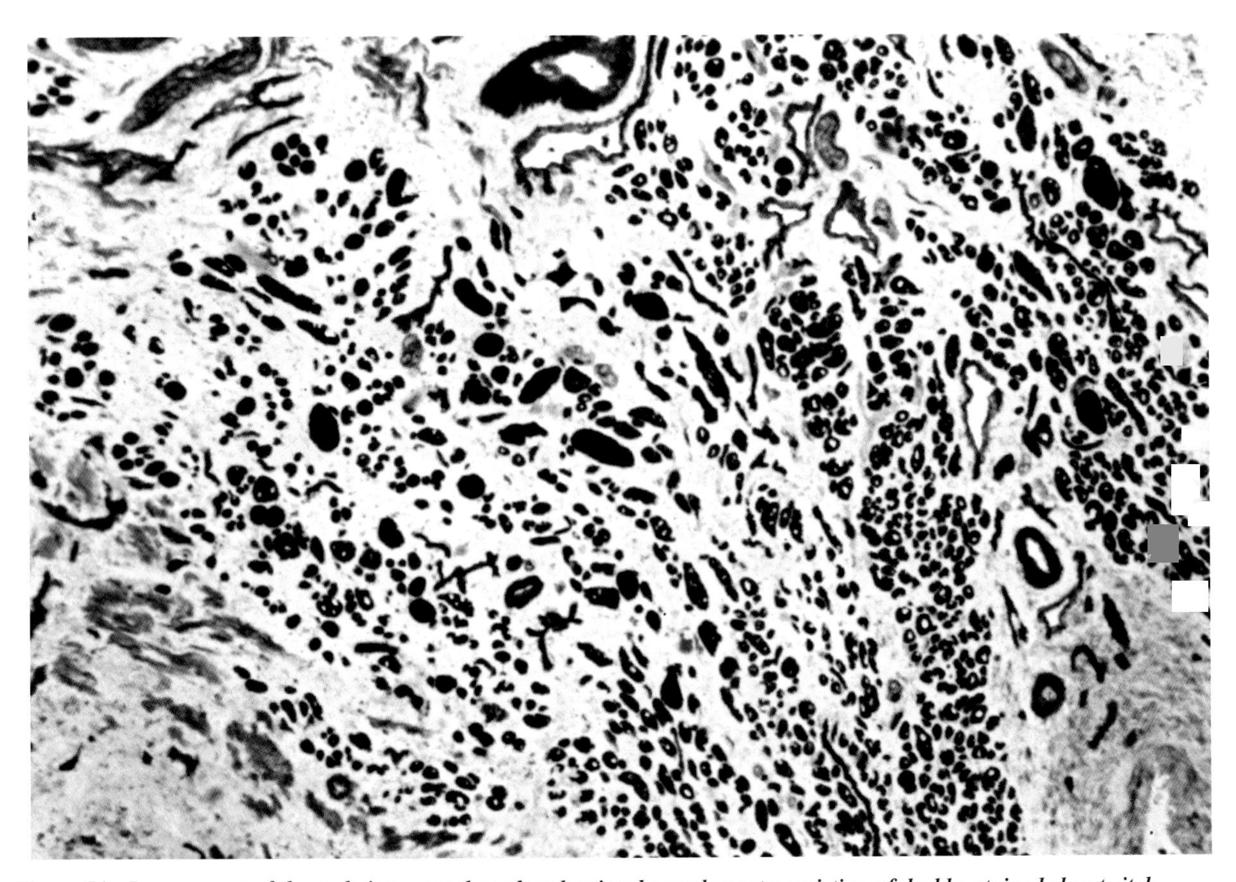

Figure 51 : Inner aspect of the male intramural uretheral striated muscle coat consisting of darkly stained slow twitch (type I) fibres. X150

VI. THE MALE URETHRA

1. Macroscopic anatomy

The male urethra (fig. 52) is a fibromuscular tube approximately 20cm long and is usually described in three parts: prostatic, membranous and spongy. The prostatic and membranous parts pass downwards while the spongy part turns forwards in the bulb of the penis. This abrupt angulation is of considerable importance when catheters or cystoscopes are being introduced. Furthermore, although the spongy and prostatic parts can be readily dilated, the external meatus and the membranous urethra are comparatively narrow.

2. Prostatic urethra

The prostatic urethra is the widest and most dilatable part of the entire male urethra. It is about 3cm long and extends through the prostate from base to apex (fig. 53). The prostatic urethra is divided into proximal and distal segments of approximately equal length by an abrupt anterior angulation of its posterior wall at the midpoint between prostate apex and bladder neck. The angle of deviation is approximately 35°, but can be quite variable and tends to be greater in men with nodular hyperplasia. The prostatic urethra lies nearer the anterior than the posterior surface of the prostate. It is widest in the middle and narrowest below, adjoining the membranous part. In cross-section it appears crescentic in outline with the convex side facing ventrally.

The characteristic crescentic shape is due to the presence on the posterior wall of a narrow median longitudinal ridge formed by an elevation of the epithelial lining and its subjacent tissue, called the urethral crest (fig. 54). On each side of the crest lies a shallow depression termed the prostatic sinus, the floor of which is pierced by the openings of the prostatic ducts. About the middle of the length of the urethral crest, the colliculus seminalis (or verumontanum) forms an elevation on which the slit-like orifice of the prostatic utricle is situated. On each side of, or just within, this orifice are the openings of the two ejaculatory ducts. The prostatic utricle is a blind-ending diverticulum about 6mm long which extends upwards and backwards within the substance of the prostate. It develops from the paramesonephric ducts or urogenital sinus and as a consequence is a remnant of the system which forms the reproductive tract in the female.

3. Membranous urethra

Emerging from the anterior aspect of the apex of the prostate, the membranous urethra (fig. 55) descends in the midline and pierces the perineal membrane. It is approximately 2cm long and its mucosa is folded, giving the lumen a stellate appearance on cross-section. Within the wall of the membranous urethra is the intrinsic striated muscle which, as in the female, is often named the external urethral sphincter (or rhabdosphincter). Lateral to the sphincter are the medial borders of the levatores ani.

The intramural muscle of the wall of the membranous urethra consists of a relatively thin inner layer of smooth muscle bundles continuous proximally with those of the prostatic urethra, and an outer layer of circularly orientated striated muscle fibres. Most of the striated muscle fibres on the inner aspect of the sphincter are unusually small in cross-section with diameters of only 15-20 μm. The majority of these fibres are slow twitch in type (fig. 51) and, unlike the female merge peripherally with larger diameter fast (type II) and slow twitch fibres. Whether these large diameter fibres represent a proximal extension of the striated muscle surrounding the bulb of the penis remains to be determined. If established, this hypothesis offers an explanation for the apparent differences in intramural striated muscle fibre size and type between females and males.

4. Spongy urethra

The spongy (or penile) urethra is approximately 15cm in length, commencing in the bulb of the penis and traversing the erectile tissue of the corpus spongiosum and glans (fig. 52). The mucosa presents numerous small recesses or lacunae and most of its lumen forms a transverse slit. Within the bulb the urethra is wider, forming the intrabulbar fossa. The lumen is also expanded within the glans to form the navicular fossa which opens at the surface as a vertical slit, the external meatus.

VII. COMPONENTS OF THE URETHRAL WALL

1. Smooth muscle

a) Basic properties

The smooth muscle cells in the urethra are small, richly supplied with afferent and efferent nerve fibres, gathered into small bundles and linked to each other by many adherens type junctions but no gap junctions. The smooth muscle bundles in the urethral wall are thinner than in the detrusor and arranged in obvious layers (fig. 56). In humans and larger mammals there is a relatively thick inner layer that is predominantly longitudinally arranged and outside this, a thinner circular muscle layer (fig. 57). In the lamina propria of the urethra scattered small bundles of only a few cells are often found. Elastic fibres are well developed in the bladder neck and urethra.

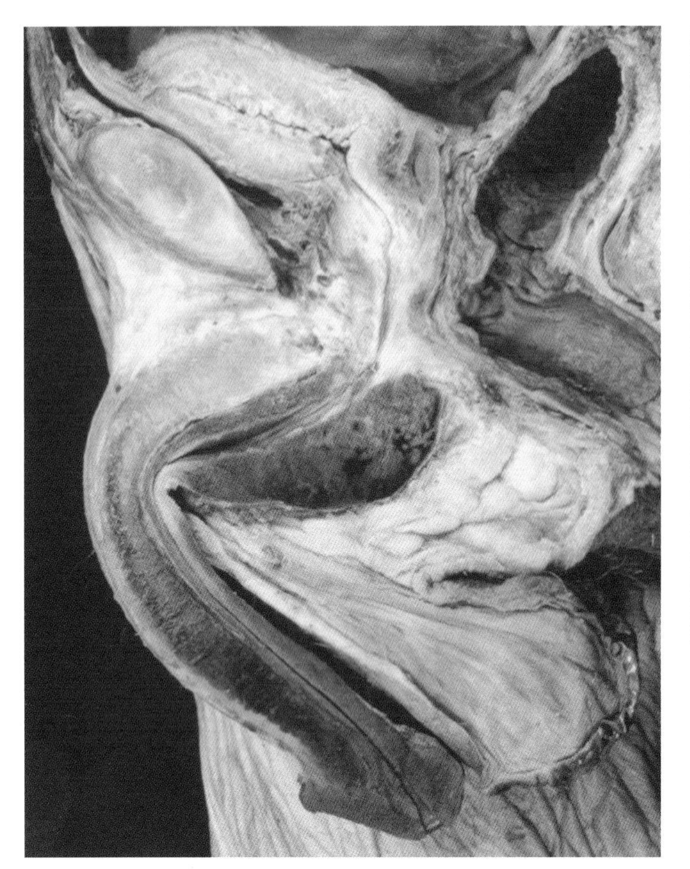

Figure 52 : Sagittal section showing the parts of the male urethra.

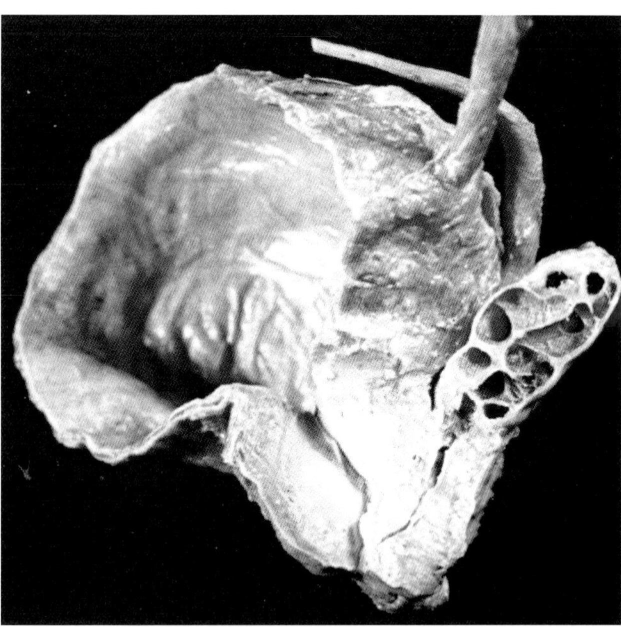

Figure 53 : Dissection of the prostate and seminal vesicle to show the prostatic urethra and ejaculatory duct.

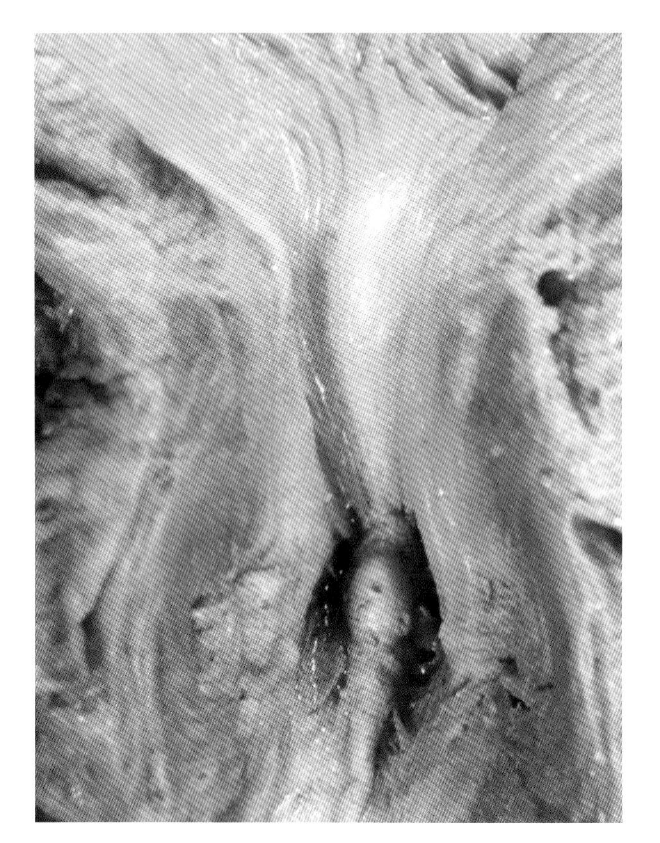

Figure 54 : Sagittal section showing the parts of the male urethra.

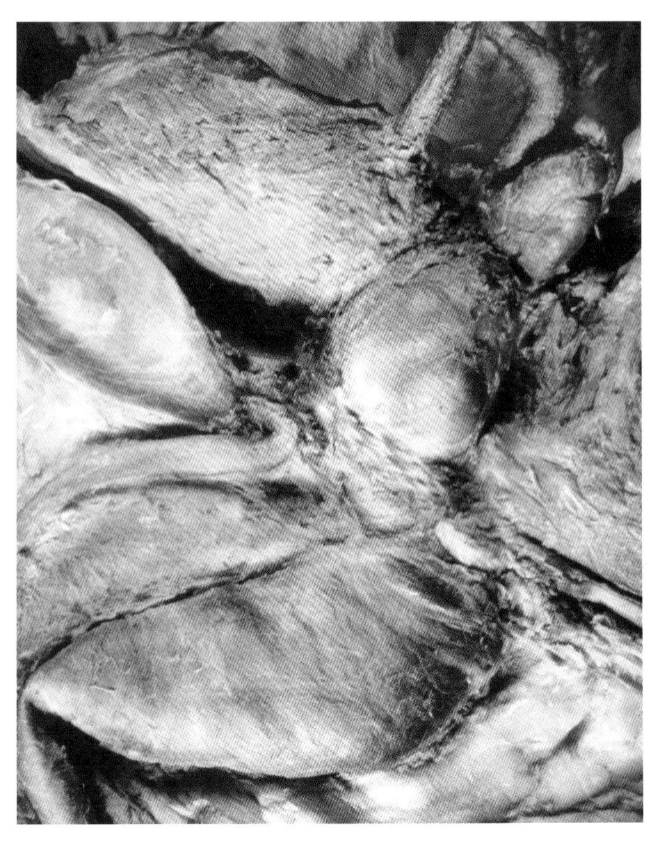

Figure 55 : The left pelvic wall and levator ani have been removed to show the prostate, membranous urethra and bulb of the penis.

In comparison with the detrusor, there is little published on the mechanical properties of the smooth muscle of the urethra. A recent study has, however, compared the force velocity relationship of circular and longitudinal smooth muscles from the rabbit urethra [190] and has shown that the maximum shortening velocity is three times higher in the longitudinal than in the circular smooth muscle. The authors conclude that the results are consistent with a tonic role for the circular smooth muscle in contracting the urethra during bladder filling, and a phasic role for the longitudinal smooth muscle in opening the urethra during micturition.

Behavioural studies demonstrate that the contractile properties of urethral smooth muscle are rather variable, depending on the region from which they are dissected, and possibly on age and hormonal status. In pig and man, smooth muscle dissected from the high pressure zone usually generates continuous sustained myogenic tone, sometimes interrupted by small oscillatory relaxations and contractions (fig. 58). A clear difference is thus seen in the contractile behaviour of smooth muscle from the detrusor and urethra. The ability of the circular elements to maintain continuous tone make it likely that there may be significant differences in their ability to develop latch bridges, or in the Ca^{2+}-sensitivity of the contractile proteins. The evoked responses are also sustained, in contrast to the detrusor, and in tissues generating tone, relaxations and contractions can be evoked by the correct stimuli.

Less work has been carried out on the electrical properties of urethral smooth muscle than on detrusor. In smaller mammals action potentials have been recorded, [191] but in the pig, which seems a better model for the human urethra, records from isolated urethral myocytes have membrane potentials of around –40 mV, and do not appear to support action potentials. They show spontaneous hyperpolarizations and possess large and small Ca^{2+}-activated $K+$ channels, and glibenclamide-sensitive ATP dependent K channels, but little evidence of voltage sensitive delayed rectifier or transient outward currents [37, 192]. There is currently no evidence about electrical coupling in urethral smooth muscle, but its in vivo ability to generate sustained myogenic tone suggests that the myocytes are well coupled.

b) Neuronal control of contractile behaviour

The innervation of the urethral smooth muscle is more complicated than the detrusor, with both excitatory and inhibitory innervation. In the pig, intramural ganglia, composed of two to 30 neurones, are found in the bladder neck and middle and distal regions of the urethra. In the smooth muscle, and in the vicinity of the striated muscle regions of the intrinsic external urethral sphincter, there are small ganglia, containing two to three neurones, which are vasoactive intestinal polypeptide-, (met) enkephalin- and somatostatin-immunoreactive [129]. Similar ganglia have been demonstrated in the human urethra, and these ganglia also contain nitric oxide synthase, (NOS) and haemoxygenase (the enzyme synthesizing CO), with various degrees of co-localization (fig. 59) [193]. Histochemically evidence demonstrates the presence of cholinesterase-positive putative cholinergic nerves, and immunohistochemical techniques show the presence of tyrosine hydroxylase-containing putative adrenergic nerves [194].

Nerves staining for acetylcholinesterase, vasoactive intestinal polypeptide, catecholamines, substance P, (met) enkephalin, gastrin and somatostatin are also found in the urethral smooth muscle in the pig urethra [129, 194]. In the rat urethra (NOS) nerves are very frequent in the smooth musculature together with cholinergic, adrenergic and neuropeptide Y (NPY)-immunoreactive (IR) nerves, whereas vasoactive intestinal peptide (VIP)-IR and calcitonin-gene-related peptide (CGRP)-IR nerves are much less abundant [195].

Acetylcholine and noradrenaline both mediate contraction in the urethra, [196, 197] and both appear to be involved in the excitatory response to intramural stimulation, although the noradrenergic component is the most significant (fig. 60). Both excitatory $\alpha 1$ and $\beta 2$ adrenoceptors are present, and there are distinct subtypes of $\alpha 1$ adrenoceptor subtypes in the human prostatic urethra (fig. 61) [198]. Nitric oxide synthase containing nerves also innervate the smooth muscle, and mediate a fast transient relaxation (fig. 62) [197-201]. In the pig, a systematic study has demonstrated that both the density of the nerves and the response to the various transmitters may vary along the length of the urethra [194].

Little information is available on the mechanisms coupling the membrane to the contractile machinery in urethral smooth muscle. In those preparations that show myogenic tone, this can be abolished by L-type Ca channel blockers, suggesting that continuous entry of calcium through these channels occurs in the resting state [197]. Depolarisation of the membrane by increasing extracellular $K+$ concentrations has variable results – small increases result in contraction, but if the concentration is increased it will often result in a biphasic response, or a pure relaxation. It has been suggested that sufficient depolarisation may result in voltage-dependent inactivation of the L-type calcium channels and relaxation [48]. Relaxation can also be mediated through activation of guanylate cyclase and elevation of intracellular cGMP, through nitrergic nerves or application of NO or NO donors (fig. 63) [3, 202]. An interesting field of research is opening up since it is likely that both the enzyme responsible for the synthesis of cGMP (guanylate cyclase) and the enzyme responsible for its

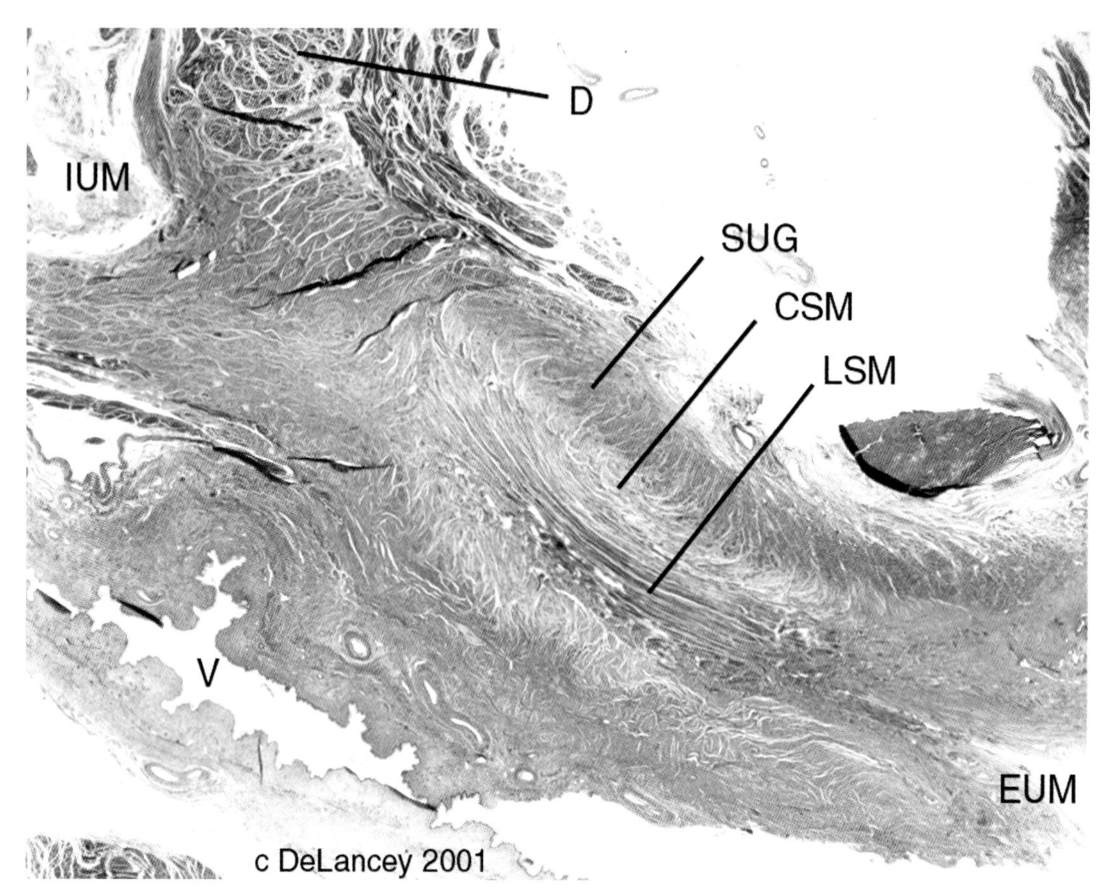

Figure 56 : Transverse section of the mid-urethra with smooth muscle stain shown on the left and trichrome stain on the right. CSM, circular smooth muscle; LSM, longitudinal smooth muscle; SUG., striated urogenital muscle; V, vagina; EUM, external urinary meatus; IUM, internal urinary meatus

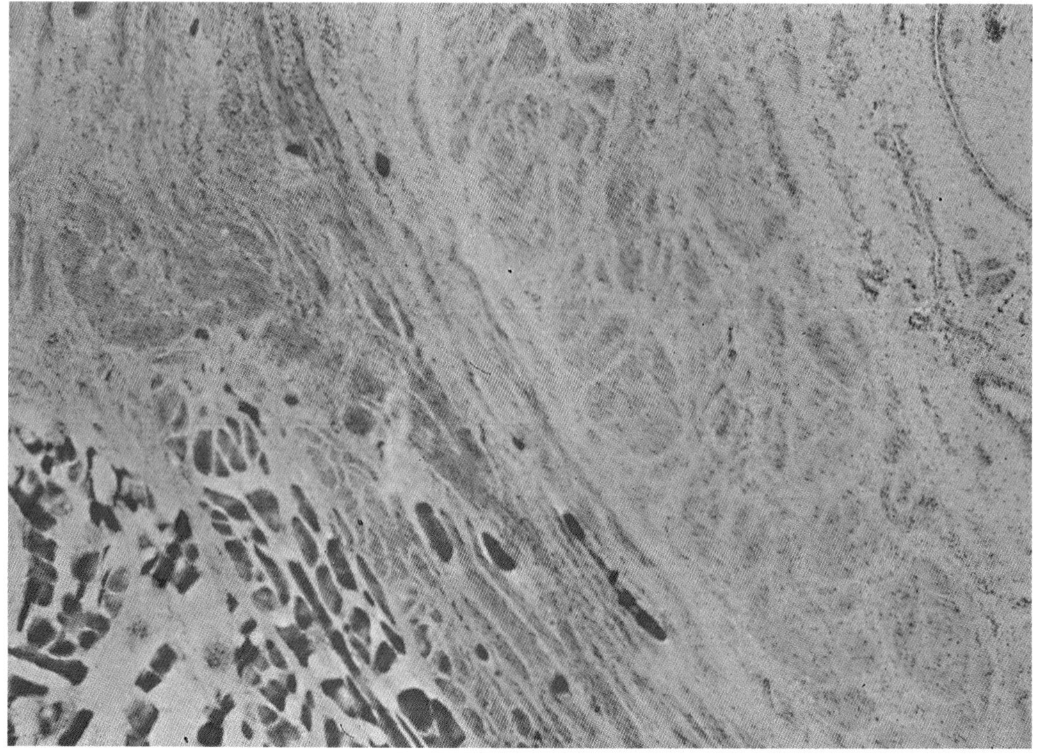

Figure 57 : Cross section of human urethra. From the outside in you can see striated muscle fibres, then a circular smooth muscle coat in which some striated muscles are intermingled. Within this is a thicker layer of longitudinally oriented smooth muscle, then the lamina propria and the urothelium.

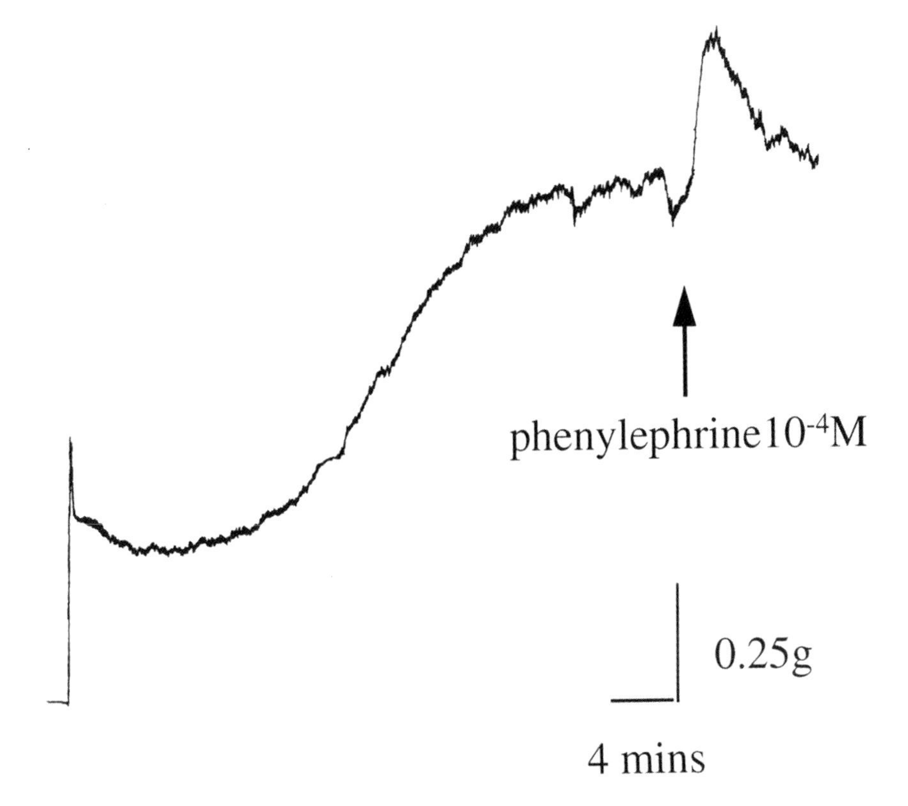

Figure 58 : Contractile behaviour of a strip of longitudinal smooth muscle dissected from the proximal third of a human female urethra. Note the development of spontaneous myogenic tone, the spontaneous transient relaxations and the contractile response to the alpha agonist, phenylephrine.

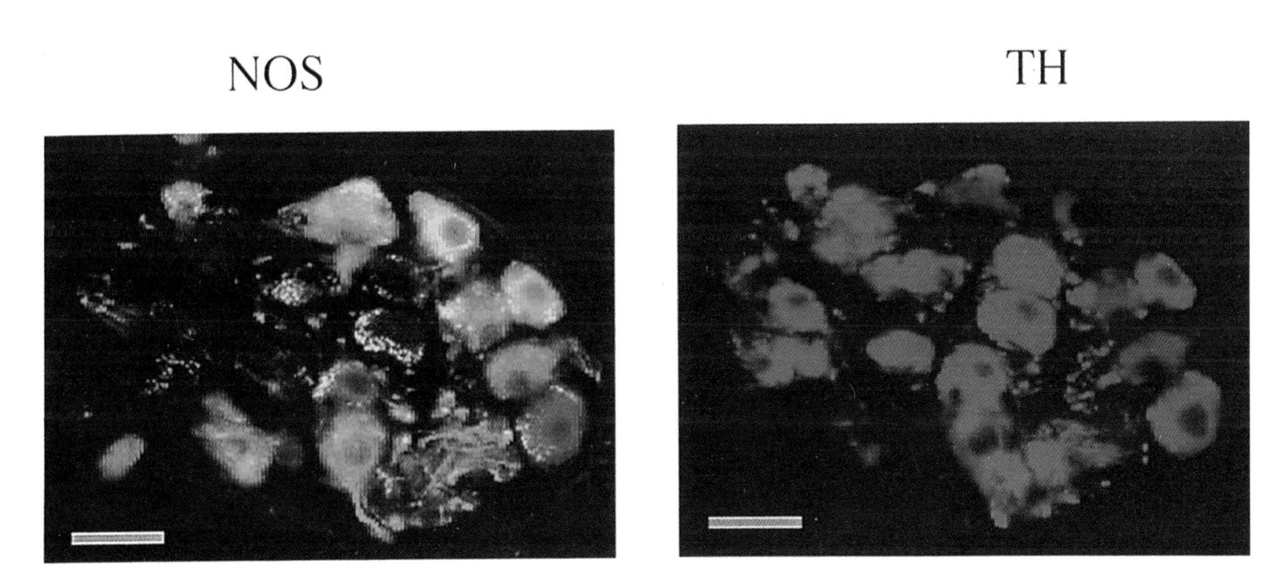

Human female urethra: proximal third, ganglion.
Bar = 100μm

Figure 59 : Intramural ganglion in the proximal female human urethra showing neurones with positive fluorescence for nitric oxide synthase immunoreactivity (green) and tyrosine hydroxylase immunoreactivity (red). Note heterogeneity of neuronal population. Most neurones are immunoreactive to both enzymes, but others for only one or other. Micrograph kindly provided by Kossen Ho.

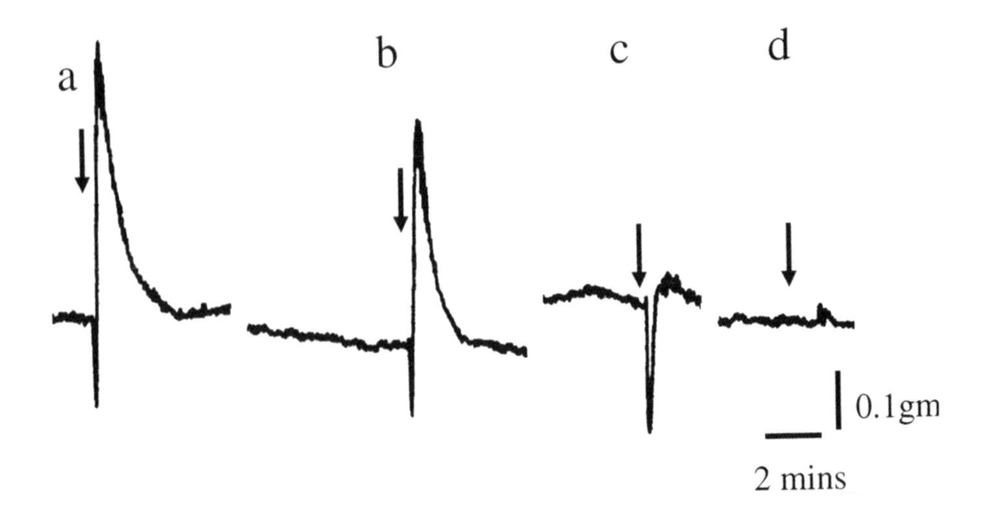

Figure 60 : Response of human female circular smooth muscle from the proximal urethra to stimulation of the intrinsic nerves (30 V, 0.2 ms, 10 Hz, 5 s). (a) control, note transient relaxation followed by contraction (b) in the presence of atropine (10^{-6} M) to block cholinergic transmission. Note reduced size of contractile response (c) in the presence of atropine and guanethidine (3.10^{-6} M) to block cholinergic and adrenergic transmission. Contractile response abolished, leaving relaxation (d) in the presence of atropine, guanethidine and NOARG (10^{-5} M) to additionally block nitrergic transmission.

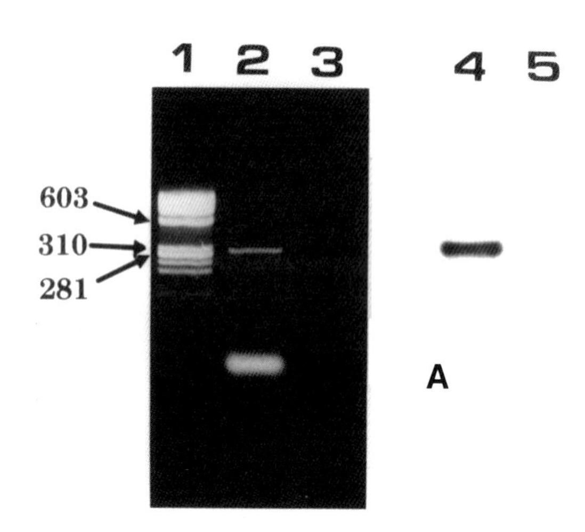

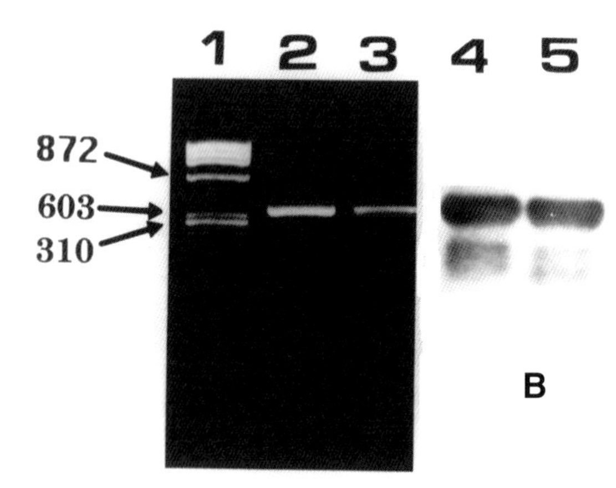

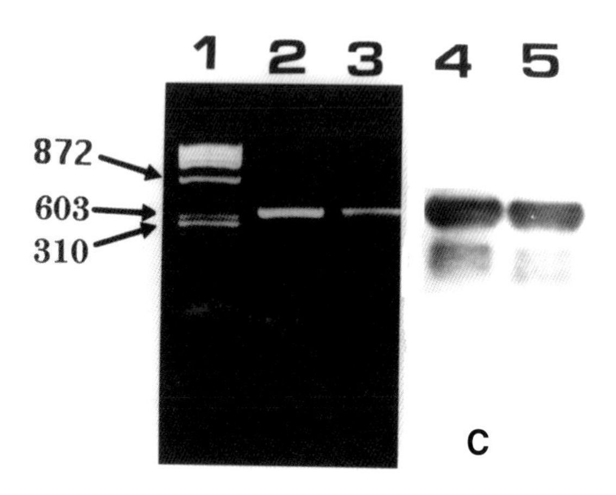

Figure 61 : Demonstration of the presence of α1a, α1b but not 1d-adrenoceptors in human prostatic urethra. Total RNA was extracted from the prostatic urethra, and amplification of the mRNA for α1a, α1b and α1d-adrenoceptors was carried out using the reverse transcription / polymerase chain reaction (RT/PCR). The figures show the results of agarose gel electrophoresis and size fractionation of the products, with Southern hybridization. Also included are results from human internal iliac artery for comparison. (a) Primers specific for α1a-adrenoceptors were used. (b) Primers specific for α1b-adrenoceptors were used. (c) Primers specific for α1d-adrenoceptors were used. From right to left, the first lanes show a size marker, the second lanes shows RT/PCR products for primers specific for α1-adrenoceptors from the prostatic urethra, the third lanes show products for primers specific for α1-adrenoceptors from the iliac artery. Lanes 4 and 5 show Southern hybridization corresponding to lanes 2 and 3, using oligonucleotide probes for the α1-adrenoceptor sequences Note the presence of α1a and α1d-adrenoceptors but no α1b in the prostate, confirmed by the Southern blots; in contrast the iliac artery shows the presence of α1b and α1d-adrenoceptors but no α1a-adrenoceptors.

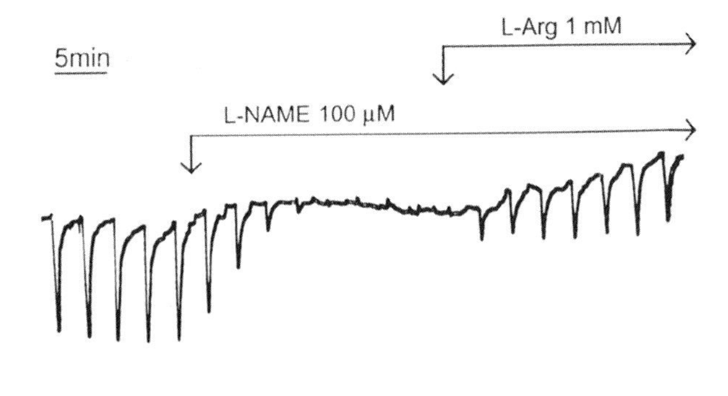

Figure 62 : Responses of the smooth muscle of the urethra to transmural nerve stimulation. The transient relaxations are abolished by addition of the nitric oxide synthase inhibitor L-NAME (100 μM), and then restored by addition of the amino acid precursor L-arginine (1 mM), suggesting that the relaxations are produced by NO synthesis.

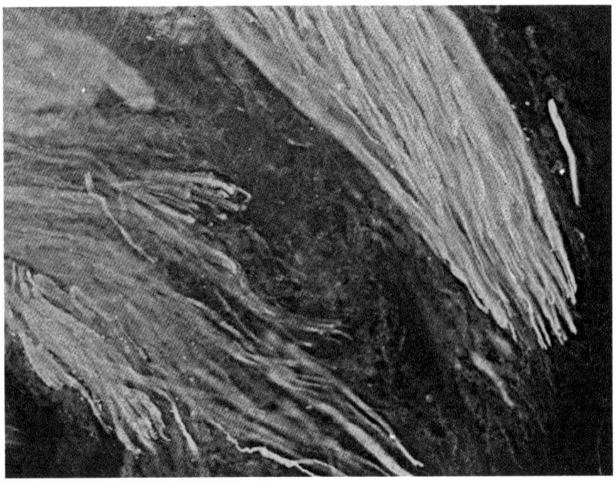

Figure 63 : Smooth muscle cells from the human prostatic urethra showing immunofluorescence to cGMP after activation of guanylate cyclase by administration of sodium nitroprusside. From Smet et al., 1996 [3].

breakdown (phosphodiesterase) may be useful targets for new drugs. Indeed inhibition of phosphodiesterase V has been shown to enhance erection in impotent men [203] and it is likely that effects on urinary outflow may be obtained by the use of similar drugs. Further studies will be necessary to investigate whether pharmacological alterations of cGMP levels may prove of importance for the development of new drugs in the treatment of voiding disorders.

c) The role of the smooth muscle

The role of the smooth muscle in the urethra is more problematic than that of the detrusor, because of its orientation. Whereas some of it is circularly oriented, and could play a role in the generation of the resting urethral pressure profile particularly since the area generating the most myogenic tone coincides with the maximum urethral pressure [197], the thickest layer is longitudinally arranged. Contraction of the longitudinal smooth muscle could play a role in stabilizing the urethra and allowing force generated by the circular muscular elements to occlude the lumen, or in aiding in the opening of the bladder neck during micturition. There is controversy about the relative roles of the urethral smooth and striated circular muscle and the lamina propria, in generating the urethral pressure profile, but it seems likely that both contribute [204]. Blocking striated sphincter activity with nicotinic neuro-muscular blocking agents has variable effects, and may reduce urethral tone, but rarely by more than 40%, suggesting that the smooth muscles are important. Blocking sympathetic tone with alpha-adrenoceptor blockers may also reduce urethral pressure by about a third [205]. There is little evidence for the involvement of the cholinergic innervation in generating urethral pressure: however, the continuous myogenic tone of the circular smooth muscle may contribute.

Damage to the innervation of the urethral smooth muscle, or changes in its properties would again be expected to significantly alter the behaviour of the urethra, and might result both in incontinence during the normal filling phase if the excitatory input is reduced, and detrusor sphincter dyssynergia if the mechanisms producing relaxation of the muscle are affected. However, the considerable difficulties in obtaining specimens of urethral smooth muscle from patients with known urethral dysfunction means that little if any work has been carried out in this area. The smooth muscle is an obvious target for pharmacological control of incontinence, as discussed in the report of the committee.

2. STRIATED MUSCLE

Striated muscle occurs in the walls of the male and female urethra, where it forms a rhabdosphincter which is separate from the periurethral skeletal muscle of the pelvic floor. In the male, the striated muscle extends from the base of the bladder and the anterior aspect of the prostate to the full length of the membranous urethra. In the female, the striated muscle extends from the proximal urethra distally. The striated sphincter is horse-shoe shaped and the muscle cells are smaller than ordinary skeletal muscle, being 15 to 20 μm in diameter.

a) Fibre type

Gosling et al [206] considered these striated muscle fibers to be slow twitch in nature. Others, however, believe that the striated sphincter is a heterogeneous population. Some [207, 208] have examined the fibre types in the striated muscle of the prostatic capsule, since this is easy to obtain, and derives from the rhabdosphincter. They have shown fast and slow fibres to be present. This has been confirmed more recently in rhabdosphincters taken from transplant donors [193]. In the male the rhabdosphincter consists of 35% fast and 65% slow twitch fibres, whereas in the female, 13% of the fibres are fast twitch (fig. 64). The slow twitch fibres could be important in developing sustained tone to occlude the urethra, whereas the fast twitch fibres could be involved in reflex contraction to elevate urethral tone when intraabdominal pressure rises. The majority of the fast twitch fibres and about a quarter of the slow twitch fibres in the intramural striated muscle of the human membranous urethral sphincter show positive staining for nitric oxide synthase in the sarcolemma [193].

b) Innervation

The urethra has a complicated neuro-anatomy, receiving as it does input from both somatic and autonomic pathways. The rhabdosphincter receives somatic input from S2-S4 nerve roots via the pudendal nerve, and the pelvic nerves also enter the muscle [209, 210]. In the cat, a triple innervation of the rhabdosphincter has been demonstrated histochemically (see [4]), with a somatic, parasympathetic and sympathetic input. Evidence for a triple innervation in the human rhabdosphincter however is not strong, and it is likely that the functional innveration is somatic, although modulation through autonomic innervation cannot be ruled out. In the pig intrinsic external urethral sphincter, vasoactive intestinal polypeptide- and gastrin-immunoreactive nerve fibres have been found bordering a small number of individual striated muscle fibres, while catecholamine-containing nerves were found predominantly in the connective tissue surrounding the striated muscle fibres. Dense populations of acetylcholinesterase-positive nerve fibres are found associated with the striated muscle fibres, with end plates on some of them [129]. It is generally agreed that the motor cell bodies of the nerves supplying the urethral striated muscle lie in a discrete area of the anterior horns of the second, third and fourth sacral segments of the spinal cord collectively known as Onuf's nucleus [50, 51].

Immunohistochemical studies have demonstrated the presence of nitric-oxide synthase containing nerve trunks and sparse fine nerve fibres running in the intramural striated muscle of the human membranous urethral sphincter, with the fine nerve fibres running parallel to and apparently innervating some striated muscle fibres [193]. Some nerve trunks containing tyrosine hydroxylase immunoreactivity course through the striated muscle, but do not seem to be specifically associated with the striated fibres, and may just been route to smooth muscle, or innervating blood vessels.

In vitro studies on the physiology of urethral striated muscles are rare. Recordings of contractile activity in rings of guinea-pig urethra have been made [211] but the results were difficult to interpret because the activity included contraction of both striated and smooth muscle activity. In vivo studies have investigated the effects of nicotinic receptor blockade on the urethral pressure in the pig [118], the dog [212] and in humans [204], demonstrating a role of the striated muscle in generating resting urethral pressure. In the dog pudendal but not pelvic nerve stimulation produces contraction of the striated muscle. Electromyography can be used to record activity in the human striated sphincter

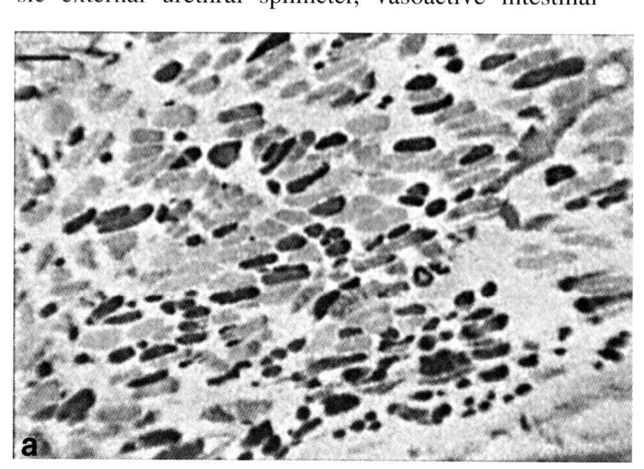

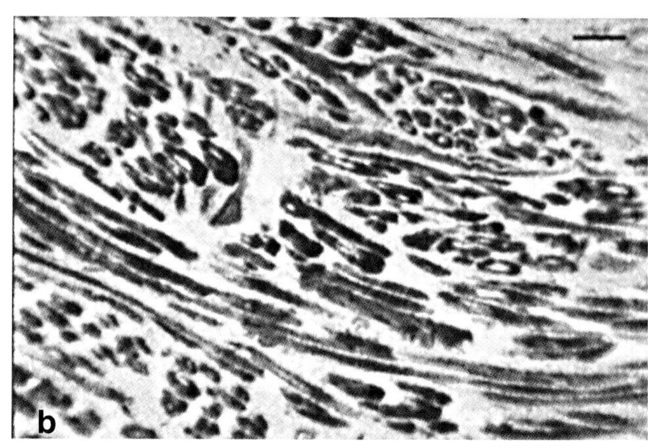

Figure 64 : Sections from the proximal third of the human male urethra (a) and (b) the female membranous urethra stained for ATPase at pH 4.3, in which the slow twitch fibres appear darkly stained. Note that most of the female striated muscle is slow twitch, whereas a significant proportion of the male fibres are fast twitch.

during filling, using concentric needle electrodes. Recordings show a steady firing of the muscle fibres at between 2-8Hz (fig. 65) [213]. Coughing, or other manoeuvres that increase intra-abdominal pressure produce a marked increase in the number of units firing. Abnormal activity can be recorded from patients with various disorders of urethral sphincter innervation [214].

c) The role of the striated muscle

The main functions of the urethral striated muscle will be in helping to generate sustained urethral pressure during bladder filling, and providing reflex increases in urethral wall pressure to prevent leakage of urine when abdominal pressure rises. It seems likely that the slow twitch fibres will be more involved in the sustained generation of urethral pressure, and the larger component of these fibres in women may be a reflection of the shorter urethral length. As with the smooth muscle, it should be remembered that failure to switch off the tonic excitation of the striated muscle during micturition can result in detrusor sphincter dyssynergia, which can be a serious problem. The fast twitch fibres, with their greater fatigueability, have the properties necessary to mediate a rapid increase in urethral pressure to prevent stress incontinence.

3. URETHRAL LAMINA PROPRIA

a) Structure

The urethral lamina propria extends from the longitudinal smooth muscle layer to the urothelium, and fills the lumen of the urethra. The lamina propria is lined proximally with a surface membrane consisting of transitional epithelium, and mucous glands have been described along its length in the female urethra [215]. Between this and the smooth muscle layer is an extensive stroma

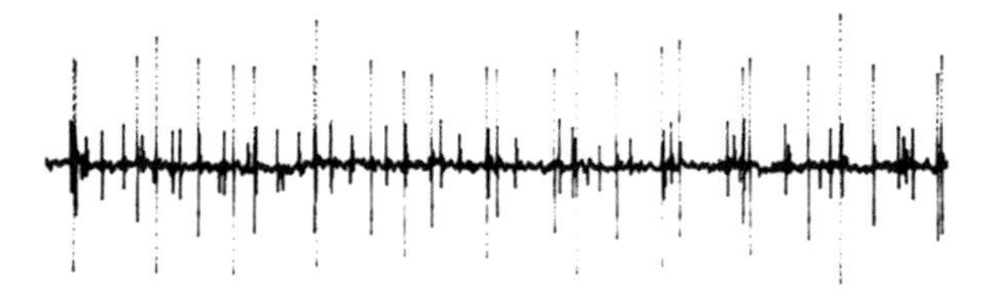

Figure 65 : Recording of the EMG of the urethral striated muscle in a normal woman during the filling phase of the micturition cycle. The recording was made with a concentric needle electrode. The electrode is picking up signals from at least four different motor units, distinguishable by the amplitude of the spikes. A large increase in the number of units firing is seen during manoeuvres that increase intra-abdominal pressure. From Fowler & Fowler, 1981 [73].

surrounding a prominent vascular plexus. The urethral stroma has been less extensively studied than the bladder stroma, but it is known to contain primarily longitudinally arranged collagen fibres and elastin fibres [216, 217]. More detailed studies have been made of the urethral stroma in female dogs, [218] and the female pig [219]. In the dog, the stroma comprises almost 80% of the total volume in the proximal urethra, and contains abundant collagen fibrils and longitudinally orientated elastic fibres. In the pig, the lamina propria is maximally developed near the vesico-urethral junction, where it occupies over 25% of the cross sectional area of the urethra. There is a dense capillary network under the mucosa in an areolar connective tissue of loose collagen fibres. The submucosa comprises a dense irregular connective tissue with collagen, elastin and fibrocytes, and an extensive vascular plexus. Small bundles of longitudinally arranged smooth muscle cells are also seen. The vascular plexus consists of predominantly longitudinally oriented blood vessels with abundant muscular arteries, large arterioles and thin-walled venules. The elastic fibres run mainly in a longitudinal direction near and amongst the longitudinal smooth muscle surrounding the mucosa. In the human female urethra the relative amount of blood vessels and striated muscle decreases with age [220]. The amount of smooth muscle remains unchanged, and the relative amount of connective tissue increases. Some stress-incontinent women seem to have a general decrease in tissue collagen concentration [221].

b) Vascular filling

The vascular filling of the urethral lamina propria is thought to be of importance for urinary continence although the magnitude of its contribution to continence is still not understood [222]. Oestrogen is known to increase the urethral blood flow and it is likely that part of the possible benefit of oestrogen on stress urinary incontinence is due to an increase in the urethral blood flow resulting in an increased distension of the lamina propria blood vessels [223, 224]. Impaired arterial blood supply to the urethra decreases the intraluminal pressure (fig. 66) [222] but it is presently not known whether it is the decrease in vascular filling or the urethral hypoxia which mediates the decrease in urethral pressure. Recently it was suggested that both these mechanisms may be involved, since it was shown that the initial drop in urethral pressure was mediated via decreased vascular filling whereas the later phase was due to an hypoxic effect on the urethral smooth muscle [224].

4. PARAURETHRAL TISSUE

Results are divergent regarding connective tissue outside the urethra. Paraurethral tissue biopsies from preme-

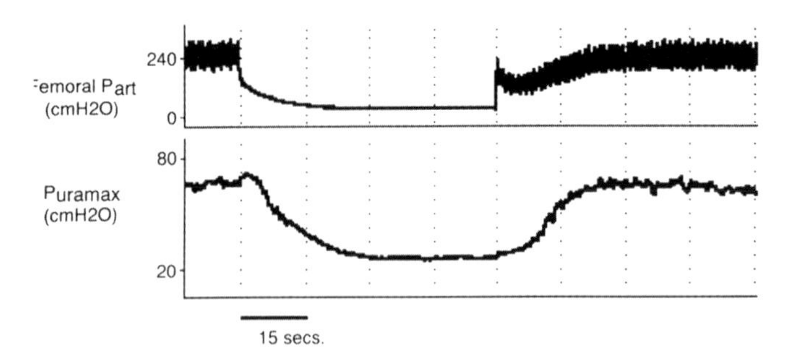

Figure 66 : In vivo recording of the urethral pressure and the left femoral artery pressure on occlusion of the terminal aorta in the pig. Note that the urethral pressure falls as the arterial inflow is cut off.

nopausal women with stress incontinence contained 30% more collagen and the diameter of the fibrils are 30% larger than in controls [225]. Postmenopausal stress incontinent women, on the other hand, have no difference in collagen concentration compared with their age controls [226]. Others have, however, found a decreased periurethral collagen concentration [227] and a decreased collagen type I to type III ratio in stress incontinent patients [228]. The macroscopic anatomy of these tissues is involved in overall support of the pelvic organs and will be discussed later in this chapter.

VIII. MODULATORY SYSTEMS

1. Nitric Oxide Syntase

In recent years, a large number of studies have shown that the gaseous molecule nitric oxide (NO) is an important signalling molecule in the urogenital tract. NO is produced by a family of isoenzymes, NO synthases (NOS) and the amino acid L-arginine is the substrate for NOS forming NO and L-citrulline in equal amounts [229]. Several types of NOS have been found and cloned. Two types have been shown to be dependent on free calcium for their NO formation and they were named endothelial (eNOS) and neuronal (nNOS), respectively after the cell type in which they were first located [229]. The third isoform which has been cloned is iNOS. It differs from the previous isoforms in that its activity is not dependent on free calcium and that it is usually only expressed after stimulation by various cytokines [229], iNOS was first found in macrophages and is known to be activated during host defense reactions.

The enzyme forming NO from L-arginine has been found in various parts of the lower urinary tract. In the bladder nNOS has been found in perivascular nerves and in nerves innervating the detrusor muscle [230]. In the vascular endothelium eNOS has been found [231]. In the urinary tract iNOS is not expressed during normal conditions but may be found in the human bladder after treatment with BCG and various cytokines [148, 149]. Thus, NOS has been found in several different cell types in the lower urinary tract and NO may serve to mediate several different functions. NO has been suggested as a mediator of nonadrenergic non-cholinergic nerve-induced relaxation in the lower urinary tract in rabbit, [232, 233] pig, [234] sheep, [235] dog [201] and man (fig. 63) [236, 237]. The opening of the bladder neck and the dilatation of urethra during the micturition reflex is also likely to be NO mediated. Although the evidence for a role of NO in the urethra and bladder neck are compelling there is still only sparse evidence for a role by NO in the detrusor muscle. Inhibition of NOS only marginally affects nerve-induced smooth muscle activity in the human detrusor [238, 239] and the detrusor has a low sensitivity to NO, making it less likely that NO has a role as a relaxant neurotransmitter in this tissue. In spite of the above, several other studies have indicated a pathophysiological role for NO in the urinary 'urge syndrome'. Thus, in rats in vivo NOS inhibitors elicit bladder hyperactivity and decreased bladder capacity [234] and in nNOS knock-out mice hypertrophic and dilated bladders and dysfunctional urinary outlets are found [231]. Increased detrusor contractions may originate from the bladder outlet region rather than from the detrusor itself [240]. Such contractions can be observed in the majority of men with outflow obstruction [241]. The mechanism behind this overactivity is not known, but it is likely that lack of an inhibitory mediator in the detrusor or the outlet region, causing an increased afferent nerve activity, may be involved. Since studies on NOS activity and NOS histochemistry have revealed a marked increase in NOS localisation in the bladder neck and urethra as compared to the detrusor it is likely that impaired NOS activity in this region may result in the development of micturition disorders. This suggests that in the detrusor NO may modulate the effects of other transmitters or that it has an afferent function as has been shown in the central nervous system. Taken together the studies indicate that a decrease in NO production leads to an increase in urinary urge symptoms. In agreement with these studies daily treatment with the NO precursor L-arginine decreases urinary symptoms in patients with interstitial cystitis [242].

NO may also be involved in the increase in voiding disorders seen in menopausal women. It is known that oestrogen treatment significantly reduces the prevalence of voiding disorders in elderly women and it has been shown that oestrogen increases the expression of both eNOS and nNOS in the uterine artery, kidney, heart, oesophagus and cerebellum [243]. Subsequent studies have also shown that oestrogen may increase the calcium-dependent NOS activity in the guinea pig urinary bladder, [244] but further studies are needed to evaluate the role of NO in voiding disorders in post-menopausal women.

In conclusion, accumulating evidence suggests that alterations in the L-arginine/NO pathway is involved in several pathophysiological mechanisms leading to voiding disorders. Further studies are needed to clarify all details of the involvement of NO in these voiding disorders but clearly the L-arginine-NO-cGMP pathway will be of great interest as a target for future drugs in this area.

2. Afferent innervation

a) Overview

Afferent nerves provide background information to the central nervous system arising from the lower urinary tract which is required for the co-ordinated activation of all reflexes related to urine storage and voiding [245, 246]. As such, afferents have potential value as targets for drug therapy for urinary incontinence [72, 247, 248]. There is ample evidence indicating that afferents are heterogenous. This heterogeneity has been verified by neurophysiological techniques, documenting the variable conduction velocities of lower urinary tract afferents and establishing the relation between this parameter and their sensitivity to applied mechanical and chemical stimuli: [249-253] these studies have revealed, among others, the existence of a population of 'silent' nociceptors which are mechanically insensitive in the normal bladder but display a novel mechanosensitivity after induction of inflammation [251]. This hereogeneity has also been documented by anatomical techniques, based on different diameters of afferent neurones and by demonstrating that primary sensory neurones innervating the lower urinary tract express a variety of transmitters/mediators in set combinations (chemical coding) [254-257].

b) Sensory-motor nerves

One of the most intriguing criteria which detects the heterogeneity of lower urinary tract afferents is a pharmacological one, based on the selective stimulant and desensitizing actions of capsaicin and related vanilloid receptor agonists [247, 248, 258-260]. The capsaicin-sensitive primary afferent neurones (CSPANs) are present in the mammalian bladder, project to the spinal cord [261, 262] and regulate the micturition threshold: [263, 264] especially important is their ability to subserve the spinal vesico-vesical reflex which, [265, 266] after chronic spinal cord transection, mediates the supraspinal vesico-vesical reflex underlying normal micturition. Moreover CSPANs are involved in signalling bladder pain [267] and activate cardiovascular reflexes arising from the lower urinary tract [268]. A further distinct feature of CSPANs is their ability to release mediators, notably peptides of the tachykinin family from their central and peripheral endings [74, 259]. Tachykinin release at spinal cord level activates micturition-related reflexes [269]. Tachykinin release from sensory nerves in the bladder wall can induce a prolonged spasm [73, 270] and inflammation (neurogenic inflammation) which is thought to be of pathogenic relevance for certain forms of cystitis [71, 271] CSPANs are present in the human bladder [71] and their pharmacological manipulation promises to have useful diagnostic and therapeutic applications [272-274].

It appears that different subtypes of the capsaicin (vanilloid) receptor may exist, and evidence has been obtained for their expression by cells other than CSPANs, such as mast cells [275] and urothelial cells. Subtype 1 of the capsaicin receptor/ion channel has recently been cloned [276].

It should be noted that CSPANs, as identified pharmacologically, [259, 277] do not overlap exactly with any of the sub-population of afferent nerves which can be distinguished on the basis of neurophysiological or anatomical criteria: although most CSPANs have axons conducting in the C-fibre range, yet not all C-fibres are capsaicin-sensitive and some CSPANs have conduction velocities in the Aδ range [278, 279]. Moreover although CSPANs have small dark, type B somata, not all primary sensory neurones of this type are capsaicin-sensitive [254].

IX. MACROSCOPIC ANATOMY OF THE MUSCULAR PELVIC FLOOR

The bony pelvic ring lies inferior to the abdominal cavity and the levator ani muscles span this space. The borders of the opening spanned by the pelvic floor are the pubic bones anteriorly, the ischial spines laterally, and the sacrum posteriorly. Between the pubis and the spines lie the tendineus arches of the levator ani and the pelvic fascia. The sacrospinous ligament and its overlying coccygeus muscles lie between the spine and the sacrum. It is this polygonal opening that must be closed by the levator ani muscles.

From an organizational standpoint, the pelvic floor consists of two specific components, namely the levator ani and the coccygeus. The latter lies in the same morphological plane as the former and completes the pelvic floor posteriorly. The coccygeus forms a triangular structure the apex of which attaches to the spine of the ischium. From the ischial spine the coccygeus forms a fibromuscular sheet which fans out medially and attaches to the lateral surface of the coccyx and the fifth segment of the sacrum. In actuality the coccygeus is nothing more than the musculotendinous internal surface of the sacrospinous ligament to which it is intimately attached. Unlike animals with mobile tails, the coccygeus is vestigial in humans and does not contribute to active movement of the pelvic floor.

1. Levator ani

In practical terms the pelvic floor is synonymous with the levator ani since this muscle forms the effective contractile support structure of the region. The muscle forms a broad thin sheet attaching anteriorly to the posterior surface of the body of the pubis and suspended laterally from the pelvic wall as far posteriorly as the ischial spine. Between the pubis and ischial spine the muscle is directly attached to (or sometimes slung from) the fascia covering the medial surface of the obturator internus. Anteriorly the levator ani is absent in the midline so that a fat-filled space containing numerous vessels lies immediately behind the pubic symphysis. That part of the muscle attaching to the pubis forms the medial component of the levator ani. In the male the most medial of these fibres from the pubis attach to the perineal body behind the prostate to form the levator prostate. In the female these medial fibres attach to the lateral vaginal wall (fig. 67) to form the so-called pubovaginalis. Other fibres from the pubis attach to the anorectal flexure where they fuse with the deep part of the external anal sphincter to form the puborectalis. More laterally placed fibres run from the pubis and the fascia covering obturator internus and are named pubococcygeus.

That part of the levator ani arising from the lateral wall of the pelvis posteriorly to the ischial spine is named the iliococcygeus. The distinction between the end of the pubococcygeus and the start of the iliococcygeus is arbitrary since one merges imperceptibly with the other as a continuous sheet of muscle. Nevertheless the fibres of iliococcygeus run medially at different angles of obliquity to merge with the component parts of the pubococcygeus.

It is generally recognized that parts of the levator ani collectively play an important role in maintaining the position of the pelvic viscera. In the female the attachments of the levator ani to the vagina and external anal sphincter are responsible, on contraction, for the anterior movement of these viscera towards the pubic symphysis [280, 281]. On contraction of the pelvic floor, this anterior movement of the vagina produces occlusive forces on the urethra resulting in its forward displacement and compression against the posterior surface of the pubis. Contraction of the levator ani is responsible for the compression of the urethra at a site distal to the anatomic location of the intramural urethral striated sphincter. Thus, the levator ani assists this sphincter not only to ensure continence, but also to produce forceful occlusion of the urethra such as occurs during coughing [282].

2. Innervation of the levator ani

The levator ani is innervated by somatic nerve fibres which emanate primarily from sacral root S3, to a lesser extent from S4 and minimally from S2 to form the pudendal nerve [283]. The pudendal nerve is a mixed nerve carrying both motor and sensory fibres and is derived from the sacral plexus. Initially the pudendal nerve lies superior to the sacrospinous ligament lateral to the coccyx. The nerve leaves the pelvis, crossing the ischial spine to gain the ischiorectal fossa via the lesser sciatic foramen. It extends forward in a fibrous tunnel (Alcock's canal) on the medial side of the obturator internus muscle and distally gives rise to branches which supply the levator ani and the membranous urethra. Some variation occurs in the pudendal nerve peripheral anatomy.

X. SUPPORT OF THE URETHRA AND PELVIC ORGANS

1. Support of the pelvic organs

In women, a special series of problems arise because the female pelvis and its supportive structures must accommodate vaginal birth. This results in a series of design compromises that must trade off the importance of pelvic organ support for the extra room needed to deliver the large-headed human fetus [284].

The pelvic organs are supported by a combination of muscle and connective tissue. The levator ani muscles have already been discussed and the connective tissue attachments will now be considered. An overview of this anatomy is shown in figure 68. The pelvic organs are attached to the pelvic walls. The connecting tissues are called the endopelvic fascia, a heterogeneous group of tissues including collagen, elastin, smooth muscle, blood vessels, and nerves [285,286]. It is common to speak of the fasciae and ligaments separately from the pelvic organs as if they had a discreet identity, yet unless these fibrous structures have something to attach to (the pelvic organs), they can have no suspensory effect.

The overall geometry of this tissue determines their mechanical function forming the endopelvic fascia attaches the uterus and vagina to the pelvic wall bilate-

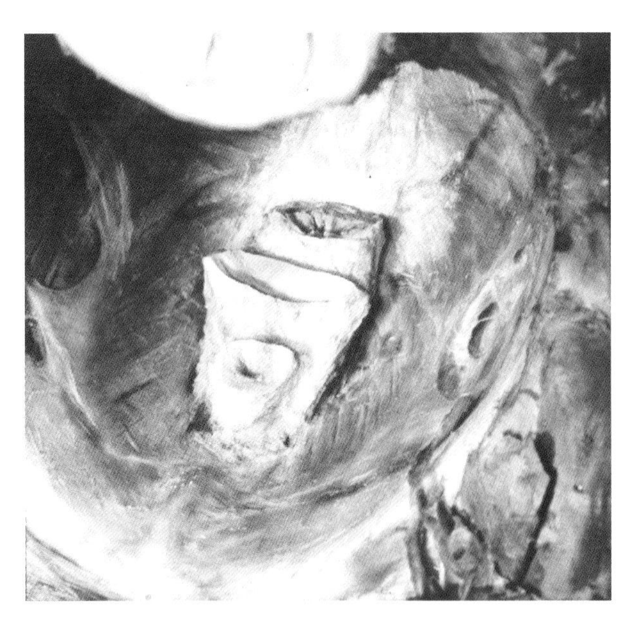

Figure 67 : Female urethra and its relationship to the vagina and the levator ani muscles.

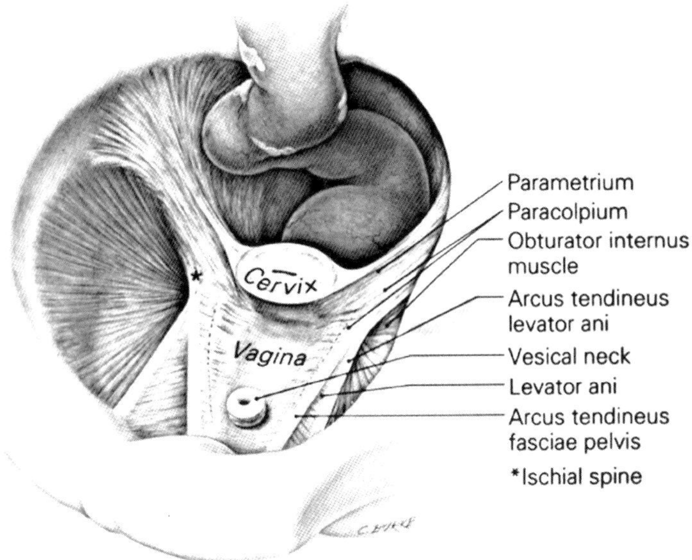

Figure 68 : Anatomical supports of the cervix and vagina after removal of the bladder and uterine corpus. (copyright DeLancey 2000).

rally. This fascia forms a continuous sheet - like mesentery extending from the uterine artery at its cephalic margin to the point at which the vagina fuses with the levator ani muscles below. The part that attaches to the uterus is called the parametrium and that which attaches to the vagina, the paracolpium.

The parametria referred to clinically the cardinal and uterosacral ligaments [285-287]. These are two different parts of a single mass of tissue. The uterosacral ligaments are the visible and palpable medial margin of the cardinal-uterosacral ligament complex and is invested with a considerable amount of smooth muscle. The paracolpium, as we will see in subsequent paragraphs, attaches the vagina to the pelvic walls in a more direct manner.

Although we name these tissues "ligaments" and "fascia" they are not the same type of tissue seen in the "fascia" of the rectus abdominus muscle or the ligaments of the knee; both of which are made of dense regular connective tissue. These supportive tissues consist of blood vessels, nerves and fibrous connective tissue and can be thought of as mesenteries that supply the genital tract bilaterally. Their composition reflects their combined function as neurovascular conduits as well as supportive structures.

There are regional variations in these tissues that explain the differences between the types of pelvic support defects seen in women with pelvic organ prolapse (fig. 69). The upper third of the vagina has the same suspensory tissues as the uterus. These long fibres elevate the upper portion of the vagina after the uterus has been removed during hysterectomy. [288]. In the middle third of the vagina the anterior and posterior vaginal walls are connected laterally to the pelvic walls. Continuous with the parametrium when the uterus remains in situ, this upper portion (Level I) consists of a relatively long sheet of tissue that suspends the vagina by attaching it to the pelvic wall. In the mid-portion of the vagina, the paracolpium attaches the vagina laterally and more directly to the pelvic walls (Level II). Ventrally, the vagina is attached to the arcus tendineus fascia pelvis. The combination of the vaginal wall and its attachments to the fascial arch comprise the structural layer that supports the bladder base and urethra. Dorsally, the vagina is attached to the inner surface of the levator ani muscles, a structural arrangement that helps to restrain the rectum from being displaced forward.

These attachments, that stretch the vagina transversely between the bladder and rectum, have functional significance. The structural layer that supports the bladder (pubocervical fascia) is composed of the anterior vaginal wall and its attachment through the endopelvic fascia to the pelvic wall. It is not a separate layer from the vagina as sometimes inferred, but is a combination of the anterior vaginal wall and its attachments to the pelvic wall. Similarly, the posterior vaginal wall and endopelvic fascia (rectovaginal fascia) form the restraining layer that prevents the rectum from protruding forward blocking formation of a rectocele as will be discussed in the next section.

In the distal vagina (Level III) the vaginal wall is directly attached to surrounding structures without any intervening paracolpium. Anteriorly the vaginal wall fuses with the urethra and is attached to the arcus tendineus,

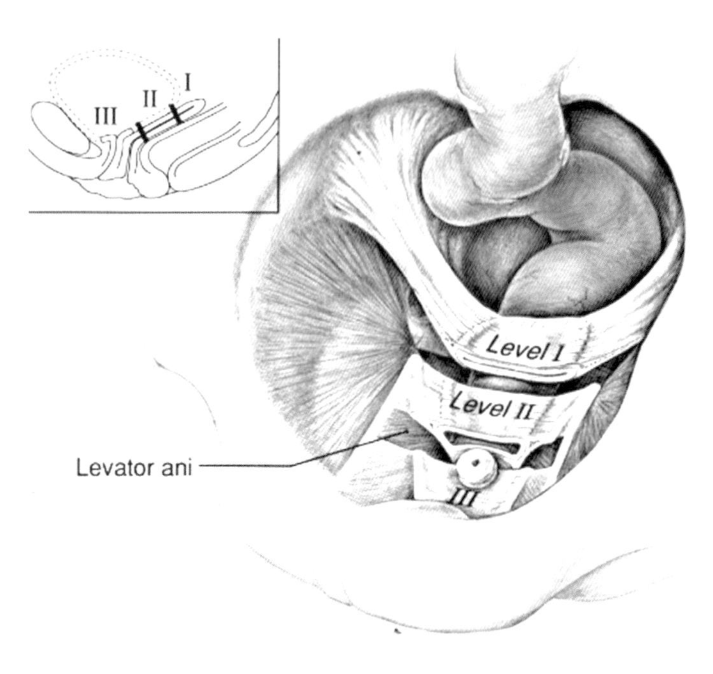

Figure 69 : Different regions of vaginal support. Note this illustration shows anatomy after hysterectomy with hysterectomy scar shown at the vaginal apex. (from DeLancey 1992)

posteriorly it fuses with the perineal body whose position is maintained through connections to the ischiopubic rami by the perineal membrane. Laterally it is attached directly to the levator ani muscles by the fibres of Luschka.

Damage to the upper suspensory fibres of the paracolpium causes a different type of prolapse from damage to the mid-level supports of the vagina. Defects in the support provided by the mid-level (pubocervical and rectovaginal fasciae result in anterior and posterior vaginal wall defects cystocele and rectocele) while loss of the upper suspensory fibres of the paracolpium and parametrium is responsible for development of vaginal and uterine prolapse. These defects occur in varying combinations and this variation is responsible for the diversity of clinical problems encountered within the overall spectrum of pelvic organ prolapse.

2. Urethral and anterior vaginal wall support

Urethral support is important to stress continence in women, as support in symptomatic women may be inadequate [289]. This support is supplied by a combination of connective tissue and muscle arranged to resist the downward force created by increases in abdominal pressure [290]. The urethra lies adjacent to and is intimately connected with the anterior vaginal wall. The connections of the vagina and urethra to the levator ani muscles and the arcus tendineus fascia pelvis determine the structural stability of the urethra.

The arcus tendineus fascia pelvis is a fibrous band that is stretched between a fine tendon-like origin from the pubic bone anteriorly to an attachment to the ischial spine. The endopelvic fascia and anterior vaginal wall form a layer that supports the urethra and vesical neck by connecting to the arcus tendineus (fig. 70). In this region, the medial portion of the levator ani muscles has a direct connection to the endopelvic fascia and vaginal wall [291]. This muscular attachment permits contraction of the levator ani muscles to stabilize the urethra during a cough.

Urethral support, therefore depends on both connective tissue and muscle action. If the connective tissue fails then the urethral supports cannot stay in their normal alignment and stress incontinence is often the result. Conversely, if the muscles are damaged, as has been shown in MR images [292] their action in supporting the urethra may be lost. Recent evidence shows that in primigravid women with stress incontinence, urethral support is preferentially lost during a cough while mobility during valsalva is no different than in continent women. [293]

3. Support of the posterior vaginal wall and rectum

The distal rectum abuts with the dense connective tissue of the perineal body [294]. The perineal body represents the central connection between the two halves of the perineal membrane (urogenital diaphragm). When the distal rectum is subjected to increased force directed caudally, the fibres of the perineal membrane become tight and resist further displacement. These fibres derive their lateral support from their attachment to the pelvic bones at the ischiopubic rami (fig. 71). The ability of this layer to resist downward displacement depends on the structural continuity between the right and left sides of the perineal membrane.

The connection between the two halves of the perineal membrane extends cranially for a distance of approximately 2 to 3 centimeters above the hymeneal ring. It is thickest and densest in the distal perineal body becoming progressively thinner towards its cranial margin. The lateral margin of the perineal body contains the termination of the bulbocavernosus muscle and terminations of the medial fibres of the levator ani muscle.

The mid-portion of the posterior vaginal wall (Level II) is attached on either side of the rectum to the inner surface of the pelvic diaphragm by a sheet of endopelvic fascia. These fascial sheets attach to the posterior lateral vaginal wall where the dorsally directed tension results in a posterior vaginal sulcus on each side of the rectum (fig. 72). These endopelvic fascial sheets prevent the ventral movement of the posterior vaginal wall. The majority of the endopelvic fascia fibres atta-

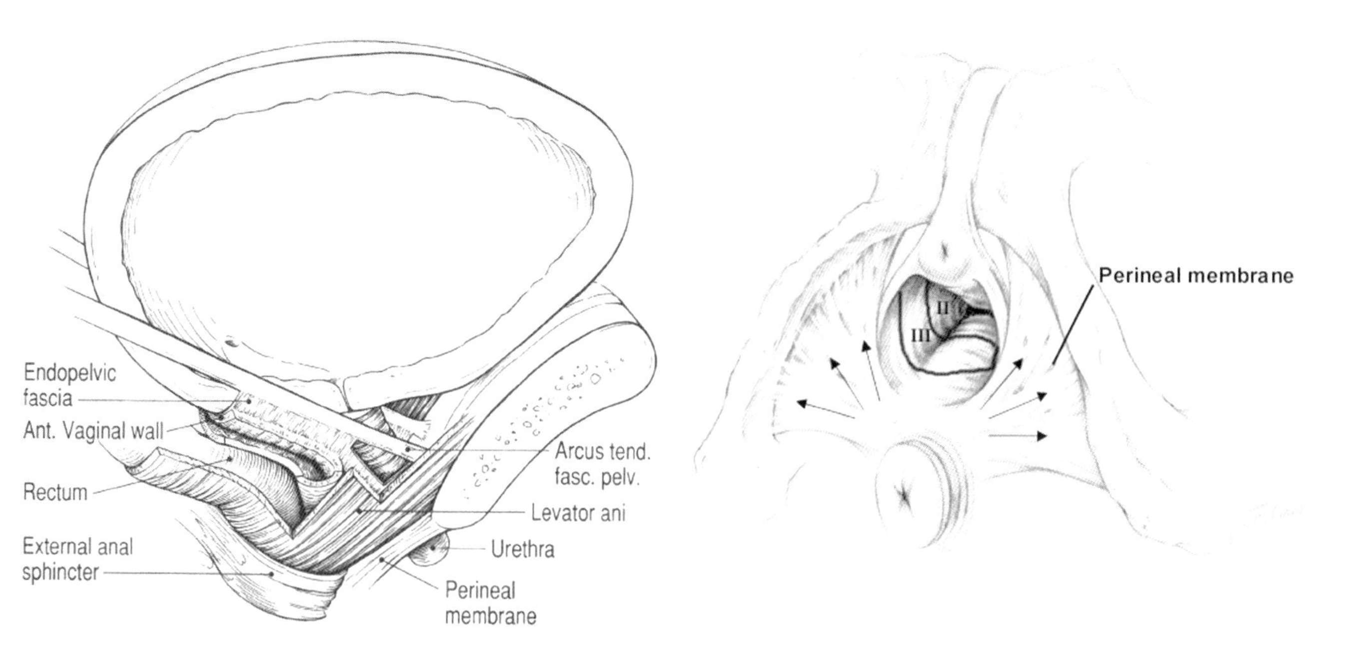

Figure 70 : Lateral view of the structures supporting the urethra and vesical neck. Portions of the levator ani, lateral vaginal wall and endopelvic fascia have been removed to show midline structures (DeLancey 1994).

Figure 71 : Support of the perineal body by the perineal membrane by its connection to the ischiopubic rami (DeLancey 1999)

ch to the vaginal wall, with only a few fibres passing from one side to the other.

The Level II and Level III supports are continuous with one another. Force applied to the anterior rectal wall in Level II is resisted by the posterior vaginal wall and its attachments to the inner surface of the pelvic diaphragm. Pressure applied to the perineal body in a caudal direction in Level III is resisted, not only by the perineal membrane, but also by the connection of the upper vaginal wall to the Level II attachments that help hold the cranial end of the perineal body (Level III) in place.

4. CONNECTIVE TISSUE OF THE PELVIC FLOOR

Considerable confusion persists with respect to the functional significance of the various fascial and ligamentous structures which have been described and implicated in the support of pelvic organs [291, 295-297]. Some authors have commented on the amount of connective tissue within human pelvic floor muscle compared with quadrapedal animals and have sought associations with the assumption of an upright posture [281]. However, the connective tissue component of the levator ani has not received the same attention as the striated muscle component, although several workers have suggested that deficient or abnormal collagen may be the cause of pelvic floor dysfunction in humans [298, 299]. A histological study of vaginal fascial connective tissue carried out in women with and without uterine prolapse reported abnormal histological changes in 7 out of 10 patients with uterine descent [300]. Other workers have shown a significantly higher incidence of pelvic organ prolapse in women with hypermobile joints compared with a control group with no clinical joint laxity, further implicating abnormalities of collagen in pelvic floor dysfunction [301]. Clearly, further studies are required in order to examine the role of contributing factors, such as age, oestrogen activity, obesity, parity and delivery, as well as sexual activity and physical work, on the structure and function of the connective tissue components of the levator ani. Data of this type may prove invaluable in furthering our understanding of the normal functioning of the pelvic floor.

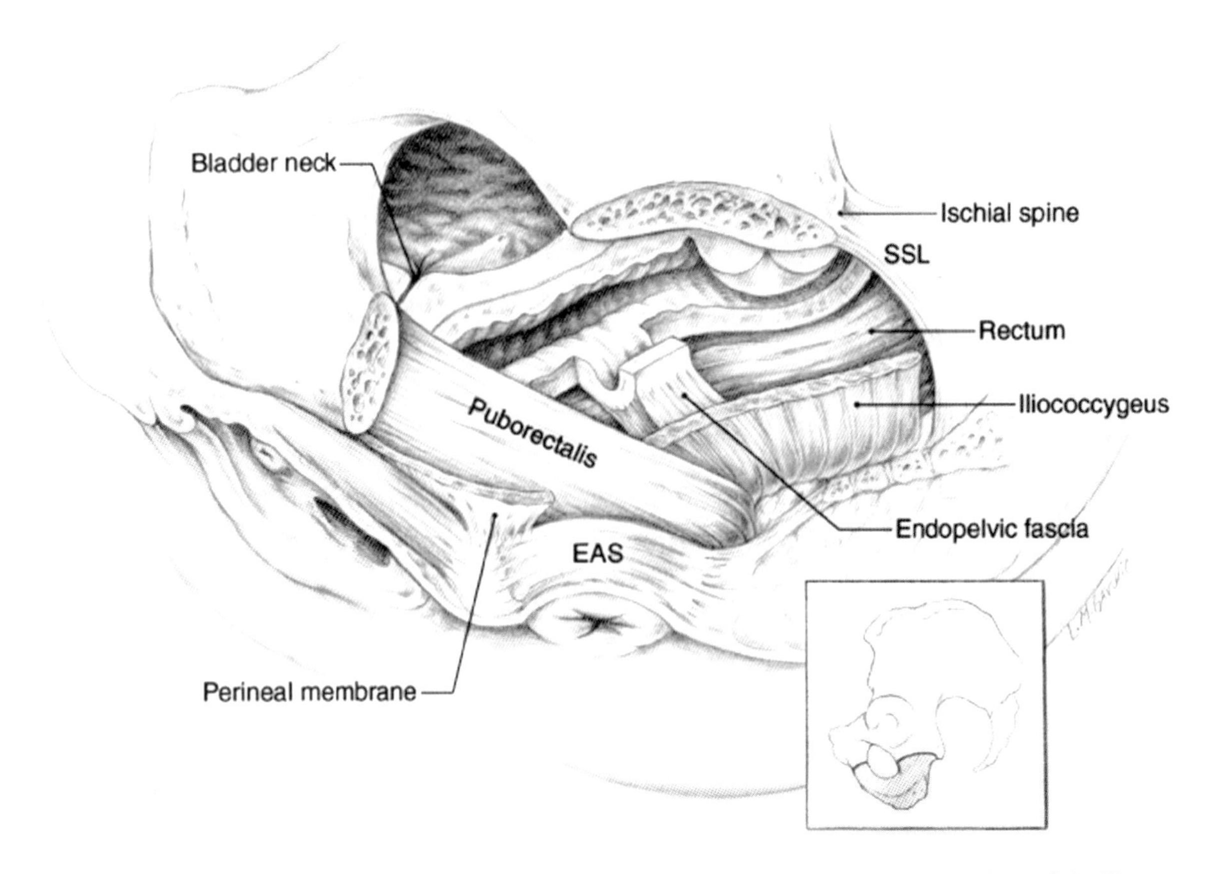

Figure 72 : Lateral view of the pelvic floor structures. The ischium has been removed as have portions of the iliococcygeus muscle and lateral vaginal wall. Note attachment of the vaginal wall by the endopelvic fascia to the inner surface of the iliococcygeal muscle. (DeLancey 1999)

XI. EFFECTS OF AGE AND PARTURITION ON PELVIC FLOOR MORPHOLOGY

Both age and vaginal delivery have been shown to affect the morphology of the pelvic floor muscles. A study on biopsy samples from a group of women with genuine stress incontinence has shown that both the number and diameters of slow and fast twitch muscle fibres decrease with increasing age [302]. Using single fibre electromyography, it has also been proposed that partial denervation of the pelvic floor may occur as a consequence of vaginal delivery [303]. Furthermore, women with urinary stress incontinence or genitourinary prolapse (or both) are more likely to demonstrate electrophysiological evidence of partial denervation of the levator ani than are asymptomatic women. These findings imply that nerve damage is an important aetiological factor responsible for weakness of the pelvic floor. Delayed nerve conduction times are indicative of damage which has been localised to the terminal branches of the pudendal nerves supplying the pelvic floor in women with stress incontinence.

Histochemical evidence for the occurrence of partial denervation and subsequent reinnervation is provided by the clustering together of fibres that are all of the same type [304]. This fibre-type clustering has been observed in biopsy samples of levator ani removed from patients with rectal prolapse and faecal incontinence [305, 306] and in patients with urinary stress incontinence and genital tract prolapse [307]. However, similar fibre-type groupings have been observed in biopsy samples from nulliparous asymptomatic women. On the assumption that these results are representative of normal, it may be that the fibre-type grouping in the levator ani is normal and thus differs from that of a typical limb skeletal muscle. In the event that such an arrangement occurs in the undamaged levator ani, it is evident that fibre-type clustering demonstrated using histochemical methods cannot be regarded as indicative of partial denervation with reinnervation. In this context a recent study [308] has failed to demonstrate histochemical evidence for partial denervation of the levator ani although structural features of muscle cell damage are reported in association with aging and with vaginal childbirth. Morphological features such as centrally placed nuclei, fibre splitting and striated cell necrosis are generally recognized as indicative of neuromuscular damage in limb skeletal muscle. Interestingly, all these features have been observed in biopsy samples of levator ani from women considered to be normal (i.e. asymptomatic and nulliparous). Thus the presence of such features in samples of levator ani cannot necessarily be interpreted as indicative of the presence of pathological damage. Nevertheless, vaginal delivery is associated with stress incontinence and urethral hypermobility, the etiology of which is probably multifactorial. Further detailed studies of the distribution of fibre types throughout the normal levator ani are essential before this uncertainty can be resolved.

XII. ANATOMY OF THE ANAL SPHINCTER COMPLEX

Faecal incontinence is a devastating condition, often associated with childbirth [309]. Because of the frequent occurrence of both faecal and urinary incontinence, this issue is covered by the consultation and a brief overview of anal sphincter anatomy provided here. The anal sphincter mechanism contains both smooth and striated muscle. Although there has been considerable conflict about sphincter nomenclature [310] the actual anatomy of this region is relatively straight forward [311-313].

There is a tubular smooth muscle sphincter that encircles the anal canal over a distance of approximately 3-4 cm above the anal verge (fig.73). It is continuous with the circular muscle layer of the intestine. The transition to the internal sphincter is marked by a thickening of the circular fibres, by an increase in the amount of collage present in the muscle, and by a change in the shape of the muscle bundles encircling the lumen [313].

The external anal sphincter surrounds the internal sphincter in its lower 2 cm by a muscular component [314] that is tethered to the coccyx through the anococcygeal rapha. Just cephalic and anterior to the external sphincter, and blending with it on its dorsal side is the puborectalis muscle. This sling-like muscle originates from the inner surface of the pubic bones and passes dorsal to the anorectum just above the external anal sphincter. Its anterior traction produces the ano-rectal angle.

Between the internal and external anal sphincter is the inter-sphincteric groove. This space receives the downward extension of the conjoined fibres of the levator ani muscles and the longitudinal smooth muscle coat of the intestine [312, 313]. These fibres suspend and elevate the anorectum preventing its downward prolapse. They terminate in the perianal skin. Their relaxation during defecation allows for eversion of the anal skin that is then pulled up into the anal canal at the end of defecation.

Much of the controversy in this anatomy has come from

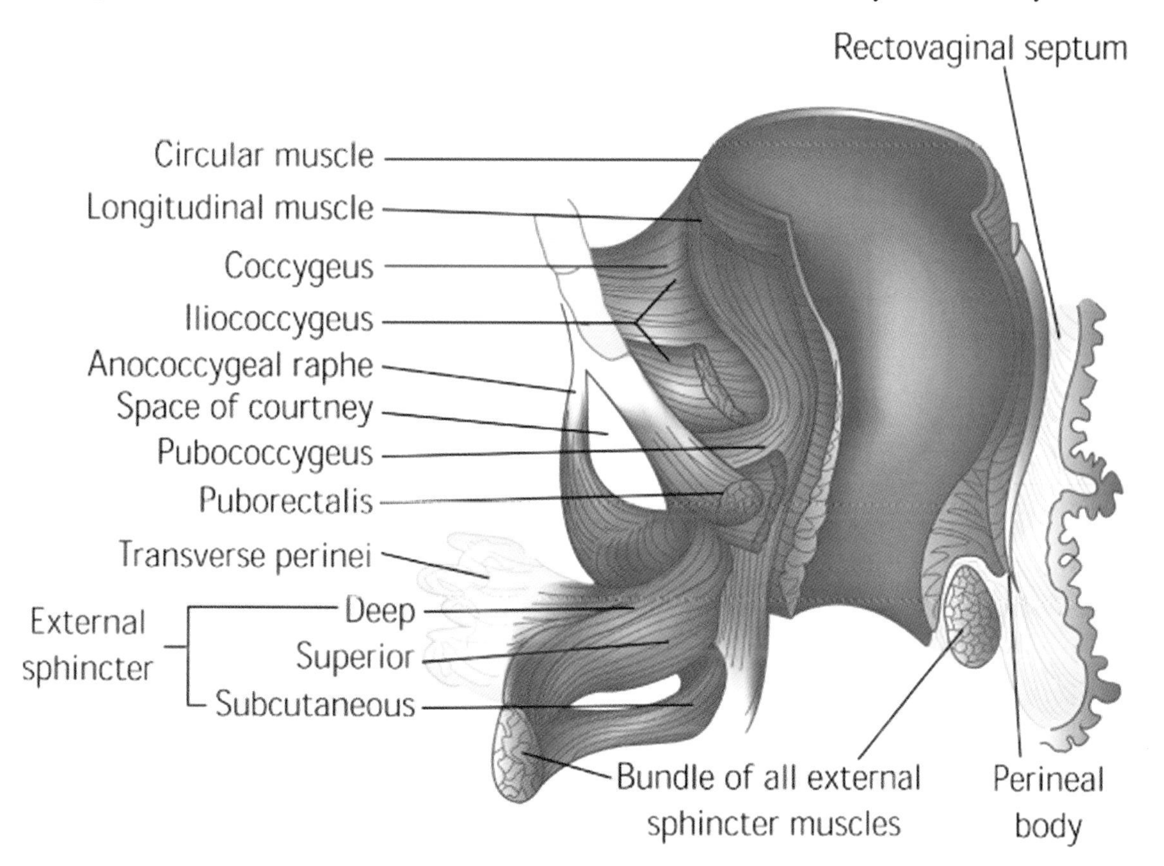

Figure 73 : Lateral view of the anal sphincter muscles after reflection of the external anal sphincter muscles. (After Oh & Kark)

differences of opinion concerning how many parts the external anal sphincter contains. It is beyond the scope of this chapter to cover this contentious issue, but may be visited in Dalley's interesting article on the subject [310]. There is little controversy about the existence of a superficial muscle associated with the perianal skin usually referred to as the subcutaneous sphincter. A larger and more robust part of the muscle lies above this platysma-like muscle. This is the external anal sphincter that encircles the anterior portion of the anal canal in the perineal body and that occasionally is lacerated during vaginal delivery. Further subdivision of this highly variable muscle into more portions has more academic than practical importance.

The external anal sphincter is innervated by S2-4 fibres that travel via the inferior hemorrhoidal portion of the pudendal nerve. While it is well accepted that childbirth leads to neurogenic damage to the innervation of the external anal sphincter [316] and to disruption of the internal and external sphincters [317] little is known on the impact of vaginal delivery on internal sphincter innervation and function even in the presence of an intact peroneum after delivery. Resting anal sphincter tonus is associated with normal internal sphincter function. Resting tone is known to be lower in women after vaginal birth complicated by a third-degree perineal tear compared to controls with rupture of the sphincters, but direct evaluation of the internal anal sphincter remains difficult.

XIII. CONCLUDING REMARKS

Urinary bladder filling and emptying involve complex mechanisms at all levels from the central nervous system down to the individual muscle cells in the bladder and urethra. Disturbed function at any level might cause incontinence. The present review is concerned with bladder and urethral anatomy. The other levels of fuction and dysfuction will be dealt with later in this volume. The urinary bladder and the urethra contain an epithelial lining surrounded by densely innervated smooth muscle and a connective tissue stroma with blood vessels and sensory nerves. We have systematically described the normal function of these tissue elements and have also given some superficial information regarding their pathophysiology. We have chosen this approach in order to give a basic research background to the more clinically-oriented descriptions of pathophysiological processes leading to incontinence that will be presented in later chapters. The reader must keep in mind that the literature on structure and function of the normal bladder and urethra is overwhelming. The papers we refer to represent only a limited (and biased) selection, but will serve as key references into the literature about the various aspects of cellular mechanisms that are involved in continence and micturition in the healthy bladder.

REFERENCES

1. Owman, C., Alm, P. And Sjöberg, N.-O.: Pelvic autonomic ganglia: Structure, transmitters, function and steroid influence. In: Autonomic Ganglia. Edited by L.-G. Elfvin. New York: John Wiley and Sons Ltd., p. 125, 1983.
2. Brading. A.F.: Physiology of bladder smooth muscle. In: The physiology of the lower urinary tract, edited by M.J. Torrens and J.F.B. Morrison, Springer Verlag: New York. p. 161,1987.
3. Smet. P.J., Jonavicius, J., Marshall, V.R. And De Vente, J.: Distribution of nitric oxide synthase-immunoreactive nerves and identification of the cellular targets of nitric oxide in guinea-pig and human urinary bladder by cGMP immunohistochemistry. Neuroscience. 71:337, 1996.
4. Elbadawi, A.: Comparative neuromorphology in animals. In: The physiology of the lower urinary tract. Edited by M. Torrens and J.F.B. Morrison. Springer-Verlag: Berlin. p. 23,1987.
5. Speakman. M.J., Walmsley. D. And Brading. A.F.: An in vitro pharmacological study of the human trigone - a site of non-adrenergic non-chloinergic transmission. Br. J. Urol., 61: 304, 1987.
6. Hai, C.M. And Murphy. R.A.: Ca2+, crossbridge phosphorylation and contraction, Ann. Rev. Physiol., 72:1334, 1989.
7. Stephens, N.L., Seow, C.Y., Halayko, A.J. And Jiang. H.: The biophysics and biochemistry of smooth muscle contraction. Canadian J. Physiol. Pharmacol., 70: 515, 1992.
8. Fuglsang, A., Khromov, A., Torok, K., Somlyo, A.V. And Somlyo, A.P.: Flash photolysis studies of relaxation and cross-bridge detachment: higher sensitivity of tonic than phasic smooth muscle to MgADP. J. Muscle Res. Cell Motility, 14: 666, 1993.
9. Harris. D.E., Work, S.S., Wright, R.K., Alpert, N.R. And Warshaw, D.M.: Smooth, cardiac and skeletal muscle myosin force and motion generation assessed by cross-bridge mechanical interactions in vitro. J. Muscle Res. Cell Motility, 15: 11, 1994.
10. Stephens, N. L.: Smooth muscle contraction: recent advances. Canadian J. Physiol. Pharmacol., 72: 1317, 1994.
11. Hellstrand. P.: Cross-bridge kinetics and shortening in smooth muscle Canadian J. Physiol. Pharmacol., 72: 1334, 1994.
12. Gunst, S.J., Wu, M.F. And Smith, D.D.: Contraction history modulates isotonic shortening velocity in smooth muscle. Am, J. Physiol, 265: C467, 1995.
13. Uchida, W., Masuda, N., Shirai, Y., Shibasaki, K., Saton, N. And Takenada, T.: The role of extra-cellular Ca2+ in

carbachol-induced tonic contraction of the pig derusor smooth muscle. Naunyn Schmiedebergs Arch. Pharmacol., 350: 398, 1994.

14. Zhao, Y., Wein, A. J. And Levin, R.M.: Role of calcium in mediating the biphasic contraction of the rabbit urinary bladder. Gen. Pharmacol., 24: 727, 1993.

15. Arner, A., Malmqvist, U. And Uvelius, B.: Cytoskeletal and contractile proteins in detrusor smooth muscle from patients with bladder outlet obstruction. Scand. J. Nephrol., 25: 262, 1991.

16. Malmqvist, U., Arner. A. And Uvelius, B.: Contractile and cytoskeletal proteins in smooth muscle during hypertrophy and its reversal. Am J Physiol., 260: C1085, 1991.

17. Malmqvist, U., Arner, A. And Uvelius, B.: Mechanics and Ca (2+) -sensitivity of human detrusor muscle bundles studied in vitro. Acta Physiol Scand., 143: 373, 1991.

18. Chiavegato, A., Scatena, M., Roelofs, M., Ferrarese, P., Pauletto, P., Passerini Glazel, G., Pagano, F. And Sartore, S.: Cytoskeletal and cytocontractile protein composition of smooth muscle cells in developing and obstructed rabbit bladder, Exp. Cell Res., 207: 310, 1993.

19. Wang, Z.E., Gopalakurup, S.K., Levin. R.M. And Chacko, S.: Expression of smooth myosin isoforms in urinary bladder smooth muscle during hypertrophy and regression, Lab. Invest., 73: 244, 1995.

20. Sjuve, R., Haase, H., Morano, I., Uvelius, B. And Arner, A.: Contraction kinetics and myosin isoform composition in smooth muscle from hypertrophied rat urinary bladder. J. Cell Biochem., 63: 86, 1996.

21. Wu, C., Kentish, J.G. And Fry, C.H.: Effect of pH on myofilament Ca 2+ - sensitivity I alpha-toxin permeabilized guinea pig detrusor muscle. J. Urol., 154: 1921, 1995.

22. Groen, J., Van Mastrigt, R. And Bosch, R.: Contractility of the guinea-pig bladder measured in situ and in vitro. Naunyn Schmiedebergs Arch. Pharmacol., 13:587, 1994.

23. Glerum, J.J., Van Mastrigt, R. And Shimada, Y.: Mechanical properties of mammalian single smooth muscle cells. III Passive properties of pig detrusor and human term uterus cells. J. Muscle Res. Cell Motility., 11:453, 1990.

24. Van Mastrigt, R., Koopal, J.W., Hak, J. And Van De Wetering, J.: Modeling the contractility of urinary bladder smooth muscle using isometric contractions. Am. J. Physiol., 251: R978, 1986.

25. Uvelius, B. And Gabella, G.: Relation between cell length and force production in urinary bladder smooth muscle. Acta Physiol. Scand., 110: 357, 1980.

26. Tammela, T. And Arjamaa, O.: Comparison of long-term and short-term stretch on rat urinary bladder in vitro. Urol. Res., 16: 277, 1988.

27. Venegas, J.G.. Viscoelastic properties of the contracting detrusor. I. Theoretical basis. Am. J. Physiol., 261: C255, 1991.

28. Finkbeiner, A.E. And O'donnell, P. D.: Responses of detrusor smooth muscle to stretch and relaxation: in vitro study. Urology., 36: 193, 1990.

29. Van Mastrigt, R.: The force recovery following repeated quick releases applied to pig urinary bladder smooth muscle, J. Muscle Res. Cell Motility., 12: 45, 1991.

30. Lin, A.T.-L., Yang, C.-H., Chen, C.-J., Chen, M.-T., Chiang, H. And Chang, I.S.: Correlation of contractile function and passive properties of rabbit urinary bladder subjected to outlet obstruction - an in vitro whole bladder study. J. Urol., 148: 944, 1992.

31. Sibley, G.N.A.: A comparison of spontaneous and nerve-mediated activity in bladder muscle from man, pig and rabbit. J. Physiol., 354: 431, 1984.

32. Creed, K.E.: Membrane properties of smooth muscle membrane of the guinea-pig urinary bladder. Pfl, ges Arch., 326: 115, 1971.

33. Klöckner, U. And Isenberg, G.: Action potentials and net membrane currents of isolated smooth muscle cells (urinary bladder of the guinea pig). Pfl, ges Archiv., 405: 329, 1985.

34. Fujii, K.: Evidence for adenosine triphosphate as an excitatory transmitter in guinea-pig rabbit and pig urinary bladder. J. Physiol., 404: 39, 1988.

35. Fujii, K., Foster, C.D., Brading, A.F. And Parekh, A.B.: Potassium channel blockers and the effects of cromakalim on the smooth muscle of the guinea-pig bladder. Br. J. Pharmacol., 99: 779, 1990.

36. Brading, A.F.: Ion channels and control of contractile activity in urinary bladder smooth muscle, Japanese J. Pharmacol., 58: 120, 1992.

37. Brading, A.F. And Turner, W.H.: Potassium channels and their modulation in the urogenital tract smooth muscles. In: Potassium channels and their modulators: from synthesis to clinical experience. Edited by J.M.Evans, et al., Taylor and Francis: London, p. 335, 1996.

38. Heppner, T.J., Bonev, A.D. And Nelson, M.T.: Ca2+-activated K+ channels regulate action potential repolarization in urinary bladder smooth muscle. Am. J. Physiol., 273: C110, 1997.

39. Bonev, A.D. And Nelson, M.T.: ATP-sensitive potassium channels in smooth muscle cells from guinea pig urinary bladder. Am. J. Physiol., 264: C190, 1993.

40. Green, M.E., G., E., Kirkup, A.J., Miller, M, And Weston, A.H.: Pharmacological characterization of the inwardly-rectifying current in the smooth muscles cells of the rat bladder. Br. J. Pharmacol., 119: 1509, 1996.

41. Foster, C.D., Speakman, M.J., Fujii, K. And Brading, A.F.: The effects of cromakalim on the detrusor muscle of human and pig urinary bladder. Br. J. Urol., 63: 284, 1989.

42. Inoue, R. And Brading, A.F.: The properties of the ATP-induced depolarization and current in single cells isolated from the guinea-pig urinary bladder. Br. J Pharmacol., 100:619, 1990.

43. Wellner, M.C. And Isenberg, G.: Properties of stretch activated channels in myocytes from the guinea-pig urinary bladder. J. Physiol., 466: 213, 1993.

44. Montgomery, B.S.I. And Fry, C.H.: The action potential and net membrane currents in isolated human detrusor smooth muscle cells. J. Urol., 147: 176, 1992.

45. Gabella, G. And Uvelius, B.: Urinary bladder of rat: fine structure of normal and hypertrophic musculature. Cell Tissue Res., 262: 67, 1990.

46. Brading, A.F. And Mostwin, J.L.: Electrical and mechanical responses of guinea-pig bladder muscle to nerve stimulation. Br. J. Pharmacol., 98: 1083, 1989.

47. Pareka, A.H., Brading, A.F. And Tomita, T.: Studies of longitudinal tissue impedance in various smooth muscles. Prog. Clin. Biol. Res., 327: 375, 1990.

48. Brading, A.F. Teramoto, T., Nakayama, S., Bramich, N., Inoue, R., Fujii, K. And Mostwin, J.: The relationship between the electrophysiological properties of lower urinary tract smooth muscles and their function in vivo. In: Smooth Muscle Excitation, Edited by T. B. Bolton. Academic Press: London. p. 403, 1996.

49. Seki, N., Karim, O.M.A. And Mostwin, L.A.: Changes in action potential kinetics following experimental bladder outflow obstruction in the guinea-pig. Urol. Res., 20:387, 1992.

50. Brading, A.F.: A Myogenic Basis for the Overactive Bladder. Urology., 50: 57, 1997.

51. Maggi. C.A., Santicioli, P. And Meli, A.: Postnatal development of micturition reflex in rats. Am. J. Physiol., 250: R926, 1984.

52. Maggi, C.A., Santicioli, P. And Meli, A.: Postnatal development of myogenic contractile activity and excitatory innervation of rat urinary bladder. Am. J Physiol., 247: R972, 1984.

53. Maggi, C.A., Manzini, S., Santicioli, P. And Meli, A.: An atropine-like inhibitory effect of DMPP on rat isolated urinary bladder. J. Auton, Pharmacol., 6: 97, 1986.

54. Maggi, C.A., Santicioli, P., Geppetti, P., Frilli, S., Spillantini, M.G., Nediani, C., Hunt, S.P. And Meli, A.: Biochemical, anatomical and functional correlates of postnatal development of the capsaicin-sensitive innervation of the rat urinary bladder. Brain Res., 471: 183, 1988.

55. Blaivis, J.G.: The neurophysiology of micturition: a clinical study of 550 patients. J. Urol., 127: 958, 1992.

56. Smet, P.J., Edyvance, K.A., Jonavicius, J. And Marshall, V.R.: Neuropeptides and neurotransmitter-synthesizing enzymes in intrinsic neurons of the human urinary bladder. J. Neurocytol., 25:112, 1996.

57. Hanani, M. And Maudlej, N.: Intracellular recordings from intramural neurons in the guinea-pig urinary bladder. J. Neurophysiol., 74: 2358, 1995.

58. Crowe, R., Light, L., Chilton, C.P. And Burnstock, G.: Vasoactive intestinal polypeptide-, somatostatin- and substance P-immunoreactive nerves in the smooth and striated muscle of the intrinsic external urethral sphincter of patients with spinal cord injury. J. Urol., 136: 487, 1986.

59. Gabella, G.: The structural relations between nerve fibres and muscle cells in the urinary bladder of the rat. J. Neurocytol., 24: 159, 1995.

60. Palfrey, E.L.H., Fry, C.H. And Shuttleworth. K.E.D.: A new in vitro microsuperfusion technique for investigation of human detrusor muscle. Br. J. Urol., 56:635, 1984.

61. Burnstock, G., Cocks, T., Crowe, R. And Kasakov, L.: Purinergic innervation of the guinea-pig urinary bladder. Br. J. Pharmacol., 63: 125, 1978.

62. Brading, A.F. And Williams, J. H.: Contractile responses of smooth muscle strips from rat and guinea-pig urinary bladder to transmural stimulation: effects of atropine and a,b-methylene ATP. Br. J. Pharmacol., 99: 493, 1990.

63. Eglen, R.M., Reddy, H., Watson, N. And Challiss, R.A.: Muscarinic acetylcholine receptor subtypes in smooth muscle. Trends Pharmacol. Sci., 15:114, 1994.

64. Kondo, D., Morita T And Tashima, Y.: Muscarinic cholinergic receptor subtypes in human detrusor muscle studied by labeled and nonlabeled pirenzepine. AFDX-116 and 4DAM. P. Urol. International. 54: 150, 1995.

65. Yamaguchi, O., Shishido, K., Tamura, K., Ogawa, T. And Fujimura. T.: Evaluation of mRNA encoding muscarinic receptor subtypes in human detrusor muscle. Neurourol. Urodyn., 13: 464, 1994.

66. Inoue, R. And Brading, A. F.: Human, pig and guinea-pig bladder smooth muscle cells generate similar inward currents response to purinoceptor activation. Br. J Pharmacol., 103: 1840, 1991.

67. Mcmurray. G., Dass, N., Ho, K.M.T. And Brading, A.F.: Purinergic mechanisms in primate urinary bladder. Br. J. Urol., 80:182, 1997.

68. Palea, S., Corsi, M., Pietra, C., Artibani, W., Calpista, A., Gaviraghi, G. And Trist, D. G.:ADP beta S induces contraction of the human isolated urinary bladder through a purinoceptor subtype different from P2X and P2Y. J. Pharmacol. Exp. Ther., 269: 193, 1994.

69. Palea, S., Pietra, C., Trist, D.G., Artibani, W., Calpista, A. And Corsi, M.: Evidence for the presence of both pre-and postjunctional P2-purinoceptor subtypes in human isolated urinary bladder. Br. J. Pharmacol., 114: 35, 1995.

70. Wammack, R., Weihe, E., Dienes, H, -P, And Hohen-Fellner, R.: The neurogenic bladder in vitro. Akt. Urol., 26: 16, 1995.

71. Eglezos. A., Giuliani, S., Viti, G. And Maggi, C.A.: Direct evidence that capasaicin-induced plasma protein extravasation is mediated through tachykinin NK-1 receptors. Eur. J. Pharmacol., 209: 277, 1991.

72. Maggi, C.A.: Therapeutic potential of capsaicin-like molecules: studies in animals and human. Life Sci., 51: 1777, 1992.

73. Meinl, S. And Maggi, C.A.: Evidence for a capsaicin-sensitive, tachykinin-mediated, component in the NANC contraction of the rat urinary bladder to nerve stimulation. Br. J. Pharmacol., 112: 1123, 1994.

74. Maggi, C.: Tachykinins and calcitonin gene-related peptide (CGRP) as cotransmitters released from peripheral ending of sensory nerves. Progress in Neurobiology, 45:1, 1995.

75. Maggi, C.: The mammalian tachykinin receptors. General Pharmacology, 26:911, 1995.

76. Schulman, C.C., Duarte-Escalante, O. And Boyarsky, S.: The ureterovesical innervation. A new concept based on a histochemical study. Br. J. Urol., 44:698, 1972.

77. Elbadawi, A. And Schenk, E.A.: A new theory of the innervation of bladder musculature. 4. Innervation of the vesicourethral junction and external urethral sphincter. J. Urol., 111:613, 1974.

78. Khanna, O.P., Barbieri, E.J., Altamura, M. And Mcmichael, R.: Vesicourethral smooth muscle: function and relation to structure. Urology, 18: 211, 1981.

79. Takeda, M., Mitzusawa, T., Obara, K., Koizumi, T., Tsutsui, T.M Hatano, A., Takahashi, H., And Takahashi, K.: Adrenergic betal, beta2, and beta3 receptor subtypes in the detrusor of human urinary bladder - evaluation by mRNA expression and isometric contraction. J. Urol., 157 suppl 4: 82, 1997.

80. Tsurusaki, M., Yoshida, M., Akasu, T. And Nagatsu, I.S.O.: Alpha 2-adrenoceptors mediate the inhibition of cholinergic transmission in parasympathetic ganglia of the rabbit urinary bladder. Synapse. 5:233, 1990.

81. Kusonoki, M., Taniyama, K. And Tanaka, C.: Neuronal GABA release and GABA inhibition of ACh release in guinea-pig urinary bladder. Am. J. Physiol., 246: R502, 1984.

82. Santicioli, P., Maggi, C.A. And Meli, A.: GABAB receptor mediated inhibition of field stimulation-induced contractions of rabbit bladder musclin-vitro. J. Pharm. Pharmacol. 36: 378, 1984.

83. Chen, T. F., Doyle, P.T. And Ferguson, D.R.: Inhibitory role of gamma-amino-butyric acid in the rabbit urinary bladder. Br. J. Urol., 69: 12, 1992.

84. Fujii, K.: Electrophysiological evidence that adenosine triphosphate (ATP) is a co-transmitter with acetylcholine (Ach) in isolated guinea-pig, rabbit and pig urinary bladder. J. Physiol., 394: 26. 1987.

85. Hashitani, H. And Suzuki, H.: Electrical and mechanical responses produced by nerve stimulation in detrusor smooth muscle of the guinea pig. Eur. J. Pharmacol., 284: 177, 1995.

86. Ganitekevich. V. And Isenberg, G.: Caffeine-induced release and reuptake of Ca2+ by Ca2+ stores in myocytes from guinea-pig urinary bladder. J. Physiol., 458: 99, 1992.

87. Chambers, P., Neal, D.E. And Gillespie, J.I.: Ca2+ mobilization in cultured human bladder smooth muscle cells in response to hypotonic stimuli. Exp. Physiol., 82: 677, 1997.

88. Yoshikawa, A., Van Breemen, C. And Isenberg, G.: Buffering of plasmalemmal Ca2+ current by sarcoplasmic reticulum of guinea-pig urinary bladder myocytes. Am. J. Physiol., 271 (C40): C833, 1996.

89. Sjögren, C., Andersson, K.E., Husted, S., Mattiasson, A. And Moller-Madsen. B.: Atropine resistance of transmurally stimulated isolated human bladder muscle. J. Urol., 128: 1368, 1982.

90. Bayliss, M And Fry, C. H.: Cholinergic and purinergic mechanisms in human detrusor from normal and obstructed bladders. Br. J. Urol., 79: 57, 1997.

91. Iacovou, J.W., Hill, S.J. And Birmingham, A.T.: Agonist-induced contraction and accumulation of inositol phosphates in the guinea-pig detrusor: evidence that muscarinic and purinergic receptors raise intracellular calcium by different mechanisms. J. Urol., 144: 775, 1990.

92. Harriss, D.R. Marsh. K.A. Birmingham, A.T. And Hill, S.J.: Expression of muscarinic M3-receptors coupled to inositol phospholipid hydrolysis: I. Human detrusor cultured smooth muscle cells. J. Urol., 154: 1241, 1995.

93. Hegda, S.S., Choppin, A., Bonhaus, D., Briaud, S., Loeb, M., Moy, T.M. Loury, D. And Eglen, R.M.: Functional role of M2 and M3 muscarinic receptors in the urinary bladder of rats: I. Vitro and in vivo. Br. J. Pharmacol., 120: 1409, 1997.

94. Rivera, L., Mcmurray, G. And Brading, A.F.: The role of calcium stores: I. The action of muscarinic agonists on mammalian urinary bladder smooth muscle. J. Physiol., 507P: 21P, 1998.

95. Abrams, P And Wein, A.J.: editor. The overactive bladder: from basic science to clinical management consensus conference. Elsevier: 1997.

96. Turner, W.H. And Brading, A.F.: Smooth muscle of the bladder in the normal and the diseased state: pathophysiology, diagnosis and treatment. Pharmacol. Ther., 75: 77, 1997.

97. Kondo, A. And Susser, J.G.: Viscoelastic properties of bladder. II. Comparative studies in normal and pathologic dogs. Invest. Urol., 11:459, 1974.

98. Cortivo, R., Pagano, F., Passerini, G., Abatangelo, G. And Castellani, I.: Elastin and collagen in the normal and obstructed urinary bladder. Br. J. Urol., 53: 134, 1981.

99. Susset. J.G., Servot-Viguier, D., Lamy, F., Madernas, P. And Black, R.: Collagen in 155 human bladders. Invest. Urol., 16: 204, 1978.

100. Uvelius, B. And Mattiasson, A.: Collagen content in the rat urinary bladder subjected to infravesical outflow obstruction. J. Urol., 132: 587, 1984.

101. Murakumo, M., Ushiki, T., Abe, K., Matsumura, K., Shinno, Y. And Koyanagi, T.: Three-dimensional arrangement of collagen and elastin fibers in human urinary bladder: scanning electron microscopic study. J. Urol., 154: 251, 1995.

102. Uvelius, B. And Mattiasson, A.: Detrusor collagen content in the denervated rat urinary bladder. J. Urol., 136:110, 1986.

103. Shapiro, E., Becich, M.J., Perlman. E. And Lepor, H.: Bladder wall abnormalities in myelodys-plastic bladders: a computer assisted morphometric analysis. J. Urol., 145:1024, 1991.

104. Lepor, H., Sunaryadi. I., Hartanto, V. And Shapiro, E.: Quantitative morphometry of the adult human bladder. J. Urol., 148: 414, 1992.

105. Levy, B.J. And Wight, T.N.: Structural changes in the aging submucosa: new morphologic criteria for the evaluation of the unstable human bladder. J. Urol., 144: 1044, 1990.

106. Macarak, E.J., Ewalt, D., Baskin, L., Coplen, D., Koo, H., Levin, R.M., J.W., D., Snyder, H., Rosenbloom, J. And Howard, P. S., The collagens and their urologic implications. Advances Exp Med. Biol., 385: 173, 1995.

107. Baskin, L.S., Constantinescu, S., Duckett, J.W., Syder, H.M. And Macarac, E.; Type III collagen decrease in normal fetal bovine bladder development. J. Urol., 152: 688, 1994.

108. Landau, E.H., Jayanthi, V.R., Churchill, B.M. Shapiro, E., Gilmour, R.F., Khoury, A.E., Macarak, E.J., Mclorie, G.A., Steckler, R.E. And Kogan, B.A.: Loss of elasticity in dysfunctional bladders. J. Urol., 152:702, 1994.

109. Macarak, E.J. And Howard, P.S.: The collagens and their urologic significance. Scand. J. Urol. Nephrol., Supp. 184: 25, 1997.

110. Rosenbloom, J., Koo, H., Howard, P.S. Mecham, R. And Macarak, E.J.: Elastic fibers and their role in bladder extracellular matrix. Advances Exp Med. Biol., 385: 173, 1995.

111. Rosenbloom, J., Abrams, W.R., Rosenbloom, J., Kucich, U., Decker, S., Mecham, R., Macarak, E. And Howard, P.: Expression of microfibrillar proteins by bovine bladder urothelium. Urology., 49: 287, 1997.

112. Kim, K.M. Kogan, B.A., Massad, C.A. And Hung, Y, -C.: Collagen and elastin in obstructed fetal bladder. J. Urol., 146: 528, 1991.

113. Takamura, S., Hiyake, K. And Takeushi, J.: Immuno-histochemical localization of proteoglycans in interstitial elements of the human bladder. Hinyokika Kiyo., 37: 329, 1991.

114. Levy, B.J. And Wigh., T.N.: The role of proteglycans in bladder structure and function. Advances Exp med. Biol., 385: 191, 1995.

115. Li, D.Y., Brooke, B., David, E.C., Mecham, P.P., Sorensen, L.K., Boaqk, B.B., Eichwala, E. And Keating M.T.: Elastin is an essential determinant of arterial morphogenesis. Nature. 393: 276, 1998.

116. Sarma, K.P.: Microangiography of the bladder in health. Br. J. Urol., 53: 237, 1991.

117. Inoue, T. And Gabella, G.; A vascular network closely linked to the epithelium of the urinary bladder of the rat. Cell Tissue Res., 263: 137, 1991.

118. Greenland, J.E. And Brading, A.F.: Urinary bladder blood flow changes during the micturition cycle in a conscious pig model. J. Urol., 156: 1858, 1996.

119. Kroyer, K., Bulow, J., Nielsen, S.L. And Kromann-Andersen, B.: Urinary bladder blood flow I. Comparison of clearance of locally injected 99m -technetium pertechnate and radioactive microsphere technique in dogs. Urol. Res., 18: 223, 1990.

120. Nielsen, K.K., Nielsen, S.L., Nordling, J. And Kromann, A.B.: Rate of urinary bladder blood flow evaluated by 133Xe wash-out and radioactive microspheres in pigs. Urol. Res., 19: 387, 1991.

121. Ohnishi, N., Kishima, Y., Hashimoto, K., Kiwamoto, H., Esa, A., Sugiyama, T., Park, Y.C. And Kurita, T.: A new method of measurement of the urinary bladder blood flow in patients with low compliant bladder. Hiyokika Kiyo., 40: 663, 1994.

122. Batista, J.E., Wagner, J.R., Azadzoi, K.M., Karane, R.J. And Siroky, M.B.: Direct measurement of blood flow in the human bladder, J. Urol., 155: 630, 1996.

123. Brading, A.F.: Alterations in the physiological properties of urinary bladder smooth muscle caused by bladder emptying against an obstruction. Scand. J. Urol. Nephrol., Suppl., 184:51, 1997.

124. Schuschke, D.A., Reed, M.W., Wingren, U.F. And Miller, F.N.: The rat urinary bladder: vasoactivity and macromolecular leakage in a new model. Microvasc. Res., 38: 23, 1989.

125. Andersson, P.O., Bloom, S.R., Mattiasson, A. And Uvelius, B.: Changes in vascular resistance in the feline urinary bladder in response to bladder filling. J. Urol., 134: 1041, 1985.

126. Guttmann, L. And Whitteridge, D.: Effects of bladder distension on autonomic mechanisms after spinal cord injuries. Brain. 70: 361, 1947.

127. Andersson, P.O., Bloom, S.R., Mattiasson, A. And Uvelius, B.: Bladder vasodilatation and release of vasoactive intestinal polypeptide from the urinary bladder of the cat in response to pelvic nerve stimulation. J. Urol., 150: 1945, 1993.

128. Hofmann, R., Gomez, R., Schmidt, R. And Tanagho, E.A.: Effects of nerve stimulation on blood flow in the urinary bladder, urethra and pelvic floor in the dog. J. Urol., 150: 1945, 1993.

129. Crowe. R. And Burnstock, G.: A histochemical and immunohistochemical study of the autonomic innervation of the lower urinary tract of the female pig. Is the pig a good model for the human bladder and urethra? J. Urol., 141: 414, 1989.

130. Levin, R.M., Brendler, K., Van Arsdalen, K.N. And Wein, A.J.: Functional response of the rabbit urinary bladder to anoxia and ischaemia. Neurourol. Urodyn., 2: 233, 1983.

131. Zhao, Y., Wein, A.J., Bilgen, A. And Levin, R.M.: The effect of anoxia on in-vitro bladder function. Pharmcology. 43: 337, 1991.

132. Pessina, F., Mcmurray, G., Wiggin, A. And Brading, A.F.: The effect of anoxia and glucose-free solutions on the contractile response of guinea-pig detrusor strips to intrinsic nerve stimulation and the application of excitatory agonists. J. Urol., 157: 2375, 1997.

133. Hossler, F.E. And Monson, F.C.: Microvasculature of the rabbit urinary bladder, Anat. Rec., 243: 438, 1995.

134. Parsons, C.L., Stauffer, C. And Schmidt, J.D.: Bladder-surface glycosaminoglycans: an efficient mechanism of environmental adaptation. Science. 208: 605, 1980.

135. Parsons, C.C., Boychuk, D., Jones, S., Hurst, R. And Callahan, H.: Bladder surface glycosaminoglycans: an epithelial permeability barrier. J. Urol., 143: 139, 1990.

136. Hicks, R.M., Ketterer, B. And Warren, R.C.: The ultrastructure and chemistry of the luminal plasma membrane of the mammalian urinary bladder: a structure with low permeability to water and ions. Phil. Trans. R. Soc. Lond., 168: 23, 1974.

137. Jost, S.P., Gosling, J.A. And Dixon, J.S.: The morphology of normal human bladder urothelium. J. Anat., 167: 103, 1989.

138. Lewis, S.A., Berg, J.R. And Kleine, T.J.: Modulation of epithelia permeability by extracellular macromolecules. Physiol. Rev., 75: 561, 1995.

139. Hurst, R.E. And Zebrowski, R.: Identification of proteoglycans present at high density on bovine and human bladder luminal surface. J. Urol., 152: 1641, 1994.

140. Donaldson, P.J., Chen, L.K. And Lewis, S.A.: Effects of serosal anion composition on the permeability properties of rabbit urinary bladder. Am. J. Physiol., 256: 1125, 1989.

141. Lewis, S.A.: The mammalian urinary bladder: it's more accommodating. News Physiol. Sci., 1: 61, 1986.

142. Ferguson, D.R., Kennedy, I. And Burton, T.J.: ATP is released from rabbit bladder epithelial cells by hydrostatic pressure changes - a possible sensory mechanism? J. Physiol., 505: 503, 1997.

143. Hohlbrugger, G.: Vesical blood-urine barrier: relevant and dynamic interface between renal function and nervous bladder control. J. Urol., 154: 6, 1995.

144. Boels, P.J., Arner, A., Malmqvist, U. And Uvelius, B.: Structure and mechanics of growing arterial microvessels from hypertrophied urinary bladder in the rat. Pflügers Arch., 426: 506, 1994.

145. Brendler, C. B., Radebaugh, L.C. And Hohler, J.L.: Topical oxybutynin chloride for relaxation of dysfunctional bladders. J. Urol., 141: 1350, 1989.

146. Mattiasson, A., Ekström, B. And Andersson, K.E.: Effects of intravesical instillation of verapamil in patients with detrusor hyperactivity, J. Urol., 141: 174, 1989.

147. Gabella, G. And Davis, C.: Distribution of afferent axons in the bladder of rats. J. Neurocytol., 27: 141, 1998.

148. Olsson, L.E., Wheeler, M.A., Sessa, W.C. And Weiss, R.M.: Bladder instillation and intraperitoneal injection of Escherichia coli lipopolysaccharide up regulate cytokines and iNOS in rat urinary bladder. J. Pharmacol. Exp. Ther., 284: 1203, 1998.

149. Jansson, O., Morcos, E., Söderhäll, M., J., A., Lundberg, J.O.N. And Wiklund, N.P.: The role of nitric oxide in BCG medicated anti tumour effects. Br. J. Cancer (in press), 1998.

150. Lundberg, J.O., Ehren, I., Jansson, O., Adolfsson, J., Lundberg, J.M., Weitzberg, E., Alving, K. And Wiklund, N.T.: Elevated nitric oxide in the urinary bladder in infectious and noninfectious cystitis. Urology, 48: 700, 1996.

151. Dixon, J.S., Jen, P.Y.P., Gosling, J.A.: The distribution of vesicular acetylcholine transporter in the human male genitourinary organs and its co-localization with neuropeptide Y and nitric oxide synthase. Neurourol. Urodynam., 19: 185-94, 2000.

152. Ek, A., Alm, P., Andersson, K.-E. And Persson, C.G.A.: Adrenergic and cholingeric nerves of the human urethra and urinary bladder. A histochemical study. Acta Physiol. Scand., 99: 345, 1997.

153. Gosling, J.A., Dixon, J.S. And Lendon, R.G.: The autonomic innervation of the human male and female bladder neck and proximal urethra. J. Urol. 118 302, 1997.

154. Sundin, T., Dahlstrom, A., Norlen. L., And Svedmyr, .N.: The sympathetic innervation and adrenoreceptor function of the human lower urinary tract in the normal state and after parasympathetic denervation. Invest. Urol., 14: 322, 1977.

155. Benson, G. S., Mcconnell, J. A. And Wood, J. G.: Adrenergic innervation of the human bladder body. J. Urol., 122: 189, 1979.

156. Kluck. P.: The autonomic innervation of the human urinary bladder. Bladder neck and urethra. A histochemical study. Anat. Rec., 198: 439, 1980.

157. Mcconnell, J., Benson, G.S. And Wood, J. G.: Autonomic innervation of the urogenital system. Adrenergic and cholinergic elements. Brain Res. Bull., 9: 679, 1982.

158. Edyvane, K. A., Smet, P.J., Jonavicius, J., And Marshall, V.R.: Regional differences in the innervation of the human ureterovesical junction by tyrosine hydroxylase, vasoactive intestinal polypeptide-, and neuropeptide Y-like immunoreactive nerves. J. Urol., 154: 262, 1995.

159. Smet, P. J. Moore, Kh. And Joavicius, J.: Distribution and colocalization of calcitonin gene-related peptide, tachykinins, and vasoactive intestinal peptide in normal and idiopathic unstable human urinary bladder. Lab. Invest., 77: 37, 1997.

160. Vaughan, C.W. And Satchell, P.M.: Urine storage mechanisms. Prog. Neurobiol., 46: 215, 1995.

161. Janig, W. And Koltzenburg, M.: On the function of spinal primary afferent fibres supplying colon and urinary bladder. J. Auton. Nerv. Syst., 30: S89, 1990.

162. Fall. M., Lindstrom, S., And Mazieres, L.: A bladder-to-bladder cooling reflex in the cat. J. Physiol., 427: 281, 1990.

163. Maggi, C.A. And Meli, A.: The sensory-efferent function of capsaicin-sensitive sensory neurons. Gen. Pharmacol., 19: 1, 1988.

164. Ferguson, D.R., Kennedy, I., And Burton, T.J.: ATP is released from rabbit urinary bladder epithelial cells by hydrostatic pressure changes - a possible sensory mechanism? J. Physiol., 505: 503, 1997.

165. Kawatani, M., Whitney, T., Booth, A.M., And Degroat, W.C.: Excitatory effect of substance P I parasympathetic ganglia of cat urinary bladder. Am. J. physiol., 257: 1450, 1898.

166. Wakabayashi, Y., Tomoyoshi, T., Fujimiya, M., Arai, R., And Maeda, T.: Substance P-containing axon terminals in the mucosa of the human urinary bladder: pre-embedding immunohistochemistry using cryostat sections for electron microscopy. Histochem., 100: 401, 1993.

167. Kumamoto, K., Ebara, S., And Matsuura, T.: Noradrenergic fibers: I. The Pacinian corpuscles of the cat urinary bladder. Acta Anat., 146: 46, 1993.

168. Dupont, M., Steers.W., Miccarty.R., And Tuttle. J.: Neural plasticity and alterations in nerve growth factor and norepinephrine in response to bladder inflammation. J. Urol., 151:284, 1994.

169. Tuttle. J. B., Steers. W. D., Albo. M., And Nataluk. E.: Neural input regulates tissue NGF and growth of the adult rat urinary bladder. J. Auton. Nerv. Syst., 49: 147, 1994.

170. Steers.W.D., Ciambotti.J., Etzel. B., Berdman. S., And De Groat. W.C.: Alterations in afferent pathways form the urinary bladder of the rat I response to partial urethral obstruction. J. Comp. Neurol., 310: 401, 1991.

171. Steers W.D., Creedon D. J., And Tuttle J.: Immunity to nerve growth factor prevents afferent plasticity following urinary bladder hypertrophy. J. Urol., 155: 375, 1996.

172. Dixon J.S., Gosling. J.A., Canning. D. A. And Gearhart. J.P.: An immunohistochemical study of human postnatal paraganglia associated with the urinary bladder. J. Anat., 181: 431, 1992.

173. Pang X., Marchand. J., Sant. G.R., Kream. R., And Theoharides.T.C.: Increased number of substance P positive nerve fibres: I. Interstitial cystitis. Br. J. Urol., 75: 744, 1995.

174. Lowe R. M., Anand. P., Terenghi.G., Williams-Chestnuts. R., Sinicropi. D., And Osborne. J.: Increased nerve growth factor levels in the urinary bladder of women with idiopathic sensory urgency and interstitial cystitis. Br. J. Urol., 79: 572, 1997.

175. Szallasi,. A., Conte, B., Goso, C., Blumberg, P. M., And Manzini, S.: Vanilloid receptors: I. The urinary bladder: regional distribution, localization on sensory nerves, and species-related differences. Naunyn Schmiedebergs Arch. Pharmacol., 347: 624, 1993.

176. Bennett, D., Dmietrieva, V., Priestley, J., Clary, D., And Mcmahon, S.: TrkA, CGRP and IB4 expression in retrogradely labelled cutaneous and visceral primary sensory neurones in the rat. Neurosci. Letts., 206: 33, 1996.

177. Yarnitsky, D. And Vardi, Y.: Bladder sensory power factor (BSPF) - a novel diagnostic tool. J. Neurol. Sci., 120: 137, 1993.

178. Sjostrand. N.O.: The adrenergic innervation of the vas deferens and accessory male genital glands. Acta Physiol. Scand., Suppl 257: 1, 1965.

179. De Groat. W. C. And Booth. A. M.: Inhibition and facilitation in parasympathetic ganglia of the urinary bladder. Fed. Proc., 39: 2990, 1980.

180. Gosling, J. A. And Thompson, S. A. Morphological and histochemical studies on developing human pelvic autonomic nerve cells and paraganglia. In: Peripheral Neuroendocrine Interaction. Edited by R.E. Coupland and W. G. Forsmann. London: Springer, pp. 37-47, 1978.

181. Thompson, S.A. And Gosling, J.A.: Histochemical light microscopic study of catecholamine-containing paraganglia in the human pelvis. Cell Tiss. Res., 170: 539, 1976.

182. Dixon, J. S., Gosling, J.A., Canning, D.A. And Gearhart, J.P.: An immunohistochemical study of human postnatal paraganglia associated with the urinary bladder. J. Anat., 181: 431, 1992.

183. Philips, M.: Fetal catecholamines. Am. J. Obstet. Gynecol., 146: 840, 1983.

184. Learmonth, J. R.: A contribution to the neurophysiology of the urinary bladder in man. Brain, 54: 147, 1931.

185. Andersson, K.-E. And Persson L.: Nitric oxide synthase and nitric oxide-mediated effects in lower urinary tract smooth muscles. World J. Urol., 12: 274, 1994.

186. DeLancey, J.O.L.: Correlative study of paraurethral anatomy. Obstet Gynecol, 68: 91-7, 1986.

187. Oelrich, T.M.: The striated urogenital sphincter muscle in the female. Anat. Rec., 205: 223-32, 1983.

188. Gosling, J.A., Dixon, J.S., Critchley, H.O.D. And Thompson, S.A.: A comparative study of the human external sphincter and periurethral levator ani muscles. Br. J. Urol., 53:35, 1981.

189. Huisman, A.B.: Aspects on the anatomy of the female urethra with special relation to urinary continence. Contrib. Gynecol. Obstet., 10: 1-31, 1983.

190. Arner.A., Mattiasson., A., Radzizewski, P. And Uvelius, B.: Shortening velocity is different in longitudinal and circular muscle layers of the rabbit urethra. Urol. Res., in press.

191. Creed, K.E., Oike, M. And Ito, Y.: The electrical properties and responses to nerve stimulation of the proximal urethra of the male rabbit. Br. J. Urol., 79: 543, 1997.

192. Teramoto, N., Creed, K.E. And Brading, A.F.: Activity of glibenclamide-sensitive K+ channels under unstimulated conditions in smooth muscle cells of pig proximal urethra. Naunyn Schmiedebergis Arch. Pharmacol., 356: 418, 1997.

193. Ho, K.M.T., Mcmurray, G., Brading, A.F., Noble. J.G., Ny, L. And Andersson, K.-E.: Nitric oxide synthase in heterogeneous population of intramural striated muscle fibres of human membranous urethral sphincter. J. Urol., 159: 1091, 1998.

194. Bridgewater, M., Davies, J.R. And Brading, A.F.: Regional variations in the neural control of the female pig urethra. Br. J. Urol., 76: 730, 1995.

195. Alm, P., Zygmunt, P.K., Iselin, C., Larsson, B., Uvelius, B., Werner, S. And Andersson, K.-E.: Nitric oxide synthase-immunoreactive, adrenergic, cholinergic and peptidergic nerves of the female rat urinary tract: a comparative study. J. Auton. Nerv. Syst. 56: 105, 1995.

196. Ek, A.: Innervation and receptor functions of the human urethra. Scand J. Urol. Nephrol. Suppl., 1997: 1, 1977.

197. Bridgewater, M., Macneil, H.F. And Brading, A.F.: Regulation of tone in pig urethral smooth muscle, J. Urol., 150: 223, 1993.

198. Hatano, A., Takahashi, H., Tamaki, M., Komeyanma, T., Koizumi, T. And Takeda, A.: Pharmacological evidence of distinct alpha I-adrenoceptor subtypes mediating the contraction of human prostatic urethra and peripheral artery. Br. J. Pharmacol., 113: 723, 1994.

199. Werkstr, M.V., Persson, K., Ny., L., Bridgewater, M., Brading, A.F. And Andersson. K.-E.: Factors involved in the relaxation of female pig urethra evoked by electrical stimulation. Br. J. Pharmacol., 116: 1599, 1995.

200. Andersson, K.-E, And Persson, K.: Nitric oxide synthase and the lower urinary tract: possible implications for physiology and pathophysiology. Scand. J. Urol. Nephrol., 175: 45, 1995.

201. Takeda, M. And Lepor, H.: Nitric oxide synthase in dog urethra: a pharmacological and histochemical analysis. Br. J. Pharmacol., 116: 2517, 1995.

202. Mcdonald, L.J. And Murad, F.: Nitric oxide and cyclic GMP signaling. Proc. Soc. Exp. Biol. Med, 211:1, 1996.

203. Boolell, M., Gepi-Attee, S., Gingell, J.C. And Allen, M. J.: Sildenafil. A novel effective oral therapy for male erectile dysfunction. Br. J. Urol., 78:257, 1996.

204. Thind, P.: The significance of smooth and striated muscles in sphincter function of the urethra in healthy women. Neurourol. Urodyn., 14: 585, 1995.

205. Torrens, M.J.: Human physiology. In: The physiology of the lower urinary tract. Edited by M. Torrens and J.F. B. Morrison. Springer-Verlag: Berlin. p. 333:1987.

206. Gosling, J.A., Dixon, J.S., Critchley, H.O. And Thomp-

son, S.A.: A comparative study of the human external sphincter and periurethral levator ani muscles. Br J. Urol., 53: 35, 1981.

207. Light, J.K., Rapoli, E. And Wheeler, T.M.: The striated urethral sphincter: muscle fibre types and distribution in the prostatic capsule. Br. J. Urol., 79: 539, 1997.

208. Elbadawi, A., Mathews, R., Light, J.K. And Wheeler, T.E.: Immunohistochemical and ultrastructural study of rhabdosphincter component of the prostatic capsule. J. Urol., 158: 1819, 1997.

209. Zvara, P., Carrier, S., Kour, N.W. And Tangho, E.A.: The detailed neuroanatomy of the human striated urethral sphincter. Br J. Urol., 74: 182, 1994.

210. Hollabaugh. R.S., Dmochowski, R.R. And Steiner, M.S.: Neuroanatomy of the male rhabdosphincter. Urology, 49: 426, 1997.

211. Von Heyden, B., Riemer, R.K., Nunes, L., Brock, G.B., Lue, T.F. And Tanagho, A.E.: Response of guinea-pig smooth and striated urethral sphincter to cromakalim, prazosin, nifedipine, nitroprusside and electrical stimulation. Neurourol. Urodyn., 14: 153, 1995.

212. Creed, K.E., Van Der Werf, B.A., Kaye, K.W.: Innervation of striated muscle of the membranous urethra of the male dog. J. Urol., 159: 1712, 1998.

213. Fowler, C.J. And Fowler, C.: Clinical neurophysiology, In: The physiology of the lower urinary tract. Edited by M. Torrens and J.F.B. Morrison. Springer-Verlag: Berlin Heidelberg. p. 309, 1987.

214. Fowler, C.J., Kirby, R.S., Harrison, M.J., Milroy, E.J. And Turner Warwich, R.: Individual motor unit analysis in the diagnosis of disorders of urethral sphincter innervation. J. Neurourol. Neurosurg. Psychiatry. 47: 637, 1984.

215. Hutch, J.A.: A new theory of the anatomy of the internal urinary sphincter and the physiology of micturition. IV. The urinary sphincteric mechanism. J. Urol., 97: 705, 1967.

216. Hickey, D.S., Phillips, J.I. And Hukins, D.W.L.: Arrangements of collagen fibrils and muscle fibers in the female urethra and their implications for the control of micturition. Br. J. Urol., 54: 556, 1982.

217. Huisman, A.B.: Aspects on the anatomy of the female urethra with special relation to urinary continence. Contrib. Gynecol. Obstet., 10: 1, 1983.

218. Augsburger, H.R., Crus-Orive, L.M. And Arnold, S.: Morphology and stereology of the female canine urethra correlated with the urethral pressure profile. Acta Anat. (Basel), 148: 197, 1993.

219. Dass, N.: Studies of the anatomy and autonomic innervation of the vesicourethral junction and urethra. D. Phil thesis in Pharmacology. Oxford University, 1997.

220. Carlile, A., Davies, I., Rigby, A. And Brocklehurst, J.C.: Age changes in the human female urethra: a morphologic study. J. Urol., 139: 532, 1988.

221. Ulmsten, U., Ekman, G., Giertz, G. And Malmstrom, A.: Different biochemical composition of connective tissue in continent and stress incontinent women. Acta Obstet. Gynecol. Scand., 66: 455, 1987.

222. Rud, T., Andersson, K.E., Asmussen, M., Hunting, A. And Ulmsten, U.: Factors maintaining the intraurethral pressure in women. Invest. Urol., 17: 343, 1980.

223. Batra, S., Bjellin, L., Sjogren, C., Iosif, S. And Widmark, E.: Increases in blood flow of the female rabbit urethra following low dose estrogens. J. Urol., 136: 1360, 1986.

224. Greenland, J.E. And Brading, A.F.: The in vivo and in vitro effects of hypoxia on pig urethral smooth muscle. Br. J. Urol., 79: 525, 1997.

225. Falconer, C., Blomgren, B., Johansson, O., Ulmsten, U., Malmström, A., Westergrenthorsson, G. And Ekman-Ordeberg, G.: Different organization of collagen fibrils in stress-incontinent women of fertile age. Acta Obstet. Gynecol. Scan., 77: 87, 1998.

226. Falconer, C., Ekman-Ordeberg, G., Blomgren, B., Johansson, O., Ulmsten, U., Westergren-Thorsson, G. And Malmström, A.: Paraurethral connective tissue in stress-incontinent women after menopause. Acta Obstet. Gynecol. Scand., 77:95, 1998.

227. Rechberger, T., Donica, H., Baranowski, W. And Jakowicki, J.: Female urinary stress incontinence in terms of connective tissue biochemistry. Eur. J. Obstet. Gynecol. Reprod. Bio., 49: 187, 1993.

228. Keane, D.P., Sims, T.J., Abrams, P. And Bailey, J.: Analysis of collagen status in premenopausal nulliparous women with genuine stress incontinence. Br. J. Obstet. Gynaecol., 104: 994, 1997.

229. Knowles, R.G. And Moncada, S.: Nitric oxide synthases in mammals. Biochem. J., 298: 249, 1994.

230. Alm, P., Larsson, B., Ekblad, E., Sundler, F. And Andersson, K. E.: Immunohistochemical localization of peripheral nitric oxide synthase-containing nerves using antibodies raised against synthesized C- and N-terminal fragments of a cloned enzyme form rat brain. Acta Physiol. Scand., 148: 421, 1993.

231. Burnett, A.L., Calvin, D.C., Chamness, S.L. Liu, J.X., Nelson, R.J., Klein, S.L., Dawson, V.L., Dawson, T.M. And Snyder, S.H.: Urinary bladder-urethral sphincter dysfunction in mice with targeted disruption of neuronal nitric oxide synthase models idiopathic voiding disorders I humans. Nature Medicine, 3: 571, 1997.

232. Andersson, K.E., Garcia-Pascual, A., Forman, A. And Tottrup, A.: Non-adrenergic, non-cholinergic nerve-mediated relaxation of rabbit urethra is caused by nitric oxide. Acta Physiol. Scand., 141: 133, 1991.

233. Dokita, S., Morgan, W.R., Wheeler, M.A., Yoshida, M., Latifpour, J. And Weiss, R.M.: NG-nitro-L-arginine inhibits non-adrenergic, non-cholinergic relaxation in rabbit urethral smooth muscle. Life Sci., 48: 2429, 1991.

234. Persson, K. And Andersson, K.E.: Nitric oxide and relaxation of pig lower urinary tract. Br. J. Pharmacol., 106: 416, 1992.

235. Garcia-Pascula, A., Costa, G., Garciasacristan, A. And Andersson, K.-E.: Relaxation of sheep urethral muscle induced by electrical stimulation of nerves: involvement of nitric oxide. Acta Physiol. Scand., 141: 531, 1991.

236. Andersson, K.E., Garcia Pascual A., Persson, K., Forman, A. And Tottrup., A.: Electrically-induced, nerve-

mediated relaxation of rabbit urethra involves nitric oxide. J. Urol., 147: 253, 1992.

237. Leone, A.M., Wiklund, N.P., Hokfelt, T., Brundin, L. And Moncada, S.: Nerve-induced release of nitric oxide in the human urogenital tract. Neuroreport., 5: 733, 1994.

238. James, M. J., Birmingham, A.T. And Hill, S.J.: Partial mediation by nitric oxide of the relaxation of human isolated detrusor strips in response to electrical field stimulation. Br J. Clin. Pharmacol., 35: 366, 1993.

239. Ehren, I., Iversen, H., Jansson, O., Adolfsson, J. And Wiklund, N.P.: Localization of nitric oxide synthase activity in the human lower urinary tract and its correlation with neuroeffector responses. Urology., 44: 683, 1994.

240. Hindmarsh, J.R., Gosling, P.T. And Deane, A.M.: Bladder instability. Is the primary defect in the urethra? Br. J. Urol., 55: 648, 1983.

241. Mcguire, E.J.: Detrusor response to outlet obstruction. World J. Urol., 2: 208, 1984.

242. Smith, S.H., Wheeler, M.A., Foster, J.H.E. And Weiss, R. M.: Improvement in interstitial cystitis symptom scores during treatment with oral L-arginine. J. Urol., 158:703, 1997.

243. Weiner, C.P. Lizasoain, I., Baylis, S.A., Knowles, R.G., Charles, I.G. And Moncada, S.; Induction of calcium-dependent nitric oxide synthases by sex hormones. Proc. Natl. Acad. Sci., 91:5212, 1994.

244. Ehren, I., Hammarstrom, M., Adolfesson, J. And Wiklund, N.P.: Induction of calcium-dependent nitric oxide synthase by sex hormones in the guinea-pig urinary bladder. Acta Physiol. Scan., 153: 393, 1995.

245. Morrison, J.F.B.: Sensations arising from the lower urinary tract. In: The physiology of the lower urinary tract. Edited by M. Torrens and J.F. B. Morrison. Springer-Verlag: Berlin. p. 89, 1987.

246. De Groat, W.C., Booth, A.M. And Yoshimura, N.: Neurophysiology of micturition and its modification in animal models of human disease. In: nervous control of the urogenital system. Edited by C.A. Maggi, Harwood Academic Publishers: Chur. p. 227, 1993.

247. Maggi, C.A.: The pharmacology of the efferent function of sensory nerves. Autonom. Pharmacol., 11:173, 1991.

248. Maggi, C.A.: The dual, sensory and efferent function of the capasaicin-sensitive primary sensory neurons in the urinary bladder and urethra. In: nervous control of the Urogenital System. Edited by C. A. Maggi, Harwood Academic Publisher: Chur. Switzerland, p. 383, 1993.

249. Bahns, E., Halsband, U. And Janig, W.: Responses of sacral visceral afferents from the lower urinary tract, colon and anus to mechanical stimulation. Pflügers Archiv., 410: 296, 1987.

250. Vera, P.L. And Nadelhaft, I.: Conduction velocity distribution of afferent fibres innervating the rat urinary bladder. Brain Res., 520: 83, 1990.

251. Habler, H.L., Janig, W. And Koltzenburg, M.: Activation of unmyelinated afferent fibres by mechanical stimulation and inflammation of the urinary bladder in the cat. J. Physiol., 425: 545, 1990.

252. Habler, H.L., Janig, W. And Koltzenburg, M.: Myelinated primary afferents of the sacral spinal cord responding to slow filling and distension of the cat urinary bladder. J. Physiol., 463: 449, 1993.

253. Sengupta, J. N. And Gebhart, G.F.: Mechanosensitive properties of pelvic nerve afferent fibres innervating the urinary bladder of the rat. J. Neurophysiology. 72:2420, 1994.

254. Lawson, S.N.: Morphology and biochemical cell types of sensory neurons. In: Sensory neurons, diversity development and plasticity. Edited by S. A. Scott, Oxford University Press: Oxford. P. 27, 1992.

255. Lawson, S.N. And Waddell, P.J.: Soma neurofilament immunoreactivity is related to cell size and fiber conduction velocity in rat primary sensory neurons. J. Physiol., 435: 41, 1991.

256. Kawatani, M., Lowe, I.P., Nadelhaft, I., Morgan, C. And De Groat, W.C.: VIP in visceral afferent pathways to the sacral spinal cord. Neuroscience. Letters. 41: 311, 1983.

257. Keast, J.R. And De Groat, W. C.: Segmental distribution and peptide content of primary afferent neuro-innervating the urogenital organs and colon of male rat. J. Comp. Neurol., 319: 615, 1992.

258. Maggi, C.A. And Meli, A.: The role of neuropetides in the regulation of the micturition reflex. J. Auto. Pharmacol., 6:133, 1986.

259. Maggi, C.A. And Meli, A.: The sensory-efferent function of capsaicin-sensitive sensory neurons. Gen. Pharmacol., 19:1, 1988.

260. Szallasi, A. And Blumberg, P.M.: Resinifentoxin and its analogs provide novel insights into the pharmacology of the vanilloid (capsaicin) receptor. L. Sci., 47: 1399, 1990.

261. Sharkey, K.A., Williams., R.G., Schultz Berga, M. And Dockray, G.J.: Sensory substance P-innervation of the urinary bladder possible site action of capsicin in causing urine retention in rats. Neuroscience. 10: 861, 1983.

262. Jansco, G. And Maggi, C.A.: Distribution of capsaicin-sensitive urinary bladder afferents I the rat spinal cord. Brain Res., 418: 371, 1987.

263. Maggi, C.A., Santicioli, P. And Meli, A.: The effects of topical capsaicin on rat urinary bladder mobility in vivo. European J. Pharmacol., 103: 41. 1984.

264. Maggi, C.A., Saticioli, P., Giuliani, S., Furio, M. And Meli, A.: The capsaicin-sensitive innervation of the rat urinary bladder: further studies on mechanism regulating micturition threshold. J. Urol., 136: 697, 1986.

265. Maggi, C.A., Santicioli, P., Geppetti, S., Furio, M., Frilli, S., Conte, B., Fanciullacci, M., Giuliani, S. And Meli, A.: The contribution of capsaicin-sensitive innervation to activation of the spinal vesico-vesical reflex in rats: relationship between substance P levels in the urinary bladder and the sensory-efferent function of capsaicin-sensitive sensory neurons. Brain Res., 415: 1, 1987.

266. De Groat. W., Kawatani, T., Hisamitsu, T. Cheng, C. L., Ma, C. P . Thor, K., Steers, W And Roppolo, J.R.: Mechanisms underlying the recovery of urinary bladder

function following spinal cord injury. J. Autonom. Nerv. Syst., 30:S71, 1990.

267. Abelli, Li., Conte, B., Somma, V., Maggi, C.S., Giuliani, S., Geppetti, S., Asessandri, M., Theodorsson, E. And Meli, Al.: The contribution of capsaicin-sensitive sensory fibers to xylene-induced visceral pain in conscious, freely-moving rats. Naunyn Schmiedeberg's Arch. Pharmacol., 337: 545, 1988.

268. Giuliani, S., Maggi, C.A. And Meil, A.: Capsaicin-sensitive afferents I the rat urinary bladder activate a spinal sympathetic cardiovascular reflex. . Naunyn Schmiedeberg's Arch. Pharmacol., 338: 1988.

269. Lecci, A., Giuliani, S., Garret, C. And Maggi, C.A.: Evidence for a role tachykinins as sensory transmitters I the activation of micturition reflex neuroscience. 54: 827, 1993.

270. Maggi, C.A., Patacchini, R., Santicioli, P. And Giuliani, S.: Tachykinin antagonists and capsaicin-induced contraction of the rat isolated urinary bladder: evidence for tachykinin-mediated cotransmission. Br. J. Pharmacol., 103: 1535, 1991.

271. Maggi, C. A., Lecci, A., Santicioli, P., Del Bianco, E. And Giulian, S.: Cyclophosphamide cysititis in rats: m involvement of capsaicin sensitive primary afferents. J. Autonom. Nerv. Syst. 38: 201, 1992.

272. Barbanti, G., Maggi, C.A., Beneforti, P., Baroldi, P. And Turini, D.: Further studies on pain relief produced by intravesical capsaicin in patients suffering from hypersensitive disorders of the lower urinary tract. Br. J. Urol., 71: 1993.

273. Fowler, C.J., Jewkes, D. Mcdonald. W.I., Lynn. B. And De Groat, W.C.: Intravesical capsaicin for neurogenic bladder dysfunction. Lancet. 339: 239, 1992.

274. Flower, C.J., Beck, R.O., Gerrard, S., Betts, C.D. And Fowler, C. G.: intravesical capsaicin for treatment of detrusor hyperreflexia. J. Neurol. Neurosurg. Psychiatry. 57: 169, 1994.

275. Biro.T., Maurer. M., Modarres. S., Lewin, N.E., Brodie, C., Cas. C., Acs. P., Paus, R. And Blimberg. P.M.: Characterization of functional vanilloid receptors expressed by mast cells. Blood. 91:1332, 1998.

276. Caterina. M.J., Schumacher. M.A., Tominaga. M., Rosen. T.A., Levine.J.D. And Julius. D.: The capsicine receptor: a heat-activated ion channel in the pain pathway. Nature. 389: 816, 1997.

277. Maggi. C.A.: The role of peptides in the regulation of the micturition reflex: an update. Gen. Pharmacol., 22: 1, 1991.

278. Szolcasanye. J.: Selective responsiveness of polymodal nociceptors of the rabbit ear to capsaicin, bradykinin and ultraviolet irradiation. J. Physiol., 388: 9, 1987.

279. Jiang, W., Kibble, A. And Morrison. J.F.B.: The effect of capsaicin on pelvic afferent inputs from the urinary bladder of anaesthetized rats. J. Physiol., 487: 119P, 1995.

280. Wilson. P.M.: Understanding the pelvic floor. S. Afr. Med. J. 47:1150, 1973.

281. Wilson. P.M.: Some observations on pelvic floor evolution in primates. S. Afr. Med. J., 47: 1203, 1973.

282. Constantinou. C., Govan.D.: Spatial distribution and timing of transmitted and reflexly generated urethral pressures in healthy women. J. Urol., 127: 964, 1982.

283. Sato, K.: A morphological analysis of the nerve supply of the sphincter ani externus, levator ani and coccygeus. Acta Anat. Nippon, 44: 187, 1980.

284. Abitbol, M.M.: Evolution of ischial spine and of the pelvic floor in the hominoidea. Amer. J. Phys. Anthropol., 75: 53, 1988.

285. Campbell, R.M.: The anatomy and histology of the sacrouterine ligaments. Am. J. Obstet. Gynecol., 59: 1, 1950.

286. Range, R.L., Woodburne, R.T.: The gross and microscopic anatomy of the transverse cervical ligaments. Am. J. Obstet. Gynecol., 90: 460, 1964.

287. Blaisdell F.E.: The anatomy of the sacro-uterine ligaments. Anat. Record, 12: 1, 1917.

288. DeLancey, J.O.L.: Anatomic aspects of vaginal eversion after hysterectomy. Am. J. Obstet. Gynecol., 166: 1717, 1992.

289. Ala-Ketola, L.: Roentgen diagnosis of female stress urinary incontinence. Roentgenological and clinical study. Acta Obstet. Gynecol. Scand. Suppl., 23:1, 1973.

290. DeLancey, J.O.L.: Structural support of the urethra as it relates to stress urinary incontinence: The hammock hypothesis. Am J. Obstet. Gynecol., 170: 1713, 1994.

291. DeLancey., J. O. L., Starr. R. A.: Histology of the connection between the vagina and levator ani muscles. J. Reprod. Med., 35: 765, 1990.

292. Kirschner-Hermanns, R., Wein, B., Niehas, S., Schaefer, W., Jakse, G.: The contribution of magnetic resonance imaging of the pelvic floor to the understanding of urinary incontinence. Br. J. Urol., 72: 715, 1993.

293. Howard, D., Miller, J.M., DeLancey, J.O.L., Ashton-Miller, J.A.: Differential effects of cough, valsalva, and continence status on vesical neck movement. Obstet. Gynecol., 95: 535, 2000.

294. DeLancey, J.O.L. Structural anatomy of the posterior compartment as it relates to rectocele. Am. J. Obstet. Gynecol., 180: 815, 1999.

295. DeLancey. J. O.L: Correlative study of paraurethral anatomy. Obstet. Gynecol., 68: 91, 1986.

296. DeLancey. J. O.L.: Structural aspects of the extrinsic continence mechanism. Obstet. Gynecol., 72: 296, 1988.

297. DeLancey., J. O. L.: The pubovesical ligament. A separate structure from the urethral supports. (pubo-urethral ligaments). Neurourol. Urodyn., 8: 53, 1989.

298. Berglas. B. , Rubin, I. C.: Histologic study of the pelvic connective tissue. Surg. Gynecol. Obstet., 97: 277, 1953.

299. Ulmsten, U., Ekman, G., Giertz. G. , Malmstrom, A.: Different biochemical composition of connective tissue in continent and stress incontinent women. Acta Obstet. Gynecol. Scand., 66: 455, 1987.

300. Makinen, J. Sonderstrom, K. O., Kiilhoma, P., Hirvonen, T.: Histological changes in the vaginal connective tissue

of patients with and without uterine prolapse. Arch. Gynecol., 239: 17, 1986.

301. Norton, P., Baker, J., Sharp, H. , Warenski, J.: Genitourinary prolapse. Relationship with joint mobility. Neurourol. Urodyn., 9: 321, 1990.

302. Koelbl, H., Strassegger, H., Riss, P. A., Gruber, H.: Morphologic and functional aspects of pelvic floor muscles in patients with pelvic relaxation and genuine stress incontinence. Obstet. Gynecol., 74: 789, 1989.

303. Smith, A.R.B., Hosker, G. L. , Warrell, D. W.: The role of partial denervation of the pelvic floor in the aetiology of genitourinary proplapse and stress incontinence of urine. A neurophysiological study. Br. J. Obstet. Gynaecol., 96: 24, 1989.

304. Dubowitz, V.: The role of histochemistry in muscle disease. In: Modern trends in Neurology. Edited by D. Williams. London: Butterworth. Pp. 189-208, 1970.

305. Bearsiek, F. Parks, A. G. Swash. M.: Pathogenesis of anorectal incontinence. A histometric study of the anal sphincter musculature. J. Neurol. Sci., 342:111, 1979.

306. Parks, A. G., Swash. M. , Ulrich. H.: Sphincter denervation in ano-rectal incontinence and rectal prolapse. Gut 18: 656, 1977.

307. Gilpin, S. A., Gosling, J. A., Smith, A.R. B., Warrell, D.W.: The pathogenesis of genito-urinary prolapse and stress incontinence of urine. A histological and histochemical study. Br. J. Obstet. Gynaecol., 96: 15, 1989.

308. Dimpfl, T.H., Jaeger, C.H., Mueller-Felber. W., Anthuber. C., Hirsch, A., Brandmaier, R., Schuessler. B.: Myogenic changes of the levator ani muscle in premenopausal women: The impact of vaginal delivery and age. Neurourol. Urodyn., 17: 197, 1998.

309. Madoff, R. D., Williams, J.G., Caushaj, P.F.: Fecal incontinence. N. Engl. J. Med., 326: 1002, 1992.

310. Dalley, A. F.: The riddle of the sphincters. The morphophysiology of the anorectal mechanism reviewed. Amer. Surgeon, 53: 298, 1987.

311. Milligan, E.T.C., Morgan, C.N.: Surgical anatomy of the anal canal with special reference to anorectal fistulae. Lancet, ii: 1150, 1934.

312. Oh, C., Kark, A.E.: Anatomy of the external anal sphincter in men. Acta Anat., 105: 25, 1979.

313. Lawson, J.O.: Pelvic anatomy. II. Anal canal and associated sphincters. Ann. R. Coll. Surg. Engl., 54: 288, 1974.

314. DeLancey, J.O.L., Toglia, M.R., Perucchini, D.: Internal and external anal sphincter anatomy as it relates to midline obstetrical lacerations. Obstet. Gynecol., 90: 924, 1997.

315. Snooks, S.J., Setchell, M., Swash, M., Henry, M.M.: Injury to innervation of pelvic floor sphincter musculature in childbirth. Lancet, 2: 546-50, 1984.

316. Snooks, S.J., Henry, M.M., Swash, M. Faecal incontinence due to external sphincter division in childbirth is associated with damage to the innervation of the pelvic floor musculature: a double pathology. Br. J. Obstet. Gynaecol., 92: 824, 1985.

317. Sultan, A.H., Kamm, M.A., Hudson, C.N., Thomas, J.M., Bartram, C.I.: Anal-sphincter disruption during vaginal delivery. N. Engl. J. Med., 329: 1905, 1993.

Committee 2

Neurophysiology and Neuropharmacology

Chairmen

J. Morrison (UAE),

W. D Steers (USA),

A. Brading (U.K.)

Members

B.Blok (The Netherlands),

C. Fry (U.K.),

W.C de Groat (USA),

H. Kakizaki (Japan),

R. Levin (USA),

K. Thor (USA)

CONTENTS

Neurophysiology and Neuropharmacology

J. Morrison, W. D Steers, A. Brading

B.Blok, C. Fry, W.C de Groat, H. Kakizaki, R. Levin, K. Thor

INTRODUCTION

It was the view of the organising committee that the work of the two former basic science committees (Cell Biology, and Neurophysiology and Neuropharmacology) should be combined and integrated into one chapter. The two chapters in the first consultation [1,2] summarise two perspectives on the science and biology of incontinence, viz (a) the central nervous mechanisms involved in micturition and incontinence, and (b) the component tissues of the bladder and urethra. This decision to combine and integrate was an important one that has caused major revisions and additions in an attempt to explain why so many components of the lower urinary tract and its innervation may change in pathological circumstances. Consequently the subcommittee of 2001 reviewed the neurosciences and cell biology together. This chapter relies heavily on the report of the first consultation publication [1,2], and some of this work will be repeated, sometimes in a condensed form, simply because the former volume is not generally available. The focus of this report is predominantly on biological factors that contribute to the overactive bladder, and special consideration is given to mechanisms that might be important in this state. This report also attempts to make an integrated approach, looking at all the tissues involved, and the interactions between them: knowledge of the urothelium and its interaction with afferent nerves and the mediators involved have increased rapidly, and a section will be devoted to this topic. Properties of the bladder smooth muscle not considered in depth in the First Consultation, including its metabolism, contraction and relaxation, excitation contraction coupling, Ca^{2+} handling and electrical connectivity that are relevant to bladder overactivity are also discussed. It will be seen that these properties affect afferent and efferent neurones in the bladder wall, and the viability of these affects reflex responses and sensation. Neurones affected in this way may be found within the intramural ganglia that are largely absent in some experimental animals, but present in humans. New information is available on the ganglia present in the human bladder wall and paraurethral tissue, and on the interstitial cells that have been found submucosally and around the smooth muscle bundles in the urethra and bladder. At the same time we will summarise and update the previous material on neuroscience and link it with cell biology and genetics in an attempt to produce a wider view against which the plasticity of cellular components of the lower urinary tract and its innervation can be considered, particularly in relation to pathological disturbances.

The overactive bladder (OAB) is a common clinical problem which may originate from dysfunction of the peripheral or central nervous pathways, the urothelium, smooth muscle and other tissue components; in inflammation or cancer there may be infiltration of inflammatory or neoplastic cells which may also influence both the function of nerve, muscle, urothelial and other cells. Much is known about the neural contribution to OAB, and much remains to be discovered. But there have also been interesting developments in recent years on non-neural factors that might contribute to bladder hyperactivity, bladder instability and altered bladder sensation. Changes in the urothelium as well as the altered responsiveness of ischaemic or denervated smooth muscle appear to be two of the most important factors in these syndromes. However, not only can the increased responsiveness of the nerves be due to changes in the urothelium or smooth muscle, conversely changes in smooth muscle and urothelium can be elicited by altered nerve activity. Furthermore, long term changes in smooth muscle (such as hypertrophy, and increased oxygen consumption) may lead to functional ischaemia and damage to neurones in the bladder wall. Because of these interactions, a vicious circle can develop in which a change in one of these components can influence the other components of the system; consequently pathophysiological changes can be described in several components of this control system when an initial (experimental) lesion has been restricted to one of these.

Models of conditions that exhibit overactive bladder and instability have been developed, and a consideration of the pathophysiology of bladder outlet obstruction, bladder inflammation, overactivity, denervation, spinal cord injury and development or aging will be presented towards the end of the report. These models have helped to produce an understanding of the pathophysiological mechanisms and are now providing a more unified hypothesis on the genesis of these conditions.

This chapter is therefore divided into four sections (a) the peripheral innervation (b) other peripheral tissues such as urothelium and smooth muscle, (c) the control of the lower urinary tract by the central nervous system, and (d) pathophysiological models of the overactive bladder.

LEVELS OF EVIDENCE

This book attempts to use Levels of Evidence throughout. The Oxford Centre for Evidence Based Medicine has laid down guidelines that apply to Levels of Therapeutic Interventions and Grades of Recommendations to patients; the existence of dispute regarding each major conclusion should be documented. These do not really apply to the basic sciences, where randomised controlled trials are not a common format of investigation, and acute studies with internal controls are more common.

Within this chapter we intend to be selective and report scientific evidence that has appropriate controls and achieves statistical significance. Other categories of evidence, e.g. uncontrolled studies, inadequate statistical support, anecdotal information, hypothesis or speculation will be referred to as such.

Of some importance in this field are species differences, and agreement or disagreement between results on different species will be made clear.

A. PERIPHERAL NERVES THAT INNERVATE THE LOWER URINARY TRACT

I. OVERVIEW

As indicated in Figure 1 and discussed in detail in chapter 1 [3], the lower urinary tract is innervated by three sets of peripheral nerves: (1) pelvic parasympathetic nerves, which arise at the sacral level of the spinal cord, excite the bladder and relax the urethra, (2) lumbar sympathetic nerves, which inhibit the bladder body and excite the bladder base and urethra in animals, (3) pudendal nerves, which excite the external urethral sphincter and associated mechanisms in the pelvic floor [3-8]. These nerves contain afferent (sensory) axons as well as efferent pathways.

The central pathways controlling lower urinary tract function are organized as simple on-off switching circuits (Fig. 2) that maintain a reciprocal relationship between the urinary bladder and urethral outlet. [2, 4-9]. The principal reflex components of these switching circuits are listed in Table 1 and illustrated in Figure 3. Intravesical pressure measurements during bladder filling in both humans and animals reveal low and relatively constant bladder pressures when bladder volume is below the threshold for inducing voiding (Fig. 4). The accommodation of the bladder to increasing volumes of urine is primarily a passive phenomenon dependent on the intrinsic properties of the vesical smooth muscle and the quiesence of the parasymapthetic efferent pathway [4-6]. In addition in some species urine storage is also facilitated by sympathetic reflexes that mediate an inhibition of bladder activity, closure of the bladder neck and contraction of the proximal part of the urethra. During bladder filling the activity of the sphincter electromyogram (EMG) also increases (Fig. 4) reflecting an increase in efferent firing in the pudendal nerve and an increase in outlet resistance which contributes to the maintanence of urinary continence. Motoneurones of the external urethral sphincter (EUS) are located in a region of the sacral ventral horn, called the nucleus of Onuf, just medial to the motoneurones of the hindlimb and lateral to those of the trunk and axial musculature. In most species motoneurones of the EUS and those of the external anal sphincter are positioned in one nucleus of [10-12], but there exists a considerable variation among species [13-15].

The storage phase of the urinary bladder can be switched to the voiding phase either involuntarily (reflexly) or voluntarily (Fig 4). The former is readily demonstrated in the human infant or in the anesthetized animal when the volume of urine exceeds the micturition threshold. At this point increased afferent firing from tension receptors in the bladder reverses the pattern of efferent outflow, producing firing in the sacral parasympathetic pathways and inhibition of sympathetic and somatic pathways. The expulsion phase consists of an initial relaxation of the urethral sphincter (Fig 4) followed in a few seconds by a contraction of the bladder, an increase in bladder pressure and the flow of urine. Relaxation of the urethral smooth muscle is mediated by activation of a parasympathetic pathway to the urethra that triggers the release of nitric oxide, an inhibitory transmitter [16,17] and by removal of adrenergic and somatic cholinergic excitatory inputs to the urethra. Secondary reflexes elicited by flow of urine through the urethra facilitate bladder emptying [4,5]. These reflexes require the integrative action of neuronal populations at various levels of the neuraxis. Certain reflexes such as those mediating excitatory outflow to the sphincters and sympathetic inhibitory outflow to the bladder are

Table 1 : Reflexes to the Lower Urinary Tract

Afferent Pathway	Efferent Pathway	Central Pathway
Urine storage Low level vesical afferent activity (pelvic nerve)	1. External sphincter contraction (somatic nerves) 2. Internal sphincter contraction (sympathetic nerves) 3. Detrusor inhibition (sympathetic nerves) 4. Ganglionic inhibition (sympathetic nerves) 5. Sacral parasympathetic outflow inactive	Spinal reflexes
Micturition High level vesical afferent activity (pelvic nerve)	1. Inhibition of external sphincter activity 2. Inhibition of sympathetic outflow 3. Activation of parasympathetic outflow to the bladder 4. Activation of parasympathetic outflow to the urethra	Spinobulbospinal Reflexes Spinal Reflex

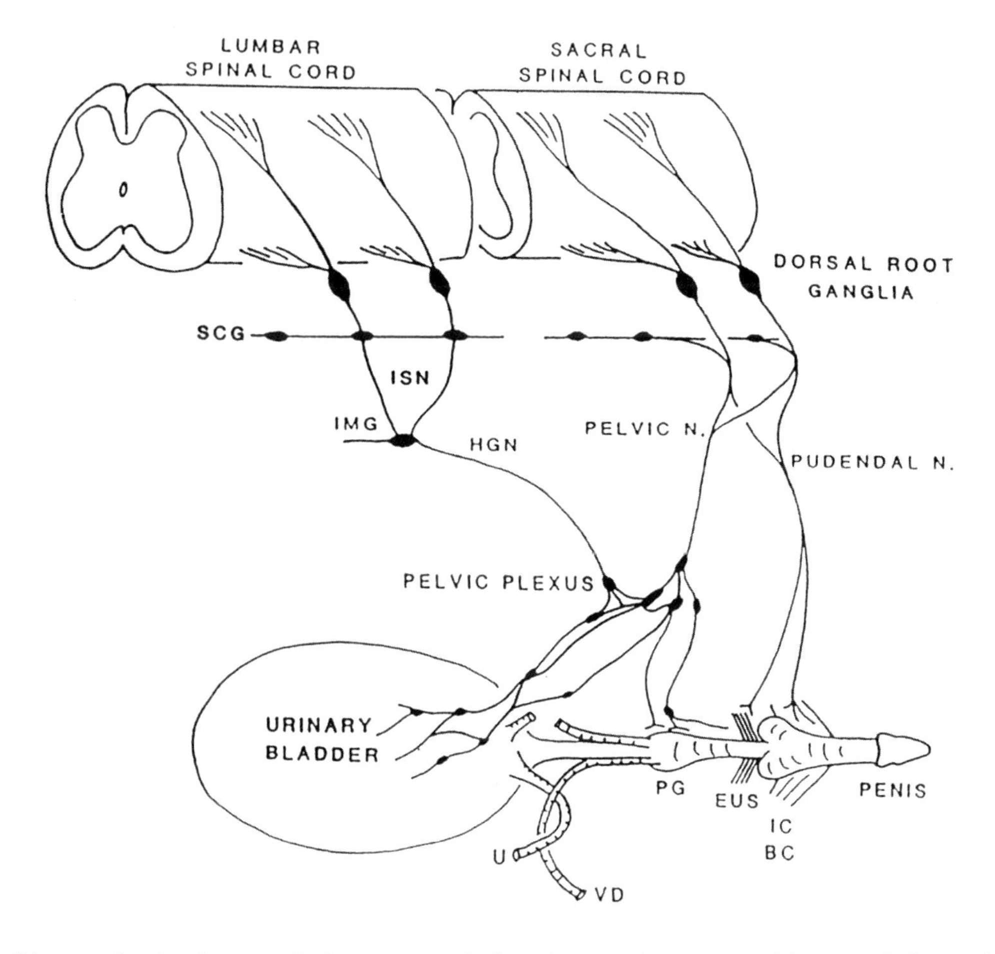

Figure 1 : Diagram showing the sympathetic, parasympathetic and somatic innervation of the urogenital tract of the male cat. Sympathetic preganglionic pathways emerge from the lumbar spinal cord and pass to the sympathetic chain ganglia (SCG) and then via the inferior splanchnic nerves (ISN) to the inferior mesenteric ganglia (IMG). Preganglionic and postganglionic sympathetic axons then travel in the hypogastric nerve (HGN) to the pelvic plexus and the urogenital organs. Parasympathetic preganglionic axons which originate in the sacral spinal cord pass in the pelvic nerve to ganglion cells in the pelvic plexus and to distal ganglia in the organs. Sacral somatic pathways are contained in the pudendal nerve, which provides an innervation to the penis, the ischiocavernosus (IC), bulbocavernosus (BC) and external urethral sphincter (EUS) muscles. The pudendal and pelvic nerves also receive postganglionic axons from the caudal sympathetic chain ganglia. These three sets of nerves contain afferent axons from the lumbosacral dorsal root ganglia. Abbreviations: ureter (U), prostate gland (PG), vas deferens (VD).

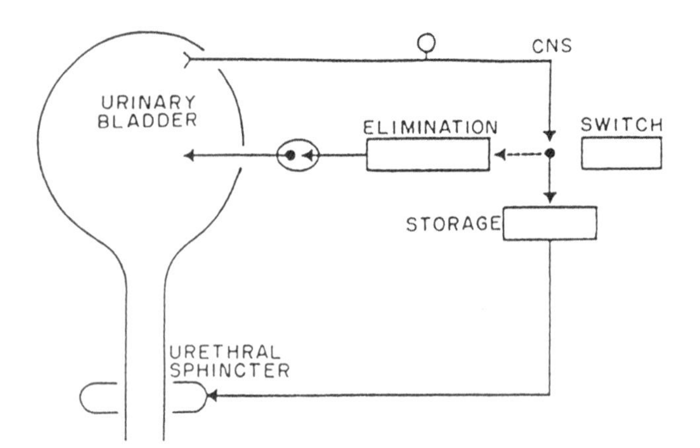

Figure 2 : Diagram illustrating the anatomy of the lower urinary tract and the switchlike function of the micturition reflex pathway. During urine storage, a low level of afferent activity activates efferent input to the urethral sphincter. A high level of afferent activity induced by bladder distention activates the switching circuit in the central nervous system (CNS), producing firing in the efferent pathways to the bladder, inhibition of the efferent outflow to the sphincter, and urine elimination.

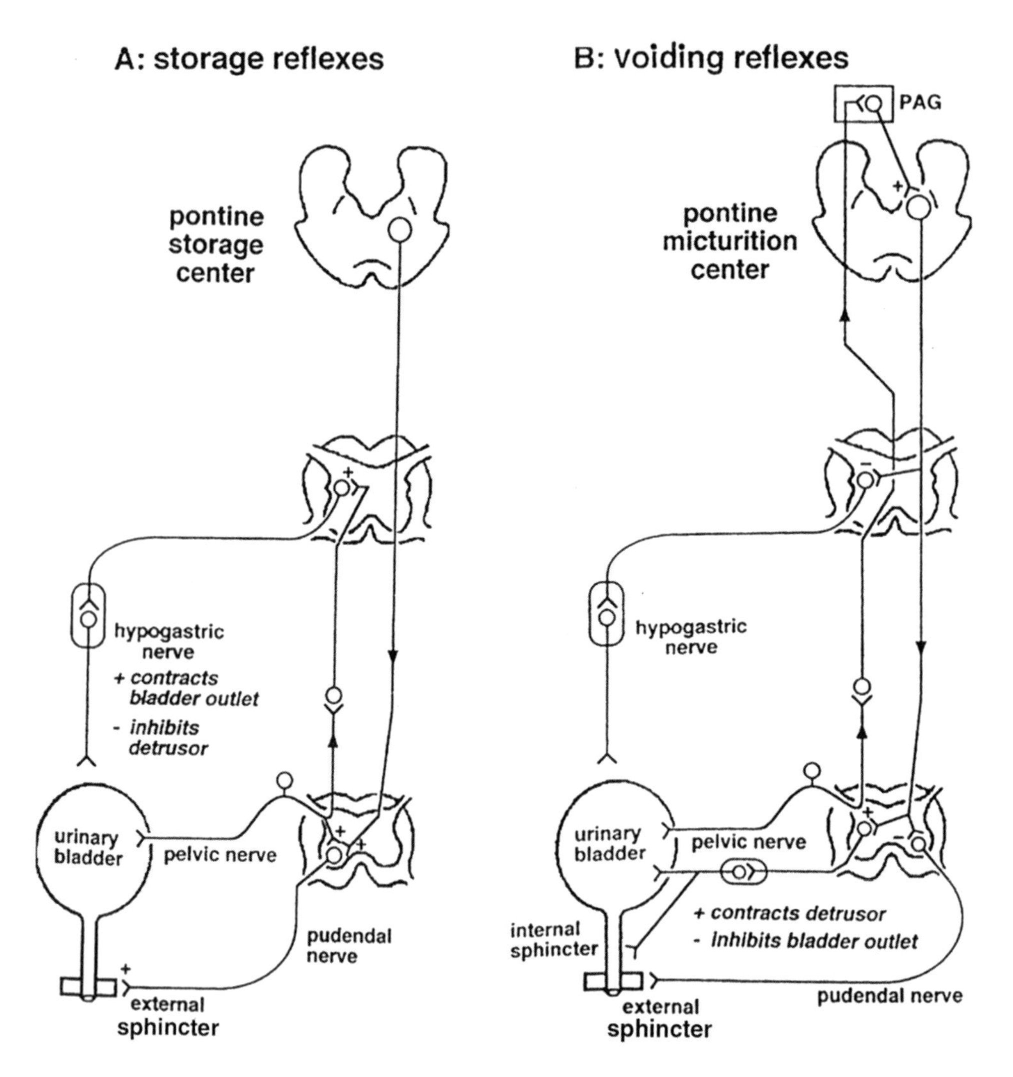

Figure 3 : Diagram showing neural circuits controlling continence and micturition. (A) Urine storage reflexes. During the storage of urine, distention of the bladder produces low level vesical afferent firing, which in turn stimulates (1) the sympathetic outflow to the bladder outlet (base and urethra) and (2) pudendal outflow to the external urethral sphincter. These responses occur by spinal reflex pathways and represent «guarding reflexes», which promote continence. Sympathetic firing also inhibits detrusor muscle and modulates transmission in bladder ganglia. A region in the rostral pons (the pontine storage center or «L» region) increases external urethral sphincter activity. (B) Voinding reflexes. During elimination of urine, intense bladder afferent firing activates spinobulbospinal reflex pathways passing through the pontine micturition center, which stimulate the parasympathetic outflow to the bladder and internal sphincter smooth muscle and inhibit the sympathetic and pudendal outflow to the urethral outlet. Ascending afferent input from the spinal cord may pass through relay neurons in the periaqueductal gray (PAG) before reaching the pontine micturition center.

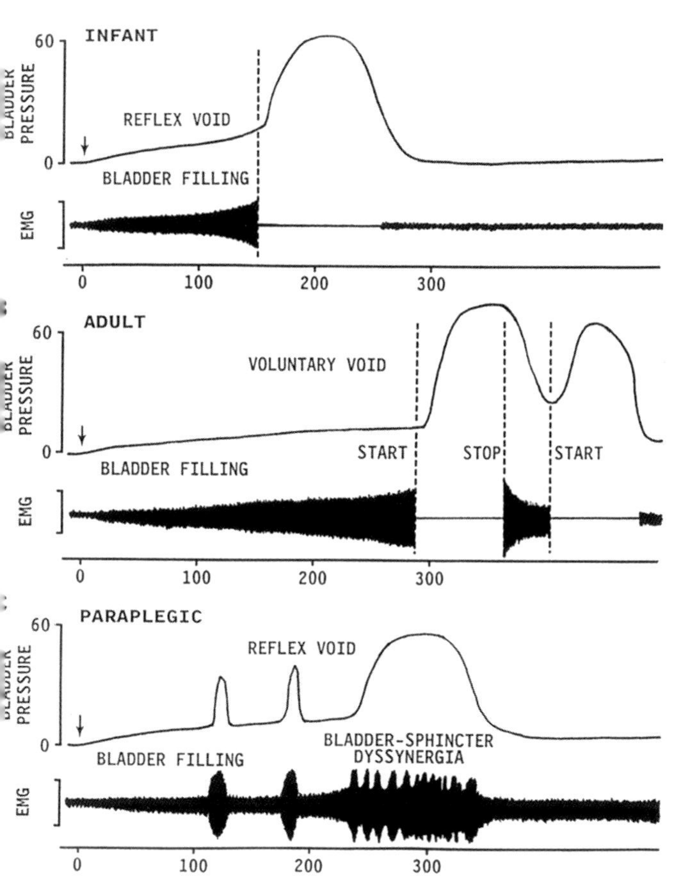

Figure 4 : Combined cystometrograms and sphincter electromyograms (EMG) comparing reflex voiding responses in an infant (A) and in a paraplegic patient (C) with a voluntary voiding response in an adult (B). The abscissa in all records represents bladder volume in milliliters and the ordinates represent bladder pressure in cm H_2O and electrical activity of the EMG recording. On the left side of each trace the arrows indicate the start of a slow infusion of fluid into the bladder (bladder filling). Vertical dashed lines indicate the start of sphincter relaxation which precedes by a few seconds the bladder contraction in A and B. In part B note that a voluntary cessation of voiding (stop) is associated with an initial increase in sphincter EMG followed by a reciprocal relaxation of the bladder. A resumption of voiding is again associated with sphincter relaxation and a delayed increase in bladder pressure. On the other hand, in the paraplegic patient (C) the reciprocal relationship between bladder and sphincter is abolished. During bladder filling, transient uninhibited bladder contractions occur in association with sphincter activity. Further filling leads to more prolonged and simultaneous contractions of the bladder and sphincter (bladder-sphincter dyssynergia).
Loss of the reciprocal relationship between bladder and sphincter in paraplegic patients interferes with bladder emptying.

organized at the spinal level (Fig 3A); whereas the parasympathetic outflow to the detrusor has a more complicated central organization involving spinal and spino-bulbo-spinal pathways (Fig 3B).

Normally, the micturition pathway is switched on five to seven times per day and this stops temporarily the tonic contraction of the pelvic floor, necessary for urinary continence. Neural structures responsible for micturition and urinary continence are located in the rostral brainstem. They coordinate motoneurons of the urinary bladder and the EUS, both groups located in the sacral spinal cord. Interruption of the descending motor fibers from the pons to the sacral cord, for example in a transected spinal cord, abolishes normal micturition and results in reflex incontinence with detrusor-sphincter dyssynergia. Patients with brain lesions rostral to the pons never show detrusor-sphincter dyssynergia. However, these patients might suffer from urge incontinence, i.e. detrusor hyperactivity and an inability to delay voiding at an appropriate place and time. Apparently, centers in the pons coordinate micturition as such, but centres rostral to the pons are responsible for the timing of the start of micturition.

II. AFFERENT NEURONES

1. Properties of bladder afferent neurons.

Afferent axons in the pelvic, hypogastric and pudendal nerves transmit information from the lower urinary tract to the lumbosacral spinal cord. [6,18,19] Pelvic nerve afferents, which monitor the volume of the bladder and the amplitude of the bladder contractions consist of myelinated (A-delta) and unmyelinated (C) axons (Table 2). Sensing bladder volume is of particular relevance during urine storage. On the other hand, afferent discharges that occur during a bladder contraction have an important reflex function and appear to reinforce the central drive that maintains the detrusor contraction. Afferents which respond both to distension and contraction, i.e., " in series tension receptors", have been identified in the pelvic and hypogastric nerves of cats and rats [20-24].

In the last decade there has been an awareness of the need to study bladder afferents under as near physiological conditions as possible to avoid sensitization or desensitization and other effects of repeated distensions on the baseline properties of afferents [24]. Single unit studies continue to have great value because there appear to be different modalities of afferent fibre in the pelvic nerve, so the search stimulus for these afferents

Table 2 : Properties of bladder afferents

Fiber-Type	Location	Normal Function	Effects of Inflammatory Mediators
A-DELTA (finely myelinated axons)	smooth muscle	Respond to muscle wall tension	Increased discharge during distension and lowered pressure thresholds
C-FIBER (unmyelinated axons)	mucosa	Respond to stretch of mucosa (Bladder Volume Sensors)	Increased discharge during distension and lowered pressure thresholds
C-FIBER (unmyelinated axons)	mucosa	Insensitive to normal bladder distension («Silent» Afferents)	Afferents become mechanosensitive thereby unmasking a new afferent pathway during inflammation
C-FIBER (unmyelinated axons)	?mucosa ?muscle ?serosa	Sensitive to overdistension (Nociceptors)	? Sensitive to some irritants

has been the electrical stimulation of the pelvic nerve at very low frequencies. This protocol avoids selecting units by repeated mechanical stimulation of the bladder, which biases the sample towards low threshold afferents and can cause damage and sensitization/desensitization of afferent endings, particularly when repeated frequently.

Afferents that respond only to bladder filling have been identified in the rat bladder, and appear to be volume receptors, possibly sensitive to stretch of the mucosa. In the cat bladder some "in series " tension receptors may also respond to bladder stretch [25]. A few afferents that can be activated at high bladder volumes or pressures have been identified in the rat and the cat [21,23,24, 26,27]. It is unclear to what extent the demonstration of these afferents depends upon sensitization induced by repeated high pressure (80 mm Hg) bladder distensions [26], which may have induced a pathological change in the bladder and affected the properties of some of the afferents that were studied later in the experiments.

Species differences as well as differences of nomenclature might account for some of the variations in reported properties of bladder afferents. For example, the conduction velocity which differentiates A-delta and C-fibres in the cat is 2 meters/sec, whereas in the rat it is 1.3 meters/sec[28]. In the cat, A-delta bladder afferents appear to be low threshold mechanoreceptors [22], whereas some C-bladder afferents [29] are mechano-insensitive ("silent C-fibers") (Table 2). Other 'silent' afferents in the cat may be nociceptive, and have been found to be sensitized by intravesical administration of chemicals [29]. However in the rat there is now evidence that a significant proportion of C fibres are active at physiological volumes , i.e. the proportion of 'silent' afferents is less than had been previously estimated [24,30], and the link between C fibres and nociception becomes more complex than previously recognised, because the 'silent' group of fibres includes some A-delta as well as some C fibres afferents. In a recent well-controlled study [31] it was found that C-fibres afferents in the rat are often mechanosensitive rather than nociceptive, and that some A-delta fibres are 'silent' afferents. Some of the afferents with high mechanical thresholds were not in the body of the bladder but at the vesico-ureteric junction; the location and the different elastic properties at this site can explain some of the differences in the functional properties. Some of the 'silent' afferents responded to capsaicin or potassium and were regarded as chemoreceptors. However, in the rat there is now evidence that C-bladder afferents behave as volume receptors and that the majority do not respond to bladder contractions. Surprisingly, in comparison to the cat, one third of the C-afferents tested behaved as "in series tension receptors", which respond to both distensions and contractions [24, 30]. There is also evidence that hormonal status can change the properies of bladder afferents [31]. Thus the division between physiological, nociceptive and 'silent' afferents is not sharp, and it would be unwise to infer function simply on the basis of conduction velocity.

2. Axon collaterals and axon reflexes

The peripheral axons of most afferent fibres divide into a series of axon collaterals in the organs they innervate, and these axons can release neurotransmitters on to various tissues, including vessels, smooth muscle, urothelium and other neurones. These axon collaterals mediate axonal reflexes, which are the basis for neurogenic extravasation and inflammation [32]. There is evidence in the human bladder that intramural neurones receive axonal contacts that contain the peptides characteristic of primary afferents (see the section on bladder ganglia and smooth muscle). Afferent and efferent fibres have close connections with mast cells in the mucosa and ganglia of the guinea-pig bladder [33] and ultrastructual evidence suggested that the communication between the cells might be bi-directional. It was suggested that these structures participate in axon reflexes that regulate normal vascular and detrusor smooth muscle function and cause vasodilatation, oedema, inflammation, and bladder hyperactivity. Other peptides that can be released by axonal reflexes include CGRP, a breakdown product of which is known to have chemotactic properties [34]. Further evidence for the involvement of mast cells in interstitial cystitis and the participation of NK-1 receptors in antigen induced cystitis indicated a mandatory participation of these receptors in the chain of events linking mast cell degranulation and inflammation [35]. In normal mice, an antigen challenge causes activation of mast cells, plasma extravasation and migration of neutrophils; however none of this occurs in the NK-1 receptor knockout mouse, which appears to be protected from inflammation induced by an antigen challenge.

3. Spinal projections of lower urinary tract primary afferent neurons

Axonal tracing experiments [18,36,37,38] have localized the segmental distribution and spinal termination of afferent pathways in the pelvic, hypogastric and pudendal nerves. The primary afferent neurons of the pelvic and pudendal nerves are contained in sacral dorsal root ganglia; whereas afferent innervation in the hypogastric arises in the rostral lumbar dorsal root ganglia. The central axons of the dorsal root ganglion neurons carry the sensory information from the lower urinary tract to second order neurons in the spinal cord. Transganglionic transport of axonal tracers has identified the spinal projections and terminal fields of visceral and somatic primary afferent neurons (Fig 5).

Visceral afferent fibers of the pelvic [37] and pudendal [38] nerves enter the cord and travel rostrocaudally within Lissauer's tract. Axon collaterals from Lissauer's tract distribute transversely around the lateral and medial edges of the dorsal horn (Figures 5 and 6). These distributions termed the lateral (LCP) and medial collateral pathways (MCP) of Lissauer's tract, respectively, carry axons to deeper layers of the spinal cord. Within the spinal gray matter, the LCP and MCP provide a dense innervation to laminae I, V, and VII and the dorsal commissure. Muscle and cutaneous afferents in the pudendal nerve terminate in different regions of the cord. Central projections of pudendal nerve afferents from the external urethral sphincter muscle have been shown to overlap with those of visceral afferents in the pelvic nerve. However, pudendal nerve cutaneous afferents innervate a terminal field within the medial third of the dorsal horn in laminae III and IV. Proprioceptive afferent fibers from the levator ani muscle are distributed most densely in medial lamina VI. This region is known to contain second order interneurons that mediate reflexes initiated by Golgi tendon organs and muscle spindles.

4. Neurotransmitters

Visceral afferent neurons contain a number of peptidergic neurotransmitters, and the central distribution of bladder afferent terminals and peptidergic immunoreactive fibers is quite similar [18,39] This similarity includes the periodic nature of their distribution in the LCP and their transverse projections through the intermediate gray matter. It has recently been shown that changes in the peptidergic nerves to the bladder occur in chemically induced cystitis [40,41]. Increased expression of CGRP, Substance P and pituitary adenylate cyclase-activating polypeptide (PACAP), a relative of VIP, are present in the spinal projections of pelvic nerve afferents following cyclophosphamide induced cystitis. Within the spinal cord, PACAP appears to facilitate micturition when administered intrathecally, and also has excitatory actions on the spinal slice preparation [42]. Electrophysiologic studies on spinal cord slices from neonatatal rats reveal that this transmitter acts on interneurons that project on to preganglionic neurons [43]. Nonpeptide neurotransmitters, such as glutamic acid [44,45] and ATP also play a role in afferent pathways from the urinary tract.

5. Urothelium : an active membrane

The urothelium is much more than the classical barrier that separates urine from the extracellular fluid. It is also an active absorptive epithelium which absorbs sodium, using amiloride sensitive sodium channels in the urothelial cell membrane. The number of these channels is controlled by the level of cAMP in the cell [46], and by the sodium balance of the animal [47]. The urothelium is also a secretory tissue that secretes urinary proteins such as tissue plasminogen activator and urokinase as well as a protease inhibitor using a Ca^{2+} regulated pathway [48].

The possibility that there may be some active control over the functional state of the urothelium has been recognised for some time. A variety of adrenergic and peptidergic receptors are present in the urothelium of the rat and other species. In the rat, β-1 receptors were predominant in the bladder neck, and β-2 receptors in the bladder dome. In addition, surgical denervation caused an increase in β-1 receptors throughout the whole bladder, which suggested that there was some functional regulation of receptor expression in response to denervation [49-51]. Neurokinin receptors (NK-1, NK-2 and NK-3 receptors) were also found in the mucosa as well as CGRP receptors in the urothelium of the bladder and urethra [50,51]. More recently the VR1 receptor which is activated by capsaicin and protons has also been found in the basal and superficial cells of rat urothelium and in nerve fibres that penetrate the urothelium [52]; the latter staining was reduced following

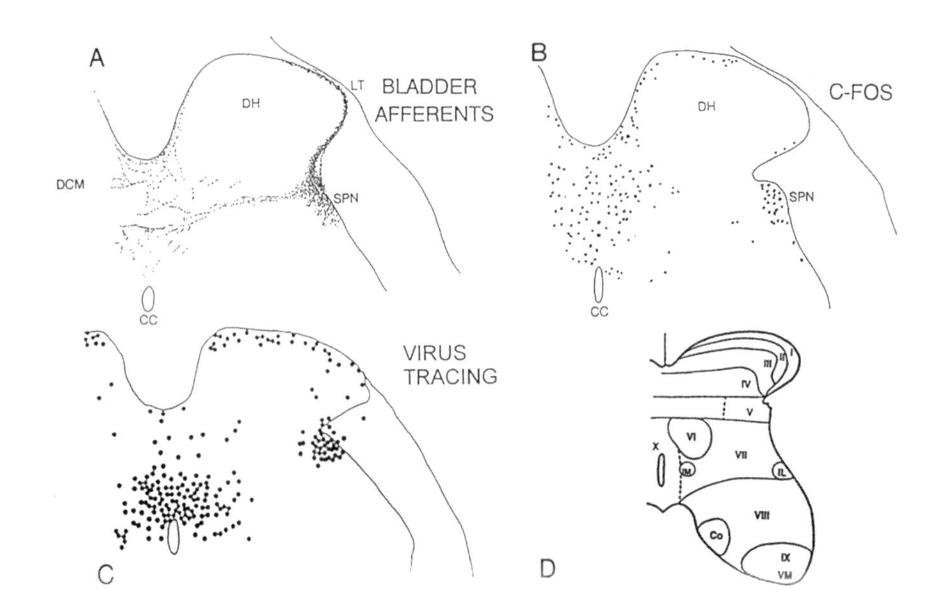

Figure 5 : Comparison of the distribution of bladder afferent projections to the L6 spinal cord of the rat (A) with the distribution of c-fos positive cells in the L6 spinal segment following chemical irritation of the lower urinary tract of the rat (B) and the distribution of interneurons in the L6 spinal cord labeled by transneuronal transport of pseudorabies virus injected into the urinary bladder (C) Afferents labelled by WGA-HRP injected into the urinary bladder. C-fos immunoreactivity is present in the nuclei of cells. DH, dorsal horn; SPN, sacral parasympathetic nucleus; CC central canal. (D) Diagram showing the laminar organization of the spinal cord.

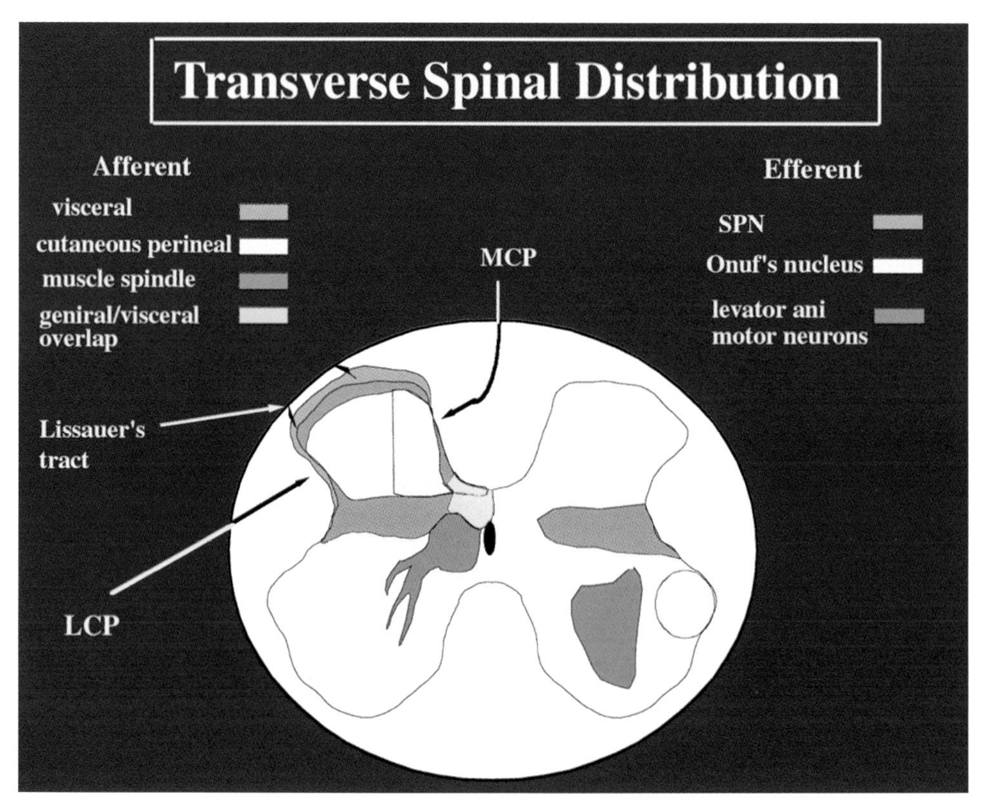

Figure 6 : Neuroanatomical distribution of primary afferent and efferent components of storage and micturition reflexes within the sacral spinal cord. For purposes of clarity, afferent components are shown only on the left, while efferent components are shown only on the right. Both components are, of course, distributed bilaterally and thus overlap extensively. Visceral afferent components (pink and green regions) represent bladder, urethral, and genital (glans penis/clitoris) afferent fibers contained in the pelvic and pudendal nerves. Cutaneous perineal afferent componets represent afferent fibers that innervate the perineal skin contained in the pudendal nerve. Muscle spindle afferent components represent Ia/b afferent fibers contained in the levator ani nerve that innervate muscle spindles in the levator ani muscle.
SPN sacral parasympathetic nucleus LCP lateral collateral projection MCP medial collateral projection

treatment with capsaicin, which suggests that these VR1 receptors were on afferent nerve endings. The VR1 receptor has also been identified in human urothelium [589]. In urothelial cells cultured from cat bladders, functional evidence of P2Y receptors was found in normal animals, and of P2X receptors in cats with feline interstitial cystitis [53]. All in all this indicates that the urothelial cells have a number of important receptors on their surface: adrenoceptors, CGRP receptors, VR1 receptors as well as neurokinin and purinergic receptor subtypes.

So there is a firm basis to the conclusion that the urothelium may be a target for the action of certain neurotransmitters including amines, purines and peptides. The responses of this tissue to such stimuli include the production of mediators that may act within the bladder wall.

6. Mucosal afferents

There is now good ultrastructural evidence that there is an afferent innervation of the epithelium which involves not only afferent endings underneath the lamina propria, but also afferent nerve endings within the urothelium itself. Intramural axons have been identified in frozen sections and in whole mount preparations of rat bladder mucosa and smooth muscle using synaptophysin-immunofluorescence and CGRP immunoreactivity as a marker for afferent axons [54]. These afferent axons were distributed over four distinct targets: (a) the base of the epithelium, (b) inside the epithelium, (c) the blood vessels (both arteries and veins) and (d) the muscle bundles. In the mucosa, all the afferent axons, except the perivascular ones, lay either inside the epithelium itself or in a subepithelial plexus very close to the basal surface of the epithelium, where multiple branching was common. The plexus was thickest in the neck of the bladder and in the initial portion of the urethra, and it became progressively less dense in the adjacent regions. It did not extend beyond the equatorial region, and therefore the mucosa of the cranial region of the bladder had no afferent axons. In contrast, the afferent innervation of the musculature was more diffuse, and appeared uniform throughout the bladder. CGRP-immunofluorescence in mucosal afferent axons was enhanced in the surviving axons 5 days after contralateral denervation, a change which may be an early sign of regeneration of these axons. In the human bladder, CGRP together with Substance P and NKA occur only infrequently in nerves in the muscle but are moderately frequent in the suburothelial layer. Also in the human there appears to be another population of CGRP-containing fibres that co-localize with NPY and galanin and some of these synapse on intramural ganglia within the bladder [55-58]. There is also recent evidence that nerve endings are found crossing the basal lamina and entering the basal layers of the human urothelium [59]. Substantial cross over of afferents from one side of the bladder to the other was present and was also found in tracing studies [60]. Nevertheless, the former authors did observe that unilateral denervation did leave some areas of the bladder wall without afferent innervation.

Levin et al [61] found that removal of the urothelium significantly and substantially increased the contractile response of the cat bladder to to electrical field stimulation, and to potassium, bethanechol and phenylephrine. They concluded that in this species, the mucosa has a significant inhibitory effect on the contractile response of the bladder to stimulation. There are a series of mediators, including nitric oxide and ATP that may be released by the mucosa, and act on the urothelium, the afferent and efferent nerves, and on the smooth muscle itself.

III. SENSITIVITY OF AFFERENT ENDINGS

1. Role of ATP and P2X3 receptors

Recent studies of mice have shown that one of the ATP receptors, the P2X3 receptor, is present in small sensory neurones innervating the bladder mucosa, and that the effects of bladder distension on these sensory endings is markedly attenuated if the gene for the P2X3 receptor is deleted. P2X3 knockout mice show major changes in sensation and in the function of the lower urinary tract, so severe that the bladder capacity is increased, the cystometrograms indicate the presence of hyporeflexia, and the frequency of urination is reduced. This receptor is one of many purinergic receptors present in the bladder and lower urinary tract, and the topic is sufficiently important to summarise the salient features of the P2X family of receptors and their distribution in rodents and humans. Of these, at least 7 subtypes of P2X receptors appear in the rat bladder [62]. Their distribution is shown in the following table, which indicates that ATP must have a major role to play within the urothelium, smooth muscle and neurones of the bladder wall.

The P2X3 receptor is of particular interest with respect to the physiology of pelvic nerve afferents because it is selectively expressed on small diameter sensory neurons, and knockout mice that do not express this receptor exhibit a marked urinary bladder hyporeflexia, characterized by decreased voiding frequency and increased bladder capacity, but normal bladder pressures [63,64]. In addition, these null mice have reduced pain-related behaviour in response to injection of ATP and formalin; and they lose the rapidly desensitizing ATP-

Table 3 : Purinergic receptors

Subtype	Distribution of Puringeric Receptor Subtypes in Rodent Bladder [62,63,76,151]
P2X1	the main purinergic receptor present in the smooth muscle cell membranes.
P2X2	present within smooth muscle
P2X3	present in nerve bundles within the detrusor and in submucosal afferents
P2X4	present in capillaries in the detrusor and lamina propria,
P2X5	a strong reaction from urothelial cell membranes
P2X6	in the basement membrane below the urothelium
P2X7	present in urothelial nuclei

induced currents in dorsal root ganglion neurons and have a reduction in the sustained ATP-induced currents in nodose ganglion neurons. Immunohistochemical studies localize P2X3 to nerve fibres innervating the urinary bladder of wild-type mice, and show that loss of P2X3 does not alter sensory neuron innervation density. Thus, P2X3 is critical for peripheral pain responses and afferent pathways controlling urinary bladder volume reflexes, which take place at physiological volumes and pressures. Antagonists to P2X3 may therefore have therapeutic potential in the treatment of disorders of urine storage and voiding such as overactive bladder.

The idea that ATP is released from urothelial cells by exposure to raised hydrostatic pressure was proposed by Ferguson et al [65] and this idea was followed up in in vitro experiments in the rat by Navasivayam et al [66]. During normal cystometry the number of impulses generated in the afferent neurons was halved after treatment with the P2X antagonist suramin, which indicated that a substantial part of the responses could be generated by the chemical purinergic signal rather than by a mechanosensitive mechanism. Suramin however is not a specific antagonist, but confirmation of the main conclusion (that mechanosensitivy is at least partly mediated by sensitivity to ATP released by stretch of the tissues) came from recent studies [67] of knockout mice, which indicated that ATP was released in the mucosa during bladder distensions, and that this release was also present and unchanged in the knockout mice. The afferent response to distension however was greatly attenuated in the knockout animals, indicating that the mechanosensitive properties of these afferents are probably largely associated with their sensitivity to ATP released within the bladder wall. Most recently, there has been a single unit analysis of bladder afferents from wild and knockout mice that also used a much more specific P2X3 receptor antagonist [68]. These studies confirmed that in this species much of the mechanoceptive response of the afferents was mediated by ATP. It appears therefore that the afferent limb of the micturition reflex is mediated to a large extent by chemoreceptors that respond to the local release of ATP

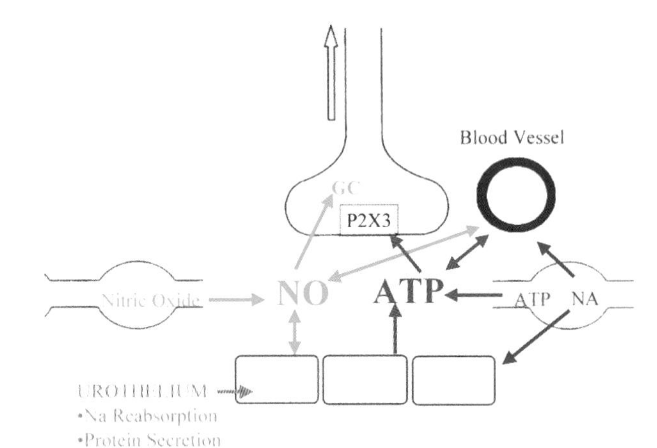

Figure 7 : This diagram of the relationship between the urothelium and an afferent nerve endings indicates the sources and effects of two important mediators – ATP and nitric oxide. The P2X3 receptor is a purinerguic receptor on afferent nerve endings that is believed to be intimately involved with the process of mechano-transduction. Noradrenaline (NA) is co-released along with ATP from sympathetic nerve endings. Nitric Oxide (NO) acts on guanylate cyclase (GC) in the afferent nerve endings.

during distensions. Furthermore, this chemosensitivity is active in the normal range of volume and pressure, and suggests that the afferent pathways of the micurition reflex arc not confined to endings in the smooth muscle layer, and that stretch of the urothelium is also involved. The P2X3 and P2X5 receptors on the smooth muscle at the site of contacts with parasympathetic neurones are lacking in patients with detrusor instability and urge [69]; some further discussion of this is contained in the section on efferent innervation of the bladder. (Fig. 7)

2. Role of nitric oxide

Nitric oxide is an important mediator that can be released from urothelium and from neurones in the submucosal plexus. The detrusor however is not very sensitive to nitric oxide in contrast to the outflow region where it effectively relaxed the smooth muscle, which suggests an involvement of nitric oxide in the decrease in urethral pressure at the start of micturition [70].

NO may be involved in the control of afferent sensitivity, and we now know that NO may in some circumstances, such as spinal cord injury, increase the activity of capsaicin-sensitive nerves within the bladder wall [71]. Basal release of nitric oxide has not been detected in the urothelium of the normal cat; however it is released in cats with feline interstitial cystitis [53], and from normal cats after the addition of agonists. Nitric oxide release from neurones and from the urothelium has been studied also in a variety of pathophysiological models using direct measurements. In one model of interstitial cystitis created by injecting DMSO into the rat bladder, there was an increase in reflex activity in pelvic efferent neurones, a decreased bladder capacity and increased afferent activity in capsaicin sensitive bladder afferents (as indicated by the development of c-fos expression in sensory pathways). In that study [72], NO was released from dorsal root ganglion cells and from urinary bladder strips by the addition of DMSO or capsaicin. In addition in normal bladders it was shown [73] that capsaicin causes NO release from the urothelium and from the bladder nerves, while norepinephrine caused NO production and release from the urothelium only. Norepinephrine of course can be released from sympathetic nerve terminals along with ATP and NPY, and this could be one mechanism by which the bladder is affected in spinal cord injury. Increased expression of neuronal NOS in bladder afferent and spinal neurones occurs following cord injury [74], and in bladder afferents following chronic bladder irritation with cyclophosphamide. Nitric oxide can act on cultures of urothelial cells to lower paracellular epithelial resistance [73], and this damaging effect on the urothelium may allow other mediators to act on sensory endings. Interestingly, the deleterious effects of nitric oxide on urothelial resistance can be blocked with GM_1 ganglioside. There is also evidence that nitric oxide can inhibit the function of primary afferent neurons [590, 591].

Nitric oxide can therefore be produced by the urothelium itself and by some of the neurones in the bladder wall and the vessels. This released NO can act on a number of targets, including sensory neurones and the urothelium itself. Knockout mice that do not have neuronal NOS appear to have normal function in the lower urinary tract ([75], and knockout animals that do not have inducible NOS are not particularly abnormal. However, the latter appear to need iNOS in the response to urinary obstruction [76]. So there is clear evidence that in certain models nitric oxide is an important mediator, but possibly not so much in normal animals.

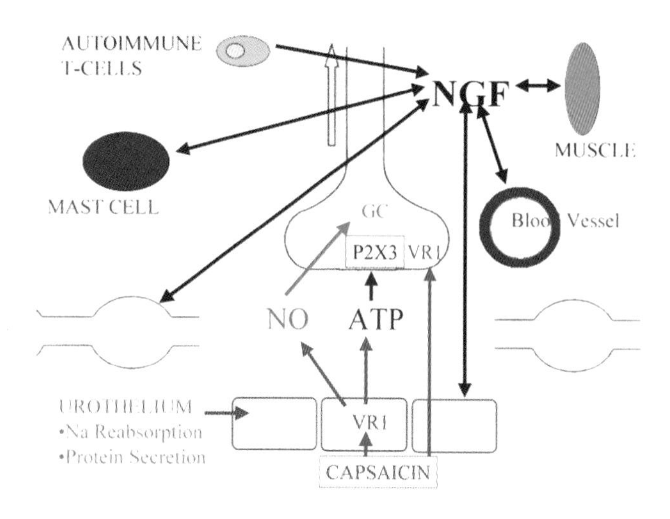

Figure 8 : This diagram of the relationship between the urothelium and an afferent nerve endings indicates the sources and effects of other important mediators – the vanilloid receptor (VR-1) ,which influences nitric oxide and ATP release, and nerve growth facto (NGF).

3. Role of tachykinins and NK-2 receptors

An electrophysiological study of pelvic nerve afferents during slow cystometry in the rat also found evidence of three types of response that characterised three classes of afferent neurones [31,77,78]. Some afferents were silent, and did not respond to distension of the bladder; most of these were C-fibres. Of those that did respond to distension, one subgroup gave the classical 'in series' type of response characterised by excitation during distension and during bladder contraction; most of these were A-delta fibres, but there was also a significant contribution from C-afferents. However, many afferents (including A-delta and C-fibres) responded only to distension, and it seems likely that these were present in the mucosa if not in the epithelium. These may be regarded as volume receptors or mucosal receptors, and significantly with respect to the latter location, they also respond to chemicals introduced within the bladder itself. These properties rather favour the view that these endings exist in the submucosa. They are probably best described as polymodal in their responses, and their excitability can be increased by a number of intravesical chemical stimuli. These nerve endings probably correspond with those described histochemically that contain CGRP, Substance P and NKA, and some of these afferents are also capsaicin-sensitive. They probably take part in axon reflexes within the bladder mucosa and release mediators including CGRP, Substance P and Neurokinin A, and are probably the source of the tachykinins that act on the NK-1 and NK-2 receptors on mast cells, smooth muscle and other nerve endings.

The view that tachykinins can sensitize sensory nerve endings is based (a) autoradiographic studies that show the disappearance of NK-2 receptors in the submucosa in capsaicin-treated rats that are deficient in sensory nerves [51], (b) on studies in which afferents can be made hypersensitive using a NKA- analogue and other intravesical chemical stimuli such as high $[K^+]$ and high osmolality, and (c) the demonstration that the development of hypersensitivity to a number of sensitizing agents including high $[K^+]$ can be blocked by an NK-2 receptor antagonist [31,77]. More recently it has been shown that rat dorsal root ganglion neurones are excited by NK2 agonists, but are inhibited by NK-3 agonists [79]. This NK2 action is on L- and N-type Ca^{2+} channels, whereas the NK-3 action is only on the L-type channels. Both of these effects are blocked by inhibition of protein kinase C.

4. Role of vanilloid (VR-1) and opiate receptor-like (ORL1) receptors

Mention has already been made of the actions of capsaicin on the urothelium and nerves. The release of NO and the increase in intracellular Ca^{2+} induced by capsaicin are blocked by the VR-1 antagonist capsazepine. The actions of capsaicin can also be facilitated by protons, which is of interest because the VR-1 receptor is known to be sensitive to protons. Whenever a membrane receptor is the site of action of an exogenous agent (for example, morphine acting on opiate receptors), the possibility of an endogenous agent (enkephalins, in the case of opiate receptors) indicates the possibility that there are new endogenous compounds that may play a role in physiology or pathophysiology. Anandamide and Nociceptin are two such compounds and are sufficiently new to deserve a mention, although much more work needs to be done to elucidate their roles.

a) Anandamide is an endogenous cannabinoid which also is an agonist of VR-1 receptors [80,81] and acts on peripheral perivascular sensory terminals in a manner that is antagonised by the capsaicin antagonist capsezepine. It can cause the release of CGRP and Substance P by increasing intracellular Ca2+, and has other actions, such as activation of G-proteins [82]. The role of anandamide in the lower urinary tract is unknown, but the identification of a naturally occurring agonist of the VR-1 receptor is worth noting. The VR-1 (capsaicin) receptor is a cation channel expressed by nociceptive neurones and can also be activated by protons or temperature greater than 43 degrees C [83,84]. Within the bladder, it may be that it is activated naturally by low pH, but such changes (e.g. in metabolic acidosis) are not usually associated with bladder pain. The expression of the VR-1 receptor in sensory neurones is regulated by Nerve Growth Factor (NGF), and concomitant with its expression, stimulation of the VR-1 receptor with capsaicin causes the release of CGRP [85].

b) Nociceptin, another endogenous ligand that binds with the opioid receptor-like 1 receptor (ORL1 receptor) has been shown to have naloxone resistant inhibitory effects on the micturition reflex. These actions are mediated at several sites including the capsaicin sensitive nerves in the bladder, and a central supraspinal site [86]. Nociceptin (100 nmol/kg) produced a long-lasting protection from capsaicin desensitization of the afferent nerves that mediate the chemoceptive micturition reflex. In fact a chemoceptive micturition reflex could be repeatedly evoked by topical capsaicin in nociceptin-pretreated rats. This is in sharp contrast to the effects of nociceptin on the local response to capsaicin which correspond to the 'efferent' function of capsaicin-sensitive afferent neurons. Taken together, these results suggest that the afferent and 'efferent' functions of capsaicin-sensitive primary afferent neurons in the rat bladder are differentiated by nociceptin, and that nociceptin has a significant action on afferent sensitivity.

Local adminsitration of kappa-opioid receptor agonists by intra-arterial injection attenuated the responses of pelvic nerve afferents from the bladder to high pressures distension of the urinary bladder [87]. These agonists had essentially the same effects whether the bladder was inflammed or not. The conclusion was that the ability of kappa opioid agonists to attenuate the responses of afferents to large bladder distensions indicated a potential use for peripherally acting kappa opioid receptor agonists in the control of urinary bladder pain.

5. Role of neurotrophins

Nerve Growth Factor (NGF; neurotrophin-1), the first of a group of growth factors called neurotrophins, is produced in larger quantities in humans with detrusor overactivity [88], interstitial cystitis and bladder cancer [89], in rats with inflammed bladders [90], spinal cord injury or chemically induced cystitis [40] or bladder outlet obstruction [91], in diabetic rats [92] and a number of other states. This protein is known to sensitize afferents from the bladder [93] and it is involved in the production of referred pain in bladder inflammation [94]. It also appears to stimulate the expression of the vanilloid receptor VR-1 [85] (Figure 9). Dmitrieva and McMahon (1996) demonstrated a role for NGF in sensitizing bladder afferents [95]. After filling the bladder with human recombinant NGF, the large majority of afferents, both myelinated and unmyelinated, became sensitised and some of the initially non-mechanosensi-

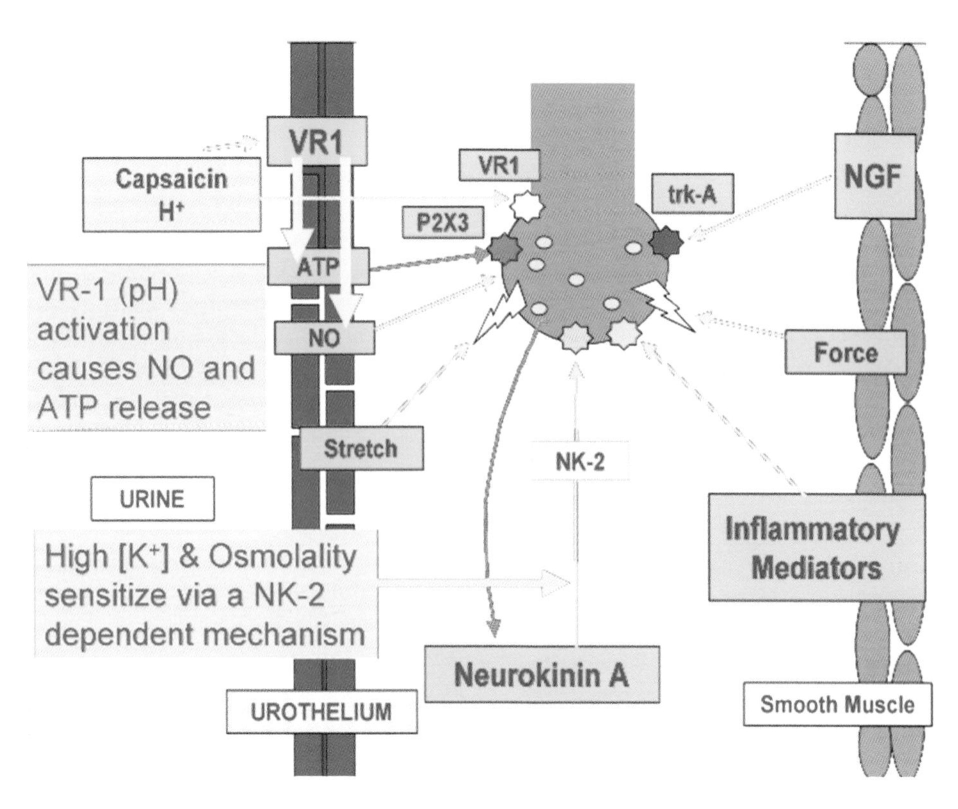

Figure 9 : This diagram summarises the relationships between different tissue component and the afferent nerve endings, and the role of different mediators.

tive became mechanosensitive. The sensitisation began within 30 min of exposure to NGF, and persisted for at least 3 hours. NGF also caused a dose-dependent extravasation of Evan's blue into the bladder, which suggests that axonal reflex mechanisms may be activated. Administration of NGF into the bladder causes bladder hyper-reactivity in Wistar, but not in Sprague-Dawley rats [96], and the effect was not influenced by pretreatment with capsaicin. This report concluded that the A-delta afferents were involved particularly in the development of hyper-reactivity. There is also evidence of referred pain following instillation of NGF into the bladder [85].

Clemow et al (2000) found that cyclic and static stretching of bladder smooth muscle cells stimulates increased NGF production. This was particularly pronounced in certain strains of rats (e.g. the spontaneously hypertensive rat and the Wistar-Kyoto Hypertensive rat). Another source of NGF is the vascular smooth muscle, and gene transcription, intracellular Ca^{2+}, protein kinase C (PKC), and autocrine release of an unknown factor appear to play a part in secretion from vascular and bladder smooth muscle. Basal cytosolic Ca^{2+} appears to be particularly involved in the regulation of NGF secretion in bladder and vascular smooth muscle cells [97].

Recently NGF gene insertion into the bladder and bladder afferent pathways as a possible treatment for diabetic cystopathy in rats, using herpes simplex virus type 1 as a vector, has been investigated [98]. The expectation was that the NGF gene may be transferred to the afferent neurones using the virus and that the expression of NGF would be increased, thus improving the availability and transport of NGF within neurones that are deficient in the protein. This experiment was successful and clearly points to one way forward in the potential treatments of this condition.

Brain Derived Neurotrophic Factor (BDNF) levels in the urinary bladder and some other epithelia are higher than those found in the brain or skin [99]. These authors concluded that visceral epithelia are a major source, but not a target, of BDNF in the adult viscera. The abundance of BDNF protein in certain internal organs suggests that this neurotrophin may regulate the function of adult visceral sensory and motor neurons. In situ hybridization experiments showed that BDNF mRNA was made by visceral epithelial cells, in several types of smooth muscle, and in neurons of the myenteric plexus. However the target receptors (trkB and p75[NTR]) were not present on the urothelium but were present in on neurons of the peripheral nervous system. Hence the neurotrophin is produced by the urothelium and can act on the nerves.

The mRNAs for NGF, BDNF and neurotrophin-3 all increase within 2 hours of bladder inflammation in the rat, and these were responsible for mediating the changes in sensory and reflex hyperactivity. However the increases in neurotrophic factor concentrations are not maintained despite an increase in their mRNAs [40,90]. These changes were most marked 4 days after acute spinal cord injury when the mRNAs for β-NGF, BDNF, Glial-Derived Growth factor [GDNF], Ciliary Neurotrophic factor [CNTF], and neurotrophins 3 and 4 [NT-3 and NT-4] were all grossly elevated. It was also concluded that these mRNAs change during development and that there is a relatively high expression of NT-3 and NT-4 protein in the adult urinary bladder, which suggests a potential importance of these factors in the adult lower urinary tract [40].

An approach to the problem of neuroprotection has been followed recently using antigen specific T-cells that target areas of damaged nerve and release neurotrophins at those sites so as to provide local neuroprotection. This mechanism is given the term neuroprotective autoimmunity [100]. In intersitital cystitis it is known that different types of inflammatory cells infiltrate the bladder wall [101,102]. These include T-cells, B-cells and macrophages, and interest has recently focused on the role of these cells in the type of inflammation found in this condition. Christmas [102] suggested that the increased numbers of CD4+, CD8+ and gamma delta cells as well as IgA+, IgG+ and IgM+ plasma cells within the urothelium and submucosa in patients with IC play an active role in the pathogenesis of the disorder. More recently there is evidence that neurotrophins can be released from autoimmune T-cells that are reactivated on meeting a specific antigen: the list of neurotrophins that can be released includes NGF, BDNF, NT-3 and NT-4/5. The mRNAs for the neurotrophin receptors TrkA, TrkB and p75 can be expressed in injured nerves, and it has been suggested that these specific receptors can mediate the effects of T-cell derived neurotrophins [103]. They also presented evidence that the neurotrophins were mediators that provided neuroprotection and suggested that T-cell intervention in the injured CNS may be a useful means of promoting protection by the supply of neurotrophins. The idea of neuroprotective autoimmunity is relatively recent in the literature [100] but is seen as a potential therapy in a number of disorders involving nerve injury. It is doubtful if T-cell mediated mechanisms are involved in most of the acute injury models studied in the lower urinary tract, but it seems quite possible that such mechanisms may be involved in chronic states such as interstitial cystitis. Recently a Japanese study using a new immunoregulator (IPD-1151T) that suppresses helper T cell mediated allergic responses has shown an improvement in symptoms and a reduction in inflammatory cell populations [104].

6. Effects of repetitive nerve stimulation on bladder activity; influence of urethral afferents

The functional properties of reflexes from the rat and cat bladder can be influenced by repetitive electrical stimulation, which causes an increased excitability of the micturition reflex and a lowering of micturition threshold. It has been known for many years that repetitive stimulation of A-delta afferents can alter the excitability of the micturition reflex in the cat [107]. It has recently been suggested that the prolonged enhancement of excitatory synaptic transmission is due to facilitation of the central micturition reflex pathway [105,106,108]. The same group also provided evidence of facilitation of the micturition reflex from stimulation of uretheral afferents, and of inhibition of bladder activity by stimulation of the dorsal nerve of the clitoris [108], which is in keeping with known interactions from the vagina and colon [4,109]. Stimulation of urethral afferents by flowing fluid through the urethra can facilitate the micturition reflex; however contraction of the urethral sphincter resulted in inhibition of bladder motility [110].

IV. EFFERENT NEURONS

1. Parasympathetic preganglionic neurons

Bladder parasympathetic preganglionic neurons (PGN) are located in the lateral part of the sacral intermediate gray matter in a region termed the sacral parasympathetic nucleus (SPN) (Old Fig. 6). The PGN are small , fusiform-shaped cells which send dendrites into lateral lamina I of the dorsal horn , the lateral funiculus and medially into the dorsal commissure. The dendritric structure very likely indicates the origin of important synaptic inputs to the cells.[5,35,36,37,114,115]. Bladder PGN send axons through the ventral roots to peripheral ganglia where they release the excitatory transmitter, acetylcholine[111]. In some species they release opioid peptide transmitters and express nitric oxide synthase [112], suggesting that they also release nitric oxide. The reflex activity and control of the parasympathetic neurones innervating the bladder is the subject of the section on Central Nervous Control.

2. External urethral sphincter motoneurons

External urethral sphincter (EUS) motoneurons are located in a circumscribed region of the sacral ventral horn, Onuf's nucleus (Fig. 6). In primates and carnivores, Onuf's nucleus is located along the lateral border of the ventral horn [38]. Within the nucleus, urethral motor neurons occupy a ventrolateral position and anal motor neurons occupy a dorsomedial position. Sphincter motoneurons exhibit tightly-bundled dendrites that run rostrocaudally within the confines of the nucleus. In addition to the rostrocaudal dendritic projections, sphincter motor neurons also exhibit transversely oriented dendritic bundles that project laterally into the lateral funiculus, dorsally into the intermediate gray matter, and dorsomedially toward the central canal. This dendritic pattern is similar to that of bladder PGN and very different from that of limb motoneurons, suggesting that EUS motoneurons and PGN receive inputs from similar regions of the spinal cord. EUS motoneurons send axons through the ventral roots and into the pudendal nerves.

• *Pudendal nerve reflexes*

The activation of urethral striated muscle sphincter neurons in response to stimulation of bladder (pelvic nerve) or urethral/perineal (pudendal nerve) afferents is part of a continence-maintaining mechanism. These reflexes recorded as efferent discharges on the pudendal nerve in chloralose-anesthetized cats were suppressed by the $\alpha1$ adrenoceptor antagonist, prazosin [113,117], but not by the $\alpha2$ blocker, idazoxan. On the other hand, clonidine, an $\alpha2$ adrenoceptor agonist suppressed the reflex in anesthetized cats [118,587]. The noradrenaline uptake blocker, tomoxetine, produced a slight inhibition alone and only a slightly greater inhibition after prazosin [586]. However, it greatly facilitated the reflex when given after idazoxan, implying that the $\alpha2$ adrenoceptor-dependent inhibitory mechanism is the dominant adrenergic modulator of this reflex under these conditions. Thus, $\alpha1$ adreneoceptor stimulation facilitates sphincter reflexes, while $\alpha2$ adreneoceptor stimulation inhibits sphincter reflexes. Stimulation of 5HT2 serotonin receptors also facilitates sphincter reflexes [115]. The pudendal nerve reflex firing in chloralose anesthetized cats was abolished by intrathecal administration of the κ-opioid agonist, ethylketocyclazocine, leaving a hindlimb reflex and bladder activity unaffected [114]. By contrast, the δ-opioid agonist, D-Ser^2-Leu^5-enkephalin-Thr^6 (DSLET), abolished bladder activity and reduced the sphincter reflex to about 60% of control, leaving a hindlimb reflex unaffected [116]. Thus the spinal opioid modulation of the external urethral sphincter has characteristics quite different from those regulating the bladder. In conclusion, the relative selectivity of monoaminergic and opioidergic modulation of this pathway offers some possibility for drug development.

3. Lumbar sympathetic outflow

Sympathetic PGN which are located in the intermediate grey matter of the rostral lumbar spinal cord have similar morphological and chemical properties to those of the parasympathetic nucleus. However, the reflex connections of the sympathetic neurones are very different from those of the parasympathetic system. There are at least two types of sympathetic postganglionic neurones that appear to be involved with the regulation of motility in the hypogastic nerve, which innervates the bladder, as well as vasoconstrictor neurones. These neurones affect transmission through the pelvic ganglia and may have direct effects on the smooth muscle and urothelium. They are regulated by afferent inputs from the bladder and the somatic domain, and by descending pathways from the brainstem and higher centres. In the chloralose-anesthetized cat, prazosin or doxazosin, $\alpha1$ adrenoceptor antagonists, suppressed spontaneous firing or the reflex discharge recorded on the hypogastric nerve in response to pelvic nerve afferent stimulation [113,587]. Clonidine, an α_2 agonist also suppresses the pelvic-to-hypogastric reflex [587] whereas idazoxan, an ?2 antagonist, had no effect. On the other hand, tomoxitine, a noradrenaline uptake blocker, inhibited the reflex, implying that the inhibitory (presumably $\alpha2$ adrenoceptor-dependent) mechanism was not very active under control conditions but could be exaggerated by elevating endogenous noradrenaline levels. This inhibition could be overcome by bladder distension. These results suggest that the lumbar sympathetic outflow is controlled by $\alpha1$ excitatory and $\alpha2$ inhibitory mechanisms. Although noradrenergic modulation of this pathway has been demonstrated in animals, it is not clear whether manipulation of the lumbar sympathetic outflow to the urinary tract can be exploited therapeutically.

V. PERIPHERAL AUTONOMIC INNERVATION AND GANGLIA

1. Localisation and histochemistry

The organisation of the peripheral autonomic nervous system supplying the lower urinary tract is not well understood and is probably considerably more complicated than suggested by the classical picture of parasympathetic and sympathetic innervation shown in most medical text-books. It is now clear that many peripheral ganglia supply post-ganglionic input to the various elements of the lower urinary tract, but it is difficult to define these ganglia unambiguously as either sympathetic or parasympathetic. Apart from the pelvic plexus, itself a diffuse and ill-defined area of nerves and ganglia, autonomic ganglia are present in the bladder, both in the suburothelium and the smooth muscle layers, and in the serosa surrounding the bladder neck and proximal urethra. An example is shown in Figure 10. A similar pattern is seen in many mammals, although the rat has a more discreet pelvic ganglion and few, if any ganglia are present in the bladder wall itself [119].

Recent studies have looked in some detail at the histochemistry and immunohistochemistry of nerves and ganglia supplying the human lower urinary tract. Panneuronal stains such as PGP 9.5 can show the full extent of the local innervation and percentages of the nerves or neurones containing the various transmitters, neuromodulators or enzymes involved in synthesising them can be assessed using specific staining techniques. Acetylcholinesterase is most commonly used to identify putative cholinergic nerves and NADPH diaphorase to localise NO synthase containing nerves. Immunoreactivity to tyrosine hydroxylase (TH), neuropeptide Y (NPY), vasoactive intestinal polypeptide (VIP), calcitonin gene-related peptide (CGRP) substance P (SubP), enkephalin (ENK), somatostatin (Som), galanin (Gal), neurokinin A (NKA), nitric oxide synthase (NOS) and haemoxygenase (HO-2), synthesising CO, have been investigated and shown to be present in nerves running in the lower urinary tract. Choline acetyltransferase (ChAT) immunoreactivity has also been studied, but it has proved difficult to get reliable staining of nerves using antibodies to this enzyme; more recently the distribution of vesicular acetylcholine transporter (VAChT) has been used to identify cholinergic nerves and neurones [120].

a) Innervation of the bladder body

There are several published studies looking at the distribution and co-localisation of markers in nerves in the normal human bladder, and Table 4 shows the results of

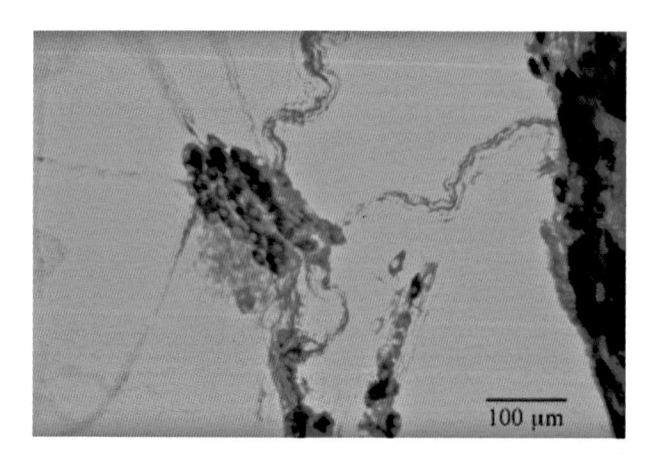

Figure 10 : Preparation of guinea-pig autonomic ganglia from bladder neck region, stained with NADPH diaphorase. Note large ganglion with many inputs. A sub-population of the cells stains positively, showing NOsynthase containing neurones.

one study looking at co-localisation of two markers in nerves in the bladder wall [121]. Sensory and motor nerves are present. Evidence suggests that SubP, CGRP and NKA are markers for sensory nerves [54,122]. In the human bladder, these markers occur infrequently in nerves running in the detrusor but are moderately frequent in the suburothelial layer [55,56,57,121]. There is clearly more than one population of CGRP immunoreactive nerves. A minor population also contains SubP and NKA, and these are suggested to be extrinsic sensory neurones (with their cell bodies in the dorsal root ganglia), but another population of nerves are found in which CGRP co-localises with Gal and NPY [57,121].

The majority of nerves running in the detrusor stain positively for acetylcholinesterase and for VAChT [120,122] and are presumptive post-ganglionic parasympathetic nerves. They run within the muscle bundles parallel with the cells and show prominent varicosities. Most of these nerves are also positive for both NPY and VIP; smaller populations show immunoreactivity to NOS and to Gal. Putative postganglionic sympathetic fibres immunoreactive for TH and NPY are seen only rarely in the detrusor, although they are moderately frequent in the suburothelium [121]. Cholinergic nerves are also present in the suburothelium; most of them in addition contain NPY and some contain NOS. Their function is uncertain, although in other organs they are thought to play a secretomotor role [120].

Neuronal cell bodies in the bladder wall ganglia are again a heterogeneous population. The ganglia are found throughout the bladder wall and can be small, consisting of only one or a few nerve cell bodies, or large with more than 30 neurones [57,123]. They show immunoreactivity to VIP, NOS, NPY and Gal in varying amounts. These neurones presumably synthesise acetylcholine, although there is a scarcity of information about ChAT immunoreactivity in human bladder. Recent results from Dixon et al (2000) [120] show that in tissue from children or neonates, 75% of the intramural ganglia show immunoreactivity to VAChT, 95% to NPY and 40% to NOS. VIP was not looked at in this study. Intramural neurones do not show immunoreactivity to ENK, SubP, CGRP or Som [57] suggesting that cell bodies of sensory neurones are not located here. Immunoreactive profiles of nerves synapsing on intramural ganglia also show distinct classes. Both populations of CGRP-containing nerves synapse on these ganglion cells - the SubP/CGRP nerves presumably being collaterals from the extrinsic sensory nerves. Postganglionic sympathetic nerves containing TH and NPY also synapse on these neurones, and the other group is the VIP/Gal/NPY containing nerve terminals, which are presumably the presynaptic cholinergic inputs. Nerve terminals immunoreactive to NOS or

Table 4 : Results of double immunolabelling of ganglia in sections cut from the proximal urethra of 4 human females. From Ho [125]

	No of ganglia examined	No of cell bodies	% showing both markers	% showing one marker only	% showing the other marker only
PGP & NOS	7	126	58	PGP 42	
TH & NOS	8	113	43	TH34	NOS 23
HO-2 & NOS	8	152	74	HO-2 25	NOS 1
VIP & NOS	6	77	69	VIP 19	NOS 12
NPY & NOS	4	68	56	NPY 37	NOS 7
NPY & VIP	4	26	69	NPY 4	VIP 27
NPY & TH	6	100	83	NPY 1	TH 14
VIP & TH	8	117	57	VIP 9	TH 34

Som do not appear to synapse with intrinsic neurones in the bladder wall.

b) Innervation of the bladder neck, trigone and urethra

Autonomic ganglia are also found in the serosa around the proximal urethra and prostate, and in the walls of the bladder neck, trigone and in the female, the proximal urethra. In the human male, however, no ganglia are found in the walls of the urethra. The bladder neck, trigone and urethra can be shown to receive a more complicated innervation than the detrusor, with functional evidence for noradrenergic and cholinergic predominantly excitatory innervation of the smooth muscle, and also non-cholinergic, non-adrenergic inhibitory innervation [124]. Histochemical and immunohistochemical examination of the ganglia and nerves again show a heterogeneous population. Table 5 gives information about paraurethral ganglia in the adult human female and co-localisation of various markers [125]. Putative sympathetic ganglia demonstrating TH immunoreactivity were common, and there was co-localisation with NPY (≈ 80%), VIP (≈ 70%), and NOS (≈ 50%). Similar co-localisation has been seen in male infants [126], and this study also showed co-localisation of TH with CGRP (≈ 50%) and Som (≈ 70%). In these male infants, ganglia not containing TH the majority showed immunoreactivity to NPY and Som (≈ 90%), others showed immunoreactivity to CGRP (≈ 65%), NOS (≈ 45%) and VIP (≈ 40%). In the proximal female urethra, virtually all of the NOS immunoreactive cells were also immunoreactive to HO-2, but of the HO-2 positive cells, 25% did not show NOS immunoreactivity [127].

c) Conclusions

The above work strongly suggests a considerable degree of complexity of the peripheral autonomic pathways controlling the lower urinary tract. Although the majority of the ganglia in the bladder wall appear to be parasympathetic, at least three classes of neurone synapse onto these cells, giving considerable scope for complex control. In the para-urethral ganglia it is impossible to classify any particular ganglion as sympathetic or parasympathetic, or to designate all the NOS containing ganglia into one or other of these classes. The situation resembles in complexity the enteric plexuses found in the gut wall, and it is impossible at present to rule out the presence of local circuits and reflexes as well as the extrinsic control coming from the central nervous system. More work is clearly needed in this area.

2. Electrophysiological Studies on Ganglia

Methods have been developed by Hanani and Maudlej [128] for visualising living ganglion cells in the guinea-pig bladder wall, and recording their electrical properties. Recently this method has been extended to the paraurethral ganglia in the same animal. Figure 10 shows one of the paraurethral ganglia stained with NADPH diaphorase, showing a ganglion containing a large number of neurones, some of which stain positively showing the presence of NOS. Preparations like this allow electrical recordings of the responses of these ganglion cells to stimulation of different preganglionic nerve fibres. Activation of most inputs results in the production of excitatory junction potentials that are blocked by nicotinic-receptor antagonists. Preliminary studies show that many of these cells appear to possess SubP receptors, activation of which enhances the sensitivity of the cells apparently through a reduction in the membrane conductance (Figure 11).

3. Interstitial Cells

Over the last few years, growing attention has been

Table 5 : Colocalization of transmitters in nerve fibres in normal bladders as assessed with confocal laser scanning microscopy. From Drake et al. [58,121]

Transmitter	Nerve site (frequency)	Proportion colocalizing second transmitter VIP	NPY	CGRP	NOS	TH	Gal	SP
VIP	Muscle (F)	-	4	0	2	NA	NA	0
	Suburo. (F)	-	4	0	2			0
NPY	Muscle (M)	4	-	1	NA	3	NA	NA
	Suburo, (M)	4	-	2		1		
CGRP	Muscle (I)	0	2	-	NA	NA	3	2
	Suburo. (M)	0	2	-			3	2
n-NOS	Muscle (M)	3	NA	NA	-	CA	NA	NA
	Suburo. (M)	3			-	0		
TH	Muscle (VI)	NA	4	NA	CA	-	NA	NA
	Suburo. MI)		4		0	-		
Gal	Muscle (M)	NA	NA	2	NA	NA	-	NA
	Suburo. (I)			2			-	
SP	Muscle (VI)	0	NA	5	NA	NA	NA	-
	Suburo. (M)	0		5				-

CA= close association observed, but transmitters not colocalised, NA= not assessed, Suburo= suburothelial plexus

0 No colocalisation present A Absent

1 1-20%	VI Very infrequent	2 21-40%	I Infrequent
3 41-60%	M Moderate	4 61-80%	F Frequent
5 81-100%	VF Very frequent		

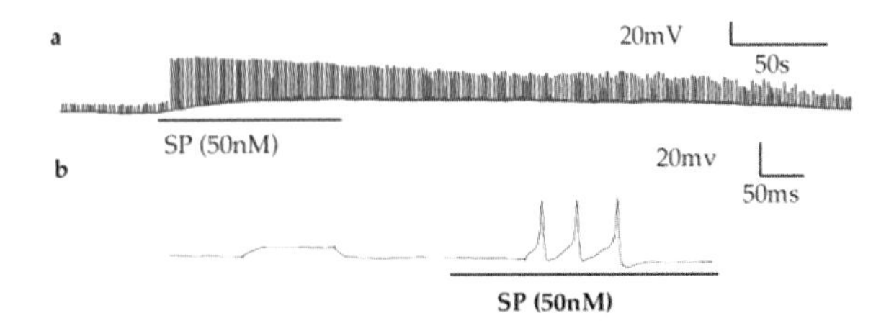

Figure 11 : Microelectrode recording from single ganglion cell. (a) on a slow time base, showing the effects of addition of substance P on the response of the cell to injection of small depolaring current. (b) recording on a faster time base of the response to a single pulse in the absence and presence of substance P.

paid to a cell type in the walls of the urinary tract that has previously received little attention, and that is the myofibroblast. Myofibroblasts are ubiquitous. They are fibroblastic cells with smooth muscle-like characteristics, and many postulated functions. They are involved in such things as growth and differentiation of tissues, formation and repair of the extracellular matrix, wound healing, secretion of growth factors and inflammatory mediators and generating the pacemaker currents underlying slow wave activity in gastrointestinal smooth muscles. Myofibroblasts have characteristic morphological features. The cells are thin and often branched or stellate. The cell membrane shows many caveolae, intermediate fibres and smooth muscle actin microfilaments are often seen in the cytoplasm but myosin is not present. The cells have well developed Golgi apparatus, and the cytoplasm is rich in endoplasmic reticulum and mitochondria. The basal lamina is poorly developed. The myofibroblasts are often linked together through gap and adherens junctions.

Many different types of myofibroblast have been distinguished by their particular locations, morphological features and staining properties. In particular classification on the basis of the cytoskeletal proteins present has been used, with immunostaining techniques. Three commonly studied proteins are vimentin (V), desmin (D) and α smooth muscle actin (A). Possibly the best known myofibroblasts are in the gastrointestinal tract, where they are known as Interstitial Cells of Cajal (ICCs). There are several types of ICC in the gut: the main pacemaking cells form a network close to the myenteric plexus and another one close to the submucosal surface. These cells express the protoocogene c-kit and can be specifically stained using antibodies to the receptor tyrosine kinase that is its gene product.

Attention focused on interstitial cells in the urinary tract following the elegant work of Smet et al [129] determining the distribution of nitric oxide synthase containing nerves and the cellular targets of nitric oxide. The latter was established using antibodies to cGMP to determine which cells responded to the nitric oxide donor sodium nitroprusside by activation of guanylyl cyclase. They showed that whereas the smooth muscle cells in the urethra responded to sodium nitroprusside with a uniform increase in cGMP levels, the smooth muscle cells in the detrusor did not. However, a class of cells in the human and guinea-pig bladder demonstrated an intense induction of cGMP immunoreactivity by sodium nitroprusside, and these were interstitial cells that morphologically appeared remarkably similar to ICCs. This was particularly interesting, since the post-ganglionic parasympathetic neurones in the bladder wall contain nitric oxide synthase, although there is no functional evidence of an inhibitory nitric innervation to the detrusor.

Recently the distribution and immunocytochemistry of myofibroblasts in the human detrusor has been examined [121]. ICC-like cells were present throughout the bladder wall, both in the laminar propria and within the smooth muscle layer. Within the detrusor they were present predominantly in the interfasicular planes and on the periphery of the muscle bundles. The cells were multipolar, with thin processes that ramified over considerable distances, and made anatomical contact with processes from other ICC-like cells, smooth muscle and varicose nerve fibres. All the ICC-like cells showed intense vimentin-like immunoreactivity, but did not show immunoreactivity to α-smooth muscle actin. The majority of cells were also weakly positive for c-kit, and co-localisation of c-kit and vimentin-like immunoreactivity was seen using confocal microscopy. The ICC-like cells did not show immunoreactivity to the pan neuronal marker PGP 9.5 or the leukocyte common antigen. The similarity between these cells in the bladder, and ICCs in the gut suggest that they may be playing some role in determining the 'myogenic' spontaneous mechanical activity seen in isolated bladder strips, and may also be involved in mediating activity between nerves and muscles as has also been suggested for ICCs [130]. It would be interesting to know whether there are differences in the numbers and distribution of the ICC-like cells in bladders from patients with acontractile or hyperactive bladders.

The possibility that ICC-like cells play a role in pacemaker activity in the urinary tract is has also been examined in the ureter and urethra. In the guinea-pig ureter, ICC-like cells have been described in the renal pelvis [131]. These cells are concentrated in the pelvi-calyceal junction with some in the renal pelvis. They spontaneously discharge action potentials which have an initial spike followed by a long plateau. It has been proposed that they act as a preferential pathway conducting and amplifying pacemaker signals to the smooth muscle cells in the ureter.

In all species studied, urethral smooth muscle develops sustained myogenic tone, and often small slow waves of contraction are superimposed on the basal tone. In the rabbit, microelectrodes have been used to record the underlying electrical slow wave activity in urethral smooth muscles [132], which was found to be similar to the smooth muscle of the gastrointestinal tract, although these workers were not aware of the presence of ICC-like cells in the urethra. Following from this observation and the observation that ICC-like cells were present in the human urethra [129], Sergeant et al [133] used collagenase to disperse cells from the rabbit urethra, and were able to demonstrate the presence of ICC-like cells, and examine both their morphology and electrophysiology. Such cells represent only a small proportion of the cells present but had morphology typical of ICCs, and as shown by Drake et al [121], in contrast to smooth muscle cells, stained strongly with anti-vimentin antibody but did not contain myosin. The ICC-like cells were non contractile, but showed spontaneous electrical activity. The authors proposed that as in the gut, the ICC-like cells may be responsible for initiating the electrical slow waves recorded from the smooth muscle cells and that the tone seen in the smooth muscles may depend on the frequency of these slow waves.

The powerful combination of immunohistochemical, ultrastructural and electrophysiological identification of ICC-like cells now makes it possible to explore the behaviour of these cells in a range of human disease conditions. In the gastrointestinal tract, prominent motility disturbances are present and evidence of involvement of ICCs in such diseases is beginning to emerge. These cells are obvious targets for future rational and effective pharmacotherapy of gut diseases. This may also be true of diseases of the urinary tract. The possibility that ICC-like cells might modulate contractile behaviour in three such different systems as (1) ureters with their distinct pacemaker region initiating synchronous phasic contractions in the smooth muscle, (2) the detrusor with little basic tone but asynchronous small tonic activity, and (3) urethral smooth muscle is intriguing. This field is clearly now one that is open for further research.

VI. PHARMACOLOGY OF PERIPHERAL PATHWAYS TO THE BLADDER

Table 6 is taken from the First Consultation [2] and summarises the various drugs that act on peripheral nerves and smooth muscle together with specific examples and their mode of action. The reader is referred to this chapter [2] and references 533-576, and the following discussion provides an update on recent advances in knowledge in this area.

1. SEROTONIN (5-HT) RECEPTORS

5-HT receptors are present in the bladder and in the central pathways controlling micturition, possibly mainly in the latter; there is some species variation in the effects of this transmitter. 5-HT is thought to act indirectly in the urinary bladder by the stimulation of

Table 6 : Drugs used for urinary incontinence and overactive bladder. This table is based on Table 4 in the First Consultation and has been updated. The conclusions are based on references 533-576.

Classification	Examples	Pharmacological Action
Anticholinergic	Atropine Tolterodine Propantheline Trospium Darfenacin*	Inhibit muscarinic receptors reducing the response to cholinergic stimulation Used to reduce intravesical pressure, increase compliance, raise volume threshold for micturition, eliminate unstable contractions. Used to treat overactive bladder with or without urge urinary incontinence
Mixed anticholinergic/smooth muscle relaxants	Oxybutynin	Blocks muscarinic receptors and directly relax smooth muscle. May possess local anesthetic properties.
Beta adrenergic agonists	FK 175*	ß3 adrenergic agonist relaxes detrusor in vitro. May be useful for overactive bladder with or without urge incontinence
Tricyclic antidepressants/ monoamine reuptake inhibitors	Imipramine Chlomipramine Amitryptiline Duloxetine*`	Multiple sites of action including peripheral anticholinergic and norepinephrine reuptake blocker with potential net action as a1 receptor agonist. Central effects to inhibit micturition through possible blockade of norepinephrine and serotonin reuptake. Thus potentially useful for overactive bladder, urge incontinence and pain disorders. Relative action at Onuf's nucleus via 5-HT1A receptors makes duloxetine potentially useful for stress incontinence.
Alpha adrenergic agonists	Ephedrine Midodrine Pseudoephedrine Phenylpropanolamine	Increase bladder outlet resistance via direct stimulation of alpha 1 receptors. Potentially useful for stress urinary incontinence.
Alpha adrenergic antagonists	Terazosin Doxazosin Alfuzosin Tamsulosin	In addition to reducing bladder outlet resistance these agents may act in central nervous system of inhibit micturition. Used for overactive bladder especially associated with benign prostatic hyperplasia. Limited data on unstable contractions and use in neuropathic bladder dysfunction.
Afferent nerve inhibitors	Lidocaine DMSO Capsaicin Resiniferatoxin*	Vanilloid receptor agonists or local anesthetics. Block sodium channels or act on vanilloid receptor expressing afferents to reduce sensation or afferent input necessary to trigger micturition. Could raise volume threshold for micturition. Thus, potentially useful for pain disorders, and overactive bladder with or without urge incontinence.
Estrogen	Estradiol	Direct application intravaginally may be useful sensory urgency. May directly increase bulk of urethra or enhance mucosal seal via urothelial hyperplasia or increased vasculature. May also up-regulate a1 receptors.

** Undergoing clinical trials. Not approved by regulatory agencies.*

presynaptic 5-HT-4 receptors on cholinergic neurones to release acetylcholine, which binds to muscarinic receptors so as to increase bladder contractility [134].

The main action of serotonin however is within the CNS, where the 5-HT-1A receptor appears to be involved in the regulation of micturition. In rats, 8-hydroxy-N,N-dipropylaminotetralin (8-OH-DPAT), the prototypical 5-HT_{1A} receptor agonist, produced a micturition contraction when bladder volume was just subthreshold for producing a physiological bladder contraction when administered intrathecally or intracerebroventricullary [135]. Furthermore, studies with the 5-HT 1A receptor antagonist, WAY100635, indicate that, in the rat, this compound can inhibit contractions evoked by bladder distension in a dose-dependent manner [136]. This action occurred only when the compound was injected intrathecally at the level of the sacral parasympathetic outflow and pelvic afferent input; the drug also blocked the contractile effects of electrical stimulation of the pontine micturition centre, which suggests that the mechanism of action is inhibition of tonic descending input to the sacral parasympathetic nucleus.

Studies of a number of 5-HT receptor antagonists in rats suggested that only the 5-HT-1A receptor antagonists had potentially useful effects on the bladder, inducing an increase in bladder capacity with no derangement of bladder contractility [137]. Two compounds were used intravenously (p-MPPI and methiothepin) and induced a dose-dependent disappearance of isovolumic bladder contractions in anaesthetized rats, and at the highest doses, the dose-response curves were bell-shaped. The amplitude of bladder contractions was not markedly altered. A consistent increase in bladder capacity was seen with p-MPPI and methiothepin, but only methiothepin decreased the voiding pressure.

In cats, it appears that 5-HT1A receptor stimulation is inhibitory to micturition contractions evoked by bladder distension [588]. In other words, the exact opposite effects seen in rats. 8-OH-DPAT increased the bladder volume threshold for inducing a contraction (i.e. increased bladder capacity) but did not inhibit the amplitude or duration of the contraction once the threshold was exceeded. Thus, these authors concluded that the site of action was on the sensory limb of the reflex. The inhibitory effects of 8-OH-DPAT were most marked when the bladder was irritated by infusion of a dilute (0,5%) solution of acetic acid. In contrast to the inhibitory effects of 8-OH-DPAT on bladder activity, it facilitated striated sphincter activity under conditions of acetic acid infusion into the bladder. Thus, 5-HT1A receptor activation has opposite effects on bladder and sphincter activity that is evoked by bladder nociception, i.e. inhibition of bladder activity and facilitation of sphincter activity. The 5-HT1A receptor antagonist WAY100635 blocked both effects.

Other 5-HT receptors are also involved in central regulation of lower urinary tract function. Steers et al . (1992) [138] reported that 5-HT2C receptor agonists inhibit bladder activity. Furthermore, it was shown [139] that 5-HT3 receptor activation inhibited supraspinal transmission of bladder afferent activity. These authors and others [140] also showed that administration of the serotonin neurotoxin, 5,7 dihydroxytryptamine (5,7 DHT) facilitated bladder activity in cats and rats, respectively. Finally, 5-HT2 receptors have been shown to facilitate reflexes to the striated sphincter muscles in cat [141].

2. α1 ADRENOCEPTORS

Much attention has focused on the role of the sympathetic nervous system and in particular α_1-adrenergic receptors (α_1ARs) which are members of the large family of G protein-coupled adrenergic receptors that mediate action of the endogenous catecholamines norepinephrine and epinephrine. cDNAs encoding three distinct α_1AR subtypes (α_{1a}, α_{1b}, α_{1d}) have been cloned, and the gene products have been expressed in cells and characterized pharmacologically [142].

α_1AR antagonists have been demonstrated to relax prostate smooth muscle and in clinical studies are capable of relieving outlet obstruction [143]. Molecular and contractility studies performed using human prostate demonstrate the α_{1a}AR is the subtype responsible for mediating contraction of prostate smooth muscle [144]. It is not surprising therefore that several highly selective α_{1a}AR antagonists have recently been demonstrated to increase urine flow in clinical settings. However, what is surprising is that while highly selective α_{1a}AR compounds are effective in relieving outlet obstruction, they do not appear to relieve irritative symptoms [145], which suggests that these symptoms may be mediated by another type of α_1AR. α_{1d}AR mRNA and protein has recently been identified in human detrusor and sacral spinal cord [146,147] some authors have hypothesized this receptor may play an important role in the development of irritative symptoms associated with bladder outlet obstruction [142,148]. Hampel et al [149] described the modulation of these receptors by bladder outlet obstruction, and Figure 12 outlines the changes in the different areas of the bladder.

3. PURINERGIC MECHANISMS

Purinergic receptors appear not to be involved to any extent in the normal function of the human bladder, although they are important in many animals. In pathological conditions of the bladder, then the purinergic mechanisms may be expressed; this topic is discussed in greater depth in the smooth muscle section. At least

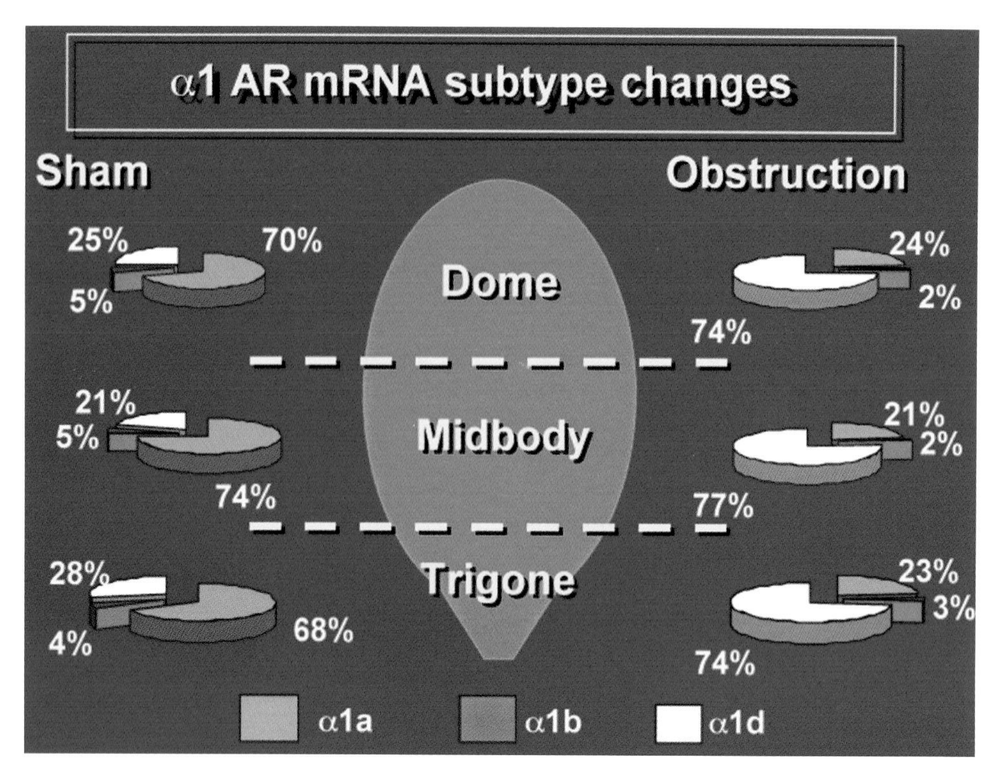

Figure 12 : The distribution of alpha-1 adrenoceptor mRNA and the effects of bladder outlet obstruction (modified from reference 149).

7 subtypes of P2X receptors appear in the rat bladder [62]. Clusters of purinergic receptor subunits can be found on the smooth muscle cell membrane beneath junctional varicosities in the detrusor muscle of the rat urinary bladder, and the P2X1 receptor appears to be the major subtype in both the rodent and human [150]. In the non-pregnant rat, clusters at junctional varicosities are principally composed of the P2X1, 2, 3 and 5 subtypes. But by day 14 of pregnancy, about 80% of theses clusters are replaced by P2X4 and 6 junctional clusters which also increase in density by more than 80% [151].

The P2X1 was found to be the predominant purinoceptor subtype in the human male bladder, consistent with pharmacological evidence [150]. These studies were performed on bladder biopsies that were obtained from nine patients undergoing prostate surgery and controls obtained from eight age-matched men undergoing routine bladder endoscopy studies and who were asymptomatic. The amount of P2X1 receptor per smooth muscle cell is greater in the obstructed than in control bladder, suggesting an increase in purinergic function in the unstable bladder arising from bladder outlet obstruction. In the foetal human bladder, P2X1 receptors, the predominant purinoceptor in adults, is expressed to a rather smaller extent. During human development, however, there are also several marked developmental changes in purinoceptor expression in the bladder, and the P2X4 subtype is expressed in developing bladders at relatively high levels. Changes in the regional distribution of purinoreceptors also occur during development, which suggests a changing role of purinergic transmission in the control of bladder motility during fetal maturation [150,152].

Changes in purinergic receptor levels have been found in the detrusor in human infant bladders, which have only low levels at 9 months or less of age but increased to approach adult levels at 2 years [69]. The association of P2X receptor subtypes and the parasympathetic nerves in the detrusor of humans was also studied [69]; levels of $P2X_4$, $P2X_6$ and $P2X_7$ subtypes in adult humans were all at least 10-fold lower than other subtypes ($P2X_1$, $P2X_2$, $P2X_3$ and $P2X_5$). In Idiopathic Detrusor Instability, these authors found a selective absence of $P2X_3$ and $P2X_5$ beneath all the parasympathetic varicosities, which was associated with a disturbance of control of detrusor contractility in this condition. It is not known whether P2X3 receptors on afferent terminals are affected (see earlier discussion).

4. Tachykinins

Bladder distension is reported to exert some contractile responses on the detrusor mediated by axonal reflexes: these sensory-motor functions of the afferent collaterals appear to involve the release of tachykinins, such as Substance P and Neurokinin A, from the afferent endings in muscle. These effects only occur when the afferents are excited by distension and can be blocked by specific NK-2 antagonists [135].

B. SMOOTH MUSCLE

The Cellular Biology chapter in First International Consultation on Incontinence [1] was concerned with the properties of the normal bladder and urethra. The properties of four components were discussed: the smooth muscle, the stroma, the blood vessels and the urothelium, and for the urethra we discussed the smooth and striated muscles and the lamina propria. In this current volume, further properties of the bladder smooth muscle, including its metabolism, contraction and relaxation, excitation contraction coupling, Ca^{2+} handling and electrical connectivity are discussed. In addition there is a new section on the ganglia present in the human bladder wall and paraurethral tissue, and on the interstitial cells that have been found submucosally and around the smooth muscle bundles in the urethra and bladder.

First, to put the rest into context, we will briefly describe some of the important functional properties that the bladder and urethra must have to fulfil their normal role.

The bladder is designed to store urine and expel it when it is socially convenient, and the urethra to prevent leakage, and yet allow voiding during micturition. To store significant amounts of urine, the bladder wall must be extremely compliant and able to stretch and rearrange itself to allow an increase in bladder volume without significant pressure rise. The bladder wall cannot, however be purely passive during filling, since initiation of a pressure rise can only occur if the shape of the bladder conforms to the minimum surface area/volume ratio possible anatomically. This constraint means that there must be continuous contractile activity in the smooth muscle cells to adjust their length during filling, but without synchronous activity that would elevate intravesical pressure and prevent filling. The smooth muscle and intrinsic nerves have to be protected from exposure to urine by the urothelium, which itself must also expand readily during filling, whilst preserving its function. Sensory nerves conveying information about the state of the bladder can, however clearly respond to the degree of distension of the bladder, and also be modulated by the composition of the urine. Bladder emptying requires relaxation of the urethral smooth muscle followed by synchronous activation of all the detrusor, since if only part of the bladder wall contracted, the uncontracted compliant areas would stretch and prevent the increase in pressure necessary for urine to be expelled through the urethra. Inhibitory nerves are necessary to switch off spontaneous tone in the urethra, and motor nerves have to innervate the detrusor smooth muscle sufficiently densely to achieve elevation of intravesical pressure in micturition and maintain it during emptying of the bladder.

1. Smooth muscle metabolism and energetics

The emphasis of this section is on the relationship between lower urinary tract function and cellular metabolism and energetics. Effective bladder and urethral function is intimately related to intracellular metabolism [153-167] Although there is an extensive information base relating cellular metabolism to vascular smooth muscle function [168- 174], there is relatively little known regarding cellular metabolism and lower urinary tract smooth muscle function.

Both bladder and urethral smooth muscle function, and the protective properties of the urothelial lining of the bladder and urethra, are dependent upon the normal delivery of oxygen and nutrients. In fact, the integrity and ability of the urothelium to protect the detrusor smooth muscle is extremely sensitive to ischaemia, acute over distension, diabetes, partial outlet obstruction, and hypoxia [175-182]. A reduction in blood flow to the urothelium has been linked to a variety of disorders including interstitial cystitis, recurrent urinary tract infections and incontinence [175,183].

Functional compartmentation refers to the observation that specific cellular functions appear to utilize energy derived from selective sources such as glycolysis, oxidative phosphorylation, or cytosolic ATP hydrolysis (*i.e.* specific compartments) [184-6]. Bladder metabolism, like that of most other smooth muscle, is characterized by substantial lactate production under aerobic, resting conditions [154-156; 161,163-165,167]. Current observations are consistent with the concept that specific enzymes and cellular functions utilize metabolic energy derived from sources other than cytosolic ATP [187-190]. Briefly, the contractile response to bethanechol (bladder body) and phenylephrine (urethra) is biphasic in nature; it consists of an initial, rapid phasic rise in tension followed by a prolonged period of sustained tension. As mentioned above, the bladder's functional ability to empty is related to the sustained phase of bladder body's response to muscarinic stimulation; in women, continence is related to the sustained urethral response to α–adrenergic stimulation [191-197]. The sustained phase of the contractile responses are lost immediately upon removal of oxygen from the bathing medium, even though the intracellular concentrations of ATP are high [189,190].

In figure 13, the effect of in-vitro anoxia on the phasic and tonic responses to bethanechol is compared to the effect on ATP concentrations. The tonic response is reduced by over 80% at a time when the phasic response and ATP concentrations are still above 80% of control. The phasic response to bethanechol and the intracellular ATP concentration are reduced at the same

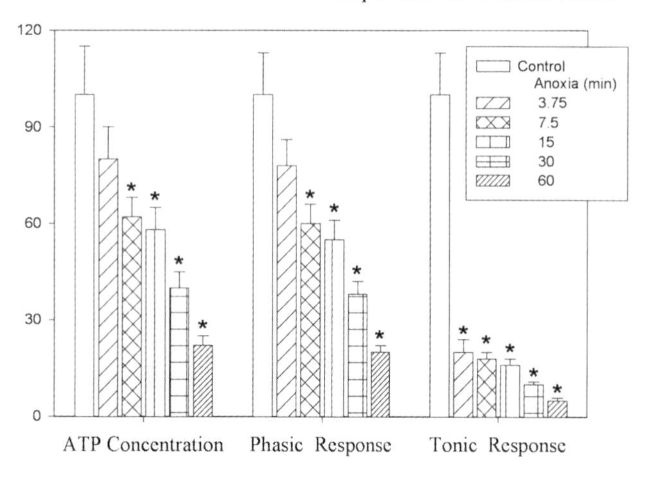

Figure 13 : Time-dependent effect of anoxia on tissue ATP concentration, and on the phasic and tonic components of the response to bethanechol. Isolated strips of rabbit detrusor were mounted in individual baths containing 30 ml Oxygenated Tyrode's solution containing glucose. A second unmounted strip was placed in each bath. The strips were incubated in for 30 minutes at which time the aeration was changed from oxygen to nitrogen for 3.75, 7.5, 15, 30, or 60 minutes. At the end of each time period the unmounted strip was removed and rapidly frozen for ATP analysis; the mounted strip was stimulated with bethanechol (250 uM) and the phasic and tonic tension determined. Control experiments were performed in oxygenated medium incubated for the same time periods. * = significantly different from control, $p < 0.05$.

rate. In similar studies, Uvelius and Arner demonstrated that the plateau response of the rat bladder to high K^+ solutions was lost rapidly upon the initiation of anoxia and restored rapidly upon re-oxygenation [198]

These observations are consistent with the concept that sustained tension is supported by high energy phosphates derived directly by oxidative phosphorylation rather than by cytosolic ATP. Further support comes from recent studies on substrate deprivation [199-201]). The urinary bladder, similar to all smooth muscles, has a low glycogen concentration [156]. Thus, in the absence of glycolytic substrates, the rate of oxidative metabolism decreases rapidly, whereas the cytosolic ATP concentration decreases at a much slower rate. Incubation of isolated bladder strips in the absence of glucose (or any other substrate) leads to an inhibition of the tonic phase (plateau phase) of the contractile response that is much faster in onset and much more pronounced than the inhibition of the phasic tension observed after substrate deprivation. Additional studies demonstrate that the tonic response to field stimulation is significantly more sensitive to glucose depletion than is the tonic responses to bethanechol or KCl; although the tonic responses to all forms of stimulation are more sensitive to glucose depletion than are their respective phasic responses [199-201]

In studies on the response of the rat bladder to glucose deprivation in the presence and absence of anoxia, the plateau phase of the response to repetitive high K^+ stimulation was significantly more sensitive to both glucose deprivation and the combination of glucose deprivation and anoxia than the peak response [198]. Thus in both rat and rabbit, the sustained responses to a variety of forms of stimulation are significantly more sensitive to glucose deprivation, anoxia, and the combination than are the peak responses. Since bladder emptying is a function of the sustained response to stimulation, these isolated strip studies support the concept that bladder emptying is significantly more sensitive to ischaemia and anoxia than is the peak voiding pressure.

2. Relationship between detrusor smooth muscle and mucosal metabolism

Several studies on acute overdistension, partial outlet obstruction, and diuresis-induced hypertrophy indicated that the mucosal layer of the bladder is significantly more sensitive to acute perturbation than the muscularis [177,178,180-182]. A comparison of the metabolism of the mucosal layer (consisting of the lamina propria, urothelium, and any connective tissue and vascular tissue within this layer) and of the muscularis layer [202] is summarised in Table 7.

The results of these metabolic studies demonstrate that the rate of glucose metabolism to lactic acid of the mucosa is more than three-fold greater than that of the smooth muscle (Table 7). The rate of CO_2 production of the mucosa is 60% greater than that of the unstimulated smooth muscle. The maximal activity of the mitochondrial enzyme citrate synthase is significantly greater in the mucosa than in the smooth muscle, while the activity of malate dehydrogenase is similar in both tissues. In separate experiments, two components of the respiratory chain were compared in smooth muscle and mucosa. The specific activities of NADH-cytochrome C reductase (NCCR) and cytochrome oxidase are similar in both tissue compartments.

The maximal activity of the enzyme creatine kinase is nearly three-fold greater in the bladder smooth muscle than in the mucosa [202], whereas the activity of adenylate kinase of the mucosa is over twice that of the smooth muscle. Although the concentrations of ATP and ADP are similar in both muscle and mucosa, the level of creatine phosphate (CP) is over four-fold greater in the bladder muscle while the level of AMP in the

Table 7 : Metabolic Comparison of Bladder Smooth Muscle and Mucosa

	Smooth Muscle	Mucosa
Glucose metabolism		
Lactic acid formation (:mol /g / h)	2.4 ± 0.2	8.0 ± 0.8**
CO2 formation (:mol / g / h)	0.15 ± 0.30	0.28 ± 0.3**
High energy phosphate content		
Creatine phosphate (nmol / mg protein)	20.0 ± 3@0	4.9 ± 0.8**
Adenosine triphosphate (nmol / mg protein)	12.8 ± 1@4	15.0 ± 1.3
Adenosine diphosphate (nmol / mg protein)	6.5 ± 0.8	5.1 ± 0.6
Adenosine monophosphate (nmol / mg protein)	8.2 ± 1@1	15.5 ± 1.2**
Enzyme activity		
Citrate synthasea (nmol /mg protein / min)	286 ± 25	421 ± 48**
Malate dehydrogenasea (nmol / mg protein / min)	464 ± 43	525 ± 60
NCCRa (nmol / mg protein / min)	406 ± 24	386 ± 58
Cytochrome oxidasea (nmol / mg protein / min)	163 ± 20	137 ± 40
Creatine kinase (nmol / mg protein / min)	582 ± 50	280 ± 20**
Adenylate kinase (nmol /mg protein / min)	50@0 ± 5.0	104 ± 10.0**
Free fatty acid content (nmol / mg protein / min)	20.5 ± 2.2	98.5 ± 15**
Endogenous lipase activity (nmol FFA (mg protein)-1 min-1)	1.75 ± 0.25	10.6 ± 1@8**

*FFA - free fatty acid; NCCR - NADH-cytochrome c reductase. a - Activity in partially purified mitochondrial preparation; All data are given as means ± SEM; **significantly different from smooth muscle (P<0.05).*

muscle is only 58% of that in the mucosa (Table 7). Creatine phosphate acts as a phosphate donor during periods of high metabolic activity (active contraction) and reduced oxygen delivery (ischaemia and hypoxia). The fact that the mucosa has a significantly lower CP concentration, and lower CK activity indicates that the mucosa would be very sensitive to reduced oxygen delivery. This hypothesis was tested by comparing the rate of ATP and CP hydrolysis for bladder smooth muscle and mucosa in the presence of anoxia [203]. The rate of ATP and CP hydrolysis for the mucosa was significantly greater than the rate of hydrolysis for the smooth muscle. This experiment confirms the fact that the mucosa has both a greater rate of oxidative metabolism, and a greater rate of high energy phosphate degradation than the smooth muscle compartment of the bladder.

Recent blood flow studies have demonstrated that blood flow to the mucosa under resting conditions is several fold higher than blood flow to the muscularis [204,205]. This correlates very well with the greater metabolic rate of the mucosa, and the greater sensitivity of the mucosa to ischaemia and hypoxia.

3. Relationship between stress incontinence and metabolism

Incontinence can be divided into two major aetiologies: urge and stress incontinence. Urge incontinence is mediated primarily by involuntary bladder contractions which occur during bladder filling (independent of whether the contractions are of myogenic or neurogenic origin). If pressure increases above urethral resistance, incontinence occurs. Stress incontinence occurs when factors such as sneezing or physical activity increase the external pressure on the bladder and further distend the bladder base area, which can give the feeling of urgency, directly produce incontinence, and stimulate urethral relaxation, thus inducing a major incontinence incident.

In men, urethral resistance is largely related to the presence of the prostate, and an external sphincter that completely encircles the urethra; active α adrenergic tone plays a relatively minor role. In women, urethral resistance, and thus continence, is much more dependent upon α-adrenergic tone [116,206-208].

A reduction of blood flow to the urethra (in pigs) resulted in rapid and parallel reductions in both urethral PO_2 and urethral pressure to very low values [209]. Restoration of blood flow resulted in an immediate and full recovery of both urethral PO_2 and urethral pressure values (Figure 14). These studies provide additional strong support for the concept that urethral tension and continence are directly related to urethral tension, which in turn is dependent upon a normal delivery of oxygen; and that urethral competency is lost rapidly during periods of ischaemia and anoxia.

Supporting this concept is an in-vitro study which demonstrates that the tonic phase of the contractile response of isolated strips of rabbit urethra to phenylephrine is lost during periods of anoxia, and restored rapidly upon re-oxygenation [193]. Figure 15 displays a representative tracing of the effect of anoxia on both isolated urethral strip tension and intracellular free calcium $[Ca^{2+}]i$ (using a surface spectrofluorometer). Phenylephrine stimulated a rapid sustained increase in tension. The rise in $[Ca^{2+}]i$ preceded the rise in tension and decayed while tension was maintained. Switching the bathing solution from 95% O_2 -5%CO_2 to 95% N-5% CO_2 resulted in immediate loss of tonic tension and increase in $[Ca^{2+}]i$ far above physiological levels. Immediately upon re-oxygenation, tension was restored and $[Ca^{2+}]i$ fell to pre-anoxia levels. These studies demonstrate that anoxia results in a loss in the tonic phase of the response to receptor-mediated contraction (both α-adrenergic and muscarinic) and a dissociation of contractile tension and $[Ca^{2+}]i$, resulting in the release of bound Ca^{2+} from intracellular storage sites.

Although there is excellent direct evidence that active α-adrenergic tension is an important factor in continence in animal models, evidence in humans comes primarily from drug studies showing that α-adrenergic stimulation is an effective therapy for specific forms of incontinence. Diokno and Taub reported that ephedrine sulfate was an effective treatment for sphincteric incontinence in 27 out of 38 patients [210]; norephedrine administration resulted in a significant increase in both maximal urethral pressure (MUP) and maximal urethral closure pressure (MUCP) [211]. Several objective clinical studies have demonstrated that the administration of phenylpropanolamine (similar to ephedrine with less central stimulation) was an effective therapy for stress incontinence and sphincteric incontinence [212,213]. Thus, there is a solid base of clinical information which demonstrates that α-adrenergic stimulation (especially via chronic slow-release therapy) increases both MUP and MUCP and significantly reduces both stress incontinence and sphincteric incontinence.

Effect of Aortic Occlusion on Urethral Pressure in the Pig

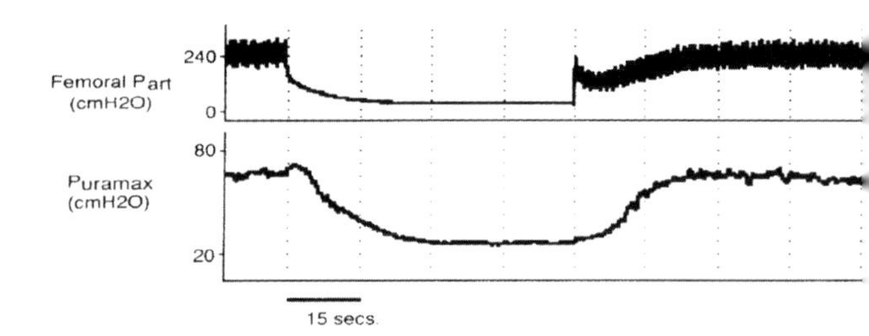

Figure 14 : In vivo recording of the urethral pressure and the left femoral artery pressure on occlusion of the terminal aorta in the pig. Note that the urethral pressure falls as the arterial inflow is cut off.

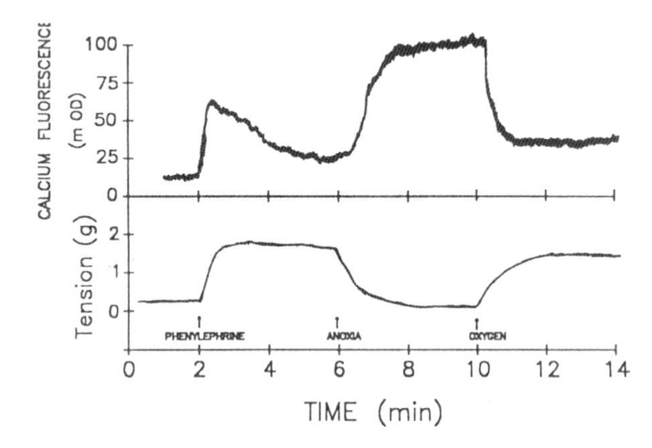

Figure 15 : Representative tracing of the effects of anoxia and re-oxygenation on the response of an isolated strip of urethral smooth muscle to phenylephrine. Isolated strips of urethral smooth muscle (rabbit) were mounted in a specially designed 1 ml flow-though chamber. A calcium probe was placed on the surface of the strip and connected to surface spectrofluorometer. One end of the strip was tied to a tension transducer. Contractile tension and intracellular free calcium were monitored simultaneously. Anoxia was induced by changing the bathing media from 95% O2 - 5% CO2 to a bathing media equilibrated with 95% N - 5% CO2 .

I. EXCITATION-CONTRACTION COUPLING

1. TENSION GENERATION

The basic mechanism of contractile activation in detrusor smooth muscle was outlined in a previous volume [1]. Briefly, motor nerves release acetylcholine and ATP that act as excitatory neurotrasmitters.

- Acetylcholine binds to a muscarinic (M_3) receptor and via a G-protein coupled mechanism leads to an increase of intracellular inositol trisphosphate (IP_3). This soluble second messenger subsequently releases Ca^{2+} from intracellular stores to elicit contraction.
- ATP binds to a purinergic ($P2X_1$) receptor that acts as a ligand-gated ion channel causing cell depolarisation, which, if great enough, opens L-type Ca^{2+} channels. The consequent Ca^{2+} influx can cause further Ca^{2+} release from intracellular stores by Ca^{2+}-induced Ca^{2+} release.

In human detrusor from stable bladders acetylcholine is the predominant neurotransmitter as contractions are abolished completely by atropine [214], whilst in most animal species (except old world monkeys) there is a dual role for acetylcholine and ATP. What has become evident recently is that in a number of pathologies affecting the human detrusor a purinergic component reappears providing an additional source of intracellular Ca^{2+} to activate the contractile proteins [215,216]. Several questions remain: i) why is ATP a functional transmitter in some bladder preparations and not others? ii) does the reappearance of purinergic neurotransmission in detrusor from pathological bladders contribute to bladder overactivity?

There are several, not mutually exclusive, reasons for the reappearance of purinergic neurotransmission in pathological human bladders:

a) the differential sensitivity of the detrusor to ATP and/or acetylcholine alters. This is unlikely, as experiments with isolated cells from stable and unstable human bladders show that the potency and magnitude of effect of these agonists, as judged by the rise of intracellular $[Ca^{2+}]$, is similar in the two groups [217]. In other words the supersensitivity to agonists such as acetylcholine that is evident at a tissue level [218] cannot be demonstrated at a cellular level.

b) Acetylcholine and ATP are hydrolysed in the synaptic cleft by acetylcholine esterase (AChE) and an ectoATPase respectively [219]. In principle a decrease in the activity of either enzyme would prolong the lifetime of the transmitter and thus enhance the magnitude of the response and increase the potency of the agonist. For example, application of the AChE inhibitor physostigmine enhances nerve-mediated contractions [214]. One study has indicated that AChE activity may be decreased in neurogenic bladders, which are often associated with unstable activity [220].

   The ectoATPase present in detrusor may be inhibited by the agent ARL 67156 (formerly FPL 67156) [221]. Application of ARL 67156 to guinea-pig bladder strips has also been shown to increase the magnitude of nerve-mediated contractions [222], indicating that the action of ATP on the muscle cell is attenuated by its extracellular hydrolysis. Moreover non-hydrolysable ATP analogues, such as α,β methylene ATP have a much greater potency than ATP itself in generating contractions. Atropine-resistant contractions in detrusor from unstable and obstructed bladders therefore may be caused by a reduced ectoATPase activity so that a proportion of released ATP would reach the detrusor cell membrane

c) The amounts of ATP and acetylcholine that are released from motor nerve terminals are different in detrusor from stable and unstable bladders. Alternatively the breakdown products of neurotransmitters may exert variable effects on transmitter release. Pre-synaptic muscarinic (M1) receptors exert an autofacilitatory effect on acetylcholine release, mediated by protein kinase C [223,224] with a possible concomitant down-regulation by M2 and M4 receptors [225,226]. There is evidence that the facilitatory mechanism at least is upregulated in animals with spinal cord transection [227,228] and represents a further site which may enhance the overall contractile state of detrusor. Less is known about the control of ATP release in detrusor nerve terminals. One study in mouse bladder has suggested that different presynaptic Ca^{2+} channels may regulate release of acetylcholine (predominantly N-type channels) and ATP (predominantly P- and Q-type channels) [229].

2. Relaxation and the relaxed state

Whilst considerable attention has been spent on mechanisms causing contraction there has been less work on the cellular physiology of tension relaxation and of the mechanisms whereby intracellular stores are refilled between successive contractions. These are equally important topics as they will influence, for example, the overall stiffness of the bladder wall and the ability of the bladder to generate consistent contractile responses.

In spite of the fact that tension generation occurs independently of membrane potential changes (and by implication the direct involvement of ion channels) the detrusor cell membrane has a very high density of Ca^{2+} channels [230]. These Ca^{2+} channels were believed originally to be all L-type channels, but recently it has been shown that about 20-25% are T-type Ca^{2+} channels [231]. The significance of this observation is that T-type Ca^{2+} channels are activated at more negative membrane potentials, and at the detrusor resting potential (about –55 to-50 mV) a significant fraction would be open.

Continuous exposure to Ca^{2+} channel antagonists does exert a negative inotropic effect on detrusor contractions [232] and when given in the interval between two exposures to cholinergic agonists reduces the response of the second exposure [233]. It has therefore been proposed that when intracellular Ca^{2+} release is terminated (and relaxation of the cell initiated), a fraction is re-accumulated into intracellular Ca-stores but a fraction is lost from the cell. The fraction that is lost is offset by Ca^{2+} influx through Ca^{2+} channels so that the cell remains in a steady-state with respect to its intracellular Ca content. This is shown in schematic form in Figure 16.

There remain a number of unanswered questions:

How is Ca^{2+} lost from the cell at the termination of the

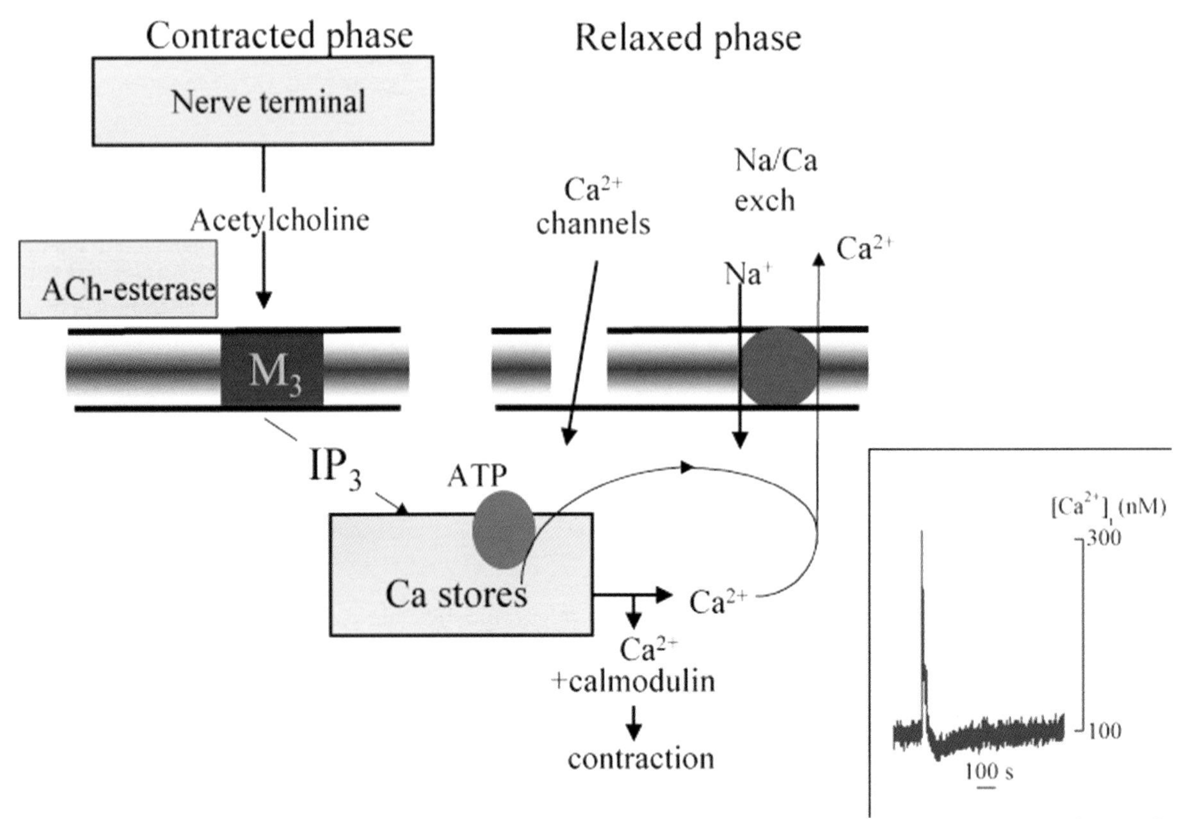

Figure 16 : A schematic diagram of the cellular events concerned with contraction (left) and relaxation (right) in human detrusor smooth muscle. To initiate contraction motor nerves release acetylcholine that binds to membrane M3 receptors. Intracellular IP3 (inositol trisphosphate) release Ca2+ from intracellular stores. The sarcoplasmic Ca2+ binds to calmodulin to initiate contraction but is also removed from the sarcoplasm by re-accumulation into the Ca-stores or removed from the cell – possibly via Na-Ca exchange. The Ca2+ lost from the cell are replaced by a Ca2+ influx, possible through Ca2+ channels. Bottom right an intracellular Ca-transient recorded during application of a muscarinic agonists to an isolated myocyte. Note the 'undershoot' of [Ca2+] after the transient .

intracellular Ca^{2+} transient? Possible routes include an ATP-driven Ca-pump or a Na^{+}-Ca^{2+} counter-exchanger. Recently evidence of Ca^{2+} extrusion through a Na^{+}-Ca^{2+} counter-exchanger has been provided [234] although it is unknown if this is the sole efflux mechanism.

Is Ca^{2+} influx through Ca^{2+} channels regulated during Ca^{2+} extrusion? If so this would enhance the efficiency whereby the cell would return to a steady-state Ca content.

A role for K^{+} channels in the regulation of detrusor function is suggested with respect to the regulation of Ca^{2+} entry via Ca^{2+} channels. The majority of K^{+} current is provided through large conductance K^{+} channels regulated by the concentration of intracellular Ca^{2+}, especially the [Ca^{2+}] immediately below the cell membrane [235, 236]. A fall of the [Ca^{2+}] would close these channels and so depolarise the membrane. These so–called BK channels are blocked by agents such as iberiotoxin and charybdotoxin. Figure 16 also shows as an inset a typical intracellular Ca^{2+} transient elicited by a cholinergic agonist. The transient rise of the [Ca^{2+}] is followed by a decline, *and an transient undershoot below the baseline*. The transient undershoot should therefore increase the closure of BK channels and hence depolarise the membrane during this phase, resulting in an increased likelihood of Ca^{2+} channel opening and thus enhancing Ca^{2+} influx. Some aspects of this scheme have been elucidated [236], however it does propose a functional role for BK channel modulators in manipulating detrusor contractility by affecting the efficiency of refilling intracellular Ca^{2+} stores.

II. THE CONTRACTILE MACHINERY

The generation of tension within a muscle cell involves the interaction of actin and myosin filaments to form a crossbridge. In detrusor smooth muscle, as in most other smooth muscles, these protein filaments are dispersed irregularly throughout the cell. This disorganised arrangement results in a less rapid contraction and one not oriented necessarily along the longitudinal axis of the myocyte. However, this suits the function of these muscles which require a more prolonged active state, and tension to be less directional within the muscle mass than are the cases in striated muscle.

Crossbridge cycling is powered by ATP hydrolysis but regulated by a transient rise of the sarcoplasmic [Ca^{2+}]. Ca^{2+} in the sarcoplasm bind to a soluble protein calmodulin (Cm), to form a complex, Ca_4Cm, which activates the contractile machinery. In smooth muscle Ca_4Cm activates the myosin molecule via activation of a myosin light chain kinase (MLCK), culminating in phosphorylation of the so-called regulatory myosin light chain (RLC) [237]. RLC phosphorylation greatly increases actin-activated myosin MgATPase activity, which results in the heavy chain of the myosin molecule forming a crossbridge with an actin filament which generates force. Crossbridge cycling - the continuous process of making and breaking of crossbridges with the consumption of ATP - can proceed as long as myosin is activated by Ca_4Cm, thus generating a contraction. Relaxation occurs when the RLC is dephosphorylated by a myosin phosphatase [238]. This generally occurs when the Ca_4Cm concentration falls due to a reduction of the sarcoplasmic [Ca^{2+}], but other Ca^{2+} independent mechanisms may also stimulate RLC dephosphorylation and also cause relaxation - an example is considered below.

Experiments with isolated contractile proteins [239] show that the Ca^{2+}-dependent regulation of the contractile apparatus in detrusor smooth muscle occurs over a range of ionised [Ca^{2+}] between 0.1 μM and 10 μM (figure 17). This is precisely the range of [Ca^{2+}] that is measured in the sarcoplasm of intact detrusor myocytes when they are relaxed and then activated by contractile agonists such as acetylcholine or its analogue, carbachol [240] (see also figure 16). Quantitative measurements such as these are important as they reinforce the importance of modulation of the sarcoplasmic [Ca^{2+}] as the key determinant of contractile regulation.

Although modulation of the sarcoplasmic [Ca^{2+}] is the most important regulator of contraction in smooth muscle such as detrusor, other factors may modulate this process. Their significance is not fully understood but they offer additional routes to fine-tune the contractile state of the muscle, both physiologically and pharmacologically. Such control points include phosphorylation of MLCK itself [241] and activation of myosin

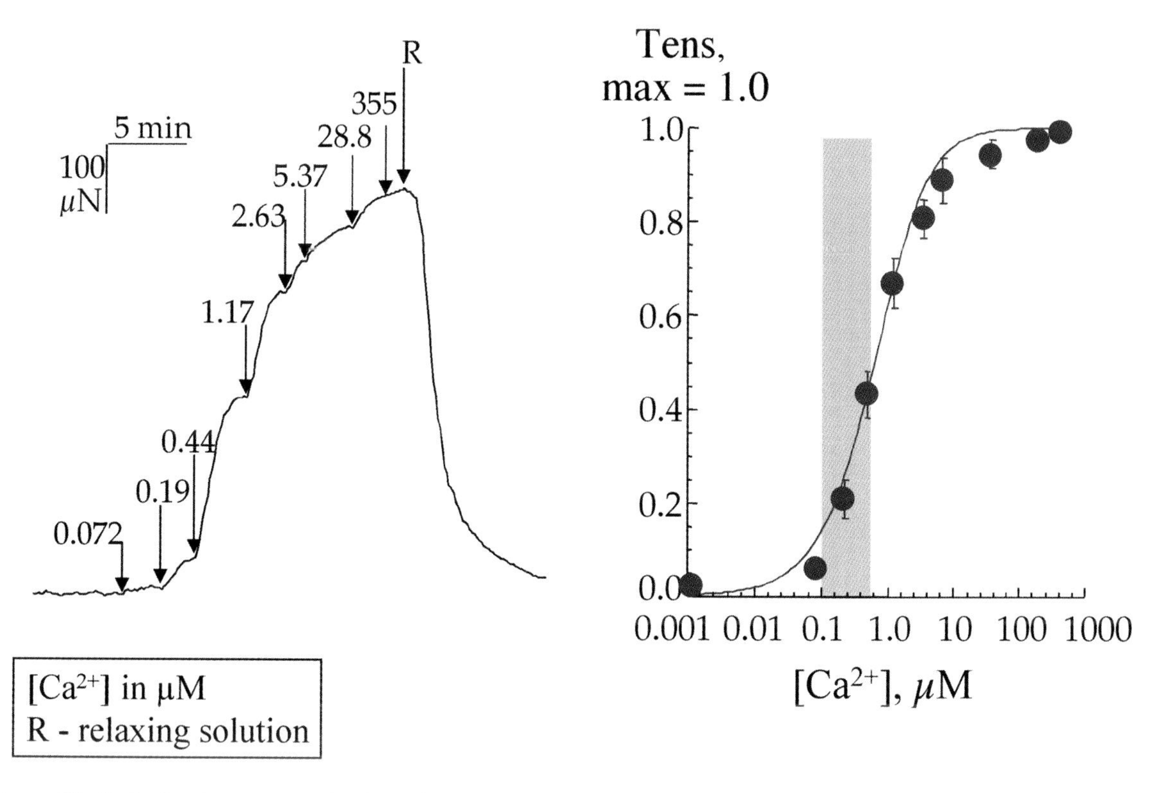

Figure 17 : Left: the change to tension in a skinned detrusor fibre when the [Ca2+] was altered between 0.072 μM and 355 μM. The fibre was 'skinned' by exposure to a solution containing a-toxin, which rendered the surface membrane freely permeable. Blockade of the intracellular organelles left a preparation of myofibrils – see [27] for details. Right: plot of the tension-[Ca2+] relationship from experiments show at left. The shaded area represents the range of intracellular [Ca2+] generated in an intact cell during exposure to a cholinergic agonist.

phosphatase [242], both of which depress myosin ATPase activity and hence contraction. Phosphorylation of MLCK suppresses its own activation by Ca_4Cm and activation of myosin phosphatase would reduce RLC phosphorylation.

An example of such modulation is given by the cyclic nucleotides, cAMP and cGMP, both of which relax smooth muscle [243]. Cellular cAMP levels are increased either by increasing the activity of adenylyl cyclase (e.g. by β-receptor activation) or by phosphodiesterase inhibition (e.g. application of caffeine). Addition of caffeine to a detrusor cell gives a good example of the relevance of the cyclic nucleotide-dependent mechanisms. Caffeine evokes a substantial rise of the $[Ca^{2+}]_i$ as it can evoke near maximal release of Ca^{2+} from intracellular stores; but paradoxically it generates little contractile activity [244], presumably by increasing cellular cAMP. cAMP activates a kinase (protein kinase A, PKA), and it was believed that PKA would mediate relaxation by for example phosphorylating MLCK [245], or myosin phosphatase. More recently it has been proposed that cAMP can also activate protein kinase G (PKG - the kinase activated by cGMP), and it is by this route that relaxation is mediated. The precise details remain to elucidated in lower urinary tract smooth muscles.

• Intercellular coupling

The importance of intercellular coupling in detrusor smooth muscle function remains an unresolved question. Connection between the sarcoplasmic space of adjacent cells is achieved by gap junctions. These are generated by the fusion of two pores in the surface membranes of contiguous cells to form a continuous sarcoplasmic bridge. The pore consists of members of a protein family called connexins and the size of the pore, and hence its physical properties, is determined by the particular connexins present [246].

In detrusor, many investigators using transmission electron microscopy have been unable to observe gap junctions, or see them only very occasionally [247], which has led to the conclusion that detrusor smooth muscle cells are not electrically coupled to a significant degree. It has been proposed that unstable activity in the bladder may be facilitated by enhanced coupling in this tissue [218]. In a subset of patients with detrusor overactivity a microscopical study showed that samples from their bladders had a greater number of so-called protrusion junctions, indicative of intercellular coupling [248]. However, more recently connexin proteins have been visualised in normal detrusor (dome and trigone) using immunohistochemical techniques or scanning electron microscopy [249,250]. However, their concentration is low and they are not clustered together, which may account for the difficulty in observing them with more conventional techniques. The immunohistochemical studies also show that the connexin subtype is connexin45 which forms relatively low conductance pores, rather than connexin 43 which is found, for example, in the myocardial intercalated disk.

These microscopical studies are in reasonable agreement with electrophysiological data. Experiments in which relatively large currents are passed through detrusor preparations demonstrate some passage of currents between several cells indicating some degree of electrical coupling [251,252]. However, the magnitude of coupling is much lower than for example in myocardium which corroborates the histological observations. Electrophysiological experiments using small currents injected into cells via microelectrodes have been unable to demonstrate significant coupling [253]. This may result from the relatively high resistance between adjacent detrusor cells which would limit the passage of such small currents, or the possibility that the detrusor mass is not a homogeneous medium but may consist of discrete and isolated bundles. The experiments passing large currents would lack the resolution to resolve any heterogeneity unlike those using microelectrodes.

The implications of these observations are important to understand why the detrusor muscle mass may behave as a functionally-coordinated tissue. If intercellular coupling is significant this will allow electrical signals to pass from cell to cell. In human detrusor, electrical events associated with contractile activation (mediated by purinergic transmitters) would be evident especially in tissue from patients with obstructed or unstable bladders [216,217]. Thus signals generated in one part of the bladder may propagate to other regions and thus contribute to the generation of an unstable contraction. The speed at which electrical signals travel, depends upon the actual magnitude of the coupling resistance: the higher the resistance the slower is the propagation velocity [254]. Approximate calculations show that an action potential could propagate at a velocity of about 5 $cm.s^{-1}$ [252]. This is probably too slow to coordinate the entire human bladder during a voiding contraction but could be sufficient to generate local contractions or a more slowly-developing contraction associated with abnormal bladder activity.

Gap junctions do not permit the passage of only electric currents but also of small molecules up to several hundred Daltons weight to ensure chemical coupling between cells. The importance of such cell-to-cell transference in harmonising the biochemical behaviour of detrusor is an unexplored subject.

• Summary

Abnormal contractile activity of tissues in the lower

urinary tract remains an important cause of adverse symptoms. The need to study the cellular physiology of the component tissues remains in order to understand the normal mechanisms that determine contractile activity as well as develop more specific agents that can target better lesions. Whilst our understanding of the individual cells that comprise the lower urinary tract is always improving, a number of themes are emerging for future work:

1. to understand in more detail the cellular pathways that determine and modulate the generation of force in lower urinary tract smooth muscle
2. to define the interaction between different cell types that may modulate each others function.
3. to identify more specifically proteins that are up- or down-regulated in abnormally functioning bladders and correlate these with changes to function
4. to investigate the precise transduction mechanisms underlying the sensory responses evoked the bladder, and the influence of surrounding tissues on the function of efferent nerves.

C. CENTRAL PATHWAYS THAT CONTROL MICTURITION

Normal micturition is controlled by neural circuits in the brain and spinal cord that coordinate the activity of visceral smooth muscle in the urinary bladder and urethra with activity of striated muscle in the urethral sphincter [4-6,8, 585]. These circuits act as on-off switches to shift the lower urinary tract between two modes of operation: storage and elimination. In infants these switching mechanisms function purely in a reflex manner to produce involuntary voiding; however, in adults urine storage and release are subject to voluntary control, presumably mediated by the cerebral cortex. Thus, the neural control of the urinary tract is distinct from that of other visceral organs such as the heart, blood vessels and the intestine that are regulated exclusively by involuntary (autonomic) reflex mechanisms.

Injuries or diseases of the nervous system in adults are some of the causes of disruption of the voluntary control of micturition causing the re-emergence of reflex micturition, resulting in bladder hyperactivity and incontinence (Fig. 18) [4-7]. Because of the complexity of the central nervous control of the lower urinary tract, incontinence can occur as a result of a variety of neurological disorders as well as changes in the peripheral innervation and smooth and skeletal muscle components.

The reflex circuitry utilised by the micurition reflex in the adult includes (1) parasympathetic pre-ganglionic neurones originating in the sacral parasympathetic nucleus (SPN), (2) somatic motoneurones innervating the external urinary sphincter (EUS) which appear to have reciprocal activity compared with SPN efferent neurones, (3) ascending and descending neurones that connect sacral primary afferents and the SPN with the the Pontine Micturition Centre (PMC), (4) and primary afferents from the lower urinary tract. There are also other central pathways that are not essential for the micturition reflex, but influence it and modulate its excitability. Most of the latter act by altering the transmission across synapses of the micturition reflex pathway within the CNS, but some also act through the lumbar sympathetic outflow.

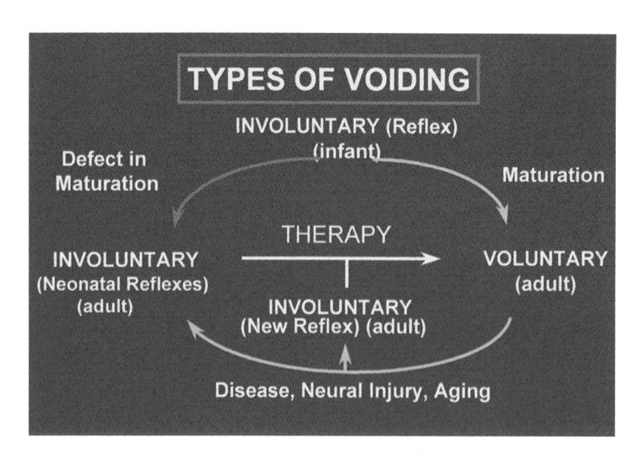

Figure 18 : Influence of postnatal maturation and pathology on voiding function. In infants, voiding is initiated and coordinated by reflex circuits. In older children and adults after maturation of central neural pathways voiding is controlled voluntarily by neural circuitry located in higher centers in the brain. A defect in neural maturation (red arrow) can allow involuntary voiding to persist in adults. Diseases, neural injury or aging can disrupt the central neural pathways mediating voluntary control of micturition and lead to the reemergence of primitive reflex mechanisms that were present in the infant or that appear as the result of synaptic remodeling and the formation of new reflex circuitry. The goal of therapy is to reverse pathology-induced involuntary micturition and to reestablish normal voluntary control of voiding.

I. SACRAL SPINAL CORD

1. SACRAL PARASYMPATHETIC NUCLEI, PUDENDAL NERVE (ONUF'S) NUCLEI AND THEIR INTERNEURONES

In the spinal cord, afferent pathways terminate on second order interneurons which relay information to the brain or to other regions of the spinal cord including the preganglionic and motor nuclei. Because bladder, urethral and sphincter reflexes are mediated by disynaptic or polysynaptic pathways but not by monosynaptic pathways, interneuronal mechanisms must play an essential role in the regulation of lower urinary tract (LUT) function.

Electrophysiological [36,255-7] and neuroanatomical techniques [258-261] including trans-synaptic tracing of pathways with pseudorabies virus (PSV) and the expression of the immediate early gene, c-fos (Fig. 5a,b) have identified LUT interneurons in the same regions of the cord that receive afferent input from the bladder (Fig. 5a). There is agreement between these techniques that interneurones concerned with bladder and/or urethral sensation and reflexes are located in the region of the sacral parasympathetic nucleus (SPN), the dorsal commissure (DCM) and the superficial laminae of the dorsal horn (Fig. 5c).

The micturition reflex can be modulated at the level of the spinal cord by interneuronal mechanisms activated by afferent input from cutaneous and muscle targets as well as inputs from other visceral organs [4,6,256, 262-4]. A potential site for modulation is at the first synapse in the reflex pathway between the bladder primary afferent and the second order projection neurons in lamina I and/or the intermediate gray matter [256,262,265,267] , a region known as the Lateral Collateral Pathway (LCP), which is likely to be one of the most important sites for the coordination of storage and voiding reflexes. Stimulation of afferent fibers from various regions (anus, colon/rectum, vagina, uterine cervix, penis, perineum, pudendal nerve) can inhibit the firing of sacral interneurons evoked by bladder distension [256]. This inhibition may occur as a result of presynaptic inhibition at primary afferent terminals or due to direct postsynaptic inhibition of the second order neurons. Direct postsynaptic inhibition of bladder PGN can also be elicited by stimulation of somatic afferent axons in the pudendal nerve or by visceral afferents from the distal bowel [266,267]. The neurons concerned contain a plethora of neurotransmitters and receptors that have been shown to inhibit afferent processing in somatic systems [5,6], and these will be considered below. Suppression of overactive bladder and of urge incontinence in patients by sacral root stimulation or other forms of neuromodulation may reflect in part activation of the afferent limb of these viscero-bladder and somato-bladder inhibitory reflexes[268-270]. Indeed, electro-stimulation of the pelvic nerve triggers changes in the sacral cord including cfos expression and alterations in neuropeptide immunoreactivity [271] .

These regions of the sacral cord also receive inputs from multiple descending supraspinal systems; e.g. from the pontine micturition center [36,272], paraventricular hypothalamus [273] , serotonergic raphe spinal neurons [274] , and adrenergic bulbospinal neurons [107]. This convergence of numerous pathways in the LCP suggests that the processing of sensory input from the lower urinary tract is likely to be subjected to complex regulation and therefore may be susceptible to various neurological diseases and thus play a critical role in the emergence of neurogenic bladder disorders.

a) Segmental Synaptic Inputs to parasympathetic preganglionic neurones (PGN)

In the neonatal rat spinal cord interneurons in the SPN and DCM regions make direct synaptic excitatory contacts with parasympathetic preganglionic neurons, and some have inhibitory effects on the motoneurones innervating the external urethral sphincter [36, 255, 257,275,276]. Interneurons dorsal and medial to the SPN make excitatory connections mediated by glutamatergic receptors [36,255,275,277]. These interneurons can in turn be activated by electrical stimulation of the LCP region of the lateral dorsal horn which contains primary afferent axons. However a minority of the medial neurons produce inhibitory synaptic responses in the PGN mediated by the release of **glycine** and gamma amino-butyric acid (**GABA**) [276]. Individual neurons release both transmitters. Glycine and GABA, and GABA-A and GABA-B agonists inhibit distension-induced firing of PGN, and inhibition of glycine receptors increases enhanced basal activity in the pudendal nerve to the urethral striated muscle sphincter and prevented the reduction in this activity associated with PMC stimulation-induced voiding in cats [278, 279]. Clinical studies have revealed that intrathecal adminstration of a GABA-B receptor agonist (baclofen) increased the volume threshold for inducing the micturition reflex [6].

b) Descending Synaptic Inputs to parasympathetic preganglionic neurones (PGN)s

As already stated, the LCP receives convergent inputs from a number of descending pathways that originate in the brainstem, Including the pontine micturition center (PMC), paraventricular, raphe-spinal neurons, and adrenergic bulbospinal neurons.

Glutamate plays an important role as a transmitter at the terminals of neurons originating from the Pontine Micturition Centre that synapse on the PGN. Glutamate exerts its affects through ionic and G-protein coupled receptors (Fig 19). Tools that have been used to investigate these actions of glutamate in the micturition reflex include the Non-NMDA glutamatergic receptor antagonists kynurenic acid or 6-cyano-7-nitroquinoxaline-2,3-dione (CNQX)) and 2-amino-5-phosphonopentanoic acid (AP5), an NMDA glutamatergic receptor antagonist.

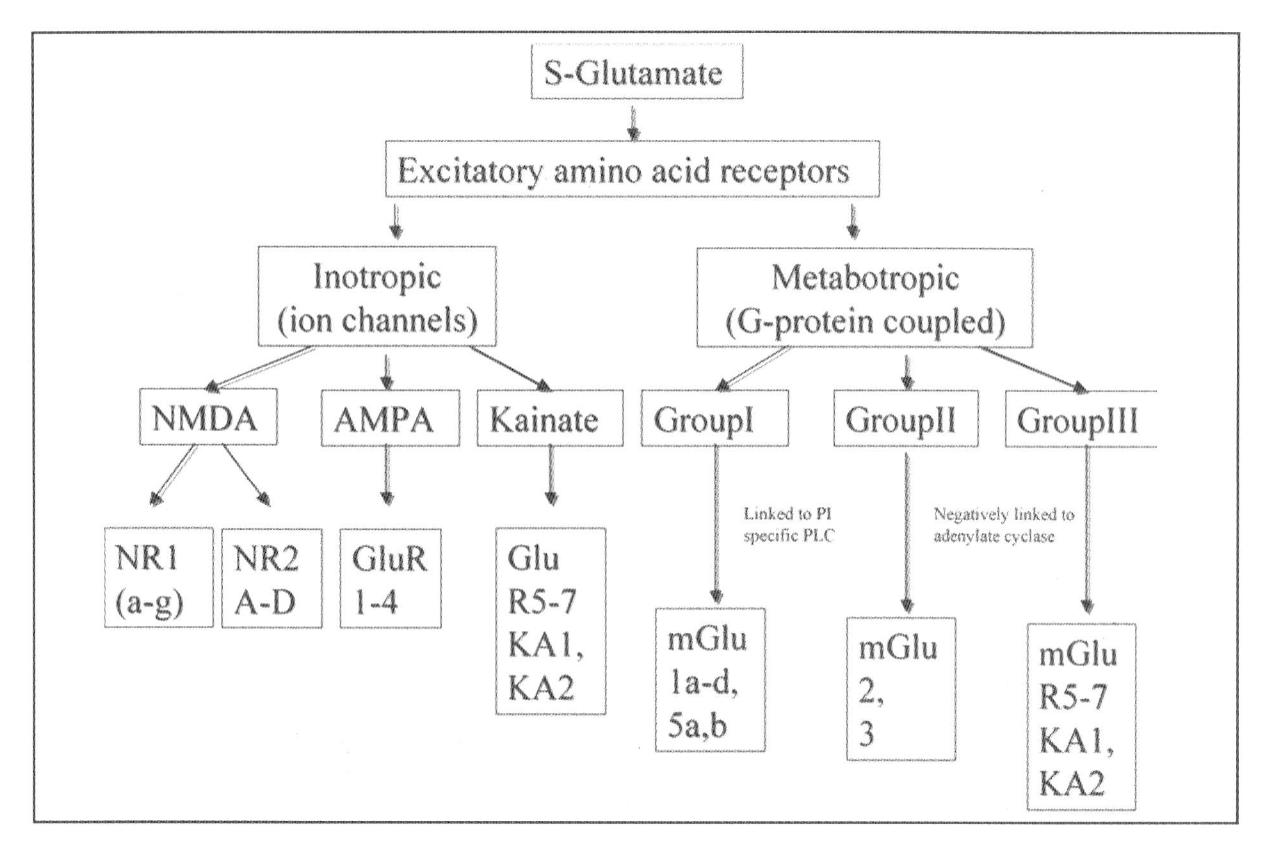

Figure 19 : Glutamate serves as an excitatory neurotransmitter in ascending, descending, interneurons and possibly afferents involved in micturition. Its actions are mediated by a wide array of receptors classified by mechanism of action. An increase in excitatory transmission could lead to OAB.

In the rat, the amplitude of (a) micturition contractions elicited by bladder distension or of (b) pelvic PGN activity elicited by stimulation of PMC is decreased by administration of NMDA (N-methyl-D-aspartate) or AMPA (α-amino-hydroxy-5-methyl-4-isoxazole propionate) receptor antagonists [277,280-283]. However in the cat, responses evoked by stimulation of the locus coeruleus are blocked by an NMDA antagonist but not by a non-NMDA antagonist [284]. It is not yet clear whether this difference represents a species difference or whether non-NMDA receptors are not significant in the direct pathway from the pontine micturition center to the PGN.

One of the main transmitters in the locus coeruleus is **noradrenaline**, but its actions, mediated by α1 adrenoceptors, on the direct pathway controlling micturition remains to be clarified. The results of experiments using α-1 and a α-2 adrenergic antagonists vary with anaesthesia, and species, and some of these drugs are not specific for adrenergic receptors [285-292]..

Opioid peptides have an inhibitory action on reflex pathways in the spinal cord. It is clear that activation of spinal δ- and probably μ-opioid receptors but not κ-opioid receptors inhibits isovolumic contractions evoked by suprathreshold distension of the bladder [293,294]. Inhibition of reflex bladder activity is mediated by δ- receptors (cat) or μ- and δ-receptors (rat) ; whereas inhibition of sphincter activity is mediated by κ-receptors [5,6]. The spinal inhibitory effect of a δ-opioid-selective agent, DPLPE, is blocked by the 5-HT antagonist, methysergide [295] ; thus the role of 5-HT in mediating the effects of spinally-administered opioid peptides is unclear. Dynorphin-B, a κ-opioid antagonist, had no effect on micturition even at 10 times its analgesic dose [294].

Therefore, a number of substances may act in the spinal cord to modulate the strength of bladder contractions, and this may be a therapeutically interesting avenue to pursue.

2. Afferent ascending pathways

Ascending Interneurons, involved in transmitting information from bladder afferents to higher centers, have been identified [296, 297,298] by combined tracing studies in which tracer substances were injected into brain stem or hypothalamus to retrogradely label spinal tract neurons and then cfos expression was used to detect neurons that responded to noxious stimulation of the bladder/urethra, or by retrograde activation using electrical stimuli. The DCM, superficial dorsal horn and SPN all contain interneurones with rostral projections that are activated during noxious [44,299] or non-noxious stimulation [258] of the rat bladder and the urethra.

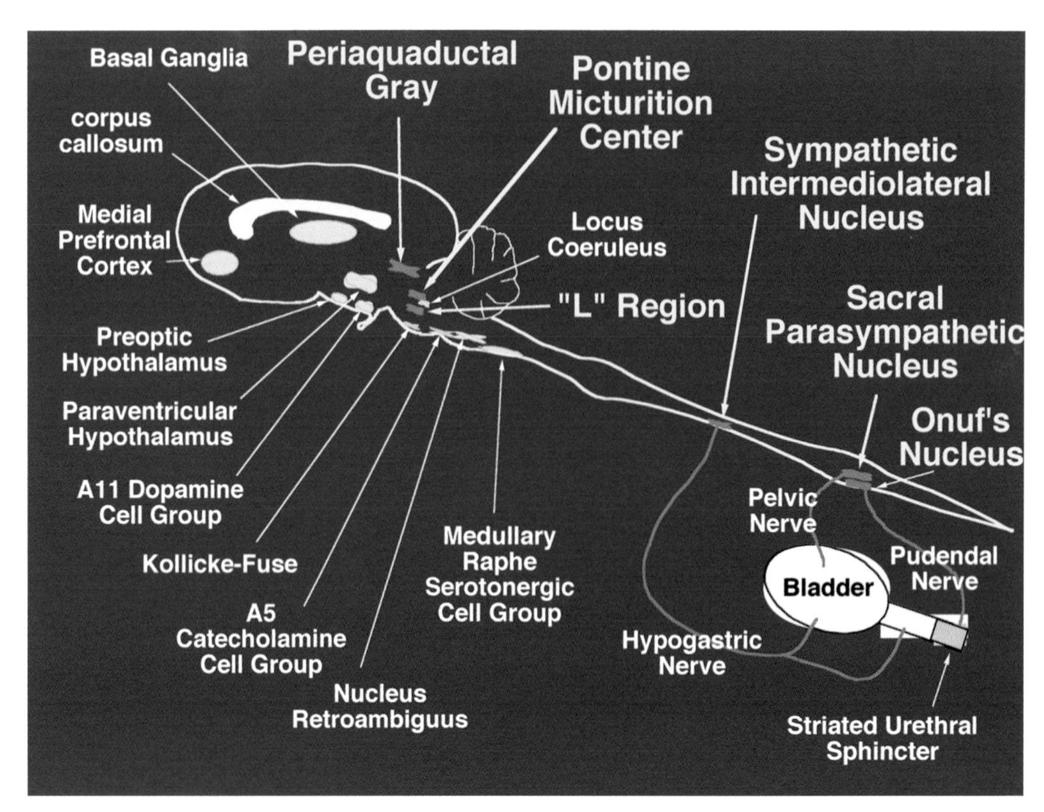

Figure 20: Diagram showing neuroanatomical distribution of brain and spinal cord nuclei involved in CNS regulation of lower urinary tract function. The primary components of the storage and micturition reflexes are shown in red and labeled in gold. The secondary (or modulatory) components are shown in pink and labeled in white.

Pharmacology of Spinal Primary Afferents and Ascending Sensory Pathways

Pharmacological experiments evaluating the effects of drugs on the central mechanisms controlling micturition have commonly used intracerebroventricular or intrathecal administration of drugs. The interpretation of results from these types of experiments is now more difficult, because recent data indicate that the micturition reflex pathway may pass the through multiple relay stations in the brain stem and be modulated by inputs from various centers in the brain (Figs. 20 & 21). Thus it is impossible to determine the exact site of action of drugs when they are administered into the cerebral ventricles or sub-arachnoid space. All that can be concluded from such an experimental design is that some central structure with access to micturition circuitry has been affected by the drug. Within the spinal cord, the action of such drugs may be on the sensory or motor components of the reflex and within the brainstem; for example cholinergic agonists are known to act on the sites within the pons and medulla to facilitate micturition [300,301] and microinjection specifically at the locus coeruleus mimics the effects of electrical stimulation at that site [5,302,303]. Details were provided by de Groat et al [2], but the main conclusions are summarized below.

Glutamate is an important excitatory transmitter in the afferent limb of the micturition reflex, and mediates its effects by means of both NMDA and nonNMDA receptors. This conclusion is based on studies of C-fos expression and the transmission of afferent activity rostrally, and the depressive effects of both NMDA and nonNMDA glutamatergic receptor antagonists [44,45,304].

The **Tachykinins** (Substance P, Neurokinin A and Neurokinin B) are structurally related peptides present in small primary afferent neurons, and their effects are mediated by the NK-1, NK-2 and NK-3 receptor subtypes of neurokinin (NK) receptors. The neurotoxin, capsaicin, which acts on the VR-1 vanilloid receptor, depletes tachykinin stores and causes degeneration of tachykinin containing primary afferents and has been used to dissect the role of these peptides. There has been considerable interest in the role of tachykinins as mediators of the first step in the spinal circuitry concerned with micturition [2]. Intrathecal treatment of adult rats with intrathecal capsaicin caused a reversible block of the micturition reflex [305]. This and other studies [306-8] suggest that substance P may play a part in transmission at the first synapse in the micturition reflex. Intrathecal administration of the NK-1 antagonists, RP 67580 and CP 96345, increased bladder capacity in conscious rats without changing micturition pressure; whereas NK-2 antagonists were ineffective [309].

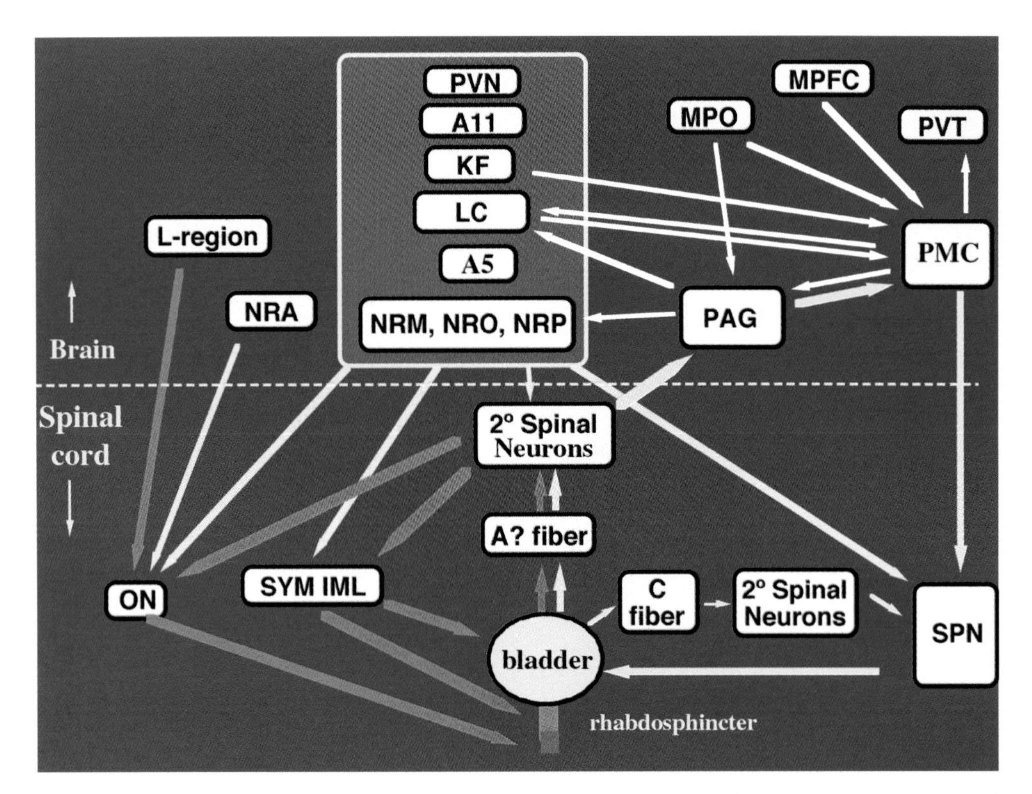

Figure 21 : Diagram of documented neuroanatomical connections of the primary and secondary components of storage and micturition reflexes. The connections of the primary components of the storage reflexes are shown in red, while the connections of the primary components of the micturition reflexes are shown in gold. The connections of the secondary (or modulatory) components of the reflexes are shown in white. Abbreviations:

- A11	*A11 group of dopaminergic neurons*	*- A5*	*A5 group of noradrenergic neurons*
- KF	*Kollicke-Fuse nucleus*	*- LC*	*locus coeruleus*
- MPFC	*medial prefrontal cortex*	*- MPO*	*medial preoptic nucleus of the hypothalamus*
- NRA	*nucleus retroambiguus*	*- NRM*	*nucleus raphe magnus*
- NRO	*nucleus raphe obscuris*	*- NRP*	*nucleus raphe pallidus*
- ON	*Onuf's nucleus*	*- PAG*	*periaqueductal gray*
- PMC	*pontine micturition center*	*- PVN*	*paraventricular nucleus*
- PVT	*periventricular thalamic nucleus*	*- SPN*	*sacral parasympathetic nucleus*
- SYM IML	*sympathetic inermediolateral nucleus*		

An inhibitory modulation by **opioid peptides** of the afferent limb of the micturition reflex at a spinal level has been suggested [2]. However the effects of morphine and its metabolites are dependent on species, anaesthesia and mode of administration, and the available data [310,311] suggest that spinal opioid mechanisms may be able to influence the afferent limb of the micturition reflex.

In addition to putative involvement in the descending limb of the micturition reflex, biogenic **monoamines** may influence the ascending limb at a spinal cord level, and may indeed be tonically active. Depletion of noradrenaline or 5-HT in the spinal cord increased micturition volume in conscious rats [287]. while blockade of noradrenaline and 5-HT re uptake in chloralose anaesthetised cats, did not affect micturition parameters unless the bladder was irritated [312]. On the other hand, intrathecal administration of blockers of 5-$HT_{1/2}$ (methysergide) or 5-HT_3 receptors (zatosetron) decreased threshold volume for perception of fullness in conscious cats [287,313] implying that descending serotonergic pathways tonically modulate afferent information at sacral spinal level.

α-1 and –2 receptor agonists and antagonists have effects that are difficult to interpret [2,288,291] because of concomitant effects on micturition pressure and residual urine volume. Intrathecal administration of a receptor subtype selective antagonists reveal that α-1A or α-1B receptors inhibit the frequency of bladder contractions on CMGs in anesthetized rats [314]. However, some α-1A receptors facilitate the descending limb of the micturition reflex pathway.

Adenosine A1 (and perhaps A2) receptor activation by intrathecal administration of the agonist produced a caffeine-sensitive increase in volume threshold in conscious rats probably because of the inhibition of excitatory interneurons, which are the presumed site of inhibitory action of the adenosine A1 agonist [315]. No studies have been reported in which the effects of adenosine receptor antagonists were evaluated, so the role of these receptors in ongoing modulation of micturition is unknown.

Intrathecally administered baclofen, a **GABA** analogue acting at GABA-B receptors, caused inhibition of distension-evoked micturition in conscious rats which appears to be independent of the release of Substance P or 5-HT. As baclofen also inhibits field stimulation evoked release of calcitonin gene-related peptide from primary afferent terminals in dorsal horn slices, one possible site for this action is suppression of primary afferent transmitter release.

Inhibitors of **Nitric Oxide** Synthase (NOS), given systemically or intrathecally, do not affect normal micturition in conscious or anesthetized rats; NOS- knockout mice also show no abnormality of micturition [316]. However, the bladder hyperreflexia that accompanies irritation with turpentine or acetic acid is ameliorated by spinal application of NOS inhibitors [317,318]. In contrast the hyperreflexia induced by intravesical administration of capsaicin is not influenced by a NOS inhibitor, although the behavioral effects of the irritation are reduced [319]. In addition to irritation, obstruction of the lower urinary tract is accompanied by increased nNOS expression in the L6/S1 DRG and dorsal horn of the spinal cord [320]. It is believed that NO is involved in mediating NMDA receptor-dependent effects but not those involving NK2 receptors. The inhibitory components of the somatovesical reflex elicited by electrical stimulation of the tibial nerve are also reduced by NOS inhibition [321]. Thus neuromodulation may operate through NO mechanisms to reduce unstable bladder contractions.

II. SUPRASPINAL PATHWAYS THAT PARTICIPATE IN THE MICTURITION REFLEX

Various studies using transections, lesions, or chemical or electrical stimulation indicate that the micturition reflex is normally mediated by a spinobulbospinal reflex pathway passing through relay centers in the brainstem (Fig. 3b) [4-6,9]. Neurons in the brain stem at or below the level of the inferior colliculus have an essential role in the control of the parasympathetic component of micturition [4-6], whereas areas of the brain above the colliculus appear to have predominantly inhibitory effects.

Although the circuitry in humans is uncertain, brain imaging studies have revealed increases in blood flow in the PMC during micturition (Figure 22) [322]. In humans it has also been confirmed that modulatory pathways exist in the caudal brainstem raphe serotonergic and coerulear noradrenergic pathways. Micturition and urinary continence are controlled by involuntary mechanisms, which have to be distinguished from the voluntary control of the pelvic floor musculature. Both mechanisms are exerting influence on the same motoneurons, but via completely separated pathways. PET scanning suggests that voluntary motor pathways involved in control of the pelvic floor originate in the most medial part of the primary motor cortex [323].

Pontine micturition center (PMC). The dorsal pontine tegmentum has been firmly established as an essential control center for micturition in normal subjects. First described by Barrington [324] it has subsequently been called "Barrington's nucleus", the "pontine micturition center" [325], or the "M region" [272,326]66,81

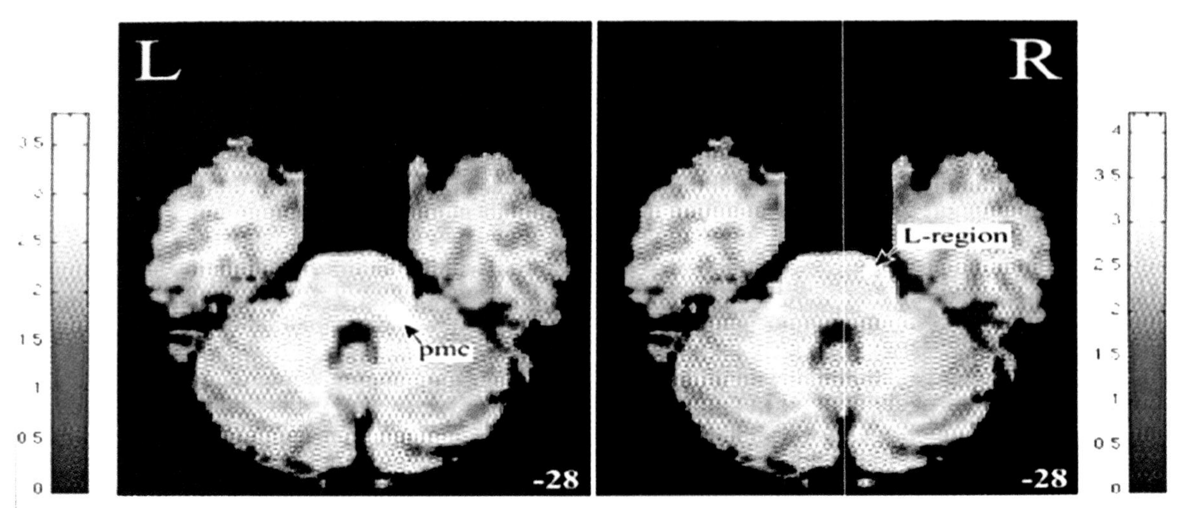

Figure 22 : PET scan of brainstem with increased activity in vicinity of pontine micturition center (PMC) during voiding. Alternatively , increased activity in L-region association with holding of urine. (after Blok et al [341])

due to its medial location. Because of its close anatomical relationship with noradrenergic cells in the locus coeruleus [327], some studies in cats have mistakenly identified the locus coeruleus as the essential region for controlling micturition [302]. The presence of reciprocal connections between the PMC and locus coeruleus [327-329] (see below), and the existence of neurons in the PMC that project to both the sacral spinal cord and the locus coeruleus via axon collaterals (Fig. 21) [328], may explain some of the difficulties distinguishing these two cell groups.

In addition to providing axonal inputs to locus coeruleus and the sacral spinal cord [328-330], neurons in the PMC also send axon collaterals to the paraventricular hypothalamic nucleus (Fig. 10), which is thought to be involved in the limbic system modulation of visceral behavior [330]. Some neurons in the pontine micturition center also project to the PAG which regulates many visceral activities as well as pain pathways [276,331]. Thus, neurons in the PMC communicate with multiple supraspinal neuronal populations that may coordinate micturition with other functons of the organism. In the rat, ascending afferent input to the pontine micturition center arises primarily from projection neurons in the lumbosacral spinal cord [332]; whereas in the cat some of the ascending input, particularly that arising form Lamina I of the dorsal horn (the LCP) seems to be relayed through the PAG [298,299, 333,334]. (Fig 21). In addition to receiving afferent input from sacral projection neurons, the dorsal and lateral PAG neurons also receive input from the medial preoptic nucleus of the hypothalamus (Fig. 10) [273], an area also implicated in sacral parasympathetic control of the bladder (see below). Neurons in the dorsal and lateral PAG project to the pontine micturition center (PMC) of the cat [334] and the rat (Fig. 21) [335,336]. Other efferent connections of the PAG include medullary serotonergic and catecholaminergic cells groups which may modulate urine storage and micturition [335,336].

Many of the neurons within the PMC of the rat contain corticotropin releasing factor (CRF) and glutamate [337]. Neurons in the PMC provide direct synaptic inputs to sacral PGN (Fig. 21) [338], as well as to GABAergic neurons in the sacral DCM [339]. The former neurons carry the excitatory outflow to the bladder, while the latter neurons are thought to be important in mediating an inhibitory influence on EUS motoneurons [276]. As a result of these reciprocal connections the PMC can promote bladder-sphincter synergy. Studies in rats indicate that activation of bladder PGN by input from the PMC can be blocked by ionotropic glutamate receptor antagonists, suggesting that neurons in the PMC utilize glutamate as a neurotransmitter [328,329].

Interestingly, the PMC also provides a dense input to lateral lamina I in the sacral cord [272,338] that overlaps with the projections of bladder primary afferent neurons [340]. It is tempting to speculate that this overlap of bladder primary afferent and supraspinal projections provides an anatomical substrate for positive feedforward facilitation of the micturition reflex to maintain an adequate excitatory outflow to the bladder in the face of decreasing levels of afferent activity as the bladder empties.

III. CENTRAL PATHWAYS THAT MODULATE THE MICTURITION REFLEX

1. PONTOMEDULLARY SYSTEMS

L-region. Axonal tracing in combination with physiological studies have identified many sites in the brain that can modulate voiding function. In the pons a region located laterally to the PMC (hence the term "L region") (Fig. 20) and just ventral to the brachium conjunctivum contains neurons that send a prominent input to EUS motoneurons in Onuf's nucleus as well as a projection to the thoracolumbar PGN (Fig 6) [15]. Bilateral lesions of the L region in the cat produce bladder hyperreflexia and incontinence [272].

Several positron emission tomography (PET) studies have provided evidence that brainstem areas involved in micturition control are comparable in cats and humans. Healthy men and women were able to micturate during scanning and showed an increased regional blood flow during micturition in the dorsal part of the pons close to the fourth ventricle (Fig. 22) [341,342]. The location of this area was similar to that of the PMC described in the cat. A second group of volunteers was not able to micturate during scanning. They showed no activation in the dorsal, but in the ventral pons, similar to the location of the PSC in cats. Apparently, the volunteers in this not successful micturition group, probably because they did not feel themselves in a safe environment, contracted their urethral sphincter and withheld their urine, although they had a full bladder and tried to urinate. Thus, in humans, increases in blood flow occur in the area comparable with the L-region of cats during periods of urinary retention suggesting that activity of neurons in this region is involved in inhibition of voiding (Fig 22) [322]

Serotoninergic raphe neurons. Bulbospinal serotonergic pathways also seem to be important in regulating voiding function. The sacral dorsal horn, SPN and Onuf's nucleus are densely innervated by serotonin (5-hydroxytryptamine, 5HT) immunoreactive (IR) terminals [274,343,344] and also exhibit moderate to high densities of various 5HT receptor subtypes. Most, if not all, of the 5HT neurons that project to the spinal cord are contained in the medullary raphe nuclei (Fig 20) [345]. Following injection of the transynaptic tracer, pseudorabies virus (PRV), into either the urinary bladder or the external urethral sphincter, numerous 5HT-IR neurons are labeled in the medullary raphe nuclei; pallidus, obscurus, and magnus; as well as in the neuropil just lateral to the pyramidal tract, the parapyramidal region [257,259-261]. Anterograde tracing studies also show direct projections from the raphe nuclei to Onuf's nucleus (Fig. 6) [346]. Electrophysiological studies have located neurons in the rostral medullary raphe (i.e. nucleus raphe magnus, NRM) that alter their firing during bladder distension [5]. 5HT neurons in nucleus raphe magnus co-express inhibitory transmitters , GABA and enkephalins; while neurons in raphe pallidus (NRP) and obscurus (NRO) (Fig. 21) co-express thyrotrophin releasing hormone and substance P, both of which have been co-localized with 5HT in individual terminals in Onuf's nucleus [343]. Chemical or electrical stimulation of the raphe nucleus [5,347] or administration of sertonergic drugs [348] inhibits reflex bladder activity.

Pontine noradrenergic pathways. The noradrenergic system in the brain stem has also been implicated in the control of lower urinary tract function [5,6,302]. Norepinephrine (NE)-containing terminals are prominent in the sacral dorsal horn, SPN and Onuf's nucleus [107,344,349]. Although the adrenoceptor subtypes on lower urinary tract neurons have not been identified it is known that $\alpha 1A$ and α_{1D} receptors are regionally distributed within the sacral spinal cord [350-353].. In the rat and human the majority of adrenergic receptors are of the α_2 type. Less prevalent are the α_1 receptors. In the rat the α_{1A} predominates. In humans based on mRNA data, the α_{1D} is predominant. Transneuronal tracing with PRV has labelled adrenergic neurons in the A5 region and in the ventral portion of locus coeruleus and subcoeruleus as well as neurons in the Kollicke-Fuse nucleus (A7 noradrenergic cell group) following injection of virus into the bladder or urethral sphincter (Fig. 21) [257-261]. Electrophysiological studies showed that bladder distension activates adrenergic neurons in locus coeruleus [331]. Neurons in the Kollicke-Fuse nucleus have been reported to project to the pontine mictrution center, as well as to autonomic centers in the spinal cord [331] The nucleus retroambiguus, located in the caudal ventrolateral medulla, contains motoneurons involved in respiration and control of abdominal musculature. In addition, this nucleus has a prominent projection to Onuf' s nucleus [346,354]. It has been speculated that this projection activates sphincter motoneurons coincident with activation of the abdominal muscles during forceful expiration such as coughing, laughing, sneezing.

2. Pharmacology of supraspinal pathways and brainstem modulatory systems

Glutamate is believed to be an excitatory neurotransmitter in the locus coeruleus or parabrachial nucleus of cats because microinjection of glutamate or its analogue DL-homocysteic acid mimics the effects of electrical stimulation at these sites (Figs 19 and 23) [355,356] . The presence of an inhibitory or mixed excitatory/inhibitory response to excitatory amino acid injection [356] may indicate that glutamate can also activate local inhibitory pathways in the pons. Injection of glutamate into the serotonergic medullary raphe nuclei which have an inhibitory function in micturition elicited only inhibitory effects [347].

Non-NMDA (N-methyl-D-aspartate) glutamatergic receptor antagonists injected intracerebroventricularly or bilaterally into the locus coeruleus blocked the activation of locus coeruleus neurons, and the EEG arousal pattern; but an NMDA glutamatergic receptor antagonist (AP-5) had no effect [357]. In conscious rats the bladder hyperactivity induced by middle cerebral artery occlusion can be aborted by pretreatment with an NMDA antagonist (MK-801) or can be suppressed by treatment after the occlusion [358]. More studies are necessary to determine the specific receptors and synapses where glutamate is functioning.

Gamma Amino-Butyric Acid GABA or GABA agonists apparently mediate a tonically active inhibitory modulation of the micurition reflex at a supraspinal level [356,358]. GABA or muscimol, a GABA-A receptor agonist, suppressed reflex bladder activity and increased the volume threshold for inducing micturition in a bicuculline-sensitive manner when injected at sites in the brainstem where electrical stimulation induced bladder contraction. Because bicuculline (a GABA antagonist) alone stimulated bladder activity and lowered the volume threshold for micturition, it was concluded that there is a tonic GABA-ergic inhibitory modulation in these region (Fig. 23) [592].

Interest in the role of dopamine in the supraspinal control of bladder function, arises from the clinical observation that patients with Parkinson's disease which is caused by degeneration of dopamine-containing neurons in the brain stem often exhibit bladder overactivity [5,6,357]. Pharmacological studies however reveal that dopamine and its agonists have mixed effects depending on the site and mode of application. In cats microinjection of dopamine into the PMC faciliated the micturition reflex [6] (Fig 24), whereas intracerebroventricular administration of dopamine or a D-1 dopamine receptor agonist (SKF38393) inhibited the micturition reflex [593].

The role of **opioid peptides** has been studied using

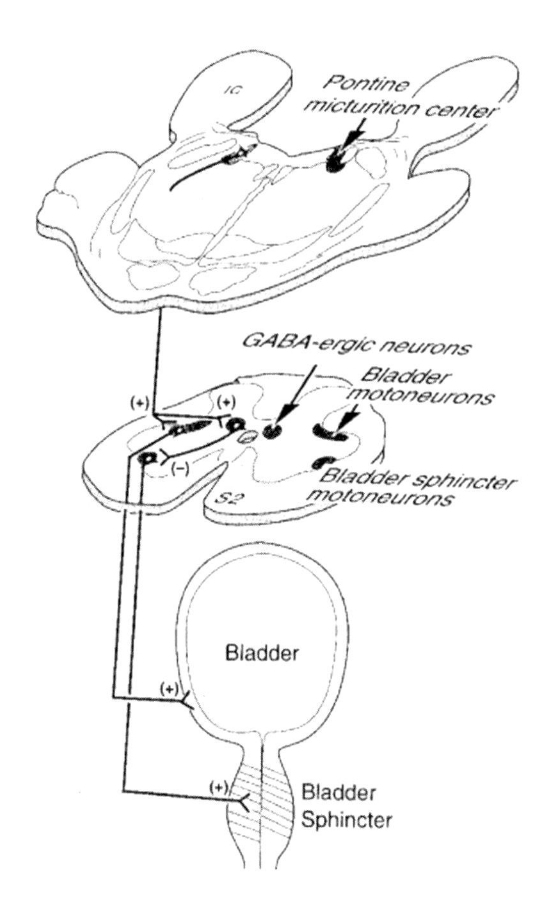

Figure 23 : Coordination of voiding with external urethral sphincter. Descending glutamatergic input to sacral spinal cord excites bladder neurons in sacral parasympathetic neurons (SPN). Simultaneous activation of GABA neurons inhibits sphinter neurons in Onuf's nucleus. Conversely, during attempts at urine storage activation of GABA neurons providing input to bladder neurons while providing excitatory input to sphincter neurons.

focal microinjections of drugs that confirm some of the results of icv injection of morphine and its antagonist naloxone [293,359] have been obtained in urethane treated rats [360]. Injection of D-Ala^2-Met^5-enkephalinamide (DAMA) into the pontine micturition center blocked isovolumic bladder contraction, an effect antagonized by systemic or local naloxone administration. Naloxone injected alone increased frequency without changing amplitude of contractions. Individual PMC neurons which were activated with bladder contraction were inhibited by fentanyl. Both μ- and δ-opioid but not κ-opioid receptors can mediate this supraspinal effect [293,361], but apparently by different mechanisms [295].

Intracerebroventricular administration of **purines** and purinergic antagonists in the rat has been used to decipher the role of ATP on supraspinal pathways involved in micturition. Recently, investigators have found that the P2X3 receptor in the brainstem facilitates micturition [362].

Conclusion

In conclusion, glutamate may be involved as an excitatory transmitter in the supraspinal circuitry controlling micturition and may be a mediator of bladder hyperactivity following neural injury, however the role of other potential excitatory transmitters needs to be examined. It is also clear that several substances can exert significant modulatory influences on these circuits (Fig. 11), and thereby have dramatic influences on micturition. The receptors for these substances therefore represent potential sites for therapeutic intervention (Fig. 24).

3. Hypothalamic systems

The paraventricular hypothalamus provides direct projections to the sympathetic intermediolateral cell column, SPN, Onuf's nucleus and the LCP in lateral lamina I in the sacral spinal cord [272], i.e. a region densely innervated by bladder primary afferent neurons [5,340]. The medial preoptic region (MPO) of the hypothalamus also appears to play a role in control of micturition since it projects to the PAG and to the PMC (Fig. 21) [272]. Further linkage between the medial preoptic nucleus and micturition has emerged from clinical brain imaging studies in patients that have revealed increases in regional blood flow in this region of the hypothalamus during micturition [322].

The paraventricular hypothalamus is one of the richest sources of neuropeptide neurotransmitters in the brain. Thus, it is possible that some of the peptidergic transmitters found in the SPN arise from the paraventricular nucleus. **Oxytocin** containing projections from the brain, presumably the hypothalamus, are found in the sacral spinal cord [363]. Oxytocin may inhibit voiding (Fig 25). Intrathecal oxytocin raises the volume threshold for micturition on awake cystometrograms. In obstructed rats, oxytocin can inhibit unstable contractions [363]. These effects can be prevented by a selective antagonist to the oxytocin receptor. Whether this transmitter and hormone acts in the dorsal horn on afferent input, interneurons or directly on autonomic preganglionic neurons is uncertain. Dopaminergic terminals which are thought to arise from **dopamine**-containing neurons of the A11 cell group in the diencephalon have been identified in the PMC as well as in the sacral spinal cord in the regions of visceral afferent projections, the SPN and Onuf's nucleus [364].

4. Cortical pathways

Although the forebrain is not essential for the micturition reflex, clinical observations suggest that it is important for the beginning of micturition. Studies on animals suggest that the prominent facilitatory effect of

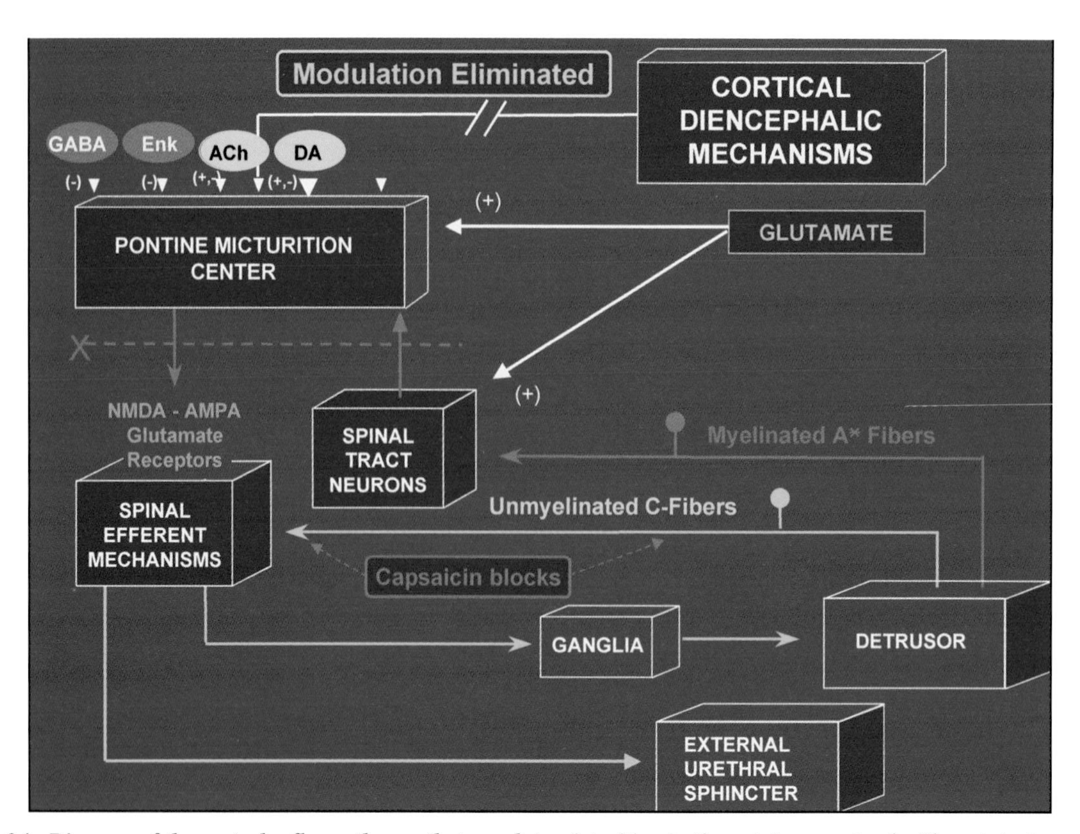

Figure 24 : Diagram of the central reflex pathways that regulate micturition in the cat. In an animal with an intact neuraxis, micturition is initiated by a supraspinal reflex pathway passing through the pontine micturition center (PMC) in the brainstem. The pathway is triggered by myelinated afferents (Aδ) connected to tension receptors in the bladder wall (detrusor). Spinal tract neurons carry information to the brain. During micturition, pathways from the PMC activate the parasympathetic outflow to the bladder and inhibit the somatic outflow to the urethral sphincter. Transmission in the PMC is modulated by cortical-diencephalic mechanisms. Interruption of the latter mechanisms leads to bladder hyperactivity. In spinal cord transected animals, connections between the brainstem and the sacral spinal cord are interrupted and micturition is initially blocked. In chronic spinal animals, a spinal micturition reflex emerges which is triggered by unmyelinated (C-fiber) bladder afferents. The C-fiber reflex pathway is usually weak or undetectable in animals with an intact nervous system. Stimulation of the C-fiber bladder afferents by instillation of ice water into the bladder activates voiding reflexes in patients with spinal cord injury. Capsaicin (20-30 mg/kg, s.c.) blocks the C-fiber reflexes in chronic spinal cats, but does not block micturition reflexes in intact cats. Intravesical capsaicin also suppresses detrusor hyperreflexia and cold-evoked reflexes in patients with neurogenic bladder dysfunction. Glutamic acid is the principal excitatory transmitter in the ascending and descending limbs of the micturition reflex pathway as well as in the reflex pathway controlling sphincter function. Glutamate acts on both NMDA and AMPA glutamatergic receptors. Other neurotransmitters that regulate transmission in the micturition reflex pathway include: gamma-aminobutyric acid (GABA), enkephalins (Enk), acetylcholine (ACh) and dopamine (DA). ACH has both excitatory and inhibitory effects on the pathway. (+) excitatory and (-) inhibitory synapse. Dopamine acts through D1 receptors on GABAergic cells and is inhibitory.

decerebration in animals with an intact neuraxis seems to be due in large part to removal of tonic inhibition originating in the cerebral cortex [5]. Various cortical areas are labeled following injection of PRV into the lower urinary tract [257-261,357]; thus, cortical control of voiding is likely to be complex. The prefrontal cortex of the rat is considered a visceromotor area, while the insular cortex is considered a viscerosensory area. Evidence for tonic cortical inhibition of bladder function was also obtained in rats in which infarction of the middle cerebral artery on one side produced a prominent decrease in bladder capacity [594]. This effect was eliminated by administering an NMDA glutamatergic receptor antagonist, indicating that glutamatergic excitatory transmission is involved in the OAB [594].

In the cat, stimulation of forebrain structures, as anterior cingulate gyrus, hypothalamus, amygdala, bed nucleus of the stria terminalis and septal nuclei, can elicit bladder contractions [366]. Although most of these regions send fibers to the brainstem, only the hypothalamic preoptic area projects specifically to the PMC [298,367].

• Studies on the Human CNS during Micturition

PET scanning studies suggests that this might also be true in humans, because the hypothalamus, including the preoptic area, was activated during micturition [341]. The direct projection from the hypothalamic preoptic area to the PMC probably conveys the "safe signal" to the PMC to start micturition. Most of the PET scanning studies on micturition [341,342,343,368] point to two cortical areas: the cingulate gyrus and the prefrontal cortex. Cerebral blood flow in the cingulate gyrus was significantly decreased during voluntary

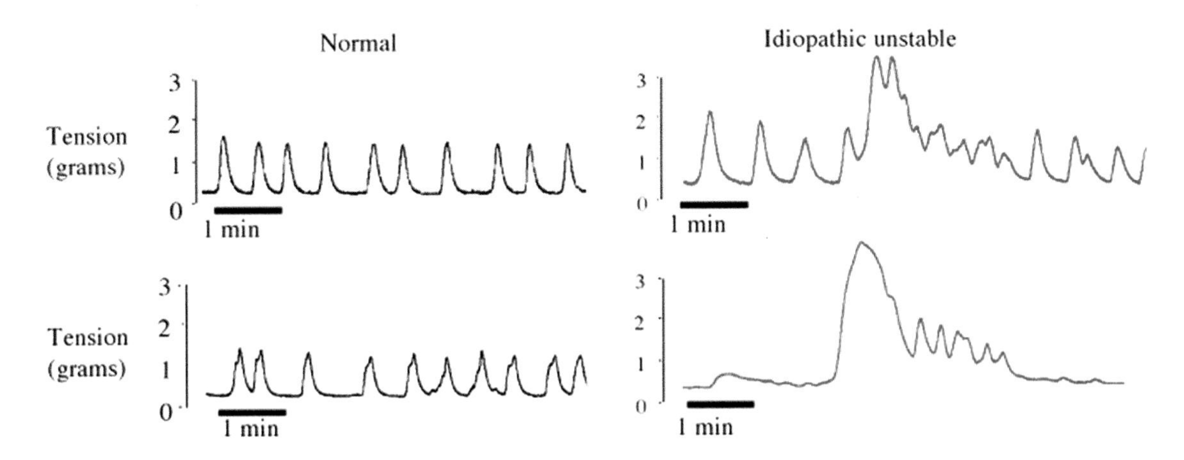

Figure 25 : Spontaneous contractile activity in detrusor strips dissected from normal (left) and idiopathically unstable (right) human bladders. Note the typical small phasic contractions of the normal detrusor strips, and the larger fused contractions in strips from unstable bladders (From [377])

withholding of urine and during the urge to void. The prefrontal cortex is active when micturition takes place and during involuntary urine withholding. Possibly, activation of the prefrontal cortex and the anterior cingulate gyrus do not reflect specific involvement in micturition, but more in general mechanisms, such as attention and response selection. The prefrontal cortex plays a role in making the decision whether or not micturition should take place at that particular time and place. Forebrain lesions including the anterior cingulate gyrus are known to cause urge incontinence [369]. The cingulate gyrus influences strongly descending pathways involved in the facilitation of motoneurons and interneurons.

PET scans were used to examine which brain areas are involved in human micturition [322]. Seventeen right-handed male volunteers were scanned during the following four conditions: 1) 15 min prior to micturition during urine holding; 2) during micturition; 3) 15 min after micturition; 4) 30 min after micturition. Ten of the 17 volunteers were able to micturate during scanning. Micturition was associated with increased blood flow in the right dorsomedial pontine tegmentum, the periaqueductal grey, the hypothalamus and the right inferior frontal gyrus [322]. Decreased blood flow was found in the right anterior cingurate gyrus when urine was withheld. The other seven volunteers were not able to micturate during scanning, although they had a full bladder and tried vigorously to micturate. In this group, during these unsuccessful attempts to micturate, increased blood flow was detected in the right ventral pontine tegmentum, which is consistent with the idea, arising from studies in cats [272,326], that this area controls the motoneurons of the pelvic floor. Increased blood flow also occurred in the right inferior frontal gyrus during unsuccessful attempts to micturate, and decreased blood flow occurred in the right anterior cingulate gyrus during the withholding of urine. The results suggest that the human brainstem contains specific nuclei responsible for the control of micturition, and that the cortical and pontine regions for micturition are predominantly on the right side. The results are in accordance with the results of a clinical analysis which was performed to determine the individual contribution of the right and left cerebral hemispheres to the frequency and urgency of micturition in 134 chronic hemiplegic patients [342,370]. A mean frequency of micturition, 9 times or more in 24 hours, was found more frequently in left than right hemiplegics. Left hemiplegics also complained more often of urgency than did right hemiplegics. A mean frequency of micturition of 9 times or more in 24 hours and urgency co-existed more frequently in left hemiplegics than in right hemiplegics. In this study dealing with the chronic sequelae of stroke, frequency and urgency of micturition occurred more commonly in patients with right hemisphere than left hemisphere lesions.

A PET study was also conducted in adult female volunteers to identify brain structures involved in the voluntary motor control of the pelvic floor during four conditions:

1) rest;

2) repetitive pelvic floor straining;

3) sustained pelvic floor straining; and

4) sustained abdominal straining.

The results revealed that the superomedial precentral gyrus, the most medial portion of the motor cortex, is activated during pelvic floor contraction and the superolateral precentral gyrus during contraction of the abdominal musculature. In these conditions, significant activations were also found in the cerebellum, supplementary motor cortex, and thalamus. The right anterior cingulate gyrus was activated during sustained pelvic floor straining.

There is general agreement on the finding that patients with lesions in only the **basal ganglia** or thalamus have normal urethral sphincter function. These patients can voluntarily contract the striated sphincter and abort or considerably lessen the effect of the abnormal micturition reflex, when an impending involuntary contraction or its onset is sensed. The patients with lesions in the cerebral cortex and/or internal capsule following a cerebrovascular accident are unable to forcefully contract the striated sphincter under these circumstances. Thus these patients have a profound abnormality in the cerebral-to-corticospinal circuitry that is necessary for voluntary control of the striated sphincter. It is intriguing that a variety of emotional (depression, anxiety) and autonomic disorders are associated with changes within the prefrontal cortex. Because many of theses emotional states are associated with OAB, it is tempting to speculate that neurochemical changes within this area of the brain have an impact on a range of voiding dysfunctions.

5. Conclusions: CNS physiology and neuropharmacology

The pathways that mediate the micturition reflex have been described: the reflex involves afferents and efferents in the pelvic nerve, and in the normal adult, the connection between these involved ascending and descending pathways that connect the sacral cord and the pontine micturition center. In some species the periaqueductal gray matter also participates in this pathway, and in humans there is now evidence of involvement of these areas as a result of PET scanning. Both glutamate and tachykinins are important in the spinal processing of afferent input from the bladder, possibly in different pathways.

Modulation of the micturition reflex – switching it off or on in appropriate circumstances – is a function of a number of important regions in the brain, ranging from the raphe nuclei in the medulla , through areas of the pons and midbrain, up to the hypothalamus, limbic system and cingulate gyrus and the frontal cortex.

Transmitters such as 5-HT, purines ,GABA, oxytocin and PACAP appear to modulate rather selectively the volume threshold by actions in the sacral spinal cord. These mechanisms, too, seem to be favorable for development of novel drug therapies. Other modulators may also prove to be useful targets for drugs, perhaps specifically in hyperreflexia, but more work is required to clarify their significance.

D. MODELS OF BLADDER OVERACTIVITY

The storage symptoms of urgency, frequency, nocturia, with or without urge incontinence usually with frequency and nocturia have recently been referred to as the overactive bladder syndrome (OAB). OAB-related problems have a devastating impact on U.S. citizens in all age groups and especially the middle-aged and elderly. In a population based European study of nearly 17,000 subjects over age 40, 16.6% (for an estimated prevalence of 22.2 million) reported symptoms consistent with OAB [371]. Only 36% had urge incontinence, and more women than men complained of OAB. Because these demographic groups are increasing in size relative to the rest of the population, the societal impact of the OAB is likely to increase in the future. Despite the projected demand for treatment, many patients are inadequately treated now. Quality of life surveys document that urinary frequency, urgency, and nocturia are some of the most bothersome aspects of voiding dysfunction. These symptoms may reflect, in part, disturbances in how the afferent threshold for micturition is regulated or how sensory information is consciously perceived. Other mechanisms for OAB may include changes in central mechanisms, efferent neural outflow, or in smooth muscle; each of these may have consequences for the functioning of other tissues concerned with micturition. In detrusor overactivity, and there is good evidence of severe changes in the function of smooth muscle and peripheral nerves.

I. PERIPHERAL MODELS OF OAB

Disturbances of the peripheral nerves and tissues can cause bladder overactivity, and models have been developed to mimic these changes. These models are relevant to neurogenic and idiopathic detrusor overactivity, bladder partial denervation, lower urinary tract obstruction, diabetes and interstitial cystitis. In some respects the division between peripheral and central causes of overactive bladder is artificial, but it serves as a useful division so that the interactions between different tissues can be seen. It must be kept in mind there are important interactions between peripheral and central neurons when there are lesions of one or other of these. There is now a greater appreciation that long-term events involving growth factors leads to plasticity in neural pathways with implications for disorders of micturition. Neurotransmitters, prostaglandins and growth factors, such as Nerve Growth Factor (NGF), are substances that provide mechanisms for communication between muscle and nerve. Disturbances in these mechanisms can cause detrusor overactivity due to alterations in either bladder smooth muscle or autonomic reflex pathways. This bladder overactivity can, in turn, lead to urge incontinence. However some of the disturbances that cause the release of nerve growth factor may also be associated with the loss of peripheral neurones, and regrowth or sprouting of affected neurones may or may not occur as a result of local NGF production.

1. Detrusor overactivity

Patients with an detrusor overactivity are defined urodynamically as demonstrating involuntary detrusor contractions during the filling phase which may be spontaneous or provoked. These patients often share a common set of symptoms, regardless of the aetiology of the condition. These are urgency (when sensations are intact), frequency, urge incontinence and nocturia. Urodynamic traces alone do not allow the determination of whether the overactivity is idiopathic or is associated with neuropathy or outflow obstruction, although in the latter case the micturition pressure is likely to be elevated. The similarity of the symptoms suggests that there may be common factors underlying the overactivity, and in this section what is known about the changes that result in involuntary contractions will be discussed, and what are the possible causative factors.

a) Common Features

Examination of the physiological properties and ultra structure of the bladder wall obtained from human or animal overactive detrusors demonstrates common changes:

- Increased spontaneous myogenic activity
- Fused tetanic contractions
- Altered responsiveness to stimuli
- Characteristic changes in smooth muscle ultra structure

Examination of the peripheral innervation and the micturition reflex in animals and humans with overactive detrusors also shows common changes:

- Patchy denervation of the bladder wall
- Enlarged sensory neurones
- Enlarged parasympathetic ganglion cells
- Increased effectiveness of a spinal micturition pathway.

All these common features make it very likely that whatever the aetiology of the condition, the underlying causative mechanisms are the same or very similar. These changes will be considered in more detail below.

b) Changes to the smooth muscle of the bladder wall.

• Changes in the unstable bladder

Smooth muscle strips dissected from overactive detrusors often show increases in spontaneous contractile activity. This has been seen in human bladder strips from obstructed overactive bladders [372] and from neuropathic unstable bladders [373]. A change in the pattern of the spontaneous activity is also seen which is very characteristic of detrusor overactivity. Strips from these bladders show fused tetanic contractions (Fig. 25), reminiscent of the activity typically shown by well coupled smooth muscles such as in the gut [374-7]. Similar fused tetanic contractions are seen in bladders from pigs with instability secondary to outflow obstruction; indeed in those with well developed overactivity, bizarre patterns are often observed [73,78] (Fig. 26).

Alterations are also seen in the responses of overactive detrusor to stimulation with agonists and to transmural electrical stimulation (either direct, or via activation of intrinsic nerves). In this case, there are differences in the patterns seen in tissues from overactive bladders of different aetiology. In obstructed bladders there is a supersensitivity to muscarinic agonists and KCl with a reduced contraction to intrinsic nerve stimulation [372,379,380]. Similar changes are seen in animal models (pig: [381,382]; rabbit: [383]). In neuropathic bladders from patients with spina bifida (Fig. 27), supersensitivity is again seen to cholinergic agonists and KCl, but there is no change in the sensitivity of the contractile response to intrinsic nerve stimulation, although the size of the response is smaller [384]. In idiopathic detrusor overactivity, bladder strips show supersensitivity to KCl, but not to muscarinic agonists and there is a reduced contractile response to intrinsic nerve stimulation (Fig. 28) [377]. There is evidence that unstable strips are more easily activated by direct electrical stimulation of the smooth muscle [384] (showing contractions elicited by transmural nerve stimulation that are resistant to the nerve blocking action of tetrodotoxin).

At an ultra structural level, a common feature seen in the overactive detrusor is the presence of protrusion junctions and ultra-close abutments between the smooth muscle cells, features occurring only rarely in normal tissue [248]. Again development of these junctions has been seen in animal models [385].

• Significance of these changes

The properties of the normal detrusor suggest that the smooth muscle bundles are not as well-coupled electrically as are most visceral smooth muscles. This poorly developed electrical coupling accounts for the small size of the spontaneous contractions in detrusor strips, since it will prevent spontaneous synchronous activation of all the smooth muscle cells. The lack of good coupling means that *in vivo* electrical activity will be able to control the length of individual cells without the risk of generating a rise in pressure. Dense innervation allows synchronous activation of the muscle and a rise in intravesical pressure during micturition.

The changes that occur in the smooth muscle of the

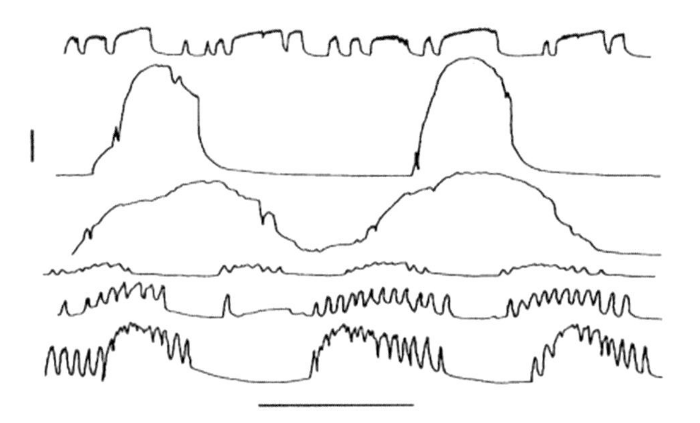

Figure 26 : Spontaneous contractile activity in a strip of smooth muscle dissected from the bladder of a pig with an unstable bladder due to partial bladder outlet obstruction.

% maximum response

Carbachol M

Neuropaths

Controls

Figure 27 : Concentration-contractile response curve to 10 sec applications of carbachol of strips from normal human bladders (round symbols) and bladders from patients with unstable bladders secondary to spina bifida (square symbols). Note the increased sensitivity of the smooth muscle to the muscarinic agonist. (From [384]).

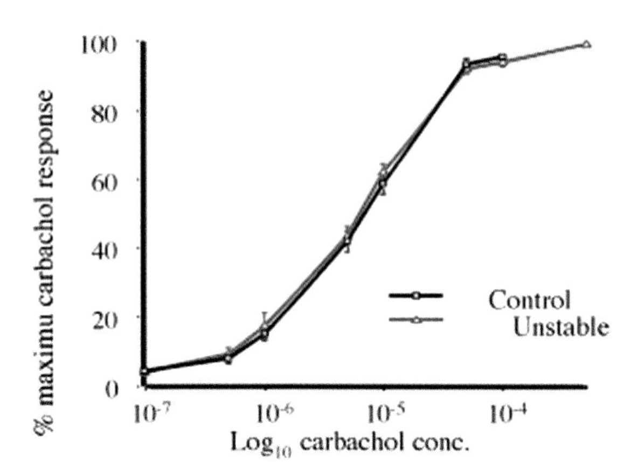

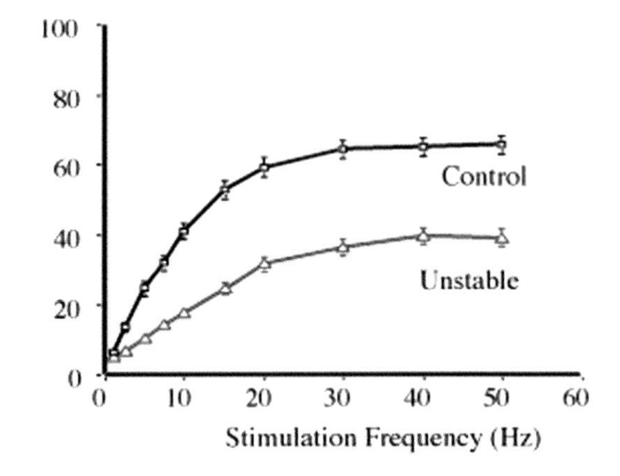

Figure 28 : Frequency-response curve to transmural nerve stimulation and concentration-contractile response curve to 10 sec applications of carbachol of strips from normal human bladders (circles) and bladders from patients with idiopathically unstable bladders (triangles). Note reduction in response to nerve stimulation, but no change in sensitivity to muscarinic agonist. (From [218]).

overactive detrusor strongly suggest that the cells are better coupled electrically, so that spontaneous electrical activity will spread and initiate synchronous contractions in many more smooth muscle cells. This would account for the fused tetanic contractions seen in the unstable bladder strips; the close abutments and protrusion junctions seen ultra structurally may be the morphological correlates of this connectivity. In the whole bladder, the increased excitability of the smooth muscle combined with the greater connectivity could result in the generation of focuses of electrical activity which could spread and produce an involuntary contraction.

Why should such changes occur in the smooth muscle of overactive bladders? Smooth muscle, along with most innervated tissues, is capable of altering its responses to changes in its pattern of activation. The types of change that are seen in the detrusor smooth muscle are reminiscent of the changes due to experimental denervation [386]. It seems very likely that the changes in detrusor properties are caused by altered patterns of activation. This will be explored below.

c) Changes in peripheral innervation and the micturition reflex

• CHANGES IN THE BLADDER WALL

Another common feature of the overactive detrusor is a change in the macroscopic structure of the bladder wall. Regardless of the aetiology of the condition, sections of the bladder wall from unstable human bladder frequently show patchy denervation of the muscle bundles. Some muscle bundles may be completely denervated, whilst neighboring ones appear normal (Figs. 29) and in other areas sparser innervation is also seen [377,384,385,387]. A similar pattern is seen in animal models (pigs: [388]; guinea-pigs: [389]; rabbit: [383]), although interestingly not in the rat [390], where the post-ganglionic neurones are all in the pelvic ganglia and not in the bladder wall. The denervated and sparsely innervated areas of the bladder wall become infiltrated with connective tissue elements such as collagen and elastin [384,385,387], and in the completely denervated areas in tissue from idiopathic and neuropathic overactive bladders, hypertrophy of the smooth muscle cells is seen [387].

• CHANGES IN NEURONAL STRUCTURE

Animal experiments (carried out mainly in the rat) have demonstrated that procedures such as spinal section or urethral obstruction, as well as leading to the development of bladder instability, also lead to an increase in size of both the afferent neurones in the dorsal root ganglia (L6 - S1, [391]) and the efferent neurones in the pelvic plexus (after obstruction: [392,393]; after spinal section: [394]). Similar increase in the size of the neurones in bladder wall ganglia in the obstructed guinea-pig has been seen.

• CHANGES IN THE MICTURITION REFLEX

Changes have also been seen in the micturition reflex in animals after recovery from spinal shock following spinal injury. Electrophysiological measurements of the central delay in the micturition reflex show a shorter delay in animals with spinal injury (for references see [395]) than in intact animals, suggesting that there has been re-organisation of the micturition pathway from a spino-bulbo-spinal pathway to a purely spinal pathway. Also, activation of specific C-fibre afferents can trigger micturition in overactive bladders, but not in normal bladders. This latter observation is thought to be true in humans, since in normal humans the ice water test (instillation of the bladder with cold water), which is thought to activate specific C-fibres, does not trigger micturition, but does so in many patients with overactive bladders [396,397]. In fact intravesical administration of selective C-fibre neurotoxins such as capsaicin and resiniferatoxin is an effective treatment in many patients with neuropathic overactivity [398].

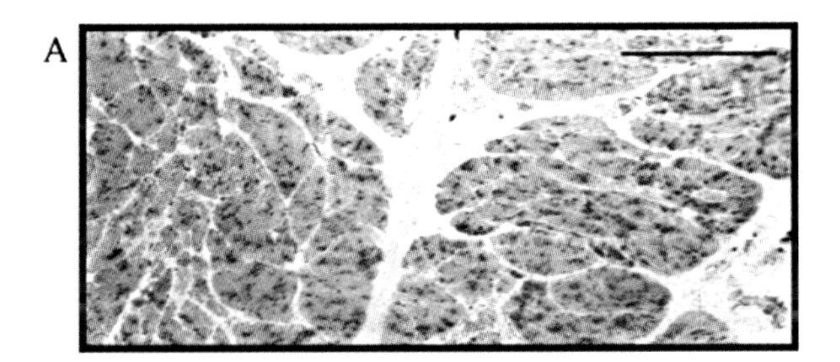

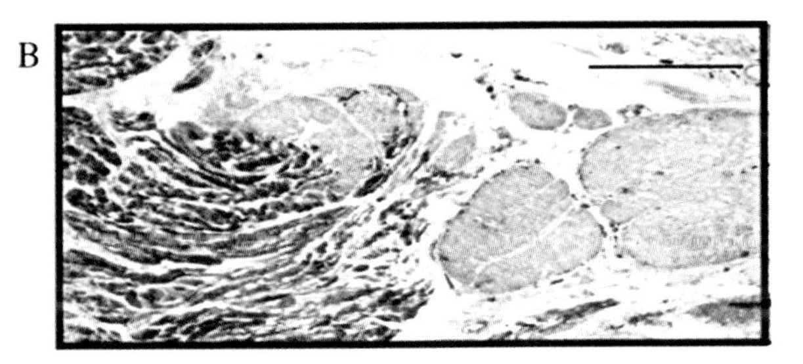

Figure 29 : Section of a normal human detrusor (A), and detrusor from a patient with idiopathic instability (B) stained to show the presence of acetylcholinesterase on the axons of intramural nerves. Note uniform dense staining of the smooth muscle bundles in normal tissue and exceptionally dense innervation of one muscle bundle adjacent to another completely denervated bundle in unstable tissue (From [218]).

d) Possible causes of these changes

It seems inherently likely that the changes associated with the overactive bladder are the result of alterations in the activity in the neuronal pathways controlling the detrusor. The sensory neurones are likely to encounter increased stimulation after outflow obstruction or inflammation of the urothelium, which could result in the hypertrophy of these neurones and also of the ganglia, since presumably increased parasympathetic activation will result. The patchy denervation suggests that there has been death of some of the intrinsic neurones in the bladder wall. The most likely cause of this is bladder wall ischaemia, which will be discussed in more detail in the next section. In brief, the bladder has been shown to be susceptible to ischaemia [124, 377, 399], since anything that raises intravesical pressure to more than 30-40cms H_2O seriously compromises blood flow in the wall. In outflow obstruction where there is a significant hypertrophy of the wall, increased metabolic demands [400] and reduced blood flow can lead to significant periods of anoxia which might result eventually in neuronal death (Fig. 30) . This could also result from detrusor sphincter dyssynergia in cases of spinal injury.

The changes in the reflex pathway that occur after spinal injury probably result from the loss of descending pathways. This may trigger the production of growth factors and the resultant sprouting of axon terminals in surviving pathways to make new and abnormal connections; for instance the C-fibres may increase their connections to the interneurones or motor neurones in the segmental spinal parasympathetic pathways. The enhanced size of the efferent post-ganglionic neurones in obstructed bladders appears to be the result of the liberation of nerve growth factor (NGF) by the detrusor, since autoimmunization of rats against NGF reduces the neuronal hypertrophy [401]. Presumably the stimulus for the production of NGF may be the increased work load of the obstructed bladder [402].

c) The problem of urgency

Everyday experience would suggest that urgency is a separate sensation from that of bladder fullness. Animal experiments recording from afferent nerves during bladder filling and contraction [19,20,403,404] have shown increased activity in a uni-modal population of small myelinated and unmyelinated (Aδ and C) fibres in response to intravesical pressure and contraction, suggesting that there are in-series stretch receptors in the bladder wall, whose activity correlates with the sensations of bladder filling and fullness. However, it seems unlikely that fibres with such properties mediate the sensation of urgency. Again from everyday experience, urgent desire to void disappears as soon as micturition starts - at a time when intravesical pressure and contractions will both be high. Unfortunately the relationship between urgency and detrusor activity cannot be investigated in animals, since we cannot know what sensations they perceive. In humans, however, it is clear from both normal and ambulatory cystometry that involuntary pressure rises may occur without eliciting any apparent sensations. A sensible theory about urgency has been proposed by Coolsaet et al [405]. They suggest that urgency is triggered by local distortions in the bladder wall, caused by activity in some muscle bundles but not others. Such a condition would arise in normal bladders if a small population of low threshold post-ganglionic parasympathetic neurones were directly activated through a spinal pathway, for instance

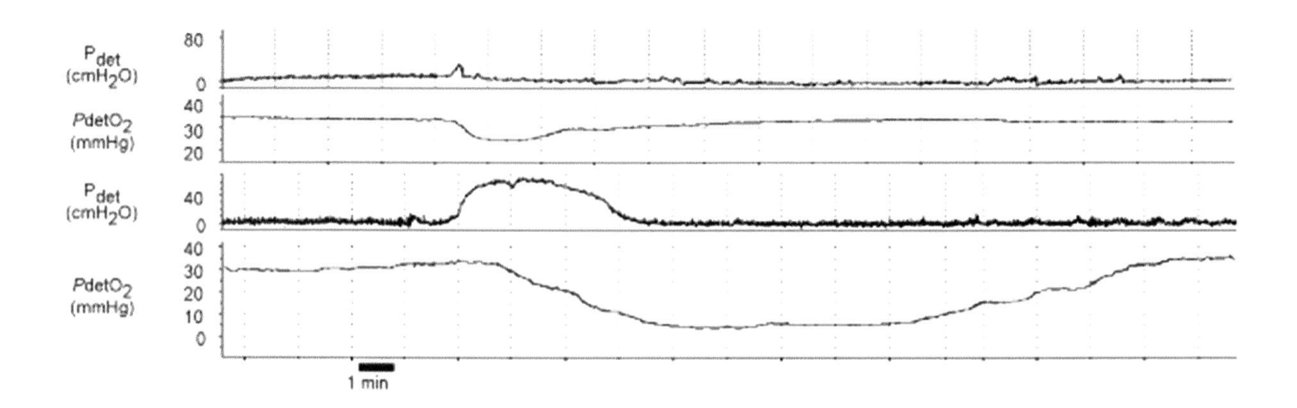

Figure 30 : Urodynamic tracings from a normal pig (upper two traces) and an obstructed pig (lower two traces). Top trace of each shows intravesical pressure, and bottom trace oxygen tension in the bladder wall. Blood flow (not shown) follows a pattern that is the inverse of the pressure rise. Note that the drop in oxygen tension significantly outlasts the rise in detrusor pressure and drop in blood flow. (From [124]).

towards the end of bladder filling. Because of relatively poor coupling between bundles, such diffuse activity would not cause a rise in intravesical pressure, but could cause sufficient local distortions in the bladder wall to activate a population of nerve fibres that might specifically mediate the sensation of urgency and play a useful role in encouraging the initiation of normal micturition. In overactive bladders, however, such diffuse activity might spread because of the increased electrical connectivity to give rise both to a premature sensation of urgency and an involuntary pressure rise. This theory would account for the efficacy of antimuscarinic drugs in the treatment of urge incontinence. If only a small number of ganglia were activated directly by the sensory nerves, suppression of their effects could eliminate both premature urgency and the involuntary contractions. Normal micturition would still occur, since this would involve recruitment of many more ganglia, and direct activation of all the smooth muscle cells. An increase in the sensitivity of fibres mediating urgency may be responsible for the enhanced urgency seen in inflammatory conditions, interstitial cystitis and other examples of sensory urgency.

f) Conclusions

It is clear that we are still some way from really understanding what causes urge incontinence. However there are sufficient clues from the observations and experimental results described above to suggest that we are dealing with the consequences of altered patterns of activation of the nerves in the micturition pathways and thus of the smooth muscle in the detrusor. In cases of severe urgency and urge incontinence, the process has probably been on-going for years, has caused periodic bladder wall ischaemia and has reached a stage in which neurones in the bladder wall have actually died; the smooth muscle in the detrusor has then become able to generate synchronous contractions and these result in the unstable pressure rises seen. What precise mechanism triggers these involuntary contractions is not yet clear, although it is likely that residual neuronal activity of some sort is often involved.

It may be that the most likely scenario for urge incontinence which is associated with overactive contractions is as follows: activity in some muscle bundles generated either by stretch or by diffuse activity in parasympathetic fibres causes local distortions of the bladder wall, this both activates the sensation of urgency and spreads to cause synchronous activation of the bladder wall resulting in an involuntary pressure rise. What happens after this may vary. If the contraction is large enough to overcome the outflow resistance, leakage will occur. This could in its turn activate receptors in the urethra and trigger secondary changes (transient opening of the bladder neck etc.), but often the pressure and sensation of urgency will subside. Synchronous detrusor contraction will itself reduce the sensation of urgency and the bladder pressure may return to normal. Activation of the detrusor smooth muscle, unless supported by continuous neural input, is self limiting, since the muscles possess Ca^{2+} activated potassium channels which ensure that the membrane hyperpolarizes and spontaneous action potentials will be switched off transiently [406]. Normally urge incontinence does not result in complete bladder emptying, but if there is a well developed segmental spinal micturition reflex and loss of any descending control, activation of the pressure/stretch receptors may reinforce the activity and produce bladder emptying.

g) Metabolic Studies related to unstable bladder contractions and outlet obstruction

In man, it is difficult to investigate the cellular mechanisms which result in progressive bladder dysfunction and overactivity. However, animal models of bladder outflow obstruction can be used to mimic the functional changes associated with benign prostatic hyperplasia (BPH) which leads in many patients to overactivity. This pathology can be induced in rat, rabbit, and pig [407,408]. Such models can be used to examine the cellular and metabolic changes occurring in the smooth muscles.

In rabbits, partial outlet obstruction induces a shift from aerobic to anaerobic metabolism as demonstrated by the shift in glucose metabolism from CO_2 to lactic acid generation (Table 8). Similarly, there is a marked decrease in the metabolism of pyruvate (mitochondrial substrate) to CO_2 [409,410]. In the rat, lactate dehydrogenase (LDH) activity (per mg wet weight) increased with the duration of obstruction, becoming statistically significant at 90 days of obstruction [409,410].

In partial outlet obstruction in rabbits, the cellular mechanism responsible for decreased oxidative metabolism involves decreased mitochondrial activity, as demonstrated by specific decreases in the enzymatic activities of citrate synthase and malate dehydrogenase and decreased ATP synthesis [166,411-413]. However, there were no effects of outlet obstruction on the activities of a variety of other enzymes including adenylate kinase, creatine kinase, hexokinase, myosin ATP'ase, and adenine phosphoribosyl transferase (Table 8) [414-416]. Further studies demonstrate that there is a dysregulation of mitochondrial genetic function[417].

In the rat, mitochondrial metabolism is not reduced to the same extent as in the rabbit model [418]. Recent studies have demonstrated that citrate synthase and malate dehydrogenase activity of the hypertrophied rat bladder (12 days following obstruction) were reduced

Table 8 : Effect of Partial Outlet Obstruction on Bladder Smooth Muscle Metabolism

	Control Smooth Muscle	**Obstructed Smooth Muscle**
Glucose metabolism		
Lactic acid formation (:mol / g / h)	1.35 ± 0.05	1.84 ± 0.10**
CO_2 formation (:mol / g / h)	0.26 ± 0.01	0.17 ± 0.01**
High energy phosphate content		
Creatine phosphate (nmol / mg protein)	18.2 ± 2.4	7.5 ± 1.0**
Adenosine triphosphate (nmol / mg protein)	8.2 ± 2.0	7.2 ± 1.3
Adenosine diphosphate (nmol / mg protein)	4.0 ± 0.3	3.2 ± 0.6
Adenosine monophosphate (nmol / mg protein)	4.0 ± 0.3	3.5 ± 0.6
Enzyme activity		
Citrate synthase [a] (nmol / mg protein) / min)	286 ± 25	140 ± 28**
Malate dehydrogenase[a] (nmol / mg protein) / min)	464 ± 43	280 ± 30
NCCR[a] (nmol / mg protein) / min)	406 ± 24	394 ± 13
Cytochrome oxidase[a] (nmol / mg protein) / min)	163 ± 20	131 ± 20
Creatine kinase (nmol / mg protein) / min)	582 ± 50	505 ± 30**
Adenylate kinase (nmol / mg protein) / min)	50 ± 5	61 ± 10**
Phosphoribosyl transferase (nmol / mg protein) / min)	33.7 ± 2.7	29.0 ± 4**
Myosin ATPase (:mol / mg protein / min)	1.61 ± 0.16	1.63 ± 0.33
Hexokinase (nmol / mg protein) / min)	11.7 ± 1.6	10.1 ± 1.0

*NCCR - NADH-cytochrome c reductase. a - Activity in partially purified mitochondrial preparation; All data are given as means ± SEM; **significantly different from smooth muscle (P<0.05).*

by 22% and 28% respectively when calculated per mg protein. No significant changes were observed if the enzyme activities were calculated per mg wet weight [418]. Additional studies on the hypertrophied rat bladder demonstrated that there was a modest reduction in the volume-fraction of mitochondria [418,419].

h) Ischaemia as an aetiological factor in obstructive dysfunction

Mild partial outlet obstruction results in an immediate increase in urethral resistance leading to an increase in voiding pressure and wall tension [399,420-424]. The increased wall tension or voiding pressure result in an increase in bladder mass (and wall thickness) [177,178,181,408,425,426]. The increase in bladder wall thickness results in cyclical periods of ischaemia-reperfusion during bladder contraction and emptying [422-4]. The relationships between intravesical pressure and blood flow, and intravesical pressure and detrusor pO_2 during and following micturition contractions are presented in figure 30. These studies have clearly demonstrated that in obstructed pigs there is a direct correlation between increased intravesical pressure (wall tension) and decreased blood flow. During the reduced blood flow, there is clearly a substantial decrease in detrusor pO_2. Although blood flow is restored rapidly after the end of the bladder contraction, detrusor pO_2 returns toward normal levels much more slowly. These same studies demonstrated that overactive bladder contractions result in a similar phasic reductions of blood flow, and pO_2. Thus, obstructed pigs that show detrusor overactivity have a greater frequency of ischaemic periods than obstructed pigs that show no overactivity.

The relationship between ischaemia and obstruction is supported by a recent study by Schröder et al. who demonstrated in rabbits that blood flow to the detrusor smooth muscle was reduced in proportion to the level of decompensation [427]. Interestingly, blood flow to the mucosa was not affected by obstruction (figure 31). Similar results have been reported [428]. During ischaemic periods there is a release of intracellular Ca^{2+} from the SR which can stimulate Ca^{2+}-activated hydrolytic enzymes such as calpain (calcium activated protease) and phospholipase A2 (Ca^{2+} activated phospholipase) [429-431]. During the reperfusion period, free radicals can be formed which stimulate lipid peroxidation. The increase in the activities of these degradative enzymes result in damage to specific membrane elements within the detrusor.

Ischaemia will damage not only smooth muscle cells but also the intrinsic neurones in the bladder wall.

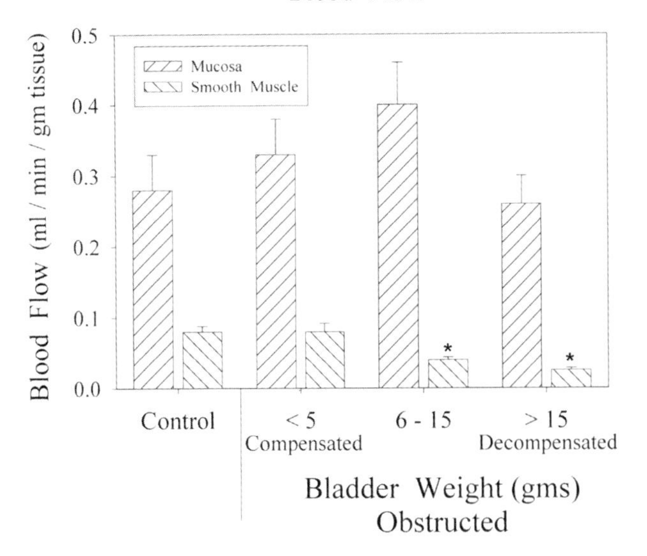

Figure 31 : Effect of partial outlet obstruction on blood flow to the detrusor smooth muscle and mucosa. 15 New Zealand White rabbits received a partial outlet obstruction by standard methods. After 4 weeks the rabbits were anaesthetized and blood flow to the muscle and mucosa were determined by a standardized fluorescent microsphere technique. A section of each detrusor was used for in vitro contractility studies. Contractile responses to field stimulation (FS), carbachol, ATP, and KCl were determined and utilized in addition to bladder weight to determine the level of decompensation present. Each bar is the mean of 5 control, 5 compensated, 5 intermediate-decompensated , and 5 decompensated rabbit bladders. * = significantly different from control, $p < 0.05$.

Indeed evidence strongly suggests that neurones are more susceptible to ischaemic damage than the detrusor smooth muscle and also that such damage is more likely to be irreversible. [189,190,200,201]. Ischaemic neuronal damage can be reduced if the tissues are treated with L-type Ca channel blockers, or exposed to ischaemic conditions in Ca-free solutions, or in the presence of free radical scavengers. The protective effect of L-type Ca channel blockers and free radical scavengers strongly suggests that free radicals produced by, and released from, the smooth muscle cells may be partially responsible for the neuronal damage, since L-type Ca channels are predominantly on the smooth muscle cells, and blockers do not prevent activation of intrinsic nerves and release of neurotransmitters [253]. Neuronal damage is commonly seen in obstructed unstable bladders and may be an important factor in causing the changes in smooth muscle properties associated with overactivity [1].

Free radicals produced in ischaemia will, through a combination of damage to neurones and to the smooth muscle itself, also begin and promote the process of decompensation. In man, there is clear clinical support for the concept that the rate of bladder deterioration in the presence of obstruction is significantly greater if involuntary bladder contractions (hyperreflexia) are present. This concept is clearly supported by experimental evidence in animal models. In both the guinea pig and rat models of partial outlet obstruction, obstructed animals that show hyperreflexia clearly show a greater level of dysfunction than animals obstructed for the same period of time that do not show hyperreflexia [432,433].

Repetitive stimulation has been used to simulate detrusor overactivity using in vitro methodologies. These studies utilized normal rabbit bladder detrusor strips mounted in individual isolated baths. The effect of repetitive stimulation using 32 Hz field stimulation on the contractile responses of the strips to field stimulation, carbachol, and KCl was determined. The results of these studies demonstrated that isolated strips that were subjected to repetitive stimulation showed a significantly greater rate of contractile failure, and show a significantly reduced ability to recover contractile function during re-oxygenation in the presence of glucose. Hypoxia exaggerated the destructive effects of repetitive stimulation [434,435]. In addition, tissues were analysed for MDA (malondialdehyde: a peroxidation product of free radical damage). There was a clear correlation between the severity of the contractile dysfunctions, the duration of the repetitive stimulation, and the concentration of MDA [434,435]. Additional studies demonstrated that the degree of dysfunction and MDA generation was directly related to the bath concentration of Ca^{2+}. Increasing calcium in the bath increased the rate and magnitude of the contractile dysfunctions and increased MDA concentration, whereas low calcium, EGTA, and the presence of Ca^{2+} blocking agents in the bath protected the contractile responses. These studies provide additional support that the detrimental effects of overactive bladder contractions are directly related to both the presence of ischaemia and Ca^{2+} cycling.

2. Aging

• Relationship between cellular metabolism and aging

Reduced energy supply (rate of ATP generation) causes a progressive decrease in the tonic response of the urethra, the loss of α"-adrenergic tonic tension, and a decreased urethral pressure, contributing to incontinence in women. In men, the decreased ability of the bladder to generate and sustain a micturition contraction would result in decreased flow rate, increased time of micturition, and increased residual volume. These symptoms are well documented to be associated with aging, even in the absence of any obstruction. This increased rate of "fatigue" in association with aging has been proposed by Lin *et al* who demonstrated that in ageing rats there was a progressive decrease in the contractile responses to repetitive autonomic stimulation (increase in fatigue) which was directly associated with both a decrease in the metabolic energy available to support the contractile responses, and a decrease in mitochondrial enzyme activities [436,437]. Thus, in association with ageing, there is a progressive reduction in the rate of high energy phosphate generation (during periods of stimulation) that significantly increases the rate of fatigue of the bladder smooth muscle. Another study demonstrated a significantly reduced ability of isolated whole bladders from aged rabbits (as compared to those from young rabbits) to generate pressure and empty efficiently [438]. The rate of power generation, the percent emptying, and the amount of work performed by bladders from old rabbits were significantly less than bladders from young rabbits. In addition, there was a marked reduction in the ability of the bladders isolated from old rabbits to respond to an increase in outlet resistance. These studies support the theory that ageing is associated with a progressive reduction in the ability of the bladder to generate metabolic energy by oxidative phosphorylation, and thus sustain increased tension. Decreased mitochondrial oxidative function in association with aging have been reported in a number of different biological systems.

a) Physical properties of the Bladder in aging

In addition to the metabolic changes, the volume and the elasticity of the bladder can change in aged humans and experimental animals.

Clinically, the frequency of micturition and the voided volume of urine, are known to increase, and there is a reduced ability to suppress the bladder once fullness has been noted. These signs and symptoms are accompanied by urodynamic changes including an increased residual volume, and a reduction in the maximum squeeze pressure generated by the urethra [439]. The increased residual urine and the lower uroflow rate found in the elderly may also reflect changes in the bladder muscle leading to less efficient and unsustained contractions [440,441]. In animal experiments it has been suggested that the volume of the bladder was similar in young and old rats, but that micturition occurred at higher pressures in the older animals [442,443] . However that is not universally accepted, and Hotta et al (1995) found that the bladders of old animals can be considerably larger than those of young animals, and the urine can be accommodated at low pressure [444].

b) Afferent and Efferent Nerve Function in Aging

Gilpin et al [445] found that the amount of nerve per mm^2 of muscle decreases with age and occurs to the same extent in males and females. Warburton and Santer [446] presented evidence which suggested a diminution in the sympathetic control of the urinary tract in aged rats; they also found however that the pattern and density of CGRP-containing afferent nerve terminals in the bladder were unchanged in old age. Thus it may be that old age causes a reduction in the innervation density of the bladder, just as it does for skeletal muscle [447].

From a functional viewpoint, micturition threshold (pressure) is reported as being unchanged [444]. However it was found that the afferents were less sensitive to volume, while retaining their sensitivity to pressure. Corresponding to this finding in rat bladders, Collas et al [448] also found a decrease in bladder sensation in association with aging in female patients with lower urinary symptoms. They found that maximum bladder capacity fell in the eighth and ninth decades; whereas the bladder capacity at first desire to void rose progressively in association with age, which is consistent with the rat data.

The responsiveness of vesical smooth muscle to neurotransmitters and other chemicals may or may not change in old age. To some extent this is dependent on what one considers 'old'; many of the changes seen in rats at >26 months of age are not seen below the age of 20 weeks. Toyoshima et al [449] found that the responsiveness to acetylcholine is reduced by aging, and suggested that the increase in intravesical pressure that occurs during stimulation with cholinergic agonists involves the participation of cholinergic M-2 receptors. Munro and Wendt [450] also found that the maximal force generated by the aged muscle strips decreased and that the maximal velocity of shortening was significantly lower in strips from aged animals as compared with those from young adults. However others have found that there was no significant age-related difference in the response to cholinergic ands other contractile stimuli [451-453]. On the other hand, there are numerous reports of aging-related changes of the detrusor response to adrenergic stimulation. Most studies showed that detrusor contractile responses to α-adrenergic stimulation increased in old male and female rats [453-5]. The detrusor response to β-adrenergic stimulation is reduced in old male rats [453,454] along with a reduction in the density of β adrenergic receptors and a decreased cyclic AMP (cAMP) production in response to β adrenergic stimulation. The combination of an increase in the α–adrenergic excitatory responses and decreased β adrenergic inhibitory responses results in a net contracting effect of noradrenaline on the aged bladders in contrast to the relaxing effect of noradrenaline in the young bladders. When noradrenaline is released by increased sympathetic activity during bladder filling [5] the enhanced adrenergic contractile response in the aged bladders might reduce functional storage capacity and thereby contribute to urinary frequency and urgency in the older persons.

In in vivo experiments, Hotta et al [444] found that both the active and the passive pressure-volume relationships were shifted to the right in the elderly animals, and that aging was associated with a reduction in the maximal pressure generated during pelvic nerve stimulation for 10 seconds at 20 /second, using square wave pulses of 10V and 1.0 msec. Also the change in intravesical pressure induced by supramaximal nerve stimulation was less in aged animals. Several studies have shown that the frequency-response curve for electrically evoked bladder contractions was similar in young and old rat bladders [442] indicating that the release of neurotransmitters from pre-synaptic nerve endings was not altered during aging.

3. OUTLET OBSTRUCTION

The development of a spinal micturition reflex with subsequent detrusor overactivity occurs in conditions other than spinal cord injury. Bladder outlet obstruction in rats causes enhancement of a spinal reflex [456,457]. Within the spinal cord obstruction stimulates an increased expression of GAP-43 which has been associated with axonal sprouting following injury [458]. These observations suggest an enhancement or *de novo* development of new spinal circuits following obstruction. Similar to spinal cord injury, obstruction causes hypertrophy of bladder afferent and efferent neurons [391,392]. Conversely, relief of obstruction is associated with the reduction of urinary frequency and reversal of these neural changes [458,459]. In animals that fail to revert to a normal voiding pattern after relief of obstruction, this neuroplasticity persists [459]. Nevertheless, these findings are not mutually exclusive of changes in the bladder smooth muscle that are also likely to participate in the development of the overactive bladder [460].

Bladder outlet obstruction also appears to initiate the morphological and electrophysiological afferent plasticity via a mechanism involving NGF (Fig.32). NGF is responsible for the growth and maintenance of sympathetic and sensory neurons and has been shown to be responsible for neuronal regrowth after injury. NGF content is increased in obstructed bladders in animals and in humans [461]. This increase in NGF content precedes the enlargement of bladder neurons and the developmental of urinary frequency [375,461]. Moreover, blockade of NGF action using autoantibodies prevents the neural plasticity and urinary frequency following obstruction [461]. In animals in whom urinary frequency persists after relief of obstruction, NGF remains elevated in the bladder. Although mechanical stretch of cultured bladder smooth muscle induces NGF expression, other insults to the bladder such as denervation and ischemia are capable of inducing NGF. These findings suggest a cause and effect relationship between NGF-mediated changes in bladder afferents and an enhanced spinal micturition reflex and urinary frequency associated with obstruction. Of interest, α-adrenoceptor and NK1 antagonists and oxytocin, administered intrathecally, can reduce unstable bladder contractions in obstructed rats [462]. These findings support the notion that changes in the spinal cord, possibly related to alterations in the processing of afferent input contribute to the bladder dysfunction after outlet obstruction.

4. INFLAMMATION

Because NGF plays such a prominent role in the development and function of afferent neurons, it is no surprise that inflammation of the urinary bladder is accompanied by neuroplasticity in sensory nerves supplying the bladder [95]. Repeated inflammatory stimuli elicits enlargement of bladder DRG neurons [463]. Following inflammation a reduction in threshold for bladder afferents occurs [595]. Likewise, it has been shown that intravesical NGF can lower thresholds for bladder afferents. Plasticity within the spinal cord may also occur. Following chemical or mechanical inflammation of the urinary bladder, increased expression of the early-immediate gene, C-fos, has been detected within the lumbosacral spinal cord [465-467] and increased expression of nitric oxide synthase occurs in bladder afferent neurons [596].

Although inflammation of the urinary bladder elevates NGF content, this rise is short lived [468]. Bladder overactivity induced by inflammation can be inhibited by a fusion protein that prevents interaction between NGF and its tyrosine-(trk-A) receptor [469]. Hence, the neuroplasticity and the potential involvement of NGF in inflammatory conditions resemble that of obstruction. Other substances including neurotrophins, prostaglandins, and tachykinins may also contribute to changes in afferent excitability [6].

II. CENTRAL MODELS OF OAB

Models of bladder overactivity involving primary lesions within the CNS have been developed in several species, and are relevant to spinal cord injury, denervation, Parkinson's disease and multiple sclerosis [5,470]. In addition, the spontaneously hypertensive rat (SHR) has provided a useful genetic model for bladder overactivity [471]. One common theme behind all of these models is that acute changes in smooth muscle can elicit long-term changes in nerves. Investigators are accustomed to examining short-term effects. However, there is now a greater appreciation that long-term events involving growth factors leads to plasticity in

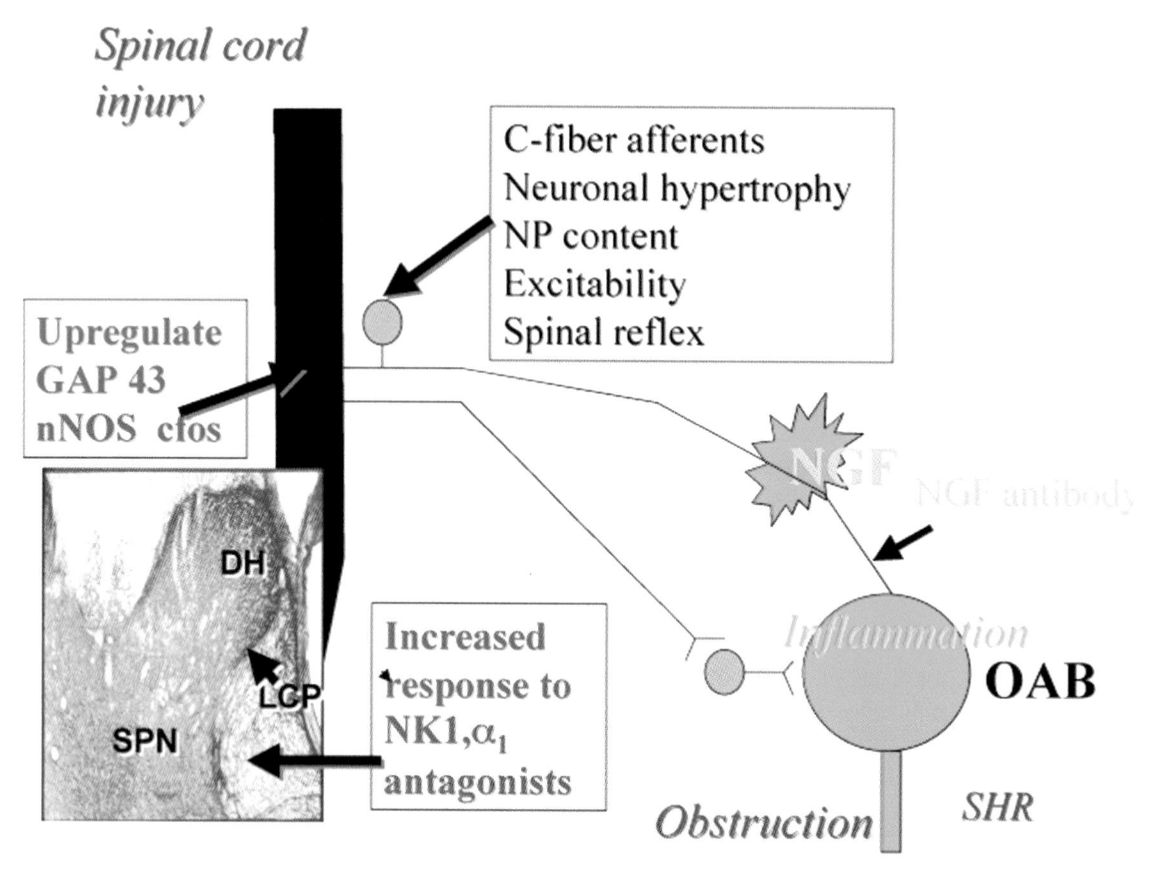

Figure 32 : Results from a wide array of pharmacological, molecular and electrophysiologic experiments suggests a similar underlying mechanisms for changes in innervation that in turn could potentially lead to afferent overactivity in variety of models for overactive bladder (OAB). Models of bladder inflammation, outlet obstruction, spinal cord injury, and the spontaneous hypertensive rat (SHR) all exhibit urinary frequency, reduction in volume threshold to micturition, and intermicturition contractions (unstable) similar to OAB in humans. All of these models are associated with elevated levels of NGF as are some clinical conditions as interstitial cystitis and obstruction. Neuronal changes occur in the dorsal root ganglia (DRG) and dorsal horn (DH) of the spinal cord. Afferent project along a lateral collateral pathway (LCP) to the sacral parasympathetic nucleus (SPN). In the DRG hypertrophy of neurons, lowered threshold for activation of neurons giving rise to C-fibers, and changes in neuropeptide (NP) content are found. In the DH, up-regulation of growth associated protein 43 (GAP43), neuronal nitric oxide synthase (nNOS), and the early immediate gene product cfos occur. Moreover, antagonists to neurokinin 1(NK1) an a1 adrenoceptors administered intrathecally inhibit OAB with these disorders. Following chemical irritation and obstruction, blockade of NGF antivity with trkA antibody or autoimmunity to NGF block neuronal plasticity and OAG.

neural pathways with implications for disorders of micturition. Neurotransmitters, prostaglandins and growth factors, such as Nerve Growth Factor (NGF), are substances that provide mechanisms for communication between muscle and nerve. Disturbances in these mechanisms can cause bladder overactivity due to alterations in either bladder smooth muscle or autonomic reflex pathways. This bladder overactivity can, in turn, lead to urge incontinence.

Cystometry and urinary frequency are commonly used to define bladder overactivity. Moreover, these measurements can monitor responses to drugs or other therapies. A multidisciplinary approach incorporating one or more biochemical, molecular, pharmacological, physiological and behavioral methods can provide insight into the pathogenesis of detrusor overactivity. (Table 9)

1. Spinal cord injury

Damage to the spinal cord cephalad to the sacral level results in bladder overactivity [472]. Acute spinal cord injury disrupts normal supraspinal circuits that control urine storage and release. Following days to weeks of urinary retention, hyperactive voiding develops. Electrophysiological data reveal that this detrusor hyperreflexia is mediated by a spinal micturition reflex that emerges in response to a reorganization of synaptic connections in the spinal cord [9,44,275,471]. In addition, bladder afferents that are normally unresponsive to low intravesical pressures become more mechanosensitive leading to the development of detrusor overactivity. Normal micturition is associated with a spinobulbo-spinal reflex mediated by lightly-myelinated A-δ afferents [5,9]. These fibers represent only 20% of blad-

Table 9 : Legend: NF = neurofilament, IB4= lectin SP= substance P CGRP=calcitonin gene related peptide, trkA-tyrosine kinase A , VR1- vanilloid receptor 1.

60% of bladder afferents are C-fibers	
Peptidergic	**Non-Peptide**
NF -	NF -
80-90% bladder C fibers	10-20% bladder C fibers
IB4 –SP/CGRP	IB4/FRAP +
Trk A-NGF	Trk B-BNDF GDNF
VR1	?VR1/ P2X3
Laminae I/II	Inner laminae II
Projection 2nd order to brainstem/thalamus	2nd order interneurons in spinal cord

der afferents in some species. Compared to A-δ fibers, the more prevalent unmyelinated C-fibers are relatively insensitive to gradual distention of the urinary bladder, at least in the cat [29]. Most C-fibers in this species remain silent during normal filling of the bladder although in the rat some studies indicate that C-fibers can fire at low pressures [26]; whereas other studies [24] showed firing at higher intravesical pressures of approximately 30 mm Hg. After spinal cord injury, a capsaicin-sensitive C-fiber-mediated spinal reflex develops (Fig 33). These C-fiber afferents are thought to play a role in the development of bladder overactivity after spinal cord injury. Capsaicin sensitive C-fibers have also been implicated in detrusor overactivity following upper motoneuron diseases such as multiple sclerosis and Parkinson's disease [473-475].

Insight into the mechanism underlying the increased mechano-sensitivity of C-fibers after spinal cord injury has been gained by examining the dorsal root ganglion (DRG) cells supplying the bladder. Plasticity in these afferents is manifested by enlargement of these cells [474] and increased electrical excitability [475]. A shift in expression of sodium (Na+) channels from a high threshold tetrodotoxin (TTX)-resistant type to a low threshold TTX sensitive type occurs after spinal cord injury.

Plasticity in bladder afferents after spinal cord injury may involve the retrograde transport of substances from either the spinal cord or bladder to the DRG neuron. Bladder DRG neurons are responsive to a variety of neurotrophins, especially NGF which has been associated with hypertrophy of bladder DRG cells in a variety of conditions (see Obstruction, Inflammation, Spontaneously Hypertensive Rat). Exposure of cultured DRG neurons to exogenous NGF promotes expression of TTX sensitive channels expressed following spinal cord injury [478]. Moreover, DRG from mice overexpressing NGF exhibit predominately TTX-S Na currents. Other trophic substances such as basic fibroblast growth factor (bFGF), brain-derived neurotrophic factor (BDNF), glial derived neurotrophic factor (GNDF),and neurotrophins-3-4 (NT-3-4) may trigger morphological and electrophysiological alterations in DRG cells after spinal cord injury. GDNF may be especially important because a small population of DRG neurons giving rise to C fibers are non-reponsive to NGF, but respond to GDNF [478]. It is worth noting that the response of other neurogenic disorders associated with urge incontinence respond to intravesical capsaicin therapy suggesting that plasticity in C-fiber afferents could form the neurogenic basis for bladder overactivity [474,475,479]. The emergence of a spinal reflex circuit activated by C-fiber bladder afferents represents a positive feedback mechanism (Fig. 34) that may be unresponsive to voluntary control by higher brain centers and thereby be able to trigger involuntary voiding.

2. Spontaneously hypertensive rat (SHR)

The spontaneously hypertensive rat (SHR) voids more frequently at lower volumes than genetic Wistar-Kyoto (WKY) controls and has overactive bladder contractions even though they produce equal amounts and concentration of urine. Urinary frequency, urgency with or without urge incontinence and involuntary bladder contractions characterize the overactive bladder (OAB) [371]. Thus the SHR may be a useful model to study either the treatment or pathophysiology of OAB. The reason for OAB in the SHR is unclear. Bladder smooth muscle from the SHR produces more nerve growth factor (NGF) than WKY [480-482]. The bladder also demonstrates a hypernoradrenergic innervation and increased responsiveness to adrenergic agonists [480,483]. However, changes in sympathetic nerves or smooth muscle responsiveness do not fully explain the OAB. The only significant in vitro finding is an enhanced β- adrenergic mediated relaxation. In vitro studies show equivalent responses to electrical stimulation, potassium chloride, cholinergic and purinergic agonists in SHR and WKY. SHR and WKY are similar in terms of histology and bladder compliance during filling. These findings do not implicate changes in smooth muscle or connective tissue. Furthermore, chemical sympathectomy with elimination of noradrenergic nerves by 6-hydroxydopamine or prevention of noradrenaline release with guanethidine fails to abolish OAB.

It can be inferred from several lines of evidence that afferents may be altered in the SHR. Published data

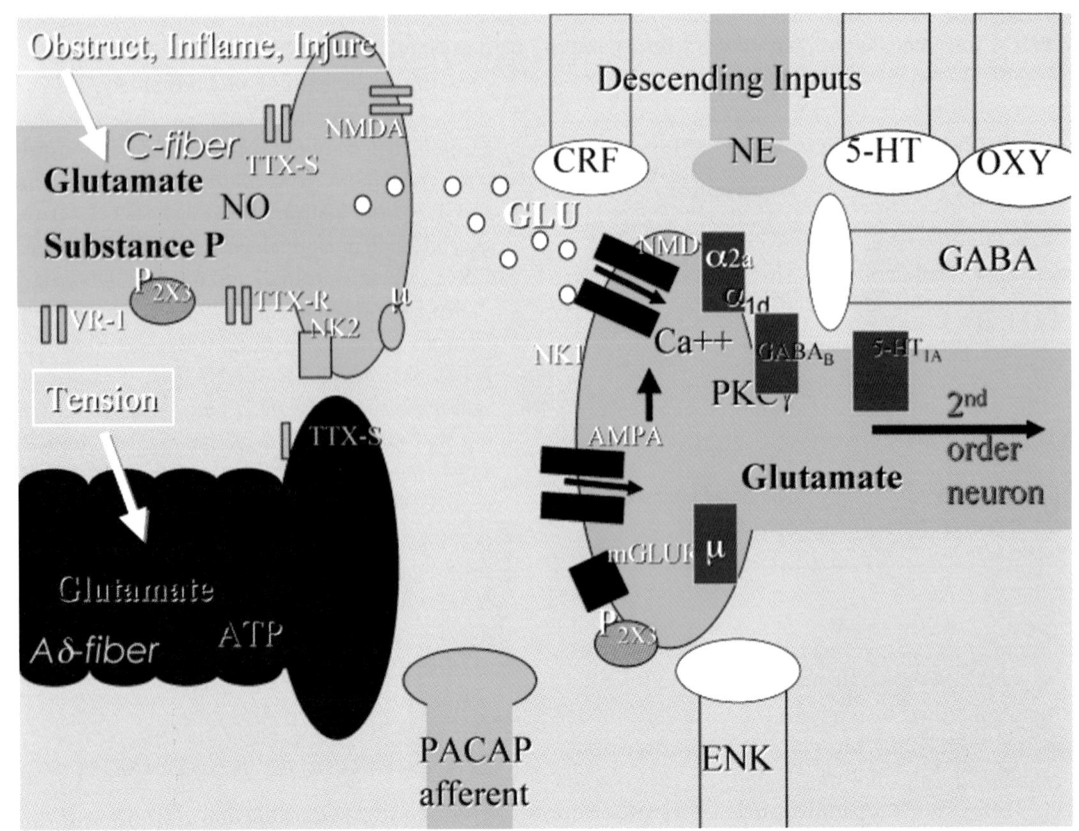

Figure 33 : Neuropharmacology within dorsal horn of sacral spinal cord. Afferents projecting to the dorsal horn are of two types Ad and C. These afferents release glutamate, substance P (SP), nitric oxide (NO), or pituitary adenlyate cyclase (PACAP) and adenosine triphosphate (ATP) among other neurotransmitters. Glutamate, SP, and PCAP are excitatory although PACAP probably modulatory. Glutamate acts at NMDA and AMPA ionotropic or metabotropic glutamate receptors. SP acts at neurokinin – (NK-1) receptors. Afferents from the lower urinary tract can synapse on second order neurons can either project rostrally to the periaqueductal gray (PAG) or on interneurons, most of which also contain glutamate. Modulatory influences on second order neurons derives from inhibitory GABAminergic interneurons (acting on predominately GABAB receptors) or descending corticotropic releasing factor (CRF), oxytocinergic (OXY), or serotonergic (5-HT2C, 5-HT1A) inhibitory neurons. Descending noradrenergic neurons acting at a1D or a2C receptors can exert either excitatory or inhibitory influences on micturition.

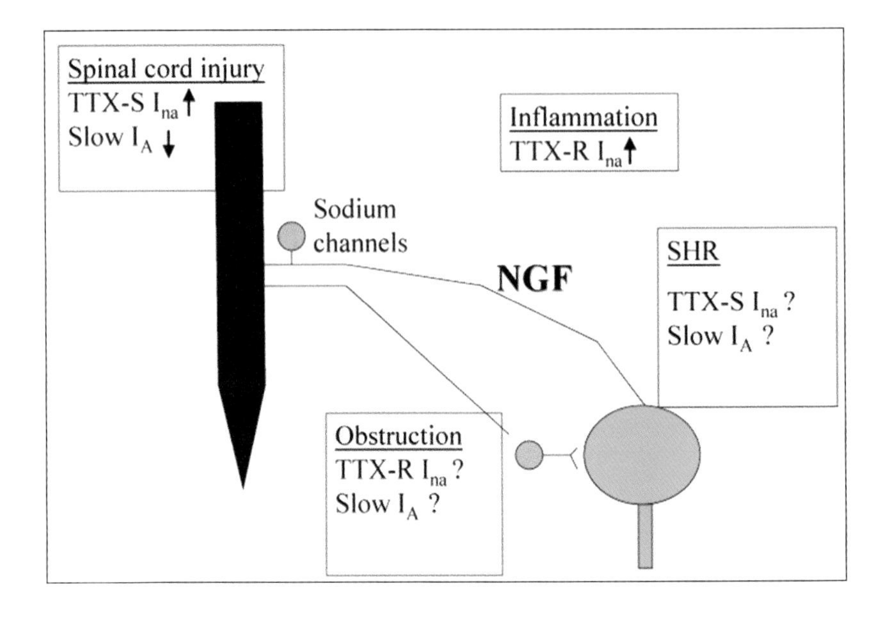

Figure 34 : Following inflammation and cystitis a rise in TTX-R Na currents is measured in bladder DRG. After spinal cord injury or in SHR increased TTX-S Na currents is seen. A reduction in slow inward delayed rectifier K currents may reduce hyperpolarization and cause increased neuronal excitability. Thus, elevated NGF may act to influence a subunit exression which affects the excitability of neurons. This excitability may be manifested in a variety of ways such as a reduction in threshold, spontaneous or burst firing of afferents. Such an increase in afferent excitability could lead to a reduction in volume threshold for micturition in OAB conditions.

reveals that DRG neurons are enlarged in SHR compared to WKY. Intrathecal administration of the α antagonist doxazosin, which may modify afferent input from the bladder, inhibits OAB in SHR. Doxazosin has no effect on bladder function in WKY. One possibility is that NGF produced in SHR influences the electrophysiologic properties of L6/S1 dorsal root ganglion (DRG) cells supplying the SHR bladder differ from other strains with regard to Na currents. These Na currents regulate the excitability of afferents. Moreover, intrathecal antisense (AS) oligonucleotides (AG) against the gene (SCN10A) encoding for $Na_V1.8$, a tetrodotoxin resistant (TTX-R) Na channel isoform raises the volume threshold for micturition and reduces unstable bladder contractions in SHR [484]. Therefore it seems reasonable to explore the differences in bladder afferents and CNS pathways in the SHR compared to WKY as a basis for OAB. The precise mechanism(s) giving rise to OAB in the SHR may not be identical to those manifested in clinical entities such as idiopathic detrusor overactivity, interstitial cystitis, and bladder outlet obstruction or spinal cord injury. However experimental manipulations including urethral ligation and chemical cystitis do not mimic the spectrum of changes seen clinically with interstitial cystitis or benign prostatic hyperplasia (BPH). Nevertheless these models have provided insight into the potential mechanisms leading to OAB. The SHR offers substantial advantages as a model for OAB. For example, animal welfare concerns are less an issue in the SHR than with surgical or chemical manipulations. Likewise, unraveling the molecular events involved in the SHR may uncover novel approaches to therapy and provide insight into the mechanisms whereby these symptoms arise.

BPH and hypertension (HTN) often coexist in the aging population. For unknown reasons the prevalence of urinary symptoms is greater in hypertensive men and women [485-490]. Recent work presented at the 5th International Consultation on BPH suggests that HTN is the major risk factor for symptoms documented by an International Prostate Symptom Score (IPSS)(P. Boyle personal communication). A subset of hypertensive patients exhibits traits indicative of an overactive autonomic nervous system. In hypertensive, but not in normotensive controls, bladder distension evokes a brisk parasympathetic response of the baroreceptor/heart rate reflex [491]. An elevated heart rate response to stress has been seen in normotensive offspring of hypertensive parents [492]. Cross breeding SHR and normotensive WKY rats creates a F1 generation in which blood pressure correlates with urinary frequency [493]. However, it is unlikely that HTN per se causes a change resulting in OAB in the SHR. Urinary frequency is present at age 3 wks in SHR at which time the animals are normotensive. Moreover, adequate control of HTN in patients does not preclude OAB symptoms. This circumstantial evidence suggests that a subtle enhancement of autonomic activity may lead to HTN and predispose to OAB. Whether a difference exists in autonomic afferents, efferents or smooth muscle between SHR and WKY and whether this difference explains altered voiding behavior is unclear.

• Plasticity in Na channel isoforms

How could NGF produced by a target tissue and then retrogradely transported to the DRG affect target organ function? Recent data suggest that membrane conductance and thus excitability of DRG neurons are altered in models associated with increased access to NGF. This altered conductance is postulated to result from changes in the structure or combination of protein subunits of Na and K channels in the cell membrane. A change in Na channel isoform appears sufficient to change the properties of afferents. NGF is known to lower the threshold for firing of bladder (hypothetical lower volume threshold for voiding)and induce spontaneous and burst firing (hypothetical overactive contractions, urgency) [95]. Examples of afferent plasticity induced by NGF include inflammation or axotomy, which trigger spontaneous firing of sensory neurons [494] (Table 10). The site of abnormal ectopic firing has been determined to be the DRG and appears to be due to changes in the isoform of the voltage gated Na channels, causing spontaneous ectopic discharges. Voltage gated Na^+ channels generate currents during the upstroke of the nerve action potential and are involved in the propagation of the nerve impulse. Tetrodotoxin (TTX) is a neurotoxin produced by puffer fish, and it binds to and inactivates voltage gated Na+ channels.

The Na+ channel is a heterotrimer of composed of α, β_1, β_2 subunits (Fig 35). Subunit composition confers electrical properties and TTX susceptibility. Distinct genes code for the voltage-gated Na+ channel subunits that control membrane excitability of DRG neurons. These genes code for α and β subunits that assemble to form channel isoforms that have been distinguished on the basis of structure, biophysical properties, and sensitivity to tetrodotoxin (TTX) [495]. The α subunit forms the pore of the Na channel. The β subunit serves as an adhesion molecule to localize the channel [597]. Loss of the β subunit may prevent TTX binding implying that β subunits can also influence function. The proportion and characteristics of Na+ currents determine the range of firing patterns and functional properties in DRG neurons.. Na channel isoforms, like those for K channels, are distinct in terms of developmental and regional expression. Most voltage-gated Na^+ channels exhibit rapid inactivation kinetics and sensitivity to nanomolar concentrations of TTX. These Na+ channels are termed TTX-sensitive (TTX-S). Small sensory neu-

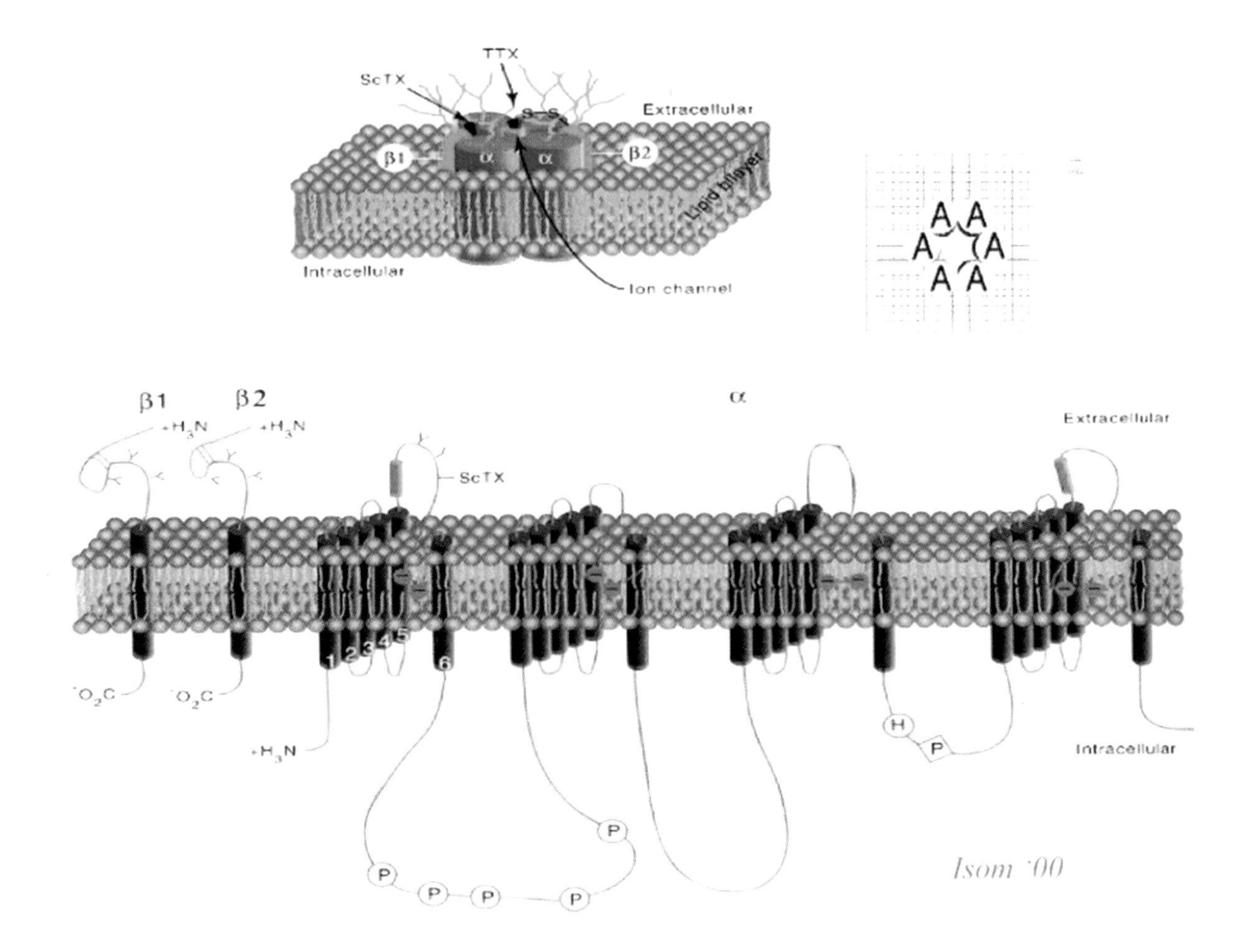

Figure 35 : Excitability of nerves is (action potential generation) attributable in part to Na currents. The Na channel is a heterotrimer composed of an a subunit forming the pore and two b subunits that anchor the channel to a membrane. Eight isoforms for the Na channel have been identified based on changes in the a subunit. Electrophysiologic properties of neuron linked to subunit expression which varies during development and with disease.

rons in the L6/S1 DRG show two types of Na^+ currents, a rapidly inactivating TTX-S I_{Na} and a slowly inactivating TTX-resistant (TTX-R) I_{Na}.

As neurons switch from a quiescent state to high frequency firing, such as with reawakening of C-fibers, they use their Na channels differently. But does DRG employ a different repertoire of Na channels? There is extensive evidence to suggest that Na+ channel subunits change in response to environmental conditions and changes in access to NGF. Two strategies are used in general to assess Na channel isoforms. First, studies can assess mRNA or protein production using in situ hybridization or immunohistochemistry for Na channel isoforms. Second, biophysical properties of cells can be assessed using patch clamp techniques. Using these methods, it has been discovered that Na channel isoforms in cells can vary by species, with disease and following acquired conditions such as inflammation and axotomy.

Does plasticity in Na channel currents occur in neurons supplying the bladder? 61% of sensory nerves innervating the rat bladder are unmyelinated C-fibers based on conduction velocities of single dorsal root fibers [31]. The remaining nerves are lightly myelinated Aδ fibers. 61% of bladder afferents respond to distension of the bladder (Shea et al 2000). 31% fail to respond to any mechanical or chemical stimuli. At least 60% of bladder DRG neurons are capsaicin-sensitive (VR-1), 95% of which give rise to C-fibers [496]. The TTX-R Na currents are present in SP/CGRP immunoreactive, trkA expressing, small DRG giving rise to C-fibers supplying the bladder [496,497]. Greater than 85% of Na currents in small diameter (C-fiber) DRG that accounted for 70% of bladder labeled cells exhibit predominately TTX-R currents. These cells demonstrate high thresholds and long duration action potentials and likely contribute to the higher thresholds for C-fibers. The remaining 30% of DRG neurons giving rise to Aδ fibers exhibit predominately TTX-S Na currents. These cells show low thresholds and short duration action potentials. After spinal cord injury, obstruction, and cystitis, an enhancement of spinal reflexes has been confirmed by abolishment with capsaicin and a positive ice-water test clinically [306,598]. Plasticity occurs in TTX-S and TTX-R Na+ channel currents in DRG neurons after spinal cord injury. With spinal cord injury 60% of dissociated bladder DRG neurons exhibit TTX-S Na currents compared to 30% in intact rats [498]. IA K currents are also postulated to be reduced causing lack of membrane relaxation. These two changes lead to enhanced excitability of C-fibers coinciding with development of a spinal micturition reflex. With cyclophosphamide cystitis, slowly inactivating I_A currents in TTX-R neurons are reduced possibly leading to OAB [498]. It has been speculated that the cellular basis for this plasticity is a change in K currents.

• CLINICAL EVIDENCE FOR ROLE OF Na CHANNELS IN OAB

Observations from use of the local anesthetic and nonselective Na channel blocker, lidocaine, suggests that Na channels can be manipulated to reduce OAB in a variety of conditions including BPH. Intravesical lidocaine at low doses blocks sensory nerve transmission from the human bladder. The effect of intravesical lidocaine may be limited to C-fibers giving rise to pathologic reflexes such as the ice water test [499]. Intravesical lidocaine increases bladder capacity and reduces involuntary contractions. In a small, uncontrolled study of elderly patients with detrusor instability, the oral Na channel blocker, mexiletine, but not intravenous lidocaine, improved or cured urge incontinence [500]. The effects of these agents vary with disease. This could indicate alterations in Na channel expression by nerves, differences in the degree of innervation or access to drug. In children with neurogenic bladders due to myelodysplasia, Lapointe and colleagues [501] found that intravesical lidocaine decreased involuntary contractions in 58% of patients but increased capacity in 71% of patients by nearly 60%. Lidocaine increases bladder capacity to the greatest degree in spinal cord injured patients (230%) compared to supraspinal neurologic conditions and BPH [502]. A reduction in involuntary detrusor contractions is only seen in the former conditions but not BPH. In contrast, Reuther and colleagues [503] found that elimination of detrusor overactivity after intravesical lidocaine was predictive of cure of symptoms after transurethral resection of the prostate. Intravesical lidocaine can even worsen detrusor overactivity in some BPH patients [504]. It is possible that the action of intravesical lidocaine is primarily limited to suburothelial nerves. This would be consistent with observations in other studies that periprostatic or subtrigonal injection of lidocaine eliminates urgency and frequency associated with BPH [505]). Regardless, bladder or prostatic afferents expressing Na channels may be involved in irritative voiding although not the cause for involuntary contractions. Differences between these small studies might be attributed to ischemia or denervation. These conditions could necessitate a higher dose of lidocaine to eliminate involuntary contractions in BPH patients. In obstructed rabbits, intravesical lidocaine but not anticholinergics, potassium channel openers or Ca^{2+} channel antagonists inhibited hyperreflexia [506]. Lidocaine eliminates pain associated with intravesical capsaicin indicating its ability to inhibit vanilloid 1 receptor (VR-1) expressing afferents probably located beneath the urothelium. In contrast, intravesical tetrodotoxin fails to block intravesical capsaicin-induced abdominal licking in rats implying that VR-1 expressing bladder afferents are TTX-R [507]. However, targeting Na channels expressed by suburothelial nerves may not be as effective as blocking those expressed by spinal nerves. Intrathecal lidocaine and especially bupivacaine eradicate urinary urgency and increase bladder capacity [508]. Therefore manipulation of Na channels expressed by spinal nerves or afferents in DRG could influence micturition. (Table 10).

3. MODELS OF PARKINSON'S DISEASE WITH OAB

Chemical or surgical lesioning of dopamine containing neurons in the basal ganglia in the rat causes changes in motor behaviors reminiscent of Parkinson's disease. CMGs in this animal demonstrate detrusor overactivity. Projections of dopamine containing fibers from the substantia nigra have opposing effects on the bladder. Activation of D2 receptors is excitatory to micturition. Conversely, release of dopamine from rostral projections results in activation of D1 receptors which elevates the threshold to micturition. This latter effect has been postulated to result from activation of D1 receptors on GABAminergic neurons which mediate inhibition of neurons involved in micturition. In a model of Parkinson's disease induced by N-methyl-4-phenyl-1,2,3,6-tetrahydropyridine (MPTP), investigators found that D1 function is reduced and D2 activity is enhanced with a net excitatory effect on micturition reflexes manifested as a reduced volume threshold for voiding and unstable bladder contractions. An animal model for Parkinson's disease has been developed in monkeys by administering a neurotoxin (N-methyl-4-phenyl-1,2,3,6-tetrahydropyridine [MPTP]) that destroys dopamine neurons [599]. Animals treated with MPTP show motor symptoms typical of Parkinson's disease and also have an overactive bladder. In these monkeys, stimulation of D-1 receptors with SKF38393 suppressed the detrusor hyperreflexia, whereas a nonselective dopamine receptor agonist (apomorphine) or a D-2 receptor agonist (quinpirole) reduced the bladder volume threshold.

Table 10 : Eight Na channel isoforms based on expression of a subunit. 6 isoforms at tetrodotoxin sensitive (TTX-S) and two are resistant (TTX-R). With conditions such as peripheral nerve axotomy, inflammation, cystitis and in the SHR changes in Na currents are measured using patch clamp methods which serve as a model for peripheral terminal function. Some TTX-R isoforms are responsive to NGF, other GDNF. In transgenic mice over-expressing NGF or in DRG cultured in the presence of NGF a rise in TTX-S currents is seen.

Channel	Previous Name	Gene Symbol	Chromosome (human)	Pharmacology	K.O. Phenotype	Abundance in Adult DRG
$Na_v1.1$	Type I	SCN1A	2q24	TTX-s		Present
$Na_v1.2$	Type II	SCN2A	2q23-24	TTX-s	lethal	Present
$Na_v1.3$	Type II	SCN3A	2q24	TTX-s		Upregulated in axotomy
$Na_v1.4$	SkM	SCN4A	17q23-25	TTX-s		Absent
$Na_v1.5$	Cardiac	SCN5A	8p21	TTX-r		Absent
$Na_v1.6$	NaCh6	SCN8A	12q13	TTX-s		Abundant
$Na_v1.7$	PN1	SCN9A	2q24	TTX-s		Abundant
$Na_v1.8$	SNS/PN3	SCN10A	3p21-24	TTX-r	Partial analgesia	Abundant

4. Stroke

Ligation of the middle cerebral artery of the rat creates brain ishemia and cerebral infarction. This animal exhibits an OAB characterized by intermicturition contractions on CMGs in conscious rats which supports the notion of tonic cortical inhibition of bladder function [354,509]. This effect was eliminated by administering an NMDA glutamatergic receptor antagonist, indicating that glutamatergic excitatory transmission is involved in the OAB [354]. Examination of other pharmacologic responses to intracerebroventricular drugs such as GABAminergic and dopaminergic agents drugs revealed an decreased GABA mediated inhibition of micturition and dopaminergic influences and glutamate transmission. Thus cerebral infarction causes plasticity in inhibitory neurons resulting in OAB.

5. OAB in clomipramine model and depression

Wolfe et al, [510] suggested that depression, anxiety, feeding disturbances, pain, irritable bowel syndrome, fibromyalgia, and changes in voiding are associated with disturbances in brain circuits using specific neurotransmitters, in particular serotonin or 5-hydroxytryptamine (5-HT). Fibromyalgia and irritable bowel syndrome are conditions seen more often in patients with interstitial cystitis (IC) than the general population [510-514], and this condition is associated with an overactive bladder and possibly to depression, which provides a potential link with 5-HT metabolism. Perhaps the strongest evidence for diminished 5-HT function in depressed patients is the remarkable efficacy of selective serotonin uptake inhibitors (SSRIs) in this group of patients. In addition, neuropharmacologic evidence indicates that some forms of depression are associated with abnormalities in the promoter for the serotonin transporter gene [515,516].

5-HT has also been implicated in the regulation of pain and also has a profound effect on bladder function. Neurons originating in the brainstem raphe nucleus synapse on visceral afferents and preganglionics in the thoracolumbar and sacral spinal cords. These neurons release 5-HT. Stimulation of raphe nuclei in the brain stem inhibits reflex bladder contractions [517]. 5-HT and its precursors, uptake blockers or 5-HT analogs inhibit bladder activity in a variety of species [518]. The actions of 5-HT are complex and mediated by over 13 different receptors. Some data suggest that 5-HT has a facilitating effect on voiding via modulation of bladder afferents, but intrathecal antagonists of $5\text{-}HT_2$ and $5\text{-}HT_3$ receptors reduce the volume threshold for voiding [519]. This latter data suggests that descending 5-HT pathways tonically depress bladder afferent input to the sacral spinal cord. Moreover, the $5HT_{2C}$ agonists MCPP and MK212 inhibit isovolumetric rhythmic bladder contractions [481,520]. On the other hand, 5-HT_{1A} antagonists inhibit bladder activity, probably on the basis of prejunctional effects [521]. Outside the CNS, 5-HT influences neurotransmission to the bladder. Presynaptic 5-HT receptors facilitate electrically evoked bladder contractions in multiple species. In humans this facilitation is mediated by 5-HT_4 receptors [522]. Taken together, the pharmacologic data suggest that 5-HT in the CNS inhibits micturition reflex pathways. By analogy, a genomic proclivity toward reduced 5-HT neurotransmission in the CNS may lead to enhanced bladder activity.

The association between emotional disorders and bladder complaints has been reported. Zorn and colleagues [523] studied 156 consecutive patients presenting to an incontinence clinic and compared their rates of depression to a cohort of continent patients. A self-administered Beck's Depression Inventory (BDI) was used to diagnose depression and subjects were queried for a history of treatment for this condition. A third of incontinent patients had an abnormal BDI (>12) and/or a history of depression, compared to only 17% of the continent cohort group. Several patients were even referred to psychiatry because of the risk of suicidal behavior. The type of incontinence was stratified by physical examination and urodynamics. Only 13% of patients with stress incontinence had depression, equivalent to the control cohort. In contrast, 42% of patients with mixed or urge incontinence had depression by history and/or BDI scoring. Most notably, 60% of patients with idiopathic urge incontinence had either undergone treatment for depression prior to the development of incontinence or scored in the depressive range on the BDI. This report suggests that the association between depression and mixed or urge incontinence is significant, but not with stress urinary incontinence. One might argue that patients with incontinence are merely more likely to be depressed or undergo psychiatric evaluation. These scenarios are unlikely because untreated patients with stress incontinence were no more likely to be depressed than controls. Moreover, a significant association between depression and urge incontinence existed regardless of whether history of treatment or BDI score was used to categorize subjects. Other causes of urge incontinence were not likely to be associated with depression.

Does correction of incontinence relieve depression? Recent studies examining BDI scores or symptoms of depression in women before and after surgery for stress incontinence revealed elevated postoperative scores even when incontinence was corrected [524,525]. Specifically, Rosenzweig and colleagues reported that depression progressed after unsuccessful surgery, but was not statistically improved with a successful procedure [524]. Together these findings suggest that incontinence itself is not the sole cause of the associated depression.

In this regard the model of depression associated with reduced levels of 5-HT in the brain has been shown to have lowered volume threshold for voiding and unstable bladder contractions. To clarify the link between emotional states, 5-HT and bladder function, we examined rats depleted of 5-HT by neonatal treatment with clomipramine. These animals develop depression and hyperactive bladder. This bladder overactivity persists in females but not males following puberty, a provocative result

6. Gender

Recent reviews suggest that urge incontinence and depression are more common in women than men, and that both conditions are commoner at times of changing hormonal levels in women [526]. Genetic, psychosocial and biological factors seem to account for this sexual dichotomy. One biological difference may be the functioning of 5-HT neurons. The serotonergic system plays a major role in depression, although there are other neurotransmitters involved. Differences in 5-HT function may explain why depression is more common in women. Women may be predisposed to depression in part because levels of 5-HT in the brain are substantially lower in women than men [527]. When the rates of 5-HT synthesis were measured in the human brain using PET, the mean rate of synthesis in normal males was found to be 52% higher than in normal females. Interestingly, estradiol (E2) administered to ovariectomized rats increases the density of 5-HT2A sites in the frontal cortex, anterior cingulated gyrus and lateral dorsal raphe. The areas with lowered 5-HT function on PET scanning correspond to areas of altered perfusion on PET scans during instructions to hold urine [342]. Taken together, these data circumstantially support a role for reduced 5-HT activity or receptor function, hormonal influences and linkage between brain sites for depression, hyperactive voiding and altered 5-HT activity.

In the CNS, estrogen modulates neuronal function by several mechanisms. One mechanism involves genomic activation through the estrogen receptor, ER-a. ER-a immunoreactive neurons are present in distinct areas of the forebrain, brainstem, and spinal cord linked with micturition. The sacral spinal cord is one of the areas involved in micturition and in primates it contains ER-a immunoreactive neurons. Also, 5-HT neurons express nuclear-estrogen receptor (ER-b) and progesterone receptors (PRs), which are gene-transcription factors. SERT mRNA decreases with estrogen treatment in primates [528]. Progesterone is without effect. Taken together, these data indicate that ovarian hormones could modify cognition, emotions, pain, and autonomic neural functions by acting on 5-HT neural pathways. Thus, the elimination of estrogens following ovariectomy might diminish the effect of neonatal clomipramine treatment.

III. GENES AND THE REGULATION OF LOWER URINARY TRACT FUNCTION

Since the last meeting there has been an exponential increase in the availability of animals in which genes have been deleted. These knockout animals provide information concerning the role of the gene products in the normal physiology and potentially in the pathophysiology of the lower urinary tract. Studies on the P2X3 receptor have been discussed above, but other important knockout animals have been studied and Table 11 indicates some of those that have been studied in normal animals.

The main conclusions from studies of knockout mice have been that the P2X3 receptor in pelvic nerve afferents that respond to physiological levels of distension is essential for normal function in the afferent limb of the micturition reflex [63,67,68]. In the autonomic ganglia, interference with the α subunit of the neuronal nicotinic receptor causes a failure of transmission through these ganglia and results in increased bladder capacity. Not surprisingly, the M3 receptor knockout suffers from urinary retention (predominantly in male animals). Of some interest also is the role of Insulin-like growth factor binding proteins, overexpression of one of which cause bladder hypoplasia, and a human syndrome linked to this is also known, if rare. Insulin-like growth factors influence the development of smooth muscle and blood vessels, and this finding is of interest to studies on development and of angiogenesis [529]. This is one example of the way in which transgenic technology and human genomics can interact. The susceptibility of humans to pathology, and the ways in which they cope with disturbances such as lower urinary tract obstruction may have its basis in their genotype. It appears that animals without neuronal nitric oxide synthase can have normal lower urinary tract function, but inducible NOS is expressed after bladder outlet obstruction, and knockout animals that do not possess inducible NOS are less able to cope with lower urinary tract obstruction [76].

Another gene (NCX) appears to control the number of neurones innervating the bladder, and its deletion actually increases the number of NADP-diaphorase staining cells in the autonomic ganglia. Bladder capacity seems unaffected by deletion of the genes for neuronal NOS, Brain Derived Neurotrophic Factor and cGMP-dependent protein kinase I (cGKI). However cGKI is involved in intracellular signaling following release of nitric oxide, and deletion of this gene abolishes NO-cGMP-dependent relaxations of urethral smooth muscle and results in hyperactive voiding [530].

The sensitivity of bladder smooth muscle to cholinergic stimulation appears to be reduced slightly in M2 receptor knockouts. Tonic, but not phasic, bladder contractions are affected by knocking out smooth muscle heavy chain myosin, whereas contractile activity appears to be unaffected by deletion of the actin-binding protein calponin.

Bladder sensation is reduced in animals that have had a deletion of the P2X3 or NK-1 receptor genes. In the former case the bladder size is increased, whereas there are no reports of this in the latter instance. Pain sensitivity generally is reduced in deletions of the P2X2, NK-1, H1 and VR-1 receptor genes, although there appears to be no information on other effects on the lower urinary tract. The significance of the P2X3 knockout in its effects on the lower urinary tract appears to relate to the significance of this receptor in normal bladder function, i.e. it is involved in the transduction of normal pressures and volumes in the mouse bladder.

So the recent data on the effects of genes on lower urinary tract function is a growth area that will affect all aspects of lower urinary tract physiology, pharmacology and pathophysiology, and considerable growth in this area can be expected.

IV. SUMMARY OF THE NEUROGENIC MECHANISMS UNDERLYING BLADDER OVERACTIVITY

Without discounting the importance of alterations in smooth muscle excitability, it appears that changes in bladder innervation orchestrated by neurotrophins manufactured by detrusor smooth muscle are temporally linked with bladder overactivity. Direct proof in humans is difficult to obtain, but circumstantial evidence is compelling . The ability of local anesthetics, intravesical afferent neurotoxins, and destruction of afferent nerves in the bladder neck and prostate to reduce urgency, frequency, and urge incontinence indicates an important role for afferent evoked reflexes [531]. The development of a spinal reflex (positive ice-water test) in patients with neurogenic bladders [479] as well as in patients with bladder outlet obstruction [598] suggests a common underlying plasticity in nerves supplying the bladder. Moreover, the association between elevated blood pressure and lower urinary tract symptoms in

Table 11 : Effects of Various knockouts on Bladder Function. The Table indicates which gene knockouts can influence Bladder size, Sensation, bladder contractions and neuronal targets in the manner indicated.

	Increased	Unchanged	Decreased
Bladder Size	P2X3 M3 (urinary retention in males) Alpha3 subunit of the neuronal nicotinic acetylcholine receptor	nNOS cGMP-dependent protein kinase I (cGKI) Brain Derived Neurotrophic Factor (BDNF)	Insulin-like growth factor-binding protein 4 (IGFBP-4) overexpression Ncx/Hox11L.1
CMG or Bladder contractions	P2X3 M3 Alpha3 subunit of the neuronal nicotinic acetylcholine receptor	M4 Calponin	(M2) Smooth muscle myosin heavy chain (tonic contraction)
Sensation			Purinergic P2X Vanilloid VR-1 Neurokinin NK1 Histamine H1
Nerve Interactions	Ncx/Hox11L.1 (Increases numbers of NADP Diaphorase-staining ganglion cells)		P2X3 (lack of response to ATP and distension) Alpha3 subunit of the neuronal nicotinic acetylcholine receptor (Decreased ganglionic transmission) NK-1 receptor (diminished axon reflexes; failure of chemo-attraction of mast cells)

Data from References 35,63,67,75,99,529,530, 577-584.

patients with BPH [532] provides a link between changes in sympathetic tone and voiding complaints. In addition the observation that aging is associated with an enhanced noradrenergic tone links the SHR model to plasticity in the lower urinary tract . Thus, common themes emerge when examining pathologic models. Urinary frequency and possibly urge incontinence are often associated with elevated neurotrophin production, an enhanced C-fiber afferent evoked bladder reflex and noradrenergic function. The realization that nerves supplying the lower urinary tract can undergo long-term changes, which possibly lead to bladder overactivity, offers a novel avenue for therapeutic intervention.

E. SUMMARY

The lower urinary tract has two main functions : storage and periodic elimination of urine. These functions are regulated by a complex neural control system located in the brain and spinal cord. This control system performs like a simple switching circuit to maintain a reciprocal relationship between the reservoir (urinary bladder) and the outlet components of the urinary tract (urethra and urethral sphincter). The switching circuit is modulated by various neurtransmitters and is sensitive to a variety of drugs. In infants the switching circuits function in a purely reflex manner to produce involuntary voiding; however in adults urine storage and release are subject to voluntary control.

Injuries or diseases of the nervous system in adults can disrupt the voluntary control of micturition causing the reemergence of reflex micturition, resulting in bladder hyperactivity and incontinence. Because of the complexity of the central nervous control of the lower urinary tract, incontinence can occur as a result of a variety of neurological disorders. Experimental studies indicate that bladder hyperactivity occurs after: (1) interruption of cortical inhibitory circuits, (2) disruption of basal ganglia function in models of Parkinson's disease, (3) damage to pathways from the brain to the spinal cord (multiple sclerosis, spinal cord injury) and (4) sensitization of bladder afferents. Various mechanisms contribute to the emergence of bladder dysfunction including reorganisation of synaptic connections in the spinal cord, changes in the expression of neurotransmitters and receptors and alterations in neural-target organ interactions mediated by neurotrophic factors.

During the past few years research in the field of Neurourology has led to the development of new concepts regarding the etiology of hyperactive bladder dysfunction and has stimulated the development of new therapeutic approaches for the treatment of incontinence, including the intravesical administration of afferent neurotoxins, such as capsaicin . In future research it will be important to focus on the development of neuropharmacologic agents that can suppress the unique components of abnormal bladder reflex mechanisms and thereby act selectively to diminish symptoms without altering normal voiding function.

F. FUTURE RESEARCH

First and foremost, more human data is required to evaluate the relative importance of mechanisms that have been demonstrated in animals. To an increasing extent, animal data is derived from studies of living cells, and that should make it easier to make the required comparisons. Nevertheless, whole animal and whole human studies will be essential if we are to extend our knowledge of pathophysiology, where the interactions between tissue components often amplify the changes seen in cells. With all animal models we should never lose sight of the question as to how closely these models really mimic the human situation.

Studies of the rat major pelvic ganglion have been and will continue to be useful in sorting out certain specific problems in neurobiology, which might be expected to lead to further relevant developments, particularly in relation to neuroplasticity. Nevertheless, the information that has been derived from such studies needs to be seen in the light of the human situation, where the ganglia are distributed within the bladder wall, and easily subjected to ischaemia and mechanical insults during obstruction, overactive bladder and other conditions that might lead to partial denervation. Denervation affects all intramural neurons and the effects of these pathophysiological changes on afferents, pre- and postganglionic autonomic neurons and on intramural neurons and their interconnections is an area open for study. The growth factors that affect nerves and vessels (including the neurotrophins and insulin-related growth factors and other trophic agents in angiogenesis and the maintenance of synaptic connectivity) each have specific targets, and it is unlikely that nerve growth factor (neurotrophin-1) will be the only important molecule in this area.

The neurotrophins however should remain a focus of activity partly because they are released by denervated tissues, but also because they show such profound changes in inflammation, spinal cord injury and other states. They are at the center of the discussion concerning the relative roles of ischaemia and partial denervation and of inflammation, cord injury and other pathologies. There are many other potential mediators as have been described earlier. In the related field of Spinal Cord Injury, there has recently been success in the use of certain neurotrophins and of stem cells in facilitating regeneration of central neurons, in some cases with some return of function. There is increasing awareness that the nature of the trauma to the spinal cord can alter the degree of damage, and new more appropriate models are being used. There is now increasing activity in this area and there can be added value in collaboration with these workers.

Genetic susceptibility to disease is being understood to a greater extent as a result of the analysis of the human genome. In this field comparisons with transgenic animals will become increasingly important in basic research and genomics will provide information about the susceptibility of humans to diseases. Transgenic animals have recently been important in the discussion of factors which cause afferent hypersensitivity, and it would be entirely appropriate to extend studies in these areas to the expression of genes in patients with related diseases. For instance, do patients with interstitial cystitis have a genetic susceptibility that might affect their urothelium, their afferent sensitivity, their smooth muscle, susceptibility of the tissues to iscahemia or a variety of other mechanisms that have been discussed in this volume. Genetic markers will be increasingly important in humans, and it is already clear from animal studies that tolerance of lower urinary tract obstruction is aided by the presence of certain genes. By the next consultation, we hope that much more will be known from animal and human studies to elucidate mechanisms and identify patients at particular risk.

These same genetic studies provide a new approach to neuropharmacology, and more specific therapies and appropriate preventive measures may become available. Studies of a more traditional nature continue to have a major role in developments in pharmacology.

In short the continuing support for basic neuroscience and cell biology, associated with the identification of genes and other factors that determine susceptibility to disease will provide a powerful approach that has, ultimately, to improve patient care. We are on the threshold of a new era of relief for patients if sufficient funding is available and if we recruit the brightest individuals to import the latest technologies to this important area.

REFERENCES

1 Brading, AF, Fry, CH, Maggi, CA, Takeda, M, Wammack, R, Wiklund, NP, Uvelius, B and Gabella, G (1999) Cellular biology in 1st international Consultation on Incontinence, Monaco 1998. Pp 105-154. In 'Incontinence' Edited by P Abrams, S Khoury and A Wein. Health Publication Ltd. ISBN 1 898452 25 3

2 de Groat, WC, Downie, JW, Levin, RM, Long Lin, AT, Morrison, JFB, Nishizawa, O, Steers, WD and Thor, KD. (1999) Basic Neurophysiology and Neuropharmacology: 1st international Consultation on Incontinence, Monaco 1998. Pp 105-154. In 'Incontinence' Edited by P Abrams, S Khoury and A Wein. Health Publication Ltd. ISBN 1 898452 25 3

3 Gosling, J., Alm,P, Bartsch, G, Bubaker, L, Creed, K, Delmas, V, Norton, P, Smet, P and Mauroy, B. Gross Anatomy of the Urinary Tract. In : Abrams, P, Khoury, S, Wein, A (Eds) Incontinence Health Publications, Ltd,., United Kingdom, pp 21-56, 1999.

4 Torrens, M.J. and Morrison, J.F.B.: The physiology of the lower urinary tract. London: Springer (1987).

5 de Groat, W.C., Booth, A.M. and Yoshimura, N.: Neurophysiology of micturition and its modification in animal models of human disease. In: The Autonomic Nervous System, Vol. 3, Chapter 8, Nervous Control of the Urogenital System. Ed.: C.A. Maggi, London, Harwood Academic Publishers, U.K., pp. 227-289, 1993.

6 Yoshimura, N., de Groat W.C.: Neural control of the lower urinary tract. Intern. J. Urol,. 4:111, 1997

7 Wein,A.J.: Neuromuscular dysfunction of the lower urinary tract. In: Campbell's Urology, 6th edition, chapter 6, Ed.: Walsh, P.C., Retik, A.B., Stamey, T.A., and Vaughan, E.D. Philadelphia, Harcourt Publishers, pp. 573-642, 1992.

8 Corcos, J and Schick, E (2001) 'The Urinary Sphincter' Pub Marcel Dekker, NY

9 de Groat, W.C.: Nervous control of the urinary bladder of the cat. Brain Res., 87: 201, 1975.

10 Sato, M., Mizuno, N., and Konishi, A.: Localization of motoneurons innervating perineal muscles: a HRP study in cat. Brain Res. 140: 149-154, 1978.

11 Roppolo, J.R., Nadelhaft, I., and De Groat, W.C.: The organization of pudendal motoneurons and primary afferent projections in the spinal cord of the rhesus monkey revealed by horseradish peroxidase. J. Comp. Neurol. 234: 475-488, 1985.

12 Kuzuhara, S., Kanazawa, I., and Nakanishi, T.: Topographical localization of the Onuf's nuclear neurons innervating the rectal and vesical striated sphincter muscles: a retrograde fluorescent double labeling in the cat and dog. Neurosci. Lett. 16:125-130, 1980.

13 Schroder, H.D.: Organization of motoneurons innervating the pelvic muscles of the male rat. J. Comp. Neurol., 192: 567-587, 1980.

14 Ulibarri, C., Popper P., and Micevych P.E.: Motoneurons dorsolateral to the central canal innervate perineal muscles in the Mongolian gerbil. J. Comp. Neurol. 356: 225-237, 1995.

15 Blok, B.F.M., Roukema, G., Geerdes, B., and Holstege, G.: Location of anal sphincter motoneurons of the female domestc pig. Neurosci. Lett. 216: 203-206, 1996.

16 Bennett, B.C., Kruse, M.N., Roppolo, J.R., Flood, H.D., Fraser, M. and de Groat, W.C.: Neural control of urethral outlet activity in vivo: role of nitric oxide. J. Urol., 153: 2004, 1995

17 Anderson, K.: Pharmacology of lower urinary tract smooth muscles and penile erectile tissues. Pharmacol. Rev., 45: 253, 1993.

18 de Groat, W.C.: Spinal cord projections and neuropeptides in visceral afferent neurons. Prog. Brain Res., 67: 165-188, 1986.

19 Jänig W, Morrison JFB. Functional properties of spinal visceral afferents supplying abdominal and pelvic organs, with special emphasis on visceral nociception, Progress in brain research 1986; 67: 87-114.

20 Iggo A. Tension receptors in the stomach and the urinary bladder, Journal of Physiology 1955; 128: 593-607.

21 Floyd, K., Hick, Verity E. and Morrison, J.F.B.: Mechano-sensitive afferent units in the hypogastric nerve of the cat. J. Physiol., 259: 457, 1976.

22 Habler, H.J., Janig, W., and Koltzenburg, M.:Myelinated primary afferents of the sacral spinal cord responding to slow filling and distension of the cat urinary bladder. J. Physiol., 463: 449, 1993.

23 Bahns, E., Ernsberger, U., Janig, W., and Nelke, A.: Functional characteristics of lumbar visceral afferent fibres from the urinary bladder and the urethra in the cat. Eur. J. Physiol., 407: 510, 1998.

24 Morrison, J.F.B. (1998) The activation of bladder wall afferent nerves. Experimental Physiology 84: 131-136

25 Downie, J.W. and Armour, J.A.: Mechanoreceptor afferent activity compared with receptor field dimensions and pressure changes in feline urinary bladder. Can. J. Physiol. Pharmacol., 70: 1457, 1992.

26 Sengupta, J.N. and Gebhart, G.F.: Mechanosensitive properties of pelvic nerve afferent fibers innervating the urinary bladder of the rat. J. Neurophysiol., 72: 2420, 1994.

27 Janig, W. and Koltzenburg, M.: On the function of spinal primary afferent fibres supplying colon and urinary bladder. J. Autonom. Nerv. Syst., 30: S89, 1990.

28 Waddell, P.J., Lawson, S.N. and McCarthy, P.W.: Conduction velocity changes along the processes of rat primary sensory neurones. Neuroscience, 30: 577, 1989.

29 Habler, H.J., Janig, W., and Koltzenburg, M.: Activation of unmyelinated afferent fibres by mechanical stimuli and inflammation of the urinary bladder in the cat. J. Physiol., 425: 545, 1990.

31 Morrison, J., Wen, J., & Kibble, A. (1999). Activation of pelvic afferent nerves from the rat bladder during filling. Scandinavian Journal of Urology & Nephrology Supplementum. 201, 73-75.

31 Shea, V. K., Cai, R., Crepps, B., Mason, J. L., & Perl, E. R. (2000). Sensory fibers of the pelvic nerve innervating the Rat's urinary bladder. J.Neurophysiol. 84, 1924-1933.

32 Koltzenburg and McMahon (1986). Plasma extravasation in the rat urinary bladder following mechanical, electrical and chemical stimuli: evidence for a new population of chemosensitive primary sensory afferents. Neurosci Lett 72:352-6

33 Keith, I. M., Jin, J., & Saban, R. (1995). Nerve-mast cell interaction in normal guinea pig urinary bladder. Journal of Comparative Neurology 363, 28-36.

34 Davies D, Medeiros MS, Keen J, Turner AJ, Haynes LW. (1992) Endopeptidase-24.11 cleaves a chemotactic factor from alpha-calcitonin gene-related peptide. Biochem Pharmacol 1992 Apr 15;43(8):1753-6

35 Saban, R., Saban, M. R., Nguyen, N. B., Lu, B., Gerard, C., Gerard, N. P., & Hammond, T. G. (2000). Neurokinin-1 (NK-1) receptor is required in antigen-induced cystitis. Am.J.Pathol. 156, 775-780.

36 de Groat, W.C., Vizzard, M.A., Araki, I. and Roppolo, J.R.: Spinal interneurons and preganglionic neurons in sacral autonomic reflex pathways. In: The Emotional Motor System. Eds: Holstege, G., Bandler, R. and Saper, C., Prog. Brain Res., Elsevier Science Publishers. 107: 97, 1996.

37 Morgan, C., Nadelhaft, I., and De Groat, W.C.: The distribution of visceral primary afferents from the pelvic nerve to Lissauer's Tract and the spinal gray matter and its relationship to the sacral parasympathetic nucleus. J. Comp. Neurol. 201: 415-440, 1981.

38 Thor, K. B., Morgan, C., Nadelhaft, I., Houston, M., and deGroat, W. C.: Organization of afferent and efferent pathways in the pudendal nerve of the female cat. J. Comp. Neurol., 288: 263, 1989.

39 de Groat, W.C.: Neuropeptides in pelvic afferent pathways. Experientia, 56: 334, 1989.

40 Vizzard, M. A. (2000). Changes in urinary bladder neurotrophic factor mRNA and NGF protein following urinary bladder dysfunction. Exp.Neurol. 161, 273-284.

41 Vizzard, M. A., Wu, K. H., & Jewett, I. T. (2000). Developmental expression of urinary bladder neurotrophic factor mRNA and protein in the neonatal rat. Brain Res.Dev.Brain Res. 119, 217-224.

42 Ishizuka O. Alm P. Larsson B. Mattiasson A. Andersson KE. Facilitatory effect of pituitary adenylate cyclase activating polypeptide on micturition in normal, conscious rats. Neuroscience. 66(4):1009-14, 1995

43 Miura A. Kawatani M. de Groat WC. Effects of pituitary adenylate cyclase activating polypeptide on lumbosacral preganglionic neurons in the neonatal rat spinal cord. Brain Research. 895(1-2):223-32, 2001

44 Birder, L.A. and de Groat, W.C.: The effect of glutamate antagonists on c-fos expression induced in spinal neurons by irritation of the lower urinary tract. Brain Res., 580:115, 1992.

45 Kakizaki, H., Yoshiyama, M., and de Groat, W.C.: Role of NMDA and AMPA glutamatergic transmission in spinal c-fos expression after urinary tract irritation. Amer. J. Physiol., 270: R990, 1996.

46 Burton, T. J., Elneil, S., Nelson, C. P., & Ferguson, D. R. (2000). Activation of epithelial Na(+) channel activity in the rabbit urinary bladder by cAMP. Eur.J.Pharmacol. 404, 273-280.

47 Frindt, G., Masilamani, S., Knepper, M. A., & Palmer, L. G. (2001). Activation of epithelial Na channels during short-term Na deprivation. Am.J.Physiol Renal Physiol 280, F112-F118.

48 Deng, F. M., Ding, M., Lavker, R. M., & Sun, T. T. (2001). Urothelial function reconsidered: a role in urinary protein secretion. Proc.Natl.Acad.Sci.U.S.A 98, 154-159.

49 Nimmo, A.J., Whitaker, E.M. and Morrison, J.F.B. (1986). The localisation of beta-adrenoreceptor subtypes in the rat urinary bladder. J. Physiol. 381, 29P.

50 Nimmo, AJ (1990) The distribution and regulation of beta-adrenergic and peptidergic receptors in the urogenital tract. PhD Thesis. University of Leeds.

51 Morrison, J. F. B., Nimmo, A. J. & Whitaker, E. M. (1990). The effect of neonatal capsaicin treatment on the distribution of neurokinin binding sites in rat bladder. J. Physiol. 423, 79P.

52 Birder, LA, Kanai, AJ, Kiss, S, Burke, N, Dineley, K, Watkins, SC, Reynolds, IJ, de Groat, WC and Caterina, MJ (2000) Evidence for functional VR1 receptors in bladder epithelial cells. Society for Neuroscience Abstracts 26:632.4.

53 Buffington, CA, Kiss, S, Kanai, AJ, Dineley, K, Roppolo, JR, Reynolds, IJ, de Groat, WC and Birder, LA (2000) Alterations in urothelium and bladder afferents in feline interstitial cystitis Society for Neuroscience Abstracts 26:349.3

54 Gabella, G. & Davis, C. (1998). Distribution of afferent axons in the bladder of rats. Journal of Neurocytology 27, 141-155.

55 Gu J, Blank MA, & Huang WM, (1984) Peptide containing nerves in human urinary bladder., Urology 24. 353-357.

56 Smet PJ, Moore KH, & Jonavicius J, (1997) Distribution and colocalization of calcitonin gene-related peptide, tachykinins, and vasoactive intestinal peptide in normal and idiopathic unstable human urinary bladder., Lab-Invest 77. 37-49.

57 Smet PJ, Edyvane KA, Jonavicius J, & Marshall VR, (1996a) Neuropeptides and neurotransmitter-synthesizing enzymes in intrinsic neurons of the human urinary bladder., J. Neurocytol. 25. 112-124.

58 Drake, M.J., Hedulnd, P., Mills, I.W., McCoy, R., McMuray, G. Gardner, B.P., Andersson, K-E. & Brading, A.F. (2000) Structural and functional denervation of human detrusor after spinal cord injury. Lab. Invest. 80, 1491-1499.

59 Landon, DN, Dasgupta, P, Hussain, IF, Brady C and Fowler, CJ (2001) Fine structure of the innervation of the lamina propria in normal human urinary bladder biopsies. BJU International (2001), 88, Suppl. 1, 4.

60 Chai, T. C., Steers, W. D., Broder, S. R., Rauçhenwald, M., & Tuttle, J. B. (1996). Characterization of laterality of innervation of the rat bladder. Scandinavian Journal of Urology & Nephrology Supplementum. 179, 87-92.

61 Levin, R. M., Wein, A. J., Krasnopolsky, L., Atta, M. A., & Ghoniem, G. M. (1995). Effect of mucosal removal on the response of the feline bladder to pharmacological stimulation. Journal of Urology 153, 1291-1294.

62 Lee, H. Y., Bardini, M., & Burnstock, G. (2000). Distribution of P2X receptors in the urinary bladder and the ureter of the rat. J.Urol. 163, 2002-2007.

63 Cockayne, D. A., Hamilton, S. G., Zhu, Q. M., Dunn, P. M., Zhong, Y., Novakovic, S., Malmberg, A. B., Cain, G., Berson, A., Kassotakis, L., Hedley, L., Lachnit, W. G., Burnstock, G., McMahon, S. B., & Ford, A. P. (2000). Urinary bladder hyporeflexia and reduced pain-related behaviour in P2X3-deficient mice. Nature 407, 1011-1015.

64 Cook , SP and McCleskie (2000) ATP, pain and a full bladder. Nature 407: 951-2

65 Ferguson, D. R., Kennedy, I., & Burton, T. J. (1997). ATP is released from rabbit urinary bladder epithelial cells by hydrostatic pressure changes--a possible sensory mechanism? Journal of Physiology 505, 503-511.

66 Namasivayam, S., Eardley, I., & Morrison, J. F. (1999). Purinergic sensory neurotransmission in the urinary bladder: an in vitro study in the rat. Bju International 84, 854-860.

67 Vlaskovska, M, Kasakov, L, Rong, W, Bodin, P, Bardini, M, Cockayne, DA. Ford, APDW and Burnstock, G (2001) P2X3 knockout mice reveal a major sensory role for urothelially released ATP. J Neuroscience 21: 5670-7

68 Rong, W, Burnstock G and Spyer, KM (2001) Purinergic modulation of mouse bladder afferent fibres: a single unit analysis. Abstracts of the International Union of Physiological Sciences, Christchurch, 2001. A1703.

69 Moore, KH, Ray, FR and Barden, JA (2001) Loss of Purinergic P2X3 and P2X5 Receptor Innervation in Human Detrusor from Adults with Urge Incontinence. J Neuroscience 21: RC166

70 Andersson, K. E. & Persson, K. (1995). Nitric oxide synthase and the lower urinary tract: possible implications for physiology and pathophysiology. Scandinavian Journal of Urology & Nephrology Supplementum. 175, 43-53.

71 Birder, L. A., Kanai, A. J., & de Groat, W. C. (1997). DMSO: effect on bladder afferent neurons and nitric oxide release. Journal of Urology 158, 1989-1995.

72 Birder, L. A., Apodaca, G., de Groat, W. C., & Kanai, A. J. (1998). Adrenergic- and capsaicin-evoked nitric oxide release from urothelium and afferent nerves in urinary bladder. American Journal of Physiology 275, F226-F229.

73 Birder, LA; Kanai, AJ; Ruiz, WG; Yoshiyama, M; de Groat, WC; and Apodaca, G. (1998b) Spinal cord injury alters nitric oxide release from urinary bladder. AUA Annual Meeting, Journal of Urology 159:20A.

74 Vizzard, M. A. (1997). Increased expression of neuronal nitric oxide synthase in bladder afferent and spinal neurons following spinal cord injury. Developmental Neuroscience 19, 232-246.

75 Sutherland, R. S., Kogan, B. A., Piechota, H. J., & Bredt, D. S. (1997). Vesicourethral function in mice with genetic disruption of neuronal nitric oxide synthase. J.Urol. 157, 1109-1116.

76 Lemack, G. E., Zimmern, P. E., Vazquez, D., Connell, J. D., & Lin, V. K. (2000). Altered response to partial bladder outlet obstruction in mice lacking inducible nitric oxide synthase. J.Urol. 163, 1981-1987.

77 Kibble, AL (1997) Modulation of Urinary Bladder Innervation by Neurokinin A. PhD Thesis, University of Leeds.

78 Jiang, W (1996) The functional properties of pelvic afferent fibres innervating the rat urinary bladder. PhD Thesis University of Leeds

79 Sculptoreanu, A and de Groat, WC. (2000) Protein kinase C is involved in neurokinin receptor modulation of the N- and L-type Ca2+ channels in dorsal root ganglion cells of the adult rat. Society for Neuroscience Abstracts 26:1645

80 Gauldie, S. D., McQueen, D. S., Pertwee, R., & Chessell, I. P. (2001). Anandamide activates peripheral nociceptors in normal and arthritic rat knee joints. Br.J.Pharmacol. 132, 617-621.

81 Tognetto, M., Amadesi, S., Harrison, S., Creminon, C., Trevisani, M., Carreras, M., Matera, M., Geppetti, P., & Bianchi, A. (2001). Anandamide excites central terminals of dorsal root ganglion neurons via vanilloid receptor-1 activation. J.Neurosci. 21, 1104-1109.

82 Howlett, A. C. & Mukhopadhyay, S. (2000). Cellular signal transduction by anandamide and 2-arachidonoylglycerol. Chem.Phys.Lipids 108, 53-70.

83 Caterina, M. J., Leffler, A., Malmberg, A. B., Martin, W. J., Trafton, J., Petersen-Zeitz, K. R., Koltzenburg, M., Basbaum, A. I., & Julius, D. (2000). Impaired nociception and pain sensation in mice lacking the capsaicin receptor. Science 288, 306-313.

84 Caterina, M. J. & Julius, D. (2001). The vanilloid receptor: a molecular gateway to the pain pathway. Annu.Rev.Neurosci. 24:487-517., 487-517.

85 Winston, J., Toma, H., Shenoy, M., & Pasricha, P. J. (2001). Nerve growth factor regulates VR-1 mRNA levels in cultures of adult dorsal root ganglion neurons. Pain 89, 181-186.

86 Giuliani, S., Lecci, A., Tramontana, M., & Maggi, C. A. (1999). Nociceptin protects capsaicin-sensitive afferent fibers in the rat urinary bladder from desensitization. Naunyn-Schmiedebergs Archives of Pharmacology 360, 202-208.

87 Su, X., Sengupta, J. N., & Gebhart, G. F. (1997). Effects of opioids on mechanosensitive pelvic nerve afferent fibers innervating the urinary bladder of the rat. Journal of Neurophysiology 77, 1566-1580.

88 Tanner, R., Chambers, P., Khadra, M. H., & Gillespie, J. I. (2000). The production of nerve growth factor by human bladder smooth muscle cells in vivo and in vitro. BJU.Int. 85, 1115-1119.

89 Okragly, A. J., Niles, A. L., Saban, R., Schmidt, D., Hoffman, R. L., Warner, T. F., Moon, T. D., Uehling, D. T., & Haak-Frendscho, M. (1999). Elevated tryptase, nerve growth factor, neurotrophin-3 and glial cell line-derived neurotrophic factor levels in the urine of interstitial cystitis and bladder cancer patients. J.Urol. 161, 438-441.

90 Oddiah, D., Anand, P., McMahon, S. B., & Rattray, M. (1998). Rapid increase of NGF, BDNF and NT-3 mRNAs in inflamed bladder. Neuroreport 9, 1455-1458.

91 Spitsbergen, J. M., Clemow, D. B., McCarty, R., Steers, W. D., & Tuttle, J. B. (1998). Neurally mediated hyperactive voiding in spontaneously hypertensive rats. Brain Res. 790, 151-159.

92 Steinbacher, B. C., Jr. & Nadelhaft, I. (1998). Increased levels of nerve growth factor in the urinary bladder and hypertrophy of dorsal root ganglion neurons in the diabetic rat. Brain Res. 782, 255-260.

93 Dmitrieva, N., Shelton, D., Rice, A. S., & McMahon, S. B. (1997). The role of nerve growth factor in a model of visceral inflammation. Neuroscience 78, 449-459.

94 Jaggar, S. I., Scott, H. C., & Rice, A. S. (1999). Inflammation of the rat urinary bladder is associated with a referred thermal hyperalgesia which is nerve growth factor dependent. Br.J.Anaesth. 83, 442-448.

95 Dmitrieva, N. & McMahon, S. B. (1996). Sensitisation of visceral afferents by nerve growth factor in the adult rat. Pain 66, 87-97.

96 Chuang, Y. C., Fraser, M. O., Yu, Y., Chancellor, M. B., de Groat, W. C., & Yoshimura, N. (2001). The role of bladder afferent pathways in bladder hyperactivity induced by the intravesical administration of nerve growth factor. J.Urol. 165, 975-979.

97 Sherer, T. B., Clemow, D. B., & Tuttle, J. B. (2000). Calcium homeostasis and nerve growth factor secretion from vascular and bladder smooth muscle cells. Cell Tissue Res. 299, 201-211.

98 Goins, W. F., Yoshimura, N., Phelan, M. W., Yokoyama, T., Fraser, M. O., Ozawa, H., Bennett, N., Jr., de Groat, W. C., Glorioso, J. C., & Chancellor, M. B. (2001). Herpes simplex virus mediated nerve growth factor expression in bladder and afferent neurons: potential treatment for diabetic bladder dysfunction. J.Urol. 165, 1748-1754.

99 Lommatzsch, M., Braun, A., Mannsfeldt, A., Botchkarev, V. A., Botchkareva, N. V., Paus, R., Fischer, A., Lewin, G. R., & Renz, H. (1999). Abundant production of brain-derived neurotrophic factor by adult visceral epithelia. Implications for paracrine and target-derived Neurotrophic functions. Am.J.Pathol. 155, 1183-1193.

100 Hohlfeld, R., Kerschensteiner, M., Stadelmann, C., Lassmann, H., & Wekerle, H. (2000). The neuroprotective effect of inflammation: implications for the therapy of multiple sclerosis. J.Neuroimmunol. 107, 161-166.

101 Erickson, D. R., Belchis, D. A., & Dabbs, D. J. (1997). Inflammatory cell types and clinical features of interstitial cystitis. J.Urol. 158, 790-793.

102 Christmas, T. J. (1994). Lymphocyte sub-populations in the bladder wall in normal bladder, bacterial cystitis and interstitial cystitis. Br.J.Urol. 73, 508-515.

103 Moalem, G., Gdalyahu, A., Shani, Y., Otten, U., Lazarovici, P., Cohen, I. R., & Schwartz, M. (2000). Production of neurotrophins by activated T cells: implications for neuroprotective autoimmunity. J.Autoimmun. 15, 331-345.

104 Ueda, T., Tamaki, M., Ogawa, O., Yamauchi, T., & Yoshimura, N. (2000). Improvement of interstitial cystitis symptoms and problems that developed during treatment with oral IPD-1151T. J.Urol. 164, 1917-1920.

105 Jiang, C. H. & Lindstrom, S. (1996). Intravesical electrical stimulation induces a prolonged decrease in micturition threshold volume in the rat. Journal of Urology 155, 1477-1481.

106 Jiang, C. H. (1998). Modulation of the micturition reflex pathway by intravesical electrical stimulation: an experimental study in the rat. Neurourology & Urodynamics 17, 543-553.

107 de Groat, W. C. and Ryall, R. W.: Reflexes to the sacral parasympathetic neurones concerned with micturition in the cat. J. Physiol. 200: 87, 1969.

108 Jiang, C. H. & Lindstrom, S. (1999). Prolonged enhancement of the micturition reflex in the cat by repetitive stimulation of bladder afferents. Journal of Physiology 517, 599-605.

109 Floyd, K., McMahon, S.B. and Morrison, J.F.B. (1982). Inhibitory interactions between colonic and vesical afferents in the micturition reflex of the cat. J. Physiol. 322, 45-52.

110 de Groat, W. C., Fraser, M. O., Yoshiyama, M., Smerin, S., Tai, C., Chancellor, M. B., Yoshimura, N., & Roppolo, J. R. (2001). Neural control of the urethra. Scand.J.Urol.Nephrol.Suppl 35-43.

111 de Groat, W.C. and Booth, A.M.: Synaptic transmission in pelvic ganglia. In: The Autonomic Nervous System, Vol. 3, Chapter 9, Nervous Control of the Urogenital System. Ed.: C.A. Maggi, Harwood Academic Publishers, London, U.K., pp. 291-347, 1993.

112 Vizzard, M.A., Erdman, S.L., Forsterman, U., and de Groat, W.C.: Differential distribution of nitric oxide synthase in neural pathways to the urogenital organs (urethra, penis, urinary bladder) of the rat. Brain Res., 646: 279, 1994.

113 Danuser, H., Bemis K. and Thor K. B.: Pharmacological analysis of the noradrenergic control of central sympathetic and somatic reflexes controlling the lower urinary tract in the anesthetized cat. J. Pharmacol. Exp. Ther., 274: 820, 1995.

114 Nadelhaft, I., de Groat, W. C.; Morgan, C.: Location and morphology of parasympathetic preganglionic neurons in the sacral spinal cord of the cat revealed by retrograde axonal transport of horseradish peroxidase. J. Comp. Neurol., 193: 265, 1980.

115 Morgan, C.W., de Groat, W.C., Felkins, L.A. and Zhang, S.-J.: Intracellular injection of neurobiotin or horseradish peroxidase reveals separate types of preganglionic neurons in the sacral parasympathetic nucleus of the cat. J. Comp. Neurol., 331:161, 19

116 Thor, K. B., Hisamitsu, T., Roppolo, J. R., Tuttle, P., Nagel, J., and de Groat, W. C.: Selective inhibitory effects of ethylketocyclazocine on reflex pathways to the external urethral sphincter of the cat. J. Pharmacol. Exp. Ther., 248: 1018, 1989.

117 Gajewski, J., Downie J. W. and Awad S. A.: Experimental evidence for a central nervous system site of action in the effect of alpha-adrenergic blockers on the external urinary sphincter. J. Urol., 132: 403, 1984.

118 Downie, J. W. and Bialik, G. J.: Evidence for a spinal site of action of clonidine on somatic and viscerosomatic reflex activity evoked on the pudendal nerve in cats. J. Pharmacol. Exp. Ther., 246: 352, 1988.

119 Gabella G, Berggren T, & Uvelius B, (1992) Hypertrophy and reversal of hypertrophy in rat pelvic ganglion neurons, J Neurocytol 21. 649-662.

120 Dixon, J. S., Jen, P. Y. P., Gosling, J.A. (2000). "The distribution of vesicular acetylcholine transporter in the human male genitourinary organs and its co-localization with neuropeptide Y and nitric oxide synthase." NU 19(2): 185-194.

121 Drake, M.J., Hussain, I.F., Hedlund, P., Brading, A.F., Fowler, C.J., & Andersson, K.E., (2000). Characterization of intramuscular myofibrioblasts in human detrusor. BJUI, 86: 367-368.

122 Ek A, Alm P, Andersson KE, & Persson CG, (1977) Adrenergic and cholinergic nerves of the human urethra and urinary bladder. A histochemical study, Acta Physiol Scand 99. 345-352.

122 Holzer P, (1988) Local effector functions of capsaicin-sensitive sensory nerve endings: involvement of tachykinins, calcitonin gene-related peptide and other neurotransmitters., Neuroscience 24. 739-768.

123 Dixon JS, Gilpin SA, Gilpin CJ, & Gosling JA, (1983) Intramural ganglia of the human urinary bladder, Br J Urol 55. 195-198.

124 Brading AF, Greenland JE, Mills IW et al. Blood supply to the bladder during filling, Scandinavian Journal of Urology and Nephrology Suppl 1999; 201: 25-31.

125 Ho KMT (2000). Neuromuscular control of the human urethral sphincter. D.Phil Thesis, Oxford University.

126 Dixon JS, Jen PY, & Gosling JA, (1997) A double label immunohistochemical study of intramural ganglia from the human male urinary bladder neck., J. Anat. 190. 125-134.

127 Ho KMT, McMurray G, Brading AF, Noble JG, Ny L & Andersson K-E (1999) Co-localisation of carbon monoxide and nitric oxide synthesising enzymes in human urethral sphincter., J Urol 161. 1968-1972.

128 Hanani M &Maudlej N, (1995) Intracellular recordings from intramural neurons in the guinea-pig urinary bladder., J Neurophys 74. 2358-2365.

129 Smet PJ, Jonavicius J, Marshall VR, & de Vente J, (1996b) Distribution of nitric oxide synthase-immunoreactive nerves and identification of the cellular targets of nitric oxide in guinea-pig and human urinary bladder by cGMP immunohistochemistry, Neuroscience 71. 337-348.

130 Sanders, K. M. (1996). "A case for interstitial cells of Cajal as pacemakers and mediators of neurotransmissionin the gastrointestinal tract." Gastroenterology 111: 492-515.

131 Klemm, M.F., Exintaris, B., & Lang, R.J., (1999). Identification of the cells underlying pacemaker activity in the guinea-pig upper urinary tract. J. Physiol. (Lond.), 519: 867-884.

132 Hashitani, H., Van Helden, D.F., & Suzuki, H., (1996). Properties of spontaneous depolarisations in circular smooth muscle cells of rabbit urethra. Br. J. Pharmac., 118: 1627-1632.

133 Sergeant, G.P., Hollywood, M.A., McClosky, K.D., Thornbury, K.D., & McHale, N.G., (2000). Specialised pacemaking cells in the rabbut urethra. J. Physiol. (Lond.), 526: 359-366.

134 Sellers, D. J., Chess-Williams, R., & Chapple, C. R. (2000). 5-Hydroxytryptamine-induced potentiation of cholinergic responses to electrical field stimulation in pig detrusor muscle. BJU.Int. 86, 714-718.

135 Lecci, A., Giuliani, S., Tramontana, M., Santicioli, P., Criscuoli, M., Dion, S., & Maggi, C. A. (1998). Bladder distension and activation of the efferent function of sensory fibres: similarities with the effect of capsaicin. British Journal of Pharmacology 124, 259-266.

136 Kakizaki, H., Yoshiyama, M., Koyanagi, T., & de Groat, W. C. (2001). Effects of WAY100635, a selective 5-HT1A-receptor antagonist on the micturition-reflex pathway in the rat. Am.J.Physiol Regul.Integr.Comp Physiol 280, R1407-R1413.

137 Testa, R., Guarneri, L., Angelico, P., Velasco, C., Poggesi, E., Cilia, A., & Leonardi, A. (2001). Effect of different 5-hydroxytryptamine receptor subtype antagonists on the micturition reflex in rats. BJU.Int. 87, 256-264.

139 Espey MJ. Du HJ. Downie JW. Serotonergic modulation of spinal ascending activity and sacral reflex activity evoked by pelvic nerve stimulation in cats. Brain Research. 798:101-8, 1998

140 Suzuki T., Kawatani, M., Erdman, S., deGroat, WC: "Role of CRF and 5-HT in Central Pathways Controlling Micturition in the Rat" Society for Neuroscience Abstracts (1990)

141 Danuser, H., Thor, K.B.: "Spinal 5-HT2 receptor-mediated facilitation of pudendal nerve reflexes in the anesthetized cat" Br. J. Pharmacol. 118:150-154 (1996)

142 Michelotti G, Price D, Schwinn D. Alpha-1 adrenergic receptor regulation: basic science and clinical implications. Pharmacol Ther 2000; 88:281-309.

143 Lepor H, Auerbach S, Puras BA, Narayan, P., Soloway, M., Lowe, F., Moon T., Leifer, G., Madsen, P. A randomized, placebo-controlled multicenter study of the efficacy and safety of terazosin in the treatment of benign prostatic hyperplasia. J Urol 1992; 148: 1467-1474.

144 Forray C, Bard J, Wetzel J., Chiu, G., Shapiro, E., Tang, R., Lepor, H., Hartig, P.R., Weinshank, R.L., Branchek, T.A., Gluchowski, C. The al-adrenergic receptor that mediates smooth muscle contraction in human prostate has the pharmacological properties of the cloned human ala subtype. Mol Pharmacol 1994; 45:703-708.

145 Blue DJ, Grino P, Jung D, Harbison M, Ford A. Evaluation of

Ro 70-0004, a selective a1a-adrenoceptor antagonist, in men with benign prostatic hyperplasia. Proceedings from the 5th International Consultation on BPH (WHO sponsored, June 25-28, 2000) Paris, France 2001:in press.

146 Malloy B., Price D., Price R., Bienstock, A., Dole, M., Funk, B., Rudner, X., Richardson C., Donatucci, C., Schwinn, D. a1-adrenergic receptor subtypes in human detrusor. J Urol 1998; 160: 937-943.

147 Stafford-Smith M, Shambra U, Wilson K, Page S, Schwinn D. a1-adrenergic receptors in human spinal cord: specific localized expression of mRNA encoding a1-adrenergic subtypes at four distinct levels. Mol Brain Res 1999; 63:254-261.

148 Schwinn D, Michelotti G. a1-adrenergic receptors in the lower urinary tract and vascular bed: potential role for the a1d-subtype in filling symptoms and effects of ageing on vascular expression. Br J Urol 2000; 85:6-11.

149 Hampel, C, Dolber, PC, Smith, MP, Savic, SL, Thüroff, JW, Thor, KB and Schwinn, DA (2001) Modulation of Bladder a1-Adrenergic Receptor Subtype Expression by Bladder Outlet Obstruction. J Urol (in press)

150 O'Reilly, B. A., Kosaka, A. H., Chang, T. K., Ford, A. P., Popert, R., Rymer, J. M., & McMahon, S. B. (2001). A quantitative analysis of purinoceptor expression in human fetal and adult bladders. J.Urol. 165, 1730-1734.

151 Yunaev, M. A., Barden, J. A., & Bennett, M. R. (2000). Changes in the distribution of different subtypes of P2X receptor clusters on smooth muscle cells in relation to nerve varicosities in the pregnant rat urinary bladder. J.Neurocytol. 29, 99-108.

152 O'Reilly, B. A., Kosaka, A. H., Chang, T. K., Ford, A. P., Popert, R., & McMahon, S. B. (2001b). A quantitative analysis of purinoceptor expression in the bladders of patients with symptomatic outlet obstruction. BJU.Int. 87, 617-622.

153 Paton, D. M. (1967). Effects of metabolic inhibitors on contraction of rabbit detrusor muscle. British Journal of Pharmacology 34, 493-498.

154 Rohner, T. J., Komins, J. I., Kirchner, P. and Adams, R. (1967). Utilization of glucose by normal, defunctionalized, and denervated bladder muscle. Investigative Urology 5, 12-18.

155 Hellstrand, P. & Vogel, H. J. (1985). Phosphagens and intracellular pH intact rabbit smooth muscle studied by 31P-NMR. American Journal of Physiology 248, C320-329.

156 Haugaard, N., Wein, A. J. & Levin, R. M. (1987). In vitro studies of glucose metabolism of the rabbit urinary bladder. Journal of Urology 137, 782-784.

157 Levin, R. M., Haugaard, N., Ruggieri, M. R. and Wein, A. J. (1987). Biochemical characterization of the rabbit urinary bladder base and body. Neurourology and Urodynamics 6, 57-61.

158 Levin, R. M., Ruggieri, M. R., Gill, H. S., Haugaard, N. and Wein, A. J. (1988). Effect of bethanechol on glycolysis and high energy phosphate metabolism of the rabbit urinary bladder. Journal of Urology 139, 646-649.

159 Levin, R. M., Hypolite, J., Ruggieri, M. R., Longhurst, P. A. and Wein, A. J. (1989a). Effects of muscarinic stimulation on intracellular calcium in the rabbit bladder: Comparison with metabolic response. Pharmacology 39, 69-77.

160 Levin, R. M., Moore, D., Ruggieri, M. R., Haugaard, N. and Wein, A. J. (1989b). Biochemical characterization of the rabbit urinary bladder: II. intracellular concentration of nucleotides. Neurourology and Urodynamics 8, 63-71.

161 Wendt, I. R. and Gibbs, C. L. (1987). Energy expenditure of longitudinal smooth muscle of rabbit urinary bladder. American Journal of Physiology 252, C88-C96.

162 Wendt, I. R. (1989). Effects of substrate and hypoxia on smooth muscle metabolism and contraction. American Journal of Physiology 256, C719-C727.

163 Arner, A., Malmqvist, U. & Uvelius, B. (1990). Metabolism and force in hypertrophic smooth muscle from rat urinary bladder. American Journal of Physiology 258, C923-C932.

164 Arner, A., Malmqvist, U., Osterman, A. & Uvelius, B. (1993). Energy Turnover and Lactate Dehydrogenase Activity in Detrusor Smooth Muscle from Rats with Streptozotocin-Induced Diabetes. Acta Physiologica Scandinavica 147, 375-383.

165 Malmqvist, U., Arner, A. and Uvelius, B. (1991). Lactate dehydrogenase activity and isoform distribution in normal and hypertrophic smooth muscle tissue from the rat. Pflüger's Archives 419, 230-234.

166 Lin, A. T.-L., Chang, L. S., Chen, M.-T., Yang, C.-H., Shiao, M.-S., Chen, C.-J. and Levin, R. M. (1992). Energetics of detrusor contraction: Effects of outlet obstruction. Neurourology and Urodynamics 11, 605-614.

167 Polyanska, M., Arner, A., Malmquist, U. and Uvelius, B. (1993). Lactate Dehydrogenase Activity and Isoform Distribution in the Rat Urinary Bladder - Effects of Outlet Obstruction and Its Removal. Journal of Urology 150, 543-545.

168 Casteels, R. & Wuytak, F. (1975). Aerobic and anaerobic metabolism in smooth muscle cells of taenia coli in relation to active ion transport. Journal of Physiology 250, 203-220.

169 Siegman, M. J., Butler, T. M., Mooers, S. U. and Davies, R. E. (1980). Chemical energetics of force development, force maintenance, and relaxation of mammalian smooth muscle. Journal of General Physiology 76, 609-629.

170 Butler, T. M. & Siegman, M. J. (1982). Chemical energetics of contraction in mammalian smooth muscle. Federation Proceedings 41, 204-208.

171 Davidheiser, S., Joseph, J. & Davies, R. (1984). Separation of aerobic glycolysis from oxidative metabolism and contractility in rat anococcygeus muscle. American Journal of Physiology - Cell Physiology 247, C335-C341.

172 Paul, R. J. (1989). Smooth muscle energetics. Annual Review of Physiology 51, 331-349.

173 Paul, R. J., Strauss, J. D. and Krisands, J. M. (1987). The effects of calcium on smooth muscle mechanics and energetics. Progress in Clinical & Biological Research 245, 319-332.

174 Scott, D. P. and Coburn, R. F. (1989). Phosphocreatine and oxidative metabolism-contraction coupling in rabbit aorta. American Journal of Physiology 257, H597-H602.

175 Ruggieri, M. R., Hanno, P. M., Samadzadeh, S., Johnson, E. W. and Levin, R. M. (1986). Heparin inhibition of increased bacterial adherence following overdistension, ischemia and partial outlet obstruction of the rabbit urinary bladder. Journal of Urology 136, 132-135.

176 Levin, R. M., Wein, A. J., Whitmore, K., Monson, F. C., McKenna, B. A. W. and Ruggieri, M. R. (1990b). Trypan blue as an indicator of urothelial integrity. Neurourology and Urodynamics 9, 269-279.

177 Monson, F. C., McKenna, B. A. W., Wein, A. J. and Levin, R. M. (1992). Effect of outlet obstruction on 3H-thymidine uptake: a biochemical and radioautographic study. Journal of Urology 148, 158-162.

178 Monson, F. C., Wein, A. J., Eika, B., Murphy, M. and Levin, R. M. (1994). Stimulation of DNA synthesis in rabbit bladder wall after partial outlet obstruction and acute observation. Neurourology and Urodynamics 13, 51-61.

179 Monson, F. C., Wein, A. J., McKenna, B. A. W., Whitmore, K. and Levin, R. M. (1991). Indigocarmine as a quantitative indicator of urothelial integrity. Journal of Urology 145, 842-845.

180 Tong, Y.-C., Monson, F. C., Eika, B. and Levin, R. M. (1992). Effects of acute in vitro overdistension of the rabbit urinary bladder on DNA synthesis. Journal of Urology 148, 1347-1350.

181 Eika, B., Levin, R. M., Monson, F. C., Murphy, M. & Longhurst, P. A. (1993). H-3-thymidine uptake by the rat urinary bladder after induction of diabetes-mellitus. Journal of Urology 150, 1316-1320.

182 Tammela, T. L. J., Levin, R. M., Monson, F. C. and Longhurst, P. A. (1994). Temporal changes in rabbit urinary bladder function and DNA synthesis during chronic treatment with furosemide. Journal of Urology 151, 503-508.

183 Irwin, P. & Galloway, N. T. M. (1993). Impaired Bladder Perfusion in Interstitial Cystitis - A Study of Blood Supply Using Laser Doppler Flowmetry. Journal of Urology 149, 890-892.

184 Campbell, J. D., Agubosim, S. & Paul, R. J. (1988). Compartmentation of metabolism and function in vascular smooth muscle: Quantitation of Na-pump activity and aerobic glysolysis. FASEB Journal 2, A755.

185 Ishida, Y. & Paul, R. J. (1989). Evidence for compartmentation of high-energy phosphagens in smooth muscle. In Muscle energetics, edn, ed. Paul, R. J., Elzinga, G. & Yamada, K., pp. 417-429. Alan R. Liss, New York.

186 Lynch, R. M. and Paul, R. J. (1989). Functional compartmentation of carbohydrate metabolism. In Microcompartmentation, edn, ed. Jones, D. P., . CRC Crit. Rev., Boca Raton.

187 Levin, R. M., High, J. and Wein, A. J. (1981). Metabolic and contractile effects of anoxia on the rabbit urinary bladder. Journal of Urology 128, 194-196.

188 van Arsdalen, K. N., Wein, A. J. and Levin, R. M. (1983). The contractile and metabolic effects of acute ischemia upon the rabbit bladder. Journal of Urology 130, 180-182.

189 Zhao, Y., Wein, A. J., Bilgen, A. and Levin, R. M. (1991). Effect of anoxia on in vitro bladder function. Pharmacology 43, 337-344.

190 Bilgen, A., Wein, A. J., Zhao, Y. & Levin, R. M. (1992b). Effects of anoxia on the biphasic response of isolated strips of rabbit bladder to fiekd stimulation, bethanechol methoxamine and KCl. Pharmacology 44, 283-289.

191 Levin, R. M., Brendler, K. and Wein, A. J. (1983). Comparative pharmacological response of an in vitro whole bladder preparation (rabbit) with response of isolated smooth muscle strips. Journal of Urology 130, 377-381.

192 Levin, R. M., Wein, A. J., Buttyan, R., Monson, F. C. and Longhurst, P. A. (1994). Update on bladder smooth-muscle physiology. World Journal of Urology 12, 226-232.

193 Levin, R. M., Levin, S. S. and Wein, A. J. (1996b). Etiology of incontinence: A review and hypothesis. Scandinavian Journal of Urology and Nephrology 30, 15-25.

194 Kato, K., Wein, A. J., Kitada, S., Haugaard, N. & Levin, R. M. (1988). The functional effect of mild outlet obstruction on the rabbit urinary bladder. Journal of Urology 140, 880-884.

195 Kato, K., Monson, F. C., Longhurst, P. A., Wein, A. J., Haugaard, N. and Levin, R. M. (1990b). The functional effects of long-term outlet obstruction on the rabbit urinary bladder. Journal of Urology 143, 600-606.

196 Chun, A. L., Wein, A. J., Gill, H. S. & Levin, R. M. (1990). Response of the whole bladder-urethra model (rabbit) to autonomic drugs. Neurourology and Urodynamics 9, 165-169.

197 Kwon, H. Y., Wein, A. J. and Levin, R. M. (1995). Effect of anoxia on the urethral response to phenylephrine. Journal of Urology 154, 1527-1531.

198 Uvelius, B. and Arner, A. (1997). Changed metabolism of detrusor muscle cells from obstructed rat urinary bladder. Scandinavian Journal of Urology and Nephrology Suppl 184, 59-65.

199 Hypolite, J. A., Wein, A. H., Haugaard, N. & Levin, R. M. (1991). Role of substrates in the maintenance of contractility of rabbit urinary bladder. Pharmacology 42, 202-210.

200 Kwon, H. Y., Longhurst, P. A., Parsons, K., Wein, A. J. and Levin, R. M. (1996). Effects of glucose deprivation on the contractile response of the rabbit bladder to repetitive stimulation. Neurourology and Urodynamics 15, 71-78.

201 Pessina, F., McMurray, G., Wiggin, A. and Brading, A. F. (1997). The effect of anoxia and glucose-free solutions on the contractile response of guinea-pig detrusor strips to intrinsic nerve stimulation and the application of excitatory agonists. Journal of Urology 157, 2375-2380.

202 Hypolite, J. A., Longhurst, P. A., Gong, C., Briscoe, J., Wein, A. J. & Levin, R. M. (1993). Metabolic studies on rabbit bladder smooth muscle and mucosa. Molecular and Cellular Biochemistry 125, 35-42.

204 Lieb, J., Chichester, P., Kogan, B., Das, A.K., Leggett, R.E., Schroeder, A., and Levin, R.M. Rabbit urinary bladder blood flow changes during the initial stage of partial outlet obstruction.(2000) J. Urol. 164, 1390-1397.

205 Awad, S. A. & Downie, J. W. (1976). Relative contributions of smoothe and striated muscles to urethral pressure profile. British Journal of Urology 48, 347-350.

205 Lieb, J., Kogan, B., Das, A.K., Leggett, R.E., Schroeder, A., and Levin, R.M .The Effect of Urine Volume and Nitric Oxide on Basal Bladder Blood Flow: Response to Catheterization and Drainage (2001) Neurourology and Urodynamics 20, 115-124.

206 Steers, W. D. (1998). Physiology and Pharmacology of the Bladder and Urethra. In Campbell's Urology, 7th edn, ed. Walsh, P. C., Retik, AB, Vaughan, ED and Wein, AJ. Published by WB Saunders, Philadelphia. ISBN 0-7216-4461-9 pp 870-915.

207 Tanagho, E. A., Meyers, F. H. and Smith, D. R. (1969a). Urethral resistance: Its components and implications: Striated muscle component. Investigative Urology 7, 195-201.

208 Tanagho, E. A., Meyers, F. H. and Smith, D. R. (1969b). Urethral resistance: Its components and implications: I Smooth muscle component. Investigative Urology J, 136-140.

209 Greenland, J. E. and Brading, A. F. (1997). The in vivo and in vitro effects of hypoxia on pig urethral smooth muscle. British Journal of Urology 79, 525-531.

210 Diakno, T. & Taub, M. (1975). Ephedrine in treatment of urinay incontinence. Urology 5, 624.

211 Ek, A., Andersson, K. E. and Gullberg, B. (1978). The effects of long term treatment with norephedrine on stress incontinence and urethral closure pressure profile. Scandinavian Journal of Urology and Nephrology 12, 105-110.

212 Awad, S. A., Downie, J. & Kiruluta, I. (1978). Alpha adrenergic agents in urinary disorders of the proximal urethra I: Stress incontinence. British Journal of Urology 50, 332-335.

213 Steward, B., Borowsky, L. and Montague, D. (1976). Stress incontintence: conservative therapy with sympathomimetic drugs. Journal of Urology 115, 558-561.

214 Sibley, G.N.A. A comparison of spontaneous and nerve-mediated activity in bladder muscle from man, pig and rabbit. Journal of Physiology 1984; 354: 431-443.

215 Palea S, Artibani W, Ostardo E, Trist DG, Pietra, C. Evidence for purinergic neurotransmission in human urinary bladder affected by interstitial cystitis. Journal of Urology 1993; 150: 2007-2012.

216 Bayliss M, Wu C, Newgreen D, Mundy AR, Fry CH. A quantitative study of atropine-resistant contractile responses in human detrusor smooth muscle, from stable, unstable and obstructed bladders. Journal of Urology 1999; 162: 1833-1839

217 Wu C, Bayliss M, Newgreen D, Mundy AR, Fry CH. A comparison of the mode of action of ATP and carbachol on isolated human detrusor smooth muscle. Journal of Urology 1999; 162: 1840-1847

218 Mills IW, Greenland JE, McMurray G, McCoy R, Ho KM, Noble JG, Brading AF. Studies of the pathophysiology of idiopathic detrusor instability: the physiological properties of the detrusor smooth muscle and its pattern of innervation. Journal of Urology 2000; 163: 646-651.

219 Crack BE, Pollard CE, Beukers MW, Roberts SM, Hunt SF, Ingall AH, McKechnie KC, Ijzerman AP, Leff P. Pharmacological and biochemical analysis of FPL 67156, a novel, selective inhibitor of ecto-ATPase. British Journal of Pharmacology 1995; 114: 475-481

220 Yoshida Y, Akimoto Y, Tatsumi H, Koda A. Experimental neurogenic bladder in rats and effect of Robaveron, a biological prepared from swine prostate, on it. Japanese Journal of Pharmacology 1986; 40: 149-159.

221 Westfall TD, Kennedy C, Sneddon P. Enhancement of sympathetic purinergic neurotransmission in the guinea-pig isolated vas deferens by the novel ecto-ATPase inhibitor ARL 67156. British Journal of Pharmacology 1996; 117: 867-872.

222 Westfall TD, Kennedy C, Sneddon P. The ecto-ATPase inhibitor ARL 67156 enhances parasympathetic neurotransmission in the guinea-pig urinary bladder. European Journal of Pharmacology 1997; 329: 169-173.

223 Somogyi GT, Tanowitz M, de Groat WC. M1 muscarinic receptor-mediated facilitation of acetylcholine release in the rat urinary bladder. Journal of Physiology 1994; 480: 81-89.

224 Somogyi GT, Tanowitz M, Zernova G, de Groat WC. M1 muscarinic receptor-induced facilitation of ACh and noradrenaline release in the rat bladder is mediated by protein kinase C Journal of Physiology 1996; 496: 245-254.

225 D'Agostino G, Bolognesi ML, Lucchelli A, Vicini D, Balestra B, Spelta V, Melchiorre C, Tonini M. Prejunctional muscarinic inhibitory control of acetylcholine release in the human isolated detrusor: involvement of the M4 receptor subtype. British Journal of Pharmacology 2000; 129: 493-500.

226 Inadome A, Yoshida M, Takahashi W, Yono M, Seshita H, Miyamoto Y, Kawano T, Ueda S. Prejunctional muscarinic receptors modulating acetylcholine release in rabbit detrusor smooth muscles Urology International 1998; 61: 135-141.

227 Somogyi GT, Zernova GV, Yoshiyama M, Yamamoto T, de Groat WC. Frequency dependence of muscarinic facilitation of transmitter release in urinary bladder strips from neurally intact or chronic spinal cord transected rats. British Journal of Pharmacology 1998; 125: 241-246.

228 Somogyi GT, de Groat WC. Function, signal transduction mechanisms and plasticity of presynaptic muscarinic receptors in the urinary bladder. Life Sciences 1999; 64: 411-418.

229 Waterman SA. Multiple subtypes of voltage-gated calcium channel mediate transmitter release from parasympathetic neurons in the mouse bladder. Journal of Neuroscience 1996; 16: 4155-4161.

230 Montgomery BSI, Fry CH. The action potential and net membrane currents in isolated human detrusor smooth muscle cells. Journal of Urology 1992; 147: 176-184.

231 Sui GP, Wu C, Fry CH. Inward Ca2+ currents in cultured and freshly isolated detrusor muscle cells - evidence of a T-type Ca2+ current. Journal of Urology 2001; 165: 627-631.

232 Rud T, Andersson K-E, Ulmsten U. Effects of nifedipine in women with unstable bladders. Urology International 1979; 34: 421-429.

233 Wu C, Fry CH. (1997). The role of the L-type Ca2+ channel in cholinergic pathways in guinea-pig detrusor smooth muscle. Journal of Physiology 1997; 499: 7-8P.

234 Wu C, Fry CH. Evidence for Na+/Ca2+ exchange and its role in intracellular Ca2+ regulation in guinea-pig detrusor smooth muscle cells. American Journal of Physiology 2001; 280: C1090-1096.

235 Markwardt F, Isenberg G. Gating of maxi K+ channels studied by Ca2+ concentration jumps in excised inside-out multi-channel patches. Journal of General Physiology 1992; 99: 841-862.

236 Wu C, Sui G, Fry CH. Characterisation of the spontaneous transient outward current in detrusor smooth muscle cells. Journal of Physiology 2000; 521: 52P

237 Stull JT, Krueger JK, Kamm KE et al. Myosin light chain kinase. In: Bárány (Ed). Biochemistry of smooth muscle contraction 1996. San Diego: Academic Press, pp 119-130.

238 Erdödi F, Ito M, Hartshorne DJ. Myosin light chain phosphatase. In: Bárány (Ed). Biochemistry of smooth muscle contraction 1996. San Diego: Academic Press, pp 131-142.

239 Wu C, Kentish JC, Fry CH. Effect of pH on myofilament Ca2+-sensitivity in alpha-toxin permeabilized guinea pig detrusor muscle. Journal of Urology 1995; 154: 1921-1924.

240 Wu C, Fry CH. The effects of extracellular and intracellular pH on intracellular Ca2+ regulation in guinea-pig detrusor smooth muscle. Journal of Physiology 1998; 508: 131-143.

241 Stull JT, Hsu LC, Tansey MG, Kamm KE. Myosin light chain kinase phosphorylation in tracheal smooth muscle. Journal of Biological Chemistry 1990; 265: 16683-16690.

242 Rembold CM. Modulation of the [Ca2+] sensitivity of myosin phosphorylation in intact swine arterial smooth muscle. Journal of Physiology 1990; 429: 77-94.

243 Denninger JW, Marletta MA. Guanylate cyclase and the NO/cGMP signalling pathway. Biochimica Biophysica Acta 1999; 1411: 334-350.

244 Hockey JS, Wu C, Fry CH. The actions of metabolic inhibition on human detrusor smooth muscle contractility from stable and unstable bladders. British Journal of Urology 2000. 86, 531-537.

245 Conti MA, Adelstein RS. The relationship between calmodulin binding and phosphorylation of smooth muscle myosin kinase by the catalytic subunit of 3':5' cAMP-dependent protein kinase. Journal of Biological Chemistry 1981; 256: 3178-3181.

246 Severs NJ. Cardiac muscle cell interaction: from microanatomy to the molecular make-up of the gap junction. Histology and Histopathology 1995; 10: 481-501.

247 Gabella G. Cells and cell junctions in the muscle coat of the bladder. Scandinavian Journal of Urology and Nephrology 1997; Suppl 184: 3-7

248 Elbadawi A, Yalla SV, Resnick NM. Structural basis of geriatric voiding dysfunction. III. Detrusor overactivity, Journal of Urology 1993; 150: 1668-1680.

249 Sui G-P, Fry CH, Dupont E, Severs NJ, Gillespie JI, Newgreen D. Intercellular electrical coupling and gap junction prevalence in detrusor from stable and unstable human bladders. Journal of Urology 2001. In the Press.

250 Wang X, Maake C, Hauri D, Hubert J. Evidence for electrical coupling of smooth muscle cells in the human trigone. Journal of Urology 2001. In the Press.

251 Seki N, Karim OM Mostwin JL. Changes in electrical properties of guinea pig smooth muscle membrane by experimental bladder outflow obstruction. American Journal of Physiology 1992; 262: F885-F891.

252 Fry CH, Cooklin M, Birns J, Mundy AR. Measurement of intercellular electrical coupling in guinea-pig detrusor smooth muscle. Journal of Urology 1999; 161: 660-664.

253 Bramich NJ, Brading AF. Electrical properties of smooth muscle in the guinea-pig urinary bladder. Journal of Physiology 1996; 492: 185-197.

254 Delmar M, Michaels DC, Johnson T, Jalife J. Effects of increasing intercellular resistance on transverse and longitudinal propagation in sheep epicardial muscle. Circulation Research 1987; 60: 780-785.

255 de Groat, W.C., Araki, I, Vizzard, M.A., Yoshiyama, M., Yoshimura, N., Sugaya, K., Tai, C., and Roppolo, J.R.: Developmental and injury induced plasticity in the micturition reflex pathway, Behav. Brain Res., 92: 127,1998.

256 de Groat, W.C., Nadelhaft, I., Milne, R.J., Booth, A.M., Morgan, C. and Thor, K.: Organization of the sacral parasympathetic reflex pathways to the urinary bladder and large intestine. J. Autonom. Nerv. Sys., 3:135, 1981.

257 Araki, I. and de Groat, W.C.: Synaptic modulation associated with developmental reorganization of visceral reflex pathways. J. Neurosci., 17: 8402, 1997.

258 Birder, L. A.; de Groat, W.C.: Induction of c-fos expression in spinal neurons by nociceptive and nonnociceptive stimulation of LUT. Am. J. Physiol., 265: R643, 1993.

259 Nadelhaft, I.; Vera, P. L.: Neurons in the rat brain and spinal cord labeled after pseudorabies virus injected into the external urethral sphincter. J. Comp. Neurol., 375: 502, 1996.

260 Vizzard, M. A., Erickson, V. L., Card, J. P., Roppolo, J. R., and de Groat, W. C.: Transneuronal labeling of neurons in the adult rat brainstem and spinal cord after injection of pseudorabies virus into the urethra. J. Comp. Neurol., 355: 629, 1995.

261 Imaizumi, M., Miura, A., Kawatani, M., and de Groat, W.C.: Excitatory postsynaptic currents elicited in lumbosacral preganglionic neurons by dorsal commissure stimulation in neonatal rat spinal cord slices. Society for Neuroscience Abstracts, 24: 1619, 19

262 de Groat, W.C.: Excitation and inhibition of sacral parasympathetic neurons by visceral and cutaneous stimuli in the cat. Brain Res., 33: 499, 1971.

263 de Groat, W.C.: Inhibitory mechanisms in the sacral reflex pathways to the urinary bladder. In: Iontophoresis and Transmitter Mechanisms in the Mammalian Central Nervous System, Eds: Ryall, R.W. and Kelly, J.S.,. Elsevier Publishers, Holland, pp. 366-36

264 Morrison, J.F.B., Sato, A., Sato, Y., and Yamanishi, T.: The influence of afferent inputs from skin and viscera on the activity of the bladder and the skeletal muscle surrounding the urethra in the rat. Neurosci. Res., 23: 195, 1995.

265 Araki, I. and de Groat, W.C.: Unitary excitatory synaptic currents in preganglionic neurons mediated by two distinct groups of interneurons in neonatal rat sacral parasympathetic nucleus. J. Neurophysiol., 76: 215, 1996.

266 de Groat W. C. and Ryall, R. W. (1969). Reflexes to the sacral parasympathetic neurones concerned with micturition in the cat. J. Physiol. 200:87-108.

267 McMahon, S. B. and Morrison, J. F. B. : Two groups of spinal interneurones that respond to stimulation of the abdominal viscera of the cat. J. Physiol., 332: 21, 1982.

268 Bosch, J.L. and Groen, J.: Sacral (S3) segmental nerve stimulation as a treatment for urge incontinence in patients with detrusor instability: results of chronic electrical stimulation using an implantable neural prosthesis. J. Urol., 154: 504, 1995.

269 Ohlsson, B.L., Fall, M. and Frankenberg-Somma, R. S.: Effects of external and direct pudendal nerve maximal electrical stimulation in the treatment of the uninhibited overactive bladder. Brit. J. Urol., 64: 374, 1989.

270 Wheeler, J.S., Walter, J.S. and Zaszczurynski, P.J.: Bladder inhibition by penile nerve simulation in spinal cord injury patients. J. Urol., 147: 100, 1992.

271 Shaker H. Wang Y. Loung D. Balbaa L. Fehlings MG. Hassouna MM. Role of C-afferent fibres in the mechanism of action of sacral nerve root neuromodulation in chronic spinal cord injury. BJU International. 85(7):905-10, 2000.

272 Holstege, G., Griffiths, D., DeWall, H., and Dalm, E.: Anatomical and physiological observations on supraspinal control of bladder and urethral sphincter muscles in cats. J. Comp. Neurol., 250: 449, 1986.

273 Holstege, G.: Some anatomical observations on the projections from the hypothalamus to brainstem and spinal cord: an HRP and autoradiographic tracing study in the cat. J. Comp. Neurol., 260: 98, 1987.

274 Kojima, M., Takeuchi, Y., Goto, M., and Sano, Y.: Immunohistochemical study on the localization of serotonin fibers and terminals in the spinal cord of the monkey (Macaca fuscata). Cell Tissue Res., 229: 23, 1983.

275 Araki, I. and de Groat, W.C.: Synaptic modulation associated with developmental reorganization of visceral reflex pathways. J. Neurosci., 17: 8402, 1997.

276 Araki, I.: Inhibitory postsynaptic currents and the effects of GABA on visually identified sacral parasympathetic preganglionic neurons in neonatal rats. J. Neurophysiol., 72: 2903, 1994.

277 Birder, L. A.; de Groat, W.C.: Induction of c-fos expression in spinal neurons by nociceptive and nonnociceptive stimulation of LUT. Am. J. Physiol., 265: R643, 1993.

278 Shefchyk, S.J., Espey, M.J., Carr, P., Nance, D., Sawchuk, M., and Buss R.: Evidence for a strychnine-sensitive mechanism and glycine receptors involved in the control of urethral sphincter activity during micturition in the cat. Exp. Brain Res., 119: 297, 1998.

279 Igawa, Y., Mattiasson A. and Andersson K. E.: Effects of GABA-receptor stimulation and blockade on micturition in normal rats and rats with bladder outflow obstruction. J. Urol., 150: 537, 1993.

280 Yoshiyama, M., Roppolo J. R. and de Groat W. C.: Effects of LY215490, a competitive alpha-amino-3-hydroxy-5-methylisoxazole-4-propionic acid (AMPA) receptor antagonist, on the micturition reflex in the rat. J. Pharmacol. Exp. Ther., 280: 894, 1997.

281 Matsumoto, G., Hisamitsu T. and de Groat W. C.: Role of glutamate and NMDA receptors in the descending limb of the spinobulbospinal micturition reflex pathway of the rat. Neurosci. Lett., 183: 58, 1995.

282 Matsumoto, G., Hisamitsu T. and de Groat W. C.: Non-NMDA glutamatergic excitatory transmission in the descending limb of the spinobulbospinal micturition reflex pathway of the rat. Brain Res., 693: 246, 1995.

283 Araki, I. and de Groat, W.C.: Unitary excitatory synaptic currents in preganglionic neurons mediated by two distinct groups of interneurons in neonatal rat sacral parasympathetic nucleus. J. Neurophysiol., 76: 215, 1996.

284 Iwabuchi, N.: Sacral glutamatergic transmission in the descending limb of the micturition reflex in the cat. Fukuoka Igaku Zasshi, 88: 30, 1997.

285 Yoshimura, N., Sasa M., Yoshida O. and Takaori S.: Mediation of micturition reflex by central norepinephrine from the locus coeruleus in the cat. J. Urol., 143: 840, 1990.

286 Yoshimura, N., Sasa M., Yoshida O. and Takaori S.: Alpha1-adrenergic receptor-mediated excitation from the locus coeruleus of the sacral parasympathetic preganglionic neuron. Life Sciences, 47: 789, 1990.

287 Espey, M. J., Downie J. W. and Fine A.: Effect of 5-HT receptor and adrenoceptor antagonists on micturition in conscious cats. Eur. J. Pharmacol., 221: 167, 1992.

288 Durant, P. A., Lucas P. C. and Yaksh T. L.: Micturition in the unanesthetized rat: spinal versus peripheral pharmacology of the adrenergic system. J. Pharmacol. Exp. Ther., 245: 426, 1988.

289 Ishizuka, O., Persson K., Mattiasson A., Naylor A., Wyllie M. and Andersson K.: Micturition in conscious rats with and without bladder outlet obstruction: role of spinal alpha 1-adrenoceptors. Br. J. Pharmacol., 117: 962, 1996.

290 Ishizuka, O., Pandita R. K., Mattiasson A., Steers W. D. and Andersson K. E.: Stimulation of bladder activity by volume, L-dopa and capsaicin in normal conscious rats--effects of spinal alpha 1-adrenoceptor blockade. Naunyn-Schmied. Arch. Pharmacol., 355: 787, 1997.

291 Ishizuka, O., Mattiasson A. and Andersson K.-E.: Role of spinal and peripheral alpha2 adrenoceptors in micturition in normal conscious rats. J. Urol., 156: 1853, 1996.

292 Kontani, H., Maruyama I. and Sakai T.: Involvement of alpha 2-adrenoceptors in the sacral micturition reflex in rats. Jpn. J. Pharmacol,, 60: 363, 1992.

293 Dray, A. and Metsch R.: Inhibition of urinary bladder contractions by a spinal action of morphine and other opioids. J. Pharmacol. Exp. Ther., 231: 254, 1984.

294 Okada, M. and Hisamitsu T.: Effects of opiate and opioid peptides administered intrathecally on the pain threshold and micturition reflex in rats. Masui, 35: 877, 1986.

295 Dray, A. and Nunan L.: Mu and delta opioid ligands inhibit reflex contractions of the urinary bladder in the rat by different central mechanisms. Neuropharmacol., 26: 753, 1987.

296 McMahon, S.B. and Morrison, J.F.B. (1982a). Spinal neurones with long projections activated from the abdominal viscera. J. Physiol. 322, 1-20.

297 Birder, L.A., Roppolo, J.R., Iadarola, M. J. and de Groat, W.C.: C-fos as a marker for subsets of visceral second order neurons in the rat lumbosacral spinal. Society for Neuroscience Abstracts, 15: 468, 1990

298 VanderHorst, V.G., Mouton, L.J., Blok, B.F., and & Holstege, G.: Distinct cell groups in the lumbosacral cord of the cat project to different areas in the periaqueductal gray. J. Comp. Neurol., 376: 361, 1996.

299 Birder, L. A. and de Groat, W.C.: Increased c-fos expression in spinal neurons after irritation of the lower urinary tract in the rat. J. Neurosci., 12: 4878, 1992.

300 O'Donnell, P. D.: Central actions of bethanechol on the urinary bladder in dogs. J. Urol., 143: 634, 1990.

301 Sillen, U., Rubenson A. and Hjalmas K.: Central cholinergic mechanisms in L-DOPA induced hyperactive urinary bladder of the rat. Urol. Res., 10: 239, 1982..

302 Sasa, M., and Yoshimura, N.: Locus coeruleus noradrenergic neurons as a micturition center. Microscopic Res. Tech., 29: 226, 1994.

303 Sugaya, K., Matsuyama K., Takakusaki K. and Mori S.: Electrical and chemical stimulations of the pontine micturition center. Neurosci. Lett., 80: 197, 1987.

304 Kakizaki, H., Yoshiyama, M., Roppolo, J.R., Booth, A.M., and de Groat, W.C.: Role of spinal glutamatergic transmission in the ascending limb of the micturition reflex pathway in the rat. J.Pharmacol. Exp. Ther., 285: 22, 1998.

305 Durant, P. A. C. and Yaksh T. L.: Micturition in the unanesthetized rat: effects of intrathecal capsaicin, N-vanillylnonanamide, 6-hydroxydopamine and 5,6-dihydroxytryptamine. Brain Res., 451: 301, 1988.

306 Cheng, C-L., Ma, C.-P. and de Groat, W.C.: Effect of capsaicin on micturition and associated reflexes in chronic spinal rats. Brain Res., 678: 40, 1995.

307 Lecci, A., Giuliani S., Garrett C. and Maggi C. A.: Evidence for a role of tachykinins as sensory transmitters in the activation of micturition reflex. Neurosci., 54: 827, 1993.

308 Santicioli, P., Maggi C. A. and Meli A.: The effect of capsaicin pretreatment on the cystometrograms of urethane anesthetized rats. J. Urol., 133: 700, 1985.

309 Lecci, A., Giuliani S., Garrett C. and Maggi C. A.: Evidence for a role of tachykinins as sensory transmitters in the activation of micturition reflex. Neurosci., 54: 827, 1993.

310 Igawa, Y., Westerling D., Mattiasson A. and Andersson K. E.: Effects of morphine metabolites on micturition in normal, unanaesthetized rats. Br. J. Pharmacol., 110: 257, 1993.

311 Booth, A. M., Hisamitsu T., Kawatani M. and De Groat W. C.: Regulation of urinary bladder capacity by endogenous opioid peptides. J. Urol., 133: 339, 1985.

312 Thor, K. B. and Katofiasc M. A.: Effects of duloxetine, a combined serotonin and norepinephrine reuptake inhibitor, on central neural control of lower urinary tract function in the chloralose-anesthetized female cat. J. Pharmacol. Exp. Ther., 274: 1014, 1

313 Espey, M. J. and Downie J. W.: Serotonergic modulation of cat bladder function before and after spinal transection. Eur. J. Pharmacol., 287: 173, 1995.

314 Yoshiyama M and De Groat WC (2001) Role of spinal alpha1-adrenoceptor subtypes in the bladder reflex in anesthetized rats. Am J Physiol Regul Integr Comp Physiol 280:R1414-9.

315 Sosnowski, M., Stevens C. W. and Yaksh T. L.: Assessment of the role of A1/A2 adenosine receptors mediating the purine antinociception, motor and autonomic function in the rat spinal cord. J. Pharmacol. Exp. Ther., 250: 915, 1989.

316 Sutherland, R. S., Kogan, B. A., Piechota, H. J., & Bredt, D. S. (1997). Vesicourethral function in mice with genetic disruption of neuronal nitric oxide synthase. J.Urol. 157, 1109-1116.

317 Rice, A.S.C. Topical spinal administration of a nitric oxide synthase inhibitor prevents the hyper-reflexia associated with a rat model of persistent visceral pain. Neurosci. Lett., 187: 111, 1995.

318 Kakizaki, H. and de Groat, W.C. Role of spinal nitric oxide in the facilitation of the micturition reflex by bladder irritation. J. Urol., 155: 355, 1996.

319 Pandita R.K., Persson, K. and Andersson, K.-E. Capsaicin-induced bladder overactivity and nociceptive behaviour in conscious rats: Involvement of spinal nitric oxide. J. Autonom. Nerv. Syst., 67: 184, 1997.

320 Zhou Y. Ling EA. Upregulation of nicotinamide adenine dinucleotide phosphate-diaphorase reactivity in the ventral horn motoneurons of lumbosacral spinal cord after urethral obstruction in the guinea pig. Neuroscience Research. 27(2):169-74, 1997

321 Morrison, J.F.B., Sato, A., Sato, Y. and Suzuki, A. The nitric oxide synthase inhibitor L-NAME reduces inhibitory components of somato-vesical parasympathetic reflexes in the rat. Neurosci. Res., 24: 195, 1996.

322 Blok, B., Willemsen, A., and Holstge, G.: A PET study on brain control of micturition in humans. Brain, 120: 111, 1997.

323 Blok. B.F.M., Sturms, L.M., and Holstege, G.: A PET study on cortical and subcortical control of pelvic floor musculature in women. J. Comp. Neurol. 389: 535-544, 1997.

324 Barrington, F.: The relation of the hindbrain to micturition. Brain, 44: 23, 1921.

325 Loewy, A. D., Saper, C. B., and Baker, R. P.: Descending projections from the pontine micturition center. Brain Res., 172: 533, 1979.

326 Blok, B.F.M. and Holstege, G.: Neuronal control of micturition and its relation to the emotional motor system. Prog. Brain Res., 107: 113, 1996.

327 Luppi, P. H., Aston, J. G., Akaoka, H., Chouvet, G., and Jouvet, M.: Afferent projections to the rat locus coeruleus demonstrated by retrograde and anterograde tracing with cholera-toxin B subunit and Phaseolus vulgaris leucoagglutinin. Neuroscience, 65:

328 Ding, Y. Q., Takada, M., Tokuno, H.; Mizuno, N.: Direct projections from the dorsolateral pontine tegmentum to pudendal motoneurons innervating the external urethral sphincter muscle in the rat. J. Comp. Neurol., 357: 318, 1995.

329 Valentino, R. J., Chen, S., Zhu, Y.; Aston, J. G.: Evidence for divergent projections to the brain noradrenergic system and the spinal parasympathetic system from Barrington's nucleus. Brain Res., 732: 1, 1996.

330 Otake, K.; Nakamura, Y.: Single neurons in Barrington's nucleus projecting to both the paraventricular thalamic nucleus and the spinal cord by way of axon collaterals: a double labeling study in the rat. Neurosci. Lett., 209: 97, 1996.

331 Valentino, R. J., Pavcovich, L. A.; Hirata, H.: Evidence for corticotropin-releasing hormone projections from Barrington's nucleus to the periaqueductal gray and dorsal motor nucleus of the vagus in the rat. J. Comp. Neurol., 363: 402, 1995.

332 Ding, Y.Q., Zheng, H.X., Gong, L.W., Lu, Y., Zhao, H., and Qin, B.Z.: Direct projections from the lumbosacral spinal cord to Barrington's nucleus in the rat: a special reference to micturition reflex. J. Comp. Neurol., 389: 149, 1997.

333 Blok, B. F., De, W. H., and Holstege, G.: Ultrastructural evidence for a paucity of projections from the lumbosacral cord to the pontine micturition center or M-region in the cat: a new concept for the organization of the micturition reflex with the peria

334 Blok, B. F.; Holstege, G.: Direct projections from the periaqueductal gray to the pontine micturition center (M-region). An anterograde and retrograde tracing study in the cat. Neurosci. Lett., 166: 93, 1994.

335 Cameron, A. A., Khan, I. A., Westlund, K. N. and Willis, W. D.: The efferent projections of the periaqueductal gray in the rat: a Phaseolus vulgaris-leucoagglutinin study. II. Descending projections. J. Comp. Neurol., 351: 585, 1995.

336 Ennis, M., Behbehani, M., Shipley, M. T., Van, B. E., and Aston, J. G.: Projections from the periaqueductal gray to the rostromedial pericoerulear region and nucleus locus coeruleus: anatomic and physiologic studies. J. Comp. Neurol., 306: 480, 1991.

337 Pavcovich LA. Valentino RJ. Central regulation of micturition in the rat the corticotropin-releasing hormone from Barrington's nucleus. Neuroscience Letters. 196:185-8, 1995

338 Blok, B. F. and Holstege, G.: Ultrastructural evidence for a direct pathway from the pontine micturition center to the parasympathetic preganglionic motoneurons of the bladder of the cat. Neurosci. Lett., 222: 195, 1997.

339 Blok, B. F., DeWeerd, H., and Holstege, G.: The pontine micturition center projects to sacral cord GABA immunoreactive neurons in the cat. Neurosci. Lett., 233: 109, 1997.

340 Steers, W.D., Ciambotti, J., Etzel, B., Erdman, S. and de Groat, W.C. Alterations in afferent pathways from the urinary bladder of the rat in response to partial urethral obstruction. J. Comp. Neurol., 310:1, 1991.

341 Blok, B.F.M., Willemsen, A.T.M., and Holstege, G.: A PET study on brain control of micturition in humans. Brain 120: 111-121, 1997.

342 Blok, B.F.M., Sturms, L.M., and Holstege, G.: Brain activation during micturition in women. Brain 121: 2033-2042, 1998.

343 Ramirez, L. V., Ulfhake, B., Arvidsson, U., Verhofstad, A. A., Visser, T. J.; Hokfelt, T.: Serotoninergic, peptidergic and GABAergic innervation of the ventrolateral and dorsolateral motor nuclei in the cat S1/S2 segments: an immunofluorescence study. J.

344 Rajaofetra, N., Passagia, J. G., Marlier, L., Poulat, P., Pellas, F., Sandillon, F., Verschuere, B., Gouy, D., Geffard, M.; Privat, A.: Serotoninergic, noradrenergic, and peptidergic innervation of Onuf's nucleus of normal and transected spinal cords of b

345 Willis, W.and Westlund, K.: Neuroanatomy of the pain system and of the pathways that modulate pain. J. Clinical Neurophysiol., 14: 2, 1997.

346 Holstege, G.; Tan, J.: Supraspinal control of motoneurons innervating the striated muscles of the pelvic floor including urethral and anal sphincters in the cat. Brain, 110: 1323, 1987.

347 Chen, S.Y., Wang, S.D., Cheng, C.L., Kuo, J.S., de Groat, W.C. and Chai, C.Y.: Glutamate activation of neurons in cardiovascular reactive areas of the cat brain stem affects urinary bladder motility. Am. J. Physiol., 265: F520, 1993.

348 Espey, M.J., Du H.-J., and Downie, J.W.: Serotonergic midulation of spinal ascending activity and sacral reflex activity evoked by pelvic nerve stimulation in cats. Brain Res., 798: 101, 1998.

349 Mizukawa, K.: The segmental detailed topographical distribution of monoaminergic terminals and their pathways in the spinal cord of the cat. Anat Anz, 147: 125, 1980.

350 Young, W.; Kuhar, M.: Noradrenergic a1 and a2 receptors: light microscopic and autoradiographic localization. Proc. Nat. Acad. Sci., 77: 1696, 1980.

351 Giuliano F. Rampin O. Alpha receptors in the central nervous system and its effects on erection. Journal of Andrology. 20(6):683-7, 1999;

352 Giroux N. Rossignol S. Reader TA. Autoradiographic study of alpha1- and alpha2-noradrenergic and serotonin1A receptors in the spinal cord of normal and chronically transected cats. Journal of Comparative Neurology. 406(3):402-14, 1999;

353 Wilson KH. Schambra UB. Smith MS. Page SO. Richardson CD. Fremeau RT. Schwinn DA. In situ hybridization: identification of rare mRNAs in human tissues. Brain Research. Brain Research Protocols. 1(2):175-85, 1997

354 Yokoyama, O., Yoshiyama, M., Namiki, M., and de Groat, W.C.: Influence of anesthesia on bladder hyperactivity induced by middle cerebral artery occlusion in the rat. Am. J. Physiol., 273: R1900, 1997.

355 O'Donnell, P. D.: Central actions of bethanechol on the urinary bladder in dogs. J. Urol., 143: 634, 1990.

356 Sillen, U., Rubenson A. and Hjalmas K.: Central cholinergic mechanisms in L-DOPA induced hyperactive urinary bladder of the rat. Urol. Res., 10: 239, 1982.

357 Marson, L.: Identification of central nervous system neurons that innervate the bladder body, bladder base, or external urethral sphincter of female rats: A transneuronal tracing study using pseudorabies virus. J. Comp. Neurol., 389: 584, 1997.

358 Yokoyama, O., Yoshiyama, M., Namiki, M., and de Groat, W.C.: Influence of anesthesia on bladder hyperactivity induced by middle cerebral artery occlusion in the rat. Am. J. Physiol., 273: R1900, 1997.

359 Hisamitsu, T. and de Groat W. C.: The inhibitory effect of opioid peptides and morphine applied intrathecally and intracerebroventricularly on the micturition reflex in the cat. Brain Res., 298: 51, 1984.

360 Willette, R. N., Morrison S., Sapru H. N. and Reis D. J.: Stimulation of opiate receptors in the dorsal pontine tegmentum inhibits reflex contraction of the urinary bladder. J. Pharmacol. Exp. Ther., 244: 403, 1988.

361 Dray, A. and Metsch R.: Opioid receptor subtypes involved in the central inhibition of urinary bladder motility. Eur. J. Pharmacol., 104: 47, 1984.

362 Rocha I. Burnstock G. Spyer KM. Effect on urinary bladder function and arterial blood pressure of the activation of putative purine receptors in brainstem areas. Autonomic Neuroscience-Basic & Clinical. 88(1-2):6-15, 2001

363 Pandita RK. Nylen A. Andersson KE. Oxytocin-induced stimulation and inhibition of bladder activity in normal, conscious rats--influence of nitric oxide synthase inhibition. Neuroscience. 85(4):1113-9, 1998

364 Holstege, J. C., Van Dijken, H., Bulis, R. M., Goedknegt, H., Gosens, T.; Bongers, C.: Distribution of dopamine immunoreac-

tivity in the rat, cat, and monkey spinal cord. J. Comp. Neurol., 376: 631, 1996.

365 Yokoyama, O., Yoshiyama, M., Namiki, M., and de Groat, W.C.: Influence of anesthesia on bladder hyperactivity induced by middle cerebral artery occlusion in the rat. Am. J. Physiol., 273: R1900, 1997.

366 Gjone, R.: Excitatory and inhibitory bladder responses to stimulation of 'limbic', diencephalic and mesencephalic structures in the cat. Acta Physiol. Scand. 66: 91-102, 1966.

367 Ding, Y.Q., Wang, D., Xu, J.Q., and Ju, G.: Direct projections from the medial preoptic area to spinally-projecting neurons in Barrington's nucleus: an electron microscope study in the rat. Neurosci. Lett. 271: 175-8, 1999.

368 Athwal, B.S., Berkley, K.J., Hussain, I., Brennan, A., Craggs, M., Sakakibara, R., Frackowiak, R.S., and Fowler, C.J.: Brain responses to changes in bladder volume and urge to void in healthy men. Brain 124: 369-377, 2001.

369 Andrew, J., and Nathan, P.W.: Lesions of the anterior frontal lobes and disturbances of micturition and defaecation. Brain 87: 233-262, 1964.

370 Kuroiwa, Y., Tohgi, H., Ono, S., and Itoh, M.: Frequency and urgency of micturition in hemiplegic patients: relationship to hemisphere laterality of lesions. J. Neurol., 234:100,1987.

371 Milsom I. Abrams P. Cardozo L. Roberts RG. Thuroff J. Wein AJ. How widespread are the symptoms of an overactive bladder and how are they managed? A population-based prevalence study. BJU International. 87(9):760-6, 2001

372 Sibley GNA. The response of the bladder to lower urinary tract obstruction, . DM thesis 1984, Oxford.

373 German K, Bedwani J, Davies J et al. What is the pathophysiology of detrusor hyperreflexia? Neurourology and Urodynamics 1993; 12: 335-336.

374 Kinder RB, Mundy AR. Atropine blockade of nerve-mediated stimulation of the human detrusor, British Journal of Urology 1985; 57: 418-421.

375 Turner WH, Brading AF. Smooth muscle of the bladder in the normal and the diseased state: pathophysiology, diagnosis and treatment, Pharmacology and Therapeutics 1997; 75: 77-110.

376 Mills IW, Greenland JG, McCoy R et al. Spontaneous myogenic contractile activity of isolated human detrusor smooth muscle in idiopathic instability, Journal of Urology 1999; 161 AUA Supplement: 253.

377 Mills IW. The Pathophysiology of Detrusor Instability and the Role of Bladder Ischaemia in its Aetiology, DM thesis 1999. University of Oxford.

378 Brading AF. Alterations in the physiological properties of urinary bladder smooth muscle caused by bladder emptying against an obstruction, Scandinavian Journal of Urology and Nephrology 1997; Suppl 184: 51-58.

379 Sibley GNA. Developments in our understanding of detrusor instability, British Journal of Urology 1997; 80,: 54-61.

380 Brading AF, Turner WH. The unstable bladder: towards a common mechanism, British Journal of Urology 1994; 73: 3-8.

381 Sibley GNA. An experimental model of detrusor instability in the obstructed pig, British Journal of Urology 1985; 57: 292-298.

382 Speakman MJ, Brading AF, Gilpin CJ et al. Bladder outflow obstruction—a cause of denervation supersensitivity, Journal of Urology 1987; 138: 1461-1466.

383 Harrison SC, Ferguson DR, Doyle PT. Effect of bladder outflow obstruction on the innervation of the rabbit urinary bladder, British Journal of Urology 1990; 66: 372-379.

384 German K, Bedwani J, Davies J et al. Physiological and morphometric studies into the pathophysiology of detrusor hyperreflexia in neuropathic patients, Journal of Urology 1995; 153: 1678-1683.

385 Brading AF, Speakman MJ, Pathophysiology of bladder outflow obstruction. In: H. Whitfield, Kirby R., Hendry WF, Duckett J (Eds) Textbook of Genitourinary Surgery Oxford: Blackwell Science, 1998; 465-479.

386 Westfall DP, Supersensitivity of smooth muscle. In: Bülbring E, Brading AF, Jones AW, Tomita T (Eds) Smooth muscle: an assessment of current knowledge. London: Arnold, 1981; 285-209.

387 Charlton RG, Morley AR, Chambers P et al. Focal changes in nerve, muscle and connective tissue in normal and unstable human bladder, British Journal of Urology 1999; 84: 953-960.

388 Speakman MJ. Studies on the physiology of the normal and obstructed bladder, . MS thesis, 1988, London.

389 Williams JH, Turner WH, Sainsbury GM et al. Experimental model of bladder outflow tract obstruction in the guinea-pig, British Journal of Urology 1993; 71: 543-554.

390 Gabella G, Uvelius B. Urinary bladder of rat: fine structure of normal and hypertrophic musculature, Cell and Tissue Research 1990; 262: 67-79.

391 Steers WD, Mackway Gerardi AM, Ciambotti J et al. Alterations in afferent pathways from the urinary bladder of the rat in response to partial urethral obstruction, Journal of Comparative Neurology 1991; 310: 401-410.

392 Steers WD, Ciambotti J, Erdman S et al. Morphological plasticity in efferent pathways to the urinary blad der of the rat following urethral obstruction, Journal of Neuroscience 1990; 10: 1943-1951.

393 Gabella G, Berggren T, Uvelius B. Hypertrophy and reversal of hypertrophy in rat pelvic ganglion neurons, Journal of Neurocytology 1992; 21: 649-662.

394 Kruse MN, Belton AL, de Groat WC. Changes in bladder and external sphincter function after spinal injury in the rat, American Journal of Physiology 1993; 264: 1157-1163.

395 de Groat WC. A neurological basis for the overactive bladder, Urology 1997; 50: 36-52.

396 Geirrson G, Lindstrom S, Fall M. The bladder cooling reflex in man - characteristics and sensitivity to temperature, British Journal of Urology 1993; 71: 675-680.

397 Geirsson G, Fall M, Lindstrom S. The ice-water test - a simple and valuable supplement to hyperreflexia: a dual center study with long-term follow-up, Journal of Urology 1997; 158.

398 Dasgupta P, Chandiramani VA, Beckett A et al. The effect of intravesical capsaicin on the suburothelial innervation in patients with detrusor hyper-reflexia. British Journal of Urology International 2000; 85: 238-45

399 Greenland JE, Brading AF. Urinary bladder blood flow changes during the micturition cycle in a conscious pig model, Journal of Urology 1996; 156: 1858-1861.

400 Levin RM, Haugaard N, Hypoilte JA et al. Metabolic factors influencing lower urinary tract function, Experimental Physiology 1999; 84: 171-194.

401 Steers WD, Creedon DJ, Tuttle JB. Immunity to nerve growth factor prevents plasticity following urinary bladder hypertrophy, Journal of Urology 1996; 155: 379-385.

402 Levin RM, Haugaard N, Levin, SS et al., Bladder function in experimental outlet obstruction: pharmacologic responses to alterations in innervation, energetics, calcium mobilization, and genetics. In: Zderic S (Ed) Muscle, Matrix, and Bladder Function. Editor. New York: Plenum Press, 1995; 7-19.

403 Morrison JFB, Sensations arising from the lower urinary tract. In: Torrens M and Morrison JFB (Eds) The physiology of the lower urinary tract, Berlin: Springer-Verlag, 1987; 89-131.

404 Namasivayam S, Eardley I, Morrison JFB. (1998) A novel in vitro bladder- pelvic nerve afferent model in the rat British Journal of Urology 82:902-905

405 Coolsaet BL, Van Duyl WA, Van Os-Bossagh P et al. New concepts in relation to urge and detrusor activity, Neurourology and Urodynamics 1993; 12: 463-471.

406 Wellner MC, Isenberg G Stretch effects on whole-cell currents of guinea-pig urinary bladder myocytes, Journal of Physiology 1994; 480: 439-448.

407 Levin, R. M., Longhurst, P. A., Monson, F. C., Haugaard, N. and Wein, A. J. (1993). Experimental studies on bladder outlet obstruction. In Prostate Diseases, edn, ed. Lepor, H. & Lawson, R. K., pp. 119-130. W.B. Saunders Co., Philadelphia.

408 Levin, R. M., Longhurst, P. A., Monson, F. C., Kato, K. and Wein, A. J. (1990a). Effect of bladder outlet obstruction on the morphology, physiology, and pharmacology of the bladder. Prostate S3, 9-26.

409 Kato, K., Lin, A. T.-L., Haugaard, N., Longhurst, P. A., Wein, A. J. and Levin, R. M. (1990a). Effects of outlet obstruction on glucose metabolism of the rabbit urinary bladder. Journal of Urology 143, 844-847.

410 Bilgen, A., Wein, A. J., Haugaard, N., Packard, D. & Levin, R. M. (1992a). Effect of outlet obstruction on pyruvate metabolism of the rabbit urinary bladder. Molecular and Cellular Biochemistry 117, 159-163.

411 Haugaard, N., Potter, L., Wein, A. J. & Levin, R. M. (1992). Effect of partial obstruction of the rabbit urinary bladder on malate dehydrogenase and citrate synthase activity. Journal of Urology 147, 1391.

412 Hsu, T. H. S., Levin, R. M., Wein, A. J. & Haugaard, N. (1994). Alterations of mitochondrial oxidative metabolism in rabbit urinary bladder after partial outlet obstruction. Molecular and Cellular Biochemistry 141, 21-26.

413 Hypolite, J. A., Longhurst, P. A., Haugaard, N. & Levin, R. M. (1997). Effect of partial outlet obstruction on C-14-adenine incorporation in the rabbit urinary bladder. Neurourology and Urodynamics 16, 201-208.

414 Haugaard, N., McKenna, B. A. W., Wein, A. J. & Levin, R. M. (1993). Effect of partial urinary outlet obstruction in the rabbit on the incorporation of adenine into adenine nucleotides in bladder smooth muscle. Neurourology and Urodynamics 12, 473-479.

415 Levin, R. M., Haugaard, N., Levin, S. S. and Wein, A. J. (1991a). Creatine kinase activity in normal and hypertrophied rabbit urinary bladder tissue (following partial outlet obstruction). Molecular and Cellular Biochemistry 106, 143-149.

416 Samuel, M., Kim, Y., Horiuchi, K. Y., Levin, R. M. and Chacko, S. (1992). Smooth muscle myosin isoform distribution and myosin ATPase in hypertrophied urinary bladder. Biochemistry International 26, 645-652.

417 Zhao, Y., Levin, R. M., Levin, S. S., Nevel, C. A., Haugaard, N., Hsu, T. H. S. and Hudson, A. P. (1994). Partial outlet obstruction of the rabbit bladder results in changes in the mitochondrial genetic system. Molecular and Cellular Biochemistry 141, 47-55.

418 Damaser, M. S., Haugaard, N. & Uvelius, B. (1997). Partial obstruction of the rat urinary bladder: Effects on mitochondria and mitochondrial glucose metabolism in detrusor smooth muscle cells. Neurourology and Urodynamics 16, 601-607.

419 Gabella, G. and Uvelius, B. (1990). Urinary bladder of rat: fine structure of normal and hypertrophic musculature. Cell and Tissue Research 262, 67-79.

420 Steers, W. D. and de Groat, W. C. (1988). Effect of bladder outlet obstruction on micturition reflex pathways in the rat. Journal of Urology 140, 864-871.

421 Karim, O., Van Koeveringe, G. & Mostwin, J. (1990). Development of abnormal voiding patterns following partial obstruction of the guinea pig urethra. Journal of Urology 143, 335A.

422 Brading, A. F. (1997b). Alterations in the physiological properties of urinary bladder smooth muscle caused by bladder emptying against an obstruction. Scandinavian Journal of Urology and Nephrology Suppl 184, 51-58.

423 Greenland, J.E., and Brading, A.F. (2001). The effect of bladder outflow obstruction on detrusor blood flow changes during the voiding cycle in conscious pigs. J Urol 165, 245_248.

424 Greenland, J.E., Hvistendahl, J.J., Andersen, H., Jorgensen, T.M., Mc Murray, G., Cortina_Borja, M., Brading, A.F., Frokiaer, J. (2000) The effect of bladder outlet obstruction on tissue oxygen tension and blood flow in the pig bladder. BJU Int, 85,1109_1114.

425 Levin, R. M., Monson, F. C., Haugaard, N., Buttyan, R., Hudson, A., Roelofs, M., Sartore, S. and Wein, A. J. (1995). Genetic and cellular characteristics of bladder outlet obstruction. Urologic Clinics of North America 22, 263-283.

426 Roelofs, M., Wein, A. J., Monson, F. C., Passerini-Glazel, G., Koteliansky, V. E., Sartore, S. and Levin, R. M. (1995). Contractility and phenotype transitions in serosal thickening of obstructed rabbit bladder. Journal of Applied Physiology 78, 1432-1441.

427 Schröder, A. Chichester, P., Kogan, B.A., Longhurst, P.A., Lieb, J., and Levin, R.M. Effect of Chronic Bladder Outlet Obstruction on the Blood Flow of the Rabbit Urinary Bladder (2001) J. Urol. 165, 640-646.

428 Lin, A. T., Chen, M. T., Yang, C. H. and Chang, L. S. (1995). Blood flow of the urinary bladder: effects of outlet obstruction and correlation with bioenergetic metabolism. Neurourology and Urodynamics 14, 285-292.

429 Tsunoo, A. and Narahashi, T. (1987). Cyclic nucleotide potentiation of muscarinic responses in neuroblastoma cells. Brain Research 407, 55-67.

430 Zhao, Y., Levin, S.S., Wein, A.J., and Levin, R.M. (1997) Correlation of ischemia / reperfusion and partial outlet obstruction induced spectrin proteolysis by calpain with contractile dysfunction in the rabbit bladder. Urology 49, 293-300.

431 Hass, M.A., Leonova, E., and Levin, R.M. (1999). Fatty Acid Profiles in Normal and Obstructed Rabbit Bladder Smooth Muscle and Mucosa. Neurourol. Urodyn. 18, 697-711.

432 van Koeveringe, G.A., Mostwin, J.L., van Mastrigt, R., van Koeveringe, B.J. (`1993) Effect of partial urethral obstruction on force development of the guinea pig bladder. Neurourol Urodyn 12,:555_566.

433 Chai, T.C., Gemalmaz, H., Andersson, K.E., Tuttle, J.B., Steers, W.D. Persistently increased voiding frequency despite relief of bladder outlet obstruction (1999). J Urol 161,1689_1693.

434 Ohnishi, N., Liu, S-P, Horan, P., and Levin, R.M. Effect of repetitive stimulation on the contractile response of rabbit urinary bladder subjected to in vitro hypoxia or in vitro ischemia followed by reoxygenation (1998) Pharmacology, 57, 139-147.

435 Levin, R.M., Whitbeck, C., and Horan, P. Effect of calcium and calcium chelators on the response of the bladder to in vitro ischemia. (1998) Br. J. Urol. 82, 882-887.

436 Lin, A-T, Yang, C.H., and Chang, L.S. Impact of aging on rat urinary bladder fatigue. (1997) J Urol 157, 1990-1994.

437 Lin, A-T, Hsu, T.H., Yang,C., and Chang, L.S. (2000). Effects of aging on mitochondrial enzyme activity of rat urinary bladder. Urol Int 65, 144-147.

438 Yu, H-J, Levin, R. M., Longhurst, P. A. and Damaser, M. S. (1997). Effect of age and outlet resistance on rabbit urinary bladder emptying. J. Urol. 158, 924-930.

439 Resnick, NM and Yalla, SV (1985) Management of urinary incontinence in the elderly. New England Journal of Medicine (1985) 313: 800-805.

440 Lin, A.T.L.: Effects of aging on mitochondrial enzyme activity of rat urinary bladder. J. Urol., 151: 447A, 1994.

441 Yu, H.J., Wein, A.J., and Levin, R.M.: Age-related differential susceptibility to calcium channel blocker and low calcium medium in rat detrusor muscle: response to field stimulation. Neurourol. Urodyn., 15: 563, 1996.

442 Chun, A.L., Wallace, L.J., Gerald, M.C., Levin, R.M., and Wein, A.J.: Effect of age on in vivo urinary bladder function in the rat. J. Urol., 139: 625, 1988.

443 Yoshida, M., Latifpour, J., Nishimoto, T., and Weiss, R.M.: Pharmacological characterization of alpha adrenergic receptors in the young and old female rabbit urethra. J. Pharmacol. Exp. Ther., 257: 1100, 1991.

444 Hotta, H, Morrison, JFB, Uchida, S and Sato, A (1995). The effects of aging on the bladder and innervation of the rat bladder. Japanese Journal of Physiology 45:823-836

445 Gilpin, SA, Gilpin, CJ, Dixon, JA, Gosling, JA and Kirby, RS (1986) The effect of age on the autonomic innervation of the urinary bladder. British Journal of Urology, 58:378-381

446 Warburton, A.L., and Santer, R.M.: Sympathetic and sensory innervation of the urinary tract in young adult and aged rats: a semi-quantitative histochemical and immunohistochemical study. Histochem. J., 26: 127, 1994.

447 McComas AJ (1977) Ageing, Chapter 12 in ' Neuromuscular Function and Disorders' Pub: Butterworths pp 101-110

448 Collas, D.M., and Malone-Lee, J.G.: Age-associated changes in detrusor sensory function in women with lower urinary tract symptoms. Int.Urogyn. J. Pelv. Floor Dysfun., 7: 24, 1996.

449 Toyoshima, A., Onodera, S., Yoshinaga, M., Takenaga, K. and Uchiyama, T. Effects of aging and the autonomic nervous system_related agents on the intravesical pressure of the bladder in situ in female rats. [Japanese]. Nippon Yakurigaku Zasshi _ Folia Pharmacologica Japonica 96:103_115, 1990.

450 Munro, D.D. and Wendt, I.R. Contractile and metabolic properties of longitudinal smooth muscle from rat urinary bladder and the effects of aging. Journal of Urology 150:529_536, 1993.

451 Saito, M., Gotoh, M., Kato, K., and Kondo, A.: Influence of aging on the rat urinary bladder function. Urol. Int., 47 Suppl 1: 39, 1991.

452 Lieu, P.K., Sa'adu, A., Orugun, E.O., and Malone-Lee, J.G.: The influence of age on isometric and isotonic rat detrusor contractions. J. Gerontol, 52: M94, 1997.

453 Lin, A.T.L., Yang, C.H., Chang, L.S., and Chen, M.T.: Aging-related changes on the adrenergic contractile response in rat urinary bladder and the prostate. Neurourol. Urodyn., 11: 304, 1992.

454 Latifpour, J., Kondo, S., O'Hollaren, B., Morita, T., and Weiss, R.M.: Autonomic receptors in urinary tract:sex and age differences. J. Pharmacol. Exp. Ther., 253: 661, 1990..

455 Nishimoto, T., Latifpour, J., Wheeler, M.A., Yoshida, M., and Weiss, R.M.: Age-dependent alterations in beta-adrenergic responsiveness of rat detrusor smooth muscle. J. Urol., 153: 1701, 1995.

456 Steers, W.D. and Tuttle, J.B. Immunity to NGF prevents afferent plasticity in the spinal cord following hypertrophy of the bladder. J. Urol., 149: 385A, 1993.

457 Steers, W.D., Ciambottti, J., Erdman, S., and de Groat, W. Morphological plasticity in efferent pathways to the urinary bladder of the rat following urethral obstruction. J. Neurosci., 10: 1943, 1990.

458 Chai, T., Baker, L., Gomez, A., Tuttle, J.B., and Steers W.D.: Hyperactive voiding in rats secondary to obstruction and relief of obstruction: Expression of a novel gene encoding for protein D123. J. Urol., 157: 349A, 1997.

459 Steers, W.D., Kolbeck, S., Creedon, D., and Tuttle, J.B.: Nerve growth factor in the urinary bladder of the adult regulates neuronal form and function. J. Clin. Invest., 88: 1709, 1991.

460 Turner, W. and Brading, A.: Smooth muscle of the bladder in the normal and the diseased state: Pathophysiology, diagnosis and treatment. Pharmacology and Therapeutics, 75: 77, 1997.

461 Steers, W.D., Kolbeck, S., Creedon, D., and Tuttle, J.B.: Nerve growth factor in the urinary bladder of the adult regulates neuronal form and function. J. Clin. Invest., 88: 1709, 1991.

462 Ishizuka, O., Mattiasson, A., Steers, W.D., and Andersson, K.-E.: Effects of spinal alpha 1-adrenoceptor antagonism on bladder activity induced by apomorphine in conscious rats with and without bladder outlet obstruction. Neurourol. Urodyn., 16: 191, 19

463 Dupont, M., Persson, K., Spitsbergen, J., Tuttle, J.B., and Steers, W.D.: The neuronal response to bladder outlet obstruction, a role for NGF., Adv. Exper. Med. Biol., 385: 41, 1995.

464 Dmitrieva, N. and McMahon, S.: Sensitization of visceral afferents by nerve growth factor in the adult rat. Pain, 66: 87, 1996.

465 Birder, L.A., de Groat, W.C., and Kanai, A.J.: Adrenergic and capsaicin evoked nitric oxide release from urothelium and afferent nerves in urinary bladder. Am. J. Physiol., 275: F226, 1998.

466 Birder, L.A., de Groat, W.C., Kanai, A.J., Truschel, S.T., and Apodaca, G.: Norepinephrine, acetylcholine and capsaicin evoked nitric oxide release in the urinary bladder epithelium, measured using a porphyrinic microsensor. Society for Neuroscience Abstracts, 24: 1619, 1998.

467 Birder, L.A., Kanai, A., Truschel, S., Ruiz, W., de Groat, W.C., and Apodaca, G.: Measurement of adrenergic and capsaicin evoked nitric oxide release from urinary bladder epithelium using a porphyrinic microsensor. FASEB Abstracts, 98: A122, 1998.

468 Dupont, M., Steers, W., and Tuttle, J.B.: Inflammation induced neural plasticity in autonomic pathways supplying the bladder depend on NGF. Society for Neuroscience Abstract, 20: 112, 1994.

469 Dmitrieva, N., Shelton, D., Rice, A., and McMahon, S.: The role of nerve growth factor in a model of visceral inflammation. Neuroscience, 78: 449, 1997.

470 Dupont, M., Steers, W.D., McCarty, R. and Tuttle, J.B.: Neural plasticity and alterations in nerve growth factor and norepinephrine in response to bladder inflammation. J. Urol., 151:284, 1994.

471 Steers, W.D., Clemow, D., Persson, K., Sherer, T., Andersson, K.-E., and Tuttle, J.B.: The spontaneously hypertensive rat: Insight into the pathogenesis of irritative symptoms in benign prostatic hyperplasia and young anxious males. Exper. Physiol. 84:137-148, 1999.

472 Kaplan, S., Chancellor, M., and Blaivas, J.: Bladder and sphincter behavior in patients with spinal cord lesions. J. Urol., 146:113, 1991.

473 Geirsson, G., Fall, M., and Sullivan, L.: Clinical and urodynamic effects of intravesical capsaicin treatment in patients with chronic traumatic spinal detrusor hyperreflexia., J.Urol., 154:1825, 1995.

474 Fowler, C., Jewkes, D., and McDonald, W.: Intravesical capsaicin for neurogenic bladder dysfunction. Lancet, 339: 1239, 1992.

475 Fowler, C., Beck, R., Gerrard, S., Betts, C., and Fowler, C.: Intravesical capsaicin for treatment of detrusor hyperreflexia. J. Neurol. Neurosurg. Psych., 57:169, 1994.

476 Kruse, M., Bray, L., and de Groat, W.: Influence of spinal cord

injury on the morphology of bladder afferent and efferent neurons. J. Autonom. Nerv. Syst., 54: 215, 1995.

477 Yoshimura, N. and de Groat, W.: Plasticity of Na channels in afferent neurons innervating the rat urinary bladder following spinal cord injury. J. Physiol., 503: 269, 1997.

478 Aguayo, L.G. and White, G.: Effects of nerve growth factor on TTX- and capsaicin-sensitivity in adult rat sensory neurons. Brain Res., 570: 61, 1992.

479 Geirsson, G.: Evidence for cold receptors in the human urinary bladder : effect of menthol on the bladder cooling reflex. J.Urol., 150: 427, 1993.

480 Spitsbergen, J., Clemow, D., MCCarty, R., Steers, W., and Tuttle, J.: Neurally mediated voiding in the Spontaneously Hypertensive Rats. Brain Res, 790:151-159, 1998.

481 Steers WD, de Groat WC (1989) Effects of m-chlorophenylpiperazine on penile and bladder function in rats. Am J Physiol 257:R1441-9

482 Steers, W., Clemow, D., Persson, K., Sherer, T., Andersson, K.-E., and Tuttle, J.B.: Observations from the spontaneously hypertensive rat: Insight into NGF regulation and noradrenergic hyper-innervation in the lower urinary tract. Adv. Exper. Cell and Biol., 462:203-292, 1999

483 Persson, K., Pandita, R., Spitsbergen, J., Steers, W.D., Tuttle, J.B., and Andersson, K-E.: Spinal and peripheral mechanisms contributing to hyperactive voiding in spontaneously hypertensive rats. Am. J. Physiol., 44:R1366-R1373, 1998

484 Lee K.S., Deaŋ-McKinney T., Tuttle, J.B., Steers W.D. (2001) Intrathecal antisense oligonucleotides against the tetrodotoxin-resistant sodium channel reduces bladder hyperactivity in the Spontaneously Hypertensive Rat. Proc International Bladder Symposium. Washington DC Mar 8-11, Pg 43,

485 Sigurdsson, J.A. and Bengtsson, C. (1983). Symptoms and signs in relation to blood pressure and antihypertensive treatment. A cross-sectional and longitudinal population study of middle-aged Swedish women. Acta Med. Scand. 213:183-90.

486 Klein, B.E., Klein, R., Lee, K.E., and Bruskewitz, R.C. (1999). Correlates of urinary symptom scores in men. Am. J. Pub. Health 89:1745-8.

487 Boyle, P. (1994). Epidemiology of benign prostatic hyperplasia: risk factors and concomitance with hypertension. Br. J.Clin. Prac. 74:18-22.

488 Boyle, P. and Napalkov, P.: The epidemiology of benign prostatic hyperplasia and observations on hypertension. Scand. J. Urol. Nephrol., 168: 7, 1995.

489 Pool, J.L. (1994). Role of the sympathetic nervous system in hypertension and benign prostatic hyperplasia. Br. J. Clin. Prac. (Symposium Supplement) 74:13-17.

490 Pool, J.L. (1996). Doxazosin: a new approach to hypertension and benign prostatic hyperplasia [Review] [70 refs]. Br. J. Clin. Prac., 50:154-163.

491 Bardelli, M., Siracusano, S., Cominotto, F, Fazio, M., Ussi, D., Fabris, B., et al. (1999). Baroreceptor-heart rate reflex sensitivity enhancement after urinary bladder distention in essential hypertensives. Urol. Res. 27:153-156.

492 Miller, S.B. (1994). Parasympathetic nervous system control of heart rate responses to stress in offspring of hypertensives. Psychophys. 31:11-16.

493 Clemow, D.B., Spitsbergen, J.M., McCarty, R. Steers, W.D., and Tuttle, J.B. (1999). Altered NGF regulation may link a genetic disposition for hypertension to altered micturition behavior. J. Urol 161:1372-1377.

494 Porreca, F., Lai, J., Bian D, Wegert, S., et al. (1999). A comparison of the potential role of the tetrodotoxin-insensitive channels, PN3/SNS and NaN/SNS2, in rat models of chronic pain. PNAS, 96:7640-7644.

495 Waxman, S.G. (1999). The molecular pathophysiology of pain: abnormal expression of sodium channel genes and its contributions to hyperexcitability of primary sensory neurons. Pain (Suppl.) 6:S133-S140.

496 Yoshimura. N., Yoshida. O., and de Groat. W.C. (1995). Regional differences in plasticity of membrane properties of rat urinary bladder afferent neurons following spinal cord injury. J. Urol. 153:262a.

497 Bennett, D.L., Dmietrieva, N., Priestley, J.V., Clary, D., and McMahon, S.B. (1996) trkA, CGRP and IB4 expression in retrogradely labelled cutaneous and visceral primary sensory neurones in the rat. Neurosci. Lett. 206:33-6.

498 Yoshimura, N., Erdman, S., Snider, W., and de Groat, W.C. (1998). Effects of spinal cord injury or neurofilament immunoreactivity and capsaicin sensitivity in rat dorsal root ganglion neurons innervating the urinary bladder. Neuroscience 83:633-643.

499 Edlund C. Peeker R. Fall M. (2001)Lidocaine cystometry in the diagnosis of bladder overactivity. Neurouro Urodyn. 20(2):147-55.

500 Castleden CM. Duffin HM. Clarkson EJ. In vivo and in vitro studies on the effect of sodium antagonists on the bladder in man and rat. Age & Ageing. 12(3):249-55, 1983

501 Lapointe SP, Wang B, Kennedy WA, Shortliffe LM: The effects of intravesical lidocaine on bladder dynamics of children with myelomeningocele. J Urol 165: 2380, 2001.

502 Yokoyama, O., Komatsu, K., Kodama, K., Yotsuyanagi, S., Nikura, S., and Namiki, M. (2000). Diagnostic value of intravesical lidocaine for overactive bladder. J. Urol. 164(2):340-3.

503 Reuther K, Aagaard J, Jensen KS: Lignocaine test and detrusor instability. Br J Urol 55: 493, 1983.

504 Sethia KK. Smith JC. The effect of pH and lignocaine on detrusor instability. British Journal of Urology. 60(6):516-8, 1987

505 Chalfin, S. and Bradley, W.: The etiology of detrusor hyperreflexia in patients with infravesical outlet obstruction. J. Urol., 127: 938, 1982.

506 Levin, R. M., Hypolite, J., Longhurst, P. A. and Wein, A. J. (1991b). Comparison of the contractile and metabolic effects of muscarinic stimulation with those of KCl. Pharmacology 42, 142-150.

507 Lecci A. Giuliani S. Lazzeri M. Benaim G. Turini D. Maggi CA. The behavioral response induced by intravesical instillation of capsaicin rats is mediated by pudendal urethral sensory fibers. Life Sciences. 55(6):429-36, 1994.

508 Kamphuis ET, Ionescu TI, Kuipers PW, de Gier J, van Venrooij GE, Boon TA: Recovery of storage and emptying functions of the urinary bladder after spinal anesthesia with lidocaine and with bupivacaine in men. Anesthesiology 88: 310, 1998.

509 Kanie S. Yokoyama O. Komatsu K. Kodama K. Yotsuyanagi S. Niikura S. Nagasaka Y. Miyamoto KI. Namiki M. GABAergic contribution to rat bladder hyperactivity after middle cerebral artery occlusion. American Journal of Physiology - Regulatory Integrative & Comparative Physiology. 279(4):R1230-8, 2000

510 Wolfe F, Russell IJ, Vipraio G, Ross K, Anderson J (1997) Serotonin levels, pain threshold, and fibromyalgia, symptoms in the general population. Journal of Rheumatology 24(3):555-559

511 O'Malley PG, Jackson JL, Santoro J, Tomkins G, Balden E, Kroenke K (1999) Antidepressant therapy for unexplained symptoms and symptom syndromes. J Family Pract 48(12):980-990

512 Neeck G (2000) Neuroendocrine and hormonal perturbations and relations to the serotonergic system in fibromyalgia patients. Scand J Rheumatol (Suppl) 113:8-12

513 Bondy B, Spaeth M, Offenbaecher M. Glatzeder K, Strats T,

Schwarts M, deJong S, Kruger M, Engel RR, Farber L, Pongratz DE, Ackenheil M (1999) The T102C polymorphism of the 5-HT2A receptor gene in fibromyalgia. Neurobiol Dis 6(5):433-439

514 Offenbaecher M, Bondy B, de Jonge S, Glatzeder K. Kruger M, Schoeps P, Ackenheil M (1999) Possible association of fibromyalgia with a polymorphism in the serotonin transporter gene regulatory region. Arthritis Rhematism 42(11):2482-2488

515 Collier DA, Stober G, Li T, Heils A, Catalano M, Di Bella D, Arranz MJ, Murray RM, Vallada HP, Bengel D, Muller CR, Roberts GW, Smeraldi E, Kirov G, Sham P, Lesch KP (1996) A Novel functional polymorphism within the promoter of the serotonin transporter gene: possible role in susceptibility to affective disorders. Mol Psych 1:453-460

516 Roy A (1999) Suicidal behavior in depression: relationship to platelet serotonin transporter. Neuropsychobiol 39:71-75

517 McMahon, S.B. and Spillane, Kathy (1982). Brainstem influences on the para-sympathetic supply to the urinary bladder of the cat. Brain Res. 234, 237-249.

518 Downie JW (1999) Pharmacological manipulation of central micturition circuitry. Current Opinion in CPNS Investigational Drugs 12:231-239

519 Espey MJ, Downie JW (1995) Serotonergic modulation of cat bladder function before and after spinal transection. Eur J Pharmacol 287:173-177

520 Steers, W.D., Albo, M., van Asselt E.: "Effects of Serotonergic Agonists on Micturition Function in the Rat" Drug Development Research 27:361-375 (1992)

521 Testa R, Guarneri L, Poggesi E, Angelico P, Velasco C, Ibba M, Cilia A, Motta G, Riva C, Leonardi A (1999) Effect of several 5-hydroxytryptamine(1A) receptor ligands on the micturition reflex in rats: comparison with WAY 100635. J Pharm Exp Ther 290:1258-1269

522 Tonini ME, Messori GP, Franceschetti CA, Rizzi AF, Castoldi AF, Coccini T, Candura SM (1994) Characterization of the 5-HT receptors potentiating neuromuscular transmission in strips of isolated human detrusor muscle. Br J Pharmacol 113:1-5

523 Zorn BH, Montgomery H, Pieper K, Gray M, Steers WD (1999) Urinary incontinence and depression. J Urol 162:82-84

524 Rosenzweig BA, Hischke D, Thomas S, Nelson AL, Bhatia NN (1991) Stress incontinence in women. Psychological status before and after treatment. J Reprod Med 36:835-838

525 Berglund AL, Lalos O (1996) The pre- and postsurgical nursing of women with stress incontinence. J Adv Nurs 23:502-511

526 Archer JS (1999) NAMS/Solvay resident essay award. Relationship between estrogen, serotonin, and depression. Menopause 6(1):71-8

527 Nishizawa S, Benkelfat C, Young SN, Leyton M, Mzengeza S, de Montigny C, Blier P, Diksic M (1997) Differences between males and females in rates of serotonin synthesis in human brain. Proc Natl Acad Sci USA 94:5308-5313

528 Pecins-Thompson M, Brown NA, Kohama SG, Bethea CL (1996) Ovarian steroid regulation of tryptophan hydroxylase mRNA expression in rhesus macaques. J Neurosci 16(21):7021-9

529 Schneider, M. R., Lahm, H., Wu, M., Hoeflich, A., & Wolf, E. (2000). Transgenic mouse models for studying the functions of insulin-like growth factor-binding proteins. FASEB J. 14, 629-640.

530 Persson, K., Pandita, R. K., Aszodi, A., Ahmad, M., Pfeifer, A., Fassler, R., & Andersson, K. E. (2000). Functional characteristics of urinary tract smooth muscles in mice lacking cGMP protein kinase type I. Am.J.Physiol Regul.Integr.Comp Physiol 279, R1112-R1120.

531 Chalfin, S. and Bradley, W.: The etiology of detrusor hyperreflexia in patients with infravesical outlet obstruction. J. Urol., 127: 938, 1982.

532 Pool, J.: Role of the sympathetic nervous system in hypertension and benign prostatic hyperplasia. Brit. J. Clinical Practice - Symposium Supplement, 74:13, 1994.

533 Morita, T., Ando, M., Kihara, K. and Oshima, H.: Species differences in cAMP production and contractile response induced by beta-adrenoceptor subtypes in urinary bladder smooth muscle. Neurourol. Urodyn., 12: 185, 1993.

534 Levin, R. M., Ruggieri, M. R., Hypolite, J. and Wein, A. J.: Beta adrenergic stimulation of cyclic AMP production in the rabbit urinary bladder. Neurourol. Urodyn., 5: 227, 1986.

535 Oshita, M., Hiraoka, Y. and Watanabe, Y.: Characterization of beta-adrenoceptors in urinary bladder: comparison between rat and rabbit. Br. J. Pharmacol., 122: 1720, 1997.

536 Strosberg, A. D. and Pietri-Rouxel, F.: Function and regulation of the beta 3-adrenoceptor. Trends Pharmacol. Sci., 17: 373, 1996.

537 Takeda, M., Mizusawa, T., Obara, K., Koizumi, T., Tsutsui, T., Hatano, A., Kanai, T. and Takahashi, K.: Adrenergic _1-, _2-, and _3-receptor subtypes in the detrusor of human urinary bladder. - Evaluation by mRNA expression and isometric contraction. Neurourol. Urodyn., 16: 365, 1997.

538 Andersson, K.E. The overactive bladder: pharmacologic basis of drug treatment. Urology, 50: 74, 1997.

539 Longhurst, P. A., Briscoe, J. A., Rosenberg, D. J. and Leggett, R. E.: The role of cyclic nucleotides in guinea-pig bladder contractility. Br. J. Pharmacol., 121: 1665, 1997.

540 Truss, M. C., Uckert, S., Stief, C. G., Forssmann, W. G. and Jonas, U.: Cyclic nucleotide phosphodiesterase (PDE) isoenzymes in the human detrusor smooth muscle. II. Effect of various PDE inhibitors on smooth muscle tone and cyclic nucleotide levels in vitro. Urol. Res., 24: 129, 1996.

541 Truss, M. C., Uckert, S., Stief, C. G., Kuczyk, M. and Jonas, U.: Cyclic nucleotide phosphodiesterase (PDE) isoenzymes in the human detrusor smooth muscle. I. Identification and characterization. Urol. Res., 24: 123, 1996.

542 Truss, M. C., Uckert, S., Stief, C. G., Kuczyk, M., Schulz-Knappe, P., Forssmann, W. G. and Jonas, U.: Effects of various phosphodiesterase-inhibitors, forskolin, and sodium nitroprusside on porcine detrusor smooth muscle tonic responses to muscarinergic stimulation and cyclic nucleotide levels in vitro. Neurourol. Urodyn., 15: 59, 1996.

543 Lepor, H., Gup, D., Shapiro, E. and Baumann, M.: Muscarinic cholinergic receptors in the normal and neurogenic human bladder. J. Urol., 142: 869, 1989.

544 Eglen, R. M., Hegde, S. S. and Watson, N.: Muscarinic receptor subtypes and smooth muscle function. Pharmacol. Rev., 48: 531, 1996.

545 Hegde, S. S., Choppin, A., Bonhaus, D., Briaud, S., Loeb, M., Moy, T. M., Loury, D. and Eglen, R. M.: Functional role of M2 and M3 muscarinic receptors in the urinary bladder of rats in vitro and in vivo. Br. J. Pharmacol., 120: 1409, 1997.

546 Wang, P., Luthin, G. R. and Ruggieri, M. R.: Muscarinic acetylcholine receptor subtypes mediating urinary bladder contactility and coupling to GTP binding proteins. J. Pharmacol. Exp. Ther., 273: 959, 1995.

547 Kondo, S. Morita, T., and Tashima, Y.: Muscarinic cholinergic receptor subtypes in human detrusor muscle studied by labeled and nonlabeled pirenzepine, AFDX-116, and 4-DAMP. Urol. Int., 54: 150, 1995.

548 Harriss, D. R., Marsh, K. A., Birmingham, A. T. and Hill, S. J.: Expression of muscarinic M3-receptors coupled to inositol phospholipid hydrolysis in human detrusor cultured smooth muscle cells. J. Urol., 154: 1241, 1995.

549 Lai, F. M., Cobuzzi, A. and Spinelli, W.: Characterization of muscarinic receptors mediating the contraction of the urinary detrusor muscle in cynomolgus monkeys and guinea pigs. Life Sci., 62: 1179, 1998.

550 Newgreen, D. T., Anderson, C. W. P., Carter, A. J. and Naylor, A. M.: Darifenacin - a novel bladder-selective agent for the treatment of urge incontinence. Neurourol. Urodyn., 14: 95, 1995.

551 Yamamoto, T., Honbo, T.,Tokoro, K., Kojimoto, Y., Kodama, R., Ohtsuka, M. and Shinomura, K.: General pharmacology of the new antimuscrinic compound vamicamide. Arzeimittel-Forschung/Drugs Res., 45: 1274, 1995.

552 Nilvebrant, L., Andersson, K. E., Gillberg, P. G., Stahl, M. and Sparf, B.: Tolterodine--a new bladder-selective antimuscarinic agent. Eur. J. Pharmacol., 327: 195, 1997.

553 Nilvebrant, L., Hallen, B. and Larsson, G.: Tolterodine--a new bladder selective muscarinic receptor antagonist: preclinical pharmacological and clinical data. Life Sci. 60: 1129, 1997.

554 Andersson, K. E.: The concept of uroselectivity. Eur. Urol., 33: 7, 1998.

555 Burnstock, G., Dumsday, and B., Smythe, A.: Atropine resistant excitation of the urinary bladder: the possibility of transmission via nerves releasing a purine nucleotide. Br. J. Pharmacol., 44: 451, 1972.

556 Palea, S., Artibani, W., Ostardo, E., Trist, D.G., and Pietra, C., Evidence for purinergic neurotransmission in human urinary bladder affected by interstitial cystitis. Urol., 150:2007, 1993

557 Burnstock, G.: P2 purinoceptors: historical perspective and classification. In P2 Purinoceptors:Localization, Function and Transduction Mechanisms. Ciba Foundation Symposium, Chichester: John Wiley and Sons, 198: 1-34, 1996: 1-34.

558 Somogyi, G. T. and de Groat, W. C.: Modulation of the release of [3H] norepinephrine from the base and body of the rat urinary bladder by endogenous adrenergic and cholinergic mechanisms. J. Pharmacol. Exp. Ther., 255: 204, 1990.

559 Braverman, A. S., Kohn, I. J., Luthin, G. R. and Ruggieri, M. R.: Prejunctional M1 facilitory and M2 inhibitory muscarinic receptors mediate rat bladder contractility. Am. J. Physiol., 274: R517, 1998.

560 Somogyi, G. T., Tanowitz, M., Zernova, G. and de Groat: M1 muscarinic receptor-induced facilitation of ACh and noradrenaline release in the rat bladder is mediated by protein kinase C. J. Physiol., 496: 245, 1996.

561 Somogyi, G. T. and de Groat, W. C.: Evidence for inhibitory nicotinic and facilitatory muscarinic receptors in cholinergic nerve terminals of the rat urinary bladder. J. Autonom. Nerv. Syst., 37: 89, 1992.

562 D'Agostino, G., Kilbinger, H., Chiari, M. C. and Grana, E.: Presynaptic inhibitory muscarinic receptors modulating [3H] acetylcholine release in the rat urinary bladder. J. Pharmacol. Exp. Ther., 239: 522, 1986.

563 Mattiasson, A., Andersson, K. E., Elbadai, A., Morgan, E. and Sjorgren, C.: Interaction between adrenergic and cholinergic nerve terminals in the urinary bladder of rabbit, cat and man. J. Urol., 137: 1017, 1987.

564 D'Agostino, G., Barbieri, A., Chiossa, E. and Tonini, M.: M4 muscarinic autoreceptor-mediated inhibition of -3H-acetylcholine release in the rat isolated urinary bladder. J. Pharmacol. Exp. Ther., 283: 750, 1997

565 Andersson, K. E.: Clinical pharmacology of potassium channel openers. Pharmacol. Toxicol., 70: 244, 1992.

566 Fry, C. H. and Wu, C.: Initiation of contraction in detrusor smooth muscle. Scand. J. Urol. Nephrol. Suppl. 184: 7, 1997.

567 Martin, S. W., Radley, S. C., Chess-Williams, R., Korstanje, C. and Chapple, C. R.: Relaxant effects of potassium-channel openers on normal and hyperreflexic detrusor muscle. Br. J. Urol., 80: 405, 1997.

568 Brading, A. F. and Inoue, R.: Ion channels and excitatory transmission in the smooth muscle of the urinary bladder. Z. Kardiol., 80: 47, 1991.

569 Levin, R. M., Kitada, S., Hayes, L., Kau, S. T., Formm-Freeck, S., Howe, B. B. and Wein, A. J.: Experimental hyperreflexia: Effect of intravesical administration of various agents. Pharmacology, 42: 54, 1991.

570 Trivedi, S., Potter-Lee, L., Li, J. H., Yasay, G. D., Russell, K., Ohnmacht, C. J., Empfield, J. R., Trainor, D. A. and Kau, S. T.: Calcium dependent K-channels in guinea pig and human urinary bladder. Biochem. Biophys. Res. Commun., 213: 404, 1995.

571 Wein, A. J.: Pharmacologic options for the overactive bladder. Urol., 51: 43, 1998.

572 Maggi, C. A., Borsini, F., Lecci, A., Giuliani, S., Meli, P., Gragnani, L. and Meli, A.: Effect of acute or chronic administration of imipramine on spinal and supraspinal micturition reflexes in rats. J. Pharmacol. Exp. Ther., 248: 278, 1989.

573 Diokno, A.C. and Taub, M.: Ephedrine in treatment of urinary incontinence. Urol., 5: 624, 1975.

574 Awad, S. A., Downie, J.W., and Kiruluta, I.: Alpha adrenergic agents in urinary disorders of the proximal urethral: I: Stress incontinence. Br. J. Urol., 50: 332, 1978

575 Dupont, M., Steers, W.D., McCarty, R. and Tuttle, J.B.: Neural plasticity and alterations in nerve growth factor and norepinephrine in response to bladder inflammation. J. Urol., 151:284, 1994.

576 Steers, W.D., Clemow, D., Persson, K., Sherer, T., Andersson, K.-E., and Tuttle, J.B.: The spontaneously hypertensive rat: Insight into the pathogenesis of irritative symptoms in benign prostatic hyperplasia and young anxious males. Exper. Physiol. In Press. 1998.

577 Xu, W., Gelber, S., Orr-Urtreger, A., Armstrong, D., Lewis, R. A., Ou, C. N., Patrick, J., Role, L., De Biasi, M., & Beaudet, A. L. (1999a). Megacystis, mydriasis, and ion channel defect in mice lacking the alpha3 neuronal nicotinic acetylcholine receptor. Proc.Natl.Acad.Sci.U.S.A 96, 5746-5751.

578 Xu, W., Orr-Urtreger, A., Nigro, F., Gelber, S., Sutcliffe, C. B., Armstrong, D., Patrick, J. W., Role, L. W., Beaudet, A. L., & De Biasi, M. (1999b). Multiorgan autonomic dysfunction in mice lacking the beta2 and the beta4 subunits of neuronal nicotinic acetylcholine receptors. J.Neurosci. 19, 9298-9305.

579 Jusuf, A. A., Kojima, S., Matsuo, M., Tokuhisa, T., & Hatano, M. (2000). Vesicourethral sphincter dysfunction in Ncx deficient mice with an increased neuronal cell number in vesical ganglia. J.Urol. 165, 993-998.

580 Matsui, M., Motomura, D., Karasawa, H., Fujikawa, T., Jiang, J., Komiya, Y., Takahashi, S., & Taketo, M. M. (2000). Multiple functional defects in peripheral autonomic organs in mice lacking muscarinic acetylcholine receptor gene for the M3 subtype. Proc.Natl.Acad.Sci.U.S.A 97, 9579-9584.

581 Matthew, J. D., Khromov, A. S., McDuffie, M. J., Somlyo, A. V., Somlyo, A. P., Taniguchi, S., & Takahashi, K. (2000). Contractile properties and proteins of smooth muscles of a calponin knockout mouse. J.Physiol 529 Pt 3:811-24., 811-824.

582 Mobarakeh, J. I., Sakurada, S., Katsuyama, S., Kutsuwa, M., Kuramasu, A., Lin, Z. Y., Watanabe, T., Hashimoto, Y., & Yanai, K. (2000). Role of histamine H(1) receptor in pain perception: a study of the receptor gene knockout mice. Eur.J.Pharmacol. 391, 81-89.

583 Morano, I., Chai, G. X., Baltas, L. G., Lamounier-Zepter, V., Lutsch, G., Kott, M., Haase, H., & Bader, M. (2000). Smooth-muscle contraction without smooth-muscle myosin. Nat.Cell Biol. 2, 371-375.

584 Stengel, P. W., Gomeza, J., Wess, J., & Cohen, M. L. (2000). M(2) and M(4) receptor knockout mice: muscarinic receptor function in cardiac and smooth muscle in vitro. J.Pharmacol.Exp.Ther. 292, 877-885.

585 Morrison, JFB (2001) Physiology of the Pelvic Floor. In 'The Urinary Sphincter' edited by J Corcos and E Schick pp 71-87 Pub Marcel Dekker, NY

586 Danuser, H., Bemis, K., and Thor, K.B. "Pharmacological Analysis of the Noradrenergic Control of Central Sympathetic and Somatic Reflexes Controlling the Lower Urinary Tract in the Anesthetized Cat" J. Pharmacol. Expt. Ther. 274:820-825 (1995)

587 Krier, J., Thor, K.B. and de Groat, W.C. Effects of Clonidine on the Lumbar Sympathetic Pathways to the Large Intestine and Urinary Bladder of the Cat. Eur. J. of Pharmacology 59: 47-53 (1979)

588 Thor, K.B., Katofiasc, M.A., Danuser, H., Springer, J.P., and Schaus, J.M. "The Role of 5HT1A Receptors in Control of Lower Urinary Tract Function in Cats" Brain Res (In press)

589 Kim, J.C., Beckel, J.M., Birder, L.A., Kiss, S., Siefried, J., Hopkins, T., Kanai, A., Dineley, K.,Reynolds, I., de Groat, W.C. Nicotinic Acetylcholine receptor subunit gene expression and functional properties of nicotinic receptors in human bladder urothelial cells. Journal of Urology, 165 (Suppl):31, 2001.

590 Yoshimura, N., Seki, S. and de Groat, W.C. Nitric Oxide modulates Ca2+ channels in dorsal root ganglion neurons innervating rat urinary bladder. Journal of Neurophysiology, 86: 304-311, 2001.

591 Ozawa, H., Chancellor, M.B., Jung, S.Y., Yokoyama, T., Yu, Y., de Groat, W.C., and Yoshimura, N., Effect of intravesical nitric oxide therapy on cyclophosphamide-induced cystitis. Journal of Urology, 162:2211-2216, 1999.

592 Mallory, BS, Roppolo, JR, and de Groat WC (1991). Pharmacological modulation of the pontine micturition center. Brain Research 546: 310-320

593 Yoshimura, N. , Sasa, M., Yoshida, O. and Takaori, S.: Dopamine D-1 receptor mediated inhibition of micturition reflex by central dopamine from the substantia nigra. Neurourol. Urodyn. 11: 535, 1992.

594 Yokoyama, O., Yoshiyama, M. Namiki, M. and de Groat, W.C. The influence of anesthesia on the

development of bladder hyperactivity following middle cerebral artery occlusion in the rat. American Journal of Physiology, 273: R1900-R1907, 1997

595 Yoshimura, N., and de Groat, W.C. Increased excitability of afferent neurons innervating rat urinary bladder following chronic bladder inflammation. Journal of Neuroscience, 19(11):4644-4653, 1999.

596. Vizzard, M.A., Erdman, S.L., and de Groat, W.C. Increased expression of neuronal nitric oxide synthase in bladder afferent pathways following chronic bladder irritation. J. Comp. Neurol., 370: 191-202, 1996.

597 Goldin, A.L. (2001) Resurgence of sodium channel research. Annu. Rev. Physiol. 63:871-94.

598 Chai, T., Gray, M., and Steers, W. D.: The incidence of a positive ice water test in bladder outlet obstructed patients: evidence for bladder neuroplasticity. J. Urol., 160: 34, 1998.

599 Yoshimura, N., Mizuta, E., Kuno, S., Sasa, M. and Yoshida, O.: The dopamine D1 receptor agonist SKF 38393 suppresses detrusor hyperreflexia in the monkey with parkinsonism induced by N-methyl-4-phenyl-1,2,3,6-tetrahydropyridine(MPTP). Neuropharmacol., 32

Committee 3

Epidemiology and Natural History of Urinary Incontinence (UI)

Chairman

S. Hunskaar (Norway)

Members

K. Burgio (USA),

A.C Diokno (USA),

A.R. Herzog (USA),

K. Hjälmås (Sweden),

M.C. Lapitan (The Philippines)

CONTENTS

Epidemiology and Natural History of Urinary Incontinence (UI)

S. Hunskaar

K. Burgio, A.C Diokno, A.R. Herzog, K. Hjälmås, M.C. Lapitan

I. INTRODUCTION

In this report we focus on the importance of understanding the epidemiology of urinary incontinence (UI) (distribution and determinants) as well as its natural history. We also discuss important topics as differences between epidemiological and clinical approach to a health problem, help seeking behaviour and methodological issues for this research.

The epidemiological population under study for this review will be community dwelling noninstitutionalized persons. The review will include discussion of the prevalence, incidence, natural history, and presence of racial and ethnic differences in the epidemiology of UI. We also reviewed correlates and potential risk factors that have been revealed in epidemiological studies.

The review examines our current state of knowledge of the epidemiology of UI, topics like the epidemiology of *fecal incontinence*, *pelvic organ prolapse* and *pelvic floor weakness* have been omitted. *Overactive bladder* (OAB) is an evolving concept with close relationship to UI. We have studied the scarce epidemiological literature on OAB, and have decided to include the urge incontinence part of OAB only (OAB with incontinence).

We have reviewed a large number of completed studies in the field of UI. We have emphasized high-quality and population based studies. We have also wanted to present studies from a broad variety of countries. Because of an abundant number of studies, only a small fraction can be presented in a text like this. Other studies not presented here may have equal standard and useful information, but lack of space precluded their inclusion.

Progress has clearly been made during the 3 years since our previous report [1]. Some important areas have been studied with increasing regularity and quality. We have searched the literature for relevant new articles from 1997 to 2000, including clinical trials that might include relevant epidemiological data on UI.

Summary points:

- This review includes discussion of the prevalence, incidence, natural history, and presence of racial and ethnic differences in the epidemiology of UI.
- Correlates and potential risk factors that have been revealed in epidemiological studies are also reviewed.

II. BASIC EPIDEMIOLOGICAL CONSIDERATIONS

1. General comments, designs and levels of evidence

In this report we emphasize the importance of understanding the epidemiology, and also give a summary of the basic concepts. Epidemiology is the scientific study of the distribution and determinants of disease in people. *Descriptive epidemiology* is the description of disease prevalence, incidence, (and mortality) by persons, place and time, while the term *analytical epidemiology* describes the search for determinants of disease risk. The discovery of risk factors and protective factors may then in turn lead to primary or secondary prevention.

In order to collect knowledge about risk factors or natural history, observational studies are needed. Cohort studies and case-control studies are the most common. However, caution are always needed when interpreting the results from such studies, as associations found in epidemiological studies may not be the same as causes. In order to strengthen the validity of epidemiological studies longitudinal designs should be preferred, and appropriate control for confounding should be done. Experimental designs will seldom be used.

Recommendations and conclusions should alway be based on a sound evidence. Levels of evidence as used for therapeutic interventions do not fit into epidemiological studies. No uniform guidelines for assessing the results of such studies excists. The level of evidence in observational studies could be judged on the soundness of the exclusion of alternative explanations by statistical and other controls.

Even in many recent studies of UI analyses are very simple. Often only proportions or percentages are used to describe differences in the prevalence of UI in different subgroups. Many analyses do not control for confounders, there is lack of stratification, or multivariate techniques are not used. There is an obvious need for more advanced epidemiological analyses of risk factors and comorbidity, and strength of associations should be determined by relative risks and odds ratios.

The *relative risk (RR)* estimates the magnitude of an association between exposure and a condition, and indicates the likelihood of having the condition in the exposed group relative to those who are not exposed (e.g. do not have the risk factor). An RR of 1.0 indicates that the rates in the exposed and nonexposed groups are identical and thus that there is no association between the exposure and the condition in that specific dataset. A value greater than 1.0 indicates a positive association or an increased risk. An RR of 2.5 for UI indicates that there is a 2.5 times increased risk or that the persons in question are 150 percent more likely to have incontinence than those without the risk factor.

The *odds ratio (OR)* is the odds for having a risk factor between persons with a condition divided by the odds among those without the condition. An OR of 2.5 for UI my be interpreted as meaning that in this sample the odds i favour of having incontinence are 2.5 times higher among those with the risk factor than among those without.

Effects may be denoted as strong when RRs or ORs are 2.0 and more, and weak when RRs or ORs are less than 2.0, but there are no generally agreed standards. For a condition with high prevalence, like UI, OR and RR will not be identical, but in practice the results can be interpreted similarly. Results should always be given with a 95% confidence interval (CI).

Words like well established and established may be used about risk factors and findings with a high level of evidence in the literature. For less documented findings words like "indications of" or "data are suggestive" may be used.

2. Definitions

Studies of disease frequency should rely on a very specific definition of the condition under investigation. The absence of a unifying definition for UI is a fundamental problem which is not resolved. The lack of such a definition leads to problems with assessing sensitivity and specificity of the findings in epidemiological studies. Variations in availability and efficacy of health care around the world may influence the prevalence of UI.

a) Incontinence

UI can be defined in several ways, and one problem when analysing the epidemiological studies is in fact that incontinence *has* been defined in many ways. However, in order to get replicable results and be able to compare different studies, widely accepted definitions are important. The International Continence Society (ICS) defines incontinence as "a condition where involuntary loss of urine is a social or hygienic problem and is objectively demonstrable". This definition may not be ideal for epidemiological purposes (will be discussed below). More common in epidemiological studies are definitions based on frequency of urine loss, e.g. "any uncontrolled urine loss in the prior year" or "more than two episodes in a month". Such definitions imply that the studies are in fact studies of period prevalence.

b) Prevalence

Prevalence is defined as the probability of being incontinent within a defined population and at a defined time point. The concept is important for establishing the distribution of the condition in the population and for projecting the need for health and medical services. Prevalence of all-cause UI is estimated as the ratio of the number of incontinent respondents identified in a cross-sectional survey to the number of all respondents in the survey (i.e., continent and incontinent). Prevalences of specific types and severity levels are estimated in an analogous manner.

c) Incidence

Incidence is defined as the probability of developing the condition under study during a defined time period. Incidence is usually reported for one-, two- or five-year time interval.

d) Type

Epidemiological surveys often must take a pragmatic approach, and therefore define incontinence type based on the symptoms alone. The classification can be done either by the researchers based on several questions, or by the respondant's confirmation of a statement or typical description. Clinical assessment allows for more differentiation of subtypes. Possible biases will be discussed below.

e) Severity

Severity of incontinence is another important factor for the prevalence estimate. Severity can be defined by factors like frequency, amount and subjective bother. Examples of how the prevalence differs when based on different definitions for severity will be shown.

Summary points:

- Descriptive epidemiology is the description of disease incidence, prevalence (and mortality) by persons, place and time.
- Analytical epidemiology describes the search for determinants of disease risk. There is a need for good longitudinal cohort studies.
- Variations in definitions and measurement issues are fundamental, and lead to problems with assessing the findings in epidemiological studies.
- There is a need for more advanced epidemiological analyses of risk factors and comorbidity using multivariate techniques, and strength of associations should be determined by relative risks and odds ratios.

III. EPIDEMIOLOGY OF ENURESIS AND UI IN CHILDREN

1. General comments and definitions

The ICS definition of UI as "a condition where involuntary loss of urine is a social or hygienic problem and is objectively demonstrable" is not quite applicable to childhood UI. "Involuntary" is very difficult to assess in children, and since bladder control is gradually developing during childhood, the standards for what is socially acceptable will vary between families and with the age of the child. The objective demonstration of UI in a child rests on assessment by the parents. Different standards and definitions make metaanalysis difficult or impossible. It is thus essential to try to reach an international consensus about the grading of severity of UI in children.

Only isolated bedwetting should be termed *enuresis* according to recommendations issued by the ICCS (International Children's Continence Society) [2]. The reason is that isolated bedwetting, *nocturnal enuresis,* is a strictly defined type of incontinence characterized by complete bladder emptyings during sleep without any symptoms pointing to bladder dysfunction. In contrast, almost all daywetting children, and children wetting both day and night, have bladder dysfunction of either a functional or organic nature and a great variety in their incontinence patterns. The one exception here is a small group of children with profuse daytime wetting due to incontinent complete bladder emptyings. Psychological factors are underlying this kind of rare childhood UI which is labelled *diurnal enuresis.*

Bedwetting should be characterized as primary or secondary, and as monosymptomatic or polysymptomatic. Monosymptomatic means that the child has no daytime symptoms. Monosymptomatic enuresis will thus be excluded if the child has day wetting, or frequency (>7 voidings per day in a 7-year-old), or infrequent voidings (<3 voidings per day), or imperative urgency. Monosymptomatic enuresis will not be excluded by moderate urgency which is found in 16% of 7-year-olds. Polysymptomatic cases are then defined as the non-monosymptomatic ones (Table 1) [3].

Nocturnal enuresis is also subdivided into *primary enuresis* (the child has not been dry for more than 6 months), and *secondary (onset) enuresis* (the bedwetting has recurred after a dry period lasting more than 6 months). Secondary enuresis may signify behavioural, neurological, infective causes, or chronic retention with overflow, and these require careful consideration.

Table 1 : Subdivision of nocturnal enuresis and diurnal urinary incontinence in children

Enuresis (nocturnal enuresis, bedwetting)
Primary
Monosymptomatic
Non-monosymptomatic
Secondary
Monosymptomatic
Non-monosymptomatic
Diurnal and nocturnal UI
Functional (detrusor overactivity)
Organic
Neuropathic
Structural
Infravesical obstruction
Epispadias
Other
Diurnal UI (day wettting only)
Functional (detrusor overactivity)
Organic
Neuropathic
Structural
Infravesical obstruction
Epispadias
Other

The healthy infant is socially incontinent but physiologically continent, because micturitions (about once every hour) are discrete and there is no leakage of urine in between micturitions [4]. Opinions regarding at what age the child is expected to become socially dry differ widely between cultures and ethnic groups. Meadow has suggested a reasonable age limit in stating that a wetting child above 5 years of age should be considered incontinent [5], although UI in children due to organic disorders is often evident already in infancy.

2. Prevalence of nocturnal enuresis

Most epidemiological studies link primary and secondary enuresis together and include also mon-symptomatic and poly-symptomatic cases. Also, enuresis is defined in different ways, and in many papers there is no frequency defined at all. The best studies are longitudinal cohort studies, but many are cross-sectional. In some cultures the parents are more complacent about the bedwetting than in others and do not regard it as a problem requiring attention. These problems in understanding epidemiology were summarized by Krantz et al. [6], who also reviewed the epidemiological studies that had been published until 1993.

Nocturnal enuresis, NE, is caused by relative nocturnal polyuria and/or nocturnal bladder overactivity combined with lack of arousal at the time when the bladder needs to be emptied. These factors have different weight in different enuretic children. The pathophysiology of NE is thus a mixed mechanism which explains difficulties encountered when trying to define enuresis in a consistent way. Stringent epidemiological studies would need to evaluate nocturnal urine production, nocturnal bladder activity, and sleep and arousal in each of the probands. Needless to say, there is no large population based study using such diagnostic evaluation.

a) Longitudinal cohort studies

A child development study has followed 1139 children born in one year in Dunedin (New Zealand) and obtained an impressive 92% follow-up 9 years later [7, 8]. It was found that primary enuresis usually remits with age (Figure 1). Another birth cohort born in 1977 in Christchurch (New Zealand) was followed up annually. By the age of 8 they found that 7% had nocturnal enuresis although this included some who had relapsed after initially becoming dry [9].

b) Survey Studies

Prevalence is defined at a specific point in time, but many studies have reported prevalence of enuresis without separately recounting data at specific ages, say seven-year-olds. Prevalence of NE at age seven is significant since many children then start school meaning more exposure to the environment and thus a greater awareness of the problem. At this age, the prevalence of nocturnal enuresis seems to be between 7 and 9 per cent (Table 2).

In more detail, the study by Hellström [10] found nocturnal enuresis in 7% of girls (of whom 3% monosymptomatic), and 12% of boys (of whom 7% monosymptomatic). Recent studies on the prevalence of nocturnal enuresis in different parts of the world are summarized in Table 3. In the early ages the prevalence in boys is reported to be higher than in girls by a 2:1 ratio in Western countries. In studies from other countries the figures are more similar in boys and girls, but there is always a predominance of boys. It seems that the sex difference diminishes by age and becomes less visible and less proven among elderly children.

In the French study [15] (Table 3), the severity and consequences of enuresis were studied in a sub-sample of 228 children (out of the 349 who had reported enuresis). In the sub-sample, 66% had more than one wet night per month, 37% more than one wet night per week, and 22% wet the bed every night. Regarding consequences, 42% of the 228 were "bothered a lot" while 15% were "not bothered at all" by their enuresis. In contrast, 92% of the 228 mothers declared that the enuresis had no effect on family life or the child's behaviour at school. Fourteen per cent of mothers punished their child and only 13% intended to seek treatment for their child. The study from The Netherlands [18] (Table 3) reported that the prevalence of enuresis was higher in the Turkish/Moroccan ethnic group (14%) than in Dutch children (6%), and higher in children in special education (especially mentally retarded, 14%) than in children in mainstream education (6%).

Even if there are some ethnic and cultural differences of enuresis prevalence, with higher rates generally reported from Eastern countries, there is nonetheless a remarkable similarity of prevalence rates of nocturnal enuresis in populations from all parts of the world.

3. Potential risk factors of nocturnal enuresis

Several risk factors have been established or suggested by epidemiological studies, the most important will be discussed here (Table 4).

a) Family history

Nocturnal enuresis is a hereditary disorder. The mode of inheritance is autosomal dominant so if both parents were enuretic as children, the risk for their offspring is 77%, while if only one parent had NE, the risk is about 45%. In the Italian study by Chiozza [17], the odds ratio was highly significant for a family history of NE in

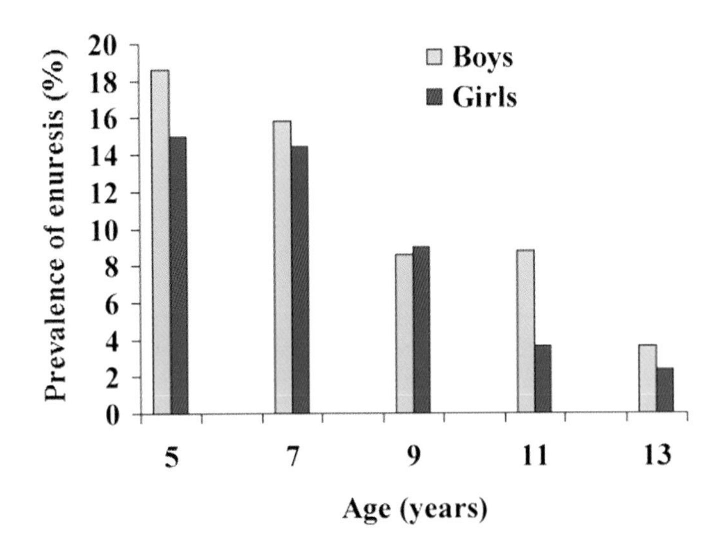

Figure 1 : Prevalence of enuresis, primary and secondary combined, for boys and girls separately. Data from [27] with permission. Comment: The prevalence in this study is higher than in most studies and the sex difference is less

Table 2 : Prevalence (% and 95% CI) of nocturnal enuresis at age seven. Results from two cross-sectional studies from Nordic countries, Hellström [10] and Järvelin [11], and one longitudinal study by Fergusson [9] from New Zealand. (Cited from Krantz et al [6]).

Author	Study period	Prevalence (% and 95% CI)
Hellström	1982	9.5 (8.5; 10.5)
Järvelin	1984	6.4 (5.3; 7.3)
Fergusson	1977-85	10.3 (8.3; 12.3)

Table 3 : Prevalence of nocturnal enuresis in recent studies. NE: Nocturnal enuresis, bedwetting. PMNE: Primary monosymptomatic nocturnal enuresis

Author	Year	Ref	Definition	Sample	Age	Prevalence (%)
Swithinbank	1994	[12]	>once/3 months	1 176	11-12	6 (boys), 4 (girls)
Bower	1996	[13]	once/month	2 292	5-12	19
Watanabe	1994	[14]	PMNE		7	15 (boys), 8 (girls)
Lottmann	1999	[15]	all NE	3 803	5-10 5-7	9 11
Nevéus	1999	[16]	once/month	1 413	6-10	8
Chiozza	1998	[17]	all NE	6 892	6-14	4
				674	7	8 (boys), 6 (girls)
Van der Wekke	1998	[18]	all NE	5 630	5-15 7-9 13-15	6 8 1
Serel	1997	[19]	all NE	5 523	7-12 7	14 (boys), 8 (girls) 16 (boys), 15 (girls)
Gümüs	1999	[20]	all NE	1 703	7-11	17 (boys), 11 (girls)
Kalo	1996	[21]	all NE	740	6-16 7	16 (boys), 14 (girls) 10 (boys), 14 (girls)
Lee	2000	[22]	all NE	7 012	7-12 7	9 14
Yeung	1997	[23]	all NE		3 521	4-12 4 7 5 (boys), 0.5 (girls)

Table 4 : Risk factors reviewed in this text

Nocturnal enuresis
Family history
Behavioural disturbances
Nocturnal polyuria
Sleep and arousal
Nocturnal bladder dysfunction
Other factors
Day and day/night wetting
Family history
Psychological disorders and sexual abuse
Disorders of bladder-sphincter nerve control
Urinary tract infections
Infravesical obstruction
Epispadias

siblings (3.1, 95% CI 1.8-5.6). By molecular genetic methods foci have been found on chromosomes 13, 12, 8, and 22 [24, 25]. A picture of pronounced heterogeneity of both genotype and phenotype is emanating [26]. The etiology of NE is thus characterized by a complex interaction of genetic and environmental factors.

b) Behavioural disturbances

Behavioural disturbances were for a long time thought to be associated with NE. Children with *secondary* enuresis may be more inclined to have associated mental health disorders later in adolescence. It is this group who might benefit from thorough assessment of any underlying emotional disturbance or psychopathology. A lack of association between *primary* NE and psychopathology in later childhood and adolescence was reported in 1990 by Feehan et al. [27] which seemed to confirm similar findings in an eight year follow-up study published in 1986 by Fergusson et al. [9]. But while it seems clear that psychopathology is not, with few exceptions, the *cause of* primary NE, evidence is accumulating that psychological consequences *caused by* enuresis should not be underestimated [28-30].

c) Nocturnal polyuria

In 1985, a virtual absence of day/night variation of vasopressin accompanied by nocturnal polyuria was found in children with NE [31]. For the first time, a coherent physiological explanation for NE, or at least a large part of the NE population, had been presented. Currently, there is a consensus that nocturnal polyuria is an important pathogenetic factor in two thirds of NE patients (those are the patients responding to desmopressin, DDAVP) while most of the remaining third have inadequate nocturnal bladder storage.

d) Sleep and arousal

Known physiological factors cannot explain why the enuretic child does not wake up to the sensation of a full or contracting bladder. Parents have expressed that enuretic children are very difficult to arouse or rather, as the parents put it, "sleeps very deeply". Some recent studies seem to support the parents' view. By using auditory signals [32], computerized EEG analysis [33], or enquiries [16], a defect in arousal has been largely validated. In the study by Nevéus, odds ratios were significantly high for high arousal threshold (2.7), pavor nocturnus (2.4), and confusion when awoken from sleep (3.4). Computerized EEG energy analysis has indicated both greater depth of sleep and impaired arousal in enuretics [34].

e) Nocturnal bladder dysfunction

Although bladder function in NE has been considered normal in many studies in the past, evidence about the bladder's pathophysiological role for NE has accumulated during recent years. As many as one third of all enuretic children may have a nocturnal detrusor overactivity. Especially non-polyuric bedwetters, those who do not respond to desmopressin, should be suspected to have a malfunctioning bladder with reduced capacity.

In this context it is interesting to note that there seems to be an association between childhood NE and adult detrusor overactivity. People with a past history of NE have a greater risk of bladder dysfunction developing in, *or remaining into,* adult life. In a random cross-section of 2613 women 30-59 years of age, 17% reported incontinence. Childhood bedwetting was associated with a prevalence of urge incontinence with odds ratios between 1.8 and 2.2 depending on the age at which dryness was achieved [35]. In another retrospective study of 1000 urodynamic records on 500 men and 500 women, 10% of the men had idiopathic detrusor instability of whom 63% had a past history of NE, while 29% of the women had detrusor instability of whom 38% had a past history of NE beyond the age of 6 [36]. The difference between men and women may reflect the gender difference in childhood bedwetting.

f) Other risk factors for nocturnal enuresis

Sleep apnoea has been associated with enuresis in some patients [37]. *Upper airway obstruction* also seems to be a cause of NE, since it is not uncommon for enuretic children to have their NE resolved after removal of large adenoids or tonsils. One study reports significant decrease or complete cure of NE in 87 (76%) of 115 enuretic children (of whom 103 with primary NE) after surgical removal of upper airway obstruction [38]. *Constipation* may cause secondary NE or make primary NE persist [39]. The important implication is that constipation has to be identified and treated in every child with NE. The polyuria in *diabetes mellitus and insipidus* increases the risk for NE which is most often of the secondary type. Children with *minor neurological dysfunction* are more vulnerable to NE, particularly if belonging to a lower social class [40]. Children *with attention deficit hyperactivity disorders (ADHD)* are 2.7 times more likely to have enuresis than the general child population [41]. Regrettably, *sexual abuse* must nowadays also count among factors that may lead to NE (most often secondary and non-monosymptomatic). A strong suspicion would prompt full investigation [42].

In addition, children with *urinary tract infection, infravesical obstruction, neuropathic bladder, psychiatric disorders*, and other conditions may be wetting their beds. Their nocturnal incontinence is, however, with very few exceptions combined with daytime symptoms, in particular daywetting. Primary monosymptomatic NE with bedwetting as the *one and only* symptom, is a well circumscribed condition that should be identified when present, thus avoiding clinical confusion generated by the huge array of childhood disorders that may have bedwetting as *one* of several symptoms.

4. Long term outcome of nocturnal enuresis

a) Remission and natural history

Longitudinal studies on the natural history of enuresis are no longer possible to perform since a large part of enuretic children receive treatment. Previous studies have confirmed the common knowledge that most children who are enuretic eventually become dry at night. The spontaneous cure rate was 14% annually between the ages of 5 and 9, 16% between 10 and 14, and 16% in the 15 to 19 year old group in the study by Forsythe and Redmond [43]. In their group there remained 33 patients who were still bedwetting at the age of more than 20 years (3%). Similar rates of prevalence relating to age were noted by Feehan et al. [27].

b) Prevalence of nocturnal enuresis in adults

The first really reliable epidemiological study on enuresis in adults in a randomly selected sample was performed in The Netherlands in 1996 [44]. To the question "Did you wet your bed at least once during the past 4 weeks?" 57 of 11 406 respondents answered "yes", thus giving an overall enuresis prevalence of 0.5%. There was no significant difference between age groups. Primary NE was reported by 50% of the men and 19% of the women, the rest had secondary enuresis.

c) Long term follow-up studies

Ten years after evaluating 3556 seven-year-olds [10], a randomly selected subsample was reinvestigated [45]. In addition, 452 teenagers out of the 461 in the original cohort who had reported symptoms (imperative urge, day wetting, emptying difficulties, or bedwetting) were contacted. Bedwetting which had been reported by 12% of boys and 7% of girls aged 7 had decreased to only one girl (0.3%) still wetting at least once a month in the randomized group, and 1 boy (0.5%) and 2 girls (1%) still wetting in the symptomatic group. Almost all of the enuretic children had received treatment starting around 7-8 years of age. Swithinbank et al found a similar decline of prevalence of NE when they investigated the original cohort of 11-12-year-old schoolchildren again at 15-16 years [12]. Nocturnal enuresis was reported by 5% of children at 11-12 years but only 1% at 15-16 years. A Finnish study [30] looked at 501 14-year-olds who had reported NE at age 8 in an original study of 5603 children. At age 14, only 16 adolescents remained enuretic (0.3% of the original total sample).

The enuresis prevalence of 0.5% in otherwise healthy adults in the Dutch study [44] refers to a largely untreated population. Fifty percent of the men had primary enuresis so they had never been consistently dry at night. Assuming a prevalence of enuresis of 8% in 7-year-old boys, this could be translated to mean that the risk for an enuretic boy to remain enuretic for the rest of his life is 3% if he does not receive active treatment during childhood. Three per cent equals the prevalence found in patients after the age of 20 years in the study by Forsythe and Redmond [43] and in the Finnish 14-year-olds [30]. It is still not clear whether active treatment of NE in childhood is able to reduce the number of adult enuretics.

5. Prevalence of day wetting, and day/night wetting

Diurnal UI as well as combined diurnal and nocturnal UI will here be reported as two manifestations of the same basic disorder; *overactive bladder* (urgency, frequency and urge incontinence). A few children have a clinical picture resembling the detrusor-sphincter dyssynergia of the neuropathic bladder, but without a neurological malformation or disease, this condition is termed *non-neuropathic bladder-sphincter dysfunction* (NNBSD) or in short *dysfunctional voiding* [46].

a) Prevalence in survey studies

Compared to nocturnal enuresis, the prevalence of diurnal or combined diurnal and nocturnal incontinence in childhood has not been extensively studied. No true longitudinal cohort studies have been published.

Prevalence of diurnal or combined diurnal and nocturnal incontinence has been reported in a few cross-sectional studies (Table 5). Diurnal or combined diurnal and nocturnal UI at least once a week seems to occur in about 2-4% of 7-year old children and is more common in girls than in boys.

6. Potential risk factors of day and day/night wetting

a) Family history

Day wetting seems to be more common in children of mothers who had diurnal UI themselves. This clinical impression has not been the object of epidemiological research. But Chiozza et al. [17] found that the highest risk for familiality of enuresis was shown by *non-monosymptomatic* NE (with diurnal frequency and urgency; OR 12.3), suggesting a hereditary background not only for bedwetting itself but also for associated bladder overactivity.

b) Psychological disorders and sexual abuse

Children in stress or with mental disorders have a higher incidence of diurnal UI as well as NE, mostly of the secondary type [48]. A special case is the rare disorder of *diurnal enuresis* which is the only kind of diurnal UI which takes place as a complete, incontinent micturition. Sexual abuse may also lead to secondary day wetting.

c) Disorders of bladder-sphincter nerve control

With few exceptions, children with *myelomeningocele* have neuropathic bladder-sphincter dysfunction with UI due to detrusor hyperreflexia and/or sphincter denervation. Skin-covered *occult spinal dysraphism* may be mistaken for non-neuropathic dysfunctional bladder. At least half of the children with *spastic cerebral palsy* have clinically silent bladder dysfunction. *Nerves* in the pelvic area may be injured by trauma such as pelvic fractures, but more common is iatrogenic trauma during surgery for imperforate anus or pelvic tumors.

d) Urinary tract infections (UTI)

Regular and complete voidings are the most efficient way to prevent urinary infection. A bacterial cystitis induces temporary detrusor overactivity. Thus, bladder dysfunction may cause UTI, and UTI may cause bladder dysfunction. The UTI may be asymptomatic. Girls with asymptomatic bacteriuria (ABU) have symptoms of an overactive bladder, such as urgency and diurnal UI, in a high percentage [49].

e) Infravesical obstruction

Boys born with posterior urethral valves are incontinent in about 20% on long-term follow up after surgical treatment [50].

f) Epispadias

Epispadias may include a malformation of the sphincter resulting in constantly dribbling UI.

7. Long term outcome of day and day/night wetting

a) Epidemiology of dryness in the day

Few studies recount the prevalence of daytime dryness. In Minnesota, 60% of children were dry in the day at two and a half years of age. Between 4 and 5 years of age, 92-95% of children in Sweden, The Netherlands and USA were dry in the day. Corresponding figures for the age group between 5 and 6 years were 95-96%, and

Table 5 : Prevalence of diurnal or combined diurnal and nocturnal UI. NNBSD: Dysfunctional voiding (see text)

Author, year	Ref	Definition	Age	Prevalence (%)
Hellstrøm 1982	[10]	Once a week Day wetting only NNBSD	7	2.1 (boys), 3.1 (girls) 0.5 (boys), 1.1 (girls) 1.0 (boys), 2.0 (girls)
Järvelin 1984	[11]	Isolated diurnal UI Diurnal/nocturnal	7	1.8 1.6
Bloom 1993	[47]	Once in 2 weeks	6-8	9.0
Neveus 1999	[16]	Diurnal UI only	6-11	4.4
Swithinbank 1994	[8]	Diurnal UI	11-12	0.2 (boys), 0.9 (girls)
Lee 2000	[22]	Diurnal UI	7-12 7	2.2 3.9
		Diurnal/nocturnal	 7	1.4 2.8

94-97 for the age group between 6 and 7 years [51]. It thus seems that children who are and remain dry in the day attain their diurnal continence already between 4-5 years of age.

b) Long term follow-up studies

Hellström et al found day wetting at least once a week at age 17 in 0.2% of boys and 0.7% of girls and as compared to 2.1% and 3.1%, respectively, at age 7 years [45]. Swithinbank et al had found a prevalence of day wetting (including also "occasional" wetting) in 12.5% in children at age 10-11 years declining to 3.0% at age 15-16 years [12]. Based on these, it seems that the prevalence of all kinds of diurnal UI will diminish with 1-2% per year of life from age 10-11 to age 15-16 years, while diurnal UI at least once a week seems to diminish with 0.2% per year of life from age 7 to age 17 years. Because of treatment the studies may not recount the true natural history.

Summary points

Nocturnal enuresis

- Primary enuresis refers to bedwetting occurring without a dry continence break of more than 6 months. Secondary enuresis refers to recurrence after a longer interval of dryness. Most epidemiological studies in the past have unfortunately combined primary and secondary enuresis together. Equally, the majority of previous studies have not kept monosymptomatic (no daytime symptoms) apart from non-monosymptomatic NE.
- The prevalence of nocturnal enuresis at age 7 in Western countries seems to be around 8%, and in an largely untreated adult population 0.5%.
- Primary nocturnal enuresis usually remits with age. The spontaneous cure rate seems to be around 15% annually between the ages of 5 and 19.
- The risk for an enuretic 7-year-old boy to remain enuretic throughout life may be calculated to 3%.
- Potential risk factors for enuresis in children reviewed in this test include family history, behavioural disturbances, nocturnal polyuria, sleep and arousal, nocturnal bladder dysfunction, sleep apnoea and upper airway obstruction, constipation, diabetes, minor neurological dysfunction and ADHD, and sexual abuse.
- It seems clear that psychopathology is not the *cause of* primary NE, while evidence is accumulating that NE has psychological consequences.
- Nocturnal polyuria seems to be the major pathogenetic factor in 2/3 of bedwetting children (those responding to antidiuretic treatment with desmopressin), while NE in the remaining third seems to be caused by bladder dysfunction that may occur only during sleep.
- There is some evidence that people with a past history of enuresis have a greater risk of bladder dysfunction developing in, or remaining into, adult life.

Day and day/night wetting

- Children who are and remain dry in the day seem to attain their diurnal continence already between 4-5 years of age.
- Diurnal UI, or combined diurnal and nocturnal UI, in children is caused by overactive bladder in the great majority of cases.
- Potential risk factors for diurnal UI in children include family history, psychological disorders, disorders of bladder-sphincter nerve control, urinary tract infections, infravesical obstruction, epispadias, and sexual abuse.
- The prevalence of diurnal UI at least once a week at age 7 seems to be around 2-4%, declining with about 0.2% per additional year of life.
- More research is needed in order to elucidate the epidemiology and genetics of childhood diurnal UI and its association with bladder dysfunction.

IV. EPIDEMIOLOGY OF UI IN WOMEN

1. PREVALENCE

A large number of epidemiological studies of UI in women have been published. Some cover a wide age span while others are surveys of a single age cohort or specific group like pregnant women. Differences in sample, definition and measurement, and survey methodology continue to make reviews challenging. Table 6 lists some of the prevalence figures reported for women sampled from community-residing populations, showing widely varying estimates. Several reviews of epidemiologic studies of UI are available, including some quite recent ones [52-58].

More epidemiologic research is available on older women of all ages because UI is considered to be a health condition of older age. A 1988 review of several European and American epidemiologic studies of older women living in the community identified a 10-40 %

Table 6 : Examples of prevalance of any UI in studies of women living in the community

First author	Ref	Year	N	Age	Prevalence (%)
Yarnell	[59]	1981	1 000	17+	45
Holst	[60]	1988	851	18+	31
Sommer	[61]	1990	414	20-79	40
Brocklehurst	[62]	1993	2 124	30+	9
Sandvik	[63]	1993	1 820	20+	29
Swithinbank	[64]	1999	2 075	18+	69
Hannestad	[65]	2000	27 936	20+	25
Temml	[66]	2000	1 262	20+	26
Bartolotti	[67]	2000	5 488	40+	11
Moller	[68]	2000	2 860	40-60	72

range of prevalence estimates of the experience of any UI and suggested a UI prevalence of 40% [55]. More recent reviews [56-58] that summarize the literature through about 1997 confirm this or even a wider range of prevalences and continue to suggest that the wide range can be attributed to the definition of UI and the sample [58] and potentially to the format of the questions about UI [55, 57]. Since these recent reviews several additional studies have been published on the prevalence of UI among older women [65-67, 69-73]. But again, a range of prevalence between 10 and 40% or even wider remains a reasonable estimate. Table 7 lists specific prevalence estimates of any urinary incontinence among older women living in the community.

The prevalence of any UI by age is addressed by several of these studies. In our previous report [1] we described the general finding of higher prevalence estimates in older ages. We also noted the intriguing suggestion of an early prevalence peak in midlife and then a steady increase among the aged. A recent study by Hannestad and her colleagues [65] of women of all ages examplifies this latter pattern. The study finds a gradual increase of prevalences across adulthood until age 50 when prevalence reaches 30%, a stabilization or even slight decline until age 70 when prevalences start rising again (Fig 2).

Prevalence has always been higher in institutions because residents in institutions tend to be older and more impaired than commuity residing women. A recent review [56] suggests a range from 6 to 72% of institutional prevalences. Several recent studies from around the world [80-87] — some of which use samples of institutions rather than individual institutions — suggest prevalences of 50% or higher.

The range of prevalences in institutions is likely a consequence of the definition and admission criteria of residential care which vary throughout the world. In Australia, for instance, they covers the spectrum from requiring very low levels of supportive care to the highest levels of assistance as found in most high level nursing homes in other countries of the world. And even within a given country definition and criteria vary from city to city and facility to facility. For this reason it is important to sample residential care facilities in the same fashion as individuals in order to obtain representative results about prevalences in such facilities.

The process underlying the relatively high prevalences in residential care facilities remains somewhat less clear. A Canadian study [77] documented a statistically nonsignificant odds ratio of 1.4 for UI among women in institutions compared to community living women after statistically controlling for age, dementia and ambulatory function. Thom and co-workers showed that existing urinary incontinence increases the risk of subsequent hospitalisation and substantially increases the risk of admission into nursing homes, independent of age, gender or the presence of any co-morbid condition [88] These investigators demonstrated that the relative risk of admission to a nursing home was two times greater for incontinent women and 3.2 times greater for incontinent men after adjustment for age, cohort factors and comorbid conditions. These findings as well as others suggest that incontinence may be a contributing factor to institutionalization. However, at this point an alternative explanation of residential care contributing in some way to the development of incontinence cannot be excluded with confidence.

2. Type

In surveys based on questionnaires or interviews only *symptoms* can be registered. Typically stress incontinence is identified when the respondent reports it to

Table 7 : Examples of prevalence of any UI in studies of older women living in the community

First author	Ref	Year	N	Age	Prevalence (%)
Yarnell	[59]	1981	1 060	65+	50
Diokno	[74]	1986	1 150	60+	38
Molander	[75]	1990	4 206	70-90	17
Sandvik	[63]	1993	1 820	60+	32
Brocklehurst	[62]	1993	840	60+	12
Holtedahl	[76]	1998	507	60-74	47
Hunskaar	[77]	1998	1 876	65+	17
Roberts	[78]	1998	762	50+	58
Chiarelli	[79]	1999	12 417	70-75	35
Iglesias	[70]	2000	486	65+	42
Maggi	[71]	2001	1 531	65+	22

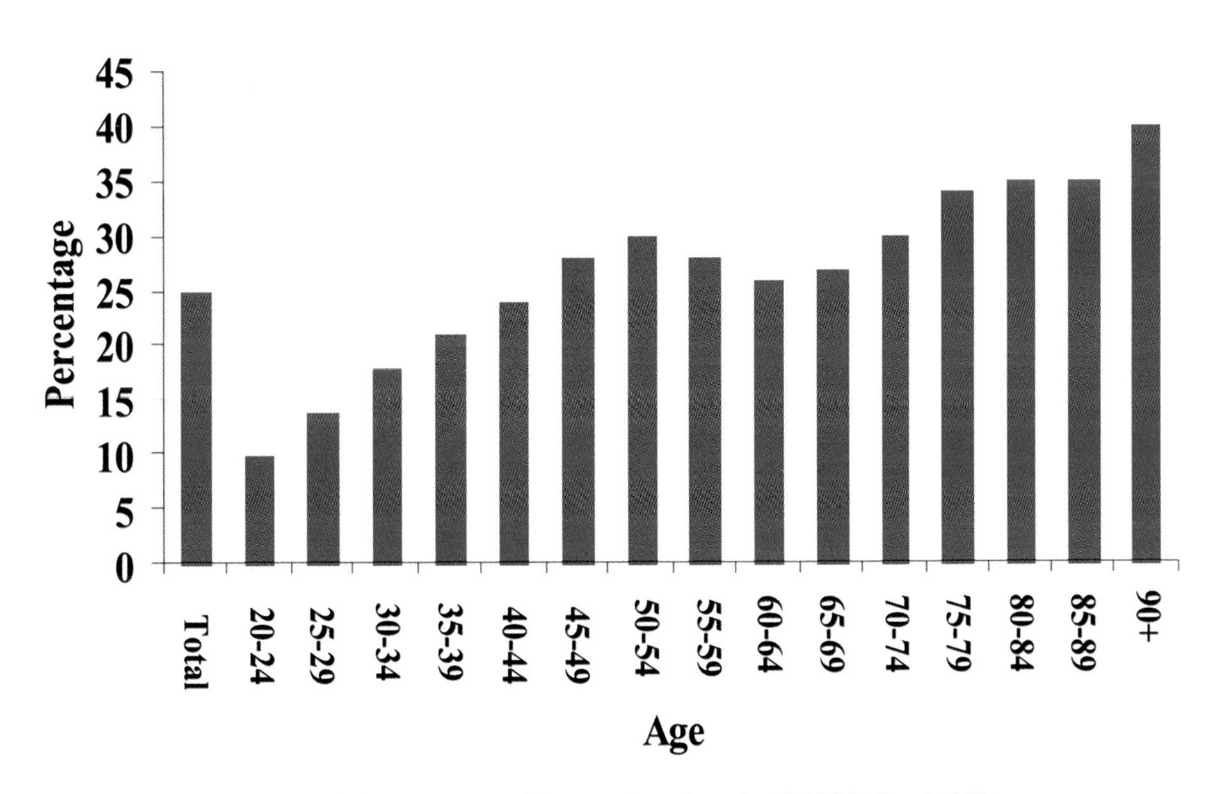

Figure 2 : Prevalence of UI (any leakage) in women 20 years+. Data from the EPINCONT study [65]

occur with physical activity, urge incontinence when it occurs in the context of a sudden urge to urinate. Diagnoses such as motor urge incontinence or genuine stress incontinence require the use of urodynamic equipment and thus cannot be made based on data from questionnaires or interviews alone.

Several authors have reported the relative proportions of stress, urge, and mixed symptoms. A few authors reported stress and urge separately without a mixed category. In Table 8 the distribution of UI types are shown, as they are found in some surveys. Overall, approximately half of all incontinent women are classified as stress incontinent, the highest proportion among urge, mixed, and stress types. A smaller proportion is classified as mixed incontinent, the smallest one as urge incontinent. The recent NOBLE telephone survey found an overall prevalence of overactive bladder with urge incontinence of 9.6% in women 18+, increasing with age from less than 5% in age group 18-44 to 19% in age group 65+ [97].

Proportions of types of UI differ by age. A survey of older women suggests that mixed incontinence predominates [74]. A survey of young and middle-aged women suggests that pure stress incontinence predominates in that age group [96]. A recent study which includes the entire age range by Hannested et al. [65] demonstrates a fairly regular increase in prevalence of mixed incontinence across the age range, and a regular decrease in prevalence of stress incontinence (Fig 3). The question has been raised about the use of self reports in epidemiological studies, and low accuracy has been found [98]. Sandvik and coauthors [95] validated diagnostic questions used in a survey against a final diagnosis made by a gynecologist after urodynamic evaluation. After using the validity (sensitivity and specificity) as basis for correcting the type distribution, the percentage of stress incontinence increased from 51 to 77 %, mixed incontinence was reduced from 39 to 11% and urge incontinence increased from 10 to 12 %. The authors warn that mixed incontinence may be overreported in epidemiological surveys, and that correction for validity indicates that a larger majority of women than hitherto reported may have pure stress incontinence. However, there are also some limitations in the use of urodynamics in documentating the presence of involuntary detrusor contractions, with both false positives and false negatives occurring. Therefore the use of urodynamic testing as a gold standard may not be entirely appropriate in establishing the true prevalence of the different types, especially urge incontinence.

Unfortunately, not all studies have carefully assessed the different types (and even fewer have examined their correlates). Therefore, proportions of stress, urge and mixed types among women are difficult to estimate and estimates vary considerably. But there are intriguing differences between the different types suggesting that the types may reflect quite different pathologies and that differentiating the types in future research might prove very fruitful.

3. Severity

Most studies have operationalized the measurement of severe incontinence by measuring frequency of urine loss. Those reporting weekly or even more frequent loss are typically assigned to the severe category. Fewer studies have also used a quantity measure by asking about amount of loss, dampening of clothes, extra laundry, restrictions in activity, or the use of protective pads. The first approach may be considered a simple attempt to operationalize the frequency of urine loss, the second approach reflects quantity but also perceptional differences, personal hygiene and coping ability. Some studies have explicitly combined a frequency and a quantity measure [63, 74]. Sandvik's Severity index [63, 99] is calculated by multiplying the reported frequency (four levels) by the amount of leakage (dichotomized to two levels). The resulting index value is further categorized into slight, moderate and severe. Typically, slight incontinence denotes leakage of drops a few times a month, moderate incontinence daily leakage of drops, and severe incontinence larger amounts at least once a week. The severity index has been validated against a 48 hour «pad weighing» test. According to this test, slight incontinence means a leakage of 6 g/24 hours (95% CI 2-9), moderate incontinence means a leakage of 17 g/24 hours (95% CI 13-22) and severe incontinence means a leakage of 56 g/24 hours (95% CI 44-67). The severity index is thus a semi-objective and quantitative measure, and does not include the woman`s subjective perception of her leakage as being a problem or not. A recent validation from Scotland concludes that the Severity index is a short, simple, valid, reliable, and sensitive measure of urinary incontinence in women, and that it can be recommended for routine use [100].

It can be shown that the prevalence is dependent on "thresholds" for diagnosis or severity For example, Sandvik [63] found that nearly half of cases were classified as having slight incontinence and only 27 % as severe. The author also investigated the "botherness" factor, and found that different levels of botherness significantly affected the prevalence estimates. If only those with moderate or severe incontinence are considered, and including only those who are bothered by

Table 8 : Relative proportions of different types of UI among women living in the community

First author	Ref	Year	Age	N	Stress (%)	Urge (%)	Mixed (%)
Yarnell	[59]	1981	18+	1 000	49	21	30
Iosif	[89]	1984	61	902	40	27	33
Diokno	[74]	1986	60+	1 955	29	10	61
Hording	[90]	1986	45	515	75	11	14
Holst	[60]	1988	18+	851	52	25	23
Elving	[91]	1989	30-59	2 631	48	7	45
Sommer	[61]	1990	20-79	414	38	33	29
Molander	[75]	1990	70-90	4 206	24	49	27
Burgio	[93]	1991	42-50	541	50	12	38
Harrison	[92]	1994	20+	314	48	9	44
Lara	[94]	1994	18+	556	48	27	21
Sandvik	[95]	1995	20+	1 820	51	10	39
Samuelsson	[96]	1997	20-60	487	68	9	23
Bartolotti	[67]	2000	40+	5 488	61	26	13
Hannestad	[65]	2000	20+	27 936	52	37	11
		Median (range)			**49 (24-75)**	**21 (7-49)**	**29 (11-61)**

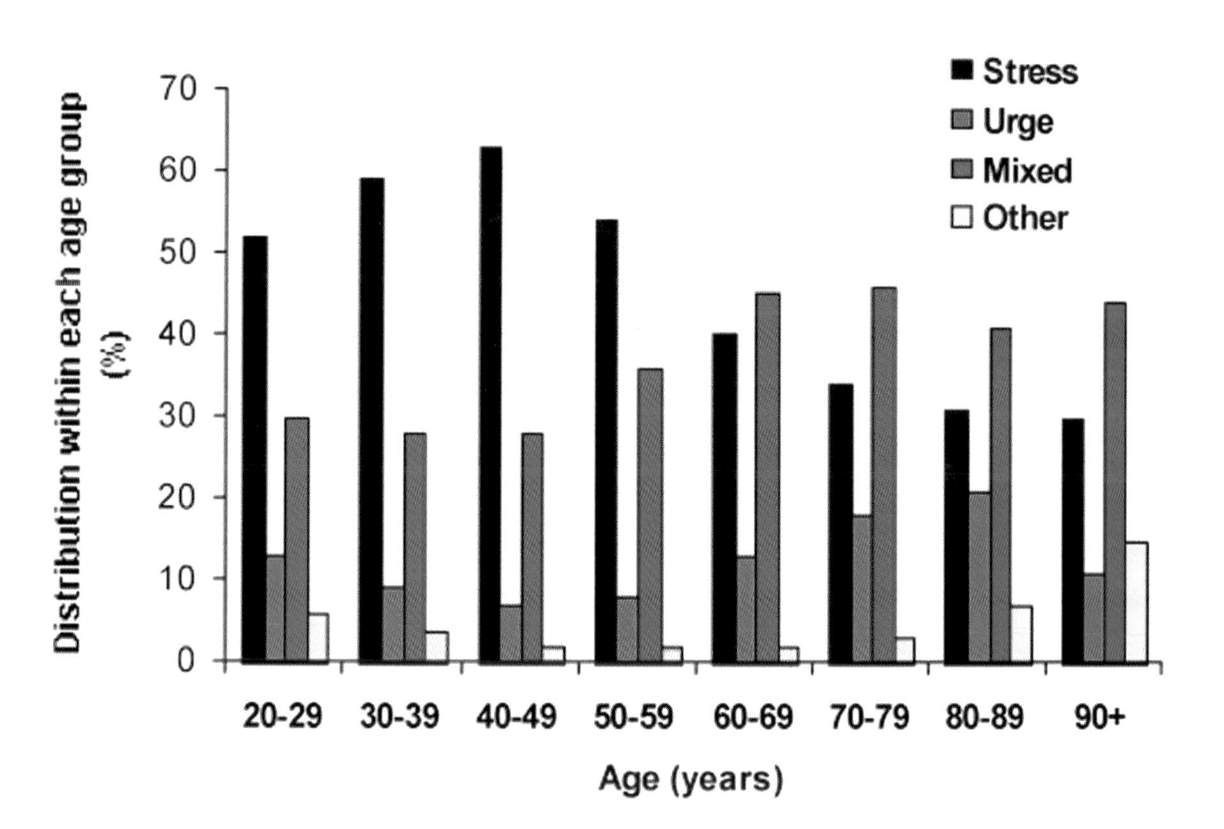

Figure 3 : Distribution of different types of UI in age groups. Data from the EPINCONT study [65]

their leakage, the findings from that study indicate that approximately one fifth of incontinent women suffer from severe incontinence. These results have recently been confirmed in the EPINCONT study [65] (Figure 4 and 5)

The severity of incontinence varies between the different types. The fraction of severe incontinence is much lower in the stress group compared to the urge and mixed groups. In the EPINCONT study [65], slight incontinence was found in 53% in the stress group, 39% in the urge group and 31% in the mixed group (Figure 6). Within each type of incontinence, severity increased with increasing age.

Even though the definition of severe or "significant" UI varies between authors, its prevalence is considerably less variable across different studies than prevalence of any UI. Prevalence estimates range between 3% and 17% (Table 9). The lesser variance among these estimates suggests that severe incontinence is less easy to deny and better understood by participants than "any incontinence" and thus may represent a more reliable figure.

Several studies found that the prevalence of significant incontinence tended to increase with advancing age [59, 61, 65, 70]. In the EPINCONT study the percentages were 2.6, 6.5, 8.6, and 13.0 for age groups 20-39, 40-54, 55-69, and 70+, respectively [65].

In summary, it is quite clear that the prevalence estimates depend on which definition of severity is used. Nevertheless, prevalence estimates of severe or significant UI display a less wide range than any UI, ranging from 3 to 17%, with a cluster between 6-10%. Moreover, it is not well established what level of severity should be regarded as clinically significant and might be indicative for treatment.

4. INCIDENCE, REMISSION AND NATURAL HISTORY

The epidemiological data are sparse about the development or the natural history of UI and its types and severity levels. Data are needed regarding the transition from continence to various levels of severity and type of incontinence.

A few studies have reported on the incidence of UI. A study of community dwelling women aged 60 years or older found that 20% of the originally continent women had developed any UI during the 1-year study period [102]. A cohort of healthy middle aged women was examined over three years [93]. Of the previously continent women 8% reported at least monthly leakage, higher rates have been found in the elderly [103]. Two recent studies of young and middle-aged women reported 1-year incidence rates of 6% and 3% [68, 104].

Likewise, rates of remission (the probability of becoming continent among previously incontinent women) vary considerable across the few studies that have investigated them, ranging over one year between 10% for older women [102], 6% [96] and 38% [68] among middle-aged and younger women. What is very clear from these findings is that substantial incidence rates are paralleled by equally substantial remission rates. It is not clear whether the level of remission reflects active treatment or intervention or whether it is part of the natural course of incontinence. Although questions

Table 9 : The prevalence of "any" and "severe" UI among older women living in the community.

First author	Ref	Year	N	Age	Any UI (%)	Severe UI (%)
Vetter	[101]	1981	1 342	70+	14	5
Diokno	[74]	1986	1 955	60+	38	3
Burgio	[93]	1991	541	42-50	58	17
Brocklehurst	[62]	1993	840	60+	12	8
Sandvik	[63]	1993	1 820	18+	29	6
Hunskaar	[77]	1998	1 876	65+	17	7
Bartolotti	[67]	2000	5 488	40+	11	6
Hannestad	[65]	2000	27 936	20+	25	7
Samuelsson	[96]	2000	487	20-60	28	8
Moller	[68]	2000	2 860	40-60	72	16
Maggi	[71]	2001	1 531	65+	22	11
		Median (range)			**29 (11-72)**	**7 (3-17)**

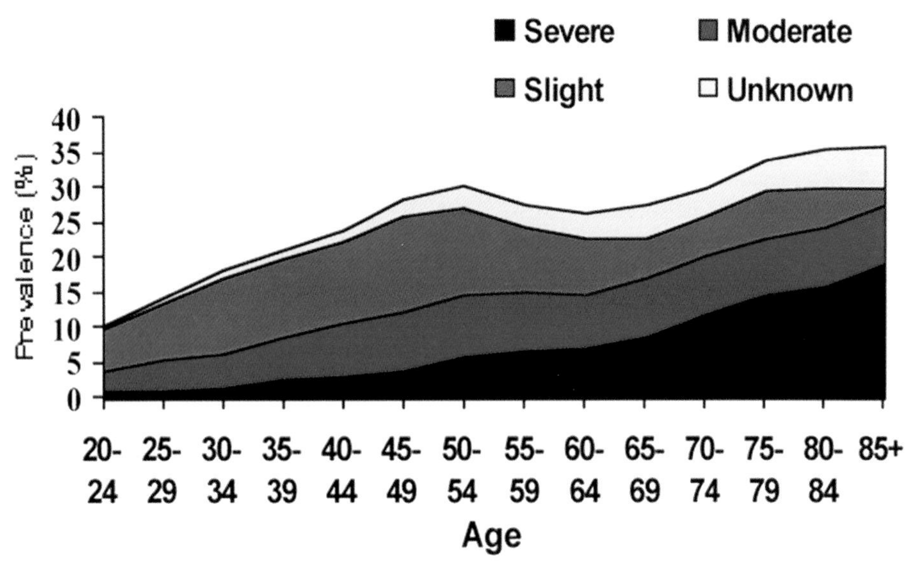

Figure 4 : Prevalence of UI by age group and severity. Data from the EPINCONT study [65]

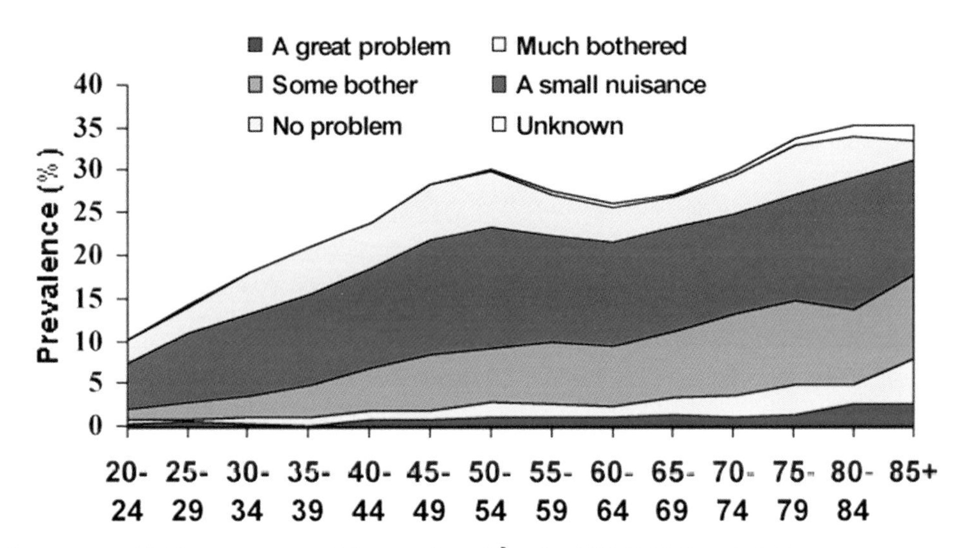

Figure 5 : Prevalence of UI by age group and impact. Data from the EPINCONT study [65]

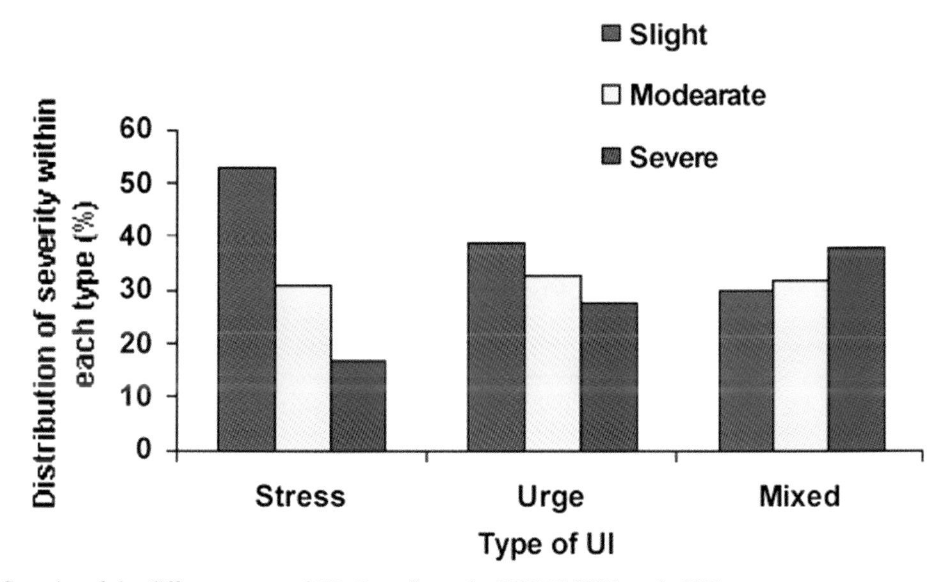

Figure 6 : Severity of the different types of UI. Data from the EPINCONT study [65]

about causal factors had been investigated in the studies, few relevant findings emerged.

In summary, longitudinal studies of incidence, remission and natural history are scarce and should be encouraged because these types of studies provide information about the course of UI and are best suited to investigate its causes and consequences. Incidence rates are not insubstantial, but it has proven difficult to establish predictors for incident UI. It is also well documented that remission can take place, but again predictors are not well understood. Remission may be related to natural recovery or to medical care, but unreliable measurements cannot be excluded either.

5. Racial and ethnic differences

Most epidemiological studies of UI have been conducted on white populations. There are several studies of non-caucasian women showing a wide variation in prevalence [72, 73, 94, 105-112]. The studies have used different methods and definitions, and the quality is heterogenious. Therefore the results are difficult to compare, and most of the studies do not lend themselves easily to crosscultural or crossnational comparisons.

Regarding black women, some data exist, and they provide some evidence that white women may be more susceptible to UI than black women. For example, some early studies examined UI predominately in the black African population. Reports by Heyn's state that black South Africans rarely developed stress incontinence and developed the related disorder of the pelvic floor prolapse at a rate 80 times lower than whites [113, 114]. Later studies of South African women attempted to explain the rarity of stress incontinence among blacks as a function of differing urethral pressures and length as well as pubococcygeal muscle strength [115, 116]. No difference in the prevalence of minor nulliparous stress incontinence among white (46 %), Indian (42 %) and black South African nurses (40 %) was demonstrated. While pelvic floor prolapse has been reported to be exceedingly rare among black South Africans it is the most common indication for major surgery in the Pokot people along the Kenyan Ugandan border [117]. In the US, Howard and her colleagues [118] report clinical data suggesting that African American women have higher uretral closure pressure, larger urethral volume, and greater vesical mobility.

Given the variability in methodology across studies, ideally comparative data are collected on different racial groups using an equivalent methodology. In the United States, the Establish Populations for Epidemiologic Studies of the Elderly reported an equal prevalence of UI among Caucasians and African American women [119]. In contrast Burgio et al. reported significant differences in regular and infrequent incontinence in African American women (18% and 15% respectively) compared to white women (32% and 28%) [93]. However only 51 of 541 women in this study were African American. In a clinical study of patients referred for evaluation of UI or prolapse, Bump and colleagues found that a larger proportion of white than African American women reported symptoms of stress incontinence (31% vs. 7%), and a larger proportion were diagnosed urodynamically as having genuine stress incontinence (61% vs. 27%) [120]. In his report, white women had a prevalence of pure genuine stress incontinence 2.3 times higher than African American women. This difference in physiologic subtypes was supported by a recent presentation of similar studies, confirming a significant difference in the predominance of stress incontinence in the white women [121]. This difference may, however, be explained by racial differences in help seeking behaviour, since it involved clinical groups. Racial differences have also been reported among pregnant women. However, the differences were evident only for stress incontinence and not for urge incontinence or other types of urine leakage [122].

Recently several large population-based studies have reported on differences between African and White American women. Fultz and her colleagues [57] found lower prevalences of urinary incontinence among African than among White Americans in well-controlled analyses; the difference was only reliable for moderate and severe forms of incontinence though. Brown and her colleagues [123, 124] showed lower prevalence of stress and mixed UI among African than White Americans, even after controlling on age and a number of health problems. Thom and his colleagues [125] reported prevalences of general UI to be higher among White Americans and were able to explain the difference by health problems and parturition factors.

In summary, there remains a paucity of information regarding UI in non-caucasian women world wide. The existing comparative data on differences between Caucasian and African American women in the US, although not entirely consistent, suggests higher prevalence of UI among Caucasian women that may be due primarily to racial differences in stress UI and attributable to pelvic and urodynamic features possibly related to childbirth. More needs to be learned about risk factors, whether they operate in a similar fashion within the different races, which ones might be able to explain racial differences, and whether and how the impact of incontinence differs by racial and cultural context.

6. Potential risk factors

Epidemiological studies conducted in various populations reveal a number of variables related to UI including several possible risk factors or contributing variables (Table 10). Most of the data regarding risk factors for the development of UI have been derived from cross sectional studies of volunteer and clinical subjects. Risk factors like smoking, menopause, restricted mobility, chronic cough, chronic straining for constipation, and urogenital surgery have not been as rigorously studied as age, parity, and obesity. This provides us with information of limited generalizability and restricts the level of inference regarding causality.

Well controlled analyses of potential risk factors and predictors are limited. Little is known about their relative and absolute value. Risk factors or causes of UI need to be investigated in a prospective or longitudinal design in order to establish the temporal ordering between risk factors and onset of UI. Unfortunately, very few longitudinal studies of UI have been conducted. Therefore this review of health-related factors is based primarily on cross-sectional studies and can only identify correlates.

Table 10 : Established and suggested risk factors for UI in women reviewed in this text

- Age
- Pregnancy
- Childbirth
- Menopause
- Hysterectomy
- Obesity
- Lower urinary tract symptoms
- Functional impairment
- Cognitive impairment
- Occupational risks
- Family history and genetics
- Other factors

a) Age

Because UI is so common among older women, it is often regarded as a normal and inevitable part of the aging process. Most studies indicate that UI is indeed correlated with age [59, 65, 71, 79, 80, 95, 103, 123, 126-130]. In one well-known study, a random sample of 842 women 17-64 years of age were interviewed [59]. The prevalence rates increased steadily with age. In another large survey, prevalence of UI in women 46-86 years old increased progressively over seven birth cohorts (1900 - 1940) from 12 % to 25 % [127]. More recent studies have yielded similar results in large samples of women. One study of 27,936 women 20+ years of age replicated the significant association between age and incontinence [65] (see Figure 2). Another study found a significant effect for age in a study of 40,155 women in three age groups: young (18 – 23), middle-aged (45 – 50), and older (70 – 75). Though age was significant, there were no differences between the middle-aged and older women [79]. Some studies have also found that age was a significant risk factor for urge incontinence, but not for stress incontinence [103, 123]. Studies that have reported a nonsignificant relationship between incontinence and age generally have had smaller sample size and more narrow age range perhaps restricting the ability to detect this effect [58, 76, 78].

Incontinence is not to be considered normal with aging; however, there are changes in the bladder and the pelvic structures that occur with age and which can contribute to UI [131, 132]. Further, UI is often attributable to medical problems or diseases that can disrupt the mechanisms of continence (e.g., diabetes mellitus), many of which are more common among older adults.

b) Pregnancy

UI in women is often assumed to be attributable to the effects of pregnancy and childbirth. The literature shows that UI is a more common occurrence among pregnant women compared with other groups of women. Prevalence rates of 31 % and 60 % have been reported [122, 133]. UI during pregnancy is a self-limiting condition for most women. Viktrup et al found a prevalence rate of 28% who developed stress incontinence during pregnancy, and 16% became free of symptoms in the puerperium [134]. However, there is some speculation that women who are incontinent during pregnancy may be predisposed to experiencing UI at later times in their lives, such as during a subsequent pregnancy, or as they age.

It is still questionable whether pregnancy itself is a risk factor for UI in later life or if it is the vaginal delivery that is the main risk factor. Iosif et al found a prevalence of 9% of persisting stress UI after cesarean deliveries [135]. Viktrup et al compared continent women having delivered vaginally with women who underwent a cesarean section and found a difference in favour of cesarean. However, three months after delivery, the difference became statistically insignificant [134].

c) Childbirth

The role of childbearing in predisposing women to UI is supported by several studies that have demonstrated a link between UI and parity [61, 91, 92, 122, 128, 136-139]. There are several explanations that may be offered [140]. First, childbirth may result in pelvic floor laxity as a consequence of weakening and stretching of the muscles and connective tissue during delivery. Second, damage may occur as a result of spontaneous lacerations and episiotomies during delivery. The result of these events can be impaired support of the pelvic organs and alteration in their positions. A third possibility is that the stretching of the pelvic tissues during vaginal delivery may damage the pudendal and pelvic nerves, as well as the muscles and connective tissue of the pelvic floor, and can interfere with the ability of the striated urethral sphincter to contract promptly and efficiently in response to increases in intra-abdominal pressure or detrusor contractions.

The evidence for the relationship between childbearing and UI is presented in several studies. For example, Thomas and colleagues reported that UI was most likely to occur in parous rather than nulliparous women at all ages (15-64 years) [141]. Furthermore, UI was most common in women who had four or more children. Others have found a threshold at one delivery [142-144]. Holst and Wilson found that UI was less common in nulliparous women but found no association with rates of UI and increasing parity [60]. However, Samuelsson et al and Jolleys suggested that the relationship between increasing rates of UI and increasing parity was linear [136, 145]. In addition, pregnant women with UI have been found in one study to have a history of more pregnancies and more births than pregnant women who were continent [122]. Vaginal delivery in particular is believed to cause pelvic neuropathy that could instigate UI [143, 146, 147].

Only 3% of women were found to have troublesome stress incontinence one year after their first vaginal birth [134]. This association between childbirth and UI diminishes with age. Foldspang found that although parity was a risk for stress incontinence, the effect decreased with age [139]. Two studies of middle-aged women have found no association between parity and UI. Hording and colleagues found that frequency of UI in 45-year-old women was not associated with frequency of births [90]. Similarly, Burgio and colleagues found that healthy perimenopausal women with UI were not any more likely to have delivered more children than continent women [93].

Until recently age as a confounder has been little focused upon when studying parity and UI. A huge study in Australia found that parity was strongly associated with UI for young women (18-23 years). For women 45-50 years there was only a modest association, and for old women (70-75 years) the association disappeared [79]. Similar results were found in a Norwegian study [144]. Nevertheless, the literature shows that age is a stronger risk factor than parity

Also there has been done little research whether time since delivery or age at delivery will influence the effect of parity. Foldspang et al found increased risk of UI with increasing age at the last childbirth for women aged 30-44 years [139]. One study found that women over 30 years old at their first delivery were at higher risk [143], while another found that increasing age at the first delivery had an influence on UI [148].

The effect of parity on the severity of UI has been little investigated. Kuh et al found a statistically significant trend for increasing severity with increasing parity [143], while Rortveit et al found no effect on severity [144]. Generally, stress UI is believed to be the incontinence type associated with parity. Kuh et al have showed such an association, but they could not find an association between urge type and parity [143].

Several obstetric factors have been explored as possible contributors to the development of incontinence. Evidence has emerged that vaginal delivery may predispose a woman to incontinence, more so than a Cesarean section. One study of incontinence in pregnancy investigated the role of prior deliveries and found that having had a prior vaginal delivery increased by 5.7 the risk of incontinence in a subsequent pregnancy compared to having no prior deliveries, but having had a Cesarean section did not increase the risk [149]. Similarly, vaginal delivery at older ages (> 30) were associated with increased risk of stress incontinence (OR=3.1) in one investigation [143]. However, Cesarean section carried an increased risk of 1.7 and there were too few respondents to make a valid comparison.

Data on other obstetric techniques and complications are inconsistent. Thom and colleagues [125] found an increased risk of UI with increased exposures to oxytocin (OR = 1.9 for one exposure, 3.1 for two exposures). Foldspang et al [129] found strong associations between incontinence and forceps delivery/vacuum extraction, episiotomy, and perineal suturing in bivariate analyses. However, the effects of these variables were insignificant in multivariate analyses possibly suggesting that they may simply have been markers for having had a vaginal delivery. In one study, 11 obstetric variables were explored [149]. Only birthweight > 4,000g and mediolateral episiotomy were associated with incontinence in subsequent pregnancy (OR=1.9 and 1.9). All other variables including perineal laceration, vaginal laceration, vacuum extraction, oxytocin stimulation, and length of 2nd stage labor were not significant. Other studies have reported no relationship between incontinence and a number of obstetric variables, including episiotomy, sphincter lesion, forceps delivery, lacerations, epidural anesthesia, long labor, and fetal birth weight [125, 145, 150, 151].

Vesico-vaginal fistula is an important cause of disastrous UI in developing countries, usually due to obstetric trauma [152]. Differences in birthing practices world wide (including route of delivery and availability of obstetric care) should be investigated to determine potential relationship to continence status.

d) Menopause

Clinically, it has long been understood that urinary symptoms are an integral part of the transition from the premenopausal to the post-menopausal state. The atrophic changes increase susceptibility to urinary tract infections and can cause storage symptoms (such as urinary frequency and urgency), dysuria, vaginal dryness, and dyspareunia. Given the evidence that atrophy of these tissues can be reversed with estrogen, and that estrogen replacement reduces UI in some cases, it seems reasonable to propose that estrogen loss contributes to the problem.

However, the literature is inconsistent in describing the role of menopause and estrogen loss as significant contributors to UI. Positive findings were reported by Rekers and colleagues, who compared premenopausal women (N=355) with postmenopausal women (N=858) and found no significant difference in the prevalence of UI between the two groups (25% versus 26%) [126]. However, there were significant differences in the frequency of incontinence episodes, indicating that postmenopausal women had more severe incontinence. Postmenopausal women were more likely to have UI on a daily basis or more frequently (7 %), compared to the premenopausal women (3 %). They were also much more likely to have urgency and nocturia. Postmenopausal women were less likely, however, to have large volume accidents, and there were no differences in the types of UI. These investigators also examined the time frame between menopause and the onset of UI. A significant increase in the incidence of UI occurred 10 years before the menopause, and an even larger increase was found at menopause. Among postmenopausal women with UI, 28% had onset before menopause, 18% around the time of menopause, and 54 % after menopause. Finally, women who experienced a surgical menopause had a higher rate of UI (36 %) compared to those who experienced a natural menopause (22 %).

Other studies have found no significant differences between postmenopausal and premenopausal women in the prevalence or the frequency of incontinence [89; 130, 143]. Some studies have even reported significantly lower prevalence rates among postmenopausal women than among premenopausal women [92, 136, 143], though in one, the effect was significant for stress incontinence but not for urge incontinence [143]. Further, recent studies of risk factors have found that incontinence is not associated with the number of years since menopause [123], age at menopause [76], nor mean age of natural menopause [125].

Related to menopause is the issue of estrogen replacement therapy. While one might expect lower rates of incontinence in women taking hormone replacement therapy, three studies have reported a two to three times increased risk of incontinence in older women taking estrogen [96, 125, 145]. In the HERS study the estrogen/progestin group worsened their UI compared to the controls [153].

e) Hysterectomy

When asked about the onset of UI, many women will report that it began immediately following hysterectomy. A hysterectomy with oophorectomy puts a woman into surgical menopause. This may imply a hormonal mechanism a cause of UI. Recently, with the development of neurophysiological investigations to measure neurologic impairment of the pelvic floor, the question has been raised whether the development of post-hysterectomy UI might be caused by nerve damage during the procedure. It may also be due to disturbances of musculo-fascial attachments of the bladder to the surrounding pelvic wall [154].

Well controlled prospective studies investigating the role of hysterectomy are scarce and results are mixed. In studies utilizing univariate analyses, some have shown significant associations between UI and hysterectomy [79, 127], as well as oophorectomy [79]. Milsom and colleagues, in a survey of 3,896 women, reported that those who had a hysterectomy were more likely to report UI than those who had not (21% vs. 16 %), and this trend occurred across five birth cohorts from 1900 to 1920 [127].

Some studies have reported no association between hysterectomy and UI in general [90] and stress incontinence in particular [143]. Others have found a significant relationship in univariate analyses but nonsignificant results after controlling for other variables in multivariate analyses [125, 143]. Studies using multivariate analysis models also yielded inconsistent results. Two studies found a positive association between hysterectomy and incontinence with odds ratios of 1.5 and 2.4 [151, 155]. In another, there was no association between UI and hysterectomy with an odds ratio of 1.07 [76].

In a review of the clinical literature on the effects of hysterectomy, Thom and Brown [156] concluded that most studies did not find an increase in UI in the first two years after surgery. Also, UI was decreased after surgery in some studies. A subsequent study of the clinical effects of hysterectomy examined the prevalence of stress and urge incontinence before and one year after hysterectomy and found no detrimental changes [157].

Thus, there is evidence to suggest that hysterectomy may place a woman at risk for UI and contradictory information to suggest that hysterectomy may not contribute to the development of UI. Thus, the role of hysterectomy remains controversial [155, 158]. Further study of the relationship of hysterectomy to UI could clarify the issue and potentially yield surgical techniques that would minimize the risks of UI.

f) Obesity

Obesity is well established as a factor that can cause UI or contribute to the severity of the condition. It is believed that the added weight of obesity, like preganancy, may bear down on pelvic tissues causing chronic strain, stretching and weakening of the muscles, nerves, and other structures of the pelvic floor. Anecdotally, patients are known to report improvement in symptoms of UI associated with weight loss and increased severity with weight gain. In addition, there is clear epidemiological support for the role of obesity in UI.

Data from several studies indicate that UI in women is associated with higher body mass index and greater weight [67, 76, 79, 93, 123, 125, 128, 137, 143, 151, 155, 159, 160]. In one study, a significant relationship was found between UI and body mass index such that women with regular UI had the highest mean body mass index and those who had never been incontinent had the lowest mean body mass index [93]. Dwyer and colleagues found that obesity was significantly more common among women with detrusor instability, as well as among those with stress incontinence, compared to continent women [161]. Similarly, in several other studies, increased body mass index was found to be an independent risk factor for incontinence [76, 103, 123, 125, 143, 149, 160]. One study found a positive "almost linear association" between BMI and both stress incontinence and urge incontinence [151]. The highest BMI quartile had a 4.2 times greater risk of stress incontinence and a 2.2 times greater risk of urge incontinence. Two studies found that increased BMI was a risk factor for stress incontinence but not for urge incontinence [123, 143].

Other investigators found no associations between UI and obesity [150, 162, 163]. One of these did find that women with a positive stress test (i.e., clinically demonstrated loss of urine with physical stress (coughing) had a higher body mass index than those who had a negative stress test [162]. The other was restricted to the study of postpartum incontinence and found that antenatal BMI did not predict postpartum UI [150]. Fischer et al [163] found a significant relationship on univariate but not on multivariate analyses. This study was limited in that there was a small range of BMI values and only 5 respondents had a BMI > 30. The possibility that the effect was dependent on a threshold value was reflected in the results of another study that found an association between UI during pregnancy and prepregnancy BMI > 35 (OR=2.5), but a lack of significance with BMI >30 (OR=1.7) [149].

In addition to the associations found between obesity, body mass index, and UI, confirmatory results have been reported for intervention studies. Bariatric surgery was used in one study to drastically reduce weight in a group of morbidly obese women [164]. As a group, the women had both subjective and objective resolution of stress as well as urge incontinence. In another study, weight reduction by bariatric surgery resulted in reduction of stress incontinence from 61 % to 12 % of the group [165]. Thus, there is strong evidence to support the causal role of excess weight in the development of UI. A link between body mass and UI supports the concept that weight gain may increase susceptibility to incontinence and suggests that weight loss may decrease incontinence.

g) Lower urinary tract symptoms (LUTS)

Irrespective of whether due to disease or normal aging, urinary tract symptoms such as blood in urine, cloudiness or foul smell in urine, burning during urination, trouble starting urine flow, inability to shut off urine flow, needing to push and strain while urinating, or needing to urinate more than once to empty bladder emerge as one of the most critical set of correlates and potential precursors of UI from the analysis of the MESA data [74]. UI is further related to fecal incontinence [74, 80]. Others have also found a strong correlation between LUTS and UI [151], and the transition from overactive bladder without incontinence to the form with incontinence should be studied.

h) Functional impairment

Another set of health-related correlates that have been substantiated in several studies are functional impairments, particularly mobility limitations [71, 74, 77, 80, 81, 103, 160, 166, 167]. Odds ratios from a recent study demonstrated the increasing likelihood of incontinence with worsening level of mobility from requiring no help with mobility to needing support (1.8), depending on care providers (5.63), and being wheelchair or bed-bound (7.38) [80]. A study of 2025 older women indicated that several measures of mobility impairment were associated with UI including inability to walk 0.5 mile (OR=2.15), inability to move heavy objects (OR=1.89) and inability to climb stairs (OR=1.66) [103]. In addition improvement in ADLs was associated with 3-year remission rates of urge incontinence (OR=0.5). Another large study of older adults 70+ years of age showed that UI was associated not only with functional impariment, but also with sensory impariment, which may contribute to mobility limitations [160]. Mobility problems include having experienced a fall during the last 12 months, being diagnosed with arthritis, currently using equipment to get around, being restricted from going out, and several performance measures of lower body physical functions.

The exact interpretation of the relationship between functional impairment and UI, however, is still being debated. At issue is whether UI is a direct consequence of difficulties in getting to the bathroom and removing clothing or whether UI is a predictor of frailty as shown in a study of 1531 older women [71]. Longitudinal information is needed to sort out the direction of causation between functional impairments and UI.

Alternatively, mobility limitations and UI may both be consequences of general frailty in older age or of an underlying systemic illness such as a stroke. There is evidence of an association between UI and stroke [79, 103, 160] as well as Parkinson's disease [71, 103]. UI may be a direct consequence of neurological damage caused by these diseases or an indirect result of the physical limitations imposed by these diseases.

i) Cognitive impairment

Studies in nursing homes have suggested a link between dementia and UI [80, 81, 84, 168-169]. Two recent studies of UI in nursing home residents have shown an association between UI and cognitive impairment using multivariate analyses. In one, patients lacking mental orientation had a 3.6 times greater risk of being incontinent than those with normal mental status [80]. In the second, the presence of dementia increased the odds of UI by 2.3 [81]. However, in a community sample, no relationship was found between mental status and difficulty holding urine [170].

In the Canadian Study of Health and Aging it was found a strong association between severity of dementia and UI in elderly women [77]. Odds ratios were 1.2, 4.0,and 12.6 for mild, moderate and severe dementia, respectively, after controling for age, residence, and ambulatory function.

A systematic review of 11 studies examining the rate of UI in persons with dementia [171] concluded that UI is common in patients with dementia and is more prevalent in demented than in nondemented older individuals.

j) Occupational risks

Currently there is a dearth of knowledge to aid medical providers in advising their patients about occupational factors that promote either the onset or recurrence of urinary incontinence.

A study of 274 female aircrew revealed that 26% experienced UI [163]. Most (89%) reported that incontinence occurred off duty, and 18% reported UI on duty while flying. Crew position affected the risk of UI, but no other occupational variables were associated with UI, including flying high performance military aircraft, the number of hours flown, or type of aircraft (high gravity vs low gravity).

k) Family history and genetics

Parallel to the developments in genetics and molecular biology, there is an interest for investigating many medical conditions for genetic components. Little is known about a genetic component for UI.

Twin studies are the best genetic studies. Only one has been identified in the literature [172]. The inheritability was significant for urge, but not for stress UI in a study of 161 MZ and 249 DZ twins aged 75+. Data suggests that about half the risk for urge incontinence is inherited in this age group.

Family studies may find evidence for familial clustering. One study found that family history was associated with stress UI [173]. Relative risks for mothers, sisters, and daughters of women with stress incontinence were 2.8, 2.9, and 2.3, respectively.

l) Other factors

Other published articles have reported correlations between UI and several other variables, including history of cystitis or urinary tract infections [80, 123, 143, 159, 174], diabetes [79, 103, 123], previous gynecological surgery [76, 92, 136], constipation [79, 151, 175], fecal incontinence [80], use of diuretics [128, 151], other drugs [103, 176], caffeine comsumption [177], perineal suturing [136], exercise [178], genital prolapse [90, 145], radiation [179], impaired function of the levator muscles [76, 90, 145], childhood enuresis [35, 143], current and former cigarette smoking [145, 180], respiratory problems [71] and nighttime awakening [71]. A recent observational study [88] reviewed the medical records of 5986 members aged 65+ of a large health maintenence organization in California. There was an increased risk of UI associated to the diagnoses of Parkinson's disease, dementia, stroke, depression, and congestive heart failure.

Summary points

- The prevalence estimates of at least some degree of UI show a wide range. The variability may be explained by factors such as variations in the definition of UI, in collection of the study samples, or variation in survey procedures, or effects of intervention.
- The median level of prevalence estimates gives a picture of increasing prevalence during young adult life (prevalence 20-30%), a broad peak around middle age (prevalence 30-40%), and then a steady increase in the elderly (prevalence 30-50%).

- Proportions of types of UI are difficult to estimate, and estimates vary considerably. Approximately half of all incontinent women are classified as stress incontinent. A smaller proportion is usually classified as mixed incontinent, and urge incontinence is the smallest category. Little is known about the risk factors and demographic correlates of the different types, but the types probably reflect different pathologies and etiologies.
- The prevalence of severe or "significant" incontinence (depending on frequency and amount of leakage, soaking of clothes, use of pads etc.), is rather consistent, and ranges between 3% and 17%, with most studies reporting between 6% and 10%.
- Incidence studies are scarce and should be encouraged. Remission can occur, but we know little about the rates of remission or its predictors. Such studies will also give a better understanding of the dynamics between risk factors and the onset of UI.
- There remains a paucity of published information regarding UI in non-caucasian women world wide. The data suggests higher prevalence of UI among Caucasian women that may be due primarily to racial differences in the prevalence of stress UI.
- A number of medical correlates of UI have been identified, but need to be investigated in a prospective, longitudinal, well controlled design in order to establish the temporal ordering between risk factors and onset of UI.
- Well controlled analyses of potential risk factors and predictors are limited. Age, childbearing, urinary symptoms, and functional impairment remain the best established risk factors.

V. EPIDEMIOLOGY OF UI IN MEN

1. General comments

The epidemiology of UI in men has not been investigated to the same extent as for females. However, progress has been made during the 3 last years. In almost all studies, the prevalence rates of UI continue to be reported to be less in men than in women by a 1:2 ratio. The type and age distribution are much different between the sexes, and risk factors, although less investigated in men, seem to be different. We have found no reviews of the epidemiological studies of male UI.

It is also important not to consider UI as an isolated problem in men, but rather as a component of a multifactorial problem. Often other urogenital symptoms such as weak stream, hesitancy, dribbling or impotence exist.

An area in male UI that is being studied and reported with increasing regularity in the last few years is post-prostatectomy incontinence. Since radical prostatectomy is being performed with increased frequency in recent years, the incidence of post-prostatectomy UI is now being scrutinized in greater detail.

2. Prevalence

Some of the major reviews also discuss the prevalence of UI in men [52, 53, 55], ranging from 3% reported by Feneley [181], 5% by Schulman [182], 9% by Thomas [141] and Malmsten [183], and 11% by Yarnell [184].

There are no studies reporting prevalences for men according to the ICS definition. But for any definition, there is a steadily increase in prevalence with increasing age (Table 11), than for women.

Due to differences in pathological anatomy and pathophysiology of UI in men, there is a different distribution in incontinence subtypes. Recent studies confirmed our previous reports of the predominance of urge incontinence (40-80%), followed by mixed forms of UI (10-30%), and stress incontinence (<10%) [55, 69, 74, 111, 182]. The increasing prevalence of UI as age increases observed in men is largely due to the contribution of the urge incontinence rather than stress incontinence. One study demonstrated an increasing rate of urge UI from 0.7% between age 50-59, 2.7% between 60-69 and 3.4% for 70 years and older respondents. Stress UI was steady at 0.5%, 0.5% and 0.1% for the above group respectively [111]. The recent NOBLE telephone survey found an overall prevalence of overactive bladder with urge incontinence of 2.6% in men 18+, increasing with age from less than 1% in age group 18-44 to 9% in age group 65+ [97].

Most studies have a large fraction of other/unclassified types. One recent study found that constant dribbling was reported by 7.4% of their respondents [111]. Terminal dribbling or postvoid dribbling is another type of leakage in men that is difficult to assign to the conventional subtypes of UI. In a recent Australian survey, 12% of respondents reported frequent terminal dribbling [185].

When it comes to severity, the sex differences do not seem to be different from those for any incontinence. Estimates for severe UI in older women tend to be about twice as high as for older men [55].

We have found no studies adressing racial or ethnic dif-

Table 11 : Examples of prevalence of UI across age spectrum in men

First author	Ref	Year	Distribution by age	Prevalence (%)
Yarnell	[184]	1979	65	9
			70 - 80	8
			80+	22
Thomas	[141]	1980	45 - 54	5
			55 - 64	9
			65 - 74	15
			75+	18
Diokno	[74]	1986	60+	19
Malmsten	[183]	1997	45	4
			50	4
			60	5
			70	7
			75	10
			80	20
			90+	28
Schulman	[182]	1997	45 - 49	2
			50 - 54	5
			60 - 64	6
			70+	14
Bartolotti	[67]	2000	51 – 60	2
			61 – 70	3
			70+	7
Ueda	[111]	2000	40 – 49	1
			50 – 59	2
			60 – 69	4
			70+	4

ferences in the prevalence of UI in men. However, unpublished data from the MESA study do not indicate differences in prevalence among white male respondents compared to African American respondents.

Literature on incidence of male UI is very scarce. The MESA study [102] found a one year incidence rate for elderly men of 9%. Substantial remission rates were also obtained, rates that were higher among men (27%) than women (11%). one likely explanation of the relative instability of male Ui focuses on the predominance of urge type incontinence among men. Urge UI is often caused by prostate gland disease, infections, or bowel dysfunction, all of which are relatively amenable to treatment or improve even without treatment.

Malmsten [183] analysed the age of onset for each age cohort. Mean debut age for all men was 63 years, mean duration was about 8-10 years in the cohorts.

3. Potential risk factors

There is relative little research concerning conditions and factors that may be associated with UI in men, and clear risk factors are more seldom scientifically documented (Table 12). However, a few available studies have identified potential risk factors which are described below.

Table 12 : Risk factors for UI in men reviewed in this text

- Age
- Lower urinary tract symptoms (LUTS)
- Functional and cognitive impairment
- Neurological disorders
- Prostatectomy
- Other Factors

a) Age

As for women increasing age is correlated with increasing prevalence of UI. There seems to be a more steadily increase in prevalence with increasing age, than for women.

b) Lower Urinary Tract Symptoms (LUTS)

In a telephone survey of 150 community-living incontinent men aged 20 years and over, about 70% had experienced a variety of other medical conditions, many of which may cause or aggravate UI [186]. About half of the men reported symptoms of bladder outlet obstruction, and almost a third had undergone prostatectomy.

In a study of 805 noninstitutionalized elderly men, Diokno and coworkers found that a variety of problems, conditions and symptoms are more prevalent among those with UI than among those without. UI was reported by only 15% of men without voiding symptoms, frequency or urgency and by 34% of those with symptoms [74]. When outlet obstruction is established, this may lead to increasing post-void residual urine which may lead to chronic retention and manifest as overflow incontinence. Established outlet obstruction may cause detrusor instability and manifest as urgency, frequency, and urge incontinence.

Recent studies reported that urinary tract infections and cystitis are strongly associated with male UI [69, 111]. Men reporting cystitis were at increased risk for UI with an odds ratio of 3.65 [111].

c) Functional and cognitive impairment

Mobility problems such as use of a wheelchair or aids to walking, as well as diagnosed arthritis or rheumatism or having a fall the last year, were significantly greater among incontinent than continent men [69, 175]. A recent report noted that UI are more likely among men whose activities of daily living (ADL) are impaired, specifically those who are unable to change clothes and unable to walk outside, with odds ratio of 17.4 and 4.36 respectively [111]. A Canadian study found odds ratios of 1.8 and 6.4 for partially and totally immobile men aged 65+, respectively, for daily UI compared to normal ambulatory function [77]. In general, most studies find similarities between men and women (see above) for functional and cognitive impairment as risk factors for UI.

d) Neurological disorders

Many specific neurological diseases may lead to UI [187]. Detrusor hyper-reflexia is seen commonly in mengingo-myelocele patients and in spinal injuries, Parkinson's disease and multiple sclerosis. Areflexic bladder dysfunction due to a cauda equina lesion or diabetes might cause overflow or a paralysed pelvic floor and hence stress incontinence. Men who had suffered a stroke were at increased risk for incontinence with an odds ratio of 7.12. Similar history of stroke did not seem to significantly increase the risk among women [111].

e) Prostatectomy

A well known iatrogenic cause of male incontinence is prostatectomy. The reported incidence of stress incontinence following TURP is about 1%. Figures from radical prostatectomy technique are much higher. As the past decade has witnessed an increased number of radical prostatectomies, and incontinence is one of the main complications of the procedure, we decided to do an indepth analysis of the postprostatectomy patient population. In addition to epidemiological studies, we included clinical trials if the report had relevant data on incontinence. Minimum follow-up and time of assessment for continence should be at 12 months from the time of surgery.

We have found overall prevalences of post-prostatectomy incontinence from 5 to well over 60%. Table 13 shows examples of recent studies on post-prostatectomy UI. The very wide range of prevalence rates may be explained by many factors, including differences in study characteristics, population characteristics, study site, and the definition used.

Incontinence rates elicited from symptoms reported by patients are generally 2-3x higher than those from physicians' observations. Studies that have performed both assessments in the same population confirm this observation that doctors underestimate postprostatectomy incontinence by as much as 75% [195-197].

Incontinence rates post-prostatectomy are observed to progressively decline with time and plateau 1 to 2 years postop [189, 191, 198]. Thus, it is important to emphasize that studies presenting incontinence rates should have a minimum follow-up of one year to establish true and reliable rates.

Modifications in the technique of radical prostatectomy have been developed primarily to minimize complications. Numerous studies demonstrate the impact of such modifications on postoperative incontinence rates. The variations associated with lower incontinence rates include the perineal approach [194, 199] and preservation of neurovascular bundle [200]. Bladder neck preservation affords earlier return to continence compared

Table 13 : Examples of prevalence of UI after radical prostatectomy

First author	Year	Ref	N	Prevalence (%)
Poon	2000	[188]	140	5.0
Walsh	2000	[189]	59	7.0
Catalona	1999	[190]	1 325	8.0
Goluboff	1998	[191]	480	8.2
Mettlin	1997	[192]	1 304 1 076	19.7 20.2
Benoit	2000	[193]	25 651	21.7
Bishoff	1998	[194]	907	44.7

to bladder neck resection although continence rates at one year post-op do not significantly differ between the two techniques [188].

Older age at time of surgery has been found to be a significant factor associated with a higher prevalence of post-prostatectomy incontinence [190, 191, 199, 200]. Catalona's work has shown that the risk for incontinence doubles for every 10 years of age beginning at age 40 years. Horie [198] further noted that rather than absolutely affecting final continence prevalence, age determined the rate at which continence would be achieved so that elderly men would take a longer time to achieve continence. Two studies however found no relation between age and incontinence prevalence [196, 201].

Other factors have been found to be associated with a higher prevalence of post-prostatectomy, although not consistently. These include : prior TURP, preoperative lower urinary tract symptoms, weight (obesity) and advanced clinical stage [200].

f) Other factors

As for women (see above) several other factors may be involved.

Summary points:

- The epidemiology of UI in men has not been investigated to the same extent as for females.
- It appears that UI is at least twice as prevalent in women as compared with men. There seems to be a more steady increase in prevalence with increasing age than for women.
- Most studies find a predominance of urge incontinence, followed by mixed forms of UI and stress incontinence the least. Most studies have a large fraction of other/unclassified types.
- Literature on incidence of male UI is still very scarce.
- Clear risk factors are more seldom scientifically documented, but several medical correlates have been reported. Risk factors reviewed in this text include age, lower urinary tract symptoms (LUTS), functional and cognitive impairment, neurological disorders, and prostatectomy.
- UI after radical prostatectomy is frequent, and should attain more attention.
- More world wide data are needed.

VI. WHY DO PREVALENCE ESTIMATES DIFFER?

1. General problems in survey research

The well documented variation in prevalence estimates is thought to result at least in part from several confounders common to survey and epidemiologic research. Herzog and Fultz [202], in a review of the prevalence and incidence of UI in community-dwelling populations, proposed that past investigations were plagued by sampling and non-response issues, by self selection and attrition, by definitional, conceptual, and measurement issues. Comprehensive reviews about measurements and methodological aspects of investigating UI are provided [52, 58, 203, 204]. It is clear that there are large methodological challenges to rigorous research in this field. In general, quality of recent large studies has undoubtly improved, but the scientific community must continous deal with methodological challenges in order to achieve progress.

2. Different definitions and measurement

A major problem in research on UI has been the use of different definitions and measurements, and this might contribute to the wide range of reported prevalence estimates. The ICS definition of UI – a condition in which involuntary loss of urine is a social or hygienic problem and is objectively demonstrable – includes objective demonstration of urine loss as one critical component. This aspect limits the ICS definition for community based epidemiologic investigations, because objective demonstration of UI is difficult to achieve outside of the clinical setting, and studies which were able to include this aspect in their assessment might have produced different prevalences. In addition, the social or hygienic aspect of the ICS definition might be problematic in epidemiologic studies because it adds a subjective aspect to an objectively defined condition and therefore confounds the investigation of prevalence, incidence, and risk factors. By the same token, the subjective definition of a problem or "bother" might be relevant in the investigation of care seeking for UI and the prediction of who is likely to become a patient for this condition.

Studies use different severity levels for defining UI. Whereas some classify any involuntary loss at all as UI, others require at least monthly, weekly og even daily loss for UI classification. Moreover, different time frames for the occurence of involuntary urine loss have been used in existing studies. Loss during the previous week, month, 6 of 12 months have been used; sometimes the time period is left unspecified. A further factor complicating the conceptualization and measurement of UI in epidemiologic studies lies in the nature of the condition. UI is a chronic condition (or set of conditions) that often starts slowly and comes and goes for a considerable time period before it become fully established [203]. If people get used to their UI or notice it less, this can interfere with valid assessment.

Ideally self-report measures are validated by clinical evaluations. However, clinical and even urodynamic investigations should be regarded as other measures, not necessarily as gold standards, because it is known to be difficult to demonstrate all urinary symptoms in the clinical setting. Diokno et al. [131] invited both continent and incontinent respondents from a community survey for extensive clinical investigations and found 83% agreement between self-reports of UI and the clinical assessment. Two Swedish studies have reported that 5% and 6% of self-reported UI could not be verified in the clinic [75, 127]. Another study [98] revealed less than satisfactory predictive validity of self-reported types of UI compared with urodynamic investigations.

Holtedahl [76] calculated prevalence estimates using different definitions of UI for the same sample of 50 to 70 year old women. The prevalence of any self-reported leakage was 47%. Self-reported regular UI with or without objective demonstration was found for 31% of women, regular incontinence according to the full ICS definition for 19%. Another study found prevalences of 69% and 30% for any UI and ICS defined UI, respectively [64]. The results indicate that the ICS definition is rather restrictive and yields prevalence estimates that are lower than many other definitions used in epidemiologic studies.

3. Sample and data collection methodology

Some surveys have selected their samples from lists of patients in general practice or in health organizations [88, 92, 101, 136, 141]. These surveys usually get good response rates, but unless such lists include all persons in the population, they are biased sampling frames. Some population based studies have included institutionalized patients [75, 127], some have excluded them [59, 65, 74], while other authors have not provided any information on this issue. The differences will obviously account for some of the variation in prevalence estimates observed among older women, as specificly shown in one study [77].

Low response rates may further bias prevalence estimates [203]. Known differences between responders and non-responders can be compensated during the analysis. The major problems is unknown differences in response rates and other characteristics. Incontinent women may not answer (or deny UI) because of embarrassment or related handicaps. But incontinent women may also find the subject particularly relevant and therefore respond to a greater extent than continent women. At present, we do not know how these factors may affect the comparision between incontinent and continent women.

Data on UI are often collected by post, while some authors have conducted personal interviews or telephone interviews. Personal interviews allow to explore issues in greater detail and they achieve generally higher response rates than postal questionnaires. There is also the possibility that responses elicited by interview are more susceptible to social desirability bias than those elicited by post.

Summary points:

- The lack of epidemiological data from populations underrepresented in research limits the world wide application of the present information.
- Many investigations are plagued by sampling and non response issues, by self selection and attrition. Many early studies were obtained from sampling patients seeking care.
- Amajor problem is the use of different definitions of incontinence. The ICS definition might be problematic in epidemiological studies because it adds a subjective aspect to an objectively verifiable definition.
- There are large methodological challenges to research in the field of UI. Unless the scientific community deals with these issues, progress will be difficult to make.

VII. HELP SEEKING BEHAVIOUR

A majority of people with UI have not sought help [59, 60, 65, 126, 182, 205-209]. In a Norwegian study 4.4 % of all women >20 years old in a community consulted their general practitioner for UI during a 3 year period [210]. Increasing age, increasing severity, increasing duration, and urge/mixed type of UI were shown to be associated with consulting a doctor [211].

The major method of actively managing UI among

community residents is the use of absorbent products [182, 205, 211-213]. Only a small proportion of incontinent community-residing women have used surgery, medication, or exercise regimens [205, 206]. The only factor that appears reliably related to whether any treatment or management is sought is the severity of the condition [205, 214], (for review see [52]). It is also probable that many primary health care providers lack confidence in managing UI, and that this contribute to undertreatment in those seeking help [215].

It is obvious that millions of men and women suffer from their UI, and that for many of them good treatment can be offered. However, for many persons with very mild or occasional UI it is probably adequate not to seek help. Others are satisfied with just information and understanding about the causes and in many cases self-care may be quite appropriate. A Danish study has also shown that simple information and advice was adequate "treatment" for 23% of the women seeking an open access incontinence clinic [216]. A recent Swedish study found that among 136 women with UI, 36% wanted clinical evaluation, and only 24% subsequently started treatment [96].

It is important to realize that many incontinent persons have never talked to a health care professional about the condition. Both epidemiological and qualitative research in this field should be encouraged in order to understand cultural, religious, and other factors for help seeking behaviour world wide [209, 214, 217].

Summary points:

- A majority of people with UI have not sought help.
- Only a small proportion of incontinent community-residing people have used surgery, medication, or exercise regimens.
- Increasing severity, increasing duration, and urge/mixed type of UI are related to consulting a health care provider.
- Health care personnell should be encouraged to approach persons at risk for UI. People with UI should be assessed so services and treatment can be offered and targeted. The patient's view of management, even denial, should be respected.

VIII. EPIDEMIOLOGY AND CLINICAL WORK: FROM RESPONDENT TO PATIENT

In this review we have emphasized some major and important differences between epidemiology and clinical work. These differences may have several implications. A selection process is most often accomplished first by self-selection (help seeking), then a referral system, which provides specialist physicians with a patient population with higher prevalence of disease, more severe disease, and often skewed type distribution, thus obtaining test results with fewer false positives, better diagnostic accuracy, and more efficient use of resources. However, such intended and purposeful selection bias has its drawbacks. There is growing evidence that this selection process introduces a serious bias into research and hampers our ability to generalize hospital based research back to general practice populations. Furthermore, it may result in recommendations and guidelines for diagnosis or therapy derived from tertiary care centres that are inappropriate at the primary care level [218]. Often guidelines, review articles or teaching material do not take into account the varying prevalence and variation in clinical picture between community and hospital. They may also emphasize use of tests or equipment that are not appropriate or relevant for general practice and primary health care, thus leading to overutilization of referrals. Data from hospitals or specialist level may also overestimate level of burden, costs and number of persons in need of treatment if such data are used for extrapolation back to community level.

One study provides substantial empirical evidence to support the existence of selection bias for UI [218]. The analyses were based on three populations of incontinent women: Community level (epidemiological survey), primary care level (prospective study), and secondary care level (university hospital, prospective study). The general practice patients were older and the hospital patients younger than those in the community. From community via general practice to hospital, there was an increase in duration, frequency of leakage, amount of leakage, severity and perceived impact of incontinence. Help-seeking at the primary care level was associated with increasing age and severity, and with urge symptoms and impact. Referral from general practice to hospital was only associated with (lower) age and urge symptoms.

Under the subtitle Severity we have given examples of how the prevalence estimates change dramatically when botherness and severity are considered. In addition, there is also selection bias through the health care system. Taken together, this emphasizes caution when epidemiological data are used in a clinical context. It concerns "level of care" in several ways; there is a large transitional zone from healthy to diseased, there is a danger of medicalization, and there is a danger of treating patients at a higher level than necessary.

Risk factors, predictors and correlates discovered in epidemiological studies are probabilistic of nature and may not be decisive in the clinical assessment of an individual patient. In addition, the attributable risk due to some known risk factors may be statistically but not clinically significant.

Summary points:

- The spectrum of severity of UI and the symptom profile of patients referred to specialist centres do not necessarily reflect the spectrum of disease seen in the community.
- The selection and referrral process may introduce bias into research and hamper the ability to generalize hospital based research back to primary care populations.
- One should be very careful with calculating numbers of patients in need of therapy based on epidemiological data.

IX. RECOMMENDATIONS FOR FURTHER RESEARCH

It is recommended to perform more sustained research on measurement of UI, its types and severity to move the research ahead. Longitudinal study designs are needed to estimate incidence of UI and describe the course of the condition and its different forms and to investigate its risk factors and possible protective factors.

There is still little knowledge as regarding prevalence, incidence, and other epidemiological data in developing countries. It is recommended that fundamental research regarding prevalence, incidence and other epidemiological data in developing countries should be encouraged, and tailored to the cultural, economic and social environment of the population under study.

Crude prevalence studies (descriptive epidemiology) from USA and Europe are abundant, and further studies should be done only with recommended and validated questionnaires or in order to combine data from the prevalence study with studies of co-factors and predictors (analytical epidemiology). Control for confounders, stratification, and multivariate techniques should be increasingly used because of the need for more advanced epidemiological analyses of risk factors and comorbidity. Strength of associations should be determined by relative risks and odds ratios, and confidence limits should be given. We have still very little knowledge of the absolute and relative importance of several risk factors, and almost no informations about the attributable risk of the factors in the society.

Some potential risk and protective factors deserve more attention. For example, the role of childbirth in the development of UI must be studied in a fashion that links population-based methods to clinical assessment of the birth trauma and follows women over many years. Such a design is necessary because the effect of childbirth may become clear only years later when the woman is older and because the woman will not be able to report the exact nature of the tear and episiotomy, etc. Other potential risk factors include overweight, various forms of stress of the pelvic floor, and smoking. Physical exercise may play protective roles. There should be more emphasis on the associations between UI and specific diseases like stroke, diabetes and genital prolapse. Genetic components should be investigated.

Primary prevention is the main goal in the management of human disease. An important strategy would thus be to identify the individuals at risk, and then take measures to reduce the risk among those individuals or in certain risk groups. Based on current knowledge there are no well documented efforts that can be done in order to avoid the occurrence of UI in large populations. Primary prevention studies should be encouraged, but the epidemiological basis for choosing appropriate interventions is weak.

The committee will again emphasize that there is merit to reconsider the definition of UI, and to move towards a standardization of measurement instruments of UI in community surveys that can be used worldwide. Developing a new definition is a scientific process requiring careful conceptualization of the condition in light of its many clinical presentations and underlying mechanisms. This will require a multi-method approach and consideration of issues such a reliability and validity. Clearly, the core of the definition is "any involuntary loss of urine". However, elaboration of this core definition may be required depending on the purpose of its use.

Table 14 : Elements in a minimum data set recommended for all epidemiological studies

- Screening question for any involuntary urine loss
- Frequency measure. For example, classification into categories of none, less than once a month, one/several times a month, one/several times a week, every day/nigth, all the time
- Quantity of urine loss for a typical episode. For example, classification into categories of none, drops, small amounts, moderate amounts, much/a great deal
- Duration. For example months, years
- Type. Based on typical description; stress, urge, mixed and other
- Severity. Either by combining excisting questions or by a validated index

In addition, it is recommended to include validated measures of bother/quality of life and urinary symptoms other than UI.

In surveys based on questionnaires or interviews symptoms can be registered.There are convincing data suggesting that the different types may reflect quite different pathologies and risk factors. Differentiating the types in future research might therefore prove very fruitful. Methodological work has still to be done in this area, but typical type descriptions should be included in new studies. Likewise, studies of risk factors should include important and known confounders as age, parity, and weight.

For the purpose of epidemiological research, it is recommended to include the following elements in the definition:

- the individual's statement of any involuntary urine loss

- the frequency of urine loss

- the quantity of urine loss

- the duration of the condition

Consistent with standard epidemiological practices, it is not recommended to include quality of life or bother in the definition of UI for epidemiological purposes. One reason to not include the patients' perceptions of the condition is that it confounds or distorts our estimates of prevalence and incidence of UI. A second reason is that it could seriously limit the detection of risk factors. Quality of life or bother may be important elements of a definition of UI for clinical purposes

Variations in definitions and measurement issues are fundamental and lead to problems with assessing the findings in epidemiological studies. We need to improve epidemiological studies by including variables that better characterize UI, so that more advanced and informative analyses may be conducted. It is therefore recommended that all epidemiological studies include ***a minimum data set*** (Table 14), including elements of screening question, frequency measure, quantity of urine loss, duration, type, and severity. In addition, it is recommended to include validated measures of bother/quality of life and urinary symptoms other than UI. We here also refer to the chapter from the committee on symptom and quality of life assessment.

ACKNOWLEDGEMENTS

We wish to acknowledge the valuable contributions of dr. Hogne Sandvik and dr. Catherine McGrother who acted as consultants for the committee. We thank several other colleagues for help, comments and suggestions.

REFERENCES

1. Hunskaar, S., Arnold, E.P., Burgio, K., Diokno, A.C., Herzog, A.R. And Mallett, V.T.: Epidemiology and natural history of urinary incontinence. In: Abrams P, Khoury S, Wein A.: Incontinence, 197-226. Plymouth: Scientific International, 1999.
2. Nørgaard, J.P., Van Gool, J.D., Hjälmås, K., Djurhuus, J.C. And Hellström, A.-L.: Standardization and definitions in lower urinary tract dysfunction in children. Br. J. Urol. Suppl., 81: 1, 1998.
3. Hjälmas, K.: Urinary incontinence in children: suggestions for definitions and terminology. Scand. J. Urol. Nephrol. Suppl., 141: 1, 1992.
4. Holmdahl, G., Hanson, E., Hanson, M., Hellström, A.-L., Hjälmås, K. And Sillen, U.: Four-hour voiding observation in healthy infants. J. Urol., 156: 1809, 1996.
5. Meadow, S.R.: Day wetting. Pediatr. Nephrol., 4: 178, 1990.
6. Krantz, I., Jylkäs, E., Ahlberg, B.M. And Wedel, H.: On the epidemiology of nocturnal enuresis: A critical review of methods used in descriptive epidemiological studies on nocturnal enuresis. Scand. J. Urol. Nephrol. Suppl., 163: 75, 1994.
7. Mcgee, R., Mackinson, T., Williams, S., Simpson, A. And Silva, P.A.: A longitudinal study of enuresis from 5-9 years. Aust. Paediatr. J., 20: 39, 1984.
8. Swithinbank, L.V., Carr, J.C. And Abrams, P.H.: Longitudinal

study of urinary symptoms in children. Scand. J. Urol. Nephrol. Suppl., 163: 67, 1994.

9. Fergusson, D.M., Horwood, L.J. And Shannon, F.T.: Factors related to the age of attainment of nocturnal bladder control: an 8-year longitudinal study. Pediatrics, 78: 884, 1986.

10. Hellström, A.-L., Hanson, E., Hansson, S., Hjalmas, K. And Jodal, V.: Micturition habits and incontinence in 7 year old Swedish school entrants. Eur. J. Pediatr., 149: 434, 1990.

11. Jarvelin, M.R., Vikevainen-Tervonen, L., Moilanen, J. And Huttenen, N.P.: Enuresis in seven year old children. Acta Paediatr., 77: 148, 1988.

12. Swithinbank, L.V., Brookes, S.T., Shepherd, A.M. And Abrams, P.: The natural history of urinary symptoms during adolescence. Br. J. Urol. Suppl., 81: 90, 1998.

13. Bower, W.F., Moore, K.H., Shephard, R. And Adams, R.: The epidemiology of childhood enuresis in Australia. Br. J. Urol., 78: 602, 1996.

14. Watanabe, H. And Kawauchi, A.: Nocturnal enuresis: Social aspects and treatment perspectives in Japan. Scand J. Urol. Nephrol. Suppl., 163: 29, 1994.

15. Lottmann, H.: Enuresis treatment in France. Scand. J. Urol. Nephrol. Suppl., 33: 66, 1999.

16. Neveus, T., Hetta, J., Cnattingius, S., Tuvemo, T., Läckgren, G., Olsson, U. And Stenberg, A.: Depth of sleep and sleep habits among enuretic and incontinent children. Acta Paediatr., 88: 748, 1999.

17. Chiozza, M.L., Bernardinelli, L., Caione, P., Delgado, R., Ferrara, P., Giorgi, P.L. Et Al.: An Italian epidemiological multicentre study of nocturnal enuresis. Br. J. Urol. Suppl., 81: 86, 1998.

18. Spee-Van Der Wekke, J., Hirasing, R.A., Meulmeester, J.F. And Radder, J.J.: Childhood nocturnal enuresis in The Netherlands. Urology, 51: 1022, 1998.

19. Serel, T.A., Akhan, G., Koyuncouglu, H.R., Öztürk, A., Dogruer, K., Ünal, S. Et Al.: Epidemiology of enuresis in Turkish children. Scand. J. Urol. Nephrol., 31: 537, 1997.

20. Gümüs, B., Vurgun, N., Lekili, M., Iscan, A., Müezzinoglu, T. And Büyüksu, C.: Prevalence of nocturnal enuresis and accompanying factors in children aged 7-11 years in Turkey. Acta Paediatr., 88: 1369, 1999.

21. Kalo, B.B. And Bella, H.: Enuresis: prevalence and associated factors among primary school children in Saudi Arabia. Acta Paediatr., 85: 1217, 1996.

22. Lee, S.D., Sohn, D.W., Lee, J.Z., Park, N.C. And Chung, M.K.: An epidemiological study of enuresis in Korean children. B.J.U. Int., 85: 869, 2000.

23. Yeung, C.K.: Nocturnal enuresis in Hong Kong: different Chinese phenotypes. Scand. J. Urol. Nephrol. Suppl., 31: 17, 1997.

24. Eiberg, H.: Nocturnal enuresis is linked to a specific gene. Scand. J. Urol. Nephrol. Suppl., 173: 15, 1995.

25. Arnell, H., Hjälmås, K., Jägervall, M., Lackgren, G., Stenberg, A., Bengtsson, B. Et Al.: The genetics of primary nocturnal enuresisi: inheritance and suggestion of a second major gene on chromosome 12q. J. Med. Genet., 34: 360, 1997.

26. Von Gontard, A., Eiberg, H., Hollman, E., Rittig, S. And Lehmkuhl, G.: Molecular genetics of nocturnal enuresis: clinical and genetic heterogeneity. Acta Paediatr. 87: 571, 1997.

27. Feehan, M., Mcgee, R., Stanton, W. And Silva, P.A.: A 6 year follow-up of childhood enuresis: Prevalence in adolescence and consequences for mental health. J. Paediatr. Child Health, 26: 75, 1990.

28. Schulpen, T.W.J.: The burden of nocturnal enuresis. Acta Paediatr., 86: 923, 1997.

29. Fergusson, D.M., And Horwood, L.J.: Nocturnal enuresis and behavioural problems in adolescence: a 15-yearlongitudinal study. Pediatrics, 94: 662, 1994.

30. Moilanen, I., Tirkkonen, T., Järvelin, M.R., Linna, S.L., Almqvist, F., Piha, J. Et Al.: A follow-up of enuresis from childhood to adolescence. Br. J. Urol. Suppl., 81: 94, 1998.

31. Rittig, S., Knudsen, U.B., Norgaard, J.P., Pedersen, E.B. And Djurhuus, J.C.: Abnormal diurnal rhythm of plasma vasopressin and urinary output in patients with enuresis. Am. J. Physiol., 25: 664, 1989.

32. Wolfish, N.M., Pivik, R.T., And Busby, K.A.: Elevated sleep arousal thresholds in enuretic boys: clinical implications. Acta Paediatr. 86: 381, 1997.

33. Kawauchi, A., Imada, N., Tanaka, Y., Minami, M., Watanabe, H. And Shirakawa, S.: Changes in the structure of sleep spindles and delta waves on electroencephalography in patients with nocturnal enuresis. Br. J. Urol. Suppl., 81: 72, 1998.

34. Hunsballe, J.M.: Increased delta component in computerized sleep electroencephalographic analysis suggests abnormally deep sleep in primary monosymptomatic nocturnal enuresis. Scand. J. Urol. Nephrol., 34: 294, 2000.

35. Foldspang, A. And Mommsen, S.: Adult female urinary incontinence and childhood bedwetting. J. Urol., 152: 85, 1994.

36. Moore, K.H., Richmond, D.H. And Parys, B.T.: Sex distribution of adult idiopathic detrusor instabilty in relation to childhood bedwetting. Br. J. Urol., 68: 479, 1991.

37. Baruzzi, A., Riva, R., Cirignotta, F., Zucconi, M,. Capelli, M. And Lugaresi, E.: Atrial natriuretic peptide and catecholamines in obstructive sleep apnoea. Sleep, 14: 83, 1991.

38. Weider, D.J., Sateia, M.J., And West, R.P.: Nocturnal enuresis in children with upper airway obstruction. Otolaryngol. Head Neck Surg., 105: 427, 1991.

39. Loening-Baucke, V.: Urinary incontinence and urinary tract infection and their resolution with treatment of chronic constipation of childhood. Pediatrics, 100: 228, 1997.

40. Lunsing, R.J., Hadders-Algra, M., Touwen, B.C. And Huisjes, H.D.: Nocturnal enuresis and minor neurological dysfunction at 12 years: a follow-up study. Dev. Med. Child Neurol., 33: 439, 1991.

41. Robson, W.L.M., Jackson, H.P., Blackhurst, D. And Leung, A.K.: Enuresis in children with attention deficit hyperactivity disorder. South. Med. J., 90: 503, 1997.

42. Forbes, F.C.: Children with enuresis. Nowadays, a strong suspicion of sexiual abuse would prompt full investigation. BMJ., 316: 777, 1998.

43. Forsythe, W.I. And Redmond, A.: Enuresis and spontaneous cure rate. Arch. Dis. Child., 49: 259, 1974.

44. Hirasing, R.A., Van Leerdam, F.J.M., Bolk-Bennink, L. And Janknegt, R.A.: Enuresis nocturna in adults. Scand. J. Urol. Nephrol., 31: 533, 1997.

45. Hellström, A.-L., Hanson, E., Hansson, S., Hjälmås, K. And Jodal, U.: Micturition habits and incontinence at age 17 – reinvestigation of a cohort studied at age 7. Br. J. Urol., 76: 231, 1995.

46. Hjalmas, K., Hoebeke, P.B. And De Paepe, H.: Lower urinary tract dysfunction and urodynamics in children. Eur. Urol., 38: 655, 2000.

47. Bloom, D.A., Seeley, W.M., Ritchey, M.L. And Mcguire, E.J.: Toilet habits and continence in children: an opportunity sampling in search of normal parameters. J. Urol., 149: 1087, 1993.

48. Järvelin, M.R., Moilanen, I., Kangas, P., Moring, K., Vikevainen-Tervonen, L., Huttunen, N.P. Et Al.: Aetiological and precipitating factors for childhood enuresis. Acta Paediatr., 80: 361, 1991.

49. Hansson, S., Hjalmas, K., Jodal, U. And Sixt, R.: Lower urinary tract dysfunction in girls with asymptomatic or covert bacteriuria. J. Urol., 143: 333, 1990.

50. Nguyen, H.T. And Peters, C.A.: The long-term complications of posterior urethral valves. B.J.U. Int. Suppl., 83: 23, 1999.

51. De Jonge, G.A.: Epidemiology of enuresis: a survey of the literature. In Kolvin I, MacKeith RC, Meadow SR (eds),: Bladder Control and Enuresis, Spastics International Medical Publications, 39-46. London: William Heinemann Medical Books Ltd., 1973

52. Fultz, N.H. And Herzog, R.: Epidemiology of urinary symptoms in the geriatric population. Geriatr. Urol., 23: 1, 1996.

53. Hampel, C., Wienhold, D., Benken, N., Eggersmann, C. And Thüroff, J.W.: Prevalence and natural history of female incontinence. Eur. Urol. Suppl., 32: 3, 1997.

54. Hampel, C., Wienhold, D., Benken, N., Eggersmann, C. And Thüroff, J,W.: Definition of overactive bladder and epidemiology of urinary incontinence. Urology, 50: 4, 1997.

55. Herzog, A.R. And Fultz, N.H.: Prevalence and incidence of urinary incontinence in community-dwelling populations. J. Am. Geriatr. Soc., 38: 273, 1990.

56. Cheater, F.M., And Castleden, C.M.: Epidemiology and classification of urinary incontinence. Clin. Obstet. Gynaecol., 14: 183. 2000.

57. Fultz, N.H. And Herzog, A.R.: Prevalence of urinary incontinence in middle-aged and older women: A survey-based methodological experiment. J. Aging. Health., 12: 459, 2000.

58. Thom, D.: Variation in estimates of urinary incontinence prevalence in community: Effects of differences in definition, population characteristics, and study type. J. Am. Geriatr. Soc., 46: 473, 1998

59. Yarnell, J.W., Voyle, G.J., Richards, C.J. And Stephenson, T.P.: The prevalence and severity of urinary incontinence in women. J. Epidemiol. Community Health, 35: 71, 1981.

60. Holst, K. And Wilson, P.D.: The prevalence of female urinary incontinence and reasons for not seeking treatment. N. Z. Med. J., 101: 756, 1988.

61. Sommer, P., Bauer, T., Nielsen, K.K., Kristensen, E.S., Hermann, G.G., Steven, K. Et Al.: Voiding patterns and prevalence of incontinence in women. A questionnaire survey. Br. J. Urol., 66: 12, 1990.

62. Brocklehurst, J.C.: Urinary incontinence in the community-Analysis of a MORI poll. BMJ., 306: 832, 1993.

63. Sandvik, H., Hunskaar, S., Seim, A., Hermstad, R., Vanvik, A. And Bratt, H.: Validation of a severity index in female urinary incontinence and its implementation in an epidemiological survey. J. Epidemiol. Community Health, 47: 497, 1993.

64. Swithinbank, L.V., Donovan, J.L., Du Heaume, J.C., Rogers, C.A., James, M.C., Yang, Q. Et Al.: Urinary symptoms and incontinence in women: Relationships between occurrence, age, and perceived impact. Br. J. Gen. Pract., 49: 897, 1999

65. Hannestad, Y.S., Rortveit, G., Sandvik, H. And Hunskaar, S.: A community-based epidemiological survey of female urinary incontinence: The Norwegian EPINCONT study. J. Clin. Epidemiol., 53: 1150, 2000.

66. Temml, C., Haidinger, G., Schmidbauer, J., Schatzl, G. And Madersbacher, S.: Urinary incontinence in both sexes: Prevalence rates and impact on quality of life and sexual life. Neurourol. Urodyn., 19: 259, 2000.

67. Bortolotti, A., Bernardini, B., Colli, E., Dibenedetto, P., Nacci, G.G., Landoni, M. Et Al.: Prevelance and risk factors for urinary incontinence in Italy. Eur. Urol., 37: 30, 2000.

68. Moller, L.A., Lose, G. And Jorgensen, T.: The prevalence and bothersomeness of lower urinary tract symptoms in women 40-60 years of age. Acta Obstet. Gynecol. Scand., 79: 298, 2000.

69. Damian, J., Martin-Moreno, J.M., Lobo, F., Bonache, J., Cervino, J., Redondo-Marquez, L. Et Al.: Prevalence of urinary incontinence among Spanish older people living at home. Eur. Urol., 34: 333, 1998.

70. Gavira Iglesias, F.J., Caridad Y Ocerin, J.M., Perez Del Molino Martin, J., Valderrama Gama, E., Lopez Perez, M., Romero Lopez, M. Et Al.: Prevalence and psychosocial impact of urinary incontinence in older people of a Spanish rural population. J. Gerontol. Biol. Sci., 55: M207, 2000.

71. Maggi, S., Minicuci, N., Langlois, J., Pavan, M., Enzi, G. And Crepalid, G.: Prevalence rate of urinary incontinence in community-dwelling elderly individuals: The Veneto Study. J. Gerontol. Med. Sci., 56A: M14, 2001.

72. Nakanishi, N., Atara, K., Naramura, H., Takashima, Y. And Fukada, H.: Urinary and fecal incontinence in a community-residing older population in Japan. J. Am. Geriatr. Soc., 45: 215, 1997.

73. Tseng, I.J., Chen, Y.T., Chen, M.T., Kou, H.Y. And Tseng, S.F.: Prevalence of urinary incontinence and intention to seek treatment in the elderly. J. Formos. Med. Assoc., 99: 753, 2000.

74. Diokno, A.C., Brock, B.M., Brown, M.B. And Herzog, R.: Prevalence of urinary incontinence and other urological symptoms in the noninstitutionalized elderly. J. Urol., 136: 1022, 1986.

75. Molander, U., Milsom, I., Ekelund, P. And Mellstrom, D.: An epidemiological study of urinary incontinence and related urogenital symptoms in elderly women. Maturitas, 12: 51, 1990.

76. Holtedahl, K. And Hunskaar, S.: Prevalence, 1-year incidence and factors associated with urinary incontinence: a population based study of women 50-74 year of age in primary care. Maturitas, 28: 205, 1998.

77. Hunskaar, S., Østbye, T. And Borrie, M.J.: Prevalence of urinary incontinence in elderly Canadians with special emphasis on the association with dementia, ambulatory function, and institutionalization. Norwegian J Epidemiol., 8: 177, 1998.

78. Roberts, R.O., Jacobsen, S.J., Rhodes, T., Reilly, W.T., Girman, C.J., Talley, N.J. Et Al.: Urinary incontinence in a community-based cohort: Prevalence and healthcare-seeking. J. Am. Geriatr. Soc., 46: 467, 1998.

79. Chiarelli, P., Brown, W. And Mcelduff, P.: Leaking urine: prevalence and associated factors in Australian women. Neurourol. Urodyn.,18:567, 1999.

80. Aggazzotti, G., Pesce, F., Grassi, D., Fantuzzi, G., Righi, E., De Vita, D. Et Al: Prevalence of urinary incontinence among institutionalized patients. a cross-sectional epidemiologic study in a midsized city in northern Italy. Urology, 56: 245, 2000.

81. Brandeis, G.H., Baumann, M.M., Hossain, M., Morris, J.N. And Resnick, N.M.: The prevalence of potentially remediable urinary incontinence in frail older people: A study using the Minimum Data Set. J. Am. Geriatr. Soc., 45: 179, 1997.

82. Sgadari, A., Topinkova, E., Bjornson, J. And Bernabei, R.: Urinary incontinence in nursing home residents: A cross-national comparison. Age Ageing, 26: 49, 1997.

83. Toba, K., Ouchi, H., Iimura, O., Sasaki, H., Nakamura, Y., Takasaki, M. Et Al.: Urinary incontinence in elderly inpatients in Japan: A comparison between general and geriatric hospitals. Aging, 8: 47, 1996.

84. Borrie, M. And Davidson, H.: Incontinence in institutions: costs and contributing factors. Can. Med. Assoc. J., 147: 322, 1992.

85. Ouslander, J.G., Palmer, M.H., Rovner, B.W. And German, P.S.: Urinary incontinence in nursing homes: incidence, remission and associated factors. J. Am. Geriatr. Soc., 41: 1083, 1993.

86. Fonda, D. And Victorian Geriatricians Peer Review Group.: Improving management of urinary incontinence in geriatric centres and nursing homes. Aust. Clin. Rev., 10: 66, 1990.

87. Peet, S.C. And Castleden, C.M.: The prevalence of urinary and faecal incontinence in hospitals and residential and nursing homes for older people. BMJ., 311: 1063, 1995.

88. Thom, D.H., Haan, M.N. And Van Den Eeden, S.: Medically

recognized urinary incontienence and risks of hospitalization, nursing home admission and mortality. Age Aging, 26: 367, 1997.

89. Iosif, C.S. And Bekassy, Z.: Prevalence of genito-urinary symptoms in the late menopause. Acta Obstet. Gynecol. Scand., 63: 257, 1984.

90. H ording, U., Pedersen, K.H., Sidenius, K. And Hedegaard, L.: Urinary incontinence in 45-year-old women. An epidemiological survey. Scand. J. Urol. Nephrol., 20: 183, 1986.

91. Elving, L.B., Foldspang, A., Lam, G.W. And Mommsen, S.: Descriptive epidemiology of urinary incontinence in 3 100 women age 30-59. Scand. J. Urol. Nephrol. Suppl., 125: 37, 1989.

92. Harrison, G.L. And Memel, D.S.: Urinary incontinence in women: its prevalence and its management in a health promotion clinic. Br. J. Gen. Pract., 44: 149, 1994.

93. Burgio, K.L., Matthews, K.A. And Engel, B.T.: Prevalence, incidence and correlates of urinary incontinence in healthy, middle-aged women. J. Urol., 146: 1255, 1991.

94. Lara, C. And Nacey, J.: Ethnic differences between Maori, Pacific Island an European New Zealand women in prevalence and attitudes to urinary incontinence. N. Z. Med. J., 107: 374, 1994.

95. Sandvik, H., Hunskaar, S., Vanvik, A., Bratt, H., Seim, A. And Hermstad, R.: Diagnostic classification of female urinary incontinence: an epidemiologic survey corrected for validity. J. Clin. Epidemiol., 48: 339, 1995.

96. Samuelsson, E., Victor, A. And Tibblin, G.: A population study of urinary incontinence and nocturia among women aged 20-59 years. Prevalence, well-being and wish for treatment. Acta Obstet. Gynecol. Scand., 76: 74, 1997.

97. Stewart, W., Herzog, A.R., Wein, A., Abrams, P., Payne, C., Corey, R. Et Al.: Prevalence of overactive bladder in the US: results from the NOBLE program. 2nd International Consultation on Incontinence, abstract no 79, Paris 2001.

98. Kirschner-Hermanns, R., Scherr, P.A., Branch, L.G., Wetle, T. And Resnick, N.M.: Accuracy of survey questions for geriatric urinary incontinence. J. Urol., 159: 1903, 1998.

99. Sandvik, H., Seim, A., Vanvik, A. And Hunskaar, S.: A severity index for epidemiological surveys of female urinary incontinence: Comparison with 48-hour pad-weighing tests. Neurourol. Urodyn., 19: 137, 2000.

100. Hanley, J., Capewell, A. And Hagen, S.: Validity study of the severity index, a simple measure of urinary incontinence in women. BMJ., 322: 1096, 2001.

101. Vetter, N.J., Jones, D.A. And Victor, C.R.: Urinary incontinence in the elderly at home. Lancet, ii: 1275, 1981.

102. Herzog, A.R., Diokno, A.C., Brown, M.B., Normolle, D.P. And Brock, B.M.: Two-year incidence, remission, and change patterns of urinary incontinence in noninstitutional older adults. J. Gerontol., 45: M67, 1990.

103. Nygaard, I.E. And Lemke, J.H.: Urinary incontinence in rural older women: Prevalence, incidence and remission. J. Am. Geriatr. Soc., 44: 1049, 1996.

104. Samuelsson, E.C., Victor, F.T. And Svardsudd, K.F.: Five-year incidence and remission rates of female urinary incontinence in a Swedish population less that 65 years old. Am. J. Obstet. Gynecol., 183: 568, 2000.

105. Ju, C.C., Swan, L.K., Merriman, A., Choon, T.E. And Viegas, O.: Urinary incontinence among the elderly people of Singapore. Age Ageing, 20: 262, 1991.

106. Shershah, S. And Ansari, R.L.: The frequency of urinary incontinence in Pakistani women. J.P.M.A., 39: 16, 1989.

107. Lee, K.S., Chan, C.J., Merriman, A., Tan, E.C. And Osborn, V.: Clinical profile of elderly urinary incontinence in Singapore: a community based study. Ann. Acad. Med. Singapore, 20: 736, 1991.

108. Brieger, G.M., Mongelli, M., Hin, L.Y. And Chung, T.K.H.: The epidemiology of urinary dysfunction in Chinese women. Int. Urogynecol. J. Pelvic Floor Dysfunct., 8: 191, 1997.

109. Kato, K. And Kondo, A.: Prevalence of urinary incontinence in working women. Jap. J. Urol., 77: 1501, 1986.

110. Fukui, J.: Urinary incontinence in women: results of questionnaires. Jap. J. Urol., 77:, 707, 1986.

111. Ueda, T., Tamaki, M., Kageyama, S., Yoshimura, N. And Yoshida, O.: Urinary incontinence among community-dwelling people aged 40 years or older in Japan: prevalence, risk factors, knowledge and self-perception. Int. J. Urol., 7: 95, 2000

112. Miles, T.P., Palmer, R.F., Espino, D.V., Mouton, C.P., Lichtenstein, M.J. And Markides, K.S.: New-onset incontinence and markers of frailty: Data from the Hispanic Established Populations for Epidemiologic Studies of the Elderly. Journal of Gerontology: Medical Sciences, 56A: M19, 2001.

113. Heyns, O.S.: Bantu Gynaecology. Johannesburg: Witwaterstrand University Press, 1956: 98.

114. Heyns, O.S.: Clin. Proc., 2: 311, 1943.

115. Skinner, D.P.: Stress Incontinence: A comparative racial study. Med. Proc., 9: 189, 1963.

116. Knobel, J.: Stress incontinence in the black female. S. Afr. J. Obstet. Gynaecol., 49: 430, 1975.

117. Cox, P.S.V. And Webster, D.: Genital prolapse amongst the Pokot. East Afr. Med. J., 52: 694, 1975.

118. Howard, D., Davies, P.S. Delancey, J.O. And Small, Y.: Differences in perineal lacerations in black and white primiparas. Obstet. Gynecol., 96: 622, 2000

119. White, L.R., Blazer, D.G. And Fillenbaum, G.: Chapter 5: Related health problems. In: Cornoni-Huntley, J., Blazer, D. G., Lafferty, M. E., Everett, D. F., Brock, D. B. and Farmer M. E., eds. Established populations for epidemiologic studies of the elderly, Volume II. National Institute on Aging, U.S. Department of Health and Human Services, Public Health Service, National Institutes of Health, NIH Publication, 1986; No. 90-495:70-6.

120. Bump, R.C.: Racial comparisons and contrasts in urinary incontinence and pelvic organ prolapse. Obstet. Gynecol., 81: 421, 1993.

121. Peacock, L.M., Wiskind, A.K. And Wall, L.L.: Clinical features of urinary incontinence and urogenital prolapse in a black inner city population. Am. J. Obstet. Gynecol., 171: 1464, 1994.

122. Burgio, K.L., Locher, J.L., Zyczynski, H., Hardin, J.M. And Singh, K.: Urinary incontinence during pregnancy in a racially mixed sample: characteristics and predisposing factors. Int. Urogynecol. J. Pelvic Floor Dysfunt., 7: 69, 1996.

123. Brown, J.S., Grady, D., Ouslander, J.G., Herzog, A.R., Varner, R.E. And Posner, S.F.: Prevalence of urinary incontinence and associated risk factors in postmenopausal women. Obstet. Gynecol., 94: 66, 1999.

124. Brown, J.S., Jackson, R.A., Kanaya, A.M., Vittinghoff, E., Resnik, H.E., Kritchevsky, S. Et At.: Urinary incontinence in elderly women: The health, aging and body composition study. 2nd International Consultation on Incontinence, Abstract nr 24, Paris 2001.

125. Thom, D.H., Van Den Eeden, S.K. And Brown, J.S.: Evaluation of parturition and other reproductive variables as risk factors for urinary incontinence in later life. Obstet. Gynecol., 90: 983, 1997.

126. Rekers, H., Drogendijk, A.C., Valkenburg, H. And Riphagen, F.: Urinary incontinence in women from 35 to 79 years of age: prevalence and consequences. Eur. J. Obstet. Gynecol. Reprod. Biol., 43: 229, 1992.

127. Milsom, I., Ekelund, P., Molander, U., Arvidsson, L. And Areskoug, B.: The influence of age, parity, oral contraception, hysterectomy and menopause on the prevalence of urinary incontinence in women. J. Urol., 149: 1459, 1993.

128. Simeonova, Z. And Bengtsson, C.: Prevalence of urinary incontinence among women at a Swedish primary health care centre. Scand. J. Prim. Health Care, 8: 203, 1990.

129. Foldspang, A., Mommsen, S. And Djurhuus J.C.: Prevalent urinary incontinence as a correlate of pregnancy, vaginal childbirth, and obstetric techniques. Am. J. Public Health, 89: 209, 1999.

130. Dolan, L.M., Casson, K., Mcdonald, P. And Ashe R.G.: Urinary incontinence in Northern Ireland: a prevalence study. B.J.U. Int. 83: 760, 1998.

131. Diokno, A.C., Brown, M.B., Brock, B.M., Herzog, A.R. And Normolle, D.P.: Clinical and cystometric characteristics of continent and incontinent noninstitutionalized elderly. J. Urol., 140: 567, 1988.

132. Staskin, D.R.: Age-related physiologic and pathologic changes affecting lower urinary tract function. Clin. Geriatr. Med., 2: 701, 1986.

133. Mellier, G. And Delille, M.A.: Urinary disorders during pregnancy and post-partum. Rev. Fr. Gynecol. Obstet., 85: 525, 1990.

134. Viktrup, L., Lose, G., Rolff, M. And Farfoed, K.: The symptom of stress incontinence caused by pregnancy or delivery in primiparas. Obstet. Gynecol., 79: 945, 1992.

135. Iosif, C.S. And Ingemarsson, I.: Prevalence of stress incontinence among women delivered by elective cesarian section. Int. J. Gynaecol. Obstet., 20: 87, 1982.

136. Jolleys, J.V.: Reported prevalence of urinary incontinence in women in a general practice. BMJ., 296: 1300, 1988.

137. Yarnell, J.W., Voyle, G.J., Richards, C.J. And Stephenson, T.P.: Factors associated with urinary incontinence in women. J. Epidemiol. Community Health, 36: 58, 1982.

138. Crist, T., Shingleton, H.M., Koch, F. And Koch, G.G.: Stress incontinence and the nulliparous patient. Obstet. Gynecol., 40: 13, 1972.

139. Foldspang, A., Mommsen, S., Lam, G.W. And Elving, L.: Parity as a correlate of adult female urinary incontinence prevalence. J. Epidemiol. Community Health, 46: 595, 1992.

140. Handa, V.L., Harris, T.A. And Ostergard, D.R.: Protecting the pelvic floor: obstetric management to prevent incontinence and pelvic organ prolapse. Obstet. Gynecol., 88: 470, 1996.

141. Thomas, T.M., Plymat, K.R., Blannin, J. And Meade, T.W.: Prevalence of urinary incontinence. BMJ., 281: 1243, 1980.

142. Faundes, A., Guarisi, T. And Pinto-Neto, A.M.: The risk of urinary incontinence of parous women who delivered only by cesarean section. Int. J. Gynaecol. Obstet. 72: 41, 2001.

143. Kuh, D., Cardozo, L. And Hardy, R.: Urinary incontinence in middle aged women: childhood enuresis and other lifetime risk factors in a British prospective cohort. J. Epidemiol. Community Health, 53: 453, 1999.

144. Rortveit, G., Daltveit, A.K. And Hunskaar, S.: Age and type dependent effects of parity on urinary incontinence. The Norwegian EPINCONT study. Obstet. Gynecol., 2001 in press

145. Samuelsson, E., Victor, A. And Svardsudd, K. Determinants of urinary incontinence in a population of young and middle-aged women. Acta Obstet. Gynecol. Scand., 79: 208, 2000.

146. Smith, A.R.B., Hosker, G.L. And Warrell, D.W.: The role of pudendal nerve damage in the aetiology of genuine stress incontinence in women. Br. J. Obstet. Gynaecol., 96: 29, 1989.

147. Snooks, S.J., Swash, M., Henry, M.M. And Setchel, M.: Risk factors in childbirth causing damage to the pelvic floor innervation. Int. J. Colorectal Dis., 1: 20, 1986.

148. Persson, J., Wolner-Hanssen, P. And Rydhstroem, H.: Obstetric risk factors for stress urinary incontinence: a population-based study. Obstet. Gynecol., 96: 440, 2000.

149. Hojberg, K.E., Salvig, J.D., Winslow, N.A., Lose, G. And Secher, N.J.: Urinary incontinence: prevalence and risk factors at 16 weeks of gestation. Br. J. Obstet. Gynaecol., 106: 842, 1999.

150. Chaliha, C., Kalia, V., Stanton, S.L., Monga, A. And Sultan, A.H.: Antenatal prediction of postpartum urinary and fecal incontinence. Obstet. Gynecol. 94: 689, 1999.

151. Moller, L.A., Lose, G. And Jorgensen, T.: Risk factors for lower urinary tract symptoms in women 40 to 60 years of age. Obstet. Gynecol., 96: 446, 2000.

152. Danso, K.A., Martey, J.O., Wall, L.L. And Elkins, T.E.: The epidemiology of genitourinary fistulae in Kumasi, Ghana, 1977-1992. Int. Urogynecol. J. Pelvic Floor Dysfunct., 7: 117, 1996.

153. Grady, D., Brown, J.S., Vittinghoff, E., Applegate, W., Varner, E. And Snyder, T.: Postmenopausal hormones and incontinence: The Heart and Estrogen /Progestin Replacement Study. Obstet. Gynecol., 97: 116, 2001

154. Brown, J.S., Sawaya, G., Thom, D.H. And Grady, D.: Hysterectomy and urinary incontinence; a systematic review. Lancet, 356: 535, 2000.

155. Brown, J.S., Seeley, D.G., Fong, J., Black, D.M., Ensrud, K.E. And Grady, D.: Urinary incontinence in older women: Who is at risk? Study of osteoporotic fractures research group. Obstet. Gynecol., 87: 715, 1996

156. Thom, D.H. And Brown, J.S.: Reproductive and hormonal risk factors for urinary incontinence in later life: a review of the clinical and epidemiologic literature. J. Am. Geriatr. Soc., 46: 1411, 1998.

157. Weber, A.M., Walters, M.D., Schover, L.R., Church, J.M. And Piedmonte, M.R.: Functional outcomes and satisfaction after abdominal hysterectomy. Am. J. Obstet. Gynecol., 181: 530, 1999.

158. Thakar, R., Manyonda, I., Stanton, S.L., Clarkson, P. And Robinson, G.: Bladder, bowel and sexual function after hysterectomy for benign conditions. Br. J. Obstet. Gynaecol., 104: 983, 1997.

159. Mommsen, S. And Foldspang, A.: Body mass index and adult female urinary incontinence. World J. Urol., 12: 319, 1994.

160. Fultz, N.H., Herzog, A.R., Raghunathan, T.E., Wallace, R.B. And Diokno, A.C.: Prevalence and severity of urinary incontinence in older African American and Caucasian women. J. Gerontol. Med. Sci., 54A: M299, 1999.

161. Dwyer, P.L., Lee, E.T.C. And Hay, D.M.: Obesity and urinary incontinence in women. Br. J. Obstet. Gynaecol., 95: 91, 1988.

162. Kolbl, H. And Riss, P.: Obesity and stress urinary incontinence: significance of indices of relative weight. Urol. Int., 43: 7, 1988.

163. Fischer, J.R. And Berg, P.H.: Urinary incontinence in United States Air Force female aircrew. Obstet. Gynecol. 94: 532, 1999.

164. Bump, R.C., Sugerman, H.J., Fantl, F.A. And Mcclish, D.K.: Obesity and lower urinary tract function in women: Effect of surgically induced weight loss. Am. J. Obstet. Gynecol., 166: 392, 1992.

165. Deitel, M., Stone, E., Kassam, H.A., Wilk, E.F. And Sutherland, D.J.A.: Gynecologic-obstetric changes after loss of massive excess weight following bariatric surgery. J. Am. Coll. Nutr., 7: 147, 1988.

166. Herzog, A.R., Fultz, N.H., Brock, B.M., Brown, M.B. And Diokno, A.C.: Urinary incontinence and psychological distress among older adults. Psychol. Aging, 3: 115, 1988.

167. Tinetti, M.E., Inouye, S.K., Gill, T.M. And Doucette, J.T.: Shared risk factors for falls, incontinence, and functional depen-

dence - unifying the approach to geriatric syndromes. JAMA., 273: 1348, 1995.

168. Ouslander, J.G., Morishita, L., Blaustein, J., Orzeck, S., Dunn, S. And Sayre, J.: Clinical, functional, and psychosocial characteristics of an incontinent nursing home population. J. Gerontol., 42: 631, 1987.

169. Ouslander, J.G., Uman, G.C., Urman, H.N. And Rubenstein, L.Z.: Incontinence among nursing home patients: clinical and functional correlates. J. Am. Geriatr. Soc., 35: 324, 1987.

170. Wetle, T., Scherr, P., Branch, L.G., Resnick, N.M., Harris, T., Evans, D. Et Al.: Difficulty with holding urine among older persons in a geographically defined community: Prevalence and correlates. J. Am. Geriatr. Soc., 43: 349, 1995.

171. Skelly, J. And Flint, A.J.: Urinary incontinence associated with dementia. J. Am. Geriatr. Soc., 43: 286, 1995.

172. Rohr, G., Kragstrup, J. And Christensen, K.: Geners indflydelse på udviklingen af urininkontinens, undersøgt blandt ældre kvindelige tvillinger. 11. Nordic Congress in General Practice, Abstract F11.143, Copenhagen 2000.

173. Mushkat, Y., Bukovsky, I. And Langer, R.: Female urinary stress incontinence. Does it have familial prevalence? Am. J. Obstet. Gynecol., 174: 617, 1996.

174. Molander, U., Arvidsson, L., Milsom, I. And Sandberg, T.: A longitudinal cohort study of elderly women with urinary tract infections. Maturitas, 34: 127, 2000.

175. Diokno, A., Brock, B., Herzog, A. And Bromberg, J.: Medical correlates of urinary incontinence in the elderly. Urology, 36: 129, 1990.

176. Montella, J. And Wordell, C.J.: The effects of drugs on the lower urinary tract. In: Ostergard, D. and Bent, A., eds.: Urogynecology and urodynamics. Baltimore: Williams and Wilkins, 1996.

177. Arya, L.A., Myers, D.L. And Jackson, N.D.: Dietary caffeine intake and the risk for detrusor instability: a case-control study. Obstet. Gynecol., 96: 85, 2000.

178. Nygaard, I., Nygaard, I.E., Thompson, F.L. Svengalis, S.L. And Albright, J.P.: Urinary incontinence in elite nulliparous athletes. Obstet. Gynecol., 84: 183, 1994.

179. Parkin, D.E., Davis, J.A. And Symonds, R.P.: Urodynamic findings following radiotherapy for cervical carcinoma. Br. J. Urol., 61: 213, 1988.

180. Bump, R.C. And Mcclish, D.K.: Cigarette smoking and urinary incontinence in women. Am. J. Obstet. Gynecol., 167: 1213, 1992.

181. Feneley, R.C., Sheperd, A.M., Powell, P.H. And Blannin, J.: Urinary incontinence: prevalence and needs. Br. J. Urol., 51: 493, 1979.

182. Schulman, C., Claesm, H. And Mattijs, J.: Urinary incontinence in Belgium: a population-based epidemiological survey. Eur. Urol., 32: 315, 1997.

183. Malmsten, U.G., Milsom, I., Molander, U. And Norlen, L.J.: Urinary incontinence and lower urinary tract symptoms: an epidemiological study of men aged 45-99 years. J. Urol., 158: 1733, 1997.

184. Yarnell, J.W.G. And St Leger, A.S.: The prevalence, severity and factors associated with urinary incontinence in a random sample of the elderly. Age Ageing, 8: 81, 1979.

185. Sladden, M.J., Hughes, A.M., Hirst, G.H. And Ward, J.E.: A community study of lower urinary tract symptoms in older men in Sydney, Australia. Aust. N.Z. J. Surg., 70: 322, 2000.

186. Hunskaar, S.: One hundred and fifty men with urinary incontinence. I. Demography and medical history. Scand. J. Prim. Health Care, 10: 21, 1992.

187. Resnick, N.M. And Yalla, S.V.: Detrusor hyperactivity with impaired contractile function: an unrecognised but common cause of incontinence in elderly patients. JAMA., 257: 3076, 1987.

188. Poon, M., Ruckle, H., Bamshad, B.R., Tsai, C., Webster, R. And Lui, P.: Radical retropubic prostatectomy: bladder neck preservation versus reconstruction. J. Urol.,163: 194, 2000.

189. Walsh, P.C., Marschke, P., Ricker, D. And Burnett, A.L.: Patient-reported urinary continence and sexual function after anatomic radical prostatectomy. Urology, 55: 58, 2000.

190. Catalona, W.J., Carvalhal, G.F., Mager, D.E. And Smith, D.S.: Potency, continence and complication rates in 1870 consecutive radical retropubic prostatectomies. J. Urol., 162: 433, 1999.

191. Goluboff, E.T., Saidi, J.A., Mazer, S., Bagiella, E., Heitjan, D.F., Benson, M.C. Et Al.: Urinary continence after radical prostatectomy: The Columbia experience. J. Urol., 159: 1276, 1998.

192. Mettlin, C.J., Murphy, G.P., Sylvester, J., Mckee, R.F., Morrow, M. And Winchester, D.P.: Results of hospital registry surveys by the American College of Surgeons : outcomes of prostate cancer treatment by radical prostatectomy. Cancer, 80: 1875, 1997.

193. Benoit, R.M., Naslund, M.J. And Cohen, J.K.: Complications after radical retropubic prostatectomy in the medicare population. Urology, 56: 116, 2000.

194. Bishoff, J.T., Motley, G., Optenberg, S.A., Stein, C.R., Moon, K.A., Browning, S.M. Et Al.: Incidence of fecal and urinary incontinence following radical perineal and retropubic prostatectomy in a national population J. Urol., 160: 454, 1998.

195. McCammon, K.A., Kolm, P., Main, B. And Schellhammer, P.F.: Comparative quality of life analysis after radical prostatectomy or external beam radiation for localized prostate cancer. Urology, 54: 509, 1999.

196. Donnellan, S.M., Duncan, H.J., MacGregor, R.J. And Russel, J.M.: Prospective assessment of incontinence after radical retropubic prostatectomy: objective and subjective analysis. Urology, 49: 225, 1997.

197. Ojdeby, G., Claezon, A., Brekkan, E., Haggman, M. And Norlen, B.J.: Urinary incontinence and sexual impotence after radical prostatectomy. Scand. J. Urol. Nephrol., 30: 473, 1996.

198. Horie, S., Tobisu, K.I, Fujimoto, H., Doi, N. And Kakizoe, T.: Urinary incontinence after non-nerve-sparing radical prostatectomy with neoadjuvant androgen deprivation. Urology, 53: 561, 1999.

199. Gray, M., Petroni, G.R. And Theodorescu, D.: Urinary function after radical prostatectomy: a comparison of the retropubic and perineal approaches. Urology, 53: 881, 1999.

200. Van Kampen, M., De Weerdt, W., Van Poppel, H., Castell Campesino, A., Stragier, J. And Baert, L.: Prediction of urinary continence following radical prostatectomy. Urol. Int., 60: 80, 1998.

201. Kao, T.C., Garner, D., Foley, J., Seay, T., Friedrichs, P., Thrasher, J.B. Et Al.: Multicenter patient self-reporting questionnaire on impotence, incontinence and stricture after radical prostatectomy. J. Urol., 163: 858, 2000.

202. Herzog, A.R. And Fultz, N.H.: Epidemiology of urinary incontinence: prevalence, incidence, and correlates in community populations. Urology Suppl., 36: 2, 1990.

203. Fultz, N.H. And Herzog, A.R.: Measuring urinary incontinence in surveys. Gerontologist, 33: 708, 1993.

204. Barry, M.J., Fowler, F.J., O'Leary. M.P., Bruskewitz, R.C., Holtgrewe, H.L. And Mebust, W.K.: Correlation of the American Urological Association symptom index with self-administered versions of the Madsen-Iversen, Boyarsky and Maine medical assessment program symptom indexes. J. Urol., 148: 1558, 1992.

205. Herzog, A.R., Fultz, N.H., Normolle, D.P., Brock, B.M. And Diokno, A.C.: Methods used to manage urinary incontinence by

older adults in the community. J. Am. Geriatr. Soc., 37: 339, 1989.

206. Seim, A., Sandvik, H., Hermstad, R. And Hunskaar, S.: Female urinary incontinence - consultation behavior and patient experiences: an epidemiological survey in a Norwegian community. Fam. Pract., 12: 18, 1995.

207. Reymert, J. And Hunskaar, S.: Why do only a minority of perimenopausal women with urinary incontinence consult a doctor? Scand. J. Prim. Health Care, 12: 180, 1994.

208. Burgio, K.L., Ives, D.G., Locher, J.L., Arena, V.C. And Kuller, L.H.: Treatment seeking for urinary incontinence in older adults. J. Am. Geriatr. Soc., 42: 208, 1994.

209. Rizk, D.E., Shaheen, H., Thomas, L., Dunn, E. And Hassan, M.Y.: The prevalence and determinants of health care-seeking behavior for urinary incontinence in United Arab Emirates women. Int. Urogynecol. J. Pelvic. Floor. Dysfunct., 10: 160, 1999.

210. Seim, A., Sivertsen, B., Eriksen, B.C. And Hunskaar, S.: Treatment of urinary incontinence in women in general practice: observational study. BMJ., 312: 1459, 1996.

211. Seim, A., Eriksen, B.C. And Hunskaar, S.: A study of female urinary incontinence in general practice: demography, medical history, and clinical findings. Scand. J. Urol. Nephrol., 30: 465, 1996.

212. Sandvik, H. And Hunskaar, S.: Incontinence pads - prevalence of use and individual consumptiom. Scand. J. Soc. Med., 21: 120, 1993.

213. Sandvik, H., Kveine, E. And Hunskaar, S.: Female urinary incontinence. Psychosocial impact, self care, and consultations. Scand. J. Caring Sci., 7: 53, 1993.

214. Dugan, E., Roberts, C.P., Cohen, S.J., Preisser, J.S., David, C.C., Bland, D.R. Et Al.: Why older community-dwelling adults do not discuss urinary incontinence with their primary care physicians. J. Am. Geriatr. Soc., 49: 462, 2001.

215. Sandvik, H., Hunskaar, S. And Eriksen, B.C.: Management of urinary incontinence in women in general practice: actions taken in the first consultation. Scand. J. Prim. Health Care, 8: 3, 1990.

216. Andersen, J.T. And Sander, P.: Minimal care - a new consept for the management of urinary incontinence in an open access, interdisciplinary incontinence clinic. The way ahead? Scand. J. Urol. Nephrol. Suppl., 179: 55, 1996.

217. Shaw, C., Tansey, R., Jackson, C., Hyde, C. And Allan, R.: Barriers to help seeking in people with urinary symptoms. Fam. Pract. 18: 48, 2001.

218. Hunskaar, S., Seim, A. And Freeman, T.: The journey of incontinent women from community to university clinic; implications for selection bias, gatekeeper function, and primary care. Fam. Pract., 13: 363, 1996.

Committee 4

Pathophysiology

Chairmen

H. Koelbl (Germany),

J. Mostwin (USA)

Members

J.P. Boiteux (France),

E. Macarak (USA),

E. Petri (Germany),

W. Schafer (Germany),

O. Yamaguchi (Japan)

CONTENTS

Pathophysiology

H. Koelbl, J. Mostwin,

J.P. Boiteux, E. Macarak, E. Petri, W. Schafer, O. Yamaguchi

A. CAUSES OF URINARY INCONTINENCE: GENERAL CONSIDERATIONS

Urinary incontinence is the most discernible manifestation of several different kinds of injuries and disease processes of the lower urinary tract or the portions of the nervous system which regulate it. Some of these diseases and injuries affect both men and women. Others are gender specific.

The most common and familiar causes of incontinence are detrusor overactivity (neurogenic and idiopathic) and sphincteric incompetence, the latter resulting from childbirth, maternal injury, pelvic weakness and post-menopausal involution of the urethra in women, or from surgical injury in men. Neurological illness and injury also remain important causes of detrusor overactivity, sphincteric weakness and incoordination.

Sphincteric incompetence and bladder dysfunction may co-exist in the same individual. They may be related or may arise by different means and require broad understanding to direct treatment. Both patient and practitioner may find it difficult to distinguish among the various causes of any one person's incontinence. This can lead to confusion in diagnosis and treatment recommendations which may then be empirical or even haphazard. Understanding the various pathways which lead to incontinence can help achieve accurate diagnosis and realistic, evidence-based treatment goals.

Understanding pathophysiology becomes more importance when the risks and cost of treatment increase, as they do when surgical correction of incontinence is considered, or when chronic use of medication, expensive programs of training, biofeedback, or implantation of devices is undertaken. Precise diagnosis also offers the greatest hope that the results of longitudinal studies will be based on solid ground.

With these issues in mind, we have considered first, the general causes of incontinence in men and women and then, the gender specific causes.

General causes (Table 1) include bladder dysfunction caused by congenital anomalies, injuries and diseases of the nervous system and abnormalities of the bladder itself: the smooth muscle, its connective tissue and innervation. Bladder innervation includes normal and abnormal sensation arising from bladder afferents and spinal coordination of bladder function with its associated sphincters. We believe these factors, although modified by age and gender, are relatively similar in men and women. These abnormalities fall under the traditional concern of the urodynamically oriented physician, the neuro-urologist, rehabilitation specialist, geriatrician or general practitioner, or the neurologist or neurosurgeon with a particular interest in bladder dysfunction.

In women, the unique problem of urethral weakness and vaginal relaxation have received special consideration (Table 2). Other gender specific issues in women include: differences in anatomy of the pelvic floor and the levator hiatus; the size and strength of pelvic muscles compared to men; the role of childbirth and maternal injury on pelvic musculature, urethra and vaginal supports; hormonal milieu of the urethra; and the effect of aging. Much attention has been directed to distinguishing detrusor from urethral factors in women's incontinence, and further, in clarifying the relative contributions of urethral dysfunction and changes in vaginal support in the development of genuine stress incontinence (GSUI). These problems have been approached by gynecologists and urologists working within the boundaries of their own specialties and more recently, across specialties in combined groups.

In men, prostatic disease or its treatment may result in incontinence from bladder or sphincteric causes (Table 3). Men with symptomatic benign prostatic hyperplasia

Table 1 : General causes of incontinence

- **Congenital anomalies**
- **Injuries and disease of the nervous system**
- **Abnormalities of bladder itself**
  - Muscle
  - Connective tissue
  - Innervation
    - *Sensory afferents*
    - *Somatosensory control and coordination of sphincter*
- **Connective tissue of lower urinary tract**
- **Aging**

Table 2 : Specific causes of incontinence in women

- **Genuine stress urinary incontinence (GSUI)**
  - Urethral weakness
  - Vaginal relaxation
- **Specific contributory factors**
  - Anatomy of pelvic floor, levator hiatus, muscle size & strength
  - Childbirth and maternal injury
  - Vaginal support of urethra
  - Aging
- **Menopause**

Table 3 : Specific causes of incontinence in men

- **Benign prostatic and infravesical outflow obstruction**
  - Bladder dysfunciton due to outflow obstruction
    - *Post-prostatectomy incontinence*
      - RESIDUAL BLADDER DYSFUNCTION
      - SPHINCTERIC INJURY
- **Radical prostatectomy for cancer**
  - sphincteric injury
  - possible bladder or urethral denervation
- **Additional prostatic surgery after cancer radiotherapy**

may develop incontinence as a result of bladder dysfunction associated with infravesical outlet obstruction (prostatic enlargement, or constriction or dysfunction of the bladder neck) or from residual bladder dysfunction or sphincteric injury after simple prostatectomy. Men undergoing radical (total) prostatectomy for treatment of localized cancer may become incontinent from sphincter injury caused or unmasked by the operation. These problems have traditionally been addressed by urologists.

We have tried to present a unified view of causes of incontinence, while recognizing the wide range of backgrounds of the members of our subcommittee. We recognize the popular tendency to consider incontinence a disease and to overlook the subtleties of etiology when assessing treatment outcomes. We note the tendency to simplify classification and treatment, and we understand the desire of both patients and practitioners for effective and satisfying treatment. Yet, while treatment options are offered and developed, we should not lose sight of the fact that our comprehensive understanding and eventual success in managing incontinence is still hampered by incomplete knowledge of pathophysiology.

B. BLADDER DYSFUNCTION AS A CAUSE OF INCONTINENCE : THE OVERACTIVE BLADDER

To the neuro-urologist, incontinence is only one symptom of bladder dysfunction. Vesico-ureteral reflux and urinary retention due to loss of contractility and detrusor-sphincter dyssynergia are also significant symptoms that may demand medical treatment. When considering bladder dysfunction as a cause in the patient's presenting symptoms, it is important to keep in mind that incontinence may be only one manifestation of a complex neurological disorder of the nervous system or the lower urinary tract.

INTRODUCTION

The most common problem with urine storage arises when the bladder fails to remain relaxed until an appropriate time for urination. The symptom syndrome is called "overactive bladder" (OAB), which refers to the symptoms of urgency, with or without urge incontinence, usually with frequency and nocturia. According to ICS terminology as of 2001, OAB symptoms are suggestive of urodynamically demonstrable detrusor overactivity (involuntary detrusor contraction) during the filling phase which may be spontaneous provoked. This may be further characterized as neurogenic when there is a relevant neurological condition. Common neurogenic causes include stroke, Parkinson's Disease, multiple sclerosis and spinal injury. Non-neurogenic etiologies may be related to outflow obstruction, aging, female anatomical incontinence, but many cases are idiopathic. This section focuses on pathophysiology of the overactive bladder and reviews studies that have provided insights into the mechanisms underlying bladder overactivity.

I. NEUROGENIC DETRUSOR OVERACTIVITY

1. SUPRAPONTINE LESIONS (FIGURE 1)

It is generally accepted that suprapontine lesions such as cerebrovascular disease and Parkinson's disease produce detrusor overactivity. The patient with suprapontine lesion loses voluntary inhibition of micturition, which corresponds to uninhibited overactive bladder according to a classification by Fall et al [1, 2].

Brain transection studies in animals with an intact neuro-axis showed that suprapontine areas generally exert a tonic inhibitory influence on the pontine micturition center (PMC) [3, 4]. In humans, the cerebral cortex(medial frontal lobes) and the basal ganglia are thought to suppress the micturition reflex. Thus, damage to the brain induces bladder overactivity by reducing suprapontine inhibition.

Recently, the mechanism of overactive bladder induced by cerebral infarction or Parkinson's disease has been further studied using animal models [5, 6]. In the central nervous system, a glutamatergic pathway is known to play a role in both excitatory and inhibitory regulation of micturition [7, 8]. Central dopaminergic pathways also have dual excitatory and inhibitory influences on reflex bladder activity [9, 10]]. It has been demonstrated that in the rat cerebral infarction model, the bladder hyperactivity is mediated by NMDA glutamatergic and D_2 dopaminergic excitatory mechanisms [6], suggesting that cerebral infarction may alter a balance between the facilitatory and inhibitory mechanism that results in up-regulation of an excitatory pathway and down-regulation of a tonic inhibitory pathway. Similarly, neuropharmacological studies in the monkey model for Parkinson's disease have shown that detrusor overactivity may result from a loss of dopaminergic inhibition mediated by D_1 receptors [9, 11].

2. SPINAL CORD LESIONS (FIGURE 2)

Spinal cord lesions above the lumbosacral level eliminate voluntary and supraspinal control of micturition, leading to bladder overactivity mediated by spinal reflex pathways [3, 12]. Disruption below the level of the pons leads to unsustained and uncoordinated detrusor contractions often associated with uncoordinated sphincter overactivity (detrusor-sphincter dyssynergia, DSD). Impairment or loss of bladder sensation is a typical feature.

Electrophysiologic studies using capsaicin have demonstrated that in chronic spinal cats, the afferent limb of the micturition reflex consists of unmyelinated C-fiber afferents, whereas in normal cats it consists of myelinated A – afferents [13-15]. Since C-fiber bladder afferents in the cat usually do not respond to bladder distension [16], a considerable reorganization of reflex connections takes place in the spinal cord following the interruption of descending pathways from the brain. In humans with spinal cord lesions, neurogenic detrusor overactivity is likely to be mediated by capsaicin-sensitive C-fiber afferents. Clinical experience with capsaicin supports the role of these C-fiber afferents in the pathophysiology of neurogenic bladder overactivity. Capsaicin has been used for the treatment of neurogenic bladder overactivity in patients with spinal cord injury or multiple sclerosis. When administered intravesically, capsaicin increased bladder capacity, reduced the micturition contraction pressure, decreased autonomic dysreflexia and reduced the frequency of incontinence [17-19]. More recently, resineferatoxin, an ultrapotent analogue of capsaicin, is also used [20, 21].

In addition to the changes in reflex pathways (i.e., C-fiber afferent-mediated micturition reflex), it has been demonstrated that a functional outlet obstruction resulting from DSD could alter the properties of bladder afferent neurons. For example, in chronic spinal animals, afferent neurons innervating the bladder increase in size, a change prevented by urinary diversion [22] . The observation suggests that some factors released in the obstructed bladder were responsible for the neural change. Subsequently, the factors were identified as nerve growth factor (NGF) [23].

Another type of plasticity in C-fiber bladder afferent neurons was evident as a change in excitability. Whole cell-patch clamp recordings revealed that hypertrophied bladder afferent neurons exhibit increased excitability due to a shift in expression of sodium channels from high-threshold tetrodotoxin (TTX)-resistant to low-threshold TTX-sensitive channels [24, 25]. In normal animals, TTX-resistant sodium channels are mainly expressed in C-fiber afferent neurons [26, 27].

II. NON-NEUROGENIC DETRUSOR OVERACTIVITY

1. OUTFLOW OBSTRUCTION (FIGURE 3)

Detrusor overactivity associated with outflow obstruction has long been recognized [28]. Sixty percent of patients with benign prostatic hyperplasia (BPH) exhibit this. On filling cystometry. Following transurethral prostatectomy (TURP), the involuntary contraction disappears in two-thirds.

The hypothesis that denervation underlies obstructed non-neurogenic detrusor overactivity comes from the

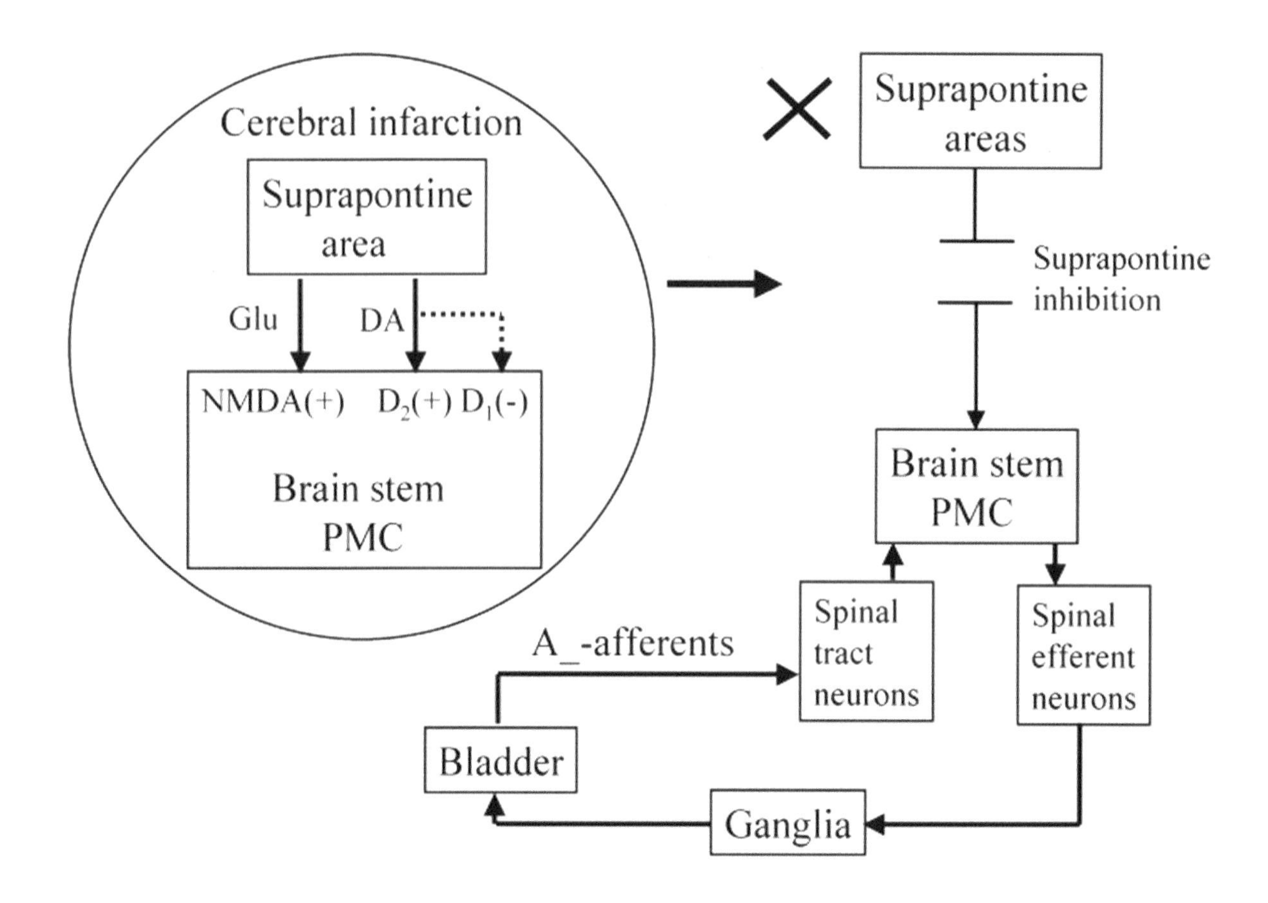

Figure 1 : Suprapontine lesions causing detrusor overactivity

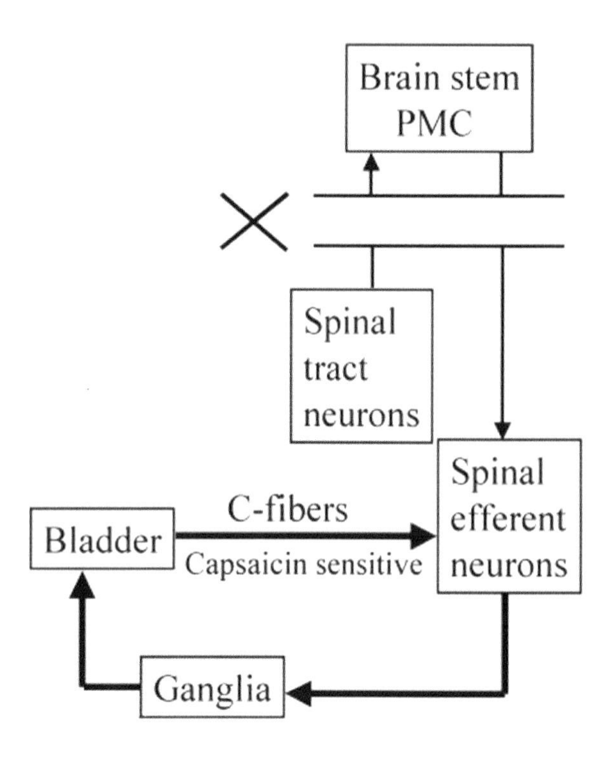

Figure 2 : causing detrusor overactivity causing detrusor overactivity

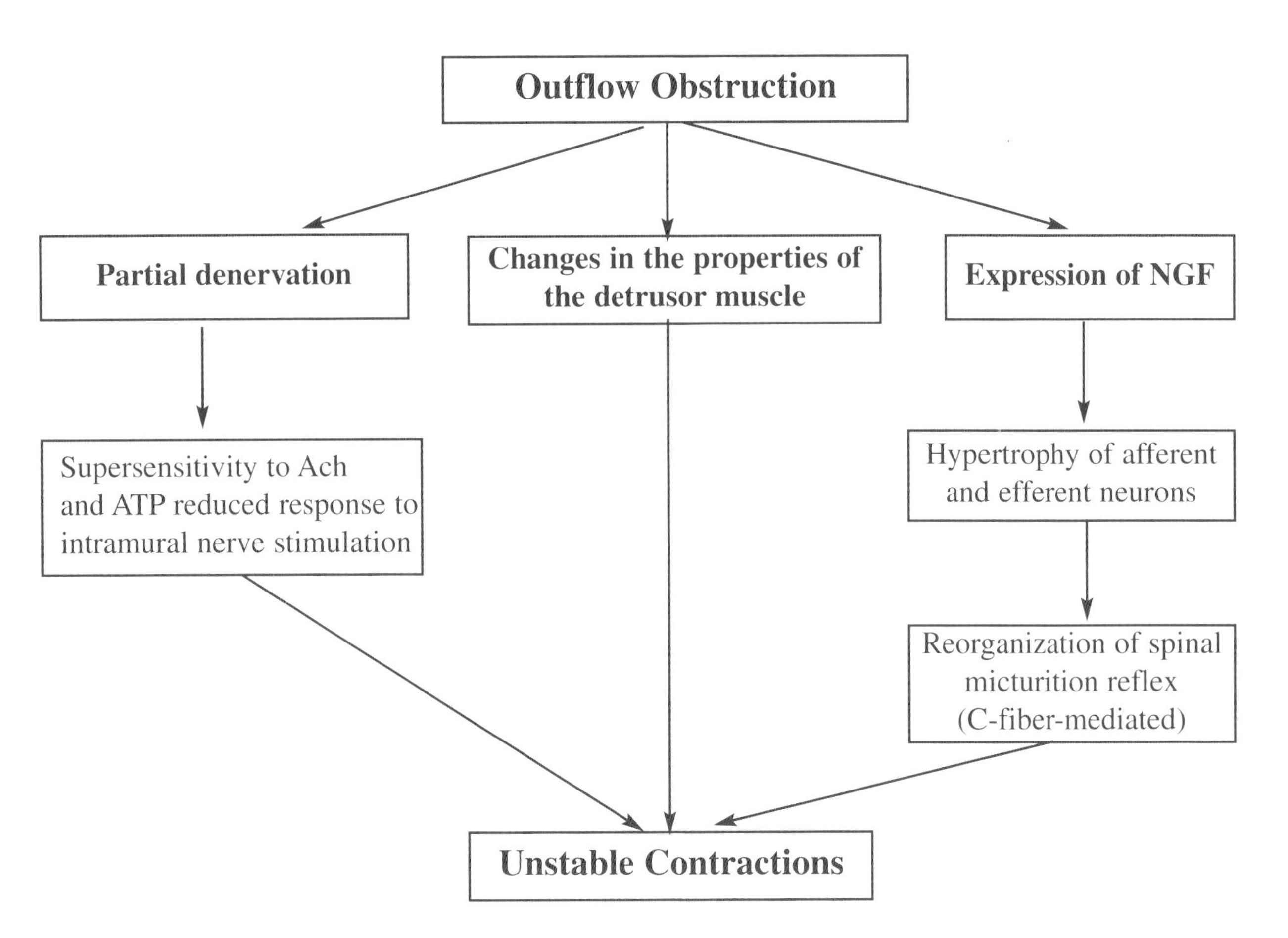

Figure 3 : Outflow obstruction causing detrusor overactivity

morphological studies of Gosling et al [29]. They observed a reduction in acetylcholinesterase staining nerves in obstructed human bladder muscle. Pharmacological studies performed on detrusor biopsies from patients with bladder outlet obstruction [30] show that muscle strips from patients with instability exhibited supersensitivity to acetylcholine (the main excitatory neurotransmitter to the human bladder) and reduction in nerve-mediated responses, as compared with strips from stable bladder. Similar pharmacological and morphological evidences of denervation were obtained from animal models of detrusor overactivity caused by urethral obstruction [31-33], demonstrating that there were significant increases in sensitivity to acetylcholine and other agonists such as high potassium, and the response to intramural nerve stimulation was significantly reduced (despite increased responsiveness of the muscle to exogenous acetylcholine), with both cholinergic and non-cholinergic (purinergic) neurotransmission being affected. These changes suggest a post-junctional supersensitivity secondary to partial denervation of the obstructed detrusor muscle, and may be the basis of the overactive bladder behavior.

However, it is not clear how denervation develops in outflow obstruction. One possibility is that there is a reduction of blood flow due to the effect of raised intravesical pressure during voiding or the increased tissue pressure of hypertrophied bladder wall during filling. Such homodynamic change was demonstrated in canine model of outlet obstruction [34]. Thus, the role of ischemia in changes in bladder function and structure following outlet obstruction has been well characterized. The recent study using iNOS knockout mice [35]suggests that generation of NO soon after obstruction is necessary to prevent detrusor dysfunction, since NO produces vasodilation and decreases platelet aggregation.

Obstruction can alter contractile properties of the detrusor muscle. In obstructed guinea pig bladder, the detrusor muscle showed a decrease in force development, suggesting a deterioration in detrusor contractility [36]. The cable properties of detrusor cells are also changed [37]. The length constant is reduced, suggesting a decrease in cell to cell propagation of electrical activity. The time constant of cell membrane is prolonged, leading to greater instability of membrane potential. This may depolarize the cell and activate L-type calcium channels. Such a mechanism could be further amplified by a depolarizing current supplied by a purinergic system, which was demonstrated to emerge in human obstructed bladder [38]. These findings may generalize that individual cells are more irritable while synchronous activation is damaged, consistent with the abnormal bladder behavior of obstructed bladder, i.e., the decreased contractility coexisting with bladder overactivity.

A different interpretation for the mechanism underlying the development of detrusor overactivity is a possible reorganization of the spinal micturition reflex following outlet obstruction. Partial urethral ligation in the rat induced hypertrophy of both bladder afferent and efferent neurons [39, 40]. This hypertrophy of bladder neurons was accompanied by increased expression of NGF in the bladder as well as in sacral autonomic centers [23], leading to facilitation of the spinal micturition reflex [39, 40]. Similarly, in patients with outflow obstruction, a spinal reflex may be responsible for the development of detrusor overactivity. This reflex is thought to be mediated by C-fibers and clinically detected as a positive response to the ice water test. C-fiber neurons are also known to contain tachykinin and other peptides as neurotransmitters. It has been suggested that in rats with bladder outlet obstruction, tachykinins can influence via NK receptors both the spinal and supraspinal control of the bladder [41, 42].

2. AGING

It has been shown recently that BPH symptom scores were not different in older men and women [43]. This suggests that lower urinary tract symptoms (LUTS) may be a similar sign of aging in both men and women. The prevalence of urgency syndromes, in particular, increases with age, independent of the presence of outflow obstruction or neurogenic disorder. A study of incontinent institutionalized elderly revealed that approximately 61% of the women and 59% of the men (without obstruction) had detrusor overactivity [44]. However, in the elderly, the boundaries between neurogenic and non-neurogenic are uncertain, since age-associated neurogenic diseases such as subclinical cerebrovascular disorders, autonomic neuropathy and chronic brain failure commonly occur. Computerized tomography, magnetic resonance imaging or SPECT sometimes can detect the presence of cerebral lesions in elderly patients with DI [45, 46]. This may distinguish neurogenic from idiopathic detrusor overactivity in a considerable number of older patients.

With regard to aging-related detrusor overactivity, Elbadawi et al. have proposed a possible pathophysiology based on detailed ultrastructural study [47-49]. Electron microscopy of detrusor biopsies revealed a characteristic structural pattern in the specimens from the elderly with this problem. The main features of this dysfunction pattern were abundant distinctive protrusion junctions and abutments which were proposed to mediate electrical coupling between the muscle cells and to be involved in generation of myogenic contraction in the overactive bladder. In addition, if the patients had impaired detrusor contractility, there was superimposed widespread degeneration of muscle cells and nerve axons, which matched the special group of elderly patients with DHIC (detrusor hyperactivity with impaired contractility) [50].

Age-dependent alterations in detrusor function also have been evaluated. Cystometry of conscious rats shows that bladder compliance decreases with aging [51]. In rat detrusor muscle, the relaxant response to noradrenalin or isoproterenol decreases with age, a change which may be related to the decreased density of beta-adrenoceptors and decreased cyclic adenosine monophosphate (AMP) production [52]. In addition, age-related changes in cholinergic and purinergic neurotransmission have been studied recently in human detrusor muscle, showing that during electrical nerve stimulation, acetylcholine release is decreased while ATP release increases with aging [53, 54]. These changes in neurotransmission may contribute to the changes in bladder function in the elderly.

3. PELVIC FLOOR DISORDERS

Detrusor overactivity is known to be associated with female stress urinary incontinence as a result of pelvic floor relaxation. After surgical correction, this disappears in approximately two-thirds of these patients [55]. This may suggest that afferent nerve activity from pelvic floor and urethra is involved in detrusor inhibition during bladder filling. Thus, the decreased afferents due to pelvic floor deficiency can lead to involuntary detrusor contraction. External and direct pudendal nerve electrical stimulation shows a good clinical results in the treatment of the overactive bladder [56, 57], thereby supporting this hypothesis.

4. HYPERSENSITIVITY DISORDERS (FIGURE 4)

Neuropeptide-containing sensory nerves have been found innervating the human bladder [58]. These sensory afferents are capsaicin-sensitive, unmyelinated C-fibers. They usually transmit sensations of bladder fullness, urgency and pain. Local release of tachykinin and other peptides from these sensory nerves in the bladder wall may produce diverse biological effects, such as bladder smooth muscle contraction, facilitation of neural transmission and increased vascular permeability [59]. These properties of bladder sensory nerves suggest that increased afferent activity can induce detrusor overactivity in patients with hypersensitive disorders. Because capsaicin suppresses C-fiber sensory neuron activity, Maggi et al [58] instilled intravesical capsaicin

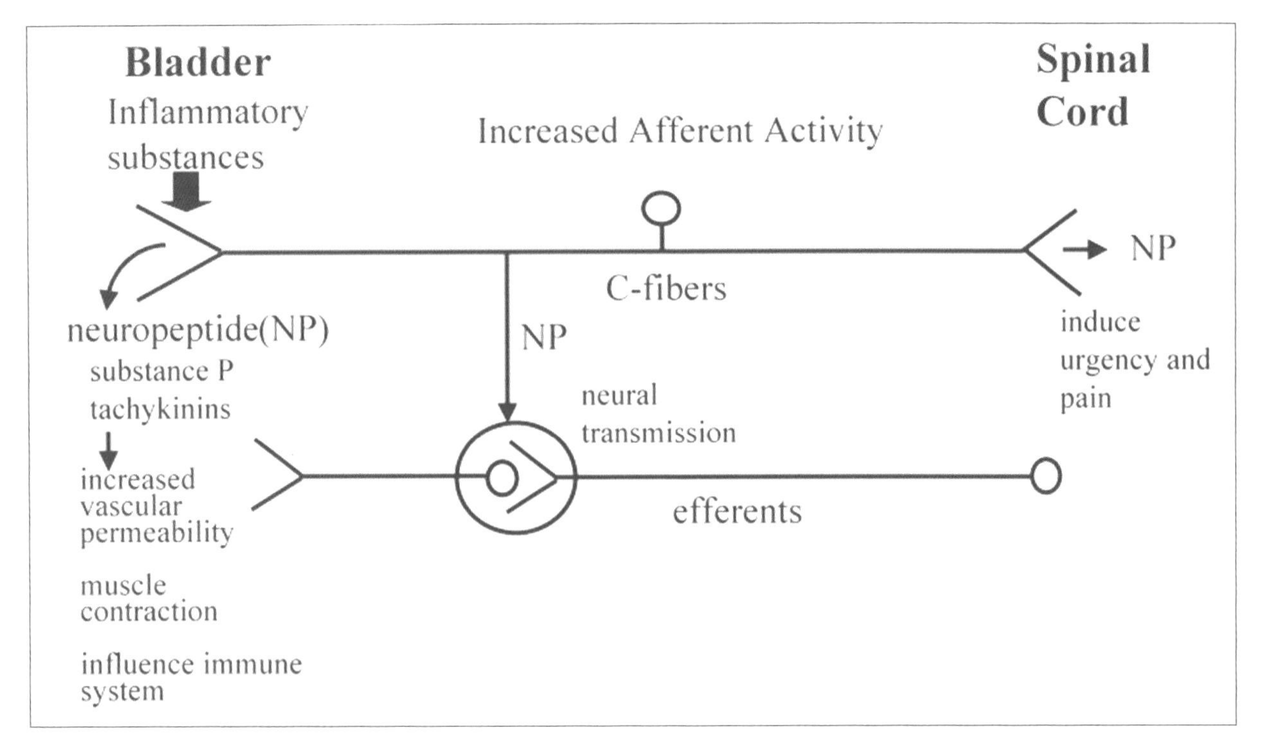

Figure 4 : Hypersensitivity causing detrusor overactivity

into patients with lower urinary tract hypersensitivity disorders, demonstrating disappearance or marked attenuation of their symptoms. More recently, a randomized placebo controlled study has shown that intravesical resiniferatoxin significantly improves the voiding pattern and pain score in patients with hypersensitivity disorder and bladder pain [60]. These results may support the above hypothesis, but knowledge about sensory functions of the human bladder is still limited.

The mechanisms of C-fiber afferent sensitization in chronic bladder inflammation have been studied using animals in which cystitis was induced by intravesical instillation of chemical agents. Inflammation is usually accompanied by a reduction in tissue pH. Protons(H^+) activate vanilloid receptors (a capsaicin-binding site) in afferent nerve terminals, resulting in Ca^{2+}-influx, and then a release of neuropeptides [61]. The electrophysiological properties of bladder afferent neurons were evaluated after chronic bladder inflammation induced by cyclophosphamide, showing that chronic inflammation increases the excitability of C-fiber afferent neurons by suppressing A-type K^+ channels [62].

Other endogenous substances such as bradykinin, histamine, prostaglandin, and ATP, which are produced by inflammation, also enhance bladder activity and neuropeptide release from C-fiber afferent neurons [61, 63] [64]. ATP receptor ($P2X_3$)-deficient mice exhibit a marked bladder hyper-reflexia as well as reduced pain-related behavior [4], suggesting that $P2X_3$ receptors in C-fiber bladder afferents may play a role in mediating bladder overactivity and bladder pain in chronic inflammatory bladder conditions such as interstitial cystitis.

5. Idiopathic detrusor overactivity (Figure 5)

The diagnosis of idiopathic detrusor overactivity requires the exclusion of all known causes, but this should include all situations where etiology is unknown. Thus, the term is used to apply to a wide range of different conditions that may have a common final pathophysiologic pathway [65].

With regard to the pathophysiology of idiopathic detrusor overactivity, Brading and Turner [66, 67] have emphasized the myogenic changes(regardless of etiology). On the basis of observation that denervation is consistently found in detrusor biopsy specimen from patients with various forms of DI [68], they have proposed that partial denervation of the detrusor may alter the properties of smooth muscle, leading to increased excitability and increased coupling between cells. Thus, local contraction (activity) that occurs somewhere in the detrusor will spread throughout the bladder wall, resulting in a coordinated myogenic contraction of the whole bladder. However, what actually triggers this local contraction is not certain. Thus, as Brading has stated [66], the changes in smooth muscle properties seem to be a necessary prerequisite for the production of unstable detrusor contraction.

It is clear from a clinical point of view that in patients

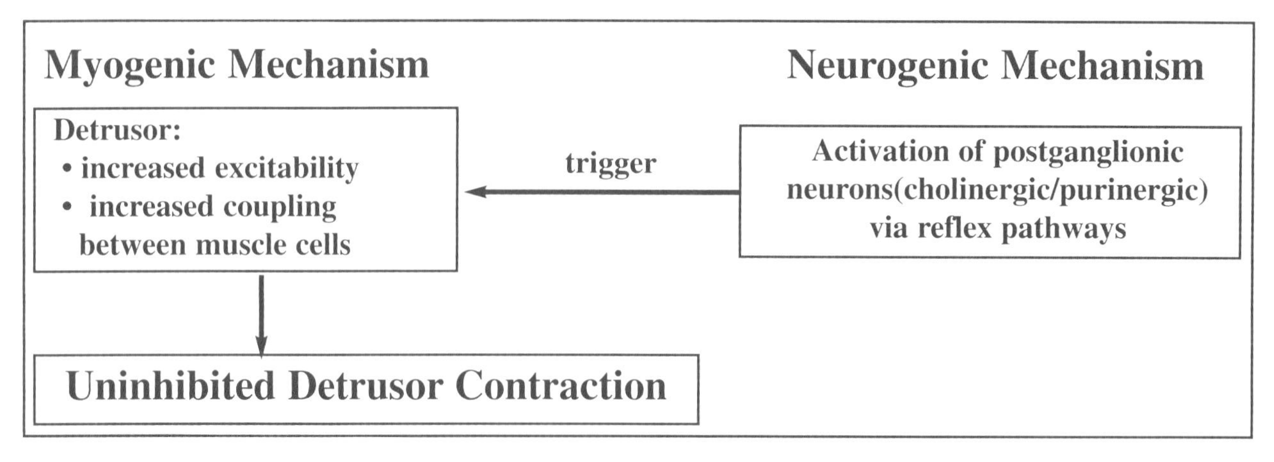

Figure 5 : Idiopathic causes detrusor overactivity

with idiopathic detrusor overactivity, antimuscarinic drugs can improve symptoms, reduce urgency and increase bladder capacity. This suggests that in these patients, there is acetylcholine (Ach) release during bladder filling, leading to an increase in detrusor tone or involuntary bladder contraction. It is speculated that Ach may be released from non-neuronal sources [69], or from postganglionic cholinergic neurons that may be activated via reorganized spinal reflex pathways or local reflex pathways in the pathologic condition. Such local release of Ach can enhance the myogenic contractile activity of the detrusor, which seems to be a trigger stimulation for inducing an involuntary contraction, as postulated in the myogenic theory of detrusor overactivity.

C. THE ROLE OF CONNECTIVE TISSUE IN THE LOWER URINARY TRACT

I. BLADDER COLLAGEN

The bladder contains large amounts of types I and III collagen. These collagens can be found in the lamina propria and in the detrusor layer. In addition to these fiber-forming collagens, type IV or basement membrane collagen can also be found in the bladder wall both beneath the urothelial layer and surrounding individual smooth muscle cells. Since collagens have the primary role of tension transfer in most tissues, it is reasonable to assume that collagen plays a similar role in the bladder.

This assumption can be supported by a number of descriptive studies that have defined the structural composition of the bladder wall at both the light and electron microscopic levels. These studies demonstrate that collagens I and III are found surrounding the muscle bundles in the detrusor layer. Immunolocalization studies with collagen-type specific antibodies to type I and III collagen demonstrate that fibers containing these collagens lie largely outside the muscle bundles with little or no localization within individual muscle bundles. In the lamina propria, the collagens form the dense irregular extracellular matrix of this layer. In addition to the collagens, there are also elastic fibers containing the protein elastin, which provides the lamina propria with its characteristic elastic nature. Thus, based upon the physical properties of the fibrous proteins, the bladder wall's tensile strength and, indeed, that of all tissues, is related to the amount and type(s) of collagen present and its arrangement.

II. TISSUE STRENGTH

For example, tendons are very strong structures capable of resisting very large tensional forces. The Achilles tendon is a good example of this type of highly organized array of fibrous type I collagen. Because the collagen molecules are arranged linearly, they easily form long strands of fibrous proteins whose diameters are substantial. The molecules within these fibers become progressively cross-linked via covalent bonds to adjacent molecules making them highly insoluble and very strong. Thus the overall mechanical strength of tissues appears to be directly related to the presence of collagen fibers, their arrangement and the way in which the collagen is associated with other structural macromolecules, e.g., proteoglycans and/or cells [70].

III. ROLE OF VITAMIN C AND METABOLIC EFFECTS

If one assumes that the tensile strength of tissues is provided by collagen, then it follows that circumstances that alter the collagen composition may, in turn, affect the overall strength of the tissue. The best known example of this modification of tissue strength is the disease scurvy. Vitamin C is a required co-factor for the enzymatic hydroxylation of proline residues in collagen by the enzyme prolyl hydroxylase. Without adequate Vitamin C, collagen is under-hydroxylated resulting in decreased rates of secretion of collagen molecules. In addition to decreased secretion of collagen, molecules that are secreted have a weaker triple helical structure and are more susceptible to proteolytic attack and thus are less durable. These molecular structural defects are reflected in lowered tissue strength and increased fragility of collagen-based structures.

In some individuals, metabolic defects or altered metabolism can account for altered tissue strength that may underlie structural defects associated with incontinence, e.g., pelvic floor laxity as discussed in the section on urethral support in this chapter.

IV. HORMONAL EFFECTS

Another potential hypothesis to explain the changes in the overall strength of connective tissues is that these changes are related to the normal aging process and/or alteration in hormones that can affect collagen metabolism. While older men experience urinary incontinence less often than do women, it is still a significant disruption in their live s [71]. During development, collagen fibril lengths and diameters increase which correlates with increased tissue strength [72]. Since genuine stress incontinence is present in a significant number of women before childbirth, these data suggest that it may result from aging, hormonal or genetic considerations. This hypothesis is further supported by the observations that many of the same structures required for preserving continence, e.g., bladder, pelvic floor, have estrogen receptors. Their activity or lack thereof may explain the increased prevalence of dysfunction in the urogenital tract in postmenopausal patients and, in particular, those not on hormone replacement therapy [73]. It has been suggested that conformational changes in the estrogen receptor are modulated by local cytokines whose levels may be dependent upon age related changes in the vaginal mucosa; however, there are little data to substantiate these hypotheses [74].

V. STRUCTURAL CHANGES IN THE BLADDER WALL

The concept that structural changes in the bladder wall and/or other structures associated with the lower tract and pelvic floor are responsible for incontinence is not entirely consistent with either biochemical data on collagen composition or clinical observations on incontinent individuals in a broad sense. It is often difficult to accurately clinically define subtle changes in voiding traits and to determine their etiology [75, 76]. For example, Gosling [77] found that smooth muscle cells in a normal bladder are closely packed together with little or no intervening connective tissue. The bundles were enervated predominantly by autonomic cholinergic nerve fibers while adrenergic nerves were observed in association with blood vessels. In the obstructed bladder, smooth muscle cells were surrounded by large amounts of connective tissue suggesting that some of the muscle cells had an altered phenotype, i.e., they converted from a contractile to a collagen synthetic phenotype. A significant reduction in the innervation of the smooth muscle cells was also observed. In contrast to those of the obstructed bladder, smooth muscle cells in the aging bladder had a normal morphology. There was a reduction in innervation although to a lesser extent than that observed in the obstructed bladder. These data suggest that the changes seen in the obstructed bladder are unlikely to be solely a consequence either of aging and/or hormonal changes. Nevertheless, information derived from morphologic evaluation of bladder tissue in concert with a diagnostic algorithm that uses age, flow-rate and post-voiding residual volumes [78] may be able to discriminate between different types of voiding dysfunctions .

VI. BLADDER FIBROSIS AND INCONTINENCE

This lack of a consensus about the cause of alterations in bladder structure is similarly evident in other studies of human patients with urodynamically proven incontinence or in animal studies of obstruction. In humans, a number of studies , either of women with stress incontinence or in men with incontinence secondary to benign prostatic hyperplasia, have been performed. Many of these studies have utilized morphometry to calculate the volumes of the muscle and connective tissue compartments in obstructed bladders and demonstrate that outlet obstruction caused histopathologic alterations in both the intervening connective tissue and the detrusor muscle. It has been suggested that, these alterations may be responsible for the occurrence of uninhibited muscle detrusor contractions and abnormal detrusor reflexes in patients with lower urinary tract obstruction [79].

Earlier studies report similar findings. In a group of 28 patients, the microscopic appearance of bladder biopsy samples was correlated with a clinical assessment that included cystoscopy and urodynamics. These results suggest an association between the severity of trabeculation and the degree of histologic change in the bladder wall, i.e., infiltration of detrusor muscle bundles by connective tissue. In patients with no outflow obstruction, mild or moderate trabeculation, as assessed cystoscopically, was not accompanied by structural alterations in the bladder wall [80].

VII. THE CAUSE OF BLADDER FIBROSIS REMAINS CONTROVERSIAL

Biopsy samples from males with proven outflow obstruction resulting from prostatic hypertrophy were compared with those from control bladder specimens. In controls, detrusor muscle bundles were composed of cells closely packed together with very little intervening connective tissue. In contrast, irrespective of age, detrusor muscle from trabeculated bladders contained many muscle bundles in which the constituent cells were of relatively small diameter and were widely separated from one another by masses of connective tissue. In the electron microscope, the dense connective tissue was seen to contain, in addition to collagen fibrils, an extensive meshwork of electron dense microfibrils apparently in continuity with the basal laminae of smooth muscle cells. [81]

Subsequent studies of detrusor muscle removed from control and urodynamically obstructed patients showed further that smooth muscle cells from obstructed patients undergo compensatory hypertrophy in response to outflow obstruction. As in their earlier studies, these investigators showed that connective tissue infiltration of detrusor muscle bundles was a characteristic morphologic change in those bladders that possess cells showing the largest increase in size [82]. Thus in human obstructed bladders, both in adult males and females, connective tissue infiltration of bladders is a consistent observation.

Another common observation, both in animal studies as well as those in human beings, is that bladder dysfunction is usually accompanied by some form of alteration in the innervation of the bladder. Although more extensive in obstructed than in aging bladder tissue, in both instances numerous investigators report a reduction in innervation of muscle cells. Thus it can be argued that initial event that predisposes a bladder to become dysfunctional is an alteration in the normal innervation pathways. How these changes are initiated is not well-understood, although there are considerable data to suggest that reduced blood flow to the bladder predisposes the tissue to nerve damage. Recent studies in the rabbit by Kazem et al [83]underscore the role that reduced blood flow and/or events associated with reduced blood flow may be a part of the process that ultimately leads to a dysfunctional bladder. In this (and many other such studies) study, it is implied that reduced blood flow likely leads to ischemia which may cause nerve damage. However, until accurate measurements of actual 0_2 levels are actually carried out in human, it remains speculative as to the mechanism underlying these changes.

In a study in which atherosclerosis was induced in rabbits, bladder fibrosis was observed. The authors suggest, based upon such experiments, that reduced blood flow to the bladder, secondary to the atherosclerosis, up-regulates TGF-beta expression in the bladder and leads to fibrosis, smooth muscle atrophy and non-compliance. Since vascular disease is a common age-associated disorder, the authors argue that reduced blood flow to the bladder may play an important role in the pathophysiology of voiding dysfunction in the elderly [83].

VIII. BLADDER FIBROSIS IN CHILDREN

Although adults represent the majority of patients with incontinence problems, obstruction in children also occurs. It has been recognized for some time that bladder collagens play important roles in governing bladder function [84, 85]. Obstruction can be the result of an anatomic congenital defect such as occurs in boys with posterior urethral valves. In addition, functional obstruction (neurogenic bladders) can result from either congenital malformations (myelomeningocele) or from spinal cord injuries. Morphometric studies of myelodysplastic bladders by Shapiro and colleagues showed an increase in connective tissue [86]. Immunohistochemistry using antibodies to collagens was used to further characterize the connective tissue response. In this study, Ewalt et al. [87] demonstrated that noncompliant bladders from children had a marked alteration in the distribution of type III collagen. Based upon these observations, these authors suggested that the lamina propria was the major capacitance layer within the bladder wall and that altered mechanical properties associated with noncompliant bladders was likely the result of the altered collagen distribution. Detrusor dysfunction is also associated with low compliance bladders. Two groups of patients were studied: neurogenics with low compliance bladders and non-neurogenics with low compliance bladders. Morphometric analysis was used to determine the proportion of connective tissue and muscle in the bladder wall samples. In the non-neurogenic group, there was a significant increase in connective tissue and a marked decrease in muscle in comparison to the control group. In the neuorgenics, there was a mild increase in connective tissue but no decrease in muscle. These investigators concluded that low bladder compliance in neurogenic patients is mainly caused by functional alterations in the bladder wall while in non-neurogenics, there is an organic change in bladder wall composition [88].

Studies on incontinent children were also performed by Landau et al [89]. Pressure specific bladder volume or the capacity of the bladder at a given pressure were measured urodynamically in patients with dysfunctional bladders. This study, unlike the earlier ones, combined morphometric as well as biochemical analyses. All patients studied were incontinent and had upper tract changes despite clean intermittent catheterization and/or pharmacotherapy. These studies demonstrated that the type III to I ratio was elevated in these patients as well as the total amount of connective tissue and the ratio of connective tissue to muscle. These authors conclude that diminished storage function of poorly compliant bladders is secondary to alteration in connective tissue content of the bladder wall.

In a study by Deveaud et al [90], a group of pediatric neurogenic and non-neurogenic patients were analyzed biochemically, immunohistologically and physiologically. These studies demonstrate that connective tissue infiltration of physically or functionally obstructed pediatric patients is characterized by an infiltration of the detrusor muscle bundles by type III collagen. This fibrotic response of the bladder results in an overall increase in collagen by approximately 10% and an increase in the type III to type I protein ratio. Analyses of mRNAs for these collagens demonstrated coordinate increases in both collagen I and collagen III mRNAs in non-neurogenic patients (largely boys with posterior urethral valves). The increase in type III collagen mRNA was in agreement with the study by Linn et al. In which type III collagen mRNA was measured by PCR [91] In neurogenic patients, there was, in contrast, an increase in the type III to type I mRNA ratio. These latter data suggest that the regulation of collagen synthesis , i.e., the molecular mechanism controlling collagen synthesis, in these two types of obstructive uropathies is likely different.

IX. ANIMAL MODELS

In addition to the studies of human patients, there are many animal models of outlet obstruction using a number of different species. Using these animal models, investigators have evaluated bladder response to outlet obstruction. The fine structure [92] and collagen content [93] of the detrusor muscle were evaluated in female rats. These studies demonstrate that bladder outflow obstruction caused an increase in voiding pressure and bladder weight and a decrease in bladder compliance [94] . Congenital bladder obstruction has also been modeled in sheep[1] and in minipigs [95] showing increased bladder weight owing to increase in both smooth muscle and collagen

SUMMARY

The studies referenced above are the synopsis of evidence accumulated over a period of approximately 25 years and suggest that bladder outlet obstruction and instability associated with it result in a series of structural changes. A common feature of these changes is an alteration in the connective tissue composition of the bladder. In addition, there are associated functional changes in compliance properties. Initially these changes are largely reversible. If the obstruction is relieved before the bladder undergoes decompensation, both structural and functional changes almost completely disappear [96]. Thus there appears to be a "window" during which intervention is beneficial to the long-term outcome of the patient. As described above, animal studies from a number of laboratories have demonstrated that the initial response of the bladder wall to obstruction can best be described as a compensatory response. That is, the bladder muscle responds to the increased work load caused by the obstruction by increasing its mass. Physiologically, the detrusor is functionally compromised and must increase its contractile force to overcome the increased resistance at the bladder neck. In response to this functional challenge, the detrusor compensates by increasing the overall amount of contractile protein. This can be observed biochemically as the level of actin and myosin increases as well as other associated contractile proteins in obstructed bladders [97]. Subsequently, there is an increase in collagen that appears to compromise the compliance properties of the bladder. The exact cause and molecular mechanism of the fibrotic response is currently unknown.

WHAT IS NOT KNOWN

Regulation of collagen synthesis is dependent upon intrinsic factors within individual cell types as well as other extrinsic factors such as cytokines, growth factors and mechanical forces. We know very little about the role of outlet obstruction and aging in altering the collagen phenotype of lamina propria fibroblasts and detrusor smooth muscle cells. Information about the intrinsic phenotype of cells both in the lamina propria and in the detrusor is needed. In addition, there are few specific markers for cells within the bladder wall. In order to understand how cell phenotype changes during aging or obstruction, it is necessary to characterize markers of individual cell types. Are all fibroblasts and muscle cells in the bladder wall the same? Do their phenotypes change with aging? What kinds of extrinsic or environmental factors alter their phenotype? Are there chemical, (e.g., hormones, cytokines) and physical,(e.g., tensional or compressive forces) factors, that can influence collagen synthesis? This is an important consideration since local and systemic factors can greatly affect the collagen phenotype of cells either within the bladder wall or within the pelvic floor. Thus it is likely that the integrity of the connective tissue in any structure is a major factor in the overall capacity of the tissue to maintain normal physiologic function. There is a paucity of information about the mechanical properties of connective tissue and how these properties can change as a function of aging. Is the process of aging different in males and females, and if so, why? Are there hormonal or other such changes that alter the tensile strength of connective tissue? Why are some connective tissues stronger than others? Are there ways to strengthen connective tissues so that they are better able to cope with aging changes? Is the collagen in fibrotic muscle bundles produced by smooth muscle cells? If so, under what conditions does their phenotype change? Are any of these intrinsic or extrinsic factors altered by aging or outlet obstruction. Similarly, little is known about how tension is transferred within the bladder wall.

While it is well appreciated that smooth muscle cells generate tension from the interaction between actin and myosin, how this tension gets distributed to other structures within the bladder wall is currently unknown. If elastic fibers store the energy released during bladder filling, how are these fibers connected to either other matrix components or structures within the bladder? Such connections surely exist or force transfer could not occur. These connections must be highly organized since the bladder fills and empties repetitively without any distortion or permanent derangement of its structure. How are these connections formed? What types of conditions can alter their normal arrangement and to what extent, if any, can they be repaired? Is physical stretching required for the normal growth of bladder tissue? More detailed studies like those of Murakumo et al [98] will be required to provide morphological evidence of the arrangement of the connective tissue elements within the bladder wall.

Likewise if one assumes that collagen fibers are the tension bearing elements, these fibers must similarly be attached to both the elastic fibers and the smooth muscle cells so that the tension generated can both be stored and transferred throughout the wall. How this is accomplished is not well understood although there are several possible mechanisms that can be inferred from studies conducted in the heart. These studies demonstrated that type III collagen fibers are arranged in a coiled configuration much like that of a coiled spring. During filling of the heart, these fibers sustain tensional forces by expanding their coiled structures [75] . A similar architecture appears to exist in the bladder . [76] As the bladder fills, tensional forces are dissipated by the thinning of the bladder wall, a rearrangement of the detrusor muscle bundles and by extension of the type III collagen coils. Thus the ability of the heart and the bladder to accommodate large distensional forces without permanent tissue damage is owing to the ability of the collagen fibers to alter both their orientation and their conformation.

The concept of anatomical repair restoring function needs to be addressed in light of what is known about cellular mechanisms of wound repair. If one assumes that progressive alteration of the connective tissue of the bladder or the pelvis for that matter can result in structural weaknesses, then it is important to understand what factors contribute to such alterations. It has been suggested that stress and urge incontinence may arise from the same anatomical defects related to connective tissue failure [99] Since any such change must have a temporal sequence, it is absolutely essential to identify the cells responsible for synthesis of the proteins that contribute to defective connective tissue and characterize the mechanism by which these cells acquire the altered synthetic phenotype. Such defects must ultimately affect the tension transfer mechanism although the nature and structural features of such a mechanism are essentially unknown. Evidence presented above and elsewhere [100] suggests that, in some individuals, compositional changes associated with incontinence are either age or hormonally related. Again, however, hard evidence of the exact cellular mechanism by which hormones, cytokines or other peptide factors can affect the mechanical properties of connective tissue is currently lacking.

Finally there is the question of the unstable bladder. What kinds of signals are generated in such bladders? Do individual cells respond to the mechanical input that is associated with overactivity? Since overactive bladders experience structural changes, what is the mechanism that initiates and sustains these changes? Bladders become accustomed to cycling early in development and it is likely that some form of mechanical stretch is required for normal physiologic function. Indeed, a number of studies have demonstrated that mechanical stretch can substantially alter gene expression and protein synthesis by bladder wall cells. What is not currently known is what happens when the normal levels or intensities of mechanical forces that the bladder experiences are replaced by those whose intensities and durations fall outside of the normal range. Are such mechanical perturbations associated with- or the result of- bladder overactivity? Both *in vitro* and *in vivo* studies have demonstrated that mechanical forces can directly affect gene transcription by promoter activation [77, 101] . Do the cells within the bladder wall respond analogously? These and other questions of a similar nature must be answered if the mechanism underlying the connective tissue changes associated with incontinence is to be understood.

The bladder is a complex organ composed of an inner storage layer (mucosa) surrounded by a smooth muscle coat whose tone is controlled by nerves. Connective tissue binds these layers together into a functional unit and permits tension generated by the smooth muscle cells to be transferred to the lamina propria layer to expel urine. Thus, although the connective tissue is passive in that it does not require energy to function, it plays a unique structural role in providing the bladder wall tissues with resilience and tensile strength. In the last several years since the first consultation on incontinence, there has been an increased awareness of the importance of understanding how connective tissues contribute to the overall physiologic function of the lower urinary tract and pelvic floor. As data accumulates on the changes that accompany normal aging, it is apparent that age-related weakening of connective tissues compromises tissue and organ function. It is likely that the increased focus of attention on connective tissues will produce new information that can help prevent or reverse such changes and thereby substantially improve the quality of life for an increasing number of affected individuals.

D. PREGNANCY, CHILDBIRTH AND THE PELVIC FLOOR

INTRODUCTION

Reduction in both perinatal and maternal mortality rates in recent decades has focused increasing attention on maternal morbidity and the long-term sequelae of childbirth. Antenatal education encourages expectant mothers to anticipate normal vaginal delivery, leading to an early restoration of normal pelvic function after the performance of routine pelvic floor exercises. Not least because of improved investigative techniques available during the past decade, the incidence and mechanisms of obstetric injury to the pelvic floor have come under scrutiny. A survey of female British obstetricians [102]revealed that one third indicated a personal preference for elective caesarean delivery of their own hypothetical uncomplicated singleton pregnancy; a general fear of pelvic floor trauma was cited as the most common reason for this choice. Despite being based on incomplete prognostic data, this sentiment may be echoed increasingly among obstetric patients and may lead to an unselective, and even misguided, increase in caesarean delivery rates.

Epidemiological studies have reported prevalence of stress incontinence ranging from 23 to 67 percent during pregnancy and 6 to 29 percent after childbirth, but little is known about how the condition affects women at this time. However, the prevalence of urinary incontinence may be to be nearly the same 8 weeks postpartum as during pregnancy.

There is a difference between self-reported symptoms and urinary incontinence as assessed by the pad test. Symptoms of fecal incontinence postpartum are reported up to 4.2%. Although many women experience physical and psychological symptoms of stress incontinence after delivery, few are looking for professional care or advice for their symptoms. Health professionals should be aware of the prevalence, and women's responses to stress incontinence so that they can initiate appropriate support and care [103, 104].

It is important that contributory obstetric factors are identified and their occurrence minimized. Vaginal birth has been recognized as being potentially traumatic to the pelvic floor. Women who have sustained significant anal sphincter injury are at greater risk of further damage of fecal incontinence with subsequent deliveries.

A more important factor is likely to be the role of pregnancy and childbirth in the development of urinary incontinence among women [105, 106].

I. EFFECTS OF PREGNANCY ON PELVIC FLOOR FUNCTION

In spite of the great advances that have been made in many areas of obstetric care, ignorance still persists regarding the fundamental physiological facts about the impact of pregnancy and delivery on lower urinary tract function. There is a striking dearth of prospective studies regarding the relationship of pregnancy and delivery to the problem of urinary incontinence among women. Further research may reveal that stress incontinence in women is related, at least in part, to the pregnant state itself, rather than to trauma sustained at delivery. If true, this has significant implications for subsequent research efforts investigating the etiology of female urinary incontinence.

Cutner and Cardozo have summarized the few papers that do exist as follows [107]: "Lower urinary tract symptoms are so common in early pregnancy that they are considered normal. Their progression throughout the antepartum period and their resolution postpartum has been documented by several authors. However, the data are confusing and the underlying causes remain uncertain. "The effects of normal pregnancy on the physiology of the lower urinary tract remain largely not investigated, in spite of the common pronouncements on this subject in the obstetrical literature [108-111].

It is commonly assumed that stress incontinence develops (at least in part) as the result of delivery trauma to the pelvic floor. However, several researchers have documented that many young nulliparous women suffer from occasional stress incontinence which is a significant clinical problem in as many as 5 % [112-114]. In a study of the relationship of pregnancy to stress incontinence, Francis [114] found that 40 % of primigravid women had a history of occasional stress incontinence before becoming pregnant, and that if such a history was present their stress incontinence invariably became worse during pregnancy. If incontinence developed during pregnancy, it tended to disappear after the puerperium, but recurred with subsequent pregnancies and became progressively worse, eventually becoming a clinical problem when these women were no longer pregnant. Francis concluded that in women who develop stress incontinence in middle life, pregnancy itself, rather than parturition, revealed the defect and made it worse. Similar conclusions have been reached by other researchers [115-117]. The prevalence of persistent stress urinary incontinence is reported to be significantly higher in grand multiparae compared with nulliparae [118].

II. PATHOPHYSIOLOGIC MECHANISMS OF BIRTH INJURY TO THE PELVIC FLOOR

Vaginal delivery, notably the first, is strongly associated with later surgery for stress incontinence, but the association is modified by maternal conditions and interventions during delivery. Vaginal delivery may initiate damage to the continence mechanism by direct injury to the pelvic floor muscles, damage to their motor innervation, or both. Additional denervation may occur with aging, resulting in a functional disability many years after the initial trauma. Physical and emotional health problems are common after childbirth, and are frequently not reported to health professionals despite the fact that many women would like more advice and assistance in dealing with them.

There would seem to exist four major mechanisms by which childbirth (vaginal delivery) might contribute to the increased risk of urinary incontinence among women:

1. injury to connective tissue supports by the mechanical process of vaginal delivery (Figure 6);
2. vascular damage to the pelvic structures as the result of compression by the presenting part of the fetus during labor;
3. damage to the pelvic nerves and/or muscles as the result of trauma during parturition;
4. direct injury to the urinary tract during labor and delivery. The physiolgic changes produced by pregnancy may make pregnant women more susceptible to injury from these pathophysiological processes (Figure 7).

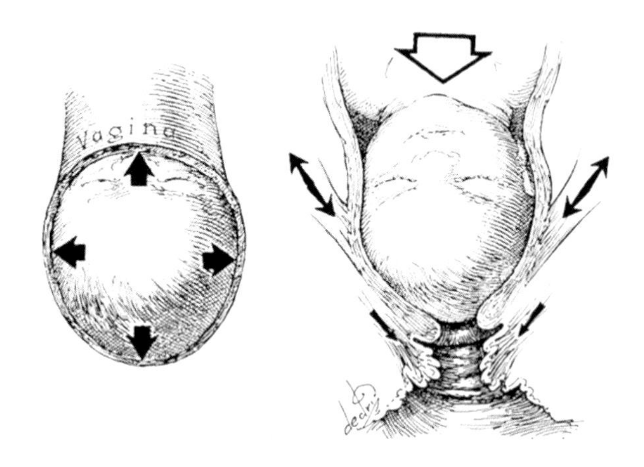

Figure 6 : Mechanisms by which the fetal head may dilate and overstretch (left) the vaginal wall or avulse cardinal and uterosacral attachments and paravaginal attachments(right). (From Nichols and Randall, Vaginal Surgery, 3rd edition, 1989, Baltimore, Williams and Wilkins (ref 205))

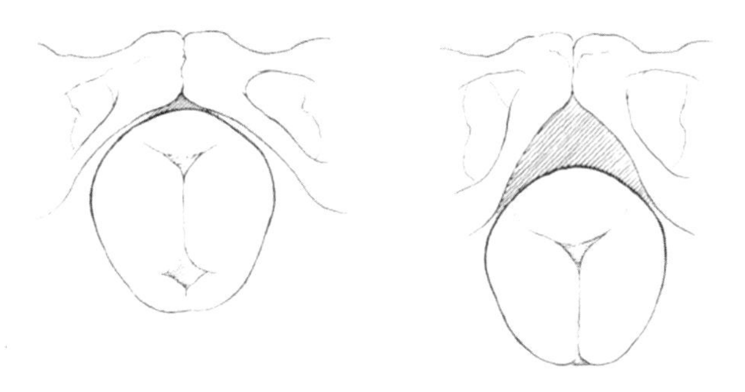

Figure 7 : Mechanisms of direct compression of the fetal head against the sub pubic urethra (left) or the paravaginal attachments (right) (From Nichols and Randall, Vaginal Surgery, 3rd edition, 1989, Baltimore, Williams and Wilkins (ref 205))

Vaginal delivery causes partial denervation of the pelvic floor (with consequent re-innervation) in most women having their first baby. Pelvic floor muscle strength is impaired shortly after vaginal birth, but for most women returns within two months. In a few this is severe and is associated with urinary and fecal incontinence. For some it is likely to be the first step along a path leading to prolapse and/or stress incontinence [119]. There is a growing body of evidence that multiparity, forceps delivery, increased duration of the second stage of labor, third degree perineal tear and high birth weight are important factors leading to pudendal nerve damage [120-122].

Peschers et al showed that pelvic floor muscle strength is significantly reduced three to eight days postpartum in women following vaginal birth but not in women after caesarean delivery. Six to ten weeks later palpation and vesical neck elevation on perineal ultrasound do not show any significant differences to antepartum values, while intravaginal pressure on perineometry remains significantly lower in primiparae, but not in multiparae. Pelvic floor muscle strength is impaired shortly after vaginal birth, but for most women returns within two months [123].

There also is EMG evidence re-innervation in the pelvic floor muscles after vaginal delivery in 80% . Mainly women who have a long active second stage of labor and heavier babies show the most EMG evidence of nerve damage. An elevation in perineal body position as well as a decrease in the area of the urogenital hiatus and of the levator hiatus at 2 weeks postpartum suggests a return of normal levator ani geometry after vaginal delivery in most patients [124].

The pudendal nerve terminal motor latency (PNTML) measured 48-72 h after delivery is increased in women delivered vaginally compared to nulliparous control subjects. Multiparity, forceps delivery, increased duration of the second stage of labor, third degree perineal tear and high birth weight are important factors leading to pudendal nerve damage [120]. Compared with spontaneous vaginal births, women having forceps or ventouse extraction have increased odds for perineal pain, sexual problems, and urinary incontinence [121]. Vaginal delivery, notably the first, is strongly associated with later surgery for stress incontinence, but the association is modified by maternal conditions and interventions during delivery [125]. Women with three or more birth deliveries were more likely to have incontinence and excessive pelvic floor descent [125]. There is no evidence to suggest that at five years after delivery use of the ventouse or forceps has specific maternal benefits or side effects [126]. Meyer et al. found that, after spontaneous and instrumental deliveries, 21% and 34% of women complained of stress urinary incontinence and 5.5% and 4% reported fecal incontinence, respectively. Substantial bladder neck hypermobility was present together with diminished functional urethral length and intravaginal and intra-anal pressures. Only 22% of patients with stress urinary incontinence during pregnancy had such incontinence after delivery [127]. Women with postpartum urinary stress incontinence have significantly greater antenatal bladder neck mobility than those women who were continent postpartum [128].

III. EPIDURAL ANALGESIA DURING LABOUR

Regional anaesthesia for the relief of labor pain has become more popular during the past 20 years. Despite interest in its possible obstetric consequences, little attention has been paid to its potential effects on the pelvic floor and perineal injury. The available published data describe conflicting results. Some studies suggest that epidural analgesia, by enabling relaxation of the pelvic floor, leads to greater control of delivery of the fetal head and consequently fewer perineal lacerations [129], but prolongation of the second stage may also increase the incidence of pudendal nerve damage [130]. Robinson et al. [131] recently examined the relationship between epidural analgesia and perineal damage, and found that the rate of significant perineal injury was higher with epidural analgesia (16,1 % compared with increased use of operative intervention .) Episiotomy and instrumental delivery were responsible for this difference. Such an association may partly explain why institutions are reporting increased rates of significant perineal injury, paralleling local increases in epidural usage [132].

IV. ROLE OF EPISIOTOMY

Episiotomy is a widely performed intervention in childbirth, despite equivocal scientific evidence regarding its benefit. It is one of the few surgical procedures performed without the patient's consent and is the most commonly performed surgical procedure in the United States. There is a widespread assumption that it may do more harm than good [132, 133]. Restrictive episiotomy policies appear to have a number of benefits com pared to routine episiotomy policies.

Proponents of routine episiotomy claim that it avoids spontaneous uncontrolled tears and long –term relaxation of the pelvic floor, but these advantages are difficult to substantiate. There is no evidence that either first- or second-degree perineal tears cause long-term consequences [109], so any argument that episiotomy prevents such spontaneous tears is inconsequential. A growing body of evidence suggests that episiotomy offers no protection against third- and forth-degree tears, which are associated with adverse sequelae. A recent overview by Myers-Helfgott and Helfgott emphasized the absence of scientific evidence to support a role for liberal elective episiotomy in the reduction of third-degree lacerations during childbirth [110]. Indeed, several reports have implicated routine episiotomy in the genesis of major perineal and anal sphincter tears, even after controlling for confounding variables [111, 112, 132, 134]. In particular, midline episiotomy is associated with significantly higher rates of third- and fourth-degree perineal tears than are mediolateral episiotomies [115-117]. Midline episiotomy is not effective in protecting the perineum and sphincters during childbirth and may impair anal continence [135]. Coats et al. [136], in a randomized controlled trial of 407 women, found that with midline episiotomy, 11,6 % of patients experienced lacerations of the anal canal versus 2 % who experienced these complications in association with mediolateral episiotomies. This association is compounded when instrumental delivery is employed, with anal sphincter injury rates of 50 % reported with the use of midline episiotomy and forceps [137]. In spite of these data, midline episiotomy is still bewilderingly widespread, presumably because it is perceived to heal better and cause less postnatal discomfort.

Restrictive episiotomy policies appear to have a number of benefits compared to routine episiotomy policies. There is less posterior perineal trauma, less suturing and fewer complications, no difference for most pain measures and severe vaginal or perineal trauma, although there was an increased risk of anterior perineal trauma with restrictive episiotomy [138, 139].

Women who have episiotomies have a higher risk of fecal incontinence at three and six months postpartum compared with women with an intact perineum. Compared with women with a spontaneous laceration, episiotomy triples the risk of fecal incontinence at three months and six months postpartum, and doubles the risk of flatus incontinence at three months and six months postpartum. A non-extending episiotomy (that is, second degree surgical incision) triples the risk of fecal incontinence and doubles the risk of flatus incontinence postpartum compared with women who have a second degree spontaneous tear. The effect of episiotomy is independent of maternal age, infant birth weight, duration of second stage of labor, use of obstetric instrumentation during delivery, and complications of labor. Therefore, midline episiotomy is not effective in protecting the perineum and sphincters during childbirth and may impair anal continence and should be restricted to specified fetal-maternal indications [140-145].

V. PELVIC FLOOR MUSCLE EXERCISE

Practice of pelvic muscle exercise by primiparas results in fewer urinary incontinence symptoms during late pregnancy and postpartum [146]. The benefits from pelvic floor muscle training are still present one year after delivery [147].

In a prospective matched controlled trial Morkved and Bo evaluated the long term effect of a postpartum pelvic floor muscle training course in the prevention and treatment of urinary incontinence. All women participated in a matched controlled study evaluating the effect of an eight-week pelvic floor muscle training program in the prevention and treatment of urinary incontinence in the immediate postpartum period and one year after delivery. Registration of continence status was assessed by structured interview and a standardized pad test. At the one year follow up, significantly more women in the control group than in the training group reported stress urinary incontinence and/or showed urinary leakage at the pad test. These investigators concluded that a specially designed postpartum pelvic floor muscle training course was effective in the prevention and treatment of stress urinary incontinence.

The benefits from pelvic floor muscle training are still present one year after delivery [147]. Sampselle et al demonstrated that practice of pelvic muscle exercise by primiparas results in fewer urinary incontinence symptoms during late pregnancy and postpartum [146]. Miller determined the characteristics of women in whom pelvic floor electrical stimulation will reduce stress urinary incontinence. They used electrical stimulation for 15 minutes twice daily or every other day for 20 weeks. At the end of 20 weeks, those with a 50% reduction in leakage episodes on voiding diary ('responders') were compared with those who did not show a 50% reduction ('non-responders'). Significant subjective and objective improvements were noted among responders by 10 and 14 weeks, respectively. Compliance was higher in responders during weeks 12-15 of the study. It was concluded that a minimum of 14 weeks of pelvic floor stimulation was necessary before significant objective improvements were seen [148].

VI. PERINEAL TRAUMA

Awareness of perineal damage after vaginal delivery has increased in recent years, due in part to better understanding of its consequences, improved methods for accurate neurophysiological evaluation and accumulation of data on prognosis. Fecal incontinence represents a distressing social handicap, and vaginal delivery is now recognized as its principal cause [149]. Obstetricians should have an awareness of the causes, symptoms, appropriate investigation and treatment options available for this complication of childbirth. Limiting episiotomy can be strongly recommended. In the absence of strong data to the contrary, women should be encouraged to engage in perineal massage if they wish and to adopt the birth positions of their choice. Factors shown to increase perineal integrity include avoiding episiotomy, spontaneous or vacuum-assisted rather than forceps birth, and in nulliparas, perineal massage during the weeks before childbirth. Second-stage position has little effect [150]. Further information on techniques to protect the perineum during spontaneous delivery is badly needed. Wherever possible , women with postpartum fecal incontinence should be assessed in a specialized clinic, which has developed a close liaison with physiotherapy, dietetic and colorectal surgical advisers.

Episiotomy, forceps use, and birth weight are important predictors of third- and fourth-degree tears. However, determinants of sulcus tears appear to be present before pregnancy. Third- and fourth-degree tears are related to physician management. Exercise mitigates the potential for severe trauma induced by episiotomy [151].

Eason et al. have systematically reviewed techniques proposed to prevent perineal trauma during childbirth and performed a meta-analysis of the evidence gathered from randomized controlled trials regarding their efficacy. The conclusion was that avoiding episiotomy decreased perineal trauma (absolute risk difference -0.23, 95% confidence interval (CI] -0.35, -0.11). In nulliparas, perineal massage during the weeks before giving birth also protected against perineal trauma (risk difference -0.08, CI -0.12, -0.04). Vacuum extraction (risk difference -0.06, CI -0.10, -0.02) and spontaneous birth (-0.11, 95% CI -0.18, -0.04) caused less anal sphincter trauma than forceps delivery. The mother's position during the second stage had little influence on perineal trauma (supported upright versus recumbent: risk difference 0.02, 95% CI -0.05, 0.09). Factors shown to increase perineal integrity include avoiding episiotomy, spontaneous or vacuum-assisted rather than forceps birth, and in nulliparas, perineal massage during the weeks before childbirth. Second-stage position has little effect. Further information on techniques to protect the perineum during spontaneous delivery is sorely needed [152].

VII. FECAL INCONTINENCE

Fecal incontinence is defined as the involuntary loss of stool at any time of life after toilet training. It is a socially and psychologically devastating condition for patients and their families, and a topic which both patients and physicians are reluctant to approach. Although the true prevalence of fecal incontinence is unknown, studies have reported it to be as high as 2, 2% in the general population, with significantly higher rates among nursing home residents and hospitalized elderly. Risk factors include advancing age, female gender and multiparity. An understanding of pelvic floor anatomy and physiology is required to appreciate how diverse medical conditions can affect mechanisms involved in normal continence.

The rectum normally serves as a storage reservoir until elimination can take place at a socially acceptable time and place. The pelvic floor muscles help to regulate the defecatory process and maintain continence. These muscles include the internal anal sphincter, the external anal sphincter and the puborectalis muscle. Each muscle contributes to normal continence, although the relative importance of each is controversial. Neurologic integrity and sensation are also key factors. Conditions associated with fecal incontinence include diarrheal states, fecal impaction, idiopathic neurologic injury, surgical and obstetric injury, pelvic trauma, collagen vascular disease, and neurologic impairment related to stroke, diabetes, or multiple sclerosis. Evaluation of the patient with fecal incontinence includes a directed history and physical examination, with particular attention paid to integrity of the perineum and rectum, and a complete neurologic evaluation. Diagnostic tools such as stool studies, anorectal manometry, defecography, electromyography, pudendal nerve conduction, and endoanal ultrasound may be employed in an outpatient setting. Fecal incontinence may be treated conservatively by employing such methods as dietary restriction, stool bulking agents, and biofeedback. Surgery may be the best option for cases refractory to medical treatment, or for those patients with rectocele or obstetrical injury [153].

Vaginal delivery may initiate damage to the anal continence mechanism by direct injury to the pelvic floor muscles, damage to their motor innervation, or both. Additional denervation may occur with aging, resulting in a functional disability many years after the initial trauma. These factors should be kept in mind when conducting vaginal birth and planning therapy for anal incontinence [154]. Vaginal delivery is related to EAS muscle EMG abnormalities. However, these are minor and seem not to indicate loss of anal sphincter function. However, some doubt exists on the commonly accepted preconception that significant damage to peripheral innervation of the EAS occurs even during uncomplicated deliveries [155].

After primary surgical repair the symptomatic patients were treated with pelvic floor exercises with or without transanal electrical stimulation. Various methods for assessing anal sphincter function were also evaluated.

One month postpartum 10 women (21%) complained of anal incontinence, 8 for flatus only; 1 patient was reoperated. After 1 year none complained of fecal incontinence, and 3 (7%) complained of flatus incontinence. We found relatively few women with anal incontinence after third- /fourth-degree laceration. The pelvic floor training program was effective, but electrical stimulation was abandoned because of anal pain. Grade IIIb lesion, dilution of the sphincter at anal ultrasonography, and sphincter weakness at palpation were significantly related to symptoms of anal incontinence. For routine follow-up after third- /fourth-degree laceration, palpation of the anal sphincter and pelvic floor seems sufficient as first-line assessment [156].

VIII. CONCLUSION

Both pregnancy and vaginal delivery are often responsible for the onset of genuine stress incontinence and pelvic floor damage. The vast majority of published data is based on analysis retrieved from questionnaires. Only a small number of prospective and investigative trials are currently available to ascertain the influences of pregnancy and childbirth responsible for the onset of urinary incontinence, fecal incontinence, and pelvic floor disorders. Longitudinal studies are needed to assess the long term consequences of pregnancy and child birth on both, lower urinary tract and pelvic floor function.

E. URETHRAL STRUCTURE, SUPPORT AND FUNCTION IN WOMEN: PATHOPHYSIOLOGY OF SUI

The factors necessary for the urethra to remain closed at rest and during increased abdominal pressure have been well characterized in recent years, but it is their functional inter-relationships which are still not fully understood. These factors include: 1) healthy, functioning striated sphincter controlled by pudendal innervation, 2) well vascularized urethral mucosa and submucosa, 3) properly aligned and functioning intrinsic urethral smooth muscle, and 4) intact vaginal wall support.

I. THE UROGENITAL DIAPHRAGM IN THE FEMALE: LOCATION OF THE URETHRAL SPHINCTER

Detailed descriptions of the urogenital diaphragm have been made by Max Brodel working with Howard Kelly [157], Oelrich [158] and further disseminated by DeLancey [159]. These reports provide clear descriptions of the urethral rhabdosphincter. The proximal one-third of the urethra is shown surrounded by a sleeve of striated muscle continuous with a longer ascending cone which extends to the vaginal introitus. Manometric and electrophysiological recordings from this proximal one-third of the urethra have shown that it generates the highest level of resting pressure and electromyographic activity (Figure 8).

This portion of the urethra is an intra-pelvic structure located immediately posterior to the pubic bone. In the past, much has been made of the loss of this intra-pelvic position in stress incontinence. It had been suggested that when the urethra descended away from its intra-abdominal position, intra-abdominal forces no longer constricted it during straining. This concept has survived and been modified into the "hammock hypothesis" [160]which suggests that the posterior position of the vagina provides a backboard against which increasing intra-abdominal forces compress the urethra. Data supporting this hypothesis are drawn from urethral pressure transmission studies showing that continent patients experience an increase in intra-urethral pressures during coughing. This pressure increase is lost in stress incontinence and may be restored following successful operations designed to stabilize or elevate the sub-urethral vaginal wall [161-164] [165-170].

The urethra is supported posteriorly and inferiorly by the anterior vaginal wall. The superior vaginal sulcus, most clearly found in nullipara, exists at this junction of the lower and middle third of the vaginal wall. This point represents the two lateral insertion points of the vaginal " hammock." Portions of the pubococcygeus muscle attach to these to sulci within the pelvis and can produce elevation during voluntary contraction.

Immediately anterior to the proximal urethra are found the reflections of the endopelvic fascia. The most prominent of these , the pubo-urethral ligaments, are sufficiently condensed to form distinct and recognizable ligaments on either side of the pubis. Although these structures form one continuous complex, they are distinguished by their names, as posterior and anterior pubo-urethral ligaments. The posterior pubo-urethral ligaments, which can be seen at the time of retropubic surgery, are the more familiar of these. These are strong fascial condensations which most likely maintain their characteristics throughout life. Previous investigators, however, have suggested that elongation of these structures may be responsible for the loss of urethral support seen in stress incontinence.

While the lower one-third of the vagina is oriented more vertically in the nullipara, the upper two-thirds of the vagina deviate horizontally. This orientation is due 1) to the posterior attachments of the cervix by the cardinal and utero-sacral ligaments and 2) to the anterior

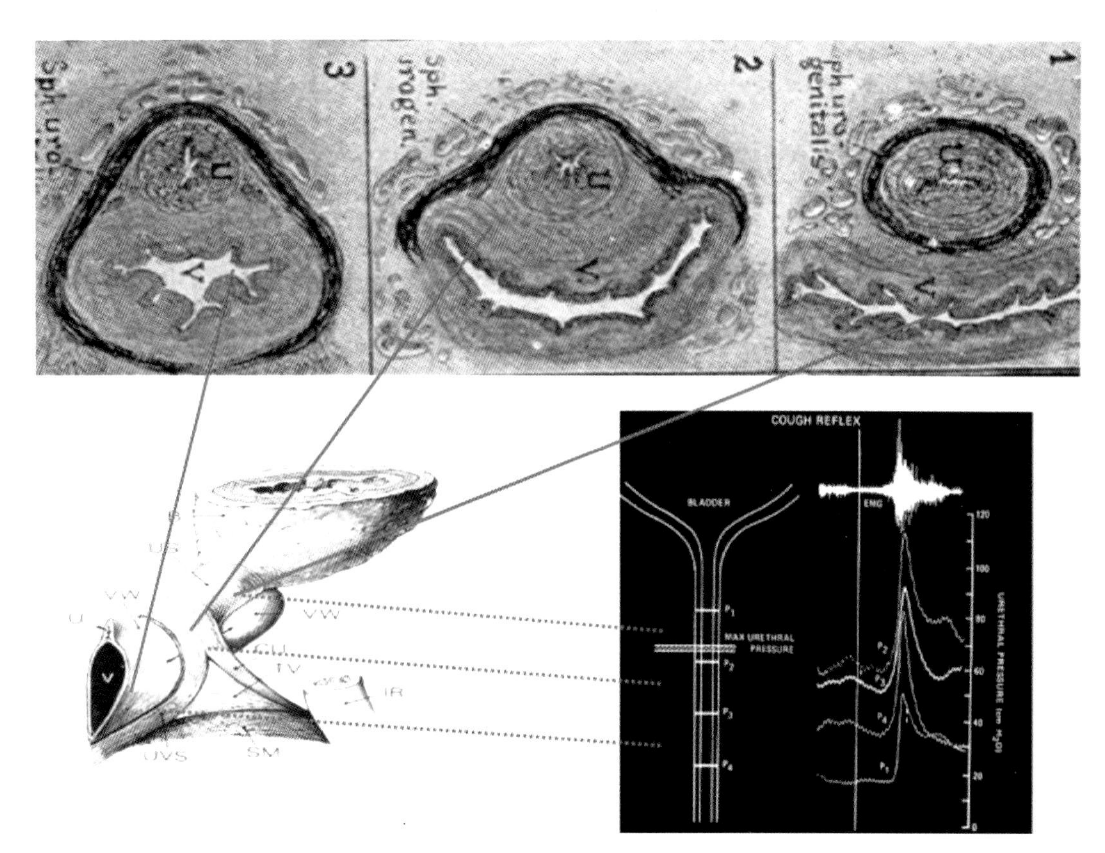

Figure 8 : Composite illustration relating transverse sections through the urethra (upper panel, (From Broedel, Archives of the Department of Art as Applied to Medicine, Johns Hopkins Medical Institutions)) to corresponding locations along the urethra (left lower panel, (From Oelrich, T.M., The striated urogenital sphincter muscle in the female. Anatomical Record, 1983. 205(2): p. 223-32, Ref 158) to the regions of high pressure and electrophysiological activity (right lower panel, From Constantinou)

position of the levator hiatus. Barium vaginograms have demonstrated this horizontal angulation of the upper two-thirds of the vagina, and show that during coughing and stressful maneuvers, the levator hiatus is shortened in an anterior direction by the contraction of the pubococcygeus muscles . Thus, the pelvic organs receive support from the shape and active contraction of the levator muscles.

A schematic diagram of the factors necessary for urogenital diaphragm support and function is provided in Figure 9.

II. EFFECT OF CHILDBIRTH, VAGINAL PROLAPSE AND URETHRAL POSITION ON URINARY CONTINENCE

Labor and delivery alter vaginal and pelvic anatomy and innervation in several ways as has been discussed in the section on maternal injuries. Each of these may contribute to the eventual development of urinary incontinence:

1. Direct crushing or traction on the pudendal nerve has been discussed above and previously suggested as a primary cause of sphincteric incompetence in stress incontinence.

2. Cardinal and utero-sacral ligaments may be stretched or torn, resulting in anterior displacement of the uterus during straining or under the influence of gravity.

3. The vagina itself may be torn away from its intrapelvic attachments with subsequent loss of the superior vaginal sulcus. There may be direct attenuation of the vaginal wall itself, manifested by loss of vaginal rugae and a thin appearance. Cullen Richardson has suggested four distinct kinds of vaginal injuries: paravaginal, central, distal, and cervical, the first two being the most commonly seen in women with stress incontinence. These defects have been identified by sonographic examination [171].

4. Finally, stretching, tearing and avulsion of the levator muscles result in a longer and wider levator hiatus. Consequently, the perineum is displaced anteriorly and posteriorly under stress and temporarily fails to support the pelvic organs. These changes in the levator hiatus with or without associated relaxa-

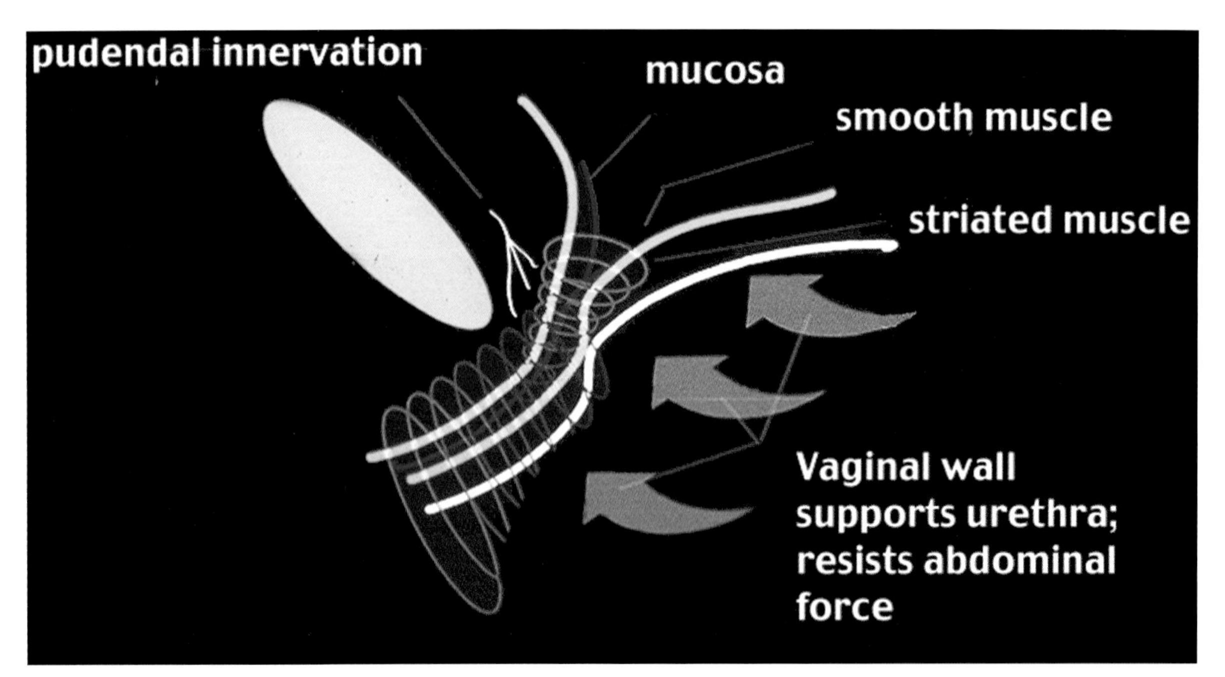

Figure 9 : Schematic illustration of the factors which are essential for urogental diaphragm support and function. These include: pudendal innervations of the urethra, mucosa and smooth muscle of the urethra, striated muscle sphincter, vaginal wall support

tion of cervical support result in chronic anterior displacement of pelvic organs with a loss of both active and passive organ support during rest and especially during straining .

In the patient with stress urinary incontinence these changes typically give rise to a rotational descent of the proximal urethra away from its retropubic position. Radiographic images of stress urinary incontinence in women have noted this and generated our earliest concepts of this condition. Jeffcoate and Roberts [172], using lateral cystourethrograms, concluded:

"...the most common characteristic anatomical change, present in four out of five cases of incontinence, is loss of the posterior urethro-vesical angle so that the urethra and trigone tend to come into line."

Hodkinson, using a suspension of barium paste placed in the bladder and a small bead chain in the urethra, produced images of the urethra at rest and during maximum straining in women with stress urinary incontinence [173, 174]. He concluded:

"...it is clear that the distinguishing topographic pathological feature is depression of the urethrovesical junction to the lowest level of the bladder during the peak of the straining effort. It is also clear that the spatial relationships of the bladder and urethra to the symphysis make no difference in either the incidence or severity of stress incontinence."

These kinds of radiographic studies, however, cannot distinguish between lateral or central defects in vaginal wall support (Figure 10). Therefore, while urethral movement can be identified as an important finding in stress incontinence, one cannot determine the exact location of the vaginal defect. Because the proximal urethra rotates out of the focal plane of ultrasonograhic probes or MRI, coronal images of vaginal relaxation have not yet shown anatomical detail at the moment of incontinence. They cannot distinguish central from paravaginal defects. For this, an examination of the patient is required.

Although we have considerable knowledge about anatomical defects in the majority of patients with GSUI, less is understood about the exact effect of these defects, and indeed, vaginal position itself, on urethral closure. Early experience with operations for stress incontinence showed that not all women with stress urinary incontinence had vaginal prolapse, that correction of vaginal relaxation did not always correct stress incontinence, and that women who redeveloped stress incontinence symptoms after apparently successful surgery did not necessarily show a recurrence of their prolapse [175]. Despite these findings, the paradigm of vaginal support as the major factor in maintaining urinary continence has prevailed, altered only recently by emerging concepts of ISD.

III. EMERGING CONCEPTS OF URETHRAL WEAKNESS AND ISD

The idea that primary urethral weakness could cause urinary incontinence independent of vaginal weakness appeared in a proposed classification by Blaivas et al [176]. In their classification, they named this Type III

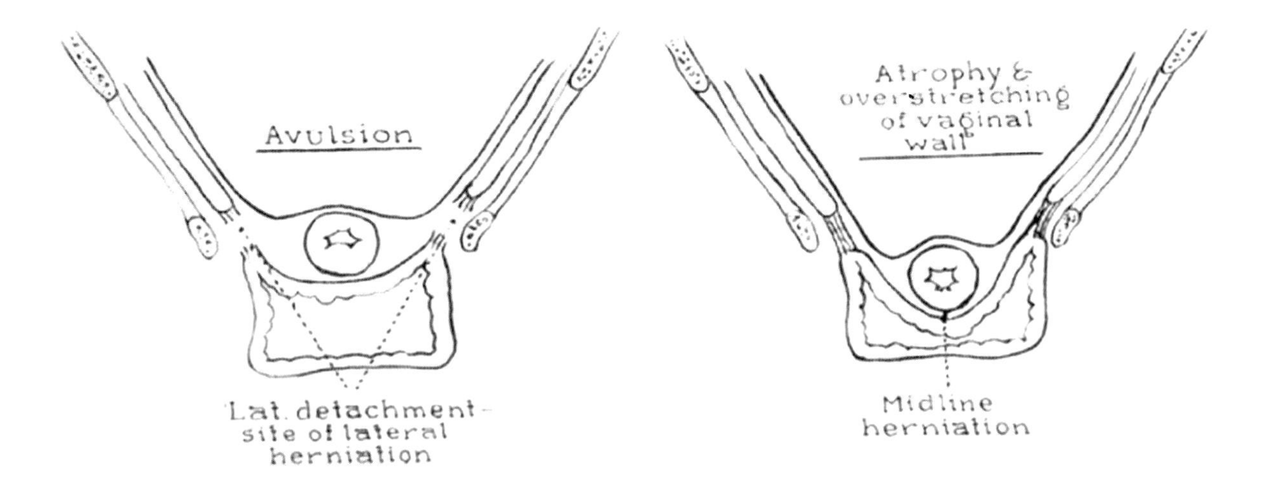

Figure 10 : Loss of urethral support may arise from defects in lateral or midline support. They may appear the same in a sagittal plane. The clinician must examine patient to determine which defect is present and to what extent. From Sanders, R.C., et al., Imaging the female urethra. Ultrasound Quarterly, 1994. 12(3): p. 167-183 (ref 202)-

incontinence to distinguish it from Types I and II, each of which showed movement, while Type III did not. This term still remains in the contemporary literature, though it is now being replaced by the term intrinsic sphincter deficiency (ISD), focusing attention on urethral elements which appear to be independent of vaginal position and mobility. These include pudendal innervation, striated sphincter mass and function, and urethral smooth muscle, mucosa and submucosal cushions.

When ISD was first introduced as a concept to explain surgical failures and the presence of stress incontinence in the absence of vaginal mobility, the diagnostic tendency was to consider the cause of stress incontinence as a dichotomy, due either to hypermobility (displacement, or prolapse of the vaginal wall) or ISD. The typical patient with ISD was described as having low urethral closure pressures, a "stovepipe" appearance on cystoscopy, and opening or funneling of the urethra under resting or minimal increases in intra-abdominal pressures on radiographic images. The common causes were thought to be surgical injury, ischemia following previous pelvic or vaginal surgery or radiation damage. It appears now, that these examples of ISD may have represented the most advanced or extreme forms.

IV. HYPERMOBILITY VS. ISD: FROM DICHOTOMY TO CONTINUUM

There has been a gradual shift away from this simple categorization of stress incontinence as being due either to hypermobility or ISD. This has arisen in part because of the development of the concept of Valsalva Leak Point Pressure (VLPP) [177, 178] and more recent analyses of long term results of stress incontinence surgery [179].

VLPP emerged as an alternative method to study urethral closure during stress for studies of urethral bulking with collagen. Investigators recognized that improvements in continence following urethral bulking did not correlate with urethral closure pressures, but did correlate with the amount of pressure required to produce leakage in the absence of intrinsic detrusor contraction. Although VLPP still lacks specific anatomic or theoretical grounding and many uncertainties related to standardization of recording methods and associated prolapse remain, low VLPP (a value of , 60 cm H_2O has been suggested) has been widely embraced as an indicator of ISD.

Just as the concept of VLPP blurred the previous distinction between simple ISD and simple hypermobility, long term outcome studies of correction of hypermobility have suggested that there may be more urethral weakness among patients with hypermobility than had been previously considered. Long term outcome studies of stress incontinence surgery have shown that there is a much greater failure rate of many of the commonly performed stress incontinence operations than had been generally appreciated, and that slings providing direct sub-urethral support seemed to provide the greatest long term protection against recurrence of incontinence [179]. Since slings had traditionally been the procedure of choice for recurrent incontinence or "Type III" (now ISD) incontinence, the possibility that ISD was more common than previously thought was more widely considered.

These two developments have led to a growing clinical impression that some degree of ISD may exist in many patients who only recently were thought to have only hypermobility as a cause of their incontinence. A typical expression of this impression is found in the conclusion of Kayigil et al. [180] following examination of 50 patients; "The high rate of intrinsic sphincteric deficiency in patients with urethral hypermobility indicates that the incidence with stress incontinence may be greater than previously believed, and may influence the apparently higher failure rates after bladder neck suspension." In contemporary clinical practice, this impression has given rise to a growing tendency to recommend suburethral sling surgery as a form of primary surgical treatment for all women with stress incontinence, where formerly this approach was reserved almost exclusively for patients with recurrent stress incontinence or significant ISD [181].

V. DIRECT STUDIES OF URETHRAL FUNCTION

As recognition of the importance of urethral function has increased, so too have the number of investigations of urethral position, urethral closure and transmission pressure profiles, Valsalva leak point pressure measurements and electromyographic examinations of the pudendal nerve and the striated sphincter. These studies are now discussed.

VI. STUDIES OF URETHRAL POSITION

Stress incontinence is frequently associated with loss of urethral position. This has been the primary pathophysiological paradigm since the observations of Hodginson and Jeffcoate and Roberts. Similar observations are still reported today [182]. Even when some displacement is seen in continent nulliparous females, incontinent women show a greater degree of mobility [183].

Successful suspensory operations, whether by sling or paraurethral suspension stabilize urethral position [175]and, when studied, increase pressure transmission during stress. It is not clear if the active contraction of urethral support seen in the female is restored after surgery, nor is it known if it is necessary for continence. It has been suggested that passive support alone is what restores continence after suspension.

VII. STUDIES OF URETHRAL PRESSURE

Stress incontinence is generally thought to be characterized by a decrease in urethral transmission profiles and resting closure pressure. Although not perfectly correlated, low resting pressures and low leak point pressures are found more commonly in patients with severe incontinence which may be more refractory to suspensory operations.

Improvement in transmission pressures is associated with successful outcomes after suspensory operations for SUI. [165, 168, 184, 185] [161, 169]. The exact mechanism for this increase in transmission is not clear. Increased exposure to intra-abdominal forces has been suggested [170, 186, 187]. Compression against the pubis by the pelvic viscera has been suggested [188]. The final position of the urethra may not be the key variable [161].

VIII. ELECTROPHYSIOLOGICAL STUDIES OF URETHRAL FUNCTION

Snooks and Swatch [120, 189-191]first brought attention to the importance of urethral denervation after childbirth and its contributions to urinary and fecal incontinence. Stress incontinence is frequently associated with a decline in the electrophysiological function of the pudendal nerve [192], the striated urethral sphincter [193], and the pelvic floor muscles [194, 195]. Electromyographic studies of normal sphincteric function show that in continent women, pressures begin to rise in the urethra before rising in the bladder, suggesting an active muscular component [196]. Most electrophysiological studies have concentrated on motor rather than sensory innervation, however, and the role of urethral sensation in GSUI is unknown.

There is a need for a hypothesis which would integrate these various observations regarding hypermobility, ISD and pudendal nerve function, place them within the context of an abnormal pelvic floor and provides a model to guide research and studies of the natural history of the condition.

IX. CONTRIBUTIONS OF IMAGING TO UNDERSTANDING OF PATHOPHYSIOLOGY

Radiographic imaging has provided considerable insight into pathophysiology of stress incontinence, ever since the advent of bead chain cystograms and simple static and straining lateral cystograms. Recently, magnetic resonance imaging (MRI) and real time ultrasonography, in addition to showing the events of stress incontinence on both a global pelvic and local urethral scale, have suggested a relationship of the proximal urethra to vaginal wall movement. It is possible to integrate these insights with the growing body of knowledge about pudendal nerve dysfunction and striated sphincter muscle mass decline in women with stress incontinence.

Dynamic fastcan MRI has been used to visualize all compartments of the female pelvis during increased intra-abdominal straining [197]. (MRI has been found comparable to standard cystography in demonstrating cystocele defects [198]). The pubococcygeal line serves as a reference marker. Normal displacement of the bladder base, the cervix or cervical cuff and the rectum can be determined and compared to women with prolapse. The urethra is shown in the context of global pelvic relaxation [199]. Most MRI studies have been descriptive rather than quantitative, but they still show far more soft tissue detail than earlier radiographic studies and thus offer new research opportunities (Figure 11 & 12).

Dynamic MRI with cine-loop reconstruction produces vivid, intuitively appealing images which can show movement of all compartments of the relaxed pelvis during straining [199]. Static MRI shows details of urethral and peri-urethral anatomy and the striated sphincter can be clearly seen [200]. Pending further improvements in resolution, MRI remains limited as a tool to study details of urethral movement. Although newer studies continue to emerge [201], at this time ultrasonogrpahy provides better visualization of moving structures.

X. REAL TIME ULTRASONOGRAPHY

Several sonographic approaches have been used for the study of stress incontinence, suprapubic, translabial and transperineal. As resolution of sonographic probes has improved, the detail previously best seen with the transrectal approach may now be seen by a transperineal approach. Studies with a trans-rectal approach have shown that funneling of the proximal urethra was the sonographic sign most-frequently associated with loss of urine [202]. In about half the patients with GSUI in this study, funneling was found to be absent at rest, appearing only with straining. In the other half, some degree of funneling was already present at rest, increasing with straining and present with actual leakage. Enhanced views of the urethra are possible with sonographic contrast material [203, 204].

The observed urethral movement and funneling resembled the rotational descent described by Nichols and

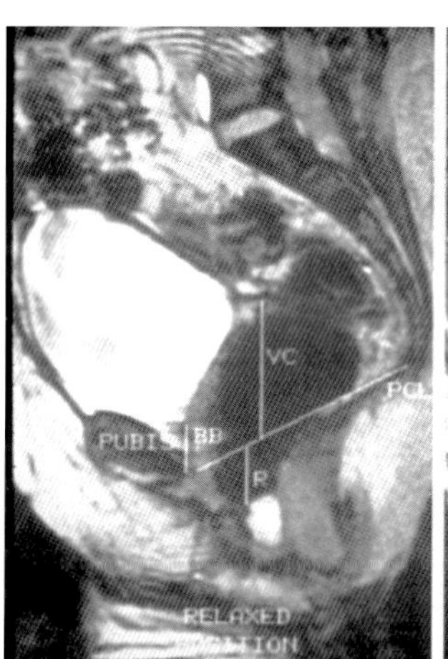

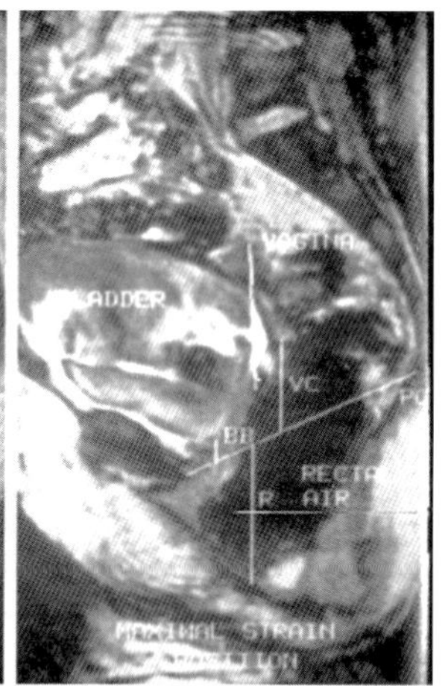

Figure 11 : MRI at rest and with straining in a healthy volunteer. Reference lines can be used to determine the degree of displacement of the three compartments of the pelvis: anterior containing bladder and urethra, middle, containing cervix, uterus and Denonvillier's fascia, and posterior, containing the rectum. From Yang, A., et al., Dynamic evaluation of pelvic floor descent using fastscan MRI and cinematic display. Radiology, 1991. 179: p. 25-33 (ref 197)

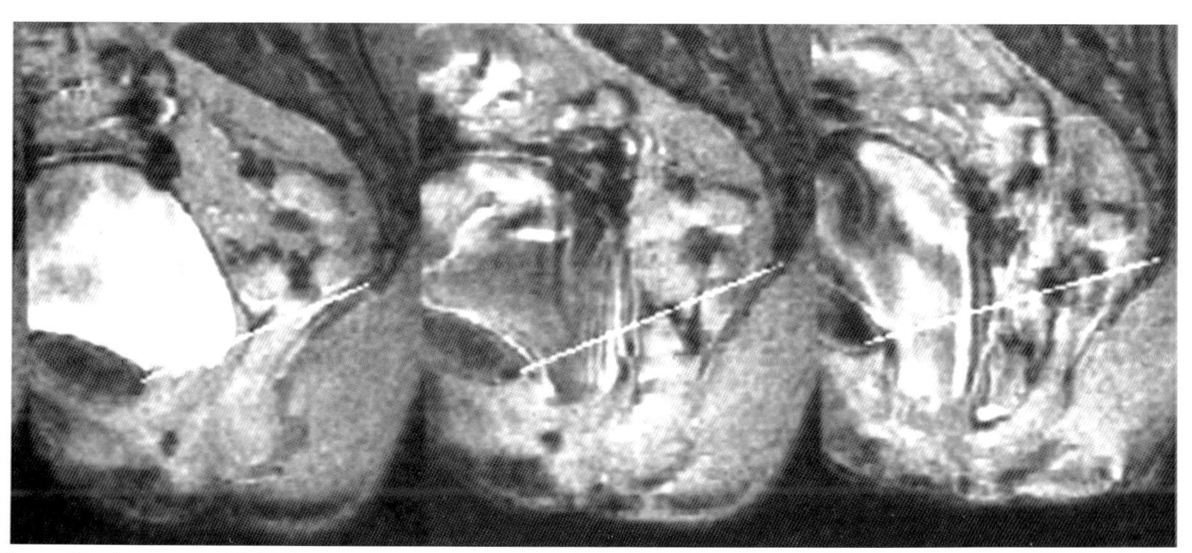

Figure 12 : Sequence of MRI images at rest and two positions of intra-abdominal straining showing the progression of an anterior compartment defect, a cystocele, as it descends out of the levator hiatus. (From Yang, A., et al., Dynamic evaluation of pelvic floor descent using fastscan MRI and cinematic display. Radiology, 1991. 179: p. 25-33 (ref 197))

Randall [205]. It was consistent with the descriptions of Jeffcoate and Roberts and Hodginson. Improved soft tissue detail seen with ultrasound permits an extension of these original observations. It appears that the anterior and posterior walls of the proximal urethra may move differently during increases in intra-abdominal pressure. At first, they appear to move together: the urethra begins its descent as a single unit. At some point, however, the anterior urethra becomes arrested in its rotational movement and appears to move more slowly. The posterior portion of the urethra continues to descend along with the vaginal wall [202, 206]. This difference in movement appears to produce a shearing apart of the two walls, leading to the appearance of funneling seen as urine leaks out of the urethra.

Examination of anatomy permits further interpretation of these observations. At the level of the pubis, the posterior portion of the ligaments travels beneath the pubis to form an anterior portion, which supports the clitoris in women, and the corpora cavernosa in men. Both Nichols and Milley [207] and Zacharin [208-210] have previously suggested that the posterior pubourethral ligaments might support the urethra, and their laxity might contribute to the descent of the urethra in stress incontinence. In these studies, longitudinal and cross-sectional views of the proximal urethra show that the ligaments travel along only the anterior portion of the urethra as they pass beneath the pubis to emerge as the anterior pubourethral ligaments. The vagina and its bilateral attachments forming the lateral sulcus support the posterior part of the urethra. It is more likely that the vaginal wall and its attachments become weaker than the strong condensations of endopelvic fascia forming these ligaments. So, the pubourethral complex, even if attenuated, probably remains stronger than the underlying vaginal wall. Sonographic examination of the prolapsing urethra thus suggests arrest of anterior urethral wall movement by the pubourethral complex, while the vaginal wall continues to rotate, pulling the posterior wall of the urethra along with it (Figure 13).

These anatomical observations, combined with current knowledge about pudendal nerve activity in normals, prolapse or stress incontinence, suggest a unifying hypothesis regarding urethral closure and vaginal movement. As intra-abdominal pressure increases, the proximal urethra begins to experience two kinds of forces, which threaten to open it. The first of these is a shearing force produced by the unequal separation of the anterior and posterior urethral walls from the pubis during straining. This is the effect of vaginal mobility on urethral closure. The second is an expulsive force, produced by the transmission of intra-abdominal forces to the bladder, which must be resisted by the urethra if opening is to be prevented. The urethra resists this primarily by intrinsic closure of the pudendally innervated striated sphincter, aided by vaginal support (Figure 14). It is likely that these shearing and expulsive forces are generated simultaneously as intra-abdominal pressure rises, one can imagine that the urethra can be brought to a point of continence threshold beyond which urethral closure cannot be maintained.

This kind of synthesis of anatomic, radiographic and physiologic observations is one example of an integrated approach. One can imagine that repeated episodes of prolapse may eventually stretch, tear or attenuate sphincter mass and contribute to a chronically weakened urethra manifested by low VLPP or low urethral closure pressures, characteristic of ISD. After severe or prolonged untreated prolapse and stress incontinence, vaginal support alone may not be sufficient to correct the deficiencies of an exhausted sphincter. Thus the possibilities that early intervention may prevent further deterioration of urethral closure mechanisms might be considered in future studies, particularly longitudinal studies, of stress incontinence.

XI. CONCLUSIONS

We are approaching a new classification of stress incontinence which will integrate hypermobility and urethral dysfunction as inter-related elements on a spectrum of change. Certain concepts have stood the test of time, and they are included below, along with conclusions:

1. Many patients with GSUI show urethral mobility, though it is not yet known what it is about that mobility which permits urethral opening during stress.
2. Some patients who present with minimal mobility or who have recurred after successful surgery have primary or residual sphincteric insufficiency.
3. Sphincteric insufficiency is related to a decline in striated sphincter muscle mass and function as measured by electrophysiological studies of pudendal nerve and sphincter function, and MRI and sonographic estimates of muscle mass. If repeated episodes of vaginal traction can be shown to enhance sphincteric damage, then the effect of early treatment of stress incontinence and prolapse on future development of ISD should be investigated, since advanced ISD remains a difficult aspect of SUI to treat.
4. Successful operations can restore urethral position but probably do not restore urethral function. A good surgical outcome probably requires a certain reserve of urethral function. It is in the area of functional understanding of urethral anatomy that the greatest progress is likely to be made.

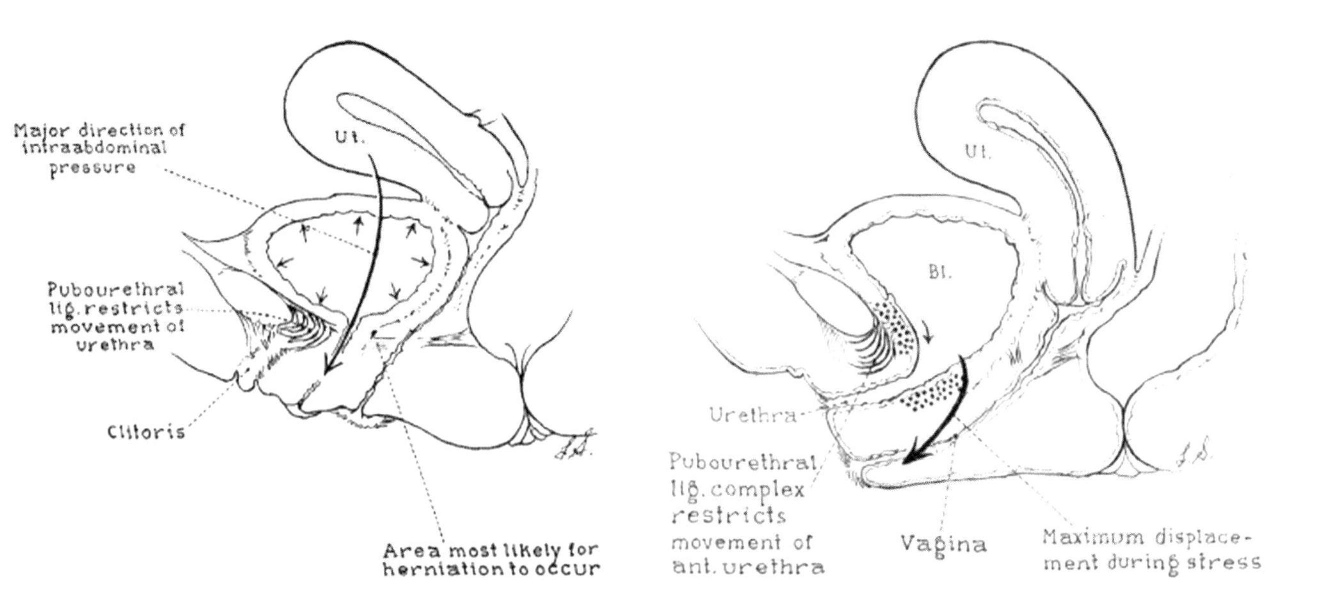

Figure 13 : How vaginal movement affects urethral closure as abdominal pressure increases. Increasing abdominal pressure forces the anterior vaginal wall out of the levator hiatus. The urethra follows. The anterior portion of the urethra can be slowed and eventually arrested in its movement while the posterior portion continues to rotate out of the pelvis with the vaginal wall. (Drawing by Leon Schlossberg, From Sanders, R.C., et al., Imaging the female urethra. Ultrasound Quarterly, 1994. 12(3): p. 167-183 (ref 202))

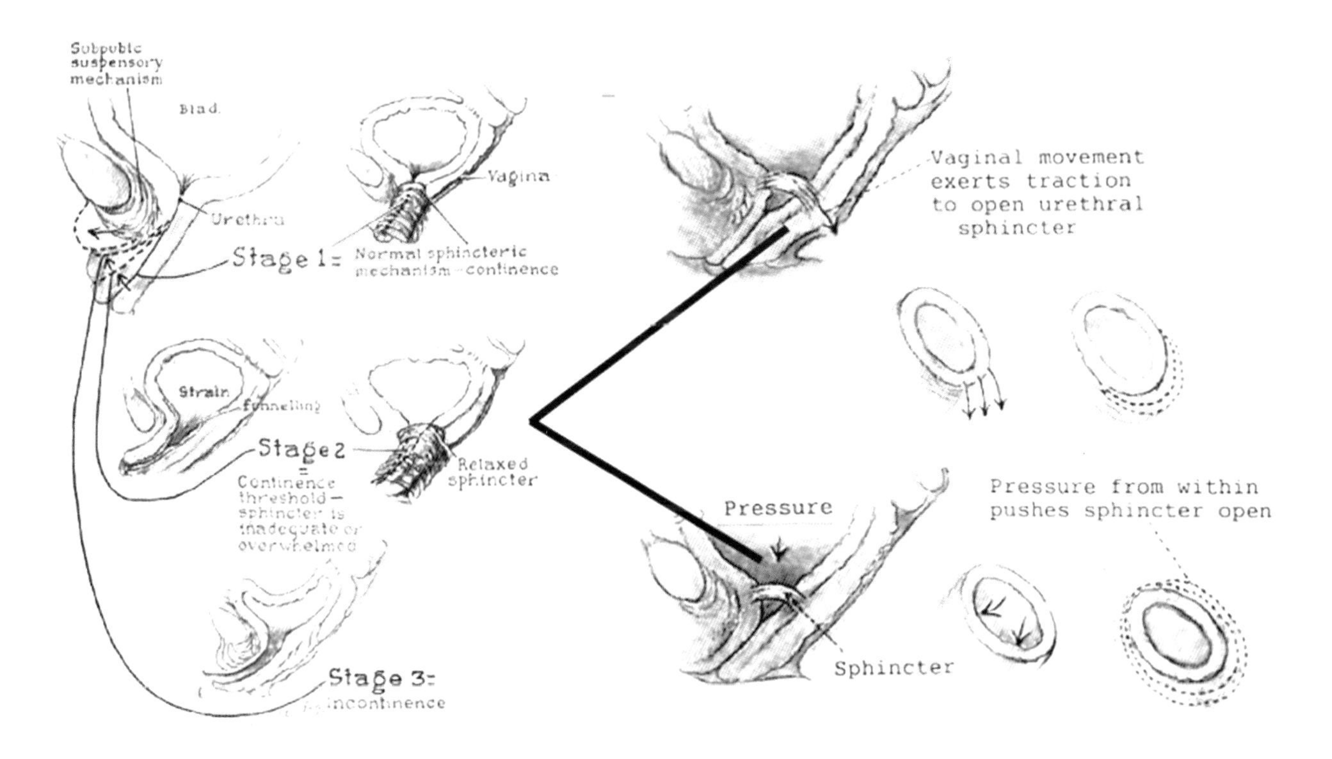

Figure 14 : How ISD and vaginal movement can interact to cause incontinence. The panel at left depicts three hypothetical stages in any given patient with vaginal relaxation and/or ISD. Stage 2 represents the point where the urethra reaches the continence threshold. There it is exposed to two simultaneous forces of differing degrees in each patient. There is a shearing force resisted by the counter-forces of vaginal support (right upper panel) and an expulsive forces resisted by the intrinsic urethral musculature (right lower panel). (Drawing by Leon Schlossberg, From Mostwin, J.L., et al., Stress incontinence observed with real time sonography and dynamic fastscan magnetic resonance imaging: insights into pathophysiology. Scan J Urol Nephrol, Suppl 207, 2000, p. 94-99. (Ref 210))

F. URINARY INCONTINENCE IN MEN: THE ROLE OF OBSTRUCTION AND PROSTATIC SURGERY

Concepts regarding male continence have arisen primarily through experience with spinal injury and neurological disease. Only recently has incontinence in aging men and women, and men with post-prostatectomy incontinence been studied more carefully. Progress has been limited by lack of knowledge about normal human anatomy and physiology and uncertainty regarding the existence and role of "internal" and "external" sphincters [211] . Urodynamic studies characterizing detrusor function and sphincter coordination in neurological injury and illness are abundant. Studies of normal and damaged sphincteric function in men have been limited, but have increased since the last report of the International Consultation on Incontinence . Urodynamic methods, electromyography and advanced imaging techniques such as magnetic resonance imaging (MRI) are powerful tools which could provide information about structure and function.

Incontinence in men may result from failure of the bladder to store, as in neurological injury or disease, or from direct sphincter injury following radical prostatectomy, or less frequently, simple prostatectomy (transurethral or open). Injury may be caused by pelvic trauma resulting in pelvic fracture with membranous urethral disruption, or by physical agents such as therapeutic radiation. Although pathophysiology may initially be classified into sphincteric and bladder causes, clinical experience underscores considerable overlap between them. We have already discussed bladder dysfunction in the elderly and in neurological illness and injury. This following section focuses on post-prostatectomy incontinence.

I. THE SPHINCTER OF THE MALE

The anatomy of the male urogenital diaphragm has been well characterized by Oelrich [212] and more recently by Myers [213, 214]. Further work by Myers since the last ICI report has grown out of experience with radical prostatectomy. Three dimensional magnetic resonance imaging reconstruction of the male urogenital diaphragm are increasing our understanding of this complex anatomical region [215]. Anatomical studies show clearly that the urogenital diaphragm is a vertically oriented tapering sleeve of striated muscle surrounding the smooth muscle of the urethra, which is itself a continuation of detrusor fibers. The structures in men and women are remarkably similar, as underscored in the work by Oelrich. The sleeve is quite narrow at the apex and wider at the base, partially open posteriorly in women to permit passage of the vagina, but completely closed in men where it is continuous with the bulbospongiosus muscle. There are slips of pubococcygeus muscle of the levator ani investing the edges of the rhabdosphincter. However, the levator ani muscles do not encircle the urethra.

These two muscle groups, levator ani and urethral rhabdosphincter, differ as to type. Levators are predominantly fast-twitch, Type II, while periurethral striated muscles are predominantly Type I, slow twitch, providing sustained tone. Thus after radical prostatectomy it is possible to interrupt the stream voluntarily by forceful contraction of the levators yet still have continuous sphincteric incompetence because of periurethral rhabdosphincter insufficiency.

The pubourethral complex stabilizes the urethra and permits the bladder to expand away from a fixed retropubic attachment and contract towards it during micturition. It seems likely that stabilization and accurate positioning of the male urethra and the ejaculatory ducts during vaginal penetration and seminal emission would be the primary function of these structures. Their presence in the female may be incidental, much as the mammary gland is in the male. It is not at all clear that pubourethral suspension by this fascial complex is essential for continence, although certain groups have recommended preservation of these structures following radical prostatectomy as a means of improving continence preservation after this operation.

II. POST-PROSTATECTOMY INCONTINENCE

In 1994, the Agency for Health Care Policy and Research published clinical guidelines for the diagnosis and treatment of benign prostatic hyperplasia [216]. The guidelines panel reviewed 27 articles regarding transurethral prostatectomy and 30 articles regarding open prostatectomy to analyze treatment outcomes. The panel reported that the risk of total incontinence, defined as complete loss of voluntary control over micturition was of great concern to patients facing a treatment decision for BPH. In an overall ranking of 15 different outcomes, the panel's proxy judges (see chapter 18) ranked total incontinence of urine as the fourth most important outcome influencing a treatment decision. "The panel's review showed stress incontinence to occur in 1.9 percent and urge incontinence in 0.5 percent of patients following open prostatectomy. Average total urinary incontinence was 0.5 percent. After TURP, 2.1 % of patients experienced stress incontinence, 1.9

% had urge incontinence, and 1.0% were reported to have total incontinence. The panel attempted to abstract data on urge incontinence, but found very few studies reporting this particular outcome, therefore a statistical analysis was not performed.

Turner-Warwick et al. [217]first directed attention to the relationship of bladder outlet obstruction, the symptoms of frequency, urgency and urge incontinence and the correlation of these symptoms with detrusor overactivity seen on cystometry. They also noted that in 75% of men, symptoms were relieved by prostatectomy. Several contemporary explanations are offered for the cause of persistent overactivity after obstruction. These include denervation supersensitivity of the bladder muscle [218-220], alterations in collagen composition of the obstructed bladder [221], emergence of altered and increased sensory reflexes mediating the micturition reflex [222, 223], and physical changes in detrusor myocytes affecting electrical transmission [224].

Causes of sphincteric damage after transurethral or open prostatectomy for BPH include direct damage to endoluminal tissue distal to the verumontanum because of surgical error or loss of landmarks, unexpected infiltration of the sphincter by carcinoma with loss of urethral compliance, and electrocautery injury to the sphincter. Incontinence after simple prostatectomy is more likely due to bladder dysfunction than pure sphincteric injury [225]. Incontinence after radical prostatectomy, an operation now being performed commonly, is more likely due to sphincteric injury.

III. RADICAL PROSTATECTOMY

Although experienced surgical centers report low rates of incontinence after radical prostatectomy, the overall prevalence in the general practicing community is unknown and may be higher. Initial urodynamic studies of incontinence after radical prostatectomy disagreed regarding etiology, although most suggest that sphincteric injury rather than bladder dysfunction was the primary cause of leakage. Further evidence has accumulated from studies since the last ICI report reinforcing the conclusion that sphincteric damage is the primary cause of incontinence after total prostatectomy.

Direct exposure and manipulation of the sphincter during radical retropubic prostatectomy (RRP) would suggest that sphincteric damage is the most likely cause of incontinence. Successful treatment with the artificial urinary sphincter prosthesis would also indirectly suggest that primary sphincteric injury is the major cause of incontinence, since outcome is usually not complicated by bladder dysfunction. Since data are gathering to show that radical prostatectomy can provide long term cancer free status with a high likelihood of cure in organ confined disease, and the operation will be considered in increasingly younger men, preservation of continence will be important in determining the acceptability of this operation in treating localized, potentially curable, cancer.

IV. ESTIMATES OF POST-PROSTATECTOMY INCONTINENCE

Initial estimates of incontinence, reviewed at the time of the first ICI report, were significant. In 1993, The American College of Surgeons Commission on Cancer reviewed the reported results of 2,122 patients treated by radical prostatectomy performed at 484 institution in 1990 [226]. (Table ***) Only 58% reported complete continence, 23% reported occasional incontinence not requiring pads, 11.2% wore 2 or fewer pads per day, 4% wore more than 2 pads per day, and 3.6% were completely incontinent. In 1992, Fowler et al published the results of an outcomes study with worse results [227]. In this series of Medicare patients (age >65) surveyed by mail, telephone, and personal interview, over 30 percent reported currently wearing pads or clamps to deal with wetness; over 40 percent said they dripped urine during cough or when the bladder was full; 23 percent reported daily wetting of more than a few drops. Six percent had surgery after the radical prostatectomy to treat incontinence.

In an editorial reviewing both reports, Walsh [228]criticized the Medicare interview studies and noted that the ACS results showed 81.1% complete continence without pads. He noted also that 40% of the men in the ACS series had Stage C or D (T3 or greater) disease which could decrease the rate of post-operative continence. In reviewing several reports from centers with broad experience, he noted that the possibility of significant urinary incontinence was low (2-5%) and the need for artificial sphincter was rare (0-0.5%) [228]. Since the previous ICI report, review of recent data indicates that centers of excellence are now reporting continence rates of approximately 88-95%.

There may be significant discrepancy between self-reported and objectively evaluated estimates of incontinence. Morten et al [229] reported on the results of 24 hour pad test at various intervals after prostatectomy: 8% of the patients were incontinent prior to surgery, 79% one month after surgery, 64% three months after surgery and 43% six months after surgery. The proportion of patients reporting problems with continence were 25% prior to surgery, 92% one month after, 81% three months after, and 50% 6 months after surgery. When directly questioned, 50% reported leaking only a few drops, a significant discrepancy between subjective perception and pad weights.

Prompted by the discrepancies between the Medicare report [227] and the reports from centers of excellence, Litweiler et al [230] reviewed continence results from 467 radical prostatectomies performed by 22 different private attending urologists in a community hospital in Texas. Of those questioned by telephone survey by an independent interviewer, 23% had been continent since surgery, 18.2% achieved delayed continence, and 58.8% were still incontinent at the time of interview. The majority of incontinent patients had stress incontinence (77.5%) while 59.8% had urge incontinence, 27.7% leaked only drops, and less than once a day. The authors concluded that these outcomes, better than the Fowler estimates, but not as good as the reports of centers of excellence were more representative of what private practitioners in America could expect with their patients.

In recent years, reports from general experience as well as centers of excellence support the initial impression that incontinence varies from 2 to 10%, being worse in men as they approach the age of 70. Catalona [231] reported that "Recovery of urinary continence occurred in 92% (1,223 of 1,325 men) and was associated with younger age ($p<0.0001$) but not with tumor stage ($p = 0.2$) or nerve sparing surgery ($p = 0.3$)." In his most recent update, Walsh [232] reported that "Urinary continence, which was defined as wearing no pads, gradually improved during the first 12 months after surgery, and at 1 2 and 18 months, 93% of the patients were dry."

Estimates of post-prostatectomy continence may thus vary widely depending on how soon after surgery the results are reported, the experience of the operating surgeons and center reporting the results, the definitions of continence, the method of interview and record retrieval, and the consideration of subjective vs. objective results. It is also important to realize that growing familiarity with the operation, its surgical anatomy, and the preservation of continence, may improve these results in the future.

V. POSSIBLE CAUSES OF SURGICAL INJURY

Anatomical studies [212, 233] have emphasized that the urethral sphincter is a tubular one which invests the urethra circumferentially from the pubis to the bladder neck unlike the frequently described planar diaphragm on which the prostate is pictured sitting like a spinning toy top. Recognizing the importance of these findings, Myers [214] has drawn attention to the variability of prostatic apical anatomy and ways of avoiding injury during the operation. Myers has also suggested that some men may have congenitally short urethral sphincters which may function well enough while supplemented by additional functional length of the prostatic urethra but when shortened after prostatectomy, these urethrae may fall below a critical level of functional length [213]. Concern about apical surgical margins prevents widespread application of these insights at this time.

The innervation of the periurethral striated sphincters is by the pudendal nerve traveling beneath the levator ani to branch within the pelvis [234] and beneath the pubis [235] The subpubic branches separate from the subpubic portion of the dorsal nerve of the penis after its division from the pudendal nerve. The branches migrate in a retrograde manner toward the sphincteric urethra. Whether these fibers are motor or sensory and what their role in post-prostatectomy incontinence might be has not yet been determined. These fibers could easily be injured by excessive cautery, suture placement into the dorsal vein complex or traction on the subpubic urethra at the time of apical dissection. Hollabaugh et all have attempted to identify and preserve these branches by modifying their surgical technique. They reported improved continence after doing so [236]. A similar approach to identify and preserve apical branches which might innervate the sphincter was reported by Kaye et al [237].

Additional recent studies suggest that denervation of the urethra or the bladder may occur during radical prostatectomy. John et al studied trigonal innervation by biochemical markers and found that "urinary incontinence was associated with decreased trigonal innervation, a high sensory threshold and low maximal urethral closure pressure" [238].

The gradual return of continence noted by many surgeons reporting from centers of excellence also suggest the possibility that denervation and re-innervation may be involved in post-prostatetcomy incontinence.

Uncertainty regarding the mechanism of post-prostatectomy incontinence has led to a number of different modifications in surgical technique. Preservation of the bladder neck is reported by some to have a better outcome, but there is concern about surgical cancer margins, despite reports indicating little difference when compared to conventional techniques [239-241]. Avoiding seminal vesicle removal during surgery has been suggested as a means to avoiding injury to sensory innervation [242], but again, there may be concerns about cancer margins and the significance of leaving these structures behind. Pubourethral ligament sparing has been advocated [243, 244]. Even intra-operative suburethral sling placement has been advocated [245]. One study compared continence after perineal and retropubic approaches, finding little difference [246].

VI. URODYNAMIC STUDIES: URETHRAL INJURY IS MORE SIGNIFICANT THAN BLADDER DYSFUNCTION

Urodynamic studies have sought to determine whether bladder or sphincter dysfunction is responsible for post-prostatectomy incontinence. In reviewing published studies, it is important to know whether patients who underwent radical prostatectomy for cancer were considered separately from those who underwent treatment for benign prostatic hyperplasia: the latter group is well known to suffer from more bladder dysfunction.

In the review of 700 patients by Walsh et al [247], no one was sufficiently incontinent to require an artificial sphincter. Eight men with the most severe incontinence requiring more than one pad per day were evaluated . The average bladder capacity was 450 cc . None of the most incontinent had uninhibited bladder contractions. There was no correlation between potency and continence and no correlation between continence and preservation or removal of one or both neurovascular bundles. The authors concluded that anatomic factors rather than preservation of autonomic innervation were responsible for post-prostatectomy incontinence.

Chao et al [247] reviewed the video-urodynamic records of 74 men referred for incontinence after radical prostatectomy. 57% had sphincter weakness alone, 39% had combined sphincter weakness and evidence of detrusor instability and/or decreased compliance. Only 4% had detrusor instability alone. 42% of the patients voided by abdominal straining without evidence of intrinsic bladder contraction. The authors concluded that detrusor abnormalities are rarely the sole cause of incontinence, with sphincter weakness being present in 96%.

In an electromyographic study of motor units of the periurethral striated sphincter in 10 men after radical prostatectomy, 7 of whom were continent, all showed loss of motor units and diminished electromyographic activity [248]. More recent reports have substantiated these early findings [249].

Hammerer et al [250] performed thorough urodynamic evaluation 6-8 weeks in 53 of 88 men who underwent radical prostatectomy. Compared to pre-operative values, they found a significant decrease in maximum urethral closure pressure (89.5 + 26.5 vs. 64.9+16.9) and also functional urethral profile length (62+11.3 vs. 26.2+8.5). Although there were slight changes in bladder capacity and threshold for voiding, there was no statistically significant change in compliance. The authors noted additionally that incontinent men showed a significantly smaller functional profile length (21.5 vs. 29.9 mm) and a lower maximal urethral closure pressure (51.3 vs. 67.7 cm H_2O).

Several recent studies have further extended earlier findings that sphincteric damage is the primary cause of post-prostatectomy incontinence, and even when associated when detrusor instability, sphincteric injury remains the primary cause [251-253]. Groutz et al examined 83 incontinent men after radical prostatectomy, concluding "sphincteric incontinence is the most common urodynamic finding in patients with post-radical prostatectomy incontinence, although other findings may coexist" [254].

One recent disturbing study reported a high incontinence rate in men undergoing relief of obstruction following brachytherapy for prostate cancer. Hu et al [255] studied 109 men who underwent brachytherapy. Ten needed surgical relief of outflow obstruction. Seven of the ten were severely incontinent afterwards. They concluded "Permanent urinary incontinence is common in patients who require a TURP or TUIP after prostate brachytherapy"

VII. ROLE OF BLADDER DYSFUNCTION IN INCONTINENCE AFTER RADICAL PROSTATECTOMY

Only two earlier studies have suggested that bladder dysfunction may be significant. Goluboff et al [256] evaluated 56 men with post-prostatectomy incontinence, 31 after transurethral, 25 after radical. Detrusor overactivity alone was present in 34 patients (61%), including 24 (77%) after transurethral resection of the prostate and 10 (40%) after radical retropubic prostatectomy. Stress incontinence alone was present in only 3 patients (5%), including 1 (3%) after transurethral resection of the prostate and 2 (8%) after radical retro pubic prostatectomy. Detrusor overactivity with stress incontinence was present in 19 patients (34%), including 6 (19%) after transurethral resection of the prostate and 13 (52%) after radical retropubic prostatectomy. Of these 19 patients 4 (21%) had poorly compliant bladders. These authors concluded that detrusor overactivity was much more likely to be the cause of incontinence than sphincteric weakness.

In an editorial, Leach drew attention to the high prevalence of detrusor overactivity and decreased compliance he had found in post-prostatectomy patients, many of whom had undergone radical prostatectomy. 33, 34. Referring to a more recent prospective study of 26 men before and 3, 6 and 12 months after radical prostatectomy, he noted a high incidence of de novo bladder overactivity in the incontinent patients [257]. These result differs from findings in patients studied an average of 3.8 years after surgery in whom a much lower incidence of bladder dysfunction was found [258].

Identification of sphincteric and bladder dysfunction preoperatively may indicate a higher risk of urinary incontinence after radical prostatectomy [259] , but it remains to be determined if such patients should be excluded form potentially curative treatment on the basis of pre-operative urodynamic testing.

VIII. EXPERIENCE WITH THE ARTIFICIAL SPHINCTER

Experience with artificial sphincter suggests that treatment of sphincteric incompetence alone can produce satisfactory results in the majority of patients with incontinence after radical prostatectomy. The experience suggests that what bladder dysfunction may co-exist has been either under-reported, or has not significantly affected the outcome with artificial sphincters [260]Perez, 1992 #214] [261] [261-267].

IX. CONCLUSIONS REGARDING POST-PROSTATECTOMY INCONTINENCE

While definitions and rates of post-prostatectomy incontinence may vary, most urodynamic analyses of post-radical prostatectomy incontinence would suggest that sphincter damage is a significant contributing factor. Emerging studies of incontinence after radical prostatectomy reinforce this conclusion. Emerging studies are suggesting that sensory denervation of the urethra may be a factor in incontinence. Two other urodynamic reports suggest that bladder dysfunction may also be present. It is important to distinguish between patients with incontinence following prostatectomy for cancer and benign disease as the latter group may have more accompanying pre-operative bladder dysfunction. Reported experience with the artificial urinary sphincter supports the conclusion that treatment of sphincteric competence results in good management of post-radical prostatectomy incontinence. There are several possible ways in which the operating surgeon can imagine injuring the sphincter, but it is less clear how the bladder itself would be injured, though the recent reports of trigonal denervation suggest that this may happen.

Even though the reported incidence of bladder dysfunction after radical prostatectomy is limited to a few studies, its potential contribution to the overall problem should not be excluded. It is possible that post-prostatectomy sphincteric incompetence facilitates bladder dysfunction in four ways: 1. A weakened sphincter may be less likely to provide the necessary recruitment and reciprocal inhibition characteristic of the storage phase of the normal bladder; 2. urine distending an incompetent proximal urethra can provoke a feeling of impending urination and a bladder contraction, 3) diminished urethral or trigonal sensitivity may diminish the normal guarding reflex, and 4) poor compliance may be evident in a chronically under-distended bladder.

Regardless of etiology, post-prostatectomy incontinence is a serious complication. If sufficiently prevalent it could lead to significant objection to surgical treatment of early prostatic cancer in younger men, the very group in whom cure is most desired and most likely to be achieved. For this reason, every effort should be made to determine the relative contributions of sphincteric and bladder damage to the etiology of this problem, and further refinements in anatomical understanding, surgical technique, accurate epidemiological reporting and further urodynamic testing of patients before and after surgery should be encouraged. Finally, improved outcome studies examining the consequences of incontinence and its true effect on quality of life must be undertaken if the problem is to be placed in a clinically useful and meaningful perspective.

X. GENERAL RECOMMENDATIONS FOR FUTURE RESEARCH

Since the last ICI report, there has been further work characterizing the anatomy and innervation of the male sphincter, but there is still no clear understanding of how injury takes place. MRI offers a promising tool for the study of male sphincteric anatomy, especially as it might be applied to comparing anatomical changes before and after surgery. It appears that sphincter damage is the main cause of incontinence after radical prostatectomy. The mechanism of injury, particularly neurological injury to the continence mechanism, should remain the primary focus of investigation. Studies of neuroanatomy and neurological function before and after surgery would be most desirable, including the effect of ischemia and physical injury on innervation and muscle function of the rhabdosphincter and the consequences of axonal regeneration on micturition reflexes.

With respect to incontinence associated with BPH or simple prostatectomy, much is already known regarding mechanisms of injury. However, little is known about the relationship of prostatic size and configuration to voiding dysfunction. Studies of the effect of prostatic growth, configuration and obstruction and sphincteric function would be valuable. Greater use of advanced imaging such as MRI and electromyographic studies of the sphincter in this population would be desirable.

REFERENCES

1. Fall, M., G. Geirsson, and S. Lindsröm, Toward a new classification of overactive bladders. Neurourol Urodyn, 1995. 14: p. 635.
2. Fall, M., B.L. Ohlsson , and C.A. Carlsson , The neurogenic overactive bladder. Classification based on urodynamics. Br J Urol, 1989. 64: p. 368.
3. DeGroat, W.C., A.M. Booth, and N. Yoshimura, Neurophysiology of micturition and its modification in animal models of human disease, in The Autonomic Nervous System: Nervous Control of the Urogenital System, C.A. Maggi, Editor. 1993, Harwood Academic Publishers: London. p. 227-290.
4. Tang, P.C. and T.C. Ruch , Localization of brain stem and diencephalic areas controlling the micturition reflex. J Comp Neurol, 1956. 106: p. 213.
5. Yokoyama, O., et al., The influence of anethesia on the development of bladder hyperactivity following middle cerebral occlusion in the rat. Soc. Neurosci. Abstracts, 1997. 23: p. 1522.
6. Yokoyama, O., et al., Glutamatergic and dopaminergic contributions to rat bladder hyperactivity after cerebral artery occlusion. Am J Physiol, 1999. 276: p. R935.
7. Yoshiyama, M., J.R. Roppolo, and W.C. De Groat, Effects of MK801 on the micturition reflex in the rat-possible sites of action. J Pharmacol Exp Ther, 1993. 265: p. 844.
8. Chen, S.Y., et al., Glutamate activation of neurons in cardiovarcular reactive area of the cat brain stem affects urinary bladder motility. Am J Physiol, 1993. 265: p. F520.
9. Yoshimura, N., et al., Dopamine D-1 receptor-mediated inhibition of micturition reflex by central dopamine from the substantia nigura. Neurourol Urodyn, 1992. 11: p. 535.
10. Kontani, H., T. Inoue, and T. Sasaki, Effects of apomorphine on urinary bladder motility in anesthetized rats. Jpn J Pharmaco, 1990. 52: p. 59.
11. Yoshimura, N., et al., The dopamine D, receptor agonist SKF 38393 suppresses detrusor hyperreflexia in the monkey with parkinsonism. Neurpharmacology, 1993. 32: p. 315.
12. Bors, E. and A.E. Comarr, Physiology of Micturition, Its Neurological Disorders and Sequelae. 1971, Baltimore: University Park Press.
13. Cockayne, D.A., et al., Urinary bladder hyporeflexia and reduced pain-related behavior in P2X3-deficient mice. Nature, 2000. 407: p. 1001.
14. De Groat, W.C., et al., Mechanisms underlying the recovery of urinary bladder function following spinal cord injury. J Auton Nervous Syst, 1990. 30(suppl): p. S71.
15. De Groat, W.C., et al., Organization of the sacral parasympathetic reflex pathways to the urinary bladder and large intestine. J Auton Nervous Syst, 1981. 3: p. 135.
16. Häbler, H.J., W. Jänig, and M. Koltzenburg, Activation of unmyclinated afferent fibres by mechanical stimuli and inflammation of the urinary bladder in the cat. J Physiol(Lond), 1990. 425: p. 545.
17. Fowler, C.J., et al., Intravesical capsaicin for treatment of detrusor hyperreflexia. J Neurol Neurosurg Psychiatry, 1994. 57: p. 169.
18. Fowler, C.J., et al., Intravesical capsaicin for neurogenic bladder dysfunction(letter). Lancet, 1992. 339: p. 1239.
19. Geirsson, G., M. Fall, and L. Sullivan, Effect of intravesical capsaicin treatment on postraumatic spinal detrusor hyperreflexia and the bladder cooling reflex. Neurourol Urodyn, 1994. 13: p. 346.
20. Chancellor, M.B. and W.C. De Groat , Intravesical capsaicin and resiniferatoxin therapy. Spicing up the ways to treat the overactive bladder. J Urol, 1999. 162: p. 3.
21. Lazzeri, M., et al., Intravesical resiniferatoxin for the treatment of detrusor hyperreflexia refractory to capsaicin. 1998. 159: p. 83.
22. Kruse, M.N., L.A. Bray, and W.C. De Groat, Influence of spinal cord injury on the morphology of bladder afferent and efferent neurons. J Auton Nervous Syst, 1995. 54: p. 215.
23. Steers, W.D., et al., Nerve growth factor in the urinary bladder of the adult regulates neuronal form and function. J Clin Invest, 1991. 88: p. 1709.
24. Yoshimura, N. and W.C. De Groat, Changes in electrophysiological and pharmacological properties of rat bladder afferent neurons following spinal cord injury. J Urol, 1995. 149: p. 340A.
25. Yoshimura, N., O. Yoshida, and W.C. De Groat, Regional differences in plasticity of membrane properties of rat bladder afferent neurons following spinal cord injury. J Urol, 1995. 153: p. 262A.
26. Arbuckle, J.B. and R.J. Docherty, Expression of tetrodotoxinresistant sodium channels in capsaicin-sensitive dorsal root ganglion neurons of adult rats. Neurosci Lett, 1995. 185: p. 70.
27. Yoshimura, N., et al., Different types of Na+ and A-typeK+ currents in dorsal root ganglion neurons innervating the rat urinary bladder. J Physiol(Lond), 1996. 494: p. 1.
28. Abrams, P.H., Detrusor instability and bladder outlet obstruction. Neurourol Urodyn, 1985. 4: p. 317.
29. Gosling, J.A., S.A. Gilpin, and J.e.a. Dixon, Decrease in the autonomic innervation of human detrusor muscle in outflow obstruction. J Urol, 1986. 136: p. 501.
30. Harrison, S.C.W., et al., Bladder instability and denervation in patients with bladder outflow obstruction. Br J Urol, 1987. 60: p. 519.
31. Sibley, G.N.A., The physiological response of the detrusor muscle to experimental bladder outflow obstruction in the pig. Br J Urol, 1987. 60: p. 332.
32. Speakman, M.J., et al., Bladder outflow obstruction-A cause of denervation supersensitivity. J Urol, 1987. 138: p. 1461.
33. Harrison, S.C.W., D.R. Ferguson , and P.T. Doyle , Effect of bladder outflow obstruction on the innervation of the rabbit urinary bladder. Br J Urol, 1990. 66: p. 372.
34. Azadzoi, K.M., et al., Canine bladder blood flow and oxygenation: changes induced by filling contraction and outlet obstruction. J Urol, 1996. 155: p. 1459.
35. Lemack, G.E., et al., Altered response to partial bladder outlet obstruction in mice lacking inducible nitric oxide synthase. J Urol, 2000. 163: p. 1981.
36. van Koeveringe, G.A., et al., Effect of partial urethral obstruction on force development of the guinea pig bladder. Neurourol Urodyn, 1993. 12: p. 555.
37. Seki, N., O.M. Karim , and J.L. Mostwin , The effect of experimental urethral obstruction and its reversal on changes in passive electrical properties of detrusor muscle. J Urol, 1992. 148: p. 1957.
38. Sjögren, C., et al., Atropine resistance of transmurally stimulated isolated human bladder muscle. J Urol, 1982. 128: p. 1368.
39. Steers, W.D., et al., Alterations in afferent pathways from the urinary bladder of the rat in response to partial urethral obstruction. J Comp Neurol, 1991. 310: p. 401.
40. Steers, W.D. and W.C. De Groat , Effect of bladder outlet obstruction on micturition reflex pathways in the rat. J Urol, 1988. 140: p. 864.
41. Ishizuka, O., et al., Role of intrathecal tachykinins for micturi-

tion in unanesthetized rats with and without bladder outlet obstruction. Br J Pharmacol, 1994. 113: p. 111.

42. Gu, B.J., et al., Role of supraspinal tachykinins for micturition in conscious rats with and without bladder outlet obstruction. Naunyn Schmiedebergs Arch Pharmacol, 2000. 361: p. 543.

43. Lepor, H. and G. Machi , Comparison of AUA symptom index in unselected males and females between fifty-five and seventy-nine years of age. Urology, 1993. 42: p. 36.

44. Resnick, N.M., S.V. Yalla, and E. Laurino, The pathophysiology of urinary incontinence among institutionalized elderly persons. New Engl J Med, 1989. 320: p. 1.

45. Griffths, D.J., et al., Geriatric urge incontinence: basic dysfunction and contributory factors. Neurourol Urodyn, 1990. 9: p. 406.

46. Kidata, S., et al., Bladder function in elderly men with subclinical brain magnetic resonance imaging lesions. J Urol, 1992. 147: p. 1107.

47. Elbadawi, A., S.V. Yalla, and N.M. Resnic, Structural basis of geriatric voiding dysfunction. ?.Aging detrusor: normal vs impaired contractility. J Urol, 1993. 150: p. 1657.

48. Elbadawi, A., S.V. Yalla, and N.M. Resnic, Structural basis of geriatric voiding dysfunction. Detrusor overactivity. J Urol, 1993. 150: p. 1668.

49. Elbadawi, A., S.V. Yalla, and N.M. Resnic, Structural basis of geriatric voiding dysfunction. Bladder outlet obstruction. J Urol, 1993. 150: p. 1681.

50. Resnick, N.M. and S.V. Yalla , Detrusor hyperactivity with impaired contractile function: an unrecognized but common cause of incontinence elderly patients. JAMA, 1987. 257: p. 3076.

51. Kohan, A.D., et al., Effect of aging on bladder function and response to outlet obstruction in female rats. Urol Res, 2000. 28: p. 33.

52. Nishimoto, T., et al., Age-dependent alterations in beta-adrenergic responsiveness of rat detrusor smooth muscle. J Urol, 1995. 153: p. 1701.

53. Yoshida, M., et al., Age-related changes in cholinergic and purinergic neurotransmission in human isolated bladder smooth muscle. Exp Gerontol, 2001. 36: p. 99.

54. Yoshida, M., et al., Age-related changes in acetylcholine and adenosine triphosphate release from human bladder smooth muscles. Neurourol Urodyn, 1999. 18: p. 346.

55. Sand, P.K., et al., The effect of retropubic urethropexy on detrusor stability. Obstet Gynecol, 1988. 71(partI): p. 818.

56. Ohlsson, B.L., M. Fall, and S. Frankenberg-Sommar, Effects of external and direct pudendal nerve maximal electical stimulation in the treatment of the uninhibited overactive bladder. Br J Urol, 1989. 64: p. 374.

57. Plevnik, S., et al., Short-term electrical stimulation: home treatment for urinary incontinence. World J Urol, 1986. 4: p. 24.

58. Maggi, C.A., et al., Cystometric evidence that capsaicin-sensitive nerves modulate the afferent branch of micturition reflex in humans. J Urol, 1989. 142: p. 150.

59. Maggi, C.A., Tachykinins and calcitonin gene-related peptide(CGRP) as cotransmitters released from peripheral endings of sensory nerves. Progr Neurobiol, 1995. 45: p. 1.

60. Lazzeri, M., et al., Intravesical resiniferatoxin for the treatment of hypersensitive disorder: a randomized placebo controlled study. J Urol, 2000. 164: p. 676.

61. Loudberg, J.M., Pharmacology of cotransmission in the autonomic nervous system: integrative aspects on amines neuropeptides adenosine triphosphate amino acid and nitric oxide. Pharmacol Rev, 1996. 48: p. 113.

62. Yoshimura, N. and W.C. De Groat, Increased excitability of afferent neurons innervating rat urinary bladder after chronic bladder inflammation. J Neurosci, 1999. 19: p. 644.

63. Maggi, C.A., et al., Evidence for the involvement of bradykinin in chemically-evoked cystitis in anesthetized rats. Naunyn-Schmiedebergs Arch Pharmacol, 1993. 347: p. 432.

64. Ishizuka, O., A. Mattiasson, and K.E. Andersson, Prostaglandin E2-indeuced bladder hyperactivity in normal conscious rats. Involvement of tachykinins? J Urol, 1995. 153: p. 2034.

65. Artibani, W., Diagnosis and significance of idiopathic overactive bladder. Urology, 197. 50(suppl 6A): p. 25.

66. Brading, A.F., A myogenic bases for the overactive bladder. Urology, 1997. 50(suppl ^A): p. 57.

67. Brading, A.F. and W.H. Turner, The unstable bladder: towards a common mechanism. Br J Urol, 1994. 73: p. 3.

68. Mills, I.W., et al., Studies of the pathophysiology of idiopathic detrusor instability: the physiological properties of the detrusor smooth muscle and its pattern of innervation. J Urol, 2000. 163: p. 646.

69. Wessler, I., C.J. Kirkpatrick , and K. Racke , Non-neuronal acetylcholine a locally acting molecule widely distributed in biological system: expression and function in human. Pharmacol Ther, 1998. 77: p. 59.

70. Silver, F.H., et al., Role of storage on changes in the mechanical properties of tendon and self-assembled collagen fibers. Conn Tissue Res, 2000. 4: p. 155-164.

71. Johnson, T. and J.G. Ouslander, Urinary incontinence in the older man. Medical Clinics of North America, 1999. 83: p. 1247-1266.

72. McBride, D.J., R.V. Trelstad, and F.H. Silver , Structural and mechanical assessment of developing chick tendon. Int. J. Biol. Macromol, 1988. 10: p. 194-200.

73. Keene, D., et al., Type III collagen can be present on banded collagen fibrils regardless of fibril diameter. J Cell Biol, 1987. 105(2393-2402).

74. Samsioe, G., Urogenital aging : a hidden problem. Am J Obstet Gynecol, 1998. 178: p. 245-249.

75. Bercovich, E., et al., A multivariate analysis of lower urinary tract ageing and urinary symptoms, the role of fibrosis. Andrologia, 1999. 71: p. 287-292.

76. Satoh, W. and T. Nakada, Characteristics of circadian change in urinary frequency, bladder capacity and residual urine volume in elderly men with lower urinary tract symptoms. Nursing and Health Sciences, 1999. 1: p. 125-129.

77. Gosling, J.A., Modification of bladder structure in response to outflow obstruction and ageing. European Urology, 1997. 32 Suppl.1: p. 9-14.

78. DuBeau, C.E., S.V. Yalla, and N.M. Resnick, Improving the utility of urine flow rate to exclude outlet obstruction in men with voiding symptoms. J Amer. Ger. Soc., 1998. 46: p. 1118-1124.

79. Hongoh, Y., et al., Morphologic changes in detrusor muscles of patients with chronic obstruction of lower urinary tract. Electronmicroscopic and immunohistochemical findings. Urology, 1991. 37(6): p. 584-589.

80. Barnard, R.J., J.S. Dixon, and J.A. Gosling, A clinical and morphological evaluation of the trabeculated urinary bladder. Progress in clinical and biological research, 1981. 78: p. 285-288.

81. Gosling, J.A. and J.S. Dixon, Structure of trabeculated detrusor smooth msucle in cases of prostatic hypertrophy. Urologia Internationalis, 1980. 35: p. 351-355.

82. Gilpin, S.A., J.A. Gosling, and R.J. Barnard, Morphological and morphometric studies of the human obstructed, trabeculated urinary bladder. Brit J Urol, 1985. 57: p. 525-529.

83. Azadzoi, K.M., et al., Atherosclerosis sinduced chronic ischemia causes bladder fibrosis and non-compliance in the rabbit. J Urol, 1999. 161: p. 1626-1635.

84. Kim K.M, et al., Collagen and Elastin in the normal fetal bladder. J Urol, 1991. 146: p. 524-527.

85. Kim K.M, Kogan B.A, and C.A. Massad, Collagen and elastin in the obstructed fetal bladder. J Urol, 1991. 146: p. 528-531.

86. Shapiro, E., et al., Bladder wall abnormalities in myelodysplastic bladders: a computer assisted morphometric analysis. J Urol, 1991. 145: p. 1024-1029.

87. Ewalt, D.H., et al., Is lamina propria matrix responsible for normal bladder compliance? J Urol, 1992. 148: p. 544-549.

88. Ohnishi, N., et al., Morphometric study of low compliant bladder. Acta Urologica Japonica, 1994. 40: p. 657-661.

89. Landau, E.H., et al., Loss of elasticity indysfunctional bladders: urodynamic and histochemical correlation. J Urol, 1994. 152: p. 702-2705.

90. Deveaud, C.M., et al., Molecular analysis of collagens in bladder fibrosis. J Urol, 1998. 160: p. 1518-1527.

91. Kaplan, E.P., et al., Type III collagen messenger RNA is modulated in non-compliant human bladder tissue. J Urol, 1997. 157: p. 2366-2369.

92. Gabella, G. and B. Uvelius, Urinary bladder of the rat: fine structure of normal and hypertrophic musculature. Cell and Tissue Research, 1990. 262: p. 67-79.

93. Uvelius, B., P. Lindner, and A. Mattiasson, Collagen content in the rat urinary bladder following removal of an experimental infravesical outlet obstruction. Urologia Internationalis, 1991. 47: p. 245-249.

94. Williams, J.H., et al., Experimental model of bladder outflow tract obstruction in the guinea pig. Brit J Urol, 1993. 71: p. 543-554.

95. Nielsen, K.K., et al., Morphological, stereological and biochemical analysis of the mini-pig urinary bladder after chronic outflow obstruction and after recovery from obstruction. Neurourology and Urodynamics, 1995. 14: p. 269-284.

96. Keane, D.P., et al., Analysis of collagen status in premenopausal nulliparous women with genuine stress incontinence. Brit. J Obstet. Gynecol., 1997. 104: p. 994 998.

97. Lin, V.K. and J.D. McConnell, Molecular aspects of bladder outlet obstruction. Advances in Experimental Medicine & Biology., 1995. 385: p. 65-74, diuscussion 75-79.

98. Murakumo, M., et al., Three dimensional arrangement of collagen and elastin fibers in human urinary bladder: scanning electron microscopy study. J Urol, 1995. 154: p. 251-256.

99. Papa Petros, P.E. and U.L. Ulmsten, An integral theory of female incontinence. Acta Obstet. Gynecol. Scand., 1990. 69: p. 7-31.

100. Peacock, E.E., Wound Repair. 3rd ed. 1984, Philadelphia: W. B. Saunders.

101. Shyu, K.G., et al., Angiotensinogen gene expression is induced by cyclical mechanical stretch in cultured rat cardiomyocytes. Biochem Biophys Res Comm, 1995. 211: p. 241-248.

102. Wall, L.L. and J.O. DeLancey, The politics of prolapse: a revisionist approach to disorders of the pelvic floor in women. Perspect Biol Med, 1991. 34(4): p. 486-96.

103. Morkved, S. and K. Bo, Prevalence of urinary incontinence during pregnancy and postpartum. Int Urogynecol J Pelvic Floor Dysfunct, 1999. 10(6): p. 394-8.

104. Mason, L., et al., The experience of stress incontinence after childbirth. Birth, 1999. 26(3): p. 164-71.

105. Beck, R.P., S. McCormick, and L. Nordstrom, Intraurethral-intravesical cough-pressure spike differences in 267 patients surgically cured of genuine stress incontinence of urine. Obstet Gynecol, 1988. 72(3 Pt 1): p. 302-6.

106. Swash, M., S.J. Snooks, and M.M. Henry, Unifying concept of pelvic floor disorders an incontinence. J Roy Soc Med, 1985. 78: p. 906-933.

107. Cardozo, L. and A. Cutner, Lower urinary tract symptoms in pregnancy. Br J Urol, 1997. 80 Suppl 1: p. 14-23.

108. Francis, W.J.A., Disturbances of bladder function in relation to pregnancy. Journal of Obstetrics and Gynecology of the British Empire, 1960. 67: p. 353-66.

109. Stanton, S.L., R. Kerr-Wilson, and V.G. Harris, The incidence of urological symptoms in normal pregnancy. Br J Obstet Gynaecol, 1980. 87: p. 897-900.

110. Hong, P.L., M. Leong, and V. Selzer, Uroflowmetric observation in pregnancy. Neurourol Urodynam, 1988. 7(61-70).

111. Parboosingh, J. and A. Doig, Studies in nocturia in normal pregnancy. J Obstet Gynaecol Br Comw, 1873. 80: p. 888-895.

112. Nemir, A. and R.P. Middleton, Stress incontinence in young nulliparous women. American Journal of Obstetrics and Gynecology, 1954. 68: p. 1166-8.

113. Wolin, L.H., Stress incontinence in young healthy nulliparous subjects. Journal of Urology, 1969. 101: p. 545-549.

114. Hojberg, K.E., et al., Urinary incontinence: prevalence and risk factors at 16 weeks of gestation. British Journal of Obstetrics andGynaecology, 1999. 106: p. 842-850.

115. Iosif, S., L. Henriksson, and U. Ulmsten, Postpartum incontinence. Urol Int, 1981. 36(1): p. 53-8.

116. Iosif, S., Stress incontinence during pregnancy and in puerperium. Int J Gynaecol Obstet, 1981. 19(1): p. 13-20.

117. Viktup, L., et al., The symptom of stress incontinence caused by pregnancy or delivery in primiparas. Obstet Gynecol, 1992. 79: p. 945-499.

118. Groutz, A., et al., Stress urinary incontinence: prevalence among nulliparous compared with primiparous and grand multiparous premenopausal women. Neurourol Urodyn, 1999. 18(5): p. 419-25.

119. Allen, R.E., et al., Pelvic floor damage and childbirth: a neurophysiological study. Br J Obstet Gynaecol, 1990. 97: p. 770-779.

120. Snooks, S.J., et al., Risk factors in childbirth causing damage to the pelvic floor innervation. Int J Colorectal Dis, 1986. 1: p. 20-24.

121. Brown, S. and J. Lumley, Maternal health after childbirth: results of an Australian population based survey. Br J Obstet Gynaecol, 1998. 105: p. 156-161.

122. Handa, V.L., T.A. Harris, and D.R. Ostergard, Protecting the pelvic floor: obstetric management to prevent incontinence and pelvic organ prolapse. [Review] [46 refs]. Obstetrics & Gynecology, 1996. 88(3): p. 470-8.

123. Peschers, U.M., et al., Levator ani function before and after childbirth. 1997. 104: p. 1004-1008.

124. Tunn, R., et al., MR imaging of levator ani muscle recovery following vaginal delivery. Int-Urogynecol-J-Pelvic-Floor-Dysfunct., 1999. 10(300-307).

125. Persson, J., -.H.P. Wolner, and H. Rydhstroem, Obstetric risk factors for stress urinary incontinence: a population-based study. Obstet Gynecol, 2000. 96(3): p. 440-5.

126. Johanson, R.B., et al., Maternal and child health after assisted vaginal delivery: five-year follow up of a randomised controlled study comparing forceps and ventouse. Br J Obstet Gynaecol, 1999. 106(6): p. 544-549.

127. Meyer, S., O. Bachelard, and G.P. De, Do bladder neck mobility and urethral sphincter function differ during pregnancy compared with during the non-pregnant state? Int Urogynecol J Pelvic Floor Dysfunct, 1998. 9(6): p. 397-404.

128. King, J. and R. Freeman, Is antenatal bladder neck mobility a risk factor for postpartum stress incontinence? Br J Obstet Gynaecol, 1998. 105(12): p. 1300-7.

129. Abitbol, M.M., Birth and human evolution: anatomical and obstetrical mechanics in primates. 1997, Westport, CT.: Bergin and Garvey.

130. Moerman, M.L., Growth of the birth canal in adolescent girls. Am J Obstet Gynecol, 1982. 143: p. 528-532.

131. Klein, M.C., et al., Relationship of episiotomy to perineal trauma and morbidity, sexual dysfunction, and pelvic floor relaxation. Am-J-Obstet-Gynecol., 1994. 171(3): p. 591-8.

132. Francis, W.J.A., The onset of stress incontinence. Journal of Obstetrics and Gynecology of the British Empire, 1960. 67: p. 899-903.

133. Cutner, A. and L.D. Cardozo, The lower urinary tract in pregnancy and the puerperium. International Urogynecology Journal, 1992. 3(312-23).

134. Wolin, L.H., Stress incontinence in young, healthy nulliparous female subjects. J Urol, 1969. 101(4): p. 545-9.

135. Signorello, L.B., et al., Midline episiotomy and anal incontinence: retrospective cohort study. BMJ, 2000. 320(7227): p. 86-90.

136. Unicef., W., Revised 1990 estimates of maternal mortality: A new approach. 1996, Geneva: World Health Organization.

137. Fortney, J.A. and J.B. Smith, The base of the iceberg: Prevalence and perceptions of maternal morbidity in four developing countries. 1996, Research Triangle Park, NC: Family Health International.

138. Carroli, P.R. and J. Belizan, Episiotomy for vaginal birth. 2000, Cochrane-Database-Syst-Rev.

139. Angioli, R., et al., Severe perineal lacerations during vaginal delivery: the University of Miami experience. Am-J-Obstet-Gynecol., 2000. 182(5): p. 1083-5.

140. Signorello, L.B., et al., Midline episiotomy and anal incontinence: retrospective cohort study. BMJ, 2000. 320(7227): p. 86-90.

141. Klein, M.C., et al., Relationship of episiotomy to perineal trauma and morbidity, sexual dysfunction, and pelvic floor relaxation. Am J Obstet Gynecol, 1994. 171(3): p. 591-598.

142. Eason, E. and P. Feldman, Much ado about a little cut: is episiotomy worthwhile? Obstet Gynecol, 2000. 95(4): p. 616-618.

143. Olayinka-Oyelese, K., W. Porter, and C. Wai, Midline episiotomy and anal incontinence. Is episiotomy ethically acceptable? [letter]. BMJ, 2000. 10(7249): p. 1602.

144. Mills, M.S. and D.J. Murphy, Midline episiotomy and anal incontinence. Results should be interpreted with caution in British context [letter]. BMJ, 2000. 320(7249): p. 1601-1602.

145. Chaliha, C. and A.H. Sultan, Midline episiotomy and anal incontinence. Training is needed in the recognition and repair of perineal trauma [letter]. BMJ, 2000. 320(7249): p. 1601.

146. Sampselle, C., et al., Effect of pelvic muscle exercise on transient incontinence during pregnancy and after birth. Obstet Gynecol, 1998. 91(3): p. 406-12.

147. Morkved, S. and K. Bo, Effect of postpartum pelvic floor muscle training in prevention and treatment of urinary incontinence: a one-year follow up. BJOG, 2000. 107(8): p. 1022-8.

148. Miller, K., et al., Pelvic floor electrical stimulation for genuine stress incontinence: who will benefit and when? Int Urogynecol J Pelvic Floor Dysfunct, 1998. 9(5): p. 265-70.

149. Cockshott, W.P., Pubic changes associated with obstetric vesico-vaginal fistulae. Clin Radiol, 1973. 23: p. 241-2247.

150. Flynn, P., et al., How can second-stage management prevent perineal trauma? Critical review. Can Fam Physician, 1997. 43(1): p. 73-84.

151. Klein, M.C., et al., Determinants of vaginal-perineal integrity and pelvic floor functioning in childbirth. Am J Obstet Gynecol, 1997. 176(2): p. 403-410.

152. Eason, E., et al., Preventing perineal trauma during childbirth: a systematic review. 2000. 95(3): p. 464-471.

153. Cooper, Z.R. and S. Rose, Fecal incontinence: a clinical approach. Mt-Sinai-J-Med, 2000. 67(2): p. 96-105.

154. Toglia, M.R. and J.O. Delancey, Anal incontinence and the obstetrician-gynecologist. Obstet Gynecol, 1994. 84(Pt 2): p. 731-740.

155. Podnar, S., A. Lukanovi&Cbreve, and D.B. WVodusek, Anal sphincter electromyography after vaginal delivery: neuropathic insufficiency or normal wear and tear? Neurourol-Urodyn, 2000. 19(3): p. 249-257.

156. Sander, P., et al., Anal incontinence after obstetric third- /fourth-degree laceration. One-year follow-up after pelvic floor exercises. Int. Urogynecol. J. Pelvic FloorDysfunct., 1999. 10(3): p. 177-81.

157. Kelly, W. and E. Burnham, Disease of the Kidneys, Ureters and Bladder, With Special reference to Women. Vol. 2. 1922.

158. Oelrich, T.M., The striated urogenital sphincter muscle in the female. Anatomical Record, 1983. 205(2): p. 223-32.

159. DeLancey, J.O., Functional anatomy of the female lower urinary tract and pelvic floor. Ciba Found Symp, 1990. 151: p. 57-69.

160. DeLancey, J.O., Structural support of the urethra as it relates to stress urinary incontinence: the hammock hypothesis. Am J Obstet Gynecol, 1994. 170(6): p. 1713-20.

161. Athanassopoulos, A., et al., Stamey endoscopic vesical neck suspension in female urinary stress incontinence: results and changes in various urodynamic parameters. International Urology & Nephrology, 1994. 26(3): p. 293-9.

162. Bump, R.C., J.A. Fantl, and W.G. Hurt, Dynamic urethral pressure profilometry pressure transmission ratio determinations after continence surgery: understanding the mechanism of success, failure, and complications. Obstet Gynecol, 1988. 72(6): p. 870-4.

163. Bunne, G. and A. Obrink, Influence of pubococcygeal repair on urethral closure pressure at stress. Acta Obstet Gynecol Scand, 1978. 57(4): p. 355-9.

164. Hilton, P. and S.L. Stanton, Urethral pressure measurement by microtransducer: the results in symptom-free women and in those with genuine stress incontinence. Br J Obstet Gynaecol, 1983. 90(10): p. 919-33.

165. Masuda, H., et al., [Analysis of continence mechanisms by stress urethral pressure profiles]. Nippon Hinyokika Gakkai Zasshi, 1994. 85(3): p. 434-9.

166. Obrink, A., G. Bunne, and A. Ingelman-Sundberg, Pressure transmission to the pre-urethral space in stress incontinence. Urol Res, 1978. 6(3): p. 135-40.

167. Penttinen, J., et al., Successful colposuspension in stress urinary incontinence reduces bladder neck mobility and increases pressure transmission to the urethra. Arch Gynecol Obstet, 1989. 244(4): p. 233-8.

168. Penttinen, J., K. Kaar, and A. Kauppila, Effect of suprapubic operation on urethral closure. Evaluation by single cough urethrocystometry. Br J Urol, 1989. 63(4): p. 389-91.

169. Rottenberg, R.D., et al., Urodynamic and clinical assessment of the Lyodura sling operation for urinary stress incontinence. Br J Obstet Gynaecol, 1985. 92(8): p. 829-34.

170. van-Geelen, J.M., et al., The clinical and urodynamic effects of anterior vaginal repair and Burch colposuspension. Am J Obstet Gynecol, 1988. 159(1): p. 137-44.

171. Martan, A., et al., [Ultrasonic evaluation of paravaginal defects before and after surgical treatment in women with urinary stress incontinence]. Ceska Gynekol, 2000. 65(3): p. 152-6.

172. Jeffcoate, T.N.A. and H. Roberts, Observations on stress incontinence of urine. Am J Obstet Gynecol, 1952. 64: p. 721.

173. Hodgkinson, C.D., Relationship of female urethra and bladder in urinary stress incontinence. American Journal of Obstetrics and Gynecology, 1953. 65: p. 560.

174. Hodgkinson, C.P., Stress urinary incontinence—1970. Am J Obstet Gynecol, 1970. 108(7): p. 1141-68.

175. Wall, L.L., et al., Bladder neck mobility and the outcome of surgery for genuine stress urinary incontinence. A logistic regression analysis of lateral bead-chain cystourethrograms. Journal of Reproductive Medicine, 1994. 39(6): p. 429-35.

176. Blaivas, J.G. and C.A. Olsson, Stress incontinence: classification and surgical approach. J Urol, 1988. 139(4): p. 727-31.

177. McGuire, E.J., R.D. Cespedes, and H.E. O'Connell, Leak-point pressures. [Review] [12 refs]. Urologic Clinics of North America, 1996. 23(2): p. 253-62.

178. McGuire, E.J., Diagnosis and treatment of intrinsic sphincter deficiency. International Journal of Urology, 1995. 2(Suppl 1): p. 7-10; discussion 16-8.

179. Leach, G.E., et al., Female stress urinary incontinence clinical guidelines panel summary report on surgical management of female stress urinary incontinence. Journal of Urology, 1997. 158: p. 875-880.

180. Kayigil, O., A.S. Iftekhar, and A. Metin, The coexistence of intrinsic sphincter deficiency with type II stress incontinence. J Urol, 1999. 162(4): p. 1365-6.

181. Chaikin, D., J. Rosenthal, and J. Blaivas, Pubovaginal fascial sling for all types of stress urinary incontinence: long-term analysis. J Urol, 1998. 160(4): p. 1312-6.

182. Kiilholma, P.J., et al., Perineal ultrasound: an alternative for radiography for evaluating stress urinary incontinence in females. Annales Chirurgiae et Gynaecologiae - Supplementum, 1994. 208: p. 43-5.

183. Meyer, S., et al., The assessment of bladder neck position and mobility in continent nullipara, mulitpara, forceps-delivered and incontinent women using perineal ultrasound: a future office procedure? International Urogynecology Journal and Pelvic Floor Dysfunction, 1996. 7(3): p. 138-46.

184. Kauppila, A., J. Penttinen, and V.M. Haggman, Six-microtransducer catheter connected to computer in evaluation of urethral closure function of women. Urology, 1989. 33(2): p. 159-64.

185. Behr, J., M. Winkler, and U. Schwiersch, [Urodynamic observations on the Marshall-Marchetti-Krantz operation]. Geburtshilfe Frauenheilkd, 1986. 46(9): p. 649-53.

186. Vanderschot, E.L., M.L. Chafik, and F.M. Debruyne, Has the suprapubic suspension operation any influence on the urethral pressure profile? Br J Urol, 1979. 51(2): p. 140-3.

187. Langer, R., et al., Continence mechanism after colpo-needle suspension for stress urinary incontinence. Journal of Reproductive Medicine, 1995. 40(10): p. 699-702.

188. Hertogs, K. and S.L. Stanton, Lateral bead-chain urethrocystography after successful and unsuccessful colposuspension. Br J Obstet Gynaecol, 1985. 92(11): p. 1179-83.

189. Snooks, S.J., P.R. Barnes, and M. Swash, Damage to the innervation of the voluntary anal and periurethral sphincter musculature in incontinence: an electrophysiological study. J Neurol Neurosurg Psychiatry, 1984. 47(12): p. 1269-73.

190. Snooks, S.J., et al., Perineal nerve damage in genuine stress urinary incontinence. An electrophysiological study. Br J Urol, 1985. 57(4): p. 422-6.

191. Swash, M., S.J. Snooks, and M.M. Henry, Unifying concept of pelvic floor disorders an incontinence. Journal of the Royal Society of Medicine, 1985. 78: p. 906-933.

192. Ismael, S., et al., Postpartum lumbosacral plexopathy limited to autonomic and perineal manifestations: clinical and electrophysiological study of 19 patients. J Neurol Neurosurg Psychiatry, 2000. 68(6): p. 771-3.

193. Takahashi, S., et al., Electromyographic study of the striated urethral sphincter in type 3 stress incontinence: evidence of myogenic-dominant damages. Urology, 2000. 56(6): p. 946-50.

194. Weidner, A., et al., Pelvic muscle electromyography of levator ani and external anal sphincter in nulliparous women and women with pelvic floor dysfunction. Am J Obstet Gynecol, 2000. 183(6): p. 1390-9; discussion 1399-401.

195. Gunnarsson, M. and A. Mattiasson, Female stress, urge, and mixed urinary incontinence are associated with a chronic and progressive pelvic floor/vaginal neuromuscular disorder: An investigation of 317 healthy and incontinent women using vaginal surface electromyography. Neurourol Urodyn, 1999. 18(6): p. 613-21.

196. Pieber, D., F. Zivkovic, and K. Tamussino, Timing of urethral pressure pulses before and after continence surgery. Neurourol Urodyn, 1998. 17(1): p. 19-23.

197. Yang, A., et al., Dynamic evaluation of pelvic floor descent using fastscan MRI and cinematic display. Radiology, 1991. 179: p. 25-33.

198. Gufler, H., et al., Comparison of cystourethrography and dynamic MRI in bladder neck descent. J Comput Assist Tomogr, 2000. 24(3): p. 382-8.

199. Yang, A., et al., Patterns of prolapse demonstrated with dynamic fastscan MRI; re-assesment of conventional concepts of pelvic floor weakness. Neurourology and Urodynamics, 1993. 12: p. 310.

200. Yang, A., et al., High resoluton magnetic resonance imaging of urethra and periurethral structures using intravaginal surface coil and quadrature phased array surface coil. Neurourology and Urodynamics, 1993. 12: p. 329.

201. Perez, N., et al., Dynamic magnetic resonance imaging of the female pelvis: radio-anatomy and pathologic applications. Preliminary results. Surg Radiol Anat, 1999. 21(2): p. 133-8.

202. Sanders, R.C., et al., Imaging the female urethra. Ultrasound Quarterly, 1994. 12(3): p. 167-183.

203. Masata, J., et al., [Ultrasonography of the funneling of the urethra]. Ceska Gynekol, 2000. 65(2): p. 87-90.

204. Schaer, G.N., et al., Improvement of perineal sonographic bladder neck imaging with ultrasound contrast medium. Obstetrics & Gynecology, 1995. 86(6): p. 950-4.

205. Nichols, D.H. and C.L. Randall, Vaginal Surgery. 1989, Baltimore: Williams and Wilkins. 463.

206. Mostwin, J.L., et al., Radiography, sonography, and magnetic resonance imaging for stress incontinence. Contributions, uses, and limitations. Urologic Clinics of North America, 1995. 22(3): p. 539-49.

207. Milley, P.S. and D.H. Nichols, The relationship between the pubo-urethral ligaments and the urogenital diaphragm in the human female. Anat Rec, 1971. 170: p. 281.

208. Zacharin, R.A., The suspensory mechanism of the female urethra. J Anatom, 1961. 97: p. 423.

209. Zacharin, R.F., The anatomic supports of the female urethra. Obstet Gynecol, 1968. 32(6): p. 754-9.

210. Mostwin, J.L., et al., Stress incontinence observed with real time sonography and dynamic fastscan magnetic resonance imaging: insights into pathophysiology. Scan J Urol Nephrol, Suppl 207, 2000, p. 94-99.

211. McGuire, E.J., Evaluation of Urinary Incontinence, in Neurourology and Urodynamics: Principles and Practice, S.V. Yalla, et al., Editors. 1988, Macmillan: New York. p. 211-220.

212. Oelrich, T.M., The urethral sphincter muscle in the male. American Journal of Anatomy, 1980. 158(2): p. 229-46.

213. Myers, R.P., Male urethral sphincter anatomy and radical prostatectomy. Urological Clinics of North America, 1991. 18(2): p. 211-225.
214. Myers, R.P., J.R. Goellner, and D.R. Cahill, Prostate shape, external striated urethral sphincter and radical prostatectomy: the apical dissection. Journal of Urology, 1987. 138(3): p. 543-50.
215. Myers, R., et al., Puboperineales: muscular boundaries of the male urogenital hiatus in 3D from magnetic resonance imaging. J Urol, 2000. 164(4): p. 1412-5.
216. U.S.DepartmentofHealthandHumanServices, Benign Prostatic Hyperplasia: Diagnosis and Treatment. Vol. N94-0582. 1994: Agency for Health Care Policy and Research.
217. Warwick, R.T., et al., A urodynamic view of prostatic obstruction and the results of prostatectomy. British Journal of Urology, 1973. 45(6): p. 631-45.
218. Brading, A.F., A myogenic basis for the overactive bladder. [Review] [52 refs]. Urology, 1997. 50(6A Suppl): p. 57-67; discussion 68-73.
219. Speakman, M.J., et al., Bladder outflow obstruction—a cause of denervation supersensitivity. Journal of Urology, 1987. 138(6): p. 1461-6.
220. Brading, A.F., et al., The role of smooth muscle and its possible involvement in diseases of the lower urinary tract. [Review] [15 refs]. Clinical Science, 1986. 70(Suppl 14): p. 7s-13s.
221. Murakumo, M., et al., Three-dimensional arrangement of collagen and elastin fibers in the human urinary bladder: a scanning electron microscopic study. J Urol, 1995. 154(1): p. 251-6.
222. Steers, W.D. and W.C. De Groat, Effect of bladder outlet obstruction on micturition reflex pathways in the rat. Journal of Urology, 1988. 140(4): p. 864-71.
223. Steers, W.D., et al., Alterations in afferent pathways from the urinary bladder of the rat in response to partial urethral obstruction. Journal of Comparative Neurology, 1991. 310(3): p. 401-10.
224. Seki, N., O. Karim, and J. Mostwin, The effect of experimental urethral obstruction and its reversal on changes in passive electrical properties of detrusor muscle. J Urol, 1992. 148(6): p. 1957-61.
225. Seaman, E.K., et al., Persistence or recurrence of symptoms after transurethral resection of the prostate: a urodynamic assessment. Journal of Urology, 1994. 152(3): p. 935-7.
226. Murphy, G.P., et al., National patterns of prostate cancer treatment by radical prostatectomy: results of a survey by the American College of Surgeons Commission on Cancer. Journal or Urology, 1993. 152: p. 1817-1819.
227. Fowler, F.J., Jr., et al., Patient-reported complications and follow-up treatment after radical prostatectomy. The National Medicare Experience: 1988-1990 (updated June 1993). Urology, 1993. 42(6): p. 622-9.
228. Walsh, P.C., Editorial: the status of radical prostatectomy in the United States in 1993: where do we go from here. Journal of Urology, 1994. 152: p. 1816.
229. Morten, J., et al., Urinary incontinence in patients undergoing radical prostatectomy. Journal of Urology, 1995. 153: p. 506A.
230. Litweiler, S.E., et al., Radical retropubic prostatectomy in a community practice setting: analysis of long-term outcomes, continence and potency rates, and retreatment rates. Journal of Urology, 1995. 193: p. 252A.
231. Catalona, W., et al., Potency, continence and complication rates in 1,870 consecutive radical retropubic prostatectomies. J Urol, 1999. 162(2): p. 433-8.
232. Walsh, P., et al., Patient-reported urinary continence and sexual function after anatomic radical prostatectomy. Urology, 2000. 55(1): p. 58-61.
233. de Leval, J., A. Chantraine, and L. Penders, [The striated sphincter of the urethra. 1: Recall of knowledge on the striated sphincter of the urethra]. [French]. Journal d Urologie, 1984. 90(7): p. 439-54.
234. Zvara, P., et al., The detailed neuroanatomy of the human striated urethral sphincter [see comments]. British Journal of Urology, 1994. 74(2): p. 182-7.
235. Narayan, P., et al., Neuroanatomy of the external urethral sphincter: implications for urinary continence preservation during radical prostate surgery [see comments]. Journal of Urology, 1995. 153(2): p. 337-41.
236. Hollabaugh, R., et al., Preservation of putative continence nerves during radical retropubic prostatectomy leads to more rapid return of urinary continence. Urology, 1998. 51(6): p. 960-7.
237. Kaye, K., et al., Urinary continence after radical retropubic prostatectomy. Analysis and synthesis of contributing factors: a unified concept. Br J Urol, 1997. 80(3): p. 444-501.
238. John, H., et al., Evidence of trigonal denervation and reinnervation after radical retropubic prostatectomy. J Urol, 2001. 165(1): p. 111-3.
239. Soloway, M. and E. Neulander, Bladder-neck preservation during radical retropubic prostatectomy. Semin Urol Oncol, 2000. 18(1): p. 51-6.
240. Poon, M., et al., Radical retropubic prostatectomy: bladder neck preservation versus reconstruction. J Urol, 2000. 163(1): p. 194-8.
241. Shelfo, S., C. Obek, and M. Soloway, Update on bladder neck preservation during radical retropubic prostatectomy: impact on pathologic outcome, anastomotic strictures, and continence. Urology, 1998. 51(1): p. 73-8.
242. John, H. and D. Hauri, Seminal vesicle-sparing radical prostatectomy: a novel concept to restore early urinary continence. Urology, 2000. 55(6): p. 820-4.
243. Jarow, J., Puboprostatic ligament sparing radical retropubic prostatectomy. Semin Urol Oncol, 2000. 18(1): p. 28-32.
244. Poore, R., D. McCullough, and J. Jarow, Puboprostatic ligament sparing improves urinary continence after radical retropubic prostatectomy. Urology, 1998. 51(1): p. 67-72.
245. Jorion, J., [Aponeurotic suspension of a vesico-urethral anastomosis after radical prostatectomy]. Acta Urol Belg, 1998. 66(2): p. 1-4.
246. Gray, M., G. Petroni, and D. Theodorescu, Urinary function after radical prostatectomy: a comparison of the retropubic and perineal approaches. Urology, 1999. 53(5): p. 881-90; discussion 890-1.
247. Walsh, P.C., A.W. Partin, and J.I. Epstein, Cancer control and quality of life following anatomical radical retropubic prostatectomy: results at ten years. Journal of Urolgy, 1994. 152: p. 1831-1836.
248. Prieto Chaparro, L., et al., [Radical prostatectomy: usefulness of selective electromyography of the periurethral sphincter in the assessment of urinary continence]. [Spanish]. Archivos Espanoles de Urologia, 1994. 47(5): p. 483-7.
249. Aanestad, O., et al., Interference pattern in the urethral sphincter: a quantitative electromyographic study in patients before and after radical retropubic prostatectomy. Scand J Urol Nephrol, 1998. 32(6): p. 378-82.
250. Hammerer, P., et al., Urodynamic parameters before and after radical prostatectomy. Journal of Urology, 1993. 149: p. 235A.
251. Ficazzola, M. and V. Nitti, The etiology of post-radical prostatectomy incontinence and correlation of symptoms with urodynamic findings. J Urol, 1998. 160(4): p. 1317-20.
252. Kleinhans, B., et al., Changes of urodynamic findings after radi-

cal retropubic prostatectomy. Eur Urol, 1999. 35(3): p. 217-21; discussion 221-2.

253. Winters, J., R. Appell, and R. Rackley, Urodynamic findings in postprostatectomy incontinence. Neurourol Urodyn, 1998. 17(5): p. 493-8.

254. Groutz, A., et al., The pathophysiology of post-radical prostatectomy incontinence: a clinical and video urodynamic study. J Urol, 2000. 163(6): p. 1767-70.

255. Hu, K. and K. Wallner, Urinary incontinence in patients who have a TURP/TUIP following prostate brachytherapy. Int J Radiat Oncol Biol Phys, 1998. 40(4): p. 783-6.

256. Goluboff, E.T., et al., Urodynamics and the etiology of post-prostatectomy urinary incontinence: the initial Columbia experience [see comments]. Journal of Urology, 1995. 153(3 Pt 2): p. 1034-7.

257. Foote, J., S.K. Yun, and G.E. Leach, Post-prostatectomy incontinence: pathophysiology, evaluation and management. Urological Clinics of North America, 1991. 18: p. 229.

258. Chao, R. and M.E. Mayo, Incontinence after radical prostatectomy: detrusor or sphincter causes [see comments]. Journal of Urology, 1995. 154(1): p. 16-8.

259. Aboseif, S.R., et al., Preoperative urodynamic evaluation: does it predict the degree of urinary continence after radical retropubic prostatectomy? Urologia Internationalis, 1994. 53(2): p. 68-73.

260. Furlow, W.L. and D.M. Barrett, Recurrent or persistent urinary incontinence in patients with the artificial urinary sphincter: diagnostic considerations and management. Journal of Urology, 1985. 133(5): p. 792-5.

261. Barrett, D.M. and W.L. Furlow, Radical prostatectomy incontinence and the AS791 artificial urinary sphincter. Journal of Urology, 1983. 129(3): p. 528-30.

262. Diokno, A.C., L.P. Sonda, and R.J. MacGregor, Long-term followup of the artificial urinary sphincter. Journal of Urology, 1984. 131(6): p. 1084-6.

263. Fishman, I.J., R. Shabsigh, and F.B. Scott, Experience with the artificial urinary sphincter model AS800 in 148 patients. Journal of Urology, 1989. 141(2): p. 307-10.

264. Gundian, J.C., D.M. Barrett, and B.G. Parulkar, Mayo Clinic experience with use of the AMS800 artificial urinary sphincter for urinary incontinence following radical prostatectomy. Journal of Urology, 1989. 142(6): p. 1459-61.

265. Kil, P.J., et al., Factors determining the outcome following implantation of the AMS 800 artificial urinary sphincter. British Journal of Urology, 1989. 64(6): p. 586-9.

266. Malloy, T.R., A.J. Wein, and V.L. Carpiniello, Surgical success with AMS M800 GU sphincter for male incontinence. Urology, 1989. 33(4): p. 274-6.

267. Webster, G.D. and S.A. Sihelnik, Troubleshooting the malfunctioning Scott artificial urinary sphincter. Journal of Urology, 1984. 131(2): p. 269-72.

Committee 5

Pelvic Organ Prolapse

Chairman

L. Brubaker (USA)

Members

R. Bump (USA),

B. Jacquetin (France),

B. Schuessler (Switzerland),

A. Weidner (USA),

P. Zimmern (USA),

R. Milani (Italy)

CONTENTS

Pelvic Organ Prolapse

L. BRUBAKER

R. BUMP, B. JACQUETIN, B. SCHUESSLER , A. WEIDNER, P. ZIMMERN, R. MILANI

I. PELVIC ORGAN PROLAPSE

Pelvic organ prolapse (POP) has a strong inter-relationship with the urinary tract. Urinary incontinence commonly co-exists with POP and the converse relationship is also true. Many studies that have been done for evaluation of urinary incontinence have not reported the effects of POP, thus limiting clinicians' ability to use the conclusions of the study for women with POP. Likewise, surgery designed to cure urinary incontinence may exacerbate POP necessitating further treatment, even further surgery. Thus, it is important for incontinence specialists to have a well-grounded understanding of POP in order to provide optimal patient care for the many women worldwide whose quality of life is impacted by pelvic floor disorders.

This chapter will provide an overview of evidence relating to POP, especially its interaction with the urinary tract. In addition, the significant gaps in knowledge will be highlighted focusing on high-priority opportunities for additional research.

II. ETIOLOGY OF PELVIC ORGAN PROLAPSE

Most of the literature regarding risk factors for POP is based on epidemiological studies (see section III), case control studies, and observational studies. A major qualification of the interpretation of epidemiological data is that association does not mean causation. Many epidemiological associations have been embraced without thoughtful confirmatory experiments.

The few studies that examine the association of POP with pregnancy implicate vaginal delivery as an important risk factor for POP. In the Oxford Family Planning Association prolapse epidemiology study parity was the strongest risk factor for the development of POP with an adjusted relative risk of 10.85 (4.65-33.81) [1]. While the risk increased with increasing parity, the rate of increase slowed after two deliveries. Samuelsson et al also found statistically significant associations of increasing parity and maximum birth weight with the development of POP [2].These same relationships relating POP to increasing parity and birth weight were observed in the case control study of women who developed prolapse under the age of 45 and in a clinical observational study of women over age 18 [3, 4]. Finally, a study of 21,449 Italian women attending menopausal clinics demonstrated a significant association between uterine prolapse and vaginal birth (OR for 3 births compared to none being 3.0 [2.1-4.3]) but not with delivery of a baby weighing >4500 grams [5]. To date, specific events of the birth process have not been studied sufficiently to identify them as risk factors for POP. Rinne & Kirkinen found no significant relationship of POP with forceps or vacuum delivery or the duration of the second stage of labor [3]. Klein et al found an association between episiotomy and diminished pelvic floor strength three months post partum but not with subjective symptoms of bulging [6]. In contrast, Taskin et al showed that routine episiotomy when combined with antepartum [7]. Kegel exercises were as effective as Cesarean delivery in avoiding advanced POP two months after delivery in a group of 100 women who had their management determined by the day of their enrollment for prenatal care.

As noted in the section on epidemiology, virtually all studies examining prolapse or surgery for prolapse demonstrate an increased prevalence with aging. Few studies look at the effect of menopause on POP risk and results are conflicting; Swift showed a significant increased risk with menopause while Olsen and the Progetto Menopausa Study Group did not [4, 5, 8].

Evidence linking constipation to POP relate to data linking POP to pelvic floor denervation and neuropathy. While vaginal childbirth has been implicated as a major inciting event for pelvic neuropathy and prolapse, chronic constipation with repeated prolonged defecatory straining efforts has been shown to contribute to progressive neuropathy and dysfunction [9-13]. In one case control study, constipation and straining at stool as a young adult before the onset of recognized POP was significantly more common in women who subsequently developed POP (61%) than in women who did not develop PFD (4%) [14]. The Swedish prolapse study provided evidence for progressive decreases in pelvic floor muscle strength with increasing age and parity. This decrease in pelvic floor muscle strength was a significant independent determinant of the risk of POP, again supporting an association between pelvic neuromuscular dysfunction and prolapse [2].

Occupational physical stress has been examined as a contributing factor for POP. One report has implicated the extreme stress associated with airborne training (including parachute jumps) with pelvic floor dysfunction and prolapse in women previously subjected to laparoscopic uterosacral ligament transection [15]. A study using the Danish National Registry of Hospitalized Patients included over 28,000 assistant nurses (who are traditionally exposed to repetitive heavy lifting) aged 20-69 and compared their risk of surgery for POP and herniated lumbar disc (a condition associated with heavy lifting at work) to the risk in over 1.6 million same-aged controls [16]. The odds ratio for the nurses compared to controls was 1.6 (1.3-1.9) for POP surgery and 1.6 (1.2-2.2) for disc surgery, suggesting that heavy lifting may contribute to POP. An Italian study demonstrated an increased risk of prolapse with lower levels of education, a possible indicator of harder physical labor, although this was not specifically investigated [5].

Obesity is another condition that is associated with chronically increased abdominal pressure [17]. Some studies have demonstrated significant relationships between increasing weight and body mass index and the risk of POP or surgery for POP [1, 5]. Others have not demonstrated this correlation or have demonstrated a loss of correlation once analysis was corrected for confounders such as age, parity, or pelvic muscle strength [2, 3]. Another medical condition associated with chronic episodic increases in abdominal pressure is chronic pulmonary disease. One case control study examined this and reported significantly more pulmonary disease (such as asthma) in women $\leq$ 45 years of age who developed prolapse (14%) compared to controls (2.4%) [3].

In the Oxford Family Planning Study the POP surgical incidence rates were higher for women who had undergone a prior hysterectomy for reasons other than prolapse (29 per 10,000) and highest for women who had undergone hysterectomy for prolapse (158 per 10,000) [1]. Marchionni et al demonstrated some degree of vaginal vault prolapse 9-13 years after hysterectomy in 11.6% of women who had the hysterectomy for prolapse and in 1.8% of women who had the hysterectomy for other benign disease [18]. Swift also demonstrated a significant association of POP with a prior history of hysterectomy or prolapse surgery [4]. While any prolapse procedure can fail for a variety of reasons, it has been suggested that certain procedures have higher risks of specific pelvic support defects. These include enterocele formation after Burch colposuspension and anterior superior segment prolapse after sacrospinous ligament fixation [19, 20, 21]. In addition, there is evidence that the vaginal route of prolapse correction is associated with damage to the pudendal nerve and results in anatomic outcomes and higher re-operation rates than abdominal route prolapse surgery [22, 23]. Finally, there have been five case reports implicating laser laparoscopic uterosacral ligament ablation for chronic pelvic pain as a cause of uterine prolapse in young women [15, 24].

There are data that link clinical, laboratory, and genetic syndromes of abnormalities of collagen to pelvic organ prolapse [25-30]. In addition, Rinne and Kirknen linked POP in young women with a history of abdominal hernias, suggesting a possible connection with abnormal collagen [3].

Finally, there is evidence from several case control studies that variations in axial and pelvic skeletal structure can be associated with increased risks of POP. These include increasing degrees of thoracic kyphosis, a decrease in lumbar lordosis and in vertical orientation of the pelvic inlet, and an increase in the transverse diameter of the pelvic inlet [31, 32, 33]. The association between early age advanced stage POP and the severe disruption of pubic bone and pelvic muscle structure in women with bladder exstrophy is well recognized [34].

III. EPIDEMIOLOGY OF PELVIC ORGAN PROLAPSE

There are few epidemiological studies of POP in contrast to urinary incontinence, probably because POP has no specific symptom complexes, especially for early state disease, and thus the condition does not lend itself well to traditional epidemiological survey techniques. Some studies utilize links to managed care, hospital, and/or surgical databases to diagnose POP rather than including a physical examination for prolapse [1, 8,35, 36]. More recently, others have used a standardized examination technique to document the status of pelvic support [2, 4, 37]. One study determined post-hysterectomy vault prolapse incidence using both approaches in the same population [18].

Appendix One shows prevalence rates for examination confirmed prolapse in four studies. The prevalence of prolapse to the level of the hymen varies from 2% to 48%. This broad range likely results from differences in sources of study populations, age, race, parity and examination techniques. Each of the four demonstrated an increased prevalence of prolapse with aging except the study by Bland et al which did not report any age analysis [37]. There is a lack of epidemiological information about POP in racial groups other than whites.

Much of our information regarding POP comes from surgical databases. Using a computerized provincial database, Allard and Rochette reported that uterine prolapse is the most frequent indication for hysterectomy in older women [35]. One third of all hysterectomies in women ≥ 50 were for prolapse in 1988 while fewer than 7% of women aged 15-49 had that indication. Eighty-one percent of vaginal hysterectomies (representing about 16% of hysterectomies) were performed for prolapse. The yearly incidence of hysterectomy for prolapse peaked in the 65-69 year age group at around 30 per 10,000 (0.3%). In a similar study from Finland, the proportion of hysterectomies for prolapse varied between 8.8 and 13.8% from 1971-1986 while the annual incidence varied from 8.0 to 12.7 per 10,000 women. Data were not stratified by age [36]. Olsen et al assessed the age-specific incidence of surgery for prolapse in a large managed care population in Oregon [8]. The annual incidence of surgery for POP varied between 0.4 per 10,000 in women aged 20-29 and 34.3 per 10,000 in women aged 70-79. When data for POP and POP + Continence Surgery (but not continence surgery alone) were combined, the surgical incidence rate in the later age group was 49 per 10,000. The Oxford Family Planning Association study followed over 17,000 women aged 25-39 from enrollment between 1968 and 1974 for up to 26 years until 1994 [1]. The annual incidence of hospital admission with a diagnosis of prolapse was 20.4 per 10,000 while the annual incidence of surgery for prolapse was 16.2 per 10,000.

The number of women with POP who are managed without hospitalization and surgery and the number with POP who never seek medical attention is unknown. Incidence and prevalence estimates based only on surgical procedure rates almost certainly underestimate the magnitude of POP. Using a surgical database, Marchionni et al estimated the 9-13 year incidence of prolapse following hysterectomy in their institution in Florence to be between 0.2 and 0.4% [18]. The incidence performing a physical exam on a random sample of the same population was over ten times greater at 4.4%

In summary, POP is a frequent indication for hysterectomy and pelvic surgery in women, with an annual age-related surgical incidence in the range of 10 to 30 per 10,000 women confirmed in several large surgical database studies. The incidence of surgery for POP increases with aging. The population prevalence for POP beyond the hymen (≥ Stage II) is probably between 2 and 4% but may be much higher in clinical populations seeking gynecological care. There is a need for well designed multi-racial and multi-ethnic random sample population based studies, which include physical examination confirmation of pelvic support, to determine the true prevalence of POP.

IV. PELVIC CO-MORBIDITIES

1. Urinary tract dysfunction and prolapse

Women with anterior vaginal wall support defects often have bladder neck hypermobility with genuine stress incontinence, as well as concurrent defects of uterine and posterior wall support. However, with greater degrees of anterior vaginal wall prolapse (Stage III and IV) fewer women have symptoms of genuine stress incontinence [38]. Severe prolapse can descend and obstruct the urethra, making assessment and management of the continence mechanism in such patients problematic [2, 38, 39, 40]. Multiple studies have described an occult incontinence rate after various methods of reducing the prolapse during preoperative testing of 23-50% [41,42,43]. However, Bump et al described an only 4% *de novo* incontinence rate in women with Stage III or IV prolapse who had been randomized to a bladder neck plication procedure as their only prophylaxis, also concluding that preoperative barrier testing was not useful in identifying women who required a urethropexy [21]. Klutke et al determined that preoperative barrier testing was most useful in identifying those women who do not leak with reduction of the prolapse, since such patients did not undergo urethropexy and had better outcomes with regard to both GSI and DI rates [44]. Because of this uncertainty, the least invasive method of bladder neck stabilization seems preferred for such patients [45].

Pelvic organ prolapse can also negatively affect voiding function, although one study noted that the majority of women with severe prolapse still void effectively [46]. Fitzgerald found that preoperative voiding studies with the prolapse reduced by a pessary was the best predictor of normalization of residuals post operatively [47].

The impact of pelvic organ prolapse on the upper urinary tract is not well described in the surveyed literature, consisting primarily of case reports of acute and acute on chronic renal failure attributed to ureteral obstruction by Stage IV uterine or vaginal vault prolapse. Hydroureter and hydronephrosis was demonstrated in such cases, resolving post repair [48,49].

2. Gastrointestinal dysfunction and POP

Repeated reports document disparities between physical exam and defecography in patients with prolapse, particularly those with large vaginal eversions. Two series of defecographies in consecutive patients with prolapse and/or evacuation disorders describe defecographic findings that changed the patient's diagnosis (though not always the management) in 46 of 62 of cases and noted enteroceles that were not found on physical exam in approximately 50% of cases [50, 51, 52]. Use of defecography as a 'gold standard' for exam in these series raises concerns, since normal asymptomatic women may have focal defecographic abnormalities, but it is clear that it is challenging to assess the posterior compartment in severe prolapse. For instance, sigmoidoceles are present in 4-11% of reported series, and are nearly always missed on physical exam [52, 53].

Relatively few of the published studies of outcomes of posterior compartment repairs provide an analysis of gastrointestinal co-morbidities as risk factors for failure. However, the prevalence of abnormal colonic transit time is approximately 20% in patients presenting with evacuation disorders [54]. An abnormal preoperative colonic transit study is the most consistently cited risk factor for failure of rectocele repair to relieve evacuatory symptoms, regardless of the surgical technique [55, 56, 57]. Recognition of the multifactorial etiology of constipation and evacuatory symptoms is advisable to help avoid disappointing surgical results.

Fecal incontinence is a more frequent complaint among women with incontinence and prolapse than in the general population, occurring in approximately 17% of patients presenting for evaluation, especially those with urinary incontinence, abnormal external anal sphincter tone, and irritable bowel syndrome [58]. There is some evidence that rectocele repair can diminish both maximal anal resting and squeeze pressures, possibly contributing to the development of incontinence in patients already at risk with abnormal preoperative manometry [60].

V. RELEVANT NOMENCLATURE

The nomenclature of POP has been troublesome for more than 100 years [59]. Brubaker and Norton summarized the impact of a non-standardized POP nomenclature [60]. The International Continence Society responded to this quandary by creating a committee to recommend a standardized nomenclature. The final approved POP terminology report of this committee was published in 1996 [61] One part of this report describes a system to describe quantitatively the position of 6 vaginal points (two anteriorly, two posteriorly, and two apically) and the length of the genital hiatus, perineal body, and vagina and is referred to as the POP-Q exam (pelvic organ prolapse – quantified). The POP-Q system has been adopted by major organizations including the International Continence Society, the Society of Gynecologic Surgeons and the American Urogynecologic Society, and the NIH as an accepted method of describing pelvic support and comparing exams over time and after interventions. The POP-Q has been shown to have reproducibility in several centers when the exam is conducted in a standardized fashion. Many aspects of physical examination are not mandated although investigators are admonished to specify their methods for determining that the full extent of the prolapse has been demonstrated. The POP-Q system has been criticized for being cumbersome and difficult to learn, although an instructional video tape available through www.augs.org facilitates the learning process. The POP description section of the POP terminology document also includes and ordinal staging system based on the quantitative POP-Q exam.

The POP-Q system itself does not include findings that some investigators believe to be essential for complete patient description, such as vaginal caliber, status of paravaginal sulci, pelvic muscle strength, or the presence of symptoms, although all of these issues are considered in three other sections of the terminology document dedicated to ancillary evaluation techniques, pelvic floor muscle testing, and symptom assessment. In summary, the POP standarization document is an important advance for researchers and clinicians who treat POP, although the POP-Q system in and of itself does not represent the sum of information needed to formulate treatment or assess the impact of treatment.

VI. NATURAL HISTORY OF PELVIC ORGAN PROLAPSE

There are no published data on POP remission. Clinically, POP does not seem to regress, although some improvement may be seen with the chronic retention of a pessary. Since prolapse is often asymptomatic until the descending segment is through the introitus, POP may not be recognized until advanced disease exists. Some women progress rapidly from mild to advanced stages of POP, while others remain stable for many years. One goal of adopting standardized systems of POP quantitation and staging is to allow clinicians and researchers to document the course of POP reliably and accurately over time. There is a need for large-scale longitudinal studies using such techniques [61].

VII. EVALUATION

Evaluation for research purposes may often be different from evaluation for clinical care. In patients seeking relief of POP-related symptoms, evaluation is often limited to physical examination, as described in the Chapter on Physical Examination. The comprehensive pelvic floor assessment should include POP examination that documents that the maximal protrusion is confirmed by the patient. Currently, most clinical care worldwide is given following simple physical examination. However, additional tools are useful in the clinical care of complex patients and essential for describing patients participating in research studies. These additional tools include various imaging modalities and urodynamic tests.

1. IMAGING

Fluoroscopy has been used throughout the world using various techniques with various goals. Probably, the most important fluoroscopic technique is the evacuation proctography or defecography, which involves imaging of rectal expulsion of a barium paste enema. It is a test of voluntary rectal evacuation and thereby yielding both anatomic and functional information.

During evacuation proctography, the wall of the rectum can be outlined by first introducing a small amount of liquid barium into the rectal cavity. A thick barium paste approximating the consistency of semi-solid feces, is then instilled into the rectum. The rectum is filled until the patient has a feeling of rectal distension, sufficient for defecation. During injection the syringe is pulled back to outline the anal canal and the skin behind the anal orifice. The vagina is filled with a small amount of contrast [62]. Lateral images are made during rest, during squeezing and on straining (without evacuation). Finally the patient is asked to evacuate the rectum. Continuous recording during the evacuation is important otherwise rapid changes or subtle findings will be missed [63]. Investigators have used a variety of techniques for rectal opacification.

As discussed previously in this chapter, POP frequently co-exists with other pelvic disorders. Therefore, many investigators prefer a combination technique that provides additional information regarding adjacent systems. This technique may include small bowel opacification with oral barium suspension and a radiopaque marker for the perineum [65]. The most comprehensive technique includes bladder filling, in order to perform a dynamic cystoproctography [64]. Advocates of this technique recommend performing the cystographic phase before rectal filling to avoid artifactual compression of the bladder secondary only to the effect of rectal filling. The cystography can be combined with urodynamic pressure measurements.

A normal rectal evacuation study has to met the five criteria of Mahieu [65].

1. Increase of anorectal angulation;

2. Obliteration of the puborectal impression;

3. Wide anal canal opening;

4. Total evacuation of contrast; and

5. Normal pelvic floor resistance.

Posterior wall prolapse is mostly seen as a bulging of the rectal wall during evacuation and, it may retain contrast after defecation [66]. The prolapse can also be filled with small bowel or sigmoid. This can be differentiated on evacuation proctography in the post-evacuation phase with an empty rectum. Accurate diagnosis of anterior wall prolapse requires bladder and vaginal contrast [66]. Pelvic organ prolapse should be described quantitatively because of the absence of normative data during fluoroscopy (Figure 1, 2).

Evacuation proctography facilitates simultaneous diagnosis of structural and functional abnormalities and allows a comprehensive, dynamic view of the pelvis. As with all tests, no single finding in isolation should be used to dictate clinical treatment when patient symptoms are inconsistent with that finding. Abnormalities of rectal configuration are common in vaginally parous

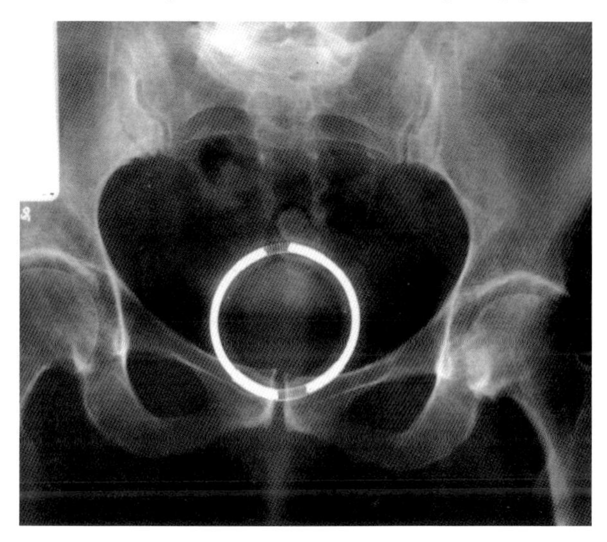

Figure 1 : The pessary is in place in the vagina, effectively reducing the pelvic organ prolapse.

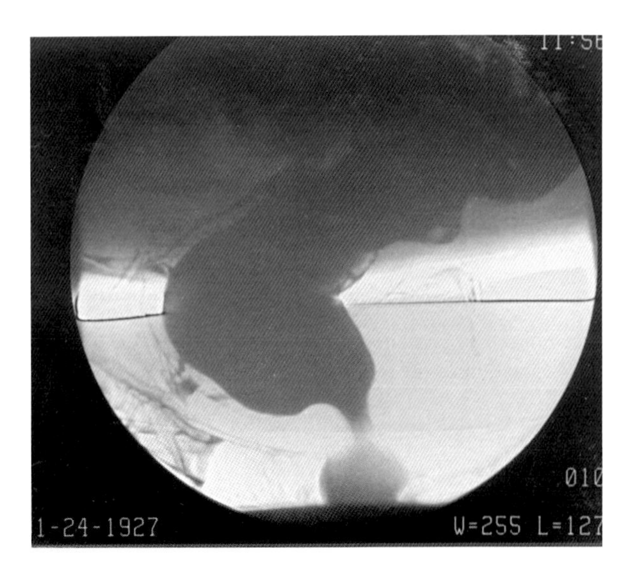

Figure 2 : During straining for defecation, the bladder vaginal apex descend abnormally. A large protrusion of small bowel is seen. Interestingly the rectum empties well indicating the absence of "rectocele".

women and may be over-interpreted, causing excessive surgical intervention in otherwise normal women [67]. Whether evacuation proctography can assist clinical understanding and management is a very relevant question. Unfortunately there is no prospective controlled study in which patient outcome with and without evacuation proctography has been evaluated.

Finally, fluoroscopy is commonly used to evaluate the bladder neck in women undergoing fluoro-urodynamic evaluation. This evaluation is more specifically addressed in other portions of this text, however, caution should be exercised when interpreting such images in women with POP. The finding of "open bladder neck" or "funneling" in women with POP should not be equated with intrinsic urethral dysfunction for purposes of treatment planning.

2. Ultrasound

Although the most important clinical results of ultrasound in urogynaecology are related to functional aspects, there are a few papers describing a clinical application of ultrasound in prolapse assessment. Perineal ultrasound can be used to assess vaginal prolapse, although only preliminary reports have been used the advantage being that it does not impede movement of the bladder neck [68, 69, 70]. A transrectal scan has been described as a useful tool in the diagnosis of enterocele [71].

It has been reported that women with a prolapse have greater bladder neck mobility than incontinent women, and the extent of the movement correlates well with the anterior wall descent [71, 72, 73].With ultrasound it is possible to visualise the pelvic floor muscles. A perineal approach has been described to image the levator ani muscle with a 5MHz probe [74,75,76]. However, a transvaginal approach with the use of a 7.5MHz transrectal probe guarantees a better and complete image of the levator ani with the possibility to visualize its full extension and to take width measurements [77]. With this technique, it is also possible to visualize lateral vaginal defects, otherwise impossible to see, and the levator hiatus, which has been found, compared to controls, to be larger in women with prolapse [78,79]. This last finding correlates well with the measurement of the urogenital hiatus using a ruler. A larger urogenital hiatus has been found in women who have a prolapse or have had unsuccessful surgical treatment. The urogenital hiatus is the same in women without a prolapse and in those treated for a prolapse with successful surgery. Finally, a renal ultrasound assessment can be used to assess the presence of hydronephrosis in women undergoing surgery for a prolapse.

3. MRI and prolapse

Dynamic cystoproctography, which includes opacification of the bladder, small bowel, vaginal lining, and a proctography, is a relatively invasive procedure involving ionizing radiation and only images the lumen of the opacified organs [80]. MRI is an alternative imaging technique. However, before MRI can be incorporated in clinical practice standardization of pelvic floor structures and of their normative variations with aging must be accomplished.

4. MRI technology

Since the classic description of the MRI of the female pelvis by Hricak in 1986, several MRI techniques have become available (vaginal, endorectal, open configuration)[80-83]. Image acquisition is improving with faster sequences (rapid sequence dynamic MRI with HASTE (Half –Fourier- acquisition single shot turbo spin echo technology) reducing the overall procedure time [84-86].

5. Normative studies

The 3D anatomy of the healthy female pelvic floor derived from MR images showed:

1. the average width of the levator hiatus, at the level of the transverse urethral ligament, is constant in the healthy female population at approximately 4 cm [87]. A widened levator hiatus was reported in association with pelvic organ prolapse.

2. In continent women, the levator plate nearly parallels the pubococcygeal line [79, 84, 88].

3. At rest, the bladder base lies above the pubococcygeal line in healthy volunteers [88, 89].

4. The mean anorectal junction position lies on the pubococcygeal line [89].

5. During pelvic floor muscle contraction, an inward cranial lift was demonstrated, confirming prior clinical observations and ultrasound findings [90]. The range of movement was from 1 to 21 mm, which is less than suggested by Kegel in 1952, although Kegel's observations were made in the supine position. A surprising finding was the movement of the coccyx during a pelvic floor muscle contraction.

6. Due to cost limitations, dynamic MRI data with Haste have not been obtained in asymptomatic nulliparous women [86,91].

6. Comparison between MRI and other studies

a. In one small study on post hysterectomy vault prolapse (13 patients), MRI was compared to intra-operative and ultrasound findings and showed no superiority towards planning a better repair [92].

b. In another study of 40 patients, dynamic MRI was found to be superior to fluoroscopic proctography because patients could be left in privacy while the images were continuously acquired without any concern for radiation exposure [93].

c. In a large study of 125 POP patients staged by dynamic MRI (image acquisition time of 2.5 minutes), prolapse was objectively graded (HMO classification), standard imaging (cystourethrography, pelvic ultrasound, or intravenous urography) was obviated, and additional pelvic pathology detected at a cost of $540 per test including interpretation [86]. Compared with intraoperative findings, MRI staging was found accurate except for rectocele [91].

7. Urodynamic testing

Presence of stress urinary incontinence (SUI) is often masked by prolapse that protrudes from the vagina. However, when the prolapse is reduced by speculum, pessary, or gauze, occult stress incontinence can thus be revealed [94-98].When a pessary can be retained for several weeks and does not obstruct the bladder and/or proximal urethra, it can be used to determine whether incontinence is present and whether it is clinically bothersome [99]. Urodynamic studies are usually performed with a prolapse reduction to determine whether an urethropexy is needed during an upcoming repair, or even during a sling procedure when sphincteric insufficiency is detected [100, 101,102,104]. Some physicians accept urodynamic information at face value and will leave the urethra unsupported if the patient did not leak during the procedure [105,106]. Conversely, some will perform a formal urethropexy or a sling depending on the valsalva leak point pressure or on the urethral closure pressure measured during the urodynamic test. Another approach is to systematically stabilize urethral support at the time of the prolapse surgery and to consider a periurethral injection or a sling procedure if SUI occurs secondarily [107].This latter approach applies particularly to older women who may have precarious lower urinary tract function, some degree of chronic retention, or who already have some urge incontinence from bladder instability. Appropriate randomized clinical trials are needed to address the utility of urodynamic testing with prolapse reduction, and the optimal surgical management for these patients.

VIII. TREATMENT

The indication for treatment of POP is uncertain. The fact that there is no standardization of this aspect of POP care is an urgent research topic.

Besides a few indications necessitating prolapse treatment (e.g. obstructed upper urinary tract and urosepsis; rectal prolapse and incarcerated bowel) the majority of interventions is based on relative indications, primarily on symptoms of the prolapse itself. The lesser the extent of prolapse the more difficult is its correlation to symptoms (e.g. bulging, difficulties during intercourse). Data on the association between the extent of a prolapse and related symptoms is weak. Furthermore, there is yet no clear cut-off between "normal" and "abnormal" anatomy especially in parous women. Based on the outcome of a recent NIH Terminology workshop on Female Pelvic Floor Disorders any pelvic organ prolapse less than Stage II needs careful assessment of the relationship between symptoms and prolapse before treatment especially surgery is applied [108].

If symptoms are not directly related to the prolapse but rather to organs involved (e.g. obstructed defecation; voiding difficulties and recurrent UTI) testing is recommended to explore the relationship between prolapse and symptoms. Treatment options are either surgery or a pessary. Physicians vary widely in their use of pessaries. Some physicians offer a pessary to all patients requesting POP treatment, whereas others never use the pessary. Most likely, there is a subgroup of women from whom the pessary is a superior option to surgery. All information regarding pessary care is anecdotal and designed for clinical care. Unfortunately, there are no randomized trials comparing the pessary with observation (natural history) or surgery. Some physicians offer a pessary to all patients requesting POP treatment, whereas never use a pessary. Most likely there is a subgroup of women for whom a pessary is a superior option to surgery (Figure 1).

Surgery is frequently offered to women with POP. The optimal procedure (or group of procedures) is not known. Experts agree that the intervention should lead to improvement of subjective outcome and quality of life. Furthermore, these issues have to be achieved with minimal complications. If preservation of specific functions are not necessary anymore (e.g. vaginal intercourse) its reconstruction may be omitted to permit a minor surgical intervention. For purposes of this chapter, surgical treatment of the relevant POP-Q sites will be addressed individually.

1. Apical prolapse (points C and D)

Simple vaginal hysterectomy is not effective to correct uterovaginal prolapse [109]. When the uterus is present, effective POP treatment requires specific steps to suspend the apex. In patients who do not want to maintain fertility or who have passed reproductive years, hysterectomy with vaginal vault suspension is commonly preferred. A wide variety of options exist and there is no clinical trial that compares one procedure against another. Expert opinion suggests that apical suspension that is performed "prophylactically" should be limited to the use of endogenous materials and aim to restore normal vaginal axis. Thus, procedures that distort the vaginal axis, such as sacro-spinous ligament suspension should not be used unless apical prolapse is present.

There is no trial that compares uterine preservation with hysterectomy when treating POP. There are significant practice differences in this regard. Uterine preserving procedures have been reported, but only in small case series. The Mancheseter procedure (amputation of the cervix with uterus suspension to the cardinal ligaments) is largely of historical interest only because of the significant rate of complications including, but not limited to, cervical incompetence, cervical stenosis, postoperative bleeding, infertility**.** Variations of the sacrospinous ligament suspension have been recommended and have the stated advantage of fertility preservation without damage to the cervix, maintenance of a normal vaginal axis, and closure of space for potential enterocele. Sutures are unilateral to preserve rectal caliber and normal defecation. A variety of abdominal approaches have been described that attach the isthmic region to the sacrum using a supportive material. The original Gilliam procedure which is known to have high failure rates when using round ligaments can be enhanced using synthetic or fascial augmentation. There are few patients represented in the reports of these procedures and no long term data. The wide variations in rate of subsequent pregnancy and term deliveries warrant extreme caution when counselling patients regarding uterine preservation for fertility indications.

Following hysterectomy, the term "post-hysterectomy" prolapse is often used. It is important to recognize that the underlying disorder may be the same, regardless of the presence of the uterus. Thus, the principles of surgical repair include repair of vaginal walls and suspension of the vaginal apex. Treatment of the apex can be effectively accomplished by a wide variety of techniques and includes both abdominal and vaginal routes of surgery. There are no published laparoscopic series of POP outcomes using a modern outcome measures, such as POP-Q with a minimum of one-year follow-up.

Surgeons generally have a preferred mode of access for treatment of apical disorders. Only one randomised trial had compared these two routes and found that the abdominal approach is superior, although this trial has been criticized for the ancillary procedures that were selected [110]. Surgeon preference for the abdominal approach may be related to patient age, although this idea is not evidence-based. Several non-randomized studies comparing sacrocolpopexy to sacrospinous fixation have been published [110,11,112,113,114]. Vaginal procedures have the surgical advantages of decreased immediate operative morbidity that must be balanced against growing concerns of surgical induced neuropathy, accelerating neuro-muscular decline. These preferences are not evidenced-based at this time (Appendix 2).

There are two retrospective clinical series dealing with vaginal length and dyspareunia after abdominal and vaginal prolapse surgery respectively (Given et al.; Anthuber et al.) [115,116]. Both conclude that vaginal length is preserved better by the abdominal approach and dyspareunia is less likely to occur.

Vaginal apical suspension can be done at the time of hysterectomy or as a separate procedure remote from the hysterectomy. These procedures include the McCall culdeplasty, the high utero-sacral suspension, the endopelvic fascia fixation, the coccygeous muscle fixation, the iliococcygeus fascia attachment and the sacrospinous ligament suspension. These procedures have been scantily reported in the literature and are listed in Appendix Two.

The sacrospinous literature reflects more patients in more institutions than any other procedure (Appendix 3). Only one trial compares two vaginal suspension methods. Colombo et al compared McCall culdeplasty with sacrospinous ligament suspension, and demonstrated an excess anterior wall recurrence with the sacrospinous (21% v 6%) [117]. Although this is consistent with expert opinion, this study has not been replicated. Overview of the existing literature gives apical (POP-Q point C) success rates between 63 and 97 %, with an associated rate of recurrent anterior failure between 0 % and 92 %.

Sacrocolpopexy has been popularised over the past forty years. This technique requires an abdominal approach, but has high cure rates which have been demonstrated by multiple surgeons in multiple institutions [118,119,120]. Aside from the need for an abdominal approach, surgeons express concern for the known risks of mesh which is frequently used in this procedure. Autologous fascia has been used, although cadaveric tissue has failed in this procedure. There is no ideal synthetic material for reconstructive pelvic surgery [121].

There is good evidence (II - 1) that the abdominal route is able to adequately fix the vaginal cuff or the vagina together with the uterus to the hollow of the sacrum or the promontory. This approach offers successful reposition of uterine or vaginal cuff prolapse even in cases with maximal extent. According to a recent systematic review success rates range in between 77,8% and 100% [122].

To bridge the distance between the vaginal cuff and the hollow of the sacrum several materials have been used (Table 1). A review of these materials was recently reported (Iglesia, et al).

Table 1 : Sacrocolpopexy materials

Homologeous
• Cadaveric Fascia lata
• Rectus sheath
Autologeous
Dura mater
Cadaveric Fascia lata
Synthetic
Prolene mesh
Mersilene mesh
Marlex mesh
Teflon
Gore Tex mesh

There is no uniformity as to the optimal site of fixation. Fixation of the cuff at the level of the promotory creates a steep unnatural vaginal axis, while fixing it at the level of S 2/3 and thus imitating natural direction of the vagina may induce high bowl outlet obstruction, if the rectal pillar with its neural supply to the rectum has to be divided [121].

One of the unresolved problems of sacrocolpopexy is the control of concomitant anterior and posterior prolapse. Results of two prospective clinical series (Baessler and Schuessler; Fox and Stanton) indicate that a double pedicle mesh advanced as far down at the anterior vaginal wall as to control for any midline defects seem to offer good results (II-1) [120, 122]. However, in these series colposuspensions and lateral repairs have also been combined.

Results for the control of posterior wall prolapse from above are much more confusing. While Fox and Stanton reported excellent results, results from Baessler and Schuessler were less promising although intraoperatively rectoceles seemed to be effectively controlled. Vaginal rectocele repair followed by abdominal colpoperineopexy concomitantly concomitantly was accompanied in one series by a disastrous mesh erosion rate especially if mesh or suture material was introduced into the abdominal cavity from below [123].

A recent overview of the existing literature on abdominal prolapse repair indicates that the use of synthetic mesh is the major source of complication inducing mesh erosion and/or infection [122]. While eroded macroporous mesh could be trimmed and closed by a layer of vaginal wall, type II and III material has to be removed if erosion/infection occurs. Besides any mesh erosion sacral osteomyelitis at the fixation site of the mesh has been reported [124].

There is no expert consensus on the definition of enterocele. A growing number of specialists believe the presence of small bowel low in the pelvis is a phenomenon secondary to the primary POP support problem. These experts believe that when the vaginal walls are reconstructed and properly suspended, no additional or specific "enterocele" repair is required. Other experts feel that specific procedures are necessary to remedy small bowel which is unusually low in the pelvic. No single procedure has been demonstrated to effectively prevent or treat enterocele, and it is unlikely that such studies will ever be done because of their complexity and the confounding effects of concomitant surgery.

2. Anterior vaginal prolapse

Experts and the majority of published literature suggest that the anterior wall is probably the most challenging part of POP cure. Several techniques for sub-diagnosis of anterior wall have been proposed, either based on specific anatomy or likely etiology. As with many aspects of POP diagnosis, such sub-categories are not evidenced-based nor have they met criteria for inter- and intra-rater reliability. However, these sub-categories are frequently used to plan the procedure(s) best suited to a particular patient. Anterior wall support defects can be primary (abnormality within the wall itself) or secondary (secondary to apical defects). The next portion of this text will discuss procedures used ***when apical suspension is adequate or being treated by a concomitant procedure.***

Anterior POP is most frequently treated by anterior colporrhaphy. Despite the high objective failure rate (approximately 50%), the procedure persists largely because of the perception of low surgical morbidity and the ease with which it is combined with other vaginal reconstructive procedures [125]. Interpretation of published results should be done with caution because of the wide variations in surgical technique. Many variations are associated with various kinds of bladder neck plications or concomittant needle suspension [126]. The recurrence rate (0 % to 50 %) is probably highly underestimated because "intravaginal" cystoceles are not taken into consideration ; for some authors, only patients needing reoperation are considered as failures, without interest for functional symptoms.

Vaginal paravaginal defect repair is more technically challenging. Since White described paravaginal repair in 1909 it has been reported to repair anterior wall support defects with success rates of 76 % - 100 % [127-133]. Appendix five lists surgical series for this procedure. This operation needs a surgeon skilled with vaginal operations according to the large opening of the paravesical space. The procedure can be accomplished abdominally, but still requires a high degree of surgical skill.

The four (or six) corner suspension was originally described by Raz for use in women with stress urinary incontinence [134,135]. Unfortunately, the anterior wall recurrence rate is unacceptably high (nearly 60 %) indicating that the procedure should not be used for anterior wall restoration [134, 136].

Some surgeons have reported case series with synthetic materials to bolster this area and reduce recurrence of the anterior wall. Overall, this effort has been limited by foreign-body complications. These case series are listed in Appendix 6 [137,138,139,140,141].

3. Posterior vaginal prolapse

Most experts believe that vaginally parous women have alterations in posterior vaginal wall support. When these become bothersome, surgical repair may be an option. Similar to the anterior wall, posterior wall support defects can be primary (defects in the posterior wall itself or its attachment to the perineal body) or secondary to a loss of apical support. This text will continue to discuss only surgery directed primarily at the posterior wall.

The indications for posterior wall repair are poorly outlined. Isolated recoceles are unusual and should raise suspicion of colonic disorders. A variety of symptoms have been attributed to "rectocele", but these symptoms are non-specific and often persist despite resolution of posterior wall anatomy. These thoughts should caution the reconstructive surgeon, since it is well known that there is a significant risk of painful intercourse following posterior vaginal wall with or without perineal reconstruction. There is some evidence that the risk of dyspareunia increases when the levator muscle is plicated. There is no consensus on the definition of rectocele, either by physical examination or by any imaging modality. However, there are a few surgical studies that use imaging for patient selection and outcome assessment of the surgery.

Retrospective comparisons of a site-specific defect posterior wall repair has been performed, but no randomized trials have been completed to date [142, 143, 144, 145,146]. The traditional posterior colporrhaphy has been studied in comparison to the trans-anal repair of rectocele.

IX. UNUSUAL FORMS OF POP

On occasion, some unusual condition may cause a mistaken diagnosis of POP. Unusual causes include, cervical elongation, wherein the apical support of the vagina is entirely intact, but the cervix has elongated and is protruding through the hymen. Certain forms of unusual cystic formation in the actual vaginal wall, or glands associated with the vagina may be mistaken for prolapse. Rarely, a prolapsed myoma can be misinterpreted for POP.

There are unusual circumstances which involve true POP including prolapse of a cervical stump, prolapse of a single loop of small bowel through an otherwise supported vaginal tube and recurrent posterior wall support defects which are related to large bowel disorders or masses, undiagnosed presacral or pelvic masses. Fortunately, these conditions are rare, but should be thought of when there is repetitive surgical failure.

X. RESEARCH TECHNIQUES FOR PELVIC ORGAN PROLAPSE

The quality of clinical research is an important issue. Because of historical traditions and the lack of regulatory requirements, evaluation of surgical procedures has not been subject to the same safety and effectiveness standards as medical therapies. The quality of the evidence supporting aspects of the surgical management of many gynecological conditions is poor. A recent systematic review found that the overwhelming majority of the literature on management of urinary incontinence did not allow any substantial assessment of the basic methodological quality of the published research [147]. The quality of research in reconstructive pelvic surgery, and the clinical care of patient based on that research would be greatly improved if certain commonly accepted principles of clinical outcomes research were routinely implemented. Basic principles have been outlined in a report of the Research Committee of the American Urogynecology Society [148].

Investigators should strive to ensure that studies are conducted and described in such a way that readers can assess the internal and external validity of the results. Internal validity refers to the conduct of the study itself—are the conclusions drawn justified by the methods used to achieve the results described? External validity refers to the generalizability of the study results—are the clinical methods and patient population similar to those used by the reader?

1. Internal validity

a) Randomization

Randomization is the preferred method for removing the effects of both intentional and unintentional bias in either the performance of the intervention or in the interpretation of the results, and significantly reduces the possibility of confounding. Important conclusions can be drawn from nonrandomized studies; however, the methodological sophistication required to overcome the inherent limitations of nonrandomized designs is in some ways greater than that required for a randomized trial. Studies where pseudo-randomization techniques are used (such as selecting patients presenting on alternating days of the week) consistently show larger effects than those where sealed envelopes or other methods based on randomly generated numbers are used [149].

b) Adequate description of patients and controls

Recruitment methods and inclusion and exclusion criteria should be specified clearly. Inclusive dates of the recruitment period, severity of the clinical condition in question, data regarding age, body mass index, and ethnicity, as well as any co-morbidities in the study population should be fully delineated. In nonrandomized study designs, criteria used to select which patients underwent the interventions being compared should be described. If these differences are not characterized, then erroneous conclusions may be drawn.

c) Description of length of follow-up

Patient and provider decision-making is dependent on the knowledge of benefits and risks over time. The duration and nature of follow-up after the study intervention is one of the most important elements of a report on management of pelvic organ prolapse, particularly if the intervention in question is surgical. The mean or median and range of duration of follow-up should be stated very clearly. In the case of a surgical intervention, the same evaluation should be performed before and after the procedure, and ideally this should occur long enough and frequently enough after the procedure to ensure adequate evaluation of results. Every effort should be made to provide follow-up of at least five years with surgical outcomes studies. Failing to account for patients lost to follow-up may lead to erroneous conclusions, especially if the loss to follow-up is related to either the underlying disease or the intervention (e.g., patients seeking care elsewhere because of continuing symptoms or unacceptable side effects of treatment). Drop out rates may reflect differences in clinically important variables, such as side effects or treatment response. Failure to account for dropouts may result in erroneous conclusions similar to those seen with failure to account for loss to follow-up. In randomized trials, patients who "dropout" of one arm and receive another intervention under study should be included in the original group for analysis (intent-to-treat analysis).

d) Recognition and description of statistical issues

Power: A considerable portion of the surgical body of literature suffers from a failure to consider the number of subjects needed to achieve results of statistical and/or clinical significance prior to embarking on the investigation. Power calculations should ideally be made prior to beginning the research to determine the feasibility of the study. While it is often difficult to estimate the magnitude of difference (the delta) likely to be found in pilot investigations, an explanation supporting the estimated difference should be described. Studies that lack power to detect differences between groups are at risk for Type II errors, which can lead investigators to erroneously conclude, for example, that important characteristics of cases and controls are not significantly different between groups. This is usually not a problem in a randomized trial of sufficient size, but is frequently seen in nonrandomized studies.

Use of appropriate statistical measures and tests: Many investigators rely on means and proportions to report summary characteristics, and t-tests and chi-square tests to assess differences. Although these are certainly appropriate in many instances, much of the type of data collected in studies of pelvic organ prolapse is not appropriate for these measures. For example, measures such as parity or number of prior surgical procedures, which are only meaningful as integers, should not be expressed as means and standard deviations—a "mean" parity of 1.75 is meaningless. Medians and ranges are more appropriate. Other measures, such as costs or length of stay, are often not distributed normally. Use of means in this case will be influenced by outliersand medians may be more appropriate.

Multivariate and survival analysis: One way to handle the effects of confounding variables is through the use of multivariate techniques such as linear or logistic regression, and these are appropriate for many nonrandomized studies of surgical outcomes. Proper statistical analysis of the time duration until failure of a procedure by any specified criterion involves use of survival analysis, a technique that has been noticeably absent from the majority surgical outcomes reports. However, investigators need to be aware of the limitations of these techniques, which are as susceptible to misuse as any other. Consultation with investigators familiar with their application is recommended.

2. External validity

a) Description of patient population

Characteristics such as age, race, prior medical, gynecological, and obstetrical history should be described, using standard terminology.

b) Characterization of baseline anatomy

The description of the methods in the study should include objective measurements of anatomy and clearly described measurement techniques. A standard, validated, and reliable method of describing subject anatomy such as the pelvic organ prolapse quantitation system should be used before and after the intervention [60].

c) Characterization of baseline symptoms

While restoration of normal anatomy may be a primary goal of the clinician, the most important goal of a patient undergoing treatment of pelvic organ prolapse is an improvement in her quality of life via a relief from the symptoms. Quality of life scales specific for urinary function, pelvic, sexual, and colorectal function are available, as well as more generic instruments that measure general social and emotional well-being such as the SF-36 or the EuroQOL [147]. Both should be utilized before and after the study intervention to adequately assess its impact on the patient.

d) Description of the timing of outcome measurement

Outcome measures may vary depending on when they are obtained. Description of when outcomes are measured facilitates comparison between studies. Ideally, the same measures will have been used prior to the intervention.

e) Description of validity and reliability of outcome measurement

Measurements of outcomes are only useful if the changes in the outcome being measured are reflected in changes in the measurement (validity) and if these changes are reasonably consistent between the same observer measuring at different times, or between different observers (reliability). References to published documentation of the reliability and validity of the measures used should be provided, or documentation provided within the text of the article.

f) Description of clinical care provided to patients

In studies involving surgical outcome, the surgical procedures involved should be described in detail. Investigations involving surgical procedures that take place over a long time period or with multiple surgeons should include an assessment of all efforts made to minimize changes or differences in technique. All investigations or examinations that are used to document surgical outcomes should be described clearly. For instance, the time until removal of a suprapubic bladder catheter is dependent on the criteria used for removal.

XI. SUMMARY

The inclusion of pelvic organ prolapse in a book on urinary incontinence emphasizes the importance of this topic for providers of continence care. The wide variations in evaluation and treatment of POP mandates worldwide attention and research efforts. Our committee was charged with reviewing a large and clinically troublesome topic. The list of evidence-based facts is strikingly short and the list of needed scientific priorities is simply the beginning of a vast research undertaking. It is our intention that with each edition of this book, the evidence-based portion will increase and the research questions will become more refined and focused. We encourage you to direct your highest quality research work to this area.

1. Evidence rating

Vaginal delivery is a major etiologic agent for POP (Level 2)

Chronic defecation disorders increase the risk of POP (Level 3)

Prior hysterectomy is associated with an increased risk for POP surgery (Level 3)

Defecography is superior to physical exam for rectocele and sigmoidocele detection (Level 4)

Women with Stage III and IV POP have fewer symptoms of genuine stress incontinence than <Stage III POP. (Level 4)

Severe prolapse can descend and obstruct the urethra (Level 2)

Occult incontinence rate may be demonstrated by various methods of POP reduction 23-50% patients. (Level 4)

Preoperative barrier testing was not useful in identifying women who required an urethropexy (Level 2)

Preoperative voiding studies with the prolapse reduced by a pessary was the best predictor of normalization of residuals post operatively (Level 4)

Sigmoidoceles are present in 4-11% of reported series, and are nearly always missed on physical exam. (Level 4)

Abnormal colonic transit time occurs in approximately 20% in patients presenting with evacuation disorders. (Level 4)

Fecal incontinence frequently coexists with POP (Level 2)

Rectocele repair can diminish both maximal anal resting and squeeze pressures, possibly contributing to the development of incontinence in patients already at risk with abnormal preoperative manometry. (Level 2).

The POP-Q system is reproducible. (Level 1)

Patient position affects severity of POP demonstrated on physical examination (Level 2)

Simple hysterectomy, without apical suspension, is ineffective for POP treatment. (Level 2) Apical suspension can be effectively accomplished by vaginal and abdominal routes (Level 3)

RECOMMENDATIONS FOR RESEARCH

Well designed multi-racial and multi-ethnic random sample population based studies, which include physician examination to determine the time prevalence of POP.

Standardization of POP-Q methodology for use in clinical trials

Longitudinal, large- scale studies to document the incidence and prevalence of POP

Determine the value of fluoroscopy (for unselected, and selected, populations of women with POP)

Determine the utility of prolapse reduction urodynamic testing

Determine the best surgical strategy to optimize urinary tract function following POP repair Standardization of indications for POP treatment

The role of hysterectomy in POP surgery requires clarification.

APPENDIX I – Prevalence Rates of POP

	Samuelsson et al 1999	Bland et al 1999	Progetto Menopausa 2000	Swift 2000
Country	Sweden	U.S.	Italy	U.S.
N	487	241	21,449	497
Age range	20-59	45-55	Around menopause 1	8 - >70
Race				
White	100%	89%	100%	47%
Black		9%		52%
Parous	54%	Unspecified	85.6%	93%
Hysterectomy	4%	28%	None	28%
Staging technique	Above, to, beyond hymen	ICS	Uterus only Baden 0, 1, ≥2	ICS
Stage ↓				
0	71.2%	73%	94.5%	6.4%
1	28.8%	23%	3.6%	43.3%
2	2%	4%	1.9%	47.7%
3	0	0		2.6%
4	0	0		0
Source of subjects	76% of every 3 year screen participants	Responded to ad for soybean supplement study	268 first-level menopause clinics in Italy	Routine gynecologic examination

APPENDIX II – Vaginal Vault Suspension Series

Technique Authors	N	Follow-up	Success rate Vaginal vault	Global success rate	Cure assessment
Attachment to iliococcygeus fascia					
- Shull (1993) (62)	42	6 weeks-5 y	95%	79%	objective
- Meeks (1994) (38)	110	up to 3 y	100%	96%	?
Coccygeus fixation					
- Thornton, Peters (1983) (68)	40	6 weeks-13 y	98%	95%	Objective
- Peters, Christenson (1995) (49)	81	mean : 37 mo	96%	95%	
Endopelvic fascia fixation					
- Symmonds (1981) (65)	160	1 – 12 y	94,5%	89%	objective subjective
Mc Call culdoplasty					
- Elkins (1995) (15)	14	3-6 mo	100%	90%	Objective
- Colombo (1998) (10)	62	4 – 9 y	95%	85%	Objective subjective
Levator Myorrhaphy (33)	36	Mean 27 mos.	94% -Apex 86% POP 1 cystocele 2 enterocele		

APPENDIX III – Sacrospinous Ligament Suspension Literature

Authors	Year	Follow-up	N° cases	Success Rate	Outcome Measure
Richter (56)	1981	1-10 y	81	70%	Objective
Nichols* (46)	1982	> 2 y	163	97%	?
Morley,Delancey (45)	1988	1 mo-11 y	92	82%	subjective objective
Brown (5)	1989	8 – 21 mo	11	91%	objective
Kettel,Herbertson (27)	1989	?	31	81%	subjective objective
Cruikshank (13)	1990	8 mo-3,2 y	48	83%	objective
Monk (44)	1991	1 mo-8,6 y	61	85%	objective
Backer (2)	1992	?	51	94%	objective
Heinonen (21)	1992	6 mo-5,6 y	22	86%	objective
Imparato* (23)	1992	?	155	90%	objective
Shull (61)	1992	2-5 y	81	65%	objective
Kaminski (25)	1993	?	23	87%	bjective
Carey (6)	1994	2 mo-1 y	63	73%	objective
Holley (22)	1995	15-79 mo	36	8% (success rate for vaginal vault only : 92% recurrent cystocele : 92%)	objective
Sauer (57)	1995	4-26 mo	24	63%	objective
Peters (49)	1995	48 mo	30	77%	subjective objective
Elkins (15)	1995	3-6 mo	14	86%	objective
Pasley* (47)	1995	6-83 mo	144	94%	subjective objective
Benson (4)	1996	12 – 66 mo (mean : 30)	42	29%	objective
Hardimann* (20)	1996	26,4 mo	125	97,6%	objective
Penalver (48)	1998	18-78 mo	160	85%	objective
Lo (34)	1998	24 – 62,4 mo (mean : 25,2)	66	80,3%	objective
Colombo (10)	1998	4 – 9 y	62	73%	Objective subjective
Meschia* (39)	1999	1 – 6,8 y (mean : 3,6)	91	94% recurrence cystocele : 16% recurrence rectocele : 10% recurrence enterocele : 6%	objective
Sze (67)	1999	7 – 72 mo (mean : 24 +/- 15)	54	67% (13/18 anterior recurrence)	objective
Cespedes (8)	2000	5 – 35 mo (mean : 17)	28	89% (1 vault prolapse, 2 cystoceles)	Subjective Objective
Giberti (19)	2001	mean : 16 mo	12	91% (1 vault prolapse, no cystocele)	Objective subjective
Lantzsch* (32)	2001	6 mo – 9 y (mean : 4,8 y)	123	96,7% for vault prolapse (other recurrence : 10 cystoceles, 1 rectocele, 1 enterocele) objective	

Except for the series of which focus primarily on vaginal vault fixation, the success rate reflect all aspects of pelvic floor reconstruction.

APPENDIX IV : Sacrocolpopexy-related observed complications From Baessler et al., in preparation

Complication	Observed cases	Number of operated patients	%
Synthetic mesh erosion/infection	45	1006	4.5
Blood loss > 500ml	41	690	5.9
Obstructive ileus	11	392	2.8
Adynamic ileus/	15	552	2.7
Pelvic haematoma	3	166	1.8

APPENDIX V – Paravaginal Repair Series

Authors	Year	N° of Patients	Cystocele Cured	recurrent	Follow-up Mean (range)	Outcome measure
White (71)	1909	19	19 (100 %)	0	Up to 3 years	?
Baden and Walker (2 bis)	1987	47	NA	NA	2-15 years	Object.
Shull et al. (63)	1994	62	47 (76 %)	15 (24 %)	1.6 (0.1-5.6 years)	Object
Grody et al (19 bis)	1995	72	71 (99 %)	1 (1 %)	(0.5-3 years)	Object
Farrel and Ling (15 ter)	1997	27	22 (80 %)	5 (20 %)	Mean 8 months	Object
Nguyen and Bhatia (46 bis)	1999	10	10 (100 %)	0	Mean 12 months	Object
Elkins et al. (15 bis)	2000	25	23 (92 %)	2 (8 %)	0.5-3 years	Object

APPENDIX VI– Synthetic Mesh for Anterior Wall Prolapse

Authors	Year	Technique	No cases	Follow-up	Recurrence	Measure outcome
Julian (24)	1996	Ant colpor + paravag repair + Marlex mesh	12 12 control (no mesh)	2 years	0 (but complications :25%) 33%	Objective (2 examiner)
Flood (16)	1998	Anterior colpor. + Marlex mesh	142	3,2y (mean)	0 (cure rate SUI = 74%)	
Mage (36)	1999	Polyester mesh (sutured to vaginal angles)	46	26 mo	0 recurrence 1 exposure	Subjective and objective
Migliari (40)	1999	4-corner + mixed fiber mesh	15	23,4 mo (mean)	1 cystocele 2 enterorectoceles (dry at follow-up = 13)	Objective
Migliari (41)	2000	Prolène mesh fixed to urethropelvic and cardinal ligaments	12	20,5 mo (mean)	3 grade 1 cystocele (asymptomatic)	Objective

APPENDIX VII – Posterior Wall Repair

Author-(Year)	Technique	N	Follow-up	Anatomic results	Symptom Resolution (of those having symptom, x % improved)
Kenton (1999) 26	Rectovaginal fascia reattachment	46	1 yr	Mean Ap value of – 2cm (-3 to 2cm) 77% improved	Protrusion : 90% Difficult defecation: 54% Constipation: 43% Dyspareunia : 92% Manual evacuation : 36%
Porter (1999) 51	Defect-specific posterior colporraphy	89	Up to 6 mo	82% improved	Stooling difficulties : 55% Vaginal mass : 74% Splinting : 65% Dyspareunia : 73%
Cundiff (1998)	Defect-specific posterior colporraphy	69	Median 12 mo (3-48)	Mean Ap and Bp –2.4 (94% improved)	Dyspareunia : 33% Constipation : 72% Splinting: 44% Fecal incontinence: 55%
Kahn (1997)	Traditional posterior colporrhaphy	140, 31 phone only	Mean 42.5 mo (11-74)	76% improved	Pressure: 37% Note: Dyspareunia incr from 30 to 47/171 post op, fecal incontinence incr from 30-47/171 post op, constipation incr from 38-56/171 post op_
Mellgran (1997) [148]	Traditional posterior colporrhaphy	25	Mean 1 Yr	96% improved	Constipation: 88% Note: Dyspareunia incr from 1 to 3/16 post op

REFERENCES

1. Mant J, Painter R. Vessey M. Epidemiology of genital prolapse: observations from the Oxford Family Planning Association study. Br J Obstet Gynaecol 1997;104:579-85
2. Samuelsson EC, Victor FTA, Tibblin G, Sv@rdsudd KF. Signs of genital prolapse in a Swedish population of women 20 to 59 years of age and possible related factors. Am J Obstet Gynecol 1999;180:299-305
3. Rinne KM, Kirkinen PP. What predisposes young women to genital prolapse? Eur J Obstet Gynecol Reprod Biol 1999; 84:23-5
4. Swift SE. The distribution of pelvic organ support in a population of female subjects seen for routine gynecologic health care. Am J Obstet Gynecol 2000;183:L277-85
5. Progetto Menopausa Italia Study Group. Risk factors for genital prolapse in non-hysterectomized women around menopause – results from a large cross-sectional study in menopausal clinics in Italy. Eur J Obstet Gynecol Reprod Biol 2000;93:125-40
6. Klein MC, Gauthier RJ, Robbins JM, Kaczorowski MA, Jorgensen SH, Franco ED, Johnson B, Waghorn RN et al. Relationship of episiotomy to perineal trauma and morbidity, sexual dysfunction, and pelvic floor relaxation. Am J Obstet Gynecol 1994;171:591-8
7. Taskin O, Wheeler JM, Yalcinoglu AI, Coksenim S. The effects of episiotomy and Kegel exercises on postpartum pelvic relaxation: a prospective controlled study. J Gynecol Surg 1996; 12:123-7
8. Olsen AL Smith VJ, Bergstrom JO, Colling JC, Clark AL. Epidemiology of surgically managed pelvic organ prolapse and urinary incontinence. Obstet Gynecol 1997;89:501-6
9. Snooks SJ, Swash M, Henry MM, Setchel M. Risk factors in childbirth causing damage to the pelvic floor innervation. Int J Colorectal Dis 1986;1:20-4
10. Gilpin SA, Gosling JA, Smith ARB, Warrell DW. The pathogenesis of genitourinary prolapse and stress incontinence of urine. A histological and histochemical study. Br J Obstet Gynaecol 1989;96:15-23
11. Smith ARB, Hosker GL, Warrell DW. The role of partial denervation of the pelvic floor in the aetiology of genitourinary prolapse and stress incontinence of urine. A neurophysiologic study. Br J Obstet Gynaecol 1989;96:24-8
12. Jones PN, Lubowski DZ, Swash M, Henry MM. Relation between perineal descent and pudendal nerve damage in idiopathic faecal incontinence. Int J Colorectal Dis 1987;2:93-5
13. Lubowski DZ, Swash M, Nichols J, Henry MM. Increases in

pudendal nerve terminal motor latency with defecation straining. Br J Surg 1988;75:1095-7

14. Spence-Jones C, Kamm MA, Henry MM, Hudson CN. Bowel dysfunction: a pathogenic factor in uterovaginal prolapse and urinary stress incontinence. Br J Obstet Gynaecol 1994;101: 147-52

15. Davis GD. Uterine prolapse after laparoscopic uterosacral transection in nulliparous airborne trainees: a report of three cases. J Reprod Med 1996;41:279-82

16. Jorgensen S, Hein HO, Gyntelberg F. Heavy lifting at work and risk of genital prolapse and herniated lumbar disc in assistant nurses. Occup Med 1994;44:47-9

17. Bump RC, Sugerman HJ, Fantl FA, McClish DK. Obesity and lower urinary tract function in women: effect of surgically induced weight loss. Am J Obstet Gynecol 1992;167:392-9

18. Marchionni M, Bracco GL, Checcucci V, Carabaneanu A, Coccia EM, Mecacci F, Scarselli G. True incidence of vaginal vault prolapse: thirteen years experience. J Reprod Med 1999;44:679-84

19. Wiskind AK, Creighton Sm, Stanton SL. The incidence of genital prolapse after the Burch colposuspension. Am J Obstet Gynecol 1992;167:399-404

20. Holley Rl, Varner RE, Gleason BP, Apffel LA, Scott S. Recurrent pelvic support defects after sacrospinous ligament fixation for vaginal vault prolapse. J Am Col Surg 1995;180:444-8

21. Bump RC, Hurt WG, Theofrastous JP, Addison WA, Fantl JA, Wyman JF, McClish DK, and the Continence Program for Women Research Group. Randomized prospective comparison of needle colposuspension versus endopelvic fascia plication for potential stress incontinence prophylaxis in women undergoing vaginal reconstruction for stage III or IV pelvic organ prolapse. Am J Obstet Gynecol. 1996;175:326-335

22. Benson JT, McClennan E. The effect of vaginal dissection on the pudendal nerve. Obstet Gynecol, 82:387-9, 1993

23. Benson JT, Lucente V, McClennan E. Vaginal versus abdominal reconstructive surgery for the treatment of pelvic support defects: a prospective randomized study with long-term outcome evaluation. Am J Obstet Gynecol ,175:1418-22, 1996.

24. Good MC, Copas PR, Doody MC. Uterine prolapse after laparoscopic uterosacral transection. J Reprod Med 1993;72:995-6

25. Al-Rawizs S, Al-Rawizs T. Joint hypermobility in women with genital prolapse Lancet. 26:1439-41, 1982.

26. Marshman D, Percy J, Fielding I, Delbridge L. Rectal prolapse: relationship with joint mobility. Aust NZ J Surg 1987;545:827-9

27. Norton P, Boyd C, Deak S. Collagen synthesis in women with genital prolapse or stress urinary incontinence. Neurourol Urodyn 1992;11:300-1

28. McIntosh LJ, Mallett VT, Frahm JD, Richardson DA, Evans MI. Gynecologic disorders in women with Ehlers-Danlos syndrome. J Soc Gynecol Invest 1995;2:559-64

29. Jackson SR, Avery NC, Tarlton JF, Eckford SD, Abrams P, Bailey AJ. Changes in metabolism of collagen in genitourinary prolapse. Lancet 1996;347:1658-61

30. Carley ME, Schaffer J. Urinary incontinence and pelvic organ prolapse in women with Marfan or Ehlers-Danlos syndrome. Am J Obstet Gynecol 2000;182:1021-3

31. Lind LR, Lucente V, Kohn N. Thoracic kyphosis and the prevalence of advanced uterine prolapse. Obstet Gynecol 1996; 87:605-9

32. Nguyen JK, Lind LR, Choe JY, McKindsey F, Sinow R, Bhatia NN. Lumbosacral spine and pelvic inlet changes associated with eplvic organ prolsape. Obstet Gynecol 2000;95:332-6

33. Sze EH, Kohli N, Miklos JR, Roat T, Karram MM: A retrospective comparison of Abdominal Sacrocolpopexy with Burch Colsuspension versus Sacrospinosus Fixation with Transvaginal Needle Suspension for the Management of Vaginal Vault Prolapse and Coexisting Stress Incontinence. Int Urogynecol J Pelvic Floor Dysfunct 10 (1999):390-393

34. Blakely Cr, Mills Wg. The obstetric and gynaecological compliations of bladder exstrophy and epispadias. Br J Obstet Gynaecol, 88:167-73, 1981.

35. Al-Allard P, Rochette L. The descriptive epidemiology of hysterectomy, province of Quebec. Ann Epidemiol 1991;1:541-9, 1981-1988.

36. Luoto R, Rutanen EM, Kaprio J. Five gynecologic diagnoses associated with hysterectomy – trends in incidence of hospitalizations in Finland,1971-1986. Maturitas 1994;19:141-52

37. Bland Dr, Earle Bb, Vitolins Mz, Burke G. Use of pelvic organ prolapse staging system of the International Continence Society, American Urogynecologic Society, and Society of Gynecologic Surgeons in perimenopausal women. Am J Obstet Gynecol,181:1324-8, 1999.

38. Richardson DA, Bent AE, Ostergard DR. The effect of uterovaginal prolapse on urethrovesical pressure dynamics. Am J Obstet Gynecol 1983; 146:901-5.

39. Bergman A, Koonings PP, Ballard CA. Predicting postoperative urinary incontinence development in women undergoing operation for genitourinary prolapse. Amer J Obst Gynec, 158:1171, 1988.

40. Zivkovic F, Ralph G, Tamussino K, Michelitsch L, Haas J. Urethral profilometry in women with uterovaginal prolapse. Intl Urogynecol J Pelvic Floor Dysfunc 1995;6:10-13.

41. Chaikin DC, Groutz A, Blaivas JG. Predicting the need for anti-incontinence surgery in continent women undergoing repair of severe urogenital prolapse. J Urol 2000;163:531-534.

42. Gallentine ML, Cespedes RD. Occult stress urinary incontinence and the effect of vaginal vault prolapse on abdominal leak point pressures. Urol 2001;57:40-44.

43. Versi E, Lyell DJ, Griffiths DJ. Videourodynamic diagnosis of occult genuine stress incontinence in patients with anterior vaginal wall relaxation. Journal of the Society for Gynecologic Investigation. 5(6):327-30, 1998.

44. Klutke JJ, Ramos S, Margolin ML, et al. Urodynamic outcome after surgery for severe prolapse and potential stress incontinence. Amer J Obstet Gynecol 2000;182:1378-1381.

45. Karram MM. What is the optimal anti-incontinence procedure in women with advanced prolapse and 'Potential' stress incontinence? Intl Urogynecol J Pelvic Floor Dysfunc 1999;10:1-2.

46. Coates KW, Harris RL, Cundiff GW, Bump RC. Uroflowmetry in women with urinary incontinence and pelvic organ prolapse. Br J Urol 1997;80:217-221.

47. FitzGerald MP, Kulkarni N, Fenner D, Postoperative resolution of urinary retention in patients with advanced pelvic organ prolapse. Amer J Obstet Gynecol 2000;183:1361-1364.

48. Barrington JW, Edwards G. Posthysterectomy vault prolapse. Intl Urogynecol J Pelvic Floor Dysfunc 2000;11:241-245.

49. Yanik FF, Akpolat T, Kocak I. Acute renal failure - An unusual consequence of uterine prolapse. Nephrol Dial Transplant 1998;13:2648-2650.

50. Altringer WE, Saclarides TJ, Dominguez JM, Brubaker LT, Smith CS. Four-contrast defecography: Pelvic 'floor-oscopy'. Dis Colon Rectum 1995;38:695-699.

51. Kelvin FM, Hale DS, Maglinte DDT, Patten BJ, Benson JT. Female pelvic organ prolapse: Diagnostic contribution of dynamic cystoproctography and comparison with physical examination. Amer J Roentgenol 1999;173:31-37.

52. Agachan F, Pfeifer J, Wexner DS. Defecography and proctography: Results of 744 patients. Dis Colon Rectum 1996;39:899-905

53. Fenner DE, Diagnosis and assessment of sigmoidoceles. Amer J Obstet Gynecol 1996;175:1438-1442.

54. Karasick S, Ehrlich SM. Is constipation a disorder of defecation or impaired motility?: Distinction based on defecography and colonic transit studies. Amer J Roentgenol 1996;166:63-66.

55. Van Dam JH, Hop WCJ, Schouten WR. Analysis of patients with poor outcome of rectocele repair. Dis Colon Rectum 2000;43:1556-1560

56. Karlbom U, Graf W, Nilsson S, Pahlman L. Does surgical repair of a rectocele improve rectal emptying? Dis Colon Rectum 1996;39:1296-1302

57. Mellgren A, Anzen B, Nilsson BY, et al. Results of rectocele repair: A prospective study. Dis Colon Rectum 1995;38:7-13

58. Jackson SL, Weber AM, Hull TL, Mitchinson AR, Walters MD. Fecal incontinence in women with urinary incontinence and pelvic organ prolapse. Obstet Gynecol 1997;89:423-427

59. Emge LA, Durfee RB. Pelvic organ prolapse: four thousand years of treatment. Clin Obstet Gynecol 1966; 9: 997

60. Brubaker L, Norton P. Current clinical nomenclature for description of prolapse. J Pelvic Surg, 1996;7:256-9

61. Bump RC, Mattiasson A, Bø K, Brubaker LP, DeLancey JOL, Klarskov P, Shull BL, Smith ARB. The standardisation of terminology of female pelvic organ prolapse and pelvic floor dysfunction. Am J Obstet Gynecol. 1996;175:10-17

62. Archer BD, Somers S, Stevenson GW, Contrast medium gel for marking vaginal position during defecography. Radiology, 1992. 182: p. 278-279

63. Hock D, Lombard R, Jehaes C, et al., Colpocystodefecography. Dis Colon Rectum, 1993. 36: p. 1015-1021

64. Kelvin FM, Maglinte D, Benson JT, Brubaker LP, Smith C, Dynamic cystoproctography: a technique for assessing disorders of the pelvic floor in women. Am J Roentgenol, 1994. 163: p. 368-370.

65. Mahieu P, Pringot J, Bodart P, Defecography. 1. Description of a new procedure and results in normal patients. Gastrointest Radiol, 1984. 9: p. 247-251.

66. Kelvin FM, Maglinte D, Hornback JA, Benson JT, Pelvic Prolapse: assessment with evacuation proctography (defecography). Radiology, 1992. 2: p. 136-140.

67. Shorvon PJ, McHugh S, Diamant NE, Somers S, Stevenson GW., Defecography in normal volunteers: results and implications. Gut, 1989. 30: p. 1737-1749.

68. Creighton, S.M., Pearce, J.M. and Stanton, S.L. (1992) Perineal video-ultrasonography in the assessment of vaginal prolapse: early observations. Br J Obstet Gynaecol 99, 310-313.

69. Wise, B.G., Khullar, V. and Cardozo, L.D. (1992b) Bladder neck movement during pelvic floor contraction and intravaginal electrical stimulation in women with and without genuine stress incontinence. Neurourol Urodyn 11, 309-311 (Abstract).

70. Clark, A., Creighton, S.M., Pearce, M. and Stanton, S.L. (1990) Localisation of the bladder neck by perineal ultrasound: methodology and applications. Neurourol Urodyn 9, 394-395(Abstract).

71. Karaus M, Neuhaus P, Wiedenmann TB. Diagnosis of enteroceles by dynamic anorectal endosonography. Dis Colon Rectum 2000; 43(12): 1683-8.

72. Bhatia, N.N., Ostergard, D.R. and McQuown, D. (1987) Ultrasonography in Urinary Incontinence. Urology 29, 90-94.

73. Boos, K., Athanasiou, S., Toozs-Hobson, P., Cardozo, L., Khullar, V. and Hextall, A. (1997) The dynamics of the pelvic floor extrinsic continence mechanism before and after Burch colposuspension. Neurourol Urodyn 16, 411-412 (Abstract).

74. Peschers, U., Schaer, G., Anthuber, C., Delancey, J.O. and Schuessler, B. (1996) Changes in vesical neck mobility following vaginal delivery. Obstet Gynecol 88, 1001-1006.

75. Bernstein, I., Juul, N., Gronvall, S., Bonde, B. and Klarskov, P. (1991) Pelvic floor muscle thickness measured by perineal ultrasonography. Scand J Urol Nephrol 137S, 131-133.

76. Bernstein, I.T. (1997) The pelvic floor muscles: muscle thickness in healthy and urinary-incontinent women measured by perineal ultrasonography with reference to the effect of pelvic floor training. Estrogen receptor studies. Neurourol Urodyn 16, 237-275.

77. Athanasiou, S., Boos, K., Khullar, V., Anders, K. and Cardozo, L. (1996) Pathogenesis of genuine stress incontinence and urogenital prolapse. Neurourol Urodyn 15, 339-340 (Abstract).

78. Nguyen JK, Hall CD, Taber E and Bhatia NN. Sonographic diagnosis of paravaginal defects: a standardization technique. Int Urogynecol 2000; 11: 341-345.

79. Delancey, J.O. and Hurd, W.W. (1998) Size of the urogenital hiatus in the levator ani muscles in normal women and women with pelvic organ prolapse. Obstet Gynecol 91, 364-368.

80. Hricak H. MRI of the female pelvis: a review. AJR 1986: 146: 1115-1122.

81. Tan IL, Stokker J, Zwamborn AW, Entius KA, Calame JJ, Lameris JS. Female pelvic floor: endovaginal MR imaging of normal anatomy. Radiology, 1998:206:777-783.

82. Nurenberg P, Forte T, Zimmern PE. Normative female urethral and supportive structural measurements determined by body coil and endorectal coil MRI. Progres en Urologie, 2000: 10: 224-230.

83. Lamb GM, deJode MG, Gould SW, Spouse E, Birnie K, Darzi A, Gedroyc WMW. Upright dynamic MR defecaeting proctography in an open configuration system. British Journal of Radiology, 2000:73:152-155.

84. Goodrich MA, Webb MJ, King BF, Bampton AEH, Compeau NG, Riederer SJ. Magnetic resonance imaging of pelvic floor relaxation: dynamic analysis and evaluation of patients before and after surgical repair. Obstet Gynecol 1993: 82:883-891.

85. Yang A, Mostwin JL, Rosenshein NB, Zerhouni EA. Pelvic floor descent in women: Dynamic evaluation with fast MR imaging and cinematic display. Radiology, 1991:19:25-33.

86. Comiter CV, Vasavada SP, Barbaric ZL, Gousse AE, and Raz, S. Grading pelvic prolapse and pelvic floor relaxation using dynamic magnetic resonance imaging. Urology, 1999: 54:454-457.

87. Fielding JR, Dumanli H, Schreyer AG, Okuda S, Gering DT, Zou KH, Kikinis R, Jolesz FA. MR-based three dimensional modeling of the normal pelvic floor in women: quantification of muscle mass. AJR, 2000:174:657-660.

88. Healy JC, Halligan S, Reznck RH, Watson S, Phillips RKS, Armstrong P. Patterns of prolapse in women with symptoms of pelvic floor weakness: assessment with MR imaging. Radiology 1997:203:77-81.

89. Goh V, Halligan S, Kaplan G, Healy JC, Bartram CI. Dynamic MR Imaging of the pelvic floor in asymptomatic subjects. AJR 2000:174:661-666.

90. Bo K, Lilleas F, Talseth T, Hedland H. Dynamic MRI of the pelvic floor muscles in an upright sitting position. NeuroUrol and Urodyn., 2001:20: 167-174.

91. Gousse AE, Barbaric ZL, Safir MH, Madjar S, Marumoto AK, and Raz, S. Dynamic half Fourier acquisition, single shot turbo spin-echo magnetic resonance imaging for evaluating the female pelvis. J.Urol. 2000: 164:1606-1613.

92. Tunn R, Paris St, Taupitz M, Hamm B, Fischer W. MR Imaging in posthysterectomy vaginal prolapse. International Urogynecology, 2000: 11:87-97.

93. Lamb GM, deJode MG, Gould SW, Spouse E, Birnie K, Darzi

A, Gedroyc WMW. Upright dynamic MR defecaeting proctography in an open configuration system. British Journal of Radiology, 2000:73:152-155.

94. Mattox TF, Bhatia NN. Urodynamic effects of reducing devices in women with genital prolapse. Int Urogynecol J 1994;5:283-6.

95. Bhatia NN, Bergman A, Gunning JE> Urodynamic effects of a vaginal pessary in women with stress urinary incontinence. Am J Obstet Gynecol 1983; 147:876-84.

96. Bump RC, Fantl JA, Hurt WG. The mechanism of urinary incontinence in women with severe uterovaginal prolapse: results of barrier studies. Obstet Gynecol 1988; 72:291-5.

97. Ramahi AJ, Richardson DA. Urodynamic changes in women using diaphragms. Neurourol Urodynam, 9: 569, 1990.

98. Hextall A, Boos K, Cardozo L, Toozs-Hobson P, Anders K, Khullar V. Videocystourethrography with a ring pessary in situ. A clinically useful preoperative investigation for continent women with urogenital prolapse? International Urogynecology Journal & Pelvic Floor Dysfunction. 9(4):205-9, 1998.

99. Sulak PJ, Kuehl TJ, Shull BL. Vaginal pessaries and their use in pelvic relaxation. J Reprod Med 1993; 38:919-23.

100. Veronikis DF, Nichols DH, Wakamatsu MM. The incidence of low-pressure urethra as a function of prolapse-reducing technique in patients with massive pelvic organ prolapse (maximum descent at all vaginal sites). American Journal of Obstetrics & Gynecology. 177(6):1305-13; discussion 1313-4, 1997.

101. Richardson DA, Bent AE, Ostergard DR. The effect of uterovaginal prolapse on urethrovesical pressure dynamics. Am J Obstet Gynecol 1983; 146:901-5.

102. Romanzi LJ, Chaikin DC, Blaivas JG. The effect of genital prolapse on voiding. Journal of Urology. 161(2):581-6, 1999.

103. Versi E, Lyell DJ, Griffiths DJ. Videourodynamic diagnosis of occult genuine stress incontinence in patients with anterior vaginal wall relaxation. Journal of the Society for Gynecologic Investigation. 5(6):327-30, 1998.

104. Fianu S, Kjaeldgaard A, Larsson B. Preoperative screening for latent stress incontinence in women with cystocele. Neurourol Urodyn 1985:4:3-8.

105. Borstad E, Rud T. The risk of developing urinary stress incontinence after vaginal repair in continent women: a clinical and urodynamic follow up study. Acta Obstet Gynecol Scand 1989; 68:545-9.

106. Bergman A, Koonings PP, Ballard CA. Predicting postoperative urinary incontinence development in women undergoing operation for genitourinary prolapse. Amer J Obst Gynec, 158: 1171, 1988.

107. Bump RC, Hurt WG, Theofrastous JP, Addison WA, Fantl JA, Wyman JF, et al. Randomized prospective comparison of needle colposuspension versus endopelvic fascia plication for potential stress incontinence prophylaxis in women undergoing vaginal reconstruction for stage III or IV pelvic organ prolapse. Am J Obstet Gynecol 1966; 175:326-35.

108. Weber AM, Abrams P, Brubaker L. The Standardization of Terminology for Researchers in Female Pelvic Floor Disorders. Int Urogynecol J 2001; 12:178-186

109. Marana HR, Andrade JM, Marana RR, Matheus de Sala M, Philbert PM, Rodriguez R. Vaginal hysterectomy for correcting genital prolapse. Long-term evaluation. J Reprod Med, 1999 ; 44 : 529-534

110. Benson JT, Lucente V, McClellan E. Vaginal versus abdominal reconstructive surgery for the treatment of pelvic support defects : a prospective randomized study with long-term outcome evaluation. Am J Obstet Gynecol, 1996 ; 175 : 1418-1421

111. Brown WE, Hoffman MS, Bouis PJ, Ingram JM, Hopes JL. Management of vaginal vault prolapse : retrospective comparison of abdominal versus vaginal approach. J Fla Med Assoc, 1989 ; 76 : 249-252

112. Hardimann PJ, Drutz HP. Sacrospinous vault suspension and abdominal colposacropexy : success rates and complications. Am J Obstet Gynecol, 1996 ;175: 612-616

113. Lo TS, Wang AC. Abdominal colposacropexy and sacrospinous ligament suspension for severe uterovaginal prolapse : a comparison. J Gynecol Surg, 1998 ; 14 : 59-64

114. Sze EHM, Kohli N, Miklos JR, Roat T, Karram MM. A retrospective comparison of abdominal sacrocolpopexy with Burch colposuspension versus sacrospinous fixation with transvaginal needle suspension for the management of vaginal prolapse and coexisting stress incontinence. Int Urogynecol J, 1999 ; 10 : 390-393

115. Given FT, Muhlendorf IK, Browing GM: Vaginal length and sexual funktion after colpopexy for uterovaginal eversion. Obstet. Gynecol 169 (1993):284-288

116. Anthuber C, Schüssler B, Hepp H: Die operative Therapie des Scheidenblindsackvorfalls. Der Gynäkologe 29 (1996):652-658

117. Colombo M, Vitobello D, Proietti F, Milani R. Randomised comparison of Burch colposuspension versus anterior colporraphy in women with stress urinary incontinence and anterior vaginal wall prolapse. BJOG, 2000 ; 107 : 544-551

118. Schettini M, Fortunato P, Gallucci M: Abdominal Sacral Colpopexy with Prolene Mesh. Int Urogynecol J Pelvic Floor Dysfunct 10 (1999): 295-299

119. Pilsgaard K, Mouritsen L:. Follow–up after repair of vaginal vault prolapse with abdominal colposacropexy. Acta Obstet Gynecol Scand 78 (1999):66-70

120. Fox SD, Stanton SL: Vault prolapse and rectocele: Assessement of repair using sacrocolpopexy with mesh interposition. BJ Obstet Gynecol;107 (2000): 1371-1375

121. Iglesia CB, Fenner DE, Brubaker L: The Use of Mesh in Gynecologic Surgery. Int. Urogynecol J 8 (1997):105-115

122. Baessler K, Schuessler B: Abdominal Sacropopexy and Anatomy and Function of the Posterior Compartment. Obstet Gynecol 97 (2001): 678-84

123. Visco AG, Weidner AC, Barber MD, Myers ER, Cundiff GW, Bump RC, Addison AW: Vaginal mesh erosion after abdominal sacral colpopexy. J Obstet Gynecol 184, (2001):297-302

124. Weidner AC, Geoffrey WC, Harris RL, Addison A: Sacral osteomyelitis: An unusual complication of abdominal sacral colopexy. Obstet Gynecol 90 (1997):689-691

125. Weber AM, Walters MD. Anterior vaginal prolapse : review of anatomy and techniques of surgical repair. Obstet Gynecol, 1997 ; 89 : 311-318

126. Kohli N, Sze EHM, Roat TW, Karram MM. Incidence of recurrent cystocele after anterior colporrhaphy with and without concomitant transvaginal needle suspension. Am J Obstet Gynecol, 1996 ; 175 : 1476-1482

127. White GR. Cystocele : a radical cure by suturing lateral sulci of vagina to white line of pelvic fascia. JAMA, 1909; 21 : 1707-1710

128. Shull BL, Baden WF. A six-year experience with paravaginal defect repair for stress urinary incontinence. Am J Obstet Gynecol, 1989 ; 160 : 1432 – 1440

129. Scotti RJ, Garely AD, Greston WM, Flora RF, Olson TR. Paravaginal repair ol lateral vaginal wall defects by fixation to the ischial periosteum and obturator membrane. Am J Obstet Gynecol, 1998 ; 179 : 1436-1445

130. NguyenJK, Bhatia NN. Transvaginal repair of paravaginal defects using the Capio suturing device: A preliminary experience. J. Gynecol Tech 1999;5:51-54

131. Baden WF, Walker T. Urinary stress incontinence: Evolution of paravaginal repair. Female Patient 1987;12:89-105

132. Grody MHT, Nyirjesy P. Kelley LM et al. Paraurethral fascial sling urethropexy and vaginal paravaginal defects cystopexy in the correction of urethrovesical prolapse. Int Urogynecol J Pelvic Floor Dysfunct 1995;6:80-85

133. Farrell SA, Ling C. Currycombs for the vaginal paravaginal defect repair.

134. Obstet Gynecol 1997;90:845-847

135. Miyazaki FS, Miyazaki DW. Raz four-corner suspension for severe cystocele : poor results. Int Urogynecol J, 1994 ; 5 : 94-97

136. Raz S, Klutke CG, Golomb J. Four-corner bladder and urethral suspension for moderate cystocele. J Urol, 1989 ; 142 : 712-715

137. Zimmern PE, Leach GE, Sirls L. Four-corner bladder neck suspension.

138. Atlas of urologic clinics of North America, 1994 ; 2 (1) : 29-36

139. Julian T. The effacacy of Marlex mesh in the repair of severe, recurrnt vaginal prolapse of the anterior midvaginal wall. Am J Obstet Gynecol, 1996 ; 175 : 1472-1475

140. Flood CG, Drutz HP, Waja L. Anterior colporraphy reinforced with Marlex mesh for the treatment of cystocèles. Int Urogynecol J Pelvic Floor Dysfunct, 1998 ; 9 : 200-204

141. Mage P. Interposition of a synthetic mesh by vaginal approach in the cure of genital prolapse. J Gynecol Obstet Biol Reprod (Paris), 1999 ; 28 : 825-829

142. Migliari R, Usai E. Treatment results using a mixed fiber mesh in patients with grade IV cystocele. J Urol, 1999 ; 161 : 1255-1258

143. Migliari R, De Angelis M, Madeddu G, Verdacchi T. Tension-free vaginal mesh repair for anterior vaginal wall prolapse. Eur Urol, 2000 ; 38 : 151-155

144. Kenton K, Shott S, Brubaker L. Outcome after rectovaginal fascia reattachement for rectocele repair. Am J Obstet Gynecol, 1999 ; 181 : 1360-1364

145. Porter WE, Steele A, Walsh P, Kohli N, Karram MM. The anatomic and functional outcomes of defect-specific rectocele repair. Am J Obstet Gynecol, 1999 ; 181 : 1352-1359

146. Cundiff GW, AC Weidner, AG Visco, WA Addison , BumpRC. An anatomical and functional assessment of the discrete defect rectocele repair. Am J Obstet Gynecol 1998;179:1451-7

147. Kahn MA, Stanton SL. Posterior colporrhaphy: its effects on bowel and sexual function. Br J Obstet Gynaecol 1997;104:82-86

148. Mellgren A, Anzen B, Nilsson BY, Johansson C, Dolk A, Gillgren P, Bremmer S, Holmstrom Results of rectocele repair; a prospective study. Dis Colon Rectum 1995;38:7-13

149. Black, NA Downs, SH. The effectiveness of surgery for stress incontinence in women: a systematic review. Br J Urol 1996; 78:497-510.

150. Wall LL, Versi E, Norton P, Bump R. Evaluating the outcome of surgery for pelvic organ prolapse. Amer J Obstet Gynecol 1998; 178:877-879.

151. Schulz KF, Chalmers I, Hayes RJ, et al. Empirical evidence of bias: dimensions of methodological quality associated with estimates of treatment effects in controlled trials. JAMA 1995;273:408-12.

Committee 6

Symptom and Quality of Life Assessment

Chair

J.L. Donovan (U.K.)

Members

X. Badia (Spain),

J. Corcos (Canada),

M. Gotoh (Japan),

C. Kelleher (U.K.),

M. Naughton (USA),

C. Shaw (U.K.)

Consultant

B. Lukacs (France)

Symptom and Quality of Life Assessment

J.L. Donovan

X. Badia, J. Corcos, M. Gotoh, C. Kelleher, M. Naughton, C. Shaw, B. Lukacs

BACKGROUND

Symptoms of incontinence are common, particularly amongst older people, and, at any age, incontinence can have a severe impact on the quality of life of some individuals. A number of treatments for incontinence are available, most of which aim to reduce the occurrence of incontinent episodes or to limit the impact of the disorder on everyday life. In research and clinical practice it is essential that the symptoms and impact of incontinence can be properly assessed and recorded. Symptoms of incontinence and their impact on patients' quality of life can be assessed in a number of ways, but the only valid way of measuring the patient's perspective of their predicament is through the use of psychometrically robust self-completion questionnaires.

In the report from the First International Consultation on Incontinence, the impact of incontinence on quality of life and methods of measuring these factors were described, and a number of questionnaires with acceptable levels of psychometric testing were recommended for use in research and clinical practice [1]. This chapter will summarise the major findings from that review, extend these with an up-dated and more systematic review of the literature, and provide more specific recommendations for questionnaires developed for use in clinical practice and research.

In addition, the developmental work for the ICIQ-SF questionnaire, launched at this Second Consultation, is detailed in Appendix I, at the end of this chapter.

LITERATURE SEARCHING STRATEGY

A number of different electronic databases were searched, limited to adults over the age of 18 years and human studies including:

Cochrane database of randomised trials for all randomised controlled trials including the word 'incontinence' from 1998 to 2001. 48 trials were identified measuring outcome of incontinence treatments.

MEDLINE and HealthSTAR between January 1990 and October 2000, using the search strategies: "Urinary Incontinence" coupled with either "Prevalence" or "Epidemiology". Additional studies were located by examining the ascending bibliography. More than 800 studies were located.

PubMed using the keywords 'incontinence' and 'quality of life'. This yielded 415 papers in total, with 109 relating to female urinary incontinence and quality of life

MEDLINE, BIDS Embase and PsychInfo databases, with supplementary searching of references lists of articles identified. Searches were carried out using MeSH headings of Urinary Incontinence and Sexual dysfunctions as well as searches on the text words Urin* and Sex* (asterisks represent wild cards). As a check further searches were carried out combining the sexual dysfunctions MeSH headings with the Questionnaires heading.

Medline and PubMed databases from 1998 – May 2001 to update literature related to the psychosocial and quality of life impact of incontinence on daily living, and the use of generic and disease-specific questionnaires to assess incontinence, using the following key words: 'urinary incontinence,' 'quality of life,' and 'psychology' crossed in various combinations. 108 articles dealt specifically with the psychological and quality of life impact of incontinence.

Symptoms of incontinence and/or its impact on quality of life can be assessed in a number of ways. Traditionally, the clinical history has been used to gain a summary view of the symptoms of incontinence experienced by patients and their impact on their lives. Increasingly, patient-completed methods of measuring incontinence are being used, including voiding diaries and questionnaires.

THE MEASUREMENT OF INCONTINENCE AND QUALITY OF LIFE

A. WHY QUESTIONNAIRES ?

Taking a thorough clinical history for patients with incontinence is an important method of assessing symptoms and degree of bothersomeness. A major concern remains, however, that it is unstandardised and probably takes a different form for each clinician and different patient encounters. The first questionnaires were an attempt to standardise the clinical history: the Boyarsky schedule for lower urinary tract symptoms, [2] and the Stamey score for incontinence [3]. These instruments have not been tested for validity or reliability, are crude, and require a clinician to mediate and interpret a patient's symptoms. This has been shown to be unreliable and often not representative of the patient's perspective of their condition [4, 5, 6, 7]. Clinicians' ratings of patients' quality of life in general tend to be lower than those given by patients themselves [7]. It is likely, with a socially embarrassing condition such as incontinence, that patients will find it difficult to describe their symptoms and difficulties fully to a clinician. The use of clinician-based measures of symptoms and quality of life is not recommended in research.

Voiding diaries (also known as frequency-volume charts or urinary diaries) are widely used to assess a limited number of lower urinary tract symptoms, usually frequency, nocturia and incontinent episodes. Patients are typically asked to complete these daily, recording frequency of urination day and night, incontinent episodes and sometimes also volume voided. They have been shown to exhibit reasonable test-retest reliability, particularly for incontinent episodes [8], but not to be able to differentiate patients with urodynamic diagnoses [9]. While voiding diaries can be helpful and may be accurate if completed regularly, they rely on recall of episodes which can be unreliable [10]. In the area of incontinence, they are also limited by the range of symptoms that can be accommodated - usually frequency, nocturia and incontinence episodes only.

For a full assessment of the symptoms of incontinence and their impact on quality of life, questionnaires completed by patients themselves and which have been shown to be valid and reliable are recommended (see below for details of recommended questionnaires).

B. QUESTIONNAIRES – THEORETICAL ASPECTS

Questionnaires can be used to record the presence and severity of urinary symptoms including incontinence, as well as the impact of incontinence on everyday activities and quality of life. They are tools to measure 'subjective' phenomena such as symptoms and impact on quality of life in an objective way. Questionnaire design and utilisation is not a simple process. In order to have confidence that the questionnaire is measuring what it is supposed to measure, that it does this reliably, and is appropriate for use in the patient or population group under investigation, a number of studies have to be conducted. There are increasing numbers of validated questionnaires in the public domain, many of which are listed in reference books, [11, 12] including some for questionnaires recommended for use in incontinence [1]. It is important to bear in mind the purpose for which any questionnaire was originally designed – the questions included will reflect the original aims. If the questionnaire is to be used in other contexts, further validation may be required.

If designed and tested thoroughly, questionnaires can have levels of precision which equal or exceed clinical measures. Of particular importance are the precision and accuracy of measures - more commonly referred to as psychometric properties.

I. PSYCHOMETRIC PROPERTIES

Empirical evidence is required to show that a questionnaire is measuring what is intended, measures this is a reproducible fashion, and is sensitive to changes over time or following interventions. These aspects are known as validity, reliability and responsiveness:

1. Validity

The validity of a questionnaire is simply whether it measures what is intended, and has three major aspects:

a) Content/face validity

Content/face validity is the assessment of whether the questionnaire makes sense to those being measured and to experts in the clinical area, and also whether all the important or relevant domains are included [13]. In particular, it is important that questions are understandable and unambiguous to the patient and that they are clinically sensible. Once the questionnaire has been developed and administered, levels of missing data can be used as an indicator of misunderstood questions.

b) Construct validity

Construct validity relates to the relationships between the questionnaire and underlying theories. This is very much an ongoing procedure which requires a number of studies of the performance of a questionnaire in a range of settings and patient groups. Each one of these studies will examine some aspect of the validity of particular constructs or 'mini-theories.'[13]. A common method of obtaining some indication of the construct validity of a questionnaire is to examine its ability to differentiate between patient groups - for example clinic attenders compared with individuals in the community, or clinic attenders with a particular diagnosis compared with those with another. Construct validity also includes the concepts of 'convergent' and 'discriminant' validity. Convergent validity involves seeing how closely a new questionnaire is related to other measures of the same construct. Discriminant validity relates to the absence of relationships between constructs that are postulated to be independent.

c) Criterion validity

Criterion validity describes how well the questionnaire correlates with a 'gold standard' measure that already exists. Such 'gold standards' may be clinical or other validated measures. While it is acknowledged that urodynamic studies represent the most accurate representation of leakage and a clinical diagnosis of incontinence, these factors are not the only ones that one would want to be reflected by a questionnaire. Questionnaires are primarily designed to measure patients' perspectives of their condition, and so the diagnosis of incontinence may be less important than the way in which urinary leakage is perceived by patients and the impact it has on their quality of life. For incontinence there is no clear gold standard but new questionnaires should be compared with existing measures using the methods suggested for construct validity.

2. Reliability

The reliability of a questionnaire refers to its ability to measure in a reproducible fashion [13]. This appears to be a simple concept, but involves the assessment of two main aspects:

a) Internal consistency

Internal consistency refers to the extent to which items within the questionnaire are related to each other. It can be assessed by statistical techniques such as item-total correlations or Cronbach's alpha coefficient [13]. If item-total correlations are used, each item should be correlated with the total score omitting that item, and items with a correlation of less than 0.2 should be eliminated or rewritten [13]. Cronbach's alpha coefficient should be calculated for the total score eliminating one item at a time, and any items which significantly increase or decrease the alpha should be re-evaluated. A Cronbach's alpha in excess of 0.70 is usually considered to show adequate internal consistency [14].

b) Reproducibility

This assesses the variability between and within observers (inter- and intra-rater reliability) for questionnaires administered by an interviewer, usually using analysis of variance (ANOVA) [13].

Particularly important for questionnaires used to examine outcome is the concept of stability - whether the questionnaire measures the same sorts of things in the same person over a period of time. A questionnaire which cannot demonstrate that responses are stable over a short period of time in a pre-treatment sample will not be able to measure change following treatment. Stability is commonly assessed by a test-retest analysis, where the questionnaire is given to the same set of respondents twice, usually with an interval of two to six weeks. For incontinence, two weeks is probably sufficient. Test-retest reliability can be assessed by the correlation between scores obtained from the two time periods. When items have more than two ratings, it is suggested that intraclass correlation coefficients are preferred [15]. These methods obscure variation from individual questions, however, and so a graphical presentation and analyses of paired differences in individual items can be helpful [16].

3. Responsiveness

There are three main aspects to the measurement of change: differentiating between those who change a lot and those who change little, the identification of factors which are associated with a good outcome, and inferring treatment effects from group differences in clinical trials [13]. Where a questionnaire results in a simple score, treatment effects can be assessed by examining pre- and post-treatment differences between the intervention and control group by unpaired t-tests or repeated measures analysis of variance [13]. Effect sizes are also commonly used. Interpreting effect sizes can be difficult, but it is suggested that 0.3 represents a small effect, 0.6 a moderate effect and 0.8 a large effect [17, 18, 19, 20]. Outside randomised controlled trials, where there may be baseline differences between treatment groups, analyses of covariance may be more appropriate. It is important to consider the thorny question of how to interpret changes. Changes may be found to be statistically significant, but this does not necessarily mean that they are of clinical significance [21].

II. METHODS OF SCORING

Questionnaires can be scored in a variety of ways,

depending on the design of the questionnaire and its particular aim. Each method will result in different patterns of scores, and so caution in interpretation should always be exercised.

- Simple additive scores where questions have high levels of internal consistency (i.e. Cronbach's alpha in excess of 0.70, preferably in excess of 0.80. More complicated questionnaires, particularly those assessing quality of life, are often constructed as profiles. Profiles contain a number of domains, each of which has its own score. Problems with such scores include that any single score may be achieved by a wide range of component scores and may give a spurious mathematical precision to scores.
- Muliplicatory scores. Here, scores from one type of question are multiplied by scores from another and then added together to reach a total score. Small changes in the aspect multiplied can have a considerable impact on the total score.
- Weighted scores. Values are assigned to items, for example by clinicians indicating that they believe that certain symptoms are more significant or severe than others. It is often difficult to justify the weights derived, and small changes in such weights can have a significant impact on scores.
- No scores assigned. In some cases, questionnaire designers advise that total or subscale scores are not developed. Questionnaires without scores can be used for descriptive purposes, for example in indicating prevalences of particular symptoms and may be useful in identifying the impact of individual items on aspects of quality of life and outcome, but the analysis may be complex.

III. INTERNATIONAL IMPLEMENTATION

Increasingly, questionnaires are required to be used in a number of different populations and settings, but psychometric properties are not necessarily transferable between populations or settings. There are particular problems with the interpretation of symptoms and aspects of quality of life in different population groups as these are likely to be influenced by cultural factors. [22 23].Guillemin et al have suggested a number of steps that should be taken to ensure that questionnaires may be used by different cultural groups: [24].

a. Translation of the questionnaire

b. Back translation into the original language

C. Committee review of translations

d. Pre-testing for equivalence using bilinguals or monolinguals

e. Re-examination of weighting of scores

There are other more recent recommendations for adapting quality of life instruments, for example, at http://www.euroqol.org and by Herdman et al [25].

Researchers who seek to translate measures for use in different languages or cultures should be advised that this can be a lengthy and complicated procedure. Whenever possible, it is advisable to use existing translated measures. Details can often be obtained from the developers of specific questionnaires.

IV. SUITABILITY/FEASIBILITY

A further issue of importance in research and clinical practice is that the questionnaire should be suitable for its purpose and feasible to be used. There is always a tension in research between having a questionnaire that encompasses all possible aspects of the condition and the necessity to avoid respondent burden and to make the instrument simple and easy to use. The majority of questionnaires so far designed in this field have a tendency to be quite long and comprehensive. There are indications, however, that shorter forms are increasingly being developed. In clinical practice (and sometimes in research), it is important for a measure to have clinical relevance, but also to be as simple and brief as possible – as, for example, with the severity index [26] and the ICIQ-SF (see below). Ultimately, the most important issue is that the most appropriate questionnaire should be used for the particular purpose intended.

V. RELATIONSHIPS BETWEEN QUESTIONNAIRES AND CLINICAL MEASURES

The relationship between urinary symptoms, the results of urodynamic investigations and quality of life impairment is complex. Each has an important role to play in the assessment of patients with urinary incontinence, and it is tempting to speculate that each would be related, in a direct and meaningful way. Quality of life assessment has become the recognised way to assess the impact of urinary symptoms on patients lives. Measuring the nature of symptoms is increasingly important if we are to accept symptom based definitions for conditions such as overactive bladder (OAB) [27].

On the whole, few and weak relationships have been found between the presence of lower urinary tract symptoms (including incontinence) and clinical measures such as urodynamics. This has been investigated amongst men with lower urinary tract symptoms and/or bladder outlet obstruction, where urinary flow rates, residual urine volumes and pressure-flow measures have been found to have very little relationship with lower urinary tract symptoms [28, 29, 30, 31, 32, 33]. The relationships between LUTS and uroflow variables have been shown to be poor [34].

Among women, the picture appears more complex. Although there is a move towards symptom based diagnoses and conservative treatments, research has shown that urinary symptoms alone inaccurately reflect the cause of lower urinary tract dysfunction. Jarvis et al, for example, compared the results of clinical and urodynamic diagnosis for 100 women referred for investigation of lower urinary tract disorders [35]. There was agreement in 68% of cases of genuine stress incontinence, but only 51% of cases of detrusor instability. The study found that although nearly all of the women with genuine stress incontinence complained of symptoms of stress incontinence, 46% also complained of urgency; and of the women with detrusor instability, 26% also had symptoms of stress incontinence [35].

Bergman and Bader evaluated 122 incontinent patients and found that a detailed urinary symptoms questionnaire had a positive predictive value of 80% for genuine stress incontinence, and only 25% for detrusor instability [36]. Versi et al, using an analysis of symptoms for the prediction of genuine stress incontinence in 252 patients found that such a system achieved a correct classification of 81% with a false positive rate of 16% [37]. Lagro Janssen et al showed that symptoms of stress incontinence in the absence of symptoms of urge incontinence had a sensitivity of 78%, specificity of 84% and a positive predictive value of 87% [38]. Kaupalla and Kujansuu tried to solve the problem of differentiating between women with detrusor instability and stress incontinence by using an urgency score composed of responses to ten structured questions [39]. They found that 81% of patients with stress incontinence had an urgency score of less than 6 compared to 26% of patients with detrusor instability [39].

Several studies have demonstrated that where stress incontinence is the only symptom reported, then genuine stress incontinence is likely to be present in over 90% of cases [40, 41]. Unfortunately, few patients present with symptoms of stress incontinence alone [42]. Individuals with diagnoses by urodynamics cannot be differentiated by questionnaires [43, 44].

Although lower urinary tract symptoms are diagnostically disappointing many patients are treated on the basis of their symptoms alone. This is particularly the case when conservative therapies are used for patients without complex pathology and when there are no contraindications to empirical treatment. Approximately 50-100 million women worldwide are thought to suffer from OAB; although many are never investigated or treated. The use of a symptom based diagnosis offers recognition that these patients have a medical condition worthy of consideration and initial treatment, without necessarily the need for complex, expensive, embarrassing and invasive urodynamic investigations.

The severity of urinary symptoms is often used as a measure of the impact of lower urinary tract dysfunction in both clinical practice and clinical trials. At its simplest severity may reflect symptom magnitude, for example the number of incontinent episodes, the number of daily voids, or the number of episodes of nocturia. Measuring the magnitude of symptoms is relatively straight forward but offers little insight into their impact.

Fraser et al showed a poor correlation between the subjective degree of incontinence measured by a visual analogue scale and leakage as measured by pad testing [45]. Kujansuu et al, demonstrated a low correlation between the physical effort for leakage and the clinical grade of incontinence [46]. Similarly, McCormack found a poor correlation between information on urinary frequency and micturition chart findings and between the measured and subjective bladder capacities [47].

Symptoms alone do not adequately assess the impact of urinary incontinence on an individual's life - this requires the use of symptom or generic/condition-specific questionnaires, although again, relationships between these measures and clinical assessments are relatively weak [48, 49, 50, 51]. Hunskaar et al used the Sickness Impact Profile to evaluate incontinent women with stress or urge incontinence [49]. Mean scores on the SIP were low for both groups, but the study concluded that the impact of incontinence on quality of life was both age and symptom dependent. [49]. Grimby et al compared the Nottingham Health Profile scores for women divided into three groups according to pad tests, a urinary diary, a cough provocation test and clinical history: urge incontinence, stress incontinence, or both [52]. A significantly higher level of emotional impairment and social isolation was found amongst those with urge and mixed incontinence than those with stress incontinence [52].

Wyman et al, using the IIQ, showed that women with detrusor instability experienced greater psychosocial dysfunction as a result of their urinary symptoms than women with genuine stress incontinence, although no relationship was found between the questionnaire score and urinary diary or pad test results [51]. Norton found a moderate relationship between clinical measures of urinary incontinence and the effect of incontinence on various aspects of daily life [48]. More recently, Kobelt has shown that the severity of symptoms of incontinence as expressed as frequency of voids and leakage correlates well with patient's quality of life and health status, as well as the amount they are willing to pay for a given percentage reduction in their symptoms [53].

Although it is of value to measure the bother caused by individual symptoms, it is important to appreciate that the majority of patients present with a multitude of different symptoms. These may change as a result of time and adaptive change, or as a result of treatment. It is accepted that patients with stress incontinence may develop frequency in order to limit stress leakage, and that these symptoms may be more problematic than the stress urinary leakage itself. Urinary symptoms and voiding dysfunction can follow surgery for genuine stress incontinence and voiding dysfunction in addition to distressing antimuscarinic side effects can follow the drug treatment of overactive bladder. Such changes can negatively impact on the overall QoL of patients. In a recent study using the King's Health Questionnaire to assess the outcome of surgery for stress incontinence it was found that two women cured of their stress incontinence had deterioration in their QoL as a result of surgery. One woman had developed the new symptom of pain attributable to the surgical procedure and the other deterioration in her irritative bladder symptoms [54].

The importance of quantifying the multidimensional effects of urinary symptoms in an objective way is incorporated into QoL questionnaires, which address the traditional domains of QoL assessment. This embraces the concept that urinary symptoms affect different people in different ways dependent on many interrelated personal attributes, values and priorities which themselves may change in response to life circumstances and experience.

In incontinence research, perhaps more so than in other diseases or conditions, morbidity is measured by proxy endpoints that are multidimensional and not always independent, such as the number of micturitions and volume voided. The relationship of these research endpoints to the lives of patients is not well understood. For example, do fewer incontinence episodes improve quality of life or is it the volume of an incontinent episode that is of most concern to patients? Incontinent patients find that many aspects of their lives are affected by the condition, including social, psychological, occupational, domestic, physical, and sexual aspects. Loss of urinary control is associated with an increased incidence of urinary tract infections, skin infections, falls and fractures as associated co-morbidities [55].

Thus, overall, there is only a weak relationship between symptomatic, QoL and objective urodynamic assessment of patients with lower urinary tract symptoms. Filling symptoms may have the greatest impact on patients, although the type, severity or number of symptoms, or the results of urodynamic investigations cannot predict the level of impairment. Few studies have, however, used validated instruments to assess the relationships between lower urinary tract symptoms, objective investigations and impairment in quality of life. It is perhaps not surprising that what is demonstrated clinically is distinct and different from what is perceived by patients in their everyday lives to be troublesome: clinical measures and validated questionnaires probably measure different but related aspects of incontinence.

VI. QUESTIONNAIRE DEVELOPMENT AND TESTING - A CONCLUSION

Self-completed questionnaires are the most suitable method for assessing the patient's perspective of their incontinence and its impact on their quality of life [56]. Questionnaires may be long and detailed for use in research, but need to be short and easy to use to be relevant for clinical practice. In addition to being valid and reliable, they need to be easy to complete, and, if they are being used to measure outcome, sensitive to change. Developing a new questionnaire and testing it thoroughly takes a great deal of time and is only necessary if there is not an existing instrument available. While there are many questionnaires available for assessing incontinence and its impact on quality of life, there is not a simple robust measure that is relevant to as wide a range of patients as possible. At the first consultation, it was decided that this committee would be charged with developing a new modular questionnaire incorporating sections on all major aspects of incontinence and its impact on quality of life for use as widely as possible in research (the modular ICIQ), with the production also of a very short measure that could be added to all studies and used in clinical practice (the ICIQ-SF). The work on the modular version is currently ongoing, but considerable progress has been made in devising the short form (see below).

A detailed review of recommended questionnaires was provided in the First Consultation document [1]. In this Second Consultation chapter, the Committee developed standardised grades of recommendation for questionnaires and applied them to evaluate all questionnaires concerned with incontinence. In the sections that follow, the grades of recommendation are explained and the recommended questionnaires are described. Questionnaires which reach the recommended standard of psychometric testing but do not include questions specifically on urinary incontinence but are in areas related to incontinence are listed in Appendix II.

A. GRADES OF RECOMMENDATION FOR QUESTIONNAIRES

Table 1 below explains the basis for the Committee's recommendations. The Committee required evidence published in peer-reviewed journal articles or book chapters to reach its decision about the grade of recommendation. The Committee decided that evidence published in abstracts or posters could be used to indicate a developing questionnaire's potential, but was not sufficiently peer-reviewed to provide the basis for a stronger recommendation.

As the developmental work for the ICIQ-SF has not yet been independently published, this questionnaire currently carries Grade C status, although will reach Grade A when the material is published.

B. QUESTIONNAIRES TO ASSESS SYMPTOMS OF INCONTINENCE

Box 1 lists the questionnaires and grades of recommendation for the assessment of symptoms of incontinence.

Questionnaires to assess symptoms of incontinence, often in the presence of other lower urinary tract symptoms, originally developed separately for men and women. However, increasingly, the questionnaires reaching the highest level of recommendation are being tested for use in both men and women (for example the UDI, King's Health Questionnaire and the ICS*male*/BFLUTS questionnaires. Each of the recommended questionnaires is described below.

Box 1. Questionnaires recommended to assess symptoms of incontinence

GRADE A : HIGHLY RECOMMENDED

Urogenital Distress Inventory [57]

UDI-6 [50]

Urge-UDI [58]

King's Health Questionnaire [59]

(Women only) **Incontinence Severity Index** [60]

(Men only) **DAN-PSS-1** [61]

(Men only) **ICS*male*.** [62]

(Men only) **ICS*male*SF** [63]

GRADE B: RECOMMENDED

Bristol Lower Urinary Tract Symptoms [64]

Symptom Severity Index [65]

GRADE C: WITH POTENTIAL

Der Inkontinenz-Fragebogen [66]

Danish LUTS [67]

Post-surgical questionnaire [3]

Voiding patterns [68]

Incontinence screening questionnaire [69]

Post-radical prostatectomy questionnaire [70]

Table 1 : Criteria for recommendation of questionnaires

Grade of recommendation	Evidence required
Highly recommended (**Grade A**)	Published data indicating that the questionnaire is **valid**, **reliable** and **responsive** to change following standard psychometric testing. Evidence must be published on all three aspects and questionnaires must be relevant for use with persons with urinary incontinence.
Recommended (**Grade B**)	Published data indicating that the questionnaire is **valid** and **reliable** following standard psychometric testing. Evidence must be published on two of the three main aspects (usually validity and reliability).
With potential (**Grade C**)	Published data (including abstracts) indicating that the questionnaire is **valid** or **reliable** or **responsive** to change following standard psychometric testing.

I. UROGENITAL DISTRESS INVENTORY (UDI) [GRADE A]

This questionnaire was developed in the US with women to assess the degree to which symptoms associated with incontinence are troubling [57]. It contains 19 lower urinary tract symptoms [57] It has been shown to have acceptable levels of validity, reliability and responsiveness in a community-dwelling population of women with incontinence [57] and in women over 60 years [71]. Results of a study with a Dutch version of the UDI have been published recently [72]. The UDI is being used increasingly in male patients, although data on its psychometric properties have not yet been reported as fully as they have in female patients.

1. UDI-6 (SHORT FORM) [GRADE A]

A short-form version of the UDI has been produced by regression analysis, with preliminary validation on samples of older adult males and females [50, 73]. It has been suggested that the UDI-6 may provide predictive information regarding urodynamic findings in women, particularly with regard to stress urinary incontinence, bladder outlet obstruction, and detrusor overactivity [74, 75]. A French language version of the UDI-6 has been reported in the literature [76].

2. U-UDI [GRADE A]

Lubeck, Brown, and colleagues in the U.S. have developed an Urge-Urinary Distress Inventory (U-UDI) to measure the symptoms and distress specific to urge incontinence in women [58, 77]. The UDI was modified by adding and deleting questionnaire items to measure symptoms associated with urge incontinence, based on focus group information [78], expert clinical opinion, and reviews of scientific literature. The final U-UDI contains 9 questions assessing frequent urination, urgency to empty your bladder, difficulty holding urine, urine leakage, urine leakage related to the feeling of urgency, urine leakage related to physical acitivity, coughing or sneezing, urine leakage not related to urgency or activity, night-time urination, and bedwetting. Participants indicate whether they have experienced these problems, and then rate the 'bothersomeness' of these symptoms on a 4 point scale from 'not at all,' 'slightly,' 'moderately,' and 'greatly.' The items in the questionnaire are averaged to form two scales: one summarising urge symptoms, and an overall score summarising the impact of mixed and urge symptoms. Higher scores indicate a higher degree of bothersomeness.

In two published studies of the U-UDI, the internal consistency reliability of the U-UDI has ranged from Cronbach alpha =.81-.84 for the urge symptoms subscale,[58, 77] and .86 for the overall score [58]. Intraclass correlation coefficients of test-retest reliability has ranged from .59 - .71 [58,77]. Guyatt's statistics assessing responsiveness to change were reported as –0.84 for participants with a stable number of incontinent episodes, and –1.71 for participants who showed an improvement in their number of incontinent episodes [58]. The scale has demonstrated acceptable convergent and discriminant validity [77]. Further work on this scale is underway.

II. KING'S HEALTH QUESTIONNAIRE [GRADE A]

The KHQ has been shown to have good reliability and validity for both males and females [59, 79, 80, 81]. Significant correlations were found with domains of the Short Form 36 health survey questionnaire. The KHQ has been translated into different language versions by MAPI Research using the IQOLA approach established for the SF-36 translations which takes the cultural aspects of health into consideration [82]. There are eight validated cultural adaptations of the questionnaire available in 26 languages, including German, Spanish, Swedish, Greek, Italian, and Japanese.).

The questionnaire is currently only available from the authors on request via e-mail at ConJK@aol.com or by writing to Professor Linda Cardozo at 8 Devonshire Place, London W1, England. In this way the use of the questionnaire and current studies employing its usage can be monitored.

The King's Health Questionnaire has been used to assess responses to clinical changes in a recent study comparing the effects of 10 weeks of tolterodine or oxybutynin therapy on OAB symptoms in 294 patients over 50 years of age [83]. Patients completed both generic instruments (SF-36 and the Euro-QoL) and the King's Health Questionnaire. Mean scores for the King's Health Questionnaire, corrected for comorbidity, were significantly higher in younger than in older women, with higher scores indicating greater impairment. Less significant effect on quality of life in older women may be a result of adaptive changes made by women over time, or possibly that younger women have more active lifestyles and thus perceive symptoms as more bothersome. Women who received either tolterodine or oxybutynin therapy during the study showed significant improvements from baseline in all domains other than health perceptions and interpersonal relationships. There were no significant differences in mean scores obtained from the SF-36 or Euro-QoL during the 10 weeks course of treatment; however, when measured with the King's Health Questionnaire, the quality of life improved significantly.

Responsiveness to clinical intervention has also recently been demonstrated in placebo controlled Phase 3 Tolterodine studies for women with overactive bladder [84]. 1529 patients with OAB were included in a randomized, parallel groups, double-blind, multinational study designed to compare the efficacy and safety of two dosage forms of tolterodine with placebo. This is the largest published QoL study of OAB patients.

Treatment comparisons were based on two primary dimensions, Role Limitations and Incontinence Impact selected *a priori* using an intent-to-treat population for whom KHQ translations were available. Multiple comparisons were corrected with Hochberg's procedure [82]. Criteria for a clinically meaningfulness difference was estimated without consideration for treatment group. The tolterodine SR group experienced significant and clinically meaningful improvement in Role Limitations scores compared with the placebo group ($p \leq 0.0002$) which means fewer limitations were imposed on their ability to perform household tasks, perform work, and carry out other normal daily activities. Patients in the tolterodine SR group also experienced significant improvement in Incontinence Impact scores compared with the placebo group ($p \leq 0.0001$), but the difference between the groups failed to meet the meaningful difference criteria.

Patients in the tolterodine SR group experienced statistically significant and clinically meaningful improvements in Severity (coping) Measures compared to placebo which means reductions in behaviours used to cope with OAB, such as wearing pads, monitoring fluid intake, and changing clothes, as well as worrying about an odour or experiencing embarrassment. Patients receiving tolterodine SR also experienced significant improvements in Symptom Severity, Physical Limitations, and Sleep and Energy versus the placebo group ($p \leq 0.006$) that did not exceed the meaningful difference criteria. HRQOL, measured by the KHQ, improved with tolterodine 4 mg SR treatment. Patients in the tolterodine group experienced statistically significant and clinically meaningful improvements in Role Limitations and Severity (coping) Measures and statistically significant improvements in Incontinence Impact, Physical Limitations, Sleep and Energy, and Symptom Severity compared with the placebo group.

The KHQ has also been used to assess the outcome of surgery for the treatment of genuine stress incontinence [85]. Bidmead et al have reported the results of both a subjective and objective follow up of patients with genuine stress incontinence treated by colposuspension. Colposuspension was performed in a standardised fashion and videourodynamic, symptom and quality of life assessment was performed before and between 6 to 12 months after surgery. 83 women completed the study of whom 51 underwent primary surgery and and 26 secondary. There was a broad general agreement between objective urodynamic changes demonstrating continence as a result of surgery and symptom and QoL score improvements. In addition pad usage pre and post operatively followed the general trend towards improved QoL. Interestingly two women had poorer QoL

Figure 1 : Difference in Mean KHQ Change Scores

KHQ	Tolterodine PR vs Placebo	Meaningful difference criteria
Incontinence Impact	-6.75*	-7.91
Role Limitations	-7.36*+	-6.29
Physical Limitations	-6.43*	-7.67
Social Limitations	-2.50	-4.44
Personal Relationships	-1.38	-2.12
Emotions	-2.40	-5.15
Sleep and Energy	-3.85*	-4.91
Severity (coping) Measures	-5.58*+	-4.49
General Health Perception	-0.13	-3.05
Symptom Severity	-1.46*	-1.68

* Statistically significant from placebo using Hochberg procedure with $p<0.05$.

+ Exceeded minimum criteria for meaningful difference.

scores after surgery, although the surgery had cured their stress incontinence. One woman had distressing irritative bladder symptoms and the second pain related to suture placement. On conventional testing both of these women would have been considered a successful surgical cure, although this was not upheld by QoL assessment. A total of 11 women had persistent stress incontinence on urodynamic testing after surgery. These women would normally be considered to have had failed surgery, although examination of their KHQ scores demonstrated a significant improvement in QoL for all women. Thie improvement in QoL compared favourably with the scores of women cured of their stress inbcontinence on urodynamic testing.

Studies are currently underway to develop a weighting system for the symptom subscale of the questionnaire, a QALY derived measure from the questionnaire and establish a clinical meaningfulness interpretation of KHQ scores. Three additional language translations are currently being performed.

III. INCONTINENCE SEVERITY INDEX (ISI) [GRADE A]

This was developed in Norway to provide a simple severity index of female incontinence for use in epidemiological surveys [60]. It comprises two questions – how often do you experience urine leakage (four levels), and how much urine do you lose (two levels). The index is calculated by multiplying the two responses together and is categorised into slight, moderate, severe and very severe [86]. The authors advocated its use routinely as a semi-objective and quantitative measure which does not include the woman's subjective perception of her leakage as being a problem or not. The index has good levels of validity, reliability and responsiveness. It was able to distinguish between women with incontinence and those without compared with pad tests, and confirmed a higher rate of prevalence in middle age [60]. It has also been shown to have good test-retest reliability and to be sensitive to change following surgery [26].

IV. DAN-PSS-1 [GRADE A]

This questionnaire was designed in Denmark to measure the degree to which men are bothered by urinary symptoms [87, 88]. It has been developed and tested for use with men only. A composite score is achieved by the multiplication of the 'symptom' by the 'bother' score, with a total range of 0 to 108 [87, 88]. The questionnaire has shown acceptable levels of validity and reliability, [88] and was shown to be responsive in the assessment of the outcome of TURP and drug therapies [88].

V. ICS*MALE* AND ICSMALESF QUESTIONNAIRES [GRADE A]

The ICS*male* and ICS*male*SF questionnaires have been developed for use with men only (although the BFLUTS questionnaire for women is almost identical). The ICS*male* questionnaire contains 22 questions on 20 urinary symptoms, and, for most questions, the degree of problem that the symptom causes. It has exhibited acceptable levels of validity, reliability and sensitivity to change following a range of treatments including surgery, minimally invasive therapies and drug treatments [62, 89,90].

Most recently, a scored short-form of the questionnaire has been produced – ICS*male*SF [63]. The developmental version of the questionnaire was subjected to a range of statistical tests including factor analysis, Cronbach's alpha and regression models within a randomised trial of treatments for men with LUTS and the questionnaire was reduced to two major sections: ICS*male*VS (voiding subscore) containing five questions (hesitancy, straining, reduced stream, intermittency, incomplete emptying), and ICS*male*IS (incontinence subscore) containing six questions(urge, stress, unpredictable and nocturnal incontinence, urgency, postmicturition dribble) [63]. The scores are obtained by simple addition. The authors indicate that questions to assess nocturia, frequency and impact on quality of life should be added to provide full data, but these questions should not be included in the score as they are separate constructs, as indicated by the statistical analysis [63].

VI. BRISTOL LOWER URINARY TRACT SYMPTOMS (BFLUTS) [GRADE B]

This questionnaire was developed for use with women only in the UK, following the pattern established for the questionnaire developed for the ICS-'BPH' study. The questionnaire covers the occurrence and bothersomeness of symptoms relating to incontinence and other lower urinary tract symptoms [64]. It has shown good levels of validity and reliability, and responsiveness and a scoring scheme are currently under development. The questionnaire has also been used to assess incontinence in both sexes in Austria [91] and is being increasingly used in epidemiological and outcome studies [92, 93, 94, 95, 96, 97, 98].

VII. SYMPTOM SEVERITY INDEX (SSI) [GRADE B]

This short questionnaire was developed in the UK for women only to assess stress incontinence [65]. It has shown acceptable levels of validity and reliability, but responsiveness has not been assessed [65].

VIII. DANISH LUTS [GRADE C]

This questionnaire was published from Denmark [67] but the layout and questions suggest that it is based on the ICS*male* and BFLUTS questionnaires [62, 64].

IX. DER INKONTINENZ-FRAGEBOGEN [GRADE C]

The aim of this questionnaire, published in German, is to differentiate between women with stress and urge incontinence (as determined by cystometry), with the intention of avoiding the need for urodynamics in all women [66].

X. POST-SURGICAL QUESTIONNAIRE [GRADE C]

A questionnaire was devised by the authors for patients to report levels of incontinence, other urinary and sexual symptoms, and satisfaction with treatment after bladder neck suspension surgery [3].

XI. VOIDING PATTERNS (DENMARK) [GRADE C]

A questionnaire was designed to assess the prevalence of incontinence and voiding patterns among women aged 29 to 79 years in Denmark but the methods of development and testing were not specified [68].

XII. INCONTINENCE SCREENING QUESTIONNAIRE (AUSTRALIA) [GRADE C]

Gunthrope and colleagues (2000) have completed preliminary validation of a screening questionnaire to assess urinary incontinence in female patients in primary care settings [69]. The resulting 5 item scale was capable of predicting almost 70% of patients who showed objective leakage of urine and misclassified fewer that 15% of these patients.

XIII. POST-RADICAL PROSTATECTOMY QUESTIONNAIRE [GRADE C]

This questionnaire was devised in the US to assess incontinence and other side-effects following radical prostatectomy for prostate cancer [70, 99]. Some preliminary testing for validity has been carried out [70, 100].

C. QUESTIONNAIRES TO ASSESS IMPACT ON QUALITY OF LIFE

The concept 'quality of life' is a complex one. A number of key domains are typically included within it, including physical, psychological and social functioning, pain overall life satisfaction, perception of health status, sometimes supplemented by others including sleep disturbance, neuropsychological functioning, sexual functioning and/or satisfaction, and participation in employment (see [1, 101] for further details). Quality of life measures can be classified into four main categories and recommended questionnaires in each category are reproduced below.

I. GENERIC MEASURES

These self-administered questionnaires aim to measure the multidimensional nature of health status and are suitable for a broad range of illnesses and populations. They do not contain specific questions on incontinence, but they have been widely used to assess the quality of life of incontinent adults on the assumption that incontinence has an impact on the general well-being of a given individual. They tend, however to be relatively insensitive to conditions such as incontinence.

All questionnaires listed have reached the highest levels of evidence relating to psychometric testing. Those highly recommended are the most commonly used for incontinence.

Box 2. Questionnaires recommended to assess generic health status in persons with incontinence

GRADE A : HIGHLY RECOMMENDED

SF-36 [102]

EuroQol EQ-5D [103]

GRADE B: RECOMMENDED

Whilst the following questionnaires have reached the highest levels of evidence relating to psychometric testing, they have only rarely been used in incontinence:

Sickness Impact Profile [104,105,106]

Nottingham Health Profile [107]

Goteborg Quality of Life [108]

1. MEDICAL OUTCOMES STUDY SHORT-FORM: SF-36 [GRADE A]

The MOS Short Form - 36 (SF-36) [102] has been used

for QoL assessment of men and women. When used with men who presented with moderate to severe urinary symptoms, the SF-36 profile was worse than that of the general population [109, 110] Kutner et al. (1994) applied the SF-36 to 352 community-dwelling elderly, of whom 14% (n=47) had urge incontinence and significantly lower scores in each of the subscales [111]. The internal consistency of the scales varied from .78 to .93 [112]. Used as an interview instead of a self-administered scale, the SF-36 has shown an internal consistency of 0.80 or better [113].

Mozes and colleagues (1999) examined the relationship between urinary symptoms and various domains of the SF-36 in 960 men taking into account their co-morbid status [114]. In the entire population, severely bothersome urinary symptoms were related to scores on three SF-36 domains: social functioning, role-emotional, and mental health. In men without co-morbidity, however, urinary symptoms were substantially related to physical functioning and general health perceptions. These findings indicated that the relative weight of the impact of urinary symptoms on quality of life may change by the presence of co-morbidities or other competing factors, such as sociodemographic characteristics.

In a study examining the use of the SF-36 to assess quality of life across six chronic disorders (incontinence, prostate cancer, COPD, AIDS, fibromyalgia, hyperlipidaemia), the measure demonstrated good discriminant and construct validity [115]. The incontinent patients were similar to the COPD and AIDS patients, in having lower physical functioning, role-physical, general health, vitality, and role-emotional domain scores than the patients with other chronic conditions. However, sample sizes within each of the six groups were low (range=n12 to n=213). In pooling the data across the six studies (n-321), the internal consistency of the subscales was very acceptable (alpha=.80 - .97). Good construct validity was also reported with the pooled data, by correlating the SF-36 with the Center for Epidemiologic Studies – Depression Scale, the Hamilton Depression Rating Scale, and several functional status and other psychological scales. These results suggest similarities in the impact of quality of life on daily life across conditions, although the factors that influcnce the individual domain scores (e.g., age, condition severity) could vary substantially by the type of chronic condition evaluated.

Test-retest reliability has been moderate to high (r = 0.60-0.80) [116]. However, responsiveness has been reported to be poor in several studies [17, 117, 118] and specifically in benign prostatitic hyperplasia (BPH) patients [119], prostate cancer patients, [120] and women with stress urinary incontinence (SUI) [121]. In an unpublished randomised trial comparing surgery and collagen injections in the treatment of stress incontinence, poor responsiveness was found with an effect size ranging from 0.13 to 0.34 for collagen injections and 0.01 to 0.35 for surgery (Corcos, unpublished data). In addition, no significant differences were found between or within groups in a community-based UI intervention for women aged 65 years or older on measured individual domains of the SF-36 [122].

In recent years, the use of the physical (PCS) and mental (MCS) health summary scores for the SF-36 have been used to assess incontinence [123]. In a study of 37,814 women from the Women's Health Australia Project, the adjusted PCS and MCS scores were lower in young (aged 18-23), middle-aged (45-50), and older (aged 70-75) women who reported leaking urine. [124] However, the greatest differences were reported in the MCS scores in the young and middle-aged women, indicating that the quality of life impact was greater among younger versus the oldest age group of women. No information was provided in the article regarding the reliability of the measures, although the adjusted means reported were comparable to the published norms for the PCS and MSC published elsewhere [123 125].

The SF-36 has been culturally adapted and/or translated into several languages, including German, Spanish and French. A derivative of the SF-36, the MOS Short Form, containing only 12 items, has been found to perform poorly with prostatectomy patients [126].

2. EuroQol/EQ-5D [Grade A]

The EQ-5D questionnaire, developed by the EuroQol group, consists of the EQ-5D self-classifier, the EQ VAS and the EQ SDQ (standard set of socio-demographic questions). Respondents are asked to describe their own health status using self-classifier [127] with a five-dimensional health state classification system of mobility, self-care, usual activities, pain/discomfort and anxiety/depression. Each of these dimensions records three levels of severity, which are indicated by numbers. No problems are coded '1', some or moderate problems '2' and extreme problems '3'. A health state can therefore be described with a five-digit number, for instance 12113. This means 'no problems' on the dimension of mobility, 'some problems' on the dimension of self-care, 'no problems' with respect to usual activities and pain/discomfort and 'severe problems' on the dimension of anxiety/depression. The classification system defines 243 health states. In addition, the states of unconsciousness and death are included. Currently there are 31 official versions of EQ-5D, of which 11 are adaptations (e.g. Spanish for Argentina). A further 19 have been completed and are awaiting official ratification by the EuroQol Group's Translation Committee.

The EQ VAS is a standard vertical 20 cm visual analogue scale for recording respondents' rating of their current health state on a 0-100 scale. A similar VAS is used when valuing hypothetically.

EQ-5D is a standardised instrument for use as a measure of health outcomes. EQ-5D is designed for self-completion by respondents and is ideally suited for use in postal surveys, in clinics and face to face interviews. It is cognitively simple, taking only a few minutes to complete. Instructions to respondents are included in the questionnaire. Applicable to a wide range of health conditions and treatments, it provides a simple descriptive profile and a single index value for heath status, from which QALY (Quality Adjusted Life Years) can be calculated, and that can be used in the clinical and economic evaluation of health care as well as population heath surveys. EQ-5D has been a specially designed to complement other quality of life measures such as the SF-36, NHP, SIP or disease-specific measures. It is one of a handful of measures recommended by the Washington Panel on Cost-Effectivenesss. In the UK, a NHS Task Group has been set up to co-ordinate the testing of EQ-5D as an outcome measure for use by clinicians and managers (www.europol.org).

Construct validity of the EQ-5D in the assessment of urinary incontinence on quality of life was tested in 1997 [53]. The study showed a good correlation between EQ-5D index and urinary symptoms. More evidence of the construct validity of the EQ-5D in urinary incontinence was demonstrated in another study which showed strong relationships between the EQ-5D index and general quality of life questions in ICS*QoL*, and a moderate relationship with the question associated with incontinence ($p=0.0022$). On the other hand, much weaker relationships were found with other specific impact questions [110].

The EQ-5D was included in an open, prospective multicenter, clinical trial conducted on 75 women with urinary incontinence with overactive bladders in order to determine the effects of trospium chloride on quality of life [128]. The results showed an improvement in quality of life and urodynamic parameters which reflect the EQ-5D sensitivity to change in the assessment of changes in urinary incontinence.

3. Sickness Impact Profile [Grade B]

The full 136-item version of the Sickness Impact Profile (SIP) was used in Norway to assess the quality of life of women with urinary incontinence [49]. Overall, the impact of incontinence was highest on sleep and rest, emotional behaviour, social interaction and recreation/past-times [49]. No new reports of the use of the SIP in observational and clinical trials of UI and BPH have been reported since the last review.

4. Nottingham Health Profile [Grade B]

The Nottingham Health Profile (NHP) has been used in Sweden to assess the quality of life of women with incontinence compared with an age-matched sample. [52]. Overall, all women with incontinence were more socially isolated than those in the general population [52]. The use of the NHP to assess incontinence has been minimal in recent years.

5. Göteborg Quality Of Life Instrument (GQL) [Grade B]

This questionnaire was designed in Sweden to assess general levels of health and their impact on well-being [108]. It was constructed originally for men, but has been tested on women. In a study of community based women in Sweden, those with incontinence were found to have significantly lower scores than continent women on four of the subscales: health, sleep, fitness and work satisfaction [129].

6. Generic measures - conclusion

In general, although several of the generic measures have achieved acceptable reliability and validity in individuals with incontinence, no measures have been shown to have sufficient sensitivity to detect changes in condition severity as a result of either treatment or a worsening/improving physical condition. The generic instruments, however, may be useful in comparing across chronic conditions or to describe the general health status of incontinent adults.

II. CONDITION-SPECIFIC MEASURES – BOTHERSOMENESS

Condition-specific measures are designed to assess the impact of incontinence on quality of life. The simplest are those concerned with the particular impact of incontinent symptoms, otherwise known as 'bothersomeness.'

For details of these questionnaires, see above – these are all highly recommended or recommended symptom questionnaires.

Box 3. Questionnaires recommended to assess bothersomeness in persons with incontinence

Grade A: Highly Recommended

DAN-PSS-1 [87]

ICS*male* [62]

Grade B: Recommended

BFLUTS [64]

III. CONDITION-SPECIFIC MEASURES - IMPACT OF INCONTINENCE ON QUALITY OF LIFE

A number of condition-specific measures have been designed to assess the wider impact of incontinence on aspects of everyday quality of life. Most have been developed for either men or women, although a small number are being evaluated for use in both sexes.

Box 4. Questionnaires recommended to assess the impact of incontinence on quality of life

GRADE A: HIGHLY RECOMMENDED

(Men and women) **Quality of life in persons with urinary incontinence (I-QoL).** [130]

(Men and women) **King's Health Questionnaire** [59]

(Women only) **Incontinence Impact Questionnaire (IIQ)** [131]

(Women only) **IIQ-7.** [50]

(Women only) **Urge-IIQ**. [58]

(Men only) **Modified IIQ and IIQ-7.** [132]

GRADE B: RECOMMENDED

(Women only) **Symptom Impact Index (SII)**. [65]

(Men only) **ICS*QoL*.** [110]

(Men only) **EORTC metastatic prostate cancer**. [133]

(Men only) **Changes in Urinary Function**.134

(Men only) **Prostate-targeted Health Related Quality of Life**. [120]

(Men only) **Functional Assessment of Cancer – Bladder/ General Scales.** [134 135]

GRADE C: WITH POTENTIAL

SEAPI QMM.136

Overactive Bladder Symptom and Health-related Quality of life (OAB-q).

(Women only) York Incontinence Perceptions Scale (YIPS). [137]

(Women only) Stress Incontinence Questionnaire (SIQ). [138]

Incontinence Stress Index. [139]

BFLUTS*QoL*. [64]

Psychosocial consequences questionnaire. [140]

Philadelphia Geriatric Center Multilevel Assessment Instrument. [141]

QOL – Synthelabo. [142]

Symptom and psychological status in stress incontinence [143]

Post-radical radiotherapy questionnaire [144]

1. QUALITY OF LIFE IN PERSONS WITH URINARY INCONTINENCE (I-QOL) [GRADE A]

This questionnaire was designed to be used in clinical trials to measure the impact of incontinence on men and women [130]. The questionnaire reaches acceptable levels of validity and reliability [130]. Reports of the use of the I-Qol in a multi-centre, double-blind placebo controlled, randomised trial confirmed the use of an overall score and three subscale scores (avoidance and limiting behaviours, psychosocial impacts, and social embarrassment) [145]. All scores achieved high internal consistency (alpha=0.87-0.93), and reproducibility (intraclass correlations – 0.87-0.91). Responsiveness statistics using changes in stress test pad weight, number of incontinent episodes, and patient global impression of the improvement of their condition ranged from 0.4-0.8. Minimally important changes ranged from 2%-5% in association with these measures and effect sizes [145].

Psychometric information on translated versions of the I-QOL have been reported for French, Spanish, Swedish, and German language versions [145]. In all countries, the use of three subscales, and an overall summary scores was confirmed. In all countries, the internal consistency (alpha=0.87-0.93) and reproducibility coefficients (intraclass correlations=0.92-0.95) were high. I-Qol scores were found to be significantly worse in all countries as perceived severity of incontinence, use of services, and the number of incontinent episodes increased. Translated versions are reported to be available in 7 other languages, but information on the psychometric properties of these instruments has not yet been published.

2. KING'S HEALTH QUESTIONNAIRE [GRADE A]

[For details, see above]

3. INCONTINENCE IMPACT QUESTIONNAIRE (IIQ) [GRADE A]

This questionnaire was developed to assess the psychosocial impact of urinary incontinence in women. It has acceptable levels of validity, reliability and responsiveness [57,131-137]. It has been used in several clinical trials,[146, 147, 148] and observational studies [149, 150, 151, 152].

A modified version has been used in men [153]. The questionnaire has also been used in Holland [72], Denmark [154], and Australia.[146] The IIQ has also been used in a study examining the use and cost of incontinence pads in the US.[155].

a) IIQ-7 (short form) [Grade A]

The IIQ has also been produced in a short form comprising 7 items, also with evidence of acceptable validity and reliability [50, 73]. A French version of the IIQ-7 was used in a study by Blanc and colleagues (1999) of stress and mixed incontinent women [76].

b) U-IIQ [Grade A]

An adapted version of the IIQ has been developed to be specific to the assessment of urge incontinence [58, 77]. The IIQ was modified by adding and deleting questionnaire items to measure symptoms associated with urge incontinence, based on focus group information, [78] expert clinical opinion, and reviews of scientific literature. The final U-IIQ contains 32 questions, arranged into 6 domains (travel, activities, feelings, physical activities, relationships, sexual function), two single items (night bladder control, and satisfaction with treatment), and a mean summary score composed of the 6 domain scales. The response categories were increased from a 4-point Likert scale to a 6-point Likert scale to allow for increased responsiveness to therapeutic changes [77]. For some questions, response categories of "never regularly do this" and "does not apply to me" were added to better characterize the impact of UI. Higher scores on the subscales and individual items indicate greater impact on daily life.

In two published reports of the U-IIQ, the internal consistency reliability of the U-IIQ has ranged from 0.74-0.96 (Cronbach alpha) for the individual subscales,[58, 77] and .90 for the overall index score [58]. Intraclass correlation coefficients of test-retest reliability has ranged from 0.68-0.88 [58, 77]. Guyatt's statistics assessing responsiveness to change were reported as –0.62 to –0.83 for participants with a stable number of incontinent episodes, and -1.00 to –1.61 for participants who showed an improvement in their number of incontinent episodes [58]. The scale has demonstrated acceptable convergent and discriminant validity [77]. Further work on this scale is reported to be underway.

c) Modified IIQ and IIQ-7 [Grade A]

A modified version of the IIQ and the IIQ-7 has been used in two studies examining the efficacy of artificial urinary sphincters in men who had developed stress incontinence after radical prostatectomy. Fleshner and Herschorn (1996) used 17 items of the IIQ to examine activities of daily living and self-perception [132]. They also changed the response choices to some of the items and added two questions from the AUA Symptoms Index. They compared 30 men receiving artificial urinary sphincters to a group of 31 men who had also undergone radical prostatectomy but who had not developed incontinence. Urinary control was similar in both groups yet several IIQ questions discriminated between groups. However, the total score was not given or analysed. The questions from the AUA Symptoms Index did not differentiate between groups (Fleshner & Herschorn, 1996) [132].

The IIQ-7 and the short form of the Urogenital Distress Inventory (UDI) were used in a study of 52 men implanted with an artificial urinary sphincter and compared to a group of 15 men with post prostatectomy incontinence. In this study, IIQ-7 scores were significantly correlated with the use of protective pads (r =.75), and the mean scores on the IIQ-7 and UDI were significantly greater after implantation of the artificial sphincter group than before [153]. Although both studies supported the validity of using the IIQ with men, it is unfortunate than none reported its reliability or responsiveness with this population.

4. Symptom Impact Index (SII) [Grade B]

This questionnaire was developed in the UK to assess the impact of stress incontinence and has acceptable levels of validity and reliability [65].

5. ICS*QoL* [Grade B]

This questionnaire is part of the ICS-'BPH' study questionnaire [89] and includes six items addressing general and specific aspects of QoL [110]. ICS*QoL* exhibits good validity but poor reliability and hence questions have to be considered independently [110].

6. EORTC metastatic prostate cancer [Grade B]

Developed in Portugal and Belgium, this questionnaire is based on other EORTC measures and aims to assess quality of life in patients with metastatic prostate cancer [133]. It has high internal consistency but test-retest reliability has not been confirmed. There is some evidence it is responsive to change following prostate cancer treatments [133].

7. Changes in Urinary Function [Grade B]

This questionnaire was tested for validity and reliability as part of a Radiation Therapy Oncology Group (RTOG) study (reported in [134]).

8. Prostate-targeted Health Related Quality of Life [Grade B]

This questionnaire consists of 20 items in three domains: sexual, urinary and bowel function and exhibits adequate validity and reliability [120].

9. Functional Assessment of Cancer Therapy - (FACT-G) and Prostate form (FACT-P) [Grade B]

A group of measures has been developed under the

general umbrella of the Functional Assessment of Cancer Therapy Scales. The FACT-BL (bladder version) has been used with patients recruited to a trial of radiation therapy in prostate cancer, and includes questions concerned with micturition, fatigue and sexuality [156].

10. SEAPI QMM Incontinence Classification System [Grade C]

This system was devised for the definition and standardisation of the measurement of incontinence in both sexes, with the aim of functioning in the same way as the TNM classification for cancers.[136] Psychometric testing is reported to have been completed, but currently this is only in the form of abstracts.

11. Overactive Bladder Symptom and Health-related Quality of life (OAB-q) [Grade C]

A questionnaire is in development by Medtap International specifically to assess the impact on quality of life of an overactive bladder in men and women. The questionnaire was developed during the National Overactive Bladder Evaluation (NOBLE) programme in the US. It contains 33 items (8 on bladder symptoms including urge incontinence and accidental loss of urine and 25 related to the impact of the symptoms on three major domains of life – concern, sleep and social. A considerable amount of work has been undertaken to evaluate the psychometric properties of this questionnaire, but it is as yet unpublished except in abstract form.

12. Stress Incontinence Questionnaire (SIQ) [Grade C]

This questionnaire, developed in the US, consists of 16 items on a four-point Likert scale to assess stress incontinence [138]. Some aspects of validity and reliability have been assessed [138].

13. York Incontinence Perceptions Scale (YIPS) [Grade C]

This questionnaire aims to evaluate psychosocial aspects of urinary incontinence and its management [137]. It has shown acceptable levels of validity, but test-retest reliability and responsiveness have not been fully assessed [137].

14. Incontinence Stress Index (ISI) [Grade C]

The original aim of this questionnaire was to measure psychological stress associated with urinary incontinence in women living in institutions [157]. but it has also been assessed for women in the community [139]. Development work using principal components and factor analyses has reduced the questionnaire to 20 items, but little data is available on psychometric properties.

15. Bristol Lower Urinary Tract Symptoms*QoL* [Grade C]

This questionnaire is the same in style as the ICS*Qol* questionnaires but only preliminary data on validity and reliability have been published [64].

16. Psychosocial Consequences Questionnaire [Grade C]

This questionnaire was developed in Norway to be used in a prospective study of the treatment of incontinence in general practice [140]. This questionnaire appears to be completed by the clinician for the patient, which has been shown to be unreliable. Test-retest reliability has not been calculated, and internal consistency is low.

17. Philadelphia Geriatric Center Multilevel Assessment Instrument (MAI) [Grade C]

This questionnaire was used to assess quality of life in housebound women in the US and has published some data indicating reliability [141].

18. QOL questionnaires concerned with incontinence (Synthelabo) [Grade C]

Questionnaires have been developed by the pharmaceutical company to assess quality of life in patients with stress and urge incontinence, but only one abstract has been published indicating these are still under development [142].

19. Symptom and psychological status in stress incontinence [Grade C]

A study was conducted in the US to assess the symptom and psychological status of women with stress incontinence but no formal evaluation of psychometric properties was undertaken [143].

20. Post-radical radiotherapy questionnaire [Grade C]

This questionnaire was developed 'ad hoc' for a specific study of radical radiotherapy and shows some evidence of adequate reliability [144].

IV. DIMENSION-SPECIFIC MEASURES – SEXUAL FUNCTION/SATISFACTION

Dimension-specific measures aim to assess just one aspect of quality of life. Questionnaires have been developed to assess aspects of sexual function and satisfaction, with a small number of these also being used to examine these factors in patients with incontinence. On the whole, these questionnaires are at the early stages of development – both psychometrically and in terms of their application to the field of urinary incontinence.

> ***Box 5. Questionnaires recommended to assess sexual function/satisfaction***
>
> **GRADE A: HIGHLY RECOMMENDED**
>
> The Psychosocial Adjustment to Illness Scale (PAIS). [158]
>
> Rust and Golombok Inventory of Sexual Satisfaction. [159]
>
> GRADE B: RECOMMENDED
>
> Brief Sexual Function Inventory. [160]
>
> BPH QOL9. [161]
>
> ICS*sex*. [162]
>
> **GRADE C: WITH POTENTIAL**
>
> BFLUTS*sex*. [163]
>
> Simple sexual function questionnaire. [164]
>
> Effect of urinary incontinence on sexuality questionnaire. [165]
>
> Effects of urinary incontinence on sexual activity questionnaire. [166]
>
> Several major symptom and quality of life questionnaires have also added single questions to assess sexual aspects. For details, see Table 2, below.

1. THE PSYCHOSOCIAL ADJUSTMENT TO ILLNESS SCALE (PAIS) [GRADE A]

This questionnaire was designed to assess the psychological and social adjustment of male and female medical patients to their illness and is in an interview or self-report format (*PAIS and PAIS-SR)* [158]. It contains a sexual relationships domain consisting of 6 items. These items assess the quality of interpersonal sexual relationships, sexual interest, frequency of sexual activity, sexual satisfaction, sexual dysfunction and interpersonal sexual conflict. Validation was carried out on groups of patients having renal dialysis, lung cancer, cardiac problems, breast cancer, and Hodgkins disease. Internal consistency of the sexual relationships domain ranged from 0.8 to 0.93 in these different clinical groups. Factor analysis confirmed the subscale structure. All 6 items in the sexual relationships domain had very marked loadings on this dimension, with no appreciable loadings from other items. Convergent validity was assessed by comparing the scale to the Global Adjustment To Illness Scale (r-0.46), the SCL-90R (r=0.13), Affect Balance Scale (r=0.42), and the Patients Attitudes, Information and Expectancies Scale (r=0.40). Discriminant validity was assessed by comparing patients screened positive and negative for lung cancer. There were differences in the mean scores between the two groups which approached significance (t=1.53, p<0.10) [101].

The PAIS has been used to investigate the impact of different types of urinary incontinence on sexual function [167] in a sample of 200 patients referred for urodynamic assessment. Compared to patients with GSI, patients having DI were significantly impaired on all items of the sexual relationships subscale, apart from the 'sexual satisfaction' item. Some aspects of validation were also carried out in a small study of 29 patients who had been treated successfully for penile cancer [168]. Internal consistency of the sexual relationships scales was good having Cronbach alpha of 0.83. Convergent and discriminant validity was shown in significant correlations with well-being scales but not with social scales. In addition, patients who had had the most radical treatments in terms of partial or total penectomy scored lower on the sexual relationships scale as did older patients (mean age 63 years) compared to younger patients (mean age 41 years), whereas having a mental disorder showed no correlation with sexual relationship scores.

2. GOLOMBOK-RUST INVENTORY OF SEXUAL SATISFACTION [GRADE A]

This questionnaire was developed systematically by sex therapists at the Maudsley Hospital Sexual Dysfunction Clinic [159]. It contains 56 items, 28 for men and 28 for women. There are four subscales covering anorgasmia, vaginismus, impotence and premature ejaculation, and 6 subscales giving separate male and female scores for avoidance, dissatisfaction and non-sensuality. A further two subscales apply to both males and females and cover infrequency and non-communication. An additional 2 items each for males and females contribute to the overall scores but are not included in the subscales. These relate to interest in sex generally.

The questionnaire was validated on a clinical sample recruited from sexual dysfunction clinics throughout the UK of 68 men and 63 women, and a control group of 29 men and 30 women randomly selected from primary care attenders. Split half reliability was 0.94 for the female scale and 0.87 for the male overall scale.

Internal consistency of subscales was, on average, 0.74. Both the overall female and male scores were found to discriminate well between clinical and non-clinical samples and scores on subscales successfully discriminated specific diagnostic groups. There was also a significant correlation between therapists ratings of severity and scores on the questionnaire. Responsiveness was assessed by comparing change in the questionnaire scores with rated improvements by sex therapists. Correlations were moderate but statistically significant (0.54 for males and 0.43 for females, $p<.005$ and $p<.01$ respectively).

This questionnaire has been used by Hunt & Moss (1996) in a small study exploring the relationship of unwanted sexual experience to detrusor instability and sexual dysfunction [169]. High levels of sexual dysfunction were found in incontinent subjects compared to other clinical groups.

3. A BRIEF MALE SEXUAL FUNCTION INVENTORY FOR UROLOGY [GRADE B]

The aim of this study was to provide a brief questionnaire concerning male sexual function that could be used for clinical and research purposes in urological settings [160]. Items were identified from the literature to produce a 50 item questionnaire which was reduced down to 22 items in a series of pilot studies for the final validation study. The questionnaire was made up of 5 subscales: libido, erectile function, ejaculation, assessment of significance of each domain and overall satisfaction. Validation was carried out on a sample of 74 men with sexual dysfunction and 60 general medical patients. Mean age was 55 and 45 years respectively. The study describes development of individual subscales down to a final questionnaire of 11 items based on measures of internal consistency and test-retest reliability. Internal consistency of the subscales ranged from 0.62 to 0.95 and ICC's from 0.79 to 0.89 for test-retest reliability. All subscales except the drive and ejaculation subscales discriminated between patients being treated for sexual dysfunction and general medical patients, but it was not expected that drive would be reduced in patients experiencing sexual dysfunction and ejaculation did not appear to be an important issue for patients.

5. QOL9 [GRADE B]

The QOL9 is a short form of the QOL20, a questionnaire previously validated in French [161]. The short form was developed using a large-scale cohort study of 7093 men with BPH who received alfuzosin for 3 months. The items were reduced by identifying questions which contributed most to establishing the global score and that reflected the structure of the questionnaire on principal components analysis.

The final, 9 item questionnaire consists of 3 items concerning general well-being, 3 items assessing BPH interferences with activities, and 3 items pertaining to patients' perceptions of their sexual life. The sexual function domain covered sexual desire, erectile function and satisfaction with sex life. The QOL9 was validated in two studies, a longitudinal study of alfuzosin, having a sample size of 4259, and a smaller cross sectional study of men having symptomatic BPH (n=48), or no symptoms of BPH (n=42), and a group of younger men (n=23). Feasibility and acceptability of the questionnaire was assessed by rates of completion of the questionnaire which was above 85%. Principal components analysis confirmed the three factor structure. Discriminant validity was measured by comparing cases and non-cases. On the sexual function domain cases scored 10.5, non-cases 15.2 and young men 26.3. The most strongly discriminating question between cases and non-cases was satisfaction with sex life. There was also a good correlation between symptom severity and the total QOL9 score. Internal consistency of the overall scale was fair with Cronbachs alpha of 0.79 for patients with BPH and 0.85 for the control groups. Test-retest reliability was good for the total score but moderate for the sexual function subscale (ICC = 0.69 - 0.88) with the quality of erection item having an ICC of 0.53. After treatment the effect size of the change in the sexual function domain was linked to age and the initial severity of symptoms but had a mean of 0.02 and 0.55 for patients treated in each of the two studies.

6. ICS*sex* [GRADE B]

The ICS*sex* is part of the ICS-BPH questionnaire. [162]. This instrument contains questions pertaining to symptoms, quality of life and sexual function. The symptom questionnaire was described in some detail in the previous consultation document but the sexual function domain has not been validated to the same extent. It consists of 4 items: to what extent sex life has been spoilt by urinary symptoms, ability to have erections, ability to ejaculate, and pain or discomfort on ejaculation. As with the other ICS questionnaires each item has an additional part to each item concerning the amount of bother the symptom causes i.e. how much of a problem is this for you?

It has been used in both clinic and community samples to assess the relationship between urinary symptoms and sexual function [162]. The strongest associations were found between storage symptoms, particularly incontinence, and sexual dysfunction. This pattern was seen in both samples. Test-retest reliability has been assessed and responses on the sexual function questions changed by one category at most, apart from the question concerning the perception that sex life has been spoilt be urinary symptoms which changed by more than one category on retest.

7. Bristol Female Lower Urinary Tract Symptoms BFLUTS*sex* [Grade C]

The BFLUTS*sex* questionnaire contains 4 questions related to sexual function: pain or discomfort due to dry vagina, whether sex life has been spoilt by urinary symptoms, pain on sexual intercourse, and leakage on intercourse. In addition to each of these items the respondent is asked how much of a problem this is for them.

Jackson et al. (1999) reported data on the sexual function questions in a study of the effects of hormone replacement therapy on post-menopausal urinary stress incontinence [163]. Sex-life spoilt by urinary symptoms was reported by around one quarter of patients and intercourse incontinence by about 10%. There was little change in these symptoms as a result of intervention, but numbers were small and the mean age was>60years with many of the sample not being sexually active. Bo, Talseth and Vinsnes (2000) also reported sexual function data using this questionnaire in a study of pelvic floor muscle training, with significant differences occurring post treatment between experimental and control groups, although this effect disappeared when baseline levels were controlled [170]. Again, however, sample sizes were small, and so responsiveness data on this questionnaire needs further evaluation.

A very similar questionnaire was devised by Bernstein et al. (1996) with some validation carried out in a clinical sample of females in Denmark [67]. This questionnaire asks whether the respondent is sexually active, whether their sex life has suffered because of urinary symptoms, leakage during intercourse and pain during intercourse. The level of accompanying bother is ascertained for 2 of the questions: impact on sex life and pain on intercourse. Missing data was found to be high for these questions, but this may reflect a low level of sexual activity in the sample. Test-retest reliability was between 69.6% and 91.1%.

8. Simple Sexual Function Questionnaire [Grade C]

Walters, Taylor and Schoenfeld (1990) used a simple, 3 item questionnaire devised by Plouffe (1985) to assess the relationship of sexual dysfunction to urodynamic diagnosis in incontinent women. The questionnaire asks if the respondent is sexually active and if so, whether there are any problems. If the respondent has problems they are asked about pain during coitus. Walters et al. (1990) added a question asking whether urinary symptoms interfered with sex [164]. Again these questions are similar to those used in the BFLUTS and the Bernstein questionnaires. Although sexual dysfunction was more prevalent in the incontinent groups there was no difference between those with GSI and those with DI.

Plouffe (1985) developed this questionnaire by comparing these three items, administered by junior interns to a sample of 57 female patients in a ward environment, to longer, more in-depth interviews carried out in private [171]. The short questionnaire was found to detect all cases of sexual dysfunction identified by in-depth interview.

9. Effect of Urinary Incontinence on Sexuality Questionnaire (EISQ) [Grade C]

This questionnaire, published in Japanese but with an English abstract, aims to evaluate the effect of incontinence on sexual function in women [165]. It exhibits good reliability and further studies are planned.

10. Effects of urinary incontinence on sexual activity [Grade C]

An eleven item questionnaire was used to assess the effects of incontinence on sexual activity in women, although no formal psychometric testing has been undertaken [166].

11. Other measures of sexual aspects

Many of the questionnaires assessing psychosocial impact of urinary symptoms contain one or possibly two questions related to sexual function. The majority of these are discussed above, either as symptom questionnaires or general quality of life questionnaires. Table 2 summarises these with particular emphasis on validation data related to the sexual activity question. Data are reported pertaining to either the subscale containing the sexual activity question or to the questionnaire as a whole when no specific information is given on the sexual activity question itself. Questionnaires containing just one question tend to focus on a general assessment of the overall impact of urinary symptoms on sexual functioning.

The Symptom Impact Index [172]. The Kings Health Questionnaire, [59] the Incontinence Impact Questionnaire, [173] and the IQOL [174] are recommended by the Committee for use as condition specific quality of life questionnaires. However, when considering the sexual items it must be borne in mind that validation of the sexual items was not always carried out e.g. Symptom Impact Index or made explicit e.g. Kings Health Questionnaire. But the questions relating to sexual function in each of the questionnaires are very similar and judgements on validity can be made by comparing questions and psychometric data between questionnaires as well as considering the psychometric properties of the scales as a whole. If more in-depth information is required concerning sexual function, the questionnaires recommended for this aspect should be used (see above).

Table 2 : Questionnaires that include one or two questions pertaining to sexual function. Questionnaires validated in women only.

Questionnaire/Authors	Sample	Topics covered in relation to sexual activity	Findings
KINGS HEALTH QUESTIONNAIRE [59]	293 women referred for urodynamics with any type of incontinence. (n=285 completed questionnaires, mean age 51.4 years))	Impact of bladder problem on sex life.	Subscale data Internal consistency -alpha =0.892 Test-retest- rho=0.87 No validation of subscale
SYMPTOM IMPACT INDEX [172]	Women undergoing surgery for Stress Incontinence (n=442 60% were between 41 and 60 years of age)	Leakage during intercourse. Impact of bladder problem on sex life.	Content validity =missing data 2.9% Validation of questionnaire did not included the sexual items
SOCIAL ACTIVITY INDEX [175]	Women with stress incontinence undergoing urodynamics (n=14, mean age 42.8 years)	Perceived ability to participate in sexual activity	Complete questionnaire data Test-retest at 1 hour - r=0.94
URGE INCONTINENCE QUALITY OF LIFE QUESTIONNAIRE [176]	Women with urge incontinence recruited from 44 investigators in France (n=98)	Anxious at the thought of sex	Internal consistency - ranged from 0.69 - 0.84 across all items Validity - total score correlated with symptom severity.
Incontinence Quality of Life Index (IQOLI) [177]	Women with urge and mixed incontinence taking part in a trial of emepronium carrageenate (n=75, aged 35-65 years)	Impact of bladder problems on enjoyment of sex life.	Complete questionnaire data Internal consistency = 0.9 Test-retest at 2 weeks - rho=0.92 Construct validity - correlation with generic QOL = 0.4 - 0.56 Responsiveness- significant difference pre and post treatment

V. INDIVIDUALISED MEASURES [GRADE C]

Individualised measures of quality of life allow patients to identify for themselves the most important aspects of their lives which constitute their appraisal of their overall quality of life. Individualised measures have not yet been used widely in the assessment of incontinence or lower urinary tract symptoms, although it is likely that measures such as the SEIQOL [179] may be useful.

VI. QUESTIONNAIRES FOR SPECIFIC PATIENT GROUPS

Most studies and questionnaires have been developed for use with members of the general population or urology/gynaecology patients with incontinence. However, some specific patient groups may experience particular problems with incontinence (for example, children or those who are severely disabled), which may require independent investigation and potentially the development of more specific measures or the addition of a new subset of items on already developed instruments [180 181].

1. QUALIVEEN: QUALITY OF LIFE RELATED TO URINARY PROBLEMS IN SPINAL CORD INJURY [GRADE B]

A questionnaire has been developed to evaluate the specific impact of urinary dysfunction on the quality of life of spinal cord injury patients in France [182]. Items were selected following patient interviews, and were then assessed for validity and reliability in 281 spinal cord injury patients with urinary difficulties. The items were reduced psychometrically and the resultant questionnaire has been named Qualiveen [182].

2. INCONTINENCE IN PATIENTS WITH MULTIPLE SCLEROSIS [GRADE C]

A study by Catanzaro explored the effects of incontinence on patients with multiple sclerosis through the use of interviews [181].

3. INCONTINENCE IN CHILDREN

Although children can be affected by urinary incontinence, no questionnaires designed specifically for use with children could be identified. One article reported on the relationship between enuresis and self-esteem [183].

Table 3 : Questionnaires validated in both women and men.

Questionnaire/Authors	Sample	Topics covered in relation to sexual activity	Findings
INCONTINENCE IMPACT QUESTIONNAIRE (IIQ) [173]	Women undergoing urodynamics who had GSI or DI (n=162, mean age 61.3 years)	Impact of leakage on ability to have sexual relations	Subscale data. Internal consistency =0.9 Construct Validity - significant correlation with generic QOL measures. Criterion validity - significant correlation with number of incontinent episodes and pad test.. Responsiveness - significant difference between pre and post treatment scores.
Wyman et al. (1987) [170]	Women with GSI and DI taking part in trial of behavioural treatment. (n=69, mean age 67.8 years)	Impact of leakage on ability to have sexual relations	Test retest of complete questionnaire r=0.73 at 1 week; r=0.65 at 6 weeks
Smoger et al. (2000) [178]	809 men recruited from primary care clinics. (n=261 with current incontinence)	Impact of leakage on ability to have sexual relations	Subscale data Significant correlation with frequency of incontinence
URGE IIQ Brown, Posner & Stewart (1999) [77]	Volunteer sample of women with urge or mixed incontinence (with predominantly urge). (n=83, mean age 63.8 years)	Impact of leakage on ability to relax and enjoy sex having an orgasm	Data on sexual function questions: Internal consistency = 0.91, Test-retest at 2 weeks ICC = 0.71, Divergent validity - weak correlation with other IIQ domains <0.1 No correlation between sexual function questions and frequency of leakage or overall ratings of impact.
Lubeck et al. (1999) [58]	Men and women with urge and mixed incontinence enrolled in a trial of oxybutynin. (n=22 male and 235 female, mean age 59.6 years))	Impact of leakage on ability to relax and enjoy sex having an orgasm	Data on sexual function questions. Content validity- 34% floor effect. Dicriminant validity - significant relationship with severity of UI. Responsiveness - Guyatt's stat=-1.07. Construct validity - i nterscale correlations were in the expected directions.
IQOL Wagner et al. (1996) [174]	62 men and women with stress, urge and mixed incontinence recruited from clinics and adverts (n=42 female and 20 male, mean age 64 years))	I worry about having sex because of my incontinence	Complete questionnaire data. Internal consistency - alpha=0.95, Test-retest at 18 days - ICC=0.93 Descriminant validity - IQOL related to severity, self perceived severity and number of medical appointments.
Patrick et al. (1999) [145]	Women with stress and mixed incontinence taking part in a trial of duloxetine.(n=288 76% were 45 years of age or older)	I worry about having sex because of my incontinence	Subscale data. Internal consistency - alpha=0.93 Test-retest at 2 weeks- ICC=0.91. Complete questionnaire data. IQOL correlated with SF36 and PGWB. and pad test, diary and self perceived severity Responsiveness statistic =0.4

USE OF QUESTIONNAIRES IN RESEARCH

The prevalence of incontinence and its impact on the quality of life of individuals varies, depending on the severity of the condition as well as other social and medical factors involved. A number of reviews of the prevalence and impact of incontinence have been published – see [1] and, since the last report. [74, 83, 97, 184 -200].

Questionnaires can be used in outcomes research and epidemiological research and it is encouraging that since the publication of the previous report,[1] an increasing number of such studies are being published which include results from validated questionnaires. It remains, however, that many studies do not include validated (recommended) questionnaires and we would strongly urge researchers to include such measures in their research. In the sections below, we update our literature review on outcome assessment (randomised trials and observational studies) and epidemiological studies.

I. RANDOMISED TRIALS

The ideal study design for assessing the outcome of treatments for incontinence is the randomised controlled trial. We would contend that the assessment of a patients' symptoms and impact on quality of life using validated self-completed questionnaires should be an essential component of any study evaluating treatments. A review of 9 trials from 1980 to 1996 concerned with electrical stimulation concluded that the standard of published trials was poor and that there was a need for more trials with larger sample sizes and using sensitive, reproducible and valid outcome measures [201]. Below, we consider the studies found relating to treatments for incontinence and their use of validated questionnaires.

Few randomised trials using recommended questionnaires were identified in the first ICI report [1] Searching of Medline and the Cochrane trials databases between 1998 and mid 2001 identified 48 randomised trials of treatments for incontinence of various sorts. Of the 48 randomised trials identified, only 19 included validated questionnaires as an outcome measure (see Table 4). Eight were undertaken in Europe, 7 in the USA, and two each in Japan and Australia. Six involved bladder training or physical therapies such as pelvic floor exercises, 5 with drug therapies, three minimally invasive therapies such as magnetic stimulation, 1 compared surgical procedures, and four involved guidelines or health care organisation. Three trials included more than 200 patients but 13 fewer than 100. Six trials were considered to reach the highest level of rigour. The trials covered a wide range of types of incontinence. Four trials employed the SF-36, 3 the IIQ, 3 the BFLUTS, 2 the QoLS-N and 4 some sort of VAS.

In the other trials, the outcome measures typically used was the frequency-volume diary (11 trials): spinal cord patients, drug trial; [202] 197 women in behavioural v. drug trial; [203] sacral nerve stimulation in 76 elderly patients; [204] 105 patients with urge or mixed incontinence, drug trial; [205] 277 with overactive bladder, drug trial; [206] 105 housebound adults, behavioural trial; [207] 361, drug trial; [208] 68 with detrusor overactivity, electrical stimulation v. sham trial; [209] 67 detrusor instability, drug trial; [210] 197 women with urge incontinence, behavioural v. drug trial; [211] 130 responders, drug type trial. [212]. In 13 trials, outcome focussed on clinical measures, with an uspecified subjective assessment by patient or clinician (unlikely to be validated) [213-225]. In a further 5 trials, the outcome measures employed were unclear [226-230].

These findings suggest that while it is encouraging that the use of validated questionnaires is increasing, far too many randomised trials still do not employ them. As these trials are evaluating the impact of treatments which aim to affect symptoms or quality of life of people with incontinence, the use of such measures should be mandatory. Without the use of valid self-completion questionnaires, the evidence from such trials should not be relied upon.

Table 4 : Randomised trials using validated questionnaires

Reference	Country	Inc. type	n	RCT	QoL measure	Result	Level evidence
Wyman [147]	USA	Stress & DI	204	Bladder training	IIQ, UDI	Combined therapy best	1
Serels [231]	US	Urge	34	Hyosya-mine v. doxazosin	Expanded AUA	Improved	2
Cammu [232]	Belgium	Stress	60	Pelvic floor v. cones	VAS, diary	No difference	2
Wikander [233]	Sweden	Post-stroke	34	Functional prog v. control	Katz ADL, FIM	Improved intervent. group	2
Moore [234]	Australia	Post-prostatec-tomy	63	Pelvic exercise v. elect. Stim. v. standard	IIQ-7, EORTC QLQC30	Inc. symptoms improved – no difference	2
Kammerer [235]	USA	Stress	35	Burch v. colporr-haphy	IIQ, own design	Lower quality of life Burch	2
Reuben [236]	USA	Any	363	Geriatric assess. v. standard	SF-36	Some improv. Intervent.	1
Jackson [93]	UK	Stress	67	HRT v. placebo	BFLUTS, SF-36, diary	No effect	2
Patric [145]	USA	Stress&mixed	288	Drug v placebo	I-QoL	Validity testing	1
Petersen [237]	Denmark	Detrusor hyper (spinal cord)	12	Casaisin v. placebo	VAS	No difference	2
Fujishiro [238]	Japan	Stress	62	magnetic stim. v. sham	Own	Sig. improve-ment	2
Bo [94]	Norway	Stress	59	Pelvic floor v. control	QoLS-N, BFLUTS	Sig. reduction in sex, social & phys problems	2
Weil [239]	Neths	Urge	44	Neuromod-ulation	Beck, SF36	QoL & UDS improved	2
Chadha [240]	Australia	Any	449	Guidelines	SF-36	No effect	1
Bo [92]	Norway	Stress	59	Pelvic floor v. control	QoLS-N, BFLUTS	Sig.Improved sex and social life	2
Choe [241]	USA	Stress	40	Mesh v. sling	VAS	Mesh better	2
Van Kampen [242]	Belgium	Post prostat-ectomy	102	Pelvic floor v. placebo	VAS	Improved intervent.	1
Fujishiro [243]	Japan	Stress	62	Magnetic stim. v. placebo	Unspec. score	Improved intervent.	2
Burgio [244]	USA	Urge	197	Biofeed-back v. oxybutynin v. placebo	Hopkins Symptom Checklist (SCL-90-R)	Psychological distress reduced in biofeedback and drug arms	1

II. OBSERVATIONAL STUDIES

Searching identified 28 observational studies, 10 of which used a prospective design with controls, 2 prospective design with historical controls, and there were 16 studies without controls (see Table 5). As these studies were not randomised, they scored poorly in terms of research quality, with 10 reaching a score of 3 but the majority (16) having the lowest rating. Most studies were small – 22 relied upon less than 100 patients. The studies spanned the various treatments – surgery, drugs, devices and conservative/physical therapies, and included the range of types of incontinence. The questionnaires used reflected the pattern for trials, with the majority including the IIQ (11 studies), six the UDI, five the SF-36, and one study each employing the BFLUTS, EuroQol, I-QOL, SIP, SII, and Beck Depression Inventory. One study used patient interviews, and four assessed incontinence using their own unvalidated measure.

Table 5 : Observational studies of outcome using questionnaires

Ref	Country	Incontinence type	n	Design	Treatment	QoL measure	Results	Level of evidence
Lemack [245]	USA	Stress	56	R	Surgery	Own	Sex func worse post op	5
Sung [95]	Korea	GSI	60	Pro	Biofeedback v pelvic floor	BFLUTS QoL	Biofeed better	3
Amunsden [246]	USA	Obstruction	32	R	Surgery post op	IIQ, UDI	Success	5
Winters [247]	USA	Stress	58	R	Collagen	Own	Improved	5
Fuertes [248]	Spain	Urge	67	Open trial	Drug	EuroQoL	Improved	5
Morgan [249]	USA	Stress	247	R Sling	surgery	UDI-SF	92% satisfaction	5
Sampselle [149]	USA	Stress	132	Pro	Pelvic floor & Bl. exercise	IIQ	Improv	5
Sander [250]	Denmark	Urge & mixed	408	Pro	Conservative clinic	SF36 and own	Signif improv	3
Filbeck [251]	Germany	Stress	105	R	Surgery	Backle QoL	Signif improv	3
Moore [252]	Australia	Stress, urge, mxd	57	Pro	Fem Assist	UDI	Equal response	3
Sand [253]	USA	Stress	63	Pro	Insert	SF36	Signif improv	3
Galloway [254]	USA	Stress	83	Pro	Innervation	1-QoL	No improv	3
Davila [150]	USA	Stress & mixed	53	Pro	Support prosthesis	IIQ	Signif improv	4
Blanc [76]	France	Stress & mixed	37	R	Bladder neck Suspension	IIQ7 UDI 6	Unclear	4
Weinberger[255]	USA	Stress & mixed	81	R	Non-surgical trial	Own	Benefit	3
Sander 154	Denmark	Stress	41	Pro	Vaginal device	IIQ, SF36	Signif improv, SF36 no diff	5
Hassouna [256]	USA	Stress	82	R	Surgery	SIP	Signif improv	5
Versi [151]	USA	Stress	14	Pro	External device	IIQ, UDI	Improved	5
Amarenco [257]	France	Urge	1701	Pro	Drug	Ditrovie	Effective	5
Versi [258]	USA	Stress & Urge	96	Pro	Device	IIQ, UDI	Signif improv	5
Rabin [259]	USA	Stress & mixed	38	Pro	Device	Own	50% improved	5
Sander [260]	Denmark	Stress	55	Pro	Device	IIQ, SF36	Signif improv, No diff	5
Black [172]	UK	Stress	442	Pro	Surgery	Black q'aire	75% improved	5
Shaker [106]	Canada	Urge	18	Pro	Sacral root	Beck, SF36	Improved	5
Wyman [146]	Australia	Stress & mixed	21	Pro	Prosthesis	IIQ	Improved	5
Siegel [152]	USA	Urge & mixed	68	Pro	Stim (elect)	IIQ	Improved	3
Richardson [261]	USA	Stress	21	Pro	Stim (elect)	IIQ	Improved only travel & physical	3
Berglund [262]	Sweden	Stress	45	Pro	Surgery	Interview	Decrease in impediments	3

III. EVALUATION OF THE IMPACT OF INCONTINENCE ON QUALITY OF LIFE

As indicated in the previous report, the term quality of life is used widely in research, often without any clear definition. It is linked to the World Health Organisation definition of health which refers to a state of physical, emotional and social well-being, and not just the absence of disease or infirmity [263]. 'Health-related quality of life' (HRQL) has been defined as including: "those attributes valued by patients including their resultant comfort or sense of well-being; the extent to which they were able to maintain reasonable physical, emotional, and intellectual function; the degree to which they retain their ability to participate in valued activities within the family, in the workplace and in the community" (Wenger and Furberg, quoted in.[101]) This definition is long, but helps to emphasise the multidimensional nature of quality of life and the importance of considering each individual's perception of their own situation in the context of non-health related aspects such as jobs, family and other life circumstances [14]. One study has shown that partners of men with LUTS can suffer because of their spouse's condition, particularly in terms of being worried about cancer or the need for surgery, and also because of disturbed sleep [264]. Quality of life measures are being increasingly used with a wide variety of patients and in many different studies, and their use has increased significantly since 1997.

Many studies have examined the impact of lower urinary tract symptoms as well as incontinence. Lower urinary tract symptoms in men have been reported to have a deleterious impact on aspects of quality of life in a great number of studies [23, 110, 126, 265-276] Symptoms causing the most bother include those associated with filling (so called 'irritative' symptoms) such as frequency, urgency, nocturia and incontinence [268, 270, 277, 278]. Increasing levels of symptoms are sometimes associated with increasing impact on everyday life [273].

Incontinence has been found to reduce social relationships and activities¨[43, 49, 52, 131, 141, 279-284] be associated with poor self-rated health, [285] impair emotional and psychological well-being, [49, 52, 283, 284, 286, 287] and impair sexual relationships [162,288, 289]. Some report that incontinence causes at least practical inconvenience, [60, 280, 290] and for many requires often elaborate planning to conceal or prepare for incontinent episodes, [138, 291] and may cause financial hardship [155]. Feelings of embarrassment or negative self-perception are common [282, 291 292]. In some studies, it is suggested that urge or mixed incontinence can have a more severe impact than stress incontinence. [72,284, 293, 294].

It is clear, however, among both men and women experiencing lower urinary tract symptoms or incontinence, that there is considerable variability in complaints of deleterious impacts. For a small proportion, these conditions seriously affect daily life including psychological and social well-being. There is a relatively large group, however, who appear to experience more limited impact or adapt to their symptoms and report only limited effects in some domains. Some are not sufficiently concerned to request treatment [295-297]. Some of this variability is likely to be related to the range of different questionnaires and measures used. More severe incontinence is seen to result in greater impact on quality of life in some studies [71]. Older women may be less affected than younger [294]. One study focused on nocturnal incontinence, showing that this symptom is more common than originally thought (present in 5.8% of women aged 19 years and older in a general practice in the UK), and that it is extremely troublesome [98].

Table 6 : Use of questionnaires to assess impact of incontinence on quality of life

No.	Country	Type of incontinence	QOL measures	Results
Simeonova [298]	Norway	stress, urge, mixed	Generic: RAND-36 disease specific:UDI and IIQ	The prevalence of urinary incontinence was 57.1%: 28.7% for stress incontinence, 5.6% for urge incontinence and 22.7% for both. Women with urge or mixed incontinence had more severe impairment of QOL as compared with only SUI.
Temml [91]	Austria	stress, urge, mixed	BFLUTS	65.7% of women and 58.3% of men stated that QOL was affected by their incontinence. A moderate or severe impairment was reported by 18.3% of women and 16.6% of men.
Simeonova [299]	Sweden	stress, urge, mixed	visual analogue scale	Women with urinary incontinence reported a poorer quality of life compared to continent women ($p<0.01$). Women with urge incontinence and women with mixed incontinence reported a poorer quality of life compared to women with stress incontinence ($p<0.05$).
O'Connor [281]	Sweden	urge, mixed	SF-36	QOL among the sample population was significantly lower in 5 of 8 dimensions compared with the general US population, and was significantly re lated to the severity of the symptoms in 6 of 8 dimensions.
Brown [300]	USA	urge	their own QOL questionnaire	Urge incontinence affects many QOL issues and contributes to limitation of activities, loss of control, and negative self-perception.
McClish [301]	USA	any type	IIQ	Cost and pad usage were significantly associated with number of incontinent episodes and QOL.
Kinn [302]	Sweden			QOL and pad use were evaluated in 460 women utilizing the free provision and home delivery of urinary incontinence pads by the Swedish health services. Satisfaction with the supplied pads was generally good, with absorptive and antiodor properties most appreciated.
DuBeau [303]	USA	urge	32 urge incontinence related QOL items obtained from literature, more than half of which were not described previously	Community-dwelling 25 women and 5 men more than 60 years of age with urge incontinence were included. Experts and patients viewed the impact of urge incontinence on QOL differently. Whereas experts focused more on functional impact, patients more often cited the impact of urge incontinence on their emotional well-being and on the interruption of activities.
Schlenk [115]	USA	any	SF-36	To examine HR-QOL as measured by the Medical Outcomes Study Short Form-36, across patient populations with chronic disorders and to compare QOL in these subjects with normative data on healthy persons. 6 disorders (urinary incontinence, prostate cancer, chronic obstructive pulmonary d isease, AIDS, fibromyalgia and hyperlipidemia. Homebound, elderly, incontinent patients had the lowest QOL for physical functioning.

Table 6 : Use of questionnaires to assess impact of incontinence on quality of life (to be continued)

No.	Country	Type of incontinence	QOL measures	Results
Robinson [304]	USA	any women over 60 ys	IIQ UDI	To determine if patient reports of urinary incontinence symptoms can predict QOL as measured by the short forms of the IIQ and UDI. The question, "Do you consider this accidental loss of urine a problem that interferes with your day-to-day activities or bothers you in other ways?" was the best predictor of the subject's responses to both QOL measures. The patients' symptoms that best correlated with both QOL measures and the report of bothersome incontinence were frequent episodes of incontinence, greater amounts of urine loss and more frequent voids.
Chiverton [287]	USA	any	no specific QOL questionnaire	To explore the incidence of depression, the correlation between mastery and depression and/or self-esteem, and depression as a mediating factor in the QOL in women with urinary incontinence. There was a higher incidence of depression in women with incontinence compared with the general popu lation. Depression did not emerge as a mediator in QOL. Mastery was the only predictor with a direct effect on QOL in women with incontinence.
Grimby [305]	Sweden	any	Nottingham Health Profile Questionnaire	Comparison between women (n=120) with urinary incontinence and an age-matched women (n=313). Women with incontinence obtained higher scores in the domains of emotional disturbance and social isolation than controls. Women with urge and mixed incontinence reported emotional disturbances more than control. But there was no difference within the domain of emotional disturbances between stress-incontinent women and the control group. Women with urge incontinence reported more disturbances of sleep than the control. Women with all types incontinence were socially more isolated.
Hunskaar [306]	Norway	urge stress	SIP	Women with incontinence obtained higher scores in the domains of emotional disturbance and social isolation than controls. Women with urge and mixed incontinence reported emotional disturbances more than control. But there was no difference within the domain of emotional disturbances between stress-incontinent women and the control group. Women with urge incontinence reported more disturbances of sleep than the control. Women with all types incontinence were socially more isolated.

IV. IMPACT OF INCONTINENCE ON SEXUAL FUNCTION AND SATISFACTION

Studies that have assessed sexual functioning in relation to urinary symptoms have shown that it is an important concept to measure when considering condition specific quality of life [1]. The majority of studies assessing the impact of incontinence on sexual life have, however, not used validated questionnaires. Most have either included one or two questions about sexual function to existing incontinence questionnaires or have relied on unvalidated instruments.

A number of studies have assessed sexual dysfunction in relation to urinary symptoms and/or surgery for incontinence (Table 7). These have been mainly carried out on female populations and the focus of questions have concerned the presence of leakage and the phase of sexual activity during which leakage occurs. The impact of urinary symptoms on sexual activity, and satisfaction with sexual activity are also commonly assessed. Studies evaluating outcomes of surgery for stress incontinence have focused on the changes in sexual activity resulting from surgery, in terms of frequency of intercourse, frequency of desire, satisfaction, pain and dyspareunia, and frequency of leakage during intercourse. Infrequently the impact of sexual dysfunction on partners is also considered.

Results of these studies are equivocal in relation to prevalence of dysfunction, differences between aetiological groups, and impact of surgery on sexual function. This points to a need for more systematic research into the aspects of sexual dysfunction that are most pertinent to quality of life and standardisation of measurement of sexual functioning with the development of well constructed and validated instruments. These instruments must take account of all aspects of sexual activity whether involving a partner or not. Consideration also needs to be given and measures developed for the impact of incontinence on partners' quality of sex life.

As can be seen, the findings from these studies are very variable and, at least in part, these variations are probably due to differences in the questionnaires and methods used. However, some studies do indicate that incontinence can have an impact on sexual matters and so this is an area requiring further investigation. It remains that the assessment of the impact of incontinence on sexual function and satisfaction is still a developing research area.

Table 7: Studies assessing sexual function and urinary symptoms using non-validated questionnaires.

Authors	Sample	Topics covered in relation to sexual activity	Findings
Lam et al. (1992) 307	Community survey of 3114 women (n=511 with UI mean age 45.1 years)	Presence of leakage during sexual intercourse.	Leakage during intercourse = 12.2% of SI, 14% of Urge, 15.3% of mixed and 7.1% of non-specific UI.
Nygaard & Milburn (1995) 308	292 Women attending routine gynaecological examination (n=224 responded, mean age 41.4 years)	UI associated with orgasm or penetration, volume of UI, whether it was a problem and if partner found it a problem.	12.9% experienced UI during sexual activity, associated with severity of UI. 45% during orgasm, 21% during intercourse and 35% during both. Only 1 woman found it a problem, and no partners did.
Sutherst & Brown (1980) 309	289 Women attending an incontinence clinic (n=208 responded, mean age 46.1 years)	Whether urinary symptoms had interfered with marital relations and sexual life in any way.	43% of those with urinary symptoms had adversely affected sexual lives. Women with DI had greater dysfunction than GSI.
Gordon et al. (1999) 310	Women attending a urogynaecology clinic (n=100 mean age 62 years)	Detailed questionnaire administered by a psychiatrist addressing desire, arousal, orgasm, and satisfaction. Also impact of urinary symptoms on sexual function.	Women with DI had worse sexual function than those with GSI or mixed incontinence.
Vierhout & Gianotten (1993) 311	254 Women attending clinic for incontinence. (n=66 with UI during sexual activity mean age 47 years)	Assessed activities during intercourse which resulted in leakage.	Deep penetration and abdominal pressure responsible in 77%, orgasm in 74%, clitoral stimulation in 50%.

Table 7 : Studies assessing sexual function and urinary symptoms using non-validated questionnaires. (CTD)

Authors	Sample	Topics covered in relation to sexual activity	Findings
Hilton (1988) 312	400 women attending urogynaecology clinic (n=79 with UI during sexual activity, mean age around 43 years)	Assessed whether leakage was associated with arousal, penetration or orgasm.	67% experienced leakage on penetration (70% GSI,4%DI and 9% mixed) and 33% on orgasm (42% GSI, 34% DI and 5% mixed)
Haase & Skibsted (1988) 313	63 Women undergoing surgery for stress incontinence and/or genital descensus. (n=55 responded, mean age 49years)	Sexual desire, dyspareunia, frequency of coitus, and any change in sex life after surgery.	24% experienced improvement, 67% no change and 9% deterioration.
Lemack & Zimmern (2000) 245	93 Women who hadundergone surgery for incontinence (n=22 sexually active Mean age 56 - 60 years)	Frequency of intercourse, satisfaction with intercourse and comparison with pre-surgery, leakage, and dyspareunia	No change after surgery
Berglund et al. (1996) 262	Women with Stress incontinence undergoing surgery (n=45 mean age 50 years)	Semi-structured interview concerning frequency of intercourse, sexual desire and sexual dysfunction	No change in frequency of intercourse post surgery. One third had increased sexual desire, slight increase in dysfunction.
Weber, Walters & Piedmonte (2000) 314	165 women undergoing surgery for UI or prolapse (n=81 sexually active, mean age 54 years)	Frequency of intercourse, incontinence during intercourse, dyspareunia, vaginal dryness	No change in frequency and vaginal dryness. 8% pre and 19% post surgery had dyspareunia. 22% pre and 26% post surgery had intercourse UI.
Iosif (1988) 315	Women undergoing surgery for UI (n=156, mean age 40.6 years)	Change in sexual relations post surgery. Frequency of intercourse, desire, enjoyment and frequency of orgasm.	1 year after surgery frequency of intercourse had increased in 15%, desire increased in 15%, enjoyment increased in 25% and orgasm frequency increased in 10%.
Clark & Romm (1993) 166	90 Women with UI evaluated by urodynamics (n=48 with completed questionnaires, mean age 41 - 48 years)	Ways in which UI affected sexual activity, satisfaction with sex life, pain, presence of orgasm, problems during sexual activity, changes that have helped problems, advice to other sufferers, advice to health professionals.	56% reported UI with sexual activity., 66% reported any urinary symptoms during sexual activity. There was little difference in prevalence rates of UI during sexual activity between diagnostic groups.
Berglund & Fugl-Meyer (1995) 316	105 Women undergoing surgery for GSI. (n=44 eligible, mean age 50 years)	Sexual activities, sexual function/ dysfunction, sexual satisfaction, impact of UI and the effects of the surgical intervention.	No significant difference between frequency of pre and post surgery coitus. Neither the magnitude of leakage nor the duration of UI influenced sexual experiences. Continence after surgery promoted sexual desire.
Macfarlane et al. (1996) 317	Community sample of 2011 men	Frequency of sexual desire and sexual intercourse, difficulties in having an erection and ejaculation, overall satisfaction	Presence of urinary symptoms and severity associated with dissatisfaction. Symptoms that most affected sex life were hesitancy, forcing, poor stream urgency and incontinence.

V. INCONTINENCE IN SPECIFIC PATIENT GROUPS

Most studies and questionnaires have been developed for use with members of the general population or urology/gynaecology patients with incontinence. Some specific patient groups may experience particular problems with incontinence, however, which may require independent investigation and potentially the development of more specific measures or the addition of a new subset of items on already developed instruments – for example for the severely disabled, [180] those with multiple sclerosis [181] or spinal cord injury.

VI. INTERNATIONAL PERSPECTIVES

The numbers of studies using validated questionnaires to assess incontinence has risen rapidly since the First ICI.[1]. The most commonly used questionnaires are the condition-specific IIQ/UDI and the generic SF-36, probably because the majority of studies originate from the USA. Increasing research into the symptom and quality of life burden of urinary incontinence is being conducted around the world.

Since 1960, searches of MEDLINE yielded the following results concerning articles about incontinence and quality of life: 0 from 1960 to 1970; 5 from 1971 to 1980; 27 from 1981 to 1990; and 209 from 1991 to 2001. The findings were similar for urinary incontinence symptoms: 5 from 1960 to 1970; 12 from 1971 to 1980; 16 from 1981 to 1990; and 47 from 1991 to 2001.

The pattern is repeated in individual countries. For example, in Japan, the study of QoL assessment in urinary incontinence was scanty before the first meeting of International Consultation on Incontinence in 1999. However, thereafter there has been a gradual increase in the assessment of quality of life with the publication of Japanese versions of IIQ, IQOL and KHQ in which linguistic validation was completed [318]. The further validation of questionnaires for reliability, validity and responsiveness is on-going using data from almost 200 patients.

APPENDIX I : DEVELOPING THE ICIQ AND ICIQ-SF

A. ICIQ

The aim of this new questionnaire is to provide a set of modules to cover all the major aspects of the assessment of incontinence and its impact on quality of life in detail. The questionnaire is currently in development and comprises eight sections: symptoms of incontinence, bothersomeness of symptoms, use of pads/protection, impact on aspects of everyday life including social and occupational factors, interference with sex life, emotional impact, follow-up after treatment, and diagnosis. The questionnaire is very long and comprehensive in this developmental phase. The content validity of the items has been established and work on construct validity and reliability is currently being undertaken.

B. ICIQ-SF

The aim of this version is to produce a brief and robust measure to evaluate the frequency, severity and impact on quality of life of incontinence among all groups: men and women, young and old, in the developed and developing world. The questionnaire was devised under the auspices of the ICI and work was initiated after the first consultation in 1999. It was launched at the Second ICI.

The developmental version comprised six major question areas covering: frequency of leakage and its bothersomeness, protection use and type, perceived quantity of leakage usually and at worst, interference with everyday life, interference with social life, and interference with sex life. There were additional questions concerned with age, sex, overall quality of life and perceived cause of leakage that were included primarily for validation purposes. The items are detailed below (figure 2).

The questionnaire has been undergoing psychometric testing and full results of this will be published in due course. As the details have not been published, the questionnaire has the official Committee rating of Grade C however, it is fully expected to reach Grade A as soon as the material is published.

Figure 2 : Items in the developmental version of the ICIQ-SF

1a. How often do you leak urine (never, about once a week or less often, 2 or 3 times a week, about once a day, several times a day, all the time).

1b. How much of a problem is this for you (0 not a problem to 10 a serious problem - VAS)

2a. Sometimes people try to protect themselves against urine loss by wearing pads, using cloth, tissue paper or other protection. In the past four weeks, have you used any protection (never, some of the time, most of the time, all of the time).

2b. If you did use protection in the past four weeks, what kind of protection did you use (tissue/toilet paper/cloth, minipads/pantliners, sanitary/incontinence/other pads, something else – please describe)

3a. We would like to know how much urine you think leaks. How much urine do you usually leak whether you wear protection or not (none, a small amount, a moderate amount, a large amount).

3b. How much was the worst leakage over the past four weeks (none, a small amount, a moderate amount, a large amount)

4. Overall, how much does leaking urine interfere with your everyday life (0 not at all to 10 a great deal - VAS)

5. How much do you feel that your social life has been spoilt by urinary leakage during the past four weeks (0 not at all to 10 a great deal - VAS)

6. How much do you feel that your sex life has been spoilt by urinary leakage during the past four weeks (0 not at all to 10 a great deal - VAS)

7. In general, how would you rate the overall quality of your life during the past four weeks (0 worst quality of life to 10 best quality of life - VAS)

I. VALIDITY

1. CONTENT VALIDITY

This was assessed following a detailed literature review, by taking soundings from the ICI committees, observation of and interviews with patients and levels of missing data. In-depth interviews with a researcher were conducted with 63 consecutive patients (46 females, 17 males) aged 18 or over, with incontinence or other lower urinary tract symptoms, attending urology clinics in the UK. Patients were observed self-completing the questionnaire and then interviewed to establish their ease of understanding, interpretation and completion of the questionnaire items.

Review by clinical and social science experts indicated that the ICIQ-SF covered all important domains and symptoms. The developmental version of the ICIQ-SF was completed in full by 87% of patients. Most items demonstrated very low levels of missing data on self-completion (the majority <2%, and only one item in excess of 4%).

2. Construct validity

Construct validity was assessed by comparing levels of incontinence as measured by the questionnaire in patients attending urology clinics and individuals in the community, with different ages and sexes. 246 males and females, registered with two UK community general practices, and 215 consecutive male and female urology clinic attenders with incontinence or other LUTS, self-completed the ICIQ-SF. As there is no clear 'gold standard' measure, further aspects of construct validity relate to the relationships between items in the ICIQ-SF and other more established questionnaires such as the ICS*male*SF and the BFLUTS questionnaires. These relationships were investigated in 118 females and 27 males attending urology clinics. Responses to comparable items were compared by crude percentage agreements and the weighted Kappa statistic.

As anticipated, the prevalence of incontinence was lower in the community (45%) than the clinic sample, with a general increase in prevalence with increasing age (P<0.05). Women in the community also reported more incontinence (59%) than men (25%) (P<0.001). In addition, there was an expected association between sex and type of incontinence in the clinic and the community sample (P<0.001 for both). As anticipated, stress incontinence was the most predominant type in community women, in contrast to men who reported more urge incontinence.

Agreement between responses to ICIQ-SF and BFLUTS items measuring the amount and frequency of incontinence were 'moderate' (85%) and 'good' (93%), with weighted kappa values of 0.42 and 0.77 respectively.

II. RELIABILITY

1. Test-retest reliability

A test-retest analysis was carried out among clinic patients who were sent a second ICIQ-SF to complete within two weeks of their first questionnaire. The data were interpreted by analyses of paired differences between test and retest responses to individual items. Agreement between responses to each item was further analysed using the weighted Kappa statistic. Data were available for 144 clinic patients (121 females, 23 males) completing both questionnaires. The reliability of a sample of 4 of these items is presented below in Figure 3.

Items assessing 'frequency of protection use' and 'amount of leakage' demonstrated excellent test-retest reliability, with a maximum difference of one response category between test and retest (out of 4-10). 'Frequency of leakage' demonstrated good test-retest reliability, with only one patient moving more than two categories. Test-retest reliability was good for the 'problem' associated with frequency of incontinence and impact on 'everyday life', 'social life' and 'sex life', with only 2-5% of patients moving more than one category. 'Overall quality of life' and 'worst leakage' were less reliable. However, whilst other items measure aspects related to incontinence alone (a condition whose status is unlikely to change significantly during the time points), the quality of life item measures other aspects of the patient's life, which cannot be assumed to remain static in the same manner. These findings were also reflected in the kappa statistics with crude agreements between test and retest responses ranging from 85-96%, and weighted Kappa values of 0.57-0.90, indicating 'good' to 'very good' agreement except 'overall quality of life' and 'worst leakage', which demonstrated 'moderate' agreement.

2. Internal consistency

Cronbach's alpha coefficient was calculated to assess the correlation between items in142 females and 104 males registered with two UK community general practices and 182 females and 41 males attending urology clinics in the UK. The alpha for the nine major items (excluding the descriptive item 2b) was 0.950, indicating a very high level of internal consistency, but also suggesting that there was considerable redundancy in the developmental version (see devising the final version below).

III. RESPONSIVENESS TO CHANGE

206 patients involved in the intervention arm of a community-based trial (MRC Incontinence Community Nurse Practitioner trial) comparing a nurse-practitioner with standard GP care completed the ICIQ-SF. All patients in this observational study were in the nurse-practitioner arm and received advice from the nurse about fluid intake, pelvic floor awareness, bladder education and other conservative therapies over a period of eight weeks (details from Dr C Shaw, committee member). Figure 4 shows the proportions of patients reporting 'any level of symptom' before and after treatment for seven items in the questionnaire. Table 8 shows the

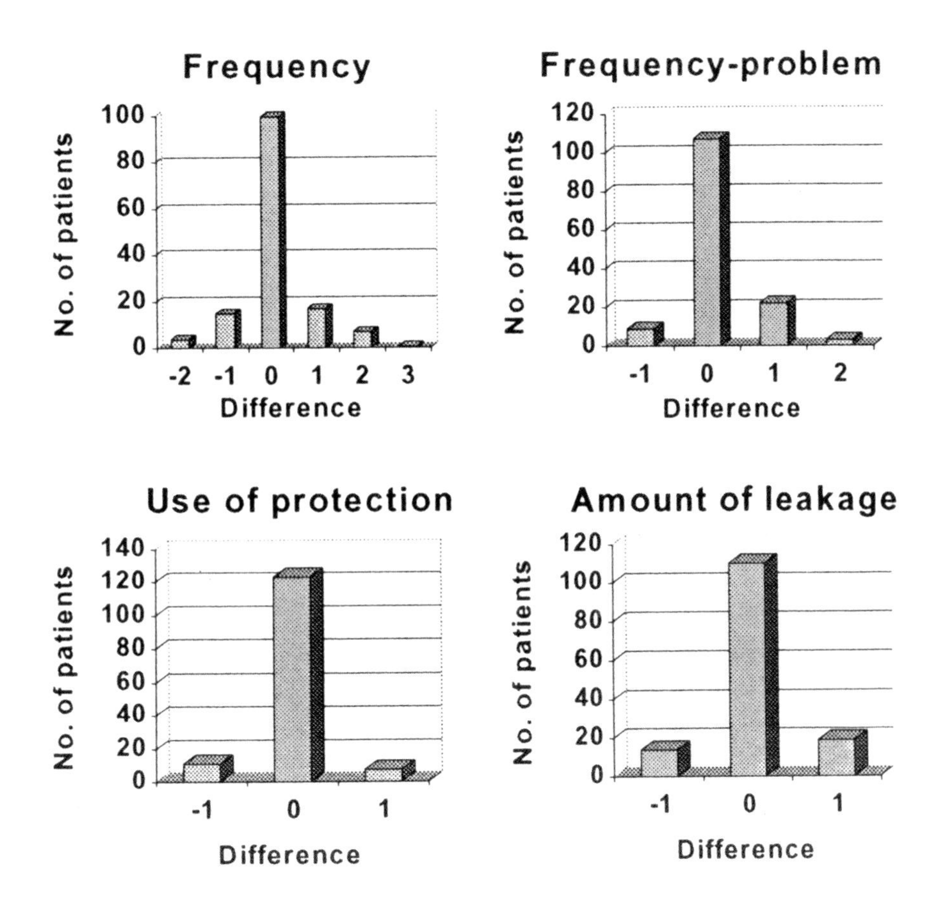

Figure 3 : Reliability of four of the developmental ICIQ-SF items

Table 8 : Change in patients reporting 'any level of symptom' (%) before and after treatment

Symptom/item	Percentage change
Frequency of leakage	-11
Frequency of leakage - problem	-15
Use of protection	-2
Usual amount of leakage	-12
Worst leakage	-7
Impact on everyday life	-12
Impact on social life	-9
Impact on sex life	-2

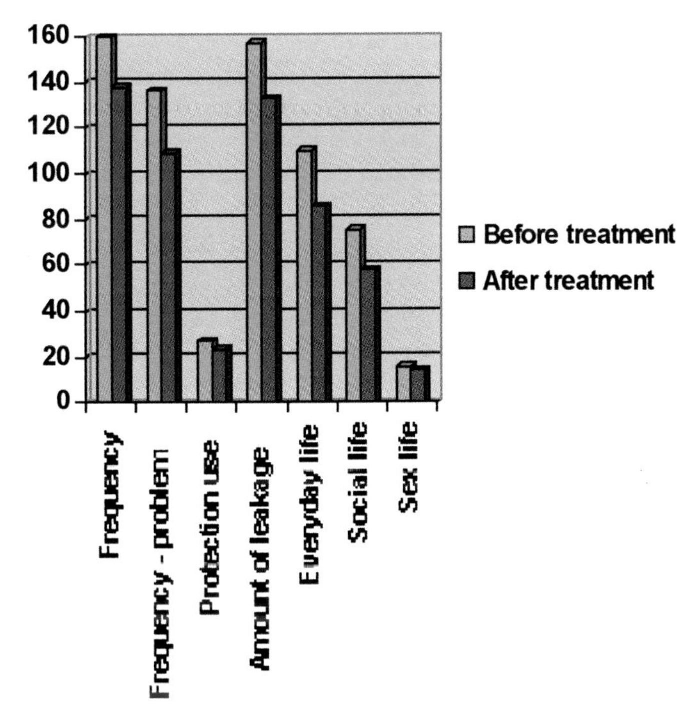

Figure 4 : Number of patients reporting 'Any level of symptom' before and after treatment

percentage change in 'any level of symptom' between baseline and follow-up. Most items were highly statistically significantly better at follow-up than baseline, i.e. 'frequency of leakage' and its associated 'problem', 'amount of leakage', 'worst leakage', impact on 'everyday life' and 'social life' ($P<0.0001$), and one item significantly better; 'impact on sex life' ($P<0.01$). There was also a decrease in the percentage of patients reporting each different type of incontinence. Following treatment, change in 'overall quality of life' and 'use of protection' did not reach statistical significance.

In a separate study, 14 consecutive patients undergoing surgery for incontinence according to normal clinical practice completed the ICIQ-SF four weeks before surgery and then approximately 12 weeks after the procedure. This work is currently ongoing, and numbers are too small for meaningful analyses of individual symptoms, but considerable improvements in all the symptoms indicated in the table above were found – with percentage changes ranging from –36 to –50. With sufficient numbers, it is likely that these changes would be found to be highly statistically (and clinically) significant for individual symptoms (as for scores, see below).

IV. INTERNATIONAL ASPECTS

There are various countries actively participating in the development of the ICIQ. Researchers at the Bristol Urological Institute, UK, acts as coordinators.

The ICIQ-SF has been translated into a number of languages for use in non-English speaking countries (by mid 2001, completed in Dutch, Japanese, Spanish and Swedish languages, and in progress for Arabic, Chinese, German, Italian, Korean, Norwegian and Portuguese) using standard methods:

Initial translation – words and sentences are literally translated and then adapted to the cultural context and lifestyle related to the language in question. This is preferably done by a bilingual native speaker(s) of the language in question who is fluent in both languages, preferably knowledgeable about the content area and aware of the intent of the questionnaire and each item.

Back translation – the final language questionnaire is translated back into the source language (English), preferably by a bilingual native speaker of the source language who was not involved with the translation stage and who is *not* knowledgeable of the content area. Items that have lost or altered their meaning are re-translated.

a) Committee review - the translations and back-translations are then reviewed to identify discrepancies in the meaning of confusing or ambiguous items/text in the questionnaire.

b) Pre-testing for equivalence – administering the questionnaire to a small sample of patients enables a researcher to probe the patient about their understanding and completion of each item, in order to confirm the face validity and acceptability of the questionnaire and to identify any discrepancies or errors in the translation.

c) Revalidation – following adaptation, the questionnaire may need revalidating because the psychometric properties of the scale may not have remained constant as a result of the adaptation process.

1. Adaptation to English-speaking populations

For predominantly English-speaking countries, such as the United States, formal translation and back-translation are not required but it is necessary to adapt the questionnaire to the cultural context. A US study group, consisting of experts and clinicians in the field of urology, was formed to adapt the ICIQ-SF to an American-English speaking population. The UK version of the ICIQ-SF was reviewed and initial minor changes were made. This adapted version is now being pre-tested on a sample of patients in the USA.

2. Japanese ICIQ-SF

The Japanese ICIQ-SF has been administered to consecutive male and female patients with incontinence attending a urology clinics. The relationship between the ICIQ-SF and the King's Health Questionnaire (Japanese version) is being investigated. In a preliminary sample of 68 patients (54 females, 14 males), agreement between ICIQ item concerned with impact on everyday life and several similar items in the KHQ (impact on life, interference with household tasks or job/daily activities) were fair (kappa 0.38, 0.24 and 0.42). Agreements between the ICIQ items on social life and sex life were fair to moderate. Agreement between the two questionnaires on the frequent use of protection was very good (kappa 0.81).

In order to assess responsiveness, patients proceeding to treatment for incontinence according to normal clinical practice were then asked to complete a second questionnaire approximately three months after treatment. Treatment included surgical or medical (drug) intervention, insertion of anti-incontinence devices and conservative management. The relationship between the ICIQ-SF and objective parameters of incontinence including the ICS pad test, abdominal leak point pressure (ALPP) and pathogenesis (including intrinsic sphincter deficiency, detrusor instability, hypermobility and so on) is being investigated in patients clinically diagnosed with stress incontinence.

V. DEVISING THE FINAL VERSION AND A SCORING SCHEME

As indicated above, the developmental version of the ICIQ-SF contained a considerable amount of redundancy. All available baseline data were used – 469 completed questionnaires – to devise the final version and scoring scheme.

The very high Cronbach's alpha statistic of 0.950 (see above) was mirrored by an initial factor analysis which showed one major factor in the developmental version with most items having loadings in excess of 0.73. The only exception was overall quality of life with a loading of 0.55. It is evident that the overall quality of life item measures aspects independent of incontinence both intuitively and as it exhibits the lowest consistency. As it also had the lowest level of test-retest reliability, the first decision made was to drop the overall quality of life item (7) from the final version.

Examination of the cross-tabulation of the frequency and problem items (Q1a, 1b) and the correlation coefficient (0.83) showed that the problem item mostly reflected the symptom frequency – that is, the degree of bothersomeness was related to the severity of the frequency. Thus the 'bother' subquestion was dropped. Similarly, the usual and worst leakage questions (3a, 3b) were also strongly related and highly correlated (0.89) and as the worst leakage had poorer test-retest reliability and higher levels of missing data, it was dropped. The questions concerned with 'impact on social life (5) and impact on daily life (4) were also very highly correlated (0.92), and since 'social life' might prove difficult to translate to other cultures, this item was also dropped.

At this stage, five items remained: 1a (frequency of leakage), 2a (use of protection), 3a (perceived quantity of leakage), 4 (impact on everyday life) and 6 (impact on sex life). The alpha for these 5 items was 0.916.

The questions concerned with protection (2a) and impact on sex life (6) were less responsive to change than the other items. In addition, the sex life item was relevant to a limited number of patients. On this basis, it was decided that the final version of the questionnaire could be reduced to three items (see Fig 5 below), and with the Cronbach's alpha being 0.917, these items could be combined into a single score.

Clinicians have also indicated that a patient's assessment of the cause of their incontinence would be useful, and so a set of questions to explore these issues is included in the final version of the questionnaire. These 'self-diagnostic' items (Fig 6) are not, however, included in the score – they are for descriptive purposes only.

VI. THE PRELIMINARY PERFORMANCE OF THE SCORES

As can be seen, the scores are not identical for each of the items and researchers are encouraged to investigate, for example by sensitivity analyses, the impact of varying the implicit weightings given to each item. The currently recommended score is shown above and ranges from 0 to 21. Table 9 shows descriptive statistics for the score using the preliminary data. Age groups were also significantly different (p<0.01).

A number of analyses have been undertaken to investigate the validity and reliability of the score. The correlation between test and retest scores was very high: 0.88 (p<0.0001), indicating excellent reliability. The correlation between ICIQ-SF and ICS*male*SF scores was also encouraging: 0.37 (p=0.065) for the voiding sub-score and 0.75 (p<0.0001) for the incontinence sub-score. There was also a reasonable correlation between the ICIQ-SF score and the ICI pad test in a Japanese study (MG, committee member): 0.40 (p=0.014). In the CNP study, there were highly statistically significant improvements in the scores between baseline and follow up: baseline mean 5.81, follow-up mean 3.88 (p<0.0001). There were similar findings in the surgical study: baseline mean 16.0, follow-up mean 5.62 (p=0.0005).

These preliminary findings suggest that the ICIQ-SF score is valid, reliable and responsive to change – but researchers are encouraged to further explore these aspects. Researchers wishing to contribute to the psychometric testing of the ICIQ-SF are encouraged to contact Jenny Donovan (jenny.Donovan@bris.ac.uk) or Kerry Avery (kerry_martin@bui.ac.uk).

Table 9 : Descriptive statistics for the ICIQ-SF score

	n	Mean	Sd	min	max	P value
All	458	7.18	6.64	0	21	
Community	245	2.36	3.26	0	16	<0.0001
Clinic	213	12.71	5.03	0	21	
Women	309	8.19	6.42	0	21	<0.0001
Men	143	4.94	6.65	0	21	

Figure 5 : Items in the final scored version of the ICIQ-SF

1. How often do you leak urine?

Never=0

About once a week or less often=1

Two or three times a week=2

About once a day=3

Several times a day=4

All the time=5

2. We would like to know how much urine you think leaks. How much urine do you usually leak whether you wear protection or not?

None=0

A small amount=2

A moderate amount=4

A large amount=6

3. Overall, how much does leaking urine interfere with your everyday life?

0 ______________________________ 10

(0 = not at all) (10 = a great deal)

Figure 6 : 'Self-diagnostic' items in the final version of the ICIQ-SF (not scored)

4. When does urine leak? (please tick all that apply to you)

Never – urine does not leak

Leaks before you can get to the toilet

Leaks when you cough or sneeze

Leaks when you are asleep

Leaks when you are physically active/exercising

Leaks when you have finished urinating and are dressed

Leaks for no obvious reaso

Leaks all the time

APPENDIX II :
VALIDATED QUESTIONNAIRES IN RELATED AREAS

A number of questionnaires reaching acceptable levels of validity and reliability have been developed for the study of related conditions such as benign prostatic disease, prostate cancer or general levels of sexual function, but which do not include incontinence *per se*. Such questionnaires may be useful in conjunction with incontinence-specific measures. Details of these questionnaires were reviewed previously [1].

For men, the following questionnaires have been tested at least to the level of the basic standard of recommended incontinence questionnaires (Committee Grade A or B):

I. ASSESSMENT OF LOWER URINARY TRACT SYMPTOMS (MEN)

AUA Symptom Index. [272]

I-PSS. [272, 319]

Patient-completed modification of the Boyarsky [2] schedule. [320]

II. ASSESSMENT OF QUALITY OF LIFE IN BENIGN PROSTATE DISEASE

BPH Health Related Quality of Life Survey. [275, 321, 322]

BPH Health Related Quality of Life (BPH-HRQOL). [323, 324, 325]

BPH Impact Index. [326]

BPH Health-related QoL survey. [321]

Mayo Health-related Quality of Life. [119, 321, 327]

III. ASSESSMENT OF QUALITY OF LIFE – PROSTATE CANCER

Cancer Rehabilitation Evaluation System - Short Form (CARES-SF) [328]

Prostate Cancer Treatment Outcome Questionnaire (PCTO-Q). [133]

PROSQOLI. [329]

IV. ASSESSMENT OF SEXUAL FUNCTION (WOMEN AND MEN)

Watts Sexual Function Questionnaire. [330]

Medical Outcomes Study (MOS) Sexual Functioning Scale. [336]

Assessment of sexual function (men)

Radiumhemmets Scale of Sexual Function. [288, 331, 332, 333, 334]

International Index of Erectile Function (IIEF). [335]

Sexual Adjustment Questionnaire (SAQ). [134]

Prostate-targeted Health Related Quality of Life. [120]

RECOMMENDATIONS - QUESTIONNAIRES

The following questions are highly recommended (Grade A) or recommended (Grade B) for use in assessing symptoms of incontinence or their impact on quality of life:

SYMPTOMS OF INCONTINENCE

GRADE A: HIGHLY RECOMMENDED

Urogenital Distress Inventory. [57]

UDI-6. [50]

Urge-UDI. [58]

King's Health Questionnaire. [59]

(Women only) **Incontinence Severity Index.** [60]

(Men only) **DAN-PSS-1.** [61]

(Men only) **ICS*male***. [62]

(Men only) **ICS*male*SF** [63]

GRADE B: RECOMMENDED

Bristol Lower Urinary Tract Symptoms.64

Symptom Severity Index. [65]

BOTHERSOMENESS

GRADE A: HIGHLY RECOMMENDED

DAN-PSS-1. [87]

ICS*male*. [62]

GRADE B: RECOMMENDED

BFLUTS. [64]

GENERIC HEALTH STATUS

GRADE A: HIGHLY RECOMMENDED

SF-36. [102]

EuroQol EQ-5D. [103]

IMPACT OF INCONTINENCE ON QUALITY OF LIFE

GRADE A: HIGHLY RECOMMENDED

(Men and women) **Quality of life in persons with urinary incontinence (I-QoL).** [130]

(Men and women) **King's Health Questionnaire**.[59]

(Women only) **Incontinence Impact Questionnaire (IIQ)**. [131]

(Women only) **IIQ-7.** [50]

(Women only) **Urge-IIQ**. [58]

(Men only) **Modified IIQ and IIQ-7.** [132]

GRADE B: RECOMMENDED

(Women only) **Symptom Impact Index (SII)**. [65]

(Men only) **ICS*QoL***. [110]

(Men only) **EORTC metastatic prostate cancer**. [133]

(Men only) **Changes in Urinary Function**. [134]

(Men only) **Prostate-targeted Health Related Quality of Life**. [120]

(Men only) **Functional Assessment of Cancer – Bladder/General Scales.** [134, 135]

SEXUAL FUNCTION/SATISFACTION

GRADE A: HIGHLY RECOMMENDED

The Psychosocial Adjustment to Illness Scale (PAIS). [158]

Rust and Golombok Inventory of Sexual Satisfaction. [159]

GRADE B: RECOMMENDED

Brief Sexual Function Inventory. [160]

BPH QOL9. [161]

ICS*sex*. [162]

RECOMMENDATIONS

RECOMMENDATIONS FOR CLINICAL PRATICE

The following recommendations were unanimous:

1. Clinicians are encouraged to include in patient evaluations, the highly recommended and recommended patient self-administered questionnaires in the appropriate language, for the assessment of urinary incontinence and its impact on patients' lives.
2. Further and detailed evaluation of the usefulness of the ICIQ-SF in clinical practice is encouraged.

RECOMMENDATIONS FOR RESEARCH

The following recommendations were unanimous:

1. Researchers are strongly encouraged to use the highly recommended questionnaires in randomised controlled trials evaluating treatments which aim to relieve symptoms or reduce impact on quality of life. Evidence from randomised trials not including such measures should not be relied upon.
2. Researchers are recommended to publish further psychometric and clinical testing of recommended and potential questionnaires to ensure their validity, reliability and responsiveness in a wide range of contexts and cultures.
3. To facilitate comparison of results across studies, researchers are strongly encouraged to include the ICIQ-SF in studies evaluating symptoms and/or impact of incontinence on quality of life, and to publish the results to allow the further evaluation of the ICIQ-SF.
4. Researchers are encouraged to conduct research into the development of questionnaires or modules of the ICIQ for specific patient groups for whom general questionnaires may not be appropriate (e.g. children, those with neurological problems, frail elderly, patients with carers).
5. Researchers are encouraged to conduct research to explore other issues of importance to patients with incontinence (e.g. the impact on sexual function and satisfaction, psychological status, economic impact) and develop modules for the ICIQ or separate questionnaires as appropriate.

REFERENCES

1. Donovan JL, Naughton M, Gotoh M, et al. Symptom and quality of life assessment. In: Abrams P, Khoury S, Wein AJ, eds. Incontinence. Plymouth: Health Publication Ltd, 1999;295-332.
2. Boyarsky S, Jones G, Paulson DF, Prout GR. New look at bladder neck obstruction by the Food and Drug Administration regulators. American Association of Genito-Urinary Surgeons 1977;68:29-32.
3. Korman HJ, Sirls LT, Kirkemo AK. Success rate of modified pereyra bladder neck suspension determined by outcomes analysis. Journal of Urology 1994;152:1453-1457.
4. Slevin ML, Plant H, Lynch D, Drinkwater J, Gregory W. Who should measure quality of life, the doctor or the patient? Cancer. 1988;57:109-112.
5. Coscarrelli-Schag C, Heinrich RL, Ganz PA. Karnofsky performance status revisited: reliability, validity and guidelines. J.Clin.Oncol. 1984;2:187-193.
6. Hutchinson TA, Boyd NF, Feinstein AR. Scientific problems in clinical scales. Journal of Chronic Diseases 1979;32:661-666.
7. Pearlman RA, Uhlmann RF. Quality of life in chronic diseases: Perceptions of elderly patients. Journal of gerontology 1988;43(2):M25-M30
8. Wyman JF, Choi SC, Harkins SW, Wilson MS, Fantl AJ. The urinary diary in evaluation of incontinent women: A test-retest analysis. Obstetrics & Gynecology 1988;71(6):812-817.
9. Barnick C. Frequency volume chart. In: Cardozo L, ed. Urogynaecology. London: Churchill Livingstone, 1997,105-107.
10. Follick M, Ahern D, Laser-Wolston N. Evaluation of a daily activity diary for chronic low back pain. Pain 1984;19:373-382.
11. Wilkin D, Hallam L, Doggett MA. Measures of Need and Outcome for Primary Health Care. Oxford: OUP, 1992;
12. Bowling A. Measuring Disease. Buckingham: Open University Press, 1995;
13. Streiner DL, Norman GR. Health Measurement Scales. Oxford: OUP, 1989;
14. Gill TM, Feinstein AR. A critical appraisal of the quality of quality-of-life measurements. JAMA 1994;272(8):619-626.
15. Kramer MS, Feinstein AR. Clinical biostatistics. Clinical Pharmacology and Therapeutics 1981;29:111-123.
16. Bland JM, Altman DG. Statistical methods for assessing agreement between two methods of clinical measurement. Lancet. 1986;i:307-310.
17. Jenkinson C, Lawrence K, McWhinnie D, Gordon J. Sensitivity to change of health status measures in a randomized controlled trial: comparison of the COOP charts and the SF-36. Quality of Life Research 1995;4:47-52.
18. Murawski MM, Meiderhoff PA. The generalizability of statistical expressions of health related quality of life instrument responsiveness: a data synthesis. Qual Life Res 1998,1:11-22.
19. Kazis LE, Anderson JJ, Meenan RF. Effect sizes for interpreting changes in health status. Med Care 1989;27:S178-189.
20. Guyatt G, Juniper EF, Walter SD, Griffith LE, Goldstein RS. Interpreting treatment effects in randomised trials. Bri Med J 1998;316:693
21. Jaeschke R, Singer J, Guyatt G. Measurements of health status: ascertaining the minimal clinically important difference. Controlled Clin Trials 1989;10:407-415.
22. Witjes WPJ, de la Rosette J, Donovan JL, et al. The ICS-'BPH' Study: International differences in lower urinary tract symptoms and related bother. Journal of Urology 1997;157:1295-1300.

23. Guess HA, Chute CG, Garraway WM, et al. Similar levels of urological symptoms have similar impact on Scottish and American men—although Scots report less symptoms. J.Urol. 1993;150:1701-1705.

24. Guillemin F, Bombardier C, Beaton D. Cross-cultural adaptation of health-related quality of life measures: literature review and proposed guidelines. J Clin Epidemiol 1993;46(12):1417-1432.

25. Herdman M, Fox-Rushby J, Badia X. A model of equivalence in the cultural adaptation of HRQoL instruments: the universalist approach. Qual Life Res 1998;7:323-335.

26. Hanley J, Capewell A, Hagen S. Validity study of the severity index, a simple measure of urinary incontinence in women. BMJ 2001;322:1096-1097.

27. Wein AJ, Rovner ES. The overactive bladder: an overview for primary care health providers. Int.J.Fertil.Womens Med. 1999;44:56-66.

28. de la Rosette JJMC, Witjes WPJ, Schäfer W, et al. Relationships between lower urinary tract symptons and bladder outlet obstruction: results from the ICS-BPH study. Neurourology and Urodynamics 1998;17(2):99-108.

29. Barry MJ, Cockett ATK, Holtgrewe HL, McConnell JD, Sihelnik SA, Winfield HN. Relationship of symptoms of prostatism to commonly used physiological and anatomical measures of the severity of benign prostatic hyperplasia. Journal of Urology 1993;150:351-358.

30. Ezz ED, Koch WFRM, de Wildt MJAM, Kiemeney LALM, Debruyne FMJ, de La R. Reliability of the International Prostate Symptom Score in the Assessment of Patients with Lower Urinary Tract Symptoms and/or Benign Prostatic Hyperplasia. Journal of Urology 1996;155:1959-1964.

31. Drutz HO. Urodynamic analysis of urinary incontinence symptoms in women. Am J Obstet Gynecol 1979;134:789

32. Cardozo L, Stanton SL. Genuine stress incontinence and detrusor instability. British Journal of Obstetrics and Gynaecology 1980; 87:893-896.

33. Shepherd AM, Powell PH, Ball AJ. The place of urodynamic studies in the investigation and treatment of female urinary tract symptoms. Journal of Obstetrics and Gynaecology 1982; 3:123-125.

34. Reynard, J. M., Yang, Q., Donovan, J. L., Peters, T. J., Schäfer, W., de la Rosette, J. J. M. C. H., Dabhoiwala, N., Osawa, D., Tong Long Lin, A., and Abrams, P.The ICS-'BPH' study: uroflowmetry, lower urinary tract symptoms and bladder outlet obstruction. British Journal of Urology 1998;82:619-623

35. Jarvis GJ, Hall S, Stamp S, Millar DR, Johnson A. An assessment of urodynamic examination in incontinent women. British Journal of Obstetrics and Gynaecology 1980;87:893-896.

36. Bergman A, Bader K. Reliability of the patient's history in the diagnosis of urinary incontinence. Int.J.Gynecol.Obstet 1990;32:255-259.

37. Versi E, Cardozo L, Anand D, Cooper D. Symptoms analysis for the diagnosis of genuine stress incontinence. British Journal of Obstetrics and Gynaecology 1991;98:815-819.

38. Lagro-Jansson AL, Debruyne FM, Van Weel C. Value of patient's case history in diagnosing urinary incontinence in general practice. Br.J.Urol. 1991;67 (6):569-572.

39. Kujansuu E, Kauppila A. Scored urological history and urethroscystometry in the differential diagnosis of female urinary incontinence. Ann.Chir.Gynaecol. 1982;71:197-202.

40. Farrer DJ, Whiteside CG, Osborne JL, Turner-Warwick RT. A urodynamic analysis of micturition symptoms in the female. Surg.Gynecol.Obstet. 1975;141:875-881.

41. Hastie KJ, Moisey CU. Are urodynamics necessary in female patients presenting with stress incontinence? Br.J.Urol. 1989;63:155-156.

42. Haylen BT, Sutherst JR, Frazer MI. Is the investigation of most stress incontinence really necessary? Br.J.Urol. 1989;64:147-149.

43. Iosif S, Henriksson L, Ulmsten U. The frequency of disorders of the lower urinary tract, urinary incontinence in particular, as evaluated by a questionnaire survey in a gynecological health control population. Acta Obstet Gynecol Scand 1981;60:71-76.

44. Frazer MI, Sutherst JR, Holland EFN. Visual analogue scores and urinary incontinence. BMJ 1987;295:582

45. Fraser MI, Haylen BT, Sutherst JR. The severity of urinary incontinence in women. Comparison of subjective and objective tests. Br.J.Urol. 1989;63:14-15.

46. Kujansuu E, Heikkinen J, Riippa P, Kauppila A. Degree of female stress urinary incontinence: an objective classification by simultaneous urethrocystometry. Gynaecology Obstetrics Investigation 1984;18:66-72.

47. McCormack M, Infante-Revard C, Schick E. Agreement between clinical methods of measurement of urinary frequency and functional bladder capacity. Br.J.Urol. 1992;69:17-21.

48. Norton C. The effects of urinary incontinence in women. International Rehabilitation Medicine 1982; 4:9-14.

49. Hunskaar S, Vinsnes A. The quality of life in women with urinary incontinence as measured by the sickness impact profile. J.Am.Geriatr.Soc. 1991;39:378-382.

50. Uebersax JS, Wyman JF, Shumaker SA, McClish DK, Fantl AJ. Short forms to assess life quality and symptom distress for urinary incontinence in women: The incontinence impact questionnaire and the urogenital distress inventory. Neurourology and Urodynamics 1995; 14:131-139.

51. Wyman JF, Harkins SW, Taylor JR, Fantl JA. Psychosocial impact of urinary incontinence in women. Obstetrics & Gynecology 1987;70(3):378-381.

52. Grimby A, Milsom I, Molander U, Wiklund I, Ekelund P. The influence of urinary incontinence on the quality of life of elderly women. Age.Ageing. 1993;22:82-89.

53. Kobelt G. Economic considerations and outcome measurement in urge incontinence. Urology 1997;50 (6A):100-107.

54. Bidmead J, Cardozo L, McLellan A, Khullar V, Kelleher C. A comparison of the objective and subjective outcomes of colposuspension for stress incontinence in women. BJOG. 2001;108:408-413.

55. Lilford RJ. The substantive ethics of clinical trials. Clin.Obstet.Gynecol. 1992;35:837-845.

56. Aaronson NK. Quality of life assessment in clinical trails: methodologic issues. Controlled Clinical Trials 1989;10:S195-S208

57. Shumaker SA, Wyman JF, Uebersax JS, McClish D, Fantl JA. Health-related quality of life measures for women with urinary incontinence: the Incontinence Impact Questionnaire and the Urogenital Distress Inventory. Quality of Life Research 1994;3:291-306.

58. Lubeck DP, Prebil LA, Peebles P, Brown JS. A health related quality of life measure for use in patient with urge urinary incontinence: a validation study. Qual Life Res 1999;1999:337-344.

59. Kelleher CJ, Cardozo LD, Khullar V, Salvatore S. A new questionnaire to assess the quality of life of urinary incontinent women. British Journal of Obstetrics and Gynaecology 1997;104:1374-1379.

60. Sandvik H, Hunskaar S, Seim A, Hermstad R, Vanvik A, Bratt H. Validation of a severity index in female urinary incontinence and its implementation in an epidemiological survey. Journal of

Epidemiology and Community Health Medicine 1993;47:497-499.

61. Hald T, Nordling J, Andersen JT, Bilde T, Meyhoff HH, Walter S. A patient weighted symptom score system in the evaluation of uncomplicated benign prostatic hyperplasia. Scand.J.Urol.Nephrol.Suppl. 1991;138:59-62.

62. Donovan JL, Abrams P, Peters TJ, et al. The ICS-'BPH' Study: the psychometric validity and reliability of the ICSmale questionnaire. British Journal of Urology 1996;77:554-562.

63. Donovan JL, Peters TJ, Abrams P, Brookes ST, de la Rosette JJMCH, Schäfer W. Scoring the ICSmaleSF questionnaire. Journal of Urology 2000;164:1948-1955.

64. Jackson S, Donovan J, Brookes S, Eckford S, Swithinbank L, Abrams P. The Bristol Female Lower Urinary Tract Symptoms questionnaire: development and psychometric testing. British Journal of Urology 1996;77:805-812.

65. Black N, Griffiths J, Pope C. Development of a symptom severity index and a symptom impact index for stress incontinence in women. Neurology and Urodynamics 1996;15:630-640.

66. Gaudenz R. Der inkontinenz-fragebogen, mit dem neuen urge-score and stress-score. Geburtsh u.Fräuenheilk 1979;39:784-792.

67. Bernstein I, Sejr T, Able J, et al. Assessment of Lower Urinary Tract Symptoms in Women by a Self-Administered Questionnaire: Test-Retest Reliability. Int Urogynecol J 1996;7:37-47.

68. Sommer P. Voiding patterns and prevalence of incontinence in women. A questionnaire survey. British Journal of Urology 1990;66:12-15.

69. Gunthrope W, Brown W, Redman S. The development and evaluation of an incontinence screening querstionnaire for female primary care. Neurology and Urodynamics 2000;19:595-607.

70. Fowler FJ, Barry MJ, Lu-Yao G, Roman A, Wasson J, Wennberg JE. Patient-reported complications and follow-up treatment after radical prostatectomy. Urology 1993;42(6):622-629.

71. Robinson D, Pearce K, Preisser J, Dugan E, Suggs P, Cohen S. Relationship between patient reports of urinary incontinence symptoms and quality of life measures. Obstet Gynecol 1998;91:224-228.

72. van der Vaart C, de Leeuw J, Roovers J, Heintz A. The influence of urinary incontenence on quality of life of community-dwelling 45-70 year old Duch women. Ned.Tijdschr.Geneeskd. 2000;6:894-897.

73. Dugan E, Cohen SJ, Robinson D, et al. The quality of life of older adults with urinary incontinence: determining generic and condition specific predictors. Quality of Life Research 1998;7 (4):337-344.

74. Gordon E, Stanton S. Urinary incontinence in elderly women. Eur Urol 1998;33:241-247.

75. Lemack GE, Zimmern PE. Predictability of urodynamic findings based on the Urogenital Distress Inventory-6 questionnaire. Urology 1999;54:461-466.

76. Blanc E, Hermieu JF, Ravery V, Moulinier F, Delmas V, Boccon-Gibod L. Value of the use of a questionnaire in the evaluation of incontinence surgery. Prog Urol 1999;9:88-94.

77. Brown JS, Posner S, Stewart AL. Urge incontinence: new health-related quality of life measures. J Am Geriatr Soc 1999:980-988.

78. Norton P, Karram M, Wall LL, Rosenzwig B, Benson JT, Fantl JA. Randomized double-blind trial of terodiline in the treatment of urge incontinence in women. Obstetrics and Gynecology 1998;84:386-891.

79. Kelleher CJ, Cardozo LD, Toozs-Hobson PM. Quality of Life and urinary incontinence. Curr Opin Obstet Gynecol 1995;7:404-408.

80. Kobelt G, Kirchberger I, Malone-Lee J. Quality of life aspects of the overactive bladder and the effect of treatment with tolterodine. Br J Urol Int 1999;83:583-590.

81. Mackillop WJ, Johnston PA. Controlled clinical trials: an ethical imperative? [letter]. J.Chronic.Dis. 1987;40:363-364.

82. Conway K, Uzun V, Marrel A, Cardozo L, Kelleher C, Haye I. Linguistic validation of the King's Health Questionnaire (KHQ) in eight languages [abstract]. Value in Health 1999;2:204

83. Kobelt G, Kirchberger I, Malone-Lee J. Quality-of-life aspects of the overactive bladder and the effect of treatment with tolterodine. BJU Int 1999;8:583-590.

84. Kelleher CJ, Pleil AM, Reese PR. Health related QoL of patients with overactive bladder receiving Tolterodine once daily. Neurourology and Urodynamics 2000;19:519-520.

85. Bidmead J, Cardozo LD, McLellan A, Khullar V, Kelleher CJ. A comparison of the objective and subjective outcomes of colposuspension for stress incontinence in women. BJOG 2001;108:408-413.

86. Sandvik H, Seim A, Vanvik A, Hunskaar S. A severity index for epidemiological surveys of female urinary incontinence: comparison with 48-hour pad-weighing tests. Neurourol.Urodyn. 2000;19:137-145.

87. Meyhoff HH, Hald T, Nordling J, Thorup A, Blide T, Walter S. A New Patient Weighted Symptom Score System (DAN-PSS-1). Scand.J.Urol.Nephrol. 1993;27:493-499.

88. Hansen BJ, Flyger H, Brasso K, et al. Validation of the self-administered Danish Prostatic Symptom Score (DAN-PSS-1) system for use in benign prostatic hyperplasia. British Journal of Urology 1995;76:451-458.

89. Abrams P, Donovan JL, de la Rosette JJMC, Schäfer W, ICS-'BPH' SG. International Continence Society 'Benign Prostatic Hyperplasia' study: background, aims and methodology. Neurology and Urodynamics 1997;16:79-91.

90. Donovan JL, Brookes ST, de la Rosette JJMC, et al. The responsiveness of the ICSmale questionnaire to outcome: evidence from the ICS-'BPH' study. British Journal of Urology International, 1999; 83: 243-48.

91. Temml C, Haidinger G, Schmidbauer J, Schatzl G, Madersbacher S. Urinary incontinence in both sexes: prevalence rates and impact on quality of life and sexual life. Neurorol Urodyn 2000;19:259-271.

92. Bo K, Talseth T, Vinsnes A. Randomized controlled trial on the effect of pelvic floor muscle training on quality of life and sexual problems in genuine stress incontinent women. Acta Obstet Gynecol Scand. 2000;79:598-603.

93. Jackson S, Shepherd A, Brookes S, Abrams P. The effect of oestrogen supplementation on post-menopausal urinary stress incontinence: a double-blind placebo-controlled trial. Br J Obstet Gynaecol. 1999;106:711-718.

94. Bo K, Talseth T, Vinsnes A. Radomized controlled trial on the effect of pelvic floor muscle training on quality of life and sexual problems in genuine stress incontinent women. Acta Obstet Gynecol Scand 2000;79:598-603.

95. Sung M, Hong J, Choi Y, Baik S, Yoon H. FES-biofeedback versus intensive pelvic floor muscle exercise for the prevention and treatment of genuine stess incontinence. J Korean Med Sci 2000;15:303-308.

96. Swithinbank LV, Donovan JL, du Heaume JC, et al. Urinary symptoms and incontinence in women: relationships between occurrence, age, and preceived impact. Br J Gen Pract 1999;49:897-900.

97. Swithinbank L, Abrams P. The impact of urinary incontinence on the quality of life in women. World Journal of Urology 1999;17:225-229.

98. Swithinbank L, Donovan JL, Rogers C, Abrams P. Nocturnal incontinence in women: a hidden problem. Journal of Urology 2000;164:764-766.

99. Fowler FJ, Barry MJ, Lu-Yao G, Wasson J, Roman AMA, Wennberg J. Effect of radical prostatectomy for prostate cancer on patient quality of life: results from a Medicare Survey. Urology 1995;45(6):1007-1015.

100. Jonler M, Madsen FA, Rhodes PR, Sall M, Messing EM, Bruskewitz RC. A prospective study of quantification of urinary incontinence and quality of life in patients undergoing radical retropubic prostatectomy. Urology 1996;48(3):433-441.

101. Naughton MJ, Shumaker SA. Assessment of health-related quality of life. In: Furberg CD, ed. Fundamentals of Clinical Trials. St. Louis: Mosby Press, 1996;185

102. Ware JE. Sf-36: Health Status Questionniare. Quality Quest Inc 1989.

103. The EG. EuroQol - a new facility for the measurement of health related quality of life. Health Policy 1990;16 (3):199-208.

104. Bergner M, Bobbett RA, Carter WB, Gilson BS. The sickness impact profile: development and final revision of a health status measure. Med Care 1981;19:787-805.

105. Gilson BS, Erickson D, Chavez CT, Bobbitt RA, Bergner M, Carter WB. A Chicano version of the Sickness Impact Profile. Cult Med Psychiatry 1980;4:137-150.

106. Shaker HS, Hassouna M. Sacral nerve root neuromudulation: an effective treatment for refractory urge incontinence. J Urol 1998;159:1516-1519.

107. Hunt SM, McEwen J, McKenna SP. Measuring health status: a new tool for clinicians and epidemiologists. Journal of the royal college of general practitioners 1985;35:185-188.

108. Sullivan M, Karlsson J, Bengtsson C, Furunes B, Lapidus L, Lissner L. The Göteborg Quality of Life Instrument - A psychometric evaluation of assessments of symptoms and wellbeing among women in a general population. Scand J Prim Health Care 1993;11:267-275.

109. Hunter JW, McKee M, Black NA. Health status and quality of life of british men with lower urinary tract symptoms: Results from the SF-36*. Urology 1995;45(6):962-971.

110. Donovan JL, Kay HE, Peters TJ, et al. Using ICSQoL to measure the impact of lower urinary tract symptoms on quality of life: evidence from the ICS-'BPH' study. British Journal of Urology 1997;80:712-721.

111. Kutner NG, Schechtman KB, Ory MG, Baker DI. Older adults' perceptions of their health and functioning in relation to sleep disturbance, falling, and urinary incontinence. J Am Geriatr Soc 1994;42:757-762.

112. McHorney CA, Ware JE, Lu R, Donald S. The MOS 36-Item Short-Form Health Survey (SF-36): III. Tests of Data Quality, Scaling Assumptions, and Reliability Across Diverse Patient Groups. Medical Care 1994;32(1):40-66.

113. Lyons RA, Perry HM, Littlepage BNC. Evidence for the validity of the short-form 36 questionnaire (SF-36) in an elderly population. Age.Ageing. 1994;23:182-184.

114. Mozes B, Maor Y, Shmueli A. The competing effects of disease states on quality of life of the elderly: the case of urinary symptoms in men. Qual.Life Res. 1999;8:93-99.

115. Schlenk E, Erlen J, Dunbar-Jacob J, et al. Health-related quality of life in chronic disorders: a comparison across studies using the MOS SF-36. Qul Life Res 1998;7:57-65.

116. Brazier JE, Harper R, Jones NMB, et al. Validating the SF-36 health survey questionniare - new outcome measure for primary care. Br.Med.J. 1992;305:160-164.

117. Jenkinson C, Lawrence K, McWhinnie D, Gordon J. Criterion validity and reliability of the SF-36 in a population sample. Quality of Life Research 1995;3:7-12.

118. Gliklich RE, Hilinski JM. Longtitudinal sensitivity of generic and specific health measures in chronic sinusitis. Quality of Life Research 1995;4:27-32.

119. Epstein RS, Deverka PA, Chute CG, et al. Validation of a new quality of life questionnaire for Benign Prostatic Hyperplasia. J.Clin.Epidemiol. 1992;45:1431-1445.

120. Litwin MS, Hays RD, Fink A, et al. Quality of life outcomes in men treated for localized prostate cancer. JAMA 1995;273(2):129-135.

121. Sand PK, Richardson DA, Staskin DR, et al. Pelvic floor electrical stimulation in the treatment of genuine stress incontinence: A multicenter, placebo-controlled trial. Am J Obstet Gynecol 1995;173:72-79.

122. McFall SL, Yerkes AM, Cowan LD. Outcomes of a small group educational intervention for urinary incontinence: health-related quality of life. J.Aging Health 2000;12:301-317.

123. Ware J, Kosinski M, Keller S. SF-36 Physical and Mental Health Summary Scales: A User's Manual. Boston, MA: 1994;

124. Chiarelli P, Brown W, McElduff P. Leaking urine: Prevalence and Associated Factors in Australian Women. Neurology and Urodynamics 1999;15:567-577.

125. Mishra G, Schofield MJ. Norms for the physical and mental health component summary scores of the SF-36 for young, middle-aged and older Australian women. Qual.Life Res. 1998;7:215-220.

126. Emberton M, Neal D, Black N, et al. The effect of prostatectomy on symptom severity and quality of life. British Journal of Urology 1996;77:233-247.

127. Brooks R. EuroQol: the current state of play. Health Policy 1996;37:53-72.

128. Fuertes ME, Garcia Matres MJ, Gonzalez Romojaro V, et al. Clinical trial to evaluate trospium chloride (Uraplex) effectiveness and tolerance in patients with detrusor instability incontinence and its impact on quality of life. Arch.Esp.Urol. 2000;53:125-136.

129. Samuelsson E, Victor A, Tibblin G. A population study of urinary incontinence and nocturia among women aged 20-59. Acta Obstet Gynaecol Scand 1997;76:74-80.

130. Wagner TH, Patrick DL, Bavendam TG, Martin ML, Buesching DP. Quality of life of persons with urinary incontinence: development of a new measure. Urology 1996;47(1):67-72.

131. Wyman JF, Harkins SW, Taylor JR, Fantl AJ. Psychosocial Impact of Urinary Incontinence in Women. Obstetrics & Gynecology 1987;70(3):378-381.

132. Fleshner N. The artificial urinary sphincter for post-radical prostatectomy incontinence: Impact on urinary symptoms and quality of life. Journal of Urology 1996;155:1260-1264.

133. da Silva FC, Reis E, Costa T, Denis L. Quality of life in patients with prostatic cancer. Cancer. 1993;71(3):1138-1142.

134. Watkins-Bruner D, Scott C, Lawton C, et al. RTOG's first quality of life study - RTOG 90-20: A phase II trial of external beam radiation with etanidazole for locally advanced prostate cancer. Int.J.Radiation Oncology Biol.Phys. 1995;33(4):901-906.

135. Cella DF, Tulsky DS, Gray G, et al. The functional assessment of cancer therapy Scale: Development and validation of the general measure. Journal of Clinical Oncology 1993;11(3):570-579.

136. Raz S, Erickson DR. SEAPI QMM Incontinece Classification System. Neurourology and Urodynamics 1992; 11:187-199.

137. Lee PS, Reid DW, Saltmarche A, Linton L. Measuring the psychosocial impact of urinary incontinence: The York Incontinence Perceptions Scale (YIPS). J.Am.Geriatr.Soc. 1995;43:1275-1278.

138. Nochajski TH, Burns PA, Pranikoff K, Dittmar SS. Dimensions of urine loss among older women with genuine stress incontinence. Neurology and Urodynamics 1993;12:223-233.

139. Yu LC, Kaltreider L, Hu T, Igou JF, Craighead WE. Measuring stress associated with incontinence. Journal of Gerontololgical Nursing 1989;15 (2):9-15.

140. Seim A, Hermstad R, Hunskaar S. Management in general practice significantly reduced psychosocial consequences of female urinary incontinence. Quality of Life Research 1997;6:257-264.

141. Breakwell SL, Noble W. Differences in physical health, social interaction, and personal adjustment between continent and incontinent homebound aged women. Journal of Community Health Nursing 1988;5(1):19-31.

142. Marquis P. Measuring quality of life in daily practice: development and validation of a short-form questionnaire in urinary urge incontinence. Poster Presentation at ICS in Yokohomo. 1997;

143. Rosenzweig BA, Hischke D, Thomas S, Nelson AL, Bhatia NN. Stress Incontinence in Women. Journal of Reproductive Medicine 1991;36(12):835-839.

144. Caffo O, Fellin G, Graffer U, Luciani L. Assessment of quality of life after radical radiotherapy for prostate cancer. British Journal of Urology 1996;78:557-563.

145. Patrick DL, Martin ML, Bushnell DM, Yalcin I, Wagner TH, Buesching DP. Quality of life of women with urinary incontincence: further development of the incontinence quality of life instrument (I-QOL). Urology 1999;53:71-76.

146. Wyman JF, Fantl JA, McClish DK, Harkins SW, Uebersax JS, Ory MG. Quality of life following bladder training in older women with urinary incontinence. Int Urolgynecol J Pelvic Floor Dysfunct 1997;8:223-229.

147. Wyman JF, Fantl JA, McClish DK, Bump RC. Comparative efficacy of behavioural interventions in the management of female urinary incontinence. Continence program for women research group. Am J Obstret Gynecol 1998;46:999-1007.

148. Brubaker L, Benson JT, Bent A, Clark A, Shott S. Transvaginal electrical stimulation for female urinary incontinence. Am J Obstet Gynecol 1997;177:536 540.

149. Sampselle CM, Wyman JF, Thomas KK, et al. Continence for women: a test of AWHONN's evidence-based protocol in clinincal practice. J Wound Ostomy Continence Nurs 2000;27:109-117.

150. Davila GW, Neal D, Horback N, Peacher J, Doughtie JD, Karram M. A bladder-neck support prosthesis for women with stress and mixed incontinence. Obstet Gynecol 1999;93:938-942.

151. Versi E, Harvey MA. Efficacy of an external urethral device in women with genuine stress incontinence. Int Urogynecol Pelvic Floor Dysfunct 1998;9:271-274.

152. Siegel SW, Richardson DA, Miller KL, et al. Pelvic floor electrical stimulation for the treatment of urge and mixed urinary incontinence in women. Urology 1997;50:934-949.

153. Habb F, Trockman BA, Zimmerin PE, Leach GE. Quality of life and continence assessment of the artificial urinary sphincter in men with minimum 3.5 years of followup. Journal of Urology 1997;158:435-439.

154. Sander P, Thyssen H, Lose G, Andersen JT. Effect of a vaginal device on quality of life with urinary stress incontinence. Obstet Gynecol 1999;93:407-411.

155. McClish D, Wyman J, Sale P, Camp J, Earle B. Use and cost of incontinence pads in female study volunteers. Continence program for women research group. J Wound Ostomy Continence Nurs 1999;26:207-208.

156. Cella D. Manual of the Functional Assessment of Chronic Illness Therapy (FACIT) Measurement System Version 4. Center on Outcomes, Research and Education (CORE), Evanston Northwestern Healthcare and Northwestern University. 1997.

157. Yu LC. Incontinence Stress Index: measuring psychological impact. Journal of Gerontological Nursing 1987;13(7):18-25.

158. Derogatis LR. The psychosocial adjustment to illness scale (PAIS). J Psychosom Res 1986;1986:77-91.

159. Rust J, Golombok S. The Golombok-Rust Inventory of Sexual Satisfaction (GRISS). Br J Clin Psych 1985;1985:63-64.

160. O'Leary MP, Fowler FJ, Lenderking WR, et al. A brief male sexual function inventory for urology. Urology 1995;46(5):697-706.

161. Lukacs B, Comet D, Grange JC, Thibault P, BPH g. Construction and validation of a short-form benign prostatic hypertrophy health-related quality of life questionnaire. British Journal of Urology 1997;80:722-730.

162. Frankel SJ, Donovan JL, Peters TJ, et al. Sexual dysfunction in men with lower urinary tract symptoms. Journal of Clinical Epidemiology 1998;51(8):677-685.

163. Jackson S, Shepherd A, Brookes S, Abrams P. The effect of oestrogen supplementaiton on post-menopausal urinary stress incontinence: a double-blind placebo-controlled trial. Br J Obstet Gynaecol 1999;1999:711-718.

164. Walters MD, Taylors S, Schoenfeld LS. Psychosexual study of women with Detrusor Instability. Obstet Gynecol 1990;1990:22-26.

165. Komatsu. Sexuality. Kango Kenkyu 1996;29:386-398.

166. Clark A, Romm J. Effect of urinary incontinence on sexual activity in women. Journal of Reproductive Medicine 1993;38(9):679-683.

167. Kelleher CJ, Cardozo LD, Wise BG, Cutner A. The impact of urinary incontinence on sexual function. Neurology and Urodynamics 1992;1992:359-360.

168. Opjordsmoen S, Fossa SD. Qualtiy of life in patients treated for penile cancer. Br J Urol 1994;1994:652-657.

169. Hunt J, Moss J. Unwanted sexual experience and female urinary incontinence. Br J Health Psychol 1996;1996:231-233.

170. Bo K, Talseth T, Vinsnes A. Randomised controlled trial on the effect of pelvic floor muscle training on quality of life and sexual problems in genuine stress incontinent women. Acta Obstet Gynecol Scan 2000;2000:598-603.

171. Plouffe L. Screening for sexual problems through a simple questionnaire. Am J Obstet Gynecol 1985;1985:166-168.

172. Black NA, Bowling A, Griffiths JM, Pope C, Abel PD. Impact of surgery for stress incontinence on the social lives of women. Br J Obstet Gynaecol 1997;315:605-612.

173. Shumaker SA, Wyman JF, Uebersax JS, McClish D, Fantl JA. Continence Program in Women (CPW) Research Group. Quality of Life Research 1994;1994:291-306.

174. Wagner TH, Patrick DL, Bavendam TG, Martin ML, Buesching DP. Quality of life of persons with urinary incontinence: development of a new measure. Urol 1996;1996:67-72.

175. Bo K. Reproductability of instruments designed to measure subjective evaluation of female stress urinary incontinence. Scand J Urol Nephrol 1994;1994:97-100.

176. Marquis P, Amarenco G, Sapede C, Josserand F, Jacquetin B, Richard F. Development and validation of a disease specific quality of life questionnaire for urinary urge incontinence. J Urol 1995;1995:

177. Renck-Hooper U, McKenna SP, Whalley D. Measuring quality of life in female urinary urge incontinence: development and psychometric properties if IQOLI. Journal of Outcomes Research 1997;1997:1-8.

178. Smoger HS, Felice TK, Kloecker GH. Urinary incontinence among male veterans receiving care in primary care clinics. Ann Intern Med 2000;2000:547-551.

179. McGee H, Hannah M, O'Boyle CA, Hickey A, O'Malley K, Joyce CRB. Assessing the quality of life of the individuals: the SEIQOL with a healthy and a gastroenterology unit population. Psychological Medicine 1991;21:749-759.

180. Parker G, Williams J. Analysis of the OPCS disability survey data on incontinence. In: Robbins D, ed. Community Care: Findings from the Department of Health Funded Research 1988-92. London: HMSO, 1993;

181. Catanzoro M. Urinary bladder dysfunction as a remedial disability in multiple sclerosis. Arch Phys Med Rehabil 1982;63:472

182. Costa P, Perrouin-Verbe B, Colvez A, et al. Quality of life in spinal cord injury patients with urinary difficulties. Eur.Urol. 2001;39:107-113.

183. Pugner K, Holmes J. Nocturnal enuresis: economic aspects and self-esteem. Scan J Urol Nephrol 1997; Supp. 183:65-69.

184. Kelleher C. Quality of life and urinary incontinence. Baillieres.Clin.Endocrinol.Metab. 2000;14:363-379.

185. Harris A. Impact of urinary incontinence on the quality of life of women. Br J Nurs 1999;8:375-380.

186. Rai G. Impact of urinary incontinence on quality of life. J Am Geriatr Soc 1998;46:1480-1481.

187. Blaivais JG. Outcome measures for urinary incontinence. Urology 1998;51:11-19.

188. Gallo M, Gillette B, Hancock R, Pelkey A, Rawlings L, Sasso K. Quality of life improvement and the reliance urinary control insert. Urol Nurs 1997;17:146-153.

189. Jackson. The patient with an overactive bladder: symptoms and quality-of-life issues. Urology 1997; 50:18-22.

190. Kujansuu E. Patient history in the diagnosis of urinary incontinence and determining the quality of life. Acta Obstet Gynecol Scand Suppl 1997;166:15-18.

191. Costa P, Mottet N. Assessing the impact of urinary incontinence in a female population. Eur Urol 1997;32:25-27.

192. Barlow D, Samsioe G, van Geelen H. Prevalence of urinary problems in European countries. Maturitas 1997;27:239-247.

193. Kelleher C. Epidemiology and classification of urinary incontinence. In: Cardozo L, ed. Urogynecology. New York: Churchill Livingstone, 1997;3-22.

194. Hampel C, Weinhold D, Benken N, Eggersmann C, Thuroff JW. Definition of overactive bladder and epidemiology of urinary incontinence. Urology 1997;50:4-14.

195. Hampel C, Weinhold D, Benken N, Eggersmann C, Thuroff JW. Prevalence and natural history of female incontinence. Eur Urol 1997;32:3-12.

196. McGrother C, Resnick M, Yalla SV, et al. Epidemiology and etiology of urinary incontinence in the elderly. World J Urol 1998;16:s3-s9

197. Thom D. Variation in estimates of urinary incontinence prevalence in the community: effects of differences in definition, population characteristics, and study type. J Am Geriatr Soc 1998;46:473-480.

198. Donovan JL. The measurement of symptoms, quality of life and sexual function. British Journal of Urology International 2000, 85 (SI):10-19

199. Donovan JL. Measuring the impact of nocturia on quality of life. British Journal of Urology International 1999;84:21-25.

200. Hunskaar S, Arnold EP, Burgio K, Diokno AC, Herzog AR, Mallett VT. Epidemiology and natural history of urinary incontinence. Int.Urogynecol.J.Pelvic.Floor.Dysfunct. 2000;11:301-319.

201. Bo K. Effect of electrical stimulation on stress and urge urinary incontinence. Clinical outcome and practical recommendations based on randomized controlled trials. Acta Obstet Gynecol Scand.Suppl 1998;168:3-11.

202. de Seze M, Wiart L, Joseph PA, Dosque JP, Mazaux JM, Barat M. Capsaicin and neurogenic detrusor hyperreflexia: a double-blind placebo- controlled study in 20 patients with spinal cord lesions. Neurourol.Urodyn. 1998;17:513-523.

203. Burgio KL, Locher JL, Goode PS, et al. Behavioral vs drug treatment for urge urinary incontinence in older women: a randomized controlled trial. JAMA 1998;280:1995-2000.

204. Schmidt RA, Jonas U, Oleson KA, et al. Sacral nerve stimulation for treatment of refractory urinary urge incontinence. Sacral Nerve Stimulation Study Group. J Urol 1999;162:352-357.

205. Anderson RU, Mobley D, Blank B, Saltzstein D, Susset J, Brown JS. Once daily controlled versus immediate release oxybutynin chloride for urge urinary incontinence. OROS Oxybutynin Study Group. J Urol 1999;161:1809-1812.

206. Drutz HP, Appell RA, Gleason D, Klimberg I, Radomski S. Clinical efficacy and safety of tolterodine compared to oxybutynin and placebo in patients with overactive bladder. Int Urogynecol.J Pelvic.Floor.Dysfunct. 1999;10:283-289.

207. McDowell BJ, Engberg S, Sereika S, et al. Effectiveness of behavioral therapy to treat incontinence in homebound older adults. J Am.Geriatr.Soc. 1999;47:309-318.

208. Millard R, Tuttle J, Moore K, et al. Clinical efficacy and safety of tolterodine compared to placebo in detrusor overactivity. J Urol 1999;161:1551-1555.

209. Yamanishi T, Yasuda K, Sakakibara R, Hattori T, Suda S. Randomized, double-blind study of electrical stimulation for urinary incontinence due to detrusor overactivity. Urology 2000;55:353-357.

210. Tincello DG, Adams EJ, Sutherst JR, Richmond DH. Oxybutynin for detrusor instability with adjuvant salivary stimulant pastilles to improve compliance: results of a multicentre, randomized controlled trial. BJU.Int 2000;85:416-420.

211. Burgio KL, Locher JL, Goode PS. Combined behavioral and drug therapy for urge incontinence in older women. J Am.Geriatr.Soc. 2000;48:370-374.

212. Birns J, Lukkari E, Malone-Lee JG. A randomized controlled trial comparing the efficacy of controlled- release oxybutynin tablets (10 mg once daily) with conventional oxybutynin tablets (5 mg twice daily) in patients whose symptoms were stabilized on 5 mg twice daily of oxybutynin. BJU.Int 2000;85:793-798.

213. Colombo M, Vitobello D, Proietti F, Milani R. Randomised comparison of Burch colposuspension versus anterior colporrhaphy in women with stress urinary incontinence and anterior vaginal wall prolapse. BJOG 2000;107:544-551.

214. Sand PK, Winkler H, Blackhurst DW, Culligan PJ. A prospective randomized study comparing modified Burch retropubic urethropexy and suburethral sling for treatment of genuine stress incontinence with low-pressure urethra. Am.J Obstet Gynecol 2000;182:30-34.

215. Gilja I, Puskar D, Mazuran B, Radej M. Comparative analysis of bladder neck suspension using Raz, Burch and transvaginal Burch procedures. A 3-year randomized prospective study. Eur.Urol 1998;33:298-302.

216. Bo K, Talseth T, Holme I. Single blind, randomised controlled trial of pelvic floor exercises, electrical stimulation, vaginal cones, and no treatment in management of genuine stress incontinence in women. BMJ 1999;318:487-493.

217. Madersbacher H, Halaska M, Voigt R, Alloussi S, Hofner K. A placebo-controlled, multicentre study comparing the tolerabili-

ty and efficacy of propiverine and oxybutynin in patients with urgency and urge incontinence. BJU.Int 1999;84:646-651.

218. Lose G, Englev E. Oestradiol-releasing vaginal ring versus oestriol vaginal pessaries in the treatment of bothersome lower urinary tract symptoms. BJOG 2000;107:1029-1034.

219. Quadri G, Magatti F, Belloni C, Barisani D, Natale N. Marshall-Marchetti-Krantz urethropexy and Burch colposuspension for stress urinary incontinence in women with low pressure and hypermobility of the urethra: early results of a prospective randomized clinical trial. Am.J Obstet Gynecol 1999;181:12-18.

220. Coleman EA, Grothaus LC, Sandhu N, Wagner EH. Chronic care clinics: a randomized controlled trial of a new model of primary care for frail older adults. J Am.Geriatr.Soc. 1999;47:775-783.

221. Dugan E, Cohen SJ, Bland DR, et al. The association of depressive symptoms and urinary incontinence among older adults. J Am.Geriatr.Soc. 2000;48:413-416.

222. Weil EH, Ruiz-Cerda JL, Eerdmans PH, Janknegt RA, Bemelmans BL, van Kerrebroeck PE. Sacral root neuromodulation in the treatment of refractory urinary urge incontinence: a prospective randomized clinical trial. Eur.Urol 2000;37:161-171.

223. Knight S, Laycock J, Naylor D. Evaluation of neuromuscular electrical stimulation in the treatment of genuine stress incontinence. Physiotherapy 1998;84:61-71.

224. Chancellor MB, Bennett C, Simoneau AR, et al. Sphincteric stent versus external sphincterotomy in spinal cord injured men: prospective randomized multicenter trial. J Urol 1999;161:1893-1898.

225. Persson J, Wolner-Hanssen P. Laparoscopic Burch colposuspension for stress urinary incontinence: a randomized comparison of one or two sutures on each side of the urethra. Obstet Gynecol 2000;95:151-155.

226. Dorschner W, Stolzenburg JU, Griebenow R, et al. Efficacy and cardiac safety of propiverine in elderly patients - a double-blind, placebo-controlled clinical study. Eur.Urol 2000; 37:702-708.

227. Wyman JF, Fantl JA, McClish DK, Bump RC. Comparative efficacy of behavioral interventions in the management of female urinary incontinence. Continence Program for Women Research Group. Am.J Obstet Gynecol 1998;179:999-1007.

228. Wilson PD, Herbison GP. A randomized controlled trial of pelvic floor muscle exercises to treat postnatal urinary incontinence. Int Urogynecol.J Pelvic.Floor.Dysfunct. 1998;9:257-264.

229. Holtedahl K, Verelst M, Schiefloe A. A population based, randomized, controlled trial of conservative treatment for urinary incontinence in women. Acta Obstet Gynecol Scand. 1998; 77:671-677.

230. Watson AJ, Currie I, Jarvis GJ. A prospective placebo controlled double blind randomised study to investigate the use of indoramin to prevent post-operative voiding disorders after surgical treatment for genuine stress incontinence. Br J Obstet Gynaecol. 1999;106:270-272.

231. Serels S, Stein M. Prospective study comparing hyoscyamine, doxazosin, and combination therapy for the treatment of urgency and frequency in women. Neurourol.Urodyn. 1998;17:31-36.

232. Cammu H, Van Nylen M. Pelvic floor exercises versus vaginal weight cones in genuine stress incontinence. Eur.J Obstet Gynecol Reprod.Biol. 1998;77:89-93.

233. Wikander B, Ekelund P, Milsom I. An evaluation of multidisciplinary intervention governed by functional independence measure (FIMSM) in incontinent stroke patients. Scand.J Rehabil.Med 1998;30:15-21.

234. Moore KN, Griffiths D, Hughton A. Urinary incontinence after radical prostatectomy: a randomized controlled trial comparing pelvic muscle exercises with or without electrical stimulation. BJU.Int 1999;83:57-65.

235. Kammerer-Doak DN, Dorin MH, Rogers RG, Cousin MO. A randomized trial of burch retropubic urethropexy and anterior colporrhaphy for stress urinary incontinence. Obstet Gynecol 1999;93:75-78.

236. Reuben DB, Frank JC, Hirsch SH, McGuigan KA, Maly RC. A randomized clinical trial of outpatient comprehensive geriatric assessment coupled with an intervention to increase adherence to recommendations. J Am.Geriatr.Soc. 1999;47:269-276.

237. Petersen T, Nielsen JB, Schroder HD. Intravesical capsaicin in patients with detrusor hyper-reflexia—a placebo-controlled cross-over study. Scand.J Urol Nephrol. 1999;33:104-110.

238. Fujishiro T, Enomoto H, Ugawa Y, Takahashi S, Ueno S, Kitamura T. Magnetic stimulation of the sacral roots for the treatment of stress incontinence: an investigational study and placebo controlled trial. J Urol 2000;164:1277-1279.

239. Weil EH, Ruiz-Cerda JL, Eerdmans PH, Janknegt RA, Bemelmans BL, van Kerrebroeck PE. Sacral root neuromodulation in the treatment of refractory urinary urge incontinence: a prospective randomised clinical trial. Eur Urol 2000;37:161-171.

240. Chadha Y, Mollison J, Howie F, Grimshaw J, Hall M, Russell I. Guidelines in gynaecology: evaluation in menorrhagia and in urinary incontinence. BJOG 2000;107:535-543.

241. Choe JM, Ogan K, Battino BS. Antimicrobial mesh versus vaginal wall sling: a comparative outcomes analysis. J Urol 2000;163:1829-1834.

242. Van Kampen M, De Weerdt W, Van Poppel H, De Ridder D, Feys H, Baert L. Effect of pelvic-floor re-education on duration and degree of incontinence after radical prostatectomy: a randomised controlled trial. Lancet 2000;355:98-102.

243. Fujishiro T, Enomoto H, Ugawa Y, Takahashi S, Ueno S, Kitamura T. Magnetic stimulation of the sacral roots for the treatment of stress incontinence: an investigational study and placebo controlled trial. J Urol 2000;164:1277-1279.

244. Burgio KL, Locher JL, Roth DL, Goode PS. Psychological improvements associated with behavioral and drug treatment of urge incontinence in older women. Journal of gerontology 2001; 56:45-51.

245. Lemack G, Zimmern PE. Sexual function after vaginal surgery for stress incontinence: results of a mailed questionnaire. Urology 2000;56:223-227.

246. Amunsden CL, Guralnick ML, Webster G. Variations in strategy for the treatment of urethral obstruction after a pubovaginal sling procedure. J Urol 2000;164:434-437.

247. Winters JC, Chiverton A, Sarpero HM, Prats LJJ. Colagen injection therapy in elderly women: long-term results and patient satisfaction. Urology 2000;55:856-861.

248. Fuertes ME, Garcia Matres MJ, Gonzelez Romojaro V, et al. Clinical trial to evaluate trospium chloride (Uraplex) effectiveness and tolerance in patients with detrusor instability incontinence and its impact on quality of life. Arch Esp Urol 2000;53:125-136.

249. Morgan TO, Westney OL, McGuire EJ. Pubovaginal sling: 4-year outcome analysis and quality of life assessment. J Urol 2000;163:1845-1848.

250. Sander P, Mouritsen L, Andersen JT, Fischer-Rasmussen W. Evaluation of a simple, non-surgical concept for management of urinary incontinence (minimal care) in an open-access, interdisciplinary incontinence clinic. Neurourol Urodyn 2000;19:9-17.

251. Filbeck T, Ullrich T, Pichlmeier U, Keil HJ, Weiland WF, Roessler W. Correlation of persistent stress urinary incontinence with quality of life after suspension procedures: is continen-

ce the only decisive postoperative criterion of success. Urology 1999;54:247-251.

252. Moore KH, Simons A, Dowell C, Bryant C, Prashar S. Efficacy and user acceptability of the urethral occlusive device in women with urinary incontinence. J Urol 1999;162 :464-468.

253. Sand PK, Staskin D, Miller J, et al. Effect of a urinary control insert on quality of life in incontinent women. Int Urogyneocol J Pelvic Floor Dysfunct 1999;10:100-1105.

254. Galloway NT, El-Galley RE, Sand PK, Appell RA, Russell HW, Carlan SJ. Extracorporeal magnetic innervation therapy for stress urinary incontinence. Urology 1999;53:1108-1111.

255. Weinberger MW, Goodman BM, Carnes M. Long-term efficacy of nonsurgical urinary incontinence treatment in elderly women. J Gerontol A Biol Sci Med Sci 1999;54:117-121.

256. Hassouna ME, Ghoniem GM. Long-term outcome and quality of life after modified pubovaginal sling for intrinsic sphincter deficiency. Urology 1999;53:287-291.

257. Amarenco G, Marquis P, McCarthy C, Richard F. Quality of life of women with stress urinary incontinence with or without pollakisuria. Presse Med 1998;27:5-10.

258. Versi E, Griffiths DJ, Harvey MA. A new external urethral device for female urinary incontinence. Obstet Gynecol 1998;92:286-291.

259. Rabin JM. Clinical use of the FemAssist device in female urinary incontinence. J Med Syst 1998;22:257-271.

260. Sander P, Thyssen HH, Lose G, Andersen JT. The effect of a vaginal device on urinary leakage and quality of life of women. J Ugeskr Laeger 2000;22:3038-3041.

261. Richardson DA, Miller KL, Siegel SW, Karram MM, Blackwood NB, Staskin DR. Pelvic floor electrical stimulation: a comparison of daily and every-other-day therapy for genuine stress incontinence. Urology 1996;48:110-118.

262. Berglund AL, Elsemann M, Lalos A, Lalos O. Social adjustment and spouse relationships among women with stress incontinence before and after surgical treatment. Soc Sci Med 2001;42:1537-1544.

263. World HO. Definition of Health. Geneva: WHO, 1978;

264. Sells H, Donovan JL, Ewings P, Macdonagh R. The development and validation of a quality of life measure to assess partner morbidity in benign prostatic enlargement. British Journal of Urology International 2000;85:440-445.

265. Lukacs B, Leplege A, Thibault P, Jardin A. Development, validation and application of a BPH - specific health related quality of life questionnaire. In: Cockett ATK, ed. Proceedings of the Third International Consultation BPH, Monaco. Jersey: Scientific International, 1996;277-280.

266. Tsang KK, Garraway WM. Impact of benign prostatic hyperplasia on general well-being of men. Prostate. 1993;23:1-7.

267. Sagnier P, MacFarlene G, Teillac P, Botto H, Richard F, Boyle P. Impact of symptoms of prostatism on level of bother and quality of life of men in the french community. Journal of Urology 1995;153:669-673.

268. Anon. A comparison of quality of life with patient reported symptoms and objective findings in men with benign prostatic hyperplasia. The Department of Veterans Affairs Cooperative Study of transurethral resection for benign prostatic hyperplasia. J.Urol. 1993;150:1696-1700.

269. Fowler FJ, Jr., Barry MJ. Quality of life assessment for evaluating benign prostatic hyperplasia treatments. An example of using a condition-specific index. Eur.Urol. 1993;24 Suppl 1:24-27.

270. Chute CG, Panser LA, Girman CJ, et al. The prevalence of prostatism: a population-based survey of urinary symptoms. J.Urol. 1993;150:85-89.

271. Fowler FJ, Jr., Wennberg JE, Timothy RP, Barry MJ, Mulley AG, Jr., Hanley D. Symptom status and quality of life following prostatectomy. JAMA 1988;259:3018-3022.

272. Barry MJ, Fowler FJ, O'Leary MP, et al. The American Urological Association Symptom Index for Benign Prostatic Hyperplasia. Journal of Urology 1992;148:1549-1557.

273. Hunter DJW, McKee CM, Black NA, Sanderson CFB. Urinary symptoms: prevalence and severity in British men aged 55 and over. Journal of Epidemiology and Community Health Medicine 1994;48:569-575.

274. Garraway WM, Russell EBA, Lee RJ, et al. Impact of previously unrecognised benign prostatic hyperplasia on the daily activities of middle-aged and elderly men. British Journal of General Practice 1993;43:318-321.

275. Girman CJ, Epstein RS, Jacobsen SJ, et al. Natural history of prostatism: Impact of urinary symptoms on quality of life in 2115 randomly selected community men. Urology 1994;44(6):825-831.

276. Doll H, McPherson K, Davies J, et al. Reliability of questionnaire responses as compared with interview in the elderly: views of the outcome of transurethral resection of the prostate. Soc.Sci.Med. 1991;33:1303-1308.

277. Jolleys JV, Donovan JL, Nanchahal K, Peters TJ, Abrams P. Urinary symptoms in the community: how bothersome are they? Br.J.Urol. 1994;74:551-555.

278. Peters TJ, Donovan JL, Kay HE, et al. The International Continence Society "Benign Prostatic Hyperplasia" Study: The bothersomeness of urinary symptoms. Journal of Urology 1997;157:885-889.

279. Kutner NG, Schechtman KB, Ory MG, Baker DI, FICSIT G. Older adults' perceptions of their health and functioning in relation to sleep disturbance, falling, and urinary incontinence. J.Am.Geriatr.Soc. 1994;42:757-762.

280. Hunskaar S, Sandvik H. One hundred and fifty men with urinary incontinence. Scand J Prim Health Care 1993;11:193-196.

281. O'Connor R, Johannesson M, Hass S, Kobelt-Nguye N. Urge incontinence, Quality of life and patients' valuation of symptom reduction. Pharmaco economics 1998;14:531-539.

282. Brown J, Sabak L, Gras J, Brown B, Kuppermann M, Posner S. Urge incontinence: the patients' perspective. J Womens Health 1998;7:1263-1269.

283. DuBeau C, Levy B, Mangione C, Resnick N. The impact of urge urinary incontinence on quality life: Importance of patients' Soc perspective and explanatory style. J Am Geriatr Soc 1998;46:683-692.

284. Grimby A, Milsom I, Molander U, Wiklund I, Ekelund P. The invluence of urinary incontinence on the quality of life of elderly women. Age Ageing 1993;22:82-89.

285. Johnson TM, Kincade JE, Bernard SL, Busby-Whitehead J, Hertz-Piciotto I, DeFreise GH. The association of urinary incontinence with poor self-rated health. Journal of the American Geriatrics Society 1998;46:693-699.

286. Herzog AR, Fultz NH, Normolle DP, Brock BM, Diokno AC. Methods used to manage urinary incontinence by older adults in the community. American Geriatrics Society 1989;37(4):339-347.

287. Chiverton P, Wells T, Brink C, Mayer R. Psychological factors associated with urinary incontinence. Clin Nurse Spec 1996;10:229-233.

288. Helgason, A. R. Prostate cancer treatment and quality of life - a three level epidemiological approach. 1997. Thesis.

289. Temml C, Haidinger G, Schmidbauer J, Schatzl G, Madersbacher S. Urinary incontinence in both sexes: prevalence rates and impact on quality of life and sexual life. Neurourol Urodyn 2000;19:259-271.

290. Sandvik H, Kveine E, Hunskaar S. Female urinary incontinence. Scand J Caring Sci 1993;7 :53-56.

291. Lagro J, Smits A, Van Weel C. Urinary incontinence in women and the effects on their lives. Scand J Prim Health Care 1992;10:211-216.

292. Ouslander JG, Hepps K, Raz S, Su HL. Genitourinary dysfunction in a geriatric outpatient population. American Geriatrics Society 1986;54:507-514.

293. Simeonova Z, Milson I, Kullendorff A, Molander U, Bengtsson C. The prevalence of urinary incontinence and its influence on the quality of life in women from an urban Swedish population. Acta Obstet Gynecol Scand 1999;78:546-551.

294. Hunskaar S, Vinsnes A. The qulity of life in women with urinary incontinence as measured by the sickness impact profile. J Am Geriatr Soc 1991;39:378-382.

295. Burgio KL, Ives DO, Locher JL, Arena VC, Kuller LH. Treatment seeking for urinary incontinence in older adults. J.Am.Geriatr.Soc. 1994;42:208-212.

296. Memel DS, Harrison GL. Urinary incontinence in women: its prevalence and its management in a health promotion clinic. British Journal of General Practice 1994;44:149-152.

297. Lagro-Janssen AL. British Journal of General Practice 1990;40:331-334.

298. Simeonova Z, Milson I, Kullendorff AM, Molander U, Bengtsson C. The influence of urinary incontinence on quality of life of community-dwelling 45-70 year old Dutch women. Ned.Tijdschr.Geneeskd. 1999;6:894-897.

299. Simeonova Z, Milson I, Kullendorff AM, Molander U, Bengtsson C. The prevalence of urinary incontinence and its influence on the quality of life in women from an urban Swedish population. Acta Obstet Gynaecol Scand 1999;78:546-551.

300. Brown JS, Subak L L, Gras J, Brown B, Kuppermann M, Posner SF. Urge incontinence: the patients persepective. J Womens Health 1998;7:1263-1269.

301. McClish DK, Wyman JF, Sale P, Camp J, Earle B. Use and cost of incontinence pads in female study volunteers. Continence program for woem research group. J Wound Ostomy Continence Nurs 1999;26:207-208.

302. Kinn AC, Zaar A. Quality of life and urinary incontinence pad use in women. Int Urogynecol Pelvic Floor Dysfunct 1998;9:83-87.

303. DuBeau CE, Levy B, Mangione C, Resnick N.M. The impact of urge urinary incontinence on quality of life: importance of patients' perspective and explanatory style. J Am Geriatr Soc 1998;46:683-692.

304. Robinson D, Pearce K, Preisser J, Dugan E, Suggs P, Cohen S. Relationships between patient reports of urinary incontinence symptoms and quality of life measures. Obstet.Gynecol. 1998;91:224-228.

305. Grimby A, Milsom I, Molander U, Wiklund I, Ekelund P. The influence of urinary incontinence of the quality of life of elderly women. Age.Ageing. 1993;22:82-89.

306. Hunskaar S, Vinsnes A. The quality of life in women with urinary incontinece as measured by the sickness impact profile. J Am Geriatr Soc 1991;378-382.

307. Lam GW, Foldspang A, Elving LB, Mommsen S. Social context, social abstention, and problem recognition correlated with adult female urinary incontinence. Dan Med Bull 1992;1992:565-570.

308. Nygaard I, Milburn A. Urinary incontinence during sexual activity: Prevalence in a gynecologic practice. Journal of Women's Health 1995;1995:83-86.

309. Sutherst J, Brown M. Sexual Dysfunction Associated with Urinary Incontinence. Urol.Int. 1980;35:414-416.

310. Gordon D, Groutz A, Sinai T, et al. Sexual function in women attending a Urolgynecology clinic. Int Urogynecol J 1999;1999:325-328.

311. Vierhout ME, Gianotten WL. Mechanisms of urine loss during sexual activity. Eur J Obstet Gynecol and Repro Biol 1993;1993:45-47.

312. Hilton P. Urinary incontinence during sexual intercourse: a common, but rarely volunteered, symptom. British Journal of Obstetrics and Gynaecology 1988;95:377-381.

313. Haase P, Skibsted L. Influence of operations for stress incontinence and/or genital descensus on sexual life. Acta Obstet Gynecol Scand 1988;1988:659-661.

314. Weber AM, Walters MD, Piedmonte MR. Sexual function and vaginal anatomy in women before and after surgery for pelvic organ prolapse and urinary incontinence. Am J Obstet Gynecol 2000;1610-1615.

315. Anonymous. Sexual function after colpo-urethrocystopexy in middle aged women. Urol Int 1988;1988:231-233.

316. Berglund AL, Fugl-Meyer KS. Some sexological characteristics of stress incontinence women. Scan J Urol Nephrol 1995;1995:207-212.

317. Holtgrewe HL, Ackermann R, Bay-Nielsen H, Coast J, Jonsson B. The economics of BPH. In: Cockett ATK, ed. Proceedings of the Second WHO International Consultation on BPH. Jersey: Scientific Communication International, 1993;35-46.

318. Homma Y, Gotoh M, Ando T, Fukuhara S. Development of the Japanese version of QOL questionnaires for urinary incontinence. Jpn J NBS 1999;10:225-236.

319. Cockett ATK, Aso Y, Chatelain C, et al. The International Consultation on Benign Prostatic Hyperplasia, Paris 1991 . Jersey: Scientific International, 1991;

320. Bolognese JA, Kozloff RC, Kunitz SC, Grino PB, Patrick DL, Stoner E. Validation of a symptoms questionnaire for benign prostatic hyperplasia. Prostate. 1992;21:247-254.

321. Epstein RS, Deverka PA, Chute CG, et al. Validation of a New Quality of Life Questionnaire for Benign Prostatic Hyperplasia. J.Clin.Epidemiol. 1992;45(12):1431-1445.

322. Panser LA, Rhodes T, Girman CJ, et al. Sexual function of men ages 40 to 79 years: the Olmsted County study of urinary symptoms and health status among men. J Am Geriatr Soc 1995;1995:1107-1111.

323. Lukacs B, Leplege A, MacCarthy C, Comet D. Construction and validation of a BPH specific health related quality of life scale including evaluation of sexuality. Urology 1995;153 Suppl:320A

324. Lukacs B, McCarthy C, Grange JC. Long-term quality of life in patients with benign prostatic hypertrophy: preliminary results of a cohort survey of 7,093 patients treated with an alpha-1-adrenergic blocker, alfuzosin. QOL BPH Study Group in General Practice. Eur.Urol. 1993;24 Suppl 1:34-40.

325. Boyle P. Cultural and linguistic validation of questionnaires for use in International studies: The Nine-item BPH-Specific Quality of Life Scale. European Urology 1997;32:50-52.

326. Barry M, Fowler F, O'Leary M, Bruskewitz R, Holtgrewe H, Mebust W. Measuring disease-specific health status in men with benign prostatic hyperplasia. Medical Care 1995;33,4:AS145-AS155

327. Epstein RS, Deverka PA, Chute CG, et al. Urinary symptom and quality of life questions indicative of obstructive benign prostatic hyperplasia. Results of a pilot study. Urology 1991;38:20-26.

328. Schag CA, Ganz PA, Heinrich RL. Cancer Rehabilitation Evaluation System - short form (Cares-SF). A cancer-specific rehabilitation and quality of life instrument. Cancer 1991;68:1406-1413.

329. Stockler MR, Osoba D, Goodwin P, Corey P, Tannock IF. Responsiveness to change in health-related quality of life in a randomized clinical trial: A comparison of the Prostate Cancer Specific Quality of Life Instrument (PROSQOLI) with analogous Scales from the EORTCQLQ-C30 and a trial specific module. J.Clin.Epidemiol. 1998;51(2):137-145.

330. Watts RJ. Sexual functioning, health beliefs and compliance with high blood pressure medication. Nursing Research 1982;5 (31):278-282.

331. Helgason AR, Fredrikson M, Adolfsson J, Steineck G. Decreased sexual capacity after external radiation therapy for prostate cancer impairs quality of life. Int.J.Radiation Oncology Biol.Phys. 1995;32(1):33-39.

332. Helgason AR, Adolfsson J, Dickman P, et al. Sexual desire, erection, orgasm and ejaculatory functions and their importance to elderly Swedish men: a population-based study. Age.Ageing. 1996;25:285-291.

333. Helgason AR, Adolfsson J, Dickman P, Fredrikson M, Arver S, Steineck G. Waning sexual function - the most important disease-specific distress for patients with prostate cancer. British Journal of Cancer 1996;73:1417-1421.

334. Helgason AR, Adolfsson J, Dickman P, Arver S, Fredrikson M, Gunnar S. Factors associated with waning sexual function among elderly men and prostate cancer patients. Journal of Urology 1997;157:1-5.

335. Rosen RC, Riley A, Wagner G, Osterloh IH, Kirkpatrick J, Mishra A. The International Index of Erectile Function (IIEF): a multidimensional scale for the assessment of erectile dysfunction. Urology 1997;49 (6):822-830.

336. Stewart AL & Ware JE, Jr. (Editors). Measuring Functioning and Well-Being: The Medical Outcomes Study Approach. Durham, NC: Duke University Press, 1992.

Committee 7

Urodynamics

Chairman

Y. HOMMA (JAPAN)

Members

J. BATISTA (SPAIN),

S. BAUER (USA),

D. GRIFFITHS (USA),

P. HILTON (U.K),

G. KRAMER (GERMANY),

G. LOSE (DENMARK),

P. ROSIER (THE NETHERLAND)

CONTENTS

Urodynamics

Y. HOMMA,

J. BATISTA, S. BAUER, D. GRIFFITHS, P. HILTON, G. KRAMER, G. LOSE, P. ROSIER

A. GENERAL REMARKS

I. INTRODUCTION

In preparing this chapter, one of the main goals of the committee has been to present evidence for the ability or inability of urodynamic investigation to improve or at least predict the outcome of treatment for incontinence. In spite of the fundamental importance of urodynamics, the committee has found that for each type of test the evidence is based either on case series (level 4 evidence) or expert opinion (level 5 evidence). For this reason it has not repeatedly restated the levels of evidence, but has graded each of its final recommendations for clinical practice on the basis of these levels of evidence. Inevitably, one of the principal recommendations is for clinical research studies to improve the quality of the evidence.

The lower urinary tract is composed of the bladder and urethra. They form a functional unit to store and evacuate urine. During the normal storage phase, as the bladder is filled with urine, a sensation of filling is perceived at a certain moment and subsequently a desire to void is felt. Normally no uncomfortable sensation such as urgency, pain or discomfort is perceived and no urinary leakage occurs. Competence of the urethra and accommodation of the bladder make it possible to store urine at a low and stable pressure. The low storage pressure insures adequate drainage of urine flow from the upper urinary tract. The normal voiding phase is characterized by the voluntary initiation of micturition followed by forceful and continuous flow with no residual urine. Coordinated relaxation of pelvic floor and external urethral sphincter as well as detrusor contraction contribute to the efficient emptying of the bladder. Urinary flow can be intentionally interrupted by voluntary contraction of urethral sphincter and pelvic floor. Nervous control mechanisms, central and peripheral as well as somatic and autonomic, integrate these functions (Figure 1).

Accordingly, two broad types of lower urinary tract dysfunction may be distinguished: dysfunction of storage and dysfunction of voiding. Clearly urinary incontinence, represents a failure to store urine adequately, but it can be associated with or aggravated by some types of voiding dysfunction of neurogenic, mechanical or functional etiology. Failure to store urine at low pressure or emptying at high pressure may affect upper urinary tract drainage and eventually its function. Occasionally, leakage may occur through channels other than the urethra. This is extra-urethral incontinence.

Urodynamic investigation is a functional assessment of the lower urinary tract to provide objective pathophysiological explanations for symptoms and/or dysfunction of the lower and upper urinary tracts. Urodynamic studies comprise a series of tests. The appropriate test(s) should be selected and performed in an attempt to answer well-defined question(s) on the target functions to be evaluated (Table 1). In the case of incontinence, the most relevant of these tests are directly related to the incontinence itself; that is, they aim to demonstrate involuntary leakage in the test setting. Cystometry with or without simultaneous imaging, ambulatory urodynamics and the measurement of leak point pressures are the primary examples of such tests. Other urodynamic tests have an indirect relation to the incontinence. The information provided by these studies may be useful in establishing etiology and may be clinically important by helping to select the most appropriate intervention. Uroflowmetry, residual urine measurement and pressure-flow studies are examples.

In the clinical work-up of an incontinent patient, urodynamic studies are indicated for the following reasons:

- to identify or to rule out the factors contributing to the incontinence and their relative importance

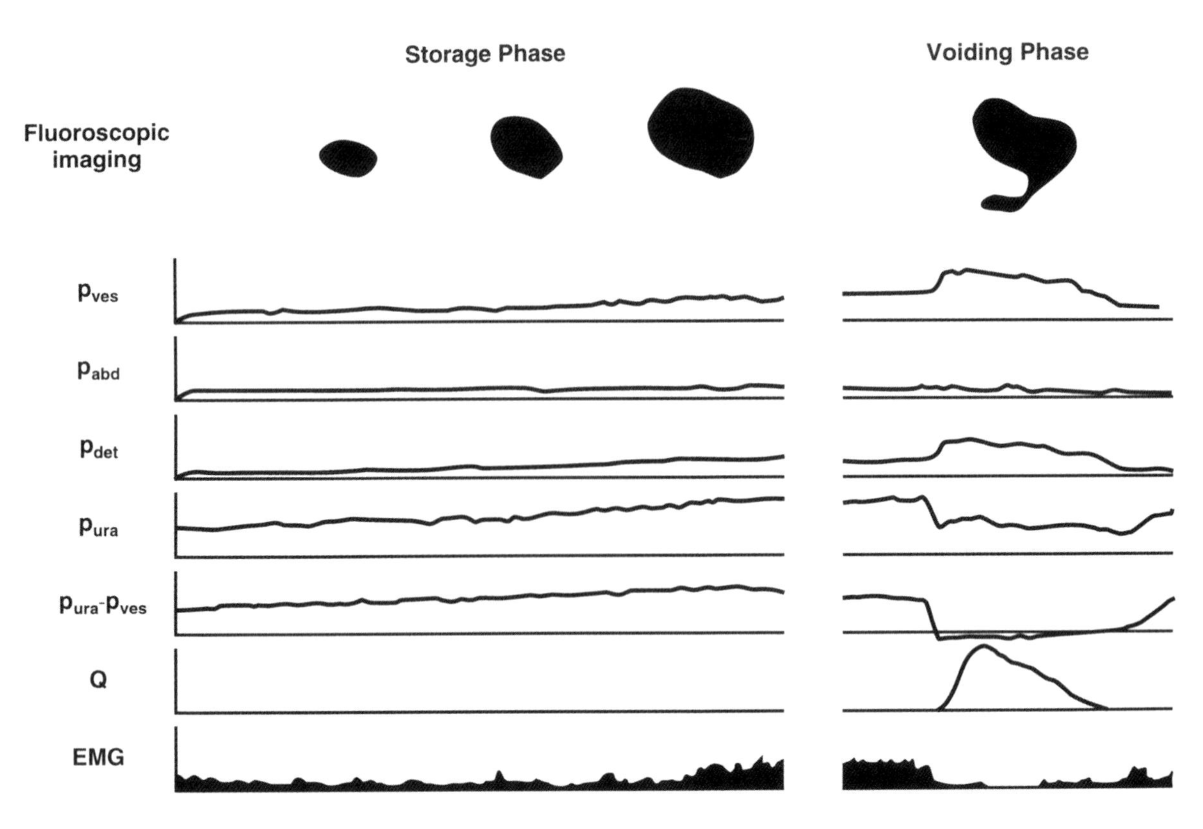

Figure 1 : Illustrative normal urodynamic findings with fluoroscopic imagings. Intravesical pressure (pves), abdominal pressure (pabd), detrusor pressure (pdet: pves-pabd), urethral pressure (pura) measured at the point of maximum urethral pressure, Pura-Pves, urinary flow (Q) and surface electromyography (EMG) during the storage and voiding phases are idealized.

Table 1 : Urodynamic Studies for Urinary Incontinence Assessment

Urodynamic study	Target function to be evaluated	Indicated patients
1. Cystometry	storage function and sensation of the bladder during the filling phase	any incontinent subjects to be investigated for their dysfunctional conditions
2. Urethral pressure measurement	urethral closing forces	subjects suspected of urethral incompetence
3. Leak point pressure measurement A. Detrusor B. Abdominal	urethral competence against pressure generated in the bladder from detrusor or abdominal forces	subjects suspected of neurogenic lower urinary tract dysfunction (A) or urethral incompetence (B)
4. Uroflowmetry, Residual urine measurement	global voiding function	any incontinent subjects (residual) or those suspected of voiding dysfunction (uroflow)
5. Pressure-flow studies	detrusor contractility and bladder outlet obstruction during the voiding phase	subjects suspected of voiding dysfunction
6. Surface electromyography	coordinated relaxation of pelvic floor during the voiding phase	subjects suspected of dysfunctional or dyssynergic voiding
7. Videourodynamics	Simultaneous observation of the morphology and function of the lower urinary tract	subjects with suspected multifactorial etiologies for incontinence or anatomical abnormalities of the lower urinary tract
8. Ambulatory urodynamic monitoring	behavior of bladder (and urethra) and leakage mechanisms during activities of daily living	subjects suspected but not proven to have incontinence or detrusor overactivity on conventional investigations

- to obtain information about other aspects of the lower urinary tract dysfunction
- to predict the consequences of the dysfunction for the upper urinary tract
- to predict the outcome, including undesirable side effects, of a contemplated treatment.
- to confirm the effects of treatment or to understand the mode of action of a particular type of treatment, especially a new one
- to understand the reasons for failure of previous treatments for incontinence

In short, urodynamic studies are indicated to objectively observe lower urinary tract function and dysfunction with the idea of choosing an appropriate treatment for the incontinence and its associated pathology. Basically, the urodynamic study should be performed and reported in accordance with the standards of the International Continence Society (ICS) [1], so as to optimize interpretation and facilitate comparison between different studies. This principle is applied hereafter; however, the chapter is not intended to simply reproduce the ICS standardization report but rather to focus on the clinical relevance of urodynamics to urinary incontinence. It includes recommendations for study procedures, interpretation of study results and the ability to predict treatment. Electrophysiological studies are treated in more detail in chapter 4.

II. THE GENERAL ASPECTS OF URODYNAMICS IN INCONTINENCE ASSESSMENT

Urodynamic investigations must be carried out in a safe, comfortable, and scientific manner, and should be reproducible within the limits of physiological variability, if repeated. This section emphasizes points that are pertinent to all urodynamic studies in the assessment of incontinence [2, 3]. These points will be repeated in other sections of this chapter where relevant to the discussion. Further details are available in textbooks [4-8].

1. Information prior to study

Prior to the urodynamic investigation a medical history, a physical examination and/or a voiding diary should be taken. Such information is absolutely necessary to select the appropriate studies and to anticipate what events might take place during the urodynamic investigation.

2. General conditions and circumstances of the study

The patient should be informed of the procedures before the studies, preferably by written leaflets but in any event by oral explanation. Any medication that may affect the patient's consciousness or that has been prescribed for lower urinary tract dysfunction should be avoided before the procedure, unless the test is specifically intended to study its effect or there is a clinical reason for not stopping medication. The nature of any such medication and the timing of its administration (especially the last dose) should be noted. Medications that affect lower urinary tract function but have been prescribed for other reasons should be taken into account when interpreting the findings.

The subject should be awake and unanesthetized during the study. In children, studies are sometimes performed under mild sedation. However, this is not desirable and can be avoided if the study is thoroughly explained to them beforehand and if care is taken to distract and calm them during the procedure (see section III.5.e).

The position of the patient during the examination (supine, sitting, standing or ambulatory) needs to be considered and should be specified in the report. In general it may be better to perform bladder filling in the sitting or standing position, or even to change the patient's position, in order to facilitate demonstration of the incontinence. If the position is changed, the pressure transducers (if external) must be repositioned at the reference level (see section I.2.e). In some cases the choice of position may be determined by the patient's condition. For example, if incontinence is due to neurological disease, demonstration of leakage during the examination is usually relatively easy, and it may be simplest to examine the patient supine.

3. The investigator

The investigator plays a crucial role in the urodynamics. The tasks of the investigator include recognition and minimization of artifacts (quality control), communication with the patient regarding sensation and intention, and direction of the whole examination. Quality control requires careful observation of the data as it is being collected. If data quality problems are identified and corrected at this time, a valid examination may be obtained. If not, the study may be uninterpretable. The investigator should talk to patients in a polite and explicit way to facilitate good communication. This is essential so that the patient understands what the investigator requires and the investigator knows how the patient feels and whether the patient is consciously inhibiting the leakage. Also he/she directs the investigation, for example, by repeating a test if the result is unclear, or introducing extra tests if needed to clarify the situation.

Thus, these tasks require diligent scrutiny throughout the progress of the study and understanding of the results while the test is being carried out. Consequently the person conducting the investigations must note and record all relevant events as well as simultaneously interpreting the findings. Simple inspection of traces after the study is completed does not yield a satisfactory interpretation [9].

Formal qualifications for urodynamic investigators have not been developed, but are being considered on a national basis in the UK and in Germany. Provided the person is experienced, the investigator conducting the study may be a physician or a nurse, or a person with a science, engineering or radiology background.

4. Catheters and transducers

Urethral catheters for bladder filling and for pressure measurement should be as small as possible in diameter so as not to interfere with observations of incontinence (leakage) and voiding. However, with a small catheter it may be difficult to drain the bladder when desired. A catheter as small as 6 or 7 French gauge reduces the voiding flow rate in both men [10] and women [11]. Even a 5 French gauge catheter increases the voiding pressure in males [12]. However, the obstructive effect of an 8 French gauge catheter is clinically acceptable in men [13], while a 10 French catheter has a more significant effect [14]. An 8 French gauge catheter tends to increase the measured Valsalva leak point pressure [15]. Thus, for adults, some authorities recommend a maximum catheter size of 8 French gauge, although others permit 10 French gauge. If external pressure transducers are employed, two small single-lumen catheters or a twin-lumen catheter should be used for bladder filling/drainage and intravesical pressure measurement, respectively. Such catheters can be left in place throughout the study so that it can readily be repeated. Optionally, a single urethral catheter with a third channel for simultaneous urethral pressure measurement may be used. If catheter-mounted transducers are employed, the catheter size and the type of transducer (e.g., strain gauge or fibre-optic) are important for interpretation and should be specified in the report. The manufacturer of the catheter and the model number or name should also be specified. Rectal catheters should be similarly described and the name of the manufacturer and the model should be specified as well.

5. Pressure measurement

The principal pressures measured during urodynamic studies are the intravesical pressure, the abdominal pressure and the urethral pressure. The difference between the intravesical and abdominal pressures is called the detrusor pressure. The symbols for these pressures are p_{ves}, p_{abd}, p_{ura} and p_{det}, respectively.

The measurement of pressure is the most important aim of urodynamic tests; nevertheless it is prone to artifacts. To monitor measurement validity, coughing at regular intervals, e.g. every 60 seconds or every 50ml infused, immediately before the examination, during the whole storage phase and immediately after the examination, is therefore essential. Coughing should consistently give similar pressure changes in p_{ves} and p_{abd} (Figure 2).

Currently, pressure is most frequently recorded by the conversion of pressure changes to the electrical properties of a strain gauge transducer. When the strain gauge is outside the body, the pressures that are generated inside the body must be transferred to it. This is possible with fluid-filled catheters and external tubing. Thus, the inserted catheter and connecting tube should be short and flexible, and should not yield to pressure change nor leak at any of connection points. All air bubbles in the system should be meticulously removed.

Transducers to measure pressure can also be mounted on a "microtip" or fiber-optic catheter that can be inserted into the body cavity. Problems related to the tubing system are not important in this case. However, hydrostatic forces inside the abdomen influence the measurement in a variable way, because the pressure reference level is not clearly defined (see *Intravesical pressure*, below) [16]. Another undesirable property of catheter-mounted transducers is that they respond not only to pressures but also to forces exerted on them by solid objects, for example, by contact with the bladder wall. Consequently, intravesical pressures measured by external transducers may differ from those measured internally by 20 cm H_2O or more [17].

Alternatively the pressure-measuring catheter can be air-filled; the catheter is provided with a small air-filled balloon to prevent entry of liquid from the bladder and is connected to external transducers by an air-filled connecting tube. As for catheter-mounted transducers, the pressure reference level is not clearly defined. The balloon must not be over-inflated (see *Abdominal pressure*, below).

In clinical urodynamic practice, absolute pressure values sometimes seem less important than pressure patterns. However, the reliability of the absolute value plays an important role in the control of measurement quality. In many clinical situations furthermore it is essential to ensure that the measured pressures are correct. For instance, when comparisons with reference values from the literature are used in clinical decision-making; or when cystometric values before and after treatment are compared in outcome analysis based on multicenter data; or when longitudinal observations on

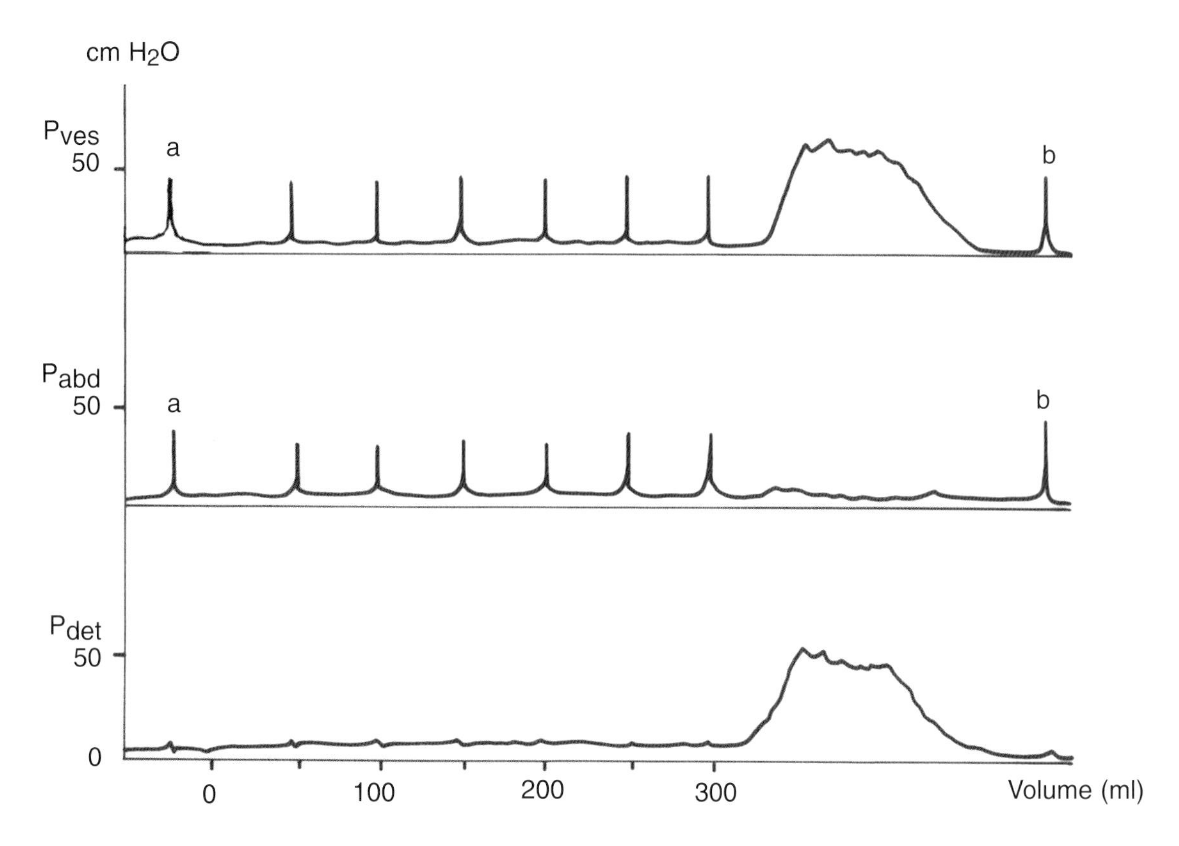

Figure 2 : Ildeal cystometric traces with coughing at regular intervals of 50ml filling. Note coughs before starting (a) and after ending the test (b).

a single patient are compared. Specific examples include leak point pressure measurement and grading of bladder outlet obstruction by pressure-flow analysis.

a) Intravesical pressure

In the physical sense p_{ves}, which is the pressure in the liquid contained within the bladder, is a true pressure. This pressure is the height, above a given reference level, to which the liquid would rise in an open catheter puncturing the bladder. p_{ves} consists of 2 components: a contribution from the internal forces in the bladder wall (p_{det}), and a contribution from the organs surrounding the bladder (p_{abd}):

i.e., $p_{ves} = p_{det} + p_{abd}$.

The standard reference level for all pressure recording is defined as the upper border of the pubic symphysis. If an external pressure transducer is used with water-filled connecting tubes, it should be zeroed to atmospheric pressure and placed at this level during the procedure. If a catheter-mounted transducer or an air-filled balloon catheter is used, the reference level for p_{ves} is at the level of the transducer or the balloon. Thus its relation to the pubic symphysis not known exactly. In these cases the transducer or balloon should be zeroed to the atmospheric pressure prior to insertion.

b) Abdominal pressure

p_{abd} represents the net effect of the forces exerted on the bladder by surrounding organs. Measuring the pressure inside the rectum or the vagina [18, 19] approximates p_{abd}.

If an external pressure transducer with water-filled tubes and catheter is used to measure p_{abd}, it should be placed at the same level as the p_{ves} transducer and zeroed in the same way, so that the same reference level is employed. If a catheter-mounted transducer is used, the reference level for $p_{abd}$is at the position of the transducer and is unlikely to be the same as for p_{ves}. This in itself can be a source of artifact.

If a water-filled balloon is inserted in the rectum for pressure measurement it is essential not to overinflate it (to no more than 50% of nominal capacity), in order to avoid an artificially elevated p_{abd}. The balloon may be punctured to prevent this possibility. Accurate measurement is not possible unless the vagina or the anal sphincter forms a tight seal around the catheter. In this regard intravaginal recording appears to be less reliable [20] unless the catheter is high in the vaginal vault. Whatever the means used to measure the abdominal pressure, its accuracy should be monitored throughout the study, by ensuring that transient pressure excursions due to coughing are recorded equally in p_{ves} and p_{abd}. Even if these conditions are met, slow rectal contractions, or an elevated tone in the rectal wall, may occur and lead to an artificially elevated and/or fluctuating value for p_{abd}.

c) Detrusor pressure

Rearranging the above equation shows that the detrusor pressure is defined as

$$p_{det} = p_{ves} - p_{abd}.$$

Therefore the detrusor pressure can be calculated from measurements of p_{ves} and p_{abd}. It represents the effect of the active and/or passive forces generated by the detrusor muscle, separate from any external pressures applied to the bladder wall. In other words it eliminates the effects of coughing and straining and shows what the detrusor itself is doing. It is difficult to distinguish the effects of straining from detrusor contractions if only p_{ves} is measured [21].

If recording is started with a nearly empty bladder, one expects the forces in the bladder wall to be very small. Consequently, provided the zeroing has been carried out correctly, p_{ves} and p_{abd} should be nearly equal and p_{det} close to zero. With catheter-mounted transducers, because the abdominal and intravesical pressures are referenced differently and to unknown reference levels, this may not be exactly correct [17]. The apparent initial value of p_{det} may be slightly greater than zero or slightly negative.

d) Urethral pressure

The pressure in the urethra may be measured during storage and/or during voiding, the former being the primary concern in this chapter. There are difficulties in the definition and measurement of p_{ura} during storage, because the urethra is collapsed during the storage phase. It contains no fluid and so p_{ura} cannot represent a true pressure in a physical sense.

Further consideration has shown that p_{ura} is the fluid pressure that would hypothetically be required to force open the collapsed urethra and so allow urine to flow [22]. The method of measurement that conforms most closely to this definition is the perfusion or Brown-Wickham method [23, 24]. In this method the liquid is slowly infused into the urethra through the sidehole port on the catheter. To accommodate the liquid, the urethra has to be forced open very slightly. The fluid pressure needed to do so is measured. The urethral pressure measured in this way varies from point to point within the urethra. Thus, a graph of urethral pressure against distance along the urethra can be drawn, the urethral pressure profile (UPP). By definition, the urethral pressure should be independent of the orientation of the catheter sidehole or transducer within the urethra. With some methods of measurement however the pressure reading does depend on the orientation (see section **II.2.a**). This is also a sign that the urethral pressure is impossible to measure correctly (by such methods) in clinical practice. Choosing a very flexible catheter [22] and a lateral orientation for the sidehole or catheter-mounted transducer minimizes the systematic error. The subtraction of p_{ves} from p_{ura} produces the urethral closure pressure.

6. Detection of leakage

Methods of detecting leakage from the bladder have not been standardized despite their critical importance in the evaluation of incontinent subjects. An electrical method of detecting urine in the urethra by measuring distal electric conductance has been shown to be a sensitive index of urine leakage [25]. Pads incorporating wire grids or temperature-sensitive diodes have been used to detect urinary leakage by the change of electric resistance or temperature. If videourodynamics is available, fluoroscopy provides a way of detecting leakage of X-ray contrast. A flowmeter placed below the patient may record leakage. In most cases, however, demonstration of a leakage relies on naked-eye observation by the investigator. If there is substantial loss, detection is easy, but loss of a few drops may be overlooked. A dry piece of cotton cloth, preferably dark-green in color, or a simple paper towel applied to the orifice [26] may help the investigator detect the urine loss.

7. Equipment for urodynamics

Urodynamic instruments intended for pressure measurement should be equipped with at least 2 pressure-measuring channels, for p_{ves} and p_{abd}, and a means of calculating and recording p_{det}. The p_{det} channel should be capable of recording slightly negative as well as positive values. A minimum sampling rate of 10 data points per second is probably necessary, although higher sampling rates have been recommended [27]. Depending on the complexity of the testing, urodynamic instruments may also have channels for infused volume, urethral pressure, voiding flow rate, voided volume, or EMG, and a means of displaying and recording these measurements together with simultaneous images. Despite such sophistication some newer systems do not allow post-processing of "automatically" analyzed data, and use recording paper with a narrow width and/or height, which can make the traces difficult to read. To rule out artifacts the examiner should inspect the traces and compare them to the data that have been automatically analyzed

The manufacturers provide data on accuracy of equipment but there is no external organization that monitors the technical and clinical data quality. Studies of intrinsic clinical and technical 'robustness,' determined by comparing different measuring techniques, are rare [28-30]. Consequently, it is not certain whether the data obtained on urodynamic equipment from different manufacturers are truly interchangeable [31]. It has also not been shown whether the data from similar equipment used in different departments are interchangeable. The intrinsic technical quality of the urodynamic equipment on the market is probably adequate; however, it should be remembered that no objective quality control exists.

The users of equipment should carefully maintain the machine in good condition, and the calibration of uroflow and pressure transducers should be checked periodically, for example, every month. If the filling volume is derived from a weight transducer this too should be checked regularly. If it is derived from counting the revolutions of a peristaltic pump, it is probably necessary to recheck or recalibrate the pump for every test, following the manufacturer's instructions.

8. Description of urodynamic study conditions

The procedures for urodynamic studies are so variable in their details that it is important to report the study conditions, so as to allow others to judge the quality of the investigations. Shown in Table 2 are the basic study conditions that should be reported in scientific articles dealing with urodynamic aspects of urinary incontinence.

9. Interpretation of study results

Urodynamic test results should be interpreted and integrated with other clinical findings to make an appropriate clinical decision. Different urodynamic findings may be present with a given clinical presentation, and the same urodynamic observations may be made in the presence of different symptoms [32-37]. The results are sometimes expressed in terms of values of selected variables. In order to attain accurate interpretation at the individual level, however, the whole chart should always be taken into account.

Table 2 : Basic Study Conditions to be Documented in Scientific Communications

- Investigator
- Circumstances during study
- Patient conditions
  - sedation, medication, position, provocation
- Equipment
  - type, calibration
- Pressure measurement
  - reference level, transducer
- Catheter
  - size, side-holes, type for microtip transducer catheter, number of channels, manufacturer
- Fluid
  - infusate, rate of infusion, temperature
- Method of leakage detection

a) Variability in urodynamic data

Lower urinary tract function has a certain physiological variability. This variation and methodological inconsistency inevitably limit the reproducibility of urodynamic investigation. For instance, uroflowmetry in symptomatic elderly men shows considerable variation in maximum flow rate [38]. Inter- and intra- observer variability in reading the maximum flow rate from a given flow curve is typically 1 ml/s or more [39]. Repeated cystometries demonstrate a tendency for capacity or volume to first contraction to increase [40, 41]. In a 3-way drug trial in women with "detrusor instability", 5/20 (25%) changed from unstable to stable after 3 weeks on placebo [42]. When cystometrograms were repeated in girls (mean age 8 years), 10% changed from stable to unstable and 14% changed from unstable to stable, from the second to the third study [43]. The proportion showing detrusor overactivity declined in successive filling cystometries, with the results of the third study showing the strongest association with symptoms [44].

b) Urodynamic classification of voiding dysfunction

When reporting or reviewing information about a urodynamic study, there is a certain minimum amount of information about the storage and voiding phases that should be described according to a well-defined terminology. The classification of lower urinary tract dysfunction shown in Table 3 is derived from the ICS, but several others have been proposed [45]. In some cases (e.g. pressure-flow studies in men) borderline (cut-off) values have been established, but in others further investigations will be needed to achieve this.

If the dysfunction observed during a urodynamic investigation is caused by an anatomical or neurological abnormality, it is advisable to add 'secondary to...' followed by a description of the dysfunction. It is sometimes better to state that the dysfunction is 'in combination with ...', if the dysfunction is of an unexpected type and/or if it is not clear whether it is attributable to the presumed primary disease.

Table 3 : Urodynamic Classification of Lower Urinary Tract Dysfunction

STORAGE PHASE	VOIDING PHASE
• Detrusor activity	**• Detrusor activity**
- normal (stable)	- normal
- overactive phasic terminal neurogenic idiopathic	- underactive - acontractile
• Bladder sensation	
- normal	
- increased (hypersensitive)	
- reduced (hyposensitive)	
- absent	
• Bladder capacity*	
• Compliance*	
• Urethral function	**• Urethral function**
- normal	- normal
- incompetent	- abnormal

**) No classification terms are given (see text 2.1.3. and 2.1.4.)*

c) Urodynamic definitions of the types of incontinence

The symptom of incontinence is usually the result of a complex spectrum of anatomical and physiological disorders of the lower urinary tract [46, 47]. Overactive detrusor contractions vary in duration and amplitude and may occur with or without concomitant urgency. Bladder sensation may be aroused by involuntary contraction of the detrusor or by other ill-defined factors. Urethral competence is maintained by urethral and para-urethral factors that become deficient in stress incontinence [48]. These deficiencies are reflected in a low maximum urethral closure pressure (MUCP, section II.2.a), a low leak point pressure (LPP, section II.3), a low pressure transmission ratio (PTR, section II.2.b), or a reduced sphincter thickness, or in pronounced urethral hypermobility and bladder descent. There is a continuous gradation of severity in these abnormalities, which is coupled with or confounded by related functions and dysfunctions. Therefore for many urodynamic variables it is impossible to provide fixed cut-off values on a clear scientific basis, so as to define any specific pathologic feature.

Nevertheless urodynamics must be taken as the gold standard that other investigations can rely upon, because incontinence is a dysfunction of the lower urinary tract and only urodynamics can describe the function or dysfunction. For this reason an explicit and unambiguous urodynamic definition of urinary incontinence and associated findings is needed.

Stress incontinence denotes a symptom and a sign: the patient's statement of involuntary loss of urine during physical exertion and the observation of leakage from the urethra synchronous with physical exertion (e.g., coughing), respectively. Urge incontinence is a symptom: an involuntary loss of urine associated with a strong desire to void (urgency). Terms for the corresponding urodynamic observations are currently under reconsideration. *Urodynamic stress incontinence* and *detrusor overactivity incontinence*, respectively, are used in this chapter. Urodynamic stress incontinence is the urodynamic observation of involuntary leakage in the absence of a detrusor contraction, with elevated intravesical pressure. Detrusor overactivity incontinence is the urodynamic observation of urine loss caused by an involuntary detrusor contraction. It may ultimately be necessary to further elaborate the terminology, since different types of urge incontinence with different etiologies exist [49-51]. Combinations of these types of incontinence, mixed stress and urge incontinence, are frequently encountered (Table 4).

Other types of incontinence are symptomatic descriptions. Various underlying urodynamic observations are possible [52]. Previously, "reflex incontinence" was defined as the loss of urine due to detrusor overactivity and/or involuntary urethral relaxation in the absence of the sensation of the desire to void. "Overflow incontinence" was defined as any involuntary loss of urine associated with over-distension of the bladder. These terms are currently being reconsidered and will probably no longer be recommended.

Nocturnal enuresis means involuntary loss of urine during sleep. It becomes clinically relevant only after the age of, for example, 5-6 years, although it is not uncommon for children to wet at night (with decreasing prevalence) until puberty.

d) Association of symptoms and urodynamic finding

It has been argued that symptoms and urodynamic findings do not match. Jensen et al reviewed 29 articles between 1975 and 1992 that addressed the clinical evaluation of urinary incontinence, and analysed the diagnostic performance of symptoms [53]. They found that the sensitivity and specificity of symptoms suggestive of either of 3 final urodynamic findings (Urodynamic stress incontinence, detrusor overactivity incontinence, or both) were 0.48 to 0.91 and 0.51 to 0.66, res-

Table 4 : Terms related to urinary incontinence that either do not (A) or do (B) need urodynamic confirmation

A	
Urinary incontinence as a symptom	the complaint of involuntary urine loss
Urinary incontinence as a sign	the objective demonstration of urine loss
Stress incontinence as a symptom	the complaint of involuntary loss of urine during coughing, sneezing, or physical exertion
Stress incontinence as a sign	the observation of urine loss from the urethra synchronous with coughing, sneezing, or physical exertion
Urge incontinence	the complaint of involuntary loss of urine associated with a sudden, strong desire to void (urgency)
Mixed incontinence	the complaint of both stress and urge incontinence
B	
Urodynamic stress incontinence	the involuntary leakage of urine during raised intravesical pressure secon dary to increased abdominal pressure, in the absence of a detrusor contraction
Detrusor overactivity incontinence	the involuntary leakage of urine during raised detrusor pressure resulting from detrusor overactivity. In patients with sensation, urgency is experienced before the leakage episode.
Urodynamic mixed incontinence	both urodynamic stress incontinence and detrusor overactivity (± incontinence)
Detrusor overactivity	the involuntary detrusor contractions during the filling phase at any time prior to "permission to void" being given. The contractions may be of any size and may be spontaneous or provoked. If contraction is observed without leakage, it may be only suggestive of detrusor overactivity incontinence. The current terminology does not distinguish overactivity accompanied by the sensation of urgency from sensation-free overactivity.

pectively, depending on the type of incontinence (Table 5). Analysis of selected or more homogenous populations did not significantly alter the validity. More recent studies on this subject have given similar results [33, 54-59]. To improve prediction most of them utilised non-urodynamic variables and a standard questionnaire or frequency-volume chart to assess the symptoms. Using voiding frequency and voided volume retrieved from frequency-volume charts, one study gave a nomogram for the probability of detrusor overactivity [60]. However, the validity of the nomogram was not confirmed in a following study [61]. The mean voided volume in frequency-volume recording was significantly smaller in detrusor overactivity incontinence (151ml, n=23) than in urodynamic stress incontinence (220ml, n=73), but there was a substantial overlap [62]. The symptom score for leakage associated with physical activity was higher for stress incontinence but other symptom scores addressing nocturia, frequency, urgency, urge incontinence or incomplete voiding did not differ between stress and urge incontinence [63]. In practice, positive predictive value and negative predictive value are of more clinical significance. Stress incontinence as the dominant symptom has a positive predictive value for urodynamic stress incontinence of more than 70% (Table 5). However, the positive predictive value of overactive bladder syndrome (frequency, urgency and/or urge incontinence) for detrusor overactivity was only 54% [64].

Thus, symptom-based diagnosis is misleading as a predictor of detrusor overactivity. It is felt, however, that stress incontinence as the dominant symptom with auxiliary evidence is specific to and predictive of urodynamic stress incontinence, especially in patients without prior surgery [55, 57].

10. Summary

- A urodynamic investigation is a functional assessment of the lower urinary tract, usually performed to provide objective pathophysiological explanations of symptoms and/or dysfunction
- Urodynamic investigations should be conducted safely in a scientific and respectful manner.
- Urodynamic measurements are prone to artifacts. They should be carefully identified and eliminated during the study whenever possible. Accurate description of study conditions and methods is essential.

Table 5 : Value of patient history for predicting urodynamic findings

Author	year	Method	Sample size	Urodynamic stress incontinence			Detrusor overactivity incontinence		Mixed incontinence	
				STV	SPT	PPV	STV	SPT	STV	SPT
Jensen	1994	Review		0.91	0.51	0.75	0.74	0.55	0.48	0.66
Handa*	1995	A	101	0.77	0.44	0.52				
Handa*	1995	B	101	0.82	0.59	0.70				
Haeusler	1995	C	1938	0.56	0.45	0.88	0.62	0.56		
Cundiff	1997	D	535	0.44	0.87	0.87	0.71	0.41	0.68	0.48
Videla	1998	E	72			0.82				
Diokno*	1999	F	76	0.83	1.0	1.0				
James	1999	G	555			0.81				
Lemack*	2000	H	174			0.92				

Abbreviations: STV; sensitivity, SPT; specificity, PPV; positive predictive value
*Predictive value for type II stress incontinence
A: limited evaluation (no urodynamics required) by AHCPR criteria [128]
B: stress incontinence dominant, no prior surgery, positive stress test, hypermobility, residual < 50ml, age < 65, no prolapse
C: Gaudenz Incontinence questionnaire
D: stress incontinence dominant
E: stress incontinence dominant, positive stress test, residual < 50ml, maximum functional capacity > 400ml
F: stress incontinence dominant, no prior surgery, hypermobility, no grade 4 prolapse and residual < 200ml
G: stress incontinence without bladder filling symptoms H: stress incontinence dominant, no prior surgery

- Appropriate examinations should be selected so as to achieve the best possible assessment of the patient's condition.
- The investigator should be well versed in the procedures and interpretation of urodynamic studies, and understand their clinical relevance in each patient.
- The limitations on the accuracy and the interchangeability of study results should be kept in mind during interpretation.

11. Future study areas

- Development of formal qualifications for investigators through certification of courses in the practice of urodynamics.
- Comparative studies of different methods of detecting urine loss during a urodynamic study.
- Standardization of equipment, instrumentation, techniques, and documentation, and adoption of a standard file format to enable interchange of results
- Determination of physiological, technical and interpretational variability for urodynamic study results.
- Better definition of the pathophysiological conditions underlying the types of incontinence and the corresponding urodynamic observations, and further refinement of the recommended terminology to reflect this.

B. URODYNAMIC STUDIES

I. CYSTOMETRY

The core test of a urodynamic investigation is cystometry. Cystometry is the continuous measurement of the pressure/volume relationship of the bladder to assess sensations, detrusor activity, bladder capacity and bladder compliance. In the context of this chapter, an important aim of cystometry is to reproduce the symptom of incontinence. For this purpose, maneuvers intended to provoke either urodynamic stress incontinence or detrusor overactivity incontinence are important.

1. Technical aspects

The bladder is most commonly filled through a transurethral catheter. The bladder can be catheterized suprapubically or it can be filled solely via (forced) renal excretion [65]. Bladder filling may be carried out with or without preliminary drainage of residual urine; whether or not this is done should be stated. If catheters are introduced using an anesthetic agent, the effect must be taken into account in the interpretation. It is important to keep in mind that *any* variations in technique may affect study results.

Historically, both liquid and gas have been used as the filling medium. Gas (carbon dioxide) is usually infused at a high rate (> 100 ml/min), allowing rapid and inexpensive performance of a study. However, it is unphysiologic and compressible, and easily provokes detrusor overactivity (see below) [66]. Rapid filling may also lead to erroneous diagnosis of reduced bladder compliance. It is not suitable for studying voiding, and leakage is very difficult to detect due to invisibility of the gas. Gas cystometry is not reliable [67] and thus not recommended.

The liquid filling medium may be physiologic saline, water, or radiographic contrast. The physical properties of the liquid, its acidity, the type of contrast medium and the concentration of ions such as K^+ and Ca^{++} may affect detrusor overactivity [68-70]. The temperature of the liquid is usually either room temperature or body temperature. Traditionally, the filling rate is referred to as 'fast' (> 100 ml/min), 'medium' or 'slow' (< 10 ml/min). Natural bladder filling is on average 1-2 ml per minute, although diuresis at up to 15 ml/min is possible for short periods. Therefore, even 'slow' urodynamic filling is already non-physiologic filling rates. For children a rate above 10% of predicted or known bladder capacity per minute might be considered a 'fast' filling rate. 'Fast' filling is considered to be provocative of detrusor overactivity (see below) and any unphysiologically 'fast' filling tends to produce lower bladder capacity and lower compliance. Stepwise cystometry, with 'fast' intermittent volume increments, has been used in research settings to determine the viscoelastic properties of the detrusor [71-73]. Particularly if 'slow' filling is used, the volume of liquid in the bladder may be considerably larger than the measured volume (i.e., the volume introduced) because of urine production during the examination.

Some authors advise that 'fast' filling rates should be used if no detrusor contractions can be elicited in the individual suffering from urge incontinence [74]. This may conflict with the aim to reproduce the symptoms experienced in daily life (see over-provocation, below). Ice water testing can be used to demonstrate the existence of a temperature-sensitive reflex detrusor contraction mediated by afferent C-fibers, The reflex is interpreted as evidence for a neurogenic abnormality [75-79]. Instructing patients not to voluntarily inhibit the urge to void, but merely to communicate sensations, increases the efficacy for identifying detrusor contractions. In a prospective study of 42 patients referred for irritative symptoms, a randomized double blind protocol asking patients to either inhibit or not inhibit micturition during cystometry showed a statistically significant increase in the presence of involuntary contractions when patients were instructed not to inhibit micturition [80].

Other provocative tests intend to demonstrate detrusor overactivity or urge or stress incontinence, include coughing (Figure 3), change of position from supine or sitting to standing, filling in the standing position, running water, handwashing, and waiting with a full bladder (sometimes when sitting on a commode). In women with incontinence, filling cystometry in the supine position without provocation demonstrates "detrusor instability" in only 38% of bladders shown ultimately to be unstable. In a further 29%, "detrusor instability" is provoked by a change of posture, and in 33% it is provoked by coughing [81].

Handwashing is another potent provocation of "detrusor instability" [82]. In women with symptoms of urge incontinence, sitting on a commode with a full bladder for 1 minute was the most provocative maneuver for "detrusor instability", being about 27 times more provocative than remaining supine [83]; the second most provocative maneuver was handwashing for 1 minute. However, these two results were based on carbon dioxide cystometry, a non-recommended method. In children, "slow" bladder filling while distracting their attention should help to evoke "detrusor instability" [84]. Since over-provocation may reveal overactive detrusor function of no clinical significance, as observed in symptom-free volunteers, the results of provocative testing must be judged in relation to symptoms.

Bladder sensation during cystometry is judged on the basis of the volume in the bladder at patient's 'first sensation of bladder filling', 'first desire to void' and 'strong desire to void'. Urgency is a compelling desire to void. A strong desire to void or urgency — depending on the patient and the investigator — usually defines the urodynamic bladder capacity (see section II.1.c *Description of study results* below). Methods of questioning the patient regarding these sensation parameters are only vaguely defined. Their reproducibility is not well documented. However, one group found that repeated bladder filling increased sensation intensity, which was more consistently related to intravesical pressure increase than to bladder volume [85]. Providing the patient with a push-button system to record sensations appears a promising way of standardizing the testing of sensation and increasing reproducibility [86].

When no equipment is available or referral is not feasible, "simple cystometry" (Figure 4) is an option [87, 88]. For the detection of detrusor overactivity, taking multichannel cystometry as the standard, simple cystometry is reported to have specificity and sensitivity of over 80% in elderly patients [89-91]. In both geriatric and female populations, the rate of detection of detrusor overactivity was not substantially different in simple and multichannel investigations [90, 91].

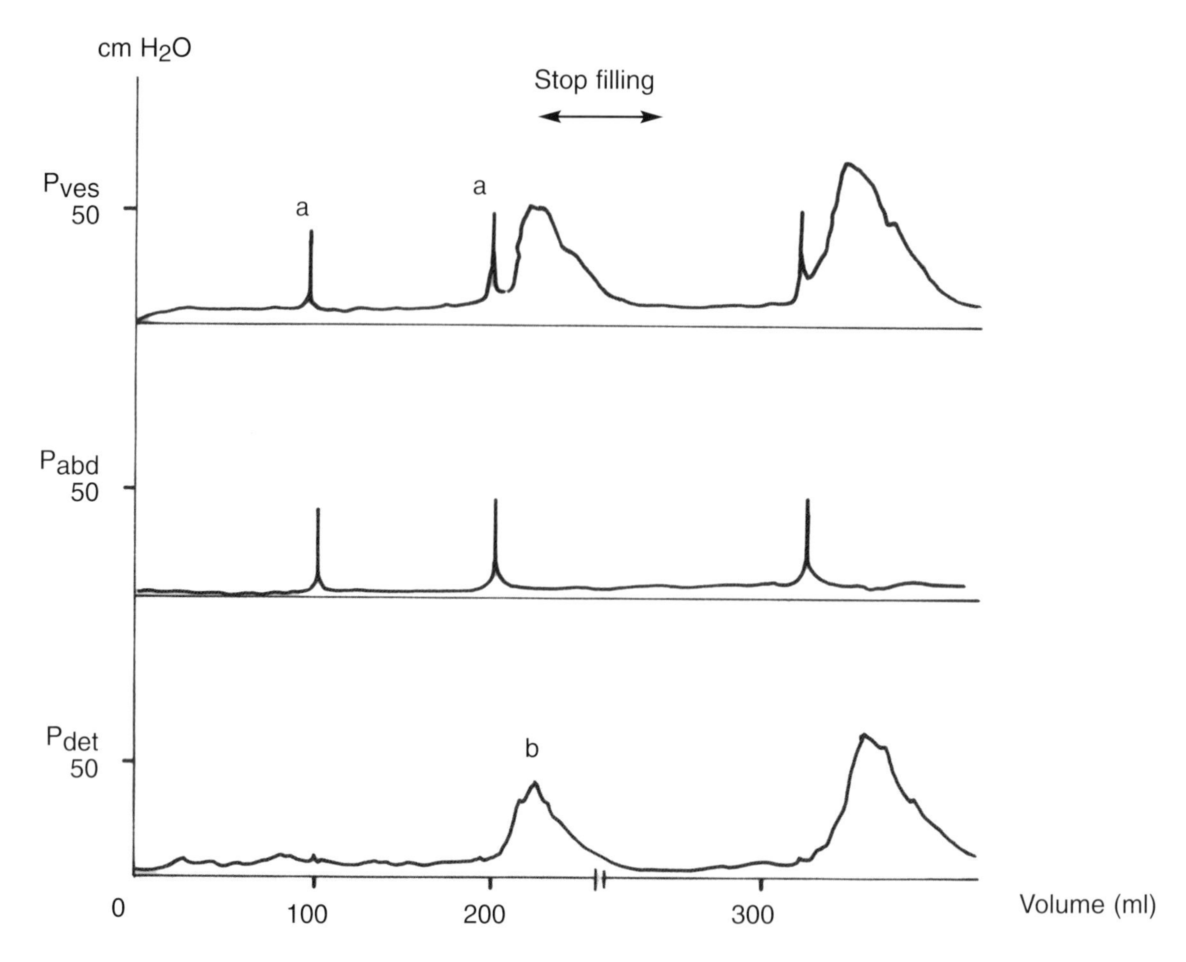

Figure 3 : Cough (a) provoked involuntary contraction (b) at 230ml.

2. SAFETY

Screening of urine for bacteriuria at the time of the test is important to rule out unrecognized infection. Antibiotics administered at or just after the study, are at the discretion of the investigator.

The main risks of cystometry are those associated with urethral catheterization. Dysuria (painful voiding) occurs in some patients after urodynamic testing, but usually disappears within 48 hours [92]. The technique used for catheterization, and for handling of transducers and connecting tubes, varies in different centers from clean to sterile. It is not known whether these variations have any effect on the infection rates. In any case, appropriate aseptic techniques should be used.

3. DESCRIPTION OF STUDY RESULTS

The study results are expressed in terms of bladder volume at various sensations or the amplitude and duration of detrusor pressure activity. Detrusor overactivity is defined as an involuntary detrusor contraction during the filling phase. It may be spontaneous or provoked and of any magnitude and duration. Sub-classification of overactive detrusor function is described below. Cystometric capacity is determined differently in different types of dysfunction. In the normal case it is the volume at which the patient states that he/she can no longer delay micturition because of strong desire to void or urgency. In urge incontinence it is the volume at which involuntary voiding occurs. In the absence of sensation cystometric capacity is the volume at which the investigator decides to terminate filling. Occasionally filling has to be terminated because of patient discomfort. The event that determines cessation of filling should be reported. Compliance is defined as volume increment per detrusor pressure increment (ml/cm H_2O). Note that all volumes should refer to the volume actually present in the bladder, not the volume introduced, and may have to be estimated.

4. INTERPRETATION OF ABNORMALITIES

In the interpretation of detrusor activity during filling, the amplitude and the duration of the contraction and the intravesical volume at which the contraction occurs should be taken into account. It should be remembered that no method of monitoring attempted suppression or inhibition has been standardized. If flow or leakage occurs, the pressure attained does not fully represent the strength of the contraction or its clinical significance.

Observation of detrusor overactivity by itself is suggestive of underlying abnormality but is not conclusive, because it is frequently observed in healthy volunteers [65, 93], especially if observations are continued for long periods, for example during ambulatory monitoring (see section II.8.c). Detrusor overactivity needs to be interpreted in the light of symptoms and signs. Observation of involuntary detrusor contraction that leads to leakage (detrusor overactivity incontinence) is more conclusive because it is clearly abnormal. However, it still requires interpretation in the light of the patient's history.

Traditionally, detrusor overactivity has been subdivided into "detrusor hyperreflexia" (overactivity with a relavant neurological condition) and "detrusor instability" (overactivity with no definite cause) [65]. These terms have been replaced by nerogenic detrusor overactivity and idiopathic detrusor overactivity, respectively. A more detailed classification of overactive bladder function, based mainly on observations of urodynamic patterns, has been proposed [94, 95]. In this classification scheme *phasic detrusor instability* describes phasic involuntary contractions of the detrusor during bladder filling; it is found commonly in younger patients with urge symptoms and no overt neurological disease. *Uninhibited overactive bladder* describes the observation of a single involuntary detrusor contraction that terminates bladder filling and causes leakage, often accompanied by reduced sensation of bladder filling; it is a common cause of urge incontinence among elderly people and appears to be associated with cortical dysfunction [50, 51, 94, 95]. These conditions have been adopted by the ICS as phasic detrusor overactivity and terminal detrusor overactivity, respectively.

Borderline (cut-off) values of volume or pressure for the various sensation are at present undetermined. However the sequence of sensations is fairly reproducible [96]. Similarly, exact reference values for normal urodynamic capacity are not available, because they depend on the technique of the investigator. The actual capacity is the total volume of fluid a patient will hold before voiding and is somewhat dependent on the rate of infusion, but changes also with repeated filling [41]. As an approximate guide, a capacity of about 300-600 ml is normal in adults. For children 30 ml+30 ml x age (in years) is an appropriate capacity [97]. As another approximate guide, 60 ml + 60 ml x age (in years) for children less than 2 years old and 180 ml+15 x age (in years) for children over 2 years old have been recently proposed [98].

Bladder compliance is influenced by infusion rates, position of the patient, the volume of fluid in the bladder and the part of cystometrogram used for compliance calculation. There is insufficient data to precisely define cut-off values between normal or abnormal compliance, but values in the range 12.5 to 30 ml/cm H_2O have been suggested as the lower limit of normal [99]. Among healthy adults, compliance is higher in women than in men [100]. Dynamic analysis of compliance, taking into account the multiple phases of bladder filling curve, has been suggested [101]. In children, the compliance determined by urodynamic investigation is an important outcome parameter [102-104]. If abnormally low compliance is observed, cystometry at a lower filling rate may lead to a different result.

Despite the differences of opinion mentioned above about the interpretation of the cystometrogram, the 'archetypal' cystometric patterns of a normal detrusor, detrusor overactivity, and low compliance are straightforward and simple to understand. It is useful to judge a cystometrogram according to these landmarks [105], even though only approximate normal values are known (Figures 4 and 5).

5. Indication for cystometry in incontinent patients

Cystometry is the basic urodynamic evaluation for incontinent patients. It may be indicated to evaluate bladder function prior to therapeutic approaches, including medical and in particular surgical interventions. Urodynamic assessment prior to surgery not only allows an accurate diagnosis but also enables a discussion with the patient of any problems that might arise

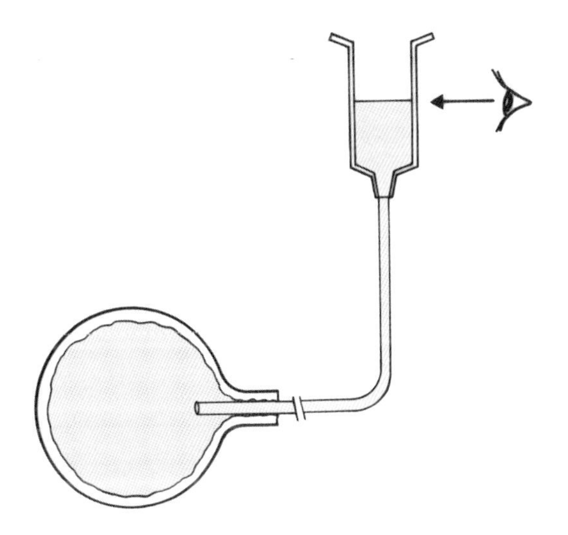

Figures 4 : Schematic diagram of simple cystometry. The height above the symphysis of the fluid meniscus in a syringe indicates intravesical pressure.

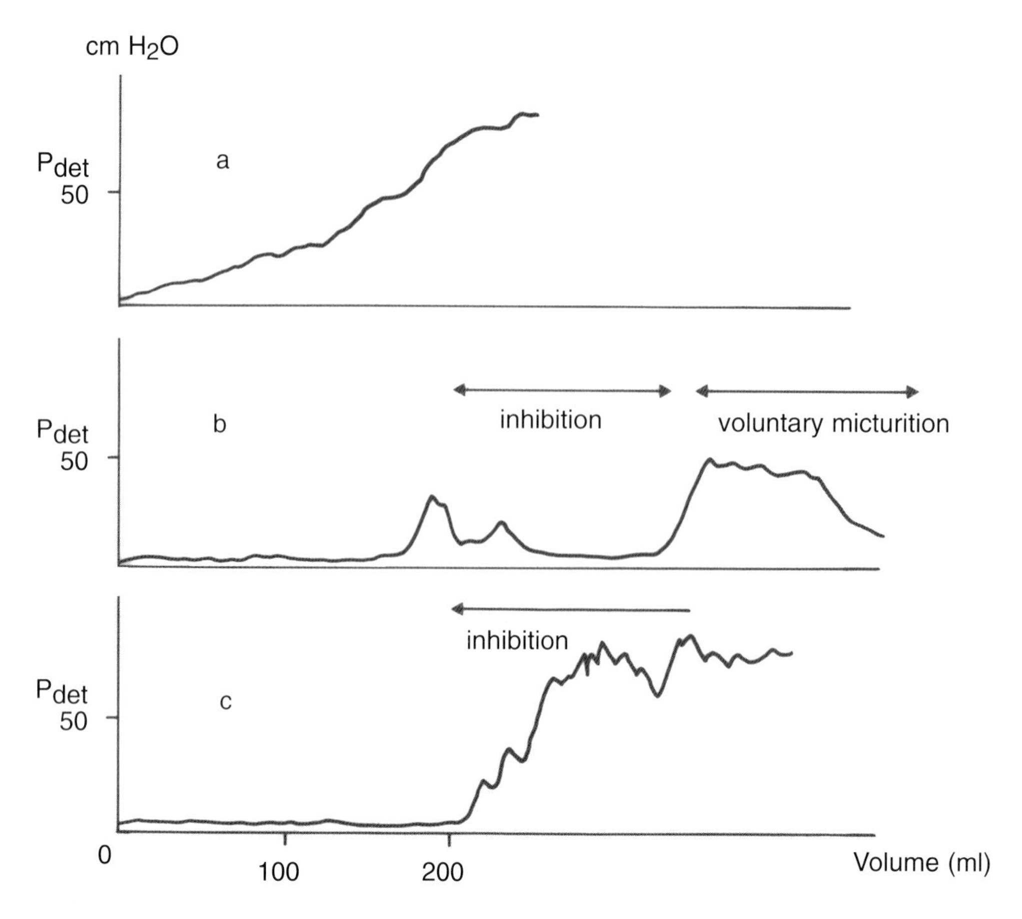

Figure 5 : Diagrams to show low compliant bladder (a), overactive detrusor with phasic pressure waves that the patient can suppress (b), and overactive detrusor with subsequent leakage that the patient cannot suppress (c).

after intervention because of other co-existing abnormalities.

From a health planning perspective, multichannel urodynamic assessment is more expensive than a cough stress test plus simple cystometry, and it appears to have a similar sensitivity for the diagnosis of urodynamic stress incontinence [106]. However, cost-effectiveness, defined in terms of treatment outcome, was not considered in this study.

6. Good urodynamic practice

- When filling cystometry is performed, intravesical (p_{ves}) and abdominal pressures (p_{abd}) should be measured and detrusor pressure (p_{det}) should be calculated; all 3 pressures should be recorded
- Initial values of p_{ves} and p_{adb} should be plausible; the initial value of p_{det} should be close to zero
- If catheter-mounted transducers are used, the initial value of p_{det} may differ from zero by up to a few cm H_2O.
- p_{ves} and p_{abd} should respond equally to coughs; frequent cough checks are essential
- Filling rates should be chosen according to the aim of the investigation
- The posture of the patient during the test is important; it is unlikely that incontinence will be consistently demonstrated in the supine position only
- To demonstrate incontinence, provocative maneuvers designed to elicit leakage should be performed
- The investigator's awareness of the patient's sensations and the instructions given to the patient are critical parameters.

7. Predictive value of filling cystometry for treatment outcome

Investigations have repeatedly shown that the success rate for surgery for stress incontinence is higher in women without detrusor overactivity [107]. A recent paper failed to show any difference in outcome in a group receiving full urodynamics as opposed to simpler methods [108]. Such investigations have usually included women both with and without symptoms of urgency and urge incontinence. An important question is therefore whether filling cystometry allows more precise selection of a group of stress-incontinent patients who will respond particularly well to surgery *in spite of* concurrent urge symptoms. Two papers suggest that surgery successfully cured urge symptoms in 91% of those with low-amplitude detrusor overactivity (peak detrusor pressure < 15 cm H_2O), but was less successful in those with no observable detrusor overactivity (cure rate 39%) [109] or those with high-amplitude overactivity (cure rate 28%) or low compliance [110]. These observations suggest an important place for filling cystometry in women with stress incontinence and urge symptoms.

Among men or patients with neuropathy detailed urodynamic examination is usually considered an essential basis for rational management. Nevertheless few studies have been undertaken to evaluate the utility of cystometry. For men, preoperative filling cystometry was unable to predict incontinence after radical prostatectomy [111] Treatment is usually conservative or medical for the elderly.

8. Summary

- Filling cystometry is the basic test for examining the aspects of bladder function concerned with the efficient storage of urine.
- Good patient-observer communication throughout the study is mandatory
- Analysis of the cystometrogram is based on pattern recognition, and evidence-based quantification of the cystometric observations is not yet possible.
- Artifacts produced by catheterization, infusion or provocation should be taken into account in the interpretation.

9. Future study areas

- Quantification of observations during cystometric investigation to achieve reliable, interchangeable and clinically relevant information
- Assessment of the reproducibility of these observations in terms of clinical outcome measurements.
- Clinical significance of involuntary detrusor contractions observed during bladder filling that do not reproduce symptoms, e.g. because they are not accompanied by sensation or leakage
- Improved methods of assessing bladder proprioception
- Confirmation of the ability of filling cystometry to predict outcome of surgery among women with stress incontinence and urge symptoms

II. URETHRAL PRESSURE MEASUREMENT

Continence is dependent on the powers of urethral resistance exceeding the forces of urinary expulsion [112, 113]. In order to maintain continence the urethral lumen should seal completely; this hermetic effect is dependent upon the softness and compressibility of the urethral wall [114]. Together, these properties determine the intraluminal *urethral pressure*. The *urethral closure pressure* represents the difference between the urethral pressure and the simultaneously recorded intravesical pressure, and conceptually, therefore, it represents the ability of the urethra to prevent urine leakage.

Urethral pressure measurements may be taken from all points along the urethra in steady-state conditions, and are reproduced in the form of a profile, e.g. the resting urethral pressure profile or the stress profile (provided the stress is maintained at a constant level, see below) (Figure 6 A, B). Alternatively the measurement may be made at one or more points along the urethra over a period of time during which conditions may be changing; the results may be presented in the form of a continuous trace, e.g. continuous urethrocystometry, or as a profile, e.g. the micturitional pressure profile.

If the lumen of the urethra is filled with fluid, the intraluminal urethral pressure is a true fluid pressure that is in equilibrium with the pressure exerted by the urethral walls [115]. In practice, however, urethral pressures are usually determined during the filling or storage phases of the micturition cycle, when the urethra is empty and collapsed; as a consequence difficulties arise in understanding, defining, and quantifying exactly what is being measured.

1. Technical aspects

Urethral pressures may be measured by perfusion techniques, by catheter-mounted microtransducers, or by catheter-mounted balloons connected to an external transducer. All 3 methods have advantages and disadvantages. One problem is that, for any technique that uses sideholes or a side-mounted transducer, the measured "pressure" is liable to show an artifactual dependence on the orientation of the sidehole(s) or transducer. This behavior depends on the stiffness of the catheter and may lead to gross artifacts. It can be minimized by choosing a very flexible catheter or a catheter with multiple sideholes or sensors.

a) Resting urethral pressure profile

In perfusion profilometry, catheters between 4 and 10 French gauge appear to give satisfactory results [116]; dimensions significantly greater than this may overestimate urethral pressure because of limited urethral dis-

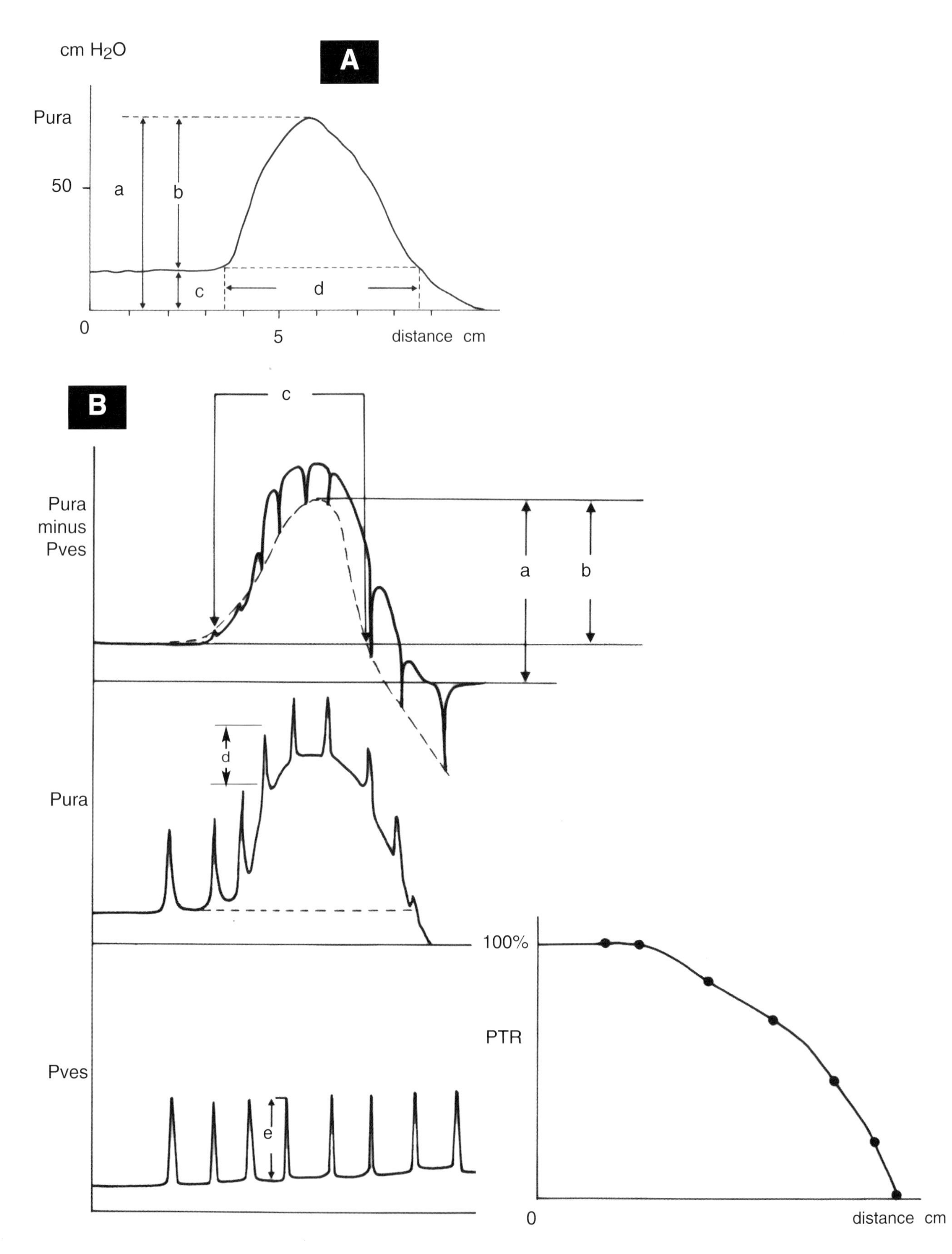

Figure 6 A : Diagram of a female resting urethral pressure profile indicating maximum urethral pressure (a), maximum urethral closure pressure (b), intravesical pressure (c), and functional profile length (d).
6B: Diagram of a female stress urethral pressure profile indicating maximum urethral pressure (stress) (a), maximum urethral closure pressure (stress) (b), and functional profile length (stress) (c). Pressure transmission ratio (PTR) is calculated as d/e.

tensibility [24, 117]. The number and location of side holes should be specified; 2 opposed holes 5 cm from the tip appear to be satisfactory, given the other limitations of the technique[24]. Orientation dependence is not usually important because the catheter is flexible, and most systems use multiple sideholes.

Perfusion is best achieved by syringe driver and not a peristaltic pump. Rates of about 1-2 ml/min can give an accurate measurement of urethral pressure [24], although higher rates may have advantages.

Liquid perfusion systems have been shown to be capable of recording a maximum rate of change of pressure of between 34 and 50 cm H_2O/s, [24] depending on the rate of perfusion, and the compliance of the perfusion system. The catheter may be withdrawn incrementally or continuously; the latter is preferred, and a mechanical or electrical device should be used. The optimal withdrawal speed is less than 7 mm/s [24, 118, 119]; typically, between 1 and 5 mm/s is chosen. Perfusion rate and withdrawal rate are important parameters which interact to determine the response time and spatial resolution of the recording. They have to be carefully chosen with this in mind.

With microtransducer systems there is little smoothing effect, and the high frequency response, estimated at over 2000 Hz [120], is more than adequate to record any physiological event in the lower urinary tract. The method is however prone to several potential methodological artifacts.

The profiles show a significant degree of directional (orientation) dependence [121-123]. Resting urethral pressure profiles recorded with the transducer face oriented anteriorly (towards the pubic symphysis) show significantly higher maximum urethral closure pressure and shorter functional urethral length than in other orientations [124]; pressure transmission ratios measured from stress profiles are significantly higher than in other orientations. Most authors have suggested profile recording with the transducer directed laterally within the urethra. It should be emphasised however that this orientation dependence is an artefact related to the presence of the catheter. Fibre-optic microtransducers have been found to show less orientation dependence but greater variability with time than conventional microtransducers [125]; they also record significantly lower pressures [125, 126], and hence may make the diagnosis of intrinsic sphincter deficiency (see below) even more problematic [126].

Balloon systems avoid any orientational dependence, but in the past it has been difficult to make the balloon small enough (a) to provide good spatial resolution along the axis of the urethra and (b) to avoid dilating the urethra so much that the urethral pressure is overestimated. However, it is possible to overcome these problems.

Urethral pressure varies with bladder volume. In continent women urethral closure pressure tends to increase with increasing volume, whereas in stress incontinent women it tends to decrease with increasing volume[127, 128]. Urethral pressure also varies with position. In continent women urethral closure pressure usually increases on assuming the erect position, whereas in stress incontinent women there is either no change or a decrease in pressure on standing [127, 129, 130].

Normal values are difficult to define. There is a dependence on age, which is discussed in section C.II.3 below.

In clinical practice the maximum value of the urethral closure pressure (MUCP), determined from the urethral pressure profile, has a standard deviation of approximately 5 cm H_2O (95% confidence limits ± 10 cm H_2O) [24, 118] or ± 5% [131]. The microtransducer technique has been shown to have greater repeatability and reproducibility [118, 121, 132]: the standard deviation of measurements made on a single occasion is approximately 3 cm H_2O (4%) and for measurements on two separate occasions it is 3.5-5 cm H_2O (depending on time separation and menstrual status) [118, 132].

b) Stress urethral pressure profiles

In the measurement of stress urethral pressure profiles the 'stress' may be provided by either repeated coughs or Valsalva manoeuvres on the part of the patient. In the latter case, asking the patient to blow into a manometer to maintain a constant level [133] can control the degree of abdominal pressure rise. The amplitude of abdominal pressure rise during coughing is more difficult to standardise. It is not clear whether the pressure transmission ratio [1] (defined in the following subsection), whilst in itself inherently variable, is dependent [134] or independent [135] of the extent of the rise in abdominal pressure. It has been shown however that the consistency of measurements is significantly greater during the 'cough profile' than the 'strain profile'[136]. The most possible flexible catheter is recommended for stress testing to prevent catheter movement and to minimise orientation artifacts.

Stress profile variables show greater variability; within-subjects standard deviations for stress MUCP and pressure transmission ratios have been reported to be 20-25% and 15-20% respectively [136, 137].

2. Description of study results

Study conditions that must be defined when urethral pressure is measured are patient position, bladder volume, rate of infusion and rate of catheter withdrawal. Descriptions especially relevant to urethral pressure measurement include functional urethral length, maximum urethral pressure, and maximum urethral closure pressure. For a stress profile, the pressure transmission ratio (PTR), defined as the ratio of increase in urethral pressure to the increase in intravesical pressure (see figure *6a*), the maximum PTR, and the pressure transmission profile are important factors. Pressure transmission ratios can be recorded at any position along the urethra; the position of the pressure sensor should be stated, e.g. in terms of quartiles of the functional urethra length or in mm from the bladder neck. For continuous measurement of urethral pressure the intrinsic variation in maximum urethral pressure should be recorded.

3. Interpretation of abnormalities

a) Urethral incompetence

Studies have consistently shown that the resting maximum urethral closure pressure falls with increasing age in both men [138] and women, and is lower in groups of stress incontinent women than in continent women; the severity of symptoms is inversely correlated with urethral pressure[113, 121, 130, 139-141]. However, significant overlap between the values found in continent and stress-incontinent women limits the discriminatory power of resting profile variables.

Most agree that the variables of the stress urethral pressure profile are of greater diagnostic value than those of the resting profile. Pressure transmission ratio [138, 142], maximum urethral closure pressure on stress, and profile area on stress [143, 144] have each been found to be the most reliable single variable by different authors, although the sensitivity even with these remains poor. Even on the basis of a discriminant analysis using a combined function of 30 resting and stress profile variables, a correct classification was possible in only 78% of patients, suggesting that the urethral pressure profile at rest and on stress is not an accurate test for the diagnosis of urodynamic stress incontinence [145].

b) Urethral pressure variations and urethral instability

During continuous urethrocystometry most patients show fluctuations in maximum urethral closure pressure of variable degree. Numerous authors have suggested that variations in excess of 10[25], 15[93, 146, 147], 20[148], or 25cmH_2O [149] might be looked on as indicating abnormality. Such pressure variations are however commonly seen in asymptomatic women [150], and it has therefore been suggested that variation in urethral pressure might more appropriately be looked on in relative terms, as a proportion of the maximum urethral pressure[119]. Several authors have suggested that variations in excess of 30-33% of the MUCP might be looked on as abnormal[149, 151, 152]. Although such variations have been reported to be associated with an increased likelihood of lower urinary tract symptoms, their clinical significance remains in some doubt[150, 153].

'Unstable urethra' is an involuntary fall in urethral pressure in the absence of detrusor activity[154]. If sufficiently pronounced it may lead to zero maximum urethral closure pressure and allow leakage of urine. It is thus distinguished from detrusor overactivity and from incompetence of the urethral sphincter against increased abdominal pressure. In the collated and revised ICS report [1] it is suggested that "terms such as 'the unstable urethra' await further data and precise definition". The authors of this chapter suggest that the term 'unstable urethra' be used only where a zero or negative closure pressure results from involuntary urethral relaxation. The term 'urethral pressure variation' should be used for lesser degrees of pressure variation, where a positive urethral closure pressure is maintained. The former would seem to be a well documented but uncommon cause of incontinence [136, 155]; the latter is undoubtedly much more common, but of doubtful significance.

4. Indications in incontinent patients

Urethral pressure measurement has been advocated in several conditions in the investigation and management of incontinent patients, especially those suspected of urethral dysfunction, although in few of these situations has its role been unequivocally established.

5. Good urodynamic practice

Good urodynamic practice must be based on an understanding of the limitations of whatever method is chosen, and the precautions required to overcome them.

If a microtransducer is used to record urethral pressure, care should be taken to use the most flexible catheter available. There should be a means of checking the orientation when the catheter is in the patient's urethra.

The orientational dependence (e.g., the differences between maximum urethral "pressures" measured with the transducer facing anteriorly, posteriorly and laterally) should be measured in typical patients, so as to establish how carefully the catheter has to be oriented in routine practice.

If a perfusion method is used, the rate of rise of pressure when the sidehole is completely blocked should be determined, and reported. This is the maximum rate of increase of urethral pressure (in cm H_2O/s) that can be measured, and it determines the response to rising pressures. A cough can result in a rate of increase of 250-

500 cm H_2O/s. To measure a "stress profile" the maximum measurable rate of pressure increase should be at least as large as this (a criterion that may be difficult to satisfy). Division of the maximum measurable rate of pressure increase by the speed of catheter withdrawal (in mm/s) yields the maximum urethral pressure gradient (in cm H_2O/mm) that can be measured. In a normal urethra the urethral pressure gradient may be as large as 5-10 cm H_2O/mm. If the system cannot measure such a gradient, the urethral pressure profile is truncated and the peak pressure is not recorded. The remedy is to increase the rate of perfusion, decrease the speed of withdrawal, or redesign the measuring system to reduce its compliance.

With a perfusion method, frequently a single channel is used both for perfusion and for measuring urethral pressure. In this case, an extra pressure, needed to drive the perfusate through the channel, is added to the measured pressure, which therefore exceeds the urethral pressure. The extra pressure may be allowed for by first measuring the apparent bladder pressure *with the perfusion running*, and then comparing urethral pressures to this artificially elevated baseline value. This method works reasonably well provided that the rate of perfusion remains constant. To minimize the problem, the perfusion channel through the catheter may be made wider (but this makes the catheter stiffer and may produce an orientation artifact); or the rate of perfusion may be decreased (but this will increase the response time and reduce the maximum measurable pressure gradient). Another solution is to use separate channels for perfusion and pressure measurement, which only come together at the sidehole; however, this may increase the stiffness and the expense of the catheter.

If a balloon is used, it should be only slightly greater in diameter than the catheter itself, and not more than 1-2 mm long. It must not be fully inflated, since inflation of the balloon requires an extra pressure over and above the urethral pressure: the balloon should appear half empty. The optimum amount of fluid (gas or air) in the balloon — sufficient to make measurements, but not enough to overinflate it — has to be determined beforehand, and meticulously adhered to.

It is often recommended that intravesical pressure should be recorded continuously throughout measurement of the urethral pressure profile. Unfortunately this requires another measuring channel; the increased catheter stiffness may cause an orientation artifact.

6. PREDICTIVE VALUE

Several studies have shown that patients undergoing *unsuccessful* surgery for urodynamic stress incontinence by several different procedures have lower pre-operative resting MUCP and functional urethral length (FUL) than those treated successfully [156-162]. In patients treated by colposuspension, those with a pre-operative resting MUCP less than 20 cmH_2O were 3 to 4 times more likely to have an unsuccessful outcome than those with higher values [163, 164]. Two recent comparative studies however, one retrospective case series[165], and one prospective randomised study[166], have shown no difference in outcome between colposuspension and sling in patients with low pre-operative maximum urethral closure pressure. Thus, whether a low maximum urethral closure pressure, suggesting intrinsic sphincter deficiency, is in fact predictive of a poorer outcome of surgery awaits further clarification.

7. SUMMARY

- The resting urethral pressure can be recorded by a number of standard techniques. All involve some degree of approximation.
- The results of both resting and stress urethral pressure measurements are highly influenced by methodological and biological factors.
- Because of the significant overlap of measured variables between different groups of patients, the diagnostic value of these variables is limited.
- Measurements of urethral pressure may have a role in the identification of intrinsic sphincter deficiency (see Section II.9).

8. FUTURE STUDY AREAS

- Development of new or improved methods of assessing urethral closure
- Developments in transducer design; especially the incorporation of sensors into finer, more flexible catheters
- Clearer definition of profile variables, especially with respect to pressure variation and correlation between these variables and other outcome measures.
- Relationship between urethral pressure variation / urethral instability and detrusor overactivity.

III. LEAK POINT PRESSURE MEASUREMENT

The bladder pressure (p_{det} or p_{ves}) at which involuntary expulsion of urine from the urethral meatus is observed is the leak point pressure (LPP). The rise in bladder pressure causing leakage may originate either from the detrusor (caused e.g. by filling a low compliant bladder or by detrusor contractions) or from an increase in abdominal pressure. Thus there are two different LPP's

— the detrusor leak point pressure and the abdominal leak point pressure — and each is a direct measure of the closure function of the entire bladder outlet under different circumstances.

The detrusor leak point pressure (DLPP) is the value of the detrusor pressure at which leakage occurs in the absence of an abdominal pressure rise. Detrusor leak point pressure measurement was introduced in myelodysplastic children as an indicator of the risk of upper urinary tract deterioration [102]. In these patients and others with neurogenic lower urinary tract dysfunction the detrusor leak point pressure [15, 102, 167, 168]is important [15, 102, 167, 169-171] [168, 172, 173] because a high value is correlated with a higher risk of upper urinary tract pathology [102, 167, 170, 171] [168, 172, 173].

In contrast, the intravesical pressure at leakage during abdominal stress in the absence of a detrusor contraction is called the abdominal leak point pressure (ALPP). The abdominal pressure increase during the test is obtained voluntarily by coughing (CLPP) or Valsalva (VLPP) [174-178] [46, 179-182] [183-186] [18, 168, 187-189] [48, 190-192]. Although higher abdominal pressures are reached on coughing [15, 170, 171, 174-177] [18, 168, 176, 179, 191, 193], the Valsalva leak point pressure (VLPP) is better controlled and less variable over time [15, 139, 178, 179, 182, 193] [46, 183-187] [18, 168, 188-190, 192]. CLPP then is used for assessing leakage in patients who fail to leak on VLPP. The abdominal leak point pressure is a diagnostic tool in patients with stress incontinence (Figure 7).

1. Technical aspects

The leak point pressure is measured by marking on the pressure recording the moment at which urine is expelled from the urethral meatus. This observation can be made by fluoroscopy [48, 102, 167, 170, 190], direct visualisation [15, 139, 174-176, 193] [180, 181, 184-187] [18, 188, 189, 191] or electric conductance measurements [194-197].

The leak point pressure depends on the calibre of the transurethral catheter [15, 168, 194, 198-200] and possibly on the method and rate of infusion [168, 198]. DLPP measurements must be made intravesically, but for ALPP measurements rectal or vaginal pressure measurement appears feasible [15, 18, 19, 194]. However, rectal or vaginal pressure measurements are inherently less reliable than intravesical measurements, and one group reported vaginal Valsalva leak point pressures to be significantly lower than those measured concurrently in the bladder [15]. Most authors now accept that the presence of a urethral catheter produces artificially high abdominal leak point pressures, and thus favour vaginal or, mostly, rectal abdominal pressure recording. This of course has the consequence that *the absence of detrusor activity and low compliance during the test* has to be documented in a different way [46, 168], and that the quality of the rectal or abdominal pressure measurement tends to be uncertain because it cannot be checked by a cough test.

Besides the influence of the catheter, VLPP is also dependent on bladder volume [15, 183-186] [18, 168, 188, 190, 201], and may be influenced by pelvic muscle contraction or urethral distortion during straining. During the test the bladder should be adequately filled: about half the cystometric capacity (200~300 ml in adults) is suggested [183, 185, 188, 194, 202] [168, 190, 191, 197]. With proper precautions the VLPP is a reasonably reproducible measurement [15, 168, 194, 197, 203]. The position of the patient at the time of measurement should be noted.

The contribution of the resting intravesical pressure to the abdominal leak point pressure is controversial. The increase in intravesical pressure from its resting level in the empty bladder was proposed originally [178]; the value of the intravesical pressure measured from its true zero is sometimes used [102, 167, 174, 177, 193] [179, 184, 186, 187, 198, 200]; the increase in intravesical pressure from its resting level immediately before straining or coughing has also been used [15, 139, 175, 176, 188, 193, 194] (Figure 8). Particularly in the sitting and standing positions, when the resting intravesical pressure may be high, there may be large differences (up to about 50 cm H_2O) between abdominal leak point pressures estimated in these different ways. CLPP is generally higher than VLPP in the same patient (Figure 8) [15, 18, 168, 189, 191].

2. Description of study results

The following study conditions should be specified: the position of patient, the type of leak point pressure assessment, the bladder volume (and its relation to the maximum bladder capacity), the location and type of the pressure sensor, the presence and size of a urethral catheter, and the method for detecting leakage. For the abdominal leak point pressure the method of applying abdominal stress and the baseline from which the pressure is measured (resting with empty bladder, resting immediately before straining or coughing, or true zero of intravesical pressure) should be specified. The results are expressed as the lowest pressure at which leakage is detected. Associated pathology, if present (e.g. cystocele) should be included in the results. It must be kept in mind that the quality of instructions given to the patient may affect the results.

3. Interpretation of abnormalities

a) Detrusor leak point pressure

The primary aim of measuring the detrusor leak point

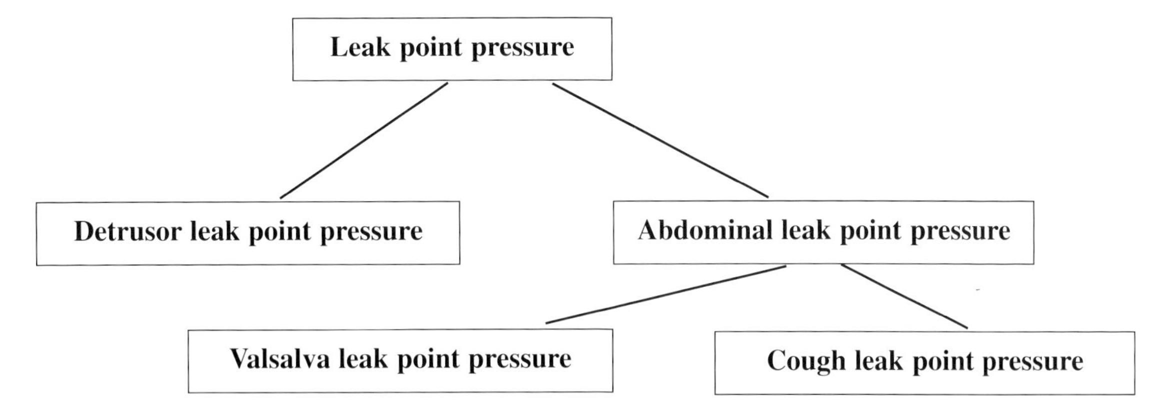

Figure 7 : Nomenclature for leak point pressures

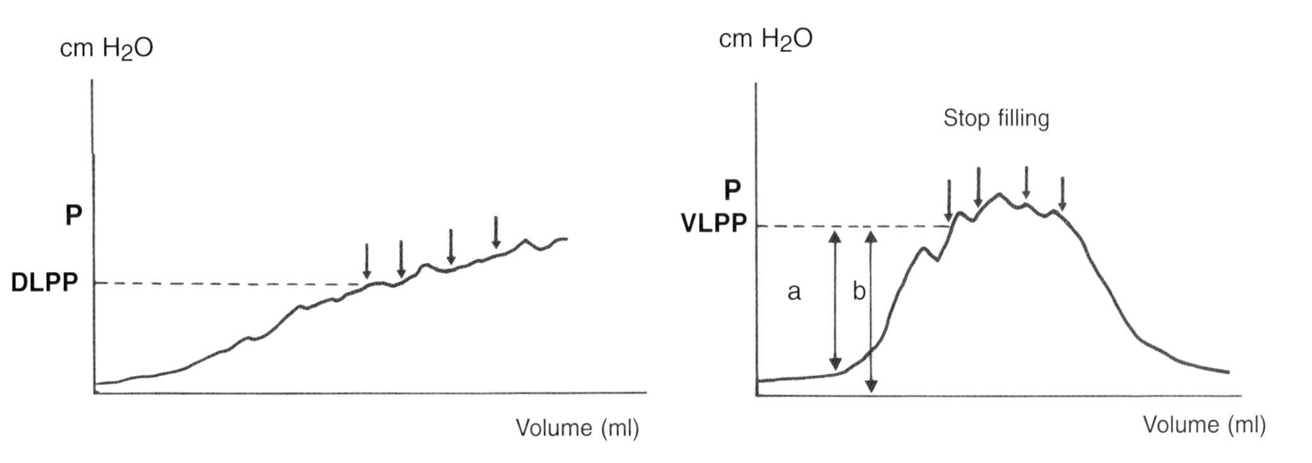

Figure 8 : Measurement of detrusor leak point pressure (DLPP: left) and Valsalva leak point pressure (VLPP: right). The rise in pressure from the base line (a) or from the zero level (b) represents VLPP depending on the investigators. Arrows indicate leakage.

pressure (DLPP) is to assess the risk to the upper urinary tract [168, 182, 183]. The critical cut-off value between high and low leak point pressure is approximately 40 cm H_2O. Patients with neurogenic bladder dysfunction and a DLPP above this level are at risk for upper urinary tract deterioration [102, 168, 172, 173, 183, 199] [177, 204-207].

b) Abdominal leak point pressure

The abdominal leak point pressure (ALPP) assesses the abdominal pressure (or pressure increase) that causes stress incontinence and thus offers a direct measure of the urethral contribution to continence [168, 182, 183]. High values (greater than 90-100 cm H_2O) suggest that stress incontinence is associated with descent of the bladder base descent or so called "hypermobility" [168, 185, 188], reflecting pelvic floor weakness. A co-existing cystocele may cause artifactually high leak point pressures and should probably be repositioned during the test [193]. Low values, less than about 60 cm H_2O, reflect more severe stress incontinence and suggest that there is intrinsic sphincter deficiency [168, 178, 183, 185, 188, 189, 202]. Low ALPP is likely to be associated with increased leakage on pad tests [191, 197, 208, 209] and increased symptomatic severity of stress incontinence [46, 48, 167, 168, 184, 202, 210, 211], but some reports contradict this association [59, 63, 212, 213]. There is a low concordance between low maximum urethral (closure) pressure and low ALPP [15, 167, 176, 178, 180, 181, 193] [48, 168, 183, 185, 197, 211, 214-216]. Thus, the gold standard method for the diagnosis of intrinsic sphincter deficiency is controversial. The value of the ALPP is related to pelvic floor muscle properties [48, 208]. A recent report has suggested that iatrogenic low ALPP might be caused by simple hysterectomy [217].

4. Indication for LPP measurement in incontinent patients

The detrusor leak point pressure should be assessed in patients with overflow incontinence, particularly of neurogenic origin. In those with neurogenic detrusor overactivity detrusor pressure should be monitored whether they are incontinent or not, particularly if coexistent detrusor-sphincter dyssynergia allows high detrusor pressures to be sustained. It is usually of no interest in those with urge incontinence without serious neuropathy[167] .

Abdominal leak point pressure measurements are used frequently to evaluate urethral function in patients with stress incontinence. A tentative diagnosis of intrinsic urethral sphincter deficiency may be made from a variety of tests [218], including X-ray classification and low resting urethral pressure profile values [168], see section II.9. At present however a low abdominal leak point pressure (< 65 cm H_2O) appears to be the most widely accepted method of diagnosis [139, 167, 178, 180, 181, 193] [183-189] [203, 214, 218-223] [48, 168, 191, 192, 210, 224-226].

5. Good urodynamic practice

a) Transurethral catheter

The catheter size must be considered in the assessment of either type of leak point pressure, since a transurethral catheter might significantly increase the pressure reading at leakage, and some patients may not leak at all with such a catheter [168, 169, 191, 194, 197-200, 224].

In the case of the detrusor leak point pressure, the effect of the catheter may be increased by the presence of urethral obstruction (for example detrusor-sphincter dyssynergia, non-relaxing urethra, urethral stricture, or prostatic obstruction). If such a catheter artefact is suspected in DLPP measurements (for which intravesical pressure measurement is essential), the "real" DLPP may be approximated by removing the urethral catheter when the leakage occurs, and replacing it immediately when this leakage stops [199]. The pressure value at this last moment may be a better estimate for the DLPP. An alternative would be to use suprapubic intravesical pressure measurement.

b) Bladder volume and filling rate

• Detrusor leak point pressure

The bladder should usually be filled at a rate that will not cause an artifactually rapid increase of detrusor pressure, since this will reduce the bladder volume at leakage. For patients with neurological pathology this is of particular importance as they may experience decreased compliance or detrusor contractions caused by too fast filling even at filling rates as low as 10-20 ml/min [227].

• Abdominal leak point pressure

When the bladder is filled for ALPP measurements, the test should be undertaken after possible detrusor reactions to the filling have subsided. The volume at which the leakage occurs should also be compared to the functional bladder volume: if the leakage volume is much higher than the regular bladder volume in everyday life, then the measured leak point pressure has little pathological impact [177, 225]. Typically the ALPP is measured at a bladder volume of 200 ml.

- Patient position

For *detrusor leak point pressure* measurement the position of the patient is not expected to have a significant influence. This test is mostly performed in the supine position.

For *abdominal leak point pressure* measurement, the patient position is of marked influence. The test should be performed in the standing position, if possible for the patient, but in any case in the position that will lead to incontinence as judged from the patient history.

- Marking of leakage

Marking the exact moment of leakage is pivotal for this assessment. As leakage is usually detected by visual or X-ray observation, the fast pressure changes that occur during coughing may easily lead to misinterpretation of the actual value of the leak point pressure. Electrical conductance recording appears to be the best method of detecting the moment of leakage, but its complexity is a drawback.

- Patient instructions

The instructions to the patient for ALPP testing (for example straining or coughing with increasing intensity) should be clear, concise, and unequivocal.

- ALPP: Absolute pressure value or increase from baseline?

Many investigators use the increase from the resting pressure (measured either at the beginning of filling or just before straining) as the value of the ALPP. This is contrary to the idea that the ALPP represents the total bladder outlet resistance. In a sitting or standing position, a resting intravesical or abdominal pressure of 20-50 cm H_2O is not uncommon [184], depending on body mass [228]. The ICS recommended use of the absolute intravesical pressure [227]. The consequence is that all reports using the pressure *increase* should be re-evaluated by adding the resting pressure to the ALPP values found (about 20 cm H_2O for sitting and 40 cm H_2O for standing patients, if the actual values are unknown). This of course raises the question of the reliability of the ALPP cut-off values, as the actual data for these values may be derived either from the absolute pressure or from the pressure increase. Fortunately, in clinical practice this difference does not seem of great importance.

6. PREDICTIVE VALUE

a) Detrusor leak point pressure

A detrusor leak point pressure > 40 cm H_2O is a definite risk factor for upper tract deterioration [29, 30, 168, 172, 173, 199] [177, 204-207] especially if incontinence occurs in everyday life [177]. Early intervention to reduce the pressure in such patients will protect the upper urinary tract [30, 168, 172, 173, 199] [177, 204-207]

b) Abdominal leak point pressure

When the diagnosis of intrinsic sphincter deficiency is based on a low ALPP the therapy of choice is a sling procedure, or the injection of bulking agents [168, 202]. The clinical outcome of these therapies for patients with low ALPP is not consistent [46, 216, 223, 229-231] [232-236] [219, 220, 237-239]. In addition, many of these authors demonstrate a post-operative increase in ALPP but not in urethral closure pressure.

7. SUMMARY

- Detrusor leak point pressure measurements are indicated for patients with neuropathic conditions and those who are unable to empty their bladder, because levels above 40 cm H_2O place the individuals at risk for upper urinary tract deterioration.
- Abdominal leak point pressure measurement is a reasonably reliable method to quantify stress incontinence, and a low value is one way of identifying intrinsic sphincter deficiency.

8. FUTURE STUDY AREAS

- Standardization and improvement of study methods and conditions [240-246], including patient position, transurethral catheter, bladder volume, and detection of leakage.
- For detrusor leak point pressure: prospective studies on the development of upper urinary tract changes (not only in neurogenic cases) with elevated DLPP. As it may be unethical to perform these studies on patients, animal models should be used.
- For abdominal leak point pressure: Further standardization of methods and conditions, sharper definition of cut-off values, more evidence for significance of cut-off values for diagnosis and for prediction of outcome.

IV. UROFLOWMETRY AND RESIDUAL URINE MEASUREMENT

Uroflowmetry is a measurement of the rate of flow of urine expelled via the urethra (the external urinary stream) during voiding. It gives an assessment of voiding in a simple, non-invasive, and relatively inexpensive way. Residual volume is the volume in the bladder immediately after voiding is completed.

1. TECHNICAL ASPECTS

A closed room where the patient can void in privacy and without interference is preferred whenever possible. Although one study in women was able to demonstrate no difference between pre- and post-instrumentation flow rates [247], uroflowmetry without previous catheterization is desirable. It is important to ensure that the micturition is representative and that an adequate volume is voided. If possible, a voided volume of at least 150 ml, and preferably 200 ml (correspondingly less in children: 50 ml or more) should be obtained. At least two uroflowmetries should be performed when obstruction is suspected, since a single flow can be misleading [248]. Home uroflowmetry by means of different portable devices has been accepted as a more accurate technique because it facilitates multiple measurements [249, 250].

For residual urine measurement in-and-out transurethral catheterization or lower abdominal ultrasonography is usually performed. The investigation must insure that the residual urine is measured accurately and completely, taking into account any urine retained due to vesicoureteral reflux or bladder diverticula. It is also important to make the measurement immediately after voiding. If catheterization is used the catheter should be withdrawn slowly to ensure complete emptying [251]. Transabdominal ultrasound is non-invasive but it requires expensive equipment. Portable ultrasound equipment is cheaper and provides a less accurate assessment, but is sufficient in most cases.

2. DESCRIPTION OF STUDY RESULTS

The traces and relevant variables should be included in the report of uroflowmetry. Uroflow traces should always be examined to rule out the errors that can occur with automatic reading [252]. The normal flow curve usually has a smooth, near-Gaussian shape, and any spikes of short duration (less than about 2 s) probably represent artifacts, due either to sphincter contraction, abdominal straining or movement of the urine stream in the funnel.

The variables include voided volume, maximum flow rate (Q_{max}), average flow rate (Q_{ave}), voiding time and flow time, which are currently displayed by most uroflowmeters. Q_{max} is the maximum measured value of the flow rate, and Q_{ave} is voided volume divided by voiding time. Flow time is the time over which measurable flow actually occurs.

Since there exists a non-linear relationship between flow rates (Q_{max} and Q_{ave}) and the voided volume, the voided volume and residual urine volume should be stated along with the values of these flow rates. The International Continence Society recommends presenting the results in a simple layout: voided volume/ Q_{max}/ residual volume [1]. Flow time and voiding time can be of interest when interpreting some patterns [253].

3. Interpretation of abnormalities

Normally, the volume of residual urine should be very small. In adults, values up to about 25 ml (measured within a few minutes of voiding) are usually considered within normal limits. Elevated residual urine (about 100 ml or more) warrants careful surveillance and/or treatment, in relation to the other parameters of measurement and the clinical situation. In children, a residual urine volume greater than about 10% of the maximum cystometric bladder capacity may be considered elevated. In the frail elderly, residual urine volumes of about 100 ml are common and may be acceptable, although they may affect choice of treatment for incontinence.

When a normal Q_{max} and a normal voided volume without residual urine are present, in either sex, infravesical obstruction or reduced detrusor contractility is unlikely. However, there is a considerable overlap in flow rates between obstructed and unobstructed patients, in males as well as females [254, 255]. Thus measurement of the flow rate alone has limited value when determining if obstruction is present in a particular patient.

Several different nomograms have been used to interpret the measured flow rates. Siroky's nomogram is used for males and the Liverpool nomograms developed using a large number of subjects have scales for males and females [254, 256]. A peak flow over the 90th percentile on the Liverpool nomogram may be suspicious for detrusor instability, but this finding is not uniformly accepted by all investigators. Flow acceleration (defined as the maximum flow divided by time to maximum flow) has also been proposed as a sign of detrusor instability [257]. However, many patients with instability have uroflow values within the normal range. Some initial work has been done on flow rates in school children [258, 259], and there is some discrepancy from adult nomograms that awaits further evaluation.

Low Q_{max} with or without residual urine is a clue to obstruction and/or to reduced detrusor contractility, although flow rate decreases with age [260]. Bladder outlet obstruction in females is rare. However, up to 30% of females with obstruction will have some degree of incontinence, although this will rarely be the only symptom. A plateau-shaped flow curve with a low Q_{max} is also suggestive of obstruction, but only pressure-flow studies can provide an accurate diagnosis. Incontinence can also be a presenting symptom in an obstructed male, due either to overflow incontinence or to detrusor instability secondary to obstruction.

A poor flow rate and elevated residual urine are more commonly due to an inadequate detrusor contraction. Repeated measurements of residual urine are needed to confirm the results [261]. They may be associated with a pronounced cystocele [262]. Residual urine may be overestimated in patients with vesicoureteral reflux, hydroureteral nephrosis, or bladder diverticula. In these conditions, X-ray or ultrasound imaging of the bladder at the completion of voiding will clarify the true post-void residual volume.

4. Indication for uroflowmetry and residual urine determination in incontinent patients

Residual urine should be determined in all patients. Although the probability of an abnormal uroflowmetry in an incontinent patient is low, several conditions that alter the voiding phase can coexist with incontinence. To exclude them, uroflowmetry is advisable for any incontinent patient. Residual urine can be conveniently determined immediately afterward.

5. Good urodynamic practice

- Flowmeter calibration should be checked regularly by following the manufacturer's instructions or, at a minimum, by pouring a known volume of water into the flowmeter at a physiological rate and checking the recorded volume.
- Patients should void with a "comfortably full bladder". Since this may be difficult to arrange, the concept of a flow clinic, where patients may drink fluids and void a number of times, may be considered.
- After voiding, patients should be asked whether the void was representative of their usual pattern
- Flow traces and the computer output derived from them should be carefully scrutinized for artifacts and corrected if necessary.

6. Predictive value

There is some evidence that poor bladder emptying, as shown by an abnormally low flow rate [263] and/or an elevated residual urine [108] may predict voiding difficulty after surgery for stress incontinence. These measurements may be useful for pre-operative counseling of patients.

7. Summary

- Uroflowmetry in privacy with the residual urine measurement should be included in the initial work-up of any incontinent subject.

- Ultrasonography is a simple noninvasive way to assess residual urine.
- Uroflowmetry should be performed prior to any urethral instrumentation.

8. Future study areas

- Development of nomograms that are easy to use and can be adjusted to a given population. (Nomograms are also required for children of various age groups, related to their sex and body size.)
- Definition of standardized flow patterns that may be associated with certain conditions related to incontinence.

V. PRESSURE-FLOW STUDIES OF VOIDING

Pressure-flow studies are concerned with voiding and therefore do not usually address incontinence directly. In a given patient, however, a pressure-flow study may shed light on the etiology of incontinence; or voiding dysfunction may be combined with incontinence; or voiding may be involuntary, so that voiding and incontinence are indistinguishable.

1. Technical aspects

The standardization report of the International Continence Society should be studied for nomenclature but it gives limited guidance about technical aspects of the test [264]. Pressure-flow studies are subject to technical as well as physiological artifacts caused by circumstances of the test. The following points should be emphasized.

The urethral catheters for the study should be 8 French gauge or smaller in size. To ensure accuracy, recording a cough immediately before and after micturition is mandatory, and more importantly, direct inspection of the raw pressure and flow data is essential to enable artifacts and unreliable data to be recognized and eliminated. If the flow pattern in the pressure-flow study is not representative of free-flow studies in the same patient, then the reliability of the interpretation may be questionable.

The stream of voided liquid should flow directly into the flowmeter (not via tubing) and the distance between the external meatus and the flowmeter should be as short as practicable.

2. Description of study results

Since the interpretation of the pressure-flow study depends on pattern recognition, a large number of different variables have been defined to help describe these patterns. Among the important variables are the maximum flow rate Q_{max} and the detrusor pressure at maximum flow ($p_{det.Qmax}$). The voided volume, the volume of post-void residual urine, the presence or absence of abdominal straining, and the flow pattern also provide useful information.

3. Interpretation of abnormalities

As long as technical artifacts have been eliminated, plotting Q_{max} and $p_{det.Qmax}$ on a nomogram provides a simple way to classify the degree of obstruction in males. The ICS obstruction nomogram is one example [264]. A similar nomogram allows the detrusor contraction to be classified in 6 grades as very weak, weak-, weak+, normal-, normal+, or strong [265]. Alternatively, similar classifications can be performed by simple calculations based on the values of Q_{max} and $p_{det.Qmax}$ [266]. However, these nomograms or calculations have limitations. They were developed primarily for analysis of voiding in males. They do not take into account any contribution from abdominal straining, nor do they indicate the etiology of any abnormality. The pressure-flow study is not a satisfactory way of estimating the maximum flow rate or the residual urine volume; free uroflowmetry is preferable.

Urethral obstruction may be due to a structural abnormality or to overactivity of the urethral closure mechanism. Structural (anatomic) abnormalities include urethral stricture, posterior urethral valve, meatal stenosis, prostatic enlargement or bladder neck contracture. Overactivity of the urethral closure mechanism may be a voluntary act (e.g., an attempt to inhibit involuntary voiding), or a physiological artifact of the examination, or a learned behavior (dysfunctional voiding) or it may be due to a neurological lesion. These possibilities can be distinguished only with the help of auxiliary information. For example, in a patient with spinal cord injury, obstruction is likely to have a neurological basis and to be due to overactivity of the striated urethral sphincter during voiding (detrusor-sphincter dyssynergia).

- ***Obstruction in women***

Recently, a number of authors have attempted to provide a urodynamic definition of obstruction applicable to women. Such a definition would be useful both pretreatment (as a possible explanation of symptoms), and post-surgery (to establish or rule out iatrogenic obstruction). Groutz et al [267] defined urethral obstruction as a persistently low *free* flow rate of less than 12 ml/s combined with a detrusor pressure at maximum flow greater than 20 cm H_2O during pressure-flow studies. The prevalence was 6.5% among consecutive women patients with various symptoms and etiologies. Lemack & Zimmern [268] examined a population of women with voiding symptoms but not necessarily with obstruction. They suggested that women with voiding detrusor pressure of 21 cm H_2O or more, together with a flow rate 11 ml/s of lower, were obstructed. The prevalence was 20%. Kuo [269] defined bladder outlet obstruction as a voiding detrusor pressure of 50 cm H_2O or greater together with a narrow urethra on voiding cystourethrography. 9.6% of their selected population of women with lower urinary tract symptoms were diagnosed with bladder outlet obstruction. Salvatore et al. [270] defined obstruction as a peak flow rate less than 15 ml/s together with a maximum voiding detrusor pressure greater than 60 cm H_2O. The prevalence in a large group of women with symptoms of urinary tract dysfunction was 1.5%. Blaivas & Groutz [271] developed an obstruction nomogram based on statistical analysis of the maximum detrusor pressure ($p_{det.max}$) during pressure-flow study of voiding, together with the maximum flow rate Q_{max} in repeated *free* uroflow studies. Patient with $p_{det.max}$ greater than 57 cm H_2O were classified as either moderately or severely obstructed. Those with p_{det} below 57 cm H_2O were classified as either mildly obstructed or unobstructed depending on the value of free Q_{max} (Figure 9). Among a group of 600 consecutive women, 6% were mildly, 2% were moderately, and fewer than 1% were severely obstructed.

These definitions use different pressures and different flow rate measurements, but Figure 9 allows an approximate comparison. It shows that there are 2 main schools of thought: some define obstruction by detrusor pressures above about 50-60 cm H_2O; others take obstruction to begin at much lower pressures of about 20 cm H_2O, provided that the flow rate is also low. The Blaivas-Groutz nomogram suggests that the lower pressure cut-off may define mild obstruction, and the higher cut-off may define moderate or severe obstruction. As one would expect, the prevalence tends to be higher in studies defining obstruction by lower cut-off pressures, although of course it depends on the patient population being studied.

Nitti et al [272] defined obstruction qualitatively as radiographic evidence of narrowing in the presence of a sustained detrusor contraction. For obstructed women the mean values of $p_{det.qmax}$ and Q_{max} were 43 cm H_2O and 9 ml/s respectively, corresponding approximately to a point near the upper boundary of the mildly obstructed region. For unobstructed women their values were 20 ml/s and 22 cm H_2O, approximately on the boundary of the unobstructed and mildly obstructed regions in the figure.

To summarize, it appears generally agreed that studies falling in the green region of Figure 9 are unobstructed, and that those falling in the amber or red regions are indeed obstructed. In the pale yellow region there is some disagreement, and this region therefore plays a role similar to that of the equivocal region in the ICS nomogram for male obstruction, outlined in blue in the figure.

There is evidence that in some types of urge incontinence voiding pressures are higher, perhaps even higher than normal [273]. Women with stress incontinence, on the contrary, tend to void at lower detrusor pressures than normal subjects. Karram et al [274] showed that 30 continent women voided at a detrusor pressure of 20 ± 14 cm H_2O (mean ± sd), while 70 women with urodynamic stress incontinence voided at a detrusor pressure of 12 ± 11 cm H_2O. Although the corresponding flow rates were not specified, and although the authors interpreted the detrusor pressure as a measure of contraction strength rather than obstruction, these figures suggest that, as one would expect, at least half of the continent women and most of those with stress incontinence were unobstructed according to Figure 9. Some of the continent women probably had pressure-flow studies in the equivocal region. Methods of assessing detrusor contractility in women have not yet been well defined.

4. INDICATIONS FOR PRESSURE-FLOW STUDIES IN INCONTINENT PATIENTS

If the free uroflow is normal with no significant residual urine there is usually no indication for a pressure-flow study. If the free uroflow is abnormal and/or there is elevated residual urine, a pressure-flow study may be performed to distinguish between urethral obstruction and detrusor underactivity (poor detrusor contractility), or to help distinguish between neuropathy and a structural urethral obstruction as the cause of detrusor overactivity and related symptoms. If incontinence surgery is being considered, a pressure-flow study may confirm suspected detrusor underactivity and thus help to warn patients who potentially may encounter post-operative voiding difficulty. However, there is no evidence that pressure-flow studies are more reliable predictors of voiding difficulty than uroflowmetry and residual urine determination [275].

In a study of women with lower urinary tract symptoms, but without a primary complaint of simple stress incontinence or overt neurological disease, pressure-flow studies demonstrated significant abnormalities in 33% [276]. The abnormalities included obstruction from various causes in 15%, dysfunctional voiding in 12%, and detrusor-sphincter dyssynergia as the initial presentation of neurological disease in 4%. Thus pressure-flow studies can provide valuable information in such cases.

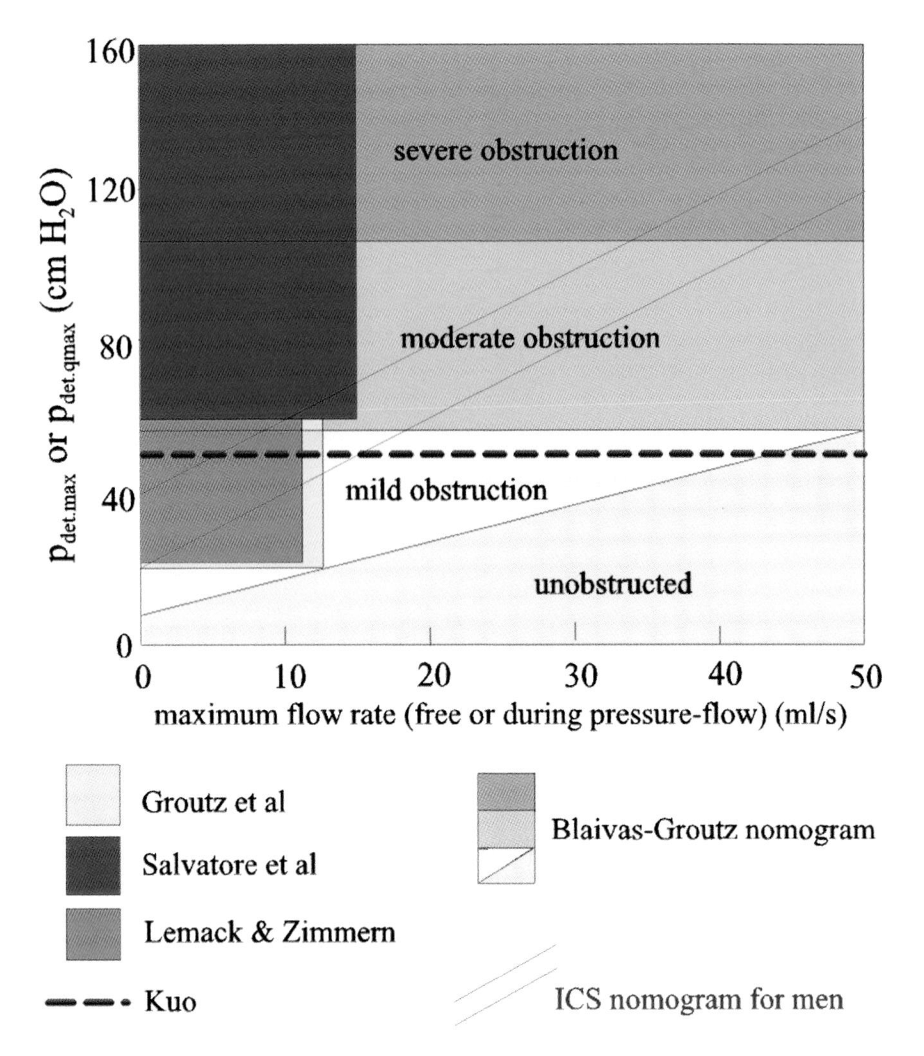

Figure 9 : Figure comparing various urodynamic definitions of obstruction in women. The ICS nomogram for the definition of obstruction (developed for males) is shown for comparison. Note that the pressure and flow rate variables plotted are not identical for all definitions.

5. Good urodynamic practice

- Measurement of pressures requires the same standards and precautions as for filling cystometry.
- Secure taping of catheters is even more important during pressure-flow studies, because the flow tends to expel the urethral catheter.
- Catheter size is especially important because too large a catheter can obstruct the urethra. 8 French gauge is the recommended maximum.

6. Predictive value

The evidence that pressure-flow studies can improve the outcome of incontinence treatment is very limited. Their main function is usually to help recognize or delineate possible neurogenic dysfunction, which would make it unlikely that standard incontinence treatment would be successful, and might rule it out entirely.

a) In women

There is little evidence that pressure-flow studies can predict success of surgery for stress incontinence. In one retrospective review of 50 patients who underwent a rectus fascia suburethral sling procedure, there was a markedly higher risk of objective failure among those who voided pre-operatively with the Valsalva maneuver (54% versus 17%) [277]. There is tentative evidence (requiring confirmation) that women who fail surgery for stress incontinence have lower opening and closing detrusor pressures in pre-operative pressure-flow studies than those in whom the surgery is successful [278]. The role of pre-operative voiding pressure in predicting outcome of surgery requires further clarification.

There is no evidence that pressure-flow studies (as opposed to uroflowmetry) can help to identify subjects with a higher risk of post-operative retention [263, 275, 279].

The evidence that urodynamics can improve outcome

for women with possible iatrogenic urethral obstruction after incontinence surgery is unclear. In a retrospective analysis of 51 women who underwent urethrolysis for voiding dysfunction post cystourethropexy, urodynamic variables were not able to predict which of them would benefit [280].

b) In men:

There is limited evidence that frail elderly men with urge incontinence do better after TURP (in particular, that their incontinence improves) if pre-operative pressure-flow study demonstrates clear obstruction [281]

7. Summary

A free uroflowmetry and a determination of post-void residual urine should always precede pressure-flow studies.

Pressure-flow studies are not required in the diagnosis of all types of urinary incontinence.

They may provide an answer to a specific question in situations where neuropathy and/or urethral obstruction are suspected.

8. Future study areas

Further refinement of nomograms for pressure-flow studies in both normal and incontinent women.

Further study of the predictive value of pressure-flow studies in incontinence treatment.

VI. SURFACE ELECTROMYOGRAPHY

Electromyography (EMG) of the urethral sphincter, the anal sphincter, or the pelvic floor is an established method for the diagnosis of lower urinary tract dysfunction [282-284]. Two types of information can be obtained from the EMG: (a) a simple indication of muscle behaviour (the kinesiological EMG); (b) an electrical correlate of muscle pathology. If one is looking for specific neuropathological information, a neurophysiological approach, based on an EMG of type (b), as described in chapter 4, is necessary. During urodynamic investigation an EMG of type (a) is usually obtained. The interpretation is mainly restricted to recording of progressively increasing EMG activity during filling of the bladder (guarding reflex), and of timely relaxation of the pelvic floor during voiding [285, 286]. While an EMG of type (b) requires needle or wire electrodes, a kinesiological EMG of type (a) can be obtained by needle electrodes or surface (patch) electrodes [286-289]. Although needle electrodes are somewhat less subject to artifacts, surface electrodes are superior for this purpose, because the signal is obtained from a larger volume of muscle and therefore is less subject to fluctuations caused by the normal physiological cycling of motor units. Surface EMG recording of this type, as an indicator of appropriate pelvic floor function or of absence of abdominal straining during voiding, has found a place in rehabilitation or biofeedback training [290-297] (e.g. flow-EMG recordings).

1. Technical aspects

The International Continence Society has published technical advice on the use of urodynamic equipment, with suggestions for EMG recording [298]. These suggestions describe methods for recording EMG activity and define the amplifier and signal-processing characteristics.

Patch or surface electrodes are often placed so as to record EMG activity in the anal sphincter because of its relatively easy access. However, this activity is not always correlated with the activity in the striated urethral sphincter [289, 299-304]. This is particularly true in patients with neurogenic lower urinary tract dysfunction [301, 302], and in patients who strain to void but relax the urethral sphincter simultaneously. In female patients, vaginal surface electromyography may offer a better approximation for the activity of the striated urethral sphincter [289].

Surface EMG recordings are highly subject to artifacts that cannot be recognised from the EMG trace provided by standard urodynamic equipment. Therefore, the EMG signal should always be monitored throughout the test via an audio or video (oscilloscope) output, to check that it has physiologically plausible characteristics. Patch electrodes in particular are subject to electrical artifacts if liquid runs over them. If this happens during voiding, it can misleadingly suggest detrusor-sphincter dyssynergia.

2. Description of study results

The surface EMG is usually obtained simultaneously with cystometry. Additional descriptive material that should be provided includes the location or type of electrode, the characteristics of the recorder, and the method of monitoring for artifacts. The amplitude of the EMG signal is measured in mV (microvolts), and the scale should be indicated on the tracing. However, the amplitude may be difficult to interpret because it depends on the distance between the electrodes and the muscle.

3. Interpretation of abnormalities

If reduced EMG activity, or none, is found in the sphincter during bladder filling, this may indicate an incompetent urethral closure mechanism [47, 294]. Normally, the EMG should become almost silent (sphincter relaxation) during voluntary voiding. If this is not the case, urethral function may be overactive. Waxing and waning of the sphincter EMG during voiding suggest a functional obstruction (detrusor-sphincter dyssynergia in neurological conditions, dysfunctional voiding in non-neuropathic patients). An increase of EMG during voiding may indicate that there is abdominal straining.

4. Indication for EMG measurement in incontinent patients

When urodynamic studies are performed in an office setting, surface EMG recording can be used to test the ability of the patient to control the pelvic floor area voluntarily and to give a gross indication of possible lack of co-ordination between the detrusor and the pelvic floor (during voiding). As a diagnostic tool, EMG in a normal urodynamic setting is probably most useful for detecting detrusor-sphincter dyssynergia [282-284, 286, 287] [290, 305-309], although this can also be inferred from fluoroscopic observations [305].

Surface EMG technique is also valuable in judging the effect of pelvic floor training therapy and can be used for biofeedback treatment.

5. Good urodynamic practice

For surface electromyography, the two signal electrodes should be placed as close as possible to the muscle involved, usually the anal sphincter.

A third (ground) electrode, attached if possible over a bony prominence, should be used.

Good mechanical adherence, resulting in good electrical contact with the skin, is vital. Preliminary skin preparation may be necessary.

It is advisable to test different types of electrode until one is found that consistently provides good electrical contact.

It is inadequate to rely only on the EMG trace provided by standard urodynamic equipment. The EMG signal should also be monitored throughout the test via an audio or video (oscilloscope) output.

6. Predictive value

There is no convincing evidence that surface EMG measurement improves the outcome of incontinence treatment.

7. Summary

- Surface electromyography has limited value in the routine urodynamic diagnostic work-up.
- A more accurate neurophysiological approach to measurement and interpretation of the sphincter EMG may be warranted in neuropathic conditions (see chapter 4).
- Therapeutic use of surface EMG may be advised in rehabilitation or biofeedback procedures to improve pelvic floor function.

8. Future study area

Definition of the most appropriate role for surface electromyography (see also chapter 4).

VII. VIDEOURODYNAMICS

Videourodynamics traditionally combines a routine urodynamic study with X-ray or ultrasound imaging [306, 310-314], although new imaging techniques such as MRI and nuclear cystometrography are coming into use. Videourodynamics is used for patients with complicated lower urinary tract dysfunction, for example lower urinary tract dysfunction due to a neurological condition [311, 313-320]. It also can offer a more accurate diagnosis in other patients [306, 312, 314, 321-323] [324-329]. Overall, the invasiveness of the study may adversely affect the functional results obtained by this method of testing; therefore, it should not be considered a first line evaluation.

Most of the advantages of videourodynamics stem from simultaneous measurement of pressure and visualization of the anatomy. Incompetent bladder neck or inadequate urethral closure during filling, or the location of urethral obstruction during voiding, can be documented directly. Descent of the bladder base, bladder base hypermobility and intrinsic sphincter deficiency can be readily distinguished. Incontinence (leakage of contrast medium) can be demonstrated fluoroscopically.

Dyssynergia between detrusor and external sphincter or bladder neck can be documented. Moreover, videourodynamics has the advantage that any sign of reflux during the filling or voiding phases can be detected immediately, and that bladder diverticula or other anatomical malformations can be documented. The disadvantages of videourodynamics are radiation exposure, high initial and running costs and less comfortable conditions for the patient.

Ultrasound videourodynamics, although it has the advantage of no exposure to radiation, requires direct contact of the ultrasound transducer with the patient's body in the area of the lower urinary tract. Large probes placed intravaginally or intrarectally may change the anatomical conditions in this area. Other disadvantages include inability to observe the upper urinary tract synchronously or to visualise the whole urethra, including the region of the striated urethral sphincter, especially in men.

1. Technical aspects

Videourodynamic investigation takes place under fluoroscopy if X-rays are used (Figure 10). It should always

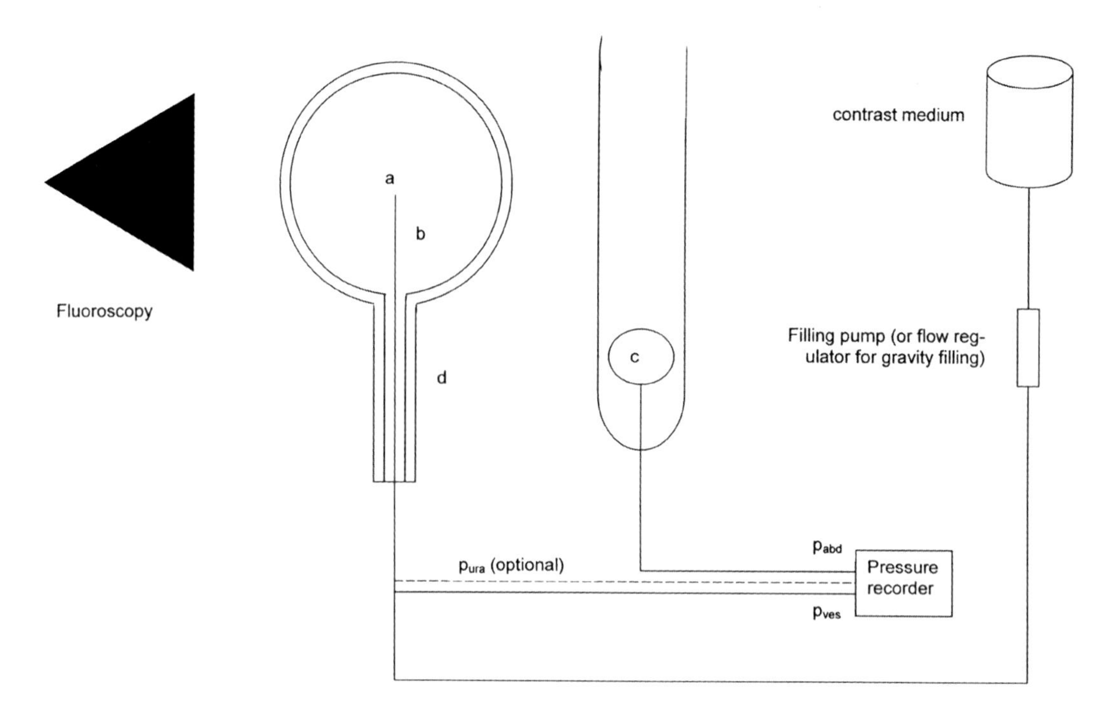

Figure 10 : Schema of videourodynamic equipment. A double lumen intravesical catheter allows bladder filling (a) and simultaneous pressure measurement of pves (b). The rectal pressure is measured for pabd (c). Optionally a triple lumen intravesical catheter will also allow simultaneous measurement of pura (d).

begin with an image taken before any contrast has been introduced. In many cases a plain film can be taken. The bladder is filled with contrast medium, which means that the flowmeter, and possibly the transducer measuring infused volume, should be adjusted to the increased density of fluid. It is of great help, when interpreting the data, if the timing of the video recording is marked on the urodynamic tracings. With modern urodynamic equipment, selected video images can be printed as part of the urodynamic recordings. If videourodynamics is not available, cystourethrograms at rest, on straining or coughing and during voiding are of potential value.

The technical aspects basically conform to regular cystometry. Videourodynamics is even more sensitive to artifacts, in particular because of its interference with lower urinary tract function (e.g. by use of a contrast medium with its higher viscosity or the difficulty of voiding under fluoroscopic monitoring) or because of potential influence on lower urinary tract anatomy (e.g. by an ultrasound transducer).

2. Description of study results

During the filling phase fluoroscopic imaging at regular intervals is necessary. Coughing and/or abdominal straining (see leak point pressure, below) should be recorded to check for descent of the bladder base, hypermobility and/or leakage. During the voiding phase, the start of voiding, the phase of maximum pressure and flow, and the end of the voiding should be documented in the video. After voiding is completed the residual urine should be recorded. Anatomical abnormalities of the bladder contour, urethra, and vesicoureteral reflux can be observed and should be documented. Reflux can occur continuously from the start of filling, at a distinct volume or pressure, during a detrusor contraction, or only during voiding. In all other respects the description of videourodynamic results is similar to that for cystometry.

3. Interpretation of abnormalities

Normally, the bladder should fill without any abnormal appearance to its contour. The normal bladder, when filled to a reasonable volume, has a smooth, more or less spherical shape. The bladder neck should be closed throughout filling and the bladder base should be approximately level with the upper border of the symphysis pubis. During coughing or abdominal straining the bladder base should remain at this level without significant movement inferiorly, the bladder neck and proximal urethra should remain closed, and there should be no observable leakage.

During voiding the bladder neck opens smoothly and widely (but with no ballooning). If it is closed during a voiding detrusor contraction, detrusor-bladder neck dyssynergia may be present. The urethra should be closed during filling and form a smooth conduit during voiding. The external urethral sphincter is open with no intermittent or sustained narrowing during voiding without proximal ballooning. If this is not the case, detrusor-sphincter dyssynergia is possible.

4. Indication for videourodynamics in incontinent patients.

In patients with neurogenic lower urinary tract dysfunction and incontinence, videourodynamics may be useful to define the cause of the incontinence. For incontinent patients with other pathology, videourodynamics is considered when the history and simpler urodynamic tests do not lead to a definite diagnosis or after failure of initial therapy based on less complicated methods of diagnosis.

5. Good urodynamic practice

Videourodynamic investigation requires the same standards and precautions as filling cystometry and pressure-flow studies. Standard radiological precautions and procedures should be followed to optimize image quality and minimize the exposure of patient and staff to radiation.

6. Predictive value

There is some evidence for clinical utility in myelodysplasia [330, 331].

7. Summary

- Videourodynamics with fluoroscopy is indicated when the diagnosis remains unclear after simpler tests are performed orwhen complicated pathology is expected from the history and symptoms.
- It has certain disadvantages; the patient is exposed to extra radiation and the technique may influence the lower urinary tract function and/or anatomy.

8. Future study area

Refinements in ultrasound imaging, and other techniques such as MRI and nuclear cystometrography, to enhance their application in videourodynamics.

VIII. AMBULATORY URODYNAMIC MONITORING

Ambulatory urodynamic monitoring (AUM) is the monitoring of leakage, flow recordings and pressure in the bladder and abdomen (rectum or vagina) with or without pressure in the urethra in an ambulatory setting [332-335]. It permits monitoring in situations where the patient usually leaks, unattended by medical staff and laboratory equipment. Detection of leakage during the recording is necessary and helps to separate clinically relevant events from artifacts [335]. If the urethral pressure is not recorded during AUM, the diagnostic sensitivity for stress incontinence may be low [336] and the diagnosis of an unstable urethra or that of low urethral closure pressure [335] is less feasible. Recording of flow during micturition enables pressure to be related to flow rate [337].

1. Technical aspects

To record bladder pressure a catheter may be introduced into the bladder transurethrally or suprapubically. Catheter-mounted microtransducers or fluid-filled catheters are commercially available. It is recommended that the urethral catheter should be 6 French gauge or less, and as soft and flexible as cooked spaghetti to avoid pressure artifacts due to bending. The catheter should be inserted only a short distance into the bladder to avoid any contact between the transducer and the bladder wall that might cause pressure artifacts. Vaginal catheters used for recording abdominal pressure should be soft and the transducer should remain in the middle of the vagina without coming in contact with the cervix. Rectal catheters are usually wrapped in a balloon. Stiff catheters in contact with the cervix and over-inflated rectal catheter balloons may cause pressure artifacts as well.

If urethral pressure is recorded, the transducer should be maintained at the maximum urethral pressure point. This may be achieved by a single stitch to the female urethral opening [335] or taping of the catheter to the vulva, penis or thigh; However, movement artifacts and catheter displacement as well as damage to the catheter, remain a problem [333]. Conduction rings on the urethral catheter outside the maximum urethral pressure point can act as a simple, cheap and sensitive leak detector [335]. The Urilos electronic nappy [338, 339] or a temperature-sensitive device [340, 341] are other methods of detecting leakage.

Recording times from 45 minutes up to 24 hours have been described [335, 342]. Starting with a partially filled bladder may reduce the overall recording time [343]. Transducers should be zeroed to atmospheric pressure and calibrated at a specified positive pressure to ensure valid recordings. Empirically, a sample frequency of around 10 Hz gives clinically adequate pressure recordings of a cough.

2. Description of study results

A portable solid state memory unit should record 2 pressures (p_{ves} and p_{abd}) and optionally the urethral pressure, together with flow and leak signals. A window should display all recorded pressures to permit monitoring of the position of the transducer. Push buttons on the solid state memory unit permit event markings when the patient perceives urgency, leakage and micturition. Drinking and voiding should also be recorded simultaneously in a diary [344].

Signals from the portable solid state memory unit are downloaded to a computer after the recording is complete and urethral closure pressure and detrusor pressure are then calculated. The time scale and signal ranges may be changed while the tracings are evaluated on the display or print-out.

3. Interpretation of abnormalities

Conventional cystometry and AUM often give different study results. In asymptomatic volunteers [345-347] as well as in symptomatic patients [339, 348-354], an increase in the number of detrusor contractions on AUM has been found, compared to conventional cystometry [355, 356]. With AUM, voiding volumes have been found to be lower [346, 347, 349, 353, 354], voiding pressures significantly greater [345, 346, 354, 357] and the micturition flow rate higher [358], than with conventional urodynamics.

During the filling phase, detrusor contractions without subsequent leakage have been found in 38 to 69% of normal volunteers undergoing AUM [345-347]. The significance of detrusor contractions not associated with leakage in asymptomatic patients is unknown. It is probably more valuable to concentrate on the detrusor contractions associated with clinical symptoms. The increased number of contractions observed during AUM may be caused by catheter irritation of the bladder wall. Microtip transducer catheters introduced deeply into the bladder cavity may record artifacts due to contact between the transducer and the bladder wall.

Patients with neuropathic conditions and low compliance during conventional cystometry were not found to have a high end-filling pressure during AUM. Instead a significantly increased frequency of phasic detrusor contractions was observed [350]. Low compliance may thus be an artifact of artificially rapid filling during conventional cystometry.

An index to classify detrusor activity observed during the filling phase of ambulatory monitoring may be useful in patients complaining of mixed incontinence [344].

The detrusor pressure recorded during the voiding phase of ambulatory monitoring is often found to consist of 2 waves, where the second is larger than the first one. The second wave or "after-contraction" may be caused by contact between the collapsed bladder wall and the microtip transducer and thus be an artifact, but it may alternatively be a physiological phenomenon [345]. The vaginal or rectal catheters used for recording the abdominal pressure may record artifacts due to kinking of the catheter in the vagina or to rectal contractions, respectively.

During recording of the urethral pressure, the closure pressure may drop to zero due to displacement of the urethral transducer out of the maximum urethral pressure zone. When no leakage is seen simultaneously with a zero closure pressure, displacement of the transducer must be presumed. A decrease in the vaginal pressure recording will cause a corresponding increase in detrusor pressure even though the bladder pressure remains stable. This may be wrongly interpreted as a detrusor contraction.

4. Indications for ambulatory monitoring in incontinent patients

Neurogenic lower urinary tract dysfunction [350], enuresis [359] in older children, evaluation of the effect pharmacotherapy [360] and electrotherapy [361], or failure of previous treatment are other possible indications for AUM.

5. Good urodynamic practice

Signals should be recorded as recommended in the ICS recommendations on ambulatory monitoring [362]. There are a number of cautions that are especially important in AUM. Stringent checks on signal quality should be incorporated in the measurement protocol. At the start of monitoring, these should include testing of recorded pressures on-line by coughing and abdominal straining in the supine, sitting and erect positions. The investigator must be convinced that signal quality is adequate before proceeding with the ambulatory phase of the investigation. Before termination of the investigation and at regular intervals during monitoring, similar checks of signal quality such as cough tests should be carried out. Such tests will serve as a useful retrospective quality check during the interpretation of traces.

The following considerations must be taken into account when using microtip transducers. They will record direct contact with solid material (the wall of a viscus or faecal material) as a change in pressure. The use of multiple transducers may eliminate this source of artefact. The transducers should be calibrated before every investigation. The zeroing to atmosphere, the difficulties with the pressure reference level, and the possibility of a negative detrusor pressure are all just as relevant as in regular cystometry (see section II.2.e, *Pressure measurement*).

Because of these difficulties, the recording of urethral pressure is usually a qualitative measurement with emphasis on changes in pressure rather than absolute values. The use of urethral electrical conductance to identify leakage in association with pressure monitoring facilitates interpretation of urethral pressure traces. Precise positioning and secure fixation of the catheters are essential to maintain signal quality. The orientation of the transducer should be documented.

6. Predictive value

The predictive value of ambulatory urodynamic studies has not been well documented.

7. Summary

- Ambulatory urodynamic monitoring is most commonly used as a second line test, especially when a conventional urodynamic investigation has failed to produce or explain the symptoms.
- It is a sensitive (but not very specific) way of detecting urine leakage, and may be indicated for patients with mixed incontinence symptoms, or those complaining of incontinence without objective evidence of leakage.
- Artifacts associated with catheter displacement may make interpretation difficult.
- A means of detecting leakage is advisable..

8. Future study areas

- Further study of the place and advantages of ambulatory monitoring
- Reproducibility of results in normal and abnormal subjects
- Clinical significance of non-symptomatic detrusor contractions and variables such as contraction number, frequency and amplitude
- Development of a mechanism for catheter fixation
- Improved quality control of recordings
- Development of automatic trace analysis related to leakage episodes

IX. INTRINSIC SPHINCTER DEFICIENCY

1. Background

Stress incontinence is believed to result from two different anomalies: (a) hypermobility of the bladder base and pelvic floor; (b) intrinsic deficiency of the urethral sphincter itself (intrinsic sphincter deficiency, ISD). The urethral pressure profile, the abdominal leak point pressure, and videourodynamics may all be used to determine the competence of the urethral closure mechanism and, if it is incompetent, to distinguish between hypermobility and intrinsic sphincter deficiency. These tests are discussed more fully in sections I.2.1, *Urethral competence and persistent stress incontinence*; II.2, *Urethral pressure measurement*; II.3, *Leak point pressure measurement*; and II.7, *Videourodynamics*.

A diagnosis of intrinsic sphincter deficiency may be based on measurements of the resting urethral pressure profile. A maximum urethral closure pressure of less than 20 - 30 cm H_2O [363] suggests intrinsic sphincter deficiency. On the other hand, a low value of the abdominal leak point pressure (below about 60 cm H_2O) is also accepted as evidence of intrinsic sphincter deficiency (ISD) [178]. Additionally, videourodynamics offers a classification of stress incontinence that covers similar ground [364]. Type I stress incontinence is leakage that occurs during stress with only slight (< 2 cm) descent of the bladder base below the upper border of the symphysis. Type II stress incontinence is leakage on stress accompanied by marked bladder base descent (> 2 cm below the same reference level); the descent may occur during the stress (type IIA) or be permanently present (type IIB). In type III stress incontinence the bladder neck and proximal urethra are already open at rest (with full bladder), with or without descent. Type II clearly corresponds to hypermobility. Types I and III represent different grades of intrinsic sphincter deficiency.

2. Concordance

The videourodynamic classification is based on direct observation of hypermobility. The urethral pressure profile provides a direct measurement of possible ISD at rest but no information about hypermobility. The interpretation of the abdominal leak point pressure in terms of ISD and/or hypermobility seems to be empirical, as there is no obvious reason why a low LPP should correspond to intrinsic sphincter deficiency or a high LPP to hypermobility. Abdominal leak point pressure measurement and urethral pressure measurement both raise difficult issues of standardization, which up to now have not been resolved (see sections II.2 and II.3).

Not surprisingly, these 3 different methods have some correlation but do not always give concordant results (see section I.2.1). ISD and hypermobility may coexist [365]; cough-induced abdominal LPP is not always consistent with urethral closure pressure measurement [197]. Therefore, at present, ISD is not a well-defined concept.

3. Predictive value

In spite of its limitations the concept of intrinsic sphincter deficiency has been used as a guide to treatment. Urethral bulking (e.g. collagen implantation) and suburethral sling operations have been recommended for use in ISD as alternatives to suspension operations that are clearly aimed at correction of hypermobility [218, 366]. However, there is little evidence that the outcome of surgery is in fact improved by patient selection based on assessment of ISD or hypermobility. Urethral bulking seems to work just as well (or as poorly) with hypermobility as without [367, 368]. Burch colposuspension and sling surgery may have similar success rates whether or not there is evidence of ISD [366].

4. Conclusion

Intrinsic sphincter deficiency (ISD) is not a clearly defined concept; different methods of assessing it give different results; it is not clear which method should be preferred. Whenever this term is used it is mandatory to specify the method used to define it, and the standards followed in applying that method.

C. CLINICAL APPLICATION OF URODYNAMIC STUDIES

I. GENERAL

As pointed out in the introduction, urodynamic studies may be performed:

- to determine the mechanism of incontinence and the relative importance of different contributory factors in complex or mixed cases.
- to obtain information about other aspects of upper and lower urinary tract function.
- to predict the outcome of treatment or no treatment, in terms of both success and side-effects, thus allowing appropriate counselling
- to determine the reasons for failure of treatment or to confirm or refute the effects of treatment

The approach to investigation depends on which of these issues is most significant in a specific patient. The approach the clinician adopts for an individual patient will vary depending on:

- the clinical presentation (i.e. type of incontinence)
- the extent of the problem (i.e. the quantity of leakage and its impact on the patient's quality of life)
- the availability of diagnostic equipment and trained personnel to interpret the findings.
- the likelihood that urodynamic investigation will influence decisions regarding treatment
- the predictive value of particular investigations in the specific circumstances presented
- the available treatment options
- the acceptability of those options to the patient
- the risk and cost associated with these investigations

Most clinicians agree that urodynamic studies should be performed in patients with complicated conditions and/or neurogenic disorders, with upper urinary tract dysfunction, or after treatment failures, especially failure of surgery. This argument is not evidence-based. Whenever correct diagnosis of the underlying type of incontinence is important, invasive urodynamic studies are essential. This is especially true in clinical research units.

In contrast, the necessity of urodynamic evaluation in non-neurogenic and uncomplicated incontinence is debatable [369]. In fact randomized trials using patients to be treated with physiotherapy demonstrated no difference in cure or improvement rate whether they had been examined with urodynamics (50 – 59%) or not (57%) [370, 371]. Surgical outcome in incontinent women aged 50 or less was not affected by prior urodynamic evaluation, if they were free of certain adverse symptoms and signs [108]. However, this is a retrospective analysis, and in reality extreme care should be taken to minimize untoward and sometimes irreversible consequences of surgery, as far as they are avoidable by pre-surgical urodynamic assessment.

Other factors which determine strategy include the probability of failure of diagnosis, based solely on signs and symptoms, the cost and invasiveness of the planned treatment, and the reversibility of the planned treatment, in particular the possible consequences of treatment failure. In the following sections, strategies for urodynamic investigation in various populations of incontinent patients will be discussed.

II. ADULTS (MALE)

Males complaining of incontinence will often have additional concerns, especially associated with the presence of benign prostatic enlargement in older men. Thus, joint evaluation of the filling and voiding phases is required for a precise diagnosis. In addition, the length of the urethra, the possibility of obstruction, and the likelihood that incontinence is of the urge type, all make it more difficult to reproduce leakage in males than in females [372]. In the case of previous surgery, evaluation of the urethra by whatever means the physician feels most comfortable (urethrography or urethroscopy) is often done, and a full urodynamic study is mandatory. Urethral or anastomotic stricture and bladder neck contracture are important concerns. Should there be a suspicion of a stricture, a uroflowmetry will provide an accurate assessment of the voiding phase. Preferably this should be followed by an ultrasound determination of the post-void residual urine volume. Strictures can cause great difficulty in passing the urodynamic catheter. In those cases, a urodynamic study using a suprapubic catheter should be considered.

1. INCONTINENCE RELATED TO OBSTRUCTION

A significant percentage of men with obstruction will present with incontinence, which may be related to detrusor overactivity or overflow incontinence. The presence of incontinence by no means rules out obstruction in the male.

There is evidence that men with infravesical obstruction (due either to prostatic enlargement or to urethral stricture) may develop detrusor overactivity and incontinence if no treatment for their obstruction is given [373]. In most men with obstruction, overactivity rather than overflow incontinence will be the mechanism involved in their leakage. In most cases, overactivity will resolve after relief of the obstruction, although this has been reported to be rarer in elderly patients [281]. A substantial number of obstructed patients will have incontinence, and the incontinence has been found to be associated with obstruction but not the residual urine volume in a large survey examining symptoms and urodynamic findings [374]. There is substantial evidence that if only overactivity without obstruction is present, the patient's incontinence can worsen after prostatic surgery [281]. A discussion of the issue may be found in the Proceedings of the 4th International Consultation on BPH. A neurogenic cause should always be sought, since there is a higher rate of incontinence after transurethral resection of the prostate in patients with Parkinson's disease who have poor voluntary sphincter control [375] and in those with clinical features of Parkinsonism who in fact have multiple system atrophy [376]. The latter findings may be suspected if urinary symptoms or erectile failure precede or present with Parkinsonism, and if there is incontinence and a high residual urine [376].

2. INCONTINENCE AFTER SURGERY

Urinary incontinence may develop in men who have undergone surgery for lower urinary tract problems other than incontinence. A thorough evaluation includes a urodynamic study, and urethrography or urethroscopy. If urodynamic evaluation reveals that there is obstruction as well as incontinence, a combined surgical treatment program can be planned [377].

The term "post-prostatectomy incontinence" is currently used in the literature to describe a wide variety of conditions (Figure 11). There are discrepancies in the reported prevalence of this type of incontinence, since the continence rate is lower when the patients are questioned by an independent observer [378]. Spontaneous recovery within the first year has been reported in a significant percentage of patients [378-380], while others advocate prompt evaluation and management [378]. Urodynamic findings are also different depen-

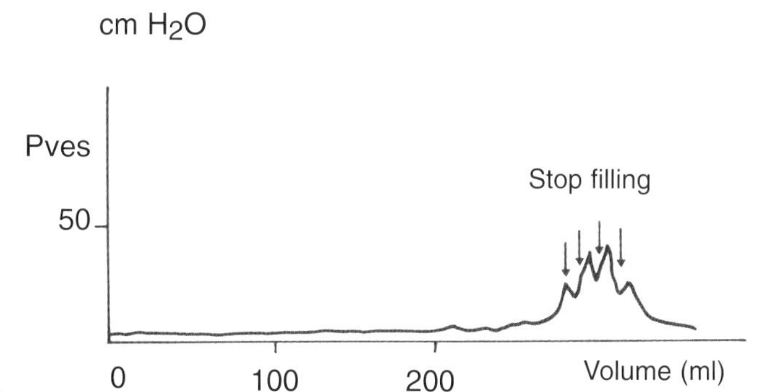

Figure 11 : A 63-year-old man with stress incontinence after a radical prostatectomy. He had a stable bladder, but leaked urine by Valsalva maneuver at pves of 30 cm H_2O or higher. Arrows indicate leakage.

ding on the type of surgery (either transurethral resection of the prostate, open prostatectomy or radical prostatectomy) [138, 379, 380]. Two factors may play a role in bladder dysfunction: 1) asymptomatic detrusor overactivity before surgery [138], and 2) an acute decrease in bladder blood flow after prostatic surgery [381]. However, sphincter incompetence seems to be the most common cause [210]. The mechanism contributing most to incontinence should be identified and managed properly.

The proliferation of techniques for orthotopic neobladder diversion has inevitably resulted in incontinence in the long term survivors, both females and males. Nocturnal incontinence is more frequent, and, as in the previous paragraph, a full urodynamic assessment is mandatory, sometimes with the aid of endoscopy, since all kind of alterations can be found. Storage problems are common and the can be managed by intermittent self catheterization [382, 383].

Post-traumatic incontinence should be examined similarly to incontinence in patients who present with it after lower urinary tract surgery. Detrusor overactivity or low compliance may be present in the filling phase, whereas obstruction or an underactive detrusor can occur in the voiding phase [384]; all of these, alone or in combination, can cause incontinence. In these patients, multiple anatomic and neurologic lesions may be present, and a complete evaluation of the bladder and urethra is necessary. Adult enuresis is also frequently associated with "detrusor instability" [385, 386].

III. ADULT (FEMALE)

This section summarises the role of urodynamic studies in commonly encountered clinical problems in the non-neuropathic adult female with urinary incontinence.

1. STRESS INCONTINENCE (AS THE ONLY SYMPTOM)

In women whose sole or main symptom is stress incontinence, the likelihood of a diagnosis of urodynamic stress incontinence approaches 100% [387, 388], particularly when the physical sign of stress incontinence is also present. Such patients are uncommon in most specialist centers; if a detailed history is taken, they represent only 2 to 10% of referrals. [389] When other symptoms are present, the likelihood of a pure diagnosis of urodynamic stress incontinence may fall to approximately 60% [32, 35].

When non-surgical treatment is being considered the most appropriate strategy would be to rely on clinical assessment. Where surgery is being considered, the role of urodynamic investigation seems to be expanding. The study is aimed not only at the confirmation of urodynamic stress incontinence but also the exclusion of detrusor overactivity and underactivity. It is geared to assessing the voiding pattern, and hence the counselling of patients about the likelihood of post-operative voiding difficulty, and the assessment of sphincter function, which may influence the choice of surgical procedure to be undertaken [390].

A stress test would be the 'gold standard' test for the diagnosis of stress incontinence. The diagnosis of urodynamic stress incontinence should be confirmed urodynamically at cystometry by the absence of involuntary contractions during leakage caused by a stress maneuver. The absence of detrusor overactivity during filling cystometry, however, may not be definitive. It would be important to perform a provocative cystometry; in ambiguous cases, videourodynamics or ambulatory urodynamics should be considered. In patients with previous unsuccessful surgery, or where marked stress incontinence is demonstrated despite limited urethral mobility, the measurement of resting urethral pressure and abdominal leak point pressure may help to identify intrinsic sphincter deficiency [163, 164, 390].

2. URGE INCONTINENCE

In general, detrusor overactivity is identified during filling cystometry in about 70% of women with complaints suggesting urge incontinence [391], although among those complaining of urge incontinence without stress, the likelihood of observing detrusor overactivity approaches 100% [388].

Therefore, if non-surgical treatment is being considered, the most appropriate strategy is to rely on clinical assessment provided other conditions have been ruled out.. Urodynamic investigation is only appropriate in urge incontinence in the research setting, or when invasive treatments are being considered after failure of drug therapy or behaviour modification techniques. Filling cystometry should allow confirmation of the diagnosis in most cases. When this proves to be inconclusive either because it fails to reproduce the patient's complaints, or fails to provide a pathophysiological explanation for the complaints, ambulatory urodynamics or urethral pressure measurement to search for urethral instability should be considered.

3. MIXED STRESS AND URGE INCONTINENCE

In patients with mixed symptoms of stress and urge incontinence the likelihood of a diagnosis of urodynamic stress incontinence varies between 30 and 60%, depending on what additional symptoms are present. Initially treatment should be conservative, either directed at the clinical 'best guess' or using combination therapy.

Where conservative treatment fails, urodynamic investigation is appropriate to direct future management (Figure 12). It is important to establish whether stress or urge incontinence is the more frequent complaint, which is the more troublesome to the patient, whether both sphincter weakness and detrusor overactivity are seen on urodynamic investigation, and whether the symptoms and the urodynamic findings correlate with one another. Filling cystometry is the investigation of choice. It should be remembered that in the presence of low urethral resistance, especially in the face of urine leakage during an investigation, detrusor pressures will give an inaccurately low value for detrusor contractility. Repeat cystometry with the bladder neck occluded, e.g. by a Foley balloon catheter, may be a useful adjunct in this situation.

4. INCONTINENCE WITH SYMPTOMS OR SIGNS OF VOIDING DIFFICULTY

Fewer than 10% of patients presenting with incontinence will complain of symptoms of voiding difficulty, although 25-90% will report such symptoms on direct

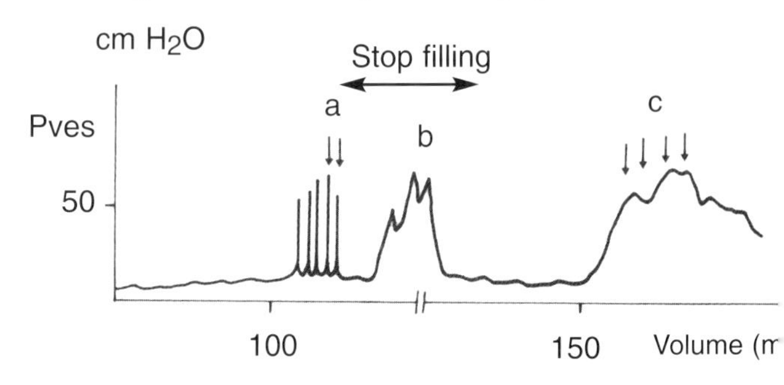

Figure 12 : Motor urge incontinence in a 69-year-old woman combined with stress incontinence. At a bladder volume of 110ml, urinary leakage was caused by sequential coughs (a) but not by Valsalva (b). Involuntary contraction at 160ml resulted in leakage (c). Arrows indicate leakage.

questioning [392, 393]. When there are significant symptoms of voiding difficulty or previous histories of anti-incontinence surgery [394], filling cystometry, uroflowmetry and pressure-flow studies would be appropriate. Since, in women, values of pressure and flow rate indicating obstruction are not clearly defined, videourodynamics may have an additional role in this field (see section II.5.c *Pressure flow studies*). Videourodynamics has no proven advantage in the absence of neurological disease. When there is evidence of increased detrusor pressure, either in the form of impaired bladder compliance during filling, or an obstructive voiding pattern, assessment of the upper urinary tract should also be undertaken.

IV. NEUROGENIC LOWER URINARY TRACT DYSFUNCTION

Neurogenic incontinence may express itself as urge incontinence, reflex incontinence, overflow incontinence or stress incontinence. Not all patients with neurogenic conditions develop typical urinary symptoms or urodynamic findings. For example, urinary symptoms associated with stroke cannot always be assumed to be due to detrusor overactivity, and the site of the lesion does not always provide convincing evidence for the expected urodynamic features. In patients with neurogenic lower urinary tract dysfunction, a specific individual diagnosis of the dysfunction is an absolute prerequisite for a correct choice of therapy [313, 395, 396].

The diagnosis is aimed at describing the (dys)function of the bladder, the urethra and the pelvic floor, their coordination during filling and voiding, and their influence on other pathologic conditions (e.g. autonomic dysreflexia); thus it always requires urodynamic investigation (Figure 13). Because many patients with this condition also show anatomical abnormalities involving the lower urinary tract and dyssynergia that can be demonstrated most easily by imaging, videourodynamics is the urodynamic test of choice [305, 313, 315, 395, 396]. Detrusor-sphincter dyssynergia or detrusor-bladder neck dyssynergia are the main neurogenic dysfunctions in the urethra. The first condition may be diagnosed by sphincter EMG recording, but it appears that videourodynamics is an equally accurate a diagnostic tool for this condition [305]. Detrusor-bladder neck dyssynergia can be diagnosed only by videourodynamics [397]. Ambulatory urodynamics might offer a better approach to recording the actual lower urinary tract dysfunction under normal circumstances. The ice water test [398-400] is believed to be specific for neurogenic detrusor dysfunction, but it must be used judiciously in young children [401].

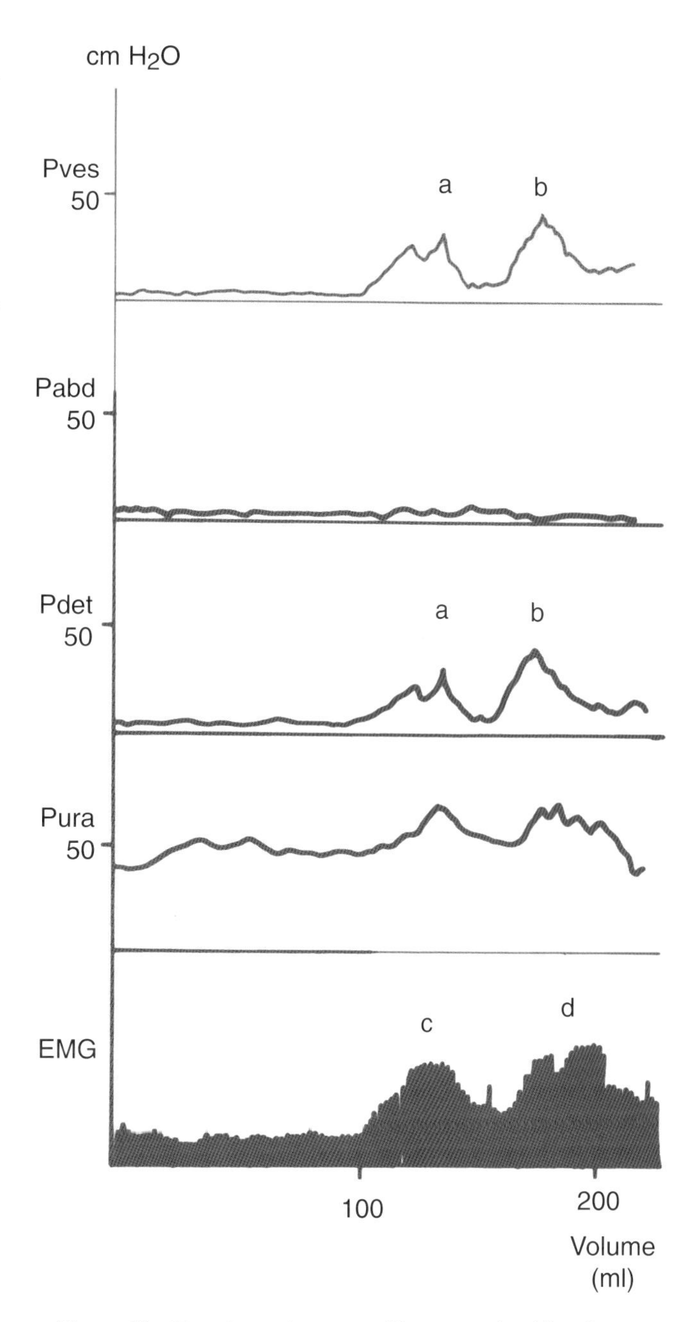

Figure 13 : Urge incontinence and interrupted voiding in a 50-year-old man with multiple sclerosis. High pressure involuntary contractions (a, b) and detrusor sphincter dyssynergia with increased surface EMG activity (c, d) were recorded. Anatomical deformity of the bladder might be present.

A comprehensive classification of neurogenic lower urinary tract dysfunction was adapted by H. Burgdörfer from the literature[402]. The neurological lesion has an immediate impact on the type of dysfunction and predicts incontinence, detrusor function, sphincteric function, and residual urine [402].

Therapy for neurogenic lower urinary tract dysfunction aims to achieve the most nearly physiological filling and voiding condition [313, 395, 396] as well as social acceptability. Timely and adequate diagnosis is of paramount importance for the patient's quality of life [395, 396, 403, 404]. Urodynamic investigation is also essential in following up the natural history of the disease or for checking the efficacy of treatment. Elevated detrusor pressure during filling or voiding puts the upper urinary tract at risk. The primary aim of therapy in patients with this condition is conversion to a low pressure bladder during filling [313, 396], even if this causes incomplete emptying. Adequate therapy depends on whether the detrusor is hyperreflexic or has reduced compliance, and only urodynamics can answer those questions unequivocally.

Since the neuropathic bladder is sensitive to the filling rate, filling may start at 10ml/min and be slowly increased slowly up to 20 or 30 ml/min. If the detrusor pressure begins to rise, the filling should be temporarily halted until the pressure falls or equilibrates. During the filling phase, patients with a neuropathy, especially those with a high spinal cord injury, may develop autonomic dysreflexia. This is a dangerous syndrome necessitating continuous blood pressure monitoring. If the blood pressure rises, the test should be terminated and the bladder should be emptied immediately.

V . CHILDREN

The indications for urodynamic evaluation in children can be divided along neurologic, anatomic and functional lines. The types of studies to be performed are based on the underlying pathologic condition rather than the presenting symptom.

1. NEUROGENIC BLADDER DYSFUNCTION

For children with myelodysplasia, urodynamic studies need to be performed soon after the back has been closed and the child is stable neurosurgically, generally within the first 2 to 3 weeks of life [266]. Cystometry looking for hyperreflexia and/or low compliance, detrusor leak point pressure, electromyography (EMG) of the external urethral sphincter and residual urine measurement are the key elements of a detailed urodynamic study. This provides not only a baseline for future comparison but also a means of determining those children at risk for deterioration of their upper urinary tract [102, 405]. Cystometry is repeated or indicated for the first time in older infants and children if they develop new onset hydronephrosis, reflux or incontinence [406, 407]. In older children on a continence program already (i.e. clean intermittent catheterization and/or drug therapy) any new incontinence not related to urinary infection nor easily treated by increasing their current regimen should be assessed by repeating cystometric, urethral pressure profilometric and EMG studies, if available [408]. A considerable number of children (40% or more) have progressive neurologic deficits as they grow up and reach puberty [409, 410]. Monitoring their external urethral sphincter EMG periodically during the first 3 to 6 years of life and then periodically with (1) any change in leg function, (2) development of incontinence despite strict adherence to current bladder and bowel continence programs, or (3) back pain or increasing scoliosis, is the most accurate way to detect a change in function. A CMG/EMG should be performed 3 months following any neurosurgical intervention to correct a tethered cord, or if scoliosis surgery has been performed that leads to changes in leg function or increased incontinence.

For children with an occult spinal dysraphism, cystometric and EMG studies are necessary preoperatively, and 3 months postoperatively following correction of the spinal defect [411, 412]. This helps the neurosurgeon to clarify the status of the sacral spinal cord pre- and postoperatively, and to use this information to determine if progressive changes occur over time, postoperatively. Twenty to 35% of infants and children under 2 have no apparent neurologic deficits grossly but suffer from upper and/or lower motor neuron injury to the bladder and urethral sphincter, preoperatively [411, 413, 414]. Less than 10% have a change in function from their surgery directly, while a variable number improve their sacral cord function, depending on the age of intervention [411, 415, 416]. With axial growth, 25 to 35% develop progressive denervation [414, 417, 418]; documenting this change and treating the incontinence problems require a detailed urodynamic study.

Sacral agenesis is a lesion that is often missed in infancy because of its subtle manifestations, with generally no loss of lower extremity motor and sensory function [419]. Urinary and/or fecal incontinence at an older age are usually the issues that lead to the diagnosis. Because both upper and/or lower motor neuron lesions of the bladder and external urethral sphincter are possible regardless of the level of absent vertebrae, a detailed urodynamic study is indicated [420-422]. The lesion tends to be non-progressive with this disorder, so characterizing its extent and treating it appropriately at the time of diagnosis is sufficient.

Spinal cord injuries in children are fortunately quite rare [423]. For those patients who regain the ability to void spontaneously, it is imperative to know if they have low filling and emptying pressures. Thus, after the initial spinal shock from the injury wears off cystometry, sphincter EMG and residual urine measurements are necessary [424-426]. Cauda equina injuries may require assessment of urethral pressure as well, due to the neurologic lesion affecting the external sphincter muscle. For those children who are continent on intermittent catheterization cystometry with sphincter EMG is needed regardless, in order to insure low bladder filling pressures and absence of hyperreflexia during filling. Balanced voiding with pressures below 40 cm H_2O will insure a stable upper urinary tract [427]. When filling and voiding pressures are elevated there is a 30% incidence of upper urinary tract deterioration [207].

Cerebral palsy is a non-progressive disease of the cerebral cortex or brainstem [428]. Affected children tend to toilet train completely, albeit at an age later than normal children [424]. Most of the time their incontinence is secondary to urgency and an inability to be toiletted on time. Dribbling in between voidings is almost never seen. Studies have shown that the children have either a normal urodynamic examination or exhibit signs of upper motor neuron dysfunction with hyperreflexia; very rarely is dyssynergia between the bladder and urethral sphincter noted during voiding [429, 430]. As a result, cystometry and sphincter EMG are needed when anticholinergic therapy fails to control the incontinence, the children are unable to empty their bladder completely when they void or an ultrasound shows hydronephrosis and a thick walled bladder.

2. Imperforate anus

Imperforate anus, as the name implies, occurs when the anal canal fails to cannulize to the surface ectoderm in the area of the future rectum. A classification system has been devised in which lesions are divided into high, intermediate or low depending on whether or not the rectum ends above, at or below the levator ani muscle. In the past imperforate anus repair for high lesions often resulted in urinary incontinence due to pudendal nerve injury that occurred from the perineal approach to bringing the rectum down to the anal verge [431]. With the advent of the posterior sagittal anoplasty this complication was eliminated as a cause for subsequent urinary incontinence, although bladder neck incompetence may be a consequence of extensive mobilization of the sigmoid colon which helps transfer the rectum to its final location. In addition, it has been noted recently, that distal spinal cord abnormalities are present on magnetic resonance imaging even in the absence of overlying skin manifestations, in 35% of children with imperforate anus [420, 432, 433]. Therefore, videourodynamics and EMG of the sphincter are indicated in any of these children who have a bony abnormality of the spine, an abnormal renal ECHO or VCUG suggestive of neurogenic dysfunction or are incontinent beyond the normally accepted toilet trained age [434].

The VATER or VACTERL association is a group of diverse abnormalities that include Vertebral bony, Anal atresia, Cardiac, Tracheo-Esophageal fistula, Renal and Limb anomalies [435]. Imperforate anus may occur as an isolated lesion or in conjunction with this association. Urinary incontinence is not common unless the spinal cord is involved (20%). Various defects of the spinal cord can be noted producing a picture of either upper and/or lower motor neuron type lesions to the lower urinary tract [420, 434, 436]. Videourodynamic studies are indicated soon after the diagnosis is made, especially if radiologic imaging demonstrates a spinal cord abnormality. These studies serve as both a reason to explore and treat any intraspinal abnormality to improve the child's chances of becoming continent of both urine and feces, and as a basis for comparison, especially if incontinence should become a problem in the future.

3. Anatomic

Anatomic abnormalities constitute a whole different set of indications for urodynamic evaluation. Boys with posterior urethral valves may present with hydronephrosis *in utero*, urinary infection in infancy and incontinence in childhood. Ablation of the valves often leads to improvement of upper urinary tract dilation and symptoms of incontinence, but in a substantial number (20 to 25%), there is no appreciable change in bladder function [437, 438]. Characterizing the bladder function during its filling and emptying phases, pre- and post resection of the valves provides the necessary parameters for improving the functional state of the lower urinary tract. [439, 440] Medical treatment may be instituted based on persistent abnormal findings of detrusor muscle function [441]. Exstrophy of the bladder can be a daunting problem to manage. Most children have their exstrophied bladder closed in the neonatal period with subsequent staged reconstruction of the bladder neck and epispadiac urethra performed at variable times in infancy and early childhood. There is a tendency now to close the bladder and complete the urethroplasty simultaneously in the newborn period. Although 15 to 20% achieve continence following the initial closure only [442], cystometry, urethral pressure profilometry and residual urine measurements are needed to characterize the status of the lower urinary tract at various stages of the reconstruction and to determine what surgical procedure or medical regimen may be needed next, in order to achieve continence [443]. Urinary incontinence following surgical excision of a ureterocele that extends down past the bladder neck to the external urethra (caecosphincteric ureterocele) may be due to an injury to the bladder neck and/or the external urethral sphincter mechanism. There is sparse evidence that this form of bladder outlet obstruction affects detrusor muscle function. Static and dynamic urethral pressure profilometry and videourodynamic studies of the bladder neck are indicated when incontinence follows treatment of this condition.

The presence of vesicoureteral reflux after apparently successful antireflux surgery warrants cystometry and a voiding pressure study. Hyperreflexia, elevated voiding pressure, significant residual urine and poor elimination habits should be determined and managed in order to help resolve the persistent postoperative reflux in a non-invasive manner. Urethral stricture disease in boys is a rare event, arising most likely from an unsuspected straddle injury in the past. A urinary flow rate pre- and postoperatively after either endoscopic or open surgery for this condition can demonstrate to the boy, the marked change in his ability to void normally. Because recurrence of a stricture may be insidious, periodic monitoring of the urinary flow rate for peak and mean values, and evaluating the characteristics of the urine stream may alert the clinician to early signs of renarrowing.

4. FUNCTIONAL

When assessing functional disorders involving the lower urinary tract in children, one must take into account the dynamics of the maturing nervous system, learned habits of elimination for bladder and bowel function and social influences that might modulate the child's behavior [444, 445].

Day and nighttime incontinence is not considered a worrisome issue until age 5 or 6. Then, most children without an unsuspected anatomic or neurologic lesion should be dry [446]. Persistent day incontinence in the absence of urinary infection and with a normal bladder and bowel emptying regimen warrants cystometry, pressure flow studies and a urinary flow rate. Stress incontinence in girls and adolescent females is rare but should be delineated with cystometry, pressure flow studies and video urodynamics or ambulatory urodynamics, if simple measures to insure regular emptying do not work.

Nighttime wetting (enuresis) is a condition that often improves over time [445-448]. Although there may be social and familial pressures to resolve the condition in various cultures before puberty, in western cultures it is generally not necessary to conduct urodynamic studies until adolescence, to determine why it has not resolved. Urodynamic testing in a home setting, such as provided by ambulatory monitoring may be an ideal method to characterize why these children have continued enuresis.

Daytime wetting as an isolated symptom in boys without nocturnal enuresis nocturna rarely warrants lower urinary tract investigation [449]. If no anatomic abnormality is present on radiologic studies it is unlikely there will be any aberration on urodynamic testing. Girls with day wetting only may have vaginal trapping of urine with subsequent postmicturition leakage. A thorough physical examination and careful questioning of when the incontinence occurs should help to define and treat the problem. Urgency or sudden incontinence throughout the day in the absence of infection should be treated with anticholinergic drugs initially; cystometry is indicated if incontinence persists despite medical therapy.

Fecal incontinence in the absence of any anatomic and/or neurologic deficit often affects lower urinary tract function and contributes to urinary incontinence in a number of ways. Constipation and fecal impaction have been shown to cause detrusor overactivity and reduced functional bladder capacity [450]. Monitoring the effectiveness of colonic emptying and assessing bowel contents during videourodynamics may provide an explanation for the lower urinary tract dysfunction noted during these studies and pose an easy, effective answer for treatment. Alternatively, fecal soiling from constipation or poor hygiene may lead to urinary infection which can then alter both detrusor and urethral function. Understanding and eliminating this etiology may normalize lower urinary tract function without the need for urodynamic studies [451].

Urinary infection is a major cause of incontinence in girls, because it can lead to low compliance, and detrusor and/or urethral instability. It can arise from a multitude of causes. As noted, bowel dysfunction may lead to its occurrence [452]. In fact, dysfunctional elimination "syndromes" are now considered the primary and not a secondary cause of recurrent urinary infection and in some cases the etiology for vesicoureteral reflux [451]. Treating these elimination disorders is paramount to surgery for reflux in many instances [451, 453]. In addition to systemic and local host factors, abnormal voiding dynamics from learned behavior patterns, aberrant voiding habits and poor hygiene are likely causes of recurrent UTI in girls [454].

Urodynamic studies in infants < 6 months of age with reflux reveal an overactive bladder in 50% and high voiding pressure in 95%[455]. With increasing age, voiding pressures diminish to normal values and overactivity resolves in most children, suggesting the presence of a transient form of bladder outflow obstruction in infants with severe reflux [456]. Similar findings were noted by several investigators assessing newborns with severe reflux [457] [458]. These studies in infants and the association of dysfunctional elimination syndromes with reflux and infection in older children strongly suggest that vesicoureteral reflux is a secondary disorder related more to abnormal bladder function than to a primary anatomic defect at the ureterovesical junction. Urodynamic studies are indicated (1) in the absence of reflux, but when voiding cystography reveals trabeculation and/or diverticulum formation, with abnormalities in the appearance of the bladder neck and urethra; (2) when there is persistent incontinence and/or recurrent infection despite long term antibiotics and anticholinergics, respectively; and (3) with an interrupted urine stream and an elevated residual urine [459]. A urinary flow rate prior to any instrumentation in a relaxed setting in order to recreate a representative flow rate is probably the single most important test to obtain [460]. An intermittent flow pattern secondary to incomplete relaxation of the sphincter throughout voiding and incomplete emptying are a likely consequence of, as well as etiology for, recurrent UTI. Videourodynamics which include bladder and urethral pressure monitoring during the filling and emptying phases of the micturition cycle can provide numerous clues, when the actual flow rate curves are normal. Sphincter EMG may be necessary as well when dyssynergia between the detrusor and sphincter is suspected.

5. Technical concerns

A reduced rate of filling, i.e. 10% of the expected bladder volume per minute, is recommended. Expected bladder volumes are noted in section 2.1.d. The smallest dual-channel urethral catheter available should be used in children for the same reasons as specified for adults. Most children can undergo studies without premedication; only the most agitated may require some degree of sedation. A suprapubic catheter placed under anesthesia the day before may make the subsequent investigations more accurate in cases of a very small caliber urethra or when a precise assessment of urethral competence is needed. It has been employed to monitor bladder pressure during natural fill cystometry.

VI. FRAIL ELDERLY

Elderly patients should not be considered differently from younger subjects simply because of their chronological age. That symptoms poorly predict urodynamic diagnosis is also true in the elderly [461, 462]. Questionnaire surveys, which have been frequently used in epidemiological studies, are known to correlate poorly with extended urodynamic testing [463]. Urodynamic findings in the elderly tend to demonstrate an overactive detrusor [464, 465], and a reduction in bladder capacity, urinary flowrate and detrusor contractility [466]. Symptoms such as urgency, frequency and incontinence are more frequently detected in aged men and women [466]. However, these changes in urodynamic and symptomatic findings associated with aging are not necessarily interrelated. For example, in a large community survey, only 12% of incontinent women and almost 5% of continent women were found to have involuntary detrusor contractions [467]. Meanwhile, other studies showed that 11% to 42% [464, 468] of continent elderly women demonstrated involuntary contractions on conventional cystometry. These observations indicate that more detailed examinations are needed to disclose the underlying pathophysiology in the incontinent elderly [461-463]. In fact diverse types of lower urinary tract dysfunction are shown to be involved in incontinence in the elderly by multichannel videourodynamics [465].

On the other hand, frail elderly patients may require special consideration. Most of them will not undergo surgical or invasive treatments for their incontinence. In this setting the Minimum Data Set and Resident Assessment Protocol [469], when administered by trained staff, provided a stepwise and non-urodynamic diagnosis of the type of incontinence without serious misclassification [470].

Among urodynamic investigations, measurement of post-void residual urine is important. If it is small, significant infravesical obstruction or detrusor underactivity or acontractility is unlikely, and a small dose of anticholinergic medication may be tried. If a large amount of residual urine is found, overflow incontinence or incontinence associated with infection is suspected, and intermittent catheterization may be indicated. The measurement is included in the Resident Assessment Protocol along with the stress test [470].

If cystometry is indicated and no equipment or referral is available, it can be modified to "simple cystometry" [87] The procedure needs only an open syringe attached to a single lumen catheter, sterile water or saline and a tape measure. Fluid is infused by gravity at a pressure head of 15-20 cm H_2O. Bladder capacity, sensation of filling, and presence of a detrusor contraction or overactivity can be semiquantified. Pressure is measured by observing the height of the column of water. These simple measures can be carried out at the bedside and may be useful for disabled patients [89-91, 471, 472]. Simple cystometry, as compared with multichannel cystometry, has a specificity of 79% or 75% and a sensitivity of 75% or 88% for the observation of detrusor overactivity [89, 90]. The accuracy can be improved by combining it with simpler tests [90, 91] or with a stress test to exclude stress incontinence [21]. Thus, simple cystometry can be helpful to assess bladder function among geriatric patients in whom formal urodynamics are either unavailable or impractical.

However, the clinical significance of these findings is limited. Detrusor overactivity is found in up to 50% of *symptom-free* elderly, while detrusor overactivity incontinence is the most likely finding in *incontinent* frail elderly in any case [465, 473]. Furthermore most of the studies recommending simple cystometry were conducted before a high prevalence of detrusor hyperactivity with impaired contractility (DHIC) was recognised [465]. This dysfunction is the most common abnormality in incontinence observed in frail elderly populations [465, 473], and is easily misdiagnosed as a stable detrusor by simple cystometry [21], because single channel cystometry is less sensitive for detecting low-pressure detrusor contractions. If a contraction coincides with a cough, the leakage may be regarded as the sign of a positive stress test. Further research is needed to estimate predictive values of non-urodynamic assessment, simple cystometry with or without simpler tests, or further referral investigation in the frail elderly.

E. CONCLUSIONS

I. GENERAL CONCLUSIONS

- Urodynamic investigation is the only means of objectively assessing lower urinary tract function or dysfunction in incontinent patients. Therefore it should be performed in clinical research and is required in clinical practice whenever detailed knowledge of lower urinary tract function is needed to decide on treatment, to help predict the outcome of treatment, or to understand the reasons for failure of treatment.
- Adherence to standardized well-documented methods is critically important to ensure the clinical and scientific reliability and reproducibility of study results. Clearly defined and widely accepted standard terminology, e.g. the terminology developed by the ICS, for describing urodynamic results facilitates straightforward and unambiguous communication.
- Urodynamic investigation by itself is inadequate to define the cause of lower urinary tract dysfunction and its consequences. Integration of symptoms, voiding diary, history, physical findings, radiologic imaging and all the results of urodynamic study are essential for the correct assessment.
- The indication for each urodynamic examination should be tailored to the individual patient in the light of the diagnostic strategy and the potential predictive value of the results it will provide.

II. RECOMMENDATIONS FOR CLINICAL PRACTICE

The following recommendations have been graded as either grade C (based on level 4 evidence from case series) or grade D (based on level 5 evidence: i.e., expert opinion). All have unanimous committee agreement.

- Investigation should only be performed in women if voiding difficulty or neuropathy is suspected, if previous surgical or non-surgical treatments have failed, or if invasive or surgical treatments are considered (Recommendation grade C).
- In men and children detailed urodynamic investigation should be undertaken (Recommendation grade D).
- Uroflowmetry with residual urine measurement and filling cystometry with and without provocation (tailored to the patient's condition) should be employed as a first-line investigation (Recommendation grade C).
- Gas cystometry is not recommended (Recommendation grade D).
- If it is necessary to estimate urethral competence during the filling phase, urethral pressure profiles and/or abdominal leak point pressure measurements are indicated (Recommendation grade C).
- Urethral function during the voiding phase should be evaluated by pressure-flow studies or videourodynamics, ± electromyography especially if neuropathy is evident (Recommendation grade D).
- Videourodynamics may be used to detect leakage and morphological abnormality simultaneously with pressure monitoring (Recommendation grade D).
- Ambulatory urodynamic monitoring might be considered for those who fail to demonstrate leakage or detrusor overactivity in other investigations (Recommendation grade D).

III. RECOMMENDATIONS FOR FUTURE RESEARCH

1. Research on clinical relevance

- To remedy the paucity of high-quality evidence for or against the utility of urodynamics in the investigation of incontinence, properly conducted, large-scale, randomized controlled trials are urgently needed to determine the role, predictive value, and effect on treatment outcomes of urodynamics, videourodynamics and ambulatory monitoring. Such trials should be conducted for various patient groups in various clinical settings
- Investigation of the predictive value of urodynamic findings for treatment outcomes

2. Research on methodological aspects

- Standardization of:

  methods for quality control of urodynamic equipment;

  techniques and instrumentation;

training and qualifications of personnel;

documentation of results.

- Development of improved techniques for assessing bladder sensation.
- Minimization of the invasiveness of urodynamic techniques (e.g., refinement of ultrasonic imaging techniques) so that they are more widely applicable and can be carried out in more natural settings, with a minimum of personnel and expense.
- Development of methods of quantification of urodynamic observations, to improve reliability, interchangeability, and clinical relevance.

3. Research on interpretational aspects

- Precise determination of physiological, technical and interpretation variability of urodynamic results.
- Revised terminology to describe urodynamic findings more precisely and clearly, especially in the field of urge incontinence, detrusor overactivity, and bladder sensation.
- Development of an improved urodynamic definition for intrinsic sphincter deficiency based on the understanding and characterization of the underlying pathophysiology.

REFERENCES

1. Abrams, P., Blaivas, J.G., Stanton, S.L. et al.: Standardisation of terminology of lower urinary tract function. Neurourol Urodyn, 7: 403,1988
2. Steers, W.D., Barrett, D.M. and Wein, A.J.: Voiding dysfunction, diagnosis, classification and management. In: Adult and Pediatric Urology, Edited by J.Y. Gillenwater, J.T. Grayhack, S.S. Howards, et al. Chicago: Year Book Medical Publishers, pp. 1220, 1996
3. Blaivas, J.G., Romanzi, L.J. and Heritz, D.M.: Urinary incontinence: pathophysiology, evaluation, treatmentoverview and nonsurgical management. In: Campbell's Urology, Edited by P.C. Walsh, A.B. Retik, E.D. Vaughan, et al. Philadelphia: Saunders, pp. 1007-1043, 1997
4. Abrams, P.: Urodynamics. London: Springer.1997
5. Blaivas, J.G. and Chancellor, M.B.: Atlas of Urodynamics. Baltimore: Williams and Wilkins.1996
6. Mundy, A.R., Stephenson, T.P. and Wein, A.J.: Urodynamics: principles, practice and application. Edinburgh: Churchill Livingstone.1994
7. Sand, P.K. and Ostergard, D.R.: Urodynamics and the evaluation of female incontinence: a practical guide. London: Springer-Verlag.1995
8. Ostergard, D.R.: Urogynecology and urodynamics: theory and practice, 4th edn. Baltimore: Williams and Wilkins.1996
9. Blaivas, J.G.: Techniques of evaluation. In: Neurourology and urodynamics: principles and practice, Edited by S.V. Yalla, E.J. McGuire, A. Elbadawi, et al. New York: Macmillan, pp. 155-198, 1988
10. Hermieu, J.F., Ravery, V., Le Coent, R. et al.: [Effects of a 6F urethral catheter on uroflowmetry in men with benign prostatic hypertrophy]. Prog Urol, 8: 1035,1998
11. Groutz, A., Blaivas, J.G. and Sassone, A.M.: Detrusor pressure uroflowmetry studies in women: effect of a 7Fr transurethral catheter. J Urol, 164: 109,2000
12. Klingler, H.C., Madersbacher, S. and Schmidbauer, C.P.: Impact of different sized catheters on pressure-flow studies in patients with benign prostatic hyperplasia. Neurourol Urodyn, 15: 473,1996
13. Reynard, J.M., Lim, C., Swami, S. et al.: The obstructive effect of a urethral catheter. J Urol, 155: 901,1996
14. Walker, R.M., Di Pasquale, B., Hubregtse, M. et al.: Pressure-flow studies in the diagnosis of bladder outlet obstruction: a study comparing suprapubic and transurethral techniques. Br J Urol, 79: 693,1997
15. Bump, R.C., Elser, D.M., Theofrastous, J.P. et al.: Valsalva leak point pressures in women with genuine stress incontinence: reproducibility, effect of catheter caliber, and correlations with other measures of urethral resistance. Continence Program for Women Research Group. Am J Obstet Gynecol, 173: 551,1995
16. Ask, P. and Hok, B.: Pressure measurement thechniques in urodynamic investigations. Neurourol Urodyn, 9: 1,1990
17. Sullivan, M.P. and Yalla, S.V.: Penile urethral compression-release maneuver as a non-invasive screening test for diagnosing prostatic obstruction. Neurourol Urodyn, 19: 657,2000
18. Miklos, J.R., Sze, E.H. and Karram, M.M.: A critical appraisal of the methods of measuring leak-point pressures in women with stress incontinence. Obstet Gynecol, 86: 349,1995
19. Theofrastous, J.P., Wyman, J.F., Bump, R.C. et al.: Relationship between urethral and vaginal pressures during pelvic muscle contraction. The Continence Program for Women Research Group. Neurourol Urodyn, 16: 553,1997
20. Wall, L.L., Hewitt, J.K. and Helms, M.J.: Are vaginal and rectal pressures equivalent approximations of one another for the purpose of performing subtracted cystometry? Obstet Gynecol, 85: 488,1995
21. Resnick, N.M., Brandeis, G.H., Baumann, M.M. et al.: Misdiagnosis of urinary incontinence in nursing home women: prevalence and a proposed solution. Neurourol Urodyn, 15: 599,1996
22. Griffiths, D.: The pressure within a collapsed tube, with special reference to urethral pressure. Phys Med Biol, 30: 951,1985
23. Brown, M. and Wickham, J.E.A.: The urethral pressure profile. Br J Urol, 41: 211,1969
24. Abrams, P.H., Martin, S. and Griffiths, D.J.: The measurement and interpretation of urethral pressures obtained by the method of Brown and Wickham. Br J Urol, 50: 33,1978
25. Plevnik, S., Vrtacnik, P. and Janez, J.: Detection of fluid entry into the urethra by electric impedance measurement: electric fluid bridge test. Clin Phys Physiol Meas, 4: 309,1983
26. Miller, J.M., Ashton-Miller, J.A. and Delancey, J.O.: Quantification of cough-related urine loss using the paper towel test. Obstet Gynecol, 91: 705,1998
27. Thind, P., Bagi, P., Lose, G. et al.: Characterization of pressure changes in the lower urinary tract during coughing with special reference to the demands on the pressure recording equipment. Neurourol Urodyn, 13: 219,1994
28. Ask, P.: Measurement techniques for urodynamic investigations. Crit Rev Biomed Eng, 17: 413,1989
29. Madersbacher, H. and Dietl, P.: Urodynamic practice in neurourological patients: techniques and clinical value. Paraplegia, 22: 145,1984
30. Kulseng-Hanssen, S.: Reliability and validity of stationary cystometry, stationary cysto- urethrometry and ambulatory cysto-urethro-vaginometry. Acta Obstet Gynecol Scand Suppl, 166: 33,1997
31. Barnes, D.G., Ralph, D., Hill, P.D. et al.: A consumer's guide to commercially available urodynamic equipment. Br J Urol, 68: 138,1991

32. Versi, E., Cardozo, L., Anand, D. et al.: Symptoms analysis for the diagnosis of genuine stress incontinence. Br J Obstet Gynaecol, 98: 815,1991

33. Haeusler, G., Hanzal, E., Joura, E. et al.: Differential diagnosis of detrusor instability and stress-incontinence by patient history: the Gaudenz-Incontinence-Questionnaire revisited. Acta Obstet Gynecol Scand, 74: 635,1995

34. Bergman, A. and Bader, K.: Reliability of the patient's history in the diagnosis of urinary incontinence. Int J Gynaecol Obstet, 32: 255,1990

35. Jarvis, G.J., Hall, S., Stamp, S. et al.: An assessment of urodynamic examination in incontinent women. Br J Obstet Gynaecol, 87: 893,1980

36. Shepherd, A.M., Powell, P.H. and Ball, A.J.: The place of urodynamic studies in the investigaton and treatment of female urinary tract symptoms. Obstet Gynecol, 3: 123,1982

37. Jackson, S.: The patient with an overactive bladder—symptoms and quality-of-life issues. Urology, 50: 18,1997

38. Golomb, J., Lindner, A., Siegel, Y. et al.: Variability and circadian changes in home uroflowmetry in patients with benign prostatic hyperplasia compared to normal controls. J Urol, 147: 1044,1992

39. Witjes, W.P., de la Rosette, J.J., Zerbib, M. et al.: Computerized artifact detection and correction of uroflow curves: towards a more consistent quantitative assessment of maximum flow. Eur Urol, 33: 54,1998

40. Thuroff, J.W., Bunke, B., Ebner, A. et al.: Randomized, double-blind, multicenter trial on treatment of frequency, urgency and incontinence related to detrusor hyperactivity: oxybutynin versus propantheline versus placebo. J Urol, 145: 813,1991

41. Homma, Y., Kondo, Y., Takahashi, S. et al.: Reproducibility of cystometry in overactive detrusor. Eur Urol, 38: 681,2000

42. Andersen, J.R., Lose, G., Norgaard, M. et al.: Terodiline, emepronium bromide or placebo for treatment of female detrusor overactivity? A randomised, double-blind, cross-over study. Br J Urol, 61: 310,1988

43. Griffiths, D.J. and Scholtmeijer, R.J.: Detrusor instability in children. Neurourol Urodyn, 1: 187,1982

44. Tubaro, A., Renzetti, R., Ranieri, M. et al.: Variability in filling cystometry results in men with LUTS and the impact on the diagnosis of an overactive bladder. Neurourol Urodyn, 19: 425,2000

45. Staskin, D., Siroky, M.B. and Krane, R.J.: Classification of voiding dysfunction. In: Clinical neuro-urology, Edited. Boston: Little, Brown and Co., pp., 1991

46. Haab, F., Zimmern, P.E. and Leach, G.E.: Female stress urinary incontinence due to intrinsic sphincteric deficiency: recognition and management. J Urol, 156: 3,1996

47. Gunnarsson, M. and Mattiasson, A.: Female stress, urge, and mixed urinary incontinence are associated with a chronic and progressive pelvic floor/vaginal neuromuscular disorder: An investigation of 317 healthy and incontinent women using vaginal surface electromyography. Neurourol Urodyn, 18: 613,1999

48. Kuo, H.: The relationships of urethral and pelvic floor muscles and the urethral pressure measurements in women with stress urinary incontinence. Eur Urol, 37: 149,2000

49. Artibani, W.: Diagnosis and significance of idiopathic overactive bladder. Urology, 50: 25,1997

50. Fall, M., Geirsson, G. and Lindstrom, S.: Toward a new classification of overactive bladders. Neurourol Urodyn, 14: 635,1995

51. Griffiths, D.J., McCracken, P.N., Harrison, G.M. et al.: Cerebral aetiology of urinary urge incontinence in elderly people. Age Ageing, 23: 246,1994

52. Blaivas, J.G., Appell, R.A., Fantl, J.A. et al.: Definition and classification of urinary incontinence: recommendations of the Urodynamic Society. Neurourol Urodyn, 16: 149,1997

53. Jensen, J.K., Nielsen, F.R., Jr. and Ostergard, D.R.: The role of patient history in the diagnosis of urinary incontinence. Obstet Gynecol, 83: 904,1994

54. james, M., Jackson, S., Shepherd, A. et al.: Pure stress leakage symptomatology: is it safe to discount detrusor instability? Br J Obstet Gynaecol, 106: 1255,1999

55. Lemack, G.E. and Zimmern, P.E.: Identifying patients who require urodynamic testing before surgery for stress incontinence based on questionnaire information and surgical history. Urology, 55: 506,2000

56. Handa, V.L., Jensen, J.K. and Ostergard, D.R.: Federal guidelines for the management of urinary incontinence in the united states: which patients should undergo urodynamic testing? Int J Gynaecol Obstet, 6: 198,1995

57. Diokno, A.C., Dimaculangan, R.R., Lim, E.U. et al.: Office based criteria for predicting type II stress incontinence without further evaluation studies. J Urol, 161: 1263,1999

58. Videla, F.L. and Wall, L.L.: Stress incontinence diagnosed without multichannel urodynamic studies. Obstet Gynecol, 91: 965,1998

59. Cundiff, G.W., Harris, R.L., Coates, K.W. et al.: Clinical predictors of urinary incontinence in women. Am J Obstet Gynecol, 177: 262,1997

60. Larsson, G., Blixt, C., Janson, G. et al.: The frequency/volume chart as a differential diagnostic tool in female urinary incontinence. Int J Gynaecol Obstet, 5: 273,1994

61. Tincello, D.G. and Richmond, D.H.: The Larsson frequency/volume chart is not a substitute for cystometry in the investigation of women with urinary incontinence. Int Urogynecol J Pelvic Floor Dysfunct, 9: 391,1998

62. Fink, D., Perucchini, D., Schaer, G.N. et al.: The role of the frequency-volume chart in the differential diagnostic of female urinary incontinence. Acta Obstet Gynecol Scand, 78: 254,1999

63. Amundsen, C., Lau, M., English, S.F. et al.: Do urinary symptoms correlate with urodynamic findings? J Urol, 161: 1871,1999

64. Digesu, G.A., Salvatore, L., Cardozo, L. et al.: Symptomatic diagnosis of the overactive bladder: Is it helpful? Neurourol Urodyn, 19: 381,2000

65. van Venrooij, G.E. and Boone, T.A.: Extensive urodynamic investigation: interaction among diuresis, detrusor instability, urethral relaxation, incontinence and complaints in women with a history of urge incontinence. J Urol, 152: 1535,1994

66. Choe, J.M., Gallo, M.L. and Staskin, D.R.: A provocative maneuver to elicit cystometric instability: measuring instability at maximum infusion. J Urol, 161: 1541,1999

67. Wein, A.J., Hanno, P.M., Dixon, D.O. et al.: The reproducibility and interpretation of carbon dioxide cystometry. J Urol, 120: 205,1978

68. Sethia, K.K. and Smith, J.C.: The effect of pH and lignocaine on detrusor instability. Br J Urol, 60: 516,1987

69. Swithinbank, L., Rogers, C., Jones, J.E. et al.: The effect of altering urinary pH on urinary symptoms in women. Neurourol Urodyn, 19: 527,2000

70. Jiang, C.H.: Influence of intravesical low pH on the micturition threshold in the rat. Neurourol Urodyn, 19: 414,2000

71. Coolsaet, B.L., van Duyl, W.A., van Mastrigt, R. et al.: Stepwise cystometry of urinary bladder. New dynamic procedure to investigate viscoelastic behavior. Urology, 2: 255,1973

72. Coolsaet, B.L., van Duyl, W.A., van Mastrigt, R. et al.: Viscoelastic properties of the bladder wall. Urol Int, 30: 16,1975

73. Kondo, A. and Susset, J.G.: Viscoelastic properties of bladder. II.

Comparative studies in normal and pathologic dogs. Invest Urol, 11: 459,1974

74. Bates, C.P., Whiteside, C.G. and Turner-Warwick, R.: Synchronous cine-pressure-flow-cysto-urethrography with special reference to stress and urge incontinence. Br J Urol, 42: 714,1970
75. Hellstrom, P.A., Tammela, T.L., Kontturi, M.J. et al.: The bladder cooling test for urodynamic assessment: analysis of 400 examinations. Br J Urol, 67: 275,1991
76. Geirsson, G., Fall, M. and Lindstrom, S.: The ice-water test—a simple and valuable supplement to routine cystometry. Br J Urol, 71: 681,1993
77. Fall, M. and Geirsson, G.: Positive ice-water test: a predictor of neurological disease? World J Urol, 14: S51,1996
78. Ronzoni, G., Menchinelli, P., Manca, A. et al.: The ice-water test in the diagnosis and treatment of the neurogenic bladder. Br J Urol, 79: 698,1997
79. Ismael, S.S., Epstein, T., Bayle, B. et al.: Bladder cooling reflex in patients with multiple sclerosis. J Urol, 164: 1280,2000
80. Blaivas, J.G., Groutz, A. and Verhaaren, M.: Does the method of cystometry affect the incidence of involuntary detrusor contractions? A prospective randomized urodynamic study. Neurourol Urodyn, 20: 141,2001
81. Arnold, E.P., Webster, J.R., Loose, H. et al.: Urodynamics of female incontinence: factors influencing the results of surgery. Am J Obstet Gynecol, 117: 805,1973
82. Mayer, R., Wells, T.J., Brink, C.A. et al.: Handwashing in the cystometric evaluation of detrusor instability. Neurourol Urodyn: 563,1991
83. Gallo, M.L., Choe, J.M., Breslin, D. et al.: Provocative testing during cystometry to elicit detrusor instability: Measured instability at maximum infusion.,1998
84. Kerr, L.A., Bauer, S.B. and Staskin, D.R.: Abnormal detrusor function precipitating hydronephrosis identified by extended voiding cystometry. J Urol, 152: 89,1994
85. Ness, T.J., Richter, H.E., Varner, R.E. et al.: A psychophysical study of discomfort produced by repeated filling of the urinary bladder. Pain, 76: 61,1998
86. Oliver, S., Susser, J., Fowler, C. et al.: Sensations during urodynamics and sensations scored in voiding diaries: are they comparable? Neurourol Urodyn, 19: 479,2000
87. Wall, L.L., Wiskind, A.K. and Taylor, P.A.: Simple bladder filling with a cough stress test compared with subtracted cystometry for the diagnosis of urinary incontinence. Am J Obstet Gynecol, 171: 1472,1994
88. Swift, S.E.: The reliability of performing a screening cystometrogram using a fetal monitoring device for the detection of detrusor instability. Obstet Gynecol, 89: 708,1997
89. Fonda, D., Brimage, P.J. and D'astoli, M.: Simple screening for urinary incontinence in the elderly: comparison of simple and multichannel cystometry. Urology, 42: 536,1993
90. Ouslander, J., Leach, G., Abelson, S. et al.: Simple versus multichannel cystometry in the evaluation of bladder function in an incontinent geriatric population. J Urol, 140: 1482,1988
91. Sutherst, J.R. and Brown, M.C.: Comparison of single and multichannel cystometry in diagnosing bladder instability. Br Med J (Clin Res Ed), 288: 1720,1984
92. Bombieri, L., Dance, D.A., Rienhardt, G.W. et al.: Urinary tract infection after urodynamic studies in women: incidence and natural history. BJU Int, 83: 392,1999
93. Vereecken, R.L. and Das, J.: Urethral instability: related to stress and/or urge incontinence? J Urol, 134: 698,1985
94. Fall, M., Ohlsson, B.L. and Carlsson, C.A.: The neurogenic overactive bladder. Classification based on urodynamics. Br J Urol, 64: 368,1989
95. Geirsson, G., Fall, M. and Lindstrom, S.: Subtypes of overactive bladder in old age. Age Ageing, 22: 125,1993
96. Wyndaele, J.J.: The normal pattern of perception of bladder filling during cystometry studied in 38 young healthy volunteers. J Urol, 160: 479,1998
97. Hjalmas, K.: Urodynamics in normal infants and children. Scand J Urol Nephrol Suppl, 114: 20,1988
98. Kaefer, M., Zurakowski, D., Bauer, S.B. et al.: Estimating normal bladder capacity in children. J Urol, 158: 2261,1997
99. Toppercer, A. and Tetreault, J.P.: Compliance of the bladder: an attempt to establish normal values. Urology, 14: 204,1979
100. Wyndaele, J.J.: Normality in urodynamics studied in healthy adults. J Urol, 161: 899,1999
101. Gilmour, R.F., Churchill, B.M., Steckler, R.E. et al.: A new technique for dynamic analysis of bladder compliance. J Urol, 150: 1200,1993
102. McGuire, E.J., Woodside, J.R., Borden, T.A. et al.: Prognostic value of urodynamic testing in myelodysplastic patients. J Urol, 126: 205,1981
103. McGuire, E.J., Woodside, J.R. and Borden, T.A.: Upper urinary tract deterioration in patients with myelodysplasia and detrusor hypertonia: a followup study. J Urol, 129: 823,1983
104. McLorie, G.A., Perez-Marero, R., Csima, A. et al.: Determinants of hydronephrosis and renal injury in patients with myelomeningocele. J Urol, 140: 1289,1988
105. Wiskind, A.K., Miller, K.F. and Wall, L.L.: One hundred unstable bladders. Obstet Gynecol, 83: 108,1994
106. Holley, R.L., Richer, H.E., Goode, P.S. et al.: Cost- effectiveness of the cough stress test with simple cystometrogram versus urodynamics in the diagnosis of genuine stress urinary incontinence. J Gynecol Techniques, 5: 135,1999
107. Griffiths, D.: Clinical aspects of detrusor instability and the value of urodynamics: a review of the evidence. Eur Urol, 34: 13,1998
108. Thompson, P.K., Duff, D.S. and Thayer, P.S.: Stress incontinence in women under 50: does urodynamics improve surgical outcome? Int Urogynecol J Pelvic Floor Dysfunct, 11: 285,2000
109. Schrepferman, C.G., Griebling, T.L., Nygaard, I.E. et al.: Resolution of urge symptoms following sling cystourethropexy. J Urol, 164: 1628,2000
110. del Campo-Rodriguez, M., Batista-Miranda, J.E., Errando-Smet, C. et al.: Outcome of colposuspension in patients with stress urinary incontinence and abnormal cystometry. Arch Esp Urol, 52: 810,1999
111. Golomb, J., Dotan, Z., Leibovitch, I. et al.: [Can preoperative urodynamic examination allow us to predict the risk of incontinence after radical prostatectomy?]. Prog Urol, 9: 288,1999
112. Barnes, A.: The method of evaluating the stress of urinary incontinence. Obstet Gynecol, 83: 108,1961
113. Enhorning, G.: Simultaneous recording of intravesical and intraurethral pressure. Acta Obstet Gynecol Scand, 176: 1,1961
114. Zinner, N., Ritter, R. and Sterling, A.M.: The mechanism of micturition. In: Scientific foundation of urology, Edited by D. Williams and G. Chisholm. London: William Heinemann, pp. 39 51, 1976
115. Griffiths, D.: Urodynamics: medical physics handbook. Bristol: Adams Hilger.1980
116. Harrison, N.W.: The urethral pressure profile. Urol Res, 4: 95,1976
117. Lose, G.: Simultaneous recording of pressure and cross-sectional area in the female urethra: a study of urethral closure function in healthy and stress incontinent women. Neurourol Urodyn, 11: 55,1992

118. Hilton, P.: Urethral pressure measurement at rest: an analysis of variance. Neurourol Urodyn, 1: 303,1982

119. Hilton, P.: Urethral pressure measurement by microtransducer: observations on methodology, the pathophysiology ofgenuine stress incontinence and the effects of treatment in the female [MD]. Newcastle upon Tyne.1981

120. Amundsen, M.: Urethrocysometry in women [MD]. Lund, Sweden: Lund.1975

121. Hilton, P. and Stanton, S.L.: Urethral pressure measurement by microtransducer: the results in symptom-free women and in those with genuine stress incontinence. Br J Obstet Gynaecol, 90: 919,1983

122. Haeusler, G., Tempfer, C., Heinzl, H. et al.: Value of urethral pressure profilometry in the female incontinent patient: a prospective trial with an 8-channel urethral catheter. Urology, 52: 1113,1998

123. Van Geelen, J.M., Doesburg, W.H. and Martin, C.B., Jr.: Female urethral pressure profile; reproducibility, axial variation and effects of low dose oral contraceptives. J Urol, 131: 394,1984

124. Teague, C.T. and Merrill, D.C.: Laboratory comparison of urethral profilometry techniques. Urology, 13: 221,1979

125. Hilton, P.: Urethral pressure measurement: a comparison of profiles obtained by conventional and fibre-optic transducers. Neurourol Urodyn, 8: 481,1989

126. Elser, D.M., London, W., Fantl, J.A. et al.: A comparison of urethral profilometry using microtip and fiberoptic catheters. Int Urogynecol J Pelvic Floor Dysfunct, 10: 371,1999

127. Awad, S.A., Bryniak, S.R., Lowe, P.J. et al.: Urethral pressure profile in female stress incontinence. J Urol, 120: 475,1978

128. Glen, E.S. and Rowan, D.: Continuous flow cystometry and urethral pressure profile measurement with monitored intravesical pressure: a diagnostic and prognostic investigation. Urol Res, 1: 97,1973

129. Hendriksson, L., Ulmsten, U. and Andersson, K.E.: The effects of changes in posture on the urethral closure pressure in stress incontinent women. Scand J Urol Nephrol, 11: 207,1977

130. Hendriksson, L., Andersson, K.E. and Ulmsten, U.: The urethral pressure profiles in continent and stress-incontinent women. Scand J Urol Nephrol, 13: 5,1979

131. Ghoniem, M., Rottenberg, J., Fretin, J. et al.: Urethral pressure profile: standardisation of technique and study of reproducibility. Urology, 5: 632,1973

132. Van Geelen, J.M., Doesburg, W.H., Thomas, C.M.G. et al.: Urodynamic studies in the normal menstrual cycle: The relationship between hormonal changes during the menstrual cycle and the urethral pressure profile. Am J Obstet Gynecol, 141: 384,1981

133. James, E.D.: The design and use of a system to investigate normal behaviour and diagnose disorders ofthe loer urinary tract [PhD]. Exter.1980

134. Schick, E.: Objective assessment of resistance of female urethra to stress. A scale to establish degree of urethral incompetence. Urology, 26: 518,1985

135. Cundiff, G.W., Harris, R.L., Theofrastous, J.P. et al.: Pressure transmission ratio reproducibility in stress continent and stress incontinent women. Neurourol Urodyn, 16: 161,1997

136. Hilton, P.: Urethral pressure measurement on stress: an anylysis of profiles abtained on coughing and straining. Neurourol Urodyn, 2: 55,1983

137. Swift, S.E., Rust, P.F. and Ostergard, D.R.: Intrasubject variability of the pressure-transmission ratio in patients with genuine stress incontinence. Int Urogynecol J Pelvic Floor Dysfunct, 7: 312,1996

138. Hammerer, P. and Huland, H.: Urodynamic evaluation of changes in urinary control after radical prostatectomy. J Urol, 157: 233,1995

139. Theofrastous, J.P., Bump, R.C., Elser, D.M. et al.: Correlation of urodynamic measures of urethral resistance with clinical measures of incontinence severity in women with pure genuine stress incontinence. The Continence Program for Women Research Group. Am J Obstet Gynecol, 173: 407,1995

140. Toews, H.A.: Intraurethral and intravesical pressures in normal and stress- incontinent women. Obstet Gynecol, 29: 613,1967

141. Low, J.A. and Kao, M.S.: Patterns of urethral resistance in deficient urethral sphincter function. Obstet Gynecol, 40: 634,1972

142. Bump, R.C., Copeland, W.E., Jr., Hurt, W.G. et al.: Dynamic urethral pressure/profilometry pressure transmission ratio determinations in stress-incontinent and stress-continent subjects. Am J Obstet Gynecol, 159: 749,1988

143. Versi, E., Cardozo, L.D., Studd, J.W. et al.: Evalution of urethral pressure profilometry for the diagnosis of genuine stress incontinence. World J Urol, 4: 6,1986

144. Meyer, S., De Grandi, P., Schmidt, N. et al.: Urodynamic parameters in patients with slight and severe genuine stress incontinence: is the stress profile useful? Neurourol Urodyn, 13: 21,1994

145. Versi, E.: Discriminant analysis of urethral pressure profilometry data for the diagnosis of genuine stress incontinence. Br J Obstet Gynaecol, 97: 251,1990

146. Ulmsten, U., Henriksson, L. and Iosif, S.: The unstable female urethra. Am J Obstet Gynecol, 144: 93,1982

147. Weil, A., Miege, B., Rottenberg, R. et al.: Clinical significance of urethral instability. Obstet Gynecol, 68: 106,1986

148. Kulseng Hanssen, S.: Prevalence and pattern of unstable urethral pressure in one hundred seventy-four gynecologic patients referred for urodynamic investigation. Am J Obstet Gynecol, 146: 875,1983

149. Versi, E. and Cardozo, L.: Urethral instability: Diagnosis based on variations of the maximum urethral pressure in normal climacteric women. Neurourol Urodyn, 5: 535,1986

150. Sorensen, S.: Urethral pressure variations in healthy and incontinent women. Neurourol Urodyn, 11: 549,1992

151. Vereecken, R.L.: Physiological and pathological urethral pressure variations. Urol Int, 57: 145,1996

152. Hilton, P.: Unstable urethral pressure-toward a more relevant definition. Neurourol Urodyn, 6: 411,1988

153. Tapp, A.J., Cardozo, L.D., Versi, E. et al.: The prevalence of variation of resting urethral pressure in women and its association with lower urinary tract function. Br J Urol, 61: 314,1988

154. Bates, C., Bradley, W., Glen, E.S. et al.: Fourth report on the standardisation of terminology of lower urinary tract function. Terminology related to neuromuscular dysfunction of the lower urinary tract. Br J Urol, 53: 333,1981

155. Sand, P.K., Bowen, L.W. and Ostergard, D.R.: Uninhibited urethral relaxation: an unusual cause of incontinence. Obstet Gynecol, 68: 645,1986

156. Behr, J., Winkler, M. and Schwiersch, U.: [Urodynamic observations on the Marshall-Marchetti-Krantz operation]. Geburtshilfe Frauenheilkd, 46: 649,1986

157. Hilton, P. and Stanton, S.L.: A clinical and urodynamic evaluation of the polypropylene (Marlex) sling for genuine stress incontinence. Neurourol Urodyn, 2: 145,1983

158. Hilton, P. and Stanton, S.L.: A clinical and urodynamic assessment of the Burch colposuspension for genuine stress incontinence. Br J Obstet Gynaecol, 90: 934,1983

159. Hilton, P.: A clinical and urodynamic study comparing the Stamey bladder neck suspension and suburethral sling procedures in the treatment of genuine stress incontinence. Br J Obstet Gynaecol, 96: 213,1989

160. Hilton, P. and Mayne, C.J.: The Stamey endoscopic bladder neck

suspension: a clinical and urodynamic investigation, including actuarial follow-up over four years. Br J Obstet Gynaecol, 98: 1141,1991

161. Weil, A., Reyes, H., Bischoff, P. et al.: Modifications of the urethral rest and stress profiles after different types of surgery for urinary stress incontinence. Br J Obstet Gynaecol, 91: 46,1984

162. Francis, L.N., Sand, P.K., Hamrang, K. et al.: A urodynamic appraisal of success and failure after retropubic urethropexy. J Reprod Med, 32: 693,1987

163. Sand, P.K., Bowen, L.W., Panganiban, R. et al.: The low pressure urethra as a factor in failed retropubic urethropexy. Obstet Gynecol, 69: 399,1987

164. Bowen, L.W., Sand, P.K., Ostergard, D.R. et al.: Unsuccessful Burch retropubic urethropexy: a case-controlled urodynamic study. Am J Obstet Gynecol, 160: 452,1989

165. Maher, C.F., Dwyer, P.L., Carey, M.P. et al.: Colposuspension or sling for low urethral pressure stress incontinence? Int Urogynecol J Pelvic Floor Dysfunct, 10: 384,1999

166. Sand, P.K., Winkler, H., Blackhurst, D.W. et al.: A prospective randomized study comparing modified Burch retropubic urethropexy and suburethral sling for treatment of genuine stress incontinence with low-pressure urethra. Am J Obstet Gynecol, 182: 30,2000

167. McGuire, E.J.: Urodynamic evaluation of stress incontinence. Urol Clin North Am, 22: 551,1995

168. Lane, T.M. and Shah, P.J.: Leak-point pressures. BJU Int, 86: 942,2000

169. Wheeler, J.S., Jr. and Walter, J.W.: Acute urologic management of the patient with spinal cord injury. Initial hospitalization. Urol Clin North Am, 20: 403,1993

170. Hernandez, R.D., Hurwitz, R.S., Foote, J.E. et al.: Nonsurgical management of threatened upper urinary tracts and incontinence in children with myelomeningocele. J Urol, 152: 1582,1994

171. Szollar, S.M. and Lee, S.M.: Intravesical oxybutynin for spinal cord injury patients. Spinal Cord, 34: 284,1996

172. Bloom, D.A., Knechtel, J.M. and McGuire, E.J.: Urethral dilation improves bladder compliance in children with myelomeningocele and high leak point pressures. J Urol, 144: 430,1990

173. Juma, S., Mostafavi, M. and Joseph, A.: Sphincterotomy: long term complications and warning signs. Neurourol Urodyn, 14: 33,1995

174. Blok, C., van Riel, M.P., van Venrooij, G.E. et al.: Continuous quantification of urethral competence with a new tube- foil sleeve catheter. J Urol, 132: 1004,1984

175. Kujansuu, E., Wirta, P. and Yla-Outinen, A.: Quantification of urethral closure function by SUI threshold after pubococcygeal sling operation. Ann Chir Gynaecol Suppl, 197: 19,1985

176. van Venrooij, G.E., Blok, C., van Riel, M.P. et al.: Relative urethral leakage pressure versus maximum urethral closure pressure. The reliability of the measurement of urethral competence with the new tube-foil sleeve catheter in patients. J Urol, 134: 592,1985

177. McCormack, M., Pike, J. and Kiruluta, G.: Leak point of incontinence: a measure of the interaction between outlet resistance and bladder capacity. J Urol, 150: 162,1993

178. McGuire, E.J., Fitzpatrick, C.C., Wan, J. et al.: Clinical assessment of urethral sphincter function. J Urol, 150: 1452,1993

179. Wan, J., McGuire, E.J., Bloom, D.A. et al.: Stress leak point pressure: a diagnostic tool for incontinent children. J Urol, 150: 700,1993

180. Swift, S.E. and Ostergard, D.R.: Evaluation of current urodynamic testing methods in the diagnosis of genuine stress incontinence. Obstet Gynecol, 86: 85,1995

181. Swift, S.E. and Ostergard, D.R.: A comparison of stress leak-point pressure and maximal urethral closure pressure in patients with genuine stress incontinence. Obstet Gynecol, 85: 704,1995

182. Griffiths, D.J. and Versi, E.: Urethral function. Curr Opin Obstet Gynecol, 8: 372,1996

183. McGuire, E.J., Cespedes, R.D. and O'Connell, H.E.: Leak-point pressures. Urol Clin North Am, 23: 253,1996

184. Nitti, V.W. and Combs, A.J.: Correlation of Valsalva leak point pressure with subjective degree of stress urinary incontinence in women. J Urol, 155: 281,1996

185. Bump, R.C., Coates, K.W., Cundiff, G.W. et al.: Diagnosing intrinsic sphincteric deficiency: comparing urethral closure pressure, urethral axis, and Valsalva leak point pressures. Am J Obstet Gynecol, 177: 303,1997

186. Desautel, M.G., Kapoor, R. and Badlani, G.H.: Sphincteric incontinence: the primary cause of post-prostatectomy incontinence in patients with prostate cancer. Neurourol Urodyn, 16: 153,1997

187. Petrou, S.P. and Kollmorgen, T.A.: Valsalva leak point pressure and bladder volume. Neurourol Urodyn, 17: 3,1998

188. Theofrastous, J.P., Cundiff, G.W., Harris, R.L. et al.: The effect of vesical volume on Valsalva leak-point pressures in women with genuine stress urinary incontinence. Obstet Gynecol, 87: 711,1996

189. Nitti, V.W., Kim, Y. and Combs, A.J.: Voiding dysfunction following transurethral resection of the prostate: symptoms and urodynamic findings. J Urol, 157: 600,1997

190. Faerber, G.J. and Vashi, A.R.: Variations in Valsalva leak point pressure with increasing vesical volume. J Urol, 159: 1909,1998

191. Peschers, U.M., Jundt, K. and Dimpfl, T.: Differences between cough and Valsalva leak-point pressure in stress incontinent women. Neurourol Urodyn, 19: 677,2000

192. Petrou, S.P. and Wan, J.: VLPP in the evaluation of the female with stress urinary incontinence. Int Urogynecol J Pelvic Floor Dysfunct, 10: 254,1999

193. Sultana, C.J.: Urethral closure pressure and leak-point pressure in incontinent women. Obstet Gynecol, 86: 839,1995

194. Siltberg, H., Larsson, G. and Victor, A.: Reproducibility of a new method to determine cough-induced leak-point pressure in women with stress urinary incontinence. Int Urogynecol J Pelvic Floor Dysfunct, 7: 13,1996

195. Plevnik, S., Brown, M., Sutherst, J.R. et al.: Tracking of fluid in urethra by simultaneous electric impedance measurement at three sites. Urol Int, 38: 29,1983

196. Sutherst, J. and Brown, M.: The fluid bridge test for urethral incompetence. A comparison of results in women with incontinence and women with normal urinary control. Acta Obstet Gynecol Scand, 62: 271,1983

197. Siltberg, H., Larsson, G., Hallen, B. et al.: Validation of cough-induced leak point pressure measurement in the evaluation of pharmacological treatment of stress incontinence. Neurourol Urodyn, 19. 591,1999

198. Decter, R.M. and Harpster, L.: Pitfalls in determination of leak point pressure. J Urol, 148: 588,1992

199. Combs, A.J. and Horowitz, M.: A new technique for assessing detrusor leak point pressure in patients with spina bifida. J Urol, 156: 757,1996

200. Belville, W.D., Swierzewski, S.J., 3rd, Wedemeyer, G. et al.: Fiberoptic microtransducer pressure technology: urodynamic implications. Neurourol Urodyn, 12: 171,1993

201. Haab, F., Dmochowski, R., Zimmern, P. et al.: [The variability of the leakage pressure threshold due to exertion "the Valsalva Leak Point Pressure" as a function of the filling volume of the bladder]. Prog Urol, 7: 422,1997

202. Cummings, J.M., Boullier, J.A., Parra, R.O. et al.: Leak point pressures in women with urinary stress incontinence: correlation with patient history. J Urol, 157: 818,1997

203. Song, J.T., Rozanski, T.A. and Belville, W.D.: Stress leak point pressure: a simple and reproducible method utilizing a fiberoptic microtransducer. Urology, 46: 81,1995

204. Wang, S.C., McGuire, E.J. and Bloom, D.A.: A bladder pressure management system for myelodysplasia—clinical outcome. J Urol, 140: 1499,1988

205. Linsenmeyer, T.A., Bagaria, S.P. and Gendron, B.: The impact of urodynamic parameters on the upper tracts of spinal cord injured men who void reflexly. J Spinal Cord Med, 21: 15,1998

206. Kurzrock, E.A. and Polse, S.: Renal deterioration in myelodysplastic children: urodynamic evaluation and clinical correlates. J Urol, 159: 1657,1998

207. Giannantoni, A., Scivoletto, G., Di Stasi, S.M. et al.: Clean intermittent catheterization and prevention of renal disease in spinal cord injury patients. Spinal Cord, 36: 29,1998

208. Takahashi, S., Homma, Y., Fujishiro, T. et al.: Electromyographic study of the striated urethral sphincter in type 3 stress incontinence: evidence of myogenic-dominant damages. Urology, 56: 946,2000

209. Pycha, A., Klingler, C.H., Haitel, A. et al.: Implantable microballoons: an attractive alternative in the management of intrinsic sphincter deficiency. Eur Urol, 33: 469,1998

210. Ficazzola, M.A. and Nitti, V.W.: The etiology of post-radical prostatectomy incontinence and correlation of symptoms with urodynamic findings. J Urol, 160: 1317,1998

211. Larosa, M., Simonazzi, M., Pozzoli, G.L. et al.: [Correlation between the leak point pressure and the clinical grade of incontinence]. Arch Ital Urol Androl, 70: 71,1998

212. Lemack, G.E. and Zimmern, P.E.: Predictability of urodynamic findings based on the Urogenital Distress Inventory-6 questionnaire. Urology, 54: 461,1999

213. Winters, J.C., Appell, R.A. and Rackley, R.R.: Urodynamic findings in postprostatectomy incontinence. Neurourol Urodyn, 17: 493,1998

214. Gudziak, M.R., McGuire, E.J. and Gormley, E.A.: Urodynamic assessment of urethral sphincter function in post- prostatectomy incontinence. J Urol, 156: 1131,1996

215. McGuire, E.J.: Diagnosis and treatment of intrinsic sphincter deficiency. Int J Urol, 2 Suppl 1: 7,1995

216. Clemens, J.Q., Bushman, W. and Schaeffer, A.J.: Urodynamic analysis of the bulbourethral sling procedure. J Urol, 162: 1977,1999

217. Morgan, J.L., O'Connell, H.E. and McGuire, E.J.: Is intrinsic sphincter deficiency a complication of simple hysterectomy? J Urol, 164: 767,2000

218. Fantl, J.A., Newman, D.K., Colling, J. et al.: Urinary incontinence in adults: acute and chronic management. Clinical practice guideline #2, 1996 Update, US Department of Health and Human Services, Public Health Service, Agency for Health Care Policy and Research,AHCPR publication # 96-0682. Rockville,1996

219. Richardson, T.D., Kennelly, M.J. and Faerber, G.J.: Endoscopic injection of glutaraldehyde cross-linked collagen for the treatment of intrinsic sphincter deficiency in women. Urology, 46: 378,1995

220. Milam, D.F. and Franke, J.J.: Prevention and treatment of incontinence after radical prostatectomy. Semin Urol Oncol, 13: 224,1995

221. McLennan, M.T. and Bent, A.E.: Supine empty stress test as a predictor of low valsalva leak point pressure. Neurourol Urodyn, 17: 121,1998

222. McGuire, E.J. and Cespedes, R.D.: Proper diagnosis: a must before surgery for stress incontinence. J Endourol, 10: 201,1996

223. Stricker, P.D.: Proper patient selection for Contigen Bard Collagen implant. Int J Urol, 2 Suppl 1: 2,1995

224. Flood, H.D., Alevizatos, C. and Liu, J.L.: Sex differences in the determination of abdominal leak point pressure in patients with intrinsic sphincter deficiency. J Urol, 156: 1737,1996

225. De Giovanni, L., Menchinelli, P., Rubino, F. et al.: Valsalva leak point pressure: how to chose the best method. Arch Ital Urol Androl, 72: 25,2000

226. Hsu, T.H., Rackley, R.R. and Appell, R.A.: The supine stress test: a simple method to detect intrinsic urethral sphincter dysfunction. J Urol, 162: 460,1999

227. Stohrer, M., Goepel, M., Kondo, A. et al.: The standardization of terminology in neurogenic lower urinary tract dysfunction: with suggestions for diagnostic procedures. International Continence Society Standardization Committee. Neurourol Urodyn, 18: 139,1999

228. Noblett, K.L., Jensen, J.K. and Ostergard, D.R.: The relationship of body mass index to intra-abdominal pressure as measured by multichannel cystometry. Int Urogynecol J Pelvic Floor Dysfunct, 8: 323,1997

229. Mikhail, M.S. and Rosa, H.: The relationship between preoperative abdominal leak point pressure and surgical outcome following retropubic urethropexy for genuine stress incontinence. Obstet Gynecol, 95: S25,2000

230. Klutke, J.J., Subir, C., Andriole, G. et al.: Long-term results after antegrade collagen injection for stress urinary incontinence following radical retropubic prostatectomy. Urology, 53: 974,1999

231. Kim, Y.H., Kattan, M.W. and Boone, T.B.: Correlation of urodynamic results and urethral coaptation with success after transurethral collagen injection. Urology, 50: 941,1997

232. McGuire, E.J. and English, S.F.: Periurethral collagen injection for male and female sphincteric incontinence: indications, techniques, and result. World J Urol, 15: 306,1997

233. Sanchez-Ortiz, R.F., Broderick, G.A., Chaikin, D.C. et al.: Collagen injection therapy for post-radical retropubic prostatectomy incontinence: role of Valsalva leak point pressure. J Urol, 158: 2132,1997

234. Kremer, C.C. and Freeman, R.M.: Which patients are at risk of voiding difficulty immediately after colposuspension? Int J Gynaecol Obstet, 6: 257,1995

235. Litwiller, S.E., Nelson, R.S., Fone, P.D. et al.: Vaginal wall sling: long-term outcome analysis of factors contributing to patients satisfaction and surgical success. J Urol, 157: 1279,1997

236. Zaragoza, M.R.: Expanded indications for the pubovaginal sling: treatment of type 2 or 3 stress incontinence. J Urol, 156: 1620,1996

237. Darson, M.F., Malizia, A.A. and Barrett, D.M.: Periurethral injection of the genitourinary spheroidal membrane. J Endourol, 10: 283,1996

238. Faerber, G.J.: Endoscopic collagen injection therapy in elderly women with type I stress urinary incontinence. J Urol, 155: 512,1996

239. O'Connell, H.E., McGuire, E.J., Aboseif, S. et al.: Transurethral collagen therapy in women. J Urol, 154: 1463,1995

240. Howard, D., Miller, J.M., Delancey, J.O. et al.: Differential effects of cough, valsalva, and continence status on vesical neck movement. Obstet Gynecol, 95: 535,2000

241. Handa, V.L., Jensen, J.K. and Ostergard, D.R.: The effect of patient position on proximal urethral mobility. Obstet Gynecol, 86: 273,1995

242. Norton, P.A. and Baker, J.E.: Postural changes can reduce leakage in women with stress urinary incontinence. Obstet Gynecol, 84: 770,1994

243. Cruikshank, S.H. and Kovac, S.R.: The functional anatomy of the urethra: role of the pubourethral ligaments. Am J Obstet Gynecol, 176: 1200,1997

244. Dietz, H.P. and Wilson, P.D.: The influence of bladder volume on the position and mobility of the urethrovesical junction. Int Urogynecol J Pelvic Floor Dysfunct, 10: 3,1999

245. Swift, S.E. and Utrie, J.W.: The need for standardization of the valsalva leak-point pressure. Int Urogynecol J Pelvic Floor Dysfunct, 7: 227,1996

246. Cummings, J.M.: Leakpoint pressures in female stress urinary incontinence. Int Urogynecol J Pelvic Floor Dysfunct, 8: 153,1997

247. Bergman, A. and Bhatia, N.N.: Uroflowmetry: spontaneous versus instrumented. Am J Obstet Gynecol, 150: 788,1984

248. Reynard, J.M., Peters, T.J., Lim, C. et al.: The value of multiple free-flow studies in men with lower urinary tract symptoms. Br J Urol, 77: 813,1996

249. Boci, R., Fall, M., Walden, M. et al.: Home uroflowmetry: improved accuracy in outflow assessment. Neurourol Urodyn, 18: 25,1999

250. Sonke, G.S., Kiemeney, L.A., Verbeek, A.L. et al.: Low reproducibility of maximum urinary flow rate determined by portable flowmetry. Neurourol Urodyn, 18: 183,1999

251. Stoller, M.L. and Millard, R.J.: The accuracy of a catheterized residual urine. J Urol, 141: 15,1989

252. Grino, P.B., Bruskewitz, R., Blaivas, J.G. et al.: Maximum urinary flow rate by uroflowmetry: automatic or visual interpretation. J Urol, 149: 339,1993

253. Jorgensen, J.B., Jensen, K.M.E., Klarskov, P. et al.: Intra and inter observer variations in classification of urinary flow curve patterns. Neurourol Urodyn, 9: 353,1990

254. Haylen, B.T., Parys, B.T., Anyaegbunam, W.I. et al.: Urine flow rates in male and female urodynamic patients compared with the Liverpool nomograms. Br J Urol, 65: 483,1990

255. Siroky, M.B., Olsson, C.A. and Krane, R.J.: The flow rate nomogram: I. Development. J Urol, 122: 665,1979

256. Haylen, B.T., Ashby, D., Sutherst, J.R. et al.: Maximum and average urine flow rates in normal male and female populations—the Liverpool nomograms. Br J Urol, 64: 30,1989

257. Cucchi, A.: Acceleration of flow rate as a screening test for detrusor instability in women with stress incontinence. Br J Urol, 65: 17,1990

258. Mattson, S. and Spangberg, A.: Flow rate nomograms in 7- to 16- year- old healty children. Neurourol Urodyn, 13: 267,1994

259. Mattson, S. and Spangberg, A.: Urine flow in healty schoolchildren. Neurourol Urodyn, 13: 281,1994

260. Madersbacher, S., Pycha, A., Schatzl, G. et al.: The aging lower urinary tract: a comparative urodynamic study of men and women. Urology, 51: 206,1998

261. Griffiths, D.J., Harrison, G., Moore, K. et al.: Variability of post-void residual urine volume in the elderly. Urol Res, 24: 23,1996

262. Coates, K.W., Harris, R.L., Cundiff, G.W. et al.: Uroflowmetry in women with urinary incontinence and pelvic organ prolapse. Br J Urol, 80: 217,1997

263. McLennan, M.T., Melick, C.F. and Bent, A.E.: Clinical and urodynamic predictors of delayed voiding after fascia lata suburethral sling. Obstet Gynecol, 92: 608,1998

264. Griffiths, D., Hofner, K., van Mastrigt, R. et al.: Standardization of terminology of lower urinary tract function: pressure-flow studies of voiding, urethral resistance, and urethral obstruction. International Continence Society Subcommittee on Standardization of Terminology of Pressure-Flow Studies. Neurourol Urodyn, 16: 1,1997

265. Schafer, W.: Analysis of bladder-outlet function with the linearized passive urethral resistance relation, linPURR, and a disease-specific approach for grading obstruction: from complex to simple. World J Urol, 13: 47,1995

266. Sidi, A.A., Dykstra, D.D. and Gonzalez, R.: The value of urodynamic testing in the management of neonates with myelodysplasia: a prospective study. J Urol, 135: 90,1986

267. Groutz, A., Blaivas, J.G. and Chaikin, D.C.: Bladder outlet obstruction in women: definition and characteristics. Neurourol Urodyn, 19: 213,2000

268. Lemack, G.E. and Zimmern, P.E.: Pressure flow analysis may aid in identifying women with outflow obstruction. J Urol, 163: 1823,2000

269. Kuo, H.C.: Videourodynamic study for diagnosis of bladder outlet obstruction in women. J Formos Med Assoc, 99: 386,2000

270. Salvatore, S., Khullar, V., Cardozo, L.D. et al.: Urodynamic parameters in obstructed women. Neurourol Urodyn, 19: 480,2000

271. Blaivas, J.G. and Groutz, A.: Bladder outlet obstruction nomogram for women with lower urinary tract symptomatology. Neurourol Urodyn, 19: 553,2000

272. Nitti, V.W., Tu, L.M. and Gitlin, J.: Diagnosing bladder outlet obstruction in women. J Urol, 161: 1535,1999

273. Griffiths, D.J.: Assesment of detrusor contraction strength or contractility. Neurourol Urodyn, 10: 1,1991

274. Karram, M.M., Partoll, L., Bilotta, V. et al.: Factors affecting detrusor contraction strength during voiding in women. Obstet Gynecol, 90: 723,1997

275. Kobak, W.H., Walters, M.D. and Piedmonte, M.R.: Determinants of voiding after three types of incontinence surgery: a multivariable analysis. Obstet Gynecol, 97: 86,2001

276. Carlson, K.V., Fiske, J. and Nitti, V.W.: Value of routine evaluation of the voiding phase when performing urodynamic testing in women with lower urinary tract symptoms. J Urol, 164: 1614,2000

277. Iglesia, C.B., Shott, S., Fenner, D.E. et al.: Effect of preoperative voiding mechanism on success rate of autologous rectus fascia suburethral sling procedure. Obstet Gynecol, 91: 577,1998

278. Diguse, G.S., Khullar, V., Cardozo, L. et al.: Pre- operative pressure- flow studies: Do they predict the outcome of cntinence surgery? Neurourol Urodyn, 19: 402,2000

279. Heit, M., Vogt, V. and Brubaker, L.: An alternative statistical approach for predicting prolonged catheterization after Burch colposuspension during reconstructive pelvic surgery. Int Urogynecol J Pelvic Floor Dysfunct, 8: 203,1997

280. Carr, L.K. and Webster, G.D.: Voiding dysfunction following incontinence surgery: diagnosis and treatment with retropubic or vaginal urethrolysis. J Urol, 157: 821,1997

281. Gormley, E.A., Griffiths, D.J., McCracken, P.N. et al.: Effect of transurethral resection of the prostate on detrusor instability and urge incontinence in elderly males. Neurourol Urodyn, 12: 445,1993

282. Massey, A. and Abrams, P.: Urodynamics of the female lower urinary tract. Urol Clin North Am, 12: 231,1985

283. Dibenedetto, M. and Yalla, S.V.: Electrodiagnosis of striated urethral sphincter dysfunction. J Urol, 122: 361,1979

284. Bump, R.C.: The urodynamic laboratory. Obstet Gynecol Clin North Am, 16: 795,1989

285. Mayo, M.E.: The value of sphincter electromyography in urodynamics. J Urol, 122: 357,1979

286. Koff, S.A. and Kass, E.J.: Abdominal wall electromyography: a noninvasive technique to improve pediatric urodynamic accuracy. J Urol, 127: 736,1982

287. Maizels, M. and Firlit, C.F.: Pediatric urodynamics: a clinical comparison of surface versus needle pelvic floor/external sphincter electromyography. J Urol, 122: 518,1979

288. Barrett, D.M.: Disposable (infant) surface electrocardiogram electrodes in urodynamics: a simultaneous comparative study of electrodes. J Urol, 124: 663,1980

289. Lose, G., Tanko, A., Colstrup, H. et al.: Urethral sphincter electromyography with vaginal surface electrodes: a comparison with sphincter electromyography recorded via periurethral coaxial, anal sphincter needle and perianal surface electrodes. J Urol, 133: 815,1985

290. Barrett, D.M. and Wein, A.J.: Flow evaluation and simultaneous external sphincter electromyography in clinical urodynamics. J Urol, 125: 538,1981

291. O'Donnell, P.D. and Doyle, R.: Biofeedback therapy technique for treatment of urinary incontinence. Urology, 37: 432,1991

292. van Gool, J.D., Vijverberg, M.A., Messer, A.P. et al.: Functional daytime incontinence: non-pharmacological treatment. Scand J Urol Nephrol Suppl, 141: 93,1992

293. McIntosh, L.J., Frahm, J.D., Mallett, V.T. et al.: Pelvic floor rehabilitation in the treatment of incontinence. J Reprod Med, 38: 662,1993

294. Gunnarsson, M. and Mattiasson, A.: Circumvaginal surface electromyography in women with urinary incontinence and in healthy volunteers. Scand J Urol Nephrol Suppl, 157: 89,1994

295. Fried, G.W., Goetz, G., Potts-Nulty, S. et al.: A behavioral approach to the treatment of urinary incontinence in a disabled population. Arch Phys Med Rehabil, 76: 1120,1995

296. Noble, J.G., Dixon, P.J., Rickards, D. et al.: Urethral sphincter volumes in women with obstructed voiding and abnormal sphincter electromyographic activity. Br J Urol, 76: 741,1995

297. Thorp, J.M., Jones, L.H., Wells, E. et al.: Assessment of pelvic floor function: a series of simple tests in nulliparous women. Int Urogynecol J Pelvic Floor Dysfunct, 7: 94,1996

298. Rowan, D., James, E.D., Kramer, A.E. et al.: Urodynamic equipment: technical aspects. Produced by the International Continence Society Working Party on Urodynamic Equipment. J Med Eng Technol, 11: 57,1987

299. Vereecken, R.L. and Grisar, P.: Perineal electromyographic patterns in urge incontinence. Arch Gynecol, 237: 235,1986

300. Siroky, M.B.: Electromyography of the perineal floor. Urol Clin North Am, 23: 299,1996

301. Rossier, A.B., Fam, B.A., Dibenedetto, M. et al.: Urodynamics in spinal shock patients. J Urol, 122: 783,1979

302. Perkash, I.: Urodynamic evaluation: periurethral striated EMG versus perianal striated EMG. Paraplegia, 18: 275,1980

303. Kaneko, S., Watabe, Y., Mizunaga, M. et al.: Automatic analysis of urethral electromyography for accurate diagnosis of voiding dysfunction. Urol Int, 47: 55,1991

304. Jost, W.H., Derouet, H. and Kaiser, T.: [Electromyography of the sphincter vesicae externus muscle. Technique, indications and outcome]. Urologe A, 36: 356,1997

305. McGuire, E.J. and Woodside, J.R.: Diagnostic advantages of fluoroscopic monitoring during urodynamic evaluation. J Urol, 125: 830,1981

306. Abdel-Rahman, M., Coulombe, A., Devroede, G. et al.: Urorectodynamic evaluation of healthy volunteers. Urology, 19: 559,1982

307. Lockhart, J.L., Shessel, F., Weinstein, D. et al.: Urodynamics in women with stress and urge incontinence. Urology, 20: 333,1982

308. Rudy, D.C., Awad, S.A. and Downie, J.W.: External sphincter dyssynergia: an abnormal continence reflex. J Urol, 140: 105,1988

309. Bo, K., Stien, R., Kulseng-Hanssen, S. et al.: Clinical and urodynamic assessment of nulliparous young women with and without stress incontinence symptoms: a case-control study. Obstet Gynecol, 84: 1028,1994

310. Koelbl, H. and Bernaschek, G.: A new method for sonographic urethrocystography and simultaneous pressure-flow measurements. Obstet Gynecol, 74: 417,1989

311. Shabsigh, R., Fishman, I.J. and Krebs, M.: Combined transrectal ultrasonography and urodynamics in the evaluation of detrusor-sphincter dyssynergia. Br J Urol, 62: 326,1988

312. Keane, D.P., Winder, A., Lewis, P. et al.: A combined urodynamic and continence unit—a review of the first 19 years. Br J Urol, 71: 161,1993

313. Rivas, D.A. and Chancellor, M.B.: Neurogenic vesical dysfunction. Urol Clin North Am, 22: 579,1995

314. McGuire, E.J., Cespedes, R.D., Cross, C.A. et al.: Videourodynamic studies. Urol Clin North Am, 23: 309,1996

315. Rickwood, A.M. and Arnold, A.J.: Current management of childhood neuropathic bladder: review of 156 cases. Z Kinderchir, 45: 238,1990

316. Perez, L.M., Khoury, J. and Webster, G.D.: The value of urodynamic studies in infants less than 1 year old with congenital spinal dysraphism. J Urol, 148: 584,1992

317. Ghoniem, G.M., Roach, M.B., Lewis, V.H. et al.: The value of leak pressure and bladder compliance in the urodynamic evaluation of meningomyelocele patients. J Urol, 144: 1440,1990

318. Kaplan, S.A., Chancellor, M.B. and Blaivas, J.G.: Bladder and sphincter behavior in patients with spinal cord lesions. J Urol, 146: 113,1991

319. Kaplan, S.A., Te, A.E. and Blaivas, J.G.: Urodynamic findings in patients with diabetic cystopathy. J Urol, 153: 342,1995

320. Chao, R. and Mayo, M.E.: Long-term urodynamic follow up in pediatric spinal cord injury. Paraplegia, 32: 806,1994

321. Saxton, H.M.: Urodynamics in the investigation of women with frequency, urgency, and incontinence, and voiding difficulties. Urol Radiol, 13: 48,1991

322. Weerasinghe, N. and Malone, P.S.: The value of videourodynamics in the investigation of neurologically normal children who wet. Br J Urol, 71: 539,1993

323. Griffiths, D.J., McCracken, P.N., Harrison, G.M. et al.: Characteristics of urinary incontinence in elderly patients studied by 24-hour monitoring and urodynamic testing. Age Ageing, 21: 195,1992

324. Passerini-Glazel, G., Cisternino, A., Camuffo, M.C. et al.: Video-urodynamic studies of minor voiding dysfunctions in children: an overview of 13 years' experience. Scand J Urol Nephrol Suppl, 141: 70,1992

325. Goluboff, E.T., Chang, D.T., Olsson, C.A. et al.: Urodynamics and the etiology of post-prostatectomy urinary incontinence: the initial Columbia experience. J Urol, 153: 1034,1995

326. Trockman, B.A., Gerspach, J., Dmochowski, R. et al.: Primary bladder neck obstruction: urodynamic findings and treatment results in 36 men. J Urol, 156: 1418,1996

327. Javle, P., Jenkins, S.A., West, C. et al.: Quantification of voiding dysfunction in patients awaiting transurethral prostatectomy. J Urol, 156: 1014,1996

328. Porter, T., Weerasinghe, N. and Malone, P.S.: Modification of therapy based on videourodynamics in neurologically normal children: Southampton 1988-1993. Br J Urol, 76: 779,1995

329. Glazier, D.B., Murphy, D.P., Fleisher, M.H. et al.: Evaluation of the utility of video-urodynamics in children with urinary tract infection and voiding dysfunction. Br J Urol, 80: 806,1997

330. Ilker, Y., Tarcan, T., Yucel, S. et al.: Re- techered cord syndorome in myelodysplasia and the importance of urological early follow- up in the early diagnosis. Neurourol Urodyn, 19: 517,2000

331. Lackner, J., Kiss, G. and Madersbacher, H.: Can early urological management improve the outcome (upper urinary tract, continence) in patients with myelomeningoceles? -Long term results. Neurourol Urodyn, 19: 532,2000

332. van Waalwijk van Doorn, E.S. and Gommer, E.D.: Ambulatory urodynamics. Curr Opin Obstet Gynecol, 7: 378,1995

333. Heslington, K. and Hilton, P.: Ambulatory urodynamic monitoring. Br J Obstet Gynaecol, 103: 393,1996

334. Bristow, S.E. and Neal, D.E.: Ambulatory urodynamics. Br J Urol, 77: 333,1996

335. Kulseng-Hanssen, S. and Klevmark, B.: Ambulatory urodynamic monitoring of women. Scand J Urol Nephrol Suppl, 179: 27,1996

336. Anders, K., Khullar, V., Cardozo, S. et al.: Ambulatory urodynamic monitoring in clinical urogynaecological practice. Neurourol Urodyn, 16: 510,1997

337. Rosario, D.J., Potts, K.L., Woo, H.H. et al.: Ambulatory pressure-flow studies in young asymptomatic males. Neurourol Urodyn, 15: 278,1996

338. James, E.D., Flack, F.C., Caldwell, K.P. et al.: Continuous measurement of urine loss and frequency in incontinent patients. Preliminary report. Br J Urol, 43: 233,1971

339. Webb, R.J., Ramsden, P.D. and Neal, D.E.: Ambulatory monitoring and electronic measurement of urinary leakage in the diagnosis of detrusor instability and incontinence. Br J Urol, 68: 148,1991

340. Wijkstra, H., van Kerrebroek, E.V.A., Koldewijn, E. et al.: The use of heat sensors in detecting urine leakage during long term urudynamic. Neurourol Urodyn, 10: 422,1991

341. Eckford, S.D., Finney, R., Jackson, S.R. et al.: Detection of urinary incontinence during ambulatory monitoring of bladder function by a temperature-sensitive device. Br J Urol, 77: 194,1996

342. van Waalwijk van Doorn, E.S. and Zwiers, W.: Ambulant monitoring to assess the efficacy of oxybutynin chloride in patients with mixed incontinence. Eur Urol, 18: 49,1990

343. Kulseng-Hanssen, S., Kristofferson, M. and Larsen, E.: Physioogical bladder filling with 2 and 4 hours recording versus 45 minutes recording with 300 ml. saline bladder? prefilling using ambulatory urodynamic equipment. Neurourol Urodyn, 14: 151,1995

344. van Waalwijk van Doorn, E.S., Ambergen, A.W. and Janknegt, R.A.: Detrusor activity index: quantification of detrusor overactivity by ambulatory monitoring. J Urol, 157: 596,1997

345. van Waalwijk van Doorn, E.S., Remmers, A. and Janknegt, R.A.: Conventional and extramural ambulatory urodynamic testing of the lower urinary tract in female volunteers. J Urol, 147: 1319,1992

346. Robertson, A.S., Griffiths, C.J., Ramsden, P.D. et al.: Bladder function in healthy volunteers: ambulatory monitoring and conventional urodynamic studies. Br J Urol, 73: 242,1994

347. Heslington, K. and Hilton, P.: A comparison of ambulatory monitoring and conventional cystometry in asymptomatic female volunteers. Neurourol Urodyn, 14: 534,1995

348. Kulseng-Hanssen, S. and Klevmark, B.: Ambulatory urethro-cysto- rectometry: A new technique. Neurourol Urodyn, 7: 119,1988

349. Styles, R.A., Neal, D.E. and Ramsden, P.D.: Comparison of long-term monitoring and standard cystometry in chronic retention of urine. Br J Urol, 58: 652,1986

350. Webb, R.J., Styles, R.A., Griffiths, C.J. et al.: Ambulatory monitoring of bladder pressures in patients with low compliance as a result of neurogenic bladder dysfunction. Br J Urol, 64: 150,1989

351. van Waalwijk van Doorn, E.S., Remmers, A. and Janknegt, R.A.: Extramural ambulatory urodynamic monitoring during natural filling and normal daily activities: evaluation of 100 patients. J Urol, 146: 124,1991

352. McInerney, P.D., Vanner, T.F., Harris, S.A. et al.: Ambulatory urodynamics. Br J Urol, 67: 272,1991

353. Heslington, K. and Hilton, P.: The incidence of detrusor instability by ambulatory monitoring and conventional cystometry pre and post colposuspension. Neurourol Urodyn, 14: 416,1995

354. Young, C.K., Godley, M.L., Duffy, P.G. et al.: Natural filling cystometry in infants and children. Br J Urol, 67: 531,1995

355. Brown, K. and Hilton, P.: The incidence of detrusor instability before and after colposuspension: a study using conventional and ambulatory urodynamic monitoring. BJU Int, 84: 961,1999

356. Groen, J., van Mastrigt, R. and Bosch, R.: Factors causing differences in voiding parameters between conventional and ambulatory urodynamics. Urol Res, 28: 128,2000

357. Webb, R.J., Griffiths, C.J., Ramsden, P.D. et al.: Measurement of voiding pressures on ambulatory monitoring: comparison with conventional cystometry. Br J Urol, 65: 152,1990

358. Webb, R.J., Griffiths, C.J., Zachariah, K.K. et al.: Filling and voiding pressures measured by ambulatory monitoring and conventional studies during natural and artificial bladder filling. J Urol, 146: 815,1991

359. McInerney, P.D., Harris, S.A., Pritchard, A. et al.: Night studies for primary diurnal and nocturnal enuresis and preliminary results of the "clam" ileocystoplasty. Br J Urol, 67: 42,1991

360. Rosario, D.J., Leaker, B.R., Smith, D.J. et al.: A pilot study of the effects of multiple doses of the M3 muscarinic receptor antagonist darifenacin on ambulatory parameters of detrusor activity in patients with detrusor instability. Neurourol Urodyn, 14: 464,1995

361. Hasan, S.T., Robson, W.A., Pridie, A.K. et al.: Outcome of transcutaneous electrical stimulation in patients with detrusor instability. Neurourol Urodyn, 13: 349,1994

362. van Waalwijk van Doorn, E., Anders, K., Khullar, V. et al.: Standardisation of ambulatory urodynamic monitoring: Report of the Standardisation Sub-Committee of the International Continence Society for Ambulatory Urodynamic Studies. Neurourol Urodyn, 19: 113,2000

363. Lose, G.: Urethral pressure measurement. Acta Obstet Gynecol Scand Suppl, 166: 39,1997

364. Blaivas, J.G. and Olsson, C.A.: Stress incontinence: classification and surgical approach. J Urol, 139: 727,1988

365. Kayigil, O., Iftekhar Ahmed, S. and Metin, A.: The coexistence of intrinsic sphincter deficiency with type II stress incontinence. J Urol, 162: 1365,1999

366. Leach, G.E., Dmochowski, R.R., Appell, R.A. et al.: Female Stress Urinary Incontinence Clinical Guidelines Panel summary report on surgical management of female stress urinary incontinence. The American Urological Association. J Urol, 158: 875,1997

367. Herschorn, S., Steele, D.J. and Radomski, S.B.: Followup of intraurethral collagen for female stress urinary incontinence. J Urol, 156: 1305,1996

368. Winters, J.C., Chiverton, A., Scarpero, H.M. et al.: Collagen injection therapy in elderly women: long-term results and patient satisfaction. Urology, 55: 856,2000

369. Vereecken, R.L.: A critical view on the value of urodynamics in non-neurogenic incontinence in women. Int J Gynaecol Obstet, 11: 188,2000

370. Ramsay, I.N., Ali, H.M., Hunter, M. et al.: A randomized controlled trial of urodynamic investigations prior to consevative treatment of urinary incontinence in the female. Int J Gynaecol Obstet, 6: 277,1995

371. Holtedahl, K., Verelst, M., Schiefloe, A. et al.: Usefulness of urodynamic examination in female urinary incontinence— lessons from a population-based, randomized, controlled study of conservative treatment. Scand J Urol Nephrol, 34: 169,2000

372. Haab, F., Ciofu, C., Pedron, P. et al.: [Feasibility of "Valsalva Leak Point Pressure". Prospective study]. Prog Urol, 7: 611,1997

373. Cucchi, A.: A possible condition of pre-instability in prostatic obstruction. J Urol, 153: 681,1995

374. de la Rosette, J.J., Witjes, W.P., Schafer, W. et al.: Relationships between lower urinary tract symptoms and bladder outlet obstruction: results from the ICS-"BPH" study. Neurourol Urodyn, 17: 99,1998

375. Staskin, D.S., Vardi, Y. and Siroky, M.B.: Post-prostatectomy continence in the parkinsonian patient: the significance of poor voluntary sphincter control. J Urol, 140: 117,1988

376. Chandiramani, V.A., Palace, J. and Fowler, C.J.: How to recognize patients with parkinsonism who should not have urological surgery. Br J Urol, 80: 100,1997

377. Mark, S., Perez, L.M. and Webster, G.D.: Synchronous management of anastomotic contracture and stress urinary incontinence following radical prostatectomy. J Urol, 151: 1202,1994

378. Ojdeby, G., Claezon, A., Brekkan, E. et al.: Urinary incontinence and sexual impotence after radical prostatectomy. Scand J Urol Nephrol, 30: 473,1996

379. Leach, G.E., Trockman, B., Wong, A. et al.: Post-prostatectomy incontinence: urodynamic findings and treatment outcomes. J Urol, 155: 1256,1996

380. Chao, R. and Mayo, M.E.: Incontinence after radical prostatectomy: detrusor or sphincter causes. J Urol, 154: 16,1995

381. Batista, J.E., Wagner, J.R., Azadzoi, K.M. et al.: Direct measurement of blood flow in the human bladder. J Urol, 155: 630,1996

382. Park, J.M. and Montie, J.E.: Mechanisms of incontinence and retention after orthotopic neobladder diversion. Urology, 51: 601,1998

383. Shimogaki, H., Okada, H., Fujisawa, M. et al.: Long-term experience with orthotopic reconstruction of the lower urinary tract in women. J Urol, 161: 573,1999

384. Woodside, J.R.: Postoperative male incontinence. In: Clinical neurourology, Edited by R.J. Krane and M.B. Siroky. Boston: Little, Brown and Co., pp. 483-491, 1991

385. McGuire, E.J. and Savastano, J.A.: Urodynamic studies in enuresis and the nonneurogenic neurogenic bladder. J Urol, 132: 299,1984

386. Torrens, M.J. and Collins, C.D.: The urodynamic assessment of adult enuresis. Br J Urol, 47: 433,1975

387. Byrne, D.J., Stewart, P.A. and Gray, B.K.: The role of urodynamics in female urinary stress incontinence. Br J Urol, 59: 228,1987

388. Farrar, D.J., Whiteside, C.G., Osborne, J.L. et al.: A urosynamic analysis of micturition symptoms in the female. Surg Gynecol Obstet, 141: 875,1975

389. Haylen, B.T., Sutherst, J.R. and Frazer, M.I.: Is the investigation of most stress incontinence really necessary? Br J Urol, 64: 147,1989

390. Hilton, P.: Surgery for genuine stress incontinence: which operation and forwhich patient? In: Micturition, Edited by J. Drife, P. Hilton and S. Stanton. London: Springer-Verlag, pp. 225, 1990

391. Jarvis, G.J.: Female urinary incontinence-which patient?-which tests? In: Urogynaecology: the invetigation and management of urinary incontinence in women, Edited by A.R.B. Smith. London: RCOG, pp. 32, 1995

392. Stanton, S.L., Ozsoy, C. and Hilton, P.: Voiding difficulties in the female: prevalence, clinical and urodynamic review. Obstet Gynecol, 61: 144,1983

393. Laor, D. and Hilton, P.: Voiding symptoms in the female: the correlation with urodynamic voiding characteristics. Neurourol Urodyn, 4: 308,1989

394. Petrou, S.P., Brown, J.A. and Blaivas, J.G.: Suprameatal transvaginal urethrolysis. J Urol, 161: 1268,1999

395. Stohrer, M.: Alterations in the lower urinary tract after spinal cord injury- diagnosis, prevention and therapy of late seqelae. World J Urol, 7: 205,1990

396. Stohrer, M., Krammer, G., Lochner-Ernst, D. et al.: Diagnosis and treatment of bladder dysfunction in spinal cord injur patients. In: Europeal Urology Update Series.1994

397. Rossier, A.B. and Fam, B.A.: 5-microtransducer catheter in evaluation of neurogenic bladder function. Urology, 27: 371,1986

398. Geirsson, G., Lindstrom, S. and Fall, M.: The bladder cooling reflex in man—characteristics and sensitivity to temperature. Br J Urol, 71: 675,1993

399. Nitti, V.W.: Ice-water test in urodynamic assessment. Lancet, 342: 1066,1993

400. Geirsson, G., Lindstrom, S. and Fall, M.: Pressure, volume and infusion speed criteria for the ice-water test. Br J Urol, 73: 498,1994

401. Geirsson, G., Lindstrom, S., Fall, M. et al.: Positive bladder cooling test in neurologically normal young children. J Urol, 151: 446,1994

402. Bors, E. and Comarr, A.E.: Neurological urology. Basel: Kager.1971

403. Bomalaski, M.D., Teague, J.L. and Brooks, B.: The long-term impact of urological management on the quality of life of children with spina bifida. J Urol, 154: 778,1995

404. Cardenas, D.D., Mayo, M.E. and Turner, L.R.: Lower urinary changes over time in suprasacral spinal cord injury. Paraplegia, 33: 326,1995

405. Bauer, S.B., Hallett, M., Khoshbin, S. et al.: The predictive value of urodynamic evaluation in the newborn with myelodysplasia. JAMA, 152: 650,1984

406. Geraniotis, E., Koff, S.A. and Enrile, B.: The prophylactic use of clean intermittent catheterization in the treatment of infants and young children with myelomeningocele and neurogenic bladder dysfunction. J Urol, 139: 85,1988

407. Teichman, J.M., Scherz, H.C., Kim, K.D. et al.: An alternative approach to myelodysplasia management: aggressive observation and prompt intervention. J Urol, 152: 807,1994

408. Bauer, S.B.: The management of spina bifida from birth onwards. In: Pediatric urology, Edited by R.H. Whitaker and J.R. Woodard. London: Butterworths, pp. 87, 1985

409. Spindel, M.R., Bauer, S.B., Dyro, F.M. et al.: The changing neurourologic lesion in myelodysplasia. Jama, 258: 1630,1987

410. Lais, A., Kasabian, N.G., Dyro, F.M. et al.: The neurosurgical implications of continuous neurourological surveillance of children with myelodysplasia. J Urol, 150: 1879,1993

411. Keating, M.A., Rink, R.C., Bauer, S.B. et al.: Neurourological implications of the changing approach in management of occult spinal lesions. J Urol, 140: 1299,1988

412. Satar, N., Bauer, S.B., Shefner, J. et al.: The effects of delayed diagnosis and treatment in patients with an occult spinal dysraphism. J Urol, 154: 754,1995

413. Yip, C.M., Leach, G.E., Rosenfeld, D.S. et al.: Delayed diagnosis of voiding dysfunction: Occult spinal dysraphism. J Urol, 124: 694,1985

414. Satar, N., Bauer, S.B., Scott, R.M. et al.: Late effects of early surgery on lipoma and lipomeningocele in children less than 1 year old. J Urol, 157: 1434,1997

415. Kondo, A., Kato, K., Kanai, S. et al.: Bladder dysfunction secondary to tethered cord syndrome in adults: is it curable? J Urol, 135: 313,1986

416. Fone, P.D., Vapnek, J.M., Litwiller, S.E. et al.: Urodynamic fin-

dings in the tethered spinal cord syndrome: does surgical release improve bladder function? J Urol, 157: 604,1997

417. Koyanagi, I., Iwasaki, Y., Hida, K. et al.: Surgical treatment supposed natural history of the tethered cord with occult spinal dysraphism. Childs Nerv Syst, 13: 268,1997

418. Pierre-Kahn, A., Zerah, M., Renier, D. et al.: Congenital lumbosacral lipomas. Childs Nerv Syst, 13: 298,1997

419. Guzman, L., Bauer, S.B., Hallett, M. et al.: Evaluation and management of children with sacral agenesis. Urology, 22: 506,1983

420. Boemers, T.M., van Gool, J.D., De Jong, T.P.V.M. et al.: Urodynamic evaluation of children with caudal regression syndrome (caudal dysplasia sequence). J Urol, 152: 1038,1994

421. Koff, S.A. and Deridder, P.A.: Patterns of neurogenic bladder dysfunction in sacral agenesis. J Urol, 118: 87,1977

422. Jakobson, H., Holm-Bentzen, M. and Hald, T.: The evaluation and management of children with sacral agenesis and dysgenesis. Neurourol Urodyn, 4: 99,1985

423. Cass, A.S., Luxenberg, M., Johnson, C.F. et al.: Management of the neurogenic bladder in 413 children. J Urol, 132: 521,1984

424. Decter, R.M., Bauer, S.B., Khoshbin, S. et al.: Urodynamic assessment of children with cerebral palsy. J Urol, 138: 1110,1987

425. Iwatsubo, E., Iwakawa, A., Koga, H. et al.: Functional recovery of the bladder in patients with spinal cord injury— prognosticating programs of an aseptic intermittent catheterization. Hinyokika Kiyo, 31: 775,1985

426. Fanciullacci, F., Zanollo, A., Sandri, S. et al.: The neuropathic bladder in children with spinal cord injury. Paraplegia, 26: 83,1988

427. Kim, Y.H., Kattan, M.W. and Boone, T.B.: Bladder leak point pressure: the measure for sphincterotomy success in spinal cord injured patients with external detrusor-sphincter dyssynergia. J Urol, 159: 493,1998

428. Steinbok, P.: Regional cerebral blood flow in pediatric moyamoya disease: age- dependent decline in specific regions. Childs Nerv Syst, 14: 688.,1998

429. Mayo, M.E.: Lower urinary tract dysfunction in cerebral palsy. J Urol, 147: 419,1992

430. Reid, C.J. and Borzyskowski, M.: Lower urinary tract dysfunction in cerebral palsy. Arch Dis Child, 68: 739,1993

431. Pena, A.: Posterior sagittal approach for the correction of anorectal malformations. Adv Surg, 19: 69,1986

432. Barnes, P.D., Lester, P.D., Yamanashi, W.S. et al.: MRI in infants and children with spinal dysraphism. AJR Am J Roentgenol, 147: 339,1986

433. Greenfield, S.P. and Fera, M.: Urodynamic evaluation of the patient with an imperforate anus: a prospective study. J Urol, 146: 539,1991

434. Kakizaki, H., Nomomura, K., Asano, Y. et al.: Preexisting neuroginic voiding dysfunction in children with imperforate anus: Problems in management. J Urol, 152: 1041,1994

435. Barry, J.E. and Auldist, A.W.: The Vater association; one end of a spectrum of anomalies. Am J Dis Child, 128: 769,1974

436. Carson, J.A., Barnes, P.D., Tunell, W.P. et al.: Imperforate anus: the neurologic implication of sacral abnormalities. J Pediatr Surg, 19: 838,1984

437. Bauer, S.B., Dieppa, R.A., Labib, K.K. et al.: The bladder in boys with posterior urethral valves: a urodynamic assessment. J Urol, 121: 769,1979

438. Mitchell, M.E.: Persistent ureteral dilation following valve resection. Dial Pediatr Urol, 5: 8,1982

439. Holmdahl, G., Sillen, U., Bachelard, M. et al.: The changing urodynamic pattern in valve bladders during infancy. J Urol, 153: 463,1995

440. Holmdahl, G., Sillen, U., Hanson, E. et al.: Bladder dysfunction in boys with posterior urethral valves before and after puberty. J Urol, 155: 694,1996

441. Peters, C.A. and Bauer, S.B.: Evaluation and management of urinary incontinence after surgery for posterior urethral valves. Urol Clin North Am, 17: 379,1990

442. Hollowell, J.G., Hill, P.D., Duffy, P.G. et al.: Bladder function and dysfunction in exstrophy and epispadias. Lancet, 338: 926,1991

443. Diamond, D.A., Bauer, S.B., Dinlenc, C. et al.: Normal urodynamics in patients with bladder exstrophy: are they achievable? J Urol, 162: 841,1999

444. Mackeith, R.L., Meadow, S.R. and Turner, R.K.: How children become dry. In: Bladder control and enuresis, Edited by I. Kolvin, R.L. MacKeith and S.R. Meadow. Philadelphia: Lippincott, pp. 3, 1973

445. Yeats, W.K.: Bladder function in normal micturition. In: Bladder control and enuresis, Edited by I. Kolvin, R.L. MacKeith and S.R. Meadow. Philadelphia: Lippincott, pp. 28, 1973

446. Bellman, N.: Encopresis. Acta Paediatr Scand, 70: 1,1966

447. Fergusson, D.M., Horwood, L.J. and Shannon, F.T.: Factors related to the age of attainment of nocturnal bladder control: an 8-year longitudinal study. Pediatrics, 78: 884,1986

448. Mueller, S.R.: Development of urinary control in children. JAMA, 172: 1256,1987

449. Lebowitz, R.L. and Mandell, J.: Urinary tract infection in children: putting radiology in its place. Radiology, 165: 1,1987

450. O'regan, S., Yazbeck, S. and Schick, E.: Constipation, unstable bladder, urinary tract infection sydrome. Clin Nephrol, 5: 154,1985

451. Koff, S.A., Wagner, T.T. and Jayanthi, V.R.: The relationship among dysfunctional elimination syndromes, primary vesicoureteral reflux and urinary tract infections in children. J Urol, 160: 1019,1998

452. Hansson, S., Hjalmas, K., Jodal, U. et al.: Lower urinary tract dysfunction in girls with untreated asymptomatic or covert bacteriuria. J Urol, 143: 333,1990

453. McKenna, P.H., Herndon, C.D., Connery, S. et al.: Pelvic floor muscle retraining for pediatric voiding dysfunction using interactive computer games. J Urol, 162: 1056,1999

454. Webster, G.D., Koefoot, R.B., Jr. and Sihelnik, S.: Urodynamic abnormalities in neurologically normal children with micturition dysfunction. J Urol, 132: 74,1984

455. Sillen, U., Hjalmas, K., Aili, M. et al.: Pronounced detrusor hypercontractility in infants with gross bilateral reflux. J Urol, 148: 598,1992

456. Sillen, U., Bachelard, M., Hermanson, G. et al.: Gross bilateral reflux in infants: gradual decrease of initial detrusor hypercontractility. J Urol, 155: 668,1996

457. Yeung, C.K., Godley, M.L., Dhillon, H.K. et al.: The characteristics of primary vesico-ureteric reflux in male and female infants with pre-natal hydronephrosis. Br J Urol, 80: 319,1997

458. Chandra, M., Maddix, H. and McVicar, M.: Transient urodynamic dysfunction of infancy: relationship to urinary tract infections and vesicoureteral reflux. J Urol, 155: 673,1996

459. Bauer, S.B., Retik, A.B., Colodny, A.H. et al.: The unstable bladder in childhood. Urol Clin North Am, 7: 321,1980

460. Van Gool, J. and Tanagho, E.A.: External sphincter activity and recurrent urinary tract infection in girls. Urology, 10: 348,1977

461. Diokno, A.C., Wells, T.J. and Brink, C.A.: Urinary incontinence in elderly women: urodynamic evaluation. J Am Geriatr Soc, 35: 940,1987

462. Ouslander, J., Staskin, D., Raz, S. et al.: Clinical versus urodynamic diagnosis in an incontinent geriatric female population. J Urol, 137: 68,1987

463. Kirschner-Hermanns, R., Scherr, P.A., Branch, L.G. et al.: Accuracy of survey questions for geriatric urinary incontinence. J Urol, 159: 1903,1998

464. Jones, K.W. and Schoenberg, H.W.: Comparison of the incidence of bladder hyperreflexia in patients with benign prostatic hypertrophy and age-matched female controls. J Urol, 133: 425,1985

465. Resnick, N.M., Yalla, S.V. and Laurino, E.: The pathophysiology of urinary incontinence among institutionalized elderly persons. N Engl J Med, 320: 1,1989

466. Homma, Y., Imajo, C., Takahashi, S. et al.: Urinary symptoms and urodynamics in a normal elderly population. Scand J Urol Nephrol Suppl, 157: 27,1994

467. Diokno, A.C., Brown, M.B., Brock, B.M. et al.: Clinical and cystometric characteristics of continent and incontinent noninstitutionalized elderly. J Urol, 140: 567,1988

468. Resnick, N.M., Elbadawi, A. and Yalla, S.V.: Ageing and the lower urinary tract: What is normal. Neurourol Urodyn, 14: 577,1995

469. Morris, J.N., Hawes, C., Fries, B.E. et al.: Designing the national resident assessment instrument for nursing homes. Gerontologist, 30: 293,1990

470. Resnick, N.M., Brandeis, G.H., Baumann, M.M. et al.: Evaluating a national assessment strategy for urinary incontinence in nursing home residents: reliability of the minimum data set and validity of the resident assessment protocol. Neurourol Urodyn, 15: 583,1996

471. Sand, P.K., Brubaker, L.T. and Novak, T.: Simple standing incremental cystometry as a screening method for detrusor instability. Obstet Gynecol, 77: 453,1991

472. Dennis, P.J., Rohner, T.J., Jr., Hu, T.W. et al.: Simple urodynamic evaluation of incontinent elderly female nursing home patients. A descriptive analysis. Urology, 37: 173,1991

473. Resnick, N.M. and Yalla, S.V.: Detrusor hyperactivity with impaired contractile function. An unrecognized but common cause of incontinence in elderly patients. Jama, 257: 3076,1987

Committee 8 A

Physical Examination

Chairman

B.L. Shull (USA)

Members

G. Hurt (USA),

J. Laycock (UK),

H. Palmtag (Germany),

Y. Yong (China),

R. Zubieta (Chile)

CONTENTS

Physical Examination

B.L. SHULL

G. HURT, J. LAYCOCK, H. PALMTAG, Y. YONG, R. ZUBIETA

I. INTRODUCTION

Urinary incontinence (UI) may be a social concern for individuals of all ages and both sexes. This chapter addresses primarily the role of physical examination in adult women who present with complaints of urinary incontinence. During the initial encounter the patient's history, urinary symptoms, urinalysis, and physical examination are all considered before initiating further evaluation or instituting therapy. In addition to urinary complaints, women may have symptoms relating to bowel function, sexual function, and pelvic organ prolapse (POP). Jackson et.al. evaluated 247 women with either UI or POP. Thirty one percent of women with UI and 7% with POP had concurrent anal incontinence (AI) [1]. In a report from Sweden, 62% of 21 consecutive women undergoing a Burch colposuspension for genuine stress urinary incontinence had concurrent fecal incontinence [2]. In a Norwegian study of women presenting with a complaint of urinary incontinence (UI), 38% of the women were found to have significant prolapse and 19% reported fecal incontinence [3]. All these aspects of the pelvic floor and pelvic floor function must be included to plan a comprehensive treatment strategy.

Presently there are few scientific data documenting the parameters of a normal pelvic examination in women of various ages and with various obstetrical histories. The components of the examination have not been universally agreed upon. It seems intuitive the examination should include an assessment of the bony architecture, pelvic floor muscle tone and muscle mass, connective tissue support, the epithelial lining of the vagina, the size, location, and mobility of the uterus, the adnexal structures, and innervation of the pelvic floor structures.

Since the first edition of this book, Samuelsson and colleagues studied the prevalence of genital prolapse and possible related factors in a general population of Swedish women ages 20-59 [4]. The prevalence of prolapse was 31%; however, only 2% of all women had a prolapse that reached the introitus. Increasing age, decreasing muscle strength, and parity were all associated with the presence of prolapse. The anterior compartment was the most frequently affected vaginal segment. DeLancey and Hurd reported that when matched for age and parity women with pelvic organ prolapse have a larger genital hiatus than women with no prolapse [5]. In addition, they found women with recurrent prolapse after pelvic surgery have a larger genital hiatus than women cured by surgery. Howard and associates tested vesical neck descent in 3 groups of women during a cough and during Valsalva's maneuver [6]. They found incontinent women have similar vesical neck mobility with both maneuvers. Continent women have less vesical neck descent with a cough than with Valsalva's maneuver.

There are few data linking bladder, bowel, or sexual function to variations in the examination of women seeking routine gynecologic care. Data on women with complaints of urinary incontinence do not include detailed, specific information about their pelvic examinations. No data exists documenting outcomes of surgical management with specific observations on preoperative physical findings such as support of the urethra and bladder, muscle function, and quantified effects of estrogen hormone on the genitourinary epithelium.

Recognizing these shortcomings in our knowledge of what is normal and how findings change with age, we presume that function and physical examination findings are related in certain individuals. For example, women with genuine stress urinary incontinence and poor support of the urethrovesical junction may respond to surgical therapy which corrects the poor support and consequently improves the function of the urethra and urethrovesical junction. On the other hand, women with genuine stress incontinence and normal support of the urethra may not respond as well to the same surgical procedure and may require a different surgical intervention [7]. In some situations, women are cured of their stress urinary incontinence, but acquire significant pelvic support defects such as enterocele, cystocele, or vaginal vault prolapse subsequent to their surgery for stress urinary incontinence [1, 8-13]. Not only do women develop postoperative support defects, they may also acquire functional complaints with urgency and emptying phase abnormalities (Table 1 [10-14] and Table 2 [9]).

Weber and associates evaluated sexual function and vaginal anatomy in 165 women before and after surgery for pelvic organ prolapse and urinary incontinence [15]. Forty-one percent were not sexually active before or after because they had no partner, had medical illnesses, or for various other reasons. In those who were sexually active, they found no clinically significant change in vaginal dimensions. Furthermore, sexual function and satisfaction improved or did not change in most women postoperatively. The exception was dyspareunia in 38% of women who had a combination of a Burch retropubic repair and a posterior colporrhaphy. But, we recognize that posterior colporrhaphy itself has a high degree of patient dissatisfaction and this is the reason for the current interest in the defect specific posterior repair [16].

It seems self evident that, women who meet the criteria for surgical therapy for genuine stress urinary incontinence should be evaluated for co-existing pelvic organ prolapse and defecatory dysfunction. They may require attention to all anatomic and function abnormalities in order to be treated in a comprehensive manner.

Table 1 : Functional and Anatomic Outcomes of Colposuspension and Paravaginal Repair

Author	**No.Patients**	**years follow up**	**% cure S.U.I**	**% new or persistent cystoceles**	**% other pelvic support defects**	**% *de novo* D.I.**
Stanton SL Cardozo LD [14]	88	1	87 obj.	11	—	6
Alcalay M Stanton SL Monga A[11]	109 of possible 366	10-20	69 obj.	7.4	27%	15
*Galloway NTM [10]	50	>3	84 obj.	—	8%	14%
**Colombo Maggioni Caruso [13]	284	>3	86 obj.	—	Approx. 30%	—
Shull BL Baden WF [12]	149	>1.5	97 subj.	5.4	10%	4%

** 44% cured with no complications ** 54% cured with no complications*

Table 2 : Anatomic Support Defects Following Colposuspension

	%Cystocele		**%Rectocele**		**%Enterocele**		**%Uterine Prolapse**	
	Preop	**Postop**	**Preop**	**Postop**	**Preop**	**Postop**	**Preop**	**Postop**
Group 1								
Mild	50	37	52	54	17	21	23	27
Marked	22	2	14	12	—	5	1	5
Group 2								
Mild	52	29	46	40	1	2	36	15
Marked	43	3	17	29	—	20	—	47

Group 1 - 96 patients who did not require additional surgery for genital prolapse after colposuspension.
Group 2 - 35 patients who did require further surgery for genital prolapse following colposuspension. [9]

Kjølhede and associates performed a prospective observational study of 21 women who underwent a retropubic colposuspension for genuine stress urinary incontinence [17]. No concomitant prolapse repair was performed. In a median time of 2 years following the colposuspension, 29% of the women had undergone subsequent surgery for pelvic organ prolapse. They concluded the colposuspension seemed to accelerate the deterioration of associated pelvic floor support defects.

Historically, one of the major deterrents to the scientific study of pelvic organ prolapse has been the lack of an accepted, objective, and validated system for describing the spectrum of pelvic support in individual patients and in study populations. In recognition of this problem, the International Continence Society (ICS) established an international, multi-disciplinary terminology standardization committee for prolapse in 1993. The committee devised a site-specific quantitative description of support that locates 6 defined points around the vagina (2 anterior, 2 posterior, and 2 apical) with respect to their relationship to the hymen (Figure 1).

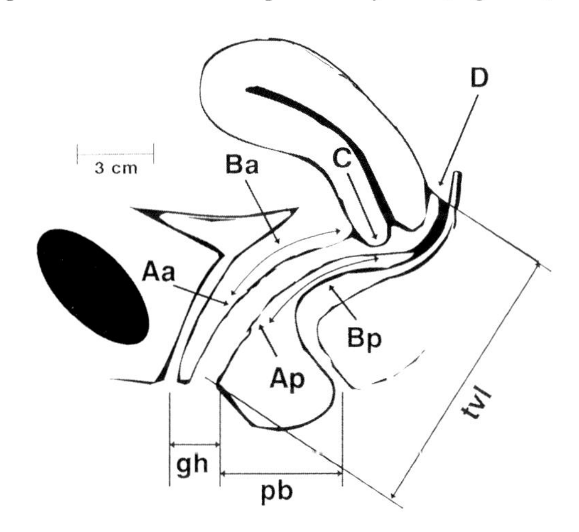

Figure 1 : Six sites (points Aa, Ba, C, D, Bp, and Ap), genital hiatus (gh), perineal body (pb), and total vaginal length (tvl)used for pelvic organ support quantitation.

Once measurements are obtained, subjects are assigned to one of five ordinal stages as follows:

Stage 0 - no prolapse is demonstrated, i.e., all points are at their highest possible level above the hymen;

Stage I - the criteria for Stage 0 are not met but the most distal portion of the prolapse is more than 1 cm above the level of the hymen;

Stage II - the most distal portion of the prolapse is 1 cm or less proximal to or distal to the plane of the hymen;

Stage III - the most distal portion of the prolapse is more than 1 cm below the plane of the hymen but protrudes no further than two centimeters less than the total vaginal length in cm; and

Stage IV - essentially complete eversion of the total length of the lower genital tract is demonstrated. In addition, the system calls for three other measurements: the anterior-posterior length of the genital hiatus and the perineal body and the total vaginal length (Figure 2).

Prior to its acceptance, reproducibility studies in six centers in the United States and Europe were completed, documenting the inter- and intra-rater reliability and clinical utility of the system in 240 women [18-22].

More recently, several authors have compared the severity of pelvic organ prolapse between examinations performed in the lithotomy position and other positions. Swift and Herring directly compared pelvic organ prolapse quantification (POPQ) measurements in the same patients examined in the dorsal lithotomy position with measurements made while the patients were in the upright position. They found a high degree of correlation between values obtained in the two positions and no significant differences in the stage of prolapse [23]. Barber and associates examined one hundred eighty-nine consecutive women in the dorsal lithotomy position and also in a birthing chair at a 45° angle in relation to the horizontal [24]. The degree of pelvic organ prolapse was assessed using the POPQ. Twenty six percent of women had a higher stage of pelvic organ prolapse when examined at a 45° angle in the birthing chair and only 4% a lower stage. There was a statistically significant increase in the degree of prolapse at all POPQ measurements except for measurement of total vaginal length. They concluded that overall a higher degree of prolapse was found in women examined at a 45° angle in the birthing chair. They also speculated that the 45° position predisposes to the greater degree of prolapse than does the standing position because sitting in the birthing chair opens the pelvic outlet and maximizes the effects of pushing. Consequently, when you can not reproduce the woman's complaints of pelvic organ prolapse when she is in the dorsal lithotomy position, consider examining her while she sits at a 45° angle.

The standardization document was formally adopted by the ICS in 1995 and by the American Urogynecologic Society and the Society of Gynecologic Surgeons in 1996. It was published in 1996[25] and is reproduced in its entirety in **Appendix I.** A 17 minute public domain video demonstrating the POPQ exam is available through the American Urogynecologic Society (www.augs.org: 2025 M Street NW, Suite 800, Washington, DC 20036-3309; phone 202-367-1167; fax 202-367-2167).

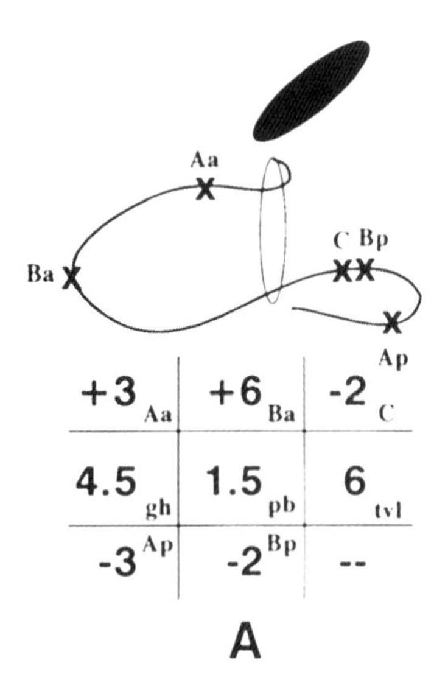

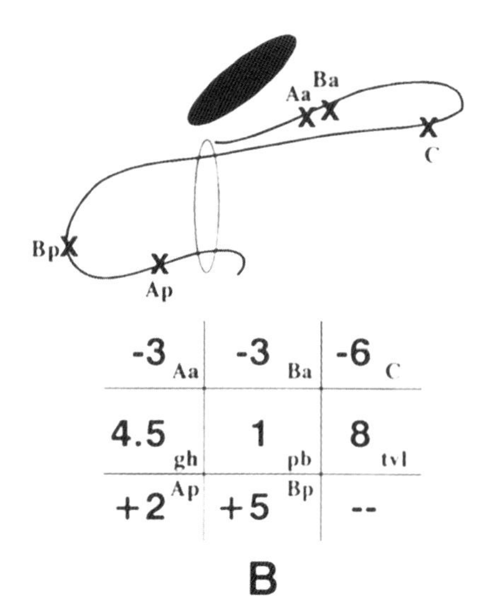

Figure 2 : Grid and line diagram of predominant anterior support defect. Leading point of prolapse is upper anterior vaginal wall, point Ba (+6). There is significant elongation of bulging anterior wall. Point Aa is maximally distal (+3) and vaginal cuff scar is 2 cm above hymen (C = -2). Cuff scar has undergone 4 cm of descent because it would be at -6 (total vaginal length) if it were perfectly supported. In this example total vaginal lenght is not maximum depth of vagina with elongated anterior vaginal wall maximally reduced but rather depth of vaginal at cuff with point C reduced to its normal full extent, as specified in text. This represents stage III Ba prolapse. B, Predominant posterior support defect. Leading point of prolapse is upper posterior vaginal wall, point Bp (+5). Point Ap is 2 cm distal to hymen (+2) and vaginal cuff scar is 6 cm above hymen (-6). Cuff has undergone only 2 cm of descent because it would be at -8 (total vaginal lenght) if it were perfectly supported. This represents stage III Bp prolapse.

The ICS POP Quantification and Staging system reliably describes the topographic position of six vaginal sites and gives information regarding perineal descent and the change in axis of the levator plate based on increases in genital hiatus and perineal body measurements. As such it is a useful tool to enhance communication among clinicians and researchers, to follow objectively changes in an individual patient over time, and to assess the success and durability of various surgical and non-surgical treatments. However, it does not identify the specific defect(s) in the pelvic support structures and mechanisms responsible for the topographic changes and cannot determine the surgical steps necessary for successful repair. Multiple ancillary procedures, including supplementary physical examination techniques, endoscopy, imaging procedures, photography, pelvic neuro-muscle testing, and intraoperative identification of discrete fascial defects [26, 27], play important roles in the formulation of a surgical strategy.

In men with urinary incontinence there frequently is an association between urethral obstruction such as prostatic enlargement, or the relief of obstruction, such as prostatectomy, and the onset of incontinence. In children congenital anomalies may be diagnosed such as spinal cord disease or abnormalities in the location of the urethral meatus. The frail, elderly population may be on medications which predispose to urinary incontinence or they may have co-existing morbidity with changes in mental status or ambulation which predispose to urinary incontinence.

II. PHYSICAL EXAMINATION

1. General clinical

The clinical assessment of patients with urinary incontinence should consist of a detailed history, a frequency/volume chart, and a physical examination. Leakage should be demonstrated objectively [28, 29].

a) History

The general history should include questions relevant to neurological and congenital abnormalities as well as information on previous urinary infections and relevant surgery. Information must be obtained on medications with known or possible effects on the lower urinary tract. The general history should also include assessment of menstrual, sexual and bowel function and obstetric history.

The urinary history (Table 3) must consist of symptoms related to both the storage and the evaçuation functions of the lower urinary tract. Many physicians have found it helpful to have the patient complete a urologic questionnaire.

This consultation has produced a working document which may be useful in evaluation of quality of life issues. ***(Note to publisher - please reference the chapter and page for Jenny Donovan=s QOL document)***

b) Frequency/volume chart

The frequency/volume chart is a specific urodynamic

Table 3 : Urologic history

- Duration and characteristics of UI
- Frequency, timing, and amount of continent and incontinent voids
- Precipitants and associated symptoms of incontinence
- Other lower urinary tract symptoms
- Fluid intake pattern
- Alterations in bowel habit or sexual function
- Previous treatment and its effects on UI
- Use of pads, briefs, or other protective devices [29].

investigation recording fluid intake and urine output per 24-hour period. The chart gives objective information on the number of voidings, the distribution of voidings between daytime and nighttime and each voided volume. The chart can also be used to record episodes of urgency and leakage and the number of incontinence pads used. The frequency/volume chart is very useful in the assessment of voiding disorders and in the follow-up treatment [28]. In patients with a high urine output per 24-hour period, it is also helpful to record the fluid intake per time. Constantly small voided volumes during day and night should arouse suspicion of a low compliance bladder. Low volumes only during daytime may be a sign of hypersensitivity (psychogenic) or of hypermobility.

c) Physical examination

Record height and weight so the body mass index (Kg/M^2) can be calculated. Perform an abdominal examination to evaluate the condition of the skin and surgical incisions and the presence of any hernias or abnormal masses (including full bladder).

2. FEMALE

a) Pelvic examination

The external genitalia should be examined for dermatologic lesions and evidence of irritative or inflammatory conditions. The internal genitalia should be examined for estrogen deficiency, abnormal vaginal secretions or urine, pelvic organ prolapse and abnormal pelvic masses. The well-estrogenized vagina has a thickened epithelium, with transverse rugae in its lower two-thirds. The poorly-estrogenized vagina has a thinned epithelium with loss of transverse rugae [30]. A number of authors have shown that vaginal pH levels are generally 5 or less in women with no infection and other definitive signs of good estrogen effect. The use of a pH indicator paper may help you evaluate the estrogen status in women with no vaginal infection [31]. The appearance of vaginal secretions may suggest a vaginal infection; urine within the vagina suggests genitourinary fistula, hypospadius or ectopic ureter. The anterior, superior, and posterior segments of the vagina should be examined for pelvic organ prolapse. The examiner can use a mirror to demonstrate the findings to the patient. The patient can confirm the examiner has identified the extent of prolapse she experiences (Figure 3).

When the patient tells you she normally has a greater amount of prolapse that you presently see, you should have her stand erect and perform any provocative maneuvers which normally are associated with her symptoms. After a period of time, repeat the examination while the patient is standing. In all women a digital rectal examination is also performed to assess sphincter tone (both resting and active) and to detect fecal impaction or a rectal mass.

Bimanual examination is performed to determine the size of the uterus and of the ovaries. Some women have co-existent pelvic disease which may require attention

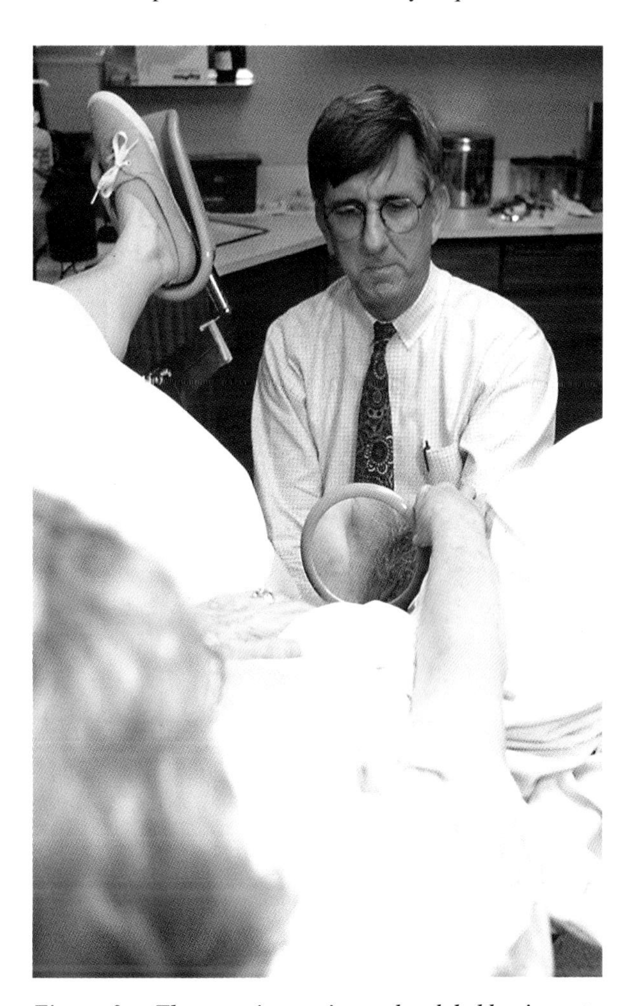

Figure 3 : The examiner using a hand held mirror to demonstrate physical findings to the patient.

in addition to the urinary incontinence. When hysterectomy or oophorectomy is indicated, there is no adverse effect on surgical success with a colposuspension procedure. Pelvic masses are rarely the cause of urinary incontinence.

Urethral diverticula are occasionally congenital but most are acquired. They may have either a simple or complex sacculation. Many patients with urethral diverticula are asymptomatic and need no treatment. Symptomatic patients report recurrent cystitis, frequency, dysuria, dyspareunia, urinary incontinence and voiding difficulties. On clinical examination a suburethral mass may be palpable; the urethra is usually tender; and, if the sacculation communicates with the urethra, it may be possible to express a purulent exudate from the urethra. Occasionally, a stone may develop within the diverticulum [32.]

b) Pelvic organ prolapse

Stress UI and pelvic organ prolapse (POP) are separate clinical entities which often coexist [1]. Significant protrusions of the vagina can obstruct voiding and defecation. Surgical repair of one pelvic support defect without repair of concurrent asymptomatic pelvic support defects appears to predispose to accentuation of unrepaired defects and new symptoms [9,11-13,17].

• ***Anterior vaginal wall descent.*** The well-supported anterior vaginal wall should not cross the longitudinal axis of the vaginal canal [33, 34]. Hypermobility of the urethrovesical junction is demonstrated by having the patient perform a maximum Valsalva effort. In women with hypermobility the increase in intra-abdominal pressure causes descent of the urethrovesical junction (bladder neck). On vaginal examination there may be loss of the transverse crease between the lower and middle thirds of the anterior vaginal wall and descent of the anterior vaginal wall (Figure 4).

Anterolateral protrusion into the vaginal canal may represent unilateral or bilateral detachment of the pubocervical fascia along the anterolateral vagina sulcus from its attachment to the arcus tendineus fascia pelvis (white line) [35]. Central protrusions of the anterior vaginal wall may represent defects in the pubocervical fascia below the trigone and base of the bladder. Advanced prolapse of the upper anterior vaginal wall may obstruct a well-supported bladder neck (Figure 5).

• ***Apical vaginal wall descent.*** Descent of the cervix, or of the vaginal apex following hysterectomy, below the level of the ischial spines is evidence of a defective vaginal suspension mechanism. In some women, the intravaginal portion of the cervix may become elongated and cause the cervix to extend into the lower vaginal canal, simulating prolapse; however the fundus may have good support. In other women the uterus may prolapse fully outside the hymen as uterine procidentia (Figure 6). Following hysterectomy the vaginal cuff may be well supported (Figure 7) or may prolapse fully outside the hymen along with other vaginal segments (Figures 8 and 9A & B).

• ***Posterior vaginal wall descent.*** The well-supported posterior vaginal wall should not cross the longitudinal axis of the vaginal canal. Posterior protrusions into the vaginal canal are most commonly caused by defects in the rectovaginal fascia allowing protrusions of the small bowel (enterocele) and/or rectum (rectocele). Normally, the anterior vaginal wall lies upon the posterior vaginal wall. Therefore, protrusions of the posterior vaginal wall can affect the function of the urethra and bladder which lie upon the anterior vaginal wall. For example, distal loss of support in the posterior segment may result in a bulge which compresses the urethra and affects voiding (Figure 10).

3. Male physical examination

The assessment and treatment algorithm focuses on the abdominal examination, digital rectal examination and neurologic testing of the perineum and lower extremities. The examination should also include external genitalia, location of the urethral meatus, retractability of the foreskin and evidence of congenital malformation. Abdominal palpation should be performed to evaluate bladder distention, specially in elderly incontinent men, who may have overflow leakage due to obstruction. Post-void residual volume should be measured in those patients.

Rectal examination should include palpation of the prostate to assess size, symmetry and consistency of the gland and its relation to the pelvic sidewall and the rectum. Detrusor instability with urge and urge incontinence are common symptoms in prostatic disease. Prostatic carcinoma must be excluded.

Incontinence combined with evacuation problems in a man often requires further investigation including urodynamics. It may be helpful to ask these patients to measure the voiding time for the first voided 100 ml on several different occasions.

Urinary incontinence is rare in men without a history of previous trauma or prostatic or pelvic surgery; therefore, neurogenic bladder dysfunction must be considered in men with no history of surgery or trauma. In those patients evaluation of perineal sensation and lower extremity reflexes is important.

Post-void dribbling is often provoked by an obstructing disease such as BPH or urethral stricture but can also be a symptom of a urethral diverticulum. Post-void residual urine volume and careful palpation of the genitalia are recommended to be performed in these patients.

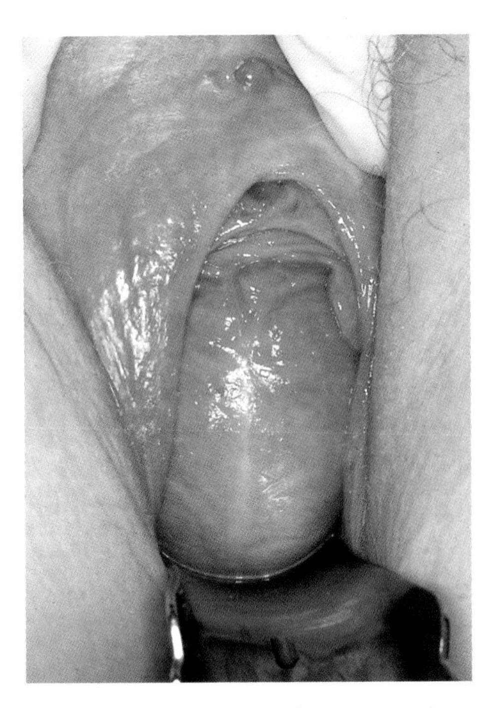

Figure 4 : The anterior vaginal segment prolapses to the hymen. A vertical scar is present from previous surgery.

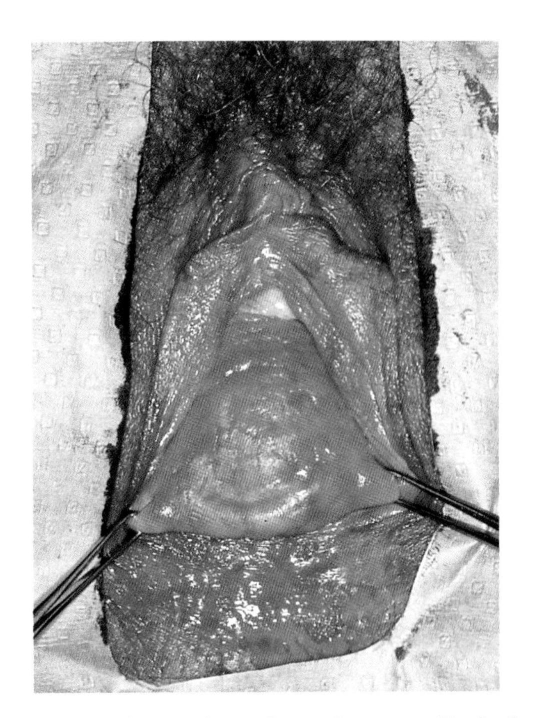

Figure 5 : The anterior vagina prolapses outside the hymen while the urethra has good support from a prior urethropexy.

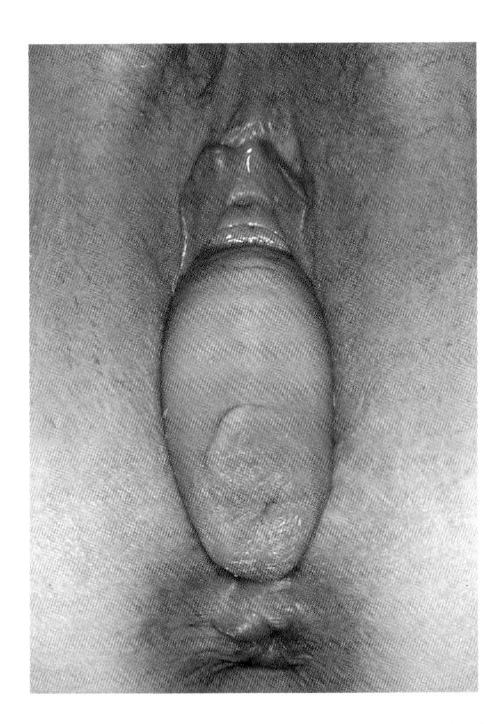

Figure 6 : The uterus prolapses fully outside the hymen, uterine procidentia.

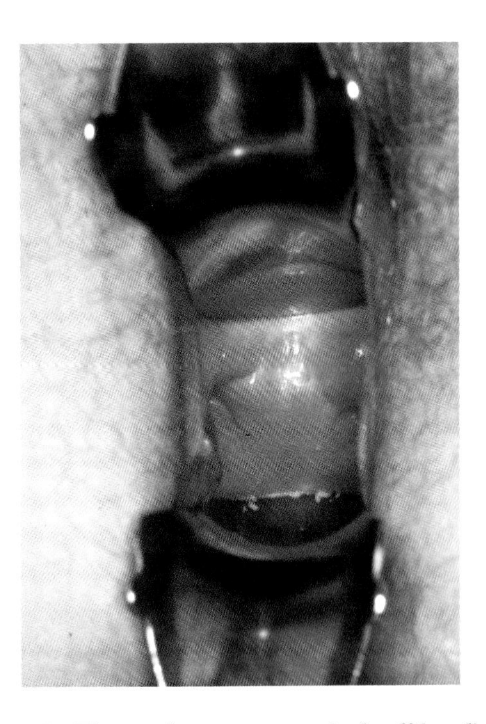

Figure 7 : The post-hysterectomy vaginal cuff has dimples at the 3 o'clock and 9 o'clock positions, the sites of the cardinal-uterosacral ligament suspension.

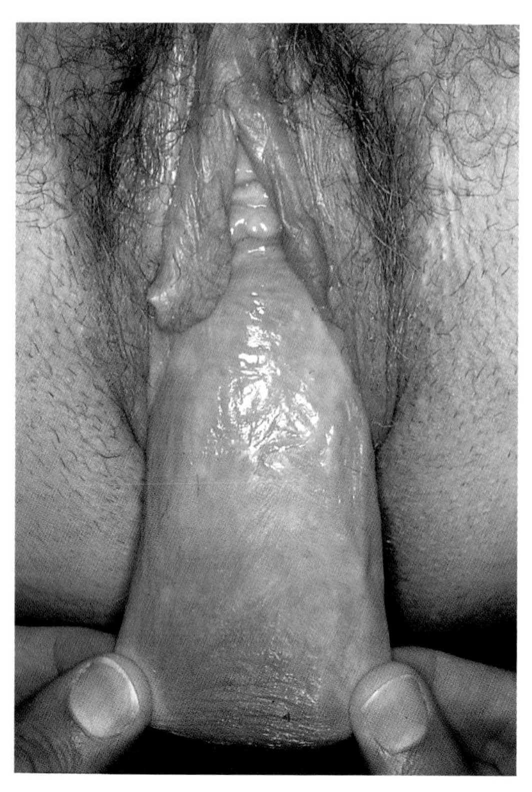

Figure 8 : Following hysterectomy the vaginal cuff may prolapse fully outside the hymen along with other vaginal segments .

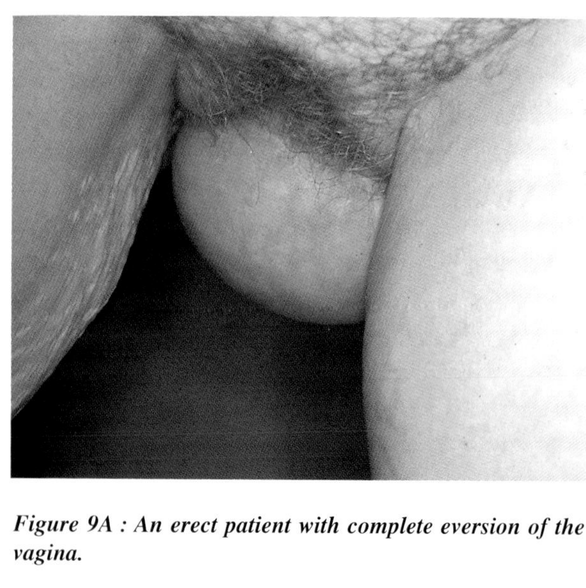

Figure 9A : An erect patient with complete eversion of the vagina.

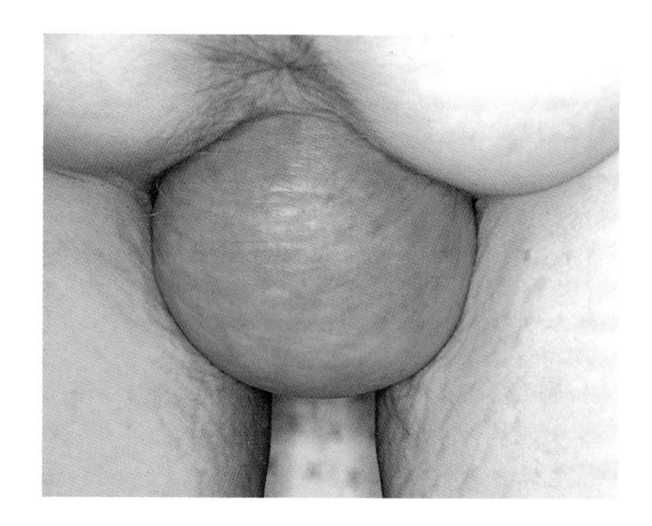

Figure 9B : A view of the same patient as seen when standing behind her.

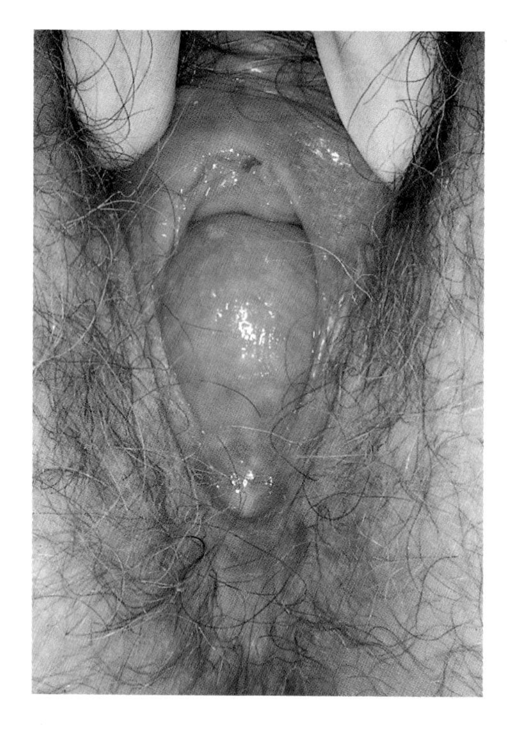

Figure 10 : The posterior vaginal segment balloons anteriorly and may affect voiding secondary to pressure in the urethra.

4. PHYSICAL EXAMINATION – CHILDREN

a) General examination

Evaluate the back and the spine for skin lesions, skeletal deformities, scars from trauma or from previous surgery. The presence of a subcutaneous fatty mass, cutaneous vascular malformation, tuft of hair, skin dimple, hyperpigmented area, hemangioma or sinus tract on the lower back may be associated with an occult spinal dysraphism, warranting further neurologic evaluation. Palpation of the coccyx may confirm absence of sacral vertebrae.

b) Pelvic examination

The labia majora and minora, introitus and perineum are examined looking for abnormalities such as bifid clitoris and labia minora adhesions. In the latter, incontinence occurs only a few minutes after voiding with no nighttime wetting. On the other hand, when the labia minora are widely separated in the inferior part or when the anus is displaced in the posterior position it may indicate a weakened, denervated perineal body.

An infrequent cause of incontinence is ectopic ureter. The most common site in girls is the posterior or lateral wall of the urethra followed by vaginal vestibule, uterus and cervix. Also look for urethral stenosis, meatal hypospadius, epispadius, or a duplicated urethra. In males it is imperative to retract the foreskin and examine the urethral meatus.

The digital rectal examination is performed to evaluate fecal impactation, rectal masses, and the external anal sphincter. The examiner evaluates motor innervation by asking the child to voluntary contract and relax the anal sphincter around the examinerэs finger. Since the abdominal straining may mimic sphincter contraction, it is useful if the examiner rests the other hand on the childэs abdomen to detect straining.

5. NEUROLOGIC EXAMINATION

A simple neurologic examination should be performed on all patients, and includes three components: (1) an assessment of anal sphincter tone, (2) an evaluation of voluntary anal contraction, and (3) an evaluation for intact perineal sensation. When abnormalities are noted, or in individuals suspected of having neurologic diseases or dysfunction, an extended neurologic examination should be performed.

An extended neurologic examination is divided into four parts: Mental Status, Sensory Function, Motor Function, and Deep Tendon Reflexes [28].

a) Mental Status is evaluated by observing the level of consciousness, orientation, speech pattern, memory, and comprehension. Urinary dysfunction may be associated with mental status changes resulting from stroke, brain tumor, degenerative neurologic diseases, or acute or chronic infection of the central nervous system.

b) Sensory Function Evaluation. Test lumbo-sacral dermatomes for position, vibration, pinprick, light touch, and temperature.

Important sensory dermatomes are L1 (base of penis, upper scrotum), L1-L2 (mid-scrotum, labia-minora), L3 (front of knee), S1 (sole and lateral area of the foot), S1-S3 (perineum and circumanal skin), and S2-S4 (sacral nerve roots which innervate both the external urethral and the anal sphincter). The sensory examination includes cutaneous sacral reflexes.

The anal reflex (S2-S5) is stimulated by light stroking of the mucocutaneous junction of the circumanal skin causing a visible contraction. Absence of this reflex suggests sacral nerve disease. In children, the disorder may be congenital. In adult women, absence of the reflex may be a consequence of trauma from vaginal childbirth.

Assess sphincter tone and volitional contraction. The presence of voluntary anal sphincter contraction indicates functioning pelvic floor innervation and sphincter muscle. Absence or decrease of the anal sphincter tone and voluntary anal contraction indicates a possible sacral or peripheral lesion. If the anal sphincter tone is present in the absence of voluntary anal contraction there may be a supra sacral lesion.

The bulbocavernous reflex (BCR) tests the innervation of all perineal striated muscles.[29] It is a local sacral spinal cord reflex arc reflecting activity in S2-S4. The BCR is elicited by squeezing the penis glands, or clitoris, which causes a reflex contraction of the external anal sphincter. Absence of the BCR could indicate sacral nerve damage. It is absent in people with a complete lower motor neuron lesion.

c) Motor Function, Look for coordination, facial asymmetry, paresis, plegias, tremor, mobility state (cane walker, wheelchair), muscle bulk for atrophy. The tibialis anterior (L4-L5), and the toe extensor (L1, S1) may be tested by dorsiflexion, plantar flexion and toe extension.

d) Deep tendon reflexes reflect the integrity of upper motor neuron (UMN) and lower motor neuron (LMN) function. The UMN lesions usually are associated with detrusor overactivity (hyper-reflexia). LMN damage results in an areflexic bladder. Hyperactive deep tendon reflexes and hypoactive deep tendon reflexes are suggestive of a UMN and LMN dysfunction respectively.

You may evaluate these deep tendon reflexes: quadriceps (L3-L4) and Achilles= tendon (L5 - S1-S2). Children with complete spinal cord lesions above the conus medullaris (UMN/ Supra sacral/ Suprasegmental) may have hyperactive deep tendon reflexes, hyper-reflexic bladder, skeletal spasticity, pathologic toe sign (Babinski), ankle clonus, and absent skin sensation below the level of the lesion. Complete spinal cord lesions at or below the level of the conus medullaris (LMN/ Sacral/ segmental) may present absent deep tendon reflexes, areflexic bladder, skeletal flaccidity, absent Babinski∍s sign, absent ankle clonus, and absent skin sensation below the level of the lesion.

6. Pelvic floor muscle strength

The continence mechanisms imply that integrity of the levator ani and external urethral sphincter is necessary to maintain continence [37,38]. It is therefore important to test the contractility of these muscles. Once the patient understands Ahow≅ to contract the pelvic floor muscles correctly, the evaluation is carried out during a maximum contraction [39].

a) Definitions:

Strength is defined as the maximum force or tension generated by a muscle or muscle group [40]. It reflects the power, endurance and functional status of the muscle.

Weakness is defined as failure to generate the expected force.

Fatigue is defined as failure to maintain the expected force with continued or repeated contraction [41].

When considering methods/devices used to measure pelvic muscle Astrength≅, cost and availability should be recognized as important factors. In this chapter only four methods are discussed (Table 4). Factors to be investigated are listed in Table 5.

Table 4 : **Methods of measurement**

Observation
Digital palpation
Perineometer
Q-tip

Table 5 : **Factors to be investigated:**

1. Right and left sided symmetry of muscle bulk
1. Right and left sided strength/endurance
2. Reflex response **with cough**
2. Functional contractility **i.e. with lifting, coughing**
3. Over-all strength
4. Displacement with contraction of muscle group. Elevation of perineal body by pubococcygeus muscles; constricting of the anus with external anal sphincter.

b) Observation

• ***Method*:** This qualitative measure can detect an in-drawing of the anus, lifting of the posterior vaginal wall and narrowing of the vaginal introitus (females); an in-drawing of the anus and slight lifting of the penis (males).

• ***Advantages*:** Suitable for both sexes and all age groups, where an internal evaluation may be in-appropriate. Inexpensive. Able to detect reflex contraction with cough, and bulbocavernosus reflex. Observe accessory muscle activity.

• ***Disadvantages*:** Subjective. Cannot distinguish right and left sides independently. Generally observing activity of the superficial perineal muscles, and assuming levators are resonding in a like manner. Difficult to observe when the patient is standing.

c) Digital palpation

• ***Method:*** - *females.* Palpation of the right and left levator ani, per vaginam. Palpation of the perineal body.

- males. Palpation of the right and left puborectalis, per ano-rectum. Palpation of the perineal body.

- Advantages: Suitable for both sexes. Inexpensive. Able to differentiate right from left. Quantitative - using modified Oxford scale or other systems [42-43]. Able to measure strength and endurance. Can detect reflex contraction with cough and patients=s ability to hold contraction during a cough. Can be used when the patient is standing.

- Disadvantages: Subjective. Not sensitive.

d) Perineometer

• ***Method*:** Manometric measure of change in a vaginal/anal pressure probe. Sensitivity depends on the device.

- Advantages: Relatively inexpensive. Able to measure strength and endurance. Quantitative [35]. Can be used when the patient is standing.

- Disadvantages: Unable to distinguish right from left. Pressure changes may be caused by increase in intraabdominal pressure, due to co-contraction of the abdominal muscles. No AGold Standard≅ device; different results with different probe sizes and materials.[44]

e) Cotton swab (Q-tip) test

• ***Method*:** Q-tip inserted into urethra (female). Downward, posterior movement of stem (measured on a goniometer) is dependent on the strength of the contraction of the pubococcygeus muscles, and mobility of the urethra.[45]

• ***Advantages:*** Inexpensive. Can measure strength and endurance.

• ***Disadvantages*:** Lacks sensitivity and specificity. Invasive. Females only.

The information learned from assessment of pelvic floor muscle strength has the following practical applications:

The patient has good pelvic floor muscles that need skill training to help maintain continence. DeLancey and associates have described knack teaching [46,47].

The patient has weak muscles that are capable of contracting but need strength and skill training. An effective exercise program should increase resting tone (Type I fibers) as well as improve the ability of fast twitch (Type II) fibers to respond to increases in intra-abdominal pressure [48.]

The patient has no perceptible contractions and needs further evaluation (EMG, MRI, neurophysiologic testing) or passive contraction therapy i.e., functional electrostimulation.

7. Others tests

a) Provocative stress testing. If stress UI is suspected, provocative stress testing (direct visualization) can be performed by having the individual relax and then cough vigorously while the examiner observes for urine loss from the urethra. Optimally these tests should be done when the patientэs bladder is full, but they should not be performed when the patient has a precipitant urge to void. They can be done in the standing or lithotomy position. If instantaneous leakage occurs with cough, then stress UI is likely; if leakage is delayed or persists after the cough, detrusor over activity should be suspected. If the test is initially performed in the lithotomy position and no leakage is observed, the test is repeated in the standing position, since the yield is increased when the test is repeated in the upright position. If bladder filling is needed to perform stress testing, this may be conveniently performed in conjunction with the catheterization being done for PVR measurement. Patients with very little urine in their bladder who leak urine during Valsalva maneuvers should be suspected of having intrinsic sphincter deficiency [49].

Bonney's original stress test was performed to demonstrate urinary leakage during coughing.[50] Subsequent modifications of the test require support of the urethrovesical junction during coughing in women who leak during a stress test. These modifications are not reliable in selecting a surgical procedure or in predicting cure.

b) Urethrovesical junction (bladder neck) mobility.

Urethrovesical junction (bladder neck) mobility should be assessed in all women with urinary incontinence. It is generally felt that women with genuine incontinence fall into several categories based **on assessment** of urethral support and urethral function. ***A 2x2 table helps to record urethral support and function (Table 6).***

Table 6 : Urethral Support and Function

Urethra	Good	Bad
Support		
Function		

The choice of therapy may be affected by the assessment of bladder neck mobility.

One method of assessing bladder neck mobility is by visual inspection. When the patient is in lithotomy position, the urethral meatus is horizontal to the floor in a woman with good bladder neck support. When she increases intra-abdominal pressure you can observe for posterior rotation of the anterior vagina and deflection of the meatus toward the ceiling, both signs of some loss of support. You may ask her to contract the pelvic muscles to determine if urethral support improves with muscle contraction, a sign pelvic floor training may be therapeutic.

A simple office procedure to quantify bladder neck mobility is the cotton swab or Q-tip test [51]. A sterile, lubricated cotton or dacron swab (Q-tip) is inserted into the urethra until it lies just within the urethrovesical junction. Using a goinometer, the angle circumscribed by the distal end of the swab is measured relative to the horizontal while the woman is performing a maximum Valsalva effort. Urethrovesical junction hypermobility is defined by a maximum strain axis exceeding +30 degrees from the horizontal (Figures 11A, 11B).

Q-tip testing does not diagnose any form of incontinence. It may be useful in differentiating stress UI due to hypermobility from that due to intrinsic sphincter deficiency. Other tests to document bladder neck mobility are used, including bead-chain cystourethrography, ultrasonography, and videocystourethrography. The chapter on imaging of the urinary tract addresses the place of these techniques.

c) Post Void Residual. Post void residual (PVR) measurement is recommended for patients with UI. Specific PVR measurement can be accomplished within a few minutes of voiding either by catheterization or by ultrasound.

Review of the literature fails to show a specific maximum PVR this is considered normal, nor is there any

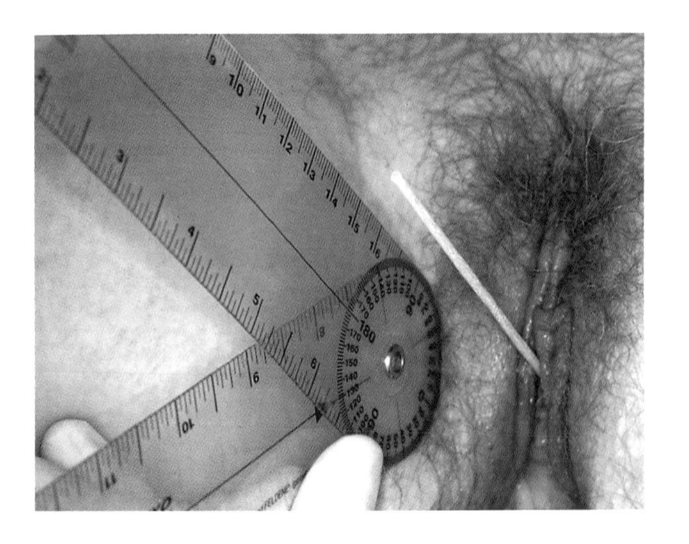

Figure 11a : A cotton tip swab (Q-tip) is located in the urethra. The angle of deflection from the horizontal is being measured with a goniometer.

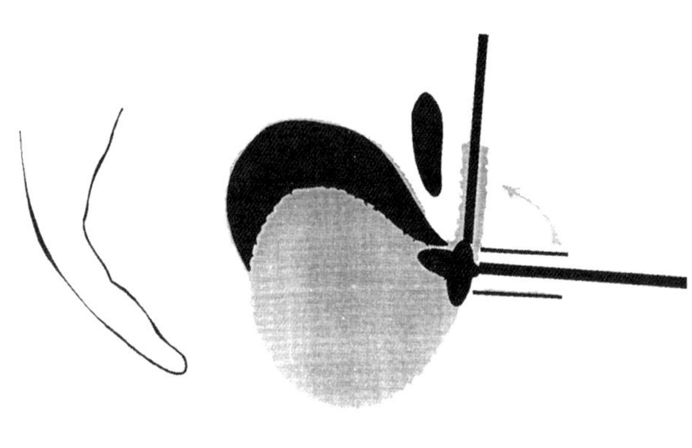

Figure 11b : A schematic representation of the cotton tip swab and the arc it will traverse with urethral mobility.

documentation of the minimal PVR that is considered abnormal. The AHCPR guidelines state that, in general, a PVR less than 50 mL is considered adequate bladder emptying and over 200 mL is considered inadequate emptying. Since PVR may vary, one measurement of PVR may not be sufficient [22].

Women with pelvic organ prolapse may have to reduce their prolapse in order to void. Women with pelvic organ prolapse and a large PVR should be evaluated for voiding phase dysfunction (e.g., outlet obstruction, detrusor hypofunction).

8. Recommendation of the Committee (Table 7)

a) Each person being evaluated for urinary incontinence should have a physical examination which includes:

- assessment of mobility and cognitive status
- abdominal examination
- sacral neurologic examination for sensory and motor function and appropriate reflex activity
- pelvic floor muscle assessment

b) Other tests:

- Attempt to demonstrate incontinence.
- Post void residual assessment.

c) In physical examination of women assess pelvic organ support

In women with pelvic organ prolapse, a standardized, validated system of pelvic organ prolapse should be the basis for the detailed pelvic examination. The ICS approved Pelvic Organ Prolapse Quantification system is an example you may use.

9. Future Research

There are 5 specific recommendations on future research regarding the physical examination of people with urinary incontinence:

a) Document natural history of changes in pelvic support and bowel and bladder function with increasing age.

b) Correlate physical examination findings with bowel and bladder function.

c) Validate findings of physical examination that are predictive of success, failure, and complications of therapy for urinary incontinence.

d) Document effects of surgical therapy for urinary incontinence on post operative pelvic support.

e) Identify the most accurate physical examination technique to correlate with other evaluation techniques.

Table 7: Recommendations for physical examination of each group of patients

Specific Groups Children	Female	Male	Frail Elderly as per other adults	Neuropatic
Psychomotor development	Pelvic examination: *-External genitalia- Vaginal epithelium*	Lower back Digital rectalsystematic examination	General examination	Complete neurologic examination
Examine lower back for spinal abnormality	*-Bladder neck mobility* *-Evidence of fistula or diverticulum—*	Sphincter tone Scrotum Urethral meatus	looking for co-morbid conditions, *i.e. heart failure*	Observe voiding
External genitalia for abnormalities				
Observe voiding	*-Size of uterus and ovaries* *-Support of the anterior, apical, and posterior segments of the vagina* *-Digital rectal examination*		Manual dexterity	

REFERENCES

1. Jackson SL, Weber AM, Hull TL, Mitchinson AR, Walters MD. Fecal incontinence in women with urinary incontinence and pelvic organ prolapse. Obstet Gynecol 1997;89:423-7.
2. Kjølhede P, Norèn B, Rydèn G. Prediction of genital prolapse after Burch colposuspension. Acta Obstet Gynecol Scand 1997; 76:266-70.
3. Seim A, Eriksen BC, Hunskaar S. A study of female urinary incontinence in general practice: demography, medical history, and clinical finding. Scand J Urol Nephrol 1996;30:465-71.
4. Samuelsson EC, Arne Victor FT, Tibblin G, Svørdsudd KF. Signs of genital prolapse in a Swedish population of women 20 to 59 years of age and possible related factors. Am J Obstet Gynecol 1999;180:299-305.
5. DeLancey JOL, Hurd WW. Size of the urogenital hiatus in the levator ani muscles in normal women and women with pelvic organ prolapse. Obstet Gynecol 1998;91:364-8.
6. Howard D, Miller JM, DeLancey JOL, Ashton-Miller JA. Differential effects of cough, valsalva, and continence status on vesical neck movement. Obstet Gynecol 2000;95:535-40.
7. Summitt RL, Bent AE, Ostergard DR, Harris TA. Stress incontinence and lower urethral closure pressure. Correlation of preoperative urethral hypermobility with successful suburethral sling procedures. J Reprod Med 1990;35:877-880.
8. Burch JC. Cooper's ligament urethrovesical suspension for stress incontinence. Am J Obstet Gynecol 1968; 100:764-774.
9. Wiskind AK, Creighton SM, and Stanton SL. The incidence of genital prolapse after the Burch colposuspension. Am J Obstet Gynecol 1992; 167:399-405.
10. Galloway NTM, Davies N, and Stephenson TP. The complications of colposuspension. Br J Urol 1987; 60:122-124.
11. Alcalay M, Monga A, Stanton SL. Burch colposuspension: a 10-20 year follow up. Br J Obstet Gynaecol 1995; 102:740-745.
12. Shull BL, Baden WF. A six-year experience with paravaginal defect repair for stress urinary incontinence. Am J Obstet Gynecol 1989;160,6:1432-1440.
13. Colombo N, Maggioni A, Caruso, et al. Adverse Effects of Burch Colposuspension. ICS proceedings, 1993. Rome.
14. Stanton SL, Cardozo LD. Results of colposuspension operation for incontinence and prolapse. Br J Obstet Gynaecol 1979; 86:693-697.
15. Weber AM, Walters MD, Piedmonte MR. Sexual function and vaginal anatomy in women before and after surgery for pelvic organ prolapse and urinary incontinence. Am J Obstet Gynecol 2000;182:1610-5.
16. Bassler K, Schuessler B. Abdominal sacrocolpopexy and anatomy and function of the posterior compartment. Obstet Gynecol 2001; 97:678-84.
17. Kjølhede P, Noren B, Ryden G. Prediction of genital prolapse after Burch colposuspension. Acta Obstet Gynecol Scand 1996; 75:849-854.
18. Athanasiou S, Hill S, Gleeson C, Anders K, Cardozo L. Validation of the ICS proposed pelvic organ prolapse descriptive system. Neurourol Urodynamics 1995;14:414-5.
19. Schussler B, Peschers U. Standardisation of terminology of female genital prolapse according to the new ICS criteria: inter-examiner reproducibility. Neurourol Urodynamics 1995;14:437-8.
20. Montella JM, Cater JR. Comparison of measurements obtained in supine and sitting position in the evaluation of pelvic organ prolapse. Int Urogynecol J 1995;6:304.
21. Kobak WH, Rosenberg K, Walters MD. Inter-observer variation in the assessment of pelvic organ prolapse. Int Urogynecol J 1996;7:121-4.
22. Hall AF, Theofrastous JP, Cundiff GC, Harris RL, Hamilton LF, Swift SE, Bump RC. Inter- and intra-observer reliability of the proposed International Continence Society, Society of Gynecologic Surgeons, and American Urogynecologic Society pelvic organ prolapse classification system. Am J Obstet Gynecol 1996;175:1467-71.
23. Swift SE, Herring M. Comparison of pelvic organ prolapse in

the dorsal lithotomy compared with the standing position. Obstet Gynecol 1998;91:961-4.

24. Barber MD, Lambers AR, Visco AG, Bump RC. Effect of patient position on clinical evaluation of pelvic organ prolapse. Obstet Gynecol 2000;96:18-22.

25. Bump RC, Mattiasson A, Bø K, Brubaker LP, DeLancey JOL, Klarskov P, Shull BL, Smith ARB. The standardisation of terminology of female pelvic organ prolapse and pelvic floor dysfunction. Am J Obstet Gynecol 1996; 175:10-17.

26. Cundiff GW, Weidner AC, Visco AG, Addison WA, Bump RC. An Anatomical and Functional Assessment of the Discrete Defect Rectocele Repair. Am J Obstet Gynecol 1998; 179:1451-7.

27. Barber MD, Cundiff GW, Weidner AC, Coates KW, Bump RC, Addison WA. Accuracy of Clinical Assessment of Paravaginal Defect in Women with Anterior Vaginal Wall Prolapse. Am J Obstet Gynecol 1999; 181:87-90.

28. Abrams P, Blaivas JG, Stanton SL, Andersen JT. The Standardization of Terminology of Lower Urinary Tract Function Recommended by the International Continence Society. Int Urogynecol J 1990;1:45-58.

29. Urinary Incontinence Guidelines Panel (1996): Urinary Incontinence in Adults: Clinical Practice Guidelines, Number 2. AHCPR Pub. No. 92-0682. Rockville, MD: Agency for Health Care Policy and Research, Public Health Service, U.S. Department of Health and Human Services, March 1996.

30. Fantl J, Cardozo L, McClish, and the Hormones and Urogenital Therapy Committee. Estrogen therapy in the management of urinary incontinence in postmenopausal women: a meta-analysis. Obstet Gynecol 1994;83:12-18.

31. Molander U, Milsom I, Ekelund P, Mellstrom D, Eriksson O. Effect of oral oestriol on vaginal flora and cytology and urogenital symptoms in the post-menopause. Maturitas. 1990;12: 113-120.

32. Fortunato P, Schettini M, Gallucci M: Diverticula of the female urethra. Br J Urol 1997;80(4):628-632.

33. Shull BL. Clinical evaluation of women with pelvic support defects. Clinical Obstet Gynecol 1993;36:939-951.

34. Baden WB, Walker TA, Lindsey JH. The vaginal profile. Tex Med 1968;64:56-8.

35. Richardson AC, Lyon JB, Williams NL. A new look at pelvic relaxation. Am J Obstet Gynecol 1976;126:568-674.

36. Blaivus JC: The bulbocavernosus reflex in urology; a prospective Study of 299 patients. J Urol 126:197, 1981.

37. Delancey JOL and Starr RA. Histology of the connection between the vagina and levator ani muscles. J Repro Med 1990;35:765-771. 11b

38. Gosling J. The structure of the bladder and urethra in relation to function. Urologic Clinic of America. 1979; 6: 31-38. 11b

39. Bump RC, Hurt WG, Fantl JA, Wyman JF. Assessment of Kegel pelvic muscle exercise performance after brief verbal instruction. Am J Obstet Gynecol 1991; 165:322-329.

40. Dinubile NA. Strength training. Clinical Sports Medicine. 1991; 10(1):33-62. 11b

41. Edwards RHT. Physiologic analysis of skeletal muscle weakness and fatigue. Clinical Science and Molecular Medicine 1978; 54:463-470.

42. Laycock J. PhD Thesis. Assessment and treatment of pelvic floor dysfunction. University of Bradford. 1992 11b

43. Brink CA, Sampselle CM, Wells TJ, Diokno AC, Gillis GL. A digital test for pelvic muscle strength in older women with incontinence. Nurs Res 1989;38:196-9.

44. Laycock J, Sherlock R. Perineometers – do we need a "Gold Standard"? Suppl, ICS (Sydney) 1995:144-145. 11b

45. Schüssler B and Hesse U. Q-Tip Testing. In: Eds. B Schüssler, J Laycock, P Norton, S Stanton. Pelvic Floor Re-education: Principles and Practice. Springer-Verlag, London. 1994. 49-50. 1V

46. Miller JM, Ashton-Miller JA, Carchidi L, DeLancey JOL. Does a three month pelvic muscle exercise intervention improve the effectiveness of the knack in reducing cough-induced urine loss in a standing stress test? American Urogynecologic Society meeting, Sept 27, 1997. Tuscon, Ariz.

47. Perucchini D, DeLancey JOL, Miller JM, Carchidi L, Krajewski K, Ashton-Miller JA. A levator ani precontraction significantly reduces bladder neck descent during coughing in women with SUI. American Urogynecologic Society meeting, Sept 27, 1997. Tuscon, Ariz.

48. Wall LL, Davidson TG. The role of muscular re-education by physcial therapy in the treatment of genuine stress urinary incontinence. Obstet Gynecol Survey 1992;47:322-331.

49. McLennan MT, Bent AE. Supine empty stress test as a predictor of low Valsalva leak point pressure. Neurourol Urodyn 1998;17:121-127.

50. Bonney V. On diurnal incontinence of urine in women. J Obstet Gynaecol 1923; N.S. 30:358-365.

51. Crystle CD, Charme LS, Copeland WE. Q-tip test in stress urinary incontinence. Obstet Gynecol 1971;38 No.2:313-315.

Committee 8 B

Clinical Neurophysiology

Chairman

C. J. Fowler

Members

J. T. Benson,

M. D. Craggs,

D.B. Vodusek,

C.C. Yang,

S. Podnar

Consultants

B. Schurch,

G. Amarenco

Clinical Neurophysiology

C. J. Fowler,

J. T. Benson, M. D. Craggs, D.B. Vodusek, C.C. Yang, S. Podnar

INTRODUCTION

Clinical neurophysiology should serve as an adjunct to the physical examination in understanding a neurological disorder. This is mostly the case in general neurological practice and with the additional problem presented by the relative inaccessibility of the pelvic floor and pelvic organs to clinical neurological examination, the expectation was that uro-neurophysiological investigations would prove to be highly valuable. The investigations have evolved over the course of 40-50 years, closely following developments in general clinical neurophysiology closely (see "Historical Background") but the reality of the situation is that few tests are currently clinically employed. Many of the investigations are now recognised to be of research value only. It is however important that the context of the development of the various investigations and their application is detailed here so that investigators can make a well informed decision about the potential benefits of using uro neu rophysiological tests.

A. GENERAL CONSIDERATIONS

I. HISTORICAL BACKGROUND

The introduction of neurophysiological techniques to investigate pelvic organ and pelvic floor function was the result of applying general clinical neurophysiological techniques to those structures as the tests became available. Sphincter EMG was first performed by Danish investigators [1] working with the founder of electromyography Buchthal, although use of kinaesiological EMG recordings during urodynamics followed some while later [2]. Latency recordings of the bulbocavernosus reflex were reported [3] soon after electrical stimulation for motor conduction studies had been described, and recordings of evoked potentials following repetitive stimulation of the pudendal nerves [4] and other pelvic sensory structures were described within a few years of other somatosensory evoked potential recordings being used in clinical practise. Cortical and root stimulation by first electrical [5] and then magnetic stimulation [6] with recording from pelvic floor musculature were carried out with some of the earliest versions of the stimulator devices.

It is interesting that the innovations of clinical neurophysiological testing were so promptly applied to investigating the pelvic floor, but there have undoubtedly been problems. One of these is that the tests have often been employed by investigators with little or no training in clinical neurophysiology who have not been aware of the importance of applying the tests only with a strong neurological understanding. This has sometimes resulted in reports of their use by uncritical observers and exaggerated claims for their usefulness. However with the passage of time those tests which have not proved to be of genuine clinical usefulness have been abandoned and an informed approach has been adopted to those tests which are still in use.

In general there have been few major innovations in general clinical neurophysiology in the last decade and thus no significant technical developments in pelvic floor neurophysiology, although an understanding of what can be learnt from the tests has continued to improve. The contributions that this specialist service can offer to understanding neurological problems is now well established both in general circumstances and as applied to the pelvic floor and bladder, and the benefits and limitations of the various tests will be discussed in this chapter.

II. CLASSIFICATION OF CLINICAL NEUROPHYSIOLOGICAL TESTS

It is possible to "classify" neurophysiological tests in different ways. As the tests are an extension of the clinical examination, a functional anatomic approach to classification makes it easiest. For the purpose of this categorisation, the nervous system is divided into "subsystems": the motor systems, divided into the somatic and autonomic, and the sensory system, both somatic and visceral. Within a particular anatomical subsystem there are central and peripheral parts. There are also important "integrative parts" (interneuronal system) at different levels of the central nervous system.

The somatic motor system comprises an upper motor neurone i.e., all neurones participating in supraspinal motor control, a lower motor neurone, which arises from spinal motor neurones to the muscle. The somatosensory system can be divided into a peripheral part with sensory receptors in skin, muscle and viscera that input into the spinal cord and a central part comprised of ascending pathways in the spinal cord and above. Sensory fibres from skin and muscle spindles are called somatic afferents whereas those, which arise from structures innervated by the autonomic nervous system are referred to as visceral afferents.

By applying this simplified model to the sacral innervation, clinical neurophysiological tests can be divided accordingly. There are those evaluating the somatic motor system (EMG, terminal motor latency measurements, and MEP) and those evaluating the sensory system (SEP). The third group comprises methods which assess reflexes. Autonomic nervous system tests relate to function of sympathetic or parasympathetic fibres.

III. GENERAL METHODOLOGICAL CONSIDERATIONS

Clinical neurophysiological tests rely on complex electronic instruments and various devices that come into contact with the patient. Equipment used is mostly standard although some specially constructed electrodes or stimulating devices have been devised to conform to uro-genito-anal anatomy. To date, there are no generally accepted guidelines for performance of individual neurophysiological tests. As when using other electromedical equipment, if standards of electrical safety are adhered to the risk to patients is negligible.

Both electrical stimulation and recording of bioelectrical activity are achieved through the use of electrodes, which are usually referred to as either "surface" or "needle". Special devices are used for magnetic and mechanical stimulation. The important neurophysiological difference between surface and needle electrodes is their selectivity, and the practical difference is their invasiveness. The choice and application of electrodes will depend mainly on the consideration of how selective a recording or stimulation is necessary.

It is recommended that the electrical stimulus is specified and characterised both in "absolute" (technical) and "relative" (physiological) terms if possible i.e. rectangular pulse, 0.2 ms, 15 mA; 3-times sensory threshold. A stimulus with defined technical parameters may have variable biological effects because of the variable influences of electrode condition, contact, tissue conductivity etc. If stimulation is applied to obtain the compound muscle action potential or sensory nerve action potential, it is usually desirable to use the so-called supramaximal stimuli [7]. Such stimuli produce responses with largest amplitudes and shortest latencies and are the least variable and most reproducible. If supramaximal stimuli are not possible or not desirable, another physiological definition of the stimulus is needed. In such cases, a threshold value (for instance sensory) is established, and then a multiple of this value is applied as the stimulus. It is common practice to define magnetic stimulus strength as the percentage of maximum output of the stimulator. The sites of placement of stimulation electrodes need to be stated using in anatomical terms.

For recording, the apparatus settings (gain, sweep speed) have to be adapted to the known range of amplitudes, latencies, duration etc. of the responses and they have to be appropriately displayed to be analysed. Particularly important is the frequency setting of filters: for surface electrode recordings it is typically 2 Hz - 1000 Hz; for needle (EMG) recordings, it is 2 5 –– 10000 Hz for concentric needle or 500 – 10000 Hz for single fibre needle.

Placement of electrodes on the scalp for evoked potential recordings are defined according to the 10-20 International EEG System. Any potential elicited by stimulation should be reproducible; therefore, as a rule, at least two consecutive recording procedures need to be performed. Some responses need to be averaged because of their small amplitude to improve the signal-to-noise ratio. Therefore, many repetitions of stimulation/recording need to be done (typically 100-200). Even such an averaged recording needs to be repeated at least twice. M-waves, MEP, sacral reflexes and SSR are recognisable after single stimuli, but, as a rule, several responses are recorded to demonstrate reproducibility. Other responses however such as the sympathetic skin responses show marked fatiguability with stimulus repetition.

For a particular stimulation procedure, the shape, latency, and amplitude of the recorded potentials are analysed. Morphologically, a particular response (or part of it) needs to be recognised as present or absent. The analysis of the shape of potentials is needed as an "identification" procedure to accurately determine the latency and amplitude of the response. The onset of the response (this is the case in M waves, MEP and sacral reflex testing) or the individual peaks of the potentials (usual in SEP assessment) is used to determine the latency. The amplitudes are analysed relative to the baseline or "peak to peak".

For further details, textbooks on clinical neurophysiology should be consulted such as Dumitru D. Electrodiagnostic Medicine. Philadelphia: Hanley & Belfus, Inc.1995, or Osselton J. Clinical Neurophysiology, Butterworth Heinemann: Oxford. 1995.

IV. CORRELATION OF NEUROPHYSIOLOGICAL PARAMETERS TO PATHOLOGY OF NERVES AND MUSCLES

1. Nerve Conduction, Evoked Potential and Reflex Studies

The electrophysiological responses obtained on stimulation are compound action potentials and relate to populations of biological units (neurones, axons, motor units, muscle fibres, etc.). It is always necessary to keep in mind which biological units one is referring to if one is characterising a lesion with the help of a neurophysiological test. If the onset of the potential is measured, the latency of a compound potential represents the fastest conduction through a particular neural channel. The amplitude of the compound potential correlates with the number of activated biological units. In theory, the amplitudes are the more relevant physiological parameter, as they tell us about the functional or structural loss of biological units. Unfortunately, amplitudes are also highly dependent on many poorly controllable technical factors. There is therefore considerable variability and as a consequence, such tests are often not sensitive. As a general rule, latency measurements depend less on technical factors but reflect little or nothing about the loss of biological units, either motor units or axons. (Figure 1).

Measurements of latencies and amplitudes of evoked potentials and reflex responses, including sympathetic skin responses, relate not only to conduction in peripheral and central neural pathways, but also to transsynaptic transmission.

2. Electromyography (EMG)

Knowledge of the structure and function of the motor unit is fundamental to understanding the application of EMG. Motor neurones, which innervate striated muscle, lie in the anterior horn of the spinal cord. Their cell bodies are relatively large and their axonal processes are correspondingly of large diameter and myelinated to allow rapid conduction of impulses. However the neurones which innervate the sphincters lie in Onuf's nucleus in the sacral spinal cord and are somewhat smaller than those innervating skeletal limb and trunk muscles. Within the muscle, the motor axon tapers and then branches to innervate muscle fibres, which are scattered throughout the muscle. The innervation is such that it is unlikely that muscle fibres, which are part of the same motor unit will be adjacent to one another (Figure 2). This dispersion of muscle fibres is said to be non-random, although the stage of development at which it occurs and the factors determi-

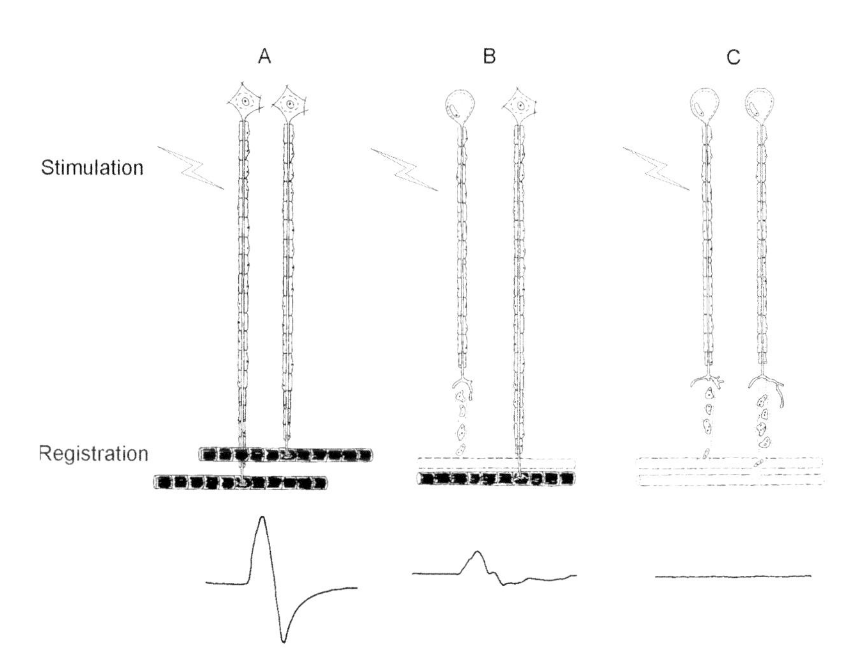

Figure 1 : Schematic representation of Compound Muscle Action Potential changes after a motor nerve lesion. On electrical stimulation of normal nerve (A) a "normal" response is obtained. In partial denervation (B) the response is smaller. In complete denervation (C) no response can be obtained. (Note that the latency of response in partial lesion may be normal due to preservation of nerve fibres with normal conduction).

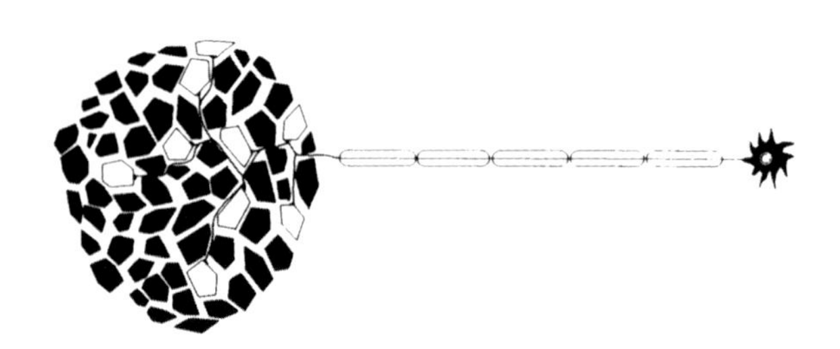

Figure 2 : Schematic representation of a motor unit. The alpha motor neuron with its cell body, its myelinated axon and the peripheral nerve endings is shown. The muscle fibres innervated by this alpha motor neuron are shown in white. (Note that the muscle fibres from one motor unit are intermingled with motor fibres from other motor units) (from [13], with permission).

ning the arrangement are not known [8]. The number of muscle fibres innervated by an axon is known as the "innervation ratio". There is no simple neurophysiological method for estimating this parameter, and the number of motor units per muscle is also difficult to estimate by clinical neurophysiological means particularly in the pelvic floor.

The contraction properties of a motor unit depend on the nature of its constituent muscle fibres. Muscle fibres can be classified according to their twitch tension, speed of contraction and histochemical staining properties. Although there is some regional variation, the pelvic floor muscles and sphincters consist predominantly of type 1 muscle fibres [9 10 11, 12]. The fatigue-resistant type 1 fibres constitute motor units, which conceivably fire for prolonged periods of time at lower firing frequencies (see below). There is no electrophysiologic method that has been shown to reliably test the presence and percentage of motor units of different muscle fibre types.

Denervated muscle fibres become hyperexcitable and start to fire spontaneously giving rise to "fibrillation" potentials, but these may take days or weeks to appear. Concentric needle EMG (CNEMG) correlates are abnormal pathologically prolonged insertion activity and pathological spontaneous activity. Completely denervated muscle may be reinnervated by axonal regrowth from the proximal nerve stump with few muscle fibres constituting "nascent" motor units. In partially denervated muscle, collateral reinnervation takes place. Surviving motor axons will sprout and grow out to reinnervate those muscle fibres that have lost their nerve supply. This results in a change in the arrangement of muscle fibres within the unit. Whereas in healthy muscle, it is unusual for two adjacent muscle fibres to be part of the same motor unit, following reinnervation, several muscle fibres, all belonging to the same motor unit, come to be adjacent to one another. CNEMG correlates are changes in motor unit potentials (MUPs) (duration, amplitude, number of phases, turns, etc); the single fibre EMG (SFEMG) correlate is increased fibre density. Early in the process of reinnervation, the newly outgrown motor sprouts are thin. Therefore, they conduct slowly such that the time taken for excitatory impulses to spread through the axonal tree is abnormally prolonged. Moreover, the neuromuscular transmission is insecure due to immaturity of the motor end-plates. CNEMG and SFEMG correlates are instability of long-duration complex potentials [13].

B. CLINICAL NEUROPHYSIOLOGICAL TESTS

The tests will be reviewed in order, looking at their aims, methods, technical performance, diagnostic performance and clinical value. Only specific issues shall be addressed herein, as others have been dealt with in the general section above or are dealt with in textbooks. Although this chapter does not attempt to be all-inclusive it does attempt to provide a substantial overview of previous and current important literature.

I. SOMATIC MOTOR SYSTEM TESTS

1. Electromyography (EMG)

The term "EMG" is often used for several different diagnostic procedures, the common denominator of which is the recording of bioelectrical activity from muscle. However used correctly the term applies to electromyographic recordings from striated muscles, often the urethral rhabdosphincter. EMG recorded to indicate the timing of a particular muscle's activity, (Figure 3) typically correlated to other urodynamic parameters such as bladder pressure and uroflow, has also been called kinesiological EMG to distinguish it from other types of diagnostic EMG procedures [14]. Kinesiological EMG signal can be recorded by various types of surface or intramuscular needle or wire electrodes.

EMG may also help in differentiating between normal, denervated, denervated and reinnervated and myopathic muscle and such EMG has also been called "motor unit" EMG which distinguishes it from "kinesiological". In the pelvic floor muscles, only neurogenic changes are well recognised and looked for in a routine evaluation.

The EMG signal may be further used to indicate that muscle has been activated through its motor nerve, either by stimulation applied to motor pathways (M wave, MEP) or to sensory pathways (reflex response).

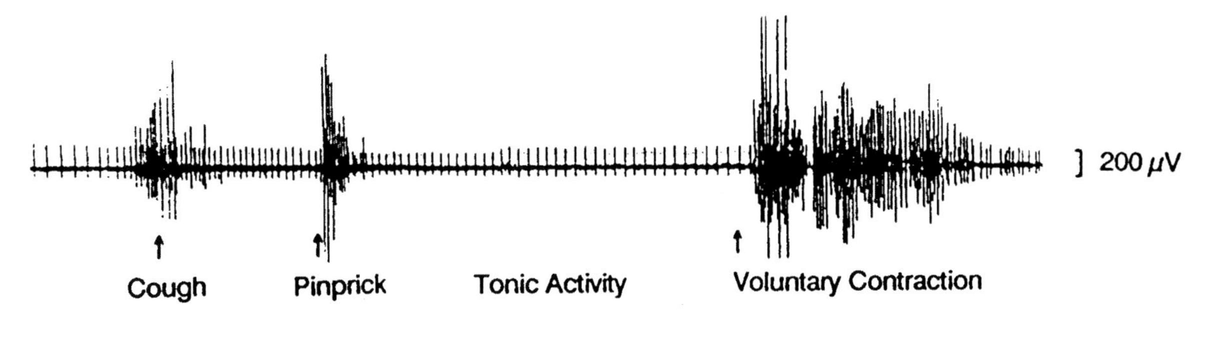

Figure 3 : Kinesiological EMG recording from the urethral sphincter muscle. Recruitment of motor units on reflex manoeuvres and on a command to contract is shown; regular continous activity of motor units represents "tonic activity". (Recorded with concentric needle electrode).

Intramuscular electrodes need to be appropriately placed in the target muscle. The external anal sphincter (EAS) is the most practical indicator muscle for lower sacral myotomes because it is easy to access, has enough muscle bulk for exact EMG analysis, and its examination is not too uncomfortable. The needle electrode should be inserted into the subcutaneous part of the EAS muscle, about 1-cm from the anal orifice, to a depth of a 3-6-mm under the mucosa non-keratinised epithelium. For the deeper part of the EAS muscle 1-3 cm deep insertions are made at the anal orifice, at an angle of about 30º to the anal canal axis [15]. Separate examination of the subcutaneous and the deeper part of the EAS muscle [16], as well as left and right EAS muscles are recommended. The needle is inserted into the middle of the anterior and posterior halves of each side ("quadrants") of the EAS muscle. The needle is – after insertion in two positions on each side – turned backwards and forwards in a systematic manner. At least 4 sites in each of the subcutaneous and/or the deeper parts of EAS muscle are thus analysed [15, 16].

The levator ani muscle can be located by transrectal or transvaginal palpation and reached transcutaneously from the perineum or transvaginally with the needle electrode. The male bulbocavernosus muscle can be inserted by needle electrode 2-3 cm in front of anal orifice, about 1 cm from middline. The female bulbocavernosus muscle can be reached either transmucosally, with a needle insertion medially to the labia minora, or through the skin lateral to the labia majora. The female urethral sphincter is anatomically separate from the pelvic floor musculature [17]. It can be approached either periurethrally, with a needle insertion 0.5 cm laterally to the urethral orifice, or it can be reached transvaginally, with the help of a speculum [18]. However a study which compared the transvaginal and periurethral route concluded that the latter is superior [19]. The male urethral sphincter is reached by the needle transcutaneously from the perineum, about 4 cm in front of anus. The needle is advanced towards the finger tip palpating the apex of prostate.

Most laboratories do not use local anaesthetics in any form before insertion of needle electrodes although some authors advocate using a local anaesthetic particularly for the examination of the female urethral sphincter from the perineum. This will prolong the examination time and interfere with concomitantly applied reflex studies.

As a rule, several sites from one or more skin penetrations are as a rule sampled in CNEMG and SFEMG. The audio output from the loudspeaker of the EMG apparatus helps in assessment of the quality of recording as well as in recognition of the electrophysiologic phenomena.

a) Kinesiological EMG

Kinesiological EMG is used to assess patterns of individual muscle activity/inactivity during defined manoeuvres (Figure 3) or during urodynamics. The diagnostic relevance of kinesiological EMG apart from polygraphic urodynamic recordings to assess detrusor/sphincter co-ordination is not yet established and there is no commonly accepted standardised method. When using surface electrodes there are problems related to validity of signal (e.g., artefacts, contamination from other muscles). With intramuscular electrodes, the procedure is more invasive, there are questions as to whether the whole muscle in large pelvic floor muscles is properly represented by the sampled muscle portions. The risks of this type of investigation relate to the type recording electrodes used; intramuscular electrodes carry a small risk of local bleeding. Infection must be avoided by following the manufacturer's recommendation for single use or sterilisation after use.

The kinesiological sphincter EMG recordings in health

show continuous activity of MUPs at rest, which may be increased voluntarily or reflexly. Such "tonic" activity has been recorded for up to two hours [20] and even after subjects have fallen asleep during the examination 21. It can be recorded in many but not all detection sites of the levator ani muscle [22], and the deeper part of the EAS muscle [16]. The urethral and anal sphincter as well as the pubococcigei can be voluntarily activated typically but only to full capacity for about 1 minute[22, 23].

Voiding in health is characterised by the cessation of all EMG activity in the urethral sphincter prior to detrusor contraction. Coordinated detrusor/sphincter activity is lost with lesions between the lower sacral segments and the upper pons so that the normal sphincter inhibition does not precede detrusor contractions but there is an increase in sphincter EMG activity during the detrusor contraction so called 'detrusor sphincter dyssynergia". On the basis of the temporal relationship between urethral sphincter and detrusor contractions, three types of dyssynergia have been described [24].

In young men with low urinary flow rates recording from the striated urethral sphincter may be helpful in demonstrating complete EMG silence during voiding, from which it may be concluded that their outflow obstruction is due to bladder neck smooth muscle.

Sphincter contraction or at least failure of relaxation during involuntary detrusor contractions was reported in patients with Parkinson's disease [25]. This neurogenic uncoordinated sphincter behaviour has to be differentiated from "voluntary" contractions that may occur in poorly compliant patients. The pelvic floor muscle contractions of the so-called non-neuropathic voiding dyssynergia may be a learned abnormal behaviour [26], and may be encountered in women and children with dysfunctional voiding [27].

The pubococcygeus in the normal female reveals similar activity patterns to the urethral and anal sphincters at most detection sites: continuous activity at rest, often some increase of activity during bladder filling, and reflex increases in activity during any activation manoeuvre performed by the subject such as talking, deep breathing, coughing. The pubococcygeus relaxes during voiding; the muscles on either side act in unison [22]. In stress-incontinent patients, the patterns of activation as well as the co-ordination between the two sides may be lost [28].

Little is known about the normal activity patterns of different pelvic floor muscles such as the urethral sphincter, urethrovaginal sphincter, anal sphincter muscle, different parts of the levator ani, although it is generally assumed that they all act in a co-ordinated fashion as one muscle. However differences have been demonstrated even between the intra- and peri-urethral sphincter in normal females [29] and co-ordinated behaviour is frequently lost in abnormal conditions; as has been shown for the levator ani, urethral, and anal sphincter [30, 31, 32, 33].

b) Concentric needle (CNE) EMG

The purpose of using CNE EMG is to differentiate normal from abnormal striated muscle.

The concentric needle electrode consists of a central insulated platinum wire which is inserted through a steel cannula and the tip ground to give an elliptical area of 580 x 150 μm. (Figure 4) This type of electrode has recording characteristics to record spike or near activity from about 20 muscle fibres [34]. The number of motor units recorded therefore depends both upon the local arrangement of muscle fibresmotor units within the motor unit muscle fascicle and the level of contraction of the muscle.

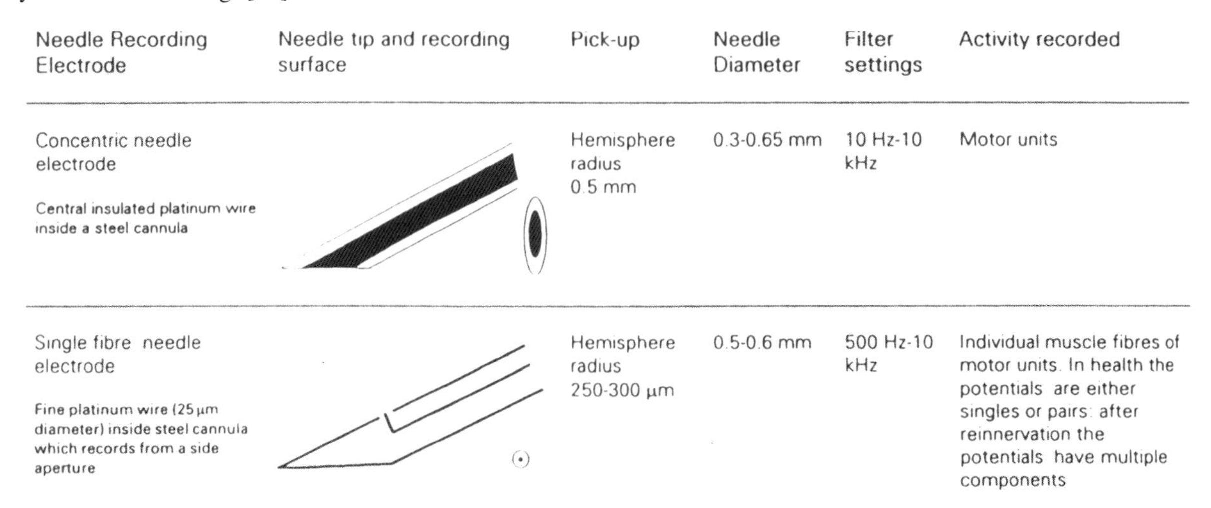

Needle Recording Electrode	Needle tip and recording surface	Pick-up	Needle Diameter	Filter settings	Activity recorded
Concentric needle electrode Central insulated platinum wire inside a steel cannula		Hemisphere radius 0.5 mm	0.3-0.65 mm	10 Hz-10 kHz	Motor units
Single fibre needle electrode Fine platinum wire (25 μm diameter) inside steel cannula which records from a side aperture		Hemisphere radius 250-300 μm	0.5-0.6 mm	500 Hz-10 kHz	Individual muscle fibres of motor units. In health the potentials are either singles or pairs: after reinnervation the potentials have multiple components

Figure 4 : The concentric needle electrode and the single-fibre needle electrode, their physical characteristics, the filter settings required for use and the nature of the activity that each records. (modified from [13]).

For the CNEMG examination one of the advanced EMG systems, which has the facility for quantitative template based MUP analysis (multi-MUP) and interference pattern (IP) analysis (turn/amplitude) is ideal. The commonly used amplifier filter settings for CNEMG are 5 Hz – 10 kHz, and need to be defined if MUP parameters are to be measured [35]. In case of published normative data, use of the filter settings employed during data acquisition is obligatory [36].

CNEMG can provide information on insertion activity, abnormal spontaneous activity, MUPs, and IP. The amount of recruitable motor units is estimated during voluntary and reflex activation. Normally, MUPs should intermingle to produce an "interference" pattern on the oscilloscope when muscle is contracted well, and during a strong cough. In addition number of continuously active MUPs during relaxation, MUP variability as well as MUP recruitment on reflex and voluntary activation can be observed.

In normal muscle, needle movement elicits a short burst of "insertion activity," which is due to mechanical stimulation of excitable membranes. This is recorded at a gain setting of 50 μV per division or cm (sweep speed 5-10 ms/division), which is also used to record spontaneous activity. Absence of insertion activity with appropriately placed needle electrode [15] will usually mean a complete atrophy of the examined muscle (after conus medullaris or cauda equina lesion, etc.).

MUPs are the only normal activity recorded with a resting electrode in sphincter muscles in a relaxed subject. This is contrast to limb muscles where complete electrical EMG silence can be achieved by relaxation. In addition to "tonic" continuously firing of motor units in sphincters, new MUPs are recruited voluntarily and reflexly. It has been shown that the two MUP populations differ in their characteristics: reflexly or voluntarily activated "high-threshold MUPs" being larger than continuously active low-threshold MUPs. As a consequence, standardised level of activity at which a template based multi-MUP analysis obtains 3-5 MUPs on a single muscle site was suggested [37].

In partially denervated sphincter muscle there is – by definition – a loss of motor units (MUs). This is difficult to establish, however, as the recruitment of MUs is dependent on patient co-operation. In women it is often achieved only with some difficulty. The parameters of a) a reduced number of activated MUs and of b) activation of MUs at increased firing rates as occurs in limb muscles has been little studied. The main obstacle to qualified assessment of these parameters is a lack of concomitant measurement of level of contraction, which although this can be readily assessed by the electromyographer when studying limb muscles requires expertise at digital examination to test power of pubococcygeus or the EAS.

There are two approaches to analysis of the bioelectrical activity of motor units, either analysis of individual MUPs or analysis of the overall activity of intermingled MUPs (the "interference pattern") (Figure 5). Generally 3 techniques of MUP analysis (manual-MUP, single-MUP and multi-MUP) and 1 technique of IP analysis (turn/amplitude – T/A) are available on advanced EMG systems.

The first technique of MUP analysis follows an algorithm similar to the original protocol used by Buchthal and his school [38], who measured MUP duration and amplitude from paper prints made from oscilloscope. In advanced EMG systems instead of measurements from the paper, MUPs are analysed from the screen. Several seconds of continuous EMG activity during relaxation or at slight reflex/voluntary activation from an individual site are "frozen" on the screen. Signals are then visually examined for the content of individual MUPs, which may then be measured automatically by the EMG system. Although duration cursors are set automatically by the EMG system, they should always be checked and reset by the operator if necessary. Using this modified "manual-MUP" analysis the highest number of MUPs (up to 10) can be obtained from the particular examination site. It takes 2-3 minutes for each site to be analysed. This technique is demanding for the operator because reproducible MUPs have to be identified, the one with the smoothest baseline chosen, and in most cases the duration cursors set by the operator manually. The technique is inevitably open to personal bias, especially the determination of MUP duration. At slightly higher levels of voluntary or reflex activation the baseline becomes unsteady, making the technique unreliable – it can be applied only at low levels of activity [39].

The introduction of the trigger and delay unit led to its widespread use for MUP analysis (Figure 6) [40]. During a constant level of EMG activity the trigger unit is set (on each examination site) on the highest amplitude steadily firing MUP. The triggered MUP is averaged until the baseline becomes smooth, which takes about 1-min for each MUP. At each site 1-3 MUPs can usually be obtained. Single-MUP analysis is quite time consuming, and provides fewer MUPs than the previously described technique. It is biased towards high amplitude and high threshold MUPs, and furthermore to personal bias as far as the choice of MUP [39]. However, single-MUP analysis is still the technique that is currently most often used in quantitative analysis of MUPs, because it is widely available for a number of years.

The most recent and sophisticated CNEMG techniques are available only on advanced EMG systems; such is the template operated "multi-MUP" analysis [41]. Here, the operator indicates – during the appropriate level of the crisp EMG activity – when the computer takes the previous (last) 4.8-sec period of the signal. From that signal MUPs are automatically extracted, quantified and sorted into 1-6 classes [41]. Each class represents consecutive discharges of a particular MUP. MUP classes are then averaged and presented (in descending order) according to the number of MUP discharges in the analysed period [41]. Cursors are set automatically using a computer algorithm. The operator has to edit the MUPs; duplicates (MUPs that appear more than once) and "problematic" MUPs (with unclear beginning or the end because of unsteady baseline) are discarded. Thus on each examination site 1-6 different MUPs can be obtained using this technique [36]. Multi–MUP analysis is the fastest and the easiest to apply of the three mentioned quantitative MUP analysis techniques. It can be applied at continuous activity during sphincter muscle relaxation, as well as at slight to moderate levels of activation [37]. Cursors are set automatically, and only exceptionally manual correction is needed. It is suggested that such problematic MUPs, with unsteady baseline and unclear beginning or end, are better discarded [36]. The multi–MUP technique has, however, difficulties with highly unstable and/or polyphasic MUPs found particularly in patients with lower motor neurone lesions; it often fails to sample them, distorts them by averaging, or sorts the same MUP to several classes (recognises it as different MUPs – duplicates). Multi-MUP samples slightly lower number of MUPs per muscle, compared to manual-MUP [39].

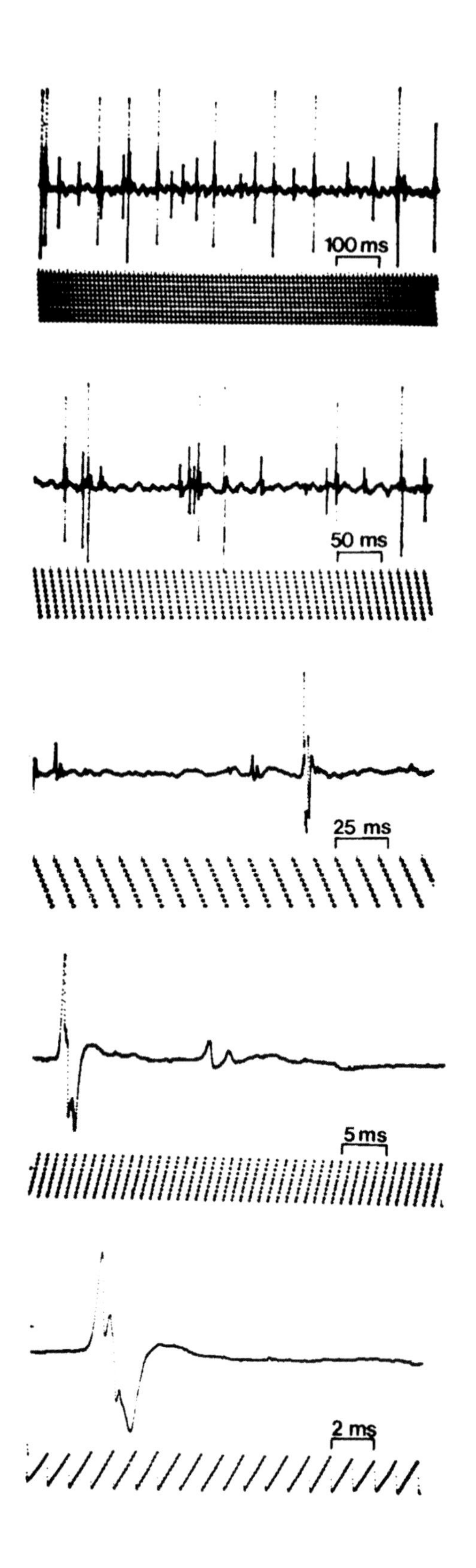

Figure 5 : EMG activity as recorded with concentric needle electrode is shown using different time scales to demonstrate how a Motor Unit Potential for analysis (lowermost row) can be "extracted" from the EMG signal. Uppermost row shows overall ("kinesiological") EMG activity in the contracting muscle. (From [13], with permission).

In the small half of the sphincter muscle collecting ten different MUPs has been said to be a minimal requirement on using "single-MUP" analysis. Using manual-MUP and multi-MUP techniques sampling of 20 MUPs (standard number in limb muscles) from each part of the EAS makes no difficulty in healthy controls [36] and most of patients [39]. Normative data obtained from the EAS muscle by standardised EMG technique using multi-MUP analysis have been published [36] (Figure 7).

Several MUP parameters have proven empirically useful in examining limb muscles in the diagnosis of neuromuscular disease. Traditionally, amplitude, duration were measured, and the number of phases counted [38]. Amplitude is the voltage (mV) difference between the most positive and most negative point on the MUP trace (Figure 6). The amplitude of MUPs is largely determined by the activity of those muscle fibres closest (within a 0.5 mm radius) to the recording electrode, where in the normal MU it is unlikely to find more than 2-3 muscle fibres [34]. It is highly sensitive to needle position and even minor adjustments of the electrode result in major amplitude changes, i.e. a change in position by 0.5 mm alters the amplitude 10-100 fold. The

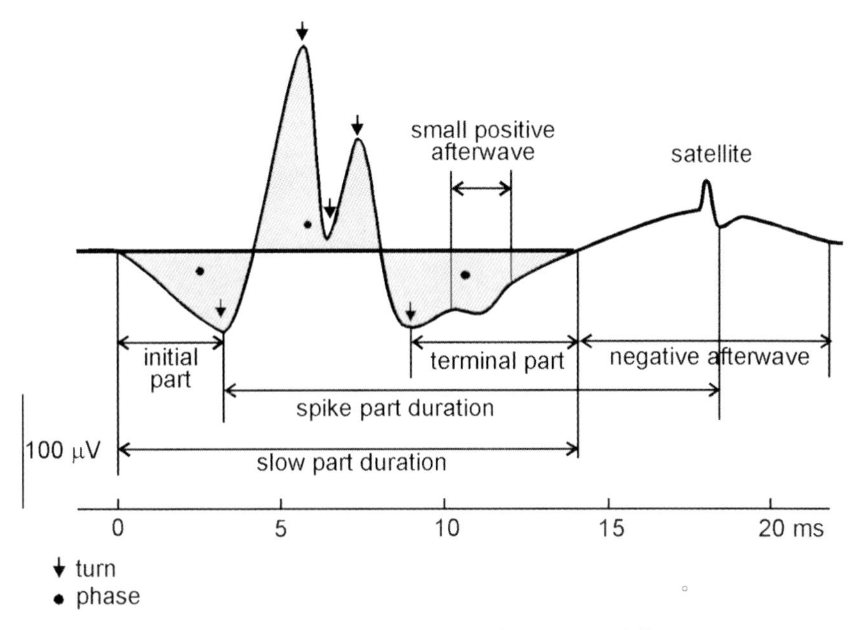

Figure 6 : Schematic representation of the Motor Unit Potential to demonstrate different components, and parameters analysed (modified from [35]).

MUP duration is the time (ms) between the first deflection and the point when MUP waveform finally returns to the baseline. It depends on the number of muscle fibres of particular MU within 2-3 mm diameter and is little affected by the proximity of the recording electrode to the nearest fibre [34]. The difficulty with duration measurement is in definition of the beginning and end of MUP. Using manual positioning of duration cursors depends on amplifier gain: at higher gain MUPs seem longer. Advanced EMG systems use algorithms including besides minimal amplitude of the trace deflection also the angle of the MUP trace towards the baseline [41]. It was agreed for automated analysis not to include late MUP components (defined "satellite" potentials" i.e. part of MUP starting at least 3 ms after the end of main part of the MUP [41], [35, 7]. However extreme prolongation of motor units by small, late potentials, often with an intervening isoelectric period are a common finding in some pathological conditions affecting the innervation of the anal sphincter and have therefore been included in manual methods of analysis [42].

The number of MUP phases is defined by the number of times the potential crosses the baseline. It is counted as "number of baseline crossings plus one" (Figure 6) [35, 43]. Number of phases or percentage of polyphasic MUPs in muscle can be determined. MUPs are usually called polyphasic when they have at least four phases (mono-, bi-, tri-, and polyphasic), although some authors have defined "polyphasic" as those MUPs having more than four [44], or even more than five phases [45]. Related to the number of phases is the MUP parameter "number of turns". A turn is defined as a change in direction of the MUP trace, which is larger than specified amplitude but not crossing the baseline. Number of turns is MUP parameter particularly sensitive to reinnervation changes in small muscles such as the EAS [36].

With the on-line computer analysis available on advanced EMG systems a number of further MUP parameters are available, including MUP area, rise time of negative peak, duration of negative peak can be measured [41 36]. In addition, "thickness" (thickness = area/amplitude) [46] and size index (size index = 2*log (amplitude (mV)) + area/amplitude) [47] can be automatically calculated. Development of these parameters resulted from studies aimed at finding MUP parameters that would better differentiate between normal and myopathic (thickness) [46], as well as normal and neuropathic muscles (size index) [47]. Thickness can be imagined as a base of the triangle, which presents a simplified MUP (its surface being area, and its height being amplitude) [46]. Myopathic MUPs are indeed distinguished from normal MUPs by their shortness and "lesser thickness" on quantitative EMG. Size index can be seen as a "normalised" thickness – in contrast to thickness it is not dependant on position of the electrode. It is formed of two parts, of which the first (logarithm of amplitude) increases, and thus counteracts the second (area/amplitude = thickness) that decreases on the electrode approach to the muscle fibres [47]. The applications of these methods to the sphincter have yet to be defined.

At higher levels of voluntary and reflex activation, normally a dense interference pattern (IP) can be seen. The IP can also be assessed using a number of automatic quantitative analyses, the turn/amplitude (T/A) analysis

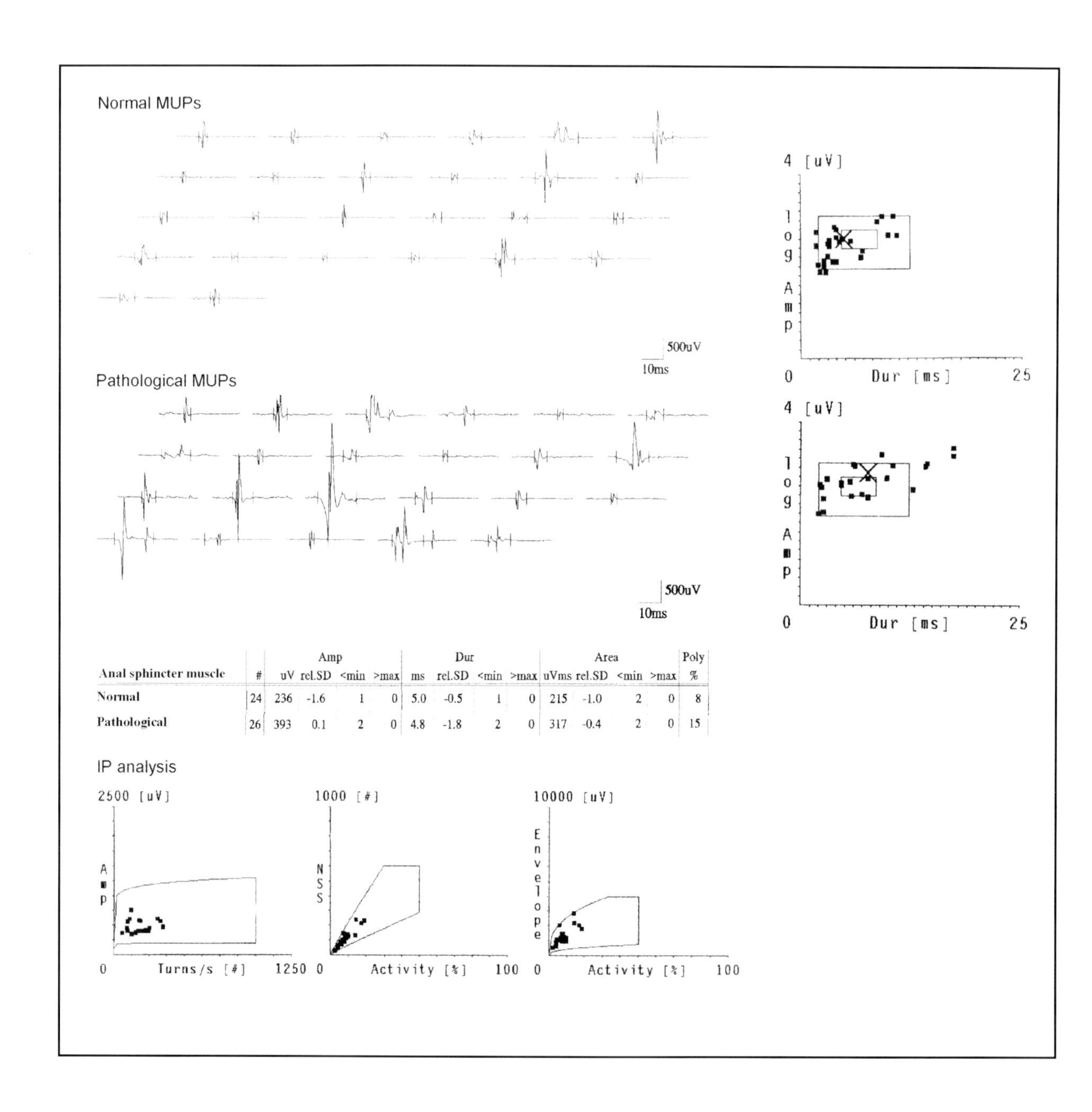

Anal sphincter muscle	#	Amp uV	Amp rel.SD	Amp <min	Amp >max	Dur ms	Dur rel.SD	Dur <min	Dur >max	Area uVms	Area rel.SD	Area <min	Area >max	Poly %
Normal	24	236	-1.6	1	0	5.0	-0.5	1	0	215	-1.0	2	0	8
Pathological	26	393	0.1	2	0	4.8	-1.8	2	0	317	-0.4	2	0	15

***Figure 7 :** Comparison of normal (above) and pathological (below) motor unit potentials (MUPs) sampled by multi-MUP analysis from the right halves of the subcutaneous parts of the external anal sphincter (EAS) muscles. To the right logarithm (amplitude) vs. duration plots of the MUPs are shown; the inner rectangle presents normative range for mean values, and the outer rectangle for "outliers". Below the MUP samples values are tabulated. Three plots on the bottom were obtained by turn/amplitude analysis in the cauda equina patient. Delineated areas ("clouds") present the normative range, and dots individual IP samples.*

The normal subject was a 45-year-old woman without pelvic floor dysfunction or abnormalities on neurological examination. Results of MUP and interference pattern (IP) analysis were normal. The pathological sample was obtained from a 36-year old man with damage of the cauda equina caused by central herniation of the intervertebral disc 13 months before the examination. On clinical examination perianal sensation was severely diminished bilaterally. No spontaneous denervation activity was present at the time of the above recording. Mean values for MUP amplitude and area are above normative range, and polyphasicity is increased. In addition, for all presented MUP parameters individual values of more than 2 MUPs are above the "outlier" limits (Table). Note that IP analysis in the patient is within normative range in spite of marked MUP abnormalities.

being the most popular [48, 49]. On applying T/A analysis, with the needle electrode in focus, subjects contract muscle voluntarily or reflexly by coughing. Examiner selects 0.5-sec time epochs of the crisp EMG signal to be analysed. IP parameters evaluated are: number of turns/second, amplitude/turn [48], % activity, number of short segments (NSS), and envelope [49]. These are measured automatically by the EMG system. "Turns" are defined as every minimum or maximum of the signal where it changes direction (i.e., constitutes a peak or trough), and the signal amplitude changes by at least 100 μV compared to the preceding and subsequent turns. Turns are counted (turns/sec; N/sec), and amplitudes between turns measured (amplitude/turn; (V) [48]. The "envelope" (μ(V) is determined as that peak-to-peak amplitude which is exceeded by only 1% of peaks and 1% of troughs in the analysed time epoch [49]. In addition, parts of the EMG signal with sharp activity (containing MUPs) are determined and NSS counted (N), and percentage of time with such sharp activity within the whole time epoch is determined ("% activity") [49]. Samples with positive values of all IP parameters are accepted for further analysis (0 values of IP parameters are interpreted as being caused by either weak contraction, or needle electrode outside the muscle). On applying T/A analysis during maximal contraction displacement of the needle electrode by a contralateral buttock is occasionally a problem, especially in muscular men. Sampling of IPs using T/A analysis is even faster than multi-MUP analysis [36]. However, sensitivity of IP analysis for detecting neuropathic changes in the EAS muscle of patients with chronic sequels after cauda equina or conus medullaris damage, is only about half of sensitivities of different MUP analysis techniques [39].

Both the template based multi-MUP analysis of MUP and T/A analysis of IP are fast (5-10 and 2-3 minutes per muscle, respectively), easy to apply, and, technically, represent clinically useful techniques. Use of quantitative MUP and IP analyses of the EAS is further facilitated by the availability of normative values [36] (Podnar et al., normative data (that can be introduced into the EMG systems' software. It has been shown that normative data are not significantly affected by age, gender [36], number of uncomplicated vaginal deliveries [50], mild chronic constipation [51], and the part i.e. subcutaneous or deeper part of the EAS muscle examined [16]. This makes quantitative analysis much simpler.

Although EMG abnormalities are detected as a result of a host of different lesions and diseases, there are in principle only two standard manifestations which can occur: a) disease of the muscle fibres themselves, and b) changes in their innervation.

• CNEMG FINDINGS DUE TO DENERVATION

After complete denervation, all motor unit activity ceases. In a denervated muscle, complete "electrical silence" is noted in the first days after such an event. The diagnosis of complete denervation also requires electrical stimulation of the relevant motor nerve to demonstrate absence of muscle response. Because motor axons take days to degenerate after injury, this proof is not available for up to 5-7 days after a denervation injury. Demonstration of complete denervation in the acute stage is rarely required because the clinical condition is usually obvious.

Ten to twenty days after the denervation, the "insertion activity" becomes longer prolonged and abnormal spontaneous activity appears in the form of short biphasic spikes (fibrillation potentials) and biphasic potentials with prominent positive deflections (positive sharp waves) (Figure 8). In perineal muscles, complete denervation can be observed after traumatic lesions to the lumbosacral spine or particularly to the pelvis but most lesions (including trauma) however, cause partial denervation [39]. In partially denervated sphincter muscle there is — by definition — a loss of motor units, but this is difficult to establish, as was already discussed.

With axonal reinnervation, MUPs appear again; first they are short, bi- and triphasic, soon becoming polyphasic, serrated and with prolonged duration [44]. In

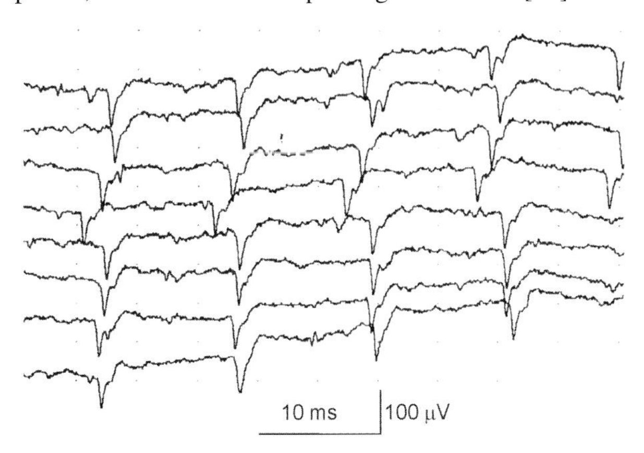

Figure 8 : Concentric needle EMG recording from right bulbocavernosus muscle of a 49-years old male. Pathological spontaneous activity (a burst of positive sharp waves) is shown.
The happily married and otherwise healthy man presented with a one year history of progressive erectile dysfunction, which became complete (no erections on attempted intercourse, masturbation; no morning erections). He recently became aware of slight gait insecurity. Signs of mild cerebellar ataxia and bilateral Babinski signs were present on examination, neuroimaging was negative. A diagnosis of possible Multiple System Atrophy was made. The diagnosis was supported by development of slight parkinsonism and urge incontinence at follow up after six months.

partially denervated muscle, some MUPs remain and mingle eventually with abnormal spontaneous activity.. In degenerative conditions, this probably begins to occurs already during the phase of subclinical sphincter involvement. As the MUPs in sphincter muscles are also short and mostly bi- or tri-phasic, as is pathological spontaneous activity, it takes some experience to differentiate fibrillations from motor unit activity. The bulbocavernosus muscle is particularly useful for examining in men with suspected recent minor partial denervation as it lacks on-going activity of low-threshold MU during relaxation although in women it can be difficult to localise the muscle and it may have more tonic activity. Therefore it is the most appropriate muscle of the lower sacral myotomes to look for fibrillation potentials and positive sharp waves. Abnormal spontaneous activity has in one report been described as the most specific marker for neuronal degeneration of Onuf's nucleus occurring in patients with Multiple System Atrophy (MSA), thus differentiating them from patients with idiopathic Parkinson's Disease [43].

Changes due to collateral reinervation are reflected by: prolongation of the wave form of the MUP (Figure 9) which may have small, late components ("satellite potentials"). MUPs show "instability" due to insecure transmission in newly formed axon sprouts and endplates. This "instability of potentials" (meaning both "jitter" and "blocking" of individual components in a complex potential) is not being assessed in routine sphincter EMG, as demonstrated in published reports.

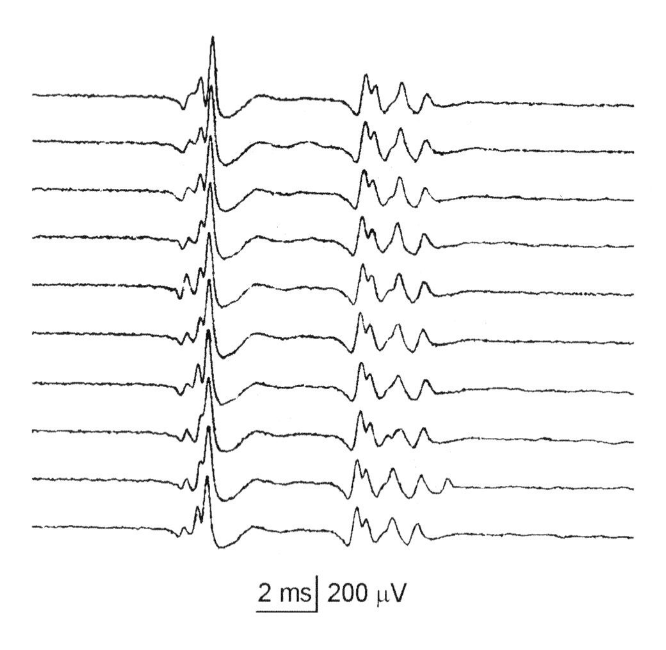

Figure 9 : Concentric needle EMG recording from the external anal sphincter from the same patient as in Fig. 8. A polyphasic motor unit potential of prolonged duration is shown. Overall, the percentage of polyphasic potentials was 50 %.

Nonetheless, it can be a helpful parameter, and may be evaluated not only by SFEMG, as originally described [52], but also by CNEMG, if a low frequency cut-off filter of 0.5 (up to 2) kHz is used along with a trigger - delay unit [53]. In skeletal muscle, with time and provided there is no further deterioration in innervation, the reinnervating axonal sprouts increase in diameter and thus increase their conduction velocity so that activation of all parts of the reinnervated motor unit become more synchronous. This increases the amplitude and reduces the duration of the MUPs towards normal measured with CNEMG. This phenomenon may be different in sphincter muscles where long duration motor units seem to be a prominent feature of reinnervated motor units in MSA [42] (Figures 9 and 10) although the effect of the relentless ongoing motor neurone atrophying process which characterises the disease may also be a factor.

c) Single fibre EMG

The SFEMG electrode has similar external proportions to a concentric needle electrode, being made of a steel cannula 0.5 - 0.6 mm in diameter with a bevelled tip (Figure 4). However, instead of having the recording surface at the tip, a fine insulated platinum or silver wire embedded in epoxy resin is exposed through an aperture on the side 1 - 5 mm behind the tip. The platinum wire forms the recording surface and has a diameter of 25 µm. It will pick up activity from within a hemispherical area 300 µm in diameter. This is very much smaller than the volume of muscle tissue from which a concentric needle electrode records, which has an uptake area of 1 mm diameter. Because of the arrangement of muscle fibres in a normal motor unit, a SFEMG needle will record only 1 - 3 single muscle fibres from the same motor unit. When recording with a SFEMG needle, the amplifier filters are set so that low frequency activity is eliminated (500 Hz - 10 kHz). Thus, the contribution of each muscle fibre appears as a short biphasic positive-negative action potential (Figure 11).

The SFEMG parameter that reflects motor unit morphology is the so-called "fibre density," which is defined as the mean number of muscle fibres belonging to an individual motor unit per detection site. To assemble this data, recordings from 20 different intramuscular detection sites are necessary [52]. The normal fibre density for the EAS is below 2.0 [54, 55, 56]. Changes with age have been reported [57], showing women, corrected for parity, have significantly greater fibre density than men [54].

The SFEMG electrode is also most suitable to record any instability of MUPs. However, this "jitter" measurement [52] is not routinely performed in pelvic floor muscles for diagnostic purposes.

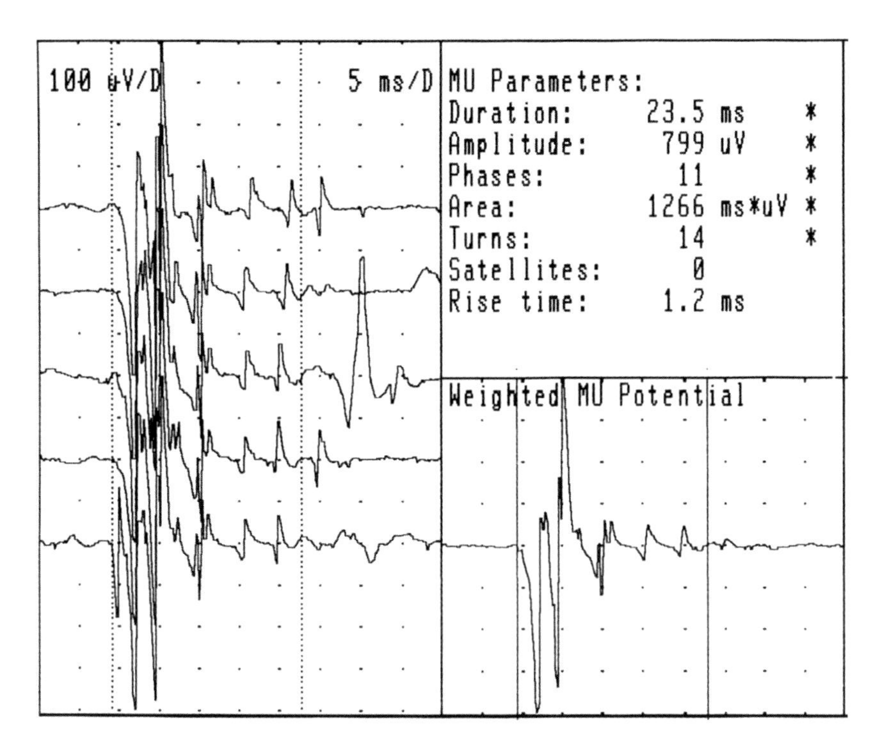

Figure 10 : A motor unit recorded from the striated anal sphincter of a woman of 53 diagnosed with probable Multiple System Atrophy. On the left the same motor unit which was captured using a trigger and delay line is shown repeatedly in falling leaf display. The insert shows the "weighted mu potential", which is a summary derived from the 5 most similar waveforms identified from a stored buffer of a large number of the recorded potential (not shown). The cursors are set to measure the duration, which in this instance is 23.5 ms.

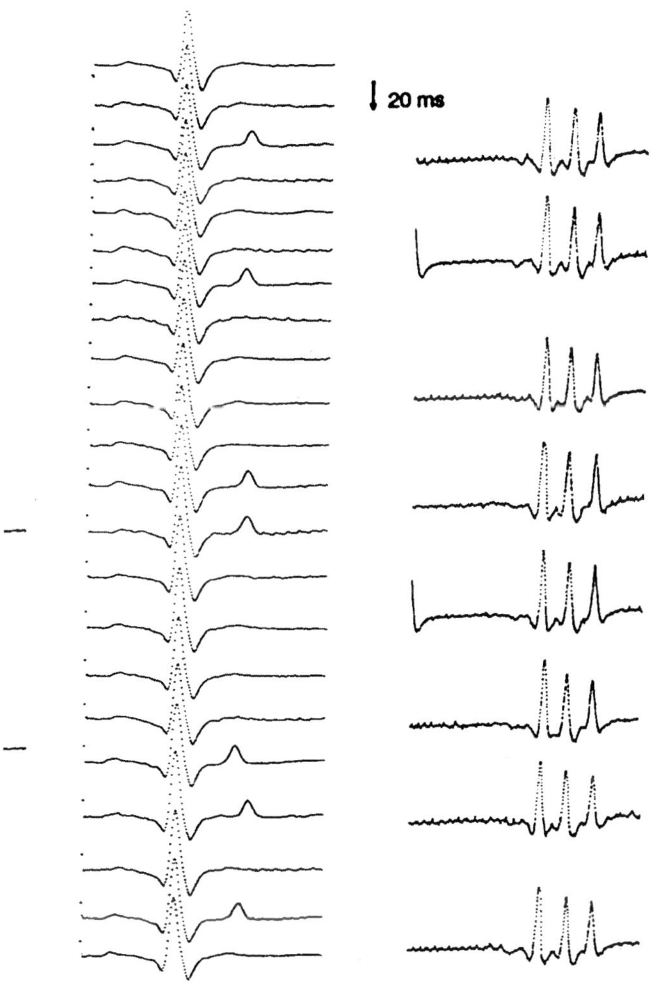

Figure 11 : Single-fibre EMG recording from the urethral sphincter of a 55 year old woman with urinary incontinence after pelvic surgery. Centre: "falling leaf" recording of a continuously firing ("tonic") motor unit, as represented by the two muscle fibre potentials. The second potential shows increased neuromuscular "jitter" and intermittent blocking; two superimpositions of ten consecutive discharges are shown on the left. Right: another "falling leaf" recording of a continuously firing motor unit, represented by three muscle fibre potentials (fibre density in this muscle was 2.2 muscle fibres per recording site). (From 14, with permission).

• **SFEMG FINDINGS IN REINNERVATED MUSCLE**

Due to the previously discussed changes in motor unit morphology, the fibre density is increased in reinnervated muscle. The method was applied to sphincter muscles in order to correlate increased fibre density findings to incontinence [56, 58].

Due to its technical characteristics, a SFEMG electrode is able to record even small changes that occur in motor units due to reinnervation, but is less suitable to detect changes due to denervation itself (i.e. abnormal insertion and spontaneous activity). SFEMG is not now widely practised in general clinical neurophysiological laboratories and the recording needles are very expensive.

d) EMG in clinical disorders

All described tests are invasive and some pain is inevitable, even with use of local anaesthetics. Additionally, all tests need considerable theoretical and practical training. It should be stressed that all abnormalities of parameters evaluated by CNEMG and SFEMG are in principle "nonspecific", i.e. almost abnormalities can occur both in neuropathic or myopathic conditions. It is the overall clinical picture, which dictates interpretation of results.

Many reports have been published on findings with either CNEMG or SFEMG in particular pathologic conditions and these will be discussed together, as the underlying pathology is the same, only reflected in a different way by the two EMG methods.

• **REINNERVATION (MULTIPLE SYSTEM ATROPHY AND CAUDA EQUINA LESIONS)**

There are several conditions in which gross changes of reinnervation may be detected in motor units of the pelvic floor. Following a cauda equina lesion, the MUP are likely to be prolonged and polyphasic [45], of increased amplitude, area, number of turns, spike duration, thickness, size index [39], and similar marked changes are seen in patients with lumbosacral myelomeningocoelae. Traumatic or surgical dissections can also affect the innervation of the sphincter and lead to loss of motor units and reinnervation of those surviving [12].

Definite "neuropathic" changes can be recorded in sphincter muscles of patients with Multiple System Atrophy (MSA), the condition formerly called "Shy-Drager syndrome" [42, 59, 60, 61, 62] (Figures 9 and 10). MSA is a progressive neurodegenerative disease, which is often, particularly in its early stages, mistaken for Parkinson's Disease. Urinary incontinence occurs early in this condition, often some years before the onset of obvious neurological features [63]. Sphincter EMG has been claimed to be of value in distinguishing between idiopathic Parkinson's Disease and MSA [42, 59, 64], but changes may be absent in the early phase of disease [65]. A recommended algorithm for neurophysiological investigation is shown in Algorithm 1. Sphincter abnormalities can also be demonstrated as a definite increase in fibre density on SFEMG, as shown by concomitant CNEMG and SFEMG recordings in patients with MSA [64]. However, CNEMG sphincter abnormalities may also be found in another parkinsonian syndrome, the Progressive Supranuclear Palsy [66].

The role of EMG in distinguishing MSA from idiopathic Parkinson's disease and other extrapyramidal diseases is thus an area of current controversy, but – bearing in mind recent data that sphincter EMG abnormalities are to a large extent absent early on in Parkinson's disease [67] – the present position of the authors is as follows. Anal sphincter EMG abnormalities (abnormal spontaneous activity or motor unit potential changes 3 standard deviations above valid control data) distinguish MSA from PD in the first five years after the onset of symptoms and signs and from pure autonomic failure, as well as from cerebellar ataxias, if other causes for sphincter denervation have been ruled out. It should be mentioned that with such criteria the sensitivity of the method is expected to be low. Extensive discussion on the subject can be found in Vodusek 2001 [68].

The sensitivity and specificity of different EMG techniques to reveal a) denervation, and b) reinnervation, have not been systematically investigated. Concerning b) analysis made from the same taped EMG signal, using reference data for mean values and "outliers" [69] revealed similar sensitivity (~ 60%) of all three mentioned MUP analysis techniques (manual-MUP, single-MUP, multi-MUP) for detecting neuropathic changes in the EAS muscle of patients with chronic sequels after cauda equina or conus medullaris lesions. Sensitivity of T/A analysis of IP was shown to be only half of this [39]. In that study muscle was regarded abnormal when any of MUP/IP parameters was outside the confidence limits [39]. This favoured MUP analysis having a higher number parameters (eight), compared to IP analysis (three T/A plots). In addition, on MUP analysis mean value, as well as use "outlier" [69] criteria for abnormality were applied [39]. A recommended algorithm for neurophysiological investigation in a case of suspected cauda equina lesion is shown in Algorithm 2.

• **EMG CHANGES IN STRESS INCONTINENCE**

Pelvic floor muscle denervation was proposed as being central in the genesis of genuine stress incontinence (GSI) [70] and EMG techniques have been used to look for lesions following childbirth and in the assessment of women with GSI. SFEMG was used to measure fibre density in the EAS and an increase was demonstrated in women with urinary stress incontinence [71]. A relationship between stress incontinence, genitourinary

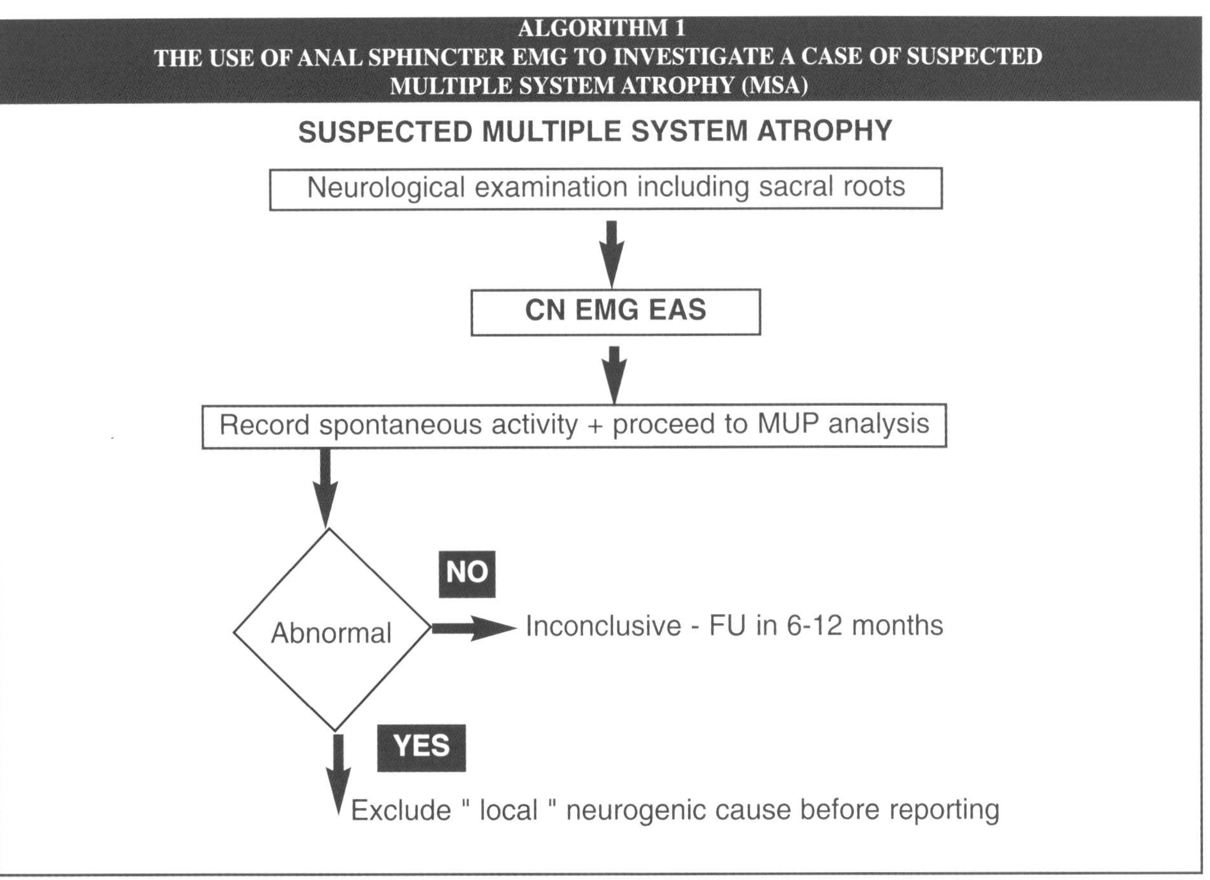
ALGORITHM 1
THE USE OF ANAL SPHINCTER EMG TO INVESTIGATE A CASE OF SUSPECTED MULTIPLE SYSTEM ATROPHY (MSA)
SUSPECTED MULTIPLE SYSTEM ATROPHY
Neurological examination including sacral roots
CN EMG EAS
Record spontaneous activity + proceed to MUP analysis
Abnormal
NO
Inconclusive - FU in 6-12 months
YES
Exclude " local " neurogenic cause before reporting

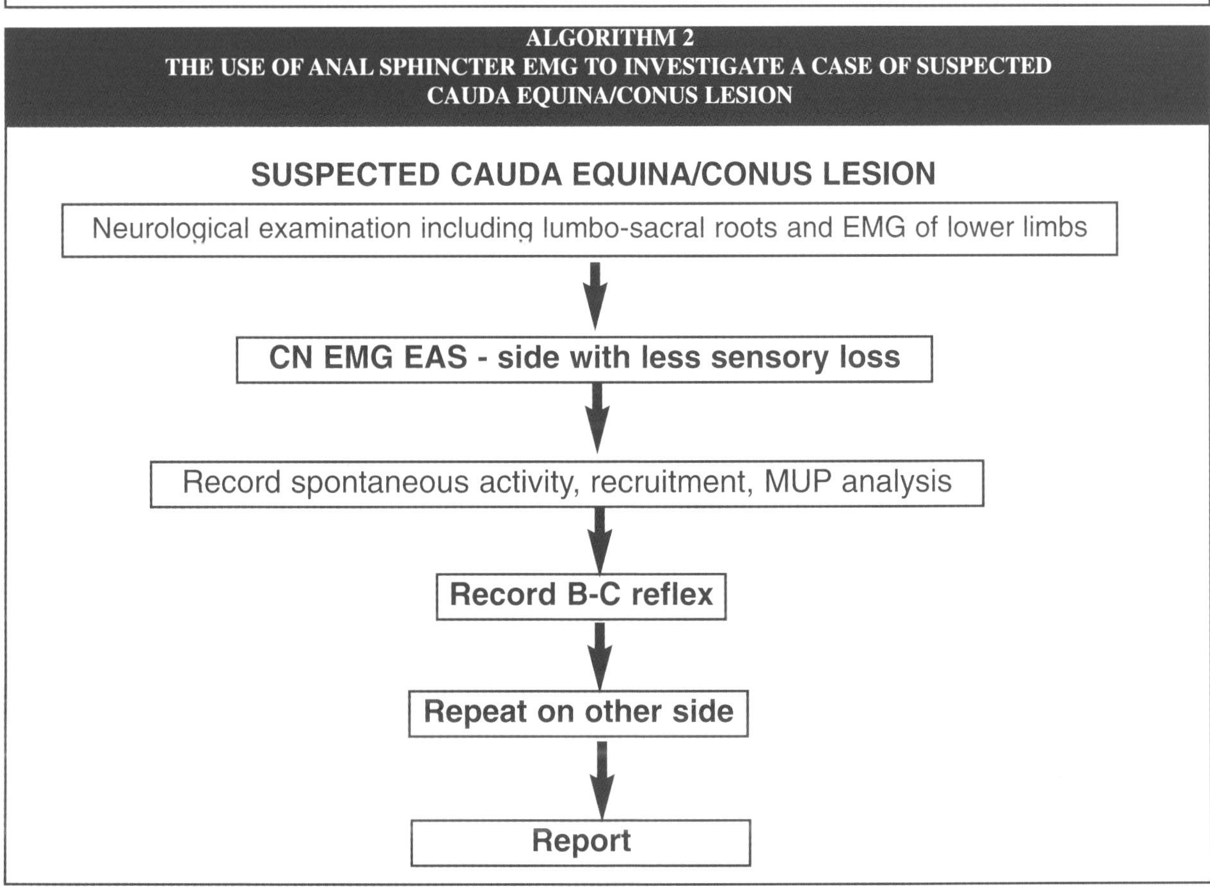
ALGORITHM 2
THE USE OF ANAL SPHINCTER EMG TO INVESTIGATE A CASE OF SUSPECTED CAUDA EQUINA/CONUS LESION
SUSPECTED CAUDA EQUINA/CONUS LESION
Neurological examination including lumbo-sacral roots and EMG of lower limbs
CN EMG EAS - side with less sensory loss
Record spontaneous activity, recruitment, MUP analysis
Record B-C reflex
Repeat on other side
Report

prolapse and partial denervation of the pelvic floor has been demonstrated, and it was concluded that pubococcygeus is partially denervated and then reinnervated in women with stress incontinence, genital prolapse or both [72]. Using CNEMG to examine pubococcygeus following childbirth, a significant increase in duration of individual motor units following labour and vaginal delivery has been found [73]. The changes were most marked in women who had urinary incontinence 8 weeks after delivery and who had had a prolonged second stage and had given birth to heavier babies.

However the practical value of the urethral sphincter CNEMG in women with urinary incontinence is not defined. Although CNEMG of the urethral sphincter seems the logical choice in patients with urinary incontinence of possibly neurogenic origin, only a small amount of pathological muscle tissue remains in many incontinent parous women [12]. This finding, as a rule, will not affect therapeutic considerations, which rely primarily on generalised involvement of pelvic floor innervation as may be revealed by CNEMG of the EAS muscle. However there have been recent reports of the use of urethral sphincter EMG to assist in the determination of the type of surgery to employ in patients with urodynamic diagnosis of intrinsic sphincter deficiency [74].

- **CNEMG FINDINGS IN WOMEN WITH URINARY RETENTION**

The striated urethral sphincter appears to be peculiarly likely to develop abnormal spontaneous complex repetitive discharge activity. This is made up of repetitively firing groups of potentials with so little "jitter" between the potentials that it is deduced the activity must be due to ephaptic or direct transmission of impulses between muscle fibres [75, 13]. Such activity may be found in chronically partially denervated sphincters with an otherwise reduced interference pattern (IP) of motor units and has been reported to be present in a proportion of asymptomatic women [76, 77]. The activity may be provoked by needle movement, or muscle contraction, or may occur spontaneously, rhythmically. However in young women with urinary retention or obstructed voiding it may be found in profuse amounts against a full background of rapidly firing motor units [78]. In these cases the pathological spontaneous activity has been called "decelerating bursts and complex repetitive discharges" [79] (Figure 12) and the similarity of the sound it produces over the audio-amplifier to the song of whales recorded under water is striking [80]. The problem for the electromyographer is to decide if the "amount" of EMG abnormality is sufficient to account for the voiding disorder. Corroborative information about the urethral sphincter function is therefore valuable and measurement of the urethral pressure profile appears to be a useful adjunct, since those with the EMG abnormality have higher mean urethral closure pressures than those who do not [81], suggesting a local disorder of contraction/relaxation. An algorithm for investigation of women in retention is shown in Algorithm 3. It has been argued that urethral sphincter EMG

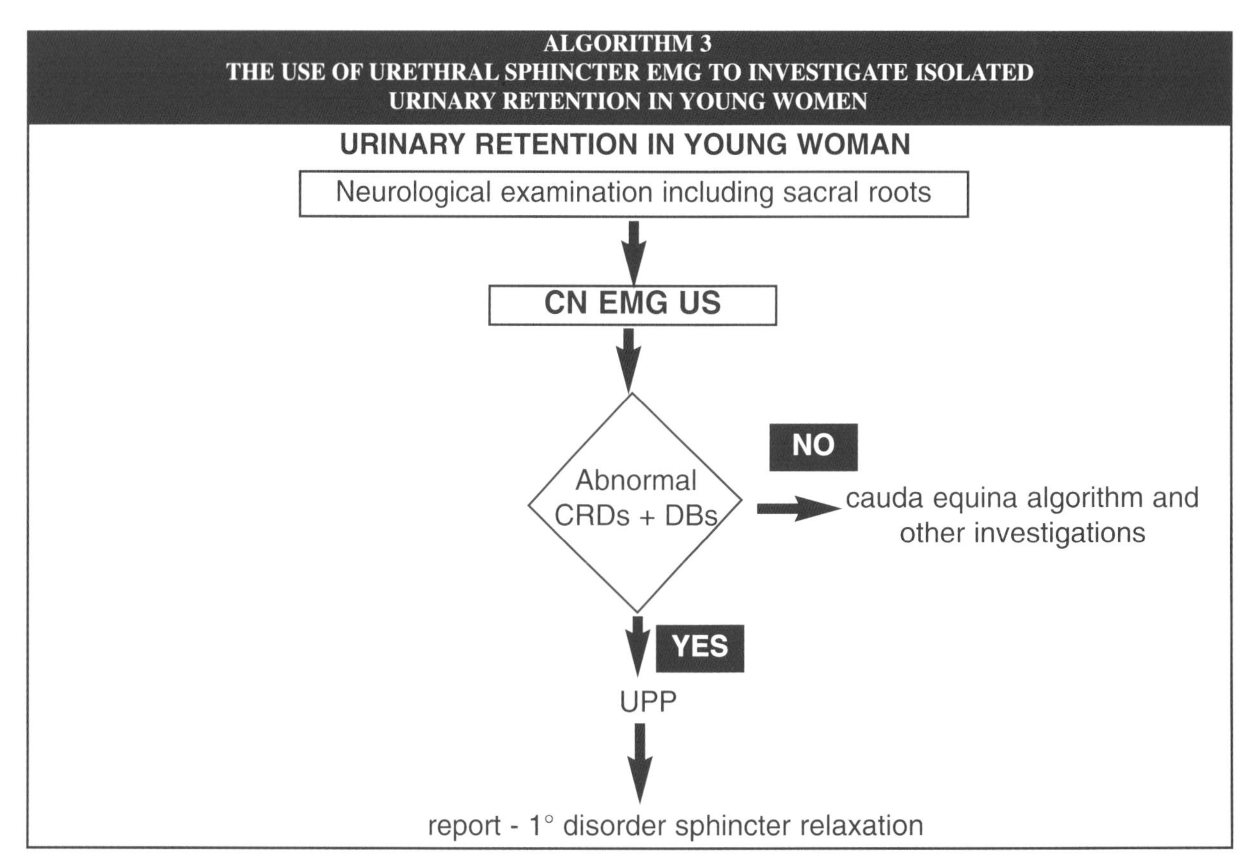

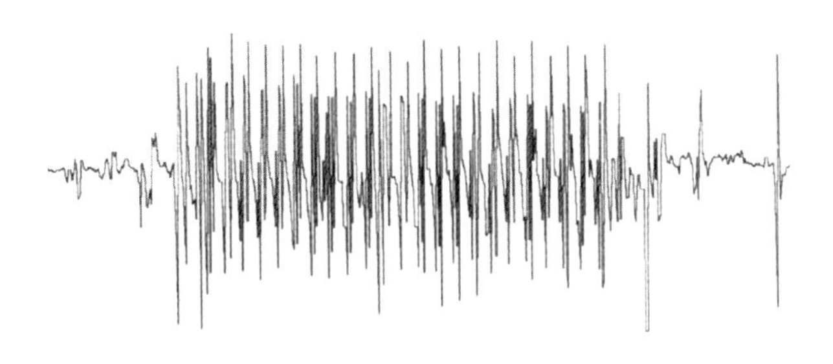

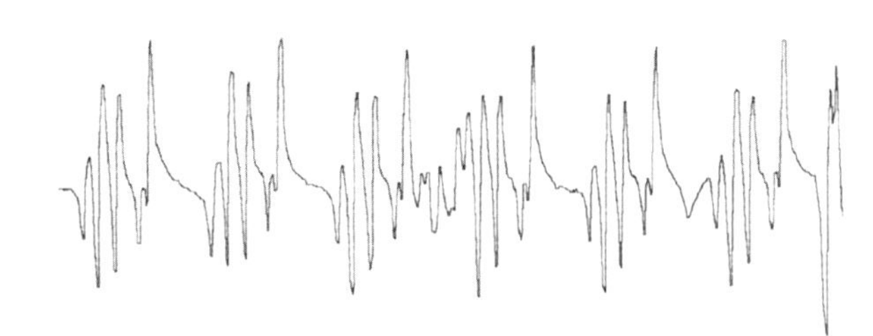

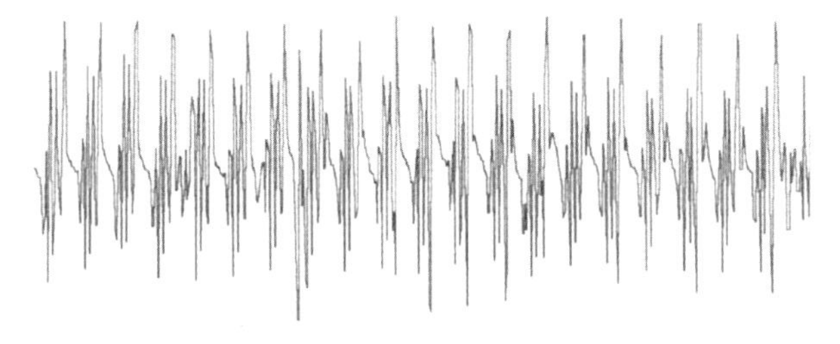

Figure 12 : EMG recording made with a CNE from the striated urethral sphincter of a young woman in urinary retention. The top panel shows a complex repetitive discharge, the details of which become clear as the time base is increasing expanded. The amplitude and time base (100uV/division and ms/division) is given by the scale bar.

is mandatory in the investigation of women with retention since the test may also detect changes of reinnervation in the presence of a cauda equina lesion [82].

The response of women in retention with profuse complex repetitive discharges and decelerating bursts to neuromodulation appears to be highly positive [83]. The extent to which women with obstructed voiding and urgency and frequency also have the same local sphincter EMG abnormality is a suggested topic for further research. It seems likely that the patients presenting clinical picture is determined by the reaction of the detrusor to the underlying sphincter abnormality which would explain why women with either retention or urgency and frequency may have the same EMG findings.

• **EMG CHANGES IN PRIMARY MUSCLE DISEASE**

There are only few reports of pelvic floor muscle EMG in generalised myopathy. In skeletal muscle, the "typical" features of myopathy are small, low amplitude polyphasic units recruited at mild effort. Such changes have not been reported in the pelvic floor even in patients known to have generalised myopathy [84]. Pelvic floor muscle involvement on histology in limb-girdle muscular dystrophy in a nulliparous female has been reported, but concentric needle EMG of her urethral sphincter was reported as normal [85]. Myopathic involvement was reported in the puborectalis and the EAS in patients with myotonic dystrophy [86].

2. PUDENDAL NERVE CONDUCTION TESTS

Measurement of motor conduction velocity is a routine method of evaluation of limb motor nerves, distinguishing between a demyelinating and axonal neuropathy, (motor conduction velocity being less than 38 m/s in the upper limb being indicative of the former condition). To make the measurement requires access to stimulation of the nerve at two well-separated points and measurement of the distance between them; a requirement that cannot be met in the pelvis. A related electrophysiological parameter to evaluate peripheral motor nerve function is the measurement of the distal (or terminal) motor latency of a muscle response, requiring only a single distal stimulation [7]. The muscle response is the compound muscle action potential (CMAP) or M-wave [7]. Pudendal nerve terminal motor latency (PNTML) can be measured by recording with a concentric needle electrode from the bulbocavernosus, the

EAS and the urethral sphincter muscles in response to bipolar surface stimulation placed perianally or perineally [87, 88, 89].

The most widely employed technique to obtain pudendal distal motor latency relies on stimulation with a special surface electrode assembly fixed on a gloved index finger, known as the St Mark's stimulator [90]. It consists of a bipolar stimulating electrode on the tip of the gloved finger with the recording electrode pair placed 3 or 5 cm proximally on the base of the finger. The finger is inserted into the rectum or vagina and stimulation is performed close to the ischial spine. Using this method, the distal motor latency for anal sphincter CMAP is typically around 2 ms, whereas with the previous method the latencies are twice longer [87, 88, 89]. The difference in latencies obtained by the perineal and transrectal method has not yet been explained, but PNTML as measured by the St Mark's electrode seems to be curiously short. Furthermore the figure for latency when recorded simultaneously with surface and needle electrodes may show some discrepancy (Figure 13). Also the traces recorded from the anal sphincter with the integral surface electrodes of the device, may be of low amplitude and marred by stimulus artefact.

Transvaginal stimulation can be applied as well and if a catheter mounted electrode is used for recording, EMG responses from the striated muscle of the urethral sphincter can be obtained. The amplitude of this response theoretically, reflects the number of excitable motor units in the striated urethral sphincter. The pudendal terminal motor latency has been found to rise with age by some studies [57, 54], but not by others [91].

Studies have shown the perineal latency was abnormally prolonged in patients with urinary stress incontinence [92, 58]. Working from the hypothesis that the pudendal nerve was stretched and injured during childbirth, several studies looked at the pudendal or perineal latency immediately post-partum. A significant increase in the mean pudendal nerve terminal motor latency was found 48-72 hours after vaginal delivery but in 60 % this had returned to normal 2 months later [93]. A follow-up study of 14 multiparous women from this group was made 5 years later [94]. The mean pudendal motor latency was found to be prolonged on both sides, fibre density of the EAS was increased, and anal manometry showed there had been a reduction in anal canal pressure during maximal squeeze contraction. From this it was concluded that occult damage to the puden-

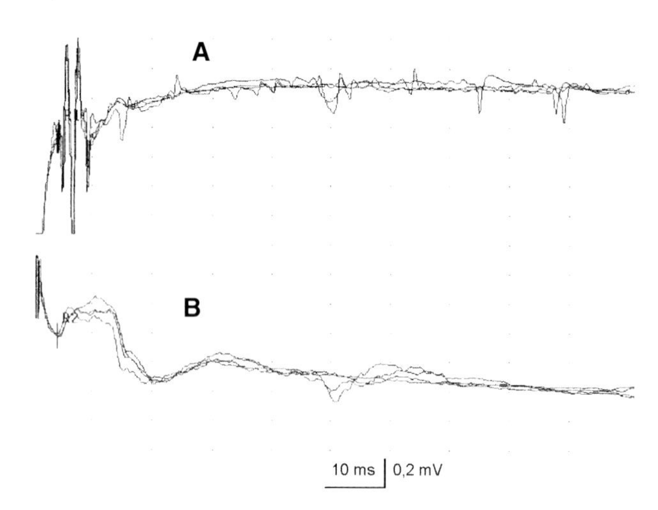

Figures 13 : Compound muscle action potentials (CMAP or M waves) of external anal sphincter on stimulation of the pudendal nerve at the ischial spine (on transrectal electrical stimulation with the St Mark's electrode) as recorded with a concentric needle (A) and surface electrode – the St Mark's electrode (B).

Simultaneous recordings show that responses can be obtained by both electrodes (Figs. C and D on the left) but the latencies may be similar (Fig. C) or significantly different (Fig. D on the left). In fact, either one or the other response may be absent (Fig. D on the right – absent response on surface recording). Responses were obtained from healthy subjects: 35-year-old male (Fig. C), 41-year-old female (Fig. D on the left) and 26-year-old male (Fig. D on the right).

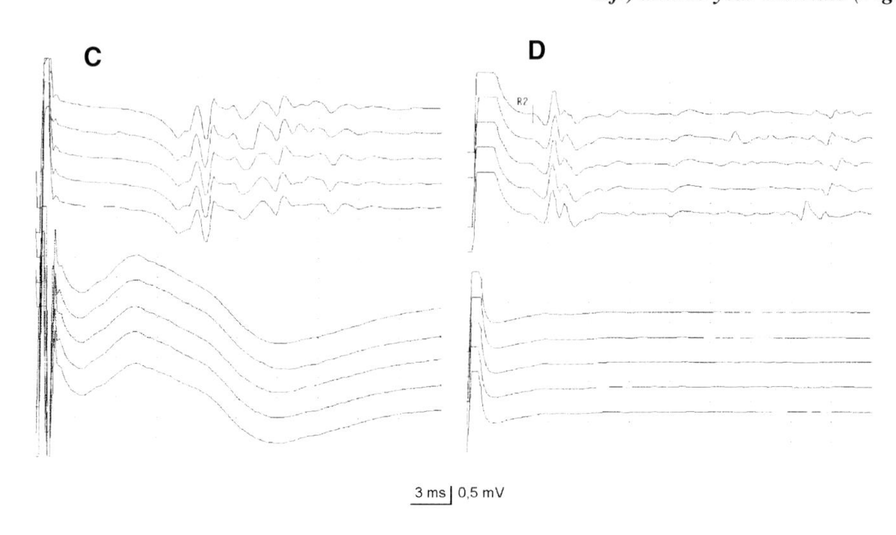

dal innervation of the EAS had persisted and worsened over the 5-year period and possibly had been exacerbated by abnormal straining patterns of defecation. No correlation of pudendal nerve terminal latency to parity was found in another study [54].

Measurement of the pudendal terminal latency has demonstrated a prolongation in women with pelvic floor prolapse [72, 95], with a further lengthening of the latency following vaginal dissection for repair or suspension procedures [95]. However the timing of reflex responses such as are involved with the recruitment of MUs on coughing or sneezing (i.e. manoeuvres which cause stress incontinence) are in the order of magnitude of tens of ms (the latency of the first component of the BCR is about 35 ms) so that the functional significance of delays of even several ms is uncertain.

Recently the PMNTL has been shown to be of value in determining the type of surgery most appropriate for patients with intrinsic sphincter deficiency, [74] and the amplitude of the response of the urethral sphincter following perineal nerve stimulation has been shown to be a predictive factor for success with sacral neuromodulation [96].

Pudendal nerve damage resulting in delayed PNTMLs in some cases may also be sustained during orthopaedic hip procedures during which a traction table is used [97].

Experts differ in their estimation of validity of the test. The pudendal motor latency, being a test of distal motor conduction cannot measure motor unit loss, denervation or reinnervation, but if using recordings from the urethral sphincter well formed, good amplitude responses can be obtained, information about the level of innervation of the sphincter will be known.

3. Anterior Sacral Root (Cauda Equina) Stimulation

Anterior root stimulation has been used to study conduction of the sacral nerve roots.

Transcutaneous stimulation of deeply situated nervous tissue became possible with development of special electrical [98] and magnetic [99] stimulators. When applied over the spine, these stimulators stimulate mainly the roots at the exit from the vertebral canal [100]. This technique was applied to sacral root stimulation soon after the device became available [5].

Electrical stimulation with needle electrodes at vertebral laminae Th12-L1 elicit M waves in the bulbocavernosus and EAS muscle [101]. Invasive percutaneous stimulation of individual roots in sacral foramina has been advocated as a diagnostic procedure before the implantation of electrodes that are to be used with implanted electrical stimulators for treatment of selected types of lower urinary tract dysfunction.

Whether or not parasympathetic efferents can be stimulated using magnetic stimulation remains controversial [102] but it is unlikely that these small diameter nerve fibres could be depolarised. It has been claimed that motor evoked potentials from the detrusor can be produced following magnetic stimulation of the cauda equina [103].

Needle EMG rather than non-selective surface electrodes should be used to record the pelvic floor and particularly the sphincter responses to electrical or magnetic stimulation of whole cauda equina. Both depolarize underlying neural structures in a nonselective fashion and activate several muscles innervated by lumbosacral segments. It has been shown that responses from gluteal muscles may contaminate recordings from the sphincters and lead to error [104].

Recording of motor evoked potentials (MEP) on magnetic stimulation is less often successful than with electrical stimulation, at least with standard coils, [6, 105] and stimulus artefacts are commonly a major problem. Positioning of the ground electrode between the recording electrodes and the stimulating coil may decrease the artefact [106].

Demonstrating the presence of a perineal MEP on stimulation over lumbosacral spine may occasionally be helpful in patients without voluntarily or reflexly activated muscles. It may help differentiate sensory from motor limb involvement of the sacral reflex arc. It also identifies the motor fibre component of a particular root if invasive stimulation is used, which is relevant before introducing therapeutic electrical stimulation procedures such as implants.

Reports on latencies from different laboratories using different types of electrodes differ. There are limited normative data and few reports, none recently, on the technique. Stimulus artefact is an acknowledged problem, and absent responses have to be evaluated with caution because of possible technical factors. The clinical value of the test has yet to be established, and there are no sensitivity and specificity data on test results in individual patients.

4. Motor evoked potentials

Magnetic brain stimulation should be used with caution in patients with a personal or family history of seizures. The stimulation has to be applied with a low frequency and single pulse magnetic brain stimulation is considered safe [107]. Using magnetic or electrical stimulation, it is possible to depolarise the motor cortex and record a response from the pelvic floor [6, 108]. Magnetic stimulation is less unpleasant than electrical stimulation, which has now been abandoned for stimulating the motor cortex in awake subjects.

The technique of magnetic stimulation is as follows:

The posterior edge of the magnetic coil is applied with direct contact to the skin 2 cm behind Cz (of the 10-20 EEG system). First, the intensity of the stimulation is progressively increased until a response is recorded from the muscle. Then the stimulation is repeated with the same intensity during a transient and moderate voluntary contraction of the pelvic floor, a procedure referred to as "facilitation". This leads to shortening of the latency. Muscle responses may be recorded from the urethral and the anal sphincters, and from the bulbocavernosus muscles using concentric needle EMG electrodes. It is advisable to use selective — i.e. needle — recording for reasons stated in III 1.3.

MEPs from the EAS [109, 110, 104], the urethral sphincter [110], the bulbocavernosus muscle [109, 104], and the levator ani muscle [109] were reported in healthy subjects.

By performing the stimulation at two different sites (brain and spinal roots), it is possible to record three different conduction times: a total conduction time, a peripheral conduction time, and a central conduction time. The total conduction time corresponds to the transit time from brain to target muscle. The peripheral conduction time is the transit time from sacral roots to the muscle. The central conduction time is obtained by subtracting the peripheral conduction time from the total conduction time. The total conduction time can be measured both at rest and during a facilitation procedure [6]. Substantially longer central conduction times have been found in patients with multiple sclerosis and spinal cord lesions as compared to healthy controls [111]. However as all of those patients had clinically recognisable cord disease, the diagnostic contribution of the method is dubious [112].

The demonstration of MEP may help in differentiating motor and sensory pathway involvement.

It is notable that a "silent period" is observed in after cortical stimulation in voluntary activated limb and also bulbocavernosus, but not EAS muscle [109].

No data as to the sensitivity and specificity of the test are available; indeed, there are no studies involving large numbers of patients. There is no established clinical use for this type of testing as yet and in general clinical neurophysiological practise practice magnetic stimulation is in little use.

II. SENSORY SYSTEM TESTS

In addition to clinical neurological testing of skin sensation of the perineum for touch, pin prick and testing of sensations of degrees of bladder filling during cystometry, there are methods of quantitative sensory testing. The function of sensory nerve pathways is also tested by clinical electrophysiological tests: peripheral sensory pathways are tested by sensory neurography, and the pathways within central nervous system by somatosensory evoked potentials (SEP).

1. Sensory testing

a) Sensory measurements during cystometry

During routine cystometry the following parameters concerning bladder sensation can be measured: first sensation of bladder filling, first desire to void and strong desire to void [113]. This is discussed in more detail in chapter 7.

In the sixth report on the standardisation of terminology of lower urinary tract function, the following is proposed regarding sensory testing: Semi-objective information on urogenital tract sensory function is obtained whenever a standard stimulus is applied and sensory thresholds are recorded [114]. The following recommendations were made: specify patient's position (supine, standing, other), bladder volume at time of testing, site of applied stimulus, number of times the stimulus was applied, number of responses recorded, sensation that was recorded (filling sensation, pulsing/throbbing sensation...), and type of applied stimulus (electrical, mechanical, chemical, others). Further the type of equipment, stimulus parameters, and absolute values as well as normal values for the specific system should be reported.

Measures of sensation during cystometry usually rely on patient-investigator dialogue and the inevitable associated prompting can lead to inaccurate descriptions by the patient of the intensity of their sensations, particularly when determining the first desire to void and grading the sensation of urge. A semi-objective technique, assessed by a psychophysical study, has been described which requires the patient to push buttons on a small key-pad device during cystometry to signal sensations of urge, thus obviating patient-investigator dialogue [115]. The utility of this technique has demonstrated and a correlation established between sensory signs and symptoms, such as urge and urgency, and cystometric findings in the urodynamic laboratory [116].

In the case of electrical stimulation, the sensory threshold has been defined. The vesical/urethral sensory threshold is defined as the least current, which consistently produces a sensation perceived by the subject during stimulation at the site under investigation. Sensory threshold measurment from the urinary bladder and the urethra using electrical current with varying amplitudes and frequencies has been reported [117], stimulating the saline filled bladder or by stimulating the bladder mucosa directly [118, 119]. Generally, the bladder has a higher threshold than the urethra or the skin of the forearm. Filling perception and electrical thresholds of the bladder mucosa have shown no correlation [120]. On the other hand urethral electrosensitivity was compared to first desire to void and cystometric bladder capacity and a statistically significant relation between the electrical sensory thresholds and cystometric findings in normal subjects has been demonstrated [121]. Applying electrical current to the proximal urethra, a study of sensory thresholds on 123 impotent males showed a statistical difference between patients with neurophysiological abnormalities and those without such abnormalities [122, 103]. Because of the wide range of actual values in both groups the overlap was so considerable that this sensory threshold measurement seemed impractical for clinical use. Significant differences were found in comparative studies of patients with proven chronic retention or stress incontinence and normal controls [123, 124], and have also been reported for anorectum [125].

Mechanical traction on the bladder trigone through an indwelling balloon catheter has been used, and the sensitivity threshold defined as the force read from a spring gauge at the moment of the first occurrence of urgency after gradually increasing the traction on the spring gauge/catheter system [126]. The value of trigonal sensitivity testing by mechanical stimulation has been questioned [127]. The outcome of a modified version of the technique was compared with cystometric findings and no correlation was found. Serious doubts were also cast on the reproducibility of this test [127]. Although it was claimed that mechanical stimulation is a more physiological stimulus to the bladder trigone than electrical stimulation [126], it should be recognised that traction applied in this way stimulates not only the trigone, but also the pelvic floor muscles and the urethra. The latter structures have an entirely different sensory innervation than the bladder trigone. The technique of trigonal sensitivity measurement by mechanical stimulation is simple to use, but it does not meet the basic criteria of a reliable test. There is uncertainty as to what is actually being tested, its outcome does not correlate with other physiological parameters and it seems to be neither reliable nor reproducible.

There is no established clinical use for any of these tests other than simple reporting of sensation during cystometry.

b) Quantitative sensory testing

Quantitative sensory testing is an extension of clinical testing of sensation. To increase the sensitivity of sensory testing and to produce quantified data, special methods and devices have been introduced. For clinical purposes, threshold is the function most conveniently measured [128]. The physiological, psychophysiological and methodological issues and controversies are not dealt with in this chapter, and in-depth reviews should be referred to [128]. Quantitative sensory testing should provide better quantified and reproducible data than routine clinical testing; in addition, if temperature sensation is tested, it provides information of thin fibre function, which is not tested by electrophysiologic tests (apart from SSR).

Only limited experience exists for testing in the urogenitoanal area; there is no commonly accepted, detailed, standardised test. Testing sensation in the lower sacral dermatomes is pertinent to lower urinary tract neurological control.

The specificity and sensitivity of the tests is not known. There is no established clinical use for any of the tests as applied to the urogenitoanal area.

• VIBRATION

Penile biothesiometry has been described as a useful screening test for evaluation of penile sensitivity in men with erectile dysfunction (ED), especially in those patients in whom an organic pathogenesis is suspected and in those patients suffering from diabetes mellitus or any other pre-existing disease with neurological implications [129]. Using a commercially available biothesiometer, vibratory stimuli are given through a 1cm wide probe at a fixed frequency of 120 cycles per minute with variable amplitude. Various stimulation sites have been used such as the tip of the index finger of the dominant hand, the penile shaft and the glans penis [130, 131]. The threshold of perception is recorded both by gradually increasing the amplitude from zero and by decreasing a strong stimulus; absence of response is also recorded. A study on 31 men with ED, concluded that biothesiometry cannot replace more elaborate methods of neurophysiological investigation [132]. No publication on patients with lower urinary tract dysfunction is known to the authors.

• TEMPERATURE

There is experimental evidence that the bladder has cold receptors [133]. This implies that the ice-water test to establish bladder sensibility and to provoke unstable bladder contractions in neuropathic or acontractile bladders is a test that depends on physiological mechanisms [134]. The bladder cooling test has been evaluated in patients with and without neurological conditions as well as in normal controls [135]. Perception of cold was normal in all control subjects and in patients with stress-incontinence. The test has also been suggested as useful in provoking bladder instability, and in determining abnormalities in bladder sensation.

Thermal testing using special thermodes is an established technique to test sensitivity of thin myelinated and nonmyelinated nerve fibre function in different body parts, particularly limbs [128]. The idea of investigating thin fibre neuropathy at the level of the urogenital organs has been challenged because peripheral neuropathy will show the earliest abnormalities distally in lower limbs. The use of thermal threshold measurements of the sole of the foot has been reported as a diagnostic tool in neurogenic ED, correlating well with other evidence [136] although there are now reports of direct genital thermal threshold testing [137]. No similar study in patients with incontinence is known to the authors.

•ELECTRICAL CURRENT

It is a common practice to establish the "threshold" for the electrical stimulus perception as applied to the penis/clitoris (or other stimulation site) at the beginning of a pudendal SEP recording session. The obtained threshold value is then used to formulate the necessary strength of stimulus used to elicit SEP. As a rule, a two to four times "threshold" current intensity is used [138]. The absolute figure however has little biological significance since resistance of the stimulating electrodes and electro-cutaneous junction are major determinants of the figure.

2. SENSORY NEUROGRAPHY

By placing a pair of stimulating electrodes across the glans and a pair of recording electrodes across the base of penis, a nerve action potential can be recorded (with an amplitude of about 10 μV) [139]. It can also be recorded by stimulating trans-rectally [140] or transperineally. The method can only be used in males.

In principle, the method would help to differentiate between sensory and motor fibre involvement and be of value in the diagnosis of sensory neuropathy. It could also help to differentiate between a supra and infraganglionary lesion in a patient with penile sensory loss.

There are few articles relating limited clinical experience with the test; however, sensitivity, specificity, and reproducibility are not known. It has no proven clinical usefulness in the incontinent patient.

3. ELECTRONEUROGRAPHY OF DORSAL SACRAL ROOTS

There is very limited literature on the subject and no routine clinical usefulness is established for the test but root recordings may be of some interest for either intraoperative or therapeutic electrical stimulation. Compound sensory root action potentials on stimulation of dorsal penile and clitoral nerve may be directly recorded intraoperatively when the sacral roots are exposed [141]. This has been found helpful in preserving roots relevant for perineal sensation in spastic children undergoing dorsal rhyzotomy and decreasing the incidence of postoperative voiding dysfunction [142]. In a study using epidural electrodes for recording, root potentials could be obtained in 4 out of 11 subjects [101] on stimulation of the dorsal penile nerve.

4. SOMATOSENSORY EVOKED POTENTIALS (SEP)

Somatosensory evoked potentials test conduction in the large fibre mediated pathways between sacrally innervated structures and the parietal sensory cortex.

a) Pudental SEP

• CEREBRAL SEP

On electrical stimulation of the dorsal penile or clitoral nerve, a cerebral SEP can be recorded [143, 144, 145 146, 4, 6, 147]. This SEP is as a rule of highest amplitude at the central recording site (Cz -2 cm : Fz of the International 10-20 EEG System [148] and is highly reproducible. (Figure 14) The first positive peak at about 40 ms (called P1 or P40) is usually clearly defined in healthy subjects using a stimulus 2-4 times the sensory threshold current strength [143, 146]. Later negative (at c. 55 ms) and then positive waves are interindividually quite variable in amplitude and expression. Similar results were obtained in many laboratories [145, 4, 6, 147].

Pudendal SEPs have been advocated in patients with neurogenic bladder dysfunction, e.g. in multiple sclerosis. However, it has been shown that even in patients with multiple sclerosis and bladder symptoms, the tibial cerebral SEP was more often abnormal than the pudendal SEP. Only in exceptional cases were the pudendal SEPs abnormal but the tibials normal, pointing to isolated conus involvement [149]. A study which looked at the value of the pudendal evoked potential when investigating uro-genital symptoms for detecting relevant neurological disease found it to be of lesser value than a clinical examination looking for signs of spinal cord disease in the lower limbs i.e. lower limb hyperreflexia and extensor plantar responses [150]. Following spinal cord injury the tibial and pudendal SEPs are of some value in predicting the degree of bladder control that may recover [151]. Cerebral SEP on penile/clitoral stimulation were reported as a possibly valuable intraoperative monitoring method in patients with cauda equina or conus at risk of a surgical procedure [152, 153].

• SPINAL SEP

Stimulating the dorsal penile nerve and recording with surface electrodes at the level of the Th12-L2 vertebrae (and the S1, Th6 or iliac spine as reference) reveals the

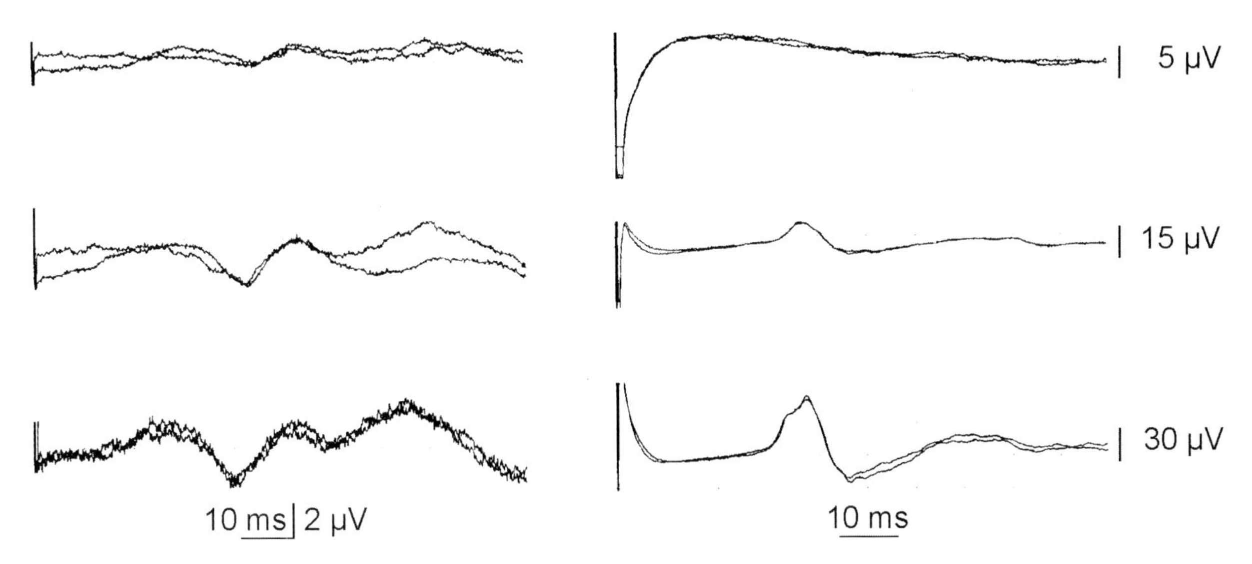

Figure 14 : SEPs (traces on the left) and sacral reflexes (traces on the right) in a healthy woman. Cerebral SEPs are recorded from Cz – 2 cm; sacral reflexes from the anal sphincter. The dorsal clitoral nerve is being stimulated with rectangular electrical pulses at 2 Hz. Stimulation and recording is performed with surface electrodes. The cerebral SEP and sacral reflex are recorded simultaneously. In the upper row the stimulation is just above sensory threshold, in the middle row the stimulation is 1.5, and in the lower row at 2-times sensory threshold (pulse duration 0.2 ms; two consecutive averages of 128 responses are superimposed). (From138, with permission).

postsynaptic segmental spinal cord activity (the spinal SEP) [146, 4, 6, 154]. Unfortunately, this spinal SEP may be difficult to record in healthy obese male subjects and in women [146 4, 6], and for this reason, such recordings are not in routine use. On stimulation of the dorsal penile nerve, even with epidural electrodes, sacral root potentials could only be recorded in 13, and cord potentials in 9 of 22 subjects [101]. Latencies of these spinal SEPs were c. 12 ms [101], substantiating the results obtained by surface recording [146, 4, 6].

• **EVOKED POTENTIAL MAPPING**

The technique of electrical brain mapping allows a functional study of the brain by recording cortical evoked potentials electrical activity over up to 32 different sites after peripheral nerve stimulation. The technique allows a bi-dimensional localisation of dipoles within the brain [148, 155, 156].

Magnetic brain mapping represents a step forward in the study of brain activity as it gives the possibility of achieving 3-dimensional source localisation on the basis of the spatial distribution of magnetic fields over the scalp. Magnetic evoked fields are recorded using a superconducting magnetometer (SQUID). For cortical sources tangential to the skull, the neuromagnetic method provides better spatial resolution than the corresponding scalp potentials recordings [155].

These techniques may be particularly informative if used in conjunction with functional brain imaging (functional MRI, which has better spatial resolution), as they have a much better time resolution. However, mapping techniques have no current clinical application in incontinent patients.

• **PUDENDAL CEREBRAL SEP ON MECHANICAL STIMULATION OF PENIS**

Mechanical stimuli, delivered to the distal penis by a custom designed electromechanical hammer triggered by an oscilloscope, have elicited cerebral SEP comparable to standard electrical stimulation in male children [157]. Painless mechanical stimulation is obviously preferable to electrical stimulation when investigating children. The method has only been introduced recently. No clinical usefulness is established.

b) Cerebral SEP on electrical stimulation of urethra and bladder

Cerebral SEP can also be obtained on stimulation of bladder mucosa [158]. SEP has also been obtained on stimulation of the anorectum [105]. When making such measurements, it is of utmost importance to use bipolar stimulation. Otherwise, somatic afferents are depolarised [159, 110]. These cerebral SEPs have been shown to have a maximum amplitude over the midline (Cz -2 cm : Fz) [159]. As the potential is of low amplitude (1 µV and less) and has a variable configuration, it may be difficult to identify in some control subjects [159, 154]. The typical latency of the most prominent negative potential (N1) has been reported to be about 100 ms, but data from different authors vary [160, 159, 161, 154]. These visceral SEPs are claimed to be more relevant to neurogenic bladder dysfunction than the pudendal SEP, as the A delta sensory afferents from bladder and proximal urethra ("visceral afferents") accompany the autonomic fibres in the pelvic nerves [159].

The introduction of a catheter and stimulating electrodes may lead to infection and possibly urethral strictures in men. The technique is painful as the urethra has to be lubricated with a jelly without anesthetics!

III. SACRAL REFLEXES

The term "sacral reflexes" refers to electrophysiologically recordable responses of perineal/pelvic floor muscles to electrical stimulation in the uro-genito-anal region. There are two reflexes — the anal and the bulbocavernosus — which are commonly clinically elicited. Both have the afferent and efferent limb of their reflex arc in the pudendal nerve, and are centrally integrated at the S2 to S4 cord levels. It is possible to use electrical [162, 160, 3, 88], mechanical [157], or magnetic [105] stimulation to elicit these. Electrical stimulation can be applied at various sites, including the dorsal penile nerve [163, 164, 162, 88, 3] the dorsal clitoral nerve [165, 143, 166,167], perianally [168, 153], via the perineum [169] and at the bladder neck/proximal urethra — using a catheter-mounted ring electrode [170, 171]. The latter reflexes are often referred to as "vesicourethral" and "vesicoanal", depending from which muscle the reflex responses are recorded. The pudendal nerve itself may be stimulated transrectally, transvaginally [172] or by applying needle electrodes transperineally [173].

The reports of sacral reflexes obtained on electrical stimulation of the dorsal penile or clitoral nerve are consistent in giving mean latencies between 31 and 38.5 ms [165, 163, 164, 162, 143, 166, 167 ,3] (Figure 15). The latency of responses on mechanical stimulation of distal penis was reported as either shorter, or longer [157] than on standard electrical stimulation. On magnetic stimulation, the latency was reported as longer [105]. These findings are most probably related to technical aspects of the stimulators used [157, 174].

Sacral reflex responses obtained on perianal or bladder neck/proximal urethra stimulation have mean latencies between 50 and 65 ms [171, 168, 88]. It is clear that the sacral reflexes obtained on bladder neck/proximal urethral stimulation have a different afferent limb. These are visceral afferent fibres accompanying pelvic nerves, which are thinner myelinated and have a slower conduction velocity than the thicker pudendal afferents. With visceral denervation (e.g. following radical hysterectomy) the viscerosomatic reflex may be lost while the sacral reflex is preserved.

The longer latency anal reflex, the contraction of the

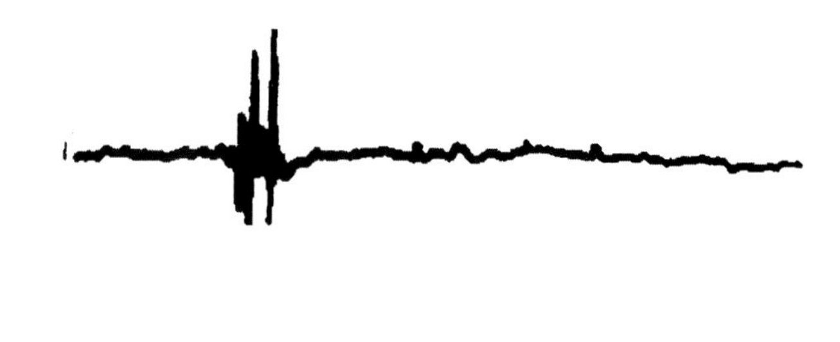

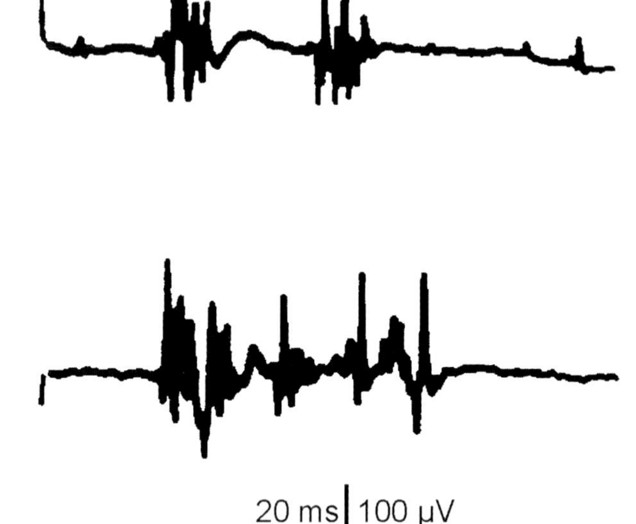

Figure 15 : Concentric needle recording from the bulbocavernosus muscle on stimulation of dorsal penile nerve (with surface electrodes) in a 67-year-old healthy man. Upper beam shows the sacral reflex on just suprathreshold stimulation, the middle beam on stimulation increased by 30 percent, and lower beam on maximal tolerable stimulation (in this case 60 percent suprathreshold). Observe the early component of the sacral reflex being joined by the second component at stronger stimulation; the division in two components is blurred at very strong stimulation. Observe also the slight shortening of latency of the first component at stronger stimulation in comparison with just suprathreshold stimulation. (From138, with permission).

EAS on stimulation of the perianal region, may also have thinner myelinated fibres in its afferent limb as it is produced by a nociceptive stimulus. On perianal stimulation, a short latency potential can also be recorded, as a result of depolarisation of motor branches to the EAS [88, 167].

EMG recording of the bulbocavernosus reflex has been shown to be more sensitive than the clinically assessed reflex response in males and particularly in females [24]. The recording of the reflex latency should increase the sensitivity to record abnormalities, but true sensitivity and specificity of the test are not known. The test has been studied extensively and a large amount of literature is available. The test is used in many laboratories in everyday practice to demonstrate "objectively" the integrity of the S2-S4 reflex arc. Several series of control data have been published, and the values are comparable. It is easy to perform and learn.

As with other tests of conduction, it is not sensitive to partial axonal lesions. Furthermore it is dependent not just on conduction through peripheral pathways, but also on transmission through the spinal cord interneuronal system and so is influenced by several factors, which may not be controlled or controllable. There are no data on sensitivity and specificity of latency or amplitude as test parameters.

1. Sacral reflex following electrical stimulation

The sacral reflex evoked on dorsal penile or clitoral nerve stimulation (the "bulbocavernosus reflex") was shown to be a complex response, often forming two components [164 , 88, 175]. The first component with a typical latency of about 33 ms, is the response that has been most often called the "bulbocavernosus" reflex. It is stable, does not habituate, and it is thought to be an oligosynaptic reflex response [175]. The second component has a latency similar to the sacral reflexes evoked by stimulation perianally or from the proximal urethra. The second component is not always demonstrable as a discreet response. The two components of the reflex may behave somewhat differently in control subjects and in patients. Whereas in normal subjects it is usually the first component that has a lower threshold, in patients with partially denervated pelvic floor muscles, often the first reflex component cannot be obtained with single stimuli, but on strong stimulation the later reflex component does occur [164]. This may cause confusion, as very "delayed" reflex responses may be recorded in patients, (implying "pathological conduction") not recognising the possibility that it is not a delayed first component but an isolated second component of the reflex. The situation can be clarified by using double stimuli, which facilitate the reflex response and may reveal in such a patient the first component, which was not obvious on stimulation with single stimuli [176]. A complete reflex arc lesion should not be inferred by absence of response if only single pulse is used for stimulation. Using paired stimuli 5-3 ms apart the second pulse arrives during the supernormal period of excitability which increases the likelihood of obtaining a response.

Sacral reflex responses recorded with needle or wire electrodes can be analysed separately for each side of the EAS or each bulbocavernosus muscle [164]. This is important because unilateral or asymmetrical lesions are common. However, unilateral stimulation of the penis is not really plausible, particularly in patients with sensory loss, unless a unilateral anaesthetic block is performed [177]. The application of stronger stimulus leads to electrical spread and bilateral depolarisation of the dorsal penile nerves cannot be excluded. Dorsal nerve of clitoris (DNC) unilateral depolarisation has recently been described in the context of sexual function [178] but no association was made between the integrity of the DNC somatosensory pathway and bladder function.

Sacral reflex responses on stimulation of the dorsal penile and clitoral nerve have been proposed to be valuable in patients with lower motor neurone lesions [162] and have been found absent or delayed in incontinent patients with conus/cauda involvement [109]. However, a reflex with a normal latency does not exclude the possibility of an axonal lesion in its reflex arc; patients with hereditary motor and sensory demyelinating neuropathy with normal bladder and sexual function have been found to have much delayed sacral reflex responses [179].

Most reports deal with abnormally prolonged sacral reflex latencies, but it has been suggested that a very short reflex latency raises the possibility of the tethered cord syndrome [180], to be due to the low location of the conus with shorter nerve roots. Shorter latencies of sacral reflexes in patients with suprasacral cord lesions have also been reported [165]. In children it has been shown that during voiding sacral reflexes are un-elicitable, but in the presence of spinal cord lesions such as myelodysplasia this normal suppression is lost [181].

Continuous intraoperative recording of sacral reflex responses on penis/clitoris stimulation is feasible if double pulses [182, 141] or a train of stimuli are used.

2. Sacral reflex on mechanical stimulation

Mechanical stimulation has been used to elicit BCR in both sexes [183] and found to be a robust technique. Either a standard commercially available reflex hammer or a customised electromechanical hammer can be used [157]. Such stimulation is painless and can be used in children or patients with pacemakers in whom electrical stimulation is contraindicated. The latency of the BCR elicited mechanically is comparable to the electrically elicited reflex in the same patients, but may be either slightly shorter or longer [157] because of the particular electromechanical device used [174]. On performing CNEMG with a needle electrode inserted into the subcutaneous part of the EAS [16] or bulbocavernosus muscle, an ipsilateral and contralateral touch or pinprick on the perineum elicits an increase in MUP firing – BCR. This manoeuvre allows the operator to evaluate efferent and afferent tracts individually.

IV. AUTONOMIC NERVOUS SYSTEM TESTS

All the uro-neurophysiological methods discussed so far assess the thicker myelinated fibres only, whereas it is the autonomic nervous system (the parasympathetic part in particular) which is most relevant for sacral functions. It has been argued that local involvement of the sacral nervous system (such as trauma, compression etc.) will usually involve somatic and autonomic fibres simultaneously. However, there are even some local pathological conditions, as a consequence of which purely isolated lesions can occur (such as mesorectal excision of carcinoma or radical prostatectomy). Methods by which the parasympathetic and sympathetic nervous system innervating the pelvic viscera could be assessed directly would be very helpful but are as yet unavailable.

Information on parasympathetic bladder innervation can to some extent be obtained by cystometry and supplemented by stimulating the parasympathetic pathway with electrical stimulation at the level of the sacral foramina with needle electrodes. However, from a clinical neurophysiological point of view direct electrophysiological testing would be desirable.

1. Tests in generalized autonomic neuropathy

In cases of suspected generalised autonomic dysfunction tests of cardiovascular innervation may be useful [13]. In cases when a general involvement of thin fibres is expected, an indirect way to examine autonomic fibres is to assess thin sensory fibre function (B.II.1.b).

Thin visceral sensory fibres are tested by stimulating the proximal urethra or bladder, and by recording sacral reflex responses or cerebral SEP.

2. Smooth muscle electromyography

The potential for smooth muscle electromyography of the detrusor may become a realistic possibility in the near future but past attempts to record such signals have in the main been thwarted by the presence of considerable movement artefact [102]. Recent experiments with a new design of electrode that minimises these artefacts has been developed and shown to record excellent 'real' electromyograms in whole animal bladders that reflect depolarisation events in detrusor muscle cells [184]. However, smooth muscle recordings associated with autonomically mediated contractions continue to be controversial with little evidence to prove their authenticity or clinical utility.

3. Sympathetic Skin Response (SSR)

The sympathetic nervous system mediates sweat gland activity in the skin. Changes in sweat gland activity lead to changes in skin resistance. On stressful stimulation such as a sudden noise, electrical pulse etc. a potential shift can be recorded with surface electrodes from the skin of the palms and the soles, and has been reported to be a useful parameter in assessment of neuropathy involving unmyelinated nerve fibres [185]. The response, known as the sympathetic skin response (SSR), can also be recorded from perineal skin and the penis [186, 187, 188, 189]. The SSR is a reflex, which consists of myelinated sensory fibres, a complex central integrative mechanism and a sympathetic efferent limb with postganglionic nonmyelinated C fibres. The stimulus used in clinical practice is usually an electric pulse delivered to an upper or lower limb (to mixed nerves), but the genital organs can also be stimulated. The latencies of SSR on the penis following stimulation of a median nerve at the wrist have been reported between 1.5 [190, 186] and 2.3 s [189] and could be obtained in all normal subjects with a large variability. The responses are easily habituated, and depend on a number of endogenic and exogenic factors including skin temperature, which should be at least above 28°C. Amplitudes (but not latencies) were reported reduced in older subjects [188]. It is commonly suggested that only an absent SSR can be taken as abnormal.

SSR is the only electrophysiological method directly testing sympathetic fibres. A correlation has been shown between the absence of the SSR response in the foot and bladder neck dyssynergia following spinal cord injury [191] and recording from the perineal region increases the diagnostic sensitivity for assessing sympathetic nerve function within the thoracolumbar cord [192]. Abnormal sympathetic skin responses in the hands are strongly predictive of autonomic dysreflexia [193].

The test is not sensitive for partial lesions as only complete absence of response can be regarded as abnormal.

C. GENERAL COMMENTS

I. CRITERIA FOR ABNORMALITY; SENSITIVITY AND SPECIFICITY OF CLINICAL NEUROPHYSIOLOGICAL TESTS

Clinical diagnosis requires that measures obtained in individual patients be compared to population norms with the intent of determining whether they are "normal" or "abnormal". Data can be classified as "abnormal" only with the understanding that they are compared to a sample from the normal population, and no precise probability is implied in predicting where these values are located relative to the normal population [171]. Predictive statements are made possible by the use of "tolerance limits". For most clinical neurophysiological tests, one-tailed tolerance limits are recommended. For any given limit of normality, there is a certain probability of falsely interpreting values (obtaining false-positives or false-negatives). Further confounding these issues is the practice of applying multiple criteria of abnormality. But ultimately, the adequacy of any given normal limit in discriminating between normal and abnormal must be supported by appropriate clinical or clinico-pathological correlations but such data are scarce, even for tests as applied in clinical neurophysiology in general.

II. USEFULNESS OF CLINICAL NEUROPHYSIOLOGICAL TESTS IN RESEARCH

Many uro-neurophysiological techniques have been applied in research. They were used to substantiate hypotheses that a proportion of patients with sacral dysfunctions, such as stress urinary and idiopathic faecal incontinence, have involvement of the nervous system [93, 72, 73, 90], to establish the function of the sacral nervous system in patients with suprasacral spinal cord injury [194], to reveal consequences of particular surgeries [195], to try to elucidate innervation of pelvic floor muscles [196 88], and to describe activation patterns of pelvic floor muscles [28, 22]. These methods have recently been introduced for intraoperative monitoring, where evoked potential studies have long since become established to help prevent lesions of the neural structures at risk from the surgical procedure [197 , 153, 141]. Neurourologic electrodiagnostic tests can be used to define reflex pathways in bladder function, demonstrating the neurologic substrate by which the central and peripheral nervous systems are integrated for co-ordinated urinary storage and voiding.

III. USEFULNESS OF CLINICAL NEUROPHYSIOLOGICAL TESTS IN EVALUATION OF INDIVIDUAL PATIENTS WITH LOWER URINARY TRACT DYSFUNCTION

Although clinical neurophysiology is practised in every neurology department, uroneurophysiological tests do not seem to be widely available even in university hospitals. They require some special expertise, but particularly additional clinical background knowledge that neurophysiology experts usually do not possess. Neurophysiologists are usually overwhelmed by other duties, and the pelvic area does not seem particularly attractive. Even in centres, which have contributed to research in the area, the tests are not routinely available for evaluation of individual patients, in whom such testing might be contributory. Lack of availability is not bothersome to most clinicians, for whom the "sophisticated " tests do not convey a readily understandable message. In the individual incontinent patient without signs or symptoms of a neurologic condition, the contribution of neurophysiological testing remains controversial; it is not expected to be either helpful or necessary in the majority of patients. Even in those patients the potential usefulness needs to be individually analysed in the overall clinical setting. The decision for testing can be said to rely on expert opinion, not on definitely established criteria derived from controlled studies.

D. RECOMMENDATIONS

I. ORGANISATION OF CLINICAL NEUROPHYSIOLOGY SERVICE FOR NEUROUROLOGY/ URO-NEUROLOGY

The information gained by clinical examination and urodynamic testing may be enhanced by uroneurophysiological tests in selected patient groups. It seems that tests have often been performed by non-neurophysiologists in research, but for routine diagnostics, an established service would seem necessary, and the physicians performing the tests should be appropriately trained, as required by national policies. As a rule, the service should be in liaison with general clinical neurophysiology. It seems optimal to create interdisciplinary programs between urology, urogynecology and neurology departments. Eventually, "neurourology" or "uroneurology" sections should provide the appropriate setting for testing of the individual patient to be performed within a wider scope of clinical evaluation, and treatment. Such specialised teams, sections, or even departments within larger institutions are as yet few, but the organisation of such teams in tertiary medical centres should be encouraged.

II. INVESTIGATION ACCORDING TO CLINICAL PROBLEM/ SUSPECTED NEUROANATOMICAL LESION

The 3 Algorithms that have been presented in the section on CN EMG describe the clinical circumstances where neurophysiological investigations are thought to be of value. All three are conditions involving the peripheral lower sacral innervation.

III. RECOMMENDATION FOR RESEARCH

Further research is recommended both to enhance the value of some current tests which appear promising, as well as to explore development of new techniques.

1. CURRENTLY USED PROCEDURE

a) Pudendal/perineal motor nerve conduction studies

a. Standardization and validation of stimulation and recording techniques

b. Reproducibility

d. Gender, age, vaginal parity effects

e. Clinical role in Stress Urinary Incontinence

f. Intraoperative monitoring

b) Sacral reflexes

a. Standardization for urethral/bladder stimulation

b. Reproducibility

c. Gender, age, vaginal parity effects

d. Clinical role definition in surgical procedures and predicting therapy outcomes.

c) EMG

a. Kinesiological EMG in SUI , urgency/frequency

b. Clinical value of recent computerised EMG analysis data

2. NEW TECHNOLOGY DEVELOPMENTS

a. Methodologies for kinesiological EMG

b. Sacral parasympathetic evaluation

c. Detrusor muscle EMG

d. Sensory nerve conduction – pudendal nerve

IV. RECOMMENDATION FOR TECHNICAL STANDARDS

Little standardisation of uroneurophysiological methods has been attempted so far. Indeed, even in "general" clinical neurophysiology there is no consensus on completely standardised tests. This is mainly due to different historical backgrounds of testing developed in different laboratories; the need to standardise methods is, however, recognized. At this stage, the authors suggest technical standards only for CNEMG and the sacral reflex on penile/clitoral stimulation (the "bulbocavernosus" reflex).

1. CNEMG

a. Type of electrode	*concentric needle;*
b. Placement of electrodes	*transcutaneous, (guided by palpation);*
c. Specifications of signal processing equipment (and its setting)	*stand. EMG equip.; filters 5 Hz - 10 kHz, 10 ms/div., 50-500 μV/div. (further defined with particular algorithm for analysis);* multi-MUP, or single-MUP analysis
d. Type and specification of decision algorithms for	*detection of pathologic spontaneous activity and* algorithms for analysis *quantification of MUPs (and/or interference pattern) -*
e. Normative data	*see* [13, 36]

2. SACRAL (BULBOCAVERNOSUS) REFLEX

a. Type of electrodes for stimulation	*surface;*
b. Type of stimulation	*electrical, 0.2 ms duration of single stimulus, "supramaximal" strength, manual triggering, 10 repetitions;*
c. Placement of stimulating electrodes	*penis / clitoris;*
d. Type of electrodes for recording	*concentric needle or surface;*
e. Placement of recording electrodes	*anal sphincter; in males also bulbocavernosus muscle;*
f. Specifications of signal	*stand. EMG equip.,*

processing equipment (and its setting)	*filters 10 Hz - 10 kHz, 10 ms/div., 50-1000 μV/div.;*
	documentation facilities;
g. Type and specification of decision	*presence;minimal latency of 10 consecutive*
	algorithms for analysis *responses (onset);*
h. Normative data	*for review see* [13].

V. SUMMARY

Lower urinary tract function relies on neurocontrol, the integrity of which is tested by clinical examination and several diagnostic methods, among them clinical neurophysiological tests. These comprise electrophysiologic methods testing conduction through motor and sensory pathways (both peripheral and central), electromyographic methods, and quantitative sensory testing. The latter include tests of sensory thresholds on mechanical stimulation, vibration, temperature, and electrical current; none of the tests (as applied to the urogenital area) have as yet proved of definite usefulness in diagnosis of patients with incontinence. The text also reviews methods and findings of electrophysiological tests including EMG, sacral reflexes, responses recorded from muscle on stimulation of motor pathways (pudendal nerve, sacral roots, motor cortex), and potentials recorded from sensory pathways (from nerve, roots, and cerebral cortex) on stimulation in the urogenital area. It is stressed that all electrophysiologic tests of conduction (terminal latency, motor evoked potentials, sensory evoked potentials, and sacral reflexes) correlate with patency of the respective neural pathway, but are not sensitive to partial neural system lesions of axonal type. The EMG signal can be used as an indicator of muscle activity patterns (kinesiological EMG), or can be analysed to reveal signs of muscle denervation (CNEMG) or signs of motor unit changes after reinnervation (CNEMG and SFEMG). Clinical neurophysiological testing should be considered only in very selected groups of incontinent patients, particularly those with suspected or known involvement of the neuromuscular system. In these, a documentation of and further characterisation of a lesion may be — in selected cases — relevant for therapeutic decisions or prognosis. At the time being, expert opinion classifies CNEMG and recording of the sacral reflex response on stimulation of

Table 1 : Neurophysiologic Studies of Pelvic Floor Muscles and Nerves

Test	Technical Aspects	Diagnostic Performance	Clinical Use for Incontinence
kEMG	Not difficult $$	Fair sensitivity	
CNEMG	Difficult $$$	Good sensitivity	
SFEMG	Difficult $$$	Good sensitivity	
PNTML	Not difficult $$	Fair sensitivity	Controversial
Anterior Sacral Root Stimulation	Moderately difficult $$$	Unknown sensitivity	
Motor Evoked Potentials (Cortical Stim)	Moderately difficult $$$	Unknown sensitivity	
Quantitative Sensory Testing	Variable (different techniques)$$	Fair sensitivity	
Pudendal Cerebral SEP	Moderately difficult $$	Good sensitivity	
Pelvic Visceral SEP	Difficult $$	Good sensitivity	
Sacral Reflex Test	Not difficult $$	Good sensitivity	
Viscero-somatic Reflexes	Moderately difficult $$$	Unknown sensitivity	
Autonomic Testing	Moderately difficult $$$	Fair sensitivity	

KEY GOOD RESEARCH POOR

the dorsal penile/clitoral nerve as optional in patients with involvement of the peripheral neuromuscular system. Other tests may be of some help in very selected patients. However, expert opinion cannot at this point recommend them for clinical practice and classifies them as investigational. Experts expect, that clinical neurophysiological tests will prove of further use particularly in research of a) correlations of test results both to the underlying lesion and disturbed function; b) pathophysiology of different types of incontinence; c) usefulness of tests in clinical practice for better diagnosis and evaluation of some physiologically based treatment modalities such as pelvic floor muscle exercises, biofeedback and electrical stimulation; d) usefulness of tests for intraoperative monitoring, and that such research will generally further insight into pathophysiology of lower urinary tract dysfunction.

A summary is given in Table 1.

GLOSSARY

BCR Bulbo-cavernosus reflex

CNEMG Concentric needle electromyography

CMAP Compound muscle action potential

DNC Dorsal nerve of Clitoris

ED Erectile dysfunction

EAS External anal sphincter

EEG Electroencephalography

EMG Electromyography

IP Interference pattern

kEMG kinesiological electromyography

MSA Multiple system atrophy

MEP Motor evoked potential

MUPs Motor unit potentials

MUs Motor units

NSS Number of short segments

PNTML Pudendal nerve terminal motor latency

SEP Somatosensory evoked potentials

SSR Sympathetic skin response

SFEMG Single fibre electromyography

SUI Stress urinary incontinence

T/A Turns / amplitude

UPP Urethral pressure profile

US Urethral sphincter

REFERENCES

1. Franksson, C.Petersen, I.: Electromyographic recording from the normal human urinary bladder, internal urethral sphincter and ureter. Acta Physiol Scan, 106: 150, 1953
2. Scott, F.B., Quesada, E.M.Cardus, C., The use of combined uroflowmetry, cystometry and electromyography in evaluation of neurogenic bladder dysfunction, in The Neurogenic Bladder, S. Boyarsky, Editor. 1967, Williams &Wilkins Company: Baltimore. p. 106.
3. Rushworth, G.: Diagnostic value of the electromyographic study of reflex activity in man. Electroenceph Clin Neurophys, S25: 65, 1967
4. Haldeman, S., Bradley, W.E.Bhatia, N.: Evoked responses from the pudendal nerve. J Urol, 128: 974, 1982
5. Swash, M.Snooks, S.J.: Slowed motor conduction in lumbosacral nerve roots in cauda equina lesions: a new diagnostic technique. J Neurol, Neurosurg Psychiat, 49: 808, 1986
6. Opsomer, R.J., Caramia, M.D., Zarola, F., et al.: Neurophysiological evaluation of central-peripheral sensory and motor pudendal fibres. Electroenceph Clin Neurophysiol, 74: 260, 1989
7. Nerve, M.A.: AAEE glossary of terms used in clinical electromyography. Muscle Nerve, G1: 10, 1987
8. Edstrom, L.Kugelberg, E.: Histochemical composition, distribution of fibres and fatiguability of single motor units. Anterior tibial muscle of the rat. J Neurol Neurosurg Psychiat, 31: 424, 1968
9. Beersiek, F., Parks, A.G.Swash, M.: Pathogenesis of anorectal incontinence: a histometric study of the anal musculature. J Neurol Sci, 42: 111, 1979
10. Gilpin, S., Gosling, J., Smith, A., et al.: The pathogenesis of genitourinary prolapse and stress incontinence of urine. A histological and histochemical study. Br J Obst Gyn, 96: 15, 1989
11. Heit, M., Benson, T., Russell, B., et al.: Levator ani muscle in women with genitourinary prolapse. Neurourol Urodyn, 15: 17, 1996
12. Hale, D., Benson, J., Brubaker, L., et al.: Histologic analysis of needle biopsy of urethral sphincter from women with normal and stress incontinence with comparison of electromyographic findings. Am J Obstet Gynecol, 180: 342, 1999
13. Fowler, C.J., Pelvic floor neurophysiology, in Clinical Neurophysiology, J. Osselton, et al., Editors. 1995, Butterworth Heinemann: Oxford. p. 233.
14. Vodusek, D.B., Electrophysiology, in Pelvic Floor Re-education, Principles and Practice, B. Schüßler, Laycock, J., Norton, P. and Stanton, S., Editor. 1994, Springer-Verlag: London. p. 83.
15. Podnar, S., Rodi, Z., Lukanovic, A., et al.: Standardization of anal sphincter EMG: technique of needle examination. Muscle Nerve, 22: 400, 1999
16. Podnar, S.Vodusek, D.B.: Standardization of anal sphincter electromyography: uniformity of the muscle. Muscle Nerve, 23: 122, 2000
17. Gosling, J.A., Dixon, J. S. And Humperson, J. R., Functional Anatomy of the Urinary Tract. Vol. 1. 1983, London: Churchill Livingstone.
18. Lowe, E.M., Fowler, C.J., Osborne, J.L., et al.: An improved method for needle electromyography (EMG) of the urethral sphincter in women. Neurourol Urodyn, 13: 29, 1994
19. Olsen, A., Benson, J.Mcclellan, E.: Urethral sphincter electromyography in women: comparison of periurethral and transvaginal approaches. Neurourol Urodyn, 17: 531, 1998
20. Chantraine, A.: EMG examination of the anal and urethral sphincters. New Developments in EMG and New Developments in EMG and Neurophysiology Ed J.E Desmedt 421, 1973

21. Jesel, M., Isch-Treussard, C., Isch, F., Electromyography of striated muscle of anal urethral sphincters, in New Developments in Electromyography and Clinical Neurophysiology, J.E. Desmedt, Editor. 1973, Karger: Basel. p. 406.
22. Deindl, F.M., Vodusek, D.B., Hesse, U., et al.: Activity patterns of pubococcygeal muscles in nulliparous continent women. Br J Urol, 72: 46, 1993
23. Vereecken, R.L., Derluyn, N.Verduyn, H.: Electromyography of the perineal striated muscles during cystometry. Urol Int, 3: 92, 1975
24. Blaivas, J.G., Sinha, H.P., Zayed, A.A.H., et al.: Detrusor-external sphincter dyssnergia. J Urol, 125: 542, 1981
25. Pavlakis, A.J., Siroky, M.B., Goldstein, I., et al.: Neurologic findings in Parkinson's Disease. J Urol, 129: 80, 1983
26. Rudy, D.C., Woodside, J. R.: Non-neurogenic neurogenic bladder: The relationship between intravesical pressure and the external sphincter electromyogram. Neurourol. Urodyn., 10: 169, 1991
27. Deindl, F., Vodusek, D., Bischoff, C., et al.: Zwei verschieddene Formen von Miktionsstorungen bei jungen Frauen: Dyssynerges Verhalten im Beckenboden oder Pseudomyotonie im externen urethralen sphinkter? Aktuelle Urologie, 28: 88, 1997
28. Deindl, F.M., Vodusek, D.B., Hesse, U., et al.: Pelvic floor activity patterns: comparison of nulliparous continent and parous urinary stress incontinent women. A kinesiological EMG study. Br J Urol, 73: 413, 1994
29. Chantraine, A., De Leval, J.Depireux, P.: Adult female intra- and periurethral sphinctre-electromyographic study. Neurourol. Urodyn 9: 139, 1990
30. Jones, P.N., Lubowski, D.Z., Swash, M., et al.: Is paradoxical contraction of puborectalis muscle of functional importance? Dis Colon Rectum, 30: 667, 1987
31. Mathers, S., Kempster, P., Swash, M., et al.: Constipation and paradoxical puborectalis contractions in anismus and Parkinson's disease: a dystonic phenomenon? J Neurol, Neurosurg Psychiat, 51: 1503, 1988
32. Vereecken, R.Verduyn, H.: The electrical activity of the paraurethral and perineal muscle in normal and pathological conditions. Br J Urol, 42: 457, 1970
33. Nordling, J.Meyhoff, H.H.: Dissociation of urethral and anal sphincter activity in neurogenic bladder dysfunction. J Urol, 122: 352, 1979
34. Nandedkar, S.D., Sanders, D.B., Stalberg, E.V., et al.: Simulation of concentric needle EMG motor unit action potentials. Muscle Nerve, 11: 151, 1988
35. Stalberg, E., Andreassen, S., Falck, B., et al.: Quantitative analysis of individual motor unit potentials: a proposition for standardized terminology and criteria for measurement. J Clin Neurophysiol, 3: 313, 1986
36. Podnar S, Vodusek D.B. : Standardisation of anal sphincter electromyography: normative data. Clin Neurophysiol, 111: 2200, 2000
37. Podnar, S.Vodusek, D.B.: Standardisation of anal sphincter EMG: high and low threshold motor units. Clin Neurophysiol, 110: 1488, 1999
38. Buchthal, F., Introduction to Electromyography. 1957, Copenhagen: Scandinavian University Press.
39. Podnar S, V.E.D., Stålberg E: Standardisation of anal sphincter electromyography: comparison of quantitative methods. Clin Neurophysiol, 111: 106, 2000
40. Czekajejewski J, E.J., Stålberg E: Oscilloscopic recording of muscle fibre action potentials. The window trigger and delay unit. Electroenceph Clin Neurophys, 27: 536, 1969
41. Stoalberg, E., Falck, B., Sonoo, M., et al.: Multi-MUP EMG analysis—a two year experience in daily clinical work. Electroenceph Clin Neurophys, 97: 145, 1995
42. Palace, J., Chandiramani, V.A., Fowler, C.J.: Value of sphincter EMG in the diagnosis of Multiple System Atrophy. Muscle Nerve, 20: 1396, 1997
43. Schwarz, J., Kornhuber, M., Bischoff, C., et al.: Electromyography of the external anal sphincter in patients with Parkinson's Disease and Multiple System Atrophy: frequency of abnormal spontaneous activity and polyphasic motor potentials. Muscle Nerve, 20: 1167, 1997
44. Brown, F.W., The Physiological and Technical Basis of Electromyoghraphy. 1984, London: Butterworth.
45. Fowler, C.J., Kirby, R.S., Harrison, M.J.G., et al.: Individual motor unit analysis in the diagnosis of disorders of urethral sphincter innervation. J Neurol, Neurosurg Psychiat, 47: 637, 1984
46. Nandedkar, S.D., Barkhaus, P.E., Sanders, D.B., et al.: Analysis of amplitude and area of concentric needle EMG motor unit action potentials. Electroenceph Clin Neurophys, 69: 561, 1988
47. Sonoo, M.Stalberg, E.: The ability of MUP parameters to discriminate between normal and neurogenic MUPs in concentric EMG: analysis of the MUP "thickness" and the proposal of "size index". Electroenceph Clin Neurophys, 89: 291, 1993
48. Stoalberg, E., Chu, J., Bril, V., et al.: Automatic analysis of the EMG interference pattern. Electroenceph Clin Neurophys, 56: 672, 1983
49. Nandedkar, S.D., Sanders, D.B.Stalberg, E.V.: Automatic analysis of the electromyographic interference pattern. Part II: Findings in control subjects and in some neuromuscular diseases. Muscle Nerve, 9: 491, 1986
50. Podnar, S., Lukanovic, A.Vodusek, D.B.: Anal sphincter electromyography after vaginal delivery: neuropathic insufficiency or normal wear and tear? Neurourol Urodyn, 19: 249, 2000
51. Podnar S, Vodusek D.B. : Standardization of anal sphincter electromyography: effect of chronic constipation. Muscle Nerve, 23: 1748, 2000
52. Stalberg, E.Trontelj, J., Single fiber electromyography. Second Edition ed. 1994, New York: Raven Press.
53. Vodusek, D.B.: Individual motor unit analysis in the diagnosis of urethral sphincter innervation [letter]. J Neurol Neurosurg Psychiat, 52: 812, 1989
54. Jameson, J.S., Chia, Y.W., Kamm, M.A., et al.: Effect of age, sex and parity on anorectal function. Br J Surg, 81: 1689, 1994
55. Vodusek, D.B., Janko, M.: SFEMG in striated sphincter muscles. Muscle Nerve, 4: 252, 1981
56. Neill, M., E., Swash, M.: Increased motor unit fibre density in the external anal sphincter in ano-rectal incontinence: a single fibre EMG study. J Neurol Neurosurg Psychiat, 43: 343, 1980
57. Laurberg, S.Swash, M.: Effects of aging on the anorectal sphincters and their innervation. Dis Colon Rectum, 32: 737, 1989
58. Snooks, S.J., Badenoch, D.F., Tiptaft, R.C., et al.: Perineal nerve damage in genuine stress incontinence. Br J Urol, 57: 422, 1985
59. Eardley, I., Quinn, N.P., Fowler, C.J., et al.: The value of urethral sphincter electromyography in the differential diagnosis of parkinsonism. Br J Urol, 64: 360, 1989
60. Sakuta, M., Nakanishi, T.Tohokura, Y.: Anal muscle electromyograms differ in amyotrophic lateral sclerosis and Shy-Drager syndrome. Neurology, 28: 1289, 1978
61. Kirby, R.S., Fowler, C.J., Gosling, J., et al.: Urethro-vesical dysfunction in progressive autonomic failure with multiple system atrophy. J Neurol, Neurosurg Psychiat, 49: 554, 1986
62. Salinas, J., Berger, Y., Delarocha, R., et al.: Urological evaluation in the Shy-Drager syndrome. J Urol, 135: 741, 1986
63. Beck, R.O., Betts, C.D., Fowler, C.J.: Genito-urinary dysfunc-

tion in Multiple System Atrophy: clinical features and treatment in 62 cases. J Urol, 151: 1336, 1994

64. Rodi, Z., Denislic, M.Vodusek, D.B.: External anal sphincter electromyography in the differential diagnosis of parkinsonism [letter]. J Neurol Neurosurg Psychiat, 60: 460, 1996
65. Stocchi, F., Carbone, A., Inghilleri, M., et al.: Urodynamic and neurophysiological evaluation in Parkinson's disease and multiple system atrophy. J Neurol Neurosurg Psychiat, 62: 507, 1997
66. Valldeoriola, F., Valls-Sole, J., Tolosa, E.S., et al.: Striated anal sphincter denervation in patients with progressive supranuclear palsy. Mov Disord, 10: 550, 1995
67. Libelius, R.Johanson, J.F.: Quantitative electromyography of the external anal sphincter in Parkinson's disease and multiple system atrophy. Muscle Nerve, 23: 1250, 2000
68. Vodusek, D.B.: Sphincter EMG and differential diagnosis of Multiple System Atrophy. Mov Dis 16; 600, 2001
69. Stoalberg, E., Bischoff, C.Falck, B.: Outliers, a way to detect abnormality in quantitative EMG. Muscle Nerve, 17: 392, 1994
70. Snooks, S.J., Barnes, P.R.H., Swash, M.: Damage to the innervation of the voluntary anal and periurethral musculature in incontinence. J Neurol Neurosurg Psychiat, 47: 406, 1984
71. Anderson, R.: A neurogenic element to urinary genuine stress incontinence. Br J Urol, 91: 41, 1984
72. Smith, A.R.B., Hosker, G.L.Warrell, D.W.: The role of partial denervation of the pelvic floor in aetiology of genitourinary prolapse and stress incontinence of urine. A neurophysiological study. Br J Obst Gyn, 96: 24, 1989
73. Allen, R., Hosker, G., Smith, A., et al.: Pelvic floor damage and childbirth: a neurophysiological study. Br J Obst Gyn, 97: 770, 1990
74. Fischer JR, Hale DS, McClellan E, Benson JT, The Use of Urethral Electrodiagnosis to select the method of surgery in women with Intrinsic Sphincter Deficiency, International Urogynecology 12, suppl 1: s33, 2001.
75. Trontelj, J., Stoalberg, E.: Bizarre repetitive discharges recorded with single fibre EMG. J Neurol Neurosurg Psychiat, 46: 310, 1983
76. Jensen, D.Stien, R.: The importance of complex repetitive discharges in the striated female urethral sphincter and male bulbocavernosus muscle. Scand J Urol Nephrol , Suppl. 179: 69, 1996
77. Fitzgerald, M., Blazek, B.Brubaker, L.: Complex repetitive discharges during urethral sphincter electromyography: clinical correlates. Neurourol Urodyn, 18: 273, 1999
78. Fowler, C.J., Christmas, T.J., Chapple, C.R., et al.: Abnormal electromyographic activity of the urethral sphincter, voiding dysfunction, and polycystic ovaries: a new syndrome? Br J Med, 297: 1436, 1988
79. Fowler, C.J., Kirby, R.S., Harrison, M.J.G.: Decelerating bursts and complex reptitive discharges in the striated muscle of the urethral sphincter associated with urinary retention in women. J Neurol Neurosurg Psychiatry, 48: 1004, 1985
80. Butler, W.J.: Pseudomyotonia of the periurethral sphincter in women with urinary incontinence. J Urol, 122: 838, 1979
81. Wiseman, O.J., Swinn, M.J., Fowler, C.J.: The maximal urethral closure pressure and urethral ultrasound in women with urinary retention. J Urol, 167 in press 2002.
82. Fowler, C.J., Kirby, R.S.: Electromyography of the urethral sphincter in women with urinary retention. Lancet, i: 1455, 1986
83. Swinn, M.J., Kitchen, N.D., Goodwin, R.J., et al.: Sacral neuromodulation for women with Fowler's syndrome. Euro Urol, 38: 439, 2000
84. Caress, J., Kothari, M., Bauer, S., et al.: Urinary dysfunction in Duchenne muscular dystrophy. Muscle Nerve, 19: 819, 1996
85. Dixon, P.J., Christmas, T.J.Chapple, C.R.: Stress incontinence due to pelvic floor muscle involvement in limb-girdle muscular dystrophy. Br J Urol, 65: 653, 1990
86. Herbaut, A.G., Nogueira, M.C., Panzer, J.M., et al.: Anorectal incontinence in myotonic dystrophy: a myopathic involvement of pelvic floor muscles [letter]. Muscle Nerve, 15: 1210, 1992
87. Rogers, J., Laurberg, S., Misiewicz, J.J., et al.: Anorectal physiology validated: a repeatability study of the motor and sensory tests of anorectal function. Br J Surg, 76: 607, 1989
88. Vodusek, D.B.Light, K.L.: The motor nerve supply of the external urethral sphincter muscles: an electrophysiologic study. Neurourol Urodyn, 2: 193, 1983
89. Pedersen, E., Klemar, B., Schroder, J., et al.: Anal sphincter responses after perianal electrical stimulation. JNeurol, Neurosurg Psychiat, 45: 770, 1982
90. Kiff, E.S. Swash, M.: Normal proximal and delayed distal conduction in the pudendal nerves of patients with idiopathic (neurogenic) faecal incontinence. J Neurol Neurosurg Psychiat, 47: 820, 1984
91. Barrett, J.A., Brocklehurst, J.C., Kiff, E.S., et al.: Anal function in geriatric patients with faecal incontinence. Gut, 30: 1244, 1989
92. Smith, A., Hosker, G.Warrell, D.: The role of pudendal nerve damage in the aetiology of genuine stress incontinence in women. Br J Obst Gyn, 96: 29, 1989
93. Snooks, S.J., Swash, M., Setchell, M., et al.: Injury to the pelvic floor sphincter musculature in childbirth. Lancet, ii: 546, 1984
94. Snooks, S.J., Swash, M., Mathers, S.E., et al.: Effect of vaginal delivery in the pelvic floor: a 5-year follow-up. Br J Surg, 77: 1358, 1990
95. Benson, T.Mclellan, E.: The effect of vaginal dissection on the pudendal nerve. Obstet Gynecol, 82: 387, 1993
96. Mastropietro M, Fuller E, Benson JT Electrodiagnostic Features of Responders and Nonresponders to Sacral Neuromodulation Test Stimulation, Internat. Urogyne 12, suppl 1; s24, 2001
97. Amarenco, G., Ismael, S.S., Bayle, B., et al.: Electrophysiological analysis of pudendal neuropathy following traction. Muscle Nerve, 24: 116, 2001
98. Merton, P.A.Morton, H.B.: Stimulation of the cerebral cortex in the intact human subject. Nature, 285: 227, 198
99. Barker, A.T., Jalinous, R.Freeston, I.L.: Non-invasive magnetic stimulation of human motor cortex [letter]. Lancet, i: 1106, 1985
100. Mills, K.R.Murray, N.M.: Electrical stimulation over the human vertebral column: which neural elements are excited? Electroenceph Clin Neurophys, 63: 582, 1986
101. Ertekin, C., Mungan, B.: Sacral Spinal Cord and Root Potentials Evoked by the Stimulation of the Dorsal Nerve of Penis and Cord Conduction Delay for the Bulbocavernosus Reflex. Neurourol Urodyn, 12: 9, 1993
102. Craggs, M.D., Shah, N., Sheriff, M., et al.: Contraction or suppresion of the bladder by magnetic stimulation of the sacral roots. Resolving the paradox. Neurourol Urodyn, 18:279, 1999
103. Bemelmans, B.L.H., Van Kerrebroeck, Ph. E. V., Debruyne, F. M. J.: Motor bladder responses after magnetic stimulation of the cauda equina. Neurourol. Urodyn., 10: 380, 1991
104. Vodusek, D.B., Zidar, J.: Perineal motor evoked responses. Neurourol Urodyn, 7: 236, 1988
105. Loening-Baucke, V., Read, N.W., Yamada, T., et al.: Evaluation of the motor and sensory components of the pudendal nerve. Electroenceph Clin Neurophys, 93: 35, 1994
106. Jost, W.H., Schimrigk, K.: A new method to determine pudendal nerve motor latency and central motor conduction time to the external anal sphincter. Electroenceph Clin Neurophys, 93: 237, 1994
107. Chokroverty, S., Hening, W., Wright, D., et al.: Magnetic brain

stimulation: safety studies. Electroenceph Clin Neurophys, 97: 36, 1995

108. Rossini, P.M., Caramia, M. D., Zarola, F.: Central motor tract propagation in man: studies with non-invasive, unifocal, scalp stimulation. Brain Res., 415: 211, 1987
109. Ertekin, C., Hansen, M.W., Larsson, L.-E., et al.: Examination of the descending pathway to the external anal sphincter and pelvic floor muscles by transcranial cortical stimulation. Electroenceph Clin Neurophys, 75: 500, 1990
110. Thiry, A.J.Deltenre, P.F.: Neurophysiological assessment of the central motor pathway to the external urethral sphincer in man. Br J Urol, 63: 515, 1989
111. Eardley, I., Nagendran, K., Lecky, B., et al.: The neurophysiology of the striated urethral sphincter in multiple sclerosis. Br J Urol, 67: 81, 1991
112. Mathers, S.E., Ingram, D.A., Swash, M.: Electrophysiology of motor pathways for sphincter control in multiple sclerosis. J Neurol Neurosurg Psychiat, 53: 955, 1990
113. Bradley, W., Timm, G.Scott, F.: Cystometry V: Bladder sensation. Urology, 6: 643, 1975
114. Abrams, P., Blaivas, J.G., Stanton, S.L., et al.: Sixth report on the standardisation of terminology of the lower urinary tract function. World J Urol, 4: 2, 1986
115. Oliver, S.E., Susser, J., Fowler, C.J., et al.: An objective measure of the sensations of urinary urge and urgency perceived by patients with detrusor instability. Br J U Int, 86 (suppl 3): 133, 2000
116. Oliver, S.E., Susser, J., Fowler, C.J., et al.: Sensations during urodynamics and sensations scored in voiding diaries: are they comparable? Neurourol Urodyn, 19 (suppl 4): 478, 2000
117. Wyndaele, J.J., Van Eetvelde, B.Callens, D.: Comparison in young healthy volunteers of 3 different parameters of constant current stimulation used to determine sensory thresholds in the lower urinary tract. J Urol, 156: 1415, 1996
118. Frimodt-Moller, C.: A new method for quantitative evaluation of bladder sensitivity. Scand J Urol Nephrol, 6: 135, 1972
119. Kieswetter, H.: Mucosal sensory threshold of urinary bladder and urethra measured electrically. Urol. Int., 32: 437, 1977
120. Wyndaele, J.J.: Study on the correlation between subjective perception of bladder filling and the sensory threshold towards electrical stimulation in the lower urinary tract. J Urol, 147: 1582, 1992
121. Powell, P.H.Feneley, R.C.L.: The role of urethral sensation in clinical urology. BJUrol, 52: 539, 198
122. Bemelmans, B., Meuleman, E., Anten, B., et al.: Penile sensory disorders in erectile dysfunction: results of a comprehensive neuro-urophysiological diagnostic evaluation in 123 patients. J Urol, 146: 777, 1991
123. Fidas, A., Macdonald, H.L., Elton, R.A., et al.: Neurophysiological measurements in patients with genuine stress incontinence of urine and the relation of neurogenic defects to the presence of spina bifida occulta. Br J Urol, 62: 46, 1988
124. Parys, B.T., Machin, D.G., Woolfenden, K.A., et al.: Chronic urinary retention—a sensory problem? Br J Urol, 62: 546, 1988
125. Rogers, J., Hayward, M.P., Henry, M.M., et al.: Temperature gradient between the rectum and the anal canal: evidence against the role of temperature sensation as a sensory modality in the anal canal of normal subjects [see comments]. Br J Surg, 75: 1083, 1988
126. Klein, L.A.: Measurement of trigonal sensitivity as a test of bladder function. J Urol, 137: 245, 1987
127. Frazer, M.I., Haylen, B.T.: Trigonal sensitivity testing in women. J Urol, 141: 356, 1989
128. Fowler, C.J., Sensory testing, in Clinical Neurophysiology, J.W. Osselton, Binnie. Editor. 1995, Butterworth-Heinemann: Oxford.
129. Padma-Nathan, H.: Neurologic evaluation of erectile dysfunction. Urol Clin North Am, 15: 77, 1988
130. Rowland, D.L., Leentvaar, E.J., Blom, J.H., et al.: Changes in penile sensitivity following papaverine-induced erection in sexually functional and dysfunctional men. J Urol, 146: 1018, 1991
131. Rowland, D.L., Greenleaf, W., Mas, M., et al.: Penile and finger sensory thresholds in young, aging, and diabetic males. Arch Sex Behav, 18: 1, 1989
132. Bemelmans, B.L., Hendrikx, L.B., Koldewijn, E.L., et al.: Comparison of biothesiometry and neuro-urophysiological investigations for the clinical evaluation of patients with erectile dysfunction [see comments]. J Urol, 153: 1483, 1995
133. Geirsson, G.: Evidence of cold receptors in the human bladder: effect of menthol on the bladder cooling reflex. J Urol, 150: 427, 1993
134. Geirsson, G., Fall, M.Lindstrom, S.: The ice-water test—a simple and valuable supplement to routine cystometry. Br J Urol, 71: 681, 1993
135. Hellstrom, P.A., Tammela, T.L., Kontturi, M.J., et al.: The bladder cooling test for urodynamic assessment: analysis of 400 examinations. Br J Urol, 67: 275, 1991
136. Fowler, C.J., Ali, Z., Kirby, R.S., et al.: The value of testing for unmyelinated fibre, sensory neuropathy in diabetic impotence. Br J Urol, 61: 63, 1988
137. Yarnitsky, D., Sprecher, E.Vardi, Y.: Penile thermal sensation. J Urol, 156: 391, 1996
138. Vodusek, D.B.: Evoked potential testing. Urol Clin North Am, 23: 427, 1996
139. Bradley, W.E., Lin, J.T.Johnson, B.: Measurement of the conduction velocity of the dorsal nerve of the penis. J Urol, 131: 1127, 1984
140. Amarenco, G., Kerdraon, J.: Pudendal nerve terminal sensitive latency: technique and normal values. J Urol, 161: 103, 1999
141. Vodusek, D.B., Deletis, V., Abbott, R., et al., Intraoperative monitoring of pudendal nerve function, in Quantitative EEG Analysis - Clinical Utility and New Methods, M. Rother, Zwiener, U., Editor. 1993, Universitätsverlag Jena: Jena. p. 309.
142. Deletis, V., Vodusek, D.B., Abbott, R., et al.: Intraoperative monitoring of the dorsal sacral roots: minimizing the risk of iatrogenic micturition disorders. Neurosurgery, 30: 72, 1992
143. Vodusek, D.: Pudendalsomatosensory evoked potential and bulbocavernosus reflex in women. Electroenceph Clin Neurophys, 77: 134, 1990a
144. Opsomer, R.J., Guerit, J.M., Wese, F.X., et al.: Pudendal cortical somatosensory evoked potentials. J Urol, 135: 1216, 1986
145. Haldeman, S., Bradley, W., Bhatia, N., et al.: Cortical evoked potentials on stimulation of pudendal nerve in women. Urol, XXL, 6: 590, 1983
146. Vodusek, D.B.: Pudendal somatosensory evoked potentials. Neurologija, 39: 149, 1990b
147. Tackmann, W., Vogel, P. And Porst, H.: Somatosensory evoked potentials after stimulation of the dorsal penile nerve: normative data and results from 145 patients with erectile dysfunction. Eur. Neurol., 27: 245, 1987
148. Guerit, J.M.Opsomer, R.J.: Bit-mapped imaging of somatosensory evoked potentials after stimulation of the posterior tibial nerves and dorsal nerve of the penis/clitoris. Electroenceph Clin Neurophys, 80: 228, 1991
149. Rodi, Z., Vodusek, D., Denislic, M.: Clinical uro-neurophysiological investigation in multiple sclerosis. Eur Neurol, 3: 574, 1996
150. Delodovici, M.L. Fowler, C.J.: Clinical value of the pudendal somatosensory evoked potential. Electroenceph Clin Neurophys, 96: 509, 1995
151. Curt, A., Rodic, B., Schurch, B., et al.: Recovery of bladder function in patients with acute spinal cord injury: significance of ASIA scores and somatosensory evoked potentials. Spinal Cord, 35: 368, 1997
152. Cohen, B.A., Major, M.R.Huizenga, B.A.: Pudendal nerve evo-

ked potential monitoring in procedures involving low sacral fixation. Spine, 16: S375, 1991

153. Vodusek, D.B., Deletis, V., Abbott, R. and Turndorf, H.: Prevention of iatrogenic micturition disorders through intraoperative monitoring. Neurourol. Urodyn., 9: 444, 1990
154. Ganzer, H., Madersbacher, H.Rumpl, E.: Cortical evoked potentials by stimulation of the vesicourethral junction: clinical value and neurophysiological considerations. J Urol, 146: 118, 1991
155. Opsomer, R.J., Guérit, J. M., Van Cangh, P. J., Rossini, P. M.: Electrical and magnetic brain mapping after pudendal nerve stimulation. J. Urol., 4: 143, 1990
156. Opsomer, R.J.Guerit, J.M.: [Electric and magnetic brain mapping following stimulation of the dorsal nerve of the penis or clitoris]. Acta Urol Belg, 59: 63, 1991
157. Podnar, S., Vodusek, D.B., Trsinar, B., et al.: A method of uroneurophysiological investigation in children. Electroenceph Clin Neurophys, 104: 389, 1997
158. Badr, G.A., Carlsson, C.-A., Fall, M., et al.: Cortical evoked potentials following the stimulation of the uyrinary bladder in man. Electroenceph Clin Neurophys, 54: 494, 1982
159. Hansen, M.V., Ertekin, C.Larsson, L.-E.: Cerebral evoked potentials after stimulation of posterior urethra in man. Electroenceph Clin Neurophys, 77: 52, 1990
160. Sarica, Y.Karacan, I.: Cerebral responses evoked by stimulation of the vesico-urethral junction in normal subjects. ECG and Clin Neurophys, 65: 440, 1986
161. Gerstenberg, T.C., Klarskov, P. And Hald, T.: Pudendal somatosensory, urethral and bladder wall evoked potentials in normals. Proceedings of ICS, 150, 1982
162. Ertekin, C.Reel, F.: Bulbocavernosus reflex in normal men and in patients with neurogenic bladder and/or impotence. J Neurol Sci, 28: 1, 1976
163. Vereecken, R.L., De Meirsman, J., Puers, B., et al.: Electrophysiological exploration of the sacral conus. J Neurol, 227: 135, 1982
164. Krane, R.J.Siroky, M.B.: Studies on sacral-evoked potentials. J Urol, 124: 872, 1980
165. Bilkey, W.J., Awad, E.A.Smith, A.D.: Clinical application of sacral reflex latency. J Urol, 129: 1187, 1983
166. Varma, J.S., A.N., S.Mcinnes, A.: Electrophysiological observations on the human pudendo-anal reflex. J Neurol, Neurosurg Psychiat, 49: 1411, 1986
167. Bartolo, D.C.C., Jarratt, J.A.Read, N.W.: The cutaneo-anal reflex: A useful index of neuropathy? Br J Surg, 7: 660, 1983
168. Pedersen, E., Harvcing, H., Klemar, B., et al.: Human anal reflexes. J Neurol, Neurosurg Psychiat, 41: 813, 1978
169. Yang, C.Bradley, W.E.: Reflex innervation of the bulbocavernosus muscle. Br J U Int, 84: 857, 2000
170. Sarica, Y.Karacan, I.: Bulbocavernosus reflex to somatic and visceral nerve stimulation in normal subjects and in diabetics with erectile impotence. J Urol, 138: 55, 1987
171. Bradley, W.E.: Urethral electromyelography. J Urol, 108: 563, 1972
172. Contreras Ortiz, O., Bertotti, A.C.Rodriguez Nunez, J.D.: Pudendal reflexes in women with pelvic floor disorders. Zentralbl Gynakol, 116: 561, 1994
173. Vodusek, D.B., Plevnik, S., Janez, J., Vrtacnik, P.: Detrusor inhibition on selective pudendal nerve stimulation in the perineum. Neurourol. Urodynam., 6: 389, 1988
174. Podnar, S., Vodusek, D.B., Trsinar, B.: Mechanically evoked bulbocavernosus reflex and pudendal somatosensory responses in children. Pflugers Arch, 431: R293, 1996
175. Vodusek, D.B., Janko, M.: The bulbocavernosus reflex. A single motor neuron study. Brain, 113: 813, 1990
176. Rodi, ZA., Vodusek D.B.: The sacral reflex studies: single versus double pulse stimulation. Neurourol. Urodyn., 14: 496, 1995
177. Amarenco, G. Kerdraon, J.: Clinical value of ipsi- and contralateral sacral reflex latency measurement: a normative data study in man. Neurourol Urodyn, 19: 565, 2000
178. Yang, C., Bowen, J., Kraft, G., et al.: Cortical evoked potentials of the dorsal nerve of the clitoris and female sexual dysfunction in multiple sclerosis. J Urol, 164: 2010, 2000
179. Vodusek, D.B., Zidar, J.: Pudendal nerve involvement in patients with hereditary motor and sensory neuropathy. Acta Neurol Scand, 76: 457, 1987
180. Hanson, P., Rigaux, P., Gilliard, C., et al.: Sacral reflex latencies in tethered cord syndrome. Am J Phys Med Rehabil, 72: 39, 1993
181. Sethi, R.K., Bauer, S.B., Dyro, F.M., et al.: Modulation of the bulbocavernosus reflex during voiding: Loss of inhibition in upper motor neuron lesions. Muscle Nerve, 12: 892, 1989
182. Deletis, V.Vodusek, D.B.: Intraoperative recording of the bulbocavernosus reflex. Neurosurgery, 40: 88, 1997
183. Dykstra, D., Sidi, A., Cameron, J., et al.: The use of mechanical stimulation to obtain the sacral reflex latency: a new technique. J Urol, 137: 77, 1987
184. Ballaro, A., Craggs, M.D.: A new approach to recording electromyographic activity from detrusor smooth muscle. J Urol, 166: in press, 2001
185. Shahani, B.T., Halperin, J.J., Boulu, P., et al.: Sympathetic skin response - a method of assessing unmyelinated axon dysfunction in peripheral neuropathies. JNeurol, Neurosurg Psychiat, 47: 536, 1984
186. Ertekin, C., Almis, S.Ertekin, N.: Sympathetic skin potentials and bulbocavernosus reflex in patients with chronic alcoholism and impotence. Eur Neurol, 30: 334, 1990
187. Ertekin, C., Ertekin, N., Almis, S.: Autonomic sympathetic nerve involvement in diabetic impotence. Neurourol Urodyn, 8: 589, 1989
188. Ertekin, C., Ertekin, N., Mutlu, S., et al.: Skin potentials (SP) recorded from the extremities and genital regions in normal and impotent subjects. Acta Neuro Scand, 76: 28, 1987
189. Daffertshofer, M., Linden, D., Syren, M., et al.: Assessment of local sympathetic function in patients with erectile dysfunction. Int J Impot Res, 6: 213, 1994
190. Opsomer, R., Boccasena, P., Traversa, R., et al.: Sympathetic skin responses from the limbs and the genitalia: normative study and contribution to the evaluation of neurourological disorders. Electroenceph Clin Neurophys, 101: 25, 1996
191. Schurch, B., Curt, A., Rossier, A.B.: The value of sympathetic skin response recordings in the assessment of the vesicourethral autonomic nervous dysfunction in spinal cord injured patients. J Urol, 157: 2230, 1997
192. Rodic, B., Curt, A., Dietz, V., et al.: Bladder neck incompetence in patients with spinal cord injury: significance of sympathetic skin response. J Urol, 163: 1223, 2000
193. Curt, A., Nitsche, B., Rodic, B., et al.: Assessment of autonomic dysreflexia in patients with spinal cord injury. J Neurol Neurosurg Psychiatry, 62: 473, 1997
194. Koldewijn, E.L., Van Kerrebroeck, P.E., Bemelmans, B.L., et al.: Use of sacral reflex latency measurements in the evaluation of neural function of spinal cord injury patients: a comparison of neuro-urophysiological testing and urodynamic investigations. J Urol, 152: 463, 1994
195. Liu, S., Christmas, T.J., Nagendran, K., et al.: Sphincter electromyography in patients after radical prostatectomy and cystoprostatectomy. Br J Urol, 69: 397, 1992
196. Percy, J.P., Neill, M., Parks, A., et al.: Electrophysiological study of motor nerve supply of pelvic floor. Lancet, i: 16, 1981
197. Gearhart, J.P., Burnett, A.Owen, J.H.: Measurement of pudendal evoked potentials during feminizing genitoplasty: technique and applications [see comments]. J Urol, 153: 486, 1995

Committee 8 C

Imaging and other Investigations

Chairman

W. ARTIBANI (ITALY)

Members

J.T. ANDERSEN (DENMARK),

J.B. GAJEWSKI (CANADA),

D.R. OSTERGARD (USA),

S. RAZ (USA),

A. TUBARO (ITALY)

Consultants

V. KHULLAR (UK),

P. KLARSKOV (DENMARK),

L. RODRIGUEZ (USA)

CONTENTS

Imaging and other Investigations

W. ARTIBANI,

J.T. ANDERSEN, J.B. GAJEWSKI, D.R. OSTERGARD, S. RAZ, A. TUBARO,
V. KHULLAR, P. KLARSKOV, L. RODRIGUEZ

INTRODUCTION

The committee was charged with reviewing and updating the chapter Imaging Techniques and Other Investigations in Urinary Incontinence (W. Artibani, J.T. Andersen, D.R. Ostergard, C.E. Constantinou, J.B. Gajewski, V.N. Nitti, P. Klarskov, G. Schaer, A. Tubaro: Incontinence, Health Publication Ltd, 1999, p. 401-445).

This revision/update was performed by the committee members and consultants, and then collegially processed to obtain a consensus.

The different techniques are categorized as imaging techniques, endoscopy, pad testing, and other investigations (urinalysis, chemical tests and tissue analysis).

They were analyzed taking into account various viewpoints as follows:

• Age (children, adults, and elderly)

• Gender

• Type of urinary incontinence:

- extra urethral/ per urethra
- congenital / acquired
- neurogenic / non-neurogenic
- stress / urge / mixed / chronic retention with incontinence/functional /other types
- postvoid dribbling

• Upper and lower urinary tract

On the basis of a peer reviewed literature review and expert opinion, the role of imaging techniques and other investigations was outlined, when possible, with regards to diagnosis, measurement of severity, indications for treatment, prognostic value, monitoring and follow-up, cost-effectiveness ratio, outcome evaluation and research interest.

For each imaging technique or investigation, general recommendations and suggested research areas are indicated.

Levels of evidence are difficult to apply to the subject of this chapter since prospective randomised trials are rarely used. We tried to follow ICUD's recommendation for issues related to assessment and investigation, by evaluating each test for technical perfomance, diagnostic performance and clinical relevance.

We used the following revised levels of evidence.

High Level Evidence : More than one prospective, comparative, blindly evaluated, trial with acceptable entry criteria, adequate statistical power, and data analysis. (Gold standard imaging techniques should be compared to new imaging modalities).

Intermediate Level Evidence: A single prospective, comparative, blindly evaluated trial with the same requirements stated for High Level, or multiple clinical trials which do not meet all the requirements for High Level (for example some are not blindly evaluated).

Low Level Evidence: Non prospective, and/or non comparative trials or prospective, comparative clinical trials with documented design flaws (e.g. insufficient patient numbers, inadequately defined entry criteria, or inadequate statistics).

No Evidence: No clinical trial data or information limited to single institution retrospective series, abstracts, or meeting presentations.

In regards with recommendations, we also defined the degree of Committee agreement as follows:

Unanimous agreement: All Committee members agree on the recommendation.

Significant Majority: At least 75 % of the Committee agree on the recommendation.

Majority: More than one-half of the Committee agrees on the recommendation. In this case, the minority opinion should be stated in the report.

No agreement.

There are places in the chapter where the degree of agreement of a recommendation is specified without indicating levels of evidence. This is the case when unanimously agreed recommendations could not be supported by data, and there should have been paradoxically a mark of no evidence or low level evidence. In case of a recommendation with high level evidence, unanimous agreement is implicit and was not specified.

A. IMAGING OF THE UPPER URINARY TRACT

I. BACKGROUND

Urinary incontinence is classically thought of as involuntary loss of urine "per uretram" as a result of sphincter and/or bladder dysfunction. Extra-urethral urinary incontinence may occur as a result of congenital anomalies such as ectopic ureters (inserting in the female distal urethra or vagina) or traumatic conditions such as fistula. Furthermore, lower urinary tract dysfunction, which may be a cause for incontinence, might compromise the transport of urine from the kidneys to the bladder resulting in hydronephrosis and renal damage. The relationship between high bladder storage pressure and renal deterioration has been well established [1].

Such damage is usually detectable at various stages by imaging of the kidneys and/or renal function tests. There are two other conditions related to urinary incontinence which may endanger the upper tract: one is chronic retention with incontinence, and the second is the presence of severe urogenital prolapse which may cause angulation of the ureters at the level of the uterine arteries with consequent hydroureteronephrosis in as many as 30% to 40% of patients [2] (Figure. 1 a,b).

II. INDICATIONS

Generally speaking, there is no need for upper tract imaging in cases of urinary incontinence with no neurological etiology.

Upper urinary tract imaging becomes an important part of the evaluation of the incontinent patient when extra-urethral urinary incontinence or potentially dangerous lower urinary tract dysfunction are known or suspected. Thus the objectives used for upper tract imaging in the incontinent patient are the following:

1. Evaluation of the ectopic ureter or ureterovaginal fistula as a cause of urinary incontinence
2. Evaluation of the kidneys in cases where urinary incontinence is related to bladder dysfunction with high storage pressures (e.g. in neurogenic voiding dysfunction, chronic retention with overflow or low-compliance bladders)
3. Exclusion of hydronephrosis in cases of urinary incontinence associated with severe uterine prolapse (Figure 2 a,b,c,d)

III. MODALITIES

The most commonly used upper tract imaging modalities include intravenous urography (IVU), ultrasonography, computerized tomography (CT scan), magnetic resonance imaging (MRI), and isotope scanning.

None of these tests have been evaluated for specificity, sensitivity, predictive value or reproducibility in connection with the diagnosis and management of urinary incontinence. There are large geographical variations concerning availability of equipment, local expertise and traditions.

Therefore, the examinations are summarized on the basis of literature review and expert opinion, and only special points with respect to urinary incontinence are mentioned.

IV. INTRAVENOUS UROGRAPHY

Intravenous urography or intravenous pyelography (IVP) is the original radiographic examination of the upper urinary tract. Successful examination is dependent upon adequate renal function. Renal dysfunction, obstruction, congenital anomalies, fistula, stones and tumors may be detected.

IVU is the appropriate first study when ureteral ectopia is suspected. Delayed films and tomography are important because the renal unit or moiety associated with an ectopic ureter is often poorly functioning. In fact, IVU is sometimes unable to detect a small, malfunctioning moiety associated with a duplication and ectopic ureter or a poorly functioning or abnormally located kidney with a single ectopic system [3-5]. In such cases where the diagnosis of ectopia is still suspected after IVU, another imaging modality such as CT, MRI (Figure 3 a,b) or isotope scanning [6-8] should be considered.

IVU is the appropriate first imaging study when uretero-vaginal fistula is suspected, usually after pelvic surgery. Typically, one sees ureteropyelocaliectasis proximal to the level of the fistula. This finding has been reported in 84-92% of cases [9,10]. Sometimes extravasation can be seen. Confirmation of the presence of the fistula, its size and exact location is often obtained with retrograde ureteropyelography.

V. ULTRASONOGRAPHY

Ultrasonography is an excellent tool for imaging of the upper urinary tracts. It is totally non-invasive, and successful imaging of the kidneys is independent of renal

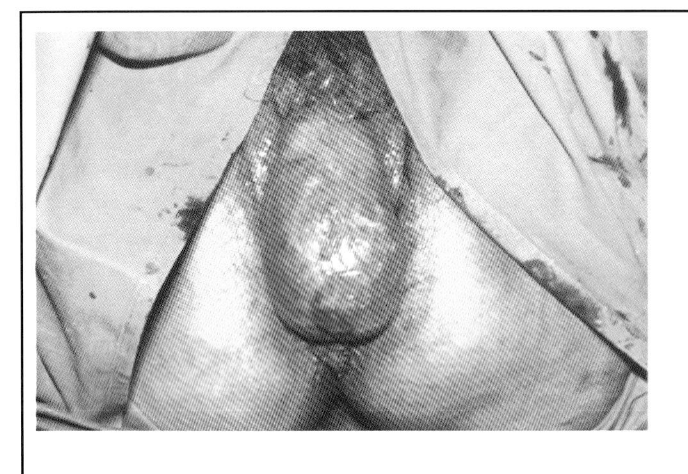

Figure 1a: Procidentia uteri.

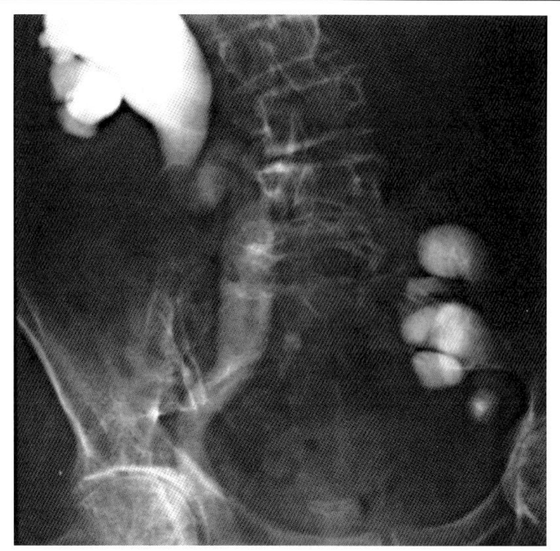

Figure 1 b: IVU: bilateral hydronephrosis. Left kidney is in sacral ectopia.

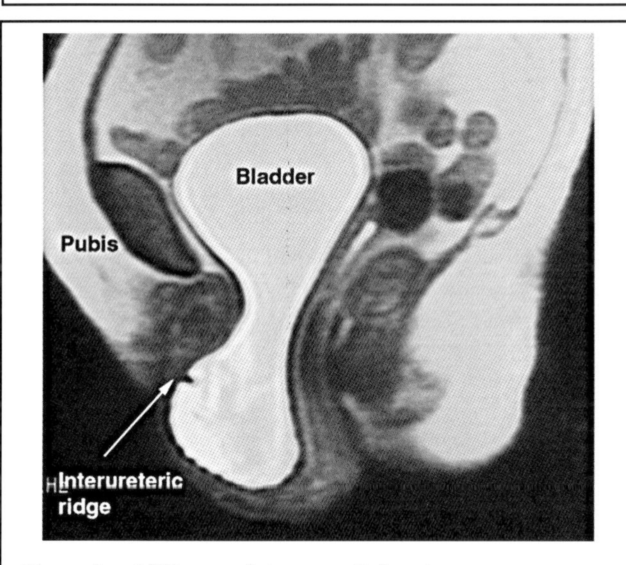

Figure 2 a: MRI: complete urogenital prolapse.

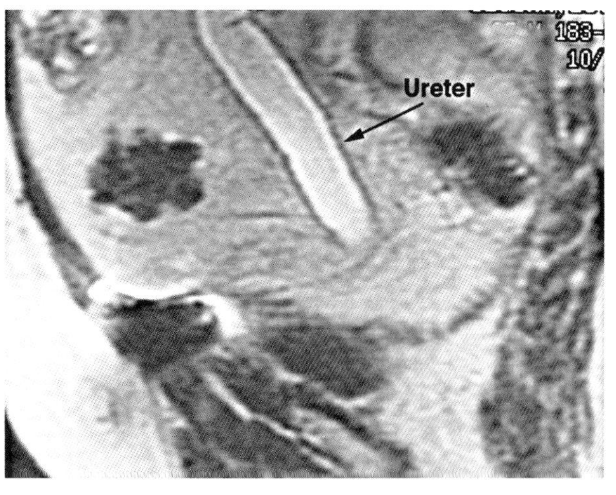

Figure 2-b: MRI: ureteral dilation

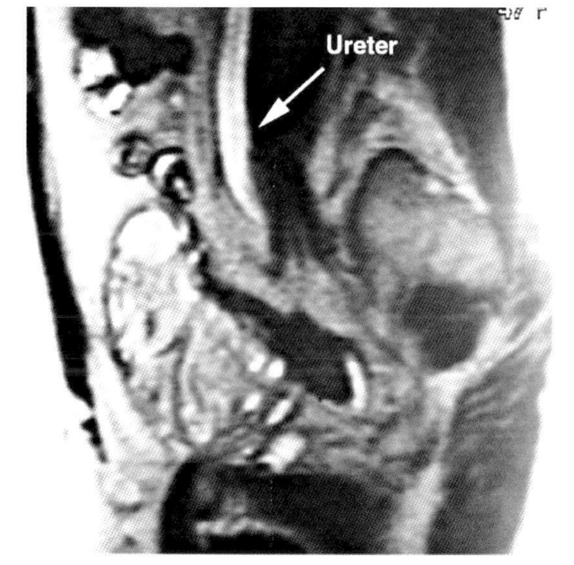

Figure 2-c: MRI: ureteral dilation

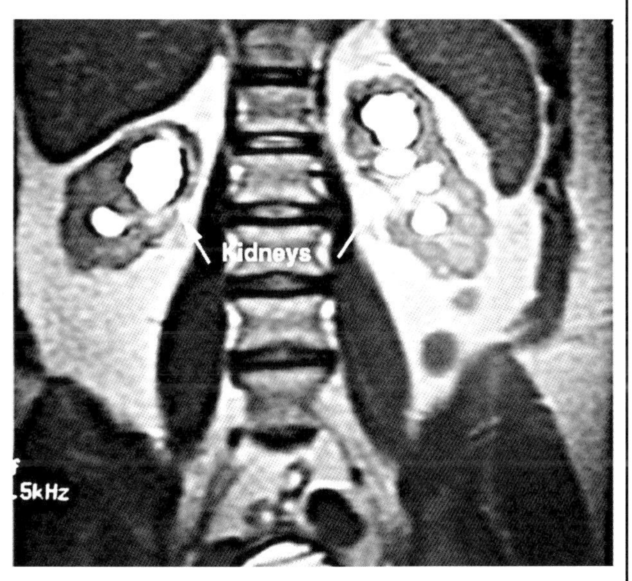

Figure 2-d:MRI bilateral hydronephrosis

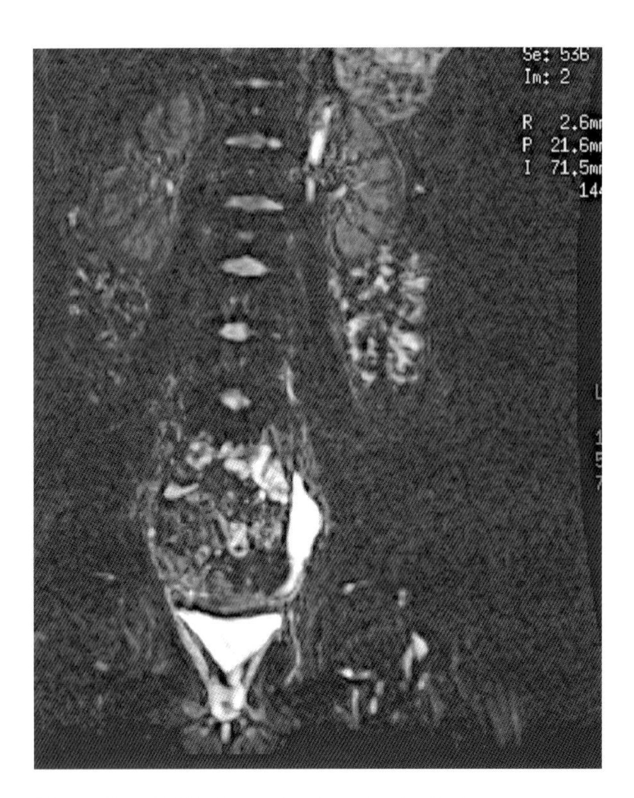

Figure 3 a : MRI diagnosis of ureteral ectopia

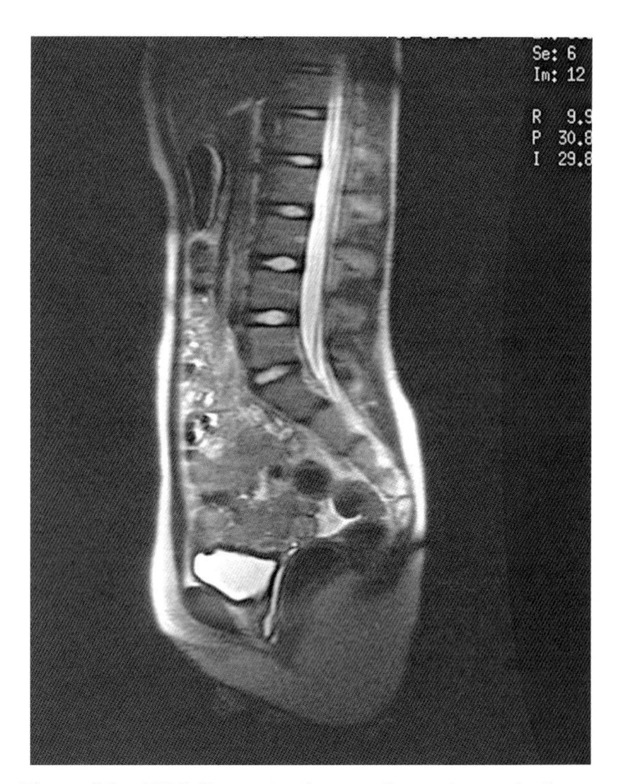

Figure 3 b : MRI diagnosis of ureteral ectopia: sagittal view

function. Ultrasound can be used to assess many features of renal anatomy including renal size and growth, hydronephrosis, segmental anomalies, stones and tumors. In the evaluation of the patient with lower urinary tract dysfunction, the detection of hydronephrosis is extremely important and may be an indication of vesico-ureteral reflux or obstruction. However, no correlation exists between the degree of dilatation and the severity of obstruction. Also renal blood flow can be detected by the doppler technique. Because ultrasonography can not predict function or degree of obstruction or reflux, other imaging modalities are often used after hydronephrosis is initially diagnosed by ultrasound.

Ultrasound is an excellent tool to follow the degree of hydronephrosis over time or the response to treatment.

VI. COMPUTERIZED TOMOGRAPHY

Computerized Tomography scan (CT) provides useful information about the anatomy of the upper urinary tract. Information can be independent of renal function, however, the addition of intravenous contrast can highlight specific anatomic characteristics (dependent upon renal function). CT scan can be used as an alternative to ultrasonography or IVP, and in many cases provides additional information, although at a higher cost. Several authors have reported the use of CT scan to detect ectopic ureter, in cases where the diagnosis is suspected, despite a normal IVU and ultrasound [11]. In these cases the small size and poor function of the ectopic moiety made diagnosis difficult by IVU.

VII. MAGNETIC RESONANCE IMAGING

Magnetic Resonance Imaging (MRI) offers some of the same benefits as CT in the evaluation of the upper urinary tracts. It has the advantage over CT in that all planes of imaging are possible. MRI may play an increasing role in the evaluation of hydronephrosis and urinary tract anomalies in the future. Its usefulness has recently been described in the diagnosis of ectopic ureter [12,13].

VIII. ISOTOPES

Isotopes are used primarily to examine functional characteristics of the upper urinary tract. Isotope scanning can be used to evaluate renal morphology and location. Renography is used to examine the differential function of the two kidneys as well as how they drain. There are many physiological factors and technical pitfalls that can influence the outcome including the choice of radionucleotide, timing of diuretic injection, state of hydration and diuresis, fullness or back pressure from the bladder, variable renal function and compliance of the collecting system [14-16].

Diuresis renography with bladder drainage is recommended when obstructive uropathy is suspected [17]. Renal scintigraphy may be useful in the evaluation of ectopic ureters in association with hypoplastic kidneys [18].

IX. CONCLUSIONS AND RECOMMENDATIONS

1. Imaging of the upper urinary tract is NOT indicated in the evaluation of non-neurogenic stress, urge or mixed urinary incontinence. (***Unanimous agreement***)
2. Imaging of the upper urinary tract is indicated in cases of (***Unanimous agreement***):
   a) neurogenic urinary incontinence with high risk of renal damage (due to high detrusor pressure, e.g. myelodysplasia, spinal cord injury, and low compliance bladders) (***High Level Evidence***)
   b) chronic retention with incontinence (***Intermediate Level Evidence***)
   c) untreated severe urogenital prolapse (***Low Level Evidence***)
   d) suspicion of extra-urethral urinary incontinence by upper tract anomaly (***High Level Evidence***)
3. The choice of the imaging techniques and their sequence depend on the clinical question and their availability. The least invasive techniques should be preferred and should precede the more invasive, also taking into consideration cost effectiveness. (***Unanimous agreement***)

X. SUGGESTED RESEARCH AREAS

1. Prevalence of upper tract deterioration in various urinary incontinence populations
2. Natural history of upper tract damage
3. Relation between upper tract dilation, renal damage and bladder function

B. LOWER URINARY TRACT (LUT) IMAGING

Radiological visualization of the position and morphology of the bladder, urethra and pelvic floor has been used mainly in connection with management of female urinary incontinence. Additional aims are to demonstrate leakage, to locate infravesical obstruction, vesicoureteral reflux, diverticula, fistula, stones, and tumours.

In males the purpose of voiding cystourethrography has been mainly to locate infravesical obstruction [1,2]. In children the diagnosis and classification of reflux and diagnosis of posterior urethral valves have been the primary goals [3]. MRI may be an alternative [4].

Positive-pressure urethrography has been designed only for the diagnosis of female urethral diverticula and was shown to be more sensitive than voiding cystourethrography [5,6,7].

B-I. IMAGING IN FEMALE URINARY INCONTINENCE AND PELVIC FLOOR DYSFUNCTION

I. FEMALE CYSTOURETHROGRAPHY

1. Background

Aspects of the history and methodology of cystourethrography in females had been reviewed by Olesen [8]. Voiding cystourethrography with lateral projection was first done by Mikulicz-Radecki in 1931 [9]. Stevens and Smith in 1937 [10] introduced a metallic bead chain into the urethra, and in 1956 Ardran, Simmons and Stewart [11] reported on a cinematographic technique with contrast media also in the vagina and rectum. During the sixties and seventies several reports emerged on combined fluoroscopy and pressure and flow recordings [12-16].

2. Methodology (projection, positioning and exposures)

Frontal and oblique projections are inferior to a straight lateral projection in diagnosing bladder descent, and in differentiating between different types of displacement. A seated position is recommended for micturition in female patients, because micturition standing or lying will increase the embarrassment and thereby the bias of the examination [8]. However, lateral projection necessitates high radiation doses with sufficiently high kV, as the central x-ray beam must penetrate the trocanteric regions and further because the urethrovesical junction sometimes is overshadowed by the lateral parts of the bladder. The position and mobility of the urethrovesical junction and leakage are supposed to be influenced by the filling volume as has been demonstrated on ultrasonography [17] and leak point pressure measurements [18]. However, in voiding cystourethrography the bladder is filled to capacity. Addition of a urethral bead chain or catheter and vaginal contrast improve the visualisation of the urethra, bladder neck and trigone. Contrast in the rectum is not necessary for urinary incontinence purposes.

Exposures at rest should be supplemented with provocative manoeuvres (coughing, straining, and squeezing) and micturition. Coughing and straining differs. Straining might be associated with relaxation or contraction of the pelvic floor, and the imaging can change accordingly. During coughing there is a reflex contraction of the pelvic floor, but coughs are of short duration and difficult to catch on spot films. Bladder suspension defects were diagnosed at rest in 49% of 420 examinations, while coughing and micturition disclosed a further number of 20% and 4% respectively [8]. Squeezing can demonstrate pelvic floor awareness and contraction [19].

3. Combined imaging and urodynamics

Videourodynamics has been by some regarded as the "gold standard" in the evaluation of lower urinary tract dysfunction [20]. However, it is controversial whether urodynamic and radiographic testing should be performed simultaneously or on separate occasions. Urodynamic examinations must be repeated several times to obtain reproducibility [21,22], and the more parameters studied the more complicated the examination will be with a corresponding risk of bias. Reproducibility of the combined examination has not been assessed, and, further, the radiation dose has to be considered [10,15,23,24]. Nevertheless simultaneous videomonitoring along with tracings of pressure and urine flow rate are important means to be sure that the exposures are made at appropriate moments so that the radiographs can be representative of the various functional states [8,13,25,26].

4. Normal and defective bladder support

The normal resting bladder has a smooth surface. The position of the internal urethral orifice is situated between the anterior and the middle third of the base just above a horizontal line through the lowermost part of the symphysis. The base is flat and slopes upwards and backwards. The urethra is straight and runs downwards and forwards giving rise to an angulation with the bladder base. The vagina lies approximately 1.5 cm behind the urethra and the trigone following a parallel course. On coughing and straining (Figure 4a) there might be a minor movement and curvation downwards, but no essential changes should occur. Squeezing should cause changes in the opposite direction. During voiding (Figure 4b) the bladder base is usually lowered about 1 cm, the angulation between the urethra and the trigone is straightened, making a funnelled appearance of the proximal urethra and the bladder base, the bladder contour is rounded and a fine sawtooth irregularity of the mucosa becomes visible above the trigone. Post voiding pictures should be interpretated with caution.

Different angles, planes, distances and morphological criteria have been used to discriminate between normal and defective bladder support.

The following parameters have been assessed for reliability:

1. The posterior urethrovesical angle (PUV) is defined by lines along the posterior urethra and the trigone [27]. Cut off values were usually 115° or more [28,29].
2. The urethral inclination is between the proximal urethral axis and the vertical plane, which is a plane outside the patient and, therefore, the angle also varies with pelvic inclination. In Green type I and type II descent the angle is less or more than 45° respectively [30].
3. The urethropelvic angle (UP) is measured during voiding as the anterior angle between a line through the middle of the internal urethral orifice and the urethral knee and a line through the posterior surface of the symphysis through the lowermost part of the obturator foramen closest to the film. In normals the mean UP is about 95° and the cut off point for bladder descent are values below 70° [8].

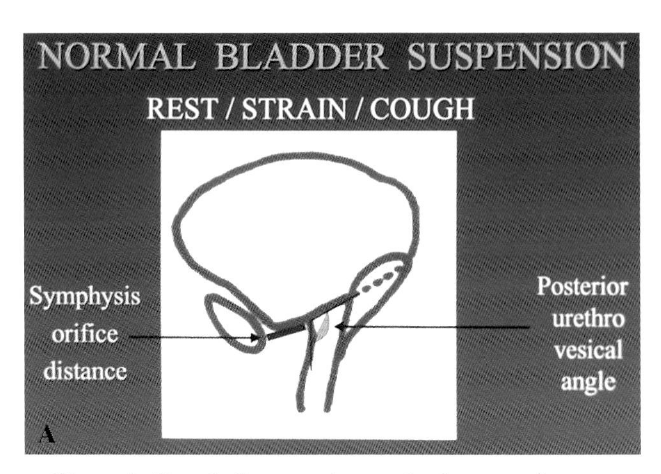

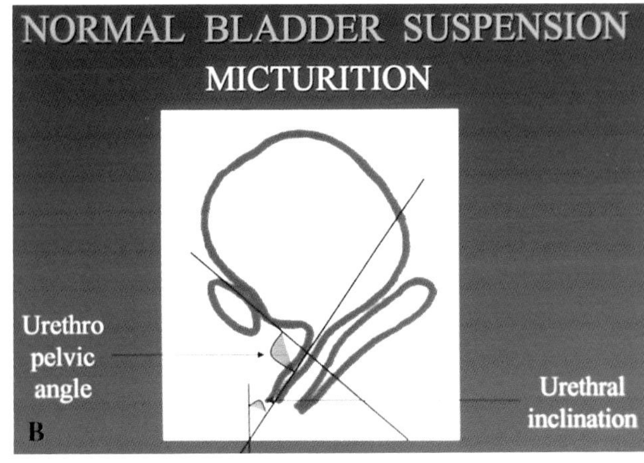

Figure 4 : Female Cysto-urethrography 1a: normal appearance on coughing, straining and squeezing 1b: normal appearance on voiding

4. Symphysis orifice distance (SO) is measured at rest as the distance on a horizontal line from the symphysis to the internal urethral orifice. Normal values are 31 +- 6 mm (mean +- SD) and values less than 20 mm are the cut off points for descent [8].

Funneling of the proximal urethra, flatness of the bladder base (both anterior and posterior to the internal urethral orifice) and the most dependent portion of the bladder base (the urethrovesical junction or a point posterior to that) are important qualitative parameters estimated on straining films [28].

Anterior bladder suspension defects or bladder base insufficiency (BBI) Figure 5 is defined as SO < 20 mm with a normally positioned vagina at rest, during coughing or micturition and/or funneling of the bladder base at rest or with coughing. The insufficiency can be graded 1-3 [8] which corresponds to Green's type I descent [30]. The supportive defect is supposed to be in the fascial and ligamentous system and their abnormal detachments (eg., paravaginal defects).

Posterior bladder suspension defects [8] Figure 6 are defined as a posterior-inferior bladder displacement and a UP of less than 70°. This corresponds to Green's type II [30]. In trigonocele (Figure 7) only the trigone and posterior part of the bladder is involved. The supportive defect is supposed to be in the muscular pelvic floor, that is, the pubo-vesical part of the pubococcygeus muscle or in paravaginal detachment.

5. Reliability

Reliability depends on both accuracy and reproducibility

The accuracy of the previously mentioned radiological criteria have been measured by comparing the test results with a final true diagnosis of genuine stress incontinence or a "gold standard" and expressed as specificity and sensitivity or as predictive values. The crux of the matter is that the diagnosis of stress urinary incontinence is controversial and might be based on subjective criteria, urodynamic tests, or measurement of leakage. Even radiological criteria have been included in the diagnosis.

Reproducibility has not been measured as test-re-test agreement, but intra- and inter-observer variation has been calculated and also adjusted for expected chance agreement (kappa coefficient). The predictive values and the kappa coefficient are supposed to depend on the prevalence [31], and therefore, comparison between different materials are difficult.

6. Specificity, sensitivity and predictive values for the diagnosis of stress incontinence and post-operative results

There is agreement in the literature that cystourethrography can not discriminate between stress incontinence and continence [29,32-34]. The specificity of 5 radiological parameters on static bead chain cystourethrography was 44-76% and the sensitivity 53-100% [35,36]. Neither was the degree of stress incontinence correlated to the type or degree of suspension defects [19,37,38]. The predictive values of demonstrating a bladder suspension defect PV-pos was 0.70 (95% c.l. 0.62-0.78) and normal appearance PV-neg was 0.52 (95% c.l. 0.41-0.63) on voiding colpo-cystourethrography [39,30]. In a later publication on 159 women PV-pos was 0.56 and PV-neg 0.74 [34].

Further, it is not possible to distinguish postoperative failures from success [8,19,31,33,36,40-43]. Colposuspension gives rise to a typical configuration, vaginal repair was usually not detectable on cystourethrography, and pelvic floor training improved the squeezing effect, but not the suspension defect [19].

7. Reproducibility

The observer variation has been evaluated in four university uro-gynecological units [19,28,38,44] (Table 1)

The inter-observer agreement was 43-79% and the intra-observer agreement was 53-99%. These figures are in the same range as has been found for other diagnostic tests [31].

8. Comparison of cystourethrography and ultrasonography

Static bead chain cystourethrography has been compared with transrectal [36] and perineal ultrasonography [45,46] and voiding colpo-cystourethrography has been compared with perineal ultrasonography [47]. The findings correlated well regarding bladder beck position and mobility, PUV, urethral inclination, SO distance and rotation angle.

Specificity, sensitivity and interobserver agreement were also comparable for the two methods. All the authors seem to prefer the sonographic modality because the imaging study can be performed at the same time as the physical examination. This has also been the case in men with neuromuscular dysfunction [2]. Simple and extensive funnelling is more easily imaged in upright patients during cystourethrography than in the supine position frequently used for ultrasound studies [48].

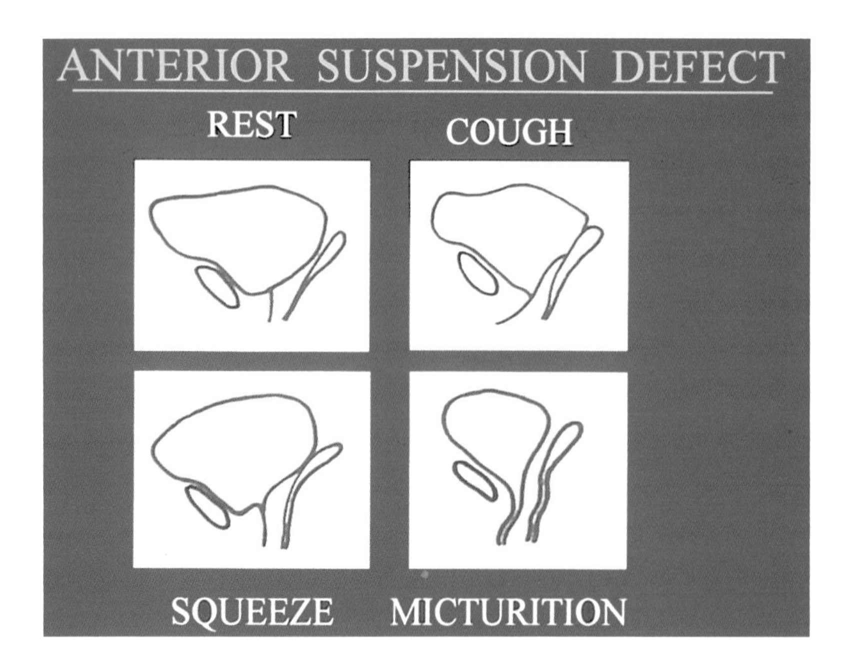

Figure 5 : Female Cysto-urethrography. Anterior bladder suspension defect

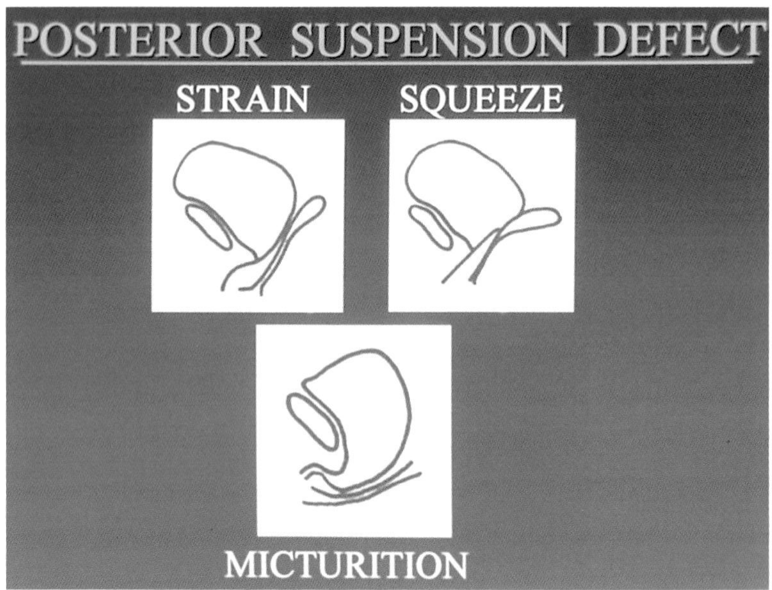

Figure 6 : Female Cysto-urethrography. Posterior bladder suspension defect

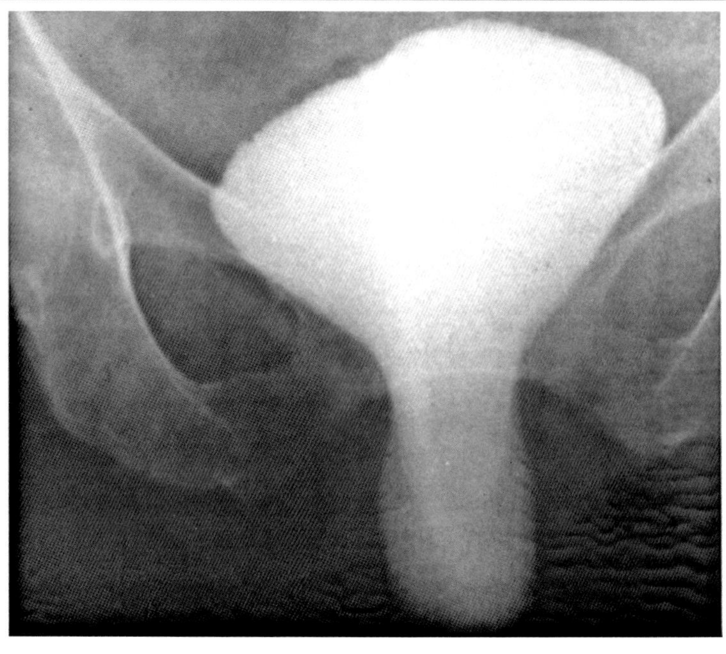

Figure 7 : Female cystourethrography: Trigonocele: The trigone herniates through the anterior vaginal wall.

Table 1 : Inter- and intra-observer variation (agreement) on cystourethrography in females with urinary incontinence.

Type of examination, patients and observers	Inter-observer variation	Intra-observer variation
Bead-chain (1) stress & urge incont. n°92 3 observers on 5 landmarks	45.8-80.7 % VCCU 2	
VCCU (2) stress incontinence n° 52 1 observer on type of descent	79% 95% c.l. 65-89	
VCCU (3) stress incontinence n° 29 2 obervers on type of descent	70% 95% c.l. 75-89	53 95% c.l. 27-78
VCCU (4) n° 93 stress & urge incont. 6 observers on type of descent	43-60% kappa 20-39%	72-99% kappa 57-98%

Legend Table 1:
1: static bead-chain cystourethrography with straining [28]. The 5 landmarks were the posterior urethrovesical angle, urethral inclination, funneling of the proximal urethra, flatness of the bladder base and most dependent position of the bladder base.
2: voiding colpo-cystourethrography (VCCU) at rest and with coughing, straining, micturition and squeezing; one observer against original diagnosis (that is, normal appearance or anterior, posterior or combined suspension defects) made by a few senior radiologists [19].
3: voiding colpo-cystourethrography at rest and with coughing, straining, squeezing and micturition. Possible diagnoses were: normal appearance or anterior, posterior or combined descent respectively [44].
4: voiding colpo-cystourethrography at rest, coughing, with holding and voiding. Possible diagnoses were: normal appearance and anterior or posterior descent respectively [38].

9. Comparison of cystourethrography and MRI

Magnetic resonance imaging and lateral cystourethrography was compared in 27 women with urinary incontinence and bladder descent [49] and with colpocystorectography in 12 women or with bead-chain cystourethrography in 20 women in a prospective study [50]. The findings on MRI were equivalent to that obtained with colpocystorectography and superior to cystourethogaphy in diagnosing rectoceles. Bias produced by difference in study position must also be considered when MRI and cystourethrography is compared.

10. Conclusions

The role of cystourethrography in the evaluation of female urinary incontinence is not yet established.

Defective bladder support can be diagnosed on voiding cystourethrography with a reliability comparable with other diagnostic tests. [***High Level Evidence***].

Dependent on local facilities the method might be considered if the choice of a surgical procedure is based on type and degree of supporting tissue insufficiency and possibly if new procedures are evaluated for the ability to restore this insufficiency. [***Low Level Evidence***].

The method can not be recommended for the diagnosis or classification of urinary incontinence. [***High Level Evidence***].

11. Recommendations

Cystourethrography is NOT indicated in primary uncomplicated stress, urge or mixed female urinary incontinence [***High Level Evidence***].

Cystourethrography may be a reasonable option in the preoperative evaluation of complicated or recurrent female urinary incontinence [***Low Level Evidence, Unanimous agreement***].

12. Suggested research areas

Standardization of technique, parameters and interpretation of cystourethrography

Possible value of cystourethrography in the evaluation of pelvic floor dysfunction (correlation of imaging to pelvic floor physical examination and to clinical outcome following therapy)

II. ULTRASOUND OF THE LOWER URINARY TRACT AND PELVIC FLOOR IN FEMALE URINARY INCONTINENCE

1. BACKGROUND

Since the 1980's reports on ultrasound evaluation of the lower urinary tract indicate that ultrasound is a valuable alternative to other imaging techniques. Studies comparing sonographic and other imaging techniques demonstrated the suitability of ultrasound [1-3]. These studies and the growing experience with pelvic floor sonography enabled the introduction of ultrasound into numerous urodynamic units as a helpful and highly informative assessment. Recent advancements in 3D ultrasonography opened new perspectives in the evaluation of incontinent female patients such as quantification of female urethral sphincter thickness and mass as well as evaluation of the urethra's submucosal vascular plexus [4-6]. A review of the international literature on urogynecology imaging shows that ultrasound studies have been predominated in recent years.

2. METHODOLOGY

Lower urinary tract ultrasound is an investigational evaluation for the study of female urinary incontinence and prolapse which allows morphological and functional documentation.

In principle two techniques should be differentiated (Figure 8):

endosonographic applications: vaginal and rectal sonography;

external applications: perineal and introital sonography.

Vaginal ultrasound is performed by introducing a linear or endfiring probe into the vagina (5 and 7.5 MHz) while ***rectal*** ultrasound uses the same probe rectally [7,8]. ***Perineal*** sonography is performed with a curved array ultrasound probe placed on the perineum (3.5 and 5 MHz) and ***introital*** ultrasound with a vaginal sector scanner placed between the labia minora (5 and 7.5 MHz) [9,10].

The decision in favour of one of the methods depends above all on local expertise and availability of the ultrasound probe although a vaginal approach has been considered to interfere with bladder neck and urethra anatomy and function [11,12]. Transrectal imaging, although invasive, does not influence urodynamic parameters during cystometry [13].

3D ultrasound imaging of the female urethra is performed with a linear 7.5 MHz probe using a transvaginal approach. Evaluation of the urethra's submucosal vascular plexus by colour Doppler can be performed by introital sonography [4, 5].

3. IMAGING

The following structures and organs can be visualised with ultrasound: urinary bladder, urethra, pubic bone, vagina, rectum and uterus. It should be emphasised that there are differences according to the ultrasound probe used, its frequency and the angle of projection. Vaginal and rectal ultrasound represent a sagittal section showing the uterus, urinary bladder, urethra and pubic bone, whereas introital and perineal sonography allow a panoramic view of the pelvis (Figure 8).

4. PICTURE ORIENTATION

The recommendation for the picture orientation is to depict cranial parts above and ventral parts on the right side. This kind of picture orientation corresponds to the representation of transvaginal ultrasound pictures preferred in European countries [14] and to the recommendations of Merz [15], Bernaschek [16] and the ICS [17] [***Level of evidence: intermediate***].

5. MEASUREMENT

Ultrasonographic examination of the bladder neck and urethra can be performed with the patients lying, sitting or standing although the study is often carried out in a supine position with the legs slightly abducted. Examination in the sitting position requires dedicated ultrasound systems to guarantee the optimal position of the probe on the perineum [18].

Bladder neck position changed little in different patient positions [19] although its mobility has been considered to be maximal in the standing position [19, 20] [Level of evidence: intermediate]. Thickness of the rhabdosphincter can be measured in transverse sections. The volume of the urethral sphincter is calculated, in female patients, using a step sectioning technique in transverse sections. Submucosal vascular plexus is imaged on a sagittal midline section with introital sonography.

Currently the retrovesical angle b and the position of the internal urethral orifice are the most important quantitative parameters [***High Level Evidence***].

The retrovesical angle β is measured as follows: one side of the angle is formed by the urethral axis, the other side by at least one-third of the bladder base near the bladder neck.

For determination of the internal urethral orifice two methods were previously investigated and their reproducibility analysed [20, 21]. Both relate to the pubic bone as a stable structure of the pelvis, which allows drawing an accurate reference line (central line of the symphysis).

Schaer et al (Figure 9) used a rectangular co-ordinate system where the x-axis is determined by the central

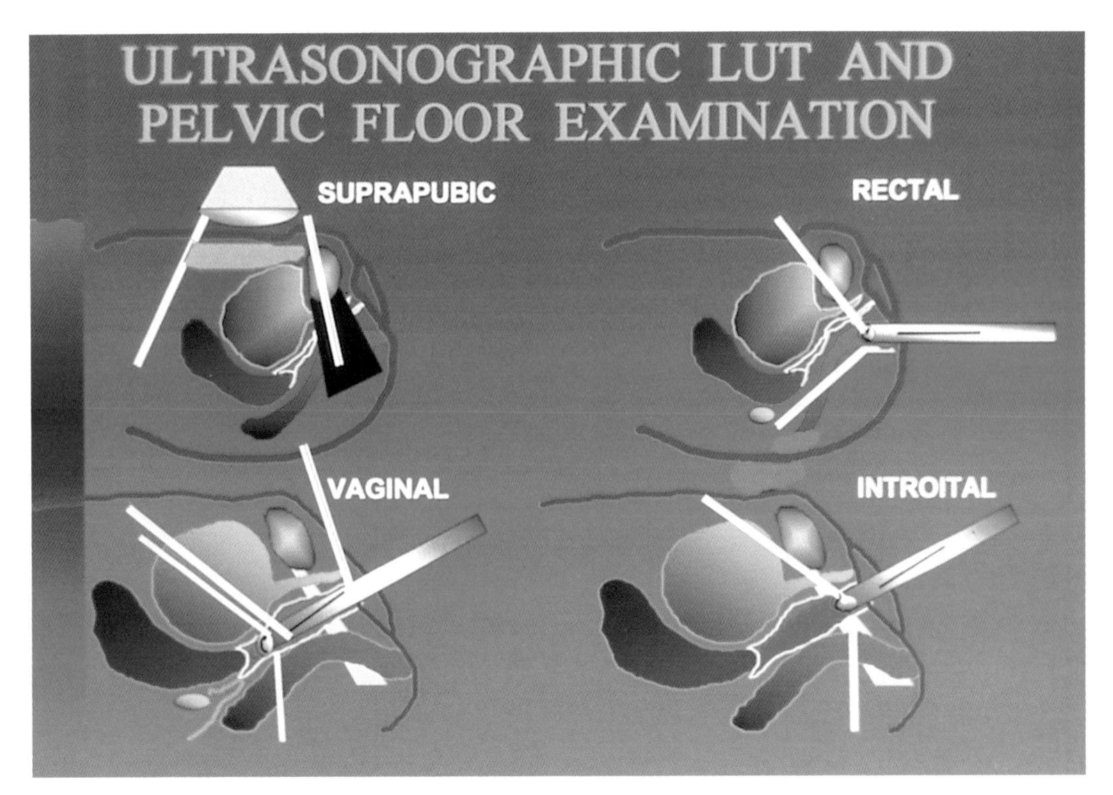

Figure 8 : Ultrasound of the lower urinary tract and pelvic floor

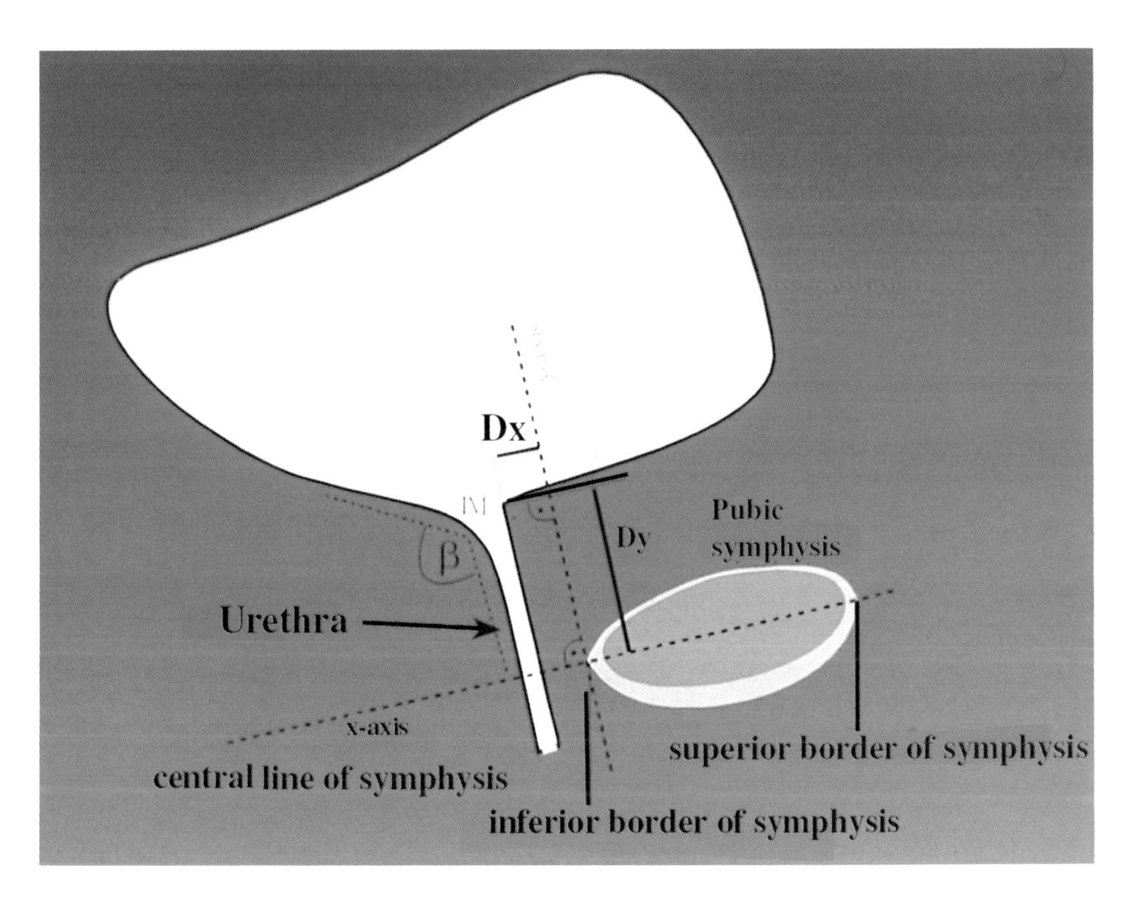

Figure 9 : Quantitative parameters of female lower urinary tract ultrasound

line of the symphysis. The y-axis is constructed perpendicular to the x-axis at the lower border of the symphysis. Dx is defined as the distance between the y-axis and the bladder neck, and Dy is defined as the distance between the x-axis and the bladder neck. For precise localisation of the bladder neck, the upper and ventral point of the urethral wall at the immediate transition into the bladder is used.

Creighton et al. measured bladder neck position with one distance and one angle. The distance is measured between the bladder neck and the inferior border of the symphysis and the angle between this distance line and the central line of the symphysis (pubourethral angle).

Qualitative parameters are bladder neck funneling (yes, no), position (high, low) and mobility (fixed, hypermobility) of the urethra and mobility of the bladder base (vertical, rotational or no descent).

6. Comparison between ultrasound and other imaging techniques

Each imaging technique has its own advantages and disadvantages (Table 2). Cystourethrography is based on projection pictures through the whole pelvis, it does not image any soft tissue except the bladder and urethra but offers several reference points. Ultrasound cuts a thin picture through the pelvis, it provides imaging of various pelvic organs and structures and provides a single reference point: the pubis. MRI produces a global view of the neuromuscular structures and organs of the pelvis which can be imaged through any plane. Ultrasound requires contact between the pelvic floor and the probe while other imaging techniques do not [1-3, 9, 22-24].

Table 2 : Advantages and disadvantages of ultrasound compared to other imaging techniques:

Advantages	Disadvantages
No irradiation	Inferior visualisation of bladder neck funneling
No catheter or wick	No representation of the entire bladder
No potentially allergenic contrast medium	No representation of pelvic muscle and adjacent structures
Availability	
Less invasive	
High acceptance (patients, physicians)	
Additional information on pelvic organs	
Therapy control	
Visual biofeedback (pelvic floor contraction)	
Less expensive	

7. Examination position

The patient's position has an influence on the measurement results. Bladder neck position at rest is relatively independent from patient position and the bladder neck to pubis distance was only slightly higher in sitting compared to supine patients (difference = 0.32 ± 0.12 cm) [25]. Examination in the sitting position resulted in bladder neck descent to a lower level compared to the supine position with an average increase of the rotation angle (β angle) by 16° [25]. If the evaluations are repeated in the same position using different imaging techniques the measured differences seem to be small and not of great importance [23, 24, 1, 2]. With the subject standing bladder neck funneling is found more frequently, and the descent of the bladder base is larger [9, 21, 26].

8. Bladder filling

Bladder volume has only slight influence on the bladder neck position and on the retrovesical angle b; with a greater bladder volume, bladder neck funneling is more often detected [25, 20, 27]. The evaluation should be performed with a bladder volume of 300 ml. Only standardised bladder volumes allow reliable comparisons of pre- and post-operative findings [***Level of evidence: high***].

9. Provocation tests

Coughing and the Valsalva manoeuvre are the most commonly used provocation tests to assess genuine stress incontinence. The results of both these tests differ as follows: during Valsalva the bladder neck lies lower and more dorsally and the angle b is larger [28, 19, 20]. Valsalva seems (physiologically) to be related to pelvic floor relaxation and coughing to contraction of the pelvic floor. Therefore, the Valsalva manoeuvre reveals descent better than coughing [29].

10. Variations caused by the ultrasound probe

Ultrasound requires body contact which differs from technique to technique. Endoluminal techniques lead to a bigger distortion of the urethrovesical anatomy than external techniques [9, 25]. The presence of the endocavitary probe can influence the bladder neck position and the angle β [21, 12, 11, 19, 30]. The evaluation should be performed with low pressure upon the visceral wall, just sufficient to obtain a good image [20].

11. Standardisation

Standardisation methodology and evaluation of ultrasound imaging of the bladder has been proposed by the German Association of Urogynecology and by the ICS [16, 17]. They recommended the following.

Picture orientation: cranial structures are to be shown above, caudal structures below and ventral structures on the right, dorsal structures on the left.

Imaging: to include urinary bladder, urethra, pubic bone, vagina, rectum, (uterus).

Measurement method: position of the internal urethral orifice should be related to the inferior border of the pubic bone (x-y co-ordinate system or pubourethral angle and distance) and retrovesical angle b.

Examination position: evaluation on the supine patient is preferable for patient comfort, bladder neck funnelling is more easily imaged in the sitting or standing position in patients with stress incontinence.

Bladder filling: 300 ml.

Provocation tests: imaging should be performed at rest and during Valsalva manoeuvre, pelvic floor contraction and coughing.

Variation caused by the ultrasound probe: beware of possible modification of bladder neck and urethral anatomy by endorectal or endovaginal ultrasound probes.

12. Role of the investigation

Ultrasound still remains an investigational technique although it is frequently used in the evaluation of female urinary incontinence and prolapse and allows functional and morphological documentation. It may not stand alone as a tool for diagnosing stress urinary incontinence because measuring bladder neck position and retrovesical angle β does not reliably predict urinary incontinence [19]. The dynamic process of bladder filling, emptying and other activities such as coughing, Valsalva and pelvic floor contraction can be illustrated helping to understand the association between anatomy and function.

Several studies have examined the reproducibility of sonographic examination of bladder neck position and no significant differences between the measurements performed by two investigators were found. A 95% CI of -4.88 to 6.29, -5.57 to 6.37, -2.93 to 5.08 was found, between 2 investigators, as regards the value of the α angle at rest, during squeezing and Valsalva respectively. No significant differences were observed in the x axis, y axis and β angle measured by two investigators [19, 24, 29, 33]

An extensive article from Bernstein [31] suggests that introital sonography provides adequate imaging of the pelvic floor; reduction of levator ani thickness with ageing was found both at rest as well as during exercise and a similar decrease of muscle mass was evident in incontinent women. Ultrasound imaging was able to show hypertrophy of pelvic floor muscles following pelvic floor training although no correlation was found with subjective and objective parameters of incontinence severity.

Pelvic floor muscle thickness has been measured by perineal ultrasonography in healthy and urinary incontinent women before and after training with 95% confidence interval of +/- 7-12%. In healthy women the median figures (and ranges) at rest, during contraction and increment during contraction were 9.8 mm (7.7-11.7), 11.2 mm (8.5-13.0) and 1.3 mm (0.2-2.0) respectively. The corresponding figures for incontinent women before training were 9.2 mm (6.7-11.3), 10.2 (7.0-12.7) and 1.1 mm (0.0-2.5) and after training 9.7 (7.8-11.7), 11.2 mm (9.2-13.2) an 1.5 mm (0.2-3.5) respectively [32].

New developments, such as, improved visualisation of funnelling by using ultrasound contrast medium [33] or depiction of structural defects with 3-D [4, 34, 35] (paravaginal defects) or intraurethral ultrasound [36] (sphincter defects) may lead to a movement of pelvic floor ultrasound from documentation of sagittal anatomy to a diagnostic tool of pelvic floor defects.

Further exploratory work is required to investigate the possible clinical benefit of ultrasound imaging in female urinary incontinence (Figures 10-17).

13. Conclusion

Lower urinary tract sonography is still regarded as an investigational technique for dynamic visualisation of urethral and bladder neck behaviour during Valsalva manoeuvre, coughing and pelvic floor contraction. Ultrasound imaging, especially with a perineal approach, can provide evidence as to urethral hypermobility and pelvic organ prolapse.

Standardisation of ultrasound technique is currently underway and is necessary to allow comparison of study protocols using ultrasound and to assure reliable and reproducible results. Evaluation of bladder neck and bladder base behaviour remains an indirect sign of pelvic floor function and integrity. Preliminary reports on new techniques, such as, intraurethral and 3-D ultrasound indicate that the future of ultrasound moves towards direct visualisation of defects, such as paravaginal or sphincteric defects.

Pelvic floor ultrasound is an investigational technique in rapid development. At present, its role in the evaluation of female urinary incontinence is not yet established. Intra-observer and inter-observer variability of ultrasound imaging of the bladder in the incontinent female patients has been tested and found to be on no statistical or clinical significance.

In conclusion, pelvic floor ultrasound does not provide a diagnosis of stress or urge incontinence, but it can be helpful in diagnosing urethral hypermobility and it can be a helpful technique to document pelvic organ prolapse (***Intermediate Level Evidence***).

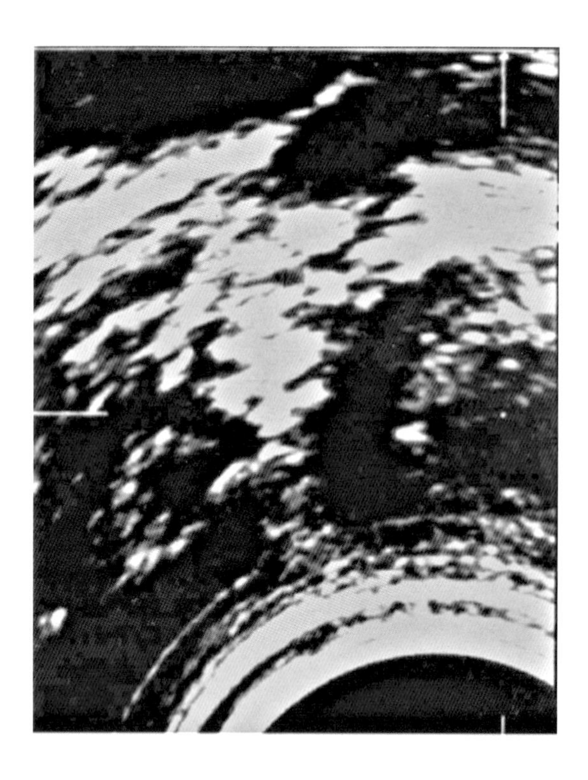

Figure 10 : Ultrasound of the female urethra

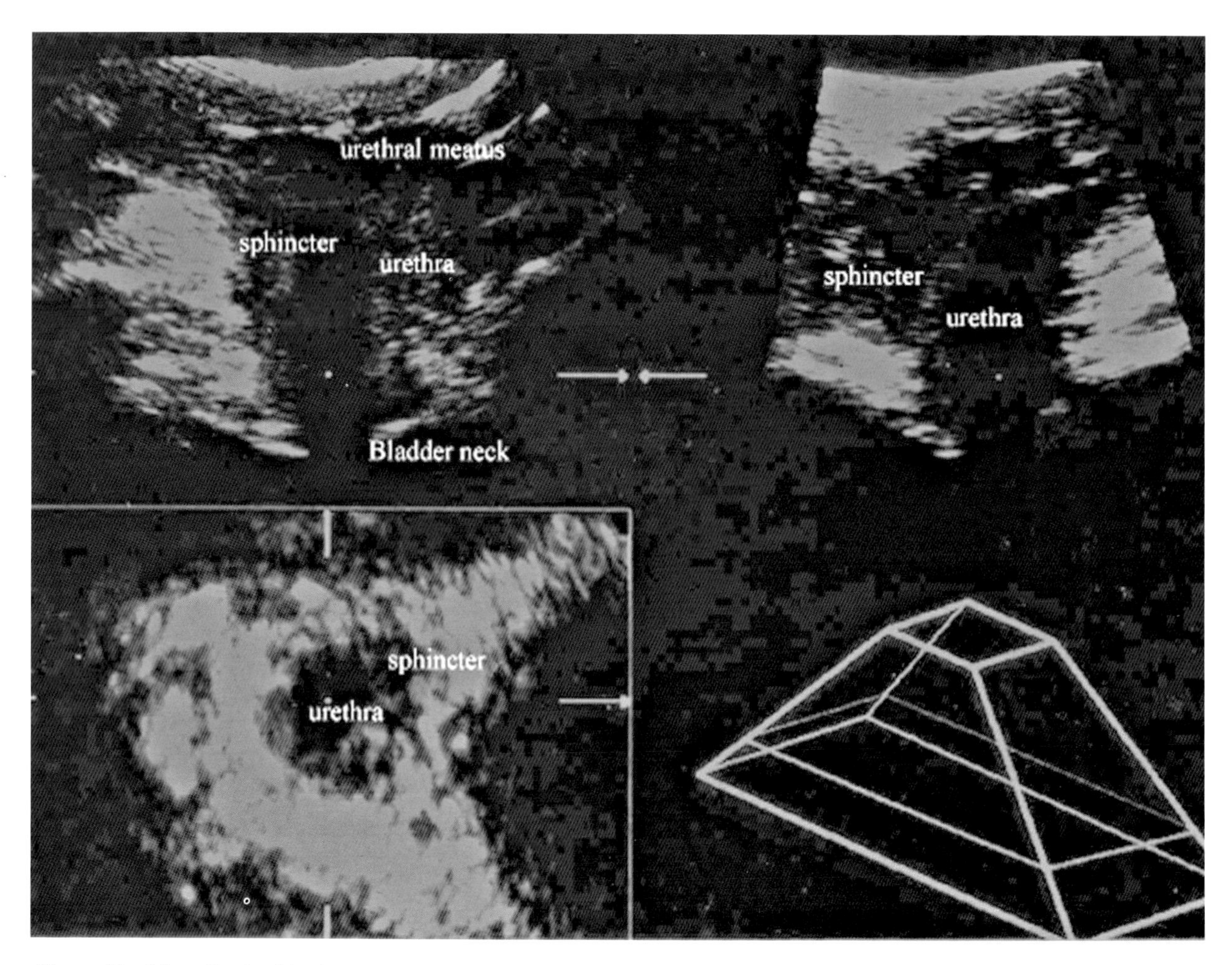

Figure 11 : 3d urethral sphincter scan

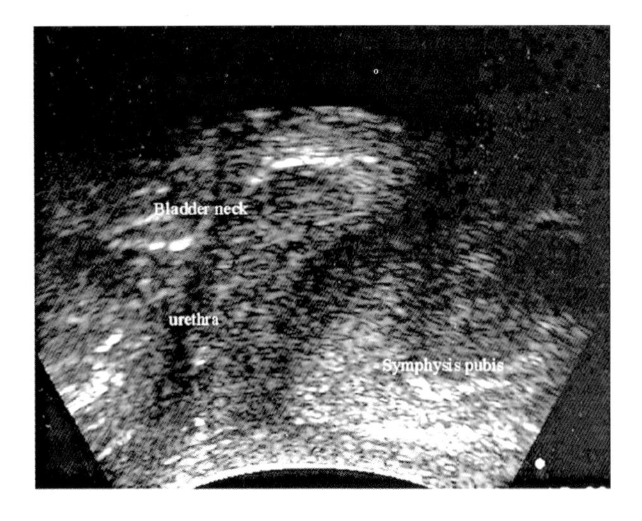

Figure 12 : Introital scan: well supported bladder neck

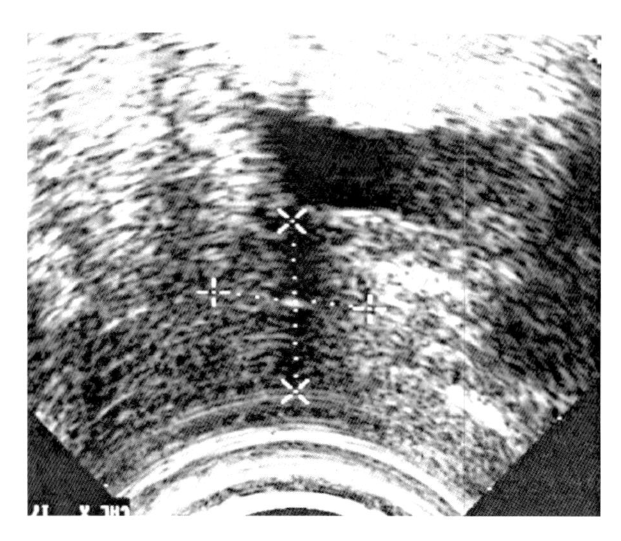

Figure 13 : Transperineal urethral sphincter at rest

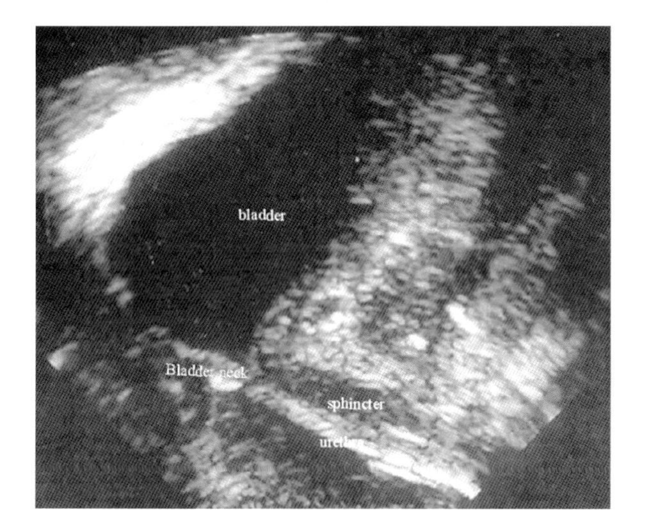

Figure 14 : Transrectal view of bladder neck and urethra

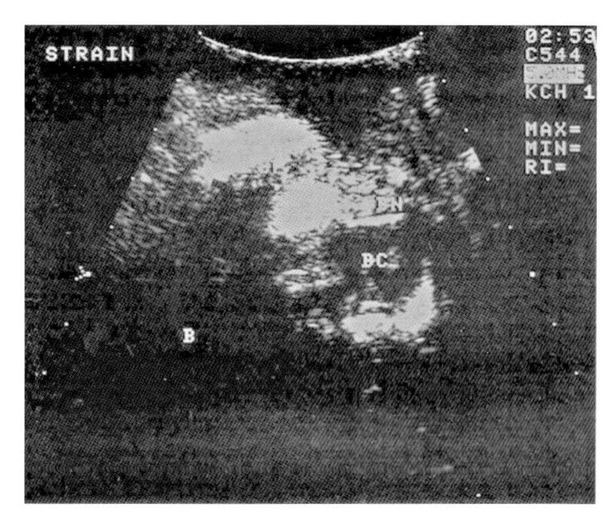

Figure 15 : Transperineal scan: bladder neck on strain

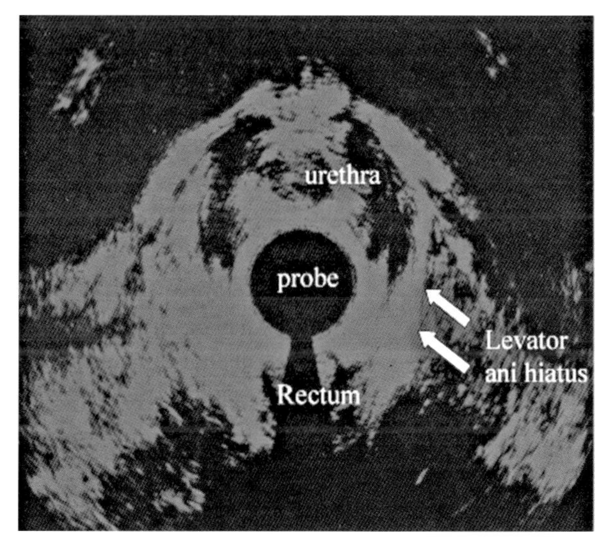

Figure 16 : Levator ani hiatus

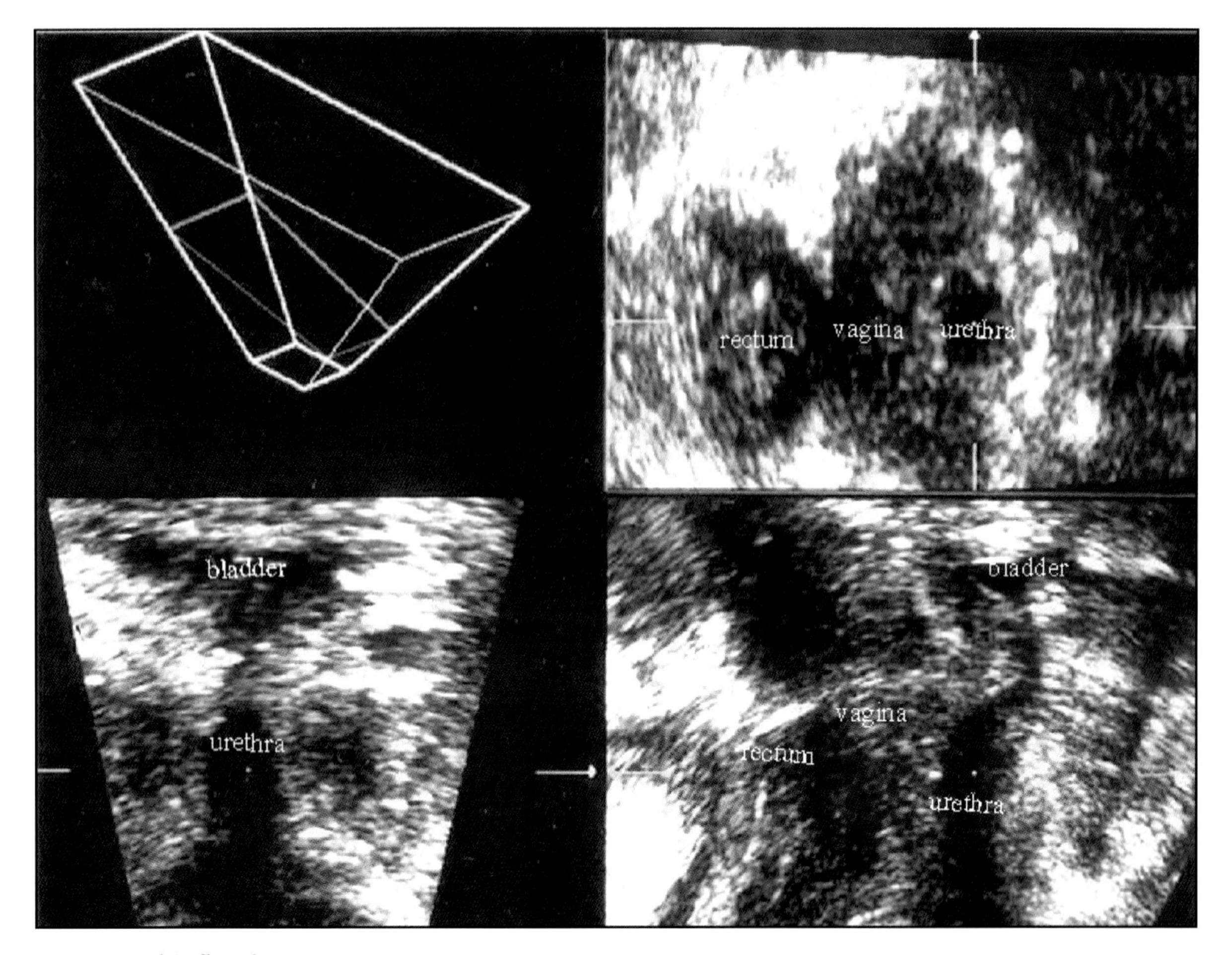

Figure 17 : Pelvic floor 3D scan

14. Recommendations

1. LUT and pelvic floor ultrasound ultrasound is NOT indicated in the evaluation of uncomplicated stress, urge or mixed female urinary incontinence (***Unanimous agreement***)

2. LUT and pelvic floor ultrasound should be considered an investigational imaging technique in the evaluation of female urinary incontinence and pelvic floor (***Unanimous agreement***)

15. Suggested research areas

1. Role of pelvic floor imaging in the evaluation of female urinary incontinence

2. Standardisation of US imaging in incontinence

Relation of ultrasound imaging to bladder neck function

3. Relation of ultrasound imaging to treatment outcome

4. New technologic developments

5. Need for proper training and full understanding of methodology

III. MRI OF PELVIC FLOOR

1. Background

Pelvic floor dysfunction encompasses a variety of fascial and anatomic defects that can affect the anterior wall, posterior wall, and apex of the vagina. Since cystocele, rectocele, uterine prolapse, enterocele, vault prolapse, and urinary incontinence tend to coexist, it is important to thoroughly evaluate all components of the pelvic floor. It has been shown that although patients might present with symptoms isolated to one pelvic floor compartment, the majority of these patients have concomitant defects in other compartments [1]. Since surgical failures have been attributed to the lack of a thorough preoperative evaluation of the female pelvis and to inadequate diagnosis and staging of pelvic floor dysfunction [2], accurate diagnosis of the coexisting abnormalities is essential in planning reconstructive and anti-incontinence procedures. In addition, up to 30% of female patients that present with stress urinary incontinence suffer from concomitant pelvic floor prolapse. Although most diagnoses of pelvic floor prolapse are made on detailed physical exam, various studies have alluded to the poor sensitivity and specificity of the pelvic exam in diagnosing various forms of pelvic floor prolapse [3-5].

Fluoroscopy has been used to evaluate the rectum and bladder and to aid in the diagnosis of cystocele and rectocele [3-4, 6]. Subsequently, pelvic ultrasonography was introduced as a less invasive alternative to fluoroscopic studies [7]. Recently, magnetic resonance imaging (MRI) has been used in the diagnostic evaluation of pelvic floor dysfunction. MRI provides anatomical detail of the pelvic floor including assessment of bladder neck and urethral mobility, rectocele, cystocele, enterocele and uterine prolapse, in a single non-invasive study which does not expose the patient to ionizing radiation [8-17]. MR imaging also provides a multiplanar thorough evaluation of the pelvic contents including the uterus, ovaries, ureters, kidneys, and levator muscles, as well as the urethra, that is unavailable by any other imaging modality [10, 12-16, 18, 19]. MRI provides useful information regarding ureteral obstruction, hydroneprosis, and uterine and ovarian pathology, which is essential in the management of women with pelvic floor disorders. In addition, at this time, MRI is the study of choice for the evaluation of urethral diverticuli (see related section).

2. Methodology

a) Conventional MRI

Advantages of MRI include lack of ionizing radiation, depiction of the soft tissues of the pelvic floor, and multiplanar imaging capability. Standard MRI consists of two dimensional image acquisition. Usually conventional T1 images and spin echo T2 weighted images are obtained. These static images provide good information on anatomy and pathological abnormalities but the long imaging time of conventional MRI has hampered its ability to evaluate pelvic organ prolapse and pelvic relaxation.The muscular anatomy of the pelvic floor, as well as the anatomy of the pelvic organs can be visualized with the use of a body coil. The use of an endovaginal coil provides superior information regarding the zonal anatomy of the urethra but the deformity of the normal anatomy by the coil itself should be considered. [20-21].

b) Ultra fast image acquisition and MR sequences

Very fast single-shot MR sequences for the evaluation of pelvic prolapse have been recently developed that allow excellent visualization of the pelvic floor in women [14, 15, 22-23]. These sequences allow a series of 1-second breath hold images to be obtained in two ways, either by obtaining a series of images covering the entire pelvis (static imaging) or repetitively in one plane while the patient is straining (dynamic imaging). The patients are placed in the supine position with legs slightly spread apart, and knees bent and supported by a pillow. There is no need for bowel preparation, premedication, instrumentation or contrast medium organ opacification. The MRI torso coil is centered at the symphysis pubis. Images are acquired in the sagittal plane using single-shot fast spin echo (SSFSE) or half Fourier acquisition, single shot turbo spin echo (HASTE) sequences. Single, mid sagittal views are obtained during 3 seconds of suspended respiration with the patient relaxed and during various degrees of progressive abdominal straining. The total MR room time is approximately 10-15 minutes.

Two sets of images are obtained. The first set consists of static sagittal and para-sagittal images covering the pelvis from left to right sidewall. These images provide information on pelvic anatomy, pathological abnormalities, and are used to select the mid-sagittal plane for the dynamic second set of images. This static sequence also allows for anatomic delineation of the pelvic sidewalls and muscular and fascial components of the pelvic floor [14, 15, 22-23] (Figure 18) The urogenital diaphragm and the levator ani musculature, as well as the anal sphincter anatomy, are also clearly demonstrated [24-25].

The static set consists of 17-20 sequential images independently acquired in a total of about 18 seconds. Static images can be acquired with a SSFSE pulse sequence using 128 x 256 matrix with repetition time (TR) of 4000 ms, echo time (TE) of 22.5 ms, 5 mm slice thickness and field of view (FOV) of 28 cm [15]. Other similar sequences have been described.

The second set of images consists of relaxed and straining mid-sagittal images used to assess the degree of pelvic floor relaxation and organ prolapse (Figure 19 a,b). One series [15, 23] describes the SSFSE parameters as 128 x 256 matrix, TR = 4000ms, TE = 90 ms, FOV = 28 cm and 5 mm slice thickness. Variations in these parameters have been described and thus the image acquisition sequences have not been standardized. Images can then be looped for viewing on a digital station as a cine stack.

This technology gives us not only the ability to look at the dynamic changes of the pelvic supporting structures, it also provides information on pelvic floor relaxation, organ prolapse, and information on the anatomical changes produced during voluntary pelvic floor contraction. Imaging studies and surgical experience have taught us that incontinence is not an isolated event but a symptom in the spectrum of pelvic floor relaxation. Christensen et al. [26] evaluated the dynamic relationship between the bladder and surrounding organs by studying the effect of voluntary pelvic floor contrac-

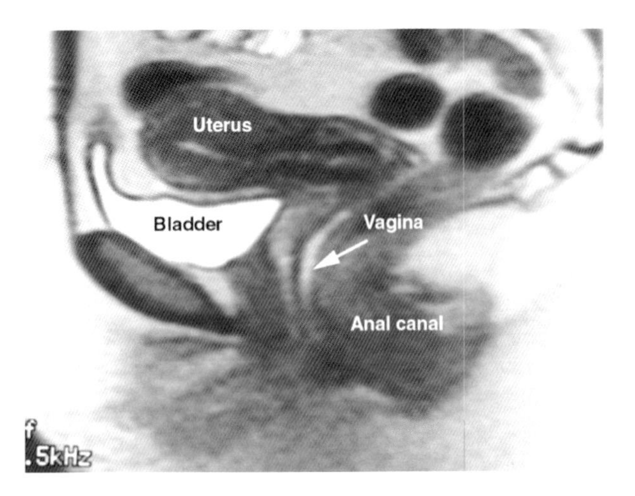

Figure 18 : Female pelvic floor MRI – sagittal view

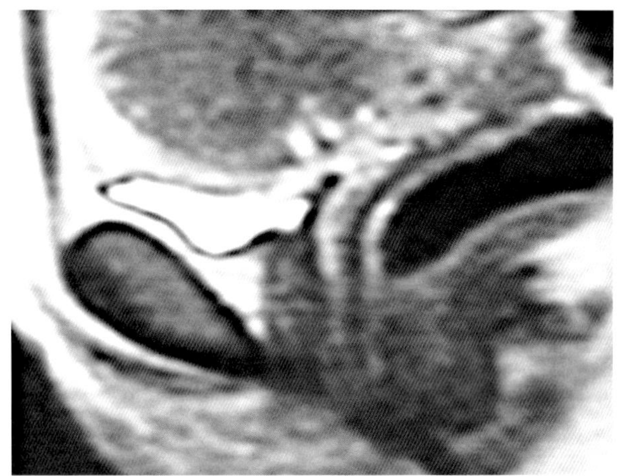

Figure 19 a : Pelvic floor MRI: Mid sagittal image - relaxed

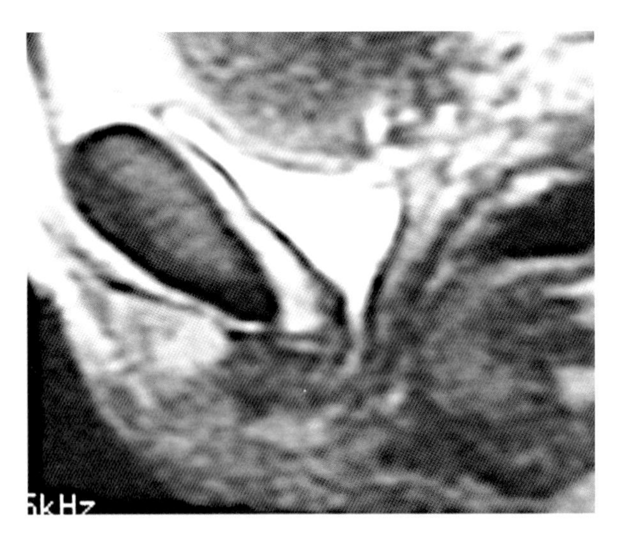

Figure 19 b : Pelvic floor MRI: midsagittal image on straining

tion on the abdominal structures. The authors quantitatively demonstrated that the displacement produced by contracting the pelvic musculature is larger in younger than older women suggesting changes due to aging. Mostwin et al. [27] found that incontinent women had significant pelvic floor displacement when compared to asymptomatic subjects.

c) Three dimensional MRI

Three dimensional (3-D) MRI provides great detail of the bony and muscular pelvic structures (Figure 20). In this technique, static or dynamic images are reconstructed using consecutive planes in the axial, sagittal and coronal dimensions. Anatomic variations of the insertion and pathway of the pubococcygeus and iliococcygeus muscles can be easily seen. Fielding et al. studied nulliparous continent female volunteers and found that the muscle morphology, signal intensity and volume are relatively uniform [28]. They described an average volume of the levator ani of 46.6 cc, width of the levator hiatus of 41.7 mm and an average posterior urethovesical angle of 143.5°. A larger range of motion of the pelvic floor is seen in younger women as compared to older women. We have also learned that in multiparous and older women the width of the levator hiatus is enlarged. This is due to the central separation of the levator musculature allowing decensus of the pelvic floor as well as the pelvic organs. Since these structures play a role on urethral support, understanding the normal anatomy as well as changes seen on the levators and pelvic floor musculature will hopefully shed light on the etiology and possible treatment of urinary incontinence. One disadvantage of 3-D MRI its that at this time it takes a relative long time to obtain the three dimensional reconstructions.

3. Standardization of anatomy

a) Normal pelvic floor support

Static, dynamic and three-dimensional MRI studies of normal subjects have enhanced our understanding of normal pelvic anatomy [28-30]. The use of MRI to analyze the pelvic floor musculature has also contributed greatly to our understanding of pelvic floor dysfunction [19, 21, 31]. MR imaging has been used to study the normal female pelvic anatomy, as well as the anatomy of the aging female and the symptomatic patient. It has been shown that in the supine position the female pelvic floor is dome shaped at rest [31-32]. During voluntary pelvic floor contractions the levator musculature straightens and becomes more horizontal. With bearing down the muscle descends, becomes basin-shaped, and the width of the genital hiatus widens. One limitation of MRI in the evaluation of the female pelvis is that the

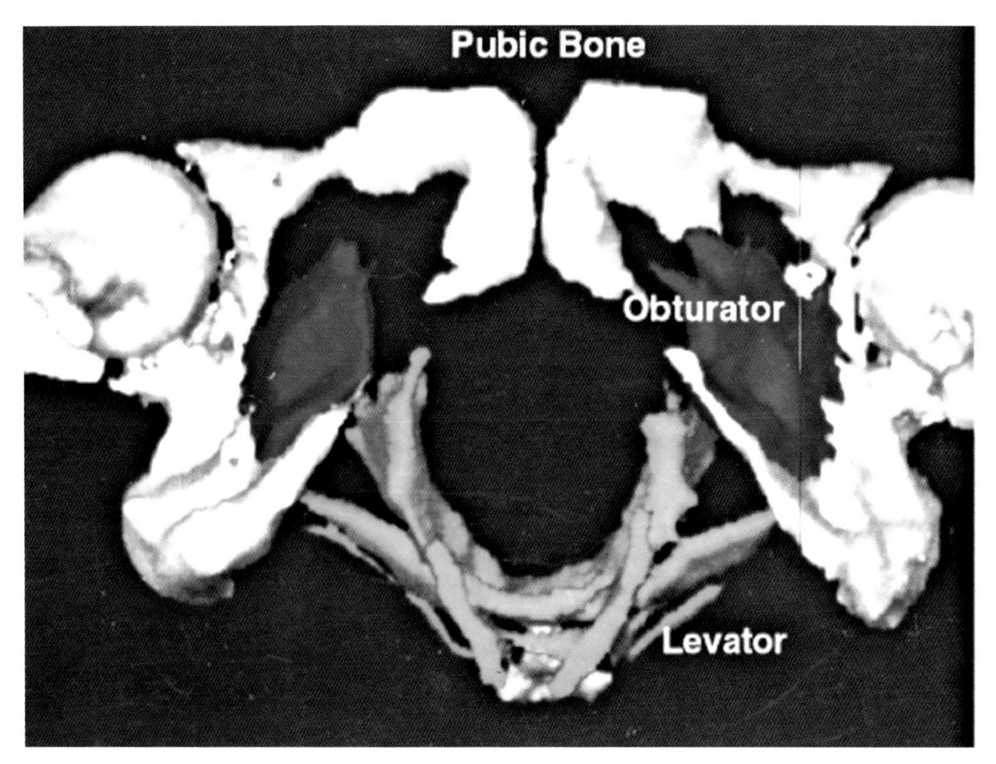

Figure 20 : 3D MRI of pelvic floor : 3D reconstruction of levator ani anatomy

studies are usually done with the patients supine. Upright dynamic MRI exists mostly as a research tool and is not widely available. Recently, Bø et al [33] evaluated the changes seen with pelvic floor contraction in continent and incontinent women using MRI in an upright sitting position. Although there was no statistical difference between the two groups, the authors demonstrated an inward movement with pelvic floor contraction (average 10.8 mm) and an outward movement with straining (average 19.1 mm). This was also reflected in the bladder neck. Interestingly, the coccyx appeared to move in the cranial direction with contraction and caudally with straining.

Another major advantage of MRI has been its ability to show the zonal anatomy of the urethra as well as the components of the intrinsic sphincteric unit. Figure 21 shows a coronal view of the urethra on a static MRI obtained with a vaginal coil. The anatomy of the urethra is clearly demonstrated. The lumen, spongy tissue and fibromuscular envelope are easily seen and correspond to the structures seen in urethral hislologic studies. A sagittal view of the urethral wall is seen in figure 22.

b) Anatomy after vaginal delivery

There are changes seen in the levator ani and pelvic floor musculature immediately after delivery which appear to change over time. Tunn et al evaluated patients on postpartum day 1 and compared the MRI images to those obtained at 1, 2, and 6 weeks and 6 months after delivery [25]. The authors evaluated levator muscle signal intensity, muscle topography, muscle thickness and pelvic floor descent. There was increased muscle signal intensity on T_2 weighted images at 1 day postpartum but the signal intensity approached normal by 6 months. The area of the urogenital and levator hiatus decreased significantly by 2 weeks postpartum. There was no statistically significant difference seen in muscle thickness over time.

c) Anatomy of urethra and bladder neck hypermobility

Saggital images obtained with the patient at rest usually show the urethra to be vertical in orientation [2a]. In patients with urethral hypermobility, with increased abdominal pressure, the proximal urethra moves inferiorly and the axis of the urethra becomes horizontal (Figure 23) [34]. In normal patients the urethral angle is usually greater than 30° and the urethrovesical angle greater than 115° . Tunn et al. [24] evaluated women with stress incontinence and compared them to controls. They found higher intensity of the levator musculature and loss of the hammock-like configuration of the anterior vaginal wall in patients with incontinence. A point of concern is that MRI is performed with the patient supine and that the lack of gravitational force might affect the anatomy seen in these images. This appears to be only a theoretical problem when evaluating patients with urethral hypermobility since both the descent of the bladder neck and the posterior urethrovesical angle do not seem to be affected by the MRI being performed in the sitting versus supine position [35].

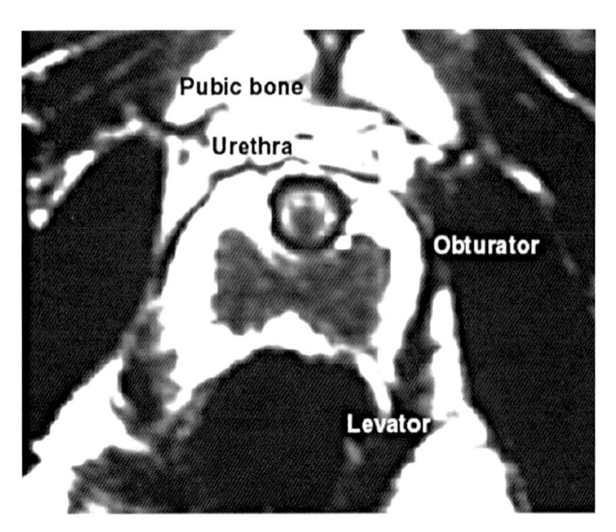

Figure 21 : MRI by vaginal coil Zonal anatomy of the urethra

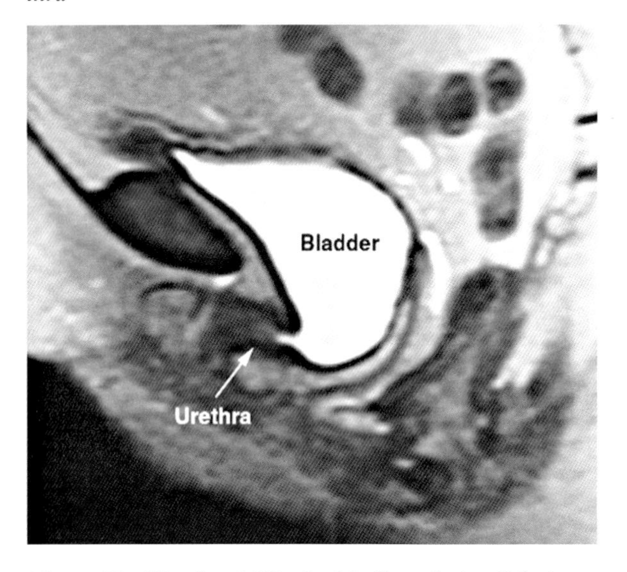

Figure 23 : Ultrafast MRI of pelvic floor during Valsalva

d) Anatomy of organ prolapse

Pelvic floor relaxation is a generalized condition involving all compartments of the pelvic floor. We can not evaluate incontinence in isolation since it is likely a result of changes in the anatomy and support of the female pelvis and is just one manifestation of pelvic floor relaxation and descent. The diagnosis of all components of pelvic prolapse is essential in surgical planning as well as in preventing surgical failures, recurrent prolapse and re-operations. Vaginal crowding due to the competition for space of the multiple organs descending into the vagina, makes the diagnosis of pelvic dysfunction difficult by physical exam alone.

Since pelvic floor dysfunction is usually generalized, the various pelvic floor compartments are best imaged simultaneously. Goose et al. evaluated the use of MRI in organ prolapse and compared the findings to physi-

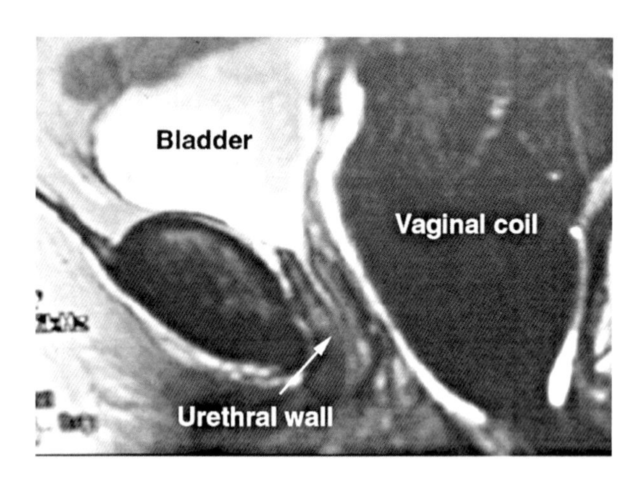

Figure 22 : MRI by vaginal coil Sagittal view

cal exam and surgical finding [15]. Pannu et al, presented a review of the anatomic changes seen with multiple forms of pelvic organ prolapse, including urethral descent and hypermobility [34]. These studies have helped clarify the muscular and anatomic changes responsible for descent.

e) Anatomy after surgery

Various studies have looked at the anatomic changes seen after surgical procedures in order to better understand how surgical therapies affect pelvic support and structures. Lineman et al. [36] evaluated women after abdominal sacrocolpopexy. The authors found that functional cine MRI identified the exact sacral fixation points after the procedure and easily identified the axis of the vagina and the exact position of the synthetic material used for the repairs. Goodrich et al used MRI to provide a dynamic analysis and evaluation of patients before and after surgical repair to evaluate structures involved in pelvic support [37]. Similar studies, will be needed in order to better evaluate the structures important for pelvic support, continence as well as the effects of surgical interventions.

f) Grading of Pelvic Floor Relaxation

A number of studies have described reference values for grading of organ prolapse [14-15, 17]. In order to evaluate descensus, certain anatomic landmarks are used. The pubococcygeal line (PCL) marks the distance from the pubis to the coccyx and serves as a fixed anatomical reference). In the nomenclature used by Comiter et al. [14], Gousse et al. [15], and others [23], the width of the levator hiatus is measured as the distance from the pubis to the pubococcygeus muscle (H-line). The hiatus is formed by the puborectalis muscle and encompasses urethra, vagina, and rectum. The M-line depicts the relaxation of the muscular pelvic floor by measuring the descent of the levator plate from the

Table 3 : Grading of hiatal enlargement, pelvic organ prolapse and pelvic floor descent using MRI.

Grade	Hiatal Enlargement	Pelvic Organ Prolapse	Pelvic Floor Descent
0	Less than 6 cm	Organ above H-line	0-2 cm
1	6-8 cm	0-2 cm below H-line	2-4 cm
2	8-10 cm	2-4 cm below H-line	4-6 cm
3	10 cm or more	4 cm or more below H-line	6 cm or more

pubococcygeal line. Using these three simple measurements, an MRI classification for degree of organ has been described [14,23]. In the normal population, during straining, the hiatus (H-line) is less than 6 cm long, and does not descend (M-line) more that 2 cm below the PCL line. The upper urethra, urethrovesical junction, bladder, upper vagina, uterus, small bowel, sigmoid colon, mesenteric fat and rectum are all above the H-line. A combination of hiatal enlargement and pelvic floor descent constitutes relaxation. As the pelvic floor descends so do the organs above it. The grading system for prolapse of any pelvic organ is based on 2 cm. increments below the H-line. By determining the degree of visceral prolapse beyond the H-line, the degree of rectocele, enterocele, cystocele, and uterine descent can be graded in a 0 to 3 scale as follows: 0 = none, 1= minimal, 2 = moderate, and 3 = severe (Table 3). Other similar systems have been described (17) and therefore there is a need for standardisation of nomenclature and grading of organ prolapse using MRI.

4. INDICATIONS

The advantages of MRI include: no need for urethral catheterization, no exposure to ionizing radiation, detailed anatomical views of the three pelvic floor compartments at rest and maximal pelvic strain, direct visualization of pelvic organs for evaluation of concomitant pathology, determination of urethral hypermobility, and evaluation of ureteral obstruction and post void residual [9-10, 13-15, 38]. Its main disadvantage at this time is that the study is performed in the supine position and, therefore, the effects of gravity have not been clearly evaluated. In addition, organ space competition in the vagina can also interfere with accurate interpretation of coexisting organ prolapse.

a) Incontinence

MRI provides information on the supporting musculature of the urethra, on the sphincteric unit, on hypermobility of the urethra, presence or absence of stress urinary incontinence and on other concomitant defects of the pelvic floor. Although urethral hypermobily and stress urinary incontinence can be evaluated with MRI, its role in the evaluation of incontinence remains one of research tool and of understanding the multiple factors affecting the continence mechanism in women. On the other hand, at this point its clinical applications for the evaluation of incontinence appear limited. A theoretical application that has been postulated is using MRI to help select patients with intact pelvic floor muscular function that could be candidates for pelvic floor exercises and biofeedback. To date no MRI series has identified a significant subgroup of patients with obvious inability to recruit the pelvic muscles and therefore the use of MRI to choose a particular therapeutic approach is limited at this time. As our understanding of the supporting structures and how their changes affect the development of incontinence increases, there might be a future role of MRI in evaluating incontinent women and determining which particular anatomic support needs to be addressed and thus directing specific surgeries for specific defects. At this time this remains only as a theoretical consideration.

b) Pelvic floor relaxation and organ prolapse

- *ENTEROCELE*

An enterocele is often missed on physical examination when it is accompanied by other significant prolapse [7]. In addition, physical examination often cannot reliably distinguish an enterocele from a high rectocele. In the past, defecography was the only available study to aid in the diagnosis of enteroceles. Enteroceles were usually only appreciated after repeated straining after evacuation and usually required opacification of the vagina in order to demonstrate the insinuation of small bowel loops between the rectum and vagina [39]. MRI has proven to be a much simpler and less invasive technique for the evaluation of enteroceles. Gousse et al. compared physical exam, intraoperative findings and MR images in women with and without prolapse [15]. The investigators found that when compared to intraoperative findings, MRI had a sensitivity of 87%, specificity of 80%, and positive predictive value of 91%. MRI was significantly superior in detecting enteroceles when compared to physical examinations. The images are obtained with the patient supine in the relaxed and straining state (Figure 24 a,b). Neither instrumentation nor invasive procedures are needed. Similarly, Lienemann et al., using MRI with opacification of organs, showed that MRI had a much higher sensitivity for detection of enteroceles when compared to physical exam and dynamic cystoproctography [40]

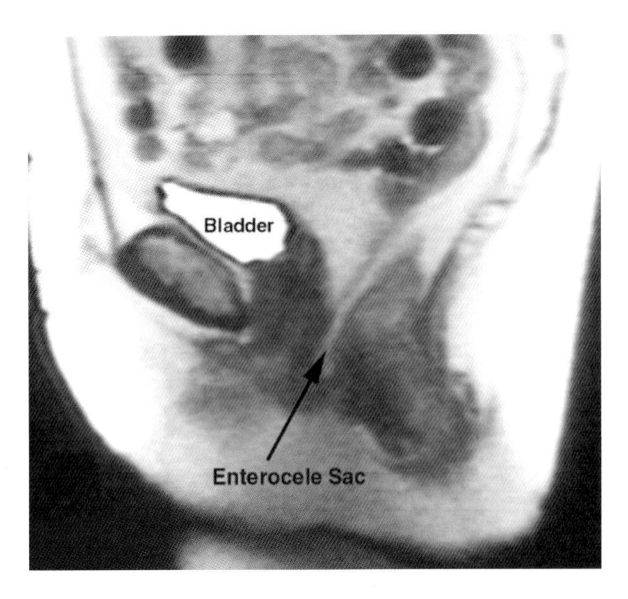

Figure 24 a : Pelvic floor MRI: enterocele a) At rest

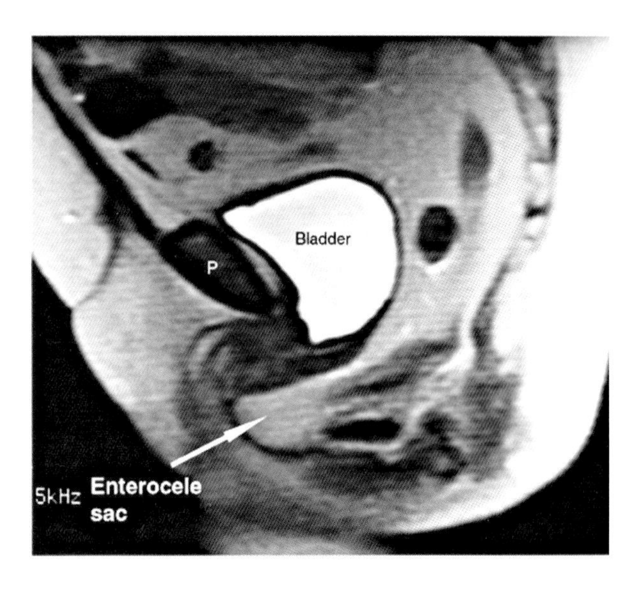

Figure 24 b : Pelvic floor MRI: enterocele b) during Valsalva

- *CYSTOCELE*

As with other forms of prolapse, high-grade cystoceles usually do not occur in isolation, and represent a spectrum of pelvic floor dysfunction [1, 3, 14]. When a large vaginal mass is present it is frequently difficult to differentiate a high-grade cystocele, from an enterocele, vaginal vault prolapse or high rectocele by physical examination alone [3-5]. In addition repair of only the cystocele without attention to the rest of the pelvic floor has been shown to predispose the patient not only to increased incidence of urinary incontinence, but also to an increase incidence of enterocele, rectocele, and/or uterine prolapse postoperatively [15]. Figures 25 a, b show an MRI of two patients with grade 2 and 3 cystocele, respectively. When compared to intraoperative findings, MRI has a sensitivity of 100%, specificity of 83%, and positive predictive value of 97% when evaluating for cystocele [15]. In addition, urethral hypermobility and post-void urine residual can be documented, as well as evaluation of ureteral obstruction and other pelvic abnormalities. Gousse et al. found that MRI was able to diagnose other type of pelvic pathology besides prolapse in 55 of 100 patients studied, including 3 with bilateral hydroureteronephrosis [15].

- *RECTOCELE*

Rectoceles are present in up to 80% of asymptomatic patients with pelvic floor dysfunction [13]. Although the diagnosis is usually made by physical exam, the reported sensitivity of pelvic examination for diagnosis of rectocele ranges from 31% to 80% [3-4, 6, 41-42]. This is usually secondary to organ competition for space in the vagina when accompanied by other significant prolapse [7]. In addition, it is often difficult to reliably distinguish an enterocele from a high rectocele. Figure 11 shows a rectocele diagnosed by dynamic MRI. A rectocele is easily seen when filled with gas, fluid, or gel. Although highly specific, when no rectal or vaginal opacification is used, MRI can miss up to 24% or rectoceles [15]. When rectal opacification is used during MRI, a correct diagnosis of rectocele can made in 100% of patients studied when compared to intraoperative findings [18]. It therefore appears that in order to increase MRI's ability to diagnose rectocele, rectal opacification is necessary. This is usually accomplished by introducing sonographic transmission gel or gadolinium into the rectum prior to MRI scanning.

- *UTERINE PROLAPSE*

The size of the uterus and the presence of concomitant uterine or ovarian pathology determine if a vaginal or abdominal hysterectomy is performed at the time of the prolapse repair. Because of the need to rule out malignancy as well as the fact that grade four uterine prolapse has been associated with insidious progressive ureteral obstruction, MRI is an excellent modality to evaluate uterine prolapse (Figure 26). It evaluates not only uterine size, position, orientation (retroversion) and pathology (fibroids, tumors, nabothian cysts, etc.), but also ovarian pathology (cyst of mass) which is essential information in determining if a vaginal of abdominal hysterectomy is indicated. In addition, MRI provides information on the presence or absence of cystocele, rectocele, urethral hypermobility and urethral diverticula, and evaluates for ureteral obstruction [9-10, 13-15, 38]. Gousse et al report a sensitivity of 83%, a specificity of 100% and a positive predictive value of 100% when comparing dynamic MR imaging to intrao-

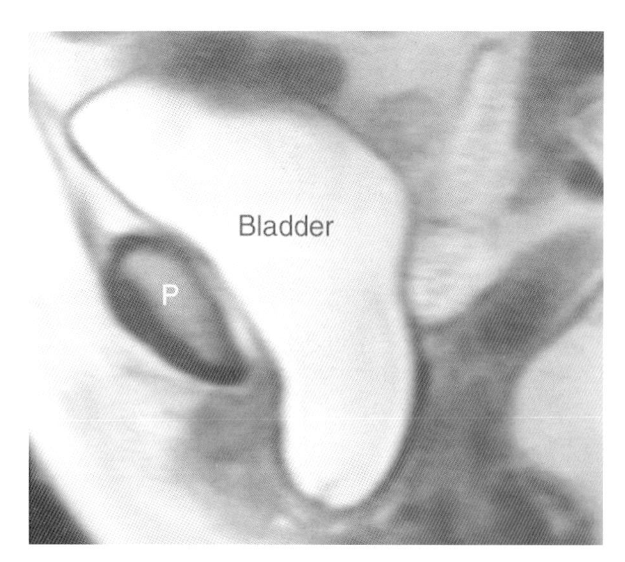

Figure 25 a : Pelvic floor MRI: grade 2 cystocele

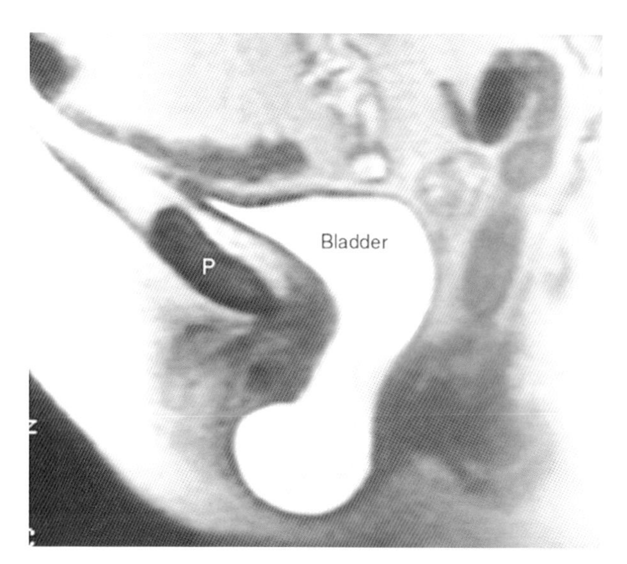

Figure 25 b : Pelvic floor MRI: grade 3 cystocele

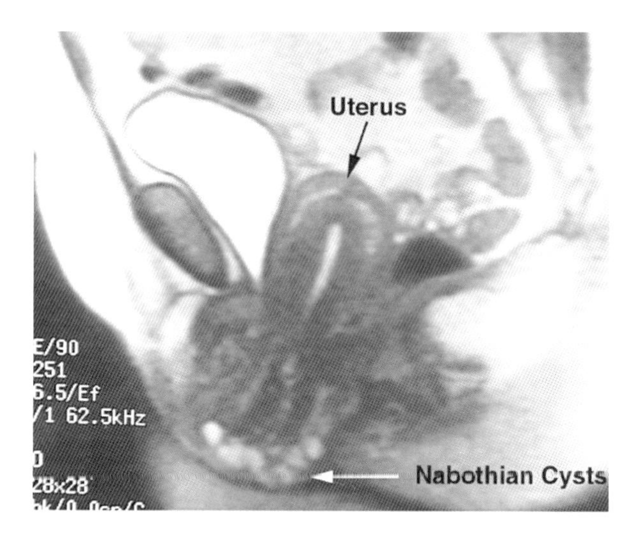

Figure 26 : Pelvic floor MRI: hysterocele

perative findings. These numbers were similar when compared to physical examination alone [15]. More importantly, MRI was able to clearly define the other compartments of the pelvic floor and diagnose uterine and/or ovarian in 30 of 100 patients evaluated [15].

5. Comparison between CT, MRI, ultrasonography, VCUG, and fluoroscopic cystocolpoproctography.

In the evaluation of incontinence and simple low-grade cystoceles, the studies of choice are the voiding cystourethrogram (VCUG) and urodynamics. VCUG is useful in determining the severity of cystocele, evaluating for urethral hypermobility and stress urinary incontinence, and documenting post void residual [6]. In addition to the above information, the evaluation of high-grade cystoceles should provide information on concomitant pelvic floor prolapse and presence or absence of urinary retention and ureteral obstruction [9-10, 13-15, 38]. Gufler et al. compared chain cystourethrography with dynamic MRI [38]. The authors found that with pelvic straining the measurements of bladder neck descent, angle of the urethra and the posterior urethrovesical angle, were not significantly different. This was not the case with perineal contraction, where the difference between the measurements was more marked. In the diagnosis of cystocele, MRI had a high degree of correlation to lateral cystourethrography with a Spearman correlation coefficient of 0.95 [38].

In urinary incontinence research, CT scanning has provided important information such as the effect of straining on the posterior component of the levator ani muscle. At this point the detail of the soft tissues obtain by MRI is superior to that of CT scanning, and therefore it has become the preferred research tool in studying the pelvic floor and its contents.

Until recently, dynamic contrast roentography and multiphasic fluoroscopic cystocolpoproctography were considered the best radiologic studies for detecting organ prolapse. These studies rely on the opacification with contrast material of the bladder, vagina, small bowel, and rectum with all organs opacified together or in phases with each organ opacified individually prior to each straining phase [4, 41, 43-44]. These studies fail to detect up to 20 percent of all enteroceles [38, 44-46]. Therefore, MRI has proven to be a much simpler and less invasive technique for the evaluation of enteroceles. In addition, MRI is able to differentiate the enteroceles according to their contents (small bowel, large bowel, rectosigmoidocele or mesenteric fat). MRI is also an excellent study to differentiate high rectoceles form enteroceles, thus allowing adequate surgical planning and safer planes of dissection [14, 15, 18, 40]. Although a recent study found that multiphasic MRI with opacification of organs and multiphasic fluoroscopic cystocolpoproctography had similar detection rates for enterocele [44], excellent images can be obtained from dynamic MRI without giving the patient oral contrast for opacification of the small bowel or giving rectal contrast. Thus the minimal added information obtained by contrast administration does not seem to warrant the invasiveness of organ opacification at this time [15, 39, 45].

In the evaluation of rectoceles, evacuation proctography has been used to diagnose enterocele, retoceles, perineal descent and rectal intussusception [36]. Dynamic contrast roentography or fluoroscopic cystocolpoproctography have also been used [4, 41-42, 43-44] to diagnosed rectoceles. The disadvantages of these techniques are the inability to visualize the soft tissue planes comprising the pelvic floor, their invasiveness, and their use of significant levels of ionizing radiation. Without the use of rectal opacification, MRI appears to be a poor choice for the evaluation of rectoceles missing up to 25% of such defects. When rectal opacification is used during MRI, Tunn et al. showed that a correct diagnosis of rectocele can made in 100% of patients studied when compared to intraoperative findings [18]. Other investigators have also shown that triphasic dynamic MRI and triphasic fluoroscopic cystocolpoproctography have similar detection rates for retocele [44]. Recently, upright dynamic MR defecating proctography has been reported [47]. Although these studies might prove to be more sensitive in detecting anorectal anomalies, their utility seems to be more pronounced in patients with disorders of defecation including anismus, intussusception, and others, and may be too invasive to justify their routine use in the evaluation of rectocele.

In the past pelvic ultrasound has been used for the evaluation of the pelvic organs specially prior to hysterectomy for uterine prolapse. MRI provides excellent information on uterine masses such as fibroids or carcinoma, as well as ovarian cystic (simple or complex) and solid masses. Hydrosalpynx and other abnormalities of the fallopian tubes as well as Nabothian cysts of the cervix and Bartholin's gland cysts are also easily seen. MRI can also be used in the evaluation of endometriosis since size and extent of edometriomas as well as pelvic organ involvement can be easily evaluated.

5. Conclusions

The use of new MR rapid sequences have allowed for the fast, detailed, and reproducible evaluation of the female pelvis including normal anatomy, pelvic floor relaxation and pelvic organ prolapse. Although MRI can provide information regarding normal anatomy, incontinence, cystocele, rectocele, uterine prolapse, enterocele and presence or absence of pelvic pathology, the main clinical contribution at this time has been in the evaluation of enterocele (***High Level Evidence***). Even though, MRI appears to provide clinically useful information related to incontinence and prolapse in a single study that does not expose patients to ionizing radiation, further studies are needed before the widespread use of MRI can be recommended (***Intermediate Level Evidence***).

6. Recommendations

1. MRI is NOT indicated in the evaluation of patients with urinary incontinence or pelvic prolapse. (**Unanimous agreement**)
2. MRI should be considered an investigational imaging technique in the evaluation of female urinary incontinence and pelvic floor dysfunction (**Unanimous agreement**).

7. Suggested research areas

1. Additional studies comparing MRI of healthy volunteers and patients with urinary incontinence and prolapse are needed to better evaluate the anatomic changes involved in urinary incontinence and pelvic floor prolapse.
2. Serial MRI of healthy volunteers are needed to better understand the effects of aging in the support structures of the pelvis and the association of these changes to the development of urinary incontinence and/or pelvic prolapse.
3. Additional studies evaluating patients before and after surgical correction and comparing anatomic changes of surgery to clinical outcomes are needed to better understand the effects of surgical intervention in the management of women with incontinence and/or prolapse.
4. Serial MRI in pre and postmenopausal women can help evaluate the influence of hormones in the pelvic support structures and the intrinsic structure of the urethra.
5. Studies of MRI with endoluminal coils might help understand the structural relationship between the spongy tissue and the fibromuscular envelope of the female urethra and evaluate their role in the intrinsic function of the urethra.

B-II. LOWER URINARY TRACT IMAGING IN POST-PROSTATECTOMY INCONTINENCE

Video-urodynamics is at present the gold standard for evaluating post-prostatectomy urinary incontinence [1-4]. The retrograde urethrogram and cystourethrography (as well as endoscopy) can have a role in identifying the presence of anastomotic strictures and possibly in defining the pathophysiology of urinary incontinence [5]. Presti et al [6], comparing 24 incontinent patients to 13 continent patients after radical prostatectomy, showed that the appearance of the bladder outlet on voiding cystourethrography was correlated with urodynamic parameters and the presence or absence of incontinence. Tubularisation above the level of the external sphincter was present in continent but absent in incontinent patients. The anatomical configuration of the reconstructed bladder outlet can influence, together with the integrity of the distal urethral sphincteric mechanism and the functional detrusor behaviour, the degree of urinary continence after radical prostatectomy.

I. RECOMMENDATIONS

Radiologic evaluation of the lower urinary tract by means of the retrograde urethrogram and voiding cystourethrography (or preferably video-urodynamics) is recommended in cases of persistent post-prostatectomy urinary incontinence. (**Low Level Evidence- Unanimous agreement**)

II. SUGGESTED RESEARCH AREA

Correlation between the morphologic appearance of the bladder outlet, functional parameters and clinical status (incontinence or continence) post-prostatectomy.

B-III.LOWER URINARY TRACT IMAGING IN NEUROGENIC INCONTINENCE

Ultrasound and cystourethrography are important tests of the lower urinary tract in patients with neurogenic dysfunction and urinary incontinence. They can provide information regarding the anatomy of the bladder and urethra, reflux, presence of diverticula, bladder wall thickness, presence of stones, and a reasonable assessment of residual urine. LUT imaging by ultrasound or cystourethrography can be performed as a separate test, but it is better performed at the time of urodynamic study (video-urodynamics) [1].

The use of ice-cooled contrast medium (iced cystourethrography) [2] can be useful in some suprasacral neurogenic patients in order to elicitate detrusor reflex and voiding.

Severe bladder trabeculation with diverticula and pseudodiverticula, reflux, wide bladder neck and proximal urethra, and narrowing at the level of the membranous urethra can suggest, mainly in children, the presence of neurogenic dysfunction of the lower urinary tract (occult spinal dysraphism, non-neurogenic neurogenic bladder) even in the absence of neurogenic symptoms and signs [3-5]. In these cases imaging abnormalities indicate the need for urodynamic evaluation, electrophysiological tests and central nervous system imaging.

I. RECOMMENDATIONS

1. Imaging of the lower urinary tract (preferably by cystourethrography) is recommended in the evaluation of evident or suspect neurogenic urinary incontinence. (***Intermediate Level Evidence-Unanimous agreement***)
2. Imaging would be preferably performed simultaneously with urodynamic evaluation (videourodynamics). However, when videourodynamics can not be performed, cystourethrography should be performed as a separate test (***Unanimous agreement***).

II. SUGGESTED RESEARCH AREA

Correlation between LUT, morphology and functional parameters.

B-IV. LOWER URINARY TRACT IMAGING: SPECIAL ISSUES

I. RESIDUAL URINE EVALUATION

Residual urine is defined as the volume of fluid remaining in the bladder immediately following the completion of micturition [1] (ICS definition).

The measurement of postvoid residual urine (PVR) can be performed by invasive and noninvasive means. Invasive means are: in-and-out catheterisation and endoscopy. Noninvasive means are transabdominal ultrasonography and radioisotope studies.

In-and-out catheterization is indicated as the gold standard for the measurement of PVR. Nevertheless the method is subject to inaccuracies, if the person performing the catheterization is not fully instructed as to the procedures and techniques to assure complete emptying (moving the catheter in and out slowly, twisting it, suctioning with syringe, suprapubic pressure), especially in cases of bladder diverticula and vesicoureteric reflux [2]. Stoller and Millard [3] showed inaccuracies in 30% of 515 male patients evaluated by full-time urological nurses with a mean difference between the initial and the actual residual volume of 76 ml in 30 % of inaccurate assessments. After further education of the nurses, inaccurate assessments were reduced to 14% with a mean difference of 85 ml.

PVR can be measured at the time of endoscopy, provided there is a blinded insertion of the instrument to avoid irrigation fluid inflow.

Both invasive means require local anaesthesia and carry the risk of urethral damage and urinary infection.

Before the era of ultrasonography, PVR was measured non-invasively by the phenolsulfonphthaleine excretion test [4] or with isotopes [5].

Ultrasound is the least invasive method of determining the PVR. There are several methods for its estimation based on transverse and longitudinal ultrasound bladder imaging. Using either three diameters (length, height, width) or the surface area in the transverse image and the length obtained in the longitudinal image, various volume formulae for a spherical or a ellipsoid body are utilised to estimate the bladder volume (Table 4).

All five formulae are equally good in assessing residual urine (93.6% concordance). Currently, no single formula can be indicated as the one best volume calculation formula.

Several studies report a sufficient accuracy in the ultrasound estimation of PVR [13-19]. False negative results are rare with PVR less than 20 ml [20] (Roherborn et al).

The intra-individual variability of PVR is high from day to day and even within a 24 hour period. This was reported in men with BPH by Birch et al [6] and by Bruskevitz et al [21]. Griffiths et al [22] examined the variability of PVR among 14 geriatric patients (mean age 77 years), measured by ultrasound at three different times of day on each of two visits separated by 2-4 weeks. Within-patient variability was large (SD 128 ml) because of a large systematic variation with time of day, with greatest volumes in early morning. The inherent random variability of the measurement was much smaller (SD 44 ml).

Several factors can influence PVR variability: voiding in unfamiliar surroundings, voiding on command with a partially filled or overfilled bladder, the interval between voiding and the estimation of residual (it should be as short as possible), the presence of vesicoureteric reflux or bladder diverticula.

Several studies [23-28] reported the questionable value of PVR as an important outcome prognosticator in male patients with benign prostatic enlargement and benign prostatic obstruction. There was no correlation of PVR with symptoms, size of the prostate and severity of outflow obstruction.

Table 4 : Comparison of different formulae to assess PVR by transabdominal ultrasound (Birch et al) in 30 men with BPH scanned three times

Author/reference	Method	Standard error	(%) 95% Confidence limits
Hakenberg et al	625 x H x W x (D1 + D2) / 2	17.5	34.3
Poston et al	7 x H x W x D1	20.0	39.2
Hartnell et al	625 x H x W x D1	17.0	33.3
Rageth & Langer	Nomogram based on areas	15.0	29.4
Orgaz et al	12.56 x H x r	12.9	25.5

Reproduced from the Proceedings of the 4th International Consultation on Benign Prostatic Hyperplasia, p. 205

Recently portable scanners were introduced, with automatic measurement of bladdder volume. In a prospective comparison [29] of one hundred measurements of PVR by portable ultrasound with measurements by catheterisation, the mean absolute error of the scanner was 52 ml. For volumes below 200 ml and 100 ml, the error was 36 ml and 24 ml respectively.

There are no specific studies on the use of PVR measurement in the assessment of urinary incontinence.

Residual urine is usually referred as an absolute value, but it can be measured also as a percentage of bladder capacity.

1. Conclusion

There is little knowledge of the aetiology and the meaning of PVR, particularly on its relation with upper tract dilation and with bacteriuria and urinary infection.

There is a lack of data on PVR in patients with various kinds of urinary incontinence.

PVR has significant intra-individual variability and is often non reproducible, due to technical errors in measurement and to still uncompletely clarified physiological variations.

Ultrasound is the least invasive method and is sufficiently accurate for clinical purposes, yet is the most expensive. In-and-out catheterization is invasive and can be inaccurate even if carefully performed.

The general opinion is that PVR measurement forms an integral part of the study of urinary incontinence, as a safety parameter to exclude a voiding efficiency disorder associated with incontinence.

2. Recommendations

1. Residual urine measurement is recommended in the initial assessment of urinary incontinence as a safety parameter and in the evaluation of treatment outcome (**Low Level Evidence- Unanimos agreement**)
2. The determination should be performed utilising realtime sonography or portable scanner or in-and-out catheterisation (**Unanimous agreement**).
3. Due to intra-individual variability, in cases where significant PVR is detected by the first measurement, several measurements should be performed (**High Level Evidence**)
4. The modality of measurement should be indicated (Unanimous agreement).

3. Suggested research areas

1. Aetiology of residual urine
2. Presence and prevalence of residual urine in various incontinent populations
3. Physiological variability and diurnal variation of residual urine
4. Validation of the role of PVR measurement in the assessment of urinary incontinence
5. Determination of the cutoff value of significant residual urine
6. Residual urine as a prognostic indicator of outcome after treatment of incontinence

II. OPEN BLADDER NECK AND PROXIMAL URETHRA AT REST

Reports in the peer reviewed literature suggest that the open bladder neck and proximal urethra at rest, during the storage phase, can be observed during cystography, videourodynamics or bladder ultrasound, both in patients with and without neurologic disease.

Distal spinal cord injury have been associated with an open smooth sphincter area, but whether this is due to sympathetic or parasympathetic decentralization or defunctionalization has never been settled [1].

Relative incompetence of the smooth sphincter area may also result from interruption of the peripheral reflex arc very similar to the dysfunction observed in the distal spinal cord injury. Twenty-one out of 54 patients with spinal stenosis were found to have an open bladder neck at rest [2].

In a review on 550 patients [3], 29 out of 33 patients with an open bladder neck had neurologic disease. Although the association was more commonly seen in patients with thoracic, lumbar and sacral lesions, the difference when compared to cervical and supraspinal lesions was not significant. Damage of sympathetic innervation to the bladder was also frequently observed in patients undergoing major pelvic surgery, such as, abdominal perineal resection of the rectum.

Patients with myelodysplasia had an inordinately high incidence of open bladder neck (10 out of 18 patients. versus 19 out of 290 having different neurological disorders).

Patients with sacral agenesis are included in the larger category of myelodysplastic patients and suffer from an open bladder neck with an areflexic bladder.

Shy-Drager syndrome is a Parkinson-like status with peripheral autonomic dysfunction. Detrusor hyperreflexia is usually found in association with an open bladder neck at rest and a denervated external sphincter [4].

Peripheral sympathetic injury results in an open bladder neck and proximal urethra from a compromised alpha-adrenergic innervation to the smooth muscle fibres of the bladder neck and proximal urethra [5]. Although it can occur as an isolated injury it is usually associated with partial detrusor denervation and preservation of sphincter EMG activity.

The loss of bladder neck closure suggests an autonomic neural deficit. The site and nature of the requisite deficit is unclear. Most of the authors agree on the importance of the sympathetic system in maintaining the integrity of the bladder neck [6-10] although the possible role of parasympathetic innervation has been proposed by others [11,12].

An open bladder neck at rest in children or in women without neurologic disease can represent a different disorder, either related to a congenital anomaly or secondary to an anatomical pelvic floor defect. Stanton and Williams [13] described an abnormality in girls with both diurnal incontinence and bed-wetting, based primarily on micturating cystourethrography, in which the bladder neck was wide open at rest. Murray et al [14] reported the "wide bladder neck anomaly" in 24.5% of the girls (35) and 9.3% of the boys (10) out of 251 children (143 girls and 108 boys) undergoing videourodynamics for the assessment of non-neuropathic bladder dysfunction (mainly diurnal incontinence). The authors considered the anomaly congenital and made the hypothesis that wide bladder neck anomaly in girls may provide a basis for the development of genuine stress incontinence in later life.

Chapple [15] reported that 21% per cent of 25 totally asymptomatic women he investigated by transvaginal ultrasound had an open bladder neck at rest. Versi [16] found a 21% prevalence of open bladder neck at rest in 147 women presenting to a urodynamic clinic and suggested that the finding is of little consequence.

Open bladder neck is a key point in defining type III stress incontinence according to the classificaton of Blaivas and Olsson [17]. This classification is based on history, imaging, and urodynamics, and distinguishes five diagnostic categories of stress incontinence. Incontinence type III is diagnosed by the presence of an open bladder neck and proximal urethra at rest in the absence of any detrusor contraction suggesting an intrinsic sphincter deficiency. The proximal urethra no longer functions as a sphincter. There is obvious urinary leakage which may be gravitational in nature or associated with minimal increase in intravesical pressure.

In pelvic fracture with membranous urethral distraction defects, when cystography (and/or cystoscopy) reveals an open bladder neck before urethroplasty, the probability of postoperative urinary incontinence may be significant, although the necessity of a simultaneous (or sequential) bladder neck reconstruction in controversial [18-20].

1. RECOMMENDATIONS

When observing an open bladder neck and proximal urethra at rest, during the storage phase, whatever imaging technique is used, it may be worthwhile to evaluate the possibility of an underlying autonomic neural deficit. (***Intermediate Level Evidence- Unanimous agreement***)

2. SUGGESTED RESEARCH AREAS

1. Relate the open bladder neck and proximal urethra at rest to the underlying neurogenic disorder
2. Longitudinal study of wide bladder neck and proximal urethra at rest in asymptomatic women
3. Evaluate the prognostic value of the open bladder neck and proximal urethra at rest

III. BLADDER WALL THICKNESS

Mean bladder wall thickness measurement of the empty bladder (< 50 ml) by means of transvaginal ultrasound has been found to discriminate between women with diagnosed detrusor instability and those with genuine stress incontinence [1] (Khullar et al, 1994) (Figure 27). All the women with detrusor instability had a mean bladder wall thickness greater than 5 mm.

Applying this test to a cohort of 180 female patients and using a bladder wall thickness greater than 5 mm as a screening test for detrusor overactivity, the sensitivity and the specificity were 84% and 89% respectively. The positive predictive value of diagnosing detrusor instability in women with a mean bladder wall thickness greater than 5 mm was 94%, compared to 61% for videourodynamics. The positive predictive value of a mean bladder wall thickness of less than 3-5 mm for diagnosing the absence of detrusor instability was 82%, compared to 76% for videourodynamics [2] (Khullar et al, 1996).

The association between thickening of the bladder wall (> 5 mm) and detrusor instability in nonobstructed women is striking and this diagnostic approach deserves confirmation of its value.

1. SUGGESTED RESEARCH AREAS

Diagnostic role of bladder wall thickness in female urinary incontinence (**Low Level Evidence**)

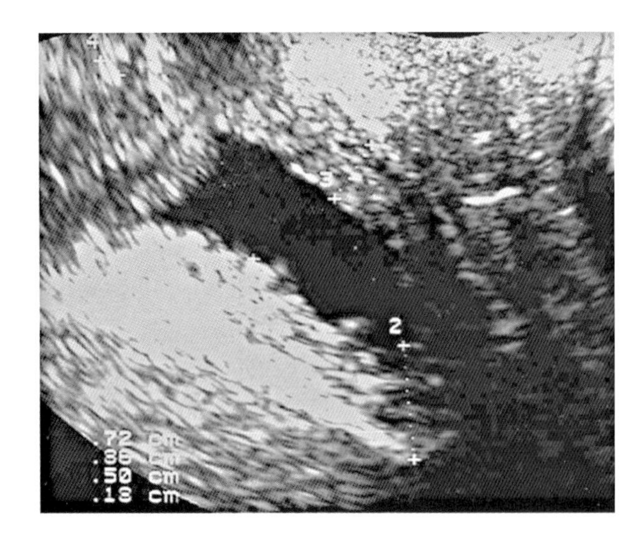

Figure 27 : Sonographic bladder wall thickness

IV. FEMALE URETHRAL DIVERTICULA

The first case of female urethral diverticulum was reported in 1805 [1].

Since the report from Davis and Cian in 1956 [2] using positive-pressure urethrography, the diagnosis has become much more common even though, despite increased clinical awareness, this pathology continues to be frequently overlooked.

Urinary incontinence is frequently associated with a urethral diverticulum. Incontinence may be a sequel to urine loss from the diverticulum itself with stress manoeuvres, genuine stress incontinence or urge incontinence [3]. Aldrige et al [4] reported urethral diverticula in 1.4% of patients with stress urinary incontinence.

The presenting symptoms of a urethral diverticulum have classically been described as the three Ds (Dysuria, postvoid Dribbling, and Dyspareunia). Since most patients present with nonspecific lower urinary tract symptoms, and the pathognomonic presentation (postvoid dribbling, urethral pain, tender periurethral mass and expression of pus form the urethra) is very uncommon, these patients undergo extensive evaluation and treatment before a correct diagnosis is established [5,6].

The diagnosis of a urethral diverticulum may be achieved by physical examination, voiding cystourethrography, positive-pressure (double-balloon) urethrography, urethroscopy, endocavitary (transurethral or transvaginal) or transperineal ultrasound sonography, urethral pressure profile or MRI.

Positive pressure urethrography is usually accomplished using a double balloon catheter according to the method described by Davis and Cian [2]. Two different models exists: the Davis-TeLinde and the Tratner catheter. Positive-pressure urethrography (and voiding urethrography) may result in a false negative study when the inflammation of the diverticulum neck prevents contrast medium to flow into the diverticulum cavity. Ultrasound sonography and MRI should be theoretically free of such false negative imaging. Chancellor et al [7] described the use of intraoperative intraluminal echographic evaluation.

A number of studies have shown that MRI is a superior image modality to both voiding cystourethrography and positive-pressure urethrography and can be considered, if available, the imaging of choice when the diagnosis of urethral diverticulum is suspected [8-13] (Figure 28 a,b). MRI provides information on location, number, extent (simple vs. saddle-bag) and size of diverticula. Endoluminal MRI with either a vaginal or rectal coil, may provide even better image quality than simple MRI [12].

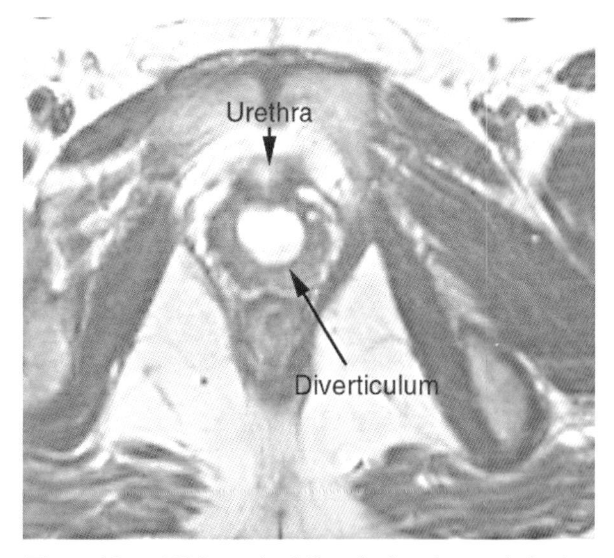

Figure 28 a : MRI: urethral diverticulum (coronal view)

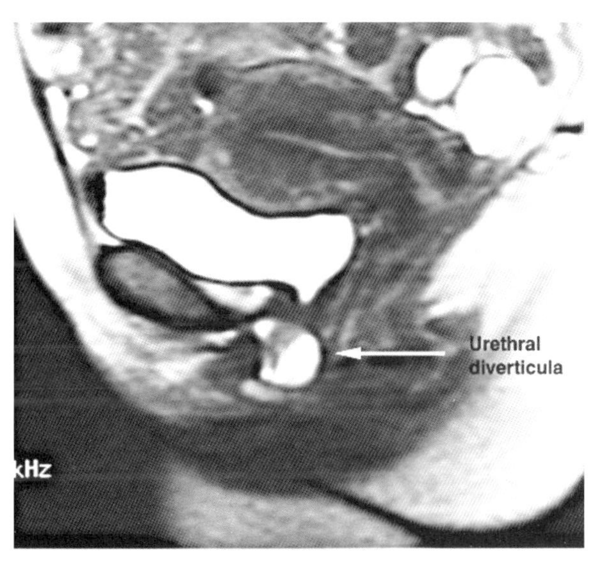

Figure 28 b : MRI: urethral diverticulum (sagittal view)

A comparison of MRI versus urethrography and urethroscopy, in a group of 20 women with urethral diverticulum, reported a 69 and 77 per cent accuracy of the two latter imaging studies versus MRI [8]. When surgical findings were compared to MRI, urethrography and urethroscopy, the diagnostic ability of the three methods was 70, 55 and 55 per cent, respectively. Diverticular ostia could not be identified by MRI study notwithstanding the use of contrast material.

Neitlich et al [9] reported in a series of 19 patients that MRI (using a fast spin echo T2-weighted pulse sequence and a dedicated pelvic multicoil) had a higher sensitivity for detecting urethral diverticula and a higher negative predictive rate in comparison with double balloon urethrography. Blander et al [11], comparing MRI and VGUG in 27 patients with urethral diverticula, found that endoluminal (endorectal or endovaginal) MRI was extremely accurate in determining the size and extent of urethral diverticula compared to VCUG; the related information can be critical when planning surgical approach, dissection and reconstruction.

In conclusion, review of the peer reviewed literature suggests that positive pressure urethrography is still a valuable tool to diagnose female urethra diverticula notwithstanding both ultrasound sonography and particularly MRI can represent valuable alternatives with a significantly higher diagnostic accuracy.

1. Recommendations

In cases of female urinary incontinence if a urethral diverticulum is suspected, appropriate imaging (positive pressure urethrography, voiding cystourethrography, urethroscopy, ultrasound, MRI) is recommended. (The choice of the type of imaging depends on their availability. Data show a higher accuracy of MRI.) **(Intermediate Level Evidence- Unanimous agreement)**

C. IMAGING OF THE NERVOUS SYSTEM (NEURO-IMAGING) IN URINARY INCONTINENCE

I. LUMBOSACRAL SPINE X-RAYS

Lower urinary tract dysfunction with urinary incontinence in children can be the expression of an underlying spinal dysraphism. In the majority of cases, abnormalities of the gluteo-sacral region and/or legs and foot are visible, but there can be cases where the abnormalities are minimal or absent. A careful evaluation of the anteroposterior and lateral film of the lumbosacral spine can identify vertebral anomalies commonly associated with nervous system anomalies.

Sacral agenesis involves the congenital absence of part or all of two or more sacral vertebrae. In the absence of two or more sacral vertebrae a neurogenic bladder is the rule.

Spina bifida occulta has a variable significance. Simple failure to fuse the laminae of the fourth and fifth lumbar vertebrae is unlikely to be important, but if the spinal canal is noticeably widened, there may be cord involvement (diastematomyelia, tethered cord syndrome).

1. Recommendations

In patients with suspected congenital neurogenic incontinence, with or without abnormalities of neurourologic physical examination, lumbosacral spine anteroposterior and lateral radiological evaluation (or MRI) is indicated. **(Intermediate Level Evidence- Unanimous agreement)**

II. CT, MRI, SPECT and PET (CNS)

Imaging of the central nervous system (CNS) is a valuable aid in the diagnosis of a variety of CNS diseases which may cause urinary incontinence.

Computerised tomography , magnetic resonance imaging , single photon emission computed tomography (SPECT), and positron emission tomography (PET) have been used and reported in the literature.

When urinary incontinence is just one of the many symptoms caused by a CNS disease, the diagnosis is made on clinical grounds and CNS imaging is carried out only to confirm it. In rare cases, urinary incontinence is the presenting symptom of an underlying neurologic disorders and CNS imaging is instrumental in the diagnosis.

The peer reviewed literature is an endless list of rare neurological conditions presenting with different symptoms including urinary incontinence in which CT scan, MRI, SPECT, and PET imaging were carried out identifying the underlying CNS disease.

After a cerebrovascular accident, the urodynamic behaviour of the lower urinary tract has been correlated to CT pictures of the brain [1,2].

The presence of significant cerebral lesions has been clearly demonstrated by CT, MRI or SPECT in the absence of clinical neurologic symptoms and signs in patients complaining of urge incontinence [3]. This can be particularly significant in elderly patients. Griffiths et al [4], studying 48 patients with a median age of 80 years, reported that the presence of urge incontinence was strongly associated (P= 0.009) with depressed perfusion of the cerebral cortex and midbrain as determined from the SPECT scan.

Kitaba et al [5] using MRI reported subclinical lesions in the brain in 40 out of 43 men more than 60 years old who complained of urinary storage symptoms; of these 40 patients, 23 (57.5%) had detrusor hyperreflexia.

Positron emission tomography (PET) studies provided information on specific brain structures involved in micturition in humans. In men and women who were able to micturate during scanning, an increase in regional blood flow was shown in the dorsomedial part of the pons close to the fourth ventricle, the pontine micturition center (PMC). PET studies showed also the activation during micturition in men and women of the mesencephalic periacqueductal grey (PAG) area. This area is known from cat experiments to project specifically to PMC and its stimulation elicits complete micturition; experimental interruption of fibers from the PAG to the PMC results in a low capacity bladder. PET studies during micturition in humans showed also an increased regional blood flow in the hypothalamus included the preoptical area which in cats can elicit bladder contractions [6,7].

These functional CNS imaging studies have a great potential to improve our knowledge on nervous functional anatomy related to vesicourethral function and dysfunction.

1. Conclusion

CNS imaging is rarely indicated in urinary incontinence.

In the advent of clinical neurological signs and/or symptoms suggestive of central nervous lesions, imaging may be indicated along with more specific neurophysiological tests (e.g. signal latency testing, evoked potential etc.).

A better knowledge of the correlation between morphologic and functional evaluation of the CNS is foreseable using present CNS functional imaging technology.

2. Recommendations

Neuro-imaging should be considered when a nervous system disorder is suspected on the basis of clinical and/or neurophysiological test findings. (**Intermediate Level Evidence-Unanimous agreement**)

3. Suggested eesearch areas

Correlation of CNS functional morphology to pathophysiology of urinary incontinence.

D. ENDOSCOPY OF THE LOWER URINARY TRACT

I. BACKGROUND

Since the introduction of the cystoscope in the early nineteenth century, endoscopy has played a growing and critical role in the evaluation of certain lower urinary tract diseases. Many investigators have recommended the routine use of urethrocystoscopy in the evaluation of urinary incontinence. In many cases these recommendations have been based on the individual investigators own feelings on the usefulness of the technique. However, rarely is specific data presented to support the recommendations.

There are four specific areas pertaining to urinary incontinence in which cystourethroscopy has been advocated:

1. Observation of the female urethral sphincteric unit to assess its ability to close and coapt. Urethrocystoscopy has been advocated in the static state to assess for intrinsic sphincter deficiency (ISD) as well as in the dynamic state, when the patient is straining, to evaluate hypermobility and urethral closure while the patient is straining. It has been reported that sluggish closure of the bladder neck during periods of a rise in intra-abdominal pressure is associated with anatomical stress urinary incontinence. Intrinsic sphincter deficiency has classically been described as a fibrotic or pipe-stem urethra. It has been suggested that endoscopy can even help to differentiate between the hypermobile urethra and the intrinsically damaged urethra.

2. Assessment of the bladder, to rule out an intravesical lesion or process that may occur concomitantly with incontinence or that may be a cause of irritability or instability.

3. Determination of extraurethral causes of urinary incontinence, such as, vesico-vaginal fistula and ectopic ureter.

4. Intraoperatively during operative correction of genuine stress incontinence

to assess for ureteral patency, intravesical foreign bodies or bladder damage.

5. Evaluation of the membranous and prostatic urethra in the male with urge incontinence (presumed to be secondary to bladder outlet obstruction or benign prostatic hyperplasia (BPH)), overflow incontinence, or post-prostatectomy incontinence.

II. EVALUATION OF THE FEMALE BLADDER OUTLET

Robertson described the procedure of dynamic urethroscopy to evaluate the bladder neck [1]. In this procedure a gas urethroscope is used to observe the urethra, bladder neck, and portions of the bladder. During visualisation manometric recording can be performed. Robertson described the appearance of true stress incontinence as a sluggish closure of the bladder neck and the appearance of the unstable bladder as a bladdder neck that closes and then opens like the shutter of a camera. This procedure was reported to be extremely useful in patients with urinary incontinence as the bladder neck can then be observed at rest, with straining, and Valsalva manoeuvres. Unfortunately, in Robertson's original description of this procedure, it was never compared to other standard methods of measuring outlet resistance. Others who advocate the technique of Robertson reported that only 43% of patients with stress incontinence actually had loss of bladder neck support on urethroscopy [2].

Scotti, et al performed a retrospective review of 204 patients who underwent dynamic urethroscopy for the evaluation of genuine stress urinary incontinence [3]. Of the 204 patients, 99 had genuine stress urinary incontinence confirmed by urodynamic testing. Urethroscopy was found to be an imprecise predictor of genuine stress urinary incontinence with a 62% sensitivity, a 74.6% positive predictive value and a specificity of 79.1%. Moreover, there were many equivocal studies. The authors concluded that urodynamic evaluation rather than urethroscopy was a more accurate predictor of genuine stress incontinence.

Horbach and Ostergard tried to predict urethral sphincter insufficiency in women with stress urinary incontinence using urethroscopy [4]. They retrospectively reviewed the records of 263 women who had a diagnosis of genuine stress urinary incontinence. They defined ISD as a maximal urethra closure pressure of 20 cm H2O or less with the patient upright with a symptomatically full bladder. They then divided patients into two groups, those with ISD and those with maximal urethral closure pressures of more than 20 cm H2O. Based on this classification, 132 women, or 50.2%, had evidence of ISD. However, when urethral function was assessed by endoscopy, only six of 132 patients with ISD were found to have an open or partially open proximal urethra and urethrovesical junction at rest during urethrocystoscopy. Clinically, these patients had very low urethral pressures and reported difficulty with continuous leakage of urine. Endoscopy appeared to have little predictive value for ISD as defined by urethral pressure profilometry.

Govier et al compared cystoscopic appearance of the female urethral sphincteric mechanism to the videourodynamic studies in 100 consecutive women with complex types of urinary incontinence [5]. Sphincteric dysfunction was classified as minimal, moderate, and severe based on the radiographic appearance of the bladder neck with straining. Urethrocystoscopy underestimated the degree of sphincter deficiency 74% of the time in patients with moderate sphincteric dysfunction and 44% of the time in patients with severe sphincteric dysfunction. The authors conclude that cystoscopy is inadequate to judge the functional integrity of the bladder outlet. Furthermore, cystoscopy alone will underestimate intrinsic sphincter deficiency in a large number of patients.

With respect to detrusor instability, characteristic urethroscopic findings of "a vesicle neck that closes and then opens like the shutter of a camera", have been described [1] Sand, and associates compared supine urethroscopic cystometry (dynamic urethroscopy) to the gold standard of multichannel urethrocystometry [6]. They found a sensitivity of only 24.6% and a positive predictive value of only 65.2% in predicting detrusor instability.

III. EVALUATION OF THE BLADDER

Is cystoscopy necessary to rule out concomitant bladder pathology in patients with urinary incontinence?

Langmade and Oliver reported on 253 patients who were operated on for stress urinary incontinence [7] They used a simple evaluation that consisted of history, stress tests, and urinalysis alone. They did, however, recommend cystoscopic evaluation if the patient also complained of symptoms of urgency. Although this dogmatic approach was recommended, it was never clearly stated if it made a difference in the treatment or outcome in these patients. Fischer-Rasmussen, et al performed extensive evaluation of women with urinary incontinence [8]. This included cystoscopy in 190 patients. They found cystoscopy to be abnormal in only 12 patients, 8 who had stress incontinence and 4 who had other types of incontinence. Abnormal findings were trabeculated bladder mucosa in five patients, benign bladder papillomas in four, and metaplasia of the trigonal mucosa in two. None of these was considered to be a significant finding. The authors concluded that cystoscopic examination did not contribute to the classification of incontinence in any case.

Cardozo and Stanton evaluated 200 patients with stress incontinence and detrusor instability [9]. Cystoscopy revealed no abnormalities amongst the 100 patients with genuine stress urinary incontinence. Fourteen of the 100 patients with detrusor instability had cystoscopic abnormalities, eg trabeculation-11, injected mucosa-1, sacculation –1, a bladder capacity of less than 100 cc-1. However, in none of these patients was the treatment affected by the results of cystoscopy.

In support of these findings, Mundy has stated that there is no direct diagnostic value of endoscopy in a patient with an unstable bladder. It may sometimes be helpful to look for and exclude a cause of hypersensitivity when this is in the differential diagnosis.[10] Dulaosal and colleagues found this necessary only in patients with hematuria. [11]. They performed urinalysis, urine cytology, and cystoscopy on 128 women who presented with urge incontinence and/or irritative voiding symptoms. Of these, 68 patients had urge incontinence, 35 of whom also had microscopic haematuria. One patient with urge incontinence and haematuria was found to have a transitional cell carcinoma of the bladder. None of the patients with urge incontinence (or irritative symptoms only) and no haematuria was found to have significant cystoscopic findings. This would support the routine use of cystoscopy for patients with urge incontinence only if hematuria is present.

IV. EXTRA-URETHRAL URINARY INCONTINENCE

Endoscopy can be an invaluable tool in the diagnosis and treatment of extraurethral incontinence due to vesico-vaginal fistula and ectopic ureter. With respect to vesico-vaginal fistula, cystoscopy can precisely localize the fistula site in the bladder and help plan surgical correction. Occasionally, a small fistula that is not seen on physical examination or by radiographic studies, can only be diagnosed by cystoscopy.

Incontinence due to ectopic ureter in the female is usually diagnosed by radiographic studies. However, the exact location of the ureteral orifice in the urethra or vagina can be identified by cystourethroscopy and/or vaginoscopy. This can be extremely helpful in the planning of corrective surgery.

V. INTRAOPERATIVE LOWER URINARY TRACT EVALUATION

Several authors have studied the value of routine cystoscopy during operative procedures for incontinence and prolapse. The approach may be transurethral [12] or transvesical [13]. The American College of OB/GYN has published a Bulletin on Operative Lower Urinary Tract Injuries [14] in which is stated "at the conclusion of the procedure, when hemostasis has been ensured, both ureters and the bladder should be inspected to confirm their integrity."

Harris, Cundiff, Theofrastous, et al [12] reported 9 unsuspected ureteral or bladder injuries during urogynecological surgery, which included 6 ureteral ligations, with four of these occurring after Burch cystourethropexy. Burch sutures were also found in the bladder as well as fascial lata from a sling procedure.

VI. EVALUATION OF THE MALE BLADDER OUTLET

Urge incontinence is one of the lower urinary tract symptoms associated with benign prostatic hyperplasia, bladder outlet obstruction, and aging in the male population. Based on the available evidence and world literature, The World Health Organization Fourth International Consultation on BPH made the following recommendation:

"Diagnostic endoscopy of the lower urinary tract is an optional test in the standard patient with LUTS (lower urinary tract symptoms) because:

1. the outcomes of intervention are unknown

2. the benefits do not outweigh the harms of the invasive study

3. the patients' preferences are expected to be divided

However, endoscopy is recommended as a guideline at the time of surgical treatment to rule out other pathology and to assess the shape and size of the prostate, which may have an impact on the treatment modality chosen [15].

Several contemporary series have described the value of urodynamics in the diagnosis of post-prostatectomy urinary incontinence [16,17,18,19,20]. However, only one describes the routine use of urethrocystoscopy. In that series 67% of patents had urethral fibrosis confirmed by endoscopy [17]. However, how this finding effected treatment was not discussed. In the study by Leach and Yun treatment of incontinence was based solely on urodynamic findings and was successful in 87% of patients [21]. Anastomotic strictures may be suspected based on uroflow and urodynamic (pressure-flow) studies and can be confirmed by voiding cystourethrogram or videourodynamics as well as by endoscopy. However, if intervention for the stricture is deemed necessary, endoscopy would be a more critical part of the evaluation. Furthermore if surgical treatment of incontinence, such as, an artificial urinary sphincter, is planned it would seem to make good clinical sense to evaluate the urethro-vesical anastomosis with endoscopy prior to surgery.

VII. RECOMMENDATIONS

1. Routine urethro-cystoscopy is NOT indicated in primary female urinary incontinence, when other pathologies are not suspected(**Intermediate Level Evidence- Unanimous agreement**).
2. Endoscopy can be considered(**Intermediate Level Evidence-Unanimous agreement**):

a) in urge incontinence to rule out other pathologies, especially in case of microscopic haematuria (e.g., bladder tumor, interstitial cystitis, etc)

b) in the evaluation of recurrent or iatrogenic cases when surgery is indicated and planned

3. Endoscopy is indicated in the evaluation of vesico-vaginal fistula and extra-urethral urinary incontinence (**High Level Evidence**).
4. Endoscopy is indicated intraoperatively in incontinence surgery to evaluate for ureteral or vesical injury (**High Level Evidence**).

VIII. SUGGESTED RESEARCH AREAS

To relate endoscopic features to diagnosis and outcome of urinary incontinence (mainly urge incontinence)

E. PAD TESTING

I. BACKGROUND

Quantitative measurement of urine leakage by using a perineal electronic nappy was first described by James et al. (1971). This innovation incorporated electrical conductivity into the nappy to facilitate estimation of the urine loss (Caldwell, 1974). Accuracy of this technique was, however, questioned by others (James & Flack, 1974; Rowan et al., 1976; Stanton, 1977; Wilson et al., 1980; Eadie et al., 1983). This was later improved by Mayne & Hilton (1988). Simple measurement of the gain in weight of perineal pads to estimate leakage was introduced by Sutherst et al. (1984) and Walsh & Mills (1981). These tests were, however, not well standardised. Bates et al. (1983) - Bristol ICS Committee on Standardization of terminology- described the one hour pad test in a more structured way and this was later endorsed by the International Continence Society in 1988 (Abrams et al.). This test, however, was shown to have poor interdepartmental correlation (Christensen 1986) and to be highly dependent on bladder volume (Lose et al., 1986). Further, 24 hour and 48 hour pad tests administered at home were developed. They showed a better estimation, but they were more cumbersome. Pyridium was also used (Wall et al. 1990). Janez et al 1993 tried to compare distal urethral electric conductance (DUEC) with the pad test (not well defined) and found both tests equal. A good review of the Pad Test was published by Ryhammer et al., in 1999.

II. DEFINITION

The pad test is a method of quantification of urine loss based on the measurement of weight gain of absorbent pads during a a test period under standardized conditions.

III. INDICATION AND METHODOLOGY

A test is indicated if quantitative analysis of the urine loss is required. Several different standards were developed. Generally tests can be divided in four groups: <1h, 1h, 24h and 48 h. (Table 5).

IV. QUALITY OF DATA

1. A SHORT PAD-TEST

a) Quantification

Jakobsen et al. (1987) found that the 40 minute test with an initial bladder volume of 75% of maximum cystometric capacity and similar activities as with a 1-hour ward test produced consistently larger amounts of urine loss as compared to a standard 1-hour ward test. The difference was attributed to significantly larger bladder volumes during performance of physical activity in a 40 minute pad test.

Kinn & Larsson (1987) reported no correlation between a short 10 minute test with fixed bladder volume and the degree of incontinence as judged from the symptoms.

Hahn & Fall (1991) in a 20 minute test with half cystometric capacity showed no false negative results in 50 women with stress urinary incontinence although there was some discrepancy (in 12% of patients) between the patients' perception of the degree of incontinence and pad test results.

Table 5 : Pad testing

Author	Time	Bladder load	Exercises
Hahn & Fall	20 min	0% of MCC	stair climbing, 100 steps, coughing (10x), running (1 min), wash hands (1 min) jumping(1 min)
ICS	1h	Drink 500 ml (15 min) before test	walking & stair climbing (30 min), standing up 10x, coughing (10x), running (1 min), bending (5x), wash hands (1 min)
Jorgensen et al	24h		Everyday activities
Jakobsen et al.	48h		Everyday activities

b) Reproducibility

The correlation factor (Pitman's nonparametric permutation test) between two separate 20 minute tests was 0.94 ($p<0.001$) (Hahn & Fall 1991). Kinn et al (1985) and Kinn & Larsson (1987) showed that the 10 minute test with a fixed pre-test bladder volume of 75% of maximal capacity was fairly reproducible ($r=0.74$).

2. One-hour test

a) Quantification

Walsh & Mills (1981) in elderly and Holm-Bentzen et al (1985) in patients with an AMS artificial sphincter showed that the one hour pad test did not correlate with subjective patient satisfaction. In an elderly population a one-hour ward test failed to demonstrate incontinence in 66% patients which complained of incontinence in comparison to a 24 hour home test which showed only a 10% false negative rate (Griffiths et al. 1991). Jakobsen et al. (1987) reported that one hour test was inferior in regard to the amount of urine loss (3 g) to 40 minute (7 g) and a 48 hour pad test (37 g). A one hour pad test was found to reflect everyday incontinence in only 48% of the patients in comparison to 81% in a 48 hour test and 77% in a 40 minute test. Jorgensen et al. (1987) remarked that only 10% did not complete the test (mean age 55 years of age) and 69% of the patients indicated that the test results correlated with daily leakage. Mayne & Hilton (1988) carried out a 1-hour pad test (n=33 patients with SUI) at a specific bladder volume (250 ml) and increased the detection rates of urine leakage (T=+92) vs. a standard 1 hour ward test (T=+62). Statistical analysis was done using Wilcoxon sign-rank test for nonparametric data. Kralj (1989) found the one-hour test to correlate with history of stress urinary incontinence in 47% (specificity 0.45) and with urge incontinence in 46%. Low correlation was attributed to small bladder volume (102 ml) during the test. Lose et al. (1989) demonstrated in 31 women a 58% correlation of the modified one-hour test (200-300 ml in the bladder) with the history of stress urinary incontinence. Mouritsen et al. 1989 (n=50) showed that a 1-hour ward pad test did not detect grade I stress incontinence in 46%, grade II in 27% and grade III in 66%. Thind & Gerstenberg (1991) compared a 1-hour ward pad test to a 24-hour home pad test and found that a 1-hour pad test had a 36% false-negative rate as compared to a 24-hour home pad test. Martan et al. (1992) found in 85 patients with incontinence that a modified 1-hour test at 75% of bladder capacity was positive in 44%.

b) Reproducibility

Klarskov & Hald (1984) demonstrated in 3 consecutive 1-hour pad tests, a correlation coefficient of 0.75 and 0.97 depending on the activity regime. The test, however, was quite demanding and a lot of patients did not complete the full testing. Christensen et al. (1986) compared a one-hour pad test in two different urological and one obstetrics & gynecological departments (20 women). The test results in two urological departments did not differ with an average pad gain of 24g and 21 g ($p>0.1$). However, pad test results between the departments of urology and gynecology differed significantly, with average pad weight gain 9g and 24 g respectively ($p<0.05$).

Kralj 1989 showed the repetitveness of a standard one-hour test to be 79%. Repetitiveness of the 2/3 bladder volume test was 84.2% and the full bladder test was 89.4% (n=418)

Lose et al. 1986 showed a significant variation between 1-hour ward test and retest in 18 patients (correlation coefficient 0.68). In about 50% of patients the degree of leakage was diverse and attributed to difference in diuresis. When the results of the 1-hour pad test were corrected for urine volume, the correlation coefficient value increased to 0.96.

c) Bladder volume

Fantl et al (1987) showed that test-retest correlation (Pearson correlation coefficient) was high and further enhanced when fluid loss was expressed as a percentage ratio of bladder volume. They used a modified one-hour test in which the bladder was filled to capacity by gravity before exercises.

Jorgensen et al (1987) showed fairly good reproducibility (r=0.68, p<0.01). When the results were calculated taking into account volume at the test start, test-retest correlation was better (r=0.93; p<0.0001). Lose et al. (1988) when using a 1-hour pad test with standardised bladder volume of 50% of maximal cystometric capacity (MCC) showed in 25 women a test retest correlation of 0.97 (p<0.001). But there was a considerable variation up to 24g between the two tests. Kralj 1989 showed that a one-hour test at 2/3 of a bladder capacity had a 73% correlation to symptoms of stress urinary incontinence and a 61% correlation to symptoms of urge incontinence. The results differed slightly when the test was done at full bladder capacity with 63% correlation for stress incontinence and 73% for urge incontinence. Jakobsen et al. (1993) compared a 1-hour pad test with a bladder filled to 50% and 75% of maximal cystometric capacity and found that the final bladder volume was equal in both groups. An increased diuresis in the 50% group accounted for an equal bladder volume in both groups. The amount of leakage in both groups was the same.

d) Diagnosis

Fluid loss was significantly greater in patients with detrusor instability in comparison to pure SUI (Fantl et al. 1987, Prajsner & Radziszewski 1998). However, the large standard deviation indicated a considerable between patient variability making the test impractical as a diagnostic tool.

3. 2-HOUR PAD TEST

A period of 60-120 minutes after a 1 litre fluid load was identified as the most optimal for the pad test because of a consistently high bladder volume (Haylen et al 1988). Han et al (1996) showed, however, that a 1-hour pad test is more practical. In children a 2-hour ward pad test yielded 70% positive results for incontinence (Hellstrom et al. 1986). Kralj 1989 showed a 2-hour pad test repetitiveness of 64.2%. Richmond et al. (1987) compared two exercise regimes with a 2-hour pad test and showed no significant differences in regard to which order the exercises were performed. They also showed that a 2-hour test is better than a 1-hour one. Only 28% had a positive test after 1 hour in comparison to 100% after 2-h. Walters et al. (1990) performed a 2-hour pad test with standard exercise in 40 women with SUI. The results showed 78% positive tests (>1g pad gain) after 1 hour and 98% after the second hour. There was no correlation between pad test results and the severity of a symptoms score.

4. 12-HOUR PAD TEST

a) Quantification

Hellstrom et al. (1986) demonstrated in 30 children with incontinence a positive 12-hour home pad test in 68%. When fluid volume (13 ml/kg) was instituted in 20 children, the frequency of the positive test increased to 80%.

5. 24-HOUR PAD TEST

a) Quantification

Jorgensen et al. (1985) showed that a 24h home test performed during daily activities is more sensitive that a 1-hour ward test with standardised bladder volume of 200-300 ml. Out of 31 patients 13 were classified as continent according to a 1-hour ward test in comparison to only 3 with a 24-hour home pad test. Klevmark et al. (1988) used s "Combined Test" of a 24h pad test and a frequency-volume chart and suggested several advantages of this combination: diuresis can be monitored and controlled better, and calculation of the percentage of urine loss with respect to a 24 hour diuresis and diagnosis of urge incontinence can be better defined. Lose et al. (1989) demonstrated 90% correlation of a 24-hour pad test with history of stress incontinence in 31 women. This was better than the results of a 1-hour test. Mouritsen et al. (1989) showed that a 24-h home test is well tolerated and as good in detecting incontinence as a 48-h test. Griffiths et al. (1991) found only a 10% false negative rate of a 24-hour pad test in an elderly population. Using non parametric coefficient of correlation, they found a significant difference between the 1-hour test and the 24 hour test. High fluid intake did not change the results of a 24-h home test, but a low fluid intake reduced a positive test by 56% (Rasmussen et al. 1994). Ryhammer et al., (1998) showed that 24-h test is superior to subjective self-reported assessment of urinary incontinence.

b) Reproducibility

Jorgensen et al. (1985) showed a significantly positive correlation (r=0.82), p<0.001) between the results of the two 24-hour home tests. Lose et al 1989 showed, however, poor correlation between a test retest with a variation of more than 100%. Groutz et al., (2000) using Lin's concordance correlation coefficient (CCC) found 24-h test very reliable instrument. Increasing test duration to 48 and 72 hours slightly improved reliability but decreased patient compliance.

6. 48-HOUR PAD TEST

a) Quantification

Jakobsen et al. (1987) showed that 48-hour pad test reflects everyday incontinence in 81% of patients. Kralj (1989) demonstrated 96% (0.92 specificity) agreement with history of incontinence but commented that it was done entirely by the patient without objective control. No statistical analysis data was given. Ekelund et al.,

Table 6 : Test-retest correlation

Author	Test	Correlation coefficient	Symptoms
Klarskov&Hald 1984	1-h	0.96	SUI&UUI
Mundt-Petterssen et al 1984	1-h F	airly good	SUI,UUI & MIX
Jorgensen et al. 1985	1-h	0.27	SUI & MIX
Lose et al 1986	1-h	0.68	SUI & MIX
Fantl et al. 1987	1-h (vol)	0.97	SUI
Fantl et al. 1987	1-h (vol)	0.84	SUI & UUI
Kinn et al. 1985	10-m (vol)	0.74	SUI
Lose et al. 1988	45-m (vol)	0.97	SUI & MIX
Victor et al. 1987	24-h	0.66	SUI
Lose et al. 1989	24-h	0.82	LUTS
Mouritsen et al. 1989	24-h	0.87	MIX
Versi et al. (1996)	24-h	0.9	LUTS
Groutz et al. (2000)	24-h	0.89	LUTS
Victor et al. 1987	48-h	0.9	SUI
Versi et al. (1996)	48-h	0.94	LUTS
Groutz et al. (2000)	48-h	0.95	LUTS

Table 7 : Pad-weight gains (g) in normal women

Author	Time	No	Mean (g)	From (g)	to (g)	SD	SEM	Note
Hahn & Fall 1991	20 min	10	0.0					
Nygaard& Zmolek, 1995	39.5 min	14	3.19	0.1	12.4	3.16		Exercise
Versi&Cardozo 1986	1h	90	0.39	0	1.15		0.04	
Sutherst et al. 1981	1 h	50	0.26	0	2.1	0.36		
Walsh & Mills, 1981	2h	6	1.2	0.1	4.0	1.35		Daily activity
Lose et al. 1989	24h	46	4.0	0	10			
Jorgensen et al., 1987	24h	23	4.0	0	10			
Mouritsen et al 1989	24h	25	2.6	0	7			
Versi et al 1996	48h	15	7.13			4.32		

(1988) found patients own weighing correlate well to control weighing at the clinic in 48-h pad test (r=0.99).

Nygaard and Zmolek (1995) in 14 continent women showed a mean pad weight, attributed to sweat for all exercises sessions of 3.19 ± 3.16 g (the Kendall coefficient of concordance of the test-retest reliability was 0.96) but there was a lot of variation between patients. Pyridium staining was not helpful in increasing specificity. Similar results with Piridium was reported by Wall et al. (1990) in a 1-hour ward test. In his study (n=18) the Pyridium test was 100% positive in patients with SUI but had false positive results in normal women (52%).

Mean pad weight loss due to evaporation or leakage (Walsh & Mills, 1981) was calculated to be 1.003 g, and ranged from -6.5 to +3.85 g (SD 1.85 g). Lose et al. (1989) showed no evidence of evaporation over 7 days if the pad was stored in a plastic bag. Versi et al. (1996) showed pads wetted with saline showed no difference in weight after 1 week and less than 10% weight loss after 8 weeks. Twelve pads were weighed by the patient and a healthcare worker with a coefficient of variance =1.55% with a mean deviation of 49%.

7. Comments

Khan & Chien (1996) eloquently pointed out that test-retest comparison should include methods of blinding and use of an appropriate index of degree of agreement which is the intra-class correlation coefficient. In most of the literature this was not implemented.

Kromann-Andersen et al (1989) argued that with considerable inter- and intra-individual variation of urine loss, the correlation of test/retest results may be overestimated and suggested different trials for small, modest and large leakage in large numbers of the patient.

8. Role of the investigation

The test has been standardised by ICS (1988) for quantification of urine loss and suggested uses for assessment and comparison of results of treatments of different types of urinary incontinence in different centers. Also, the AUA report on Surgical Management of Female Stress Urinary Incontinence includes a pad test (pretreatment evaluation) as a standard of efficiency for clinical trials (Leach et al., 1997). The Urodynamic Society included a pad test in a Standards of Efficacy for Evaluation of Treatment Outcomes in Urinary Incontinence (Blaivas et al., 1997). No suggestion was made in the last two reports of which test to use.

9. Summary

The 1-hour pad test is not very accurate unless a fixed bladder volume is applied

The sequence of exercises has little effect on test results

A pad weight gain ≥ 1 g = positive 1h test

A 24 hour test correlates well with symptoms of incontinence

A 24-hour test has good reproducibility

A pad weight gain >= 4g = positive 24 h test

A test lasting longer than 24 h has little advantage

A pad test cannot distinguish between stress and urge incontinence

V. RECOMMENDATIONS

1. The pad test is useful as an optional investigative tool in routine evaluation of urinary incontinence **(Intermediate Level Evidence- Unanimous agreement)**
2. Pad test is useful in clinical trials and research studies.

The following standards are suggested:

a) 20 min-1 h ward test with fixed bladder volume (pad weight gain >= 1g = positive test) **(Intermediate Level Evidence- Unanimous agreement)**

or

b) 24 h home pad test during daily acitivity (pad weight gain >= 4g/24h = positive test) **(Intermediate Level Evidence- Unanimous agreement)**

VI. SUGGESTED RESEARCH AREAS

1. Proper validation
2. Evaluation of the ability to detect all the spectrum of urinary incontinence (from mild to severe)
3. Sensitivity to change in time of incontinence status

F. OTHER INVESTIGATIONS

I. URINALYSIS IN THE EVALUATION OF THE INCONTINENT PATIENT

" The urinalysis is a fundamental test that should be performed in all urological patients. Although in many instances a simple dipstick urinalysis provides the necessary information, a complete urinalysis includes both chemical and microscopic analysis" [1]

In relation to urinary incontinence, urinalysis is not a diagnostic test, but a screening test, important in order to detect haematuria, glucosuria, pyuria and bacteriuria. Even in the absence of controlled studies, there is general expert consensus that the benefits of urinalysis clearly outweigh the costs involved, although the use of urinalysis should always be associated with prognostic significance [2]. A positive urinalysis will prompt infection treatment and/or the use of additional tests such as endoscopy and urinary tract imaging.

In the evaluation of urinary incontinence in the female, urinalysis is recommended since 60% of women with stable bladder will develop detrusor overactivity at the time of urinary tract infection (UTI). Pyuria was found to be common among incontinent but otherwise asymptomatic, female patients. Pyuria was not necessarily associated with UTI, the significance of sterile pyuria in the elderly population is still unclear [3]

A Norwegian survey of general practitioners' management of female urinary incontinence suggested that urinalysis is the most frequently performed test (73%) and is far more frequent than gynaecological examination (54%) [4]. Another survey suggested that urinalysis is one of the three-part assessment of UI together with patient history and physical examination [5]. The same apply, according to Stricker, for patient selection for collagen implant [6]. A minority of the reviewed papers suggested that urine culture should be carried out together with urinalysis [7,8]. Urinalysis is also considered of importance in the evaluation of nursing home residents who are incontinent [9], in peri- and postmenopausal women [10], in older women reporting urinary incontinence [11]. Belmin J, et al, suggested than significant urine samples can even be obtained from disposable diapers in elderly incontinent women [12].

It is recommended that geriatric incontinent patients undergo history, physical examination, tests of lower urinary tract function and urinalysis. The latter test is proposed to rule out the presence of UTI [13].

The clinical relevance of asymptomatic bacteriuria in the elderly is controversial, although many suggest this condition does not deserve any treatment. DuBeau and Resnick suggest the use of urinalysis in the diagnostic algorithm to identify asymptomatic bacteriuria in incontinent residents of nursing homes [14].

1. Recommendation

1. It is considered standard to perform a urinalysis either by using a dipstick test or examining the spun sediment. (***Unanimous agreement***)
2. If a dipstick test is used, it is recommended chosing of a "multiproperty" strip that includes fields for haematuria, proteinuria, glucose and ketones, leukocytes esterase (indicating the presence of leukocytes in the urine) and nitrite tests (suggesting bacteriuria). (***Unanimous agreement***)

2. Suggested research areas

Determine the role of urinalysis as a screening test in various incontinent populations.

Determine the prognostic significance of urinalysis in urinary incontinence

II. CHEMICAL TESTS

The prevalence of renal damage or of biochemical abnormalities in the general population of patients with urinary incontinence is very low, but there are subgroups of patients where the prevalence can be higher (e.g., neurogenic incontinence, overflow incontinence).

The routine use of a battery of common chemical and/or haematological tests in patients with urinary incontinence appears to be a prudent rule of good clinical practice in the following situations:

a) chronic retention with incontinence

b) neurogenic LUT dysfunction

c) when surgery is contemplated

d) when there is a clinical suspicion.

The cost of performing a single test can be similar to the cost of a battery of tests.

Special tests such as ADH and measurement of atrial natriuretic polypeptide have proven useful in research of enuresis in childhood and nocturia in the elderly [1,2]. Changes in the circadian rhythm of these, and probably also other hormones regulating the renal excretion of water, will in the future contribute to a better understanding of pathophysiology. Synthetic ADH-analogues have already come into clinical use for the treatment of nocturnal enuresis. However, the clinical value of these specific tests remains to be established.

Sex hormones exert physiological effects on the female urinary tract, with estrogens having an additional influence on the structures of the pelvic floor [3]. High affinity estrogen receptors have been identified in the bladder, trigone, urethra and pubococcigeus muscle of women. Oestrogen pretreatment enhances the contractile response of animal detrusor muscle to alpha-adrenoceptor agonists, cholinomimetics and prostaglandins, as well as enhances the contractile response to alpha-agonists in the urethra.

The dependence on oestrogens of the tissues of the lower urinary tract contributes to increased urinary problems in postmenopausal women.

Usually oestrogen deficiency is clinically evaluated on the basis of the presence of atrophic urethritis and vaginitis. Estrogen status can be ascertained via plasma estradiol and estrone levels, as well as from parabasal and superficial cell counts from both the urethra and the vagina [4].

Recently, Ayshek et al [5] developed a method of determining the ability of plasma to inhibit purified elastase activity and showed that the plasma from 30 women with urinary stress incontinence had a reduced capacity to inhibit the activity of purified elastase compared to 30 age-matched control women. The loss of inhibition of elastase activity might result in increased elastin degradation in connective tissues supporting the bladder and the urethra and contribute to the development of stress incontinence.

1. Recommendation

Standard chemical tests for renal function are recommended in patients with urinary incontinence and a high probability of renal damage [***Intermediate Level Evidence- Unanimous agreement***].

2. Suggested research areas

search for plasma markers of defective pelvic floor connective tissue

III. TISSUE ANALYSIS

Microscopic, morphometric, histochemical and ultrastructural analysis of specimens from various sites (skin, vagina, levator ani and detrusor) of patients with urinary incontinence is an exciting research line. This was applied mainly but not only to female urinary incontinence with or without genital prolapse.

A defect in connective tissue can be the cause of female stress urinary incontinence, possibly associated with defective support due to concomitant genital prolapse.

Brincat et al [1-3] intensively studied skin collagen in relation to menopause, concluding that skin collagen is influenced by sex hormones status and declines after menopause. Skin collagen content from skin biopsy specimens was found to be significantly greater (48%, $p< 0.01$) in a group of postmenopausal women (29) treated with sex hormone implants, compared to an untreated group of women (26) who were matched for age.

Versi et al [4] hypothesized skin collagen as a model of urethral collagen and concluded that collagen may be the pivot through which oestrogens have their beneficial effect on sphincteric function.

Norton et al [5,6] showed that collagen synthesis is altered in recurrent inguinal haernia and in recurrent genital prolapse. They reported also that joint hypermobility, a clinical marker for abnormal collagen, was prevalent in women with genital prolapse but not in women with stress incontinence. They were not able to show differences in collagen synthesis in women with stress incontinence.

Keane et al [7] compared the collagen content, the type I:III collagen ratio and the collagen cross-link content in specimens obtained from periurethral vaginal biopsies in 36 premenopausal nulliparous women with urodynamically proven genuine stress incontinence, with 25 continent controls. The nulliparous women with genuine stress incontinence had significantly less collagen in their tissues ($P < 0.0001$) compared with the continent controls. There was also a decreased ratio of type I to type III collagen ($P= 0.0008$) and a decrease of the collagen cross-link content.

The concept at the basis of this research line is that there is an active and dynamic ongoing process of turnover and remodeling of the pelvic connective tissue which can explain acquired or congenital, general or sectorial disorders.

Decreased innervation in female stress incontinence is another point of interest. Gilpin, Gosling et al [8] compared histological and histochemical analysis of biopsy samples of pubococcygeus muscle obtained from asymptomatic women and from women with stress urinary incontinence. In incontinent women there was a significant increase in the number of muscle fibres and changes in the diameter of type I (slow-twitch) and type II (fast twitch) fibres showing pathological damage, attributable to partial denervation of the pelvic floor.

Hanzal et al [9] claimed prognostic importance for the outcome of patients with genuine stress incontinence undergoing anteroposterior vaginal repair depending on the presence of striated muscle tissue in biopsies from pubococcygeal muscle. The absence of striated muscle tissue in 19 patients was associated with poor clinical and urodynamic outcome in comparison with 11 patients with the presence of striated muscle tissue in the specimen.

Helt et al [10] found no evidence of denervation or reinnervation in levator ani muscle biopsies from incontinent and/or prolapse patients compared to asymptomatic women.

Falconer et al [11] studied transvaginal biopsies near the external meatus from 11 stress incontinent women of fertile age and from 10 comparable controls, processed for indirect immunochemistry using protein b gene product 9.5 (PGP 9.5) as a general neuronal marker. Nerve fibre profiles/mm of projected epithelial area were significantly lower in the incontinent group, suggesting decreased innervation.

Elbadawi et al [12-14] in an extensive study program showed distinctive ultrastructural features of muscles, nerves and interstitium of the detrusor in various urodynamic conditions (detrusor overactivity, impaired contractility, outflow obstruction, aging bladder). These findings need to be reproduced by different groups.

In conclusion, tissue analysis in urinary incontinence is an interesting and promising research line. There is a need for further studies on pelvic floor components (connective and muscular tissue) and on detrusor.

G. CONCLUSIONS

Only a few of the imaging techniques and other investigations we considered have been properly evaluated in the literature with respect to reproducibility, specificity, sensitivity and predictive value in connection with the diagnosis and the management of urinary incontinence.

The routine clinical use of imaging techniques and other investigations is often based on expert opinion, common sense or local expertise and availability, rather than on evidence based clinical research.

The assessment methods we considered can be subdivided into safety tests, tests with specific indications and investigational tests.

Safety tests are indicated in all patients complaining of urinary incontinence. This refers to urinalysis and residual urine evaluation. While for urinalysis there is easy agreement, the role of PVR measurement as a safety test, proposed at the level of basic assessment in many algorithms, needs to be confirmed in terms of validity and cost effectiveness by means of prospective studies.

Tests with specific and selected indications follow.

Upper urinary tract imaging (as well as renal function assessment) may be indicated in cases of neurogenic urinary incontinence with risk of renal damage, chronic retention with incontinence, incontinence associated with severe genitourinary prolapse and suspicion of extraurethral incontinence.

The role of imaging techniques in the study of female urinary incontinence and of the pelvic floor is not yet established.

Cystourethrography has been well studied in terms of intra- and inter-observer variability, but cannot be recommended for the diagnosis or classification of urinary incontinence, while it is a reasonable option in the preoperative evaluation of complicated and/or recurrent cases.

Pelvic floor ultrasound is widely used in some countries. This technique is in rapid and continuous technologic and methodologic evolution. Pelvic floor ultrasound is very promising, but it should still be considered investigational, although standardisation is already in process.

In female urinary incontinence, as well as in neurogenic and postprostatectomy incontinence, the gold standard remains the simultaneous performance of imaging and urodynamics (videourodynamics). Some morphological findings, such as, open bladder neck and proximal urethra at rest, bladder wall thickness, diverticula and pseudodiverticula, membranous urethral narrowing, can have clinical and diagnostic relevance.

Lumbosacral spine X-rays have specific indications in children with suspect neurologic incontinence without gluteo-sacral stigmata.

Imaging of the CNS should be considered when a neurologic disorder is suspected on the basis of clinical, imaging and neurophysiological findings.

Urethrocystoscopy is indicated in cases of incontinence with microscopic haematuria, in the evaluation of recurrent or iatrogenic cases, in the evaluation of vesico-vaginal fistula and extra-urethral urinary incontinence.

The following tests were considered ***investigational***: ultrasound and MRI of the pelvic floor, MRI and functional neuro-imaging, and tissue analysis.

MRI of the female pelvic floor is to be considered the most promising research tool with potential future clinical applications, due to the tremendous amount of simultaneous information it can provide. Its main present limitation is that MRI is not available everywhere and cost effectiveness studies are needed.

Functional neuroimaging is going to provide new insight on functional anatomy of CNS related to vesicourethral function and dysfunction.

Many of these tests promise improvemements in our knowledge of pathophysiology of urinary incontinence and possibly better management.

The content of the draft inevitably reflects the composition of the Committee. The members are all clinicians, users of imaging techniques, without being necessarily experts of technology. Specific experts in imaging methods, like MRI and functional imaging of the CNS should be involved in the future.

The main goal of clinical research in the field we covered remains the prospective evaluation of accuracy, efficacy and cost-effectiveness of imaging techniques and other investigations and the validation of their role in the assessment flow charts of various types of urinary incontinence.

REFERENCE

A. IMAGING OF THE UPPER URINARY TRACT

1. McGuire EM, Woodside JR and Borden TA: Prognostic value of urodynamic testing in myelodysplasic children. J Urol 126:205, 1981.
2. Kontogeorgos L, Vassillopoulos P, Tentes A: Bilateral severe hydroureteronephrosis due to uterine prolapse. Br J Urol, 57:360, 1985
3. Braverman, R.M. and Lebowitz, R.L.: Occult ectopic ureter in girls with urinary incontinence: diagnosis using CT. Am J Roentgen, 156: 365, 1991.
4. Utsunomiya, M., Itoh, H., Yoshoika, T., Okuyama, A.. and Itatani, H.: Renal dysplasia with a single vaginal ectopic ureter: the role of computerized tomography. J. Urol., 132;98, 1984.
5. Prewitt, L.H. and Lebowitz, R.L.: The single ectopic ureter. Am J Roentgen, 127:941, 1976.
6. Borer, J.C., Bauer, S.B., Peters, C.A. et al: A single system ectopic ureter draining an ectopic dysplastic kidney: delayed diagnosis in the young female with continuous urinary incontinence. Br. J. Urol., 81(3):471, 1998.
7. Bozorgi, F.; Connolly, L.P., Bauer, S.B. et al: Hypoplastic dysplastic kidney with a vaginal ectopic ureter identified by technetium-99m.DMSA scintigraphy. J Nucl Med 39(1):113, 1998.
8. Carrico, C. and Lebowitz, R.L.: Incontinence due to an intrasphincteric ectopic ureter: why the delay in diagnosis and what the radiologist can do about it. Pediatr Radiol, 28:942, 1998.
9. Mandal, A.K., Sharma, S.K., Vaidyanathan, S. and Goswami, A.K.: Ureterovaginal fistula: summary of 18 years' experience. Br. J. Urol., 65:453, 1990.
10. Murphy, D.M., Grace, P.A. and O'Flynn, J.D.: Ureterovaginal fistula: a report of 12 cases and review of the literature. J. Urol., 128:924, 1984.
11. Pantuck, A.J., Barone, J.G., Rosenfeld, D.L. and Fleisher, M.H.: Occult bilateral ectopic ureters causing urinary incontinence: diagnosis by computed tomography. Abdominal Imaging, 21:78, 1996.
12. Avni, E.F., Matos, C., Rypens, F and Schulman, C.C.: Ectopic vaginal insertion of an upper pole ureter: demonstration by special sequences of magnetic resonance imaging. J. Urol., 158:1931, 1997.
13. Kaneko, K., Ohtsuka, Y., Suzuki, Y., Yabuta, K., Yamataka, A. and Miyano, T.: Masked ureteral duplication with ectopic ureter dectected by magnetic resonance imaging. Acta Paediatrica Japonica, 38(3):291, 1996.
14. Conway, J.J.: "Well-tempered" diuresis renography: it's historical development, physiological and technical pitfalls, and standardized technique protocol. Seminars in Nuclear Med., 22:74, 1992.
15. Hvistendahl, J.J., Pedersen, T.S., Schmidt, F., Hansen, W., Djurhuus, J.C. and Frokier, J.: The vesico-renal reflex mechanism modulates urine output during elevated bladder pressure. Scand. J. Urol. Nephrol., 186 (31 suppl.) 24, 1997.
16. O'Reilly, P.H.: Diuresis renography. Recent advances and recommended protocols. Br. J. Urol., 69:113, 1992.
17. Ruikka, I.: Residual urine in aged women and its influence on the phenolsulfonphthaleine excretion test. Geront. Clin., 3:65, 1963.
18. Pattaras, P.J., Rushton, H.G. and Majd,M: The role of 99mtechnetium dimercapto-succinic acid renal scans in the evaluation of occul ectopic ureters in girls with paradoxical incontinence. J. Urol,, 162:821, 1999

B. LOWER URINARY TRACT (LUT) IMAGING

B-I. IMAGING IN FEMALE URINARY INCONTINENCE AND PELVIC FLOOR DYSFUNCTION

1. Andersen JT. Prostatism: Clinical, radiological and urodynamic aspects. Neurourol Urodyn 1982; 1:241-293.
2. Shapeero LG, Friedland GW, Perkash I. Transrectal sonographic voiding cystourethrography: studies in neuromuscular bladder dysfunction. A J R 1983; 141:83-90.
3. Bellinger MF. The management of vescicoureteric reflux. Urol Clin N Amer 1985; 12:23-29.
4. Nolte-Ernsting CC, Glowinski A, Katterbach FJ, Adam G, Rasche V, Gunther RW. MR-micturating cystourethrography using radical k-space sampling. Rofo Fortschr Geb Rontgenstr Neuen Bildgeb Verfahr 1998;168:385-389.
5. Fortunato P, Schettini M, Gallucci M. Diverticula of the female urethra. Br J Urol 1997; 80:628-632.
6. Jacoby K, Rowbotham RK. Double balloon positive pressure urethrography is a more sensitive test than voiding cystourethrography for diagnosing urethral diverticulum in women. J Urol 1999;162:2066-2069.
7. Romanzi LJ, Groutz A, Blaivas JG. Urethral diverticulum in women: diverse presentations resulting in diagnostic delay and mismanagement. J Urol 2000;164:428-433.
8. Olesen KP. Descent of the female urinary bladder. A radiological classification based on colpo-cysto-urethrography. Dan Med Bull 1983; 30:66-84.
9. Mikulicz-Radecki F. Röntgenologische studien zur ätiologie der urethralen inkontinenz. Zbl Gynäk 1931; 55:7-95-810.
10. Stevens WE, Smith SP. Roentgenological examination of the female urethra. J Urol 1937; 37:194-201.
11. Ardran GM, Simmon CA, Stewart JH. The closure of the female urethra. J Obstet Gynaec Brit Emp 1956; 63:26-35.
12. Enhörning G, Miller ER, Hinman F Jr. Urethral closure studied

with cineroentgenography and simultaneous bladder-urethra pressure recording. Surg Gynec Obstet 1964; 118:507-516.

13. Palm L. Bladder Function in women with diseases of the lower urinary tract. Thesis. Munksgaard, Copenhagen 1971: 1-226.

14. Shopfner CE. Cystourethrography: Methodology, normal anatomy and pathology. J Urol 1970; 103:92-103.

15. Bates CP, Whiteside CG, Turner-Warwick R. Synchronous cine/pressure/flow/cysto- urethrography with special reference to stress and urge incontinence. Br J Urol 1970; 42:714-723.

16. Olesen KP, Walter S. Colpo-cysto-urethrography: a radiological method combined with pressure-flow measurements. Dan Med Bull 1977; 24:96-101.

17. Dietz HP, Wilson PD: The influence of bladder volume on the position and mobility of the urethrovesical junction. Int Urogynecol J 1999; 10:3-6

18. Theofrastous JP, Cundiff GW, Harris RL, Bump RC: The effect of vesical volume on Valsalva leak-point pressure in women with genuine stress urinary incontinence, Obstet Gynecol 1996; 87:711-714

19. Klarskov P, Jepsen PV, Dorhp S. Reliability of voiding colpo-cysto-urethrography in female urinary stress incontinence before and after treatment. Acta Radiol 1988; 29:685-688.

20. Barnick CG, Cardozo LD, Beuness C. Use of Routine videocystourethrography in the evaluation of female lower urinary tract dysfunction. Neurourol Urodyn 1989; 8:447-449.

21. Sorensen S, Knudsen VB, Kirkeby HJ, Djurhuus JC Urodynamic investigations in healthy fertile females during the menstrual cycle. Scand J Urol Nephrol, Suppl, 1988, 114:28-34.

22. Hansen F, Olsen L, Atan A, Jakobsen H, Nordling J. Pressure-flow studies: an evaluation of within-testing reproducibility-validity of the measured parameters. Neurourol Urodyn 1997; 16:521-532.

23. Pick EJ, Davis R, Stacey AJ. Radiation dose in cine-cystourethrography of the female. Br J Radiol 1960; 33:451-454.

24. Westby M, Ulmsten U, Asmussen M. Dynamic urethrocystography in women. Urol Int 1983; 38:329-336.

25. Rud T, Ulmsten U, Westby M. Initiation of micturition: a study of combined urethrocystometry and urethrocystography in healthy and stress incontinent females. Scand J Urol Nephrol 1979; 13:259-264.

26. de Goeij WBKMV. Incontinence of urine in women: Thesis. Krips Repro, Meppel 1976:1-253.

27. Jeffcoate TNA, Roberts H. Stress incontinence of urine. J Obstet Gynaec Brit Emp 1952; 59:685-697.

28. Fantl JA, Hurt G, Beachley MC, Bosch HA, Konerding KF, Smith PJ. Bead-chain cystourethrogram: an evaluation. Obstet Gynecol 1981; 58:237-240.

29. Drutz HP, Shapiro BJ, Mandel F. Do static cystourethrograms have a role in the investigation of female incontinence? Am J Obstet Gynecol 1978; 130:516-520.

30. Green TH. Development of a plan for the diagnosis and treatment of urinary stress incontinence. Am J Obst Gynec 1962; 83:632-468.

31. Gjorup T. Reliability of diagnostic tests. Acta Obstet Gynecol Scand 1997; Supp. 166:76:9-14.

32. Greenwald SW, Thornbury JR, Dunn LJ. Cystourethrography as a diagnostic aid in stress incontinence. An evaluation. Obstet Gynecol 1967; 29:324-327.

33. Kitzmiller JL, Manzer Ga, Nebel WA, Lucas WE. Chain cystourethrography and stress incontinence. Obstet Gynecol 1972; 39:333-340.

34. Pelsang RE, Bonney WW. Voiding cystourethrogaphy in female stress incontinence. Am J Roentgenol 1996;166:561-565.

35. Bergman A, McKenzie C, Ballard CA, Richmond J. Role of cystourethrography in the preoperative evaluation of stress urinary incontinence in women. J Reprod Med 1988; 33:372-376.

36. Bergman A, McKenzie CJ, Richmond J, Ballard CA, Platt LD. Transrectal ultasound versus cystography in the evalaution of anatomical stress urinary incontinence. Br J Urol 1988; 62:228-234.

37. Christ F, Meyer-Delpho W. Röntgendiagnostik bei der weiblichen harninkontinenz. Fortschr Röntgenstr 1981; 134:551-556.

38. Mouritsen L, Strandberg C, Jensen AR, Berget A, Frimodt-Moller C, Folke K. Inter and intra-observer variation of colpo-cysto-urethrography diagnoses. Acta Obstet Gynecol Scand 1993; 72:200-204.

39. Fischer-Rasmussen W, Hansen RI, Stage P. Predictive values of diagnostic tests in the evaluation of female urinary stress incontinence. Acta Obstet Gynecol Scand 1986; 65:291-294.

40. Stage P, Fischer-Rasmussen W, Hansen RI. The value of colpo-cysto-urethrography in female stress and urge incontinence and following operation: Acta Obstet Gynecol Scand 1986; 65:401-404.

41. Ala-Kretola L, Kauppila A, Jouppila P, Ylikorkala O. Pre and postoperative bead chain urethrocystography in female stress urinary incontinence. Acta Obstet Gynecol Scand 1981; 60:369-374.

42. Thuneborg P, Fischer-Rasmussen W, Jensen SB. Stress urinary incontinence and posterior bladder suspension defects. Results of vaginal repair versus Burch colposuspension. Acta Obstet Gynecol Scand 1990; 69:55-59.

43. Meyhoff HH, de Nully MB, Olesen KP, Lindahl F. The effects of vaginal repair on anterior bladder suspension defects. Acta Obstet Gynecol Scand 1985; 64:433-435.

44. Thind Po, Lose G, Falkenlove P, Egeblad M. Vurdering af miktionscystourethrografi. Intra-og interobservatorvariation. Ugeskr Læger 1991; 153:338-340.

45. Gordon D, Pearce M, Norton P, Stanton SL. Comparison of ultrasound and lateral chain urethrocystography in the determination of bladder neck descent. Am J Obstet Gynecol 1989; 160:182-185.

46. Kölbl H, Bernaschek G, Wolf G. A comparative study of perineal ultrasound scanning and urethrocystography in patients with genuine stress incontinence. Arch Gynecol Obstet 1988; 244:39-45.

47. Mouritsen L, Strandberg C. Vaginal ultrasonography versus colpo-cysto-urethrography in the evaluation of female urinary incontinence. Acta Obstet Gynecol Scand 1994; 73:338-342.

48. Dietz HP, Wilson PD : Anatomical assessment of the bladder outlet and proximal urethra using ultrasound and videocystourethrography. Int Urogyn J 1998 ; 9:365-369

49. Gufler H, DeGreorio G, Allmann KH, Kundt G, Dohnicht S. Comparison of cystourethrography and dynamic MRI in bladder neck descent. J Comput Assist Tomogr 2000;24:382-388.

50. Gufler H, Lauenberger J, DeGregorio G, Dohnicht S, Langer M. Pelvic floor descent: dynamic MR imaging using a half-Fourier RARE sequence. J Magn Reson Imaging 1999;9:378-383.

II. ULTRASOUND OF THE LOWER URINARY TRACT AND PELVIC FLOOR IN FEMALE URINARY INCONTINENCE

1. Koelbl H, Bernascheck G, Wolf G: A comparative study of perineal ultrasound scanning and urethrocystography in patients with genuine stress incontinence. Arch Gynecol Obstet, 244(1):39-45, 1988.

2. Gordon D, Pearce M, Norton P, Stanton SL: Comparison of ultrasound and lateral chain urethrocystography in the determi-

nation of bladder neck descent. Am J Obstet Gynecol, 160(1):182-185, 1989.

3. Schaer GN, Koechli OR, Schuessler B, Haller U: Perineal ultrasound for evaluating the bladder neck in urinary stress incontinence. Obstet Gynecol, 85(2):220-224, 1995]

4. Athanasiou S, Khullar V, Boos K, Salvatore S, Cardozo L. Imaging the urethral sphincter with three-dimensional ultrasound. Obstet Gynecol 1999; 94:295-301.

5. Beco J, Leonard D, Leonard F. Study of the female urethra's submucous vascular plexus by color Doppler. World J Urol 1998; 16:224-228

6. Kondo Y, Homma, Y, Takahashi S, Kitamura T and Kawabe K. Transvaginal ultrasound of urethral sphincter at the mid urethra in continent and on continent women. J. Urol, 165;149-152, 2001]

7. Quinn MJ, Beynon J, McMortensen NUJ, Smith PJB. Transvaginal endosonography: a new method to study the anatomy of the lower urinary tract in urinary stress incontinence. BJU 1988;62:414-417.

8. Nishizawa O, Takada H, Sakamoto F. Combined urodynamic and ultrasonic techniques: a new diagnostic method for the lower urinary tract. Tohoku J Exp Med. 1982;136:231-232.

9. Kohorn E, Scioscia AL, Jeanty P, Hobbins JC: Ultrasound cystourethrography by perineal scanning for the assessment of female stress urinary incontinence. Obstet Gynecol, 68:269-272, 1986.

10. Koelbl H and G. Bernaschek. A new method for sonographyc and urethrocystography and simultaneous pressure-flow measurements. Obstetrics & Gynecology, 1989;74, 417-422

11. Wise BG, Burton G, Cutner A, Cardozo LD: Effect of vaginal ultrasound probe on lower urinary tract function. Br J Urol 1992, 70:12-16.

12. Beco J, Leonard D, Lambotte R: Study of the artefacts induced by linear array transvaginal ultrasound scanning in urodynamics. World J Urol 1994, 12:329-332.

13. Richmond DH and J. Sutherst. Transrectal ultrasound scanning in urinary incontinence: the effect of the probe on urodynamic parameters. BJU 1989;64:582-585].

14. Bernaschek G: Current status of vaginal ultrasound – a worldwide survey. Geburt u. Frauenheilk, 51:729-733, 1991

15. Merz E: Current status of vaginal sonography. Part I: Basic principles and gynecologic diagnosis. Ultraschall Med, 15:2-10, 1994

16. Bernaschek G: Endosonography in obstetrics and gynecology: the importance of standardized image display. Obstet Gynecol, 74:817-820, 1989.

17. Tubaro A, and Carter for the ICS subcommittee on the standardisation of imaging. The standardisation of ultrasound imaging of the bladder. www.icsoffice.org

18. Schaer GN, Siegwart R, Perucchini D, DeLancey JO. Examination of voiding in seated women using a remote-controlled ultrasound probe. Obstet Gynecol 1998; 91:297-301

19. Hol M, Van-Bolhuis C, Vierhout ME: Vaginal ultrasound studies of bladder neck mobility. Br J Obstet.Gynaecol. 1995, 102:47-53

20. Schaer GN, Koechli OR, Schuessler B, Haller U: Perineal ultrasound: determination of reliable examination procedures. Ultrasound.Obstet.Gynecol. 1996, 7:347-352.

21. Creighton SM, Pearce JM, Stanton SL: Perienal video-ultrasonography in the assessment of vaginal prolapse: early observations. Br J Obstet Gyneacol, 93:310-313, 1992

22. Voigt R, Halaska M, Michels W, Voigt P, Martan A, Starker K: Examination of the urethrovesical junction using perineal sonography compared to urethrocystography using a bead chain. Int Urogynecol J, 5:212-214, 1994.

23. Bergman A, McKenzie CJ, Richmond J, Ballard CA, Platt LA: Transrectal ultrasound versus cystography in the evaluation of anatomical stress urinary incontinence. Br J Urol, 62:228-234, 1988.

24. Mouritsen L, Strandberg C: Vaginal ultrasonography versus colpocystourethrography in the evaluation of female urinary incontinence. Acta Obstet Gynecol Scand, 73:338-342, 1994]

25. Mouritsen L, Bach P. Ultrasonic evaluation of bladder neck position and mobility: the influence of urethral catheter, bladder volume and body position. Neurourol Urodyn 1994; 13:637-646

26. Fielding JR, AJR Am J Roentgenol 1998, 171:1607-1610

27. Dietz HP, Wilson PD. The influence of bladder volume on the position and mobility of the urethrovesical junction. Int Urogynecol J Pelvic Floor Dysfunct 1999; 10:3-6.

28. Schaer GN, Koelbli H, Voigt R, Merz E, Anthuber C, Niemeyer R, Ralph G, Bader W, Fink D, Grischke E. Recommendations of the German Association of Urogynecology on functional sonography of the lower female urinary tract. Int Urogynecol J Pelvic Floor Dysfunct, 7(2):105-108, 1996.

29. Peschers UM, Fanger G, Schaer GN, Vodusek DB, DeLancey JO, Schuessler B. Bladder neck mobility in continent nulliparous women. BJOG 2001; 108:320-324

30. Mouritsen L, Strandberg C, Frimodt MC: Bladder neck anatomy and mobility: effect of vaginal ultrasound probe. Br J Urol 1994, 74:749-752.

31. Bernstein I, The pelvic floor muscles; muscle thickness in healthy and urinary-incontinent women measured by perineal ultrasonography with reference to the effect of pelvic floor training. Estrogen receptor studies. Neurourol Urodyn, 1997, 16(4): 237-275.

32. Bernstein I, Juul N, Gronvall S, Bonde B, Klarskov P: Pelvis floor muscle thickness measured by perineal ultrasonography. Scand J Urol Nephrol, Suppl, 137:131-133, 1991

33. Schaer GN, Koechli OR, Schuessler B, Haller U: Improvement of perineal sonographic bladder neck imaging with ultrasound contrast medium. Obstet Gynecol, 86(6):950-954, 1995

34. Boos K, Athanasiou S, Salvatore S, Cardozo L: The assessment and measurement of paravaginal defects using transvaginal ultrasound. Int Urogynecol J, 7(3):163, 1996.

35. Nerstrom H, Holm HH, Christensen NE, Movild AF, Nolsoe C: 3-dimensional ultrasound based demonstration of the posterior urethra during voiding combined with urodynamics. Scand J Urol Nephrol, suppl, 137:125-129, 1991

36. Schaer GN, Schmid T, Peschers U. DeLancey JOL: Intraurethral ultrasound correlated with urethral histology. Obstet Gynecol, 1998; 91(1):60-4.

III. MRI OF PELVIC FLOOR

1. Maglinte DD, Kelvin FM,Fitzgerald K, et al. Association of compartment defects in pelvic floor dysfunction. AJR Am J Roentgenol, 172:439-444, 1999.

2. Safir MH, Gousse AE, Rovner ES, et al. 4-Defect repair of grade 4 cystocele. J Urol, 161:587-594, 1999.

3. Kelvin FM, Maglinte DD. Dynamic cystoproctography of female pelvic floor defects and their interrelationships. AJR Am J Roentgenol, 169:769-774, 1997.

4. Kelvin FM, Hale DS, Maglinte DD, et al. Female pelvic organ prolapse: diagnostic contribution of dynamic cystoproctography and comparison with physical examination. AJR Am J Roentgenol, 173:31-37, 1999.

5. Stovall DW. Transvaginal ultrasound findings in women with chronic pelvic pain. Obstet Gynecol, 95(4 Suppl 1):S57, 2000.

6. Raz S, Erickson D, Sussman E. Operative repair of rectocele, enterocele and cystocele. Adv Urol, 5:121-144, 1992.

7. Siproudhis L, Ropert A, Vilotte J, et al. How accurate is clinical examination in diagnosing and quantifying pelvirectal disorders? A prospective study in a group of 50 patients complaining of defecatory difficulties. Dis Colon Rectum, 36:430-438, 1993.
8. Klutke C, Golomb J, Barbaric Z, et al. The anatomy of stress incontinence: magnetic resonance imaging of the female bladder neck and urethra. J Urol, 143:563-566, 1990.
9. Yang A, Mostwin JL, Rosenshein NB, Zerhouni EA. Pelvic floor descent in woman: dynamic evaluation with fast MR imaging and cinematic display. Radiology, 179:25-33, 1991.
10. Goodrich MA, Webb MJ, King BF, et al. Magnetic resonance imaging of pelvic floor relaxation: dynamic analysis and evaluation of patients before and after surgical repair. Obstet Gynecol, 82:883-891, 1993.
11. Strohbehn K, Ellis JH, Strohbehm JA, DeLancey JO. Magnetic resonance imaging of the levator ani with anatomic correlation. Obstet Gynec, 87:277-285, 1996.
12. Ozasa H, Mori T, Togashi K. Study of uterine prolapse by magnetic resonance imaging: topographical changes involving the levator ani muscle and the vagina. Gynecol Obst Invest, 34:43-48, 1992.
13. Lienemann A, Anthuber C, Barron A, et al: Dynamic MR colpocystorectography assessing pelvic-floor descent. Eur Radiol, 7:1309-1317, 1997.
14. Comiter CV, Vasavada SP, Barbaric ZL, et al. Grading pelvic floor prolapse and pelvic floor relaxation using dynamic magnetic resonance imaging. Urology, 54:454-457, 1999.
15. Gousse AE, Barbaric ZL, Safir MH et al. Dynamic half fourier acquisition single shot turbo spin-echo magnetic resonance imaging for evaluating the female pelvis. J Urol, 164:1606-1613, 2000.
16. Rouanet JP, Mares P, Courtieu C, Maubon A. Static and dynamic MRI of the normal and pathological female pelvic floor. J Gynecol Obstet Biol Reprod, 164:1606-1613, 2000.
17. Lienemann A, Sprenger D, Jansen U, et al. Functional MRI of the pelvic floor. The methods and reference values. Radiologie, 45:458-464, 2000.
18. Tunn R, Paris S, Taupitz M, et al. MR imaging in posthysterectomy vaginal prolapse. Int Urogynecol J Pelvic Floor Dysfunct, 11:87-92, 2000.
19. Healy JC, Halligan S, Reznek RH et al. Patterns of prolapse in women with symptoms of pelvic floor weakness: assessment with MR imaging. Radiology, 203:77-81, 1997.
20. Tan IL, Stoker J and Lameris JS. Magnetic resonance imaging of the female pelvic floor and urethra: body coil versus endovaginal coil. Magma, 5(1):59-63, 1997.
21. Tan IL, Stoker J, Zwamborn AW, et al. Female pelvic floor: endovaginal MR imaging of normal anatomy. Radiology, 206:777-783, 1998.
22. Busse RF, Riederer SJ, Fletcher JG, et al. Interactive fast spin-echo imaging. Magn Reson Med, 44:339-48, 2000
23. Barbaric ZL Marumoto AK, and Raz S. Magnetic resonance imaging of the perineum and pelvic floor. Topics in Magnetic Resonance Imaging, 12(2):83-92, 2001.
24. Tunn R, Paris S, Fischer W, Hamm B, and Kuchinke J. Static magnetic resonance imaging of the pelvic floor muscle morphology in women with stress urinary incontinence and pelvic prolapse. Neurourol and Urodyn, 17:579-589, 1998.
25. Tunn R, DeLancey JO, Howard D, Thorp JM, Ashton-Miller JA and Quint LE. MR imaging of levator ani muscle recovery following vaginal delivery. Int Urogynecol J Pelvic Floor Dysfunct, 10(5): 300-307, 1999.
26. Christensen LL, Djurhuus JC, Lewis MT, Dev P, Chase RA, Constantinou PS and Constantinou CE. MRI of voluntary pelvic floor contractions in healthy female volunteers. Int Urogynecol J Pelvic Floor Dysfunct, 6:138, 1995.
27. Mostwin JL, Genadry R, Sanders R and Yang A. Anatomic goals in the correction of female stress urinary incontinence. J Endourol, 10(3):207-212, 1996.
28. Fielding JR, Dimanli H, Schreyer AG, et al. MR-based three-dimensional modeling of the normal pelvic floor in women: quantification of muscle mass. AJT Am J Roentgenol, 174:657-660, 2000.
29. Goh V, Halligan S, Kaplan G, et al. Dynamic MR imaging of the pelvic floor in asymptomatic subjects. AJR Am J Roentgenol, 174:661-666, 2000.
30. Myers RP, Cahill DR, Kay PA, et al. Puboperineales: muscular boundaries of the male urogenital hiatus in 3D from magnetic resonance imaging. J Urol, 164:1412-1415, 2000.
31. Hjartardottir S, Nilsson J, Petersen C, Lingman G. The female pelvic floor: a dome — not a basin. Acta Obstet Gynecol Scand, 76:567-571, 1997.
32. Hugosson C, Jorulf H, Lingman G and Jacobsson B. Morphology of the pelvic floor. Lancet, 337:367, 1997.
33. Bø K, Lilleås F, Talseth T, and Hedland H. Dunamic MRI of the pelvic floor muscles in an upright sitting position. Neurourol and Urodyn, 20:167-174, 2001.
34. Pannu HK, Kaufman HS, Cundiff GW, Genadry R, Bluemke DA, and Fishman EK. Dynamic MR imaging of pelvic organ prolapse: spectrum of abnormalities. Radiographics, 20:1567-1582, 2000.
35. Fielding JR, Griffiths DJ, Versi E, Mulkern RV, Lee M-LT, Jolesz FA. MR imaging of pelvic floor continence mechanisms in the supine and sitting positions. AJR Am J Roentgenol, 171:1607-1610, 1998.
36. Lienemann A, Sprenger D, Anthuber C, Baron, A, and Reiser M. Functional cine magnetic resonance imaging in women after abdominal sacrocolpopexy. Magnetic Resonance Imaging, 97(1):81-85, 2001
37. Goodrich MA, Webb MJ, King BF, Bampton AE, Campeau NG, Riederer SJ. Magnetic resonance imaging of pelvic floor relaxation: dynamic analysis and evaluation of patients before and after surgical repair. Obstetrics and Gynecology, 82(6):883-891, 1993.
38. Gufler H, DeGreforio G, Allman KH et al. Comparison of cystourethrography and dynamic MRI in bladder neck descent. J Comput Assist Tomogr, 24:382-388, 2000.
39. Weidner AC, Low VHS. Imaging studies of the pelvic floor. Obstet Gynecol Clin North Am, 25:825-848, 1998.
40. Linemann A, Anthuber C, Baron A, Reuser M. Diagnosing enteroceles using dynamic magnetic resonance imaging. Dis Colon Rectum, 43:205-212, 2000.
41. Altringer WE, Saclarides TJ, Dominguez JM, et al. Four-contrast defecography: pelvic "floor-oscopy". Dis Colon Rectum, 38:695-699, 1995.
42. Cundiff GW, Nygaard I, Bland DR, Versi E. Proceedings of the American Urogynecologic Society Multidisciplinary Symposium on Defecatory Disorders. Am J Obstet Gynecol, 182:S1-S10, 2000.
43. Takano M, Hamada A. Evaluation of pelvic descent disorders by dynamic contrast roentography. Dis Colon Rectum, 43:205-212, 2000.
44. Kelvin FM, Maglinte DDT, Hale DS, Benson JT. Female pelvic organ prolapse: a comparison of triphasic dynamic MR imaging and triphasic fluoroscopic cystocolpoproctography. AJR Am J Roentgenol, 174:81-84, 2000.
45. Brubaker L, Retzky S, Smith C, Saclarides T. Pelvic floor evaluation with dynamic fluoroscopy. Obstet Gynecol, 82:863-868, 1993.
46. Hock D, Lombard R, Jehaes C, et al. Colpocystodefecography. Dis Colon Rectum, 36:1015-1021, 1993.

47. Lamb GM, Jode MG, Gould SW, et al. Upright dynamic MR defaecating proctography in an open configuration MR system. Br J Radiol, 73:152-155, 2000.

B-II. LOWER URINARY TRACT IMAGING IN POST-PROSTATECTOMY INCONTINENCE

1. Leach GE, Vip C and Donovan BJ: Post-prostatectomy incontinence: the influence of bladder dysfunction. J Urol, 138:574, 1987
2. Leach GE and Yun SK: Post-prostatectomy incontinence:part I. The urodynamic findings in 107 men. Neurourol Urodyn, 11:91-97, 1992
3. Leach GE and Yun SK: Post-prostatectomy incontinence:part II. The results of treatment based on urodynamic evaluation. Neurourol Urodyn, 11:99-105, 1992
4. Leach GE, Trockan B, Wong A, Hamilton J, Haab F and Zimmern PE: Post-prostatectomy incontinence: urodynamic findings anf treatment outcomes. J Urol, 155: 1256- , 1996
5. McCallum RW, Alexander MW and Rogers JM: Etiology and method of investigation of male urinary incontinence. J Can Assoc Radiol, 36:4-11, 1985
6. Presti JC, Schmidt RA, Narayan PA, Carroll PR and Tanagho EA: Pathophysiology of urinary incontinence after ardical prostatectomy. J Urol, 143: 975-978, 1990

B-III.LOWER URINARY TRACT IMAGING IN NEUROGENIC INCONTINENCE

1. Webster DG and Kreder KJ: The neurourologic evaluation, in Campbell's Urology, seventh edition, WB Saunders Company, 1998, pp: 927-952
2. Bors E and Comarr AE: Neurological Urology, Physiology of Micturition, Its Neurological Disorders and Sequelae, Karger 1971, pp. 157
3. Hinman F: Urinary tract damage in children who wet. Pediatrics, 54:142- ,1974
4. Allen TD: The non-neurogenic bladder. J Urol, 117:232- ,1977
5. Williams DI, Hirst G, Doyle D: The occult neuropathic bladder. J Pediatr Surg, 9:35- , 1975

B-IV .LOWER URINARY TRACT IMAGING: SPECIAL ISSUES

I. RESIDUAL URINE EVALUATION

1. ICS Standardization Of Terminology Of Lower Urinary Tract Function. Neurol Urodyn, 7:403,1998
2. Purkiss, S.F.: Assessment Of Residual Urine In Men Following Catheterization. Br J Urol, 66(3):279, 1990
3. Stoller, M.L. And Millard, R.J.: The Accuracy Of A Catheterized Residual Urine. J Urol, 1741:15,1989
4. Ruikka, I.: Residual Urine In Aged Women And Its Influence On The Phenolsulfonphthaleine Excretion Test. Geront. Clin., 3:65, 1963
5. Mulrow, P.J., Huvos, A. And Buchanan, D.L.: Measurement Of Residualurine With I-131-Labeled Diodrast. J. Lab. Clin. Med.,57 :1961
6. Birch, N.C., Hurst, G. And Doyle, P.T.: Serial Residual Volumes In Men With Prostatic Hypertrophy. Br J Urol, 62:571,1998
7. Hakenberg. O.W., Ryall, R.L., Langlois, S.L. And Marshall, V.R.: The Estimation Of Bladder Volume By Sonocystography. J Urol, 130:249,1983
8. Poston, G.J., Joseph, A.E.A. And Riddle, P.R.: The Accuracy Of Ultrasound In The Measurement Of Changes In Bladder Volume. Br J Urol, 55:361,1983
9. Hartnell, G.G., Kiely, E.A. And Williams, G.: Real-Time Ultrasound Measurement Of Bladder Volume: A Comparative Study Of Three Methods. Br J Radiol,60:1063,1987
10. Rageth, J.C. And Langer, K.: Ultrasonic Assessment Of Residual Urine Volume. Urol Res, 57:57,1982
11. Orgaz, R.E., Gomez, A.Z., Rmirez, C.T. And Torres, J.L.M. : Application Of Bladder Ultrasonography. Bladder Content And Residual. J Urol, 125:164,1981
12. 4 Th International Consultation On Benign Prostatic Hyperplasia, Proceedings, Pp.205, 1998
13. Piters, K., Lapin, S. And Bessman, A.N.: Ultrasonography In The Detection Of Residual Urine. Diabetes, 28:320, 1979
14. Pedersen, J.F., Bartrum, R.J. And Grytter, C.: Residual Urine Detection By Ultrasonic Scanning. Am J Roengtenol Radium Ther Nucl Med, 125:474, 1975
15. Griffiths, C.J., Murray, A. And Ramsden, P.D.: Accuracy And Repeatibility Of Bladder Volume Measurement Using Ultrasonic Imaging. J Urol, 136:808,1986
16. Beacock, C.J.M., Roberts, E.E., Rees, R.W.M. And Buck, A.C.: Ultrsound Assessment Of Residual Urine. A Quantitative Method. Br J Urol,57:410,1985
17. West, K.A.: Sonocistography. A Method For Measuring Residual Urine. Scand J Urol Nephrol,1:68,1967
18. Mclean,G.K. And Edell, S.L.: Determination Of Bladder Volumes By Gray Scale Ultrasonography. Radiology, 128:181,1978
19. Widder, B., Kornhuber, H.H. And Renner, A.: Restharnmessung In Der Ambulanten Versorgung Mit Einem Klein- Ultrashallgerat. Dtsch Med Wochen-Schr,108:1552,1983
20. Roehrborn, C.G., Chinn, H.K., Fulgham, P.F., Simpkins, K.L. Nd Peters, P.C.: The Role Of Transabdominal Ultrasound In The Preoperative Evaluation Of Patients With Benign Prostatic Hypertrophy. J Urol, 135:1190,1986
21. Bruskewitz, R.C., Iversen,P And Madsen, P.O.: Vlue Of Post-Void Residual Urine Determination In Evaluation Of Prostatism. Urology, 20:602, 1982
22. Griffiths, D.J., Harrison, G., Moore, K. And Mccracken, P.: Variability Of Post-Void Residual Urine Volume In The Elderly. Urol Res,24(1):23, 1996
23. Andersen, J.T.: Prostatism. Detrusor Hyperreflexia And Residual Urine. Clinical And Urodynamic Aspects And The Influence Of Surgery On The Prostate. Scan J Urol, 16:25,1982
24. Dunsmuir, W.D., Feneley, M., Corry, D.A., Bryan, J. And Kirby, R.S.: The Day-To-Day Variation (Test-Retest Reliability) Of Residual Urine Measurement. Br J Urol, 77(2):192,1996
25. El Din, K.E., Kiemeney, L.A.L.M., De Wildt, M.J.A.M., Debruuyne, F.M.J. And De La Rosette, J.J.M.C.H.: Correlation Between Uroflowmetry, Post-Void Residue And Lower Urimary Tract Symptoms As Measured By The International Prostate Symptom Score. Urology,48:393,1996
26. Abrams, P.H. And Griffiths, D.J.: The Assessment Of Prostatic Obstruction From Urodynamic Measurements And From Residual Urine. Br J Urol,51:129,1979
27. Leblanc, G., Tessier, J. Ad Schick, E. : The Importance And Significance Of Post-Micturitional Bladder Residue In The Estimation Of Prostatism. Prog Urol, 5(4):511, 1995
28. Barry, M.J., Cockett, A.T., Holtgrewe, H.L., Mcconnel, J.D., Sihelnik, S.A. And Winfield, H.N.: Relationship Of Symptoms Of Prostatism To Commonly Used Physiological And Anatomical Measures Of The Severity Of Benign Prostatic Hyperplasia. J Urol, 150:351,1993
29. Ding, Y.Y., Sahadevan, S., Pang, W.S. And Choo, P.W.: Clinical Utility Of A Portable Ultrasound Scanner In The Measurement Of Residual Urine Volume. Singapore Med J, 37(4):365, 1996

II. OPEN BLADDER NECK AND PROXIMAL URETHRA AT REST

1. Wein, A.J., Levin, R.M. And Barrett, D.M.: Voiding Dysfunction:Relevant Anatomy Physiology And Pharmacology. In Gillenwaterjy, Grayhack Jt, Howards Ss And Duckett Jw (Eds): Adult And Pediatric Urology. Cichago, Y Ear Book Medical Publisher, Inc: 1987, Pp.800-62
2. Wein, A.J. :Neuromuscular Dysfunction Of The Lower Urinary Tract. In: Campbell's Urology, Pc Walsh, Ab Retik, Ta Stamey, Ed Vaughan (Eds). W.B. Saunders Company, 1992, Pp 573-642
3. Barbalias, G.A. And Blaivas, J.G. : Neurologic Implications Of The Pathologically Open Bladder Neck. J Urol, 129(4):780, 1983.
4. Salinas, J.M., Berger, Y., De La Roche, R.E. And Blaivas, J.G.: Urological Evaluation In The Shy Drager Syndrome. J Urol, 135 (4) :741, 1986
5. Blaivas, J.G. And Barbalias, G.A.: Characteristics Of Neural Injury After Abdominoperineal Resection. J Urol, 129(1): 84,1983
6. De Groat, W.C And Steers, W.D. : Autonomic Regulation Of The Urinary Bldder And Sexual Organs. In Loewry Ad, Spyers Km, Eds: Central Regulation Of The Autonomic Functions,1st Ed Oxford University Press. P.313,1990
7. Nordling , J: Influence Of The Sympathetic Nervous System On Lower Urinary Tract In Man. Neurol Urodyn, 2:3,1983
8. Woodside, J.R. And Mcguire, E.J.: Urethral Hypotonicity After Suprasacral Spinal Cord Injury. J Urol, 121 (6):783, 1979
9. Mcguire, E.J.: Combined Radiographic And Manometric Assessment Of Urethral Sphincter Function. J Urol, 118(4):632, 1977
10. Mcguire, E.J.: The Effects Of Scral Dervation On Bladder And Urethral Function. Surg Gyecol Obstet, 144(3):343,1977
11. Nordling, J. ,Meyhoff, H.H. And Olesen, K.P.: Cysto-Urethrographic Appearance Of The Ladder And Posterior Urethra In Neuromuscular Disorders Of The Lower Urinary Tract. Scand J Urol Nephrl, 16(2):115,1982
12. Gosling, J.A., Dixon, J.S. And Lendon, R.G.: The Autonomic Innervation Of The Human Male And Female Bladder Neck And Proximal Urethra. J Urol, 118(2):302,1977
13. Stanton, S.L. And Williams, D.: The Wide Bladder Neck In Children. Br J Urol, 45:60,1973
14. Murray, K., Nurse, D., Borzyskowski, M. Anm Mundy, A.R.: The 2congenital" Wide Bldddер Neck Anomaly: A Common Cause Of Incontinence In Children. Br J Urol, 59(6):533,1987
15. Chapple, C.R., Helm, C.W., Blease, S., Milroy, E.J.G., Richards, D. And Osborne, J.L.: Asymptomatic Bladder Neck Incompetence In Nulliparous Females. Br J Urol, 64(4): 357,1989
16. Versi, E.: The Significance Of An Open Bladder Neck In Women. Br J Urol, 68(1):42,1991
17. Blaivas, J.G. And Olsson, C.A.: Stress Incontinence: Classification And Surgical Approach. J Urol, 139:737,1988
18. Macdiamid, S., Rosario, D. And Chapple, C.R: The Importance Of Accurate Assessment And Conservative Management Of The Open Bladder Neck In Patients With Post-Pelvic Fracture Membranous Urethral Distraction Defects. Br J Urol, 75:65, 1995
19. Isekin, C.E. And Webster, G.D.: The Significance Of The Open Bladder Neck Associated With Pelvic Fracture Urethral Distraction Defects. J Urol, 162:347, 1999
20. Shivde, S.R.: The Significance Of The Open Bladder Neck Associated With Pelvic Fracture Urethral Distraction Defects. J Urol, 163:552, 2000

III. BLADDER WALL THICKNESS

1. Khullar V, Salvatore S, Cardozo LD, Kelleher CJ, Bourne TH: A novel technique for measuring bladder wall thickness in women using transvaginal ultrasound. Ultrasound Obstet Gynecol, 4:220-223, 1994
2. Khullar V, Cardozo LD, Salvatore S, Hill S: Ultrasound: a non invasive screening test for detrusor instability. Br J Obstet Gynaecol, 103:904-908, 1996

IV. FEMALE URETHRAL DIVERTICULA

1. Hey W: Practical Obervations in Surgery. Philadelphia. J. Humphries, 1805
2. Davis HJ and Cian LG: Positive pressure urethrography: a new diagnostic method. J Urol, 75:753, 1956.
3. GE Leach, BA Trockmann: Surgery for vesicovaginal and urethrovaginal fistula and urethral diverticulum, in Campbell's Urology, Seventh Edition, WB Saunders Company, 1998, pp:1135-1153//1145-1153
4. Aldrige CW, Beaton JH, Nanzig RP: A review of office urethroscopy and cystometry. Am J Obstet Gynecol, 131:432-435, 1978
5. Ganabathi K, Leach GE, Zimmern PE, Dmochowski R. Experience with management of urethral diverticulum in 63 women. J Urol, 152:1445-1452, 1994.
6. Romanzi LJ, Groutz A, Blaivas JG. Urethral diverticulum in women: diverse presentations resulting in diagnostic delay and mismanagement. J Urol, 164:428-433, 2000.
7. Chancellor MB, Liu JB, Rivas DA, Karasick S, Bagley DH and Goldberg BB: Intraoperative endo-luminal ultrasound evaluation of urethral diverticula. J Urol, 153:72, 1995
8. Kim B, Hricaaak H and Tanagho EA: Diagnosis of urethral diverticula in women: value of MR imaging. Am J Roentgenol, 161(4): 809-15, 1993
9. Neitlich JD, Foster HE, Glickman MG, Smith RC. Detection of urethral diverticula in women: comparison of a high resolution fast spin echo technique with double balloon urethrography. J Urol, 159:408-410, 1998.
10. Daneshgari F, Zimmern PE, Jacomides L. Magnetic resonance imaging detection of symptomatic noncommunicating intraurethral wall diverticula in women. J Urol, 161:1259-1262, 1999.
11. Blander DS, Broderick GA, Rovner ES. Magnetic resonance imaging of a "saddle bag" urethral diverticulum. Urology, 53:818-819, 1999.
12. Blander DS, Rovner ES, Schnall MD, et al. Endoluminal magnetic resonance imaging in the evaluation of urethral diverticula in female. Urology, 57:660-665, 2001.
13. Takano M, Hamada A. Evaluation of pelvic descent disorders by dynamic contrast reontography. Dis Colon Rectum, 43:205-212, 2000.

C. IMAGING OF THE NERVOUS SYSTEM (NEURO-IMAGING) IN URINARY INCONTINENCE

I. LUMBOSACRAL SPINE X-RAYS

1. Jacobson, H., Holm-Bentzen, M. And Hage, T.: Neurogenic Bladder Dysfunction In Sacral Agenesis And Dysgenesis. Neurol Urodyn, 4:99,1985
2. Boemers, T.M., Vangool, J.D., Dejorg, T.P.V.M. And Bax, K.M.A.: Urodynamic Evaluation Of Children With Caudal Regression Syndrome (Caudal Dysplasia Sequence) J Urol, 151:1038, 1994
3. Anderson, F.M.: Occult Spinal Dysraphism: A Series Of 73 Cases.Pediatrics, 55:826, 1975
4. Flanigan, R.F., Russel, D.P. And Walsh, J.W.: Urologic Aspects Of Tethered Cord. Urology, 33:80,1989

5. Kaplan, W.E., Mclone, D.G. And Richards, I: The Urologic Manifestations Of The Tethered Spinal Cord. J Urol, 140:1285,1988

6. Kondo, A., Kato, K., Kanai, S. And Sakakibara, T.: Bladder Dysfunction Secondary To Tethered Cord Syndrome In Adults: Is It Curable? J Urol, 135:313,1986

7. Scheible, W., James, H.E., Leopold, G.R. And Hilton, S.W.: Occult Spinal Dysraphism In Infants: Screening With High-Resolution Real-Time Ultrasound. Radiology, 146:743, 1983

8. Trcey, P.T. And Hanigan, W.C.: Spinal Dysraphism. Use Of Magnetic Resonance Imaging In Evaluation. Clin Pediatr, 29:228, 1990

II. CT, MRI, SPECT and PET (CNS)

1. Tsuchida S, Noto H, Yamaguchi O, Itoh M: Urodynamic studies in hemiplegic patients after cerebrovascular accidents. Urology, 21:315, 1983

2. Khan Z, Starer P, Yang WC, Bhola A: Analysis of voiding disorders in patients with cerebrovascular accidents. Urology, 32:256, 1990

3. Andrew J, Nathan PW: Lesions of the frontal lobes and disturbances of micturition and defecation. Brain, 87:233-262, 1964

4. Griffiths DJ, McCracken PN, Harrison GM, McEwan A: Geriatric urge incontinence: basic dysfunction and contributory factors. Neurourol Urodyn. 9:406-407, 1990

5. Kitada S, Ikel Y, Hasui Y, Nishi S, Yamaguchi T, Osada Y: Bladder function in elderly men with subclinical brain magnetic resonance imaging lesions. J Urol, 147:1507-1509, 1992

6. Blok BFM, Willemsen ATM and Holstege G: A PET study on brain control of micturition in human. Brain, 120:111, 1997

7. Blok BFM and Holdstege G: The central control of micturition and continence: implications for urology. B J Urol Int, 83, suppl 2: 1, 1999

D. ENDOSCOPY OF THE LOWER URINARY TRACT

1. Robertson, J.R.: Urethroscopy - the neglected gynecological procedure. Clin. Obstet. Gynecol., 19:315, 1976.

2 Aldridge, C.W. Jr., Beaton, J.H. and Nanzig, R.P.: A review of office cystoscopy and cystometry. Am. J. Obstet Gynecol., 131:432, 1978.

3 Scotti, R.J., Ostergard, D.R., Guillaume, A.A. and Kohatsu, K.E.: Predicative value of urethroscopy compared to urodynamics in the diagnosis of genuine stress incontinence. J. Reprod. Med., 35:772, 1990.

4 Horbach, N.S. and Ostergard, D.R.: Predicting intrinsic sphincter dysfunction in women with stress urinary incontinence. Obstet. Gynecol., 84: 188, 1994.

5 Govier, F.E., Pritchett, T.R. and Kornman, J.D.: Correlation of the cystoscopic appearance and functional integrity of the female urethral sphincteric mechanism. Urology, 44:250, 1994.

6 Sand, P.K., Hill, R.C. and Ostergard, D.A.: Supine urethroscopic and standing cystometry as screening methods for the detection of detrusor instability.

7 Langmade, C.F. and Oliver, J.A.: Simplifying the management of stress incontinence. Am. J. Obstet. Gynecol., 149: 24, 1984.

8 Fischer-Rasmussen, W., Hansen, R.I. and Stage, P.: Predicative value of diagnostic tests in the evaluation of female urinary stress incontinence. Acta Obstet. Gynecol. Scand., 65:291, 1986.

9 Cardozo, L.D. and Stanton, S.L.: Genuine stress incontinence and detrusor instability-a review of 200 patients. Br. J. Obstet. Gynecol., 87:184, 1980.

10 Mundy, A.R.: The unstable bladder. Urol. Clin. N.A., 12:317, 1985.

11 Duldulao, K.E., Diokno, A.C. and Mitchell, B: Value of urinary cytology in women presenting with urge incontinence and/or irritative voiding symptoms. J. Urol., 157:113, 1996.

12 Harris, R.L.,Cundiff, G.W.,Theofrastous, J.P., Yoon, H., Bump, R.C. and Addison, W.A.: The value of intraoperative cystoscopy in urogynecologic and reconstructive pelvic surgery. Am J Obstet Gynecol 177:6, 1997.

13 Timmons, C. and Addison, A.: Suprapubic teloscopy: extraperitoneal intraoperative technique to demonstrate ureteral patency. Obstet Gynecol 75:1, 1990.

14 Lower urinary tract operative injuries. ACOG Technical Bulletin, No.238, July 1997.

15 World Health Organization proceedings of the 3rd consultation on benign prostatic hyperplasia (BPH), Monaco, June 26-28, 1995, pp. 191-193.

16 Leach, G.E., Trockman, B., Wong, A., Hamilton, J., Haab, F. and Zimmern, P.E.: Post-prostatectomy incontinence: urodynamic findings and treatment outcomes. J. Urol. 155: 1256, 1996.

17 Desautel, M.G., Kapoor, R., and Badlani, G.H.: Sphincteric incontinence: the primary cause of post-prostatectomy incontinence in patients with prostate cancer. Neurourol. Urodyn., 16:153, 1997.

18 Gudziak, M.R., McGuire, E.J. and Gormley, E.A.: Urodynamic Assessment of urethral sphincter function in post-prostatectomy incontinence. J. Urol., 156, 1131, 1996.

19 Chao, R. and Mayo, M.E.: Incontinence after radical prostatectomy: detrusor or sphincter causes. J. Urol., 154:16, 1995.

20 Goluboff, E.K., Chang, D., Olsson, C.A. and Kaplan, S.A.: Urodynamics and the etiology of post-prostatectomy urinary incontinence: the initial Columbia experience. J. Urol., 153:1034, 1995.

21 Leach, G.E., and Yun, S.K.: Post-prostatectomy incontinence: Part II. The results of treatment based on urodynamic evaluation. Neurourol. Urodyn., 11:99, 1992.

E. PAD TESTING

1. Abrams P, Blaivas JG, Stanton SL, Andersen JT (Chairman) (1988): The standardization of terminology of lower urinary tract function. Scand J Urol Nephrol Suppl 114:5.

2. Abrams P, Blaivas JG, Stanton SL, Andersen JT (Chairman) (1988): The standardization of terminology of lower urinary tract function. International Continenece Society Committee on Standardisation of Terminology. Neurourol Urodyn 7:403-427

3. Anand D, Versi E, Cardozo L (1985): The predictive value of the pad test. "Proceedings of the International Continence Society," 15th meeting, London, pp 290-298.

4. Bates P, Bradley W, Glen E, Griffiths D, Melchior H, Rowan D, Stanton S, Sterling A, Sundin T, Thomas D, Torrens M, Warwick RT, Zinner N, Hald T (1983): Fifth Report on the standardisation of terminology of lower urinary tract function. Bristol International Society Committee on Standardisation of Terminology.

5. Batista MJE, Arano BP, Errando SC, Puigpelat FT, Granda CM, Da Silvia VF (1997) Quantification of urine leaks: standardized one-hour pad test. Actas Urol Esp 21(2):111-116.

6. Blaivas JG, Appell RA, Fanti JA, Leach G, McGuire EJ, Resnick NM, Raz S and Wein AJ. (1997) Standards of efficacy for evaluation of treatment outcomes in urinary incontinence: Recommendations of the Urodynamic Society, Neurourol Urodyn 16:145-147.

7. Caldwell KPS (1974) Clinical use of recording nappy Urol Int 29:172-173
8. Christensen SJ, Colstrup H, Hertz JB, Lenstrup C, Frimodt-Møller C (1986): Inter- and intra-departmental variations of the perineal pad weighing test. Neurourol Urodyn 5:23-28.
9. Eadie AS, Glen ES, Rowan D (1983) The Urilos recording nappy system Be J Urol 55:301-303
10. Eadie AS, Glen ES, Rowan D (1984) Assessement of urinary loss over a two-hour test period: A comparison between the Urilos recording nappy system and the weighed perineal pad method. Proc 14th Ann Meeting, ICS Innsbruck, pp 94-95.
11. Ekelund P; Bergstrom H; Milsom I; Norlen L; Rignell S. Quantification of urinary incontinence in elderly women with the 48-hour pad test. Arch Gerontol Geriatric 1988 Dec; 7 (4): 281-7
12. Elser DM, Fanti JA, McClish DK, and the Continence Program for Women Research Group: Comparison of "Subjective" and "Objective" measures of severity of urinary incontinence in women. (1995) 14:311-316.
13. Fantl JA, Harkins SW, Wyman JF, Choi SC, Taylor JR (1987) Fluid loss quantitation test in women with urinary incontinence: A test-retest analysis. Obstet Gynecol 70:739-743.
14. Griffiths DJ, McCracken PN, Harrison GM (1991) Incontinence in elderly: Objective demonstration and quantitative assessment Br J Urol 67:467-471.
15. Groutz A; Blaivas JG; Chaikin DC; Resnick NM; Engleman K; Anzalone D; Bryzinski B; Wein AJ. Noninvasive outcome measures of urinary incontinence and lower urinary tract symptoms: a multicenter study of micturition diary and pad tests. J Urol 2000 Sept; 164 (3 Pt 1): 698-701.
16. Hahn I, Fall M (1991): Objective Quantification of stress urinary incontinence: A short reproducible, provovative Pad-Test. Neurourol Urodyn 10:475-481
17. Hald T: Quantitation of urine loss (1989) Neurourol Urodyn 8:543-544.
18. Han HC (1996): One-hour or two-hour perineal pad test, which would you choose?. Proceedings ICS Athens pp 382
19. Haylen BT, Sutherst JR (1987): The classification and treatment of genuine stress incontinence based on the results of pad testing. "Proceedings of the International Continence Society," 17th meeting, Bristol, p 63-64.
20. Haylen BT, Frazer MI, Sutherst JR (1988): Duretic response to fluid load in women with urinary incontinence: Optimum duration of pad test. Br J Urol 62:331-333.
21. Hellstrom A-L, Andersson K, Hjalmas K, Jodal V. (1986) Pad test in children with incontinence. Scand J Urol Nephrol 20:47-50.
22. Holm-Bentzen MH, Klarskov P, Opsomer RJ, Maegaard EM, Hald T (1985) Objective assessement of urinary incontinence after successful implantation of AMS artificial urethral sphincter. Neurourol Urodyn 4:9-13.
23. Jakobsen H, Vedel P, Andersen Jt (1987): Objective assessment of urinary incontinence. An evaluation of three different pad-weighing tests. Neurourol Urodyn 6:325-330.
24. Jakobsen H, Kromann-Andersen B, Nielsen KK, Meagaard E: (1993) Pad weighing tests with 50% or 75% bladder filling. Does it matter. Acta Obstet Gynecol Scan 72:377-381.
25. James ED, Eng C, Flack FC, Caldwell KPS, Martin MR (1971) Continous measurement of urine loss and frequency in incontinence patients. Br J Urol 43:233-237.
26. James ED, Flack FC. (1974) Assessment of recording nappy, Urol Int 29:174-175.
27. Janez J, Rodi Z, Mihelic M, Vrtacnik P, Vodusek DB, Plevnik S: Ambulatory distal urethral electric conductance testing coupled to a modified pad test. (1993) Neurourol Urodyn 12:324-325.
28. Jørgensen L, Steen A, Bagger PV, Fisher-Rasmussen W (1985) The one-hour pat-weighing test for assessment of the result of female incontinence surgery. Proc 15th Ann Meeting ICS, London pp 392-393.
29. Jørgensen L, Lose G, Andersen JT (1987a): One hour pad-weighing test for objective assessment of female urinary incontinence. Obstet Gynecol 69:39-41.
30. Jørgensen L, Lose G, Thunedborg P (1987b): Diagnosis of mild stress incontinence in females: 24-hour home pad weighing test versus the 1-hour ward test. Neurourol Urodyn 6:165-166.
31. Khan KS, Chien PF (1996): Comments on "Evaluation of the home pad test in the investigation of female urinary incontinence" Br J Obstet Gynaecol 103(7):720
32. Kinn A-C, Larsson B. Nielsson E (1985): Pad test in urinary stress incontinence-standardisation and reliability. Sacn J urol Nephrol, Suppl 101, p 15,
33. Kinn A-C, Larsson B. (1987) Pad test with fixed bladder volumen in urinary stress incontinence. Acta Obstet Gynecol Scand 66:369-371.
34. Klarskov P, Hald T (1984): Reproducibility and reliability of urinary incontinence assessment with a 60 min test. Scand J Urol Nephrol 18:293-298.
35. Klevmark B, Talseth T, Eri LM: Objective assessment of urinary incontinence. The advantage of relating 24 hours pad-weighing test to frequency volume chart ("Combine test").(1988) Neurourol Urodyn 7:155-160.
36. Kralj D (1989): Comparative study of pad tests-reliability and repetitiveness. Neurourol Urodyn 8: 305-306.
37. Kromann-Andersen B, Jakobsen H, Andersen T: Pad-weighing tests: A literature survey on test accuracy and reproducibility. (1989) Neurourol Urodyn 8:237-242
38. Leach GE, Dmochowski RR, Appell RA, Blaivas JG, Hadley HR, Luber KM, Mostwin JL, O'Donnell PD and Roehrborn CG: (1997) Female stress urinary incontinence clinical guidelines panel summary report on surgical mangement of female stress urinary incontinence. J Urol 158:875-880.
39. Lose G, Gammelgaard J, Jørgensen TJ (1986): THE ONE-HOUR PAD-WEIGHING TEST: Reproducibility and the correlation between the test result, the start volume in the bladder, and the diuresis. Neurourol Urodyn 5.17-21.
40. Lose G, Rosenkilde P, Jørgensen TJ, Schroeder T, Gammelgaard J, (1986) The pad test performed with standardized bladder volume. Proc 16th Ann Meeting ICS, Boston, pp 474-476.
41. Lose G, Rosenkilde P, Gammelgaard J, Schroeder T (1988): Pad-weighing test performed with standardized bladder volume. Urology 32:78-80.
42. Lose G, Jørgensen L, Thunedborg P (1989): Twenty-four hour pad weighing test versus 1-hour ward test in the assessement of mild stress incontinence. Acta Obstet Gynecol Scand 68:211-215.
43. Lose G, Versi E. (1992) Pad-weighing tests in the diagnosis and quantification of incontinence. Int Urogynecol 3:324-328.
44. Martan A, Halaska M, Voigt R. (1992): Our experience with modified pad weight test. Proceedings ICS Halifax, pp233-234.
45. Martan A, Koleska T, Halaska M. (1993) Personal experience with the modified pad-weight test, Cesk Gynekol 58(1):3-5
46. Mayne CJ, Hilton P: Short Pad Test: Standardisation of method and comparison with 1-hour test (1988) Neurourol Urodyn 7:443-445.
47. Mayne CJ, Hilton P: The distal urethral electrical conductance test: Standardisation of method and clinical reliability (1988) Neurourol Urodyn 7:55-60.
48. Mouritsen L, Berild G, Hertz J (1989): Comparison of different methods for quantification of urinary leakeage in incontinent women. Neurourol Urodyn 8:579-587.

49. Mulder AFP, Vierhout ME: Combine ambulatory urodynamics and pad testing. (1991) Neurourol Urodyn 10:420-421.

50. Mundt-Pettersen B, Mathiasson A, Sundin T (1984): Reproducibility of the 1 hour incontinence test proposed by the ICS standardization committee. Proc 14th Ann Meeting ICS, Innsbruck, pp 90-91.

51. Nygaard I, Zmolek G: Exercise pad testing in continent exercisers: Reproducibility and correlation with voided volume, pyridium staining and type of exercise. (1995) Neurourol Urodyn 14:125-129.

52. Prajsner A; Radziszewski P. Ambulatory diagnosis of urinary incontinence among women: the role of a one-hour pad weight test."/ "Diagnostyka ambulatoryjna nietrzymania moczu u kobiet: rola jednogodzinnego testu wkladkowego. Wiad Lek 1998; 51 (5-6): 254-9

53. Rasmussen A, Mouritsen L, Dalgaard A, Frimodt-Moller C:(1994) Twenty-four hour pad weighing test: Reproducibility and dependency of activity level and fluid intake. Neurourol Urodyn 13:261-265.

54. Richmond DH, Sutherst JR, Brown MC (1987): Quantification of urine loss by weighing perineal pads. Observation on the exercise regimen. Br J Urol 59:224-227.

52. Rowan D, Deehan C, Glen E. (1976) Detection of urine loss using the Exeter Recording Nappy and other similar devices. Urol Int 31:70-77.

53. Ryhammer AM; Laurberg S; Djurhuus JC; Hermann AP. No relationship between subjective assessment of urinary incontinence and pad test weight gain in a random population sample of menopausal women. J Urology 1998 March; 159 (3): 800-3.

54. Ryhammer AM; Djurhuus JC; Laurberg S. Pad testing in incontinent women: a review. Int Urogynecol J Pelvic Floor Dysfunction 1999; 10 (2): 111-5.

55. Siltberg H, Victor A, Larson G. (1997) Pad-weighing tests: the best way to quantify urine loss in patients with incontinence. Acta Obstet Gynecol Scan; Suppl 166:26-32

56. Stanton SI, Ritchie D (1977) Urilos: The practical detection of urine loss. Am J Obstet Gynecol 128:461-463.

57. Sutherst J, Brown M, Shawer M (1981): Assessing the severity of urinary incontinence in women by weighing perineal pads Lancet 1:1128-1130.

58. Sutherst J, Brown M, Richmond D:(1986) Analysis of the pattern of urine loss in women with incontinence as measured by weighing perineal pads. Br J Urol 58:273-278

59. Thind P, Gerstenberg TC: One-hour ward test vs. 24-hour home pad weighing test in the diagnosis of urinary incontinence. (1991) Neurourol Urodyn 10:241-245

60. Versi E, Cardozo LD (1984): One hour single pad test as a simple screening procedure. Proc 14th Ann Meeting ICS Innsbruck, pp 92-93.

61. Versi E, Cardozo LD (1986): Perineal pad weighing versus videographic analysis in genuine stress incontinence. Br J Obstet Gynecol 93:364-366.

62. Versi E, Anand D, Smith P, Seddon G, Hardy E, Orrego G (1996) Evaluation of the home pad test in the investigation of female urinary incontinence Br J Obstet Gynaecol 103(2):162-167.

63. Victor A, Larsson G, Åsbrink A-S (1987): A simple patient-administered test for objective quantitation of the symptom of urinary incontinence. Scand J Urol Nephrol 21:277-279.

64. Victor A (1990): Pad weighing test - a simple method to quantitate urinary incontinence. Ann Med 22:(6) 443-447

65. Wall LL, Wang K, Robson I, Stanton SL (1990): The pyridium pad test for diagnosing urinary incontinence. A comparative study of asymptomatic and incontinent women. J Reprod Med 35:682-684.

66. Walsh JB, Mills GL (1981) Measurement of urinary loss in elderly incontinent patients. A simple and accurate method. Lancet, I:1130-1131.

67. Walters MD, Dombroski RA, Prihoda TJ (1990) Perineal pad testing in the quantitation of urinary incontinence. Int Urogynecol J, 1:3-6.

68. Wilson PD, Al Samarrai MT, Brown ADG, (1980) Quantifying female incontinence with particular reference to the Urilos System Urol Int 35:298-302.

F. OTHER INVESTIGATIONS

I. URINALYSIS IN THE EVALUATION OF THE INCONTINENT PATIENT

1. C.B. Brendler, Evaluation of the Urologic Patient, History, Physical Examination and Urinalysis, in Campbell's Urology Seventh Edition, vol. 1, pp. 144, 1998

2. European Urinalysis Guidelines – Summary, Scand J Clin Lab Invest, 60:1-96, 2000

3. Ouslander, J.G., Schapira, M., Schnelle, J.F. and Fingold, S: Pyuria among chronically incontinent but otherwise asymptomatic nurding home residents. J Am Geriatr Soc, 44(4):420, 1996

4. Sandvick, H. and Hunskaar, S.: General practitioners' management of female urinary incontinence. Medical records do not reflect patient's recall. Scand J Prim Health Care, 13(3):168, 1995

5. Kennedy, K.L., Steidle, C.P. and Letixia T.M.; Urinary incontinence: the basics. Oostomy Wound Manage, 41(7):16, 1995

6. Stricker, P.D.: Proper patient selection for Contigen Bard collagen implant. Int. J Urol, supll 1:2, 1995

7. Stein, M., Discippio, W., Davia, M. and Taub, H.: Biofeedback for the treatment of stress and urge incontinence. J Urol, 153:641, 1995

8. Wall, L.L., Wiskind, A.K. and Taylor, P.A.: Simple bladder filling with a cough stress compared with subtracted cystometry for the diagnosis of urinary incontinence. Am J Obstet Gynecol, 17(6):1472, 1994

9. Ouslander, J.G. and Schnelle, I.F.: Incontinence in the nursing home. Ann Intern Mad, 122(6):438, 1995

10. Young, S.B. and Pingeton, D.M.: A practical approach to perimenopausal and postmenopausal urinary incontinence. Obstet Gynecol Clin North Am, 21(2):357, 1994

11. McIntosh, L.J. and Richardson, D.A.: 30-minute evaluation of incontinence in the older woman. Geriatrics, 49(2):35, 1994

12. Belmin, J., Hervias, Y., Avellano, E., Oudart, O. and Durand, I.: Reliability of sampling urine from disposablediapersin elderly incontinent women. J Am Geriatr Soc, 41(11):1182, 1993

13. Ouslander, J.G.:Geriatric urinary incontinence. Dis Mon, 38(2):65, 1992

14. Dubeau, C.E. and resnick, N.M.: Evaluation of the causes and severity of geristric incontinence. A critical appraisal. Urol Clin North Am, 18(2):243, 1991

II. CHEMICAL TESTS

1. Rittig, S., Knudsen, U.B., Norgaard, J.P., Pedersen, E.B. and Djurhuus, J.C.: Abnormal diurnal rythm of plasma vasopressin and urinary output in patients with enuresis. Amer J Physiol, part 2, 256:F664, 1989

2. Matthiesen, T.B., Rittig, S., Norgaard, J.P., Pedersen, E.B. and

Djurhuus, J.C.: Nocturnal polyuria and natriuresis in male patients with nocturia and lower urinary tract symptoms. J Urol, 156:1292, 1996

3. Miodrag, A., Castleden, C.M. and Vallance, T.R.: Sex hormones and the female urinary tract. Drugs, 36:491, 1988)

4. Fantl, J.A., Wyman, J.F., Anderson, R.L., Matt, D.W. and Bump, R.C.: Postmenopausal urinary incontinence: comparison between non-estrogen-supplemented and estrogen-supplemented women. Obstet Gynecol, 71: 823, 1988

5. AybeK, Z., Mathrunbutham, M., Rao, S., Badlani, G. and Kushner, L.: Capacity of plasma to inhibit elastase is reduced in patients with stress urinary incontinence. J.Urol., 159:5 ab 57, p 15, 1998

III. TISSUE ANALYSIS

1. Brincat, M., Moniz, C.F., Studd, J.W.W., Magos, A And Cooper, D.. Sex Hormones And Skin Collagen Content In Postmopausal Women. Br Med J, 287:1337,1983

2. Brincat, M., Moniz, C.F., Studd, J.W.W., Darby, A., Magos, A ., Emburey, G. And Versi, E.: Long-Term Effects Of The Menopause And Sex Hormones On Skin Thickness. Br J Obstet Ginaecol, 92:256, 1985

3. Brincat, M., Moniz, C.F., Kabklan, S., Versi, E., O'dowd, T., Magos, A.L., Montgomery, J. And Studd, J.W.W.: Decline In Skin Collagen Content And Metacarpal Index After Menopause And Its Prevention With Sex Hormone Replacement. Br J Obstet Ginaecol, 94:126, 1987

4. Versi, E., Cardozo, L., Brincat, M., Montgomery, J. And Studd, J.W.W.: Correlation Of Urethral Physiology And Skin Collagen In Postmenopausal Women. Br J Obstet Ginaecol, 95:147, 1988

5. Norton, P., Boyd, C. And Deak, S.: Collagen Synthesis In Wmnen With Genital Prolapse Or Stress Urinry Incontinence. Neurol Urodyn, 11:3,1992 Et Al 1987

6. Norton, P.A.: Etiology Of Genuine Stress Incontinence. I: The Femle Pelvic Floor. Disorders Of Function And Support. By L.T. Saclarides, F.A. Davis Company, Philadelphia, Pp.153, 1996

7. Keane, D.P., Sims, T.J., Balley, A.J. And Abrams, P.: Analysis Of Pelvic Floor Electromyography And Collagen Status In Pre-Menopausal Nulliparous Females With Geenuine Stress Incontinence. Neurol Urodyn, 8 :308, 1997

8. Gilpin, S.A., Gosling, G.A., Smith, A.R.B. And Warrell, D.W.: The Pathogenesis Of Genotourinary Prolapse And Stress Incontinence Of Urine Br J Obstet Ginaecol, 96:15,1989

9. Hanzai, E., Berger, E. And Koelbl, H.: Levator Ani Muscle Morphology And Recurrent Genuine Stress Incontinence. Obstet Ginaecol, 81(3):426, 1993

10. Helt, M., Benson, J.T., Russell, B. And Brubaker, L.: Levator Ani Muscle In Women With Genitourinary Prolapse: Indirect Assessment By Muscle Histopatology. Neurol Urodyn, 15(1):17, 1996

11. Falconer, C., Ekman-Orderberg, G., Hilliges, M. And Johanson, O.: Decreased Innervation Of The Paraurethral Epithelium In Stress Urinary Incontinent Women. Eur J Obstet Gynaecol Reprod Biol, 72(2):195, 1997

12. Elbadawi. A., Yalla, S.V. And Resnick, N.M.: Structural Basis Of Geriatric Voiding Dysfunction. Iii Detrusor Overactivity. J Urol, 150:1668, 1993

13. Elbadawi. A.: Pathology And Pathophysiology Of Detrusor Incontinence. Urol Clin North Am, 22(3):499, 1995

Committee 9

Pharmacological Treatment of Urinary Incontinence

Chairman

K-E. ANDERSSON (SWEDEN),

Members

R. APPELL (USA),

S. AWAD (CANADA),

C. CHAPPLE (U.K.),

H. DRUTZ (CANADA),

A. FINKBEINER (USA),

J. FOURCROY (USA),

F. HAAB (FRANCE),

A. WEIN (USA)

CONTENTS

Pharmacological Treatment of Urinary Incontinence

K-E ANDERSSON,

R. APPELL, S. AWAD, C. CHAPPLE, H. DRUTZ, A. FINKBEINER, J. FOURCROY, F. HAAB, A. WEIN

I. INTRODUCTION

The functions of the lower urinary tract, to store and periodically release urine, are dependent on the activity of smooth and striated muscles in the urinary bladder, urethra, and external urethral sphincter. These structures constitute a functional unit which is controlled by a complex interplay between the central and peripheral nervous systems and local regulatory factors (Andersson 1993, de Groat et al. 1999, de Groat and Yoshimura 2001). Malfunction at various levels may result in bladder control disorders disorders, which roughly can be classified as disturbances of filling/storage or disturbances of emptying (Wein 2001a). Failure to store urine may lead to various forms of incontinence (mainly urge and stress incontinence), and failure to empty can lead to urinary retention, which may result in overflow incontinence. Theoretically, a disturbed filling/storage function can be improved by agents that decrease detrusor activity, increase bladder capacity and/or increase outlet resistance (Wein 2001a).

Many drugs have been tried, but the results are often disappointing, partly due to poor treatment efficacy and/or side effects. The development of pharmacologic treatment of the different forms of urinary incontinence has been slow, and the use of some of the currently prescribed agents is based more on tradition than on evidence based on results from controlled clinical trials (Andersson et al 1999, Wein 2001a).

In this report, we update the recommendations from the previous International Consensus meeting. The most relevant information obtained since the last meeting is reviewed and summarised. Agents specifically used for treatment of urinary tract infections and interstitial cystitis have not been included. Drugs have been evaluated using different types of evidence (Table 1). Pharmacological and/or physiological efficacy evidence means that a drug has been shown to have desired effects in relevant preclinical experiments or in healthy volunteers (or in experimental situations in patients). This information has been considered in our clinical drug recommendations, which are based on evaluations made using a modification of the Oxford system, in which emphasis has been given to the quality of the trials assessed.

Table 1 : Types of evidence

PHARMACODYNAMIC
In vitro
In vivo
PHARMACOKINETIC
Absorption
Distribution
Metabolism
Excretion
PHYSIOLOGICAL
Animal models
Clinical phase I
CLINICAL
Oxford guidelines

II. CENTRAL NERVOUS CONTROL

The normal micturition reflex in the adult individual is mediated by a spinobulbospinal pathway, passing through relay centers in the brain (Figure 1). In infants, the central pathways seem to be organized as on-off switching circuits, but after the age of 4-6 years, voiding is initiated voluntarily by the cerebral cortex (de Groat et al 1999). Studies in humans and animals have identified areas in the brainstem and diencephalon that are specifically implicated in micturition control, namely Barrington's nucleus or the pontine micturition center (PMC) in the dorsomedial pontine tegmentum, which directly excites bladder motoneurons and indirectly inhibits urethral sphincter motoneurons via inhibitory interneurons in the medial sacral cord; the periaqueductal grey (PAG) receiving bladder filling information, and the pre-optic area of the hypothalamus, which is probably involved in the initiation of micturition. According to PET-scan studies in humans, these supraspinal regions are active during micturition (Blok et al 1998, Nour et al 2000).

III. PERIPHERAL NERVOUS CONTROL

Bladder emptying and urine storage involve a complex pattern of efferent and afferent signalling in *parasympathetic*, *sympathetic* and *somatic* nerves (Figures 1 and 2). These nerves are parts of reflex pathways which either maintain the bladder in a relaxed state, enabling urine storage at low intravesical pressure, or which initiate micturition by relaxing the outflow region and contracting the bladder smooth muscle. Contraction of the detrusor smooth muscle and relaxation of the outflow region result from activation of *parasympathetic* neurones located in the sacral parasympathetic nucleus (SPN) in the spinal cord at the level of S2-S4 (de Groat *et al.*, 1993). The postganglionic neurones in the pelvic nerve mediate the excitatory input to the human detrusor smooth muscle by releasing acetylcholine (ACh) acting on muscarinic receptors. However, an atropine-resistant component has been demonstrated, particularly in functionally and morphologically altered human bladder tissue (see below). The pelvic nerve also conveys parasympathetic fibres to the outflow region and the urethra. These fibres exert an inhibitory effect and thereby relax the outflow region. This is mediated partly by release of nitric oxide (Andersson & Persson, 1993), although other transmitters might be involved (Bridgewater & Brading, 1993; Hashimoto *et al.*, 1993; Werkstrom *et al.*, 1995).

Most of the *sympathetic* innervation of the bladder and urethra originates from the intermediolateral nuclei in

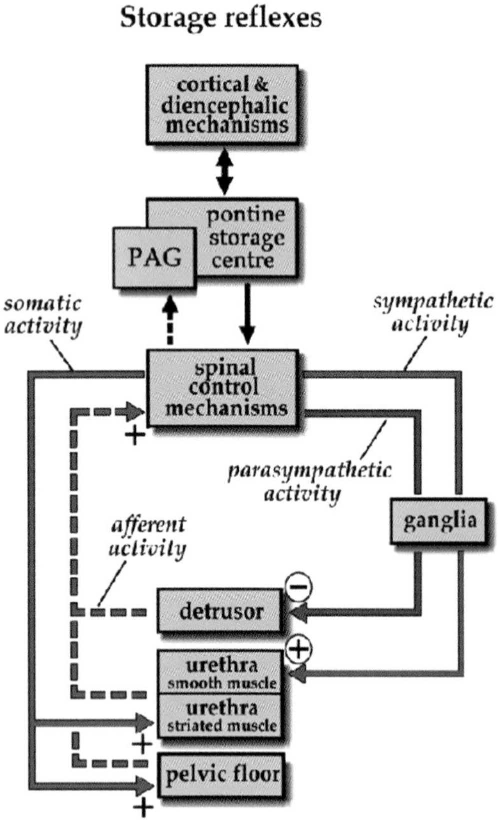

Storage reflexes

cortical & diencephalic mechanisms
PAG
pontine storage centre
somatic activity
sympathetic activity
spinal control mechanisms
parasympathetic activity
afferent activity
ganglia
detrusor
urethra smooth muscle
urethra striated muscle
pelvic floor

Figure 1 : During filling, there is continuous and increasing afferent activity from the bladder. There is no spinal parasympathetic outflow that can contract the bladder. The sympathetic outflow to urethral smooth muscle, and the somatic outflow to urethral and pelvic floor striated muscles keep the outflow region closed. Whether or not the sympathetic innervation to the bladder (not indicated) contributes to bladder relaxation during filling in humans has not been established.

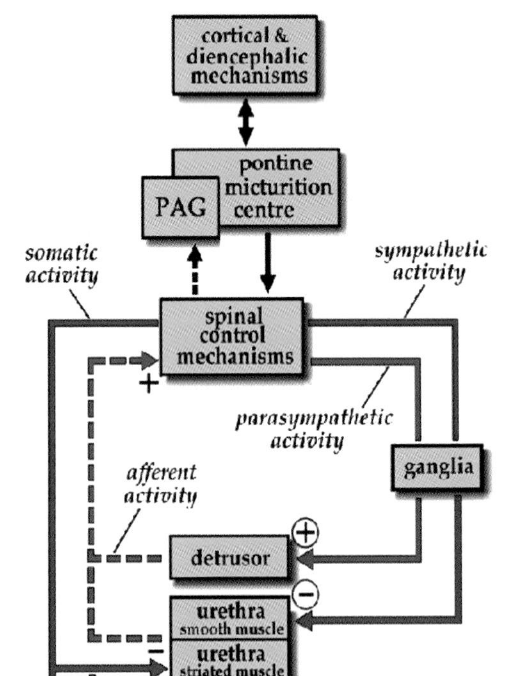

Figure 2 : Voiding reflexes involve supraspinal pathways, and are under voluntary control. During bladder emptying, the spinal parasympathetic outflow is activated, leading to bladder contraction. Simultaneously. the sympathetic outflow to urethral smooth muscle, and the somatic outflow to urethral and pelvic floor striated muscles are turned off, and the outflow region relaxes.

the thoraco-lumbar region (T10-L2) of the spinal cord. The axons travel either through the inferior mesenteric ganglia and the hypogastric nerve, or pass through the paravertebral chain and enter the pelvic nerve. Thus, sympathetic signals are conveyed in both the hypogastric and pelvic nerves (Lincoln & Burnstock, 1993).

The predominant effects of the sympathetic innervation of the lower urinary tract in man are inhibition of the parasympathetic pathways at spinal and ganglion levels, and mediation of contraction of the bladder base and the urethra. However, in several animals, the adrenergic innervation of the bladder body is believed to inactivate the contractile mechanisms in the detrusor directly (Andersson 1993). Noradrenaline is released in response to electrical stimulation of detrusor tissues *in vitro*, and the normal response of detrusor tissues to released noradrenaline is relaxation (Andersson 1993).

Most of the *sensory* innervation of the bladder and urethra reaches the spinal cord via the pelvic nerve and dorsal root ganglia. In addition, some afferents travel in the hypogastric nerve. The sensory nerves of the striated muscle in the rhabdosphincter travel in the pudendal nerve to the sacral region of the spinal cord (Lincoln & Burnstock, 1993). The most important afferents for the micturition process are myelinated Aδ-fibres and unmyelinated C-fibres travelling in the pelvic nerve to the sacral spinal cord, conveying information from receptors in the bladder wall to the spinal cord. The Aδ-fibres respond to passive distension and active contraction, thus conveying information about bladder filling (Janig & Morrison, 1986). C-fibres have a high mechanical threshold and respond primarily to chemical irritation of the bladder mucosa (Habler *et al.*, 1990) or cold (Fall *et al.*, 1990). Following chemical irritation, the C-fibre afferents exhibit spontaneous firing when the bladder is empty and increased firing during bladder distension (Habler *et al.*, 1990). These fibres are normally inactive and are therefore termed "silent fibres".

IV. PATHOGENESIS OF BLADDER CONTROL DISORDERS

As pointed out previously, bladder control disorders can be divided into two general categories: disorders of filling/storage and disorders of voiding (Wein 2001). Storage problems can occur as a result of weakness or anatomical defects in the urethral outlet, causing stress urinary incontinence, which may account for one-third of cases. Failure to store also occurs if the bladder is unstable or overactive, and this may affect > 50 % of incontinent men and 10-15% of incontinent young women. Overactive bladder can occur as a result of sensitization of afferent nerve terminals in the bladder or outlet region, changes of the bladder smooth muscle secondary to denervation, or to damage to CNS inhibitory pathways as can be seen in various neurological disorders, such as multiple sclerosis, cerebrovascular disease, Parkinson's disease, brain tumors, and spinal cord injury. Overactive bladder may also occur in elderly patients due to changes in the brain or bladder during aging. Urinary retention and overflow incontinence may occur in patients with urethral outlet obstruction (e.g. prostate enlargement), neural injury, and/or diseases that damage nerves (e.g. diabetes mellitus) or in those who are taking drugs that depress the neural control of the bladder (Wein 2001).

V. BLADDER CONTRACTION

Normal bladder contraction in humans is mediated mainly through stimulation of muscarinic receptors in the detrusor muscle. Atropine resistance, i.e. contraction of isolated bladder muscle in response to electrical nerve stimulation after pretreatment with atropine, has been demonstrated in most animal species, but seems to be of little importance in normal human bladder muscle (Andersson 1993, Bayliss et al 1999; Figure 3). However, atropine-resistant (non-adrenergic, non-cholinergic: NANC) contractions have been reported in normal human detrusor and may be caused by ATP (Hoyle et al. 1989, Luheshi and Zar 1990, Ruggieri et al. 1990). ATP acts on two families of purinergic receptors: an ion channel family (P2X) and a G-protein-coupled receptor family (P2Y). Seven P2X subtypes and eight P2Y subtypes have been identified. In several species (rabbit, cat, rat, and human), various studies suggested that multiple purinergic excitatory receptors are present in the bladder (de Groat and Yoshimura 2001). Immunohistochemical experiments with specific antibodies for different P2X receptors showed that $P2X_1$ receptors are the dominant subtype in membranes of rat detrusor muscle and bladder vascular smooth muscle. Excitatory receptors for ATP are present in parasympathetic ganglia, afferent nerve terminals, and urothelial cells (de Groat and Yoshimura 2001). $P2X_3$ receptors, which have been identified in small-diameter afferent neurons in dorsal root ganglia, have also been detected immunohistochemically in the wall of the bladder and ureter in a suburothelial plexus of afferent nerves. In $P2X_3$ knockout mice, afferent activity induced by bladder distension was significantly reduced (Cockayne et al 2000). These data indicate that purinergic receptors are involved in mechanosensory signaling in the bladder.

A significant degree of atropine resistance may exist in morphologically and/or functionally changed bladders

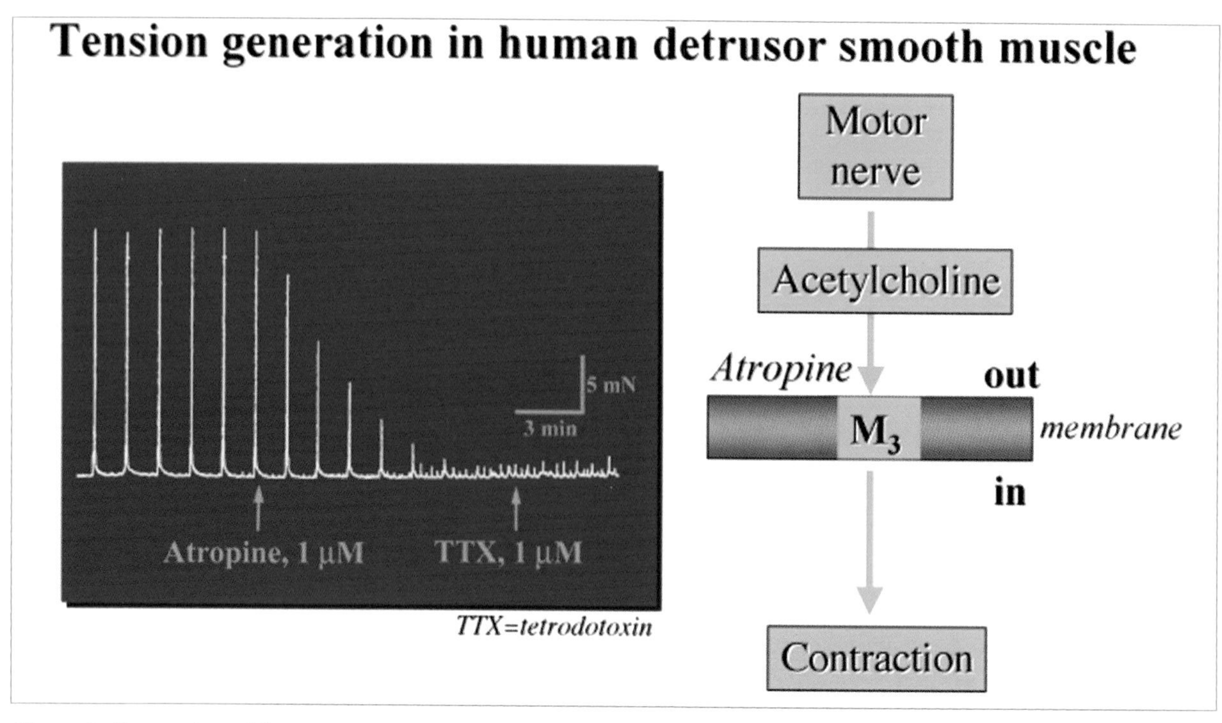

Figure 3: Contraction of the normal human bladder. Acetylcholine is released from cholinergic motor nerves and binds to the main contraction-mediating muscarinic (M_3) receptor (see also Figure 5). Note that there is prcatically no atropine resistance. Modified from Bayliss et al (1999).

(Figure 4), and has been reported to occur in hypertrophic bladders (Sjögren et al. 1982, Smith and Chapple 1994), interstitial cystitis (Palea et al. 1993), neurogenic bladders (Wammack et al. 1995), and in the aging bladder (Yoshida et al 2001). The importance of the NANC component to detrusor contraction in vivo, normally, and in different micturition disorders, remains to be established.

1. Muscarinic Receptors

Molecular cloning studies have revealed five distinct genes for muscarinic ACh receptors in rats and humans, and it is now generally accepted that five receptor subtypes correspond to these gene products (Eglen et al. 1996, Caulfield and Birdsall 1998). Muscarinic receptors are coupled to G-proteins (Figure 5). The signal transduction systems involved varies, but M_1, M_3, and M_5 preferentially couple to phosphoinositide hydrolysis leading to mobilization of intracellular calcium, wheras activation of muscarinic M_2 and M_4 receptors inhibits adenylyl cyclase activity. It has been suggested that muscarinic receptor stimulation may also inhibit K_{ATP} channels in smooth muscle cells from urinary bladder through activation of protein kinase C (Bonev and Nelson 1993).

2. Bladder muscarinic receptors

Detrusor smooth muscle from various species contains muscarinic receptors of the M_1 and M_3 subtype (Hegde and Eglen 1999). In the human bladder, the occurrence of mRNAs encoding M_2 and M_3 subtypes has been demonstrated, whereas no mRNA encoding M_1 receptors was found (Yamaguchi et al 1996). The M_3 receptors in the human bladder are believed to cause a direct smooth muscle contraction through phosphoinositide hydrolysis (Harriss et al 1995), whereas the role for the M_2 receptors is not clarified. However, it has been suggested that M_2 receptors may oppose sympathetically (via β-ARs) mediated smooth muscle relaxation, since in rats activation of M_2 receptors results in an inhibition of adenylyl cyclase (Hegde et al 1997). Contractile mechanisms involving M_2 muscarinic receptors, such as activation of a non-specific cationic channel and inactivation of potassium channels, may be operative in the bladder (Hegde and Eglen 1999). However, there is general agreement that M_3 receptors are mainly responsible for the normal micturition contraction (Hegde and Eglen 1999). Even in the obstructed rat bladder, M_3 receptors were found to play a predominant role in mediating detrusor contraction (Krichevsky et al 1999). On the other hand, in certain disease states, M_2 receptors may contribute to contraction of the bladder. Thus, in the denervated rat bladder, M_2 receptors, or a combination of M_2 and M_3 receptors mediated contractile responses (Braverman et al 1998, 1999). Also in patients with neurogenic bladder dysfunction, detrusor contraction can be mediated by M_2 receptors (Braverman et al 2001).

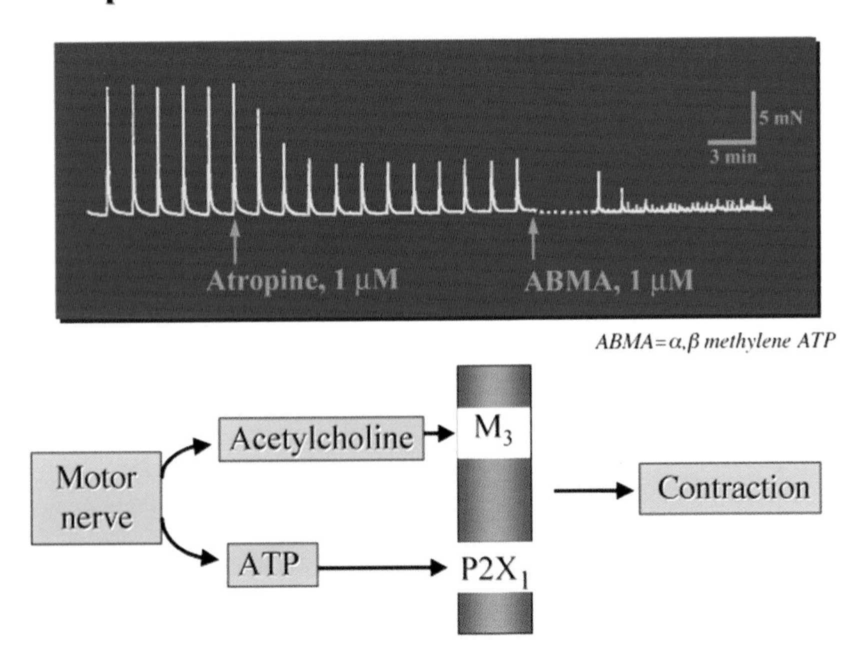

Figure 4 : Atropine resistance in the human bladder. The contraction remaining after addition of atropine is caused by ATP, and can be abolished by α,β methylene ATP, which causes desensitization of P2X receptors. Modified from Bayliss et al (1999).

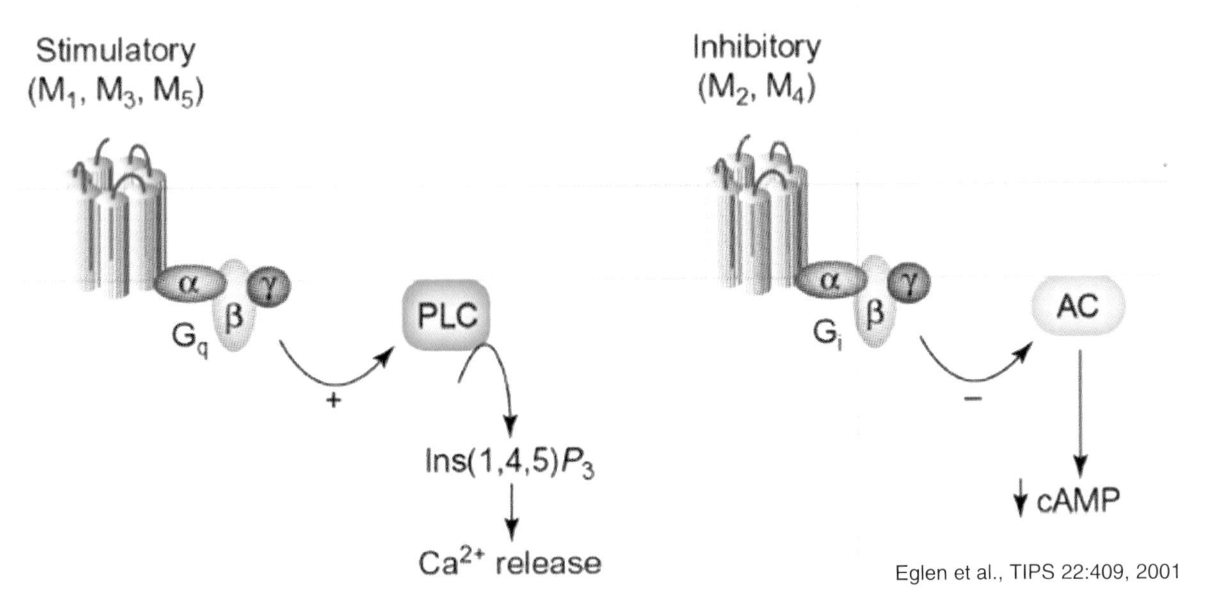

Figure 5 : Acetylcholine (ACh) is released from cholinergic nerve terminals, and acts on muscarinic receptors (M_1 and M_5) in the detrusor. Both M2 and M3 receptors are coupled to G-proteins (G-p) and may contribute to bladder contraction, but different signal transduction pathways are involved. M2 receptors inhibit adenylyl cyclase (AC), which leads to a diminished intracellular level of cyclic AMP (cAMP). cAMP mediates bladder relaxation. Stimulation of M3 receptors activates phospholipase C (PLC) to generate inositol triphosphate (IP3). IP3 can release calcium ions (Ca2+) from the sarcoplasmic reticulum and this Ca2+ will activate the contractile machinery within the cell with resulting bladder contraction. The voiding contraction is believed to be mediated mainly through M3 receptors.

Muscarinic receptors may also be located on the presynaptic nerve terminals and participate in the regulation of transmitter release. The inhibitory pre-junctional muscarinic receptors have been classified as muscarinic M_2 in the rabbit (Tobin and Sjögren 1995) and rat (Somogyi and de Groat 1992), and M_4 in the guinea-pig (Alberts 1995) and human (d'Agostino et al 2000) urinary bladder. Pre-junctional facilitatory muscarinic receptors appears to be of the M_1 subtype in the rat and rabbit urinary bladder (Tobin and Sjögren 1995, Somogyi and de Groat 1992). Prejunctional muscarinic facilitation has also been detected in human bladders (Somogyi and de Groat 1999). The muscarinic facilitatory mechanism seems to be upregulated in hyperactive bladders from chronic spinal cord transected rats. The facilitation in these preparations is primarily mediated by M_1 muscarinic receptors (Somogyi and de Groat 1999).

The muscarinic receptor functions may be changed in different urological disorders, such as outflow obstruction, neurogenic bladders, bladder overactivity without overt neurogenic cause, and diabetes. However, it is not always clear what the changes mean in terms of changes in detrusor function.

VI. DRUGS USED FOR TREATMENT OF BLADDER OVERACTIVITY

It has been estimated that more than 50 million people in the developed world are affected by urinary incontinence, and even if it affects 30-60% of patients older than 65 years, it is not a disease exclusive to aging. It appears that detrusor overactivity may be the result of several different mechanisms, both myogenic (Brading 1997) and neurological (de Groat 1997). Most probably, both factors contibute to the genesis of the the disease.

An abundance of drugs has been used for the treatment of the hyperactive detrusor (Table 2). However, for many of them, clinical use is based on the results of preliminary, open studies rather than randomized, controlled clinical trials (RCTs; for discussion of clinical research criteria, see addendum). It should be stressed that in many trials on both detrusor instability and detrusor hyperreflexia, there has been such a high placebo response that meaningful differences between placebo and active drug cannot be demonstrated (Thüroff et al 1998). However, drug effects in individual patients may be both distinct and useful.

As underlined by several other subcommittees, drugs may be efficacious in some patients, but they do have side effects, and frequently are not continued indefinitely. Hence it would be worth to consider them as an adjunct to conservative therapy. The role of pharmacotherapy is even more contentious in older, and particularly frail older people (see report from Committee no 10).

1. Antimuscarinic (anticholinergic) drugs

Voluntary, but also involuntary, bladder contractions are mediated mainly by ACh –induced stimulation of muscarinic receptors on bladder smooth muscle. Antimuscarinic drugs will therefore depress both types of contraction, irrespective of how the efferent part of the micturition reflex is activated. In patients with involuntary bladder contractions, the volume to the first contraction is increased, the amplitude of the contraction is decreased, and total bladder capacity is increased (Jensen 1981). However, the "warning time", i.e., the time between the perception of an involuntary contraction about to occur and its occurrence, and the ability to suppress are not increased.

Several studies have supported that antimuscarinics can depress involuntary bladder contractions (Low 1977, Cardozo and Stanton 1979, Blaivas et al. 1980, Naglo et al. 1981). On the other hand, there are several reports of insufficient efficacy of antimuscarinics given orally to patients with unstable detrusor contractions (Ritch et al. 1977, Walther et al. 1982, Bonnesen et al, 1984, Zorzitto et al. 1986). It is unclear to what extent this can be attributed to low bioavailability of the drugs used, side effects limiting the dose that can be given, or to atropine resistance.

Atropine and related antimuscarinics are tertiary amines. They are well absorbed from the gastrointestinal tract and pass into the central nervous system (CNS) well. CNS side effects may therefore limit their use. Quaternary ammonium compounds are not well absorbed, pass into the CNS to a limited extent, and have a lower incidence of CNS side effects (Pietzsko et al. 1994). They still produce well-known peripheral antimuscarinic side effects, such as accommodation paralysis, constipation, tachycardia and dryness of mouth. All antimuscarinic drugs are contraindicated in narrow angle glaucoma.

Antimuscarinics are still the most widely used treatment for urge and urge incontinence (Andersson et al 1999). However, currently used drugs lack selectivity for the bladder (Eglen et al. 1996), and effects on other organ systems may result in side effects which limit their usefulness. Theoretically, drugs with selectivity for the bladder could be obtained, if the subtype(s) mediating bladder contraction, and those producing the main side effects of antimuscarinic drugs, were different. One way of avoiding many of the antimuscarinic side effects is to administer the drugs intravesically. However, this is practical only in a limited number of patients.

Table 2 : Drugs used in the treatment of detrusor overactivity. Assessments according to the Oxford system

	Level of evidence	Grade of recommendation
ANTIMUSCARINIC DRUGS		
Tolterodine	1	A
Trospium	1	A
Propantheline	2	B
Atropine, hyoscyamine	2	D
(Darifenacin, solifenacin)	UNDER INVESTIGATION	
DRUGS ACTING ON MEMBRANE CHANNELS		
Calcium antagonists	UNDER INVESTIGATION	
Potassium channel openers	UNDER INVESTIGATION	
DRUGS WITH MIXED ACTIONS		
Oxybutynin	1	A
Propiverine	1	A
Dicyclomine	4	C
Flavoxate	4	D
ALPHA-ADRENOCEPTOR ANTAGONISTS		
Alfuzosin	4	D
Doxazosin	4	D
Prazosin	4	D
Terazosin	4	D
Tamsulosin	4	D
BETA-ADRENOCEPTOR AGONISTS		
Terbutaline	4	D
Clenbuterol	4	D
Salbutamol	4	D
ANTIDEPRESSANTS		
Imipramine	2	C*
PROSTAGLANDIN SYNTHESIS INHIBITORS		
Indomethacin	4	C
Flurbiprofen	4	C
VASOPRESSIN ANALOGUES		
Desmopressin	1	A
OTHER DRUGS		
Baclofen	2**	C**
Capsaicin	3	C
Resiniferatoxin	UNDER INVESTIGATION	

** SHOULD BE USED WITH CAUTION ** INTRATHECAL USE*

Several antimuscarinic drugs have been used for treatment of bladder overactivity. For many of them, documentation of effects is not based on RCTs satisfying currently required criteria, and some drugs can be considered as obsolete (e.g. emepronium). Information on these drugs has not been included, but can be found elsewhere (Andersson et al 1999, 2000).

a) Atropine

Atropine (dl-hyoscyamine) is rarely used for treatment of detrusor overactivity because of its systemic side effects, which preclude its use. However, in patients with detrusor hyperreflexia, intravesical atropine may be effective for increasing bladder capacity without causing any systemic adverse effects, as shown in open pilot trials (Ekström et al. 1993, Glickman et al. 1995, Deaney et al 1998, Enskat et al 2001).

The pharmacologically active antimuscarinic half of atropine is l-hyoscyamine. Although still used, few clinical studies are available to evaluate the antimuscarinic activity of l-hyoscyamine sulfate.

b) Propantheline

Propantheline bromide is a quaternary ammonium compound, non-selective for muscarinic receptor subtypes, which has a low (5 to 10%) and individually varying biological availability (Andersson 1988). It is usually given in a dose of 15 to 30 mg 4 times daily, but to obtain an optimal effect, individual titration of the dose is necessary, and often higher dosages. Using this approach in 26 patients with uninhibited detrusor contractions, Blaivas et al. (1980) in an open study obtained a complete clinical response in all patients but one, who did not tolerate more than propantheline 15 mg 4 times daily. The range of dosages varied from 7.5 to 60 mg 4 times daily. In contrast, Thüroff et al. (1991) comparing the effects oxybutynin 5 mg x 3, propantheline 15 mg x 3, and placebo, in a randomized, double-blind, multicenter trial on the treatment of frequency, urgency and incontinence related to detrusor overactivity (154 patients with idiopathic detrusor instability or detrusor hyperreflexia), found no differences between the placebo and propantheline groups. In another randomized comparative trial with crossover design (23 women with idiopathic detrusor instability), and with dose titration, Holmes et al. (1989) found no differences in efficacy between oxybutynin and propantheline. The AHCPR (Agency of health Care policy and Research) Clinical practice Guidelines (Urinary Incontinence Guideline Panel) lists 5 randomized controlled trials reviewed for propantheline, showing a reduction of urge (percent drug effect minus percent effect on placebo) between 0 to 53 %. Controlled randomized trials (n=6) were also reviewed by Thüroff et al (1998), who confirmed a positive, but varying response.

Although the effect of propantheline on detrusor overactivity has not been well documented in controlled trials satifying standards of today, it can be considered effective, and may, in individually titrated doses, be clinically useful.

c) Trospium

Trospium chloride is a quaternary ammonium compound with antimuscarinic actions on detrusor smooth muscle, but also with effects on ganglia (Antweiler 1966). However, the clinical importance of the ganglionic effects has not been established. In isolated detrusor muscle, it was more potent than oxybutynin and tolterodine to antagonize carbachol-induced contractions (Ückert et al 1998). Trospium has no selectivity for muscarinic receptor subtypes. Its biological availability is low, approximately 5% (Schladitz-Keil et al 1986, Füsgen and Hauri 2000), and it does not cross the blood-brain barrier. It seems to have no negative cognitive effects (Füsgen and Hauri 2000, Todorova et al 2001, Wiedemann et al 2001). Several open studies have indicated that the drug may be useful in the treatment of detrusor overactivity (Lux and Widey 1992, Madersbacher et al 1991, Stöhrer et al. 1991). In a placebo-controlled, double-blind study on patients with detrusor hyperreflexia (Stöhrer et al. 1991), the drug was given twice daily in a dose of 20 mg over a 3-week period. It increased maximum cystometric capacity, decreased maximal detrusor pressure and increased compliance in the treatment group, whereas no effects were noted in the placebo group. Side effects were few and comparable in both groups. In a randomized, double-blind multicentre trial in patients with spinal cord injuries and detrusor hyperreflexia, trospium and oxybutynin were equieffective; however, trospium seemed to have fewer side effects (Madersbacher et al. 1995.

The effect of trospium in urge incontinence has been documented in placebo-controlled, randomized studies. Allousi et al (1998) compared the effects of the drug with those of placebo in 309 patients in a urodynamic study of 3 weeks duration. Trospium 20 mg was given b.i.d. Significant increases were noted in volume at first unstable contraction and in maximum bladder capacity. Cardozo et al (2000) investigated 208 patients with bladder instability, who were treated with trospium 20 mg b.i.d. for two weeks. Also in this study, significant increases were found in volume at first unstable contraction and in maximum bladder capacity in the trospium treated group. Trospium was well tolerated with similar frequency of adverse effects as in the placebo group. Höfner et al. (2000) compared the effects of oxybutynin 5 mg b. i.d. with those of trospium 20 mg b.i.d. in a double-blind, randomized study over 12 months in 358 patients with urge symptoms or urge incontinence. The urodynamic improvements after the two drugs were comparable, but oxybutynin produced a significantly higher rate of side effects, and the drop-out rate was higher in the oxybutynin group.

Jünemann et al (2000) compared trospium 20 mg b.i.d with tolterodine 2 mg b.i.d in a placebo-controlled double-blind study on 232 patients with urodynamically proven bladder overactivity, sensory urge incontinence or mixed incontinence. Trospium reduced the frequency of micturition, which was the primary endpoint, more than tolterodine and placebo, and also reduced the number of incontinence episodes more than the comparators. Dry mouth were comparable in the trospium and tolterodine groups (7 and 9%, respectively).

Trospium chloride has a documented effect in detrusor overeractivity, and seems to be well tolerated.

d) Tolterodine

Tolterodine is a potent and competitive antagonist at muscarinic receptors, developed for treatment of urinary urgency and urge incontinence (Nilvebrant et al. 1997a, b, Hills et al. 1998, Clemett and Jarvis 2001). The drug has no selectivity for muscarinic receptor subtypes, but still shows some selectivity for the bladder over the salivary glands in an animal model (Nilvebrant et al. 1997a, and possibly in man (Stahl et al. 1995). Tolterodine has a major active metabolite with a similar pharmacological profile as the mother compound (Nilvebrant et al. 1997 c). This metabolite significantly contributes to the therapeutic effect of tolterodine (Brynne et al. 1997, 1998). Tolterodine is rapidly absorbed and has a half-life of 2-3 h, but the effects on the bladder seem to be more long-lasting than could be expected from the pharmacokinetic data. The main metabolite also has a half-life of 2-3 h (Brynne et al. 1998). In healthy volunteers, orally given tolterodine in a high dose (6.4 mg) had a powerful inhibitory effect on micturition and also reduced stimulated salivation 1 h after administration of the drug (Stahl et al. 1995). However, 5 h after administration, the effects on the urinary bladder were maintained, whereas no significant effects on salivation could be demonstrated.

The relatively low lipophilicity of tolterodine implies limited propensity to penetrate into the CNS, which may explain a low incidence of cognitive side effects (Chapple 2000, Clemett and Jarvis 2001)

Several randomised, double-blind, placebo-controlled studies, both on patients with idiopathic detrusor instability and detrusor hyperreflexia, have documented a significant reduction in micturition frequency and number of incontinence episodes (see Hills et al. 1998, Clemett and Jarvis 2001). Tolterodine seems to be well tolerated when used in the dosage range 1 to 4 mg a day. Chancellor et al (2000) reported the results of a double-blind randomized study on 1022 patients comparing tolterodine 2 mg b.i.d. to placebo. Active drug reduced urge incontinence episodes by 46% versus base-line, and the effect compared to placebo was also significant. Withdrawals were essentially the same between the two treatment groups.

A once daily formulation of tolterodine has recently been developed, and the first large scale (1529 patients) clinical trial compared the effects of this agent to placebo and the twice daily formulation (van Kerrebroeck et al 2001). Tolterodine extended release 4 mg once daily and tolterodine immediate release 2 mg twice daily both significantly reduced the mean number of urge incontinence episodes per week compared with placebo. The median reduction in these episodes as a percentage of the baseline values was 71% for tolterodine ER, 60% for tolterodine IR, and 33% for placebo. Treatment with both formulations of tolterodine was also associated with statistically significant improvements in all other micturition diary variables compared with placebo. The rate of dry mouth (of any severity) was 23% for tolterodine ER, 30% for tolterodine IR, and 8% for placebo. The rates of withdrawal were comparable for the two active groups and the placebo group. No safety concerns were noted.

In a placebo-controlled study, comparing tolterodine 2 mg bid and oxybutynin 5 mg t.i.d in 293 patients with detrusor instability, both drugs were found to be equally effective in reducing frequency of micturition and number of incontinence episodes. However, tolterodine appeared to have a better efficacy/tolerability profile (Abrams et al. 1998). These findings were largely confirmed by other investigators (Drutz et al 1999, Malone-Lee et al 2001). Malone-Lee et al (2001) compared oxybutynin and tolterodine in 378 patients 50 years and older with symptoms of overactive bladder. They received 10 weeks of treatment with tolterodine 2 mg b.i.d. or oxybutynin 5 mg b.i.d (final doses). Patients treated with tolterodine had significantly fewer adverse events (69% versus 81%), notably dry mouth (37% versus 61%), than those in the oxybutynin group. Each agent had comparable efficacy for improving urinary symptoms. The authors concluded that tolterodine was as effective as oxybutynin for improving the symptoms of overactive bladder, but had superior tolerability. These data contrast with those of Appell et al (2001) comparing extended-release oxybutynin chloride and immediate release tolterodine in a 12-week randomized, double-blind, parallel-group study in 378 patients with overactive bladder. Participants who had between 7 and 50 episodes of urge incontinence per week and 10 or more voids in 24 hours received extended-release oxybutynin, 10 mg once daily, or tolterodine, 2 mg b.i.d. The outcome measures were the number of episodes of urge incontinence, total incontinence, and micturition frequency at 12 weeks adjusted for baseline. At the end of the study, extended-release oxybutynin was found to be significantly more effective than tolterodine in each of the main outcome measures adjusted for baseline. Dry mouth, the most common adverse event, was reported by 28.1% and 33.2% of participants taking extended-release oxybutynin and tolterodine, respectively. Rates of central nervous system and other adverse events were low and similar in both groups. The authors concluded that extended-release oxybutynin was more effective than tolterodine and that rates of dry mouth and other adverse events were similar in both treament groups.

No comparative trials between extended release tolterodine and the extended release form of oxybutynin have so far been reported. However, comparison of the immediate release forms would seem to indicate that efficacy is no different, whereas the side effect profile of tolterodine is favorable (Chapple 2000, Wein 2001b). Head to head comparisons between the two extended release preparations are required to adequately compare efficacy and tolerability between the two agents.

Tolterodine, in both the immediate and extended release forms, has a well documented effect in detrusor overactivity, and the side effect profile seems acceptable.

e) Darifenacin

Darifenacin is a selective muscarinic M_3 receptor antagonist developed for treatment of bladder overactivity (Alabaster 1997). In vitro, it is selective for human cloned muscarinic M_3 receptors relative to M_1, M_2, M_4 or M_5. On theoretical grounds, it may be argued that M_3

vs M_1 receptor selectivity may provide an advantage over non-selective agents, since both M_3 and M_1 receptors have been implicated in salivary mucous secretion (Culp et al 1996), and in an anesthetized dog model model, selectivity for the urinary bladder over the salivary gland has been demonstrated (Newgreen et al. 1995, Wallis et al. 1995). M_3 vs M_1 selectivity may be associated with a low rate of cognitive impairment (M_1; Pavia et al 1998). M_3 vs M_2 selectivity can provide little effect on heart rate (M_2), and M_3 vs M_5 selectivity may reduce impairment of visual accommodation (M_5; Eglen and Nahorski 2000, Choppin and Eglen 2000). However, the clinical importance of these potential advantages has not been established.

Published clinical information on the effect of darifenacin is scarce. In a pilot study on patients with detrusor instability, the drug was found to reduce the total number, maximum amplitude, and duration of unstable bladder contractions (Rosario et al. 1995). In a randomised, double-blind trial of 25 patients with detrusor instability, the effects of darifenacin 15 mg and 30 mg o.d. and oxybutynin 5 mg t.i.d. on ambulatory urodynamic monitoring and salivary flow were compared (Mundy et al 2001). Both drugs had similar urodynamic efficacy, but oxybutynin reduced salivary flow significantly more than darifenacin. In another controlled study, on 27 healthy male subjects, the effects of darifenacin 7.5 and 15 mg o.d., dicyclomine 20 mg q.d.s, and placebo on cognitive and cardiac functions were investigated (Nichols et al 2001). Unlike dicyclomine, darifenacin had no detectable effects on cognitive or cardiovascular function.

Darifenacin is currently being evaluated in a phase III global clinical evaluation programme for the treatment of bladder overactivity, to identify the optimal dose regimen and to assess its potential clinical benefits.

f) Solifenacin (YM-905)

Solifenacin (YM905) is a long acting muscarinic receptor antagonist developed for the treatment of overactive bladder.

In guinea-pig urinary bladder smooth muscle preparations, solifenacin inhibited cholinergic responses with nanomolar potency. When tested in anaesthetised mice, both solifenacin and oxybutynin potently inhibited carbachol-induced increase of urinary bladder pressure. However, only oxybutynin was associated with potent inhibition of carbachol-stimulated salivary secretion (Ikeda et al. 1998). In cellular systems, solifenacin appears to be more potent as a muscarinic receptor antagonist for bladder smooth muscle than for salivary gland when compared with reference molecules like oxybutynin or tolterodine, indicating a potentially beneficial efficacy/tolerability profile (Ikeda et al. 1999). The clinical relevance of these findings is currently being investigated in phase III clinical studies.

2. Drugs acting on membrane channels

a) Calcium antagonists

Activation of detrusor muscle, both through muscarinic receptor and NANC pathways, seems to require influx of extracellular Ca^{2+} through Ca^{2+} channels, as well as via mobilization of intracellular Ca^{2+} (Andersson 1993). The influx of extracellular calcium can be blocked by calcium antagonists, blocking L-type Ca^{2+} channels, and theoretically, this would be an attractive way of inhibiting detrusor overactivity (Andersson and Forman 1978). However, there have been few clinical studies of the effects of calcium antagonists in patients with detrusor overactivity (see Andersson et al 1999). Intravesical instillation of verapamil was found to increase bladder capacity and decrease the degree of leakage during cystometry in patients with detrusor hyperreflexia (Mattiasson et al. 1989). The effect was less pronounced in patients with non-neurogenic overactivity (Babu et al. 1990).

Available information does not suggest that systemic therapy with calcium antagonists is an effective way to treat detrusor overactivity, but controlled clinical trials are lacking. However, the possibility that intravesical therapy with these drugs could be useful should not be ignored, nor the fact that calcium antagonists may enhance the effects of antimuscarinic agents (Andersson et al. 1986). Oral nifedipine has been used effectively as prophylaxis for autonomic hyperreflexia during urologic instrumentation in spinal cord injured patients (Wein 2001b).

b) Potassium channel openers

Opening of K^+channels and subsequent efflux of K^+ will produce hyperpolarization of various smooth muscles, including the detrusor (Andersson 1992, Shieh et al 2000). This leads to a decrease in Ca^{2+} influx by reducing the opening probability of Ca^{2+} channels with subsequent relaxation or inhibition of contraction. Theoretically, such drugs may be active during the filling phase of the bladder, abolishing bladder overactivity with no effect on normal bladder contraction. K^+ channel openers, such as pinacidil and cromakalim, have been effective in animal models (Andersson 1992), but clinically, the effects have not been encouraging.

The first generation of openers of ATP-sensitive K^+ channels, such as cromakalim and pinacidil, were found to be more potent as inhibitors of vascular preparations than of detrusor muscle, and in clinical trials performed with these drugs, no bladder effects have been found at doses already lowering blood pressure (Hedlund et al.

1991, Komersova et al. 1995). However, new drugs with K_{ATP} channel opening properties have been described, which may be useful for the treatment of bladder overactivity (Howe et al. 1995, Masuda et al. 1995, Butera et al 2000, Gilbert et al. 2000, Shieh et al 2000).

K^+ channel opening is an attractive way of treating bladder overactivity, since it would make it possible to eliminate undesired bladder contractions without affecting normal micturition. However, at present there is no evidence from controlled clinical trials to suggest that K^+ channel openers represent a treatment alternative.

3. Drugs with "mixed" actions

Some drugs used to block bladder overactivity have been shown to have more than one mechanism of action. They all have a more or less pronounced antimuscarinic effect and, in addition, an often poorly defined "direct" action on bladder muscle. For several of these drugs, the antimuscarinic effects can be demonstrated at much lower drug concentrations than the direct action, which may involve blockade of voltage operated Ca^{2+} channels. Most probably, the clinical effects of these drugs can be explained mainly by an antimuscarinic action. Among the drugs with mixed actions was terodiline, which was withdrawn from the market because it was suspected to cause polymorphic ventricular tachycardia (torsade de pointes) in some patients (Conolly et al. 1991, Stewart et al. 1992).

a) Oxybutynin

Oxybutynin has several pharmacological effects, some of which seem difficult to relate to its effectiveness in the treatment of detrusor overactivity. It has both an antimuscarinic and a direct muscle relaxant effect, and, in addition, local anesthetic actions. The latter effect may be of importance when the drug is administered intravesically, but probably plays no role when it is given orally. In vitro, oxybutynin was 500 times weaker as a smooth muscle relaxant than as an antimuscarinic agent (Kachur et al. 1988). Most probably, when given systemically, oxybutynin acts mainly as an antimuscarinic drug. Oxybutynin has a high affinity for muscarinic receptors in human bladder tissue and effectively blocks carbachol-induced contractions (Nilvebrant et al. 1985, Waldeck et al. 1997). The drug was shown to have higher affinity for muscarinic M_1 and M_3 receptors than for M_2 receptors (Nilvebrant et al. 1986, Norhona-Blob and Kachur 1991), but the clinical significance of this is unclear.

Oxybutynin is a tertiary amine that is well absorbed, but undergoes an extensive first-pass metabolism (biological availability 6% in healthy volunteers). The plasma half-life of the drug is approximately 2 hours, but with wide interindividual variation (Douchamps et al 1988, Hughes et al. 1992). Oxybutynin has an active metabolite, N-desethyl oxybutynin, which has pharmacological properties similar to those of the parent compound (Waldeck et al. 1997), but which occurs in much higher concentrations (Hughes et al. 1992). Considering this, it seems reasonable to assume that the effect of oral oxybutynin to a large extent is exerted by the metabolite. The occurrence of an active metabolite may also explain the lack of correlation between plasma concentration of oxybutynin itself and side effects in geriatric patients reported by Ouslander et al. (1988).

Several controlled studies have have shown that oxybutynin is effective in controlling detrusor overactivity, including hyperreflexia (Thompson and Lauvetz 1976, Moisey et al. 1980, Hehir and Fitzpatrick 1985, Gajewski and Awad 1986, Cardozo et al. 1987, Zeegers et al. 1987, Holmes et al 1989, Thüroff et al. 1991, More et al. 1990, Tapp et al. 1990, Iselin et al. 1997, see reviews by Yarker et al. 1995, Thüroff et al 1998, Wein 2001). The recommended oral dose of the immediate release form is 5 mg t.d. or q.i.d., even if lower doses have been used. Thüroff et al (1998) summarized 15 randomized controlled studies on a total of 476 patients treated with oxybutynin. The mean decrease in incontinence was recorded as 52% and the mean reduction in frequency for 24 h was 33%. The overall "subjective improvement" rate was reported as 74 % (range 61% - 100%). The mean percent of patients reporting side effects was 70 (range 17% - 93%). Oxybutynin 7.5 to 15 mg/day significantly improved quality of life of patients suffering from overactive bladder in a large open multicenter trial. In this study, patients compliance was 97% and side effects - mainly dry mouth - was reported by only 8% of the patients (Amarenco et al. 1998).

In nursing home residents (n=75), Ouslander et al. (1995) found that oxybutynin did not add to the clinical effectiveness of prompted voiding in a placebo-controlled, double blind, cross-over trial. On the other hand, in another controlled trial in elderly subjects (n=57), oxybutynin with bladder training was found to be superior to bladder training alone (Szonyi et al. 1995).

Several open studies in patients with spinal cord injuries have suggested that oxybutynin, given orally or intravesically, can be of therapeutic benefit (Szollar and Lee 1996, Kim et al. 1997).

The therapeutic effect of immediate release oxybutynin on detrusor overactivity is associated with a high incidence of side effects (up to 80% with oral administration). These are typically antimuscarinic in nature (dry mouth, constipation, drowsiness, blurred vision) and are often dose-limiting (Baigrie et al. 1988, Jonville et al. 1992). Oxybutynin passes the blood-brain barrier and may have effects on the central nervous system

(Pietsko et al 1994, Todorova et al 2001). The drug can cause cognitive impairment (Katz et al, Ferrara et al. 2001), and this side effect may be particularly troublesome in the geriatric population (Ouslander et al 2000).The effects on the electrocardiogram of oxybutynin were studied in elderly patients with urinary incontinence (Hussain et al. 1994); no changes were found. It cannot be excluded that the commonly recommended dose 5 mg x 3 is unnecessarily high in some patients, and that a starting dose of 2.5 mg x 2 with following dose-titration would reduce the number of adverse effects (Malone-Lee et al. 1992, Amarenco et al. 1998).

Once daily formulations of oxybutynin have been developed. The oxybutynin ER (Ditropan XL) uses an innovative osmotic drug delivery system to release the drug at at a controlled rate over 24 h. This formulation overcomes the marked peak to trough fluctuations inplasma levels of both drug and the major metabolite, which occurs with immediate release oxybutynin (Gupta and Sathayan 1999). A trend towards a lower incidence of dry mouth with oxybutynin ER was attributed to reduced first pass metabolism and to the maintenance of lower and less fluctuating plasma levels of drugs. Clinical trials on oxybutynin ER have concentrated primarily on comparing this drug with immediate release oxybutynin. Anderson et al (1999) reported on a multicenter, randomized, double-blind study on 105 patients with urge incontinence, or mixed incontinence with a clinically significant urge component. Urge urinary incontinence episodes were the primary efficacy parameter. The number of weekly urge incontinence episodes decreased from 27.4 to 4.8 after controlled and from 23.4 to 3.1 after immediate release oxybutynin, and total incontinence episodes decreased from 29.3 to 6 and from 26.3 to 3.8, respectively. Weekly urge incontinence episodes from baseline to end of study also decreased to 84% after controlled and 88% after immediate release oxybutynin. Since only patients who had previously responded to treatment with oxybutynin were selected for treatment, these figures do not represent what can be considered normal in clinical practice. Dry mouth of any severity was reported by 68% and 87% of the controlled and immediate release groups, respectively, and moderate or severe dry mouth occurred in 25 and 46%, respectively.

Another controlled study comparing efficacy and safety of controlled release oxybutynin with conventional immediate-release oxybutynin, included 226 patients with urge incontinence (Versi et al 2000). They were known to respond to anticholinergic therapy and had seven or more urge incontinence episodes per week. Reductions in urge urinary incontinence episodes from baseline to the end of treatment were 18.6 to 2.9 per week (83% mean decrease) and 19.8 to 4.4 per week (76% mean decrease) in the controlled- and immediate-release oxybutynin groups (differencc non-significant), respectively. The incidence of dry mouth increased with dose in both groups, but there was no difference in dry mouth rates between the groups: 47.7% and 59.1% for the controlled- and immediate-release. However, a significantly lower proportion of patients taking controlled-release oxybutynin had moderate to severe dry mouth or any dry mouth compared with those taking immediate-release oxybutynin.

As referred to previously, Appell et al (2001) compared extended-release oxybutynin chloride 10 mg/day and tolterodine 2 mg b.i.d in a 12-week randomized, double-blind, parallel-group study in 378 patients with overactive bladder. Extended-release oxybutynin was found to be significantly more effective than tolterodine in each of the main outcome measures (number of episodes of urge incontinence, total incontinence, and micturition frequency at 12 weeks) adjusted for baseline, and the rates of dry mouth and other adverse events were similar in both treatment groups.

A different extended release form of oxybutynin was utilized by Birns et al (2000), who reported comparable efficacy of a 10 mg preparation with 5 mg b.i.d. of immediate release oxybutynin. Efficacy was similar, but the extended release formulation was better tolerated, patients only reporting approximately half the total number of adverse effects than with the immediate release preparation. Nilsson et al (1997), however, failed to demonstrated improved tolerability with this controlled release tablet.

Other administration forms of oxybutynin have been introduced. Rectal administration (Collas and Malone-Lee 1997, Winkler and Sand 1998) was reported to have fewer adverse effects than the conventional tablets. A transdermal preparation is in clinical trials.

Administered intravesically, oxybutynin has in several studies been demonstrated to increase bladder capacity and produce clinical improvement with few side effects, both in hypereflexia and in other types of bladder overactivity, and both in children and adults (Brendler et al. 1989, Madersbacher and Jilg 1991, O'Flynn and Thomas 1993, Weese et al 1993, Mizunaga et al. 1994, Buyse et al. 1995, Enzelsberger et al. 1995, Madersbacher and Knoll 1995, Kaplinsky et al. 1996), although adverse effects may occur (Kasabian et al. 1994, Palmer et al. 1997). Cognitive impairment can also occur in children treated with intravesical oxybutynin. Since it was reported that these effects may differ from those with oral administration (Ferrarra et al, 2001), these patients should be closely monitored.

Oxybutynin has a well-documented efficacy in the treatment of detrusor overactivity, and is, together with tolterodine, the drug of first choice in patients with this disorder.

b) Dicyclomine

Dicyclomine has attributed to it both a direct relaxant effect on smooth muscle and an antimuscarinic action (Downie et al. 1977). Favorable results in detrusor overactivity have been demonstrated in several studies (Beck et al. 1976, Awad et al. 1977, Fischer et al. 1978, Castleden et al. 1987), performed more than a decade ago and which do not satisfy current criteria of good quality RTCs.

Even if published experiences of the effect of dicyclomine on detrusor overactivity are favourable, the drug is not widely used, and RTCs documenting its efficacy and side effects are scarce.

c) Propiverine

Propiverine has been shown to have combined anticholinergic and calcium antagonistic actions (Haruno et al. 1989, Haruno 1992, Tokuno et al. 1993). The drug is rapidly absorbed, but has a high first pass metabolism. Several active metabolites are formed (Haustein and Hüller 1988, Muller et al. 1993), whose pharmacological characteristics remain to be established. It seems most probable that these metabolites contribute to the clinical effects of the drug.

Propiverine has been shown to have beneficial effects in patients with detrusor overactivity in several investigations. Thüroff et al (1998) collected 9 randomized studies on a total of 230 patients, and found reductions in frequency (30%) and micturitions per 24 h (17%), a 64 ml increase in bladder capacity, and a 77% (range 33-80%) subjective improvement. Side effects were found in 14 % (range 8-42%). In patients with hyperreflexia, controlled clinical trials have demonstrated propiverine´s superiority over placebo, showing symptomatic improvement in approximately 50% and 25% of cases, respectively (Takayasu et al. 1990, Richter et al. 1997). Propiverine also increased bladder capacity and decreased maximum detrusor contractions. Controlled trials comparing propiverine, flavoxate and placebo (Wehnert and Sage 1989), and propiverine, oxybutynin and placebo (Wehnert and Sage 1992, Madersbacher et al. 1999), have confirmed the efficacy of propiverine, and suggested that the drug may have equal efficacy and fewer side effects than oxybutynin.

Stöhrer et al (1999) reported a double-blind, randomised, prospective, multicentre trial comparing propiverine 15mg t.i.d. to placebo in 113 spinal cord injury patients with detrusor hyperreflexia. Maximal cystometric capacity increased significantly in the propiverine group, by an average of 104 ml. Changes in bladder capacity at first contraction and in maximum bladder contraction were likewise statistically significant. Bladder compliance showed a more pronounced increase under propiverine in comparison to placebo. Sixty-three per cent of the patients expressed subjectively an improvement under propiverine in comparison with 23% of the placebo group. Dryness of the mouth (37% in the propiverine and 8% in the placebo group), and accommodation disorders (28% and 2% respectively) were reported side effects.

Madersbacher et al (1999) compared the tolerability and efficacy of propiverine (15 mg t.i.d.) oxybutynin (5 mg b.i.d.) and placebo in 366 patients with urgency and urge incontinence in a randomized, double-blind placebo-controlled clinical trial. Urodynamic efficacy of propiverine was judged similar to that of oxybutynin, but the incidence of dry mouth and the severity of dry mouth were judged less with propiverine than with oxybutynin.

Dorschner et al (1999) investigated in a double-blind, multicentre, placebo-controlled, randomized study, the efficacy and cardiac safety of propiverine in 98 elderly patients (mean age 68 years), suffering from urgency, urge incontinence or mixed urge-stress incontinence. After a 2-week placebo run-in period, the patients received propiverine (15 mg t.i.d.) or placebo (t.i.d.) for 4 weeks. Propiverine caused a significant reduction of the micturition frequency (from 8.7 to 6.5) and a significant decrease in episodes of incontinence (from 0.9 to 0.3 per day). Resting and ambulatory electrocardiograms indicated no significant changes. The incidence of adverse events was very low (2% dryness of the mouth under propiverine – 2 out of 49 patients).

Propiverine has a documented beneficial effect in the treatment of detrusor overactivity, and seems to have an acceptable side effect profile. Its complex pharmacokinetics with several active, not very well characterized metabolites, needs more attention.

d) Flavoxate

The main mechanism of flavoxate's effect on smooth muscle has not been established. The drug has been found to possess a moderate calcium antagonistic activity, to have the ability to inhibit phosphodiesterase, and to have local anesthetic properties; no anticholinergic effect has been found (Guarneri et al. 1994). It has been suggested that pertussis toxin-sensitive G-proteins in the brain are involved in the flavoxate-induced suppression of the micturition reflex in rats (Oka et al 1996). Its main metabolite (3-methylflavone-8-carboxylic acid, MFCA) has been shown to have low pharmacological activity (Cazzulani et al. 1988, Caine et al. 1991).

The clinical effects of flavoxate in patients with detrusor instability and frequency, urge and incontinence have been studied in both open and controlled investigations, but with varying rates of success (Ruffman 1988). Stanton (1973) compared emepronium bromide and flavoxate in a double-blind, cross-over study of patients with detrusor instability and reported improvement rates of 83% and 66% after flavoxate or emepronium bromide, respectively, both administered as 200 mg 3 times daily. In another double-blind, cross-over study comparing flavoxate 1200 mg/day with that of oxybutynin 15 mg daily in 41 women with idiopathic motor or sensory urgency, and utilising both clinical and urodynamic criteria, Milani et al. (1993) found both drugs effective. No difference in efficacy was found between them, but flavoxate had fewer and milder side effects. The lack of placebo arm in these studies, reduces the value of the efficacy conclusions.

Other investigators, comparing the effects flavoxate with those of placebo, have not been able to show any beneficial effect of flavoxate at dosages up to 400 mg 3 times daily (Briggs et al. 1980, Chapple et al. 1990, Dahm et al. 1995).

In general, few side effects have been reported during treatment with flavoxate. On the other hand its efficacy, compared to other therapeutic alternatives, is not well documented.

4. α-ADRENOCEPTOR ANTAGONISTS

The normal human detrusor responds to noradrenaline by relaxing (Perlberg and Caine 1982, Åmark 1986), probably because of the effect on both α- and β-adrenoceptors (ARs). Stimulation of α_2-ARs on cholinergic neurons may lead to a decreased release of acetylcholine, and stimulation of postjunctional β-ARs to direct relaxation of the detrusor muscle (Andersson 1993, 1997).

Drugs stimulating α-ARs have hardly any contractile effects in isolated, normal human detrusor muscle. However, there is evidence that this may change in bladder overactivity associated with for example hypertrophic bladder and outflow obstruction (Perlberg and Caine 1982) and neurogenic bladders (Andersson 1993). A significant subtype selective α_{1D}-AR mRNA upregulation was found in rats with outflow obstruction (Schwinn and Michelotti 2000), but functional correlates were not reported. It cannot be excluded that factors such as the degree and duration of obstruction have an important influence on the α-ARs in the detrusor, but the functional consequences have not been established.

Even if it is well known that α-AR antagonists can ameliorate lower urinary tract symptoms in men with BPH (Andersson et al. 1997), and occasionally can abolish detrusor overactivity in these patients (Perlberg and Caine 1982, Caine 1986, Eri and Tveter 1995), there are no controlled clinical trials showing that they are an effective alternative in the treatment of bladder overactivity in this patient category. In an open label study, Arnold (2001) evaluated the clinical and pressure-flow effects of tamsulosin 0.4 mg once daily in patients with lower urinary tract symptoms (LUTS) caused by benign prostatic obstruction. He found that tamsulosin can produce a significant decrease in detrusor pressure, increase in flow rate and a symptomatic improvement in patients with LUTS and confirmed obstruction.

α-AR antagonists have been used to treat patients with neurogenic bladders and bladder overactivity (Jensen 1981, Petersen et al. 1989, Åmark and Nergård 1991, Abrams 2001); however, the success has been moderate. Abrams (2001) reported results from a placebo-controlled study (4 weeks duration) on the effects of tamsulosin in 263 patients with supra-sacral spinal cord lesions and neurogenic lower urinary tract dysfunction. There was a trend, but no statistically significant reduction of maximum urethral pressure with tamsulosin after 4 weeks. In 134 patients who completed a 1-year open-label treatment, significant positive effects, urodynamic as well as symptomatic, were found. At present no definitive conclusions can be drawn on the efficacy of α_1-AR antagonists in the treatment of neurogenic bladders until further information is available.

Lower urinary tract symptoms in women have been reported to respond favorably to treatment with α-AR antagonists (Jollys et al 1993, Lepor and Machi 1993). In a prospective open study of 34 women with urgency and frequency, evaluated by an expanded AUA symptom score, a combination of doxazosin and hyoscyamine was found to be more effective than either drug given alone (Serels and Stein 1998). The value of such a combination should be evaluated in a controlled clinical trial.

Although α-AR antagonists may be effective in selected cases of bladder overactivity, convincing effects documented in RCTs are lacking. In women, these drugs may produce stress incontinence (Dwyer and Teele 1992, Marshall and Beevers 1996).

5. β–ADRENOCEPTOR AGONISTS

In isolated human bladder, non-subtype selective β-AR agonists like isoprenaline have a pronounced inhibitory effect, and administration of such drugs can increase bladder capacity in man (Andersson 1993). However, the β-ARs of the human bladder were shown to have functional characteristics typical of neither β_1-, nor β_2-ARs, since they could be blocked by propranolol, but not by practolol or metoprolol (β_1) or butoxamine (β_2) (Nergårdh et al. 1977, Larsen 1979). On the other hand, receptor binding studies using subtype selective ligands, suggested that the β-ARs of the human detrusor are primarily of β_2 subtype (Levin et al. 1988), and favourable effects on bladder overactivity were reported in open studies with selective β_2-AR agonists such as terbutaline (Norlén et al. 1978, Lindholm and Lose 1986). In a double-blind investigation clenbuterol 0.01

mg 3 times daily was shown to have a good therapeutic effect in 15 of 20 women with motor urge incontinence (Grüneberger 1984). Other investigators, however, have not been able to show that β-AR agonists represent an effective therapeutic principle in elderly patients with unstable bladder (Castleden and Morgan 1980), or in young patients with myelodysplasia and detrusor overactivity (Naglo et al. 1981).

Atypical β-AR-mediated responses, reported repeatedly in early studies of β-AR antagonists, have been shown to be mediated by a β_3-AR, which has been cloned, sequenced, expressed in model system, and extensively characterized functionally (Lipworth 1996, Strosberg and Pietri-Rouxel 1997). Both normal and neurogenic human detrusors were shown to express β_1, β_2-, and β_3-AR mRNAs, and selective β_3-AR agonists effectively relaxed both types of detrusor muscle (Igawa et al. 1999, 2001, Takeda et al 1999). Thus, it seems that the atypical β-AR of the human bladder may be the β_3-AR. Whether or not this is of importance in humans, and whether β_3-AR stimulation will be an effective way of treating the overactive bladder, has yet to be shown in controlled clinical trials.

6. Antidepressants

Several antidepressants have been reported to have beneficial effects in patients with detrusor overactivity (Martin and Schiff 1984, Lose et al. 1989). However, imipramine is the only drug that has been widely used clinically to treat this disorder.

Imipramine has complex pharmacological effects, including marked systemic antimuscarinic actions (Baldessarini 1985) and blockade of the reuptake of serotonin and noradrenaline (Maggi et al. 1989a), but its mode of action in detrusor overactivity has not been established (Hunsballe and Djurhuus 2001). Even if imipramine 25 to 75 mg, given intramuscularly to 11 patients with uncontrolled detrusor contractions (Diokno et et al. 1972), had no effect, several investigators have found that the drug can be effective in the treatment of bladder overactivity. Thus, in elderly patients with detrusor instability, who received oral imipramine in doses up to 150 mg daily, good effects were reported (Castleden et al. 1981, 1986). Raezer et al. (1977) found that a combination of propantheline and imipramine was particularly useful. Even if it is generally considered that imipramine is a useful drug in the treatment of detrusor overactivity, no good quality RCTs that can document this have been retrieved.

It has been known for a long time that imipramine can have favourable effects in the treatment of nocturnal enuresis in children with a success rate of 10-70 % in controlled trials (Miller et al. 1987, Hunsballe and Djurhuus 2001).

It is well established that therapeutic doses of tricyclic antidepressants, including imipramine, may cause serious toxic effects on the cardiovascular system (orthostatic hypotension, ventricular arrhythmias). Imipramine prolongs QTc intervals and has an antiarrhythmic (and proarrhythmic) effect similar to that of quinidine (Bigger et al 1977, Giardina et al 1979). Children seem particularly sensitive to the cardiotoxic action of tricyclic antidepressants (Baldessarini 1985).

The risks and benefits of imipramine in the treatment of voiding disorders do not seem to have been assessed. Very few studies have have been performed during the last decade (Hunsballe and Djurhuus 2001), and no good quality RCTs have documented that the drug is effective in the treatment detrusor overactivity. However, a beneficial effect has been documented in the treatment of nocturnal enuresis.

7. Prostaglandin synthesis inhibitors

Human bladder mucosa has the ability to synthesize eicosanoids (Jeremy et al. 1987), and these agents can be liberated from bladder muscle and mucosa in response to different types of trauma (Downie et al. 1984, Leslie et al. 1984). Even if prostaglandins cause contraction of human bladder muscle (Andersson 1993), it is still unclear whether prostaglandins contribute to the pathogenesis of unstable detrusor contractions. More important than direct effects on the bladder muscle may be sensitization of sensory afferent nerves, increasing the afferent input produced by a given degree of bladder filling. Involuntary bladder contractions can then be triggered at a small bladder volume. If this is an important mechanism, treatment with prostaglandin synthesis inhibitors could be expected to be effective. However, clinical evidence for this is scarce.

Cardozo et al. (1980) performed a double-blind controlled study of 30 women with detrusor instability using the prostaglandin synthesis inhibitor flurbiprofen at a dosage of 50 mg 3 times daily. The drug was shown to have favourable effects, although it did not completely abolish detrusor overactivity. There was a high incidence of side effects (43%) including nausea, vomiting, headache and gastrointestinal symptoms. Palmer (1983) studied the effects of flurbiprofen 50 mg x 4 versus placebo in a double-blind, cross-over trial in 37 patients with idiopathic detrusor instability (27% of the patients did not complete the trial). Active treatment significantly increased maximum contractile pressure, decreased the number of voids and decreased the number of urgent voids compared to baseline. Indomethacin 50 to 100 mg daily was reported to give symptomatic relief in patients with detrusor instability, compared with bromocriptine in a randomized, single-blind, cross-over study (Cardozo and Stanton 1980). The incidence of side effects was high, occurring in 19 of 32 patients. However, no patient had to stop treatment because of side effects.

The few controlled clinical trials on the effects of prostaglandin synthesis inhibitors in the treatment of detrusor overactivity, and the limited number of drugs tested, makes it difficult to evaluate their therapeutic value. No new information has been published during the last decade.

8. Vasopressin analogues

a) Desmopressin

Desmopressin (1-desamino-8-D-arginine vasopressin; DDAVP) is a synthetic vasopressin analogue with a pronounced antidiuretic effect, but practically lacking vasopressor actions (Andersson et al. 1988). It is now widely used as a treatment for primary nocturnal enuresis (Nevéus et al 1999). Studies have shown that one of the factors that can contribute to nocturnal enuresis in children and probably in adults, is lack of a normal nocturnal increase in plasma vasopressin, which results in a high nocturnal urine production (Rittig et al. 1989, Matthiesen et al. 1996, Nørgaard et al. 1997, Hjälmås 1999). By decreasing the nocturnal production of urine, beneficial effects may be obtained in enuresis and nocturia. However, the drug may also have stimulatory effects on the CNS, as found in rats (DiMichele et al. 1996).

Several, controlled, double-blind investigations have shown intranasal administration of desmopressin to be effective in the treatment of nocturnal enuresis in children (Miller et al. 1992, Moffat et al. 1993, Nevéus et al 1999). The dose used in most studies has been 20 µg intranasally at bedtime. However, the drug is orally active, even if the bioavailability is low (less than 1% compared to 2 to 10% after intranasal administration), and its oral efficacy in primary nocturnal enuresis in children and adolescents has been documented in randomized, double-blind, placebo controlled studies (Janknegt et al 1997, Skoog et al 1997).

Positive effects of desmopressin on nocturia in adults have been documented. Nocturnal frequency and enuresis due to bladder instability responded favourably to intranasal desmopressin therapy even when previous treatment with "antispasmodics" had been unsuccessful (Hilton and Stanton 1982). Also in patients with multiple sclerosis, desmopressin was shown in controlled studies to reduce nocturia, and micturition frequency (Hilton et al. 1983, Kinn and Larsson 1990, Eckford et al. 1994, Fredrikson et al. 1996). Furthermore, desmopressin was shown to be successful in treating nocturnal enuresis in spina bifida patients with diurnal incontinence (Horowitz et al. 1997). Oral desmopressin has proved to be effective in the treatment of nocturia with polyuric origin. In addition to prolonging sleep duration to first void, desmopressin reduced the number and frequency of nocturnal voids and nocturnal urine volume in both men and women (Weiss et al 2001, van Kerrebroeck et al 2001).

Desmopressin is a well documented therapeutic alternative in paediatric nocturnal enuresis, and seems to be effective also in adults with nocturia with polyuric origin. Even if side effects are uncommon, there is a risk of water retention and hyponatremia during desmopressin treatment (Robson et al. 1996, Schwab and Ruder 1997), and due consideration should be given to this potential side effect, particularly in elderly patients.

9. Other drugs

a) Baclofen

Baclofen is considered to depress monosynaptic and polysynaptic motorneurons and interneurons in the spinal cord by acting as a $GABA_B$ receptor agonist, and has been been used in voiding disorders, including detrusor hyperreflexia secondary to lesions of the spinal cord (Andersson 1988, Wein 1995). The drug may also be an alternative in the treatment of idiopathic detrusor overactivity (Taylor and Bates 1979). However, published experience with the drug is limited.

Intrathecal baclofen may be useful in patients with spasticity and bladder dysfunction, and increase bladder capacity (Kums and Delhaas 1991, Steers et al. 1992, Bushman et al. 1993).

10. Capsaicin and resiniferatoxin

Capsaicin, the pungent ingredient of red peppers, has identified a pharmacological classification of subpopulations of primary afferent neurons innervating the bladder and urethra, the "capsaicin-sensitive nerves". Capsaicin exerts a biphasic effect on sensory nerves: initial excitation is followed by a long-lasting blockade which renders sensitive primary afferents (C-fibres) resistant to activation by natural stimuli (Maggi 1993). It is believed that capsaicin exerts these effects by acting on specific receptors, "vanilloid" receptors (Szallasi 1994). It is possible that capsaicin at high concentrations (mM) has additional, non-specific effects (Kuo 1997).

Cystometric evidence that capsaicin-sensitive nerves may modulate the afferent branch of the micturition reflex in humans was originally presented by Maggi et al. (1989b), who instilled capsaicin (0.1-10 µM) intravesically in five patients with hypersensitivity disorders; with attenuation of their symptoms a few days after administration of capsaicin. Intravesical capsaicin, given in considerably higher concentrations (1-2 mM) than those administered by Maggi et al. (1989b), has since been used with success in detrusor overactivity associated with neurological disorders such as multiple sclerosis, or traumatic chronic spinal lesions (Igawa et al. 1996). The effect of treatment may last for 2 to 7 months (Fowler et al. 1992, Geirsson et al. 1995, Chandiramani et al. 1996, Cruz et al. 1997, De Ridder et al 1997, Cruz 1998, Wiart et al. 1998 de Ridder and Baert 2000, Fowler 2000). However, negative results have also been reported (Petersen et al (1998). de Ridder et al. (1997) recommended that the drug should not be given to severely disabled, bedridden patients.

Side effects of intravesical capsaicin include discomfort and a burning sensation at the pubic/urethral level during instillation, an effect that can be overcome by prior instillation of lidocaine, which does not interfere with the beneficial effects of capsaicin (Chandiramani et al. 1996). No premalignant or malignant changes in the bladder have been found in biopsies of patients who had repeated capsaicin instillations for up to 5 years (Dasgupta et al. 1998).

Resiniferatoxin is a phorbol related diterpene, isolated from some species of Eurphorbia, a cactus-like plant. It has effects similar to those of capsaicin. Given intravesically, resiniferatoxin has been shown to be approximately 1000 times more potent than capsaicin in stimulating bladder activity (Ishizuka et al. 1995b). Moreover, resiniferatoxin seems able to desensitize bladder sensory fibers with less C-fos expression in the rat spinal cord (Craft et al. 1995, Cruz et al. 1996). Craft et al. (1995) reported that resiniferatoxin, instilled intravesically, produced a desensitization of bladder afferents that lasted approximately 2 months in a rat behavioral model. The authors also suggested that resiniferatoxin may be superior to capsaicin as an agent for desensitization therapy. Lazzeri et al. (1997), instilled resiniferatoxin intravesically in 15 subjects, including 8 normals and 7 with bladder over activity (6 with hyperreflexia). Resiniferatoxin (10 nM concentration) did not produce any warm or burning sensation suprapubically. In the patients with bladder overactivity, but not in the normal patients, the mean bladder capacity increased significantly immediately after resiniferatoxin treatment. However, this effect remained in only 2 out of the 7 patients 4 weeks after the instillation. Higher doses (50 and 100 nM) were used by Cruz et al. (1997) who treated 7 patients with hyperreflexia with intravesical resiniferatoxin. They found no temporary deterioration of urinary symptoms, as seen with capsaicin, and found improvement in urinary frequency in 5 of the patients that lasted up to 3 months. The beneficial effect of resiniferatoxin has been confirmed in other studies (Lazzeri et al 1998, Silva et al 2000). These observations make resiniferatoxin an interesting alternative to capsaicin, but further investigations are needed to explore its clinical potential. Currently it is not in clinical development owing to formulation problems.

VII. DRUGS USED FOR TREATMENT OF STRESS INCONTINENCE

Many factors seem to be involved in the pathogenesis of stress urinary incontinence: urethral support, vesical neck function, and function of the urethral muscles (DeLancey 1977). Such anatomical factors cannot be treated pharmacologically. However women with stress incontinence have lower resting urethral pressures than age-matched continent women (Henriksson et al. 1979, Hilton and Stanton 1983), and since it seems likely that there is a reduced urethral closure pressure in most women with stress incontinence, it seems logical to increase urethral pressure to improve the condition.

Factors which may contribute to urethral closure include urethral smooth muscle tone and the passive properties of the urethral lamina propria in particular the vascular submucosal layer. The relative contribution to intraurethral pressure of these factors is still subject to debate. However, there is ample pharmacological evidence that a substantial part of urethral tone is mediated through stimulation of α-ARs in the urethral smooth muscle by released noradrenaline (Andersson 1993). A contributing factor to stress incontinence, mainly in elderly women with lack of estrogen, may be lack of mucosal function. The role of striated urethral and pelvic floor muscles has not yet been established.

The pharmacological treatment of stress incontinence (Table 3) aims at increasing intraurethral pressure by increasing tone in the urethral smooth muscle, or by affecting tone of the striated muscles in the urethra and pelvic floor (see below). Although several drugs may

Table 3 : Drugs used in the treatment of stress incontinence Assessments according to the Oxford system

ALPHA-ADRENOCEPTOR AGONISTS		
Ephedrine	3	C
Norephedrine (phenylpropanolamine, PPA)	2	NR
OTHER DRUGS		
Imipramine	4	C*
Clenbuterol	4	C
(Duloxetine)	UNDER INVESTIGATION	
Hormones		
Estrogens	2	D

NR = NOT RECOMMENDED
* SHOULD BE USED WITH CAUTION

contribute to such an increase in intraurethral pressure, including β-AR antagonists and imipramine (see Andersson 1988, Wein 1995), only α-AR agonists and estrogens (see below), alone or together, have been more widely used.

a) α-Adrenoceptor agonists

Although several drugs with agonistic effects on α-ARs have been used in the treatment of stress incontinence, for example midodrine (Jonas 1982, Gnad et al. 1984) and norfenefrine (Lose and Lindholm 1984), ephedrine and norephedrine seem to be the most widely used drugs (Andersson 1988, Wein 1995). Ephedrine, pseudoephedrine (a stereoisomer of ephedrine), and norephedrine (phenylpropanolamine, PPA) directly stimulate α- as well as β-ARs, but can also release noradrenaline from adrenergic nerve terminals. They have all been reported to be effective in stress incontinence, as found in open and controlled clinical trials (Diokno and Taub 1975, Awad et al. 1978, Ek et al. 1978, Collste and Lindskog 1987, Siltberg et al 1999), ephedrine at a dose of 25 to 50 mg 3 to 4 times daily, and PPA at a dose of 50 to 100 mg 2 to 3 times daily. These drugs lack selectivity for urethral α-ARs, and may increase blood pressure. They also can cause sleep disturbances, headache, tremor and palpitations (Andersson 1988, Wein 1995). Long-term experience with the drugs is lacking. It has been pointed out that individuals taking PPA might have an initial increase in blood pressure that can be dangerous (Vick et al 1994), and it should be noted that the FDA has asked manufacturers to voluntarily stop selling PPA-containing drugs and replace the ingredients with a safer alternative. Judging from the clinical benefit documented with PPA and the possible risks, this drug (and probably drugs with similar action) should not be used.

Radley et al (2001) evaluated the effect of the selective α_1-AR agonist, methoxamine, in a randomised, double-blind, placebo-controlled, crossover study on a group of women with genuine stress incontinence, while measuring maximum urethral pressure (MUP), blood pressure, heart rate, and symptomatic side effects. Methoxamine evoked non-significant increases in MUP and diastolic blood pressure, but caused a significant rise in systolic blood pressure and a significant fall in heart rate at maximum dosage. Systemic side effects including piloerection, headache, and cold extremities were experienced in all subjects. The authors suggested that the clinical usefulness of direct, peripherally acting subtype-selective α_1-AR agonists in the medical treatment of stress incontinence may be limited by side effects.

Attempts have been made to develop agonists with selectivity for the human urethra. Among the three high affinity α_1-AR subtypes identified in molecular cloning and functional studies (α_{1A}, α_{1B}, α_{1D}), α_{1A} seems to predominate in the human lower urinary tract (Andersson 2001). However, the receptor with low affinity for prazosin (the α_{1L}-AR), which has not been cloned and may represent a functional phenotype of the α_{1A}-AR, was found to be prominent in the human male urethra. In the human female urethra, the expression and distribution of α_1-AR subtypes were determined by in situ hybridisation and quantitative autoradiography. mRNA for the α_{1A} subtype was predominant, and autoradiography confirmed the predominance of the α_{1A}-AR (Nasu et al 1998).

No drug with appropriate sub-type selectivity is currently available, and the role of α-AR agonists in the treatment of stress incontinence has yet to be established.

α-AR agonists has been used used in combination with estrogens (Kinn and Lindskog 1988, Ahlström et al. 1990), and with other nonsurgical treatments of stress incontinence, such as pelvic floor exercises and electrical stimulation. Beisland et al (1984) treated 24 women with genuine stress incontinence using PPA (50 mg twice daily) and estriol (1 mg per day vaginally) separately and in combination. They found that the combination cured 8 women and improved further 9 and was more effective than either drug given alone. Hilton and collegues (1990) used (estrogen vaginal or oral) alone or in combination with PPA to treat 60 postmenopausal women with genuine stress incontinence in a double-blind, placebo controlled study. Subjectively the symptom of stress incontinence improved in all groups, but objectively only in the women given combination therapy. Even if this type of treatment can be effective in women with mild stress incontinence or in those not suitable for surgery, the risks with PPA and related compounds (see above) do not seem to motivate their use as single drug therapy or in combination with estrogen. In carefully selected patients, selective α_1-AR antagonists may be used on an "on demand" basis in certain situations known to provoke leakage.

b) β-Adrenoceptor antagonists

The theoretical basis for the use of β-AR antagonists in the treatment of stress incontinence is that blockade of urethral β-ARs may enhance the effects of noradrenaline on urethral α-ARs. Even if propranolol has been reported to have beneficial effects in the treatment of stress incontinence (Gleason et al 1974, Kaisary 1984), there are no RCTs supporting such an action.

c) Imipramine

Imipramine, among several other pharmacological effects, inhibits the re-uptake of noradrenaline and serotonin in adrenergic nerve ending. In the urethra, this can be expected to enhance the contractile effects of noradrenaline on urethral smooth muscle. Theoretically, such an action may also influence the striated muscles in the urethra and pelvic floor by effects at the spinal cord level (Onuf´s nucleus).

Gilja et al (1984) reported in an open study on 30 women with stress incontinence that imipramine, 75 mg daily, produced subjective continence in 21 patients and increased mean maximal urethral closure pressure (MUCP) from 34 to 48 mm Hg. Lin et al (1999) assessed the efficacy of imipramine (25 mg imipramine three times a day for three months) as a treatment of genuine stress incontinence in forty women with genuine stress incontinence. A 20-minute pad test, uroflowmetry, filling and voiding cystometry, and stress urethral pressure profile were performed before and after treatment. The efficacy of successful treatment was 60% (95% CI 44.8-75.2). No RCTs on the effects of imipramine seem to be available.

d) Clenbuterol

Since β-AR antagonists have been used as a treatment of stress incontinence, it seems paradoxical that the selective β_2-AR agonist, clenbuterol, was found to cause significant clinical improvement and increase in MUCP in 165 women with stress incontinence (Yasuda et al 1993). The study was double-blind and placebo-controlled. The number of patients reporting any degree of improvement was 56 (out of 77) in the clenbuterol group and 48 (out of 88) in the placebo group, and the changes in MUCP was 3.3 cm H_2O in the clenbuterol and -1.5 cm H_2O in the placebo group. The positive effects were suggested to be a result of an action on urethral striated muscle and/or the pelvic floor muscles.

Ishiko et al (2000) investigated the effects of clenbuterol on 61 female patients with stress incontinence in a 12-week randomized study, comparing drug therapy to pelvic floor exercises and a combination of drug therapy and pelvic floor exercises. The frequency and volume of stress incontinence and the patient´s own impression were used as the basis for the assessment of efficacy. The improvement of incontinence was 76.9 %, 52.6 %, and 89.5 % in the respective groups. In an open study, Noguchi et al (1997) reported positive results with clenbuterol (20 mg b.i.d for 1 month) in 9 of 14 patients with mild to moderate stress incontinence after radical prostatectomy. Further well-designed RTCs documenting the effects of clenbuterol are needed to adequately assess its potential as a treatment for stress incontinence as it is possible that this agent may have a novel as yet undefined mechanism of action.

e) Duloxetine

Duloxetine, a combined noradrenaline and 5-HT reuptake inhibitor, has been shown, in animal experiments, to increase the neural activity to the external urethral sphincter, and increase bladder capacity through effects on the central nervous system (Thor and Katofiasc 1995). In a double-blind, placebo-controlled study in women with stress (n=140) or mixed (n=146) incontinence, duloxetine (20-40 mg q.d.) was shown to cause significant improvements in several efficacy measures (ICS 1 h stress pad test, 24h pad weight, number of incontinence episodes, quality of life assessment; Zinner et al 1998). The drug was well tolerated and there were few discontinuations due to side effects (8% for duloxetine, 3% for placebo).

The drug is still undergoing clinical trials.

VIII. DRUGS USED FOR TREATMENT OF OVERFLOW INCONTINENCE

According to the definition of the ICS (1997), overflow incontinence is "leakage of urine at greater than normal bladder capacity. It is associated with incomplete bladder emptying due to either impaired detrusor contractility or bladder outlet obstruction". Two types of overflow incontinence are recognized, one as a result of mechanical obstruction, and the other secondary to functional disorders. Occasionally both types can coexist.

The clinical presentation of overflow incontinence may vary depending on the age of the patient and the cause of the incontinence. In children, overflow incontinence can be secondary to congenital obstructive disorders (e.g., urethral valves) or to neurogenic vesical dysfunction (myelomeningocele, Hinman syndrom). In adults, overflow incontinence may be associated with outflow obstruction secondary to BPH or can be a consequence of diabetes mellitus. Mixed forms may be seen in disorders associated with motor spasticity (e.g., Parkinson´s disease).

Pharmacologic treatment (Table 4) should be based on previous urodynamic evaluation. The aim of treatment is to prevent damage to the upper urinary tract by normalizing voiding and urethral pressures. Drugs used for increasing intravesical pressure, i.e.,"parasympathomimetics" (acetylcholine analogues such as bethanechol, or acetylcholine esterase inhibitors), or β-AR antagonists, have not been documented to have beneficial effects (see, Finkbeiner 1985, Wein et al 1994). Stimulation of detrusor activity by intravesical instillation of prostaglandins have been reported to be successful; however, the effect is controversial and no RCTs are available (Andersson 1988, Wein et al. 1994, Wein, 2001a).

The "autonomous" contractions in patients with para-

Table 4 : Drugs used in the treatment of overflow incontinence. Assessments according to the Oxford system

ALPHA-ADRENOCEPTOR ANTAGONISTS		
Alfuzosin	4	C
Doxazosin	4	C
Prazosin	4	C
Terazosin	4	C
Tamsulosin	4	C
*(Phenoxybenzamine)	4	NR
MUSCARINIC RECEPTOR AGONISTS		
Bethanechol	4	D
Carbachol	4	D
ANTICHOLINESTERASE INHIBITORS		
Distigmine	4	D
OTHER DRUGS		
Baclofen	4	C
Benzodiazepines	4	C
Dantrolene	4	C

NR = NOT RECOMMENDED

sympathetic decentralisation are probably caused by α-AR mediated bladder activity, since they can be inhibited by α-AR antagonists (Sundin et al 1977). The α-AR antagonist that has been most widely used is probably phenoxybenzamine (Hachen 1980, Krane and Olsson 1973, McGuire et al 1976). However, uncertainties about the carcinogenic effects of this drug, and its side effects (Caine 1986) have focused interest on selective α_1-AR antagonists such as prazosin (Andersson et al 1991).

Other means of decreasing outflow resistance in these patients, particularly if associated with spasticity are baclofen, benzodiazepines (e.g., diazepam) and dantrolene sodium (see Wein et al 1994, Wein 2001a).

IX. HORMONAL TREATMENT OF URINARY INCONTINENCE

1. ESTROGENS AND THE CONTINENCE MECHANISM

The estrogen sensitive tissues of the bladder, urethra and pelvic floor all play an important role in the continence mechanism. For a woman to remain continent the urethral pressure must exceed the intravesical pressure at all times except during micturition (Abrams et al 1990). The urethra has four estrogen sensitive functional layers which all play a part in the maintenance of a positive urethral pressure:

1 epithelium,

2 vasculature,

3 connective tissue,

4 muscle.

a) Estrogens in the treatment of urinary incontinence

There are a number of reasons why estrogens may be useful in the treatment of women with urinary incontinence. As well as improving the "maturation index" of urethral squamous epithelium (Bergman et al 1990), estrogens increase urethral closure pressure and improve abdominal pressure transmission to the proximal urethra (Hilton et al 1983, Bhatia et al 1989, Karram et al 1989). The sensory threshold of the bladder may also be raised (Fantl et al 1988). Salmon et al (1941) were the first to report the successful use of estrogens to treat urinary incontinence over fifty years ago. Intramuscular estrogen therapy was administered to 16 women with dysuria, frequency, urgency and incontinence for 4 weeks. Symptomatic improvement occurred in 12 women until treatment was discontinued, at which time the symptoms recurred. Further studies on larger numbers of patients (Musiani 1972, Schleyer-Saunders 1976) also showed impressive subjective improvement rates of between 39-70%.

There are a number of different causes of lower urinary tract disorders in postmenopausal women (Bent et al 1983). It is well recognized that there is a poor correlation between a woman´s symptoms and the subsequent diagnosis following appropriate investigation (Jarvis et al 1980). Unfortunately, initial trials took place before the widespread introduction of urodynamic studies and therefore almost certainly included a heterogenous group of individuals with a number of different pathologies. Lack of objective outcome measures also limit their interpretation.

Lose and Englev (2000) evaluated the effect of estrogens in two hundred and fifty-one postmenopausal women, with a mean age of 66 years, reporting at least one bothersome lower urinary tract symptom in an open, randomised, parallel group trial. One hundred and thirty-four women were treated with an oestradiol-releasing ring for 24 weeks; 117 women were treated with oestriol pessaries 0.5 mg every second day for 24 weeks. Subjective scores of urgency, frequency, nocturia, dysuria, stress incontinence and urge incontinence were evaluated. The two treatments were equally efficacious in alleviating urinary urgency (51% vs 56%), urge incontinence (58% vs 58%), stress incontinence (53% vs 59%) and nocturia (51% vs 54%). The authors concluded that low dose vaginally administered oestradiol and oestriol are equally efficacious in alleviating lower urinary tract symptoms which appear after the menopause. The lack of a placebo group makes the improvement rates difficult to evaluate.

b) Estrogens for stress incontinence

The role of estrogen in the treatment of stress incontinence has been controversial, even though there are a number of reported studies (see, Hextall 2000). Some have given promising results but this may be because they were observational, not randomized, blinded or controlled. The situation is further complicated by the fact that a number of different types of estrogen have been used with varying doses, routes of administration and durations of treatment. Fantl et al (1996) treated 83 hypo-estrogenic women with urodynamic evidence of genuine stress incontinence and/or detrusor instability with conjugated equine estrogens 0.625 mg and medroxyprogesterone 10 mg cyclically for 3 months. Controls received placebo tablets. At the end of the study period the clinical and quality of life variables had not changed significantly in either group. Jackson et al (1996) treated 57 postmenopausal women with genuine stress incontinence or mixed incontinence with estradiol valerate 2 mg or placebo daily for 6 months. There was no significant change in objective outcome measures although both the active and placebo group reported subjective benefit.

There have been two meta-analyses performed which have helped to clarify the situation further. In the first, a report by the Hormones and Urogenital Therapy (HUT) committee, the use of estrogens to treat all causes of incontinence in postmenopausal women was examined (Fantl et al 1994). Of 166 articles identified which were published in English between 1969 and 1992, only six were controlled trials and 17 uncontrolled series. The results showed that there was a significant subjective improvement for all patients and those with genuine stress incontinence. However, assessment of the objective parameters revealed that there was no change in the volume of urine lost. Maximum urethral closure pressure did increase significantly, but this result was influenced by only one study showing a large effect. In the second meta-analysis, Sultana and Walters (1990) reviewed 8 controlled and 14 uncontrolled prospective trials and included all types of estrogen treatment. They also found that estrogen therapy was not an efficacious treatment of stress incontinence, but may be useful for the often associated symptoms of urgency and frequency.

Estrogen when given alone therefore does not appear to be an effective treatment for stress incontinence. However, several studies have shown that it may have a role in combination with other therapies (for combination with α-AR agonists, see above). In a randomized trial, Ishiko et al (2001) compared the effects of the combination of pelvic floor exercise and estriol (1mg/day) in sixty-six patients with postmenopausal stress incontinence. Efficacy was evaluated every three months based on stress scores obtained from a questionnaire. They found a significant decrease in stress score in mild and moderate stress incontinence patients in both groups three months after the start of therapy and concluded that combination therapy with estriol plus pelvic floor exercise was effective and capable of serving as first-line treatment for mild stress incontinence.

c) Estrogens for urge incontinence

Estrogen has been used to treat postmenopausal urgency and urge incontinence for many years, but there are few controlled trials confirming that it is of benefit (Hextall 2000).

A double blind multi-center study of 64 postmenopausal women with the "urge syndrome" has failed to confirm its efficacy (Cardozo et al 1993). All women underwent pre-treatment urodynamic investigation to establish that they either had sensory urgency or detrusor instability. They were then randomized to treatment with oral estriol 3 mg daily or placebo for 3 months. Compliance was confirmed by a significant improvement in the maturation index of vaginal epithelial cells in the active but not the placebo group. Estriol produced subjective and objective improvements in urinary symptoms, but it was not significantly better than placebo. Grady et al (2001) determined whether postmenopausal hormone therapy improves the severity of urinary incontinence in a randomized, blinded trial among 2763 postmenopausal women younger than 80 years with coronary disease and intact uteri. The report included 1525 participants who reported at least one episode of incontinence per week at baseline. Participants were randomly assigned to 0.625 mg of conjugated estrogens plus 2.5 mg of medroxyprogesterone acetate in one tablet daily (n = 768) or placebo (n = 757) and were followed for a mean of 4.1 years. Severity of incontinence was classified as improved (decrease of at least two episodes per week), unchanged (change of at most one episode per week), or worsened (increase of at least two episodes per week). The results showed that incontinence improved in 26% of the women assigned to placebo compared with 21% assigned to hormones, while 27% of the placebo group worsened compared with 39% of the hormone group (P =.001). This difference was evident by 4 months of treatment and was observed for both urge and stress incontinence. The number of incontinent episodes per week increased an average of 0.7 in the hormone group and decreased by 0.1 in the placebo group (P <.001). The authors concluded that daily oral estrogen plus progestin therapy was associated with worsening urinary incontinence in older postmenopausal women with weekly incontinence, and did not recommend this therapy for the treatment of incontinence. It cannot be excluded that the progestagen component had a negative influence on the outcome of this study.

Estrogen has an important physiological effect on the female lower urinary tract and its deficiency is an etiological factor in the pathogenesis of a number of conditions. However, the use of estrogens alone to treat urinary incontinence has given disappointing results.

ADDENDUM 1

CLINICAL RESEARCH CRITERIA

The Committee has included a section on clinical research criteria to encompass general considerations relating to design of clinical trails and appropriate assessments of efficacy of pharmacotherapy for incontinence (see also Blaivas et al 1997).

Existing pharmacotherapies are designed to reduce symptoms and improve quality of life and we therefore feel that these measures should, wherever possible, be considered to be primary efficacy parameters. It is obviously important to document as secondary endpoints the mechanistic aspects of any therapy and for this reason it is essential that objective urodynamic parameters are measured including data relating to frequency and volumes voided (the frequency volume chart), urgency and degree of urgency, number of urge incontinent episodes and wherever possible data relating to volume at first unstable contraction and amplitude of unstable contractions.

It is important that therapies should be administered for adequate lengths of time to allow a steady state situation to be established and also bearing in mind the existing literature base which suggests that drugs may take up to 2 months to produce optimum efficacy often as a consequences of the concomitant bladder retraining and behavioural aspects relating to improvement of symptoms which occur on treatment.

It is important to provide long term follow up data and to appreciate the relevance of data relating to real life practice as well as the essential randomised control data.

The limitations of both approaches however should be adequately taken into account and interpretation of data. Whenever possible pragmatic study designs should be used. It is essential that both cost benefit and cost efficacy should be adequately addressed at an early stage in development of any new therapy.

Whenever a new therapeutic modality is being introduced then the limitations of in vitro and in vivo pharmacological data particularly when based on animal models should be recognised and appropriate proof of concept studies conducted. The role of innovative clinical investigative approaches is to be encouraged including the use of ambulatory urodynamic assessment using a cross-over design.

Adequate patient selection criteria should be utilised which reflect the nature of the population to be treated with particular reference to not excluding the specific population groups which will be a principle target of future therapy. For instance many studies exclude the frail elderly and those with concomitant medical problems. These groups are often in particular risk of being troubled by incontinence.

It is essential that randomised placebo controlled study designs are used wherever possible and that the studies are adequately powered. Peer reviewed journals should be strongly encouraged not to publish studies which do not stick to these criteria. Studies utilising symptoms as an inclusion criterion require greater numbers of patients than those using specific criteria with a clearly identifiable disease entity; therefore studies using overactive bladder criteria require larger numbers than those using detrusor instability.

It may be recommended that all future studies stratify for age, taking into consideration age-related changes in bladder function. Future research with drugs should consider a conservative arm in the study design.

ADDENDUM 2

PLACEBO

A placebo response refers to the change that may occur in response to the administration of an inactive drug, also called a dummy drug. The placebo effect is defined as the difference between the response with the placebo versus the changes that occur without the administration of any drug. This change may be due to spontaneous remission of the disease, regression toward the mean, life changes, the passage of time, or factors as subtle as the value of more frequent interaction with the provider and the expectancy of a result. The patient's expectations of what is going to happen can lead to self-cure.

The origin of placebo controlled trials probably began with Cornell Conference on Therapy in 1946 and advocacy for the use of placebos in randomized controlled trials (RCT) is generally credited to Dr. Harry Gold. At this conference Dr. Eugene F DuBois noted "If you take three groups, one given no treatment, a second given placebo, and a third given the test drug, you will very often find that the group given the placebos get along very much better, have a much higher percentage of cures than those without treatment, and perhaps, almost as many as those with the test drug, in some cases more".

Today the results of adequate and well-controlled investigations provide the primary basis for determining whether there is 'substantial evidence' to support the claims of effectiveness for new drugs and antibiotics. Well-designed clinical trials allow investigators to distinguish the effect of active drug from other influences such as a spontaneous change in the course of the disease, the placebo effect, or even biased observations. Adverse effects caused by a drug can be separated from those resulting from underlying disease.

It is now over fifty years since the first paper that looked at the 'powerful placebo' response and a wide range of clinical studies have reported a placebo response averaging 32 percent (Beecher, 1955). Recently this placebo response has been questioned by Hrobjartsson and Gotzsche (2001), who suggested that the reported large effects of placebo could therefore, at least in part, be artifacts of inadequate research methods. These authors, using Cochrane techniques, found little evidence in general that placebos had powerful clinical effects. However, it is believed that the "uncompromising condemnation of placebos is a bit too sweeping" (Bailer, 2001). There is still evidence that placebo benefits are demonstrable in these studies especially in the treatment of pain.

The use of placebo controlled clinical trials is not required by most regulatory agencies. What is required is adequate and well controlled investigations. By regulation, the Food and Drug Administration (FDA) has described these as placebo control, dose-comparison studies; no treatment concurrent controls, active treatment concurrent controls; and even historical controls (from www.fda.gov/cderCommittee for Advanced Scientific Education Seminar, 1999). (This document lists examples of studies where you cannot do placebo control trials.) Active control trials are to be used "when the condition treated is such that the administration of placebo, or no treatment would be contrary to the interests of the patient." When a new treatment is tested for a condition for which no effective treatment is known, there is usually no ethical problem with a study comparing the new treatment to placebo. Many placebo-controlled trials are conducted as add-on-trials where all patients receive a specified standard therapy or therapy left to the choice of the treating physician or institution.). Even when placebo or a no-treatment control arm is used this does not imply that the patient does not get any treatment at all. For example, in cases of oncology trials when no active drug is approved the patient will still receive standard of care palliative therapy.

Use of a placebo control may raise problems of ethics, acceptability, and feasibility, when an effective treatment is available for the condition under study in a proposed trial. In cases, where an available treatment is known to prevent serious harm, such as death or irreversible morbidity in the study population, it is generally inappropriate to use a placebo control. There are occasional exceptions, however, such as cases in which standard therapy has toxicity so severe that many patients have refused to receive it (FDA Guidance). The use of placebos is not acceptable or ethical in most instances for assessing and managing pain as stated by most professional organizations.

One should also consider the possibility of an increased risk of adverse events during the treatment cycle, e.g. 12 weeks or longer if patients are not receiving the active therapeutic intervention.

It is estimated that more placebos have been administered to participants in clinical trials than any single experimental drug, which should provide a wealth of substantial knowledge that almost no one evaluates. Traditionally, most studies of a new molecular entity for the treatment of urge and mixed incontinence have used a placebo arm in the clinical trials for the approval process or a comparator arm. In some cases the placebo response in the 12-week studies have made it difficult to detect significant differences between the active drug and the placebo. One possibility is that there is a bladder training effect developing with the completion of multiple frequency-volume charts resulting in this 'placebo' response.

It is difficult to compare the placebo response between different studies since the inclusion criteria and severity of disease may not be comparable. The planning of these studies must take into consideration this placebo response in order to adequately detect statistical significant differences between drug and placebo.

Variability of individual responses and response to inactive drug in each of these studies must be considered in the planning of future trials. Most studies are 12 weeks in duration and do not provide long term data on the outcome of patients on placebo. In addition data is not separated by severity of disease. Most importantly there is a learning response probably associated with the patient's beliefs and expectations that must be considered in any of these clinical trials.

REFERENCES

Abrams P and The European Tamsulosin NLUTD Study Group. Tamsulosin efficacy and safety in neurogenic lower urinary tract dysfunction (NLUTD). J Urol 165 Suppl:276 (abstract 1137)

Abrams P, Blaivas JG, Stanton SL et al. The standardisation of terminology of lower urinary tract function. Br J Obstet Gynecol 97:1, 1990

Abrams P, Freeman R, Anderstrom C et al. Tolterodine, a new antimuscarinic agent: as effective but better tolerated than oxybutynin in patients with an overactive bladder. Br J Urol 81:801, 1998

Ahlström K, Sandahl B, Sjöberg B et al. Effect of combined treatment with phenylpropanolamine and estriol, compared with estriol treatment alone, in postmenopausal women with stress urinary incontinence. Gynecol Obstet Invest 30:37, 1990

Alabaster VA. Discovery & development of selective M3 antagonists for clinical use. Life Sci 60:1053, 1997

Alberts P. Classification of the presynaptic muscarinic receptor that regulates 3H-acetylcholine secretion in the guinea pig urinary bladder in vitro. J Pharmacol Exp Ther 274:458, 1995

Allousi S, Laval K-U, Eckert R. Trospium chloride (Spasmo-lyt) in patients with motor urge syndrome (detrusor instability): a double-blind, randomised, multicentre, placebo-controlled study. J Clin Res 1:439, 1998

Amarenco G, Marquis P, McCarthy C et al. Qualité de vie des femmes souffrant d´impériosité mictionelle avec ou sans fuites: étude prospective aprés traitement par oxybutinine (1701 cas). Presse Medicale 27:5, 1998

Åmark P, Nergårdh A. Influence of adrenergic agonists and antagonists on urethral pressure, bladder pressure and detrusor hyperactivity in children with myelodysplasia. Acta Paed Scand 80:824, 1991

Åmark P. The effect of noradrenaline on the contractile response of the urinary bladder. Scand J Urol Nephrol 20:203, 1986

Anderson RU, Mobley D, Blank B et al. Once daily controlled versus immediate release oxybutynin chloride for urge urinary incontinence. OROS Oxybutynin Study Group. J Urol 161:1809, 1999

Andersson KE, Appell R, Cardozo LD et al. Pharmacological treatment of urinary incontinence. In: Incontinence, 1st International Consultation on Incontinence. Abrams P, Khoury S & Wein A (eds), Plymbridge Distributors Ltd, UK, pp447-486, 1999

Andersson KE, Appell R, Cardozo LD et al. The pharmacological treatment of urinary incontinence. BJU Int 84:923, 1999

Andersson K-E, Bengtsson B, Paulsen O. Desamino-8-D-Arginine vasopressin (DDAVP): Pharmacology and clinical use. Drugs of Today 24:509, 1988

Andersson K-E, Ek A, Hedlund H et al. Effects of prazosin on isolated human urethra and in patients with lower motor neuron lesions. Invest Urol 19:39, 1981.

Andersson K-E, Forman A. Effects of calcium channel blockers on urinary tract smooth muscle. Acta Pharmacol Toxicol Suppl II: 90, 1978

Andersson K-E, Fovaeus M, Morgan E et al. Comparative effects of five different calcium channel blockers on the atropine resistant contraction in electrically stimulated rabbit urinary bladder. Neurourol Urodyn 5:579, 1986

Andersson K-E, Lepor H, Wyllie M. Prostatic α1-adrenoceptors and uroselectivity. Prostate 30:202, 1997

Andersson KE, Persson K. The L-arginine/nitric oxide pathway and non-adrenergic, non-cholinergic relaxation of the lower urinary tract. Gen Pharmacol 24:833, 1993.

Andersson K-E. Clinical pharmacology of potassium channel openers. Pharmacol Toxicol 70:244, 1992

Andersson K-E. Current concepts in the treatment of disorders of micturition. Drugs 35:477 1988

Andersson KE. Neurotransmission and drug effects in urethral smooth muscle. Scand J. Urol. Nephrol. Suppl. 207: 26, 2001.

Andersson K-E. The pharmacology of lower urinary tract smooth muscles and penile erectile tissues. Pharmacol Rev 45: 253, 1993

Antweiler H. Zur Pharmakologie und Toxikologie von Azoniaspiranen in der Nortropin- bzw. Pseudonortropin-Reihe. Arzneimittel Forsch/Drug Res 16: 1581, 1966

Appell RA, Sand P, Dmochowski R et al. Prospective randomized controlled trial of extended-release oxybutynin chloride and tolterodine tartrate in the treatment of overactive bladder: results of the OBJECT Study. Mayo Clin Proc 76:358, 2001

Arnold EP. Tamsulosin in men with confirmed bladder outlet obstruction: a clinical and urodynamic analysis from a single centre in New Zealand. BJU Int 87:24, 2001

Awad SA, Bryniak S, Downie JW et al. The treatment of the uninhibited bladder with dicyclomine. J Urol 117:161, 1977

Awad SA, Downie JW, KirilutaHG. Alpha-adrenergic agents in urinary disorders of the proximal urethra, part I: sphincteric incontinence. Br J Urol 50: 332, 1978

Babu R, Vaidyanathan S, Sankaranarayan A et al. Effect of intravesical instillation of varying doses of verapamil (20 mg, 40 mg, 80 mg) upon urinary bladder function in chronic traumatic paraplegics with overactive detrusor function. Int J Clin Pharmacol 28:350, 1990

Baigrie RJ, Kelleher JP, Fawcett DP et al. Oxybutynin: is it safe? Br J Urol 62: 319, 1988

Bailer J C. The powerful placebo and the wizard of Oz. New England Journal of Medicine 344:21, 2001

Baldessarini KJ. Drugs in the treatment of psychiatric disorders. In: Gilman et al. (Eds.) The pharmacological basis of therapeutics, 7th ed., McMillan Publishing Co., pp 387-445,1985

Bayliss M, Wu C, Newgreen D et al. A quantitative study of atropine-resistant contractile responses in human detrusor smooth muscle, from stable, unstable and obstructed bladders. J Urol 162:1833, 1999

Beck RP, Arnausch T, King C. Results of treating 210 patients with detrusor overactivity incontinence of urine. Am J Obstet Gynecol 125:593, 1976

Beecher H K. The powerful placebo. JAMA 159:1602, 1955

Beisland HO, Fossberg E, Moer A et al. Urethral insufficiency in postmenopausal females:treatment with phenylpropanolamine and estriol separately and in combination. Urol Int 39:211, 1984

Bent AE, Richardson DA, Ostergard DR. Diagnosis of lower urinary tract disorders in postmenopausal patients. Am J Obstet Gynecol 145:218, 1983

Bergman A, Karram MM, Bhatia NN. Changes in urethral cytology following estrogen administration. Gynecol Obstet Invest 29:211, 1990

Bhatia NN, Bergman A, Karram MM. Effects of estrogen on urethral function in women with urinary incontinence. Am J Obstet Gynecol 160:176, 1989

Bigger JT, Giardina EG, Perel JM et al . Cardiac antiarrhythmic effect of imipramine hydrochloride. N Engl J Med 296: 206, 977.

Birns J, Lukkari E, Malone-Lee JG. A randomized controlled trial comparing the efficacy of controlled-release oxybutynin tablets (10 mg once daily) with conventional oxybutynin tablets (5 mg twice daily) in patients whose symptoms were stabilized on 5 mg twice daily of oxybutynin. BJU Int 85:793, 2000

Blaivas JG, Appell RA, Fantl JA et al. Standards of efficacy for evaluation of treatment outcomes in urinary incontinence: Recommendations of the Urodynamic Society. Neurourol Urodyn 16:145, 1997

Blaivas JG Labib KB, Michalik J et al. Cystometric response to propantheline in detrusor hyperreflexia: therapeutic implications. J Urol 124:259, 1980

Blok BF, Sturms LM, Holstege G.Brain activation during micturition in women. Brain 121: 2033, 1948.

Bonev AD, Nelson MT. Muscarinic inhibition of ATP-sensitive K+ channels by protein kinase C in urinary bladder smooth muscle. Am J Physiol 265:C1723, 1993

Bonnesen T, Tikjøb G, Kamper AL et al. Effect of emepronium bromide (Cetiprin) on symptoms and urinary bladder function after transurethral resection of the prostate. A double-blind randomized trial. Urol Int 39:318, 1984

Brading AF. A myogenic basis for the overactive bladder. Urology 50 (Suppl 6A):57, 1997

Braverman A, Legos J, Young W et al. M2 receptors in genito-urinary smooth muscle pathology. Life Sci 64:429, 1999.

Braverman AS, Luthin GR, Ruggieri MR. M2 muscarinic receptor contributes to contraction of the denervated rat urinary bladder. Am J Physiol 275:R1654, 1998

Braverman, AS, Ruggieri MR, Pontari MA. The M2 muscarinic receptor subtype mediates cholinergic bladder contractions in patients with neurogenic bladder dysfunction. J Urol 165 Suppl:36 (abstract 147)

Brendler CB, Radebaugh LC, Mohler JL. Topical oxybutynin chloride for relaxation of dysfunctional bladders. J Urol 141:1350, 1989

Bridgewater M, MacNeil HF, Brading AF. Regulation of tone in pig urethral smooth muscle. J Urol 150:223, 1993.

Briggs KS, Castleden CM, Asher MJ. The effect of flavoxate on uninhibited detrusor contractions and urinary incontinence in the elderly. J Urol 123:665, 1980

Brynne N, Dalen P, Alvan G. Influence of CYP2D6 polymorphism on the pharmacokinetics and pharmacodynamics of tolterodine. Clin Pharmacol Ther 63:529, 1998

Brynne N, Stahl MMS, Hallén B. Pharmacokinetics and pharmacodynamics of tolterodine in man: a new drug for the treatment of urinary bladder overactivity. Int J Clin Pharmacol Ther 35:287, 1997

Bushman W, Steers WD, Meythaler JM. Voiding dysfunction in patients with spastic paraplegia: urodynamic evaluation and response to continuous intrathecal baclofen. Neurol Urodyn 12:163, 1993

Butera JA, Antane MM, Antane SA et al. Design and SAR of novel potassium channel openers targeted for urge urinary incontinence. 1. N-Cyanoguanidine bioisosteres possessing in vivo bladder selectivity. J Med Chem 43:1187, 2000

Buyse G, Verpoorten C, Vereecken R et al. Treatment of neurogenic bladder dysfunction in infants and children with neurospinal dysraphism with clean intermittent (self)catheterisation and optimized intraversical oxybutynin hydrochloride therapy. Eur J Pediatr Surg 5 Suppl 1: 31, 1995

Caine M, Gin S, Pietra C et al. Antispasmodic effects of flavoxate, MFCA, and Rec 15/2053 on smooth muscle of human prostate and urinary bladder. Urology 37:390, 1991

Caine M. The present role of alpha-adrenergic blockers in the treatment of benign prostatic hyperplasia. J Urol 136:1, 1986

Cardozo L, Chapple CR, Toozs-Hobson P et al. Efficacy of trospium chloride in patients with detrusor instability: a placebo-controlled, randomized, double-blind, multicentre clinical trial. BJU Int 85:659, 2000

Cardozo L, Rekers H, Tapp A et al. Oestriol in the treatment of postmenopausal urgency: a multicentre study. Maturitas 18:47, 1993

Cardozo LD, Cooper D, Versi E. Oxybutynin chloride in the management of idiopathic detrusor instability. Neurourol Urodyn 6:256, 1987

Cardozo LD, Kelleher CJ. Sex hormones, the menopause and urinary problems. Gyn Endocrinol 9:75, 1995

Cardozo LD, Stanton SL, Robinson H et al. Evaluation on flurbiprofen in detrusor instability. Br Med J 280:281, 1980

Cardozo LD, Stanton SL. A comparison between bromocriptine and indomethacin in the treatment of detrusor instability. J Urol 123:399, 1980

Cardozo LD, Stanton SL. An objective comparison of the effects of parenterally administered drug in patients suffering from detrusor instability. J Urol 122:58, 1979

Castleden CM, Duffin HM, Gulati RS. Double-blind study of imipramine and placebo for incontinence due to bladder instability. Age Ageing 15:299, 1986.

Castleden CM, Duffin HM, Millar AW. Dicyclomine hydrochloride in detrusor instability: A controlled clinical pilot study. J Clin Exper Gerontol 9:265, 1987

Castleden CM, George CF, Renwick AG et al. Imipramine - a possible alternative to current therapy for urinary incontinence in the elderly. J Urol 125: 318, 1981

Castleden CM, Morgan B. The effect of ß-adrenoceptor agonists on urinary incontinence in the elderly. Br J Clin Pharmacol 10:619, 1980

Caulfield MP, Birdsall NJ. International Union of Pharmacology. XVII. Classification of muscarinic acetylcholine receptors. Pharmacol Rev 50:279, 1998

Cazzulani P, Pietra C, Abbiati GA et al. Pharmacological activities of the main metabolite of flavoxate 3-methylflavone-8-carboxylic acid. Arzneim Forsch /Drug Res 38:379, 1988

Chancellor M, Freedman S, Mitcheson HD et al. Tolterodine, an effective and well tolerated treatment for urge incontinence and othe overactive bladder symptoms. Drug Invest 19:83, 2000

Chandiramani VA, Peterson T, Duthie GS et al. Urodynamic changes during therapeutic intravesical instillations of capsaicin. Br J Urol 77:792, 1996

Chapple CR, Parkhouse H, Gardener C et al Double-blind, placebo-controlled, cross-over study of flavoxate in the treatment of idiopathic detrusor instability. Br J Urol 66:491, 1990

Chapple CR. Muscarinic receptor antagonists in the treatment of overactive bladder.Urology (Suppl 5A):33, 2000

Choppin A, Eglen RM. Pharmacological characterisation of muscarinic receptors in feline and human isolated ciliary muscle. Br J Pharmacol 129:206P, 2000

Clemett D, Jarvis B. Tolterodine a review of its use in the treatment of overactive bladder. Drugs Aging 18:277, 2001

Cockayne DA, Hamilton SG, Zhu QM et al. Urinary bladder hyporeflexia and reduced pain-related behaviour in P2X3-deficient mice. Nature 407:1011, 2000

Collas D, Malone-Lee JG. The pharmacokinetic properties of rectal oxybutynin - a possible alternative to intravesical administration. Neurourol Urodyn 16:346, 1997

Collste L, Lindskog M. Phenylpropanolamine in treatment of female stress urinary incontinence. Double-blind placebo controlled study in 24 patients. Urology 40:398, 1987

Connolly MJ, Astridge PS, White EG et al. Torsades de pointes complicating treatment with terodiline. Lancet 338:344, 1991

Craft RM, Cohen SM, Porreca F. Long-lasting desensitization of bladder afferents following intravesical resiniferatoxin and capsaicin in the rat. Pain 61: 317, 1995

Cruz F, Avelino A, Coimbra A. Desensitization follows excitation of bladder primary afferents by intravesical capsaicin, as shown by c-fos activation in the spinal cord. Pain 64:553, 1996

Cruz F, Guimaraes M, Silva C et al. Desensitization of bladder sensory fibers by intravesical capsaicin has long lasting clinical and urodynamic effects in patients with hyperactive or hypersensitive bladder dysfunction. J Urol 157:585, 1997

Cruz F, Guimaraes M, Silva C et al. Suppression of bladder hyperreflexia by intravesical resiniferatoxin. Lancet 350:640, 1997

Cruz F. Desensitization of bladder sensory fibers by intravesical capsaicin or capsaicin analogs. A new strategy for treatment of urge incontinence in patients with spinal detrusor hyperreflexia or bladder hypersensitivity disorders. Inter Urogynecol J Pelvic Floor Dysfunct 9: 214, 1998.

Culp DJ, Luo W, Richardson LA et al. Both M1 and M3 receptors regulate exocrine secretion by mucous acini. Am J Physiol 271:C1963, 1996

D'Agostino G, Bolognesi ML, Luchelli A et al. Prejunctional muscarinic inhibitory control of acetylcholine release in the human isolated detrusor : involvement of the M_4 receptor serotype. Br J pharmacol 129: 493, 2000.

Dahm TL, Ostri P, Kristensen JK et al Flavoxate treatment of micturition disorders accompanying benign prostatic hypertrophy: a double-blind placebo-controlled multicenter investigation. Urol Int 55:205, 1995

Dasgupta P, Chandiramani V, Parkinson MC et al. Treating the human bladder with capsaicin: is it safe? Eur Urol 33:28, 1998

de Groat WC, Booth AM, Yoshimura N. Neurophysiology of micturition and its modification in animal models of human disease. In: The Autonomic Nervous System. Vol. 6, Chapter 8, Nervous Control of the Urogenital System, ed. by C.A. Maggi. Harwood Academic Publishers, London, U.K., pp. 227-89, 1993

de Groat WC, Downie JW, Levin RM et al. Basic Neurophysiology and Neuropharmacology. In Incontinence, 1st International Consultation on Incontinence, Abrams P, Khoury S, Wein A (eds), Plymbridge Distributors Ltd, UK, pp 105-154, 1999.

de Groat WC, Yoshimura N. Pharmacology of the lower urinary tract. Annu Rev Pharmacol Toxicol 41:691, 2001

de Groat WC. A neurological basis for the overactive bladder. Urology 50 (Suppl 6A):36, 1997

De Ridder D, Baert L. Vanilloids and the overactive bladder. BJU Int 86:172, 2000

De Ridder D, Chandiramani V, Dasgupta P et al. Intravesical capsaicin as a treatment for refractory detrusor hyperreflexia: a dual center study with long-term followup. J Urol 158:2087, 1997

Deaney C, Glickman S, Gluck T et al. Intravesical atropine suppression of detrusor hyperreflexia in multiple sclerosis. J Neurol Neurosurg Psychiatry 65:957, 1998

DeLancey JOL. The pathophysiology of stress urinary incontinence in women and its implications for surgical treatment. World J Urol 15:268, 1997

DiMichele S, Sillén U, Engel JA et al. Desmopressin and vasopressin increase locomotor activity in the rat via a central mechanism: implications for nocturnal enuresis. J Urol 156:1164, 1996

Diokno AC, Hyndman CW, Hardy DA et al. Comparison of action of imipramine (Tofranil) and propantheline (Probanthine) on detrusor contraction. J Urol 107:42, 1972

Diokno AC, Taub M. Ephedrine in treatment of urinary incontinence. Urology 5: 624, 1975

Dorschner W, Stolzenburg JU, Griebenow R et al. Efficacy and cardiac safety of propiverine in elderly patients - a double-blind, placebo-controlled clinical study. Eur Urol 37:702, 2000

Douchamps J, Derenne F, Stockis A et al. The pharmacokinetics of oxybutynin in man. Eur J Clin Pharmacol 35:515, 1988

Downie JW, Twiddy DAS, Awad SA. Antimuscarinic and noncompetitive antagonist properties of dicyclomine hydrochloride in isolated human and rabbit bladder muscle. J Pharmacol Exp Ther 201:662, 1977

Downie, JW, Karmazyn M. Mechanical trauma to bladder epithelium liberates prostanoids which modulate neurotransmission in rabbit detrusor muscle. J Pharmacol Exp Ther 230:445, 1984

Drutz HP, Appell RA, Gleason D et al. Clinical efficacy and safety of tolterodine compared to oxybutynin and placebo in patients with overactive bladder. Int Urogynecol J Pelvic Floor Dysfunct 10:283, 1999

Dwyer PL, Teele JS. Prazosin: a neglected cause of genuine stress incontinence. Obstet Gynecol 79: 117, 1992.

Eckford SD, Swami KS, Jackson SR et al. Desmopressin in the treatment of nocturia and enuresis in patients with multiple sclerosis. Br J Urol 74:733, 1994

Eglen RM, Hegde SS, Watson N. Muscarinic receptor subtypes and smooth muscle function. Pharmacol Rev 48:531, 1996

Eglen RM, Nahorski SR. The muscarinic M5 receptor: a silent or emerging subtype? Br J Pharmacol 130:13, 2000

Ek A, Andersson K-E, Gullberg B et al. The effects of long-term treatment with norephedrine on stress incontinence and urethral closure profile. Scand J Urol Neprol 12:105, 1978

Ekström B, Andersson K-E, Mattiasson A. Urodynamic effects of intravesical instillation of atropine and phentolamine in patients with detrusor hyperactivity. J Urol 149:155, 1992

Enskat R, Deaney CN, Glickman S. Systemic effects of intravesical atropine sulphate. BJU Int 87:613, 2001

Enzelsberger H, Helmer, H, Kurz C. Intravesical instillation of of oxybutynin in woman with idiopathic detrusor instability: a randomised trial. Br J Obstet Gynaecol 102:929, 1995

Eri L M, Tveter K J. α-Blockade in the treatment of symptomatic benign prostatic hyperplasia. J Urol 154:923, 1995

Fall M, Lindstrom S, Mazieres L. A bladder-to-bladder cooling reflex in the cat. J Physiol 427:281, 1990

Fantl JA, Bump RC, Robinson D et al. Efficay of estrogen supplementation in the treatment of urinary incontinence. Obstet Gynecol 88:745, 1996

Fantl JA, Cardozo LD, McClish DK et al. Estrogen therapy in the management of urinary incontinence in postmenopausal women:a meta-analysis. First report of the Hormones and Urogenital Therapy Committee. Obstet Gynecol 83:12, 1994

Fantl JA, Wyman JF, Anderson RL et al. Postmenopausal urinary incontinence: comparison between non-estrogen and estrogen supplemented women. Obstet Gynecol 71:823, 1988

Ferrara P, D'Aleo CM, Tarquini E et al. Side-effects of oral or intravesical oxybutynin chloride in children with spina bifida. BJU Int 87:674, 2001.

Finkbeiner AE. Is bethanechol chloride clinically effective in promoting bladder emptying : a literature review. J Urol 134:443, 1985

Fischer CP, Diokno A, Lapides J. The anticholinergic effects of dicyclomine hydrochloride for uninhibited neurogenic bladder dysfunction. J Urol 120:328, 1978

Fowler CJ, Jewkes D, McDonald WI et al. Intravesical capsaicin for neurogenic bladder dysfunction. Lancet 339:1239, 1992

Fowler CJ. Intravesical treatment of overactive bladder. Urology 55(Suppl 5A):60, 2000

Fredrikson S. Nasal spray desmopressin treatment of bladder dysfunction in patients with multiple sclerosis. Acta Neurol Scand 94:31, 1996

Fusgen I, Hauri D. Trospium chloride: an effective option for medical treatment of bladder overactivity. Int J Clin Pharmacol Ther 38:223, 2000

Gajewski JB, Awad SA. Oxybutynin versus propantheline in patients with multiple sclerosis and detrusor hyperreflexia. J Urol 135:966, 1986

Geirsson G, Fall M, Sullivan L. Clinical and urodynamic effects of intravesical capsaicin treatment in patients with chronic traumatic spinal detrusor hypereflexia. J Urol 154:1825, 1995

Giardina EG, Bigger JT Jr, Glassman AH et al. The electrocardiographic and antiarrhythmic effects of imipramine hydrochloride at therapeutic plasma concentrations. Circulation 60:1045, 1979

Gilbert AM, Antane MM, Argentieri TM et al. Design and SAR of novel potassium channel openers targeted for urge urinary incontinence. 2. Selective and potent benzylamino cyclobutenediones. J Med Chem 43:1203, 2000

Gilja I, Radej M, Kovacic M et al. Conservative treatment of female stress incontinence with imipramine. J Urol 132: 909, 1984

Gleason DM, Reilly SA, Bottacini MR et al. The urethral continence zone and its relation to stress incontinence. J Urol 112:81, 1974

Glickman S, Tsokkos N, Shah PJ. Intravesical atropine and suppression of detrusor hypercontractility in the neuropathic bladder. A preliminary study. Paraplegia 33:36, 1995

Gnad H, Burmucic R, Petritsch P et al. Conservative therapy of female stress incontinence. Double-blind study with the alpha-sympathomimetic midodrin. Fortschr Med 102:578, 1984 (in German)

Grady D, Brown JS, Vittinghoff E et al. Postmenopausal hormones and incontinence: the Heart and Estrogen/Progestin Replacement Study. Obstet Gynecol 97:116, 2001

Grüneberger A. Treatment of motor urge incontinence with clenbuterol and flavoxate hydrochloride. Br J Obstet Gynaecol 91:275, 1984

Guarneri L, Robinson E, Testa R. A review of flavoxate: pharmacology and mechanism of action. Drugs Today 30:91, 1994

Gupta SK, Sathyan G. Pharmacokinetics of an oral once-a-day controlled-release oxybutynin formulation compared with immediate-release oxybutynin. J Clin Pharmacol 39: 289, 1999.

Habler HJ, Janig W, Koltzenburg M. Activation of unmyelinated afferent fibres by mechanical stimuli and inflammation of the urinary bladder in the cat. J Physiol 425:545, 1990

Hachen HJ. Clinical and urodynamic assessment of alpha adrenolytic therapy in patients with neurogenic bladder function. Paraplegia 18:229, 1980

Harriss DR, Marsh KA, Birmingham AT et al. Expression of muscarinic M3-receptors coupled to inositol phospholipid hydrolysis in human detrusor cultured smooth muscle cells. J Urol 154:1241, 1995

Haruno A, Yamasaki Y, Miyoshi K et al. Effects of propiverine hydrochloride and its metabolites on isolated guinea pig urinary bladder. Folia Pharmacol Japon 94:145, 1989

Haruno A. Inhibitory effects of propiverine hydrochloride on the agonist-induced or spontaneous contractions of various isolated muscle preparations. Arzneim-Forsch /Drug Res 42:815, 1992

Hashimoto S, Kigoshi S, Muramatsu I. Nitric oxide-dependent and -independent neurogenic relaxation of isolated dog urethra. Eur J Pharmacol 231:209, 1993

Haustein KO, Huller G. On the pharmacokinetics and metabolism of propiverine in man. Eur J Drug Metab Pharmacokinet 13:81, 1988

Hedlund H, Andersson K-E, Mattiasson A. Effects of pinacidil on detrusor instability in men with outlet obstruction. J Urol 146:1345, 1991

Hegde SS, Choppin A, Bonhaus D et al. Functional role of M2 and M3 muscarinic receptors in the urinary bladder of rats in vitro and in vivo. Br J Pharmacol 120:1409, 1997

Hegde SS, Eglen RM. Muscarinic receptor subtypes modulating smooth muscle contractility in the urinary bladder. Life Sci 64:419, 1999

Hehir M, Fitzpatrick JM. Oxybutynin and prevention of urinary incontinence in spina bifida. Eur Urol 11:254, 1985

Henriksson L, Andersson K-E, Ulmsten U. The urethral pressure profiles in continent and stress incontinent women. Scand J Urol Nephrol 13:5, 1979

Hextall A. Oestrogens and lower urinary tract function. Maturitas 36:83, 2000

Hills CJ, Winter SA, Balfour JA. Tolterodine. Drugs 55:813, 1998

Hilton P, Hertogs K, Stanton SL. The use of desmopressin (DDAVP) for nocturia in women with multiple sclerosis. J Neurol Neurosurg Psychiatry 46: 854, 1983

Hilton P, Stanton SL. The use of intravaginal oestrogen cream in genuine stress incontinence. Br J Obstet Gynecol 90:940, 1983

Hilton P, Stanton SL. The use of desmopressin (DDAVP) in nocturnal frequency in the female. Br J Urol 54:252, 1982

Hilton P, Stanton SL. Urethral pressure measurement by microtransducer: the results in symptom-free women and in those with genuine stress incontinence. Br J Obstet Gynaecol 90:919, 1983

Hilton P, Tweddel AL, Mayne C. Oral and intravaginal estrogens alone and in combination with alpha adrenergic stimulation in genuine stress incontinence. Int Urogyn J 12:80, 1990

Hjalmas K. Desmopressin treatment: current status. Scand J Urol Nephrol Suppl. 202:70, 1999.

Höfner K, Halaska M, Primus G et al. Tolerability and efficacy of Trospium chloride in a long-term treatment (52 weeks) in patients with urge-syndrome: a double-blind, controlled, multicentre clinical trial. Neurourol Urodyn 19:487, 2000.

Holmes DM, Montz FJ, Stanton SL. Oxybutinin versus propantheline in the management of detrusor instability. A patient-regulated variable dose trial. Br J Obstet Gynaecol 96:607, 1989

Horowitz M, Combs AJ, Gerdes D. Desmopressin for nocturnal incontinence in the spina bifida population. J Urol 158:2267, 1997

Howe BB, Halterman TJ, Yochim CL et al. ZENECA ZD6169: A novel KATP channel opener with in vivo selectivity for urinary bladder. J Pharmacol Exp Ther 274:884, 1995

Hoyle CHV, Chapple C, Burnstock G. Isolated human bladder: evidence for an adenine dinucleotide acting on P2X-purinoceptors and for purinergic transmission. Eur J Pharmacol 174:115 1989

Hrobjartsson A, Gotzsche C. Is the Placebo Powerless? New England Journal of Medicine 344:1594, 2001

Hughes KM, Lang JCT, Lazare R et al. Measurement of oxybutynin and its N-desethyl metabolite in plasma, and its application to pharmacokinetic studies in young, elderly and frail elderly volunteers. Xenobiotica 22:859, 1992

Hunsballe JM, Djurhuus JC. Clinical options for imipramine in the management of urinary incontinence. Urol Res 29:118, 2001

Hussain RM, Hartigan-Go K, Thomas SHL et al. Effect of oxybutynin on the QTc interval in elderly patients with urinary incontinence. Br J Clin Pharmacol 37:485P, 1994

Igawa Y, Komiyama I, Nishizawa S et al. Intravesical capsaicin inhibits autonomic dysreflexia in patients with spinal cord injury. Neurourol Urodyn 15: 374, 1996

Igawa Y, Yamazaki Y, Takeda H et al. Functional and molecular biological evidence for a possible beta3-adrenoceptor in the human detrusor muscle. Br J Pharmacol 126:819, 1999

Igawa Y, Yamazaki Y, Takeda H et al. Relaxant effects of isoproterenol and selective beta3-adrenoceptor agonists on normal, low compliant and hyperreflexic human bladders. J Urol 165:240, 2001

Ikeda K, Kobayashi S, Suzuki M et al. Effect of YM905, a novel muscarinic receptor antagonist, on salivary gland and bladder. Japan J Pharmacol 76 (Suppl1):243, 1998.

Ikeda K, Suzuki M, Kobayashi S et al. YM905, a novel antimuscarinic agent displays tissue preference for the urinary bladder M3 receptor. FASEB J 13: A157, 1999.

Iselin CE, Schmidlin F, Borst F et al. Oxybutynin in the treatment of early detrusor instability after transurethral resection of the prostate. Br J Urol 79: 915, 1997

Ishiko O, Hirai K, Sumi T et al. Hormone replacement therapy plus pelvic floor muscle exercise for postmenopausal stress incontinence. A randomized, controlled trial. J Reprod Med 46:213, 2001

Ishiko O, Ushiroyama T, Saji F et al. beta(2)-Adrenergic agonists and pelvic floor exercises for female stress incontinence. Int J Gynaecol Obstet 71:39, 2000

Ishizuka O, Mattiasson A, Andersson K-E. Urodynamic effects of intravesical resiniferatoxin and capsaicin in conscious rats with and without outflow obstruction. J Urol 154:611, 1995

Jackson S, Shepherd A, Abrams P. The effect of oestradiol on objective urinary leakage in postmenopausal stress incontinence; a double blind placebo controlled trial. Neurourol Urodyn 15:322, 1996

Janig W, Morrison JF. Functional properties of spinal visceral afferents supplying abdominal and pelvic organs, with special emphasis on visceral nociception. Prog Brain Res 67:87, 1986

Janknegt RA, Zweers HMM, Delaere KPJ et al. Oral desmopressin as a new treament modality for primary nocturnal enuresis in adolescents and adults: a double-blind, randomized, multicenter study. J Urol 157:513, 1997

Jarvis GJ, Hall S, Stamp S et al. An assessment of urodynamic investigation in incontinent women. Br J Obstet Gynecol 87:184, 1980

Jensen D Jr. Pharmacological studies of the uninhibited neurogenic bladder. II. The influence of cholinergic excitatory and inhibitory drugs on the cystometrogram of neurological patients with normal and uninhibited neurogenic bladder. Acta Neurol Scand 64:175, 1981

Jensen D. Uninhibited neurogenic bladder treated with prazosin. Scand J Urol Nephrol 15:229, 1981.

Jeremy JY, Tsang V, Mikhailidis DP et al. Eicosanoid synthesis by human urinary bladder mucosa: pathological implications. Br J Urol 59:36, 1987

Jollys JV, Jollys JC, Wilson J et al. Does sexual equality extend to urinary symptoms? Neurourol. Urodyn 12:391, 1993

Jonas D. Treatment of female stress incontinence with midodrine: preliminary report. J Urol 118:980, 1982

Jonville AP, Dutertre JP, Autret E et al. Effets indésirables du chlorure d´oxybutynine (Ditropan®). Therapie 47:389, 1992

Jünemann KP, Al-Shukri S. Efficacy and tolerability of trospium chloride and tolterodine in 234 patients with urge-syndrome: a double-blind, placebo-controlled multicentre clinical trial. Neurourol Urodyn 19:488, 2000

Kachur JF, Peterson JS, Carter JP et al. R and S enantiomers of oxybutynin: pharmacological effects in guinea pig bladder and intestine. J Pharmacol Exp Ther 247: 867, 1988

Kaisary AV. Beta-adrenoceptor blockade in the treatment of female stress urinary incontinence. J d´Urol (Paris) 90:351, 1984

Kaplinsky R, Greenfield S, Wan J et al. Expanded followup of intravesical oxybutynin use in children with neurogenic bladder. J Urol 156:753, 1996

Karram MM, Yeko TR, Sauer MV et al. Urodynamic changes following hormone replacement therapy in women with premature ovarian failure. Obstet Gynecol 74:208, 1989

Kasabian NG, Vlachiotis JD, Lais A et al. The use of intravesical oxybutynin chloride in patients with detrusor hypertonicity and detrusor hyperreflexia. J Urol 151:944, 1994

Katz IR, Sands LP, Bilker W et al. Identification of medications that cause cognitive impairment in older people: the case of oxybutynin chloride. J Am Geriatr Soc 46:8, 1998

Kim YH, Bird ET, Priebe M et al. The role of oxybutynin in spinal cord injured patients with indwelling catheters. J Urol 158:2083, 1996

Kinn A-C, Larsson PO. Desmopressin: a new principle for symptomatic treatment of urgency and incontinence in patients with multiple sclerosis. Scand J Urol Nephrol 24:109, 1990

Kinn AC, Lindskog. Estrogens and phenylpropanolamine in combination for stress urinary incontinence in postmenopausal women. Urology 32:273, 1988

Komersova K, Rogerson JW, Conway EL et al. The effect of levcromakalim (BRL 38227) on bladder function in patients with high spinal cord lesions. Br J Pharmacol 39:207, 1995

Krane RJ, Olsson CA. Phenoxybenzamine in neurogenic bladder dysfunction, part II: clinical considerations. J Urol 104:612, 1973

Krichevsky VP, Pagala MK, Vaydovsky I et al. Function of M3 muscarinic receptors in the rat urinary bladder following partial outlet obstruction. J Urol 161:644, 1999

Kums JJM, Delhaas EM. Intrathecal baclofen infusion in patients with spasticity and neurogenic bladder disease. Preliminary results. World J Urol 9: 99, 1991

Kuo H-C. Inhibitory effect of capsaicin on detrusor contractility: Further study in the presence of ganglionic blocker and neurokinin receptor antagonist in the rat urinary bladder. Urol Int 59:95, 1997

Larsen JJ. a- and ß-Adrenoceptors in the detrusor muscle and bladder base of the pig and ß-adrenoceptors in the detrusor of man. Br J Urol 65:215, 1979

Lazzeri M, Beneforti P, Spinelli M et al. Intravesical resiniferatoxin for the treatment of hypersensitive disorder: a randomized placebo controlled study. J Urol 164:676, 2000

Lazzeri M, Beneforti P, Turini. Urodynamic effects of intravesical resiniferatoxin in humans: preliminary results in stable and unstable detrusor. J Urol 158:2093, 1997

Lepor, H., Machi, G. Comparison of the AUA symptom index in unselected males and females between 55 and 79 years of age. Urology 42:36, 1993

Leslie CA, Pavlakis AJ, Wheeler JS et al. Release of arachidonate cascade products by the rabbit bladder: neurophysiological significance? J Urol 132:376, 1984

Levin RM, Ruggieri MR, Wein AJ. Identification of receptor subtypes in the rabbit and human urinary bladder by selective radioligand binding. J Urol 139:844, 1988

Lin HH, Sheu BC, Lo MC et al. Comparison of treatment outcomes for imipramine for female genuine stress incontinence. Br J Obstet Gynaecol 106:1089, 1999

Lincoln J, Burnstock G. Autonomic innervation of the urinary bladder and urethra. In: The Autonomic Nervous System. Vol. 6, Chapter 2, Nervous Control of the Urogenital System, ed. CA Maggi, London: Harwood Academic Publisher, pp 33-68, 1993

Lindholm P, Lose G. Terbutaline (Bricanyl®) in the treatment of female urge incontinence. Urol Int 41:158, 1986

Lipworth BJ. Clinical pharmacology of ß3-adrenoceptors. Br J Clin Pharmacol 43:291, 1996

Lose G, Englev E. Oestradiol-releasing vaginal ring versus oestriol vaginal pessaries in the treatment of bothersome lower urinary tract symptoms. 107:1029, 2000

Lose G, Jorgensen L, Thunedborg P. Doxepin in the treatment of female detrusor overactivity: A randomized double-blind crossover study. J Urol 142: 1024, 1989

Lose G, Lindholm D. Clinical and urodynamic effects of norfenefrine in women with stress incontinence. Urol Int 39:298, 1984

Low JA. Urethral behaviour during the involuntary detrusor contraction. Am J Obstet Gynecol 128:321977

Luheshi GN, Zar MA. Presence of non-cholinergic motor transmission in human isolated bladder. J Pharm Pharmacol 42:223, 1990

Lux B, Wiedey K D. Trospium chloride (Spasmex ®) in the treatment of urine incontinence. Therapiewoche 42:302, 1992

Madersbacher H, Halaska M, Voigt R et al. A placebo-controlled, multicentre study comparing the tolerability and efficacy of propiverine and oxybutynin in patients with urgency and urge incontinence. BJU Int 84:646, 1999

Madersbacher H, Jilg G. Control of detrusor hyperreflexia by the intravesical instillation of oxybutynin hydrochloride. Paraplegia 29:84, 1991

Madersbacher H, Knoll M. Intravesical application of oxybutynin: Mode of action in controlling detrusor hyperreflexia. Eur Urol 28:340, 1995

Madersbacher H, Stöhrer M, Richter R et al. High-dose administration of trospium chloride in the treatment of detrusor hyperreflexia. Urologe Ausg A 30: 260, 1991

Madersbacher H, Stöhrer M, Richter R et al. Trospium chloride versus oxybutynin: a randomized, double-blind, multicentre trial in the treatment of detrusor hyper-reflexia. Br J Urol 75:452, 1995

Maggi CA, Barbanti G, Santicioli P et al. Cystometric evidence that capsaicin-sensitive nerves modulate the afferent branch of micturition reflex in humans. J Urol 142:150, 1989

Maggi CA, Borsini F, Lecci A et al. The effect of acute and chronic administration of imipramine on spinal and supraspinal micturition reflexes in rats. J Pharmacol Exp Ther 248:278, 1989

Maggi CA. The dual, sensory and "efferent" function of the capsaicin-sensitive primary sensory neurons in the urinary bladder and urethra. In: The Autonomic Nervous System, vol. 3, Nervous control of the urogenital system. Chapter 11, p 227, Maggi, C. A. (ed.) Harwood Academic Publishers, Chur, Switzerland, pp 383-422, 1993

Malone-Lee J, Lubel D, Szonyi G. Low dose oxybutynin for the unstable bladder. Br Med J 304:1053, 1992

Malone-Lee J, Shaffu B, Anand C et al. Tolterodine: superior tolerability than and comparable efficacy to oxybutynin in individuals 50 years old or older with overactive bladder: a randomized controlled trial. J Urol 165:1452, 2001

Marshall HJ, Beevers DG. Alpha-adrenoceptor blocking drugs and female urinary incontinence: prevalence and reversibility. Br J Clin Pharmacol 42:507, 1996

Martin MR, Schiff AA. Fluphenazine/nortriptyline in the irritative bladder syndrome: a double-blind placebo-controlled study. Br J Urol 56:178, 1984.

Masuda N, Uchida W, Shirai Y et al. Effect of the potassium channel opener YM934 on the contractile response to electrical field stimulation in pig detrusor smooth muscle. J Urol 154:1914, 1995

Matthiesen TB, Rittig S, Norgaard JP et al. Nocturnal polyuria and natriuresis in male patients with nocturia and lower urinary tract symptoms. J Urol 79:825, 1996

Mattiasson A, Ekström B, Andersson K-E. Effects of intravesical instillation of verapamil in patients with detrusor hyperactivity. J Urol 141:174, 1989

McGuire EJ, Wagner FM, Weiss RM. Treatment of autonomic dysreflexia with phenoxybenzamine. J Urol 115:53, 1976

Milani R, Scalambrino S, Milia R et al. Double-blind crossover comparison of flavoxate and oxybutynin in women affected by urinary urge syndrome. Int Urogynecol J 4:3, 1993

Miller K, Atkin B, Moody ML. Drug therapy for nocturnal enuresis. Drugs 44: 47, 1992

Mizunaga M, Miyata M, Kaneko S et al. Intravesical instillation of oxybutynin hydrochloride therapy for patients with a neurogenic bladder. Paraplegia 32:25, 1994

Moffat ME, Harlos S, Kirshen AJ et al. Desmopressin acetate and nocturnal enuresis: how much do we know? Pediatrics 92:420, 1993

Moisey CU, Stephenson TP, Brendler CB. The urodynamic and subjective results of treatment of detrusor instability with oxybutynin chloride. Br J Urol 52:472, 1980

Moore KH, Hay DM, Imrie AE et al. Oxybutynin hydrochloride (3 mg) in the treatment of women with idiopathic detrusor instability. Br J Urol 66:479, 1990

Mullcr C, Siegmund W, Huupponen R et al. Kinetics of propiverine as assessed by radioreceptor assay in poor and extensive metabolizers of debrisoquine. Eur J Drug Metab Pharmacokinet 18:265, 1993

Mundy AR, Abrams P, Chapple CR et al. Darifenacin, the first selective M3 antagonist for overactive bladder: comparison with oxybutynin on ambulatory urodynamic monitoring and salivary flow. International Continence Society 2001.

Musiani U. A partially successful successful attempt at medical treatment of urinary stress incontinence in women. Urol Int 27:405, 1972

Naglo AS, Nergårdh A, Boréus LO. Influence of atropine and isoprenaline on detrusor hyperactivity in children with neurogenic bladder. Scand J Urol Nephrol 15:97, 1981

Nasu K, Moriyama N, Fukasawa R et al. Quantification and distribution of alpha1-adrenoceptor subtype mRNAs in human proximal urethra. Br J Pharmacol 123:1289, 1998

Nergårdh A, Boréus LO, Naglo AS. Characterization of the adrenergic beta-receptors in the urinary bladder of man and cat. Acta Pharmacol Toxicol 40:14, 1977

Neveus T, Lackgren G, Tuvemo T et al. Enuresis--background and treatment. Scand J Urol Nephrol Suppl 206:1, 2000

Newgreen DT, Anderson CWP, Carter AJ et al. Darifenacin - a novel bladder-selective agent for the treatment of urge incontinence. Neurourol Urodyn 14:95, 1995

Nichols D, Colli E, Goka J et al. Darifenacin demonstrates no effect on cognitive and cardiac function: results from a double-blind, randomised, placebo controlled study. International Continence Society 2001

Nilsson CG, Lukkari E, Haarala M et al. Comparison of a 10-mg controlled release oxybutynin tablet with a 5-mg oxybutynin tablet in urge incontinent patients. Neurourol Urodyn 16:533, 1997

Nilvebrant L, Andersson K-E, Gillberg P-G et al. Tolterodine - a new bladder selective antimuscarinic agent. Eur J Pharmacol 327:195, 1997a

Nilvebrant L, Andersson K-E, Mattiasson A. Characterization of the muscarinic cholinoceptors in the human detrusor. J Urol 134: 418, 1985

Nilvebrant L, Gillberg PG, Sparf B. Antimuscarinic potency and bladder selectivity of PNU-200577, a major metabolite of tolterodine. Pharmacol Toxicol 81:169, 1997c

Nilvebrant L, Hallén B, Larsson G. Tolterodine - A new bladder selective muscarinic receptor antagonist: preclinical pharmacological and clinical data. Life Sci 60:1129, 1997b

Nilvebrant L, Sparf B. Dicyclomine, benzhexol and oxybutynin distinguish between subclasses of muscarinic binding sites. Eur J Pharmacol 123:133, 1986

Noguchi M, Eguchi Y, Ichiki J et al. Therapeutic efficacy of clenbuterol for urinary incontinence after radical prostatectomy. Int J Urol 4:480, 1997

Nørgaard JP, Djurhuus JC, Watanabe H et al. Experience and current status of research into the pathophysiology of nocturnal enuresis. Br J Urol 79:825, 1997

Norhona-Blob L, Kachur, JF. Enantiomers of oxybutynin: in vitro pharmacological characterization at M1, M2 and M3 muscarinic receptors and in vivo effects on urinary bladder contraction, mydriasis and salivary secretion in guinea pigs. J Pharmacol Exp Ther 256:562, 1991

Norlén L. Sundin T, Waagstein F. Effect of beta-adrenoceptor stimulation on the human bladder in vivo. Urol Int 33:355, 1978

Nour S, Svarer C, Kristensen JK et al. Cerebral activation during micturition in normal men. Brain 123:781, 2000.

O´Flynn K J, Thomas D G. Intravesicular instillation of oxybutinin hydrochloride for detrusor hyperreflexia. Br J Urol 72:566, 1993

Oka M, Kimura Y, Itoh Y et al. Brain pertussis toxin-sensitive G proteins are involved in the flavoxate hydrochloride-induced suppression of the micturition reflex in rats. Brain Res 727:91, 1996

Ouslander JG, Blaustein J, Connor A et al. Pharmacokinetics and clinical effects of oxybutynin in geriatric patients. J Urol 140:47, 1988

Ouslander JG, Schnelle JF, Uman G et al. Does oxybutynin add to the effectiveness of prompted voiding for urinary incontinence among nursing home residents? A placebo-controlled trial. J Am Geriatr Soc 43:610, 1995

Ouslander JG, Shih YT, Malone-Lee J et al. Overactive bladder: special considerations in the geriatric population. Am J Manag Care 6(11 Suppl):S599, 2000

Palea S, Artibani W, Ostardo E et al. Evidence for purinergic neurotransmission in human urinary bladder affected by interstitial cystitis. J Urol 150:2007, 1993

Palmer J. Report of a double-blind crossover study of flurbiprofen and placebo in detrusor instability. J Int Med Res 11 Supplement 2:11, 1983

Palmer LS, Zebold K, Firlit CF et al. Complications of intravesical oxybutynin chloride therapy in the pediatric myelomeningocele population. J Urol 157:638, 1997

Pavia J de Ceballos ML, Sanchez de la Cuesta F. Alzheimer's disease: relationship between muscarinic cholinergic receptors, beta-amyloid and tau proteins. Fundam Clin Pharmacol 12:473, 1998.

Perlberg S, Caine M. Adrenergic response of bladder muscle in prostatic obstruction. Urology 20:524, 1982

Petersen T, Husted S, Sidenius P. Prazosin treatment of neurological patients with detrusor hyperreflexia and bladder emptying disability. Scand J Urol Nephrol 23:189, 1989

Petersen T, Nielsen JB, Schroder HD. Intravesical capsaicin in patients with detrusor hyper-reflexia--a placebo-controlled cross-over study. Scand J Urol Nephrol 33:104, 1999

Pietzko A, Dimpfel W, Schwantes U et al. Influence of trospium chloride and oxybutynin on quantitative EEG in healthy volunteers. Eur J Clin Pharmacol 47: 337, 1994

Radley SC, Chapple CR, Bryan NP et al. Effect of methoxamine on maximum urethral pressure in women with genuine stress incontinence: a placebo-controlled, double-blind crossover study. Neurourol Urodyn 20:43, 2001

Raezer DM, Benson GS, Wein AJ et al. The functional approach to the management of the pediatric neuropathic bladder: a clinical study. J Urol 177: 649, 1977

Richter R, Madersbacher H, Stohrer M et al. Double-blind, placebo-controlled clinical study of propiverine in patients suffering from detrusor hyperreflexia. International Medical Society of Paraplegia, 36th Annual Scientific Meeting, May 14-16, 1997, Innsbruck

Ritch AES, Castleden CM, George CFet al. A second look at emepronium bromide in urinary incontinence. Lancet 1:504, 1977

Rittig S, Knudsen UB, Nørgaard JP et al. Abnormal diurnal rhythm of plasma vasopressin andurinary output in patients with enuresis. Am J Physiol 256:F664, 1989

Robson WL, Nørgaard JP, Leung AK. Hyponatremia in patients with nocturnal enuresis treated with DDAVP. Eur J Pediatr 155:959, 1996

Rosario DJ, Leaker BR, Smith DJ et al. A pilot study of the effects of mutiple doses of the M3 muscarinic receptor antagonist darifenacin on ambulatory parameters of detrusor activity in patients with detrusor instability. Neurourol Urodyn 14:464, 1995

Ruffmann R. A review of flavoxate hydrochloride in the treatment of urge incontinence. J Int Med Res 16:317, 1988

Ruggieri MR, Whitmore KE, Levin RM. Bladder purinergic receptors. J Urol 144:176, 1990

Salmon UL, Walter RI, Gast SH. The use of estrogens in the treatment of dysuria and incontinence in postmenopausal women. Am J Obstet Gynecol 14:23, 1941

Schladitz-Keil G, Spahn H, Mutschler E. Determination of bioavailability of the quaternary ammonium compound trospium chloride in man from urinary excretion data. Arzneimittel Forsch/Drug Res 36:984, 1986

Schleyer-Saunders E. Hormone implants for urinary disorders in postmenopausal women. J Am Geriar Soc 24:337, 1976

Schwab M, Ruder H. Hyponatraemia and cerebral convulsion due to DDAVP administration in patients with enuresis nocturna or urine concentration testing. Eur J Pediatr 156:668, 1997

Schwinn DA, Michelotti GA. alpha1-adrenergic receptors in the lower urinary tract and vascular bed: potential role for the alpha1d subtype in filling symptoms and effects of ageing on vascular expression. BJU Int 85 Suppl 2:6, 2000

Serels, S., Stein M. Prospective sydy comparing hyoscyamine, doxazosin, and combination therapy for the treatment of urgency and frequency in women. Neurourol Urodyn 17:31, 1998

Shieh C, Feng J, Buckner SA et al. Functional implication of spare ATP-sensitive K(+) channels in bladder smooth muscle cells. J Pharmacol Exp Ther 296:669, 2001

Siltberg H, Larsson G, Hallen B et al. Validation of cough-induced leak point pressure measurement in the evaluation of pharmacological treatment of stress incontinence. Neurourol Urodyn 18:591, 1999

Silva C, Rio ME, Cruz F. Desensitization of bladder sensory fibers by intravesical resiniferatoxin, a capsaicin analog: long-term results for the treatment of detrusor hyperreflexia. Eur Urol 38:444, 2000

Sjögren C, Andersson K-E, Husted S et al. Atropine resistance of the transmurally stimulated isolated human bladder. J Urol 128:1368, 1982

Skoog SJ, Stokes A, Turner KL. Oral desmopressin: a randomized double-blind placebo controlled study of effectiveness in children with primary nocturnal enuresis. J Urol 158:1035, 1997

Smith DJ, Chapple CR. In vitro response of human bladder smooth muscle in unstable obstructed male bladders: a study of pathophysiological causes? Neurourol Urodyn 134:14, 1994

Somogyi GT, de Groat WC. Evidence for inhibitory nicotinic and facilitatory muscarinic receptors in cholinergic nerve terminals of the rat urinary bladder. J Auton Nerv Syst 37: 89, 1992

Somogyi GT, de Groat WC. Function, signal transduction mechanisms and plasticity of presynaptic muscarinic receptors in the urinary bladder. Life Sci 64:411, 1999

Stahl MMS, Ekström B, Sparf B et al. Urodynamic and other effects of tolterodine: a novel antimuscarinic drug for the treatment of detrusor overactivity. Neurourol Urodyn 14:647, 1995

Stanton SL. A comparison of emepronium bromide and flavoxate hydrochloride in the treatment of urinary incontinence. J Urol 110:529, 1973

Steers WD, Meythaler JM, Haworth C et al. Effects of acute bolus and chronic continuous intrathecal baclofen on genitourinary dysfunction due to spinal cord pathology. J Urol 148:1849, 1992

Stewart DA, Taylor J, Ghosh S etv al. Terodiline causes polymorphic ventricular tachycardia due to reduced heart rate and prolongation of QT interval. Eur J Clin Pharmacol 42:577, 1992

Stöhrer M, Bauer P, Giannetti BM et al. Effect of trospium chloride on urodynamic parameters in patients with detrusor hyperreflexia due to spinal cord injuries: a multicentre placebo controlled double-blind trial. Urol Int 47:138, 1991

Stohrer M, Madersbacher H, Richter R et al. Efficacy and safety of propiverine in SCI-patients suffering from detrusor hyperreflexia--a double-blind, placebo-controlled clinical trial. Spinal Cord 37:196, 1999

Strosberg D, Pietri-Rouxel F. Function and regulation of the ß3-adrenoceptor. Trends Pharmacol Sci 17:273, 1997

Sultana CJ, Walters MD. Estrogen and urinary incontinence in women. Maturitas 20:129, 1990

Sundin, T., Dahlström, A., Norlén et al. The sympathetic innervation and adrenoreceptor function of the human lower urinary tract in the normal state and after parasympathetic denervation. Invest Urol 14:322, 1977

Szallasi A. The vanilloid (capsaicin) receptor: receptor types and species differences. Gen Pharmacol 25:223, 1994

Szollar SM, Lee SM. Intravesical oxybutynin for spinal cord injury patients. Spinal Cord 34:284, 1996

Szonyi G, Collas DM, Ding YY et al. Oxybutynin with bladder retraining for detrusor instability in elderly people: a randomized controlled trial. Age Aging 24:287, 1995

Takayasu H, Ueno A, Tuchida S et al. Clinical Effects of propiverine hydrochloride in the treatment of urinary frequency and incontinence associated with detrusor overctivity: A double-blind, parallel, placebo-controlled, multicenter study. Igaku no Ayumi 153:459, 1990 (in Japanese)

Takeda M, Obara K, Mizusawa T et al. Evidence for beta3-adrenoceptor subtypes in relaxation of the human urinary bladder detrusor: analysis by molecular biological and pharmacological methods. J Pharmacol Exp Ther 288:1367, 1999

Tapp AJS, Cardozo LD, Versi E et al. The treatment of detrusor instability in post menopausal women with oxybutynin chloride: a double blind placebo controlled study. Br J Obstet Gynaecol 97:521, 1990

Taylor MC, Bates CP. A double-blind crossover trial of baclofen - a new treatment for the unstable bladder syndrome. Br J Urol 51:504, 1979

Thompson IM, Lauvetz R. Oxybutynin in bladder spasm, neurogenic bladder, and enuresis. Urology 8:452, 1976

Thor KB, Katofiasc MA. Effects of duloxetine, a combined serotonin and norepinephrine reuptake inhibitor, on central neural control of lower urinary tract function in the chloralose-anesthetized femal cat. J Pharmacol Exp Ther 274:1014, 1995

Thuroff JW, Bunke B, Ebner A et al. Randomized, double-blind, multicenter trial on treatment of frequency, urgency and incontinence related to detrusor hyperactivity: oxybutynin versus propantheline versus placebo. J Urol 145: 813, 1991.

Thuroff JW, Chartier-Kastler E, Corcus J et al. Medical treatment and medical side effects in urinary incontinence in the elderly. World J Urol 16 Suppl 1:S48, 1998

Tobin G, Sjögren C. In vivo and in vitro effects of muscarinic receptor antagonists on contractions and release of [3H]acetylcholine in the rabbit urinary bladder. Eur J Pharmacol 28:1, 1995

Todorova A, Vonderheid-Guth B, Dimpfel W. Effects of tolterodine, trospium chloride, and oxybutynin on the central nervous system. J Clin Pharmacol 41:636, 2001

Tokuno H, Chowdhury JU, Tomita T. Inhibitory effects of propiverine on rat and guinea-pig urinary bladder muscle. Naunyn-Schmiedeberg´s Arch Pharmacol 348:659, 1993

Ückert S, Stief CG, Odenthal KP et al. Responses of isolated normal human detrusor muscle to various spasmolytic drugs commonly used in the treatment of the overactive bladder. Arzneimittelforschung 50:456, 2000

Van Kerrebroeck P, Bäckström T, Blaivas JG et al. Oral desmopressin (Miririn, DDAVP) in the treatment of nocturia in women. J Urol 165 Suppl:250 (abstract 1031)

Van Kerrebroeck P, Kreder K, Jonas U et al. Tolterodine once-daily: superior efficacy and tolerability in the treatment of the overactive bladder.Urology 57:414, 2001

Versi E, Appell R, Mobley D et al. Dry mouth with conventional and controlled-release oxybutynin in urinary incontinence. The Ditropan XL Study Group. Obstet Gynecol 95:718, 2000

Vick J, Weiss L, Ellis S. Cardiovascular studies of phenylpropanolamine. Arch Int Pharmacodyn Ther 327; 13, 1994

Waldeck K, Larsson B, Andersson K-E. Comparison of oxybutynin and its active metabolite, N-desethyl-oxybutynin, in the human detrusor and parotid gland. J Urol 157:1093, 1997

Wallis RM, Burges RA, Cross PE et al. Darifenacin, a selective muscarinic M3 antagonist. Pharmacol Res 31suppl:54, 1995

Walther S, Hansen J, Hansen L et al. Urinary incontinence in old age. A controlled trial of emepronium bromide. Br J Urol 54:249, 1982

Wammack R, Weihe E, Dienes H-P et al. Die Neurogene Blase in vitro. Akt Urol 26:16, 1995

Weese DL, Roskamp DA, Leach GE et al. Intravesical oxybutynin chloride: experience with 42 patients. Urology 41:527, 1993

Wehnert J, Sage S. Comparative investigations to the action of Mictonorm (propiverin hydrochloride) and Spasuret (flavoxat hydrochloride) on detrusor vesicae. Z Urol Nephrol 82:259, 1989

Wehnert J, Sage S. Therapie der Blaseninstabilität und Urge-Inkontinenz mit Propiverin hydrochlorid (Mictonorm®) und Oxybutynin chlorid (Dridase®) - eine randomisierte Cross-over-Vergleichsstudie. Akt Urol 23: 7, 1992

Wein AJ, Longhurst PA, Levin RM. Pharmacologic treatment of voiding dysfunction. In Urodynamics, Principles, Practice, and Application, ed by Mundy A.R., Stephenson T.P., Wein, A.J. 2nd ed., pp 43-70, 1994

Wein AJ. Neuromuscular dysfunction of the lower urinary tract and its treatment. In Campbells Urology 8th ed, 2001a

Wein AJ. Pharmacological agents for the treatment of urinary incontinence due to overactive bladder. Exp Opin Invest Drugs 10:65, 2001b

Weiss J, Blaivas JG, Abrams P et al. Oral desmopressin (Miririn, DDAVP) in the treatment of nocturia in men. J Urol 165 Suppl:250 (abstract 1030)

Werkstrom V, Persson K, Ny L et al. Factors involved in the relaxation of female pig urethra evoked by electrical field stimulation. Br J Pharmacol 116:1599, 1995

Wiart L, Joseph PA, Petit H et al. The effects of capsaicin on the neurogenic hyperreflexic detrusor. A double blind placebo controlled study in patients with spinal cord disease. Preliminary results. Spinal Cord 36:95,1998

Wiedemann A, Füsgen I, Hauri D. New aspects of therapy with trospium chloride for urge incontinence. Eur J Geriatrics 3:41, 2001

Winkler HA, Sand PK. Treatment of detrusor instability with oxybutynin rectal suppositories. Int Urogynecol J Pelvic Floor Dysfunct 9:100, 1998

Yamaguchi O, Shisda K, Tamura K et al. Evaluation of mRNAs encoding muscarinic receptor subtypes in human detrusor muscle. J Urol 156:1208, 1996

Yarker YE, Goa KL, Fitton A. Oxybutynin: A review of its pharmacodynamic and pharmacokinetic properties, and its therapeutic use in detrusor instability. Drugs Aging 6:243, 1995

Yasuda, K., Kawabe, K., Takimoto et al., and the Clenbutrol Clinical Research Group. A double-blind clinical trial of a b2-adrenergic agonist in stress incontinence. Int Urogynecol J 4: 146, 1993

Yoshida M, Homma Y, Inadome A et al. Age-related changes in cholinergic and purinergic neurotransmission in human isolated bladder smooth muscles. Exp Gerontol 39: 99, 2001

Zeegers AGM, Kiesswetter H, Kramer AEJ et al. Conservative therapy of frequency, urgency and urge incontinence: a double-blind clinical trial of flavoxate hydrochloride, oxybutinin chloride, emepronium bromide and placebo. World J Urol 5:57, 1987

Zinner N, Sarshik S, Yalcin I et al. Efficacy and safety of duloxetine in stress urinary incontinent patients: double-blind, placebo-controlled multiple dose study. ICS 28th Annual Meeting, Jerusalem, Israel, September 14-17, 1998

Zorzitto ML, Jewett MAS, Fernie GRet al. Effectiveness of propantheline bromide in the treatment of geriatric patients with detrusor instability. Neurourol Urodyn 5:133, 1986

Committee 10 A

Conservative Management of Urinary Incontinence in Childhood

Chairman

R. JM NIJMAN (THE NETHERLANDS)

Members

R. BUTLER (U.K.),

J. VAN GOOL (THE NETHERLANDS),

C.K YEUNG (HONG KONG, CHINA),

W. BOWER (AUSTRALIA)

Consultant

K. HJÄLMÅS (SWEDEN)

CONTENTS

Conservative Management of Urinary Incontinence in Childhood

R. JM NIJMAN

R. BUTLER, J. VAN GOOL, CK YEUNG, W. BOWER

K. HJÄLMÅS

I. INTRODUCTION

In this chapter the different conservative treatment modalities of urinary incontinence in childhood will be discussed. In order to understand the pathophysiology of the most frequent encountered problems in children the normal development of bladder and sphincter control will be discussed briefly.

Most children present with either nocturnal enuresis or day and nighttime incontinence: the underlying pathophysiology will be outlined and the specific investigations for children will be discussed. For general information on epidemiology and urodynamic investigations the respective chapters are to be consulted. Specific information on those conditions that require surgical treatment such as epispadias and ectopic ureter is provided in the chapter on surgical management.

1. NORMAL DEVELOPMENT OF BLADDER AND SPHINCTER CONTROL

Normal bladder storage and voiding involve low-pressure and adequate bladder volume filling followed by a complete and succinct detrusor contraction associated with adequate relaxation of the sphincter complex. This process requires normal sensation and adequate bladder outlet resistance. The neurophysiological mechanisms involved in normal bladder storage and evacuation include a complex integration of sympathetic, parasympathetic and somatic innervation which is ultimately controlled by a complex interaction between spinal cord, brain stem, midbrain and higher cortical structures [1].

Achievement of urinary control is equally complex and as yet not fully understood; various developmental stages have been observed [2].

In newborns the bladder has been traditionally described as uninhibited, and it has been assumed that micturition occurs automatically by a simple spinal cord reflex, with little or no mediation by the higher neural centres. However studies have indicated that even in full-term fetuses and newborns, micturition is modulated by higher centres and the previous notion that voiding is spontaneous and mediated by a simple spinal reflex is probably an oversimplification. Fetal micturition seems to be a behavioural state-dependent event: intrauterine micturition is not randomly distributed over various behavioural (sleep and arousal) states, but occurs almost exclusively while the fetus is awake [3].

During the last trimester the intra-uterine voiding frequency is approximately 30 times every 24 hours [4]. Immediately after birth voiding is usually very infrequent during the first few days of life. The first void may only take place after 12 to 24 hours. After the first week frequency increases rapidly and peaks at the age of 2 to 4 weeks to an average of once per hour. It then decreases and remains stable after 6 months to about 10 to 15 times per day. After the first year it decreases to 8 to 10 times per day, while voided volumes increase by three- to fourfold.

During the postnatal period micturition control mechanisms undergo further changes and extensive modulation. Using ambulatory bladder monitoring techniques in conjunction with polysomnographic recordings it has been shown that even in newborns the bladder is normally quiescent and stable and micturition does not occur during sleep [5]. This inhibition (or lack of fascilitation) of detrusor contractions during sleep is also observed in infants with neurogenic bladder dysfunction who have marked detrusor overactivity while they are awake. In response to bladder distension during sleep, an infant nearly always exhibits clear electroencephalograhic evidence of cortical arousal, facial grimaces or limb movements, or actual awakening. Sleeping infants are always seen to wake up before bladder activity returns and voiding occurs. This arousal period may be transient and the infant may cry and move for a brief period before micturition and then shortly afterward go back to sleep. Because this wakening response is already well established in newborns, it follows that the control of micturition probably involves more complicated neural pathways and higher centres than has been appreciated. There is also strong evidence that a pronounced reorganisation of pre-existing synaptic connections and neural pathways involved in bladder control occurs during the early postnatal period.

In newborns micturition occurs at frequent intervals, may be *intermittent*, but bladder emptying efficiency is usually good. In over 80 percent of voids it is complete after voiding or quick succession of small voidings [6]. During infancy voiding pressures are much higher than in adults. It has also been noted that these pressures are higher in boys than in girls (mean Pdet max of 118 vs. 75 cm H_2O, respectively, P<.03) [7, 8]. These higher detrusor pressures decrease progressively with increasing age. Besides in 20-70 percent of infants with normal lower urinary tracts, intermittent voidings were observed. They tend to disappear with increasing age, and are thought to represent variations between individual infants in the maturation of detrusor and sphincteric co-ordination during the first 1 to 2 years of life. Videourodynamic studies have confirmed these findings [5,7,8,9,10].

Between the age of 1 and 2, conscious sensation of bladder filling develops. The ability to void or inhibit voiding voluntarily at any degree of bladder filling commonly develops in the second and third years of life. Central inhibition is crucial to obtain continence.

During the second or third year of life, there is progressive development towards a socially conscious continence and a more voluntary type of micturition control develops. The child becomes more aware of the sensation of bladder distension and the urge to urinate, as well as social norms and embarrassment associated with urinary incontinence. Through an active learning process, the child acquires the ability to voluntarily inhibit and delay voiding until a socially convenient time, then actively initiates urination even when the bladder is not completely full and allow urination to proceed to completion. During the first years of life, gradual development to an adult type of voluntary micturition control that conforms to the social norms depend on an intact nervous system in addition to at least three other events occurring concomitantly: a progressive increase in functional storage capacity, maturation of function and control over the external urinary sphincter and most importantly achievement of volitional control over the bladder-sphincteric unit so that the child can voluntarily initiate or inhibit a micturition reflex [11].

The final steps are usually achieved at the age of 3 to 4 years when most children have developed the adult pattern of urinary control and are dry both day and night. The child has learned to inhibit a micturition reflex and postpone voiding and voluntarily initiate micturition at socially acceptable and convenient times and places. This development is also dependent on behavioural learning and can be influenced by toilet training which in turn depends on cognitive perception of the maturing urinary tract.

It is understandable that this series of complex events is highly susceptible to the development of various types of dysfunction. Various functional derangements of the bladder-sphincter-perineal complex may occur during this sophisticated course of early development of normal micturition control mechanisms. These acquired functional disorders overlap with other types of bladder functional disturbances that may have a more organic but congenital underlying pathophysiological basis.

2. NORMAL VALUES

a) Normal bladder capacity

The bladder capacity increases during the first 8 years of life roughly with 30 ml per year, so with an average capacity of 30 ml in the neonatal period, a child's bladder volume can be calculated as Y = 30 + 30 X, where Y = capacity in ml and X = age in years (Fig 1) [12].

Hjälmås described a linear correlation that could be used up to 12 years of age: in boys, Y = 24.8 X + 31.6, in girls Y = 22.6 X + 37.4, where Y is capacity in ml, and X is age in years (13). It should be noted that these data were obtained during cystometric investigations and not necessarily reflect normal bladder volumes. Obviously, the relation between age and bladder capacity is not linear for all ages, nor is the relation between body weight and bladder capacity [14].

Another formula to calculate functional bladder capacity in infants is: bladder capacity (ml) = 38 + (2.5 x age (mo)) [10].

Kaefer and co-workers demonstrated that a non-linear model was the most accurate for the relation between age and bladder capacity, and they determined two practical linear equations:

Y = 2 X + 2 for children less than 2 years old, and Y = X/2+6 for those 2 years old or older; Y = capacity in ounces, X = age in years (Fig. 2) [15].

Girls were found to have a larger capacity than boys, but the rate of increase with age was not significantly different between them. Data on 'normal' bladder capacity have been obtained in continent children undergoing cystography, with retrograde filling of the bladder.

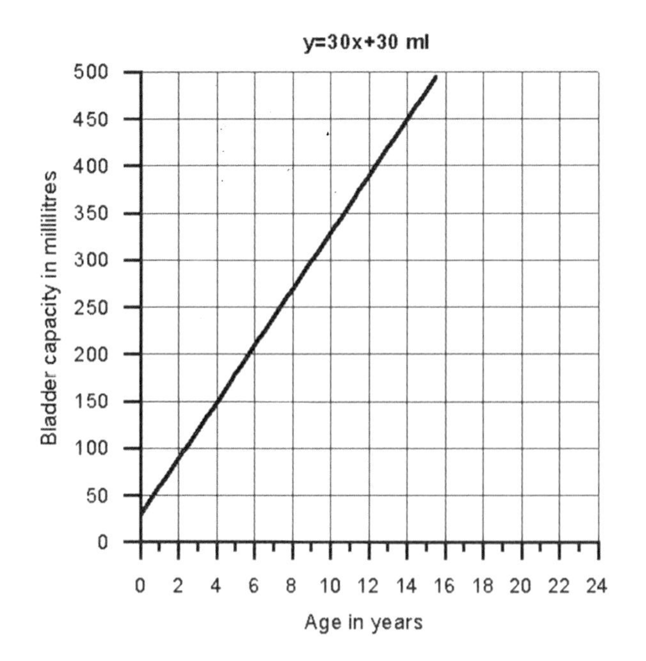

Figure 1 : Bladder capacity using the formula Y = 30 + 30 X (Y= capacity in ml, X = age in years)

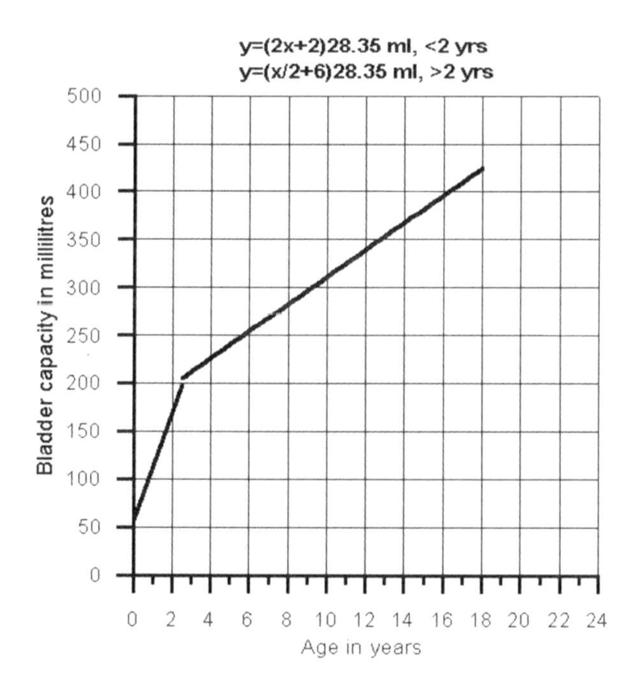

Figure 2 : Bladder capacity using the formula described by Kaefer et al. Y = (2 X + 2) x 28.35 ml < 2 years Y = (X/2+6) x 28.35 ml > 2 years (Y = capacity in ml, X is age in years)

Data obtained from the International Reflux Study indicate that there is not a linear relation between age and capacity and that there is a huge variability. (Fig 3).

b) Normal voiding pattern

The micturition frequency of the fetus during the last trimester is approximately 30 per 24 hours. It decreases

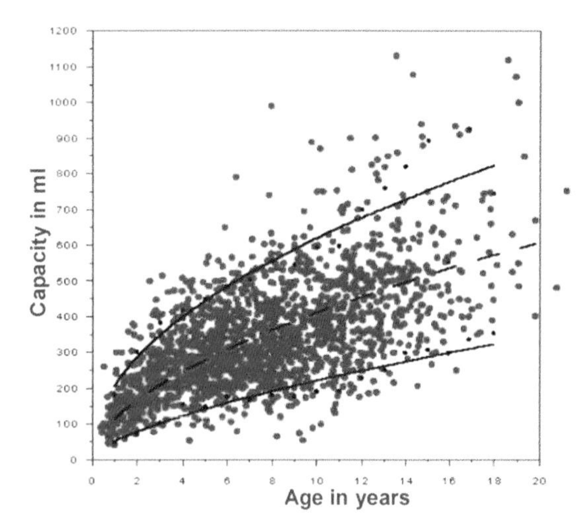

Figure 3 : Bladder capacities determined by VCUG in the International Reflux Study

to 12 during the first year of life, and after that it is reduced to an average of 5±1 voidings per day [10,15].

Thus, the normal range for the micturition frequency at age seven is 3 to 7 [16].

By age 12, the daily pattern of voiding includes 4-6 voids per day [17].

Mattson and Lindström emphasize the enormous variability of voiding frequencies in children: in individual children, the weight-corrected diuresis could vary up to 10-fold [18].

c) Normal pressures at voiding

Bladder dynamics in children have demonstrated developmental changes with age. Bladder pressures at voiding in children are similar to adults, with a mean maximum pressure of 66 cm H_2O in boys, and 57 cm H_2O in girls [19].

These pressures are lower than those reported in infancy by Yeung et al, who found boys having pressures of 118 cm H_2O, girls 75 cm H_2O [5].

d) Normal urinary flow rates

Urinary flow rates in normal children have been only minimally described. Szabo et al Published nomograms for flow rates vs age in normal children [20].

As in adults, flow rates are clearly dependent upon voided volume, and normal values can only be applied to flow rates that have been registered when voiding at a bladder volume approximating the normal capacity for age [18,21].

The definitions in this chapter comply with "Standardisation and definitions in lower urinary tract dysfunction in children", published in the British Journal of Urology in 1998 on behalf of the International Children's Continence Society (ICCS) [22].

II. EVALUATION IN CHILDREN WHO WET

Even with clear definitions, the approach to history-taking and physical examination has to be structured. The child's complaints at presentation are not synonymous with the signs and symptoms that have to be checked to arrive at a diagnosis. Also, sociocultural aspects and psychomotor development will distort the presentation. Validated questionnaires are very helpful in structuring the history-taking; they at least provide checklists [23].

With a structured approach the diagnosis of monosymptomatic nocturnal enuresis can be made with confidence.

When ultrasound imaging of kidneys and bladder, recording of urinary flow, and measurement of post-void residual are added to history and physical examination, the clinical entities caused by non-neurogenic detrusor-sphincter dysfunction can be diagnosed accurately in the majority of cases, and a high level of suspicion can be maintained towards incomplete bladder emptying in both neurogenic detrusor-sphincter dysfunction and structurally caused incontinence. This is important in view of the potential these conditions have to cause irreversible loss of kidney function.

In a minority of incontinent children the non-invasive assessment yields dubious results, or results suggesting gross deviations from normal function. Only in these situations there is an indication for invasive investigations, such as:

- Voiding cystourethrography.
- Invasive urodynamics (cystometry, pressure-flow, EMG studies, videocystometry).
- Renal scans or intravenous urography.
- Cystourethroscopy.

1. History taking

For the pediatric age group, where the history is jointly obtained from parents and child, and where the development of bladder control generates specific problems, a structured approach is recommended, with a questionnaire [23].

Many signs and symptoms pertaining to voiding and wetting are new to the parents, and they should be specifically asked for, with the questionnaire as checklist. If possible the child should be addressed as a collaborator and questioned directly, as the symptoms prompting the parents to seek consultation may be different from that which is problematic for the child.

A voiding diary is mandatory to determine a child's voiding frequency and voided volumes. Checklists and voiding dairy can be filled out at home, and checked at he first visit to the clinics. History-taking should also include assessment of bowel function; a similar pro-active procedure with a questionnaire should be followed for defecation and fecal soiling [24].

The general history-taking should include questions relevant to familial disorders, neurological and congenital abnormalities, as well as information on previous urinary infections, relevant surgery and menstrual and sexual functions. Information should be obtained on medication with known or possible effects on the lower urinary tract.

At times it is helpful to more formally evaluate the child's psychosocial status and the family situation e.g. using validated question forms such as CBCL (Achenbach) or the Butler forms [25,26].

Child abuse is very often signalled first by symptoms of bladder-sphincter dysfunction [27].

2. Physical examination

Apart from a general pediatric examination, the physical examination should include the assessment of perineal sensation, the perineal reflexes supplied by the sacral segments S1-S4 (standing on toes, bulbocavernosus) and anal sphincter tone and control. Special attention should be paid to inspection of the male or female genital region, and of the urethral meatus. Asymmetry of buttocks, legs or feet, as well as other signs of *occult neurospinal dysraphism* in the lumbosacral area (subcutaneous lipoma, skin discoloration, hair growth and abnormal gait) should be looked for specifically.

In examining the abdomen, the presence of a full sigmoid colon or descending colon is a significant finding with a history of constipation.

Detailed questioning of the parents' observation of the child's voiding habits is essential as is direct observation of the voiding, if possible. Children may have their voiding dysfunction ameliorated or even eliminated by correcting anomalies of body position detected when observing the child's micturition. Children may void in awkward positions, e.g. with their legs crossed or balancing on the toilet without proper support of the legs, thereby activating the pelvic floor and obstructing the free flow of urine (Fig. 4) [28].

3. Urinalysis

In order to be comprehensive, physical examination should include urinalysis to identify any infection and glucosuria.

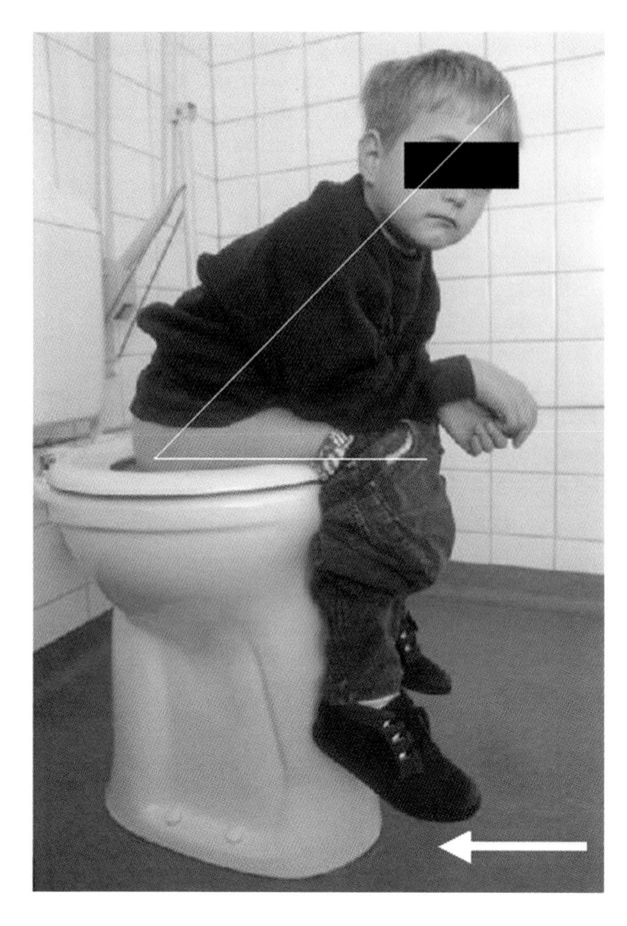

Figure 4 : Improper position for voiding: the feet are not supported (unbalanced position) and the boy is bent forward. Support of the feet will correct this and will the pelvic floor muscles allow to relax properly.

4. Non-invasive diagnostic techniques

a) Frequency/volume charts: bladder diary

The frequency/volume chart is a detailed diary recording fluid intake and urine output over 24-hour periods. The chart gives objective information on the number of voidings, the distribution of day and night voids, along with the voided volumes and episodes of urgency and leakage, or dribbling. In order to obtain a complete picture defecation frequency and/or soiling are often recorded.

From the frequency/volume chart the child's "functional" bladder capacity may be assessed as the largest voided volume, with the exception of the morning micturition which actually represents nighttime bladder capacity. Whenever possible, filling out the chart is the responsibility of the child: the parents provide assistance and support. Ideally the chart should cover 3 complete days, but in reality completion over a weekend restricts the record to 2 days.

The frequency volume chart is a reliable non-invasive measure of maximum bladder storage capacity and can be used as an outcome measure in children with bladder dysfunction if care is taken to minimise confounding factors and sources of error during chart completion [29].

The amount of urine voided by a non-supervised child during the day varies considerably since the child's voidings are dictated more by social circumstances and /or bladder activity rather than by bladder capacity. Children with bladder symptoms void smaller volumes of urine than may be expected from traditional estimates [29]. This is unrelated to either gender, type of presenting incontinence or a positive family history of bladder dysfunction. The only significant influence upon voided volumes recorded on a frequency volume chart is the age effect, and voided volumes in incontinent children increase incrementally with age. The frequency volume chart is useful when comparing the mean voided volume and SD by a child's age.

Validation and test/retest data on frequency/volume charts whilst scarce indicate that voiding interval is the most variable parameter [29]. Data in normal children and in children with different categories of incontinence are available for comparison [29,30,31].

In order to obtain a complete picture it is better to ask for a bladder diary: fluid intake as well as voiding frequency, voided volumes, incontinence episodes and defecation frequency and/or soiling are recorded.

Test/retest evaluation is not available; trend analyses of frequency/volume charts can be extracted from currently available data.

b) Quantification of urine loss

Subjective grading of incontinence may not indicate reliably the degree of dysfunction. For objective grading, 12-hour pad test and frequency/volume charts are validated instruments [30,31].

In children, the 12-hour pad test should also give information about fluid intake. The pad test is complementary to the bladder diary, which denotes more the frequency of incontinence and the distribution of wetting episodes than the quantities of urine lost.

The amount of urine lost during sleep can be determined by weighing diapers or absorbent pads, before and after sleep. To obtain a measure of the total nocturnal urine output, the volume of the early-morning voiding should be added to the amount lost during sleep.

c) Quantification of constipation

In grading constipation, scoring a plain X-ray of the abdomen (Barr score) yields inconsistent results [33,34,35].

A better way to match clues from the medical history with signs and symptoms is the measurement of colonic transit time. As many children with non-neurogenic detrusor-sphincter dysfunction habitually use their pelvic floor as emergency brake, anomalous defecation frequency and constipation have a high prevalence in this group. Overt constipation should be dealt with before embarking on treatment of incontinence or detrusor-sphincter dysfunction [36].

d) Urinary flow

Voiding should be analysed in detail in all incontinent children with the exception of monosymptomatic bedwetting where voiding, as far as we know, is normal.

Graphic registration of the urinary flow rate during voiding is becoming a standard office procedure. Flow patterns and rates should be consistent to allow for evaluation, and several recordings are needed to obtain consistency.

Approximately 1% of school children have a voiding that can be labelled abnormal with flattened or intermittent flow curves. The remaining 99% have a bell-shaped flow curve [21].

Flow recordings with a voided volume of less than 50% of the functional capacity are not consistent: they represent voiding on command, and many children will try to comply by using abdominal pressure. A helpful tool in this respect is the bladder scan: before micturition the bladder volume can be assessed. If the bladder is still nearly empty the child should be asked to drink some water until the bladder is full enough for a reliable flow.

Urinary flow may be described in terms of rate and pattern and may be continuous, intermittent (in fractions), or staccato.

Measurement of urinary flow is performed as a solitary procedure, with bladder filling by diuresis (spontaneous or forced), or as part of a pressure/flow study, with bladder filling by catheter. Patterns and rates should be consistent to allow for evaluation, and several recordings are needed to obtain consistency [37].

The same parameters used to characterise continuous flow may be applicable, if care is exercised, in children with intermittent, or staccato flow patterns. In measuring flow time, the time intervals between flow episodes are disregarded. Voiding time is total duration of micturition, including interruptions.

5. Ultrasound imaging of upper and lower urinary tract

In most clinical settings, ultrasound imaging techniques are routinely used in children with incontinence. Upper tract abnormalities such as duplex kidney, dilatation of the collecting system, and gross reflux nephropathy can be readily detected, but detection of the more subtle expressions of these abnormalities require urological expertise on the part of the ultrasound operator.

Lower urinary tract abnormalities are even more difficult to assess for the inexperienced, aside from bladder wall thickness: a bladder wall cross-section of more than 3-4 milimeters, measured at 50% of expected bladder capacity, is clinically suspect for long-standing detrusor overactivity [38].

a) Post-void residual volume

Except in small infants, the normal bladder will empty completely at every micturition [39].

The identification or exclusion of post-void residual is therefore an integral part of the study of micturition. However, an uneasy child voiding in unfamiliar surroundings may yield unrepresentative results, as may voiding on command with a partially filled or overfilled bladder. When estimating residual urine, voided volume and the time interval between voiding and estimation of post-void residual should be recorded. This is of particular importance if the patient is in a diuretic phase. In patients with gross vesicoureteral reflux urine from the ureters may enter the bladder immediately after micturition and may falsely be interpreted as residual urine. The absence of residual urine is an observation of clinical value, but does not exclude infravesical obstruction or bladder-sphincter dysfunction with absolute certainty. An isolated finding of residual urine requires confirmation before being considered significant, especially in infants and young children.

b) Ultrasound-flow-ultrasound

This combination of imaging and non-invasive urodynamics is a standardised procedure to obtain representative data on both flow rate and flow pattern, as well as on post-void residual volumes. With ultrasound, bladder filling is assessed and compared with the functional or expected bladder capacity for age—when these values correspond, the child is asked to void in the flowmeter. After recording the flow, post-void residual is assessed again. This procedure avoids the registration of flow rates at unrealistic bladder volumes.

6. Invasive diagnostic techniques

The important question (for the incontinent child) whether invasive diagnostic procedures are necessary is decided by the results of the non-invasive procedures. The diagnostic information needed is that which is necessary to find the correct treatment. Indicators include voiding frequency of 3 or less per day, straining or manual expression during voiding, a weak urinary stream, previous febrile urinary tract infection, continuous dribbling incontinence or pronounced apparent stress incontinence, or previously identified dilating vesicoureteral reflux.

The finding of genitourinary abnormalities or signs of occult spinal dysraphism at physical examination also indicate the need for further diagnostics. Urinary flow registration will detect the plateau-shaped flow curve typical for structural infravesical obstruction, and the intermittent flow suggesting detrusor-sphincter dyscoordination [37].

A clinically significant post-void residual at repeated occasions clearly points to incomplete bladder emptying. The pad test will detect the cases with obvious stress incontinence, or continuous dribbling. Ultrasound imaging will raise suspicion for extravesical ectopic ureters, even when history and pad test do not point to dribbling incontinence.

In short, invasive diagnostics are indicated when the non-invasive program raises suspicion on neurogenic detrusor-sphincter dysfunction (occult spinal dysraphism), infravesical anatomical obstruction (especially posterior urethral valves), genitourinary abnormalities (e.g. epispadias), advanced non-neurogenic bladderdetrusor-sphincter dysfunction (as in children with dilating vesicoureteral reflux and/or febrile urinary tract infections), or significant post void residuals.

To diagnose the complex of non-neurogenic detrusor-sphincter dysfunction, recurrent urinary tract infections and vesicoureteral reflux, urodynamic studies are needed in only a minority of all incontinent children.

• TECHNIQUE

Cleanse and rinse the external genitalia with lukewarm water: do not use detergents. Use a feeding tube with side holes and a rounded tip (Ch 06-08) or balloon catheter to catheterise the bladder; check the urine for infection. Empty the bladder completely before filling. Use a radio-opaque dye of maximum 30% concentration, at body temperature, and fill the bladder by slow-drip infusion, with a hydrostatic pressure of not more than 40 cm H_2O. Note the volume of the contrast medium instilled. Use fluoroscopy during filling at regular intervals.

Take spot-films (70mm or 90mm camera) supine, with partial filling and at the end of filling, in AP projection, of the complete urinary tract. Upper tracts and lower tract should be visible.

When voiding is imminent, change the position of the child so that spot films of bladder and urethra in 3/4 projection during actual voiding can be taken. Also take a spot film during voiding of the upper urinary tract: the degree of vesicoureteral reflux (VUR) may change with the pressure generated by the detrusor muscle during voiding. Post-void residual volumes are a very inconsistent finding with VCUG. The voiding phase is critically important to VCUG, both for reflux detection and for assessment of voiding dynamics. Without a voiding phase, the VCUG is incomplete.

Prophylactic antibiotics are indicated, to minimise the risk for post-VCUG urinary tract infection especially in children with an anatomic abnormality.

• INDICATIONS FOR VCUG

A VCUG is an invasive procedure and should only be done if the outcome will influence the management. It is indicated in children with recurrent urinary tract infections to detect reflux and in children with an abnormal flow pattern to detect infravesical abnormalities (like valves, strictures or a syringocele).

In children with incontinence the lateral projection during voiding is the most important part of the study. Especially in children with stress incontinence or a neuropathic bladder the position and configuration of the bladder neck during filling and voiding should be noted.

In children with non-neurogenic detrusor-sphincter dysfunction as well as in children with neurogenic detrusor-sphincter dyssynergia, the proximal urethra may show the so-called 'spinning top' configuration, during filling and during voiding. With detrusor and pelvic floor muscles contracting at the same time, the force of the detrusor contraction will dilate the proximal urethra down to the level of the forcefully closed striated external sphincter. The resulting 'spinning top' configuration used to be seen as a sure sign of distal urethral stenosis, a concept held responsible for recurrent urinary tract infections in girls, with urethral dilatation or blind urethrotomy as the obvious therapy. However, urodynamics made it clear that the 'spinning top' will only appear when detrusor and pelvic floor contract synchronously, which makes it a functional anomaly, not an anatomical one [40,41].

Women often recall their experience with VCUG as young girls in terms bordering to abuse. The use of VCUG in children should be limited to the absolutely necessary.

a) Urodynamics

Especially in children urodynamic investigations should only be performed if the outcome will have consequences for treatment. Both children and parents need careful preparation and adequate information before the study is done. It is an invasive procedure and artefacts may occur. Because of the invasiveness of the investigations all children are anxious and this may reflect in the outcome of the study. Especially during the first filling cycle, when the child does not know what to expect, instability may be seen and the voiding phase can be incomplete due to contraction of the pelvic floor muscles during voiding. Once the child knows that filling and voiding are not painful a subsequent filling and voiding cycle may show a completely different pattern. The study should be repeated at least 2 or 3 times. Still the results may not always be reproducible and it should be stressed that the primary objective is to treat the child and not a "urodynamic abnormality" per se.

Special attention should be given to a pleasant surrounding for the child: one or both parents should be present and young children may be given a bottle. Older children may be distracted by watching a video movie. The child should be awake, unanaesthetised and neither sedated nor taking any drugs that affect bladder function

During the study the investigator has the opportunity to observe the child and discuss various findings and correlate them to what the child feels and/or normally would do in such circumstances.

In children, the transition from filling phase to voiding phase is not as marked as in adults. To avoid missing this important transition, cystometry and pressure-flow/EMG measurements are performed as one continuous study in paediatric urodynamics.

Electromyography of pelvic floor muscles evaluates the activity of the striated urethral sphincter, in the filling phase and in the voiding phase. Surface skin electrodes are usually used to record the EMG. In children the pelvic floor EMG is probably of much more importance than in adults as it helps to differentiate the different voiding disorders.

Filling the bladder can be achieved by diuresis (natural fill cystometry) or retrograde by catheter. For retrograde filling by catheter, saline 0.9% or contrast medium at body temperature is recommended in children, without additives; CO_2 is not recommended.

When filling by catheter, slow fill cystometry (5 – 10 percent of expected bladder capacity per minute) is recommended in children, as certain cystometric parameters, notably compliance, may be significantly altered by the speed of bladder filling.

Involuntary detrusor contractions may be provoked by rapid filling, alterations of posture, coughing, walking, jumping, and other triggering procedures.

The presence of these contractions does not necessarily imply a neurologic disorder. In infants, detrusor contractions often occur throughout the filling phase.

Bladder sensation is difficult to evaluate in children. Only in toilet-trained cooperative children is it a relevant parameter. *First desire to void* is not relevant in the infant, but can be used as a guideline in children of 4 years and older. *Normal desire to void* should be considered the volume at which some unrest is noted, e.g. wriggling with the toes; this usually indicates voiding is imminent. In the older child, the volume may be small with the first cystometry, for fear of discomfort. This is the reason that in pediatric urodynamics several cycles of filling are recommended. The difference between strong desire to void and urgency may be too subtle for children to perceive.

Maximum cystometric capacity (CBC) is the volume in the bladder at which the infant or child starts voiding. The value for maximum cystometric capacity is derived from volume voided plus residual volume. Values for CBC should be interpreted in relation to normal values for age.

Compliance indicates the change in volume for a change in pressure. For children with neuropathic bladder-sphincter dysfunction, data are available relating poor compliance to the risk of upper urinary tract damage [41].

The urethral closure mechanism during storage may be normal or incompetent. The normal urethral closure mechanism maintains a positive urethral closure pressure during filling, even in the presence of increased abdominal pressure or during detrusor overactivity (guarding reflex) [42]. Immediately prior to micturition the normal closure pressure decreases to allow flow.

Infravesical obstruction, recorded with a pressure/flow study, may be anatomical or functional in nature. An *anatomical obstruction* creates a urethral segment with a small and fixed diameter, that does not dilate during voiding. As a result, the flow pattern will be plateauing, with a low and constant maximum flow rate, despite high detrusor pressure and complete relaxation of the urethral sphincter. In a *functional obstruction*, it is the active contraction of the urethral sphincter during passage of urine that creates the narrow urethral segment, constantly or intermittently. To differentiate anatomical from functional obstruction, information is needed about the activity of the urethral sphincter during voiding. This information can be obtained, and recorded together with pressure and flow, by monitoring the urethral pressure at the level of the urethral sphincter, or by recording a continuous electromyogram of the striated urethral sphincter sensu stricto. For clinical purposes, in patients where the urethral sphincter is not readily accessible, the electromyogram of the external anal sphincter is often used to monitor activity of the striated urethral sphincter. This corresponds to activity of the pelvic floor muscles (Fig. 5). Also the use of video

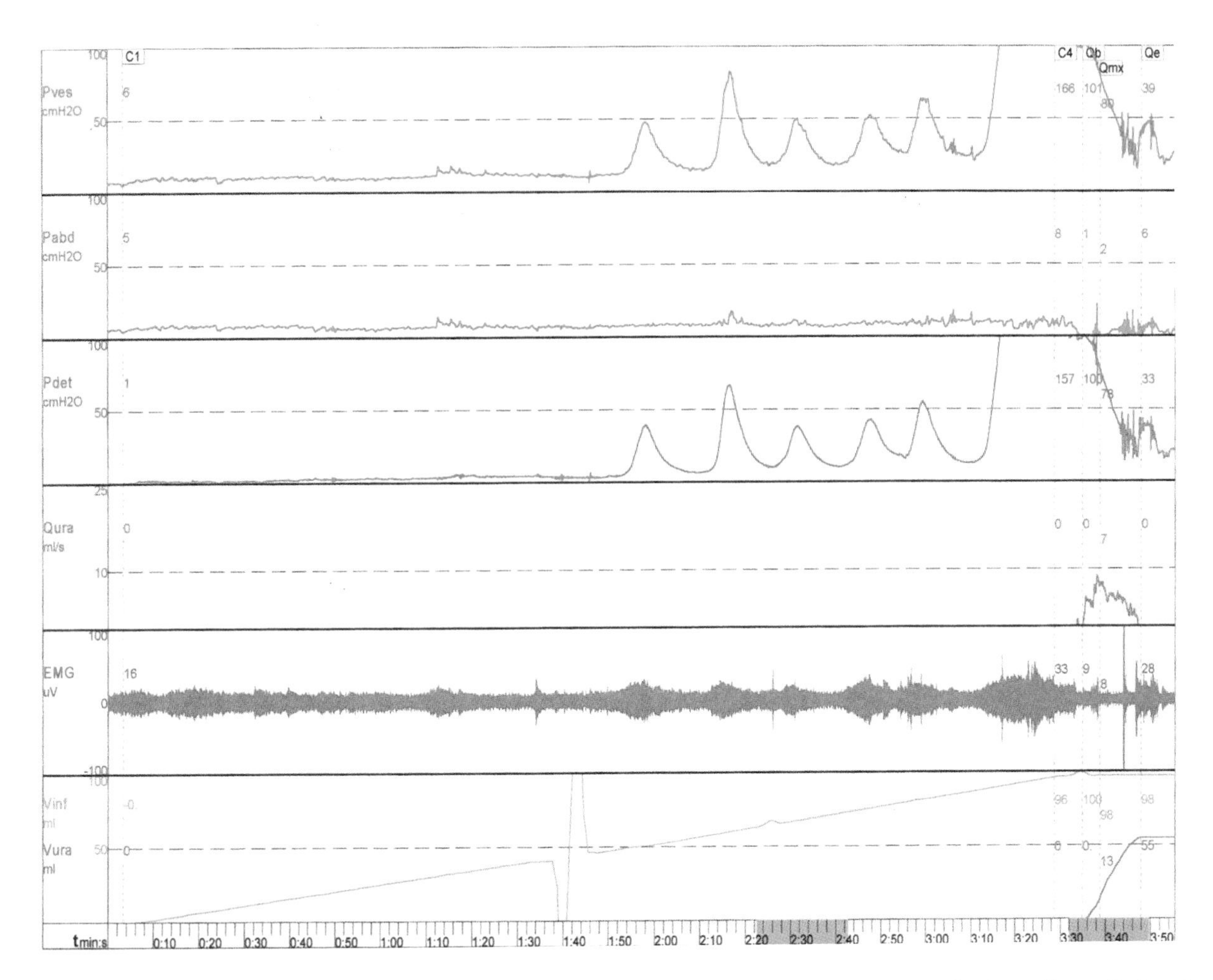

Figure 5 : Urodynamic study illustrating bladder overactivity, counter action of pelvic floor muscles (guarding reflex) and incomplete relaxation during voiding resulting in post void residual urine (bladder instability + dysfunctional voiding).

urodynamics can be very helpful in this respect, as contractions of the pelvic floor muscles can actually be seen during the voiding phase.

In infants and small children, pelvic floor muscle overactivity during voiding (with post-void residuals) is not uncommon: in all probability it is a normal developmental feature [5,7].

(Over) activity of the urethral sphincter may occur during the voiding contraction of the detrusor in neurologically normal children; this set of events is termed dysfunctional voiding.

Grade of recommendation: for all diagnostic procedures level 2

III. NOCTURNAL ENURESIS

1. Definition

Nocturnal enuresis can be defined as an involuntary voiding of urine during sleep, with a severity of at least three times a week, in children over 5 years of age in the absence of congenital or acquired defects of the central nervous system [44].

It has been argued that parental concern and child distress should also play a part in determining the clinical significance of the problem [45].

Although there is general consensus about the core descriptors of nocturnal enuresis, divergent opinions flourish over many specific aspects of the definition [46].

Age is one such issue. Most definitions refer to 5 years as the watershed although occasionally the child's 'mental age' is taken into account. The age criteria is somewhat arbitrary but reflects the natural course of bladder acquisition. It has been contested that 5 years is appropriate as it is around this time that a child normally is able to start micturition at will and has thus developed cognitive control over voiding [47].

Verhulst et al argue for flexibility in age criteria due to different rates of acquisition for boys and girls. Extrapolation from Verhulst's figures suggests that the prevalence rate for 8 year old boys is equivalent to that for girls at 5 years [48].

2. Severity

Children manifestly vary in wetting frequency. Only some 15 percent of children wet every night although most children wet more than once a week [49,48].

In a population survey of nearly 1,800 Irish children aged 4 –14 year olds, Devlin found the frequency of wetting as follows: less than once per week in 33 percent, once per week in 11 percent and 2 to 4 times per week in 25 percent [50].

Epidemiological surveys may seek to define the problem if bedwetting occurs more than once a month whereas, in contrast, most trials of treatment effectiveness work to a more severe criteria of perhaps at least 4 wet beds per week. In clinical practice, parental and child concern over the bedwetting, rather than severity itself, seems the relevant issue. Some children and parents are concerned over an occasional wet bed, while others will accept regular wetting. Clinically severity can be defined as: infrequent (1-2 wetting episodes per week), moderately severe (3 – 5 wetting episodes per week) or severe (6 – 7 wetting episodes per week).

3. Prevalence

The extent of bedwetting is widespread. It has been argued that nocturnal enuresis is the most prevalent of all childhood problems [51].

In the United Kingdom estimates suggest around 750,000 children and young people over 7 years will regularly wet the bed. In the USA recent evaluations of prevalence suggest some 5 to 7 million children regularly experience primary nocturnal enuresis [52,53,54].

Epidemiological surveys tend to adopt 'lenient' criteria in defining nocturnal enuresis. They survey a sample or the whole community asking parents to check against a list should their child wet the bed. Such surveys (including any episodes of nocturnal enuresis) undertaken in Great Britain, Holland, New Zealand and Ireland suggest that the prevalence for boys is around: 13-19% at 5 years, 15-22% at 7 years, 9-13% at 9 years and 1-2% at 16 years. For girls the prevalence rates are reported to be:

• 9-16% at 5 years, 7-15% at 7 years, 5-10% at 9 years and 1-2% in the late teenage years [48,50,55,56].

All surveys suggest the rate of bedwetting reduces with advancing age. The rate of decline in incidence with the child's age has been assessed as around 14% for 5-9 year olds and 16% for those 10-18 years old. A small percentage of individuals each year do therefore establish nocturnal bladder control. It might be construed that rather than 'growing out of the problem', they are able to develop improved nocturnal bladder control through maturational processes (Fig. 6).

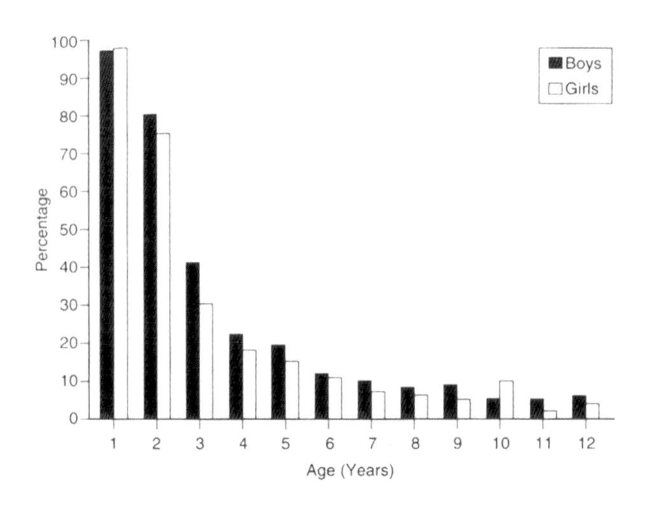

Figure 6 : Prevalence of nocturnal enuresis by age, redrawn from Verhulst et al.

Many adults will be reluctant to come forward or admit to currently having a problem of bedwetting. Hirasing et al sampled over 13,000 adults [18-64 years] and found an overall prevalence rate of nocturnal enuresis at 0.5% [57]. Of these, 12 percent of men and 29 percent of women had daytime incontinence. Fifty percent of men and 35 percent of the women had never consulted a health professional about their bedwetting. Thirty eight percent of the men and 26 percent of the women had never done anything to try and become dry.

The enuresis prevalence of 0.5% in otherwise healthy adults in this study refers to a largely untreated population. Fifty percent of the men had primary enuresis so they had never been consistently dry at night. Assuming a prevalence of enuresis of 8 percent in 7-year-old boys, this could be translated to mean that the risk for an enuretic boy to remain enuretic for the rest of his life is 3 percent if he does not receive active treatment during childhood. Three per cent equals the prevalence found in patients after the age of 20 years in the study by Forsythe and Redmond and in the Finnish 14-year-olds as described by Moilanen [58,59]. It is still not clear whether active treatment of nocturnal enuresis in childhood is able to reduce the number of adult enuretics.

4. Inheritance

In most children bedwetting is a familial problem. Sporadic bedwetting with no affected relatives is found in 30 percent of children.

The mode of inheritance is autosomal dominant, so if both parents were nocturnal enuretics as children, the risk for their offspring is 77 percent. If only one parent had nocturnal enuresis the risk is about 45 percent. As a genetically determined disorder, nocturnal is unusual as the great majority of patients show a spontaneous resolution of their enuresis with time. Thus the hereditary trait leads to a delay of maturation of the mechanisms responsible for sleeping without wetting the bed, not to a permanent disorder in most cases.

With linking analysis, foci have been found on chromosomes 8, 12, 13 and 22 [60,61,62].

It is conceivable that more than 10 chromosomes are involved. With increasing knowledge a picture of pronounced heterogeneity of both genotype and phenotype is emanating. The etiology of nocturnal enuresis is characterised by a complex interaction of genetic and environmental factors.

5. The gender difference

In a population survey of 706 families in London ,Weir found a higher prevalence for boys than girls at age 3 years with 56 percent of boys and 40 percent of girls being wet at night more than once a week [63].

A recent survey of over 2900 three year old twin pairs born in England and Wales in 1994 found a significant difference between boys and girls in development of nocturnal bladder control with 54.5 percent of girls and 44.2 percent of boys being dry at night [64].

Historically girls have been reported as more likely to experience secondary enuresis and associated daytime incontinence, urinary frequency, emotional and behavioural problems, urinary tract infections, along with tolerant mothers, and a high level of concern about their enuresis [50,55,65,66,67].

Girls have also been reported to be less likely to have a family history or genetic pre-disposition to bedwetting [64,68].

6. Classification

The traditional classification is based on the child's history of enuresis. Children who have never achieved a period of up to 6 months free of bedwetting are considered to have primary nocturnal enuresis. There may be indications of slight maturational delay in primary nocturnal enuresis with low birth weight, soft signs of neurological delay, delayed motor development and shorter height [65,69,70,71,72].

However children with primary nocturnal enuresis do not have an increased likelihood of behavioural problems compared with children who are not bedwetters or former bedwetters [57,73,74,75].

Secondary or onset nocturnal enuresis is the re-emergence of wetting after a period of being dry. The time period is usually considered to be a minimum of 6 months, although some take 1 year to be the specified enuresis-free period. A birth cohort of 1265 New Zealand children studied over 10 years by Fergusson et al found an increased risk of secondary enuresis with age [76]. They found the proportion of children who developed secondary enuresis were: 3.3 percent at 5 years, 4.7 percent at 6 years, 6.2 percent at 7 years, 7.0 percent at 8 years, 7.5 percent at 9 years and 7.9 percent at 10 years.

Secondary nocturnal enuresis appears to be associated with a higher incidence of stressful events particularly parental separation, disharmony between parents, birth of a sibling, early separation of the child from parents and psychiatric disturbance in a parent [76,77,78].

Von Gontard and colleagues found children with secondary enuresis had significantly more emotional difficulties compared to those with primary nocturnal enuresis [78]. Their evidence also suggests children with secondary enuresis, compared to those with primary enuresis, are significantly more likely to have behavioural problems, a finding which corresponds to that of McGee et al [73].

Both Jarvelin and Fergusson et al compellingly argue that primary and secondary enuresis are aspects of the same problem [69,76]. They claim the two classifications share a common etiological basis. The rate at which a child acquires primary control influences his or her susceptibility to secondary enuresis. The primary form is regarded as being the consequence of a delay in maturation of the physiological mechanisms. The child's capacity to sustain and maintain nocturnal bladder control is manifest in the rate at which control is acquired. On the other hand this capacity determines the child's susceptibility to lapsing when exposed to stress.

a) Mono-symptomatic versus non-mono-symptomatic

Mono-symptomatic nocturnal enuresis refers to those children who report no bladder or voiding problems associated with their wetting. Non-mono-symptomatic nocturnal enuresis refers to bedwetting which is associated with bladder instability and voiding problems such as urgency and postponement during the day, but no daytime wetting [79].

This classification becomes extremely important in considering the most appropriate treatment intervention.

Many parents are unaware of daytime symptoms when seeking help for bedwetting and when identified these symptoms should be treated prior to intervention for the nocturnal enuresis.

Between 10-28% of children with nocturnal enuresis have associated daytime problems and if they have urinary incontinence during the day these children should not be regarded as having nocturnal enuresis: they should be considered to be incontinent. The night time incontinence is not any longer an isolated phenomenon but part of the symptomatology of functional incontinence. They are more resilient to treatment and more vulnerable to relapse [58,80].

7. Understanding nocturnal enuresis

The pathophysiology of nocturnal enuresis has been studied extensively and is still not fully understood. A conceptual model has been proposed for understanding nocturnal enuresis, envisaging it as a problem or delayed maturation in one or more of the following systems: a lack of stability in bladder functioning, a lack of arginine vasopressin release and an inability to wake from sleep to full bladder sensations (Fig. 7) [81].

The clinical benefits of employing this model are extensive:

1. It provides an explanation, for both child and parents, as to the reasons for the ongoing problem
2. It assists the assessment process in that the focus is on which aspect[s] of the system is letting the child down
3. Following from the assessment, the model enables the appropriate treatment interventions to be selected
4. Having an understanding as to why a particular treatment might be advocated, improves compliance with treatment
5. Because the model emphasises the child's difficulty in acquiring processes that are outside of his or her control, it removes the child from blame

This is supported by the work of Neveus et al, who sought to evaluate differences in sleep factors between children with wetting problems and dry children [82].

Children with nocturnal enuresis aged between 6 and 10 years were found to have both impaired arousal and bladder instability.

a) Lack of nocturnal vasopressin release

Normal subjects have a marked circadian variation in urine output, leading to a significant reduction of urine excretion and a corresponding increase of urine osmo-

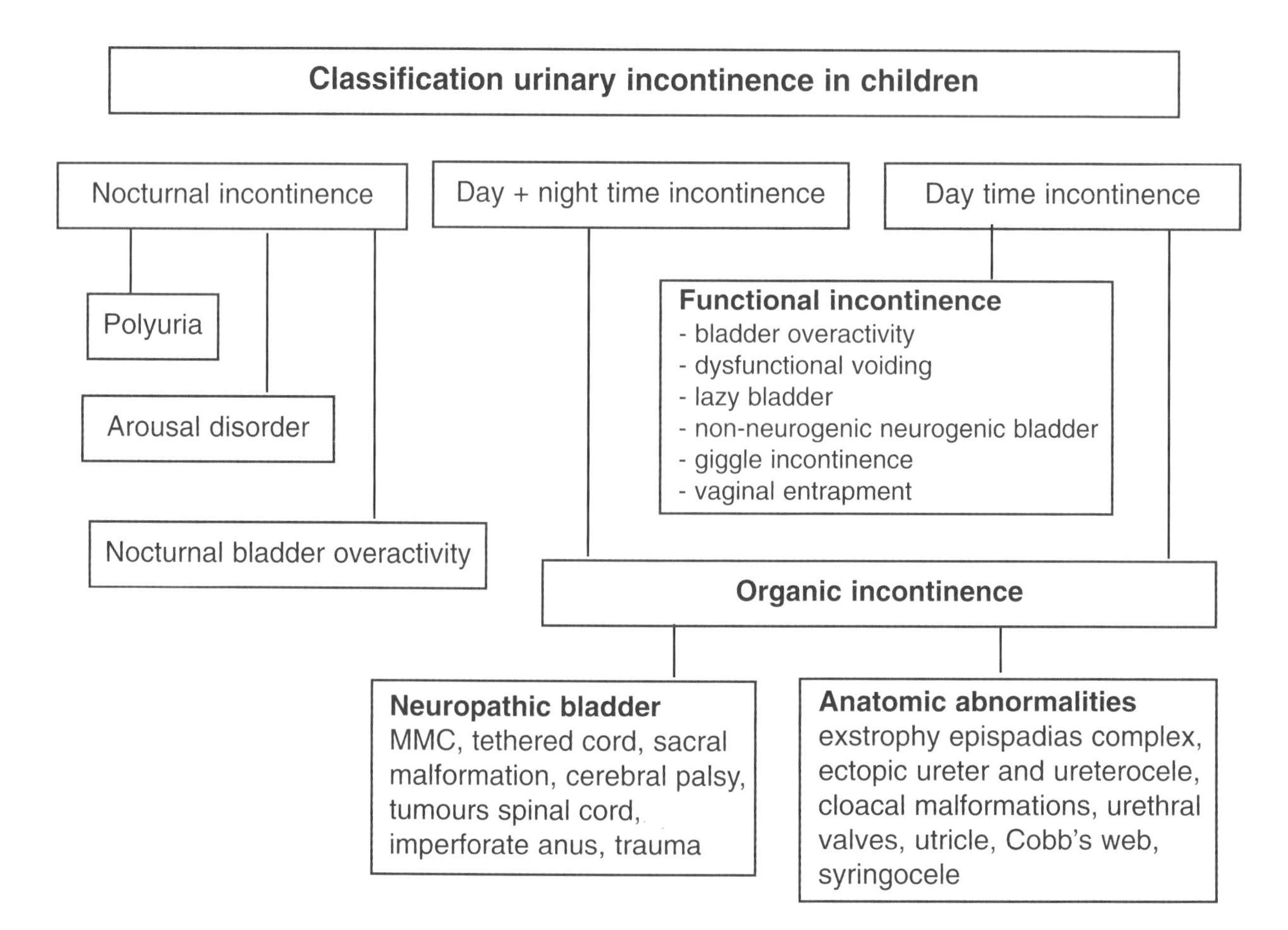

Figure 7 : Classification of urinary incontinence in children. Most causes of anatomic abnormalities need surgical treatment and are not discussed in this chapter.

lality during sleep [83]. Decrease of renal urine production during the night allows for sleep not disturbed by a full bladder. In children this is the result of nocturnal increase of plasma vasopressin (a polypeptide containing nine amino acids, produced in the hypothalamus and stored in the posterior pituitary gland), which results in increased urine concentration and reduced urine volume during sleep. This could explain why most children who are not enuretic tend to sleep through the night without being wet [30].

In adolescence and adult age there is no diurnal rhythm of plasma vasopressin concentration, and the changes in urine production occur entirely owing to a decrease in the urinary sodium excretion [84].

Two thirds of patients with mono-symptomatic nocturnal enuresis have been found to have a lack of circadian rhythm of vasopressin, resulting in high nocturnal urine production which exceeds bladder capacity [85, 86,87].

Detection of low plasma vasopressin levels cannot realistically be considered as part of a routine clinical assessment. Alternatively we can look for clinical signs of low vasopressin during the assessment interview. Weighing the diapers and adding the first morning void provides the total nocturnal urine output: if this total exceeds the child's functional bladder capacity it could be an indication for nocturnal polyuria.

Wolfish et al interestingly found that most nocturnal enuretic episodes occur in the first third of the night and many studies report that the enuretic episode is most likely to occur in the first 2 hours of sleep [88,89].

There may be a small sub-group of children with impaired renal sensitivity to vasopressin or desmopressin [90,91] Recent work by Devitt et al suggests that 18 percent of children have 'normal' levels of plasma vasopressin release but remain enuretic [87]. These children all failed to respond to therapeutic dosage of desmopressin. This finding could indicate renal insensitivity to vasopressin but could also be indicative for bladder overactivity or a small functional bladder capacity. Total urine output during the night could be helpful in differentiating between the two conditions (is there really nocturnal polyuria?).

b) Bladder overactivity during the night

The bladder, in order to function appropriately, needs to be stable during filling and have an appropriate functional capacity. Bladder instability usually causes functional bladder capacity to be decreased [92].

Watanabe and his colleagues, employing EEG and cystometry recording during sleep, discovered that in 32 percent of children with nocturnal enuresis uninhibited bladder contractions occurred resulting in enuresis [93,94,95]. These children had smaller functional bladder capacities at the point of wetting, than children with enuresis who did not have bladder instability.

Yeung et al have recently reported that 44 percent of treatment failures [with desmopressin or the enuresis alarm] have normal daytime bladder functioning but marked unstable bladder contractions during sleep resulting in enuresis [96]. Almost none of these children had nocturnal polyuria.

It is important clinically to be aware of the possibility of bladder instability as a cause of the child's nocturnal enuresis. Under the new classification system, such children might be described as having non-monosymptomatic nocturnal enuresis.

The following signs are indicative of bladder instability [85,96,97]:

In the daytime: frequency (more than 7 times per day), urgency, (unsuccessful) holding manoeuvres such as squatting and low or variable functional bladder capacity (small voided volumes)

At night: multiple wetting episodes, variability in the amount of urine in the diaper and waking during or immediately after wetting

c) Lack of arousal from sleep

The fundamental mechanism resulting in nocturia or nocturnal enuresis is that the bladder fills to its capacity during sleep and needs to be emptied. Bladder fullness is due to nocturnal polyuria and/or a reduction of the bladder capacity due to improper relaxation of the detrusor during sleep. These factors can not by themselves explain why the enuretic child does not wake up during the night to the sensation of a full or contracting bladder.

Whether the child has bladder instability or lack of vasopressin release resulting in over production of urine, the enuresis event results from the child's inability to awaken from sleep (Fig. 8).

Non-enuretic children are more likely to wake to void than enuretic children [98].

This might explain why the most heavily endorsed view of both children and parents, regarding the aetiology of nocturnal enuresis is a belief in deep sleep [99].

However a raft of evidence counters such a belief. Sleep patterns of children with nocturnal enuresis are no different from children who do not have nocturnal enuresis [85].

Enuretic episodes occur during all stages of sleep in proportion to the amount of time spent in that stage and appear to occur independent of sleep stage but when the

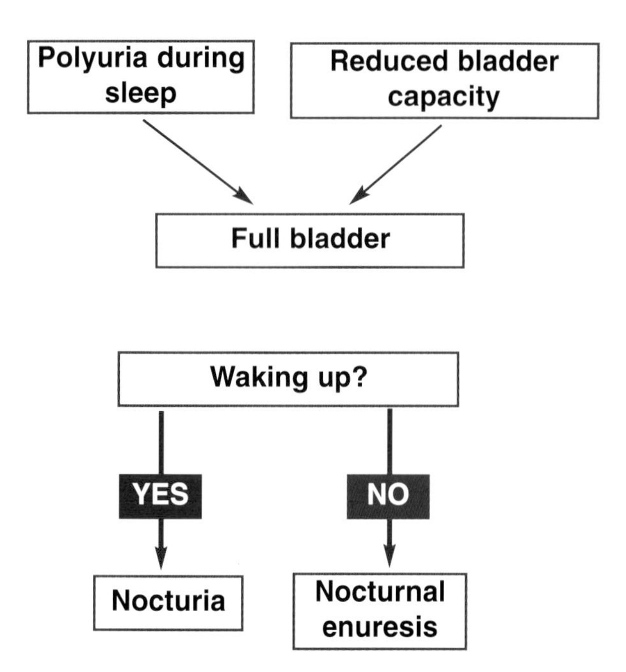

Figure 8 : Basic pathophysiology of nocturnal enuresis or nocturia. When the bladder is full because of (relative) polyuria and/or a reduced bladder capacity, the child either wakes up to void (nocturia) or voids while sleeping (nocturnal enuresis).

bladder is filled to the equivalent of maximal daytime functional capacity [88,100,101,102].

Bedwetting children sleep normally but are unable to suppress nocturnal bladder contractions or awaken in response to them or to bladder fullness.

The issue is one of the child's inability to arouse from sleep when the bladder reaches its maximum capacity, which Watanabe and colleagues have demonstrated in a series of EEG studies. Watanabe et al make the distinction between two forms of arousal difficulty based on EEG recordings. They suggest 'Type I' is a mild disturbance of arousal where the full bladder creates changes in arousal so the child moves to a lighter stage (1 or 2) of sleep, but the child does not waken. This accounts for 57 % of the enuretic population. 'Type IIa' is much less common (9 percent of the enuretic population) and caused by a more severe 'disturbance in arousal'. They found no EEG changes in response to the full bladder and no arousal from sleep in 'Type IIa' enuresis, whereas in 'Type IIb' (34 percent) in addition continuous detrusor overactivity is found during sleep.

Wolfish et al suggest the most difficult part of the night for all children to arouse from sleep, is the first third [88].

Waking becomes easier as the night progresses. However, Norgaard, Mikkelsen et al and Wolfish et al have all found that children with nocturnal enuresis are also more likely to wet in the first third of the night, often in the first two hours following sleep [88,100,101]. Thus the point of bladder fullness for most enuretic children coincides with a time of night where they find it most difficult to wake from sleep.

It is possible to gauge a child's level of arousability by asking about their ability to arouse to the external signals such as bad weather, noise or unusual sounds, internal signals such as illness worry or self instructions, full bladder signals.

Some children demonstrate an ability to wake but fail to complete voiding in the toilet. They may find leaving bed difficult because of the cold, a fear of the dark, or practical reasons such as the toilet being not readily accessible. Such children benefit from practical ways of help, such as warmth in the room, a torch or a receptacle for urination in the bedroom.

8. Treatment of nocturnal enuresis

The normal annual resolution rate of monosymptomatic nocturnal enuresis is not always accounted for in cure rates reported. When reporting is done with survival analysis, the resolution rate remains visible throughout follow-up [58,79,103].

The outcome of pharmacological treatment for nocturnal enuresis is expressed as either full response or partial response, while on the prescribed medication. A ***full response*** is defined as a reduction in wet nights of at least 90%, ***partial response*** is defined as a reduction in wet nights of 50%-90%; less than 50% reduction in wet nights is considered to be non-response [45,104,105].

A ***lasting cure*** is defined as a full response, still present 6 months or longer after discontinuation of pharmacotherapy. With other forms of therapy (alarm treatment, dry-bed training), full response or partial response are noted immediately after the actual intervention.

With a follow up of at least 6 months, response can become a *lasting cure* (>90% reduction) or a *lasting improvement* (50%-90% reduction). In reports on the outcome of nocturnal enuresis, it should be ascertained if nocturia did replace the nighttime wetting [106].

Nocturia occurs when a child wakes up at night to void.

The older definition of full response, 1 wet night or less per month, correlates closely with a reduction of 90% or more in the number of wet nights.

The 90 percent cut-off point has been chosen in order to allow for the occasional wetting that can occur up to 2 years after otherwise successful treatment during a night when the child sleeps very deeply after a tiring day or runs a fever.

For the individual patient who has achieved a significant reduction in wet nights, the occasional wet episodes (eg once or twice a month) still remain a problem not to be underestimated, especially in the adolescent and adult patient population. Therefore the 90 percent cut-off point should really only apply to the pre-pubertal child.

It is essential to explain the problem to children with mono-symptomatic nocturnal enuresis and their parents and give general advice such as to eat, drink and void regularly during the day, abstain from drinking too much during the late afternoon and evening and have relaxed routines at bedtime. It should be stressed that the condition is common and usually a benign delay in maturation without any psychopathological undertone. A positive attitude towards the child should be utilised and explained that the bed-wetting eventually will cease "but nobody knows exactly when that will happen". Up to 19 percent of children will become dry within the next 8 weeks without any further treatment [107].

The management of Nocturnal enuresis (Figs. 9 and 10) depends on:

- the child's motivation to participate in treatment
- exclusion of confounding psychosocial factors
- providing information and instruction about daily habits underlining the importance of having regular fluid intake and voidings and relaxed routines at bedtime
- regular review of intervention

Although treatment modalities like lifting, fluid restriction, dry-bed training, retention control training, psychotherapy, acupuncture, hypnosis all have been used, there is not sufficient data in the literature to recommend any of these.

Comparison of treatment outcome and cure rates is difficult because of the inconsistent use of definitions and the inclusion of children with daytime symptoms and variable follow-up periods in most studies.

a) Enuresis alarm

The enuresis alarm is the most effective way to treat mono-symptomatic nocturnal enuresis [103]. Intervention with an alarm is associated with nine times less likelihood of relapse than antidiuretic therapy [108].

Alarm therapy has been shown in a meta-analysis to have a 43 percent lasting cure rate [109,110].

Alarm treatment is slow in the beginning so it should be continued at least 6 to 8 weeks before it is considered

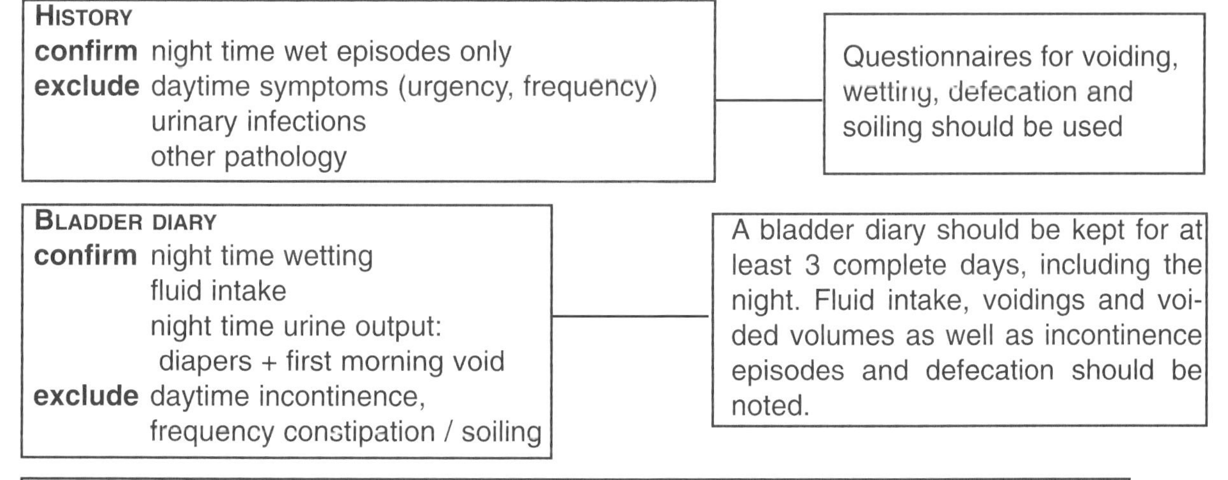

Diagnostic work-up nocturnal enuresis
HISTORY
confirm night time wet episodes only
exclude daytime symptoms (urgency, frequency)
urinary infections
other pathology
Questionnaires for voiding, wetting, defecation and soiling should be used
BLADDER DIARY
confirm night time wetting
fluid intake
night time urine output:
diapers + first morning void
exclude daytime incontinence,
frequency constipation / soiling
A bladder diary should be kept for at least 3 complete days, including the night. Fluid intake, voidings and voided volumes as well as incontinence episodes and defecation should be noted.
PHYSICAL EXAMINATION
confirm normal anatomy, psychomotor development
exclude anatomical abnormalities (genital area and back), neurological abnormalities (reflexes)
Additional and invasive diagnostic procedures are only indicated in selected cases with suspicion of other pathology

Figure 9 : Schematic work-up in patients presenting with nighttime wetting only.

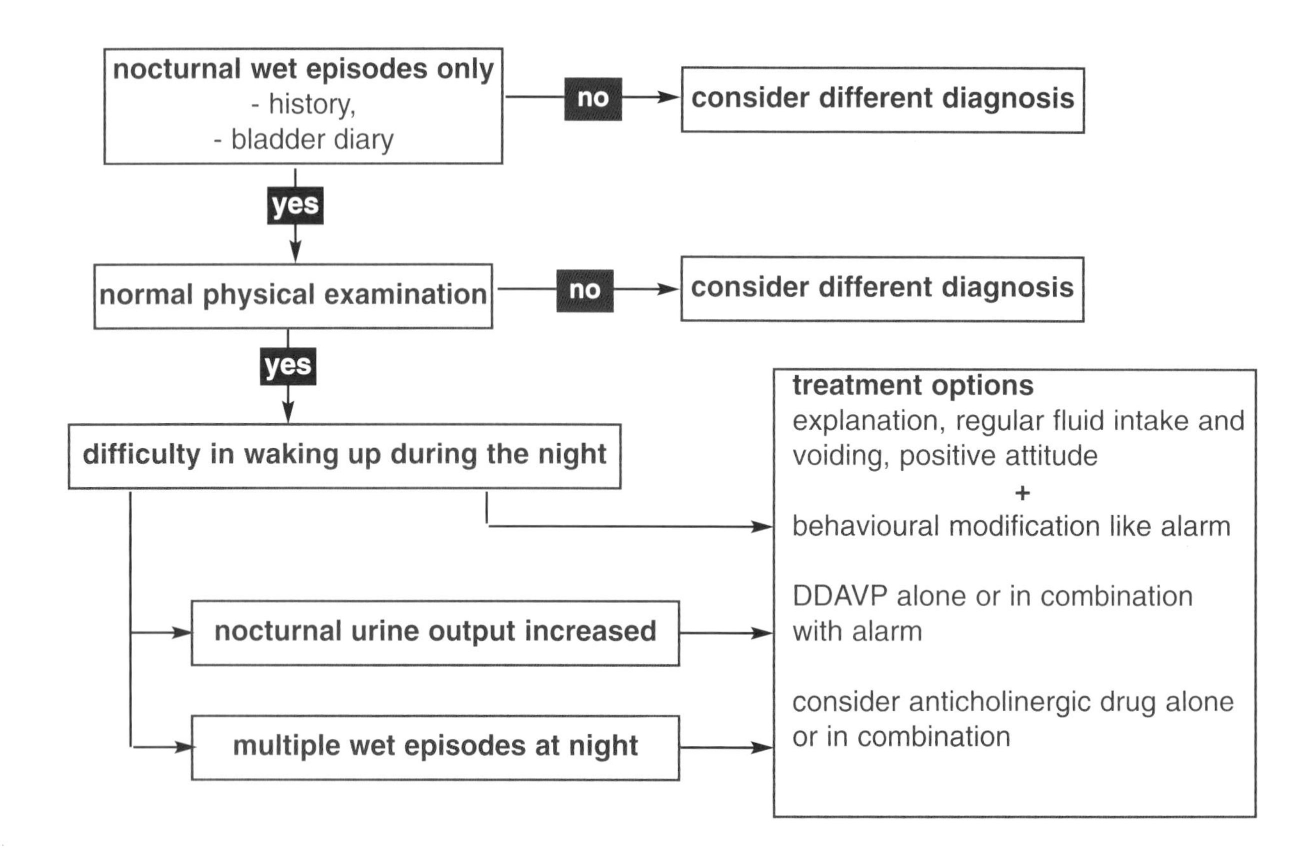

Figure 10 : Pragmatic approach to diagnosing and treatment of nocturnal enuresis.

effective or not. Compliance remains a problem: dropout rates are rarely disclosed in reported studies. Proper guidance and instructions are mandatory.

The mode of action of the alarm has been believed to be an amelioration of arousal to a full bladder, which may be true but lacks scientific validation (see also section IV.3). An interesting finding is that alarm increases nocturnal bladder capacity, which may explain why children after successful treatment are often able to sleep dry without nocturia [111].

Possible future alarm design could include a small ultrasound transducer to monitor bladder volume during the night, so that at a predetermined volume a sound signal is emitted, thus waking the child before the enuresis occurs. ***Level of evidence: 1***

b) Desmopressin

Placebo controlled studies have shown that the antidiuretic drug DDAVP is significantly more effective than placebo [112,113]. Patients on desmopressin were 4.6 times more likely to achieve 14 consecutive dry nights compared with placebo [114]. However, there was no difference after treatment was finished.

In most trials a response rate (more than 50 percent reduction of wet nights) of 60 to 70 percent is found. This corresponds with the number of patients who have nocturnal polyuria as main factor responsible for their nocturnal enuresis.

It has also been established that responders have in fact nocturnal polyuria

Relapse after short-term treatment is rather the rule, whereas long-term treatment may yield better cure rates [115].

Long-term results have been found to be 23 percent of children treated and 31 percent of those who responded to treatment. The 23 percent is not significantly better than spontaneous resolution [116].

Because DDAVP is a potent antidiuretic drug, there have been reports on severe water retention with hyponatremia and convulsions, but these are sporadic [117,118]. ***Level of evidence: 1***

c) Combined treatment with alarm and Desmopressin

Combined treatmen is superior to alarm alone especially for nonresponders of each individual treatment. Both treatments are started at the same time : the vast action of DDAVP is believed to fascilitate the child's adaptation to the alarm [119]. After 6 weeks the DDAVP is discontinued while the alarm treatment is continued until the child becomes completely dry. Compared with either therapy alone, the combination has been found to be particularly effective in children with psychosocial problems. ***Level of evidence: 1***

d) Anticholinergic drugs

In those children who have bladder overactivity during the night, treatment with anticholinergic drugs should be considered [120]. Because it is difficult to perform a nighttime cystometry in these children it may be tried in children who not respond to DDAVP or given in combination with alarm. At present no studies have been performed to demonstrate its efficacy.

e) Tricyclic antidepressants

Because Imipramine and other drugs of the same family have potential lethal side effects they can not be generally recommended for treatment of this non-lethal disorder [121].

Although treatment with tricyclic drugs is associated with a decrease of one wet night per week, the lasting cure rate of only 17 percent restricts the use of these drugs.

Only in selected cases (like adolescent boys with Attention Deficit Hyperactivity Disorder and persistent nocturnal enuresis) it could be considered. ***Level of evidence: 2***

f) Inhibitors of prostaglandin synthesis

Because nocturnal polyuria in children with Nocturnal enuresis may not be entirely attributed to a defect in free water excretion, but rather to an increase in nocturnal excretion of sodium, cyclooxygenase inhibitors (like diclofenac) which reduce urinary sodium excretion, have been tried and in a randomised double blind placebo controlled study proved to be effective [122]. Further studies need to be done to elucidate the role of these drugs.

Full response (while on medication) and cure rates (6 months after cessation of treatment) of Nocturnal Enuresis are summarisez in table 1.

Table 1 : Full response (while on medication) and cure rates (6 months after cessation of treatment) of Nocturnal Enuresis.

	Full response	Cure
Alarm treatment	65 %	43 %
Desmopressin	31 %	22 %
Dry-bed training	40%	18 %
Imipramine		17 %

g) Non responders

About one third of children do not respond to treatment with alarm and/or DDAVP. This should arouse suspicion on nocturnal detrusor overactivity. Prescription of anticholinergics should be considered although evidence from the literature is lacking.

On the other hand some of these children may have functional incontinence (lazy bladders , children with overdistended bladders and infrequent voiding), which was not discovered during the initial workup. They should be given a strict voiding regimen and a combination of DDAVP with the alarm [92].

IV. BEHAVIOUR THERAPY

Behaviour therapy can be considered to be an approach that seeks to change behaviour patterns through altering the individual's environmental contingencies. Its theoretical roots lie in behaviourism which suggests that behaviour derives from contingencies of reinforcement and particular responses made in the presence of stimulus situations.

The focus is on the behaviour itself, rather than any underlying dynamics possibly causing the behaviour. Behaviour is now considered to include an individual's thinking processes and thus the emergence of cognitive behaviour therapy.

Effective treatment within a behaviour therapy tradition aims to modify behaviour which the individual finds distressing or inappropriate. Behaviour therapy is technique driven and includes a range of procedures which can assist the individual in altering their behaviour patterns.

Techniques that have been advocated in treating nocturnal enuresis include:

- positive reinforcement
- cognitive re-structuring
- arousal training
- normalised voiding
- positive practice
- retention control training
- dry bed training
- full spectrum home training

1. Positive reinforcement

Positive reinforcement of a behaviour increases the frequency or strength of that behaviour. Rewards and star charts for 'dry beds' has been traditionally adopted by many parents and health professionals yet they tend to be largely unsuccessful. Children quickly loose faith in them. Generally this is because such reward schedules focus on the outcome (dry night), which the child has little, if any, control over. For most children the dry night is a reward in itself.

There are no reported studies on the effectiveness of such contingent positive reinforcement with nocturnal enuresis. However, there is one study where the alarm has been coupled with 'tangible rewards' contingent on outcome. Kaplan et al described a study of 70 children aged over 6 years with severe nocturnal enuresis (75 percent had tried other methods unsuccessfully) [123]. They allocated 38 children to the alarm plus rewards and 32 were treated with alarm monotherapy in a non-randomised process. Success rates (14 consecutive dry nights) were 87 percent with alarm + rewards compared to 65 percent for alarm monotherapy. The combination of alarm + rewards tended to produce higher success rates but there were no significant differences across the treatment methods on any of the outcome measures.

Rewarding dry nights raises theoretical and ethical concern over the issue of control. A child experiences little control over whether they are wet or dry during sleep and the three main causes (bladder overactivity, lack of vasopressin release and failure to arouse) responsible for nocturnal enuresis are not conceptualised as within the child's control or will [81].

However rewarding a dry night implies that the mechanisms responsible for being dry (bladder stability, release of vasopressin and waking to a full bladder during sleep) are within their control. It might be argued that being dry itself is the intrinsic reward and Harter has argued that tangible rewards for actions the child wishes to engage in will decrease or undermine intrinsic motivation by decreasing the child's sense of self-determination and competence [124].

Current thinking suggests the process, not the outcome, should be rewarded. This means rewarding what is controllable. Rewarding the behaviour or efforts the child makes towards improving the chances of being dry. Thus stars or small rewards might be made contingent on:

- increased daytime drinking
- regular daytime voiding
- waking up to go to the toilet
- voiding before sleep
- waking quickly to an alarm triggering

2. Cognitive re-structuring

There are anecdotal reports concerning the promotion of 'appropriate' thought processes to facilitate improved bladder control. Butler suggested three cognitive processes – auto-suggestion, restructuring beliefs and visualisation. Few studies have however, investigated cognitive change directly [45].

With auto-suggestion the individual is encouraged to cue self statements to a particular event. Thus when passing a toilet door, a child may be taught to think to him or herself 'I can only wee in the toilet'. An investigation by Edwards and van der Spuy found that self instructions were more important than the trance state during hypnotherapy but with a success rate of only 19 percent, autosuggestion cannot be considered a primary form of treatment for nocturnal enuresis [125].

Re-structuring beliefs focuses on enhancing the child's belief that they are active and responsible for behaviour change. Thus an internal attribution for success, it is argued, fosters the child's belief that 'dryness' is due to a change in their functioning, not due to the treatment intervention. Butler et al found that with a structured withdrawal programme over 70 percent of children remained dry when medication was withdrawn [126,127].

They argue that the effective element was that children were encouraged to internalise the success rather than consider the medication as the reason for success.

Visualisation is the employment of imagery as a vehicle for establishing improved bladder control. Only one case study can be found in the literature [128].

An immediate response was noted in this case with a child who had become dependent on the enuresis alarm to wake him.

3. Enuresis alarm

The enuresis alarm remains the most effective means of facilitating arousal form sleep. The essential principle is to alert and sensitise the child to respond quickly and appropriately to a full bladder during sleep, converting the signal from one of urination to that of inhibition of urination and waking. The child usually reacts to the alarm triggering by contracting the muscles of the pelvic floor (and thus stopping urination) and waking. The key to success is not the stimulus intensity of the alarm triggering, but the child's preparedness to awake and respond to the signal [88].

There are variables that coincide with the use of the alarm that may enhance its effectiveness:

- an expectation of success [99],
- avoidance conditioning, whereby the child seeks to avoid the unpleasantness of the noise by spontaneous waking or contraction of the pelvic floor muscles [129],
- increased functional bladder capacity [130],
- increased production of vasopressin in response to the stress of waking to the alarm, which might explain why some 80% of children who become dry with the enuresis alarm are able to sleep through the night and [52],
- a conditioned response whereby waking after urina-

tion serves as an unconditioned stimulus while the startle response of pelvic floor contractions which stops urination is the unconditioned response [131]. With repeated triggerings the alarm produces a conditioned response of inhibition of urination in the presence of detrusor contractions during sleep. Learning to control the pelvic floor muscles during the night, it is argued enables the child to sleep through the night.

Given such possible mechanisms of action it may be postulated that enhanced effectiveness might be facilitated by a positive expectation of success, an emphasis on the importance of waking when the alarm is triggered, reinforcement for waking quickly to the alarm triggering, increasing the child's understanding of the process and keeping detailed records of progress

Reviews of alarm treatment effectiveness suggest a success rate of between 65-75% on undifferentiated samples of children with nocturnal enuresis, where the duration of treatment was between 5 and 12 weeks [103,132,133].

Relapse rates in the 6 months following treatment are in the order of 15 - 30 % [103].

Children successfully treated with an enuresis alarm are less likely to relapse compared with pharmacological interventions [134].

Comparison of the different types of alarm did not show significant outcomes [103].

In general it can be stated that alarm treatment is more effective than other forms of treatment and the lasting cure rate about twice as high [135].

Alarm treatment appears to result in the child learning to sleep through not wake to a full bladder as expected. Monda and Husmann found that during treatment children did wake up to void but following treatment, 70 percent of those who became dry, successfully slept through the night [136]. ***Level of evidence: 1***

4. Arousal training

Arousal training entails reinforcing appropriate behaviour [waking and toileting] in response to alarm triggering. The aim is to reinforce the child's rapid response to the alarm triggering, not on 'learning to keep the bed dry'.

The instructions involve:

- setting up the alarm before sleep
- when the alarm is triggered the child must respond by turning it off within 3 minutes
- the child completes voiding in the toilet, returns to bed and re-sets the alarm
- when the child reacts in this fashion he is rewarded with 2 stickers
- when the child fails to respond in this way the child pays back one sticker

Van Londen et al first described this procedure with a group of 41 children, aged 6-12 years, with predominantly primary enuresis [137]. They reported 98 percent success (14 consecutive dry nights) compared to 73 percent success with alarm monotherapy.

The difference was significant ($p<0.001$). Ninety two per cent remained dry after $2^{1/2}$ years suggesting very low relapse rate. An extraordinary aspect of this study was the lack of contact between therapist and parents. All those included were parents who had ordered an alarm from a rental agency and were given the instructions with the alarm. The authors conclude that arousal training is 'definitely the treatment of choice for non-clinical enuretic children between 6 and 12 years'. Compared with other studies and considering experience of daily practise one may question the very high success rate in this particular group of patients.

5. Normalised voiding

Normalised voiding involves:

- increasing daytime fluid intake
- increasing the frequency of micturitions during the day by voiding regularly at pre-determined times [every 2-3 hours] and
- avoidance of postponing urination.

This is usually used in combination with other treatment modalities. It is an attempt to normalise voiding, whereas many of the children postpone voiding. Although this form of treatment in itself may be the cornerstone of success, it has never been tested as a stand-alone treatment. In a study by Kruse et al, a small group of patients (n=5) was described, aged 10 years and older, all of whom had a history of several treatment failures and who tended to hold in the daytime [92].

Most children also had a small functional bladder capacity and day-time urgency: most likely due to detrusor overactivity. They found using an alarm with normalised voiding was successful (<1 wet per fortnight) with two individuals at 1 month; successful with another child at 5 month and a further success at 9-12m. The 1 'failure' reduced wetting frequency to twice a fortnight, from 50 percent wet at baseline after 1 month of treatment.

6. Positive practice

The aim of positive practice is to develop an alternative response to bedwetting. Following a wet bed, the child is encouraged to practice the following, both immediately and prior to bed-time the next night:

- the child is encouraged to lie in bed with the lights off,
- count to 50,
- go to the toilet and attempt to urinate,
- repeat this 20 times.

For younger children the procedure is reduced to 10 repetitions counting to 20. Bollard and Nettelbeck in their component analysis of dry bed training employed this strategy with 12 individuals with a success rate of 83 percent [138].

It may be clear that this can only be attempted in motivated children and good parental support.

7. Retention control training

The aim is to assist the detrusor muscles in adapting to increased bladder pressure and volumes and make the child aware of to full bladder sensations [139].

Once a day the child is asked to drink 3 glasses of water. When the child indicates a need to void, he/she is asked to hold (postpone micturition) for increasing amounts of time (in 3 minute increments). Rewards are given for each increase and the process discontinued when the child is able to postpones for 45 minutes. When used with children with nocturnal enuresis it has been combined with the enuresis alarm. Houts et al found a success rate of 87 percent with 15 children when combined with an enuresis alarm [131].

There has been an attempt to use night time retention control training in combination with an alarm. The aim is to increase functional bladder capacity and practice inhibiting urination. Before bedtime the child is given a large drink (at least 2 glasses). Every hour during sleep, the child is woken and directed to the toilet (see next section *scheduled waking*) At the toilet door the child is then asked if he/she can hold for another hour. If the child elects to hold, he or she is praised, but if the child elects to void, he or she is encouraged to hold for a few minutes before voiding. At the bedside the child is given another large drink. This procedure was discontinued after one night with Bollard & Nettelbeck finding a success rate of 92 percent in 12 children [138]. Motivation and parental support are essential in this type of training.

8. Scheduled waking

The aim is to encourage arousability from sleep. As originally described, there are two aspects: hourly waking on the first night and scheduled waking thereafter [129].

With the hourly waking on one night only, the child is:

- woken each hour with a minimal prompt,
- asked to void in the toilet and
- praised for having kept the sheets dry.

On subsequent nights, scheduled waking involved waking the child three hours after sleep and encouraging him or her to void. For every dry night the waking time is brought forward by a 1/2 hour until it is timed to occur one hour after going to sleep.

Bollard & Nettelbeck found this procedure was 100% effective when combined with the alarm in 12 children [138].

9. Dry bed training

This is a package of behavioural procedures used in conjunction with the enuresis alarm first described by Azrin et al [129]. It incorporates:

- the enuresis alarm,
- positive practice (practice of waking),
- cleanliness training (encouraging the child to take responsibility for removing of wet night clothes and sheets, re-making the bed and resetting the alarm),
- waking schedules – to ease arousability from sleep as described above and involving:

1. for the first night, waking the child each hour, praising a dry bed, encouraging the child to decide at the toilet door whether he or she needed to void, and on returning to bed the child is encouraged to have a further drink and
2. on the second night the child is woken and taken to the toilet 3 hours after going to sleep. For each dry night the waking time is brought forward by 30 minutes. If wet on any night the waking time stays at the time of the previous evening. The waking schedule was discontinued when the waking time reached 30 minutes following sleep. The waking schedule is resumed if the child begins wetting twice or more in any week, starting again 3hours after sleep.

- social reinforcement and
- increased fluid intake.

High success rates and low drop out have been reported although relapse rates are no different to enuresis alarm treatment. Modifications have been advocated to remove some of the more punitive elements of the programme but it remains a complex, time consuming and demanding procedure.

Hirasing et al found 80 percent success with group administered dry bed training. Girls responded better than boys [140]. The majority of parents were satisfied with the programme but opinions of the children were divided. Factors not related to success were the child's age, bedwetting frequency, secondary enuresis or family history.

An important component analysis by Bollard & Nettelbeck found that the enuresis alarm accounted for most of the success achieved through dry bed training, that a large proportion of the components of the procedure could be eliminated without sacrificing much of its overall effectiveness and that the waking schedule coupled with the enuresis alarm was as effective as the complete dry bed training programme [138]. ***Level of evidence: 3***

10. Full spectrum home training.

This programme incorporates:

- the enuresis alarm,
- retention control training,
- cleanliness training and
- overlearning,

Whelan and Houts claim a 75 percent success rate after an average of 12 weeks. This is not dissimilar to success rated with the alarm on its own. As with dry bed training, the enuresis alarm has proved to be by far the most effective component of the programme leading some clinicians to consider all the other procedures to be adjuncts to the alarm and employed for specific situations [140].

The enuresis alarm remains the most effective means of facilitating arousal from sleep. The key to success is not the stimulus intensity of the alarm triggering, but the child's preparedness to awake and respond to the signal.

V. DAY AND NIGHT TIME INCONTINENCE

1. Introduction

Urinary incontinence in children may be caused by a congenital anatomical or neurologic abnormality, such as ectopic ureter, bladder extrophy or myelomeningocele (MMC). Many children, however, do not have such an obvious cause for their incontinence and they are referred to as having 'functional incontinence'.

The process of gaining control over bladder and sphincter function is complex and it is understandable that this series of complex events is highly susceptible to the development of various types of dysfunction. These acquired functional disorders overlap with other types of bladder functional disturbances that may have a more organic but congenital underlying pathophysiological basis.

The desire to void is a sensation which, in the developing child, is incorporated into daily life so that voiding takes place at an appropriate time and place. Problems with training or psychological difficulties can have a great impact on the results of training: some parents send their child to the toilet many times, though his/her bladder may be empty [142].

Voiding in these circumstances can only be achieved by abdominal straining. As the child will be rewarded when he or she produces even the smallest amount of urine, the result may be an abnormal voiding pattern. The same is true when children receive negative feedback related to voiding [143].

Functional urinary incontinence in children may be due to disturbances of the filling phase, the voiding phase or a combination of both. Detrusor overactivity may cause frequency and urgency, with or without urge incontinence. Girls present with symptoms of detrusor overactivity more often than boys, but sometimes other symptoms, such as urinary tract infections or constipation, prevail. Incomplete or no relaxation of the sphincteric mechanism during voiding results in intermittent voiding. When incontinence is the result of urethral overactivity during voiding the term 'dysfunctional voiding' is used [144].

Bladder function during the filling phase in these children may be essentially normal, but instability may be present. In children with a lazy bladder, voiding occurs without detrusor contractions, and post-void residuals and incontinence are the main characteristics.

Diagnosis is based on the medical and voiding history, a physical examination, bladder diaries and uroflowmetry. The upper urinary tract should be evaluated in children with recurrent infections and dysfunctional voiding (reflux). Uroflowmetry can be combined with pelvic floor electromyography to demonstrate overactivity of the pelvic floor muscles. Urodynamic studies are usually reserved for patients with dysfunctional voiding and those not responding to treatment [145].

Treatment is usually a combination of 'standard therapy' (see below), behaviour therapy, bladder training, physiotherapy and medical treatment. The importance of treatment during childhood was pointed out in a general population study of 1333 adult women. Fifty percent reported symptoms of stress incontinence and 22 percent reported symptoms of urge incontinence. Eight percentage had severe symptoms. Women who at age six years had wet episodes during the day or several nights a week were more likely to suffer severe incontinence and report urge symptoms: occasional bedwetting was not associated with an increased risk in adult life [146].

The role of α-blockers needs to be evaluated further. Also, neuromodulation may have a place in treatment but the exact indications need to be defined. Clean intermittent self-catheterization is sometimes necessary in children with a lazy bladder and large residuals who do not respond to a more conservative approach.

2. PREVALENCE

For detailed information on the prevalence of daytime incontinence the Chapter on Epidemiology should be consulted, where an overview is presented on the currently available data. The main problem is that it is impossible to draw any conclusions from the presented data as different studies have used definitions and criteria that differ from others. Daytime or combined daytime and nighttime incontinence at least once a week seems to occur in about 2-4 percent of 7-year old children and is more common in girls than in boys [17].

Overall the rates of prevalence vary from 1 to 10 percent, but in general for 6 to 7 year old children the prevalence is somewhere between 2 and 4 percent, and rapidly decreases during the following years [65,66,98, 147,148,149,150,151].

Children with daytime or mixed wetting were found to suffer from urgency in 50.7 percent of the cases, with 79.1 percent wetting themselves at least once in 10 days [65].

Urge symptoms seem to peak at age 6–9 years and diminish towards puberty, with an assumed spontaneous cure rate for daytime wetting of about 14% per year [58,193].

Most children are toilet-trained by the age of 3 years, though there is a huge social and cultural variation. In a recent study by Bloom et al, the mean age ranged from 0.75 to 5.25 years, with girls being trained earlier (2.25 years) than boys (2.56 years) [147].

Hellström et al found day wetting at least once a week at age 17 in 0.2% of boys and 0.7% of girls and as compared to 2.1% and 3.1%, respectively, at age 7 years [152].

Swithinbank et al had found a prevalence of day wetting (including also "occasional" wetting) in 12.5% in children at age 10-11 years declining to 3.0% at age 15-16 years [153].

Based on these, it seems that the prevalence of all kinds of daytime incontinence diminishes with 1-2% per year of life from age 10-11 to age 15-16 years, while daytime incontinence at least once a week seems to diminish with 0.2% per year of life from age 7 to age 17 years. Because of treatment the studies may not recount the true natural history.

By the age of 5 years, unless organic causes are present, the child is normally able to void at will and to postpone voiding in a socially acceptable manner. By this age, night-time and daytime involuntary wetting become a social problem and a cause for therapeutic intervention.

Some children are diagnosed with an urge syndrome or dysfunctional voiding, but are actually victims of child abuse. This is difficult to prove but should be kept in mind, especially when invasive diagnostic and therapeutic procedures are contemplated. Of adult women with complex urinary symptoms, a significant proportion report sexual abuse as a child [154].

3. BLADDER-SPHINCTER DYSFUNCTION, RECURRENT URINARY TRACT INFECTION AND VESICOURETERIC REFLUX

The relationship between bladder dysfunction and VUR was first described by Allen and Koff and since confirmed by several authors [155,156,157,158] (Fig. 11).

In a study by Sillen of children with gross bilateral reflux, extreme detrusor overactivity without signs of infravesical obstruction was found in boys. Infant girls with gross bilateral reflux did not show the same degree of detrusor overactivity [159].

Similar findings were noted by other investigators assessing newborns with severe reflux. These studies in infants and the association of dysfunctional elimination syndromes with reflux and infection in older children strongly suggest that vesicoureteral reflux is a secondary disorder related more to abnormal bladder function than to a primary anatomic defect at the ureterovesical junction.

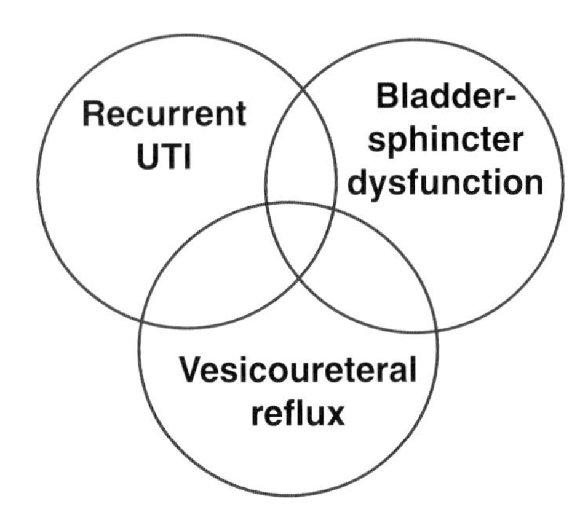

Figure 11 : Association of recurrent UTI, bladder-sphincter dysfunction and vesicoureteral reflux: each occurs separately, but the combination increases the risk of renal damage.

It has recently been shown that increased intravesical pressure, without reflux may be detrimental for the upper tracts: renal scarring without reflux was described by Vega at al recently [160].

Vesicoureteric reflux is a common finding in children with a neuropathic bladder and detrusor-sphincter dyssynergia: with the institution of clean intermittent catheterisation combined with anticholinergic drugs, reflux disappears in a high percentage of cases. It is believed that the decrease of detrusor overactivity and restoration of functional capacity in combination with regular and complete emptying of the bladder are the responsible co-factors [161].

In a prospective non-randomised clinical series of daywetting children a strong correlation was found between recurrent urinary tract infections and bladder-sphincter dysfunction [162,163]. Girls with asymptomatic bacteriuria were found to have symptoms of an overactive bladder, such as urgency and daytime incontinence in a high percentage [164].

In the majority of children with detrusor-sphincter dysfunction the recurrent infections disappeared following successful treatment of the bladder dysfunction. This finding confirms the hypothesis that detrusor-sphincter dysfunction is the main factor responsible for the infections (and to a lesser extend vice versa) [165,166].

At present, current opinion is that vesicoureteral reflux as such does not predispose to UTI: however it may facilitate renal involvement (causing pyelonephritis) once bacteriuria has been established in the bladder. This concept has not been scientifically validated and the incidence of renal scars as a consequence of pyelonephritis is reportedly the same, regardless of whether reflux has been documented or not [167].

In clinical studies there is a strong association between bladder-sphincter dysfunction, recurrent UTI and reflux, but the causal relationships still need to be scientifically investigated. Because of this association, bladder-sphincter dysfunction in combination with vesicoureteral reflux and infection is a potentially hazardous situation for the upper urinary tract and should be treated with appropriate care and sometimes even aggressively [23,168,169,170].

4. Classification

Several classifications have been used for children who present with varying degrees of 'functional' urinary symptoms unrelated to apparent disease, injury or congenital malformation. Some are based on urodynamic patterns, others on clinical presentation. The majority of children present with frequency, urgency and infections, with or without incontinence. Although the correlation between urodynamic findings and presenting symptoms does not seem to be very high, urodynamic investigations have given us more insight into the pathophysiology behind the symptoms and signs, and made the clinical expression of non-neurogenic bladder–sphincter dysfunction more specific [171,172].

On the basis of urodynamic studies, the functional dysfunctions can be termed unstable bladder, bladder-sphincter dyscoordination, lazy bladder and occult neurogenic bladder. According to the definition of the International Children's Continence Society, incontinence as a result of a filling phase dysfunction (mainly bladder instability) is called urge syndrome and urge incontinence [22]. When incontinence is the result of a voiding phase dysfunction it is called dysfunctional voiding, being subdivided into staccato voiding, interrupted voiding and lazy bladder syndrome.

The term 'non-neurogenic detrusor–sphincter dysfunction' is used to describe the whole spectrum, from simple detrusor instability to severe cases with deterioration of the upper tracts. The fact that we cannot demonstrate a neurologic deficit, however, does not exclude the possibility that a neurologic abnormality was present at the onset of the problem. It has been postulated that detrusor instability may eventually lead to lazy bladder syndrome or severe dys-coordination between detrusor and sphincter. However, the natural history of many of these children does not confirm this hypothesis, nor the early onset of severe pathology in some of them.

Hoebeke et al found no evidence for this dysfunctional voiding sequence: children with functional incontinence have different primary diseases, but all have a common risk of incontinence, UTI (especially in girls with a lazy bladder), reflux (15%) and constipation (17%) [173] (Fig. 12).

a) Urge syndrome and urge incontinence

Clinically, this condition is best characterised by frequent episodes of an urgent need to void, countered by contraction of the pelvic floor muscles (guarding reflex) and hold manoeuvres, like squatting. The symptoms are caused by detrusor overactivity during the filling phase, causing the imperative urge to void. These detrusor contractions are countered by voluntary contraction of the pelvic floor muscles to postpone voiding and minimise wetting. The detrusor contractions can be demonstrated urodynamically, as can the increased activity of the pelvic floor muscles during each contraction. The voiding phase is essentially normal, but detrusor contraction during voiding may be extremely powerful. The flow rate reaches its maximum quickly and may level off ('tower shape').

Depending on fluid intake and urine production, the complaints of incontinence become worse towards the

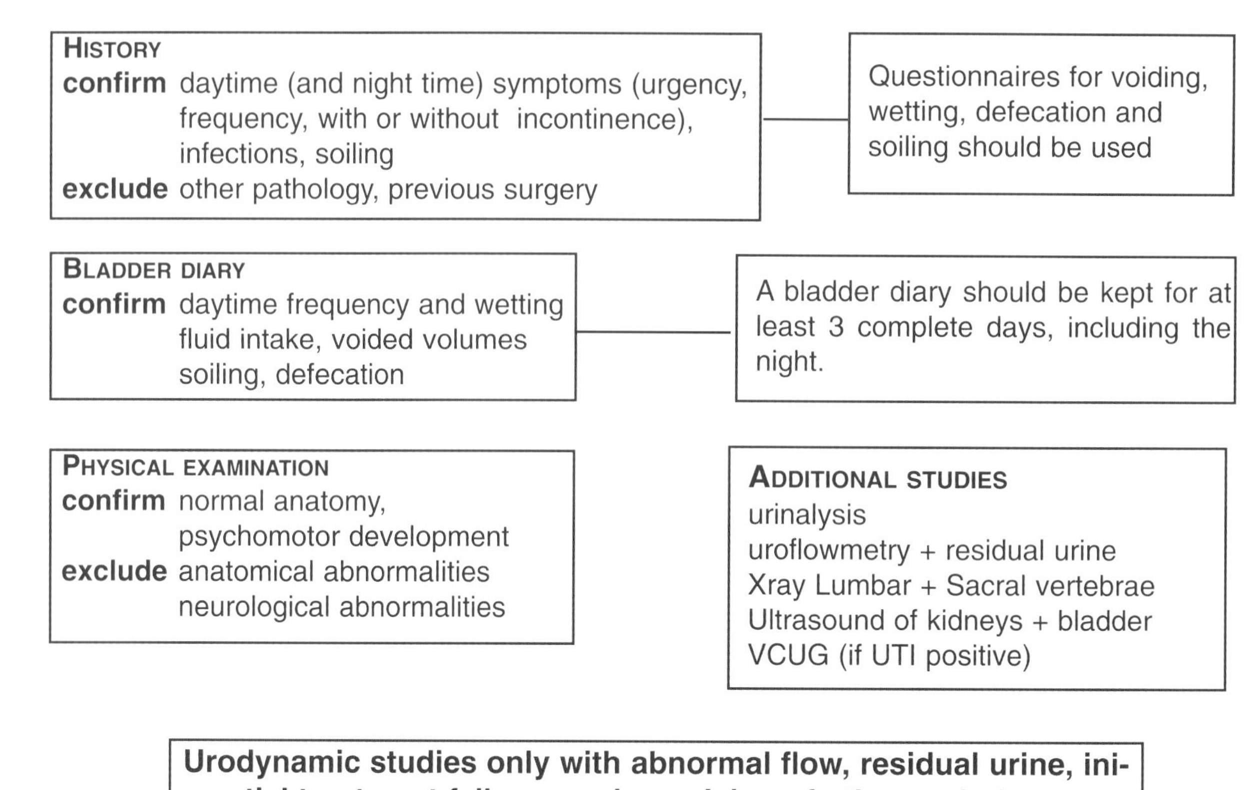

Diagnostic work-up functional incontinence
HISTORY
confirm daytime (and night time) symptoms (urgency, frequency, with or without incontinence), infections, soiling
exclude other pathology, previous surgery
Questionnaires for voiding, wetting, defecation and soiling should be used
BLADDER DIARY
confirm daytime frequency and wetting fluid intake, voided volumes soiling, defecation
A bladder diary should be kept for at least 3 complete days, including the night.
PHYSICAL EXAMINATION
confirm normal anatomy, psychomotor development
exclude anatomical abnormalities neurological abnormalities
ADDITIONAL STUDIES
urinalysis
uroflowmetry + residual urine
Xray Lumbar + Sacral vertebrae
Ultrasound of kidneys + bladder
VCUG (if UTI positive)
Urodynamic studies only with abnormal flow, residual urine, initial treatment failures and suspicion of other pathology.
Cystoscopy is rarely indicated

Figure 12 : Schematic work-up of children presenting with daytime (and night time incontinence)

end of the day, due to loss of concentration and fatigue and may also occur during the night. Children usually diminish their fluid intake to minimise wetting, and therefore incontinence may not be the main complaint or symptom. Urge syndrome should also be considered in "continent" children with recurrent UTI and vesicoureteral reflux: the bladder diary will usually demonstrate that fluid intake is minimal and voided volumes are smaller than expected.

Some children with bladder overactivity are not incontinent during the day but only at night: during the day they usually also demonstrate the symptoms of bladder overactivity and should be treated accordingly. They do not have monosymptomatic nocturnal enuresis but "incontinence".

The powerful flow resulting from urge syndrome can cause further problems, particularly when the pelvic floor muscles have become overactively trained and act as a bladder outlet funnel. It has been postulated that in children with recurrent urinary tract infections this may damage the mucosa and be the cause of pain and more infections.

Frequent voluntary contractions of the pelvic floor muscles inevitably lead to postponement of defecation, and constipation and faecal soiling are common signs in children with overactive bladder [174]. The constipation is worsened by diminished fluid intake. Constipation may be the leading symptom.

By adopting a structured approach to history and physical examination, the diagnosis of urge syndrome can be made in the majority of patients with confidence, without the need for invasive diagnostic procedures. Urine flow rate registration and post-void residual urine measurement can be helpful. Children with recurrent urinary tract infections require an ultrasound evaluation of the upper tracts as well as a voidingcystourethrograph (VCUG) to assess reflux [23,175].

The primary mode of therapy in urge syndrome is antimuscarinic medication. Attention should however also be given to explanation and demystification of the problem, together with voiding instructions, treatment of concomitant constipation and urinary infections.

By adopting a structured approach to history and physical examination, the diagnosis of urge syndrome can be made in the majority with confidence, without the need for invasive diagnostic procedures.

There is no evidence that medical treatment is better than standard therapy.

b) Dysfunctional voiding

Children with dysfunctional voiding usually present with incontinence, urinary tract infections and constipation. It is primarily believed to be a voiding disorder, but detrusor dysfunction is common.

No clear data are available on the possible causes of dysfunctional voiding. It may be that overactive bladder eventually leads to overactivity of the pelvic floor muscles, with subsequent insufficient relaxation during voiding. Alternatively, poor relaxation of the pelvic floor muscles during voiding may be a learned condition.

In some girls anatomical anomalies of the external urethral meatus seem to be associated with a higher incidence of dysfunctional voiding. The stream may be deflected anteriorly and cause stimulation of the clitoris with subsequent reflex activity of the bulbocavernosus muscle causing intermittent voiding [176].

In those children with poor or no coordination between detrusor contraction and sphincter relaxation, there may be many similarities with true detrusor–sphincter dyssynergia, which by definition is a neurologic problem.

Several forms of abnormal flow patterns in children with dysfunctional voiding have been described, inclu ding the following:

- Staccato voiding: characterised by periodic bursts of pelvic floor activity during voiding, with prolonged voiding time and sometimes residual urine. The flow is still continuous.
- Interrupted voiding: characterised by incomplete and infrequent voiding, with micturition in several separate fractions. Bladder volume is usually enlarged and unsustained contractions can be seen during voiding. Residual urine is usually present.

Detrusor instability may be seen in both forms of dysfunctional voiding during urodynamic studies, but it may be absent [23,162,166,172,177].

Diagnosis should be based on a careful history and physical examination, complemented by bladder diaries, renal ultrasound studies, and urinary flow and residual urine measurements. The pattern of the flow curve is usually indicative. The combination of uroflowmetry with pelvic floor electromyography (EMG) registration and post-void measurement of residual urine may obviate the need for an invasive urodynamic study.

Primary aim in the treatment of dysfunctional voiding is relaxation of the pelvic floor muscles: if bladder overactivity is present as well, anticholinergic drugs can be added to relax the detrusor muscle and increase functional capacity. Recurrent urinary infections and constipation should be treated and prevented during the treatment period. Rehabilitation of the pelvic floor aims at complete relaxation of the pelvic floor muscles and complete emptying of the bladder.

c) Lazy Bladder syndrome

Children with a lazy bladder void infrequently, and usually present with urinary tract infections and overflow incontinence. Urodynamically, the bladder has a greater than normal capacity, a normal compliance and there is no detrusor contraction during voiding. Abdominal pressure is the driving force for voiding.

A correct diagnosis can only be made through urodynamic investigation. Renal function studies, renal ultrasound and VCUG should be performed to assess the extent of renal damage and reflux. Long-standing overactivity of the pelvic floor may in some children be responsible for decompensation of the detrusor, leading to a non-contractile detrusor. However, no data are available to support this theory.

Treatment is aimed at optimising bladder emptying after each void. Clean intermittent (self) catheterisation is the method of choice in combination with treatment of infections and constipation (which may be extreme in these patients). Intravesical elctrostimulation has been described, but is as yet not recommended as a routine procedure in these children.

d) Non-neurogenic neurogenic bladder

This condition has been described by Hinman and Bauman, and was looked upon as an acquired personality disorder [178,179,180].

It is also referred to as 'occult neuropathic bladder' [181].

The psychogenic model has since been abandoned and the condition is now considered to be the extreme endstage of dysfunctional voiding, though no studies confirm this pathophysiological chain of events.

Urodynamically, non-neurogenic neurogenic bladder is characterised by diminished bladder volume and compliance. Bladder instability is usually present (resembling hyperreflexia in the neuropathic bladder) and overactivity of the pelvic floor muscles occurs during voiding. Videourodynamics or a VCUG usually shows all the features of a true neuropathic bladder. It is believed that long-standing detrusor overactivity in combination with pelvic floor overactivity may lead to this condition.

Although physical and neurologic examination, as well as an MRI of the spinal cord, may be completely normal, a hidden neurologic disorder must be considered. This is because, in many patients, the early onset of the problems and severe renal impairment make the 'end-stage theory' less likely.

Treatment is complex in these patients. Sometimes anticholinergic drugs in combination with clean intermittent (self) catheterisation is sufficient, but occasionally surgical bladder augmentation to safeguard the upper urinary tract and promote continence is necessary.

e) Giggle incontinence

Laughter can trigger partial to complete bladder emptying in some children well into their teenage years, and intermittently into adulthood [182].

The condition occurs in both boys and girls and is generally self-limiting. The exact mechanism of leakage is poorly understood as demonstrable urodynamic studies do not reveal abnormality, there is no anatomical dysfunction and both urinalysis and upper tract visualisation are normal.

It has been postulated that laughter induces a general hypotonic state with urethral relaxation, thus predisposing an individual to incontinence, however the effect has not been demonstrated on either smooth or skeletal muscle [183]. It has also been suggested that giggle incontinence is due to laughter triggering the micturition reflex and overriding central inhibitory mechanisms.

Suffererers are neurologically normal but display physiological variations in response or control [184,185].

Treatment is notoriously difficult and often long term, such that positive results may simply reflect a natural history of the disorder. There are reports of positive results with conditioning training, methylphenidate, and Imipramine [183,184,186].

There is no acceptable evidence that any of these treatments are better than no intervention.

f) Vesicovaginal entrapment

Urinary leakage that occurs in girls within a short time following micturition to complete bladder emptying and is not associated with any urge to void may be associated with entrapment of urine in the vagina. The hymen can be funnel shaped or the labia partially fused or functionally unable to be spread during voiding. The classic presentation is of a girl who does not spread her legs during voiding or who on questioning has a posterior pelvic tilted position on the toilet. Alteration of voiding mechanics results in an immediate improvement in post-void continence.

5. NON-PHARMACOLOGICAL TREATMENT

The main objectives of treatment are to normalise the micturition pattern, normalise bladder and pelvic floor overactivity and cure the incontinence, infections and constipation.

Traditional therapy for day-wetting children is cognitive and behavioural, using explanation of bladder function, learning to recognise the sensation of urge, and eradication of holding manoeuvres (i.e. immediate micturition without postponement). Micturition charts and diaries are established aids for bladder retraining, sometimes in combination with alarm clocks, reminding the child to urinate every 3–4 hours. Ultrasound can be used as a biofeedback mechanism to aid reduction of residual volume.

"Bladder training" is used widely, but the evidence that it works is variable [168,187,188]. Some authors contend that in less severely affected children a thorough explanation of the underlying causes and the expected progress of resolution is sufficient treatment in itself [149]. More active conventional management involves a combination of cognitive, behavioural, physical and pharmacological therapy methods. Common modes of treatment include parent and child reassurance, bladder retraining (including timed toileting), pharmacotherapy, pelvic floor muscle relaxation and the use of biofeedback to inhibit rises in detrusor pressure associated with urinary incontinence [189,190,191,192, 193]. Further treatment options include suggestive or hypnotic therapy and acupuncture.

A combination of bladder training programs and pharmacological treatment, aimed specifically at reducing detrusor contractions, is often useful and sometimes necessary.

Curran et al described the long term results of conservative treatment of children with idiopathic bladder overactivity [194]. Of 30 patients follow-up was long enough to draw conclusions; it showed complete resolution in 21 and markedly improvement in five patients. The average time to resolution of symptoms was 2.7 years. Children with very small or large bladders were less likely to benefit from this treatment. Age and gender were not significant predictors of resolution although girls were more likely to have resolution than boys.

a) Bladder rehabilitation

Urotherapy is used in the rehabilitation of the dysfunctional bladder and is a combination of cognitive, behavioral and physical therapy methods. The program is based on careful evaluation of bladder function and knowledge about normal development of bladder control. The evaluation also includes how the child itself handles the situation.

The aim of urotherapy is to normalise the micturition pattern and prevent further functional disturbances: it is an integrated concept, from filing to the emptying phase.

Although the concept of urotherapy dates back to the late 1970's, clinical studies are still scarce and describe compound therapies rather than single interventions, which makes it difficult to evaluate the results [169,190,191].

Rehabilitation of bladder and pelvic floor muscles using different modalities, such as explanation and instructions, in combination with medical treatment of constipation and infections, physiotherapy and biofeedback play a major role in the treatment of children with bladder and sphincter dysfunctions.

1. Standard therapy

Once the child is interested in its own bladder and voiding problem, careful instructions can be given to the child. The function of the bladder and sphincteric mechanism is explained and the child has to learn how to void again. This can obviously be done in several ways and much depends on the child's abilities and parental support.

The main points are:

- explanation and demystification
- instructions on how and when to void (at regular intervals and in a good position)
- bladder diaries
- treatment of concomitant constipation
- treatment of concomitant infections and antibiotic prophylaxis

Regular voidings, sufficient fluid intake and dietary measures to promote easy defecation are of utmost importance. Also voiding in such a way that the pelvic floor muscles can relax completely during voiding is important. Bladder diaries are filled in by the child to follow the daily life of the child. Children with urge syndrome start with shorter intervals, gradually increasing them as soon as urgency attacks disappear. Children with dysfunctional voiding have to learn how to decrease the intervals.

During the treatment period it is important to have the child frequently visit the clinic in order to offer sufficient support to the child and parents and to discuss the diaries and check for residual urine. Home training programs, including reminders, are designed for use between the visits to the clinic.

This standard approach is always used as a first step. Although this method has been described by several authors, there are no prospective randomised studies available to evaluate the success rate. ***Level of evidence: 2***

2. Physiotherapy

In children with urge syndrome and dysfunctional voiding the pelvic floor muscles are almost always overactive: the primary objective of physical therapy therefore should be to teach the children to relax the pelvic floor muscles during voiding.

Success rates vary between 50 and 80 percent: all studies describe a heterogenous group of children, use more than one treatment modality (like standard therapy in combination with physical therapy and biofeedback) and outcome is defined inconsistently [196,197].

The cited studies describe physiotherapy exercises in an excellent way and show definite improvement of signs and symptoms. Controlled studies about pelvic floor exercises are still missing. The finding of these studies that children who previously had been treated unsuccessfully with biofeedback or standard therapy alone responded to the comprehensive package suggests that the comprehensive program is more effective. ***Level of evidence: 3***

b) Biofeedback

Biofeedback implies perception to some degree of detrusor contraction (filling phase) or pelvic floor relaxation (emptying phase). This achieved by monitoring continuously a signal that carries information about detrusor or pelvic floor muscles. The feedback loop enables the child to influence the process provided cognitive capabilities are developed normal. The feedback loop also graphically demonstrates the habitual non-physiological response of children with urge syndrome or dysfunctional voiding. Training with biofeedback can be used as a single treatment [198, 199], or in conjunction with a comprehensive rehabilitation program [195,196,200].

An overactive detrusor contraction with imperative urge should be inhibited before it escalates. With central inhibition, the emergency brake of forceful pelvic floor muscle contraction need not be applied.

Cystometric biofeedback is used to teach the child how to recognise and inhibit overactive detrusor contractions by watching the pressure curve during cystometry: this is invasive and time consuming and therefore has limited use and is not used as a routine treatment.

Using the flowpattern as biofeedback, with or without EMG of pelvic floor muscles, will teach the child how to relax the pelvic floor during micturition: the child sits on a toilet with a flow transducer, watching the flow curve and EMG on line on a computer display, trying to empty completely in one relaxed voiding. Ultrasound can be used to determine residual urine. Sometimes interactive computer games are used to make it more attractive to children [201].

The results of biofeedback are reported only in a few studies. In one study the results were classified as good in 68%, improved in 13 % and not improved in 29%: the positive effect of biofeedback is confirmed by others. In most studies no information is provided on residual urine. Also inclusion criteria and outcome measures vary considerably between the various studies [202,203,204,205]. ***Level of evidence: 2-3***

In its most simple form it can be regarded as a self-disciplinary measure to correct a long-standing bladder habit. The principle of "re-education" using biofeedback has also been used to train individual children to inhibit inappropriate rises in detrusor pressure during bladder filling. The practice of biofeedback can help children learn both inhibition of vesical pressure increase and improved recruitment of skeletal muscle urethral closure mechanisms [206].

c) Clean intermittent (self) catheterisation

In children with a lazy bladder, when the detrusor contractions are minimal or absent, bladder emptying can be achieved with timed and double voiding. If this does not provide adequate results, clean intermittent self-catheterization (CISC) may be tried. This requires careful guidance for both the child and the parents. Sometimes it is necessary to give the child a suprapubic catheter for a while and gradually prepare him/her to accept CISC. Once the infections have cleared and the child is continent it will become easier for both the parents and the child to accept. The frequency of CISC depends on the severity of the problem and may vary between four times a day and once a day before going to bed.

d) Electrostimulation

Neuromuscular electrical stimulation may be directed at the pelvic floor or the detrusor. However, the invasive nature of the procedure makes it less attractive, particularly for children. A recently described technique using transcutaneous stimulation with surface electrodes stimulating the sacral root (S3) provided promising results but needs further validation [207]. Stimulation of 2 Hz was applied for 2 hours daily over 6 weeks in 16 children with proven detrusor instability. Two did not respond at all, but bladder capacity increased in nine patients and incontinence decreased in six.

At present there is insufficient data available to justify intravesical electrostimulation or transcutaneous neuromodulation routinely in children. Some centres are using different modalities to test their efficacy in children [208,209,210,211].

e) Alarm treatment

This modality is not frequently used for daytime wetting, but occasionally individual patients may benefit. Only one randomised clinical trial has been published to establish the efficacy of this form of treatment. Halliday et al compared a contingent alarm (which sounded when the child wet) with a non-contingent alarm system (which sounded at intermittent intervals) [212]. The trial included 44 participants half of whom were assigned to each of the two types of alarm by a quota allocation system that considered age, sex, type and frequency of daytime wetting. After 3 months of treatment success was measured as 6 consecutive weeks without daytime wetting. All children who failed to achieve this dryness were said to be persistently wetting during the day. By this definition 9 children in the non-contingent group and 6 children in the contingent group had persistent wetting. Although the risk of persistent wetting with the contingent alarm was 67 percent of the risk of persistent wetting with the non-contingent alarm, the difference in reduction in wetting between the two groups was not significant (RR 0.67, 95% CI 0.29 to 1.56).

f) Conclusion

Most clinical studies describe compound therapies rather than single interventions, which makes it difficult to evaluate the results. Physiotherapy and biofeedback both focus on the pelvic floor. Relaxation of the pelvic floor during voiding is essential for normal voiding and most of these patients are unable to relax their pelvic floor muscles. Biofeedback is important for showing the children the effect of their efforts.

Most studies only state the clinical responses, and do not provide information on urodynamic parameters before and after treatment. A 'normal' flow curve does not mean normal voiding if no information is provided on post-void residual urine. In most papers the inclusion and exclusion criteria are not clearly documented, and it may very well be that the more difficult patients with both storage and voiding dysfunction were included in the study population. Furthermore, different series may describe different groups of patients due to poor definitions and an inadequate classification system.

In children with a suspected infravesical anatomic obstruction or abnormality, endoscopic investigations should be performed. Most often the abnormality can be treated at the same time. In girls, a meatal web may cause a deflection of the stream upwards (causing stimulation of the clitoris and bulbocavernosus reflex). A meatotomy may cure this problem, though no information on the long-term effects is available [176].

6. PHARMACOLOGICAL THERAPY

Many clinicians use adjunctive anticholinergic drug therapy to decrease detrusor contractility and facilitate greater functional bladder storage. Detrusor overactivity is believed to play an important role in many children with functional incontinence, vesicoureteral reflux and urinary infections [213].

In the presence of moderate to severe daytime incontinence some clinicians bypass bladder training and institute pharmacotherapy alone [169].

The outcome of pharmacological treatment for incontinence during the day is "unpredictable and inconsistent" and few randomised studies have been performed to evaluate safety and efficacy.

Currently, the drug most widely used to relax the overactive detrusor is oxybutynin-HCl. It has antimuscarinic, local anaesthetic and muscle relaxant properties [214].

If oral medication is poorly tolerated, it may be administered intravesically, but in these children this is rarely an option, whereas in children with neuropathic bladder dysfunction who are catheterised at regular intervals it may be a good alternative [215].

Side-effects are common – up to 10 percent of children have to discontinue the drug because of intolerable side-effects, such as headache, blurred vision, constipation, altered behaviour, dry mouth and flushed cheeks. Reduced saliva production may induce tooth decay, and constipation may worsen [170,182]. The incidence of side effects seems to be a dose related, both for oral and intravesical administration [216].

Oxybutynin crosses the blood–brain barrier and psychological and personality changes may be seen. Anecdotal documentation of dramatic improvement in school achievements following withdrawal of the drug in MMC patients further supports the need for more sophisticated drugs with fewer side-effects.

A novel drug, tolterodine, with a more pronounced and specific antimuscarinic effects on the detrusor has become available and is currently being evaluated in children. Preliminary results from a dose finding/pharmacokinetics study show that the optimal dosage in children aged 5–10 years is 1 mg b.d. No safety concerns have been noted [217,218,219].

The only drug which has been investigated in a randomised placebo controlled way is terodiline [220,221].

Because of serious cardiac side effects terodiline has been withdrawn from the market.

Other drugs like trospium and propiverine have been used in children, but results are variable and inclusion and outcome criteria were not in accordance with ICCS definitions which make comparison with other studies difficult [222,223,224].

Treatment of the overactive pelvic floor and sphincter is much more difficult. Recently the results of α-adrenergic blockade were presented[224].The initial results are promising but further studies are needed to define the place of alpha-blockers.

To evaluate the efficacy of different treatment modalities a prospective multi-centre trial (European Bladder Dysfunction Study (EBDS, EEC Biomed I, CT 94-1006) has been designed, in which pharmacotherapy (oxybutynin vs placebo) is compared with biofeedback and standard therapy. Although preliminary results are available, final outcome results will become available in 2002.

In preparation of this chapter an extensive review of the literature has been performed: only 6 studies (out of 1013) qualified for analysis. But the limited number of identified randomised controlled trials does not allow a reliable assessment of the benefits and harms of different methods of management in children. Further studies on the different behavioural (bladder training, psychotherapy), physical (pelvic floor muscle relaxation), electrical stimulation and drug therapies that are currently being used in children as standard treatment are required.

7. CONCLUSION

Although the condition of urinary incontinence in children is distressing, significantly effective treatment has not been identified. Of the studies reviewed the only treatment found to be beneficial was the drug terodiline, an anticholinergic with calcium agonist properties. Although the particular study did not demonstrate adverse effects on blood pressure, subsequent work established an association with ventricular arrhythmia and terodiline was ultimately withdrawn.

Three specific problems were identified concerning the evaluation of interventions for children with daytime urinary incontinence.

Firstly, few trials exist and of those identified three were of historical interest only. The most recent trial (EBDS) concerns current clinical intervention, namely the use of biofeedback and oxybutynin, and is therefore clinically relevant, but the final results are not yet available. Other interventions in routine clinical use, such as the combination of education, bladder training, physical therapies, bowel management and antibiotic prophylaxis have never been evaluated with respect to no intervention or placebo. New trials are warranted to evaluate these and other interventions which are commonly used by clinicians to treat childhood incontinence. It would be ideal if randomised and controlled trials were conducted when an intervention is first identified rather than after the unproven treatment has become routine practice. It is acknowledged that many clinicians feel an ethical dilemma about randomising children to a study arm that offers no genuine assistance. However, if routine conservative treatment has a proven benefit, randomised controlled trials can use this therapy as the control arm.

The second problem involves the size and design of existing trials being inappropriate to allow identification of the true effects of interventions studied. As is well known the power of the trial to detect effects of interventions is proportional to the event rates in the groups and the number of patients in the trial. Small trials may miss modest but clinically important effects. In our systematic review four of the five trials enrolled 61 patients or fewer. Other design parameters that warrant particular attention include randomisation of participants, control for intervention, and blinding for each of the subjects, assessors and data analysts. Since problems in trial design and reporting may bias the observed intervention effects, editors of the major biomedical journals have published guidelines for the reporting of trials in the form of CONSORT statement (Consolidated Standards for Reporting of Trials).

Finally, standardised outcome measures would be beneficial and allow synthesis of data from different studies. Four areas of quantification can be identified: severity of incontinence, bladder storage, features of bladder emptying, and quality of life. In measuring incontinence a clinician may be interested in either the severity or the frequency of episodes. Bladder storage has routinely been evaluated by both cystometry and the bladder diary, while bladder emptying requires data from uroflowmetry in addition to estimates of pre and post void urine volumes. Measures of quality of life in children with childhood incontinence are also rare. In summary, studies to establish reliable valid outcome measures would inform higher quality clinical trials.

In conclusion, further work is required in this difficult clinical area. Firstly, the establishment of outcome measures is warranted, thence randomised controlled trials of routine therapy to allow the use of such management in a control capacity for other studies. Such interventions that would reward further investigation include: bladder and voiding education, bladder drill, retention training, bowel management, hypnotherapy and alternative therapies, psychology, prophylactic antibiotic medication, neuromodulation, biofeedback therapy and pelvic floor muscle awareness and specific relaxation. Only then can the efficacy of new interventions be measured in children with voiding dysfunction or the urge syndrome.

In summary, while there is a wide therapeutic choice available to clinicians, many of the commonly used treatments are of dubious value and have not been rigorously evaluated in careful clinical trials with an appropriate study design.

Children who suffer this distressing condition, and their families, and those who care for them clinically, need clear guidance as to which treatments are of proven value. They need access to treatments which work, and they need protection from treatments which do not work.

VI. NEUROGENIC DETRUSOR-SPHINCTER DYSFUNCTION

1. INTRODUCTION

Although significant advances have been made in the diagnosis and management of children with incontinence secondary to neurogenic detrusor-sphincter dysfunction, the primary objective of treatment has remained the same i.e. preservation of the upper urinary tract and renal function.

Most neuropathic bladders are encountered in children with Myelomeningocele (MMC), tethering of the cord or sacral anomalies. Traumatic spinal lesions in children are less frequent.

In most cases the defect will be apparent at birth: only occasionally children with tethering of the cord will come to the attention of the physician with minor defects, such as Spina bifida occulta with slight discoloration of the skin, abnormal hair growth or a sacral dimple.

At birth the majority of these patients have normal upper tracts: without proper management urinary tract infections and secondary changes of the bladder may cause upper tract deterioration in up to 60 percent within 5 years [226,227].

Treatment of the bladder dysfunction is therefore primarily aimed at preservation of the upper urinary tract and secondarily at gaining continence and improvement of quality of life.

Management goals are directed at promoting a low pressure reservoir and regular emptying (in the first years of life), while later in life, as the child grows up, promoting continence is added.

2. Pattern recognition

In children with neuropathic bladder dysfunction the detrusor may be normal, overactive or inactive. The urethral sphincter may be normal, overactive or paralysed. These conditions may exist in any combination [228,229,230].

Urodynamic evaluation (preferably in combination with fluoroscopy) makes pattern recognition possible. Four major types are usually used to describe the detrusor-sphincter dysfunction:

1. Detrusor overactivity (hyperreflexia) with overactivity of the sphincter,
2. Detrusor hyperreflexia with underactivity of the sphincter,
3. Detrusor underactivity with sphincter overactivity and
4. Detrusor underactivity with sphincter underactivity.

Urodynamic investigations make it possible to establish a management plan for each individual patient. For the very young child the combination of an overactive detrusor and sphincter is potentially dangerous because of the high intravesical pressures, which will put the upper tract at risk (vesicoureteral reflux and hydronephrosis), whereas an inactive detrusor and paralysed sphincter is relatively safe, providing low pressure reservoir [231]. ***Level of evidence: 2***

3. Management

The urological problems in children with a neuropathic bladder are either associated with high intravesical pressures or insufficiency of the sphincteric mechanism.

In the first years of life the kidneys are highly susceptible to back-pressure and infection. In this period emphasis will be on documenting the pattern of neurogenic detrusor- sphincter dysfunction and assessing the potential for functional obstruction, vesicoureteral reflux. Ultrasound studies and a VCUG to exclude reflux have to be performed soon after birth. A urodynamic evaluation can be done after some weeks and needs to be repeated at regular intervals, in combination with evaluation of the upper tracts [232]. ***Grade of recommendation: 2***

Initial treatment consists of oral or intravesical anticholinergic treatment in combination with clean intermittent catheterisation, to start soon after birth.

At present Oxybutynin, Tolterodine, Trospium and Propiverine are the most frequently used drugs: some clinical studies are available, but no randomised placebo controlled studies have been performed [218,233,234,235,236,237,238,239]. ***Level of evidence: 2***

As fecal evacuation is also impaired in most patients, colonic lavage may have to be started even at this very young age.

In children the early institution of intermittent catheterisation has the advantage that it becomes an integral part of daily routines and is well accepted by the parents.

Children with a good response to anticholinergic treatment and an overactive sphincter may be continent in between catheterisations. Bladder pressure and development of the upper tracts will determine whether additional treatment is necessary.

Therapy resistant overactivity of the detrusor, or small capacity and poor compliance will usually need to be treated by bladder augmentation.

It has been postulated that overactivity of the sphincter in combination with an overactive detrusor (classical detrusor sphincter dyssynergia) causes secondary changes of the bladder wall, due to the frequent increased intravesical pressures. These bladder wall changes (collagen deposition in the muscular layer) may cause further loss of elasticity and compliance: resulting in a small non-compliant bladder with continuously elevated pressures. It is believed that early institution of intermittent catheterisation and anticholinergic drugs may prevent this in some patients [233].

At present there is not enough evidence that this management protocol indeed decreases the need for later augmentation. No prospective trials have been described.

Children with detrusor overactivity (hyperreflexia) but without sphincter activity will fare better in terms of their upper tracts, but they will be severely incontinent. Initial treatment will be intermittent catheterisation (as it may reduce the degree of incontinence and offers a much better control over urinary infections) with anticholinergic drugs: at a later age the outlet resistance has to be increased in order to render them continent [240].

No validated medical treatment is available to enhance the bladder outlet, although some authors have advocated alpha-receptor stimulation of the bladderneck. For permanent continence surgical procedures need to be considered [241,242,243,244,245,246].

It is important to establish adequate bowel emptying before attempting to correct bladder dysfunction surgically or medically.

REFERENCES

I. NORMAL DEVELOPMENT AND VALUES

1. Steers WD. Physiology and pharmacology of the bladder and urethra. In Walsh PC, Retol AB, Vaughan ED, Wein AJ (eds): Campbell's Urology, 7th ed. Philadelphia, WB Saunders, 870-916, 1997
2. Muellner SR: Development of urinary control in children, some aspects of the cause and treatment of primary enuresis. JAMA 172: 1256-1261, 1960
3. Ohel G, Haddad S, Samueloff A: Fetal urine production and micturition and fetal behavioral state. Am J Perinatol 12:91-92,1995
4. Goellner MH, Ziegler EE, Fomon SJ: Urination during the first 3 years of life. Nephron 28:174-178, 1981
5. Yeung CK, Godley ML, Ho CKW, Ransley P, Duffy PG, Chen CN, Li AKC: Some new insights into bladder function in infancy. Br J Urol 6:235-240, 1995
6. Yeung CK, Godley ML, Duffy PG, Ransley PG: Natural filling cystometry in infants and children. Br J Urol 75: 531-537,1995
7. Yeung CK, Godley ML, Dhillon HK, Duffy PG, Ransley PG: Urodynamic patterns in infants with normal lower urinary tracts or primary vesico-ureteric reflux. Br J Urol 81: 461-467, 1998
8. Bachelard M, Sillen U, Hansson S, Hermansson G, Jodal U, Jacobsson B: Urodynamic pattern in asymptomatic infants: siblings of children with vesico-ureteric reflux. J Urol 162: 1733-1737,1999
9. Sillen U, Solsnes E, Hellstrom Al, Sandberg K: The voiding pattern of healthy preterm neonates. J Urol 163:278-281, 2000
10. Holmdahl G, Hansson E, Hansson M, Hellstrom A-L, Hjälmås, Sillen U: Four hour voiding observation in healthy infants. J Urol 156: 1809-1812, 1996
11. Yeates WK: Bladder function in normal micturition. In Kolvin I, MacKeith RC, Meadow SR (eds): Bladder Control and Enuresis. London, W Heinemann Medical, 28-365, 1973
12. Koff SA: Estimating bladder capacity in children. Urology 21:248-251, 1983
13. Hjälmås K: Micturition in infants and children with normal lower urinary tract: a urodynamic study. Scand J Urol Nephrol 37:9-17, 1976
14. Zerin JM, Chen E, Ritchey ML, Bloom DA: Bladder capacity as measured at voiding cystourethrography in children-relationship in toilet training and frequency of micturition. Radiology 187: 803-806, 1993
15. Kaefer M, Zurakowsky D, Bauer SB, Retik AB, Peters CA, Atala A, Treves ST: Estimating normal bladder capacity in children. J Urol 158:2261-2264, 1997
16. Berk LB, Friman PC: Epidemiological aspects of toilet training. Clin Paediatrics, 29:278-282, 1990
17. Hellström A.L, Hanson E, Hansson S, Hjälmås K and Jodal U: Micturition habits and incontinence in 7-year old Swedish school entrants. Eur J Paediatr 149:434-437, 1990
18. Mattsson S, Lindström S: Diuresis and voiding pattern in healthy schoolchildren. Br. J. Urol. 76: 783-789, 1995
19. Wen JG, Tong EC: Cystometry in infants and children with no apparent voiding symptoms. Br. J. Urol. 81: 468-473, 1998
20. Szabo L, Fegyvernski S: Maximum and average urine flow rates in normal children- the Miskolc nomograms. Br J Urol 76:16020, 1995
21. Mattson S , Spangberg A: Urinary flow in healthy school children. Neurourol Urodyn 13: 281-296, 1994
22. Nørgaard JP, van Gool JD, Hjälmås K, Djurhuus JC, Hellström A-L. Standardization and definitions in lower urinary tract dysfunction in children. Br J Urol 81:1-16, 1998

II. EVALUATION IN CHILDREN WHO WET

23. Van Gool JD, Hjälmås K, Tamminen-Möbius T and Olbing H: Historical clues to the complex of dysfunctional voiding, urinary tract infection and vesicoureteral reflux—the International Reflux Study in Children. J Urol 148:1699-1702, 1992
24. Benninga MA, Büller HA, Staalman CR, Gubler FM, Bossuyt PM, Plas RN van der, and Taminiau JAJM: Defecation disorders in children, colonic transit time versus the Barr-score. Eur J Pediatr 154:277-284, 1995
25. Butler RJ: Establishment of working definitions in nocturnal enuresis. Arch Dis Child 66:267-271, 1991
26. Achenbach TM: Manual for the child behavior checklist 4-18 and 1991 profile. Burlington, Vt: University of Vermont, 1991
27. Bloom D A: Sexual abuse and voiding dysfunction [editorial]. J Urol 153:777, 1995
28. Wennergren HM, Öberg BE and Sandstedt P: The importance of leg support for relaxation of the pelvic floor muscles. A surface electromyography study in healthy girls. Scand J Urol Nephrol 25:205-213, 1991
29. Bower WF, Moore KH, Adams RD, Shepherd R: Frequency volume chart data from 3222 incontinent children. Br J Urol. 80:658-662, 1997
30. Mattson S: Voiding frequency, volumes and intervals in healthy schoolchildren. Scand J Urol Nephrol 28:1-11, 1994
31. Kirk J, Rasmussen PV, Rittig S and Djurhuus JC: Micturition habits and bladder capacity in normal children and in patients with desmopressin-resistant enuresis. In: Nørgaard JP, Djurhuus JC, Hjälmås K, Hellström A.-L and Jørgensen TM (eds.). Proceedings, Second International Workshop, International Enuresis Research Center, Aarhus. Scand J Urol Nephrol 173:49-50, 1995
32. Hellström A.-L, Andersson K, Hjälmås K and Jodal U: Pad tests in children with incontinence. Scand J Urol Nephrol 20:47-50, 1986
33. Barr RG, Levine MD, Wilkinson RH and Mulvihill,D: Chronic and occult stool retention—a clinical tool for its evaluation in school-aged children. Clin Pediatr 18:674-676, 1979
34. Blethyn AJ, Verrier Jones K, Newcombe R, Roberts GM and Jenkins HR: Radiological assessment of constipation. Arch Dis Child 73:532-533, 1995
35. Rockney RM, McQuade WH and Days AL: The plain abdominal roentgenogram in the management of encopresis. Arch Pediatr Adolesc Med 149:623-627, 1995
36. Van der Plas RN, Benninga MA, Buller HA, Bossuyt PM, Akkermans LM, Redekop WK and Taminiau JA: Biofeedback training in treatment of childhood constipation: a randomised controlled study [see comments]. Lancet 348:776-780, 1996
37. Hannson S, Hellström A-L, Hermansson G and Hjälmås K: Standardisation of urinary flow patterns in children. In: Nørgaard JP, Djurhuus JC, Hjälmås K, Hellström A-L and Jørgensen TM, eds. Proceedings of the Third International Children's Continence Symposium. Royal Tunbridge Wells: Wells Medical 159-161; 1996
38. Müller L, Bergström T, Hellström, Svensson E, Jacobsson B: Standardised ultrasound method for assessing detrusor muscle thickness in children. J Urol 164: 134-138, 2000
39. Roberts DS and Rendell B: Postmicturition residual bladder volumes in healthy babies. Arch Dis Child 64:825-828, 1989
40. Lyon RP and Smith DR: Distal urethral stenosis. J Urol 89:414-421, 1963

41. Saxton HM, Borzyskowski M and Robinson LB: Nonobstructive posterior urethral widening (spinning top urethra) in boys with bladder instability. Radiology 182:81-85, 1992

42. McGuire EJ, Woodside JR, Borden TA and Weiss RM: Prognostic value of urodynamic testing in myelodysplastic patients. J Urol 126:205-209, 1981

43. Park JM and Bloom DA: The guarding reflex revisited. Br J Urol 80:940-945, 1997

III. NOCTURNAL ENURESIS

44. WI, Butler RJ. Fifty years of enuresis alarms. Arch Dis Child 64: 879-85, 1989

45. Butler RJ. Nocturnal Enuresis: The Child's Experience. Oxford: Butterworth Heinemann;1994

46. Butler RJ. Annotation: night wetting in children: psychological aspects. J Child Psychol Psychiat 39: 1-11, 1998

47. Crawford JD. Introductory comments. J Paediatrics 114: 687-690, 1989

48. Verhulst FC, Vander Lee JH, Akkerkuis GW, Sanders-Woudstra JAR, Timmer FC, Donkhorst ID. The prevalence of nocturnal enuresis: do DSM-III criteria need to be changed? J Child Psychol Psychiat 26: 989-93, 1985

49. Foxman B, Burciaga Valdez RB, Brook RJ. Childhood enuresis: Prevalence, perceived impact and prescribed treatments. Paediatrics 77: 482-487, 1986

50. Devlin JB. Prevalence and risk factors for childhood nocturnal enuresis. Irish Medical Journal 84: 118-120, 1991

51. Collins RW. Enuresis and encopresis. In RH Woody [Ed.] Encyclopedia of clinical assessment; San Fransisco; Jossey-Bass, 1980

52. Houts AC. Nocturnal enuresis as a biobehavioural problem. Beh Ther 22: 133-151, 1991

53. Miller K . Concomitant nonpharmacologic therapy in the treatment of primary nocturnal enuresis. Clinical Paediatrics 7: 32-37, 1993

54. Warzak WJ Psychosocial implications of nocturnal enuresis. Clinical Paediatrics 7; 38-40, 1993

55. Rutter ML, Yule W, Graham PJ. Enuresis and behavioural deviance: some epidemiological considerations. In I Kolvin, RC McKeith [Eds] Bladder Control and Enuresis; London; Heinemann, 1973

56. Feehan M, McGee R, Stanton W, Silva PA. A 6 year follow up of childhood enuresis: prevalence in adolescence and consequences for mental health. J Paed Child Health 26: 75-79, 1990

57. Hirasing RA, van Leerdam FJM, Bolk-Bennick l, Janknegt RA. Bedwetting in adults; ICCS Abstracts, Paris; 84, 1997

58. Forsythe WI, Redmond A. Enuresis and spontaneous cure rate: study of 1129 enuretics. Arch Dis Childhood 49: 259-263, 1974

59. Moilkanen I, Tirkkonen T, Järvelin MR, Linna SL, Almqvist F, Piha J, Räsänen E, Tamminen T; A follow-up of enuresis from childhood to adolescence. Br J Urol, 81, 94-97, 1998

60. Eiberg H, Berends I, Mohr J: Assignment of dominant inherited nocturnal enuresis (ENUR) to chromosome 13q. Nat Genet 10:354-356, 1995

61. Arnell H, Hjälmås K,Jägervall M et al: The genetics of primary nocturnal enuresis: Inheritance and suggestion of a second major gene on chromosome 12q. J Med Genet 34: 360-365, 1997

62. Von Gonthard A, Eiberg H, Hollman E, Rittig S, Lehmkuhl G: Molecular genetics of nocturnal enuresis: Linkage to a locus on chromosome 22. In Djurhuus JC, Hjälmås K, Jörgensen TM et al (eds): proceeedings, Fourth International Workshop, International Research Centre, Aarhus, Scand J Urol Nephrol 33 (Suppl 202):76-80, 1999

63. Weir K: Night and day wetting among a population of three year olds. Devel Med Child Neurol 24: 479-484, 1982

64. Butler RJ, Galsworthy MJ, Rijsdijk F, Plomin R: Genetic and gender influences on nocturnal bladder control. Scand J Urol and Nephrol 35: 177-183, 2001

65. Jarvelin MR, Vikevainen-Tervonen L, Moilanen I, Huttunen NP: Enuresis in seven year old children. Acta Paediatrica Scand 77: 148-153, 1988

66. De Jonge GA: Epidemiology of enuresis: a survey of the literature. In I Kolvin, RC McKeith, SR Meadow [Eds] Bladder Control and Enuresis. Heinemann, London, 1973

67. Butler RJ, Brewin CR, Forsythe WI: Maternal attributions and tolerance for nocturnal enuresis. Behaviour Research and Therapy 24: 307-312, 1986

68. Bakwin H: Enuresis in twins. American J of Disease in Childhood 121: 222-225, 1971

69. Jarvelin MR: Developmental history and neurological findings in enuretic children. Develop Med and child Neurology; 31: 728-736, 1989

70. Fergusson DM, Horwood LJ, Shannon FT: Factors related to the age of attaining bladder control: An 8-year longitudinal study. Paediatrics 78: 884-890, 1986

71. Essen J, Peckham C: Nocturnal enuresis in childhood. Delop Med and Child Neurology; 18: 577-589, 1976

72. Jarvelin MR, Moilanen I, Kangas P, Morring K, Vivekainen-Tervonen L, Huttunen NP, Seppanen J: Aetiological and precipitating factors for childhood enuresis. Acta Paediatrica Scandanavica; 80: 361-369, 1991

73. McGee R, Makinson T, Williams S, Simpson A, Silva PA: A longitudinal study of enuresis from five to nine years. Aust Paed J 20: 39-42, 1984

74. Wagner WG, Geffken G: Enuretic children: How they view their wetting behaviour. Child Study Journal 16:13-18, 1986

75. Friman PC, Handwerk ML, Swearer SM, McGinnis JC, Warzak WJ: Do children with primary nocturnal enuresis have clinically significantly behaviour problems? Arch Pediatr Adol Med; 152: 537-539, 1998

76. Fergusson DM, Horwood LT, Shannon FT: Secondary enuresis in a birth cohort of New Zealand children. Paediatric & perinatal Epidemiology; 4: 53-63,1990

77. Jarvelin MR, Moilanen I, Vikevainen Tervonen L, Huttunen NP: Life changes and protective capacities in enuretic and non-enuretic children. J Child Psychol Psychiat; 31: 763-774,1990

78. Von Gontard A, Hollman E, Eiberg H, Benden B, Rittig S, Lehmkuhl G. Clinical enuresis phenotypes in familial nocturnal enuresis. Scand J Urol Nephrol 183: 11-16, 1997

79. Van Gool JD, Nieuwenhuis E, ten Doeschate IOM, Messer TP, de Jong TPVM: Subtypes in monosymptomatic nocturnal enuresis. Scand J Urol Nephrol 202: 8-11, 1999

80. Fielding D: The response of day and night wetting children and children who wet only at night to retention control training and the enuresis alarm. Behaviour Research and Therapy 18; 305-317, 1980

81. Butler RJ, Holland P: The three systems: a conceptual way of understanding nocturnal enuresis. Scand J Urol and Nephrol; 34: 270-277, 2000

82. Neveus T, Hetta J, Cnattingius S, Tuvemo T, Läckgren G, Olsson U, Stenberg A: Depth of sleep and sleep habits among enuretic and incontinent children. Acta Pædiatr, 88:748-52, 1999

83. Rittig S, Matthiesen TB, Hunsballe JM et al: Age related changes in the circadian control of urine output. In Djurhuus JC, Hjälmås K, Jörgensen TM et al (eds): proceeedings, Second International Workshop, International Research Centre, Aarhus, Scand J Urol Nephrol Suppl 173:71-74, 1995

84. Rittig S, Matthiesen TB, Pedersen EB et al: Sodium regulating hormones in enuresis. In Djurhuus JC, Hjälmås K, Jörgensen TM et al (eds): proceeedings, Fourth International Workshop, International Research Centre, Aarhus, Scand J Urol Nephrol Suppl 202:45-46, 1999

85. Norgaard JP, Pedersen EB, Djurhuus JC.:Diurnal antidiuretic hormone levels in enuretics. J Urol 1985; 134: 1029-1031, 1985

86. Rittig S, Knudsen UB, Norgaard JP, Pedersen EB, Djurhuus JC: Abnormal diurnal rhythm of plasma vasopressin and urinary output in patients with enuresis. Amer J Physiol ; 256: 664-667, 1989

87. Devitt H, Holland P, Butler RJ, Redfern E, Hiley E, Roberts G: Plasma vasopressin and response to treatment in primary nocturnal enuresis. Arch Dis Child 80: 448-451, 1999

88. Wolfish N: Sleep arousal function in enuretic males. Scand J Urol Nephrol 202: 24-26, 1999

89. Norgaard JP, Rittig S, Djurhuus JC: Nocturnal enuresis: an approach to treatment based on pathogenesis. J Paediatrics114: 705—710, 1989

90. Norgaard JP, Jonler M, Rittig S & Djurhuus JC: A pharmacodynamic study of desmopressin in patients with nocturnal enuresis. J Urol 153: 1984-1986, 1995

91. Medel R, Dieguez S, Brindo M, Ayuso S, Canepa C, Ruarte A: Monosymptomatic primary enuresis: differences between patients responding or not responding to oral desmopressin. Br J Urol 81: 46-49, 1998

92. Kruse S, Hellstrom A-L, Hjälmås K: Daytime bladder dysfunction in therapy resistant nocturnal enuresis. Scand J Urol and Nephrol 33: 49-52, 1999

93. Watanabe H, Kawauchi A, Kitamori T, Azuma Y: Treatment systems for nocturnal enuresis according to an original classification system. Euro Urol 25: 43-50, 1994

94. Watanabe H, Imada N, Kawauchi A, Kotama Y, Shirakawa S: Physiological background of enuresis Type I: a preliminary report. Scand J Urol and Nephrol Suppl 183: 7-10, 1997

95. Watanabe H: Sleep patterns in children with nocturnal enuresis. Scand J Urol Nephrol Suppl 173: 55-58, 1995

96. Yeung CK, Chiu HN, Sit FKY: Sleep disturbance and bladder dysfunction in enuretic children with treatment failure: fact or fiction? Scand J Urol Nephrol 202: 20-23, 1999

97. Lettgen B: Differential diagnosis for nocturnal enuresis. Scand J Urol Nephrol Suppl 183: 47-49, 1997

98. Bower WF, Moore KH, Shepherd RB, Adams RD: The epidemiology of childhood enuresis in Australia. Br J Urol 78: 602-606, 1996

99. Butler RJ, Redfern EJ, Holland P: Children's notions about enuresis and the implications for treatment. Scand J Urol Nephrol 163: 39-47, 1994

100. Mikkelsen EJ, Rapoport JL, Nee L, Gruenau C, Mendelson W, Gillin JC: Childhood enuresis 1: sleep patterns and psychopathology. Arch Gen Psychiat 37: 1139-1144, 1980

101. Norgaard JP, Djurhuus JC: The pathophysiology of enuresis in children and young adults. Clin Paediatrics 7: 5-9, 1993

102. Norgaard JP: Pathophysiology of nocturnal enuresis. Scand J Urol and Nephrol Suppl 140; 1-35, 1991

103. Forsythe WI, Butler RJ: Fifty years of enuresis alarms. Arch Dis Child 64:879-885, 1989

104. Butler RJ: Establishment of working definitions in nocturnal enuresis. Arch Dis Child 66:267-271, 1991

105. Djurhuus JC, Nørgaard JP, Hjälmås K: What is an acceptable treatment outcome? In: Djurhuus JC, Hjälmås K, Jørgensen TM, Nørgaard JP, Rittig S, eds. Proceedings, Third International Workshop, International Enuresis Research Center, Aarhus. Scand J Urol Nephrol, Suppl 183: 75-77, 1997

106. Blaivas JG, Appell RA, Fantl JA, Leach G, McGuire EJ, Resnick NM, Raz S, Wein AJ: Standards of efficacy for evaluation of treament outcomes in urinary incontinence: recommendations of the Urodynamic Society. Neurourol Urodyn 16:145-147, 1997

107. Devlin JB, O'cathain C : Predicting treatment outcome in nocturnal enuresis. Arch Dis Child 65 :1158-1161, 1990

108. Glazener CMA, Evans JHC: Alarm interventions for nocturnal enuresis in children (Cochrane Review). In: The Cochrane Library, Issue 2, 2001

109. Houts AC, Berman JS, Abramson H: Effectiveness of psychologicl and pharmacological treatments for nocturnal enuresis. J Consult Clin Psychol 30: 737-745, 1994

110. Bengtsson B, Bengtsson M: Childhood enuretics in adult age: A longterm prospective follow-up of 88 children. In Nørgaard JP, Djurhuus JC, Hjälmås K et al (eds): Proceedings of the Third International Children's Continence Society Symposium, Royal Turnbridge Wells, England, Wells Medical, 61-63, 1996

111. Oredsson AF, Jørgensen TM: Changes in nocturnal bladder capacity during treatment with the bell and pad for monosymptomatic nocturnal enuresis. J Urol 160: 166-169, 1998

112. Terho P: Desmopressin in nocturnal enuresis. J Urol 145:818-820, 1991

113. Tullus K, Bergstrom R, Fosdal I, Winnergard I, Hjalmas K: Efficacy and safety during long-term treatment of primary monosymptomatic nocturnal enuresis with desmopressin. Swedish Enuresis Trial Group. Acta Paediatr;88:1274-1278, 1999

114. Glazener CMA, Evans JHC: Desmopressin for nocturnal enuresis in children (Cochrane review). In the Cochrane Library, Issue 2, 2000

115. Miller K, Klauber GT: Desmopressin acetate in children with severe primary nocturnal enuresis. Clin Ther 12:357-366, 1990

116. Hjälmäs K, Hanson E, Hellström A-L, Kruse S, Sillen U: Longterm treatment with desmopressin in children with primary monosymptomatic nocturnal enuresis: an open multicentre study. Br J Urol, 82:704-709, 1998.

117. Robson WLM, Nørgaard JP, Leungn AKC: Hyponatremia in patients with nocturnal enuresis treated with DDAVP. Eur J Pediatr 155: 959-962, 1996

118. Lane WM, Robson M, Shashi V, Nagaraj S, Nørgaard JP: Water intoxication in a patient with the prader-willi syndrome treated with desmopressin for nocturnal enuresis. J. Urol. 157:646-647, 1997

119. Bradbury MG, Meadow SR: Combined treatment with enuresis aarm and desmopressin for nocturnal enuresis. Acta Paediatr 84:1014-1018, 1995

120. Nijman JM: Paediatric voiding dysfunction and enuresis. Curr Opin Urol 10:365-370, 2000

121. Geller B, Reising D, Leonnard HL, Riddle MA, Walsh BT: Critical review of tricyclic antidepressants use in children and adolescents. J Am Acad Child Adolesc Psychiatry 38:513-516, 1999

122. Natochin YV, Kuznetsova AA: Nocturnal enuresis: correction of renal function by desmopressin and diclofenac. Pediatr Nephrol 2000;14:42-47, 2000

IV. BEHAVIOUR THERAPY

123. Kaplan SL, Breit M, Gauthier B, Busner J: A comparison of three nocturnal enuresis treatment methods. J Amer Acad Child Adol Psychiatry; 28: 282-286, 1989

124. Harter S: Pleasure derived from challenge and the effects of receiving grades on children's difficulty level choices. Child Development 49: 788-799, 1978

125. Edwards SD, Van der Spuy HI: Hypnotherapy as a treatment for enuresis. J Child Psychology and Psychiatry; 26: 161-170, 1985

126. Butler RJ, Holland P, Hiley E, Redfern E: Preventing relapse following medication for the treatment of childhood nocturnal enuresis. Paed Today 6: 30-35, 1998

127. Butler RJ, Holland P, Robinson J: An examination of the structured withdrawal programme to prevent relapse in nocturnal enuresis. J Urol: in press ,2001

128. Butler RJ: Establishing a dry run: a case study in securing bladder control. Br J Clinical Psychology 32: 215-217, 1993

129. Azrin NH, Sneed TJ, Foxx RM: Dry-bed-training: rapid elimination of childhood enuresis. Beh Res Ther 12: 147-156, 1974

130. Fly Hansen A, Jorgensen TM: Treatment of nocturnal enuresis with the bell and pad system. Scand J Urol Nephrol Suppl 173: 101-102, 1995

131. Houts AC: Behavioural treatment for enuresis. Scand J Urol and Nephrol 1995; Suppl 173: 83-88, 1995

132. Doleys DM: Behavioural treatments for nocturnal enuresis in children: a review of the recent literature. Psychol Bull 84: 30-54, 1977

133. Johnson SB: Enuresis. In: Daitzman RD, editor. Clinical behaviour therapy and behaviour modification. London: Garland STPM Press 81-142, 1980

134. Wille S.:Comparison of desmopressin and enuresis alarm for nocturnal enuresis. Arch Dis Child 61: 30-33,1986

135. Houts AC, Peterson JK, Whelan JP: Prevention of relapse in full-spectrum home training for primary enuresis: a component analysis. Behaviour Therapy17: 462-469, 1986

136. Monda JM, Husmann A: Primary nocturnal enuresis: a comparison among observation, imipramine, desmopressin acetate and bed-wetting alarm systems. J Urol 154: 745-748, 1995

137. van Londen A, Van Londen-Barentsen MW, Van Son MJ, Mulder GA: Arousal training for children suffering from nocturnal enuresis: a 2_ year follow up. Beh Res Ther 31: 613-615, 1993

138. Bollard J, Nettelbeck T: A component analysis of dry bed training for treatment of bedwetting. Beh Res Ther 20: 383-390, 1982

139. Fielding D: The response of day and night wetting children and children who wet only at night to retention control training and the enuresis alarm. Behaviour Research & Therapy 18; 305-317, 1980

140. Hirasing RA, Bolk-Bennick L, Reus H: Dry bed training by parents: results of a group instruction program. J Urology 156: 2044-2046, 1996

141. Whelan JP, Houts AC: Effects of a waking schedule on primary enuretic children treated with full-spectrum home training. Health Psychology 9: 164-176, 1990

V. DAY AND NIGHT INCONTINENCE

142. Jeffcoate TNA, and Francis WJA: Urgency incontinence in the female. Am J Obst Gyn 94:604–618, 1966

143. Straub LR, Ripley HS, and Wolf S: Disturbances of bladder function associated with emotional states. JAMA 141:1139–1143, 1949

144. Hjälmås K, Hoebeke PB, de Paepe H: Lower urinary tract dysfunction and urodynamics in children. Eur Urol, 38:655-65., 2000

145. Pfister C, Dacher JN, Gaucher S, Liard-Zmuda A, Grise P, Mitrofanoff P: The usefulness of a minimal urodynamic evaluation and pelvic floor biofeedback in children with chronic voiding dysfunction. BJU Int 84:1054–1057, 1999

146. Kuh D, Cardozo L, Hardy R. Urinary incontinence in middle aged women: childhood enuresis and other lifetime risk factors in a British prospective cohort. J Epidemiol Community Health 53:453–458, 1999

147. Bloom DA, Seeley WW, Ritchey ML, McGuire EJ: Toilet habits and continence in children: an opportunity sampling in search of normal parameters. J Urol 149:1087-1090, 1993

148. Bloomfield JM, Douglas JWB: Bedwetting: prevalence amongst children aged 4-7 years. Lancet 1:850-852, 1956

149. Mattsson S: Urinary incontinence and nocturia in healthy schoolchildren. Acta Paediatrica 83:950-954, 1994

150. Meadow SR: Day wetting. Pediatr Nephrol 4:178-184, 1990

151. Sureshkumar P, Roy LP, Knight JF, Craig JC: Prevalence of urinary incontinence, urinary tract infection and other voiding symptoms in Australian primary school children (abstract). Proc RACP Annual Scientific Meeting, Perth, May, 1999

152. Hellstrom A-L, Hanson E, Hanson S, Hjälmås K and Jodal U: Micturition habits and incontinence at age 17 – reinvestigation of a cohort studied at age 7. Br J Urol, 76:231-234, 1995

153. Swithinbank LV, Brookes ST, Shepherd Am and Abrams P: The natural history of urinary symptoms during adolescence. Br J Urol 81, 90-93, 1998

154. Ellsworth PI, Merguerian PA, and Copening ME: Sexual abuse: another causative factor in dysfunctional voiding. J Urol 153:773–776, 1995

155. Allen TD: Vesicoureteral reflux as a manifestation of dysfunctional voiding. In: Hodson CJ and Kincaid-Smith P (eds). Reflux nephropathy. New York: Masson, 171-171, 1979

156. Koff SA, Lapides J and Piazza DH: Association of urinary tract infection and reflux with uninhibited bladder contractions and voluntary sphincteric obstruction. J Urol 122:373-376, 1979

157. Scholtmeijer RJ, Griffiths DJ: The role of videourodynamic studies in diagnosis and treatment of vesicoureteral reflux. J. Ped. Surg. 25: 669-671, 1990

158. Soygür T. Arikan N, Ye_illi, Gö_ü_: Relationship among pediatric voiding dysfunction and vesicoureteral reflux and renal scars. Eur Urol.54: 905-908,1999

159. Sillen U, Hjälmås K, Aili M, Bjure J, Hanson J and Hansson S: Pronounced detrusor hypercontractility in infants with gross bilateral reflux. J Urol: 148: 598-599,1992

160. Vega-P JM, Pascual LA: High pressure bladder: an underlying factor mediating renal damage in the absence of reflux? BJU Int. 87: 581-584, 2001

161. Lindehall B, Claesson I, Hjalmas K and Jodal U: Effect of clean intermittent catheterisation on radiological appearance of the upper urinary tract in children with myelomeningocele. Br J Urol 67:415-419, 1991

162. Van Gool JD and Tanagho EA. External sphincter activity and recurrent urinary tract infections in girls. Urology 10: 348-353, 1977

163. Van Gool JD, Vijverberg MAW and de Jong TPVM: Functional daytime incontinence clinical and urodynamic assessment. Scan J Urol Nephrol Suppl 141: 58-69, 1992

164. Hansson S, Hjälmås K, Jodal U and Sixt R: Lower urinary tract dysfunction in girls with asymptomatic or covert bacteriuria. J Urol, 143:333-335, 1990

165. Van Gool JP, Kuijten RH, Donckerwolcke RA, Messer AP and Vijverberg MAM: Bladder-sphincter dysfunction, urinary infection and vesico-ureteral reflux with special reference to cognitive bladder training. Contrib Nephrol 39: 190-210, 1984

166. Bachelard M, Sillen U, Hansson S, Hermansson G, Jacobson B, Hjälmås: Urodynamic patterns in infants with urinary tract infection. J Urol 160: 522-526, 1998

167. Rushton GH, Majd M: Dimercaptosuccinic acid renal scintigraphy for the evaluation of pyelonephritis and scarring-a review of experimental and clinical studies. J Urol 148:1726-1732, 1992

168. Varlam DE and Dippell J: Non-neurogenic bladder and chronic renal insufficiency in childhood. Paed Neph 9:1-5, 1995

169. van Gool JD, Vijverberg MAW, Messer AP: Functional daytime incontinence: non-pharmacological treatment. Scand J Urol Nephrol Suppl 141:93-103, 1992

170. Hjälmås K, Passerini-Glazel G, Chiozza ML: Functional daytime incontinence: pharmacological treatment. Scand J Urol Nephrol 141:108-114, 1992

171. Weerasinghe N, and Malone PS: The value of videourodynamics in the investigation of neurologically normal children who wet. Br J Urol 71:539–542, 1993

172. Glazier DB, Murphy DP, Fleisher MH, Cummings KB and Barone JG. Evaluation of the utility of video-urodynamics in children with urinary tract infection and voiding dysfunction. Br J Urol 80: 806-808, 1997

173. Hoebeke P, Laecke van E, Camp van C, Raes A, Walle van de J: One thousand video-urodynamic studies in children with non-neurogenic sphincter dysfunction. BJU Int. 87: 575-580, 2001

174. Loening-Baucke: Urinary incontinence and urinary tract infection and their resolution with treatment of chronic constipation of childhood. Pediatrics, 100:228-32, 1997

175. Koff SA: Relationship between dysfunctional voiding and reflux. J Urol 148:1703–1705, 1992

176. Hoebeke P, Laecke E van, RaesA, Gool JD van, Walle J vande: Anomalies of he external urethral meatus in girls with non-neurogenic bladder sphincter dysfunction. BJU Int 83:294–298, 1999

177. Vereecken RL, Proesmans W:Urethral instability as an important element of dysfunctional voiding. J Urol 163:585–588, 2000

178. Hinman F, and Bauman FW: Vesical and ureteral damage from voiding dysfunction in boys without neurologic or obstructive disease. J Urol 109:727, 1973

179. Ochoa B: The urofacial (Ochoa) syndrome revisited. J Urol 148:580-583, 1987

180. Bauer SB: Neuropathology of the lower urinary tract. In Kelalis PP, King LR and Belman AB (eds.): Clinical Pediatric Urology, ed. 3. Philadelphia, WB Saunders pp 399, 1992

181. Williams DI, Hirst G and Doyle D: The occult neuropathic bladder. J Paediatr Surg 9:35-41, 1974

182. Maizels M, Ghandi K, keating B, Rosenbaum D: Diagnosis and treatment for children who cannot control urination. Current Prob Paed 402-450, 1993

183. Sher PK, Reinberg Y: Successful treatment of giggle incontinence with methylphenidate. J Urol 156:656-658), 1996

184. Arena MG, Leggiadro N: Enuresis rissoria: evaluation and management. Funct Neurol 2: 579-582, 1987

185. Glahn BE: Giggle incontinence (enuresis rissoria). A study and an aetiological hypothesis. Br J Urol 51:363-366, 1979

186. Elinza-Plomp A, Boemers TM: Treatment of enuresis rissoria in children by self-administered electric and imaginary shock. Br J Urol 76:775-778, 1995

187. I Cigna RM, Chiaramonte C, Lo Gaglio C, Milazzo M, Lo Piparo M and De Grazia E: Enuresis in children. Diagnostic assessment and treatment. Minerva Pediatrica 41: 371-373, 1989

188. Cochat P, Colombe M: Instabilitie uretrale. In Enuresie et troubles mictionnels de l'enfant. Ed. Cochat P. Elsevier Paris; 204-207, 1997

189. Fernandes E, Vernier R, Gonzalez R: The unstable bladder in children. J Paediat ;118: 831-837, 1991

190. Hellstrom A-L, Hjälmås K and Jodal U: Rehabilitation of the dysfunctional bladder in children: method and three year follow up. J Urol;138:847-849, 1987

191. Himsl KK, Hurzwitz RS: Paediatric urinary incontinence. Urol Clin N Am;18:283-293, 1991

192. Hinman F: Urinary tract damage in children who wet. Paediatrics;54: 142 –150, 1974

193. van Gool JD, de Jong GA: Urge syndrome and urge incontinence. Arch Dis Child 64:1629-1634, 1989

194. Curran MJ, Kaefer M, Peters C, Logigian E, Bauer SB: The overactive bladder in childhood: long-term results with conservative management. J Urol; 163:574–577, 2000

195. Vijverberg MA, Elzinga-Plomp A, Messer AP, Van Gool JD, de Jong TPVM: Bladder rehabilitation: the effect of a cognitive training programme on urge incontinence. Eur Urol 31:68–72, 1997

196. Hoebeke P, Walle van de J, Theunis M, Paepe de H, Oosterlinck W, Renson C: Outpatient pelvic-floor therapy in girls with daytime incontinence and dysfunctional voiding. Eur Urol; 48:923-928, 1996

197. Paepe de H, Renson C, Laecke van E, Raes A, Walle van de J, Hoebeke P: Pelvic-floor therapy and toilet training in young children with dysfunctional voiding and obstipation. BJU Int 85: 889-893, 2000

198. Maizels M, King LR, Firlit CF: Urodynamic biofeedback – a new approach to treat vesical sphincter dyssynergia. J Urol 122: 205-209, 1979

199. Nørgaard JP, Djurhuus JC: Treatment of detrusor-sphincter dyssynergia by biofeedback. Urol Int 37:326-329,1982

200. Paepe de H, Hoebeke P, Renson C and Walle van de J: Pelvic-floor therapy in girls with recurrent urinary tract infections and dysfunctional voiding. Br J Urol 81: 109-113, 1998

201. McKenna PH, Herndon CD, Connery S, Ferrer FA: Pelvic floor muscle retraining for pediatric voiding dysfunction using interactive computer games. J Urol; 162:1056–1062, 1999

202. Combs AJ, Glassberg AD, Gerdes D, Horowitz. Biofeedback therapy for children with dysfunctional voiding. Urology 52: 312-315, 1998

203. Glazier DB, Ankem MK, Ferlise V, Gazi M, Barone JG: Utility of biofeedback for the daytime syndrome of urinary frequency and urgency of childhood. Urology; 57: 791-794, 2001

204. Porena M, Costantini E, Rociola W, Mearini E: Biofeedback successfully cures detrusor-sphincter dyssynergia in pediatric patients. J Urol 163:1927-1931, 2000

205. Yamanishi T, Yasuda K, Murayama N, Sakakibara R, Uchiyama T, Ito H: Biofeedback training for detrusor overactivity in children. J Urol 164: 1686-1690, 2000

206. Hoebeke PB, Renson C, Vanden Broecke H, Theunis M, Van Laecke E, Vande Walle J: Ambulatory pelvic floor training in dysfunctional voiding. Proc 3rd Int Child Cont Symp, Sydney, Oct;86-87, 1995

207. Klingler HC, Pycha A, Schmidbauer , Marberger M:Use of peripheral neuromodulation of the S3 region for treatment of detrusor overactivity: a urodynamic-basic study. Urol. 2000; 56: 766-771, 2000

208. Hoebeke P, De Paepe H, Renson C, Van Laecke E, Raes A, Everaert K and Vande Walle J: Transcutaneous neuromodulation in non-neuropathic bladder sphincter dysfunction in children: preliminary results. BJU Int 83, Suppl. 3: 93-94, 1999

209. Kaplan WE: Intravesical electrical stimulation of the bladder: pro. Urololgy 56:2-4, 2000

210. Decter RM: Intravesical electrical stimulation of the bladder: con. Urology 56: 5-8, 2000

211. Gladh G, Mattson S, Lindström S: Anogenital electrical stimulation as treatment of urge incontinence in children. BJU Int. 87: 366-371, 2001

212. Halliday S, Meadow SR, Berg I: Successful management of daytime enuresis using alarm procedures: a randomly controlled trial. Arch Dis Child 62:132-137, 1987

213. Homsy YL, Nsouli I, Hamburger B, Laberge I, Schick E: Effects of oxybutynin on vesicoureteral reflux in children. J Urol 134:1168–1171, 1985

214. Dikno Al, Lapides J: A new drug with analgesic and anticholinergic properties. J Urol 108:307-310, 1972

215. Aubert D, Cencig P, and Royer M: Oxybutynin chlorhydrate for treatment of urinary incontinence and hyperactive bladder in children. Ann Pediatr 33:629–634, 1986

216. Kaplinsky R, Greenfield S, Wan J, Fera M: Expanded follow up on intravesical oxybutynin chloride used in children with neurogenic bladder. J Urol 156:753-756, 1996

217. Hjälmås K , Hellström AL, Mogren K, Läckgren G, Stenberg A: The overactive bladder in children: a potential future indication for tolterodine. BJU Int., 87:1-7, 2001

218. Goessl C, Sauter T. Michael T, Bergé B, Staehler M, Miller K: Efficacy and tolerability of tolterodine in children with detrusor hyperreflexia. Urol; 55: 414-418, 2000

219. Munding M, Wessells H, Thornberry B, Riben D: Use of Tolterodine in children with dysfunctional voiding: an initial report. J Urol 165:926-928, 2001

220. Hellstrom AL, Hjalmas K, Jodal U: Terodiline in the treatment of children with unstable bladders. Br J Urol 63: 358-362, 1989

221. Elmer M, Norgaard JP, Djurhuus JC, Adolfsson T: Terodiline in the treatment of diurnal enuresis in children. Scand J Prim Health Care 6: 119-124, 1988

222. Gesch R, Schönberger B (1992) Instabile Blase und Enuresis im Kindesalter. Vortrag, 4. Deutscher Kongress der GIH, Berlin, November 06-07, 1992

223. Siegert J, Schubert G, Nentwich H-J: Pharmakotherapie der Enuresis mit Urge-Symptomatik. Klinische Untersuchungen zur Wirksamkeit und Verträglichkeit der Kinderform von Propiverin-Hydrochlorid (Mictonetten®). In: Jonas U (ed) Jahrbuch der Urologie, Biermann-Verlag, Zülpich, pp 177-181, 1994

224. Hoashi E, Yokoi S, Akashi S, Muramatsu Y, Aikawa T, Inoue H, Awaya Y, Usui N, Miyamoto R: Safety and efficacy of propiverine hydrochloride (BUP-4® tablets) in children. A study focussed on nocturia. Jpn J Paediat 51: 173-179, 1998

225. Austin PF, Homsy YL, Masel J, Cain MP, Casale AJ, Rink RC: Alpha-adrenergic blockade in children with voiding dysfunction. BJU Int 83(Suppl 3):93, 1999

VI. NEUROPATHIC BLADDER AND SPHINCTER

226. Wilcock AR, Emery JL: Deformities of the renal tract in children with myelomeningocele and hydrocephalus, compared with those children showing no such deformities. Br J Urol 42:152-159, 1970

227. Hunt GM, Whitaker RH: The pattern of congenital renal anomalies associated with neural tube defects. Dev Med and Child Neurol 29:91-95, 1987

228. Van Gool JD: Spina Bifida and neurogenic bladder dysfunction-a urodynamic study . Impress, Utrecht, 1986

229. Van Gool JD: Neuropathic and non-neuropathic bladder-sphincter dysfunction in children. Pediatr Adoles Med 5:178-192, 1994

230. Baskin LS, Kogan A, Benard F: Treatment of infants with neurogenic bladder dysfunction using anticholinergic drugs and intermittent catheterisation. Br J Urol 66:532-534, 1990

231. Tanaka H, Kakizaki H, Kobayashi S, Shibata T, Ameda K, Koyanaqi T: The relevance of urethral resistance in children with myelodysplasia: the impact on upper urinary tract deterioration and the outcome of conservative management. J. Urol. 161: 929-932, 1999

232. Sillén U, Hansson E. Hermansson G, Hjälmås, Jacobsson B, Jodal U: Development of the urodynamic pattern in infants with myelomeningocele. Br J Urol 78: 596-601, 1996

233. Ghoneim GM, Bloom DA: Bladder compliance in myelomeningocele children. J Urol 141: 1404-1407, 1989

234. Greenfield SP, Ferra M: The use of intravesical oxybutynin in children with neurogenic bladder. J Urol 146:532-534, 1991

235. Joseph DB, Bauer SB: Clean intermittent catheterisation of infants with neurogenic bladder. Pediatrics 84:78-82, 1989

236. Drago JR, Weller L: The role of intermittent catheterisation in the management of myelomeningocele. J Urol 118:92-94, 1977

237. Edelstein RA, Bauer SB: The long-term urological response to of neonates with myelodysplasia treated proactively with intermittent catheterisation and anticholinergic therapy. J Urol 154:1500-1504, 1995

238. Åmark P, Bussman G, Eksborg S. Follow-up of long-time treatment with intravesical oxybutynin for neurogenic bladder in children. Eur Uro. 34: 148-153, 1998

239. Grigoleit U, Mürtz G, Goepel M, Kramer G, Stöhrer M: Efficacy and safety of propiverine hydrochloride in children with detrusor hyperreflexia due to myelomeningocele - A retrospective analysis. Submitted to: 31st Annual Meeting of the International Continence Society, Seoul, September 18-21, 2001

240. Van Gool JD, de Jong TPVM, Boemers TM: Einfluss des intermittierenden Katheterismus auf Harnweginfekte und Inkontinenz bei Kindern mit Spina Bifida. Monatschr Kinderh 139: 592-596, 1991

241. Naglo AS: Continence training of children with neurogenic bladder and hyperactivity of the detrusor. Scan J Urol Nephrol 16:211-217, 1982

242. Austin PF, Westney OL, Leng WW, McGuire EJ, Ritchey ML:Advantages of rectus fascial slings for urinary incontinence in children with neuropathic bladder. J Urol: 165; 2369-2371, 2001

243. Guys JM, Fakhro A, Louis-Borrione C, Prost J, Hautier A: Endoscopic treatment of urinary incontinence: long-term evaluation of the results. J Urol: 165; 2389-2391, 2001

244. Kassouf W, Capolicchio G, Bernardinucci G, Corcos J: Collagen injection for treatment of urinary incontinence in children. JUrol: 165; 1666-1668, 2001

245. Kryger JV, Leverson G, Gonzalez R: Long-term results of artificial urinary sphincters in children are independent of age at implantation. J Urol: 165; 2377-2379 ,2001

246. Holmes NM, Kogan BA, Baskin LS: Placement of artificial urinary sphincter in children and simultaneous gastrocystoplasty. J Urol: 165; 2366-2368 , 2001

Committee 10 B

Conservative Manag

Chairman

A. Kondo (Jap

Members

TL. Lin (Taiwan, China),

J. Nordling (Denmark),

M. Siroky (USA),

T. Tammela (Finland),

Conservative Management in Men

A. Kondo

TL. Lin, J. Nordling, M. Siroky, T. Tammela

I. INTRODUCTION

Urinary incontinence jeopardizes the dignity and health of patients. In addition to consuming considerable resources, it is associated with embarrassment, stigmatization, isolation, depression, loss of morale, and/or increased risk of institutionalization. Furthermore, it constitutes a considerable burden to families and caregivers [1-3] and predisposes the patient to perineal rashes, pressure ulcers, urinary tract infection, falls and bone fractures. The prevalence of urinary incontinence is about 10% among men who reside in the community and are otherwise healthy and about 30% among women [4].

Male incontinence may result from inappropriate life styles, disturbances in bladder or sphincter function, distorted environmental parameters, and/or a combination of these disorders. The major causes of male incontinence are nocturnal enuresis, post-prostatectomy incontinence and post-micturition dribbling. These vesicourethral dysfunctions may be caused by detrusor overactivity, chronic infection, irradiation, bladder outlet obstruction, bladder malignancy or neurologic lesions. Unlike the female, in men sphincteric incompetence occurs rarely but may be due to trauma, surgery to the prostate or neurologic disorders. We herewith discuss incidence, risk factors, and management of urinary incontinence in adult males by means of conservative treatment modalities. Since the elderly population has been increasing rapidly especially in the developed countries, there is increasing need for devices for containment of urinary incontinence. These devices must be evaluated from the therapeutic and economical point of view.

When we looked for references, we have been cautious not to be much involved in urinary incontinence among frail, elderly people wherever possible, since that is discussed in other committees.

II. LIFESTYLE INTERVENTIONS IN MALE ADULTS

1. Background

There are no prospective, randomized studies on the effect of life style interventions on urinary incontinence in males. Most of our information comes from epidemiological studies that have investigated associations between life style and urinary incontinence.

2. Reduction in body weight

In women a significant correlation between body mass index and urinary incontinence has been reported [5] but no similar study has been reported in males. In a cross-sectional study in male patients, body weight and body mass index did not correlate with lower urinary tract symptoms (LUTS) (C) [6].

3. Reduction in cigarette smoking

In animal models, nicotine has been demonstrated to produce phasic contractions of the urinary bladder [7, 8]. Although an association between cigarette smoking and incontinence in adult women has been described [9, 10], not until quite recently have there been reports on the association of cigarette smoking and LUTS in males. Koskimäki et al. [11] reported an association between smoking and LUTS as measured by the Danish Prostatic Symptom Score–1, especially bothersomeness including urgency and urge incontinence. Compared with individuals who had never smoked, age-adjusted odds ratios of LUTS were 1.47 (95% CI 1.09-1.98) for current smokers and 1.38 (1.08-1.78) for former smokers. The association of cigarette smoking with LUTS was confirmed by Haidinger et al. [6] who observed a highly significant positive correlation between the numbers of cigarettes smoked per day and the irritative score of the International Prostatic Symptom Score (IPSS). In addition, in a population of 528 men aged 60-89 the odds ratio of urgency for current smokers was 2.55 (95% CI 1.13-5.73) and for former smokers 1.28 (0.68-2.41) compared with those who had never smoked [12]. These findings support the suggestion that smoking may cause urge incontinence and that the adverse effects of smoking are to some extent reversible once smoking ceases. These facts imply that smoking should be discouraged.

4. Reduction in caffeine intake

It has been demonstrated that, following administration of caffeine, a statistically significant increase in detrusor pressure occurs during bladder filling in patients with detrusor instability whereas in normal patients no cystometric abnormality is noted [13]. However, there are conflicting data on the clinical significance of coffee or tea drinking in urinary incontinence. Some studies have not found any relation between caffeine intake and urinary incontinence [5, 12, 14, 15] whereas others have reported an association between high caffeine intake and detrusor overactivity [16]. Although decreased caffeine intake has often been advocated for the treatment of urinary incontinence [17], the evidence for that is weak (C).

5. Reduction in fluid intake

Urine loss has been shown to be significantly related to fluid intake in geriatric patients [18, 19] (B). Overhydration was found in the majority of the elderly who complained of pollakisuria when frequency-volume charts were utilized [20] (C). Although reduction in fluid intake has been recommended in the treatment of urinary incontinence [17], no relation was found between reduction in fluid intake and outcome in treating urinary incontinence in frail, elderly people [14] or older women living at home [15]. In fact, completely opposite findings recommending increased fluid intake have also been reported [21]. There is no strong evidence to recommend reduction in fluid intake for the treatment of urinary incontinence (C).

6. Reduction in alcohol

In a cross-sectional study, regular alcohol consumption resulted both in higher total IPSS (p=0.01) and irritative scores (p=0.02) (B) [6]. However, in a population based survey involving 1059 people aged 60-89, alcohol use did not predict urgency [12].

7. Summary

Several studies have reported the effects of life style on urinary incontinence. Cigarette smoking and regular alcohol consumption have been identified to be significantly correlated with urgency and urge urinary incontinence (B). It is suggested that smoking should be discouraged (D). On the other hand there are conflicting reports of caffeine intake and fluid intake on urinary incontinence (C). Body mass index does not correlate with LUTS in male adults (C).

III. NOCTURNAL ENURESIS IN MALE ADULTS

1. Background

Nocturnal enuresis in adults may not only lead to embarrassment and discomfort but also affect careers, social life and personal relationships. Enuresis can be defined as any involuntary loss of urine; it may be nocturnal, both nocturnal and diurnal, or diurnal alone. Primary nocturnal enuresis refers to the patient who has never been dry at night, and secondary or acquired nocturnal enuresis refers to the patient who has been dry for at least a year before the onset of present enuresis. High pressure chronic retention is an uncommon but important cause of leakage at night (nocturnal enuresis) in old men. Other pathologic conditions such as detrusor overactivity, low compliance and chronic retention, will lead to upper urinary tract dilation and impair renal function. Reasons for secondary enuresis include psychosomatic factors such as dysfunctional voiding [22-24], sleep disorders, organic factors such as tethered cord syndrome [25], diabetes mellitus, constipation [26], abnormal diurnal rhythm of plasma vasopressin [27], and certain abnormalities manifested by abnormal ECG patterns [28, 29].

2. Primary nocturnal enuresis

Although it is believed that the majority of enuretics will easily and spontaneously cure as they grow older, a large-scale survey of bedwetting in the Netherlands found that 0.6% of male adults still suffered from nocturnal enuresis [30]. In a large Finnish study of 11220 subjects aged 33-60 years, the corresponding number was 0.3% [31]. The latter study involved twins and confirmed the central role of genetic liability in adult enuresis. Treatment modalities for primary enuresis include an alarm bell [32], desmopressin (DDAVP) at bedtime [33] and antimuscarinic agents such as oxybutynin [34]. Secondary enuresis should be treated according to the causative factors involved. Strategies for this pathology will be covered in more detail by the children's committee.

Hirasing et al. [30] studied a random sample of 4527 non-institutionalized Dutch male adults (18-64 years old) in 1997 and found that 0.6% of them had nocturnal enuresis at least once in the past 4 weeks. Fifty percent of the enuretic patients had primary enuresis nocturna and never consulted a care provider. Previously, Forsythe and Redmond [35] observed that 33 (3%) of 1129 former patients who attended the Enuretic Clinic were still wetting after 20 years. Torrens and Collins [36] studied 54 adults having enuresis with the largest number of them being in their 20's. Seventy percent (70%) demonstrated either detrusor overactivity or low bladder compliance. Whiteside and Arnold [37] urodynamically investigated 50 patients with persistent primary enuresis 25 of whom were >20 years old. They found that nocturnal enuresis was associated mainly with normal detrusor function while nocturnal plus diurnal enuresis was mainly associated with detrusor overactivity McGuire and Savastano [38] studied 55 adults with enuresis, 13 of whom (24%) were adults. They observed detrusor overactivity was the predominant clinical finding in these patients. Fidas et al. [39] studied 25 primary adult enuretics with a mean age of 28 years by means of urodynamic assessment and neurophysiological measurements of static EMG and sacral reflex latencies (SRL). Detrusor overactivity was present in 15 patients (60%) and abnormal neurophysiological measurements were found in 88% of them. Hunsballe [40] found increased delta activity in electroencephalography among adult primary enuretics compared to normal controls indicating increased depth of sleep.

3. Secondary nocturnal enuresis

a) Diabetic cystopathy

Diabetic cystopathy refers to the spectrum of voiding dysfunction in patients with diabetes mellitus. This is marked by insidious onset and progression with minimal symptomatology. Although the common urodynamic findings are impairment of bladder sensation, increased post-void residual volume and decreased detrusor contractility, involuntary contractions are frequently observed in these patients [41]. Kitami [42] studied 173 diabetic patients. Of the patients, 32 (18%) suffered from urinary incontinence and detrusor overactivity was observed in 13 of the 32 patients (41 %). Starer & Libow [43] observed an even higher rate of urinary incontinence in elderly patients. Of 23 patients with mean age of 80, 17 (74%) suffered from urinary incontinence and detrusor instability was found in 13 (76%) of them. In experimental animals Andersson et al. [44] observed in a cystometric study of diabetic rats, that there was an increased compliance, a higher threshold volume for initiating a micturition reflex without residue and spontaneous rhythmic contractions.

b) Outlet obstruction

Sakamoto et al [45] found that in 8 males without day-time incontinence, nocturnal enuresis was due to severe bladder outlet obstruction and resolved after treatment of obstruction. In a group of patients with delayed presentation of posterior urethral valves the most common presenting symptom was diurnal enuresis in 60% [46].

c) Endocrine disease

Goswami et al [47] studied 30 consecutive patients with active Graves' disease (thyrotoxicosis) whose age averaged 31 years. Of the patients 12 (40%) had some bladder symptoms and 4 (13%) had nocturnal enuresis. These pathologies resolved after euthyroidism was achieved.

d) Sleep apnea

In the elderly obstructive sleep apnoea might be a cause of nocturnal enuresis [48]. Treatment with nasal continuous positive airway pressure was more effective than conservative treatment (B).

e) Drug induced enuresis

It has been known for some time that some patients suffer from drug-induced enuresis and/or retention for a certain period of time. Since resolution of this pathology is directly associated with cessation of taking the drug(s), it is essential to identify medications such as thioridazine for psychiatric patients [49], risperidone for schizophrenia [50], and prazosin for hypertension [51].

4. Summary

The incidence of nocturnal enuresis in the male adult-population is 0.3-0.6% (B). The majority of those with primary enuresis suffered from detrusor overactivity (50-70%) (C). Etiologies of secondary enuresis include bladder outlet obstruction, diabetic cystopathy, obstructive sleep apnea, Graves' disease, anti-psychotic medication, alpha-antagonists for hypertension, and so on (C). If one finds causative factors of underlying diseases or medications, the treatment should be directed to these pathologies (C). Strategies for managing this condition will be covered in more detail by the children's committee.

IV. POST- PROSTATECTOMY INCONTINENCE

1. Background

We are here concerned with conservative treatment of post-prostatectomy incontinence, defined as any treatment strategy not involving surgical intervention. Prostatectomy, especially when performed for control of cancer, continues to be an important cause of incontinence in the male. Incontinence rates following radical prostatectomy vary widely among different series due to disparities in patient selection and in the definition of incontinence (some degree of incontinence versus total incontinence). Greater understanding of the anatomy of the prostatic apex and the perineal floor, as well as attention to details of surgical technique, have all contributed to improvements in continence rates. If further improvement is to be achieved, we shall have to increase our understanding of the mechanisms, risk factors and preventive strategies related to post-prostatectomy incontinence.

2. Quality of studies

There are 4 recent randomized controlled trials of pelvic floor training dealing with urinary incontinence following radical prostatectomy [52-55] in a total of 318 patients. In this section, evidence for the efficacy of various conservative approaches to this distressing problem is reviewed.

3. Non-surgical incontinence

In men without a prior history of surgery, pelvic surgery or trauma, incontinence is almost always due to abnormalities of bladder function. Sphincteric incompetence in men who have not had surgery is usually due to a neurological deficit (cauda equina or lower cord injury, myelomeningocele). Continuous or unconscious incontinence may mimic stress incontinence and may occur secondary to bladder outlet obstruction, impaired contractility or a combination of the two. Loss of storage function may be due to detrusor overactivity, neurogenic detrusor overactivity, and diminished bladder compliance.

a) Detrusor overactivity

This pathology increases with aging in both men and women [56]. In males bladder outlet obstruction is an additional etiologic factor. Relief of obstruction reverses detrusor overactivity in 50-60% of cases, although reversal is less common in the elderly [57]. The mechanism of detrusor overactivity is incompletely understood at present. Increased electrical coupling between muscle fibers [58] as well as denervation supersensitivity [59] may play a role. Detrusor overactivity has been produced in an animal model of pelvic ischemia [60].

b) Neurogenic detrusor overactivity

This is caused by neurological conditions, most commonly stroke [61], dementia [62] and Parkinson's disease or multiple system atrophy [63, 64]. Even mild hypoperfusion of the cerebral cortex has been shown to be associated with neurogenic detrusor overactivity [65].

c) Diminished bladder compliance and capacity

These findings seem to accompany the aging process (56]. Severe diminution of bladder capacity may follow pelvic irradiation [66]. Ischemic changes of the detrusor muscle may play a role in the loss of bladder compliance [67].

4. Mechanisms of post-prostatectomy incontinence

The table analyzes 573 patients described in 8 articles [68-75] who suffered urinary incontinence after undergoing surgery for benign prostatic hyperplasia or prostatic cancer. Urodynamic studies identified 34% of patients as having sphincter incompetence, 26% as having detrusor overactivity and 33% of mixed incontinence. Other factors such as low compliance were responsible for the remaining 7%. Figure 1 schematically illustrates the proportion of these findings.

a) Transurethral (TURP) and open prostatectomy

The incidence of incontinence following transurethral prostatectomy continues to be low, approximately 1% (76]. Patient continence following TURP depends on a normal bladder filling and an intact distal striated muscle sphincter. The pelvic floor muscles normally provide additional closure during periods of increased abdominal pressure such as during coughing or laughing as well as during periods of detrusor overactivity. Kahn et al. reported [71] that sphincteric incompetence alone accounted for approximately 25% of incontinence patients following TURP. The remaining 60-75% of patients had detrusor overactivity, either alone or in combination with sphincteric incompetence. Although it is well known that detrusor overactivity fol-

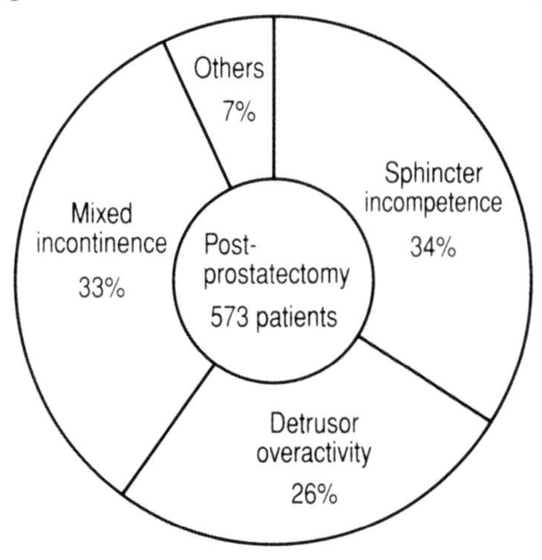

Figure 1 : A pie chart represents 4 major etiologies of post-prostatectomy incontinence.

Table 1 : Etiologies of post-prostatectomy incontinence are analyzed based on 573 patients reported in 8 articles [9-76].

Authors	Sphincter incompetence	Detrusor overactivity	Mixed incontinence	Others
Andersen (68) (n=34, 1978)	24%	44%	26%	6%
Fitzpatrick (69) (n=68, 1979)	26%	16%	38%	19%
Leach (70) (n=38, 1987)	40%	19%	42%	0
Kahn (71) (n=63, 1991)	22%	49%	25%	3%
Goluboff (72) (n=56, 1995)	5%	61%	34%	0
Chao (73) (n=74, 1995)	57%	4%	39%	0
Leach (74) (n=201, 1996)	41%	10%	25%	24%
Desautel (75) (n=39, 1997)	59%	3%	35%	3%
Mean	34%	26%	33%	7%

lowing TURP is common, it is unclear why postoperative detrusor overactivity causes incontinence in some patients but not in others.

b) Radical prostatectomy

In comparison to TURP, incontinence is much more common after radical prostatectomy, whether performed by the retropubic or the perineal route. In patients who have had radical prostatectomy, the striated urinary sphincter may play a more important role (Table 1). In physician reported studies, the incidence of total incontinence is 0-5% and the incidence of stress incontinence requiring some degree of protection is 5-15% [77-79]. In studies based on patient self-report, the incidence of any degree of incontinence is 66% and the incidence of pad use is 33% [80]. Many studies have indicated - somewhat surprisingly - that urethral incompetence alone is present in only about one third of cases [72, 74]. Detrusor overactivity alone accounts for 20% and the remainder are due to a combination of these two factors. In contrast, more recent studies have found that sphincteric incompetence rather than bladder overactivity is the predominant factor causing post-radical prostatectomy incontinence [73, 75, 81]. Patients who undergo a nerve-sparing radical prostatectomy appear to have a better chance of achieving continence than those undergoing standard radical prostatectomy [82]. Recent enhancements to the nerve-sparing prostatectomy may preserve external sphincter function and shorten the time to achieve post-operative continence [83].

5. Risk factors for post-prostatectomy incontinence

a) Neurological Disease

Patients with neurological disorders associated with detrusor hyperreflexia are at increased risk of incontinence following all types of prostatectomy. Such disorders include cerebrovascular disease, multiple sclerosis and Parkinson's disease. Staskin et al noted that patients with Parkinson's disease who had poor voluntary sphincter control suffered a significantly higher post-prostatectomy incontinence rate than did those who had preserved voluntary control [84]. Recent studies have confirmed this and pointed out that many severely debilitated patients with parkinsonism actually suffer from multiple system atrophy. Chandiramani et al stated that these patients should not undergo prostatectomy because urinary incontinence is unavoidable postoperatively [63]. Peripheral neuropathy affecting the external sphincter is often mentioned as a risk factor [71] but good studies are difficult to find.

b) Age

Whenever it is specifically mentioned, increased age appears to be correlated with increased risk after radical prostatectomy incontinence. For example, in the study by Steiner et al, patients in the fifth decade had an incontinence rate of 2% in comparison to 14% for patients in the eighth decade [82].

c) Radiation therapy

Radical prostatectomy following radiation therapy to the prostates is rarely performed and is associated with markedly higher incontinence rates [85].

d) Prior TURP

Although prior prostatectomy was reported to be associated with higher rates of incontinence in the past, modern series appear to show that prior TURP does not affect incontinence rates following radical prostatectomy [65].

6. Treatments of post-prostatectomy incontinence

a) Patient selection

Detrusor overactivity is an important contributing factor to postoperative incontinence. In patients with symptoms of urge incontinence, pre-operative urodynamics may be used to identify patients with severe overactivity or loss of bladder compliance who may do poorly in terms of regaining continence. Patients with severe parkinsonism or multiple system atrophy may be at particular risk and should be managed non-operatively if possible [71, 84].

b) Modification of surgical technique

During radical prostatectomy, careful anatomic dissection of the apex to preserve urethral length and fixation are important factors in reducing post-operative incontinence. Preservation of the anterior attachments of the urethra, including the puboprostatic ligaments, seems to aid in rapid achievement of post-operative continence [86]. This result may be due to preservation of the external sphincter complex.

c) Peri-operative pelvic floor training

In males the effects of pelvic floor muscle training (PFMT) and electrical stimulation (ES) have been evaluated in patients suffering from post-prostatectomy incontinence. PFMT has been the mainstay of therapy and improvement has been reported in men who follow an intensive exercise regimen in nurse-run or physiotherapy clinics [87, 88]. Some have proposed that continence is regained more rapidly when PFMT is augmented with ES [89, 90], biofeedback [91, 92] or transcutaneous electrical stimulation [93]. Most studies suggest that these treatments are successful but control groups are missing, sample sizes are small, objective measures of incontinence are not included and long-term follow-up is lacking. Moreover, the uncontrolled nature of the studies does not account for a placebo effect that was reported to be as high as 25 % in women with incontinence [94, 95] or for spontaneous improvement that may occur up to 12 months after surgery [96, 97]. Subjective improvement rates have varied between 60 and 82 %.

So far four randomized controlled trials evaluating PFMT and ES have been reported. Porru et al [55] randomly assigned a total of 58 patients about to undergo TURP into a control group or an investigational group. The latter was instructed to contract the perineal muscles 45 times a day after the removal of the urethral catheter. Urge incontinence, terminal dribbling and voiding interval in those with PFMT significantly improved up to 3 weeks after surgery compared to the control. However this difference ceased to be significant after 4 weeks suggesting recovery of the muscle was substantial in patients of the control group. Since the exercise is simple and easy to perform, this should be recommended to all patients who undergo TURP.

Van Kampen et al [53] compared effects of PFMT and sham stimulation of placebo electrotherapy in those with radical prostatectomy. One hundred and two men following radical prostatectomy were randomized after catheter removal into two equal sized groups. A trained physiotherapist instructed PFMT in combination with initial ES and biofeedback in 50 men. Urinary continence was achieved after 3 months in 88% of the treatment group and 56% in the control group. At 1 year, continence rate was 95% and 81%, respectively, reducing the difference in proportion between treatment and control group being 14 % (95 % CI 2-27). In the treatment group, improvement in both duration and degree of incontinence was significantly better without side effects or risks from therapy than in the control group during the first 4 months.

Moore et al. [52] randomized 58 patients after radical prostatectomy to 3 groups: control group (short instructions on PFMT before surgery), intensive pelvic floor muscle training, and PFMT and electrostimulation. Although the patients were recruited 8 weeks after surgery, their urine loss averaged 463g/24 hours and was much more than that reported by van Kampen et al [53]. The authors found no effects of either PFMT alone or in combination with ES compared with control treatment. The inconsistent conclusion may be explained by the degree of incontinence being very severe in their patients, the small number of patients in each group and the initial rapid spontaneous improvement of the sphincter component (463g at baseline to 115g 12 weeks after treatments) that masked any treatment benefits.

Bales et al. [54] randomly allocated 100 men who were scheduled to undergo radical prostatectomy to a group of intensive pelvic floor muscle trainings with biofeedback and to a control group that received only brief explanations of pelvic floor muscle trainings. Continence rates were not significantly different between the two group at 1, 2, 3, 4, and 6 months after surgery. There were some shortcomings in the study design compared to that of van Kampen et al. For instance, those assigned to PFMT had only one 45-min session of muscle training prior to surgery in Bale's patients compared to regular, frequent attendance to training programme in Van Kampen's patients. It is quite likely that it is not PFMT itself but insufficient exposure to adequate and meaningful PFMT that led to treatment failure.

Although sphincter muscle function recovers spontaneously after TURP in one month, PFMT enhances recovery of continence during the first few weeks. In patients who undergo radical prostatectomy, after an initial period of rapid improvement, incontinence continues to improve even beyond three months following surgery. Only a small minority of men had incontinence by 6 to 12 months. Therefore, there is an argument for delaying formal conservative management for at least three months and focusing intensive therapy on those with persistent incontinence. The data available suggest that PFMT and ES are beneficial in the management of post-prostatectomy urinary incontinence but the correct timing remains unclear.

d) Pharmacotherapy for post-prostatectomy incontinence

Urinary incontinence following transurethral or open prostatectomy for benign prostatic obstruction may be due to sphincter incompetence, detrusor overactivity, or combination of both factors [74, 75]. Stewart et al. [98] used phenylpropanolamine, a sympathomimetic agent, in patients with stress incontinence after prostatectomy. They found this agent to have low efficacy, particularly for severe incontinence. Khanna used ephedrine, phenylephrine or propranolol in patients with post-prostatectomy incontinence and achieved cure or improvement in 73% patients. However, Khanna's paper did not describe the type of incontinence and the study was not placebo-controlled [99]. The true effect of sympathomimetics in treating post-prostatectomy stress incontinence is questionable (C).

Detrusor overactivity following prostatectomy can be managed pharmacologically. Theodorou et al used oxybutynin on post-prostatectomy detrusor overactivity and found that 8 of 13(61.5%) patients either were cured or significantly improved [100]. Leach et al found that 59% of incontinent patients following prostatectomy for benign prostatic obstruction were mainly due to "high-pressure bladder dysfunction," which included detrusor overactivity and/or low compliance. They treated bladder dysfunction with oxybutynin or propantheline initially followed by adding imipramine if initial medication failed. Although they reported an improvement in pad scores, which decreased from 2.69 to 1.69, there was no information on the efficacy of individual drugs [74]. Iselin et al reported an interesting paper on managing early detrusor overactivity after TURP. They used oxybutynin 2 days after TURP and discovered that, compared with placebo, oxybutynin significantly decreased frequency, urgency and detrusor pressure at first sensation of filling (C) [101].

7. Summary

Detrusor overactivity is a major contributing factor in post-prostatectomy incontinence. It is, however, not possible to predict whether this pathology will subside after TURP or radical prostatectomy. Urodynamically, 34% of incontinent patients suffered sphincter incompetence, 26% suffered detrusor overactivity, and 33% suffered mixed incontinence (B). Pelvic floor muscle training is beneficial in the treatment of post-prostatectomy incontinence (B), although different study designs arrived at conflicting conclusions. Research on detrusor overactivity in association with prostatic surgery is strongly needed.

V. POST-MICTURITION DRIBBLING

1. Mechanism and Incidence

Post-micturition dribbling is characteristic of male patients and is usually unrelated to either urethral stricture or urethral obstruction [102-104]. This pathology is due to pooling of urine in the bulbous urethra after micturition, which later drains by gravity or body movement. In rare cases a urethral diverticulum may be the cause. Since this symptom itself is minor and does not threaten one's life, not many patients visit urologists for treatments. Furuya et al. [105] reported their study on incidence, frequency, and severity by sending questionnaires to 3034 healthy male subjects. Of the patients 2839 (94%) sent replies. The incidence of this condition was found to be 17%, which increased from 12% in those in their 20's to 27% in those in their 50's. One third of the patients experienced the dribbling once a week or more. Although 94% of them noted spotting or slight wetting of their underwear, 22% noticed their pants got considerably wet. Sommer et al. [106] found in 572 men from 20 to 79 years of age a similar incidence but no increase with age. Peterson et al. [107] evaluated the incidence of post-micturition dribbling in 1251 men with lower urinary tract symptoms (LUTS) by questionnaires in the ICS «BPH» study. They found that post-micturition dribbling was present in 67% of 1250 men but did not increase with age (69% in those < 60 years, 69% in those of their 60's and 65% in those > 70 years) and that post-micturition dribble bothered men the most among 19 subjective symptoms.

2. Treatments

Furuya and his associates [105] mentioned that younger men prefer fashionable trunks which lack a front exit and inevitably compress the bulbous urethra from below during micturition. If this is the reason for this symptom, one should abandon this type of the underwear and put on a conventional one instead. Paterson et al. [107] compared treatment with counselling, urethral milking and pelvic muscle exercise in a prospective, randomised study. They found counselling without effect, while both urethral milking and pelvic floor exercise were effective with pelvic floor exercise being the most effective.

In any case, it is advisable to recommend those who wet their underwear after voiding to thoroughly milk the anterior urethra, which is illustrated in figure 2, and/or to shake their pelvis rhythmically. If a wetting episode persists, urinary flowmetry and cystourethrography are suggested to rule out possible lower urinary tract pathology.

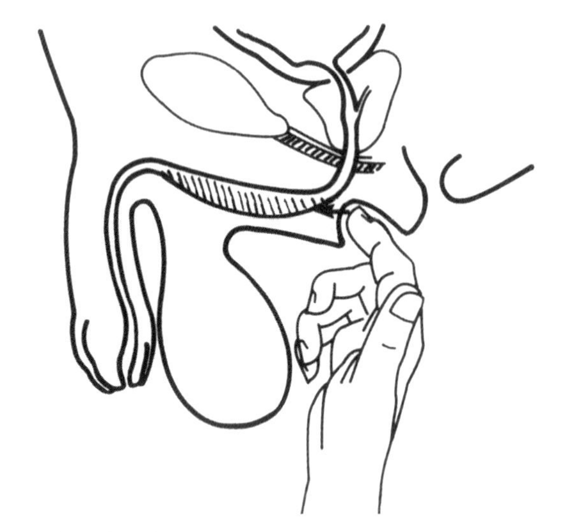

Figure 2 : This shows how to milk the bulbous urethra of those with post-voiding dribbling.

3. Summary

Post-micturition dribbling is a minor condition which does not hamper health but is a nuisance and causes discomfort and embarrassment (B). This symptom is present in 17% of healthy adults and 67% of those with LUTS (B). Since this condition is usually due to urine pooled in the bulbous urethra, it is advisable to thoroughly milk the urethra (B) and/or to rhythmically shake one's pelvis prior to putting back the penis (D). Pelvic floor training might be even better treatment (B).

VI. PHARMACOTHERAPY FOR STORAGE SYMPTOMS AND NOCTURIA

1. Background

Drugs managing lower urinary tract dysfunction have been applied on both the female and the male. There is no evidence of different effects of these drugs depending on sex. As for drugs for detrusor overactivity, the reader is referred to a chapter on the pharmacologic treatment prepared by other committee.

2. Drug therapy for storage symptoms in men

Overactive detrusor symptoms in men are usually due to detrusor overactivity associated with bladder outlet obstruction. About 60% of symptomatic older men have bladder storage symptoms, including urgency, frequency and urge incontinence [108]. Investigators have proposed several mechanisms explaining bladder outlet obstruction-induced overactivity. Steers et al. demonstrated an increased incidence of short latency spinal reflex in obstructed rats [109]. Sibley et al. showed a partial denervation with resulting supersensitivity to cholinergic stimulation in obstructed pig bladders [110]. Both findings indicated a neurogenic origin of obstruction-induced overactivity. Another proposed mechanism is increased alpha-adrenergic responses in the obstructed detrusor, as reported by Perlberg et al. [111].

Theoretically, drugs aiming at reducing bladder outlet obstruction may concurrently improve storage LUTS. However, reports on pharmacotherapy of BOO usually compare the effects by a total symptom score, instead of emptying and storage symptoms, respectively. It is difficult to identify or compare the effects of these drugs on damaged storage functions, particularly for urge incontinence. Although storage LUTS associated with BOO can be improved by drugs targeting outlet obstruction, the improvement in symptoms is often not enough to satisfy the patient. An addition of an anticholinergic agent may improve storage LUTS, but at the same time may compromise bladder emptying, particularly in the presence of severe outlet obstruction or weak detrusor contractility. A recent study, however, describing the use of tolterodine in men with BOO showed no increase in voiding dysfunction [112]. Dahm et al. [113] used flavoxate and placebo to treat storage symptoms of patients with "benign prostatic hyperplasia". They found that flavoxate was not more effective than placebo for relieving symptoms. Chapple et al. have proposed a combination of alpha-1 adrenergic antagonist and anticholinergics to further ameliorate storage LUTS of patients with suspected BPO [114]. Well-controlled studies are necessary to demonstrate the value of this combination therapy.

3. Drugs for nocturia

Urinary frequency (nocturia) and even urge incontinence at nighttime is one of the more debilitating urinary symptoms in males, greatly affecting sleep and quality of life, particularly for the elderly. Nocturia can be caused by nocturnal polyuria and/or decreased functional bladder capacity. Nocturnal polyuria may be due to aging-associated loss of renal concentrating ability, increased sodium excretion, decreased nocturnal production of anti-diuretic hormone or disturbance of renin-angiotensin-aldosterone axis. Decreased nocturnal functional capacity may be due to idiopathic or obstruction-induced detrusor overactivity, or due to increased residual urine. Sleep disorders may also contribute to nocturia [115].

Pharmacotherapy of nocturia is based on the etiology. Theoretically, if nocturia is due to BPH-induced outlet obstruction, alpha-adrenergic antagonists and/or 5 alpha reductase inhibitors may decrease outlet obstruction and reduce nocturnal urinary frequency. However, there are no available data specifically addressing the effects of these drugs on nocturia. Encouraging urine excretion before sleep or decreasing urine production at nighttime are other techniques to manage nocturnal polyuria. In a double blind placebo-controlled study, Reynard et al. used the diuretic frusemide 6 hours before bedtime to reduce urine excretion at nighttime. Nocturnal voiding frequency and urinary production were significantly reduced [116] (B).

Several reports have demonstrated that desmopressin (DDAVP) before bedtime may decrease nocturnal urinary production with a reduction of nocturnal urinary frequency, particularly for patients with higher nocturnal urinary volume [117, 118] (B). Since desmopressin increases urine concentration and reduces total urine output, it has been shown to be effective and well tolerated in the treatment of nocturia in male adults [119]. However, the optimal dosage is not determined yet. Some investigators suggested 0.1mg is enough [120], while others advised 0.4mg [121]. Side effects of DDAVP should be balanced with the benefits. With fluid retention induced by DDAVP, hyponatremia, edema, or even heart failure may occur [122] and care should be exercised when used in the older men. The serum sodium should be checked 3 days after starting the treatment or changing the dose.

In young adult enuretics, bedtime imipramine may decrease nocturnal urinary output curing nocturnal enuresis. The antidiuretic effect of imipramine may come from its alpha-adrenergic actions on proximal renal tubules with increased urea and water reabsorption more distally in the nephron [123]. Whether imipramine also has similar effects in older individuals with nocturnal polyuria deserves further clinical investigation.

4. Summary

Drugs for storage symptoms are to be chosen depending on etiology of the condition. Anti-cholinergics in addition to drugs targeting outlet obstruction may be beneficial for those with outlet obstruction, urgency and urge incontinence (A). Nocturia due to nocturnal polyuria was favorably treated with frusemide or desmospressin (DDAVP) (B).

VII. BEHAVIORAL THERAPY FOR MALE ADULTS

1. Background

Behavioral therapy refers to several techniques that modify patients' voiding behavior to achieve urinary continence. These techniques include bladder training, timed voiding and prompted voiding. They are frequently combined to achieve maximum benefits.

2. Bladder training

In bladder retraining, the focus of treatment is on changing the patient's bladder habits. The goal is to reduce urinary incontinence by increasing bladder capacity and restore normal bladder function. This is accomplished by providing the patient with a voiding schedule and by gradually increasing the intervals between voids. In women [124], there is some evidence for the efficacy of bladder training in the treatment of urge incontinence but in men that information is missing. Oxybutynin with bladder training was superior to bladder training alone in reducing frequency due to detrusor overactivity in very elderly people (mostly women) living at home [125]. Bladder training may be helpful for the treatment of urge incontinence in males, but at this time there is insufficient evidence to come to any conclusion (D).

3. Timed (Scheduled) voiding

The patients are scheduled to void at a fixed interval, usually 2 to 4 hours. This technique allows the bladder to remain at a lower volume and thus avoid provoking involuntary detrusor contractions, particularly in the elderly patient with impaired mobility. The number of reports on using this technique specifically in male patients is limited. Sogbein et al. applied timed voiding in incontinent men in a geriatric hospital with an 85% improvement rate [126]. Timed voiding may also help stress incontinence in men. Burgio et al. instructed timed voiding with 2-hour interval on 20 men with post-prostatectomy incontinence [127] which initially resulted in 33.1% increase in urge incontinence and 28.5% decrease in stress incontinence. When biofeedback was subsequently taught to control the sphincter muscle and to inhibit the detrusor overactivity, urge and stress incontinence decreased 80.7% and 78.3%, respectively. Since this technique is simple and harmless, it can be recommended as an initial management for urinary incontinence in men (C).

4. Prompted voiding

This technique gives positive social reinforcement when patients, who are checked by caregivers at regular intervals, request toileting assistance. In contrast to timed voiding, the toileting is not scheduled in advance. This technique is mainly for the elderly with impaired cognitive function [128,129]. There are no articles reporting this method specifically in men. Although published studies generally concluded the technique had a favorable effect, these studies are usually not adequately controlled. Other disadvantages of this method are that it requires considerable manpower and compliance from nursing staff [130] (C).

5. Summary

Bladder training, timed voiding and prompted voiding have been studied in male adults suffering from urinary incontinence. Due to lack of well-controlled studies, clinical effects are not convincing (C or D).

VIII. PELVIC FLOOR MUSCLE TRAINING AND ELECTRO-STIMULATION

1. Urge incontinence

The rationale behind the use of pelvic floor muscle training (PFMT) or electrical stimulation (ES) to treat urge incontinence is the observation that ES of the pelvic floor muscle inhibits detrusor contraction [131]. The aim of therapy is to inhibit detrusor muscle contraction by voluntary contraction of the PFMs when urgency is present and to prevent sudden falls in urethral pressure [132]. Several randomized, controlled studies have demonstrated that PFMT is more effective than no treatment [133, 134] and more effective than other conservative methods in treating genuine stress incontinence in women [134, 135] (A). In PFMT with biofeedback, the biofeedback is intended to increase the patient's motivation by demonstrating positive effects of their efforts. Hence the combination of biofeedback with PFMT may increase the effectiveness of the training and improve the outcome of treatment (C).

2. Stress incontinence

This pathology in adult males is rare and mostly caused by surgery or trauma. PFMT following TURP or radical prostatectomy is effective and was discussed in the section on post-prostatectomy incontinence.

3. Chronic pelvic pain syndrome

In a descriptive study, Clemens et al [136] applied PFMT supplemented with EMG biofeedback plus bladder training to 19 male patients with chronic pelvic pain syndrome. AUA symptom score and urgency score were significantly reduced by the therapy. However, only 10 patients completed full treatment sessions and the follow-up period was short (5.8 months). Whether the therapeutic benefits come from PFMT remains unclear (C).

4. Geriatric patients

In geriatric patients PFMT and ES have been used as part of a combination of several therapies and interventions which makes it difficult to evaluate their roles in the treatment. In a randomized control study, McDowell et al. randomized 105 subjects comprising 95 females and 10 males aged 60 and older to either biofeedback-assisted PFMT or the control group. They observed that subjects treated with active treatments resulted in a clinically significant reduction in urinary incontinence in homebound older adults despite high levels of co-morbidity and functional impairment [137]. This suggests that PFMT may be beneficial in the treatment of urinary incontinence in geriatric patients (B).

5. Summary

PFMT or ES can be offered as a first-line treatment for those with urge incontinence (C) and stress incontinence (B).

IX. DEVICES FOR CONTAINMENT OF URINARY INCONTINENCE

1. Background

For patients with intractable urinary incontinence, the goals of management should be 1) protection of skin, 2) protection of clothing and bedding, and 3) control of odor. The methods available may be divided into absorbent products, collecting devices and occluding devices. Figure 3 illustrates various kinds of absorbent products, collecting devices and occlusive devices available in the market.

2. Absorbent products

Absorbent products are of three general types:

1. products designed to be worn inside underwear (pads, liners, shields, inserts),
2. diapers, both disposable and reusable, and
3. underpads for bedding.

a) Pads and liners are worn inside conventional underwear or inside a built-in pouch. Their construction is similar to that of diapers [138].

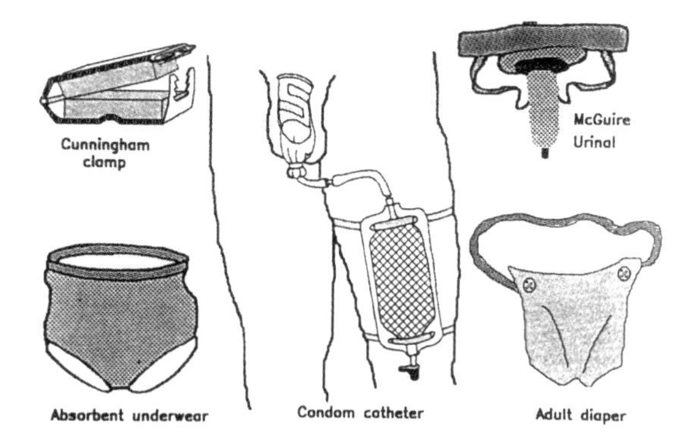

Figure 3 : Absorbent and collecting devices available on the market.

b) Disposable diapers are convenient and popular but expensive [139]. They are generally constructed of a soft inner lining, an absorbent middle layer and a waterproof outer layer [140]. The absorbent middle layer is made of cellulose fibers with or without the addition of polymers that gel with urine. The waterproof outer layer is made of rayon, polyester, polypropylene or polyethylene. Skin sensitization from rosin allergens in diapers has been described [141].

c) Since wet bed sheets have a markedly increased coefficient of friction, increasing the risk of skin abrasion, the use of effective bedding underpads is important in protecting the skin of incontinent patients [142]. The polymer underpad seems to be the most effective in containing urine [143-145].

d) Failure of absorbent products occurs when the absorbing material is saturated beyond its capacity. Improper fitting at the legs is also a common reason for failure. Skin irritation or reaction (diaper rash) remains a major problem [146].

3. Collecting devices

Urine collecting devices are used by 10-15% of all nursing home residents and by about 50% of those who are bedridden [147]. A variety of devices are available, including the condom sheath, the McGuire urinal and the drip collector. The condom sheath is the most widely used because of convenience, low cost and disposability. However, there are risk factors associated with these devices, including dermatitis [148], penile ischemia/necrosis, urethral erosion and increased incidence of urinary infection [149]. Guarding against excessive pressure on the penis is especially important in patients with impaired sensation. Limiting factors may include small penile size and redundant foreskin. It may be necessary to perform a circumcision or penile implant to facilitate placement of a condom sheath [150].

4. Occluding devices

The most common device in this category is the Cunningham clamp. Another version of the penile clamp is the C3 clamp made by Timm Medical. The Cunningham clamp consists of an adjustable clamp lined with soft foam-like material as a cushion. The C3 device is a Styrofoam urethral cushion held in place with a Velcro strap. The Cunningham clamp has the advantage of low cost, simplicity of use and effectiveness. However, it is unsightly and for many patients it is uncomfortable to wear. The C3 device is smaller and lighter than the Cunningham but is somewhat less effective as an occluding device. The Cunningham clamp should be put around the penis and closed only tight enough to occlude the urinary leak. Problems arise when the clamp is worn too long or closed too tightly, leading to skin necrosis, urethral erosion or peri-urethral abscess.

5. Summary

Disposable pads and diapers are effective but costly to purchase. This cost difference is ameliorated by savings in labor costs and better skin protection in incontinent patients. Though level of evidence is low, it is common knowledge that the condom catheter is by far the most commonly used external collecting device in males. Careful attention to its use should be paid to enhance its effectiveness and reduce complications. Our society where the elderly have been rapidly increasing depends heavily on these products to deal with urinary and fecal incontinence. Consequently it is important that these products have to be prepared and evaluated from the therapeutic and economic point of view.

X. GENERAL CONCLUSIONS

- Urinary incontinence in male adults cab be satisfactorily cured or managed provided pathologies and etiologies are clearly identified.
- Smoking habits increase the prevalence of lower urinary tract symptoms 1.5 times compared to non-smokers and stopping smoking decreases odds ratios (B). Accordingly, it is advised that cigarette smoking should be discouraged (D). Reductions in body weight, in caffeine intake, in fluid intake or in alcohol consumption are not known to significantly improve urinary incontinence (C).
- The prevalence of nocturnal enuresis is 0.3 to 0.6% in large randomly sampled population studies and 2.9% in former enuretics. Although the cause of nocturnal enuresis is multifactorial, a majority of patients suffer from detrusor overactivity (C). Secondary nocturnal enuresis should be treated by looking for underlining causative factors.

- Risk factors related to post-prostatectomy incontinence have to be investigated prior to surgery (C). Urodynamic studies of patients with post-prostatectomy incontinence show this to have several causes, including sphincter incompetence, detrusor overactivity, or mixed incontinence (B). Pelvic floor muscle training (PFMT) is beneficial in the treatment of post-prostatectomy incontinence (B), although different study designs arrived at conflicting conclusions.
- Post-micturition dribbling is present in 17 to 51% of male adults. The etiology is pooling of urine in the bulbous urethra. Clinical managements include pelvic floor muscle training and milking the bulbous urethra immediately after micturition, (B).
- Storage LUTS with BOO was shown to be successfully treated by anti-cholinergics (A). Desmopressin and frusemide (B) were of effect for the treatment of urinary frequency and nocturia.
- The effects of behavioral treatments such as bladder training, timed voiding and prompted voiding are not supported by strong evidence (C).
- Pelvic floor muscle training and electro-stimulation are effective for those suffering from stress incontinence (B) or urge incontinence (C).
- Devices for containment of incontinence are effective but lack well-controlled studies.

XI. FUTURE RESEARCH AND RECOMMENDATIONS

Randomized controlled trials (RCTs) are necessary to assess the effectiveness of lifestyle interventions. Further studies on the pathophysiology of detrusor overactivity especially associated with bladder outlet obstruction are needed. RCTs of pelvic floor muscle training (PFMT) for those having post-prostatectomy incontinence are necessary in large randomized samples in order to identify its real value and to assess the correct time to initiate PFMT. Pharmacological research is needed to satisfactorily treat nocturia caused by nocturnal polyuria. Devices for the containment of urinary incontinence should be produced and evaluated from the therapeutic and economic point of view.

REFERENCES

1. Resnick NM. Geriatric incontinence. Urol Clin North Am 23: 55-74, 1996.
2. Herzog AR, Diokno AC, Fultz NH. Urinary incontinence: Medical and psychological aspects. Ann Rev Gerontol Geriatr 9: 74-119, 1989.
3. Wyman JF, Harkins SW, Fantl JA. Psychological impact of urinary incontinence in the community-dwelling population. J Am Geriat Soc 38: 282-8, 1990.
4. Kondo A, Saito M, Yamada Y, Kato T, Hasegawa S, Kato K. Prevalence of hand-washing urinary incontinence in healthy subjects in relation to stress and urge incontinence. Neurourol Urodyn 11: 519-23, 1992.
5. Burgio KL, Matthews KA, Engel BT. Prevalence, incidence and correlates of urinary incontinence in healthy, middle aged women. J Urol 146:1255-9, 1991.
6. Hadinger G, Temml C, Schatzl G, Brossner M, Schmidbauer CP, Madersbacher S. Risk factors for lower urinary tract symptoms in elderly men. Eur Urol 37: 413-20, 2000.
7. Koley B, Koley J, Saha Jk. The effects of nicotine on spontaneous contractions of cat urinary bladder in situ. Br J Pharmacol 83: 347-55, 1984.
8. Hisayama T, Shinkai M, Takayanagi I, Toyoda T. Mechanism of action of nicotine in isolated bladder of guinea-pig. Br J Pharmacol 95: 465-72, 1988.
9. Bump & Mcclish DM.Cigarette smoking and pure genuine stress incontinence of urine: a comparison of risk factors and terminants between smokers and non-smokers. Am J Obstet Gynecol 170: 579-82, 1994.
10. Tampakoudis P, Tantanassis T, Grimbitzis G, Papaletsos M, Mantalenakis S. Cigarette smoking and urinary incontinence in women: a new calculative method of estimating the exposure to smoke. Eur J Obstet & Gynecol and Reprod Biol 63: 27-30, 1995.
11. Koskimäki J, Hakama M, Huhtala H, Tammela TLJ. Association of smoking with lower urinary tract symptoms. J Urol 159: 1580-2, 1998.
12. Nuotio M, Jylhä M, Koivisto A-M, TammelaTLJ. Association of smoking in urgency in older people. Eur Urol, in press (2001).
13. Creighton Sm, Stanton SL. Caffeine: does it affect your bladder? Br J Urol 66: 613-4, 1990.
14. Fried GW, Goetz G, Potts-Nulty S, Cioschi Hm, Staas WE, JR. A behavioral approach to the treatment of urinary incontinence in a disabled population. Arch Phys Med Rehabil 76: 1120-4, 1995.
15. Tomlinson BU, Dougherty Mc, Pendergast JF, Boyington AR, Coffman MA, Pickens SM. Dietary caffeine, fluid intake and urinary incontinence in older rural women. Int Urogynecol J Pelvic Floor Dysfunct 10: 22-8, 1999.
16. Arya LA, Myers DL, Jackson ND. Dietary caffeine intake and the risk for detrusor instability: a case-control study. Obstet Gynecol 96: 85-9, 2000.
17. Iqbal P, Castleden CM. Management of urinary incontinence in the elderly. Gerontology 43: 151-7, 1997.
18. Griffiths DJ, Mccracken PN, Harrison GM, Gormley EA. Relationship of fluid intake to voluntary micturition and urinary incontinence in geriatric patients. Neurourol Urodyn 12: 1-7, 1993.
19. Griffiths DJ, Mccracken PN, Harrison GM, Moore KN. Urge incontinence in elderly people: factors predicting the severity of urine loss before and after pharmacological treatment. Neurourol Urodyn 15: 53-7, 1996.
20. Saito M, Kondo A, Kato T, Yamada Y. Frequency-volume charts: Comparison of frequency between elderly and adult patients. Br J Urol 72: 38-41, 1993.
21. Dowd TT, Campbell JM, Jones JA. Fluid intake and urinary incontinence in older community-dwelling women. J Community Health Nurs 13: 179-86, 1996.
22. Hinman F, Baumann FW. Vesical and ureteral damage from voiding dysfunction in boys without neurologic or obstructive disease. J Urol 109:727-732, 1973.
23. Baumann FW, Hinman F. Treatment of incontinent boys with non-obstructive disease. J Urol 111:114-116,1974.
24. Hinman F, Jr. Nonneurogenic neurogenic bladder (the Hinman syndrome): 15 years later. J Urol 136:769-777, 1986.

25. Kondo A, Kato K, Kanai S, Sakakibara T. Bladder dysfunction secondary to tethered cord syndrome in adults: is it curable? J Urol 135:313-316, 1986.

26. O'Regan S, Yazbeck S, Hamberger B, Schick E. Constipation a commonly unrecognized cause of enuresis. Am J Dis Child 140:260-261, 1986.

27. Ritting S, Knudsen UB, Norgaard JP, Pedersen EB, Djurhuus JC. Abnormal diurnal rhythm of plasma vasopressin and urinary output in patients with enuresis. Am J Physiol 256:F664-71, 1989.

28. Campbell EW, Jr., Young JD, Jr. Enuresis and its relationship to electroencephalographic disturbances. J Urol 96:947-9, 1966.

29. Watanabe H, Kawauchi A, Kitamori T, Azuma T, Azuma Y. Treatment system for nocturnal enuresis according to an original classification system. Eur Urol 25:43-50, 1994.

30. Hirasing RA, Van Leedam FJ, Bolk-Bennink L, Janknegt RA. Enuresis nocturna in adults. Scand J Urol Nephrol 31:533-536, 1997.

31. Hublin C, Kaprio J, Partinen M, Koskenvuo M. Nocturnal enuresis in a nationwide twin cohort. Sleep 21:579-585, 1998.

32. Elinder G, Soback S. Effect of Uristop on primary nocturnal enuresis. A prospective randomized double-blind study. Acta Paediatr Scand 74:574-578, 1985.

33. Vandersteen DR, Husmann DA. Treatment of primary nocturnal enuresis persisting into adulthood. J Urol 161:90-2, 1999.

34. Hjalmas K. Pathophysiology and impact of nocturnal enuresis. Acta Paediatr 86: 919-22,1997.

35. Forsythe WI, Redmond A. Enuresis and spontaneous cure rate. Study of 1129 enuretics. Arch Dis Child 49:259-63, 1974.

36 Torrens MJ, Collins CD. The urodynamic assessment of adult enuresis. Br J Urol 47: 433-40, 1975.

37. Whiteside CG, Arnold EP. Persistent primary enuresis: a urodynamic assessment. Br Med J 1:364-367, 1975.

38. Mc Guire EJ, Sabastano JA. Urodynamic studies in enuresis and the nonneurogenic neurogenic bladder. J Urol 132:299-302, 1984.

39. Fidas A, Galloway NT, Mcinnes A, Chisholm GD. Neurophysiological measurements in primary adult enuretics. Br J Urol 57:635-640,1985.

40. Hunsballe JM. Increased delta component in computerized sleep electroencephalographic analysis suggests abnormally deep sleep in primary monosymptomatic nocturnal enuresis. Scand J Urol Nephrol 34:294-302, 2000.

41. Kaplan SA, Blaivas JG. Diabetic cystopathy. J Diabet Complications 2: 133-39, 1988.

42. Kitami K. [Vesicourethral dysfunction of diabetic patients]. Nippon Hinyokika Gakkai Zasshi 82:1074-83, 1991.

43. Starer P, Libow L. Cystometric evaluation of bladder dysfunction in elderly diabetic patients. Arch Intern Med 150:810-813, 1990.

44. Andersson PO, Malmgren A, Uvelius B. Cystometrical and in vitro evaluation of urinary bladder function in rats with streptozotocin-induced diabetes. J Urol 139: 1359-62, 1988.

45. Goswami R, Seth A, Goswami AK, Kochupillai N. Prevalence of enuresis and other bladder symptoms in patients with active Graves' disease. Br J Urol 80:563-6, 1997

46. Sakamoto K, Blaivas JG. Adult onset nocturnal enuresis. J Urol 165: 1914-7, 2001.

47. Bomalaski MD, Anema JG, Coplen DE, KooHP, Rozanski T, Bloom DA. Delayed presentation of posterior urethral valves: a not so benign condition. J Urol 162: 2130-2132, 1999.

48. Kiely JL, Murphy M, Mcnicholas WT. Subjective efficacy of nasal CPAP therapy in obstructive sleep apnoea syndrome: a prospective controlled study. Eur Respir J 13: 1086-90, 1999.

49. Berrios GE. Temporary urinary incontinence in the acute psychiatric patient without delirium or dementia. Br J Psychiatry 149: 224-7, 1986.

50. Poyurovsky M, Weizman A. Risperidone-induced nocturnal enuresis. Isr J Psychiatry Relat Sci 34:247-8, 1997.

51. Mathew TH, McEwen J, Rohan A. Urinary incontinence secondary to prazosin. Med J Aust 148:305-6, 1988.

52. Moore KN, Griffiths D, Hughton A. Urinary incontinence after radical prostatectomy: a randomized controlled trial comparing pelvic muscle exercises with or without electrical stimulation. Brit J Urol 83: 57-65, 1999.

53. Van Kampen M, Deweerdt W, Van Poppel H, De RidderD, Feys H, Baert L. Effect of pelvic-floor re-education on duration and degree of incontinence after radical prostatectomy: a randomised controlled study. Lancet 355: 98-102, 2000.

54. Bales GT, Gerber GS, Minor TX, Mhoon DA, McFarland JM, Kim HL, Brendler CB. Effect of preoperative biofeedback/pelvic floor training on continence in men undergoing radical prostatectomy. Urology 56: 627-30, 2000.

55. Porru D, Campus G, Caria A, Madeddu G, Cucci A, Rovereto B, Scarpa RM, Pili P, Usai E. Impact of early pelvic floor rehabilitation after transurethral resection of the prostate. Neurourol Urodyn 20: 53-9, 2001.

56. Madersbacher S, Pycha A, Schatzi G, Mian C, Klingler CH, Marberger M.The aging lower urinary tract: A comparative urodynamic study of men and women. Urology 51:206-12, 1998.

57. Gormley EA, Griffiths DJ, McCracken PN, Harrison GM, McPhee MS. Effect of transurethral resection of the prostate on detrusor instability and urge incontinence in elderly men. Neurourol Urodyn 12:445-453, 1993.

58. Elbadawi A, Yalla SV, Resnick N. Structural basis of geriatric voiding function. III. Detrusor overactivity. J Urol 150: 1668-80, 1993.

59. Speakman MJ, Brading AF, Gilpin CJ, Dixon JS, Gilpin SA, Gosling JA. Bladder outflow obstruction: a cause of denervation supersensitivity. J Urol 138:1461-6, 1987.

60. Azadzoi KM, Tarcan T, Kozlowski R, Krane RJ, Siroky MB. Overactivity and structural changes in the chronically ischemic bladder. J Urol 162:1768-78, 1999

61. Marinkovic S, Badlani G. Voiding and sexual dysfunction after cerebrovascular accidents. J Urol 165: 359-70, 2001.

62. Griffiths DJ, Mccracken PN, Harrison GM, Gormley EA, Moore K, Hooper R, McEwan AJ, Triscott J. Cerebral aetiology of urinary urge incontinence in the elderly people. Age Ageing 23:246-250, 1994.

63. Chandiramani VA, Palace J, Fowler CJ. How to recognize patients with parkinsonism who should not have urological surgery. Br J Urol 80:100-104, 1997.

64. Singer C. Urinary dysfunction in Parkinson's disease. Clin Neurosci 5:78-86, 1998.

65. Griffiths D. Clinical studies of cerebral and urinary tract function in elderly people with urinary incontinence. Behav Brain Res 92:151-155, 1998.

66. Schultheiss TE, Lee WR, Hunt MA, Hanlon AL, Peter RS, Hanks GE. Late GI and GU complications in the treatment of prostate cancer. Int J Radiat Oncol Biol Phys 37:3-11, 1997.

67. Azadzoi KM, Tarcan T, Siroky MB, Krane RJ. Atherosclerosis-induced chronic ischemia causes bladder fibrosis and non-compliance in the rabbit. J Urol 161: 1626-1635, 1999.

68. Andersen JT, Nordling J. Urinary incontinence after transvesical prostatectomy. Urol Int 33: 191-8, 1978.

69. Fitzpatrick JM, Gardina RA, Worth PHL. The evaluation of 68 patients with post-prostatectomy incontinence. Br J Urol 51: 552-5, 1979.

70. Leach GE, Yip CM, Donovan BJ. Post-prostatectomy incontinence: the influence of bladder dysfunction. J Urol 138: 574-8, 1987.

71. Khan Z, Mieza M, Starer P, Singh VK. Post-prostatectomy incontinence. Urology 38: 483-488, 1991.

72. Goluboff ET, Chang DT, Olsson CA, Kaplan SA. Urodynamics and postprostatectomy urinary incontinence: The initial Columbia experience. J Urol 153: 1034-7, 1995.

73. Chao R, Mayo ME. Incontinence after radical prostatectomy: detrusor or sphincter causes. J Urol 154:16-18, 1995.

74. Leach GE, Trockman B, Wong A, et al: Post-prostatectomy incontinence: urodynamic findings and treatment outcomes. J Urol 155:1256-1259, 1996.

75. Desautel MG, Kapoor R, Badlani GH. Sphincteric incontinence: the primary cause of post-prostatectomy incontinence in patients with prostate cancer. Neurourol Urodyn 1997;16:153-60, 1997.

76. Mebust WK, Holtgrewe HL. Current status of transurethral prostatectomy: a review of the AUA National Cooperative Study. World J Urol 6:194, 1989.

77. Catalona WJ, Basler WJ. Return of erections and urinary continence following nerve sparing radical retropubic prostatectomy. J. Urol 150:905-907, 1993.

78. Geary ES, Dendlinger TE, Freiha FS, Stamey TA. Incontinence and vesical neck strictures following radical perineal prostatectomy. Urology 45:1000, 1995.

79. Krane RJ. Urinary incontinence after treatment for localized prostate cancer. Mol Urol 4:279-286, 2000.

80. Kao TC, Cruess DF, Garmer D, et al: Multicenter patient self-reporting questionnaire on impotence, incontinence and stricture after radical prostatectomy. J Urol 163:858-864, 2000.

81. Gudziak MR, McGuire EJ, Gormley EA. Urodynamic assessment of urethral sphincter function in post-prostatectomy incontinence. J Urol 156: 1131-1134, 1996.

82. Steiner MS, Morton RA, Walsh PC. Impact of anatomical radical prostatectomy on urinary incontinence. J Urol 145: 512-515, 1991.

83. Steiner MS. Anatomic basis for the continence-preserving radical retropubic prostatectomy. Semin Urol Oncol 18:9-18, 2000.

84. Staskin DS, Vardi Y, Siroky MB. Post-prostatectomy continence in the Parkinsonian patient: The significance of poor voluntary sphincter control. J Urol 140:117-8, 1988.

85. Rainwater LM, Zincke H. Radical prostatectomy after radiation therapy for cancer of the prostate: feasibility and prognosis. J Urol 140:1455-9, 1988.

86. Lowe BA. Preservation of the anterior urethral ligamentous attachments in maintaining post-prostatectomy urinary continence: a comparative study. J Urol 158: 2137-2141, 1997.

87. Joseph AC, Chang MK. A bladder behavior clinic for post prostectomy patients. Urol Nursing 9: 15-9, 1989.

88. Meaglia JP, Joseph AC, Chang M, Schmidt JD. Post-prostatectomy urinary incontinence: response to behavioural training. J Urol 144: 674-6, 1990.

89. Hirakawa S, Hassouna M, Deleon R. ElHilali M. The role of combined pelvic floor stimulation and biofeedback in post-prostatectomy urinary incontinence. J Urol 149: 235A, 1993.

90. Salinas CJ, Virseda CM, Salomon MS, Bravo Derueda C, Aristizabal JM, Resel EL. Results of electrical stimulation in the treatment of post-prostatectomy urinary incontinence. Actas Urolog Espanol 20: 544-50, 1996.

91. Burgio K, Stutzman RE, Engel BT. Behavioral training for post-prostatectomy urinary incontinence. J Urol 141: 303-6, 1989.

92. Jackson J, Emerson L, Johnson B, Wilson J, Morales A. Biofeedback: a non-invasive treatment for incontinence after radical prostatectomy. Urol Nursing 16: 50-4, 1996.

93. Krauss DJ, Lilien OM. Transcutaneous electrical nerve stimulator for stress incontinence. J Urol 125: 790-3, 1981.

94. Laycock J, Jerwood D. Does pre-modulated interferential therapy cure genuine stress incontinence? Physiotherapy 78: 553-60, 1993.

95. Sand PK, Richardson DA, Staskin DR, Swift SE, Appell RA, Whitmore KE. Pelvic floor electrical stimulation in the treatment of genuine stress incontinence: a multicenter, placebo-controlled trial. Am J Obstet Gynecol 173: 72-9, 1995.

96. Jonler M, Madsen FA, Rhodes PR, Sall M, Messing EM, Bruskewitz RC. A prospective study of quantification of urinary incontinence and quality of life in patients undergoing radical retropubic prostatectomy. Urology 48: 433-40, 1996.

97. Donnellan SM, Duncan HJ, Macgregor A, Russell JM. Prospective assessment of incontinence after radical prostatectomy: objective and subjective analysis. J Urol 49: 225-30, 1996.

98. Stewart BH, Banowsky LH, Montague DK. Stress incontinence: conservative therapy with sympathomimetic drugs. J Urol 115:558-559, 1976.

99. Khanna OP. Disorders of micturition: neuropharmacologic basis and results of drug therapy. Urology 8: 316-28, 1976.

100. Theodorou C, Moutzouris G, Floratos D, Plastiras D, Katsifotis C, Mertziotis N. Incontinence after surgery for benign prostatic hypertrophy: the case for complex approach and treatment. Eur Urol 33: 370-375, 1998.

101. Iselin CE, Schmidlin F, Borst F, Rohner S, Graber P. Oxybutynin in the treatment of early detrusor instability after transurethral resection of the prostate. Br J Urol 79:915-919, 1997.

102.Stephenson TP, Farrar DJ. Urodynamic study of 15 patients with postmicturition dribble. Urology 9: 404-406, 1977.

103. Furuya S, Yokoyama E. [Urodynamic studies on postmicturition dribble] Hinyokika Kiyo 29:395-400, 1983.

104. Corcoran M, Smith G, Chisholm GD. Indications for investigation of post-micturition dribble in young adults. Br J Urol 59:222-223, 1987.

105. Furuya S, Ogura H, Tanaka M, Masumori N, Tsukamoto T. [Incidence of postmicturition dribble in adult males in their twenties through fifties]. Hinyokika Kiyo 43 :407-410, 1997.

106. Sommer P, Nielsen KK, Bauer T, Kristensen ES, Hermann GG, Steven K, Nordling J. Voiding patterns in men evaluated by a questionnaire survey 2. Br J Urol 1990: 65(2):155-160.

107. Paterson J, Pinnnock CB, Marshall VR. Pelvic floor exercises as a treatment for post-micturition dribble 1. Br J Urol 79:892-7, 1997.

108. Abrams PH, Farrar DJ, Turner-Warwick RT, Whiteside CG, Feneley RC. The results of prostatectomy: a symptomatic and urodynamic analysis of 152 patients. J Urol 121:640-642, 1979.

109. Steers WD, De Groat WC. Effect of bladder outlet obstruction on micturition reflex pathways in the rat. J Urol 140:864-871, 1988.

110. Sibley GN. The physiological response of the detrusor muscle to experimental bladder outflow obstruction in the pig. Brit J Urol 60:332-336, 1987.

111. Perlberg S, Caine M. Adrenergic response of bladder muscle in prostatic obstruction. Its relation to detrusor instability. Urology 20:524-527, 1982.

112. Abrams P, Kaplan S, Millard R. Tolterodine treatment is safe in men with bladder outlet obstruction (BOO) and symptomatic detrusor overactivity (DO). Neurourol Urodyn 20: 547, 2001.

113. Dahm TL, Ostri P, Kristensen JK, Walter S, Frimodt-Moller C, Rasmussen RB, Nohr M, Alexander N. Flavoxate treatment of micturition disorders accompanying benign prostatic hypertrophy: a double-blind placebo-controlled multicenter investigation. Urol Int 55:205-208, 1995.

114. Chapple CR, Smith D. The pathophysiological changes in the bladder obstructed by benign prostatic hyperplasia. Br J Urol 73:117-123, 1994.

115. Pressman MR, Figueroa WG, Kendrick-Mohamed J, Greenspon LW, Peterson DD. Nocturia. A rarely recognized symptom of sleep apnea and other occult sleep disorders. Arch Intern Med 156:545-550, 1996.

116. Reynard JM, Cannon A, Yang Q, Abrams P. A novel therapy for nocturnal polyuria: a double-blind randomized trial of frusemide against placebo. Br J Urol 81:215-218, 1998.

117. Asplund R, Sundberg B, Bengtsson P. Oral desmopressin for nocturnal polyuria in elderly subjects: a double-blind, placebo-controlled randomized exploratory study. BJU Int 83:591-595, 1999.

118. Miller M. Nocturnal polyuria in older people: pathophysiology and clinical implications. JAGS 48: 1321-9, 2000.

119. Weiss J, Blaivas JG, Abrams P, Mattiasson A, Robertson G, Van Kerrebroeck P, Walter S. Oral desmopressin (Minirin, DDAVP) in the treatment of nocturia in men. J Urol 165: Suppl 250, 2001.

120. Asplund R, Sundberg B, Bengtsson P. Desmopressin for the treatment of nocturnal polyuria in the elderly: a dose titration study. Br J Urol 82:642-646, 1998.

121. Cannon A, Carter PG, Mcconnell AA, Abrams P. Desmopressin in the treatment of nocturnal polyuria in the male. Br J Urol Int 84:20-24, 1999.

122. Bernstein SA, Williford SL. Intranasal desmopressin-associated hyponatremia: a case report and literature review. J Fam Pract 44:203-208, 1997.

123. Hunsballe JM, Rittig S, Pedersen EB, Olesen OV, Djurhuus JC. Single dose imipramine reduces nocturnal urine output in patients with nocturnal enuresis and nocturnal polyuria. J Urol 158:830-836, 1997.

124. Fantl JA, Wyman JF, McClish DK, Harkins SW, Elswick RK, Taylor JR, Hadley EC. Efficacy of bladder training in older women with urinary incontinence. JAMA 265: 609-13, 1991.

125. Cazzulani P, Panzarasa R, Luca C, Oliva D, Graziani G. Pharmacological studies on the mode of action of flavoxate. Arch Int Pharmacodyn Ther 268:301-312, 1984.

126. Sogbein SK, Awad SA. Behavioural treatment of urinary incontinence in geriatric patients. Can Med Assoc J 127:863-864, 1982.

127. Burgio KL, Stutzman RE, Engel BT. Behavioral training for post-prostatectomy urinary incontinence. J Urol 141: 303-306, 1989.

128. Schnelle JF, Traughber B, Sowell VA, Newman DR, Petrilli CO, Ory M. Prompted voiding treatment of urinary incontinence in nursing home patients. A behavior management approach for nursing home staff. J Am Geriatr Soc 37:1051-1057, 1989.

129. O'Donnell PD. Behavioral modification for institutionalized individuals with urinary incontinence. Urology 51: 40-42, 1998.

130. Remsburg RE, Palmer MH, Langford AM, Mendelson GF. Staff compliance with and ratings of effectiveness of a prompted voiding program in a long-term care facility. J Wound Ostomy Continence Nurs 26:261-269, 1999.

131. Godec C, Cass A, Ayala G. Bladder inhibition with functional electrical stimulation. Urology 6: 663-6, 1975.

132. Bo K, Berghams LCM. Nonpharmacologic treatments for overactive bladder – pelvic floor exercises. Urology 55 (Suppl 5A): 7-11, 2000.

133. Largo-Janssen TLM, Debruyne FMJ, Smits AJ, VanWeel C. Controlled trial of pelvic exercises in the treatment of urinary stress incontinence in general practice. Br J Gen Pract 41: 4445-9, 1991.

134. Bo K, Talseth T, Holme I. Single blind, randomised controlled trial of pelvic floor exercises, electrical stimulation, vaginal cones and no treatment in management of genuine stress incontinence in women. BMJ 318: 487-493, 1999.

135. Henalla S, Hutchins C, Robinson. Non-operative methods in the treatment of female stress incontinence of urine. J Obstet Gynecol 9: 222-5, 1989.

136. Clemens JQ, Nadler RB, Schaeffer AJ, Belani J, Albaugh J, Bushman W. Biofeedback, pelvic floor re-education, and bladder training for male chronic pelvic pain syndrome. Urology 56: 951-955, 2000.

137. McDowell BJ, Engberg S, Sereika S, Donovan N, Jubeck ME, Weber E, Engberg R. Effectiveness of behavioural therapy to treat incontinence in homebound older adults. J Am Geriatr Soc 47: 309-18, 1999.

138. Cottenden AM: Incontinence pads: clinical performance, design and technical properties. J Biomed Eng 10:506-514, 1988.

139. Kozakov S, Shats V. Cost-effectiveness of disposable diapers versus catheters in dependent patients. Harefuah 124:258-261, 1993.

140. Biesecker JE, Edlich JE, Thomas HL, Steers WD. Recent advances in absorbent products for the incontinent patient with burns. J Burn Care Rehabil 16:146-153, 1995.

141. Karlberg AT, Magnusson K. Rosin components identified in diapers. Contact Dermatitis 34:176-180, 1996.

142. Biesecker JE, Thomas HL, Thacker JG, Blackwood HS, Edlich RF. Innovations in the design and performance of underpads for patients with burns. J Burn Care Rehabil 16:66-73, 1995.

143. Rbown DS. Diapers and underpads, Part 1: Skin integrity outcomes. Ostomy Wound Manage 40:20-22, 24-26, 28, 1994.

144. Brown DS: Diapers and underpads, Part 2: Cost outcomes. Ostomy Wound Manage 40:34-36, 38, 40, 1994.

145. Leiby DM, Shanahan N. Clinical study: assessing the performance and skin environments of two reusable underpads. Ostomy Wound Manage 40:30-32, 34-37, 1994.

146. Boiko S. Diapers and diaper rashes. Dermatol Nurs 9:33-39, 43-46, 1997.

147. Hebel JR, Warren JW. The use of urethral, condom, and suprapubic catheters in aged nursing home patients. J Am Geriatr Soc 38:777-784, 1990.

148. Harmon CB, Connolly SM, Larson TR. Condom-related allergic contact dermatitis. J Urol 153:1227-1228, 1995.

149. Johnson ET. The condom catheter: Urinary tract infection and other complications. South Med J 76:579-582, 1983.

150. Perkash I, Kabalin JN, Lennon S, Wolfe V. Use of penile prostheses to maintain external condom catheter drainage in spinal cord injury patients. Paraplegia 30:327-332, 1992.

Committee 10 C

Conservative Treatment in Women

Chairman

P. D. Wilson (New Zealand)

Members

K. Bo (Norway),

J Hay-Smith (New Zealand),

I. Nygaard (USA),

D. Staskin (USA),

J. Wyman (USA),

Consultant

A. Bourcier (France)

CONTENTS

Conservative Treatment in Women

P. D. WILSON,

K. BO, J HAY-SMITH, I. NYGAARD, D. STASKIN, J. WYMAN,

A. BOURCIER

I. INTRODUCTION

Conservative treatment is any therapy that does not involve pharmacological or surgical intervention. In women, it includes principally, lifestyle interventions, physical therapies, bladder retraining (all encompassed by the term "behavioural therapy" used in some countries) and anti-incontinence devices. On the whole these treatments are simple, low cost remedies with a low risk of adverse effects and do not prejudice other subsequent treatment options. As the prevalence of female urinary incontinence is high, and with the current constraints on the healthcare economy, conservative treatment constitutes the principal form of management at primary care level. It is the first line of treatment for women with stress and/or urge incontinence. It is also indicated for those women for whom other treatments, in particular surgery, are inappropriate, for example, those who are unwilling to undergo or who are not medically fit for surgery, and those who plan future pregnancies (as these may adversely affect surgery). Other indications include patients awaiting or who wish to delay surgery and women whose symptoms are not serious enough for surgical intervention.

To date, however, only a relatively small number of objective clinical comparative studies of adequate patient numbers have been carried out to assess the effectiveness of conservative treatment of urinary incontinence. This chapter reviews the main types of conservative treatment particularly with regard to their effectiveness. This information assists the counselling of neurologically "normal" adult women regarding these treatment options (readers are directed to the chapters on men, children, the elderly and neuropathic patients for discussion on the effect of these conservative treatments in these specific groups). A systematic review of the literature has been carried out, comment made on the quality of all relevant studies identified, and recommendations on efficacy made on the best available level of evidence reviewed. ***(see Introduction to Management Chapters Reference .....)***

To date, only a relatively small number of objective clinical comparative studies with large numbers have been carried out to assess the effectiveness of conservative treatment.

II. LIFESTYLE INTERVENTIONS

1 BACKGROUND

Various lifestyle factors may play a role in either the pathogenesis of, or later, the resolution of incontinence. While published literature about lifestyle factors and incontinence is sparse, alterations in lifestyle are frequently recommended by health care professionals and lay people alike. However, to date, most studies about lifestyle report associations only and do not assess the actual effect of applying or deleting the behaviour in question on incontinence. Currently, only a relatively small number of randomized trials have been carried out to assess the effect of a specific lifestyle on incontinence. This section will examine the evidence for the association and use of lifestyle interventions in the management of female urinary incontinence. A summary of the search strategy and inclusion/exclusion criteria is given in Appendix 1.

Regarding lifestyle interventions, most studies to date have reported associations only and have not assessed the actual effect of applying or removing the behaviour in question.

2. WEIGHT LOSS

a) Quality of data

One randomized pilot study was found [1]. Two prospective cohort studies [2],[3] evaluated the effect of weight loss. Other study designs were cross-sectional, retrospective cohort, or case-control studies.

Sample sizes for the interventional trials were 12 [2], [3], and 10 [1]. Sample sizes for studies which assessed the association between obesity and incontinence, but in which no intervention was done, ranged from 193 [4] to 7949 [5]. The case control study had a sample size of 108 cases and 108 controls [6].

The outcome measure in all studies with the exception of Bump [2] and Subak [1] was subjective, as determined by a self-administered questionnaire. Bump also utilized objective measures including urodynamics, bladder diary and standardized fluid loss quantification test. Subak also utilized a 7-day urinary diary.

Follow-up periods for the interventional studies were one year after gastroplasty surgery [2] , 6 months after completion of weight reduction, either by means of low calorie liquid or reduced calorie solid diet [1] and not stated [3].

b) Results

Many researchers [7], [6], [8] [9], [4], [10], [11], [5] and [12] reported an association between increased weight, or increased body mass index, and urinary incontinence. This association held after controlling for age and parity. In one multivariate analysis, Brown [11] reported that the prevalence of daily incontinence increased by an odds ratio of 1.6 per 5 BMI (body mass index, kg/m2) units. In a multivariate analysis of a different population, Brown [5] found that the prevalence of at least weekly stress incontinence increased by 10% (OR 1.1) per 5 units BMI. Similarly, Foldspang [13] reported an odds ratio of 1.07 for incontinence prevalence per BMI unit, after controlling for other factors.

Two groups [2], [3] reported resolution of incontinence in the majority of cases after massive weight loss in morbidly obese women undergoing surgical weight reduction procedures. While obesity is commonly considered a risk for stress incontinence, in Bump's [2] study, women with urge incontinence were as likely to experience post-operative continence as women with stress incontinence. In Subak's [1] pilot study of 10 women, all six of the women achieving a weight loss of at least 5% had at least a 50% reduction in incontinent episodes compared to one out of the four women with <5% weight loss.

In a cross-sectional study of 1800 `Swedish women [14], 15% incontinent women reported at least a 5 kg weight loss in the preceding 5 years, compared to 11% of continent women (p=.05). This may be secondary to intentional weight loss as a treatment for urinary incontinence, rather than some effect of weight loss itself.

c) Summary

Obesity is an independent risk factor for the prevalence of urinary incontinence. Massive weight loss significantly decreases incontinence in morbidly obese women. Preliminary evidence suggests that moderate weight loss may also result in decreased incontinence. (Level of Evidence: 1/2).

d) Recommendation

Weight loss is an acceptable treatment option for morbidly obese women. At this time, there is scant information on whether weight loss resolves incontinence in women who are moderately obese. At least one such larger trial is now ongoing. Based on the current evidence, maintaining normal weight through adulthood may be an important factor in the prevention of the development of incontinence. Given the high prevalence of both incontinence and obesity in women, the dual issues of weight loss and prevention of weight gain should receive high research priority.

GRADE OF RECOMMENDATION: B

Obesity is an independent risk factor for urinary incontinence. There is level 2 evidence that weight loss in morbidly obese women decreases incontinence, and scant preliminary level 1 evidence that moderately obese women who lose weight have less incontinence than those who do not.

3. Physical forces (exercise, work)

a) Quality of data

No randomized trials exist in which incontinence prevalence is compared between subjects assigned to heavy work or high impact activity versus sedentary activities. One case-control study compared the incidence of surgery for incontinence and/or prolapse [15], while a second compared nulliparous women with and without stress incontinence symptoms [16]. Bø [17] and Nygaard [18] evaluated the difference in incontinence prevalence between women engaged in high versus low impact activities. Davis [19] described a series of women who became incontinent after parachute jumping. In a retrospective cohort study, Nygaard [18] compared incontinence prevalence in high-impact versus low-impact former athletes. Bø [20] compared incontinence prevalence between Norwegian Olympians and controls.

Sample sizes range from 144 [18] to 305 [17] for the cohort studies. One case series had nine subjects [19]. The population-based case control study compared 28,619 cases with 1,652,533 controls. The recent study by Bø [17] compared 572 athletes, ages 15-39 years, with 574 controls.

b) Results

Minimal stress incontinence is common in young exercising women [21], [17], [16]. College athletes participating in high impact activities are more likely to report the symptom of stress incontinence during exercise than those participating in low impact exercise [18]. Bø [20] found no difference in incontinence prevalence between elite athletes and controls. However, the prevalence of stress and urge incontinence symptoms was higher in athletes who had a diagnosed eating disorder than those without such a diagnosis. There is little available information on whether strenuous exercise or activity causes the condition of incontinence later in life. In a study which questioned women who were Olympians approximately 25 years ago, those who competed in gymnastics or track and field were not more likely to currently report daily or weekly incontinence than Olympians who competed in swimming [22] Nygaard 1997. Certain provocations may cause stress incontinence: a recent report described nine nulliparous infantry trainees who developed stress incontinence and pelvic floor defects for the first time during airborne training, which included parachute jumping [19]. The precise number of total trainees is unknown but is estimated to be approximately 500.

Surprisingly little information is available on the relationship between stressors in the workplace and urinary incontinence. Danish nursing assistants, who are exposed to frequent heavy lifting, were 1.6 fold more likely to undergo surgery for genital prolapse and/or incontinence than women in the general population; the study did not control for parity nor weight [15].

c) Summary

Strenuous exercise is likely to unmask the symptom of stress incontinence during the provocation. There is no evidence that strenuous exercise causes the condition of incontinence. In a small number of women without other known risk factors, extreme provocations such as parachute jumping may cause incontinence. There is scant uncontrolled data that suggests that women engaged in occupations with heavy lifting may be predisposed to genital prolapse and/or incontinence. (Level of Evidence: 2/3). The data is insufficient to draw any firm conclusions. In spite of the fact that healthcare professionals commonly advise restricting exercise and heavy lifting following incontinence or prolapse surgery, there is no published evidence that this improves surgical outcome.

d) Recommendations

Given the large proportion of women who are employed in various occupations that require heavy lifting and the paucity of scientific data about the association of such exertions and incontinence, this association should be investigated further. Specifically, research must establish whether heavy exertion is an etiologic factor in the pathogenesis of incontinence, and whether changing exertions can alleviate established incontinence.

GRADE OF RECOMMENDATION: C

There is scant level 2 and 3 evidence that suggests that active women may be more likely to report incontinence than sedentary women, and that heavy occupational work may be associated with pelvic organ prolapse and urinary incontinence. However, there are no trials that assess the role activity plays in treating urinary incontinence.

4. Smoking

a) Quality of data

One case-control study compared incontinent smokers with incontinent non-smokers [23], while a second compared smoking behaviour between continent and incontinent women [24]. Three large cross sectional studies evaluated multiple risk factors for incontinence, including smoking [11], [25], [26]. In vitro studies assessed the effects of nicotine on bladder muscle contraction.

Sample sizes were 189 [23], 160 [24], 7949 [11], 7338 [26], and 1761 [25].

b) Results

Smokers were more likely to report incontinence than non-smokers in two studies [24], [26], but not in two others [11],[25]. After adjusting for age, parity, type of delivery, and pre-pregnancy BMI, smokers had a 1.3 fold higher risk (95% CI 1.0-1.8) of reporting incontinence at 16 weeks gestation than non-smokers [26]. Incontinent smokers were found to have stronger urethral sphincters and lower overall risk profiles than incontinent non-smokers [23] therefore, it was proposed that more violent coughing promotes anatomic defects which allow incontinence. In potential support of nicotine as a risk factor for incontinence, Hisayama and Koley [27] found that nicotine produces phasic contraction of isolated bladder muscle probes in vitro. However, Milson [28] reported an apparent paradoxical local estrogenic effect of nicotine on the vagina, resulting in a decrease in vaginal pH and an increase in lactobacilli.

c) Summary

The data relating to the association of smoking and

incontinence is conflicting. Smokers may have a different mechanism causing their incontinence than non-smokers (Level of Evidence 3/4). No data has been reported examining whether smoking cessation resolves incontinence.

d) Recommendations

Further prospective studies are needed to determine whether smoking cessation prevents the onset, or promotes the resolution, of incontinence.

GRADE OF RECOMMENDATION: C.

No data has been reported examining whether smoking cessation resolves incontinence.

5. Dietary factors

a) Quality of evidence

Preliminary results (in abstract form) of a randomized trial on the effects of caffeine upon frequency, urgency and urge incontinence are available [29]. One randomized trial has assessed the efficacy of fluid management in the treatment of incontinence. No randomized trial was identified that addressed dietary changes.

One study compared women with detrusor overactivity with continent women who received caffeine tablets [30], while another compared caffeine intake between women with detrusor overactivity and those without [31]. The effect of decreasing caffeine intake in a small cohort of incontinent women was examined in a prospective fashion [32]. One large epidemiologic trial analyzed the effect of coffee drinking in a multivariate fashion [11].

Sample sizes were: 26 [29] (target sample size is 90 subjects); 30 [30], 128 [33], 126 [34], 7949 [11], 6037 [35], 159 [31], and 34 [32].

b) Results

- **Caffeine:**

Following caffeine intake, women with detrusor overactivity had increased detrusor pressure on bladder filling, while continent women had no such abnormality [30]. In a population of 259 consecutive women presenting for urodynamics [31], 131 women with detrusor overactivity had a significantly higher mean caffeine intake (484 +/- 123 mg/day) than women without this diagnosis (194 +/- 123 mg/day). This association persisted after controlling for age and smoking. In 34 women with symptoms of urinary incontinence (mostly mixed) who decreased caffeine intake (from 900 mg/day to 480 mg/day), episodes of daily urine loss also decreased (from 2.33 to 1.0 per day) [32]. In the initial group of adults enrolled in the randomized trial [29] subjects who reduced caffeine intake to <100 mg per day decreased daily incontinent episodes by 74% compared to a 32% reduction in those who continued normal caffeine intake during the one-month study period. No difference was seen in urgency or number of voids between the groups (though, as noted, the final sample size has not yet been achieved). In a multivariate analysis, [11] found no association between coffee drinking or alcohol drinking and daily incontinence.

- **Decrease fluid intake:**

In a geriatric population, there was a strong relationship between evening fluid intake, nocturia, and nocturnal voided volume; this relationship was weaker for diurnal intake and voiding [33]. In incontinent women over age 55 years, there was a modest positive relationship between fluid intake and severity of incontinence in women with stress incontinence; fluid intake accounted for 14% of the explained variability in number of incontinent episodes [34]. No such correlation was found in women with detrusor overactivity. In a randomized trial [36], 32 women were assigned to one of three groups: increase fluid intake by 500 cc over baseline, decrease by same amount, or maintain baseline level. While non-adherence to the protocol made results difficult to interpret, the authors reported that 20 women who had fewer incontinent episodes at the end of the trial attributed this to drinking more fluids.

- **Alcohol:**

After adjusting for age and gender, no association was found between urinary incontinence and consumption of alcohol [35].

- **Diet:**

Anecdotal evidence suggests that eliminating dietary factors such as artificial sweeteners and certain foods may play a role in continence.

c) Summary

Fluid intake plays a minor, if any, role in the pathogenesis of incontinence. The data on caffeine intake and incontinence are conflicting. While large cross-sectional surveys indicate no association, small clinical trials do suggest that decreasing caffeine intake improves continence (Level of Evidence: 2/3).

d) Recommendations

Given the fact that decreasing fluids may lead to urinary tract infections, constipation, or dehydration, this intervention should be reserved for patients with abnormally high fluid intakes.

Caffeine consumption is pervasive in many societies and may play a role in exacerbating urinary incontinence. Larger randomized trials to assess the effect of caffeine and other dietary factors are feasible and important.

GRADE OF RECOMMENDATION: B

Fluid intake would appear to play a minor, if any, role in the pathogenesis of incontinence.

Level 2 and 3 evidence is conflicting on whether caffeine intake is associated with urinary incontinence. There is scant level 1 evidence that decreasing caffeine improves continence.

6. CONSTIPATION

a) Quality of data

No published trials were found which assess the effect of regulating bowel function on incontinence. An observational study compared the self-report of straining as a child with urogynecologic symptoms as an adult. Population-based studies assessed multiple risk factors for incontinence [37], [38].

Sample sizes range from 73 for the observational study [39] to 213 in a study correlating the surrogate measures of perineal descent and pudendal neuropathy [40] to 1154 and 1051 in the population-based studies [37], [38] respectively.

b) Results

In a small observational study, 30% of women with stress incontinence and 61% of women with uterovaginal prolapse reported straining at stool as a young adult, compared to 4% of women without urogynecologic symptoms [39]. In a large population-based study of 1154 women over age 60 years, those with urinary incontinence were slightly more likely to report constipation than those who were continent of urine (31.6% vs 24.7%) [37]. After adjusting for demographic and obstetric confounders, women who reported straining at stool were 1.9 times (95% CI 1.3, 2.6) and 1.7 times (95% CI 1.2, 2.4) more likely to report stress incontinence and urgency, respectively [38]. There appears to be an association between straining and pudendal nerve function. The mean pudendal nerve terminal motor latency (PNTML) increased after straining, correlated with the amount of descent, and returned to resting by four minutes after a strain [41]. Others found evidence of pudendal neuropathy in only 25% of women with abnormal perineal descent; in this large group of patients with defecating dysfunction no relationship was seen between neuropathy and pelvic descent, leading to the conclusion that pelvic descent and neuropathy may be two independent finding [40].

c) Summary

There is fair data to suggest that chronic straining may be a risk factor for the development of incontinence. (Level of Evidence:2/3). There are no intervention trials that address the effect of resolving constipation on urinary incontinence.

d) Recommendations.

Further research is needed to delineate the role of straining in the pathogenesis of incontinence. If the association holds, public education, particularly of parents and pediatricians, is needed to make an impact on the common problem of straining in children.

GRADE OF RECOMMENDATION: C

Chronic straining may be a risk factor for pelvic organ prolapse and urinary incontinence

(level 2 and 3 evidence). No intervention trials have examined the impact of resolving constipation on urinary incontinence.

7. OTHER

a) Quality of data

One study rigorously assessed urine loss during various postural changes (crossing legs and bending forward) [42]. No study has evaluated whether postural changes are a satisfactory form of treatment outside of the laboratory setting. Timed voiding and relaxation techniques, particularly for urge incontinence, are discussed in (Chapter…). There are many other lifestyle interventions suggested either by health care professionals or the lay press for the treatment of urinary incontinence, including reducing emotional stress, wearing non-restrictive clothing, utilising a bedside commode, decreasing lower extremity edema, treating allergies and coughs, wearing cotton underwear, and increasing sexual activity. These interventions are, however, all anecdotal in nature.

b) Results

Postural changes: Urine loss during provocations can be significantly decreased by crossing the legs or by crossing the legs and bending forward [42].

c) Summary

There is no scientific evidence about whether other lifestyle changes except for some postural changes, affects either the treatment of, or the prevention of, urinary incontinence. (Level of Evidence 2/3).

d) Recommendations

As various lifestyle interventions are recommended by

physicians, studies evaluating the effect of implementing these factors on incontinence are warranted. While some lifestyle changes may prove beneficial for individual patients, it is unlikely that manipulating these factors will have a major effect on the overall incontinence problem.

GRADE OF RECOMMENDATION: C.

There is level 2 evidence that postural changes may decrease urinary incontinence. There is no evidence whether other such lifestyle changes decrease urinary incontinence.

III. PHYSICAL THERAPIES

1. Introduction

Graded muscle training alone, or in combination with other physical adjuncts such as biofeedback, electrical stimulation, and vaginal cones, is used to rehabilitate and strengthen the pelvic floor muscles. The physical therapy (physiotherapy) profession has a long tradition in the use of these physical agents for the prevention and treatment of incontinence [43],[44].

This section will examine the evidence for the use of pelvic floor muscle training with and without adjuncts, electrical stimulation and vaginal cones in the prevention and management of adult female stress, urge and mixed urinary incontinence, and makes recommendations for effective treatment based on the findings. In order to present the best possible evidence and in an attempt to differentiate specific treatment effects from a host of other variables the review is restricted to the findings from systematic reviews of randomised clinical trials (RCTs), or the findings of RCTs where systematic reviews were not available. A summary of the search strategy used to identify systematic review and randomised trial reports is given in Appendix 1.

As the focus of this section was to present the evidence on the effect of physical therapies in neurologically 'normal' adult women, readers are directed to the chapters on men, children, the elderly, and neuropathic disorders for discussion on the effects of physical therapies in these specific groups.

2. Pelvic Floor Muscle Training (PFMT)

a) Background

In 1948 Arnold Kegel reported on the successful treatment of 64 cases of female urodynamic stress incontinence using pelvic floor muscle exercises, with a perineometer for resistance and biofeedback [45]. The biological rationale for the use of PFMT in the management of stress incontinence is based on the reasoning that a strong and fast pelvic floor muscle (PFM) contraction will clamp the urethra, increasing the urethral pressure and preventing leakage during an abrupt increase in intra-abdominal pressure[46]. DeLancey [47] has also suggested that an effective contraction of the PFM may press the urethra against the pubic symphysis, creating a mechanical pressure rise. The timing of the pelvic floor muscle contraction may also be important. It has been suggested that a well-timed, fast and strong PFM contraction may prevent urethral descent during abrupt intra-abdominal pressure rise [48] and there is some evidence that the PFM "reflex" contraction is a feed-forward loop, as it may precede the bladder pressure rise by 200-250 milliseconds [49].

Miller et al [50] have demonstrated that voluntary contraction of the PFM before or during cough can effectively prevent urinary leakage after only a week of training. However in healthy continent women, co-contraction of the pelvic floor muscles before or during physical exertion is an automatic response and does not require conscious effort. Pre-contractions may be possible before single bouts of physical exertion but it is unlikely that women would be able to voluntarily contract the PFM throughout prolonged activities such as running or dancing. Therefore one aim of PFMT is to build the muscles to reach the automatic response level.

The objective of PFMT in the management of stress incontinence is usually to improve strength and/or timing of the pelvic floor muscle contraction. Regular strength training increases the number of activated motor units, frequency of excitation (neural adaptation) and muscle volume (hypertrophy) [51], [52]. However, muscle fiber hypertrophy is a slow process and begins only after regular and intense strength training for more than eight weeks [52]. With increased resistance, training hypertrophy may continue for years and a prolonged training period is needed to increase muscle volume.

The use of PFMT (or voluntary pelvic floor muscle contraction to control urge as part of a bladder training program) in the management of urge incontinence has a less substantial biological rationale. Godec et al demonstrated reflex inhibition of the detrusor muscle with an electrically stimulated contraction of the PFM. Godec et al [53], De Groat [54] and Morrison [55] have both shown inhibition of the detrusor by unconscious contraction of the PFM experimentally. It has been suggested that reflex inhibition of detrusor contractions may accompany repeated voluntary pelvic floor muscle contraction or maximum contractions [44], [48], [56].

For the purposes of this review PFMT was defined as any program of repeated voluntary pelvic floor muscle contraction taught by a health care professional. This definition includes variations in the purpose of PFMT (e.g. PFMT for strengthening or urge suppression), the teaching of PFMT (e.g. individual or group teaching), the types of contractions (e.g. quick or held), and the number of contractions per day, etc.

Pelvic floor muscle training has been used in preference to other previously used terms such as Kegel's exercises, pelvic exercises, pelvic floor exercises and pelvic floor muscle exercises. The use of the term Kegel's exercises no longer seems appropriate as current practice is very different to the program originally suggested by Kegel in 1948 [45]. Descriptions that fail to include the word muscle seem equally inappropriate, as it is the muscular component of the pelvic floor that is the focus of any exercise program. Any term used should also state that the pelvic floor muscles, not the pelvic muscles in general, are the targets of the intervention. Further, the authors of this sub-chapter suggest that the use of the term training is more appropriate than exercise as exercise is commonly interpreted as one episode of training whereas training means repeated exercise over time. The effect of training is dependent on four factors; the type of exercise, frequency, intensity and duration of the training period [57]. The dose response curve for training suggests that there is a baseline (or floor) below which training is ineffective, and an upper limit (or ceiling) above which over-training syndromes are created [58]. The use of the term pelvic floor muscle training (PFMT) is proposed and used throughout.

This section reviews the evidence comparing PFMT with no treatment, placebo treatments, or any other single intervention (e.g. electrical stimulation, surgery, medication, etc). It also includes comparisons of different PFMT programs although PFMT with or without biofeedback or intravaginal resistance is reviewed separately in this section. There are four published systematic reviews pertinent to this section [59], [60], [61], [62]. The Cochrane review by Hay-Smith et al [62] was the most up to date of these reviews, and included meta-analysis of trial data where appropriate. Therefore the following summary of results and the recommendations are based upon the rigorous review of trials of PFMT identified by Hay-Smith et al. Readers are encouraged to seek out the full report for details of the method, results and further discussion.

b) Quality of data

A brief summary of the quality of the trials included in the systematic review by Hay-Smith et al is presented below [62]. It is worth noting that there is one further trial awaiting assessment for possible inclusion in the Cochrane Review of PFMT [56] that is relevant to this section. Readers may wish to locate this most recent trial to determine if the results are likely to alter the findings given below.

• Random allocation concealment

Of the 31 trials contributing to this section, random allocation concealment was adequate in five [63], [64], [65], [7], [66] and probably inadequate in two [67], [68], and in the remainder it was either unclear if allocation was adequately concealed, or the authors stated simply that allocation was at "random".

• Masking of participants and assessors

As in any physical intervention it can be difficult or impossible to adequately mask participants to the intervention. Only one trial [69], a comparison of PFMT and placebo PFMT, attempted this. Masking of outcome assessors was clearly stated in nine of the 31 trials [64], [70], [71], [68], [50], [72], [73],[69], [66]. Two trials stated that outcome assessors were not masked [74], [75] and in the remainder this was not reported.

• Sample size and power calculation

In six trials the size of the study population was based on a power calculation [63], [64], [67], [22], [66], [75]. Six trials randomised more than 50 women to each comparison group [70], [68], [73], [76], [7], [75], in 13 trials the group sizes ranged from 25 to 49 [63], [64], [71], [65], [67], [77], [78], [79], [80], [72], [81], [66], [82], and the remaining 19 trials allocated less than 25 women to each comparison group.

• Losses to follow up

Eight studies had no dropouts or losses to follow up [83], [84], [85], [79], [50], [69], [86], [82]. The proportion of dropouts was less than 10% in six trials [63], [71], [78], [68], [73], [81] and in the remainder it varied from 12% [64], [75] to 37% [66]. Only four trials clearly reported some or all of their analysis on the basis of intention to treat principles [64], [70], [65], [72].

• Post treatment follow-up

Nine of the 31 trials followed women up beyond the post treatment evaluation [78], [71], [87], [72], [66], [60], [74], [83], [79]. Length of follow up ranged from three months [71] to five years [87], [60]. Overall, data from long-term follow up was sparse and difficult to interpret. Often trial participants for whom treatment had not been successful had gone on to receive alternative treatment. Therefore follow up data were usually presented for all women participating in the study rather than by original group allocation (e.g. [72]), or only one of the comparison groups was followed up (e.g. [63]).

c) Results

• PFMT programs

There was considerable variation in the PFMT programs used in the included trials. The length of the training period was between six weeks [85] and six months

[63], [83], [76]. Some programs included hourly contractions [78]; others used sets of contractions repeated three times per day [63]. The number of contractions per day ranged from 36 [63] to 200 [71], and the length of hold from three [71] to 40 seconds [83]. One program specifically included strength and endurance training elements [83]. Individual teaching, training and supervision was a feature of some programs [71], [78], [68] whilst group teaching was used in others [79], [73], and two trials used individual teaching followed by group exercise [63], [64]. In general, many PFMT programs were poorly reported and other advice/education given concurrently was rarely detailed.

In 1995 Bø reviewed PFMT programs reported in the literature and compared these with existing evidence on the physiology of strength training in 'normal' voluntary muscle [48]. Few studies had used programs that reflected current understanding of effective strength training. Similarly, the current review found considerable variability in the content of PFMT programs, which suggests there is still little knowledge, or consensus between practitioners, about what constitutes an effective PFMT program. While the following paragraphs make recommendations for PFMT based on the exercise science literature these should be viewed with caution. The extrapolation is based on the equivalence between the PFM of women with urinary incontinence and 'normal' skeletal muscle. As there is a growing body of research that documents nerve, muscle and connective tissue changes in women with urinary incontinence this equivalence is in doubt. However, as some women (e.g. nulliparous women) experience urinary leakage without any obvious signs of this damage it is possible that in these women the muscles are 'untrained' rather than damaged. Similar training principles are used for untrained, damaged and healthy muscles, with training adapted to the needs and tolerance of each individual.

Success of PFMT will depend on ability to perform a correct voluntary pelvic floor muscle contraction initially [88], [89], [45]. Therefore it seems appropriate that all women should be taught how to perform a voluntary pelvic floor muscle contraction by a person with skills in the assessment and training of pelvic floor muscles, and examined to check that a correct contraction is taking place, before PFMT is undertaken.

Prior to PFMT, a woman should be assessed by a person with skills in the assessment and training of pelvic floor muscles to ensure that a correct voluntary pelvic floor muscle contraction is being performed, and to determine if any facilitation techniques or adaptations are required to the recommended training program.

Effective strength training relies on specificity (i.e. training reflects the functional activity of the muscle) and overload (i.e. increasing resistance to, or duration of, muscle contraction). To encourage specificity Bø suggests that co-contraction of other related muscles (e.g. glutei, hip adductors) should be minimized so that the PFM are targeted and contraction of the PFM is not masked by strong contractions of other muscle groups [48] . Research suggests that it is not possible to maximally contract the PFM without co-contraction of Transversus Abdominus [63], [90]. Contraction of Transversus Abdominus can be observed as a tucking in or bracing of the lower abdominal wall with no movement of the pelvis, and should be allowed in order to facilitate maximum contractions. In addition, PFMT in a variety of 'functional' positions such as sitting and standing, rather than the traditional supine lying [63], and the use of voluntary pelvic floor muscle contraction prior to anticipated rises in intra-abdominal pressure (e.g. with cough or sneeze) are more recent additions to many PFMT programs [83], [91], [50].

Effective overload strategies are likely to include close to maximal voluntary pelvic floor muscle contraction, increased length of contraction, increased number of contractions and reduced rest periods. Strength training theory suggests that near maximal contractions are the most significant factor in increasing strength [92] and ideally contractions need to be sustained for 6-8 seconds to recruit an increasing number of motor units and fast twitch fibers [93]. There is a fixed recruitment pattern during voluntary contraction. Slow twitch (ST) fibers are recruited first but with increasing resistance more and more fast twitch fibers (FT) are recruited. Fast twitch fibers possess low oxidative capacities and fatigue easily. However, they are needed during rapid movements and close to maximal contractions. All types of muscle fibers will hypertrophy in response to strength training but FT fibers have a greater potential for hypertrophy than ST fibers. As the strongest stimulation for strength increase is the intensity of the contraction (as close to maximum as possible), the main objective in training is to recruit as many motor units as possible, regardless whether they are ST or FT fibers. To improve the potential for strength gains, PFMT should be conducted over sufficient time that both neural adaptation and hypertrophy can occur. Thus, training periods of at least 20 weeks have been recommended (American College of Sports Medicine 1992).

Extrapolation from research in other skeletal muscle groups indicates that PFMT should include three sets of eight to 12 slow velocity maximal contractions, three to four times a week [52] and training needs to be continued for 15 to 20 weeks (American College of Sports Medicine 1992). However, indiscriminate use of this protocol may have adverse effects due to muscle fatigue unless women are individually assessed to determine the strength/weakness of their PFM. Depending on assessment findings of fatigability a modified PFMT program may be needed initially, progressing to meet the above recommendations. The need for modification relates to the dose response curve for training. For example, a woman who is able to perform only four near maximal contractions will begin her training at this level. To recommend more than four near maximal contractions at the outset may result in problems associated with over training. Alternatively, an insufficient training dose inhibits progression and fails to maximize training effect.

There is a marked lack of consistency in PFMT programs used in clinical practice. On the basis of extrapolation from exercise science literature, PFMT programs should include three sets of eight to 12 slow velocity maximal voluntary pelvic floor muscle contraction sustained for six to eight seconds each, performed three to four times a week and continued for at least 15 to 20 weeks.

• PFMT versus no treatment

Seven trials, that randomised a total of 679 women, have compared PFMT with no treatment [71], [78], [84], [50], [73] or a control treatment (i.e. Bø et al offered women use of the Continence Guard and Lagro–Janssen et al provided advice on absorbent products) [64], [68]. Three trials included women with only urodynamic stress incontinence [64], [78], [84]. One trial included women with urodynamic diagnoses of urodynamic stress or mixed incontinence [71]. The three remaining trials included women with symptoms of urine leakage [68], [50], [73].

The meta-analysis by Hay-Smith et al [62] found that PFMT was significantly better than no treatment for self reported cure, self reported cure/improvement and leakage episodes in 24 hours in women with stress and/or mixed incontinence. A sensitivity analysis in women with stress incontinence alone (symptom or urodynamic) found that PFMT was significantly better than no treatment for the rate of self reported cure/improvement. The review also found that women in PFMT groups also had consistently greater reductions in urine leakage on short pad test, and greater improvements in measures of pelvic floor muscle activity [62]. It also suggested that self-reported cure/improvement was a more common outcome of PFMT than cure alone. Women in the PFMT groups were 7.25 times more likely to be cured than women in no treatment groups (RR 7.25, 95% CI 1.99, 26.49), and this increased to 23.04 times for combined cure/improvement (RR 23.04, 95% CI 7.56, 70.22).

Follow up data was reported by three trials, at three months [71], nine months [78]) and five years [87]. The most complete and best quality data comes from the follow up study undertaken by Lagro-Janssen and Van Weel [87]. Data from 88 of the original sample of 110 women was reported. The number of continent women (25%) was the same after five years but a significant number of women reported their condition had worsened. Women with urge or mixed incontinence were less likely to be satisfied with the outcome of treatment at five years, although two thirds of all the women followed up remained satisfied with the outcome of treatment and did not want any further intervention. Nearly half (43%) of the women who had received PFMT were no longer training at all. For women with stress incontinence continued training was the only significant predictor of outcome at five years.

The PFMT programs used in these seven trials varied considerably and yet Hay-Smith et al [62] reported a consistent effect of PFMT. This raises a number of questions about which element, or combinations of elements, of training are most effective. The recent trial by Miller et al [50] suggests for example that simply teaching a correct voluntary pelvic floor muscle contraction and the use of this contraction prior to an anticipated change in intra-abdominal pressure (i.e. "The Knack") may be one element of an effective training program. Anecdotally, contact with a health care professional with special training in continence management includes considerable advice/education on the anatomy and physiology of the bladder and pelvic floor, lifestyle advice, and information about good bladder habits. These elements of intervention are rarely reported and their effect has not been investigated. Where PFMT has been combined with other lifestyle and behavioural interventions it is difficult to determine if the effect of PFMT in comparison to 'no treatment' reflects the effect of PFMT, the effect of the advice/education, or a combination of both. Other issues worthy of consideration include the expertise of the person providing the PFMT, and the 'intensity' of the PFMT program. There is some evidence that the latter is a factor (see below – "*Standard versus intensive PFMT*").

There is level 1 evidence that PFMT is better than no treatment for women with stress and/or mixed incontinence.

• PFMT versus placebo treatments

Three trials, that randomised a total of 208 women, compared PFMT with placebo treatments. The placebos were placebo PFMT [69], placebo medication [70], and placebo electrical stimulation [85]. The trials included women with symptoms of stress incontinence only [69], urodynamic stress incontinence [85]) and women with detrusor overactivity with or without urodynamic stress incontinence [70]. The meta-analysis by Hay-Smith et al [62] found a consistent effect, namely that PFMT was significantly better than placebo treatment for self reported cure, self-reported cure/improvement and leakage episodes in 24 hours. There were not sufficient data available to make sensitivity analysis by diagnostic group appropriate.

There is level 1 evidence that PFMT is better than placebo treatments for women with stress, urge or mixed incontinence.

• 'Standard' versus 'intensive' PFMT programs

Six trials, that randomised 1080 women, compared 'standard' versus 'intensive' PFMT programs. Two trials compared a standard home based training program with the same program reinforced on audiotape in women with urodynamic stress incontinence [67] and women with urodynamic stress incontinence, detrusor overactivity and mixed incontinence [72]. Two trials, in postnatal women with urine leakage, compared standard postnatal care with an individualized postnatal PFMT program [7], [66]. The two remaining trials, both in women with urodynamic stress incontinence, compared home-based training with a program that included more contact with a physiotherapist [63], [82]. One of the six trials in this comparison did not report any urinary outcomes [67] and another did not present the data by group allocation but by diagnosis [72]. Consequently neither trial contributed data to the meta-analysis. Hay-Smith et al [62] found that 'intensive' training was significantly better than 'standard' training for self reported cure and self reported cure/improvement in women with postnatal urine leakage and women with stress incontinence. A sensitivity analysis in women with urodynamic stress incontinence also found that 'intensive' PFMT was significantly better than 'standard' training for self reported cure. The findings from short pad tests and measures of pelvic floor muscle activity did not consistently favour one group over the other. For both these outcomes Bø et al [63] reported significantly greater improvement in the 'intensive' therapy group versus the 'standard' treatment group, whereas Wong et al [82] and Wilson and Herbison [66] reported improvements in both standard and intensive groups with no significant differences between the groups.

Follow up beyond post treatment assessment was reported by three trials, at six months [72], 15 to 35 months [66] and five years [63]. There were difficulties interpreting the data from the two former trials, and the latter trial followed up only the women from the 'intensive' training group. Fourteen of the 23 women followed up by Bø & Talseth continued to be satisfied with the outcome of PFMT and did not want any further treatment and 70% were continuing to train at least once a week five years after supervised training ceased [60].

While not strictly a comparison of 'standard' and 'intensive' PFMT a single trial comparing inpatient and outpatient conservative management of urinary incontinence in women was found [94]. Management included PFMT, bladder training, advice etc and the researchers found symptoms of both groups significantly improved with no clear benefit of inpatient over outpatient treatment. Ramsay et al [94] concluded outpatient management was the more cost-effective option.

There is level 1 evidence to suggest that 'intensive' PFMT is better than 'standard' training programs for women with stress incontinence, and postnatal women with symptoms of urine leakage.

• PFMT versus electrical stimulation (ES)

Hay-Smith et al combined data from eight trials, in 295 women with urodynamic stress incontinence that compared PFMT and electrical stimulation [62]. Interferential therapy was used in three trials [78], [95], [74], four trials used some other form of pulsed alternating current [64], [83], [86], [96], and in one trial the type of stimulation was not specified [85].

However the clinical heterogeneity (i.e. considerable variation in the types of electrical stimulation used, and the stimulation protocols) made it difficult to combine the findings of these studies in a meaningful way. Hay-Smith et al [62] did not find any significant differences between PFMT and electrical stimulation groups for self reported cure although this comparison was extremely close to favouring PFMT. Similarly rates of self reported cure/improvement was not significantly different between the groups, However when the data from the two trials [64], [83] that compared PFMT with long term intravaginal stimulation in women with stress incontinence were combined this was statistically in favour of PFMT for self reported cure/improvement. The findings from a variety of pad tests were not consistent.

Three trials reported follow up beyond post treatment evaluation, at nine months [78], approximately two years [74] and four years [83]. The most complete and best quality data comes from the study by Hahn et al [83] who followed up 19 of the 20 women who participated in the original trial. Five had incontinence surgery, four were further improved, eight were unchanged and two had recurrent symptoms. Three women were not doing any PFMT, six were training "now and then", and five were doing PFMT "regularly".

Due to the variation in electrical stimulation types and protocols tested in the existing trials it was difficult to combine the findings in a meaningful way. At present there is insufficient evidence of the effect of PFMT versus electrical stimulation in women with stress incontinence.

• PFMT versus weighted vaginal cones

PFMT and vaginal cones were compared in seven trials that randomised a total of 539 women. Five trials included women with urodynamic stress incontinence [64], [65], [77], [97], [81], one trial included women with symptoms of stress incontinence only [80] and one trial was in postnatal women with symptoms of urine leakage [66]. Hay-Smith et al [62] found that women with urodynamic stress incontinence had significantly fewer leakage episodes in 24 hours after PFMT than cones. All other outcomes were less clear-cut; with some trials favouring neither treatment while others favoured PFMT or cones.

One trial [66] included long-term follow up, at 15 to 32 months post treatment. It was difficult to interpret the findings as data from three of the comparison groups was combined (three groups received treatment from a physiotherapist but not all three groups received training with vaginal cones) and compared with the standard postnatal care group.

There is a lack of consistency in the findings from trials comparing PFMT and weighted vaginal cones. At present there is insufficient evidence of the effect of PFMT versus vaginal cones in women with stress incontinence or postnatal women with symptoms of urine leakage

• PFMT versus bladder retraining (behavioural therapy)

(Please refer to the section on bladder retraining, Section IV)

• PFMT versus medication

PFMT has been compared with topical oestrogens [78], [84] with anticholinergic (oxybutynin chloride) [70], and with alpha adrenergic (phenylpropanolamine) [76]. Both oestrogen trials, in women with urodynamic stress incontinence, found that the PFMT group was more likely to be cured or improved on short pad test. PFMT was better than oxybutynin chloride for self-reported cure/improvement and the number of leakage episodes in 24 hours for women with detrusor overactivity with or without urodynamic stress incontinence, although there was no significant difference in the rate of self reported cure between the groups. The findings from the trial comparing PFMT with phenylpropanolamine in women with stress or mixed incontinence did not clearly favour one group over the other.

Only the trial by Henalla et al [84] included follow up beyond the end of treatment. At nine months three of 17 women in the PFMT had recurrent leakage whereas all three women who had initially improved with topical oestrogens had recurrent symptoms when oestrogen therapy was discontinued.

• PFMT versus surgery

Two trials, in 94 women with urodynamic stress incontinence, compared surgery with PFMT. The surgical procedure varied in one trial depending on the basis of voiding cystourethrogram [79] and in the other trial all women randomised to surgery had an open Burch colposuspension [98]. Unfortunately the trial by Tapp et al [98] has only been reported in two abstracts. As there were inconsistencies in the data reporting between the abstracts the data were excluded from consideration. On the basis of one trial, in women with urodynamic stress incontinence, many more women in the surgery group reported cure post treatment, although there was no significant difference in the rate of self reported cure/improvement between the groups. Women in the surgery group also had significantly fewer leakage episodes in 24 hours post treatment.

For comparisons of PFMT with medication or surgery only a single trial was found for each comparison and/or the trial reporting was very poor. The following statements should be viewed only as hypotheses that require further testing. In women with stress and mixed incontinence there may be no difference between PFMT and phenylpropanolamine, but in women with detrusor overactivity with or without urodynamic stress incontinence PFMT may be better than oxybutynin chloride. In women with urodynamic stress incontinence PFMT may be better than topical oestrogens, but surgery may be better than PFMT.

d) Summary

There is a lack of consistency in PFMT programs that implies an underlying lack of understanding of the physiological principles of rehabilitating (pelvic floor) muscle, or differences in muscle training philosophies. However, there is Level 1A evidence to suggest that in women with stress or mixed incontinence PFMT is better than no treatment, and placebo treatments. There is also Level 1 evidence that 'intensive' PFMT programs are more effective than 'standard' training programs. There is conflicting evidence and/or difficulties in combining the findings of trials comparing the effects of PFMT with electrical stimulation, vaginal cones, medications and surgery. Thus, the effectiveness of PFMT versus electrical stimulation, vaginal cones, medication and surgery is unclear. The long-term outcome of PFMT is also unclear, although on the basis of limited data women may continue to be satisfied with the outcome of training for up to five years.

e) Recommendations

PFMT should be offered as therapy to women with stress and mixed incontinence (Grade of recommendation – A). For women with mixed and urge incontinence it may be appropriate to offer PFMT in combination with bladder training.

On the basis of extrapolation from the exercise science literature Bø suggests that PFMT programs include three sets of eight to 12 slow velocity maximal voluntary pelvic floor muscle contractions, sustained for six to eight seconds each, performed three to four times a week, and continued for 15 to 20 weeks [48].

The addition of voluntary pelvic floor muscle contraction in a variety of functional positions and prior to anticipated changes in intra-abdominal pressure is also recommended. Prior to PFMT a person with skills in the assessment and training of pelvic floor muscles should assess each woman to ensure that a correct voluntary pelvic floor muscle contraction is being performed and to determine what facilitation techniques or adaptations, if any, are required to the recommended training program to ensure an appropriate training intensity. (Grade of recommendation - C).

More high quality RCTs, with long term follow up, are needed to investigate the effectiveness of PFMT relative to other physical therapies, conservative management strategies, pharmaceuticals and surgery. Further comparisons of different types of PFMT to determine which components, or combinations of components, are most effective are also required.

3. Biofeedback and/or Intravaginal Resistance

a) Background

Biofeedback (BF) is commonly used in conjunction with PFMT to assist with training. Intravaginal resistance devices (IVRD) are less common but have also been used to enhance the training process. BF involves the use of monitoring instruments to detect and amplify the various internal physiologic events or conditions of which the person is usually unaware [99]. BF may involve vaginal or anal probes using pressure or electromyographic sensors with information produced in visual and/or auditory form (Figures 1, 2) Information about how the PFM are functioning is presented to the patient to facilitate awareness and co-ordination, and to provide motivation during strength training. Intravaginal resistance devices (e.g. balloon catheters, perineometers etc) provide resistance to enhance strength training (Figure 3) but may also give simultaneous BF. Presumably combination therapies have become popular as they are thought to be more effective than PFMT alone.

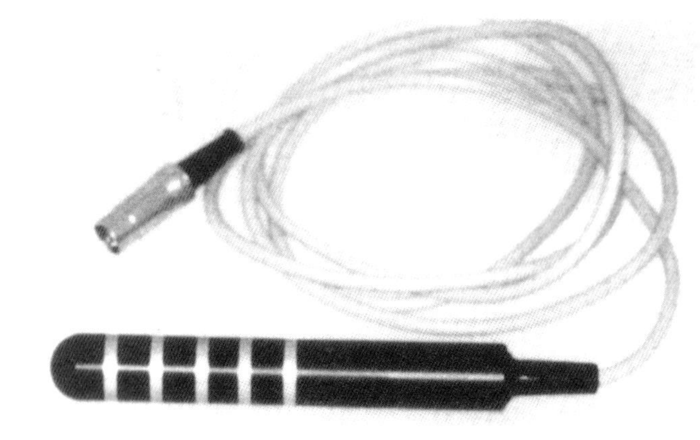

Figure 1 : Surface EMG electrodes on vaginal probe

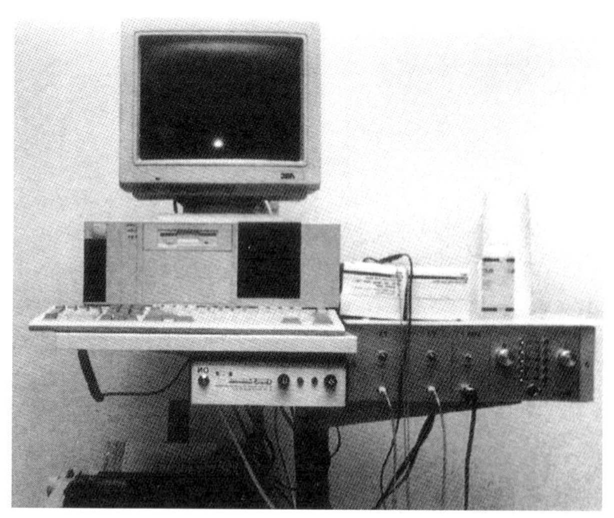

Figure 2 : Vaginal biofeedback (pelvic floor muscle contractility reflected on a lighted scale on the screen)

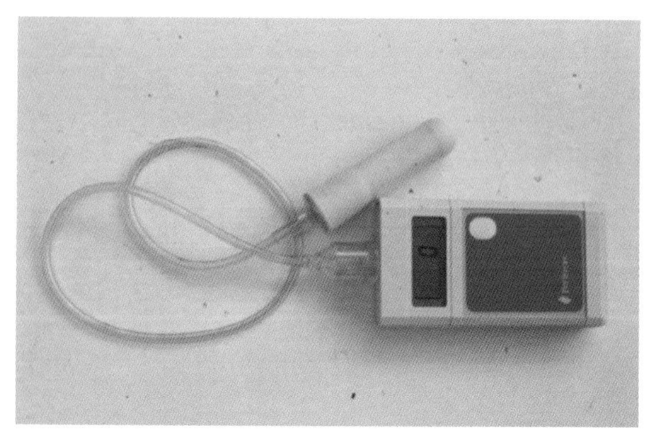

Figure 3 : Perineometer

For the purposes of this review all forms of BF were included, e.g. pressure perineometers with visual or auditory display, electromyography from vaginal probes, etc. To be classified as a trial including BF, repeated use of the BF device was required. This excluded trials where the sole purpose of BF was to assist in the teaching of correct voluntary pelvic floor muscle contraction and was not used thereafter (e.g. [70]). IVRDs that used a pressure filled vaginal probe (e.g. water or fluid filled) were included. While weighted vaginal cones might be considered as a resistance-training device they have been reviewed separately as their proposed mode of action differs from that of pressure devices (see Weighted Vaginal Cones, Section III.5) (Figure 4).

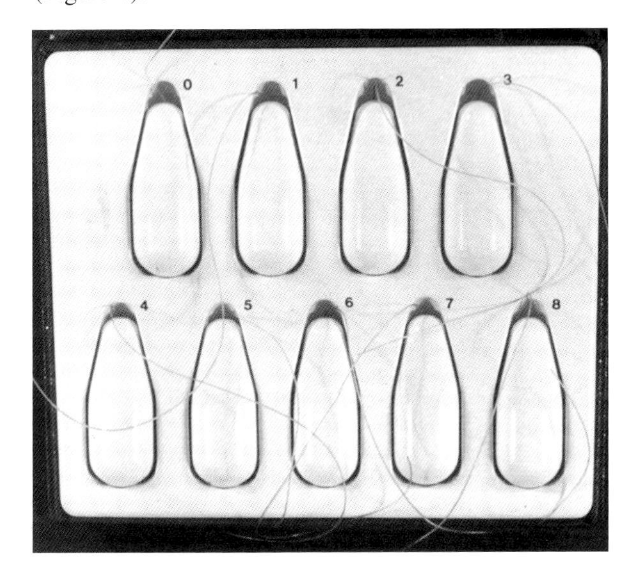

Figure 4 : Vaginal Cones

This section reviews the trials comparing PFMT alone with BF assisted PFMT, or PFMT resisted by an intra-vaginal pressure device. Five systematic reviews that included trials comparing PFMT with or without BF and IVRD were identified [59], [100], [101], [102], [62]. The Cochrane review by Hay-Smith et al was the most up to date of these reviews, and included meta-analysis of trial data where appropriate. Therefore the following summary of results and the recommendations are based upon the rigorous review of trials of PFMT (with or without BF or IVRD) identified by Hay-Smith et al [62]. Readers are encouraged to seek out the full report for details of the method, results and discussion.

b) Quality of Data

A brief summary of the quality of the trials included in the systematic review by Hay-Smith et al [62] is presented below. It is worth noting that there is one further trial, published as an abstract of a study in progress [103] awaiting assessment for inclusion in the review by Hay-Smith et al. Readers may wish to locate this paper in order to judge for themselves if the results would affect the findings presented below.

- **Random allocation concealment**

Of the 11 trials contributing to this section the random allocation concealment was adequate in two [102], [91], and in the remainder it was either unclear if allocation was adequately concealed or the authors stated simply that allocation was at "random" [71], [104], [105], [106], [80], [107], [108], [109], [110].

- **Masking of participants and assessors**

Two trials clearly stated that outcome assessors were masked to group allocation [102], [71] and in the remainder this was not reported.

- **Sample size and power calculation**

None of the 11 trials reported the power calculation used to estimate the size of the study population. None of the trials was large. Only two trials randomised more than 25 women to each comparison group [71], [80] and in both cases the comparison groups number less than 50. The remaining trials all included less than 25 women per comparison group.

- **Losses to follow up**

Four trials had no dropouts or losses to follow up [102], [104] , [105], [106]. The proportion of dropouts was less than 10% in two trials [71], [109] and in the remainder it varied from 14% [107] to 33% [80]. None of the studies clearly stated that the analysis was on the basis of intention to treat.

- **Post treatment follow-up**

Two trials followed women up beyond the post treatment assessment, at three months [71]) and two to three years [91].

c) Results

- **BF protocols**

There is some variation in the types of BF used. Five trials used BF from a vaginal probe with EMG electrodes [102], [71], [91], [108], [110]. The other five trials used a vaginal probe sensitive to pressure changes [104], [106], [80], [107], [109]. Visual feedback was provided in all the trials, and two devices provided auditory feedback too [102] , [106]. Four trials used clinic only BF [102], [71], [91], [110], and three recommended daily BF at home [104], [80], [107]. Two trials used a mix of both clinic and home BF [106], [108], and the remaining trial compared home and clinic BF [109]. The number of treatments with BF and the overall length of treatment varied considerably, and in one trial the PFMT group had fewer clinic visits than the biofeedback group [91].

• BF assisted PFMT versus PFMT alone

Ten trials, which randomised a total of 389 women with urodynamic stress (four trials), stress (four trials) or urodynamic stress incontinence with or without detrusor overactivity (two trials), compared BF assisted PFMT with PFMT alone. The meta-analysis by Hay-Smith et al [62] found no statistically significant differences between the groups for rates of self reported cure or cure/improvement, or the number of leakage episodes in 24 hours. A similar trend was seen in the pad test data and measures of pelvic floor muscle activity. There were insufficient data in any of the comparisons to make sensitivity analysis on the basis of diagnostic group appropriate. However the data that suggested no difference between the groups for self reported cure/improvement all came from trials in women with urodynamic stress incontinence alone.

Data from one trial [102] suggested that the BF group improved more quickly than the PFMT only group (at six weeks), although there were no significant differences either at six weeks or post treatment (12 weeks) but this has not been investigated or confirmed by any other BF study to date. A group that are, anecdotally, reported to benefit from BF are those women who are not able to voluntarily contract their PFM initially but this hypothesis has not been investigated to date.

Only two trials included follow up post treatment, and the most complete and best quality long-term follow up data was provided by Glavind et al [91]. The BF group, who had more clinic visits than the women receiving PFMT alone, were more likely to report continued cure or improvement at two to three years, and were also more likely to be doing regular PFMT.

There is level 1 evidence that BF assisted PFMT is no more effective than PFMT alone for women with stress and mixed incontinence. At present there is insufficient evidence to determine the effect of IVRD in women with stress incontinence.

• PFMT with IVRD versus PFMT alone

Four small trials, in women with stress incontinence, were included in this comparison. Two trials clearly stated that an IVRD was used with PFMT [105], [109]. The two remaining trials used a pressure device to 'exercise' the pelvic floor muscles [107], [106] and this device also provided BF. As the primary intent of the intravaginal device in the latter two trials was not clear (i.e. resistance versus biofeedback) these two trials were included in both the BF and IVRD sections. Neither of the two trials that were clearly investigating the effect of IVRD [105], [109] included any data that were able to contribute to the meta-analysis by Hay-Smith et al [62]. Overall, there were not any significant differences between the IVRD and PFMT groups.

d) Summary

There is some variation in BF protocols that may reflect availability of BF equipment and the ongoing technical developments in this area. There is Level 1 evidence to suggest that BF assisted PFMT is no more effective than PFMT alone in women with urodynamic stress or mixed incontinence. There is insufficient evidence to make a judgment about the effectiveness of IVRD in women with stress incontinence.

e) Recommendations

There is no apparent difference in the effectiveness of PFMT with or without BF (Grade of recommendation - A) although clinicians may find occasions when BF is a useful adjunct to treatment for the purposes of teaching, motivation, compliance, etc.

Further large, high quality RCTs are required to investigate the effectiveness of BF assisted PFMT. Two areas requiring attention are women who are not able to voluntarily contract their PFM or have a very poor quality (intensity) of contraction at initial assessment, and the rate of improvement in BF assisted training versus PFMT alone. The effect of intravaginal pressure devices to assist PFMT has not been adequately investigated to date.

4. Electrical stimulation

a) Background

The literature concerning electrical stimulation in the management of urinary incontinence is very difficult to interpret. Perhaps the primary cause is the lack of a well-substantiated biological rationale underpinning the use of electrical stimulation. However, the theoretical basis of stimulation interventions is emerging with increasing understanding of the neuro-anatomy and physiology of the central and peripheral nervous systems. It is also becoming clear that the mechanisms of action may vary depending on the cause(s) of incontinence and the structure(s) being targeted by electrical stimulation, e.g. pelvic floor muscle or detrusor muscle, peripheral or central nervous system. In general, the aim of electrical stimulation for women with stress incontinence appears to be to improve the function of the pelvic floor muscles, while for women with urge incontinence the objective seems to be to inhibit detrusor overactivity. Overall, studies poorly report the biological rationale underpinning the application of electrical stimulation being tested.

Electrical stimulation is provided by clinic based mains powered machines (i.e. those that need to be plugged into a wall socket) but also more recently portable battery powered stimulators (Figure 5). Electrical stimulation also offers a seemingly infinite combination of current types, waveforms, frequencies, intensities, electrode placements etc. Without a clear biological rationale it is difficult to make reasoned choices of electrical stimulation parameters. Additional confusion is created by the relatively rapid developments in the area of electrical stimulation and a wide variety of stimulation devices and protocols have been used even for the same condition. For example, in the last 15 years or so women with stress incontinence have been treated using anything from a single episode of maximal stimulation under general anaesthetic for 20 minutes with vaginal and buttock electrodes [111], to 10 sessions of Interferential therapy at 10 to 40 Hz with perineal body and symphysis pubis electrodes [74], to six months of low intensity stimulation at 10 Hz using a vaginal electrode [112].

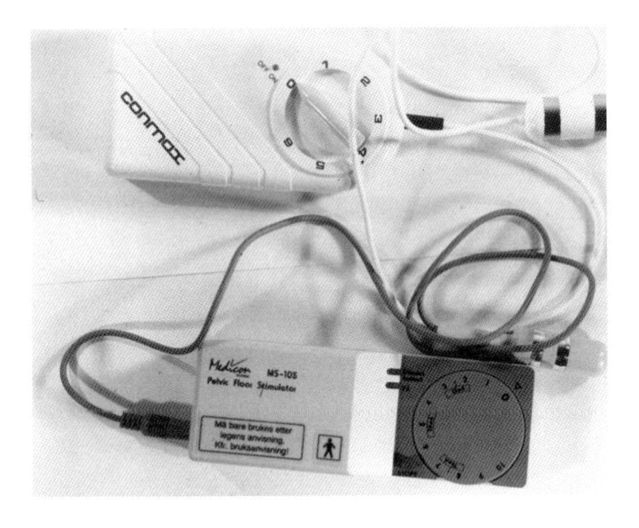

Figure 5 : Electrostimulator with vaginal probe

Finally the nomenclature used to describe electrical stimulation has been inconsistent. Stimulation has sometimes been described on the basis of the type of current being used (e.g. Faradic stimulation, Interferential therapy), but is also described on the basis of the structures being targeted (e.g. neuromuscular electrical stimulation), the current intensity (e.g. low-intensity stimulation, or maximal stimulation), and the proposed mechanism of action (e.g. neuromodulation). In the absence of agreement of how best to classify electrical stimulation the authors of this chapter have made no attempt to do so. The authors were also reluctant to use any existing system to group the electrical stimulation protocols in the trials as many were poorly described and could therefore be erroneously classified.

This section reviews the evidence comparing electrical stimulation (ES) with no treatment, placebo ES and comparisons of different ES protocols. It also includes trials comparing ES with any other single intervention (e.g. surgery, medication etc) except (a) ES versus PFMT, which is included in the section on PFMT, and (b) ES versus weighted vaginal cones, which is included in the section on vaginal cones. Three systematic reviews [61], [56], [62] have been published that include trials relevant to this section. However none of the reviews appeared to include a complete record of all the available trials. The following qualitative summary of the evidence regarding electrical stimulation is based on the trials included in both of the previous systematic reviews with addition of trials located through additional searching (see Appendix 1). To be included in this section a trial needed to (a) be a RCT, (b) include women with urinary incontinence, and (c) investigate the effect of electrical stimulation versus no treatment, placebo treatment, any other single treatment, or compare different electrical stimulation protocols. Abstracts reporting trials in progress were excluded.

b) Quality of data

One of the trials located [113] was excluded from the analysis as it was a preliminary report of a trial in progress. Readers should also note that the trials by Yamanishi et al [114] included men and women with urinary incontinence. It is possible that the effects of stimulation might be different between sexes (due to difference in electrode placement for example) so these studies have not contributed to the analysis where they do not differentiate the effects of treatment in women versus men.

• Random allocation concealment

Of the 20 trials contributing to this section random allocation concealment was adequate in three [56], [64], [112], and in the remainder it was either unclear if allocation was adequately concealed or the authors simply stated that allocation was at "random".

• Masking of participants and assessors

Masking of assessors was clearly stated in nine of the 20 trials [56], [64], [115], [116], [117], [118], [111], [114], [119]. Two trials stated that outcome assessors were not masked [74] , [78], and in the remainder this was not reported.

• Sample size and power calculation

In five studies the size of the study population was based on a power calculation [56], [64], [116], [117], [118]. Two trials randomised more than 50 women to each comparison group [120], [111]. In six trials the group sizes ranged from 25 to 49 [64], [78], [116], [117], [98] , [119], and the remaining 12 trials allocated less than 25 women to each comparison group.

• **Losses to follow up**

Four trials had no dropouts or losses to follow up [118], [85], [74] , [121]. The proportion of dropouts was less than 10% in four trials [115], [78], [86], [114], and in the remainder it varied from 12% [56], [64], [111], [122], [119]) to 21% [123].

• **Post treatment follow-up**

Nine of the 20 trials followed women up beyond the post treatment evaluation [115], [78], [85], [112], [74] ,[122], [111], [114], [119]. The length of follow-up ranged from 6 weeks [111] to six months [115], [78], [85], [112]. Yamanishi et al [114], [119] only followed up those participants who had improved with treatment, monthly for several months.

c) Results

• **ES protocols**

Some ES protocols were poorly reported, lacking detail of stimulation parameters, devices and methods of delivery. However, on the basis of the details that have been reported it appeared that there was considerable variation in ES protocols with no consistent pattern emerging.

1. ES PROTOCOLS FOR WOMEN WITH STRESS INCONTINENCE

Few trials clearly stated whether direct or alternating currents were being used. Two earlier trials [121], [98], used faradic current (low frequency interrupted direct current) but it is assumed that most if not all of the remaining trials used alternating currents. In those trials using alternating current only one trial described the pulse shape – a bipolar square wave [120].

The most commonly used descriptors were frequency and pulse duration. Four trials used a single frequency, ranging from 20 Hz [120] to 50 Hz [64], [116] . Two trials included stimulation at both 10 Hz and 35 Hz [115], [112] although the protocols were different. Other protocols included stimulation at 12.5 Hz and 50 Hz [117], 10-50 Hz [111]), 0 to 100 Hz [78], and finally a 30 minute treatment including 10 minutes at 1 Hz, 10 minutes 10 - 40Hz and 10 minutes at 40 Hz [74] . Pulse durations ranged from 0.08 milliseconds [115] up to 100 milliseconds [120]. Six trials also detailed the duty cycle used during stimulation. The ratios ranged from 1:3 [64], and 1:2 [120] , [116], to 1:1 [115] , [112]) and one trial alternated between a ratio of 1:1 and 1:2 [117].

Four trials asked women to use the maximum tolerable intensity of stimulation [64] , [120] , [74] , [117] and one trial increased output until there was a noticeable muscle contraction [85]. The trial by Knight et al [112] compared "low intensity" and "maximal intensity" protocols. Both the trials by Hofbauer et al [85] and Knight et al [112] also asked women to add a voluntary PFM contraction to the stimulated contraction, although in the latter trial this was only for the maximal intensity group.

Current was most commonly delivered via a single vaginal electrode [64], [120], [112], [116], [117], [121]. One trial used both vaginal and buttock electrodes [111]. In two trials external electrodes were used, perineal body and symphysis pubis [74], perineal and buttock [115], and in two studies the electrode placement was not clearly described [78], [85].

The length and number of treatments was also highly variable. The longest treatment periods included daily treatment at home for six months [64], [112]. Medium length treatment periods were based on twice-daily treatment at home for eight [120] to 12 weeks [116], [117]. The shortest treatment periods were all for clinic-based stimulation, ranging from 10 [78], [74], to 16 [112], and 18 sessions in total [85].

2. ES PROTOCOLS FOR WOMEN WITH URGENCY, URGE INCONTINENCE, DETRUSOR OVERACTIVITY

Although it appeared all the ES trials in this section used alternating current only three trials specifically stated this, biphasic [56]; bipolar [120]; biphasic pulsed current [86]. These same three trials were the only ones to detail the pulse shape, rectangular [56]; square [120]; asymetric [86].

Four trials gave details of the frequencies used and these ranged from 10 Hz [118] to 20 Hz [120] , a combination of 12.5 & 50 Hz [86] , and 10 to 40 Hz [56]. Pulse durations were reported in four trials, and these were 0.1 microseconds [120] , 200 microseconds [56], [118], and 300 microseconds [86]. Two trials used a duty cycle ratio of 1:2 [120], [86].

Intensity of stimulation progressed from five to 25 mA in the trial by Smith [86]. Three trials used the maximum tolerable intensity [56], [118], [120] , and one study increased intensity up to the pain threshold [123]. Current was most commonly delivered by a vaginal electrode [56], [120], [86] or vaginal and anal electrodes [123], [122] although one trial used external surface electrode placements with two electrodes over S2-3 sacral foramina or two electrodes just above the symphysis pubis [118].

The length and number of treatments was also highly variable. The longest treatment period was four months of daily stimulation [86]. Medium length treatment periods were based on twice daily stimulation for eight [120] , nine [124] or 12 weeks [123]. The shortest treatment period consisted of a single episode of stimulation after the voiding phase of cystometry before filling was repeated [118]. One trial compared clinic based stimulation once a week versus twice a week for five and up to 10 weeks [122].

There is a marked lack of consistency in the electrical stimulation protocols used in clinical practice to treat women with stress, urge and mixed incontinence. This seems likely to continue until the infinite variation of stimulation parameters available to researchers and clinicians is narrowed by further investigation into the biological rationale underpinning electrical stimulation.

• ES versus no treatment or control treatment

1. Women with stress incontinence

A single, small trial has compared ES with no treatment in women with stress incontinence [78]. Eight of the 25 women receiving ES were 'objectively' cured or improved (negative pad test or more than 50% reduction in pad test) at three months, versus none of the 25 women in the no treatment group. One trial has compared ES with control intervention (women were offered use of the Continence Guard (Coloplast AS, used infrequently by 14 out of 30 controls) in women with stress incontinence [64]. Bø et al found that ES was better than control intervention for change in leakage episodes over three days, using Social Activity Index and Leakage Index. However, only one of these measures (change in leakage episodes over three days) remained significant ($p=0.047$) with intention to treat analysis. PFM activity was significantly improved in the ES group after treatment, but the change in activity was not significant when compared with controls. Two of 30 controls were cured (≤ 2 g leakage) on pad test with standardized bladder volume on pad test) compared to 7/25 in the ES group. One of 30 women in the control group reported the condition was "unproblematic" after treatment versus 3/25 in the ES group, but 28/30 and 19/25 wanted further treatment respectively.

2. Women with urgency/frequency, urge incontinence, retention/voiding difficulty

Rosier et al (1997) investigated the effect of sacral neuromodulation for urgency/frequency an/or urge incontinence and/or retention/voiding difficulties [125]. Unfortunately the abstract only reports the quality of life data from 35 people (all women) who took part in a larger multicentre study, and the data were not presented by comparison group.

In a four arm RCT in women with detrusor overactivity Berghmans et al [56] investigated the effect of no treatment, lower urinary tract exercises alone (reclassified as PFMT for the purposes of this review), electrical stimulation alone, and electrical stimulation in combination with lower urinary tract exercises. The two main outcome measures were change in the Detrusor Overactivity Index (DAI) and the Incontinence Impact Questionnaire (IIQ). Neither the no treatment or combination therapy groups showed any significant change pre to post treatment. There were significant improvements in the electrical stimulation alone and PFMT alone groups for the DAI and a positive (but not significant) trend towards improvement in the IIQ. When the data from women with 'proven' detrusor overactivity at baseline (DAI ≥ 0.5) were analysed separately the most significant improvements in the DAI were seen in the electrical stimulation group. Overall it appeared that electrical stimulation was better than no treatment.

There are only single trials of good quality investigating the effect of electrical stimulation versus no treatment (or control treatment) in women with urodynamic stress incontinence or women with detrusor overactivity. Consequently there is insufficient evidence to judge whether electrical stimulation is better than no treatment for women with urodynamic stress incontinence or detrusor overactivity.

• ES versus placebo ES

In three of the 11 trials the placebo stimulation devices provided a limited output that the trialists considered would have no treatment effect [115], [85], [117]. In the other eight trials the placebo device appeared as though it was working but in fact there was no electrical output [123], [118], [120], [74] , [116], [111], [114], [119]. Seven of the 11 trials specifically reported that some attempt was made to remove the participants' expectations of the physical sensations that might accompany stimulation in an effort to mask participants to their allocation to active or placebo stimulation [118], [120], [74], [116], [117], [114], [119]. In one trial the stimulation was delivered under general anaesthesia [111].

1. Women with stress incontinence

Four trials compared ES with placebo ES in women with urodynamic stress incontinence [85], [74], [116], [117]. One trial compared ES with placebo ES in men and women with urodynamic stress incontinence [114]. One further trial compared [115] compared ES/PFMT versus placebo ES/PFMT in women with urodynamic stress incontinence and for the purposes of analysis this trial was considered to be a comparison of ES with placebo ES. Hofbauer et al [85] provided minimal detail of participants, methods and stimulation parameters. Laycock & Jerwood [74] used clinic based, short-term (10 treatments) maximal stimulation with an Interferential current applied with external surface electrodes. Four trials were based on daily home stimulation for four [114], six [115] or 12 weeks, [116], [117].

The two most comparable trials in terms of stimulation parameters reported contrasting findings. Sand et al [117] found that the ES group has significantly greater changes in the number of leakage episodes in 24 hours, number of pads used, amount of leakage on pad test, and PFM activity (perineometry) than the placebo stimulation group. In addition the ES group had significantly improved subjective measures (e.g. visual analogue measure of severity) than the placebo group. Neither group demonstrated significant change in the quality of life measure (SF 36). In contrast Luber & Wolde-Tsadik [116], did not find any statistically significant differences between ES and placebo ES groups for rates of self reported cure or improvement, objective cure (negative stress test during urodynamics), number of incontinence episodes in 24 hours, or valsalva leak point pressure.

The other trials generally favoured ES over placebo ES. Yamanishi et al [114] reported significant improvement in a range of outcomes in the ES group but not the placebo ES group (i.e. number of leakage episodes, number of pad changes, disturbance in activities of daily living, self report of improvement, pad test). Laycock & Jerwood [74] generally found significantly greater improvements in the ES group (pad test, PFM activity, self reported severity) although the decrease in incontinence episodes was not significantly different between the groups post treatment. Blowman et al [115] found a significant decrease in the number of leakage episodes in the ES group only. Hofbauer et al [85] reported that 3/11 women in the ES group were cured/improved (not defined) versus 0/11 in the placebo ES group.

One further trial [120] that compared ES with placebo ES in a group of women with urodynamic stress incontinence, detrusor overactivity or both, conducted a subgroup analysis on the basis of diagnosis and did not find any changes in urodynamic measures for women with USI in either ES or placebo ES groups.

2. Women with urgency, sensory urgency, detrusor overactivity, urge incontinence

Three trials were identified. Due to the considerable difference in stimulation parameters and sample populations it does not seem appropriate to try and combine the findings of these trials in any way.

Abel et al [123] randomized 28 postmenopausal detrusor overactivity incontinent women to either active stimulation (maximal anal and vaginal stimulation for 20 minutes once a week for 12 weeks) or placebo stimulation (no current). The results showed a significant improvement in subjective parameters (VAS) but not in objective measurements (24 hour pad test and incontinence episodes per day).

Bower et al [118] used a single stimulation episode given after the voiding phase of cystometry and before bladder filling was repeated. The results were reported separately for women with detrusor overactivity and those with sensory urgency. For women with detrusor overactivity both stimulation groups (10 Hz, sacral electrodes and 150 Hz, symphysis pubis electrodes) showed significant improvements in urodynamic measures when compared with the placebo stimulation group (i.e. reduction in maximum detrusor pressure, increase in first desire to void, proportion of women with a stable bladder). However there were no significant differences between stimulation and placebo groups for change in maximum cystometric capacity or detrusor pressure at first desire to void. Fewer measures were reported for women with sensory urgency. The only significant findings were a significant increase in first desire to void in the 150 Hz group, and a significant increase in the maximum cystometric capacity in the placebo ES group.

Yamanishi et al [119] investigated maximum intensity stimulation delivered daily for four weeks in men and women with detrusor overactivity. There was significantly more improvement in a number of outcomes in the ES group compared with the placebo ES group post treatment (i.e. nocturia, number of leakage episodes, number of pad changes, quality of life score, urodynamic evidence of improvement in detrusor overactivity, self report of cure or improvement). For a single outcome, self report of cure/improvement, subgroup analysis on the basis of sex was reported. Women in the active ES group were much more likely to report cure/improvement than women in the placebo ES group.

One further trial [120] that compared ES with placebo ES in a group of women with urodynamic stress incontinence, detrusor overactivity or both, conducted a subgroup analysis on the basis of diagnosis and found that women with pretreatment detrusor overactivity who received active stimulation were significantly less likely to have urodynamic evidence of detrusor overactivity post treatment.

3. Women with stress, urge or mixed incontinence

ES and placebo stimulation were compared in two trials that included women with symptoms [111] or urodynamic [120] diagnoses of stress, urge or mixed incontinence. Neither trial found any significant differences between the stimulation and placebo stimulation groups post treatment for a range of outcomes including frequency, number of leakage episodes, self report of cure or improvement and quality of life. Brubaker et al [120] did include a subgroup analysis by diagnosis and these findings have been reported previously.

Due to the variation in stimulation protocols it is difficult to interpret the findings of trials comparing electrical stimulation with placebo stimulation. For women with urodynamic stress incontinence the findings of two good quality trials using similar stimulation protocols are contradictory. For women with detrusor overactivity there is a trend in favour of active stimulation over placebo stimulation.

• ES with PFMT versus PFMT alone

1. Women with stress incontinence

Four trials compared ES in combination with PFMT versus PFMT alone in women with stress incontinence [85], [112] , [121], [98]. As both arms in these trials received the same PFMT the trials are essentially investigating the effect of ES. Two small trials, using faradic stimulation, were reported only as abstracts [121], [98] and another small trial gave minimal detail of participants, methods and stimulation parameters [85]. In a three arm RCT Knight et al [112] compared PFMT versus PFMT with home based low intensity ES versus PFMT with clinic based maximal intensity stimulation. Ten of 21 women in the PFMT group, 9/25 women in the low intensity stimulation group, and 16/24 in the maximum intensity stimulation group reported cure or great improvement. All three groups had significant improvements in pad test after treatment, with no significant differences in the percentage reduction between the groups. Similarly all three groups had improvements in vaginal squeeze pressure, but there were no significant differences in improvement.

Overall Knight et al [112] did not find any clear benefits of ES in addition to PFMT. This finding is similar to that of the three small poorly reported trials [85], [121], [98], which found no significant differences between the groups receiving combined ES/PFMT and PFMT alone.

2. Women with detrusor overactivity

In a four arm RCT in women with detrusor overactivity Berghmans et al [56] investigated the effect of no treatment, lower urinary tract exercises alone (reclassified as PFMT for the purposes of this review), electrical stimulation alone, and electrical stimulation in combination with lower urinary tract exercises. The two main outcome measures were change in the Detrusor Overactivity Index (DAI) and the Incontinence Impact Questionnaire (IIQ). The combination therapy group did not demonstrate any significant changes pre to post treatment. There were significant improvements in the PFMT group for the DAI and a positive (but not significant) trend towards improvement in the IIQ. These findings do not suggest added benefit from stimulation.

It is important to note that Berghmans et al [56] theorise that the combination of stimulation/PFMT used in their trial may be counterproductive because the former is targeted at the supraspinal reflexes while the latter may work on central inhibition.

For comparisons of electrical stimulation with PFMT versus PFMT alone the reporting was very poor in three of the four trials in women with stress incontinence, and only a single trial was found for women with detrusor overactivity. At present it seems that there is no extra benefit in adding electrical stimulation to PFMT but this hypothesis needs to be investigated in further high quality trials.

• Comparisons of different methods of ES

1. Women with stress incontinence

A single trial [112] compared low intensity with maximal electrical stimulation in women with urodynamic stress incontinence. Both groups also received PFMT. There was a trend, across a range of outcomes including self report of cure or improvement, pad test, and perineometry, for women who received clinic based maximal stimulation to benefit more than women in the low intensity stimulation group although most differences were not significant. Long term follow up (12 months) suggested that women in both groups continued to improve subjectively, and this was most noticeable in the group of women who had received the combination of PFMT and low intensity stimulation. The trialists speculated that the combination of PFMT and low intensity stimulation was counterproductive, as the low intensity stimulation had resulted in conversion of fast to slow twitch fibers to the detriment of fast-twitch fibre activity required in response to rapid changes in intra-abdominal pressure.

2. Women with detrusor overactivity

Bower et al [118] compared the effect of 10 Hz sacral stimulation via two surface electrodes versus 150 Hz stimulation via two surface electrodes placed just above the symphysis pubis. The findings for women with detrusor overactivity and sensory urgency were presented separately. Both stimulation groups (10 Hz, sacral electrodes and 150 Hz, symphysis pubis electrodes) showed significant improvements in the urodynamic measures of first desire to void and maximum detrusor pressure although neither group showed any significant change in maximum cystometric capacity. The same proportion (44%) of women in each stimulation group demonstrated a 'stable' bladder post stimulation and only the 150 Hz group show a significant improvement in the threshold volume.

Lobel et al [122] compared once a week and twice weekly stimulation in women with detrusor overactivity and did not find any significant differences in any outcome measured (including leakage episodes and quality of life) between the groups. Although more than half the women in the study were improved symptomatically post treatment only 25% were sufficiently satisfied with outcome that they did not wish for further treatment.

When reviewing electrical stimulation trials in general, and trials comparing electrical stimulation protocols in particular, it appears that some electrical stimulation protocols may be more effective than others AND/OR some populations of women receive more benefit from electrical stimulation than others. Both these variables require further investigation.

- **ES versus medication**

1. WOMEN WITH STRESS INCONTINENCE

A single trial [78] compared electrical stimulation (Interferential) with vaginal oestrogens (Premarin). Eight of 25 women in the stimulation group reported they were cured or improved versus 3/24 in the oestrogen therapy group. There was a significant reduction in leakage on pad test in the stimulation group but not the oestrogen group. In contrast the maximum urethral closure pressure was significantly increased in the oestrogen group but not the stimulation group. Long-term follow-up (nine months) found that subjectively one of the eight women in the stimulation group who had reported cure/improvement post treatment had recurrent symptoms, as did all three women in the oestrogen group once oestrogen therapy ceased.

2. WOMEN WITH DETRUSOR OVERACTIVITY

The single trial [86] that compared electrical stimulation and medication (propantheline bromide) in women with detrusor overactivity with or without urodynamic stress incontinence did not find any statistically significant differences in outcome (self reported improvement and urodynamic parameters) between the two groups.

With only single small trials comparing electrical stimulation with medication there is insufficient evidence to determine if electrical stimulation is better than vaginal oestrogens in women with urodynamic stress incontinence, or electrical stimulation is better than anticholinergic therapy in women with detrusor overactivity.

d) Summary

There is a lack of consistency in ES protocols that implies a lack of understanding of the physiological principles of rehabilitating urinary incontinence through electrical stimulation, and this inconsistency means direct comparison between studies is extremely difficult. Overall there is insufficient evidence to determine if ES is better than no treatment in women with urodynamic stress incontinence or detrusor overactivity. In trials comparing ES with placebo ES in women with urodynamic stress incontinence the findings of the two good quality trials using similar stimulation protocols were contradictory. In women with detrusor overactivity there is a trend in favour of ES but the trials are small and not easily comparable. There is also insufficient evidence to determine if ES is better than medication for women with urodynamic stress incontinence or detrusor overactivity. There may be no benefit in adding ES to PFMT although three of the four trials in this section were small, poorly reported, and used electrical stimulation protocols that have been superseded by developments in the understanding of electrical stimulation effects.

It is not clear if any particular ES protocol is more effective than any other. The variability in the findings of the trials included in this section may in part be due to differences in the effectiveness of the wide range of protocols that have been tested. There are many differences in clinical application that have not yet been investigated. For example, some clinicians suggest that 'active' ES (i.e. the patient voluntarily contracts the PFM during stimulation) is better than 'passive' ES but the effect of these two approaches has not yet been evaluated.

Equally it may be that some populations or subgroups of women benefit from ES more than others. For example, anecdotal evidence suggests that ES is used with particular effect for women who are unable to perform a voluntary pelvic floor muscle contraction on initial assessment. However, this observation has not been investigated to date.

e) Recommendations

Further high quality RCTs, in larger samples and with long term follow up, are urgently required to investigate all aspects of the use of ES in the treatment of urinary incontinence in women.

5. WEIGHTED VAGINAL CONES

a) Background

Weighted vaginal cones were developed as a method of strengthening and testing the function of the PFM [126] (Figure 5). Theoretically, the sensation of 'losing the cone' from the vagina might provide strong sensory feedback and prompts a PFM contraction in order to retain the cone. Since their introduction a variety of cones have been developed (i.e. different sizes, shapes and weights), they have been in widespread use, and directly marketed to women through mail order companies. A review that questions the theoretical framework and effects of vaginal cones on PFM strength has been published [127].

This section reviews the evidence comparing vaginal cones with no treatment, placebo treatment, or any other single treatment (e.g. electrical stimulation). For trials comparing cones and PFMT readers are referred to the section on PFMT. A rigorous Cochrane systematic review of weighted vaginal cones (VC) has been published [128]. The following summary of results and the recommendations are based upon the systematic review. Readers are encouraged to seek out the full report for details of method, results and discussion.

b) Quality of data

A brief summary of the quality of the trials included in the systematic review by Herbison et al [128] is presented below.

• Random allocation concealment

Of the five trials contributing to this section allocation concealment was adequate in two [64], [66], and in the remainder [129], [130], [96] it was either unclear if allocation was adequately concealed or the authors simply stated that allocation was at "random".

• Masking of participants and assessors

Masking of participants was not possible in any of the included trials. Masking of outcome assessors was clearly stated in two of the five trials [64], [66]. In the remainder this was not reported.

• Sample size and power calculation

In two trials the size of the study population was based on a power calculation [64], [66]. One trial randomised more than 50 women to each comparison group [66], in three trials the group sizes ranged from 25 to 49 [64], [129], [130], and the remaining trial allocated less than 25 women to each comparison group [96].

• Losses to follow up

The proportion of dropouts was 10% or less in one trial [129], and in the remainder it varied from 12% [64] to 37% [130], [66].

• Long term follow-up

Two of the five trials followed women up beyond the post treatment evaluation [129] six months, [66] two to four years.

c) Results

• VC protocols

Unlike PFMT and ES, the VC protocols were relatively similar. Three trials asked women to retain the heaviest cone possible for 15 minutes twice a day [129], [66], [96]. The other two trials recommended 15 minutes [130] and 20 minutes [64] per day. The trials used sets of cones that included nine [129], [66], five [130], [96] and three weighted cones [64]. The minimum cone weight was 20 grams in four trials [64], [129], [130], [66] and the maximum cone weight was 70 [64], [130] or 100 grams [129], [66].

1. VC VERSUS NO TREATMENT OR TREATMENT

Two trials compared VC with control interventions in women with urodynamic stress incontinence [64], and postnatal women with symptoms of urinary incontinence [66]. In the trial by Bø et al [64] women in the control group were offered the use of the Continence Guard (Coloplast AS), and in the trial by Wilson & Herbison [66] women in the control group continued their "normal" postnatal care. The meta-analysis by Herbison et al [128] reported that VC were significantly better than control treatment for self reported cure and cure/improvement, although other measures such as leakage episodes and pad test did not show significant differences between the groups. Bø et al [64] found that VC were better than control for the Leakage Index, but the groups were not significantly different with regard to the proportion wanting further treatment.

There is level 1 evidence that weighted vaginal cones are better than control treatments for self reported cure/improvement women with urodynamic stress incontinence or postnatal women with symptoms of urine leakage.

2. VC WITH PFMT VERSUS PFMT ALONE

Two trials compared combined VC/PFMT with PFMT alone [130], [66] and these trials were considered to have investigated the effect of VC. The systematic review of Herbison et al [128] found that there was no overlap in the outcomes measured in these trials and that no significant differences between groups was found in either study.

There is level 1 evidence that there is no benefit in the addition of weighted vaginal cones to a PFMT program.

3. VC VERSUS PFMT

(Readers are referred to the section on PFMT. Section III. 2C)

4. VC VERSUS ES

Three trials have compared VC with ES in women with urodynamic stress incontinence [64], [96] and women with symptoms of predominantly stress incontinence

[129]. In addition to VC or ES women in both arms of the RCT by Olah et al were given a PFMT program. The meta-analysis by Herbison et al [128] did not find any significant differences between the VC and ES groups with respect to self-report of cure/improvement, leakage episodes, or improvement in pad test. Bø et al [64] also reported no differences between the groups for additional outcomes such as the Social Activity Index, Leakage Index, or the proportion wanting further treatment.

There is level 1 evidence that weighted vaginal cones are no better than electrical stimulation in the treatment of women with urodynamic stress incontinence or symptoms of stress incontinence.

d) Summary

While there is considerable similarity in the trials investigating the effect of VC, there were few trials in total. Most of the trials were small and some were of poor to moderate quality. While treatment with VC may be better than control treatment, it seems that it may be no better or worse than electrical stimulation. The addition of VC to a PFMT program may add no further benefit over PFMT alone.

e) Recommendations

Further high quality, large RCTs, are required to substantiate the effect of training with VC in the management of female urinary incontinence.

f) Adverse effects

All trials referred to in this section were scanned for records of adverse events associated with treatment. Thirty-seven trials made no statement about adverse effects [123], [63], [118], [71], [120], [104], [105], [67],[91], [78], [84], [85], [106], [112], [95], [74] , [50], [72], [73], [97], [130], [69], [125], [107], [111], [108], [109], [121], [98], [81], [76], [7], [66], [96], [82], [75].

One trial had recorded adverse events but these were not reported in the abstract of the trial [80].

Five trials stated that no participant reported adverse events associated with treatment [102], [115], [116], [114].

Three trials reported adverse events but only in the non physical therapy groups, i.e. surgery [79], medication [70], and anti-incontinence device [131].

Ten trials did report adverse events associated with physical therapy treatments [64], [65], [83], [77], [68], [122], [129], [117], [86], [119]. Six women reported adverse effects associated with PFMT (e.g. uncomfortable feeling during exercise) in the trial by Lagro-Janssen et al [68].

Six trials [64], [83], [122], [117], [86], [119], investigating electrical stimulation or placebo stimulation reported 44 adverse events in ES groups (e.g. leg tremor, vaginal discomfort or bleeding) and nine adverse events in placebo ES groups (e.g. disagreeable feeling). Four trials that included comparisons of VC reported 39 adverse events associated with treatment including aesthetic dislike of the device, discomfort associated with prolapse or insertion, and problems maintaining motivation [64], [65], [77], [129].

Overall, recording and/or reporting of adverse events was poor. From the evidence available it appears that adverse events associated with PFMT were rare, but more common with VC, ES or placebo ES.

6. Other factors affecting outcome

All included studies were examined for analysis of factors that may have affected the outcome(s) of intervention. Eighteen studies discussed one or more characteristics of the sample population that might have affected outcome [132], [120], [71], [65], [133], [105], [83], [78] , [85], [79] , [112] , [74], [116] , [50], [73], [117], [76], [119].

The three most commonly mentioned factors (five trials each) were initial severity of incontinence, age of participants and motivation/compliance with intervention. Three trials found that severity did not predict response to treatment [71], [83], [78], the findings of one trial suggested that women with more severe leakage were less likely to improve [85], and one further trial found that responders to intensive PFMT were women with more severe incontinence [132] . Three trials suggested that there was no association between age and outcome [78], [85], [68], another found that cure/improvement was less likely in older women [73], while another trial found that responders to intensive PFMT were likely to be older [132] .

With regard to motivation/compliance all five trials found a similar association. That is, responders either seemed to be more motivated [132] or showed greater levels of compliance [68], [73], [117], [76]. Two trials, included in the comparison of intensive versus standard PFMT, compared groups that did or did not receive audiotapes to assist with home training. One of these trials found that the audiotape group was more compliant with PFMT [67] whereas the other did not [72]. Authors of another trial, comparing ES with PFMT, commented that women appeared to be more compliant with clinic based ES than home PFMT and speculate that this is because women are impressed by the stimulator used in treatment [74].

Duration of symptoms and urodynamic parameters were discussed by four trials each. Two trials found that women with a longer history of symptoms responded better to intensive PFMT [132] or maximal electrical stimulation [112], whereas Hofbauer et al [85] and Lagro-Jansen et al [68] reported that duration of symptoms had no effect on outcome. Such a wide range of urodynamic parameters has been reported it is difficult to see any pattern emerging to date. Ferguson et al [105] did not find that initial maximum urethral closure pressure was associated with outcome, however Bø & Larsen (1992) [132] reported that responders to intensive PFMT were more likely to have a negative closure pressure initially. Neither of these trials found an association between functional urethral length and outcome. Elser et al (1999) [133] reported that the outcome of their trial comparing behavioural training, PFMT or combined therapy in women with detrusor overactivity with or without urodynamic stress incontinence was independent of urodynamic diagnosis. In the course of searching for trials for inclusion in this review an abstract of an RCT, comparing the outcome of conservative management based on urodynamic or symptom diagnosis, was located [134]. Ramsay found that there was no difference between the groups for cure/improvement post treatment.

Three trials each referred to the effect of previous surgery or initial PFM strength. No effect was found for previous surgery (type unspecified) [85], urethral suspensions [71], or previous pelvic floor repair or hysterectomy [78]. In the trial by Miller et al [50] reduction in leakage one week after beginning PFMT (the 'Knack') was not related to the initial findings from digital assessment of PFM. In contrast Knight et al [112] found that women who responded best to maximal electrical stimulation had weaker PFM, and Bø & Larsen [132] reported that women who responded to intensive PFMT had stronger PFM initially.

A range of other factors was reported by one or two studies. Henalla et al [78] found that mild genito-urinary prolapse seemed to have no effect on outcome, as did Hofbauer et al [85]. Lagro-Janssen et al [68] stated that psychological features appeared to have no effect on outcome. Bø & Larsen [132] reported that responders to intensive PFMT had higher BMI, but that the following factors had no effect – parity, maximum birthweight of babies, maternal weight gain in pregnancy, menopausal status, previous PFMT, and family history of stress incontinence.

In summary, many of the factors traditionally supposed to affect outcomes of physical therapy interventions (e.g. age, severity of incontinence) might be less crucial than previously thought. From the trial reports available the single factor that consistently appeared to be associated with positive outcome was greater motivation and/or compliance with the intervention. It should be noted that the association between compliance with physical therapy interventions and improvement might not be due to the effect of the intervention alone but some other unknown factor. For example, trial participants who are compliant with active or placebo drug do better than those who are not compliant with either active or placebo medication (The Coronary Drug Project Research Group, 1980). Essentially, further investigation of all the above factors is required in subsequent high quality RCTs before any real conclusions may be drawn.

DeLancey [135] makes a compelling argument for intervention for urodynamic stress incontinence to be based on accurate diagnosis of the underlying pathology, whether it be neurological, ligamentous/fascial, or muscular. For example, he suggests that PFMT may be inappropriate where innervation of the muscles is not intact or where the muscles have been detached from their fascial connections. A similar argument (for a different set of underlying pathologies) could be made for urge incontinence. Accurate diagnostics may be more important than other factors for predicting success of physical therapies. However current diagnostic procedures, such as urodynamics, do not seem to be able to reliably predict outcome.

Many of the factors traditionally supposed to affect the outcomes of physical therapy interventions (e.g. age, severity of incontinence) may be less crucial than previously thought. The single factor that is consistently associated with positive outcome is greater motivation and/or compliance with the intervention. At present there is no convincing evidence of the need for urodynamic evaluation to confirm diagnosis prior to conservative management.

7. Prevention

a) Background

PFMT has long been recommended to prevent or delay the onset of both urinary and faecal incontinence, in particular during pregnancy and after childbirth [44], [43]. However there are few published reports of trials investigating the effectiveness of PFMT and/or other physical modalities for the primary prevention (preventing incontinence occurring by removing its causes) or secondary prevention (detecting asymptomatic dysfunction early and treating it to stop progression) of incontinence.

This subsection will examine the evidence for PFMT and/or other physical modalities used for the primary or secondary prevention of incontinence. A rigorous Cochrane systematic review of 10 trials investigating physical therapies for the prevention of incontinence is currently in press [128]. The following summary of results and the recommendations is based on the findings of the currently unpublished review. Readers are encouraged to seek out the full publication in the Cochrane Library for details of the method, results and discussion.

b) Quality of data

A brief summary of the quality of ten [136], [137], [138], [139], [140], [42], [141], [142], [143], [144] of the 11 trials included in the systematic review by Herbison and Hay-Smith [128] is presented below. One trial, included by Herbison & Hay-Smith, has been excluded from the summary presented here, as it was a study undertaken in men [145].

• Random allocation concealment

Of the ten trials random allocation concealment was adequate in two [142], [144] and in one it was inadequate (i.e. alternation) [140]. The remaining seven trials stated only that group allocation was at random.

• Masking of participants and assessors

Two trials stated that assessors of outcome were masked to group allocation [142], [144], and in one trial assessors were not masked [143]. None of the remaining seven trials stated whether the assessor was masked or not.

• Sample size and power calculation

One trial reported a power calculation [143]. Trials varied in size, and in four there were less than 25 participants per comparison group [136], [138], [42], [144]. Three trials randomised more than 50 participants per group [139], [141], [143] and one of these was a large trial with 900 women in each comparison group [143].

• Losses to follow up

Two trials had no losses to follow up or withdrawals [136], [137]. In one trial the drop out rate was less than 10% [138] and in six trials the drop out rates ranged from 11% [140], [143] to 36% [142]. Data on drop outs were not available from the remaining trial [141] as it was reported as a study in progress.

• Post treatment follow-up

Three trials assessed women at trial entry and then once after intervention, at six weeks [144], 12 weeks [137] and six months [138]. Dougherty et al [136] and Nielsen et al [140] assessed women after six and eight week intervention periods respectively, but also followed up a proportion of their sample later at two to 18 months [136] and eight months [140]. The abstract by Norton & Baker [42] implied that women were assessed after a four week intervention period, and that follow up was also undertaken at six months but no data was reported [42]. Four trials had baseline, intermediate and end-point measures [139], [141], [143] and three of these studies recruited women during pregnancy [139], [141], [142]. Meyer et al recruited women during pregnancy, randomised them to intervention or control groups at two months after delivery, and evaluated outcome at 10 months postpartum [139]. In the trial by Reilly et al [141] antenatal women were recruited at 18-20 weeks gestation, and then followed up at 34 weeks gestation and three months postpartum. Sampselle et al recruited women at 20 weeks gestation and repeated their measures at 35 weeks gestation, six weeks, six and twelve months postpartum [142]. Finally, Sleep & Grant [143] recruited women within 24 hours of delivery and followed them up at both ten weeks and three months postpartum. With respect to these four trials the findings reported in the results are those from the last assessment point.

c) Results

Only four of the 10 trials reported urinary or faecal incontinence as an outcome measure [141], [143], [142], [139] and the remainder assessed principally changes in PFM 'strength' [140], [144], [137], [138], [136], [42].

• Preventing incontinence

All four trials investigated the effect of PFM rehabilitation on the prevalence of postpartum incontinence. Sampselle et al [142] enrolled primigravid women at 20 weeks gestation, and randomised them to receive tailored PFMT program (a correct voluntary pelvic floor muscle contraction was checked and 30 contractions per day at or near maximal intensity recommended) or routine antenatal and postnatal care. Controlling for baseline incontinence the prevalence of urinary incontinence was significantly less in the PFMT group than the control group at 35 weeks gestation (p=0.043), six weeks postpartum (p=0.032) and six months postpartum (p=0.044). By 12 months there was no significant difference in the prevalence of urinary incontinence between the groups. In the trial by Sleep & Grant [143] postnatal women were recruited within 24 hours of vaginal delivery and randomised to receive either a reinforced PFMT program (daily visits by midwifery co-ordinator while in hospital to reinforce PFMT instruction) or routine care. Routine care included small group teaching on PFMT run by obstetric physiotherapists on the postnatal wards, any information received on PFMT during antenatal education, and leaflets on PFMT. More women in the reinforced PFMT group gave a history of antenatal incontinence symptoms (32% versus 29% in the routine care group) and reported doing antenatal PFMT (57% versus 46% in the routine care group). At three months 180/816 women (22%) in the reinforced PFMT group and 175/793 women (22%) in the routine care group had urine leakage symptoms. Twenty one and 22 women from each group respectively had occasional faecal loss. Meyer et al [139] recruited primparae during pregnancy, and then at two months postpartum randomised them to receive either routine care or 12 sessions of biofeedback and electrostimulation with physiotherapists trained in pelvic floor re-education. No details of the routine care, biofeedback or electrical stimulation are reported in the abstract. At two months postpartum nine women in the control group and 26 women in the re-education group had symptoms of stress incontinence. At 10 months postpartum the figures were eight and six respectively. At 10 months the number of women with faecal incontinence was three and two in each group respectively. In an abstract of a trial in progress Reilly et al [141] reported on data from 53/150 primigravid women three months postpartum. Only primigravid women without any previous urinary incontinence or neurological disorder were included in the trial, and randomized to receive a PFMT program supervised by a physiotherapist or no treatment. In the preliminary analysis subjective reports of stress incontinence were more common in the no treatment group (14/33) than the PFMT group (2/20) at three months postpartum.

In summary, only one of the trials [141] is a purely primary or secondary prevention trial. As the full report of this study was not available at the time of writing no further interpretation of the findings is possible. The other three trials in this section included women with existing incontinence symptoms. In some respects these trials might be better classified as early intervention studies rather than prevention studies.

As yet, it is not clear what effect PFMT or (undefined) pelvic floor re-education has on the prevention of urinary or faecal incontinence in antenatal or postnatal women. Sampselle et al [142] appeared to show benefit of PFMT over routine care in the early postpartum period but the difference in prevalence of incontinence between groups was no longer significant at 12 months. This was the only one of the three trials to state specifically that a correct voluntary pelvic floor muscle contraction was checked prior to training. In contrast, the large trial by Sleep & Grant [143] did not show any difference between reinforced PFMT and routine care (that did include usual advice on PFMT) on the prevalence of urinary or faecal incontinence at three months postpartum. It is possible that there was not sufficient difference between the interventions to demonstrate differences in effect on incontinence. Overall Meyer et al [139] did not show that there was any difference in prevalence of urinary or faecal incontinence between routine care and pelvic floor re-education groups. However at 10 months postpartum 20/26 women in the re-education group no longer had stress incontinence symptoms versus 1/9 in the control group.

• Measures of PFM activity

1. PFMT VERSUS CONTROL TREATMENTS

In a small trial of 35 nulliparous women, without any indication of pelvic floor muscle dysfunction and no history of incontinence, Thorp et al [144] investigated the effect of a six week thrice daily PFMT program (versus no intervention) on surface EMG measures from vaginal and anal plug electrodes. There were no differences between the groups for either maximal or sustained vaginal or rectal EMG measurements after training.

Nielsen et al [140] recruited primiparous women at 33 weeks gestation and randomised them to receive usual antenatal/postnatal care (including encouragement to perform daily voluntary pelvic floor muscle contraction) or a PFMT comprising 50 brief maximal contractions twice a day for the last eight weeks of pregnancy. The trial report did not state if any of the women had previous incontinence symptoms. Both groups had significant improvements in vaginal squeeze pressure over the last weeks of pregnancy, and a significant decrease at eight weeks postpartum compared with the baseline measure. At eight weeks postpartum the PFMT group had significantly greater vaginal squeeze pressure than the control group. This finding remained in a subgroup of women (rural women) who were followed up at eight months postpartum.

Norton & Baker [42] randomised postnatal women six weeks after vaginal delivery to one of three arms, control (posture and lifting taught), PFMT (control intervention plus single teaching session and home program of 100 contractions per day) or vaginal cones. No participant had pre pregnancy leakage, half had leakage in pregnancy, and a third postpartum leakage. It was difficult to extract any useful data from the abstract of this trial in progress. From the third of participants who had completed the study it appeared that there were no significant changes in introital and vaginal squeeze pressures in the control group but a significant improvement in introital pressure in the PFMT group after four weeks of training.

In a small three arm trial Dougherty et al [136] randomised [45] postpartum women six to seven weeks after vaginal delivery to control (sitting with intravaginal resistance device insitu with no voluntary pelvic floor muscle contraction, although these were allowed at other times), PFMT (alternating days of strength and endurance training six days a week for six weeks), or PFMT with intravaginal resistance device in situ. All groups demonstrated improvement in maximum and sustained vaginal squeeze pressure after six weeks.

Although there were greater improvements in both PFMT groups there were no significant differences between the three groups.

To date, the trials in this area are small. In addition one trial was in progress at the time of reporting and data were therefore incomplete. It is difficult to combine the findings from the individual studies. The following statements should be viewed only as hypotheses to be tested, that (a) there may not be significant gains in PFM 'strength' in nulliparous women without incontinence symptoms or other pelvic floor dysfunction, (b) that PFMT is better than control treatment (no treatment or routine care) to increase PFM 'strength' in women after vaginal delivery.

2. PFMT VERSUS WEIGHTED VAGINAL CONES

Three trials compared PFMT with weighted vaginal cones in postnatal women [137], [138], [42]. Jonasson et al [137] recruited women at eight weeks postpartum and randomised them to a 12 week program of either PFMT (voluntary pelvic floor muscle contraction in a variety of positions progressing to a maximum of 90 contractions twice a day) or vaginal cones (retain heaviest cone possible in standing/walking for 15 minutes twice a day). There was no statement in the trial report about previous incontinence symptoms. The heaviest cone that could be retained was chosen as the measure of PFM 'strength'. Women in both groups, who could initially retain 20 to 30g cones initially, had significant improvements in 'strength' with greater improvements in the cones group. Among women who could initially retain cones weighing 40g or more, only the cones group showed significant improvements in 'strength'. In a later trial, Jonasson et al [138] randomised health postnatal women following vaginal delivery to a six month program of either PFMT (program as previously) or cones (retain heaviest 'ball' possible for 30 minutes per day). Once again, the heaviest cone that women were able to retain during two minutes of standing/walking measured PFM 'strength'. 'Strength' improved significantly in both groups with greater improvement in the cones group. Norton & Baker [42] randomised postnatal women six weeks after vaginal delivery to one of three arms, control (posture and lifting taught), PFMT (control intervention plus single teaching session and home program of 100 contractions per day) or vaginal cones (no details given). It was not clear from the abstract if the cones group also received the control and PFMT interventions. Norton & Baker [42] did state that no participant had pre pregnancy leakage, half had leakage in pregnancy, and a third postpartum leakage. It was difficult to extract any useful data from the abstract of this trial in progress. From the third of participants who had completed the study it appeared that introital and vaginal squeeze pressures might be significantly greater in the cones group after four weeks of training, although the difference between the groups might disappear by six months.

In summary, it is not clear if there is any difference in the effectiveness of PFMT or training with cones to increase PFM 'strength' in postnatal women. Although it appears both methods of training may result in improvements in 'strength' two of the trials use cone weight as the measure of strength and this may advantage the groups training with cones. As these women have 'practiced' the action of retaining a cone, this measure may be of familiarity and practice with the device, rather than 'strength'.

d) Summary

There is lack of evidence about the effectiveness of PFMT or other PFM rehabilitation programs (e.g. electrical stimulation) for the prevention of urinary or faecal incontinence. The absence of long term follow-up in any of the included RCTs is disappointing. There are some trials investigating the effect of PFMT and/or vaginal cones on PFM 'strength'. These trials are evaluating, at best, a surrogate end point. PFMT may be better than control treatments (no treatment or routine care) at improving PFM 'strength' in postnatal women but this should be considered a hypothesis to be tested further. It is not clear if there are greater improvements in 'strength' after PFMT or training with vaginal cones in postnatal women.

e) Recommendations

Further high quality RCTs, with long term follow-up, investigating the effectiveness of physical therapies for the prevention of urinary incontinence in women at risk, or in the general female population, are urgently required. It is worth noting that the Cochrane Review by Herbison & Hay-Smith [128] has identified two trials in progress investigating the effect of PFMT in the prevention of incontinence and readers are referred to the review for further details.

IV. BLADDER RETRAINING

1. INTRODUCTION

The section examines the evidence on the use of bladder retraining in cognitively intact, noninstitutionalized women with urge, stress, and mixed incontinence, and provides recommendations for its effective use in clinical practice. A summary of the search strategy and inclusion/exclusion criteria for selecting studies for review is provided in the Appendix. See the section on conservative therapy in the elderly for a detailed discussion of the other types of scheduled voiding regimens that are used in management of urinary incontinence in women who are cognitively impaired and/or institutionalized.

Several systematic reviews on bladder retraining with qualitative synthesis have been published [146], [147], [148]. Recently, the Cochrane Collaboration published an updated review of *Bladder Training for Urinary Incontinence in Adults* which graded the quality of the included studies with respect to treatment of urge incontinence only [149]. To date, there has been no other published meta-analysis (quantitative synthesis).

2. Bladder retraining

a) Background

Bladder retraining (also referred to as a bladder discipline, bladder drill, bladder training, and bladder re-education) is a term used to describe the educational and behavioral process used to re-establish urinary control in adults. It was first described by Jeffcoate and Francis in 1966 as "bladder discipline" which involved a program of patient education and a scheduled voiding regimen used to manage functional disorders of the lower urinary tract in women [150]. Later, Frewen in a series of articles published from 1972 to 1982 brought widespread attention to the role of bladder retraining in the treatment of urge incontinence with or without associated detrusor overactivity and sensory-urgency problems without incontinence [151], [152, 153], [154]. Evidence indicating that bladder retraining was also effective in women with urodynamic stress incontinence [147] led to clinical practice guidelines in the United States recommending its use for women with urge, stress, and mixed incontinence as a first-line of therapy [155]. These recommendations did not require that urodynamic evaluation be performed prior to the initiation of therapy.

Specific goals of bladder retraining include correcting faulty habit patterns of frequent urination, improving ability to control bladder urgency, prolonging voiding intervals, increasing bladder capacity, reducing incontinent episodes, and building patient confidence in controlling bladder function. The underlying mechanism of how bladder retraining achieves its effects is poorly understood. Several hypotheses have been proposed including improved cortical inhibition over detrusor contractions; improved cortical facilitation over urethral closure during bladder filling, improved central modulation of afferent sensory impulses; altered behavior resulting from better individual awareness of the lower urinary tract function and circumstances that cause incontinence, and increasing the "reserve" capability of the lower urinary tract system [147], [156], [75].

Bladder retraining programs typically involve several key elements: patient education on the mechanisms underlying continence and incontinence; a scheduled voiding regimen with gradually progressive voiding intervals; urgency control strategies using distraction and relaxation techniques; self-monitoring of voiding behavior; and positive reinforcement provided by a clinician [156]. Bladder retraining requires a cognitively intact and motivated patient who is capable of independent toileting and can adhere to the scheduled voiding regimen.

A previous systematic review by Roe, Williams, and Palmer [149] involving seven trials on bladder retraining in the management of urge incontinence alone concluded that the evidence suggests bladder retraining may be helpful when compared to no treatment. However, Roe et al cautioned interpretation of this conclusion because it was based on limited data. The review also concluded that there was not enough evidence to show whether drug therapy was better than bladder retraining or useful as a supplement to it.

b) Quality of included studies

This updated review from that reported at the First International Consultation on Incontinence, focuses only on randomized and nonrandomized controlled trials. (See the previous review for a comprehensive listing of clinical series evaluating bladder retraining.) Since the last review, there have been three reports on bladder retraining; two were not included as they were retrospective analyses [157], [158].

Six clinical trials have been published on the efficacy of bladder retraining alone in women. Of these, five are randomized clinical trials (RCTs) [159], [160], [147], [161], [75] involving a total of 626 women; and one was a nonrandomized controlled trial with a long-term follow-up [68], [87].

Of the RCTs, two compared bladder training to an untreated control group [159], [147], one RCT compared bladder retraining to two other behavioral interventions (pelvic floor muscle training augmented with biofeedback or a combination of both therapies) [75]; and two RCTs compared bladder retraining to anticholinergic drug therapy [160], [161]. Two of these RCTs [147], [75] published additional papers reporting on different treatment outcomes [162], [163], [133]. The nonrandomized trial compared bladder retraining for those with urge incontinence alone or bladder retraining with pelvic floor muscle training for those with mixed incontinence to a no-treatment control group [68]. However, due to the small number of subjects receiving bladder training alone (N=9) and the method of reporting, these results will not be presented [68].

The age of the study populations ranged from 17 [160]

to 90 years [147]. All studies investigated the effect of bladder retraining in women with detrusor overactivity, low compliance bladder, or sensory bladder. Two RCTs also included women with urodynamic stress incontinence with or without detrusor overactivity [147], [75] and the nonrandomized trial included women with urge or mixed incontinence [68]. Sample sizes ranged from 50 [160] to 204 women [75]. Only one study reported a power calculation [75]. All trials had intervention groups containing 25 or more subjects.

Follow-up periods were variable with all studies conducting at least on post-treatment assessment within 4-12 weeks of treatment initiation. Several trials included an additional evaluation at 3 to 12 months post-treatment. One study conducted a 5-year follow-up [87]. Outcome measures used included self report of benefit (e.g., cure or improvement) [159], [160], [68], [87], [161], [75], a urinary diary [147], [68], [161], [75]), pad tests [147], [75] quality of life instruments [147], [163], [75], and urodynamic measures [159], [162], [161], [133]. Compliance with the bladder retraining protocol was reported in only one study [75].

c) Results

• Bladder Retraining Programs

Several variations may occur in how bladder retraining programs are implemented. Variation in the scheduled voiding protocols range from a mandatory regimen with restriction of voiding in between assigned toileting times to a self-scheduling regimen with no restriction of voiding if urgency becomes unbearable. The initial assigned voiding interval may vary from 30 minutes to 2 hours with 1 hour being the most common interval; with the increase in voiding interval from 15 to 60 minutes. Generally, voidings are not required during sleeping hours. Other variations in retraining programs involve the setting in which bladder retraining is conducted; use of adjunctive treatments such as pelvic floor muscle training or drug therapy; type of urgency control techniques used; and whether fluid modifications are incorporated into the program. Early protocols in the United Kingdom required hospitalization for 5-13 days to ensure strict protocol adherence [159], [160]. Later protocols implemented bladder retraining as an outpatient treatment program lasting from 6 to 12 weeks [147], [75]. Techniques of urgency control include a variety of distraction and relaxation techniques such as deep breathing exercises, mathematical problem solving and other attention tasks, positive self-statements, perineal pressure, and use of pelvic floor muscle contraction to control a specific urge. Fluid modifications such as an increase or decrease of fluid intake or a change in timing of fluid intake were not generally recommended. Most bladder retraining protocols required self-charting of voiding patterns.

Results of treatment typically occur within two weeks after commencing treatment [160], [75]. The reported cure rates for reducing urinary incontinence ranges from 12% to 90% [147]Fantl et al., 1991; [159] depending on how efficacy is measured. Subjective improvement rates measured by the patient's self-report are 73% to 90% [159], [161]. When using urinary diaries to evaluate cure rates, the rates range from 12% to 16% [147], [75]. Studies reporting on the long-term effect of bladder retraining are limited [87].

1. Bladder Retraining Versus No Treatment

Bladder retraining as the sole therapy has been used in the treatment of detrusor overactivity, urodynamic stress incontinence, mixed incontinence, and urge incontinence with a stable bladder.

There is Level 1 evidence that bladder retraining is an effective treatment for women with urge, stress, and mixed urinary incontinence.

Two RCTs reported significant improvements in the bladder retraining group as compared to an untreated control group [159], [147]. Jarvis and Millar [159] investigated the effect of an in-patient bladder retraining program in women with a diagnosis of detrusor overactivity, whereas Fantl et al.,[147] studied the effect of an outpatient program in women with urodynamic stress incontinence, detrusor overactivity, and mixed incontinence. Reported cure/improvement rates varied between the two trials which may have reflected the different follow-up periods, the type of outcome measures used, or the bladder retraining protocol. Jarvis and Millar [159] reported that 90% of the treatment group were continent and 83.3% were symptom free at 6 months; whereas, in the control group 23.3% were continent and symptom free. All women who were symptom free after treatment reverted to a normal cystometrogram.

Fantl et al [147] reported that 12% of the treatment group were continent and 76% had reduced their incontinent episodes at least 50% or more at 6-weeks as measured by a 7-day urinary diary. These results were maintained at 6 months. They also reported a 55% improvement in quality of life measured by the Incontinence Impact Questionnaire at 6-weeks which was maintained over a 6-month period; however, there was not a direct correlation between improvements on a urinary diary and the Incontinence Impact Questionnaire [163]. Significant reductions were also observed with diurnal and nocturnal frequency and pad weights. While some women did revert back to normal bladder function following training, no relationship was found between changes in urodynamic variables and the number of incontinent episodes [162]. Women with detrusor overactivity with and without urodynamic stress incontinence had similar reductions in incontinent episodes and improvements in quality of life.

2. Bladder Retraining Versus Pelvic Floor Muscle Training

One trial that compared bladder retraining with pelvic floor muscle training augmented with biofeedback found that both interventions were equally effective in reducing incontinent episodes and improving quality of life in women with urodynamic stress incontinence, detrusor overactivity, or both diagnoses. In a multicentre RCT, [75] cure rates determined by a 7-day urinary diary, were reported to be 18% and 16% in the bladder retraining group at 3 and 6 months post-randomization, respectively, versus 13% and 20% in the pelvic floor muscle training group. Improvement rates (i.e., percent of patients achieving greater than 50% reduction of incontinent episodes) in the bladder retraining group was 52% and 46% at 3 and 6 months, respectively, versus 57% and 56% in the pelvic floor muscle training group. Women with detrusor overactivity with and without urodynamic stress incontinence has similar reductions in incontinent episodes. Changes in incontinence severity were unrelated to urodynamic changes [133].

One RCT has indicated that bladder retraining and pelvic floor muscle training have similar efficacy in women with urge, stress and mixed incontinence and this finding requires further investigation.

3. Bladder Retraining Versus Medication

Two RCTs concluded that bladder retraining was superior to anticholinergic drug therapy in women with detrusor overactivity. Jarvis [160] found that inpatient bladder retraining was superior to an outpatient program of combined drug therapy of 200 mg (three times a day) flavoxate hydrocholoride and 25 mg (three times a day) imipramine. Cure/improvement rates in the bladder retraining group were 84% subjectively continent and 76% symptom free versus 56% continent and 48% symptom free in the drug therapy group. Patients who were symptom free at 4 weeks were able to maintain their effects at 12 weeks. Cystometric changes in both groups were related to the clinical changes.

Columbo and his associates [161] reported that a 6-week course of oxybutynin had a similar clinical cure rate (e.g., self-reported total disappearance of urge incontinence, no protective pads, or further treatment) as bladder retraining (74% versus 73% respectively). Oxybutynin clinically cured 93% of patients with detrusor overactivity, 67% of those with low-compliance bladder, and 60% of those with sensory bladders. Bladder retraining clinically cured 62% of those with detrusor overactivity, 75% of those with low compliance bladders, and 81% of those with sensory bladders. However, the relapse rate at 6-months was higher for the oxybutynin group, whereas, those in the bladder retraining group maintained their results better. Changes in bladder stability corresponded to symptom improvement in both groups.

There is Level 1 evidence to suggest that bladder retraining has similar benefits in women with detrusor overactivity as drug therapy available prior to 1996, and may have greater long term benefit.

d) Summary

There appears to be Level 1 evidence to suggest that for women with urge, stress, and mixed urinary incontinence that bladder retraining is more effective than no treatment. Evidence is inconsistent about expected cure rates which may be dependent on when and how the outcome was measured or reflect differences in the bladder retraining protocol. Findings on objective (cystometric) changes do not always correspond to successful subjective change.

One RCT has indicated that bladder retraining and pelvic floor muscle training have similar efficacy; this finding requires further investigation. Bladder retraining appears to have similar benefits as drug therapy available prior to 1996 and may have greater long term benefit.

e) Recommendations

Bladder retraining should be offered as therapy to women with urge, stress, and mixed urinary incontinence.

GRADE OF RECOMMENDATION: A

There is a lack of consistency in bladder retraining protocols. On the basis of extrapolation from the bladder retraining literature, an outpatient retraining protocol should include an initial voiding interval typically beginning at 1 hour during waking hours, which is increased by 15-30 minutes per week depending on tolerance of the schedule (i.e., fewer incontinent episodes than the previous week, minimal interruptions to the schedule, and the woman's feeling of control over urgency), until a 2-3 hour voiding interval is achieved. A shorter initial voiding interval, i.e., 30 minutes or less, may be necessary for women whose baseline urinary diaries reveal an average voiding interval of less than 1 hour. Education should be provided about normal bladder control and methods to control urgency such as distraction and relaxation techniques and pelvic floor muscle contraction. Self-monitoring of voiding behavior using urinary diary or treatment log should be included in order to determine adherence to the schedule, evaluate progress, and determine whether the voiding interval should be changed (Figure 6). Clinicians should monitor progress, determine adjustments to the voiding interval, and provide positive reinforcement to women undergoing bladder retraining at least weekly during the training period. If there is no reduction in incontinent episodes after three weeks of bladder retraining, the patient should be re-evaluated and other treatment options considered. Inpatient bladder retraining programs may follow a more rigid scheduling regimen with progression of the voiding interval on a daily basis.

GRADE OF RECOMMENDATION: C

Further RCTs are needed that compare bladder retraining alone to lifestyle interventions, pelvic floor muscle training, and drug therapies in the management of stress, urge, and mixed incontinence. Studies are also needed to determine the long-term efficacy of bladder retraining.

3. Bladder retraining in combination with other adjuncts (pelvic floor muscle training and medications)

a) Background

Bladder retraining has been used in combination with pelvic floor muscle training, bladder biofeedback, estrogen replacement therapy, and anticholinergic drug therapy in the management of urge, stress, and mixed incontinence. Refer to Section 2 (c) for discussion of bladder retraining protocols.

b) Quality of the data

Seven studies were reviewed that compared bladder retraining with other interventions including placebo interventions. Of these, five are RCTs [164], [165], [166], [94], [75] involving 394 women; and two are nonrandomized controlled trials [167], [68].

One RCT compared bladder retraining with pelvic floor muscle training to bladder retraining alone or pelvic floor muscle training alone [75]; one RCT compared bladder retraining with pelvic floor muscle training to psychotherapy and anticholinergic drug therapy [164] two RCTs compared bladder retraining with anticholinergic drug therapy to bladder retraining with placebo [165], [166] and one RCT compared an inpatient to an outpatient program consisting of bladder retraining and pelvic floor muscle training [94]. One non-randomized controlled trial compared anticholinergic drug therapy with bladder retraining to bladder retraining with placebo [167], and the other compared bladder retraining for women with urge incontinence and bladder retraining and pelvic floor muscle training for women with mixed incontinence to a control group [68].

The age of the study population ranged from 26 [94] to 98 [166]. Some trials included a few men, and it was not possible to determine the effect on women only [166]; 56 women and 4 men. All studies with the exception of one trial [75] investigated the combined effect of bladder retraining with another intervention which may have included a placebo treatment in women with detrusor overactivity, urge incontinence with stable detrusor function, or urge incontinence without known detrusor dysfunction, or sensory bladder. In the one exception, women with urodynamic stress incontinence, detrusor overactivity and/or both diagnoses were included in the study population [75]. Sample sizes ranged from 20 [79] to 204 women [75]. All but one RCT had intervention groups containing 25 or more subjects [164]. Two studies reported power calculations [79], [75], but only one study achieved statistical power [75]. Outcome was measured most frequently by subjective report of cure or improvement [164], [165], [166], [68], [94], [75] and urinary diary [79], [164], [165], [87], [94], [75], followed by urodynamic measures [79], [164], [133], quality of life evaluation [75], pad test [94], and cost [94]. Three studies reported on compliance in the assessment of treatment outcome [68], [166], [75].

Follow-up periods were variable with most studies conducting at least one post-treatment assessment within five days to three months following treatment initiation. One trial included an additional evaluation at six months post-randomization[75]. Longer-term follow-up was completed in one study [87].

c) Results

- **Bladder Retraining with Pelvic Floor Muscle Training Versus Bladder Retraining Alone, Psychotherapy, or Drug Therapy**

Only one trial was found that compared bladder retraining to a combination behavioral intervention program (bladder retraining and pelvic floor muscle training). Although combination therapy resulted in greater reductions in incontinent episodes and improvements in quality of life at three months post-randomization, the results suggest that bladder retraining is as effective as combination therapy when evaluation occurs six months post-randomization. In Wyman's previously cited study [75] cure rates as determined by a 7-day urinary diary

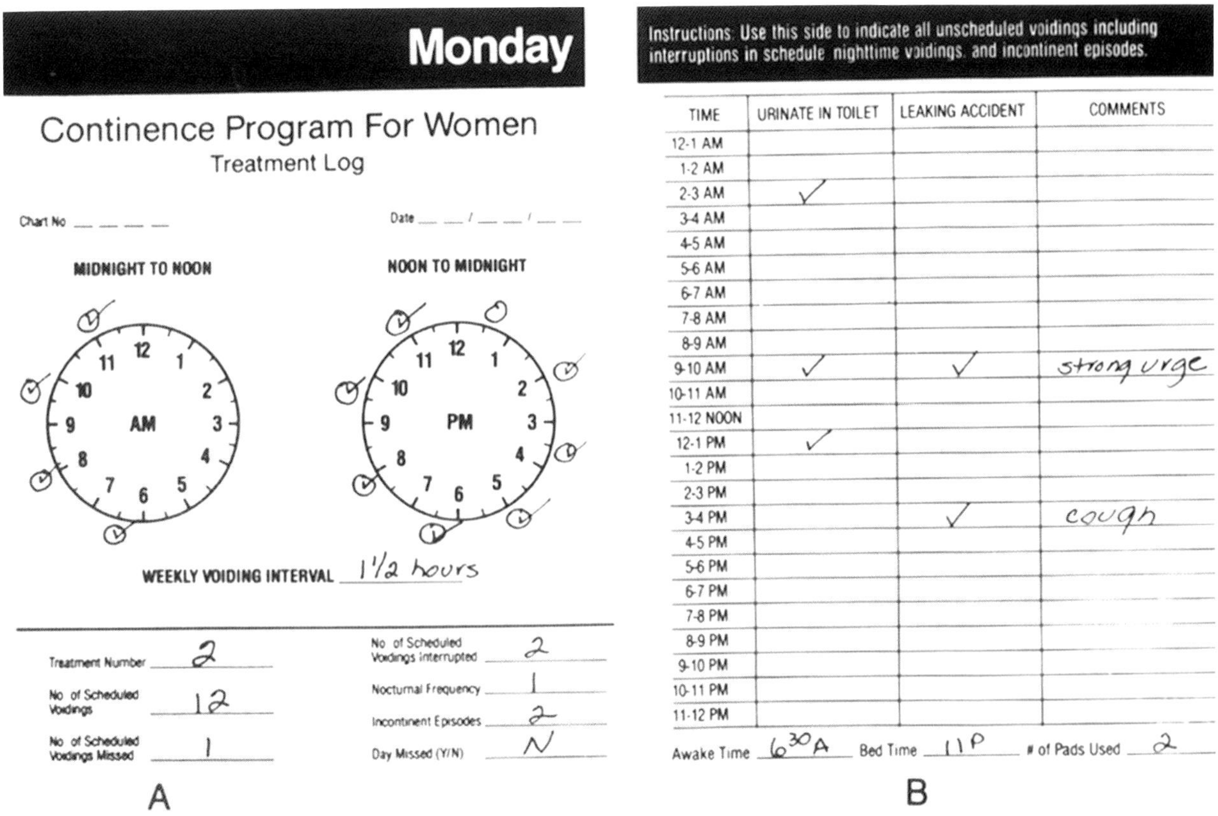

Monday

Continence Program For Women

Treatment Log

Chart No __ __ __ __ Date __ / __ / __

MIDNIGHT TO NOON — NOON TO MIDNIGHT

WEEKLY VOIDING INTERVAL 1 1/2 hours

Treatment Number	2	No of Scheduled Voidings Interrupted	2
No of Scheduled Voidings	12	Nocturnal Frequency	1
No of Scheduled Voidings Missed	1	Incontinent Episodes	2
		Day Missed (Y/N)	N

A

Instructions: Use this side to indicate all unscheduled voidings including interruptions in schedule nighttime voidings, and incontinent episodes.

TIME	URINATE IN TOILET	LEAKING ACCIDENT	COMMENTS
12-1 AM			
1-2 AM			
2-3 AM	✓		
3-4 AM			
4-5 AM			
5-6 AM			
6-7 AM			
7-8 AM			
8-9 AM			
9-10 AM	✓	✓	strong urge
10-11 AM			
11-12 NOON			
12-1 PM	✓		
1-2 PM			
2-3 PM			
3-4 PM		✓	cough
4-5 PM			
5-6 PM			
6-7 PM			
7-8 PM			
8-9 PM			
9-10 PM			
10-11 PM			
11-12 PM			

Awake Time 6^30 A Bed Time 11 P # of Pads Used 2

B

Figure 6 a, b : Bladder retraining self-monitoring

at 3 months post-randomization were 31% in the combination therapy group, whereas it was 18% in the bladder retraining group. Improvement rates (i.e., 50% or greater reduction in incontinent episodes) were 70% in the combination therapy group, whereas they were 51% in the bladder retraining group. However, by 6 months post-randomization, both cure and improvement rates in combination therapy had dropped (27% and 59%, respectively), whereas cure and improvement rates were better maintained in the bladder retraining group (16% and 41%, respectively). Women with urodynamic stress incontinence or detrusor overactivity with and without stress incontinence had similar reductions in incontinent episodes at the 3 and 6 months post-randomization evaluations.

The effectiveness of bladder retraining in combination with pelvic floor muscle training as compared to bladder retraining alone is as yet unclear and further investigation is warranted (Level 1).

In another RCT, bladder retraining with pelvic floor muscle training was compared to brief psychotherapy or drug therapy (propantheline) in women with detrusor overactivity and sensory-urgency syndrome [164]. Incontinent episodes and nocturia as measured by a 7-day urinary diary were significantly reduced in the psychotherapy group but not in the bladder retraining or drug therapy groups at 12 weeks post-treatment initiation. Improvement in the bladder retraining group was associated with cystometric improvements in detrusor pressure.

An RCT that compared an impatient to an outpatient program of bladder retraining and pelvic floor muscle training reported that an outpatient program was as effective and could be conducted at less cost [94]. Subjective cure/improvement rates were 63% in both groups, dry pad testing had similar rates in inpatients (70%) as outpatients (77%), and cure rates at 3 months (defined as no incontinent episodes on a urinary diary) were similar in inpatients (63%) versus outpatients (53%).

• Bladder Retraining with Drug Therapy

Three trials comparing anticholinergic drug therapy with bladder retraining to bladder retraining with placebo [167], [165], [166] were not consistent with respect to the additive benefit when combining bladder retraining with anticholinergic drug therapy in the treatment of detrusor overactivity. Szonyi et al., [166] using a double-blind placebo controlled, parallel group design found no difference between 2.5 mg of oxybutynin twice daily with bladder retraining versus the placebo group (bladder retraining and placebo) in reducing incontinent episodes or nocturia. However, the investigators concluded that the drug group was superior to the placebo (bladder retraining) group because it had greater subjective benefit (86% versus 55%). Another study using a similar research design reported no difference between the placebo (bladder retraining and placebo) and 25 mg of terodiline with bladder retraining in reducing incontinent episodes [165]. In contrast, one nonrandomized, double-blinded placebo controlled design found that terodiline with bladder retraining was superior to bladder retraining and placebo [167] on both objective and subjective measures.

The effectiveness of adding bladder retraining to drug therapy and vice versa is unclear, and requires further investigation (Level 1/2).

d) Summary

The effectiveness of bladder retraining in combination with pelvic floor muscle training in comparison to bladder retraining alone is unclear, and further investigation is warranted (Level 1). The one RCT available suggests that the long-term benefit of bladder retraining alone may be similar to that of bladder retraining combined with pelvic floor muscle training. Additional benefit of combining bladder retraining with drug therapy available prior to 1996 was not consistently noted.

e) Recommendations

Further RCTs are needed that compare the additive benefit of bladder retraining to lifestyle interventions, pelvic floor muscle training, and drug therapies in the treatment of urinary incontinence. In addition, research is needed to determine subgroups of patients who will derive the greatest benefit from bladder retraining alone or in combination with pelvic floor muscle training or drug therapy.

4. Factors affecting outcomes of bladder retraining

Analysis of factors affecting treatment outcome is problematic in most published studies due to low power with relatively small subgroups. Nine of the 12 trials reported on factors affecting the outcomes of bladder retraining. Of these, three trials reported on factors affecting outcomes associated with bladder retraining as the sole therapy [147], [161], [75]. One study reported that age was not a factor in treatment outcome [147]. Compliance was mentioned as a factor affecting treatment outcome in a small study [68] but not in a larger study comparing the efficacy of bladder retraining to pelvic floor muscle training alone and combination behavioral therapy [75].

There is conflicting evidence of whether symptomatology, urodynamic diagnosis, or urodynamic parameters affect treatment outcome. Two RCTs found that urodynamic diagnosis (urodynamic stress incontinence, detrusor overactivity, or both) had no effect on treatment outcome whether measured by urinary diaries or standardized quality of life instrument, and change back to normal function did not correlate to an improvement in incontinence severity [147], [162],[75], [133]. However, two other RCTs found that those patients who became subjectively continent reverted back to normal detrusor function [159], [160]. One trial found that patients with sensory bladders did better than those with detrusor overactivity or low compliance bladders [161]. One trial conducting a five-year follow-up found subjects with urge or mixed incontinence were least likely to maintain their results [87].

5. Adverse effects associated with bladder retraining

Four of the 12 studies reviewed made a statement about adverse effects associated with bladder retraining [159], [160], [147], [161]. In these studies, there were no reported adverse effects. Although the reporting of adverse effects was poor across studies, it appears that bladder retraining is safe and acceptable to patients.

V. ANTI-INCONTINENCE DEVICES IN THE FEMALE PATIENT

1. Introduction

Urinary loss in the female patient may be the result of overactivity or underactivity of the detrusor or outlet, alone or in combination. Devices may act to correct, compensate for, or circumvent the pathology of the detrusor or outlet, in order to improve urinary storage and/or emptying. Varying levels of manual dexterity are required of the patient, depending on the type of device. For some devices, health care provider intervention may be necessary for device sizing, training, prescribing, and/or device insertion and replacement at regular intervals.

The devices reviewed in this section are not permanently implanted into the female patient, but are extra-urethral, intra-vaginal or intra-urethral. The devices may be disposable or re-usable following each voiding episode, or may be replaced daily, after several days, or may be left indwelling for up to 28 days. The Food and Drug Association (United States FDA) defines a device as 'non-implant' only if it is left indwelling for less than 28 days. Devices designed for chronic intra-urethral usage must be replaced within this time interval.

Pessaries, the most commonly utilized devices for prolapse and incontinence, have never been subjected to an

RCT or compared to other devices. Most reports of device usage, prior to 1995 are descriptive or laboratory based, but more recent studies have provided more subjective and objective data, and have incorporated quality of life assessment.

There are four RCTs (two articles and two abstracts) among the reports published in this section. Device protocols rarely have employed a non-treatment group, cannot easily employ a 'placebo' model, and are usually designed as open longitudinal studies, utilizing the patients' baseline data as the control. Comparison studies between devices are needed, which ideally should be randomized and 'crossover' designed, and one such study is included. There is only one abstract and one paper which compares two different devices, no studies which compare device use to other forms of conservative or surgical therapy, and no publications which report cost-effectiveness data.

Urinary incontinence is a 'quality of life' issue, and physician and patient "acceptability", in addition to the literature reports of efficacy and safety, have been a major determinant of clinical and commercial success. Of note, many devices have demonstrated higher efficacy and quality of life scores during laboratory observation and clinical trial settings, than in clinical practice. A simple explanation may be that health care provider support, during clinical trials, may improve patient willingness to complete the protocol and improve satisfaction. Patient willingness to perform instrumentation may vary by device type, the anatomic location of placement, and the perceived level of invasiveness. Prashar [131] utilized a ten item questionnaire, given to 104 consecutive women, and reported attitudes to becoming familiar with genital anatomy and placing devices into the vagina or upon the urethra. Only 30% of the women were quite comfortable about the concept of touching their genitalia and this attitude was age dependent. Only 21% were willing to insert a continence device into their vagina, varying weakly with age but significantly affected by previous tampon or diaphragm usage. Only 15% felt very comfortable about placing a continence device on to their urethra, and this was not affected by age and was only slightly more common in previous tampon users. Older women were less likely to understand the anatomy of their genitalia or to be comfortable about the idea of exploring it, but age was no barrier to willingness to employ a urethral or vaginal continence device.

Additionally, the denominator for 'patient satisfaction' may not reflect device acceptance in clinical use, since 'intent to treat' patients, who are initially screened, but do not want to utilize the device, may not be included in the patient satisfaction data, and patients who 'drop out' of the study due to adverse events or dissatisfaction, may be included in safety data, but are often excluded from efficacy and quality of life assessments at the termination of the study. Consequently, many of the devices which have performed adequately in clinical studies have not achieved acceptance by physicians and patients in clinical practice, or attained commercial success. Many of the devices which are included in the review, have been approved by regulatory agencies but are no longer marketed.

This sub-chapter will examine the evidence for the management of urinary incontinence using non-implanted devices in the non-neurogenic female patient. A summary of the search strategy is given in Appendix 1.

There are an increasing number of more carefully designed studies since the initial review, including 4 RCTs (2 abstracts and 2 papers), but to date, there is only one abstract and one paper comparing two different non-implant devices. There are no studies comparing device use to pad use or other forms of conservative therapy, or to surgical intervention. Although there is increasing data supporting the efficacy and tolerability of intra-vaginal support, extra-urethral occlusive, and intra-urethral devices, there has not been wide clinical acceptance by physicians or patients for device use in the ambulatory female population for the treatment of urodynamic stress incontinence.

2. Devices that treat incontinence secondary to failure to empty (detrusor underactivity / outlet overactivity) in the non-neurogenic adult female

a) Background

Failure to empty the bladder decreases functional bladder capacity. The non-neurogenic adult female may demonstrate the symptoms and signs of overflow incontinence. The acute and chronic management of these patients and the indications for catheterisation are reviewed in the section on treatment of the neurogenic patient.

b) Quality of included studies

Treatment for urinary retention may involve an indwelling catheter, intermittent catheterisation, or the monitoring of clinical parameters during continued overflow voiding. There have been no published studies on the use of catheter drainage in the ambulatory population. In a descriptive study of 15 patients, without controls, Nativ [168] described a sphincter-pump prosthesis, composed of a self retaining silicone catheter with a self contained urinary pump (flow 10-12 cc/sec), which is activated by a small hand-held control device for bladder emptying (Figure 7 (In-Flow / SRS Medical). A physician must change the device.

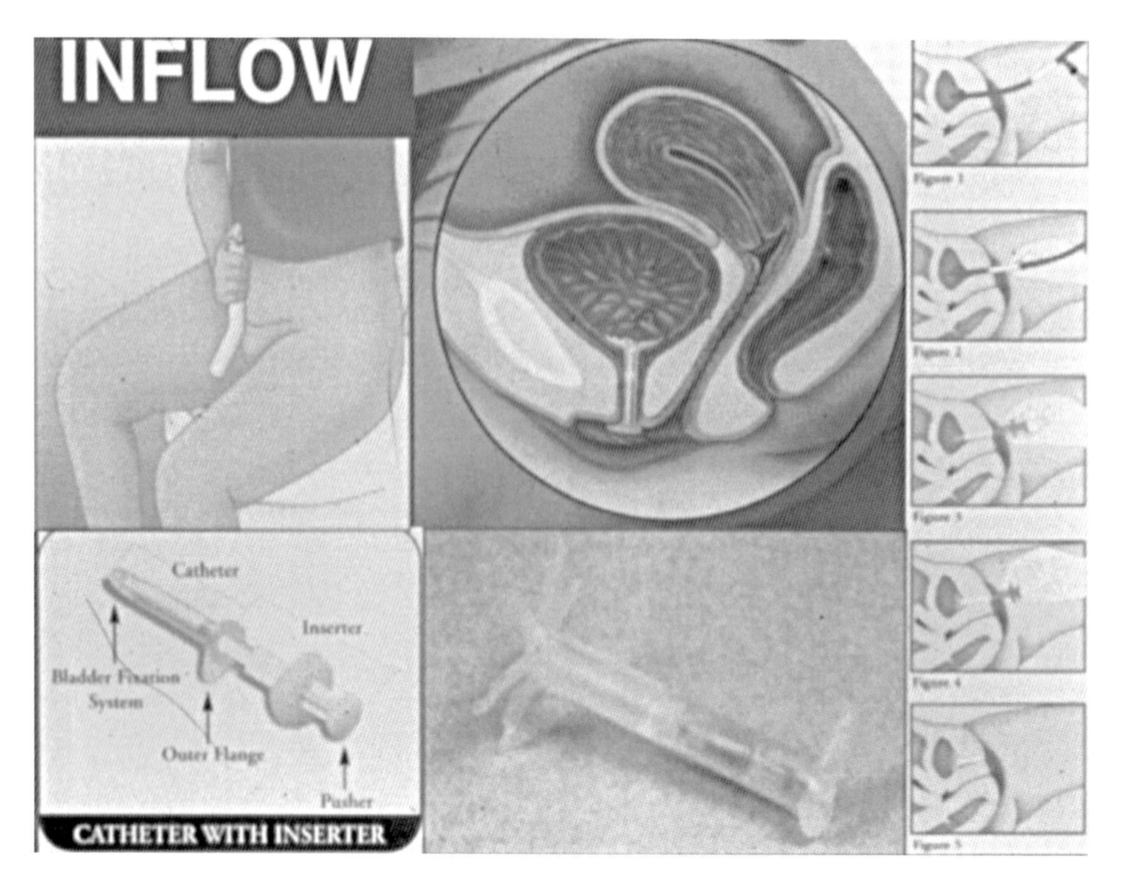

Figure 7 : Inflow device (clockwise from upper left: hand held control device, device in place, device insertion, device open, device prior to insertion

c) Results

The In-Flow device improved continence and bladder emptying in this single report, with minimal morbidity, but the study was short term, and there were no specific comments on effects of the device on urethral integrity.

d) Summary

Treatment of urinary retention may be accomplished by observation, indwelling or intermittent catheterisation. Newer technologies for bladder emptying will require further study. (Level of evidence: 4).

e) Recommendations

Newer technologies, which do not require external collection of urine, utilizing indwelling mechanical urethral valves and pumps, may provide an alternative for carefully selected patients. This area should be identified as an important topic for future research.

GRADE OF RECOMMENDATION: D.

3. Devices that treat failure to store (outlet underactivity) in the non-neurogenic ambulatory adult female population

Introduction

Failure to store secondary to decreased outlet activity may be manifested in the symptoms and signs of urodynamic stress incontinence (USI). Treatment of this condition with devices has been reported utilizing:

1) External urinary collection,

2) Intravaginal support of the bladder neck, and

3) Blockage of urinary leakage by occluding egress,

- **i) at the external meatus, or**
- **ii) with an intraurethral device.**

1) External collection devices

a) Background

The use of pads, diapers and incontinence pants are discussed in page 666. Female external collecting devices are placed over the urethral meatus or within the introital area, are secured by straps, adhesive or suction, and empty into an external drainage bag. These devices can be utilized for failure to store secondary to an underactive outlet or an overactive bladder. These devices have been developed, tested, and a few reports on their use have been published, but they have not been widely distributed or sold.

b) Quality of included studies

Studies describing devices for the collection of urine in female patients are descriptive, and were performed on patients in a rehabilitation center or nursing home, and not in the ambulatory population. Edwards [169], Bonnar [170], and Cardozo [171] reported on devices of historical interest, which are not commercially available.

c) Summary

External collecting devices for the ambulatory female patient are cumbersome and have demonstrated low efficacy. There are no devices in clinical use.

Previous devices have failed to solve the problems of: 1) sizing, due to variations in anatomy, 2) providing an effective and comfortable meatal or vaginal locator, 3) developing an anchoring method with suction and/or adhesion, that coapts without tissue injury, 4) allowing duration of usage, and 5) adjusting to the degree of mobility of the patients (Level of evidence: 5).

d) Recommendation

The development of a product for the external collection of urine in the ambulatory and non-ambulatory female patient is a very important area for future research.

GRADE OF RECOMMENDATION :D

There are currently no adequate collection devices for the ambulatory female population.

2) Intravaginal devices which support the bladder neck

a) Background

Support of the bladder neck to correct urodynamic stress incontinence has been achieved, with varying success utilizing traditional i) tampons, ii) pessaries and contraceptive diaphragms, and iii) intravaginal devices specifically designed to support the bladder neck.

b) Quality of included studies

• Tampons/pessaries:

Nygaard[172] performed a prospective, randomized, single blind, and laboratory based study testing 18 patients (age 33-73) with three 40 minute standardized aerobics sessions, utilizing either a Hodge pessary, a super tampon, or no device and measuring urinary loss by pad weight (PdWt).

• Diaphragms / Pessaries:

Realini [173]analyzed the benefit for one week, in 10 selected patients of a coil-type diaphragm ring, which was softer than a pessary, utilizing diaries and a two hour pad test. Suarez [174] included urodynamic testing in his evaluation of a contraceptive diaphragm in 12 patients. Bhatia [175], [176] reported on the urodynamic effects of a Smith Hodge pessary, and suggested this as a modality to predict the outcome for bladder neck support surgery.

• Specific bladder neck support devices:

Included in this category are:

1. Removable reusable intra-vaginal ring, composed of silastic, and constructed with two prongs which are placed behind the symphysis to support the bladder neck (Introl, no current distributor) Biswas [177], Davila [178], [179], Moore [180],[181] and Kondo [182] (Figure 8).

   The pilot study by Biswas [177], the developer of the device, was a laboratory study, which employed a straining cystogram. Following this study, the number of device sizes was increased from 8 to 25. A variety of different protocols were employed to study efficacy, safety and satisfaction by Davila [178],[179], Moore [180],[181] and Kondo [182]. In general, a voiding diary which specified voiding and leakage episodes and a one hour pad weight test (PdWt-1hr) were utilized as the primary pre and post device use objective parameters, and a quality of life (QOL) instrument was utilized by all investigators. Of specific interest, is that in the trial by Moore [181] one third of the women were identified as having undergone previous vaginal surgery or colposuspension, and the three gynaecologists who fitted the patients had no prior knowledge of how to fit the device. Study periods varied from three to four weeks [177, 179], 12 weeks ([181] and 6 months [182].

2. Three different single use disposable devices:

- a clam-type device composed of polyurethrane foam, which is folded up upon its long axis and placed into the sagittal plane in the vagina, and when moistened, its dimensions expand by 30% and create a supportive cushion under the urethrovesical junction (Conveen Continence Guard, Coloplast, Denmark) (Figure 9a, 9b) ([183],[184],[185]
- a newer version of the expanding polyurethrane design, with similarities to a tampon, recently reported in an abstract (Coloplast, Denmark) (Figure 10) [124], and
- an expanding polyvinyl alcohol sponge (Ladycon, Home Care Engros, Norway) [124]

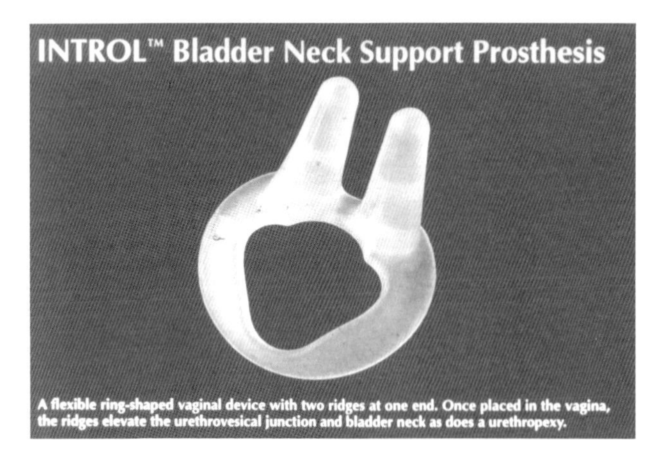

INTROL™ Bladder Neck Support Prosthesis
A flexible ring-shaped vaginal device with two ridges at one end. Once placed in the vagina, the ridges elevate the urethrovesical junction and bladder neck as does a urethropexy.

FIgure 8 : Introl bladder neck support prosthesis

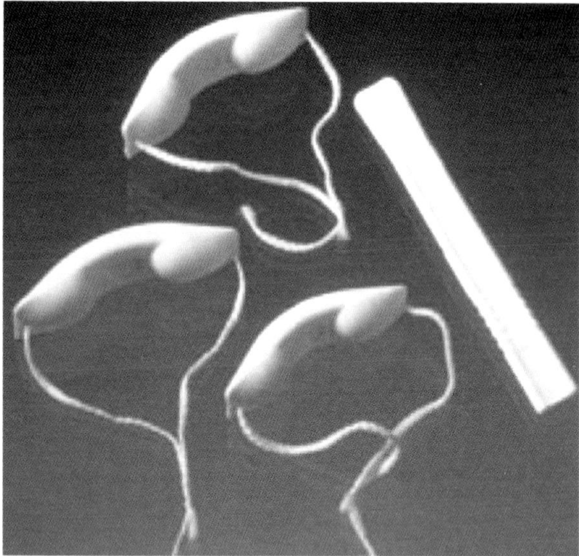

Figure 9 a : Conveen "clam" type devices with inserter

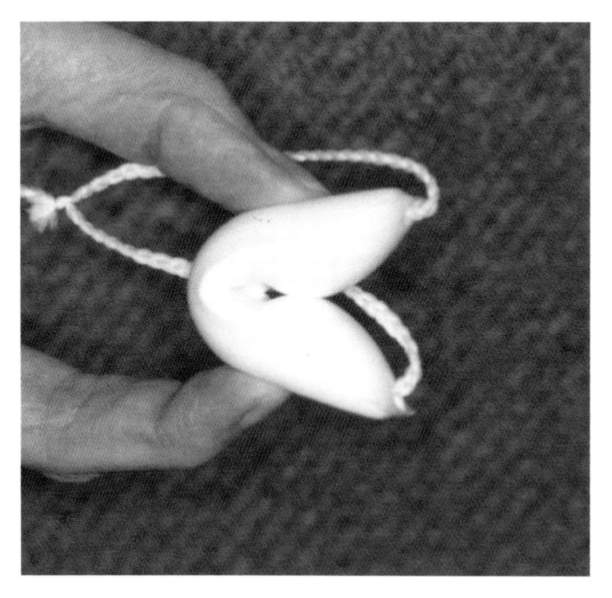

Figure 9 b: Conveen device (compressed by fingers) into functional position assumed in vagina.

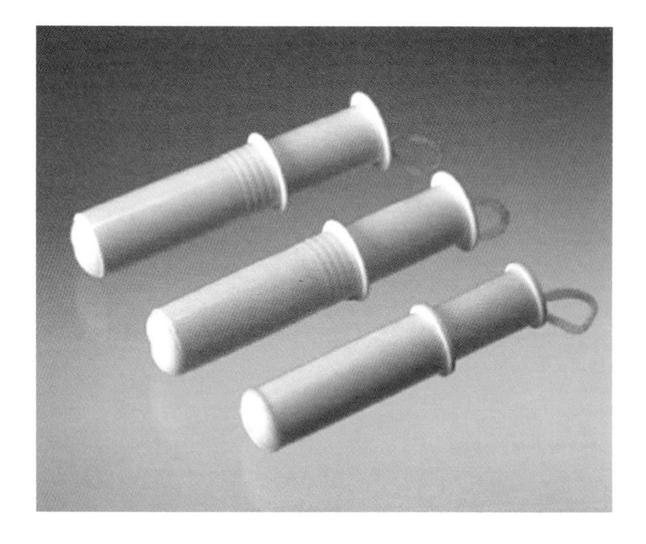

Figure 10 : Conveen "tampon" types within inserters.

Thyssen [184], [183], Hahn [185] and Bidmead [124] utilized PdWt and diary data as objective parameters and employed QOL instruments. Of specific interest, the abstract by Bidmead [124] which reported a new version of the device described as a continence "tampon", utilized a crossover design, employing two five week trials comparing the original and newer device. The report on the polyvinyl sponge, by Glavind[186] was an acute laboratory study of only six women utilizing a PdWt measurement during 30 minutes of aerobic exercise.

c) *Results*

• Tampons and Diaphragms:

Continence rates were 6/14 cured and 2/14 improved with tampons [172], 4/10 improved with a diaphragm [173], and 9/12 with an oversized contraceptive diaphragm [174].

• Specific bladder neck support prostheses:

Due to significant differences in device design, the outcomes for the studies of the silastic device should not be compared with the polyurethrane and polyvinyl devices, which share similar modes of function. Of note, all studies demonstrate an improvement in continence by the methods employed. Studies performed in the acute setting, regardless of the device type, demonstrate better performance than diary based studies performed over time. Efficacy is also higher in patients with minimal to moderate urinary leakage.

• Reusable intra-vaginal silastic device.

Biswas [177] determined that 86% of the patients were continent with the device in place on cystogram.

Davila [179] in the intial study demonstrated that (83%) of patients were dry on PdWt. On further and more detailed study, Davila found a statistically significant reduction in incontinence on PdWt (USI, mean 46.6 to 16.6g; mixed incontinence, mean 31.9 to 6.8 g) and in the bladder diary, mean 28.6 to 7.8 losses per week; mixed incontinence, mean 30.2 to 15 losses per week). QOL improved in both groups. Side effects included five urinary tract infections and 23 cases of vaginal mucosal soreness or mild irritation[178].

Moore[181] detailed problems with both sizing and efficacy. Of the 80 recruits, four could not be fitted, and 11 did not satisfy all entry criteria. Of the 65 participants, 39 (60%) withdrew; 20 for distorted vaginal anatomy which made fitting difficult, five for lack of efficacy, four for constipation, and ten for unrelated patient events. In the remaining 26 patients, PdWt decreased from a baseline median of 19 g to 2 g ($p<0.001$), 62% were continent, and 15% were >50% improved, and wished no further therapy. Moore concluded that the device was difficult to fit in women who have had multiple vaginal surgeries or were oestrogen deficient. Long-term follow-up showed that 18 of 26 (from the original 65) continued to wear the device at six months (interim dropouts being due to intercurrent illness in half, the remainder had declining efficacy). Of these, 78% continued to wear the device for a minimum follow-up of two years. In a separate study of patients with mixed incontinence by Moore [181], of the 21 recruits, five never wore the device home, leaving 16 participants. A further two did not reach week four, because of poor efficacy or inability to fit the device. In the 14 who reached week four, the median number of leaks/day declined from 4.3 to 1.0 ($p = 0.002$). Median PdWt loss fell from 53 to 7g ($p = 0.012$). Cystometry showed an increase in maximum bladder capacity ($p < 0.05$) and a modest reduction in severity of detrusor overactivity, with no evidence of outflow obstruction. Three women discontinued because of poor efficacy or a poorly fitting device, leaving 11 of 16 participants (69%) at week eight, when median PdWt decreased to 2mL.

Kondo [182] found no urinary flow obstruction with the device in place. Urine loss decreased from 20.6 to 4.8 gm. per hour ($p < 0.001$) on the 60-minute PdWt. Twenty two patients (29%), reported complete continence, and 39 (51%) had decreased severity of incontinence by more than 50%. Minor adverse effects occurred in 26% of the patients. According to the global usefulness rating which was employed, 62 patients (81%) had some or maximum benefit.

• Disposable polyurethane and polyvinyl devices:

Thyssen [183],([42]) reported on 19/22 women with stress incontinence, subjectively and objectively cured or improved in a short-term study, and who then continued the treatment with the device for one year. All 19 completed the study, 13 (68%) were subjectively dry, (26%) were improved and one (5%) reported unchanged incontinence. All but one had decreased leakage at the 24-PdWt, and 67% a greater than 50% decrease. Subjectively cure was 41%, and 36% were dry on 24 hour pad test. Overall reduced leakage was statistically significant ($p < 0.0005$) No significant changes were found in the other urodynamic measurements, specifically, urinary flow rate.

Hahn [185] reported on 121 women, in a four week study. Patients dropped out because of vaginal irritation (25%), other product related reasons (6%), lack of time (6%), or failure to complete a user questionnaire. Of the remaining 90 (mean age 47.5), 85 performed a 24 PdWt, which showed that baseline leakage of 42 ml/ 24h decreased to 14 ml/ 24h ($p <0.001$). Of these, 39 (46%) were continent. The device was considered unpleasant by 8%, and caused some local discomfort in 62% on direct questioning: 75% of these wished to continue using the device. The authors noted that older women (age 56-65) tolerated the device and appeared more motivated to continue. Coexistent atrophic vaginitis and the use of topical oestrogen was not discussed.

In the third study, by Thyssen [184] subjective cure in 11/55 women (20%) and improvement in 27/55 (49%) was reported. The 24-hour PdWt mean leakage and episodes in the voiding diary significantly decreased. After three months, 55 (58%) of patients desired to continue device usage. The IOQ showed highly significant improvement, as well as two additional incontinence related quality of life questionnaires. Responses to the SF-36 general health questionnaire showed no significant changes.

Bidmead[124] reported on 61 women recruited in a RCT , which compared the "clam" to the "tampon" device. Only 38 (62%) completed the study due to discomfort or lack of efficacy. Thirty-six women desired to continue device use following the study, with 73% preferring the "tampon" type design for its ease of use.

d) Summary

Support of the bladder neck resulting in improved continence is possible with intravaginal devices without causing significant lower urinary tract obstruction or morbidity.

Efficacy with the Introl silastic pronged "pessary" device ranged from 65-90% reduction in PdWt with 29-83% dry and 15-50% improved [179], [178], [182], [181], [180]. At six months 32%, and at two years 22% of patients continued device use [182]. The major problem appears to be with sizing, especially in patients with prior vaginal surgery or with vaginal atrophy [182]. The device is re-usable so a fix cost following purchase is to be expected. The device is not currently marketed.

Efficacy with the Conveen polyurethrane expanding "clam" device ranged from 20-68% of patients subjectively dry [185], [124] and 49% improved [184]. There was a 66% reduction in PdWt, with 46% of patients continent. At one month 75% of patients [185] and at three months 58% [124] continued device use, with 73% preferring the "tampon" type device. The device is worn for 24 hours and is disposable. Difficulty with insertion is improved with the "tampon" over the "clam" version. The device is currently marketed (Coloplast – www.coloplast.com). The polyvinyl tampon device was tested only in the laboratory during aerobic exercise [186]. It is currently marketed (Home Care Engros).

Patients must accept the mode of treatment and have proper anatomy and manual dexterity. Relatively high drop-out rates in monitored studies, during which patient support is provided, indicates the need for proper patient selection and patient and provider education. (Level of Evidence = 2)

e) Recommendation

Vaginal support devices should be included in the treatment options when managing women with stress urinary incontinence, dependent upon the availability of product, patient acceptance, and cost and especially in younger patients who may be contemplating further pregnancies. However, long-term results are not available and studies comparing these therapies to other forms of conservative therapy or surgery have not been performed.

GRADE OF RECOMMENDATION B

Support of the bladder neck, resulting in improved continence, is possible with intravaginal devices without causing significant lower urinary tract obstruction or morbidity, but require patient acceptance and a degree of manual dexterity for use.

3) Blockage of urinary leakage by occluding egress - occlusive devices

i) Blockage at the external meatus

a) Background

Devices have been developed which block urinary leakage at the external urethral meatus. Several devices have utilised either adhesive or mild suction to occlude urinary loss at the urethral meatus. In addition to a simple barrier effect, compression of the wall of the distal urethra has been hypothesized to contribute to continence.

Miniguard (no current distributor) (Figure 11) is a triangularly shaped foam device which utilizes an adhesive hydrogel to adhere to the peri-meatal area. The device is single use, removed prior to voiding, and disposable.

FemAssist (no current distributor) (Figure 12 - FemAssist) is a hat-shaped silicone device, that adheres by applying an adhesive gel to the edge of the device, squeezing the central dome and creating a vacuum. The device is then placed over the urethral meatus, and upon release the meatal mucosa is drawn up into the device and the urethral lumen is occluded. Designed and tested in three sizes (3 x 2.5 cm, 2.5 x 2 cm 2 x 2 cm) it may be worn for up to four hours or until voiding, after which the device is washed in hot soapy water and then reapplied. The device is reusable for one week.

CapSure (C. R. Bard, Inc but not currently marketed) is applied and retained by suction. A petroleum based lubricant is applied prior to device use. The device is removed for voiding and re-utilized for up to 2 weeks.

b) Quality of included studies

Urinary diaries and PdWt were employed in all studies

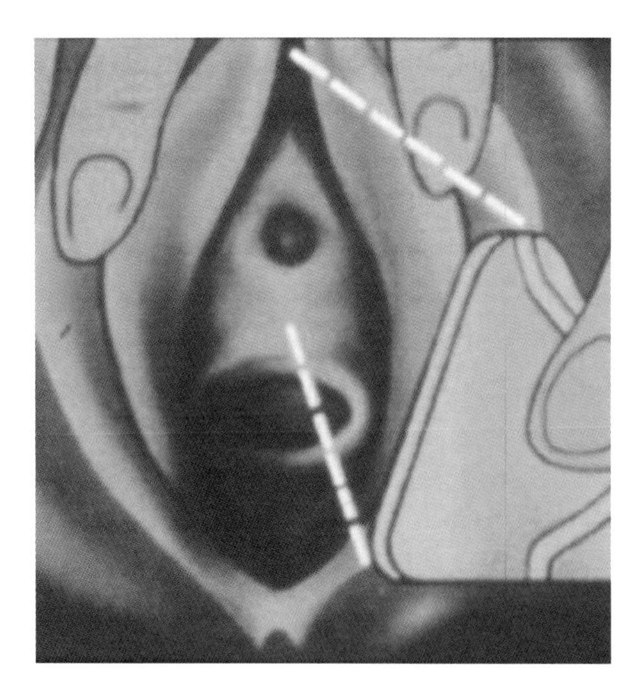

Figure 11: Miniguard

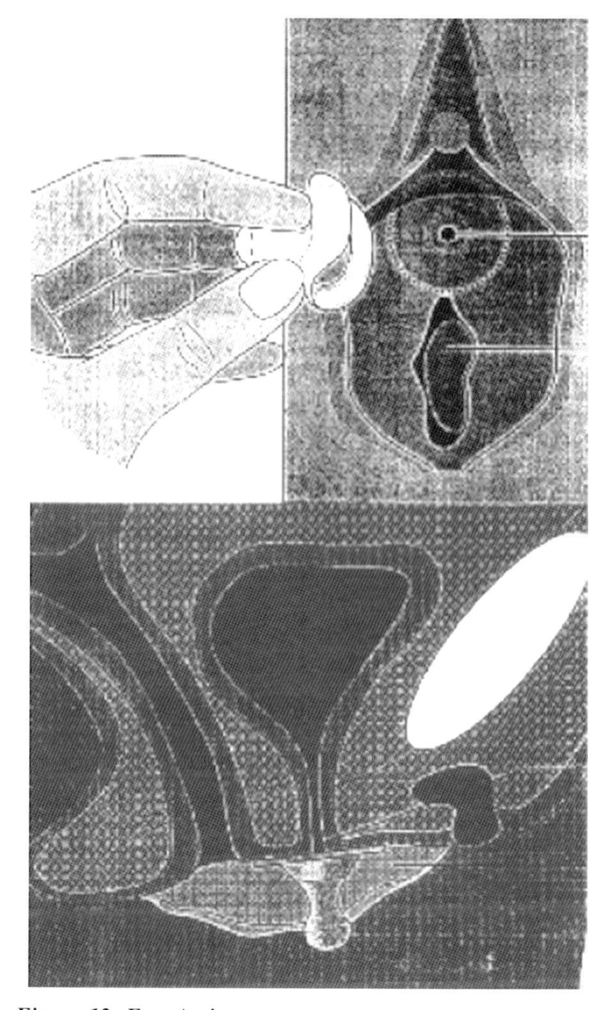

Figure 12: Fem Assist

for objective efficacy measurements [187] (Minguard), [188] (Miniguard), [189] (FemAssist), [181] (FemAssist), [190],[191] (FemAssist), [192] (CapSure).

Incontinence input questionnaires (IIQ), visual analogue score (VAS), QOL, and / or urogenital distress inventory (UDI) were also employed [188], [193], [189], [194], [190], [191], [192].

Study lengths differed from laboratory [190], four weeks [193], [189], [194] to three months [188], [191], [192]. There were no RCT's. Study designs were open and longitudinal.

c) Results

• Miniguard

Eckford[187] analyzed the efficacy of a single application of this device during a one hour pad test which reported that 25% of patients were continent, 50% were improved, but 25% had worse incontinence. Brubaker [188] studied 648 recruited, 411 enrolled, 390 utilizing, and 346 completing patients. Of the 65 women who did not complete the trial, 21 withdrew before device use, 17 were lost to follow-up, 12 withdrew for device related reasons, nine developed an unrelated condition, and there were six protocol violations. Brubaker reported statistically significant objective (12 hour PdWt 15.8g +/- 26.5 to 6.9g +/- 11.5 p<.001) and subjective (leakage questionnaire 10.1 +/- 5.1 to 3.5 +/- 4.3 p<.001 with similar IOQ scores) improvement and no significant change in urinary tract infections, postvoid residual urine volume and cystometric indices. Symptoms of vulvar irritation or lower urinary tract discomfort occurred in a small percentage of subjects but were generally transient, and only three women discontinued using the device. The protocol employed a unique self-instruction method by the patients. Also noted was a persistence of efficacy (p<.001) 4 weeks following device discontinuation.

• FemAssist

Versi [189] reported that the mean pad weight decreased by 47% (P=0.056). Of the nine women who had a positive pad test (>2 g) without the device, five were dry (<2 g) with the device (P<0.05). VAS scores showed a significant improvement for the symptom of stress incontinence (P<0.05). QOL scores improved significantly by 38% (P<0.05) for the IIQ and and 29% (P<0.01) for UDI. Versi [189] studied 155 women with stress or mixed leakage, of whom 133 attempted to use it and 96 enrolled in a four week study. The mean pad test loss fell from 27 g to 9.4 g (p< 0.001) and 49% were dry. Cure was more likely in those with mild incontinence.

Moore [181] reported on 57/100 recruited women who completed a one-month trial. Reduction of incontinence was statistically significant for pad testing, which revealed that 47% of the patients became continent and 33% had more than 50% benefit, while 9% had worse leakage. Those with severe baseline leakage were equally likely to respond as those with mild or moderate pad test loss. Women with stress, urge or mixed incontinence appeared to respond equally well. Dropouts included 13% who were unwilling to utilize the device [188].

Tincello [190] found the median (range) loss with and without the device was 4.9 (0-65) ml and 21 (1-94), respectively (P< 0.01); and 20 patients were less wet when using the device. The median (range) VAS scores were; discomfort 35 (4-93), embarrassment 11 (0- 75), and acceptability 65 (3-100). Discomfort was greater among the women with a greater loss. The acceptability correlated negatively with discomfort (r = -0.53) and negatively with embarrassment (r = 0.39); 15 patients (56%) reported that they would use the device in the long-term. Tincello [191] reported that 10/41 women (24.4%) declined to participate and six (14.6%) withdrew before two weeks. Ten (24.4%) failed to attend for two-week follow-up and 11 (26.8%) did not continue for three months. Two (4.9%) did not attend three-month follow-up. Only two women (4.9%) completed the study. There was no difference in pad test results or in results from voiding diaries. The urinary incontinence device had low acceptability and was ineffective, and we cannot recommend it for nonsurgical management of urodynamic stress incontinence.

• **Capsure**

Bellin [192] reported on 88/100 completers after 12 weeks, with 82% elimination of leakage on Pad- Wt, 91% continent on provocative stress test (single cough assessment of leakage), and 48 percent dry and 40% improved on urinary diaries. Pad-Wt leakage decreased from 6.67 gm (.55-25.95 range) to .19 gm (0-2.5 range) by week 12. Five patients withdrew secondary to vaginal irritation and three due to poor device fit.

d) Summary

External urethral occlusive devices were found to be of varying efficacy, with minimal morbidity. Efficacy of the combined studies reveals a continence rate of approximately 50% dry and 2/3 of patients improved. Of note, the studies by Tincello [190],[191] suggested poorer efficacy and patient satisfaction with the FemAssist device, in distinction to other studies utilizing this device.

Adherence to the peri-meatal area is essential, as all devices are occlusive, achieving the effect by either blocking at the meatus or compressing the distal urethral lumen, as opposed to absorptive. However, the method and degree of adherence is the determining factor for the type and severity of local irritation. Patient selection based on motivation, appropriate anatomy, and manual dexterity, in combination with efficacy and morbidity will determine overall satisfaction. There is no data which compares one extra-urethral device to another, or to incontinence pads. A single RCT comparing extra-urethral and intra-urethral devices is reviewed in the section on intra-urethral devices (see below). Cost comparisons for disposable versus short-term reusable devices are not available. Efficacy for different grades of incontinence has not been established. The objective degree of continence improvement in the clinical laboratory (pad and stress tests) is greater than in community use (diaries). (Level of evidence = 3/4)

e) Recommendation

Further research of the role of devices which block urinary leakage at the external urinary meatus are recommended. One half of patients utilizing these devices in monitored studies were dry and 2/3 of the patients were improved with minimal morbidity. These devices have a role in the algorithm of conservative treatment based on patient acceptance, availability and cost, especially in those patients with mild or moderate stress incontinence who prefer to avoid pads or surgery. (Grade of Recommendation C).

External patch in cup devices placed over the urethral meatus, and held in place by an adhesive or mild suction have demonstrated efficacy with minimal morbidity.

ii) Intraurethral devices

a) Background

Similarities among the devices which are inserted into the urethra to prevent urinary leakage include a method to prevent intravesical migration with a meatal plate, enhance retention within the urethra, (by utilizing spheres, dilations, inflatable balloons, or flanges), and accomplish bladder emptying, by removal of the device. None of the devices are recommended for re-use after removal. The FemSoft (Rochester Medical Corporation) (Figure 13) is currently distributed, but the Viva and Reliance (Figure 14, 15) devices, which are also reviewed in this sub-section, are not currently marketed.

b) Quality of included studies

Neilsen [140],[195] and Pechers [196] studied patients who utilized a disposable plastic device composed of an oval meatal plate, a soft stalk with a removable semi-rigid guide, and spheres along the stalk (Viva). Peschers screened 53 patients with USI and 21 patients accepted treatment with the two sphere device. During a four month study, the investigators analyzed subjective improvement and performed pad-weight and cough tests [196].

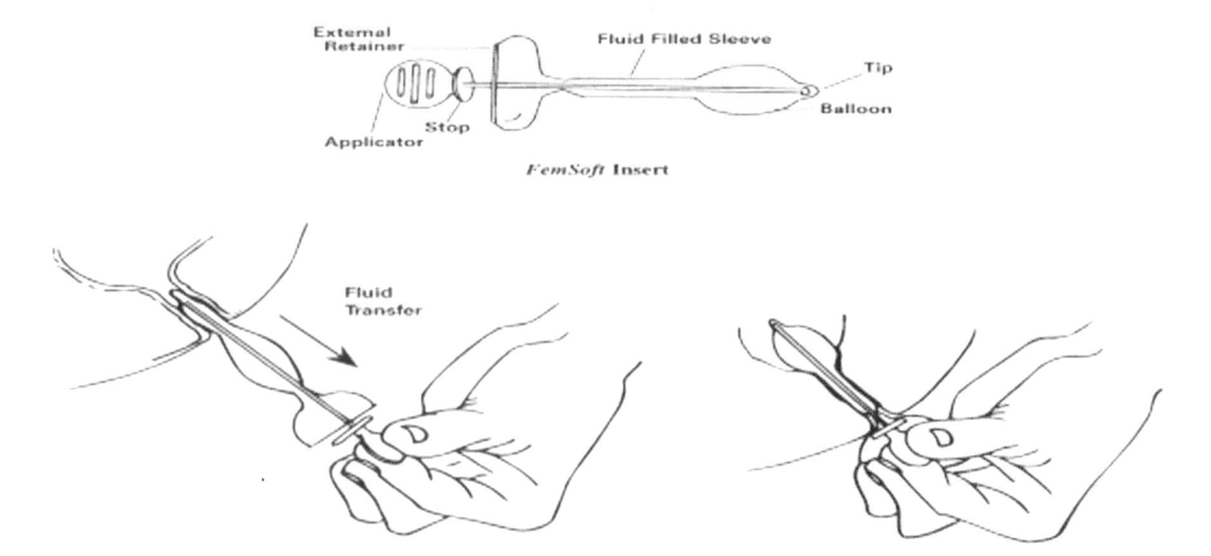

Figure 13 : Femsoft – Urethral Insert

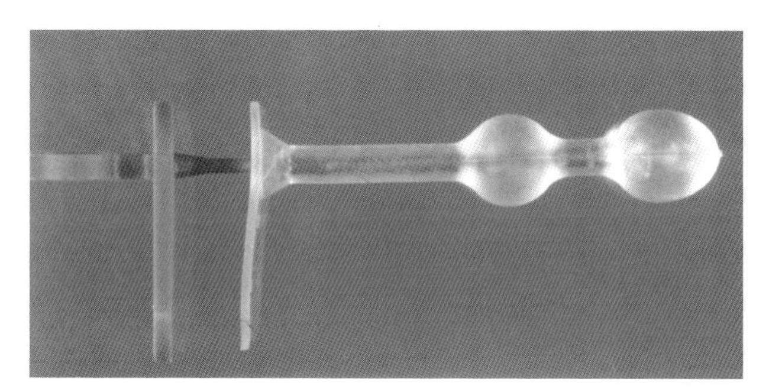

Figure 14 : Urethral plug

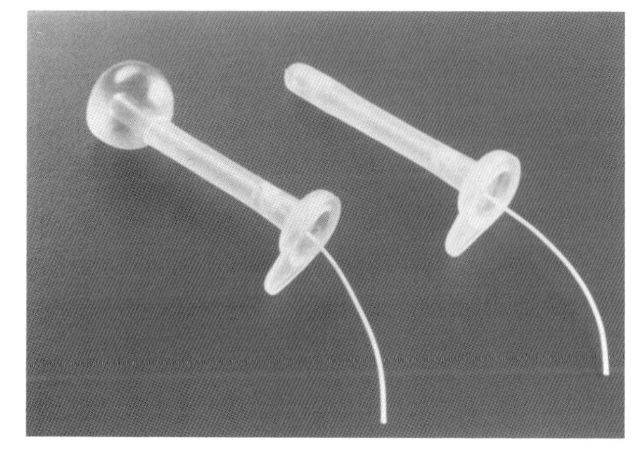

Figure 15 : Reliance insert

Staskin [197] reported on a four month study of 135 of 215 patients who utilized a disposable balloon tipped urethral insert made from thermoplastic elastomer, inflated with an applicator on insertion and deflated by pulling a string at the meatal plate for removal during voiding (Reliance). Primary outcome included a laboratory PdWt-1hr. The patients reported on diary and quality of life questionaires. Miller [198] and Sand [199] reported on 63 of the 135 patients from the above cohort who continued to utilize the balloon tipped intra-urethral insert for one year.

Boos [200] reported in an abstract, a randomized prospective parallel group trial comparing the Reliance [197], [198], [199] intra-urethral insert versus the Femassist [193], [189], [194], [190], [191] external meatal occlusive device. Assessments at baseline, one month, and three months included subjective efficacy, seven day diary, and PdWt-1hr.

At the time of this report, results from a prospective two-year follow-up study of the FemSoft urethral insert are not yet available. In a small, randomized pilot study assessing the efficacy of the FemSoft in preventing incontinence during strenuous exercise, Dunn [201] measured pad weights during four standardized aerobics sessions during which six subjects were randomly assigned to exercise twice with the insert and twice without it. The medians of the averaged pad weights for the two different types of sessions were compared.

c) Results

Most patients who utilize intra-urethral devices report dryness or improvement in the laboratory and on diaries. The major morbidities are discomfort, urinary tract infections and hematuria. Most patients who completed the studies were subjectively and objectively continent or improved, Viva demonstrating 94.4% improvement in leakage for Neilsen [195], the ord 66.7% for Peschers [196]. The Reliance device provided 72% complete dryness with 17% improvement on diary, and 80% complete dryness and 15% improvement on pad weight testing for Staskin [197], 79% complete dryness and 16% significant improvement on objective pad weight studies consistent with the improvement in subjective diaries (p<.0001) for Miller [198]. The patients reported improved comfort and ease of use over time, with sensation of device presence decreasing from 35% at week one to 7% at 12 months for ([58]). The volume of urine lost during exercise decreased from a median of 20 gram (range 4.9-80.2 grams) without the insert to 2.6 grams (1.3-6.8) when the insert was worn (p=.03). On a 5-point scale in which 1 represented very comfortable and 5 very uncomfortable, subjects rated the mean comfort for the sessions performed with the insert in place as 2.1.

Treatment for positive urine cultures was undertaken in 20% of symptomatic and 11% of asymptomatic patients, 39% of patients had positive cultures which were not treated and 30% had negative cultures at all monthly intervals for the four month study. The main reason for drop-out were discomfort [197]. One or more episodes of gross hematuria (24%), cystoscopic findings of mucosal irritation at 4 or at 12 months (9%) and asymptomatic bacteruria (30%) on monthly cultures were also documented [198].

In the only comparative study, by Boos [200] the superior efficacy of the intraurethral device (Reliance) versus an extraurethral device (FemAssist) was mitigated by the higher incidence of side effects. Of the 102 women who were enrolled, 80 patients completed the study with a reduction in incontinence, Reliance 28.6 cc (1-99) to 0.8 cc (0-4.6) 40.8% subjectively dry, and the remainder improved, versus Femassist 36 cc (1.1-128) to 4.3 cc (0-30) 28.3% subjectively dry, 60.4 % improved, 9.4% unchanged and 1 patient worse. Urinary tract infections were seen in approximately 7% in both groups at three months. The authors concluded that both devices were efficacious, the Femassist being more comfortable but requiring greater skill to achieve continence, and the Reliance to be significantly better in controlling incontinence but with a higher degree of "nuisance" side effects.

d) Summary

Intraurethral inserts have demonstrated superior efficacy to other forms of devices used in the control of urinary incontinence [88]. The common morbidities associated with the use of these devices are urinary tract infection, hematuria and discomfort. Bacteruria, without symptomatic infection, was similar to extraurethral device use [88] which approaches screening urinalysis data [188], or may be similar to the rates seen with self catheterization [197]. Hematuria, microscopic or gross, presents a diagnostic dilemma for a patient undergoing screening urinalysis. Device migration into the bladder, which requires endoscopic intervention for removal, is the most serious reported problem. Long term results are limited, although data on patients with 4 months to one year of intra-urethral device use do not appear to demonstrate an increase in urinary loss by objective testing, after device discontinuation [197], [198], [199]. Patient and physician acceptance of this form of therapy has been limited, and the only device reviewed in this section, which is currently commercially available is the FemSoft (Rochester Medical Corporation, 1800-FEMSOFT.com). (Level of Evidence: 3)

e) Recommendation

Further development and study of the use of intraurethral devices for the treatment of urodynamic stress incontinence is recommended. The role of intraurethral devices in patients who do not achieve the desired efficacy with other forms of conservative therapy, and wish to avoid surgery, requires further study. The placement of this therapy in the algorithm of conservative intervention has not been evaluated in relation to other forms of conservative therapy and other devices (except in one RCT abstract), with respect to short and long term efficacy and safety, cost, and quality of life, and comparative RCT's are needed.

GRADE OF RECOMMENDATION: C

Intraurethral devices have demonstrated the highest efficacy, but have been associated with higher incidence of urethral irritation, haematuria, and urinary tract infection in comparison to other devices.

VI. GENERAL CONCLUSIONS & SUMMARY OF RECOMMENDATIONS

Conservative treatment (lifestyle interventions, physical therapies, bladder retraining and devices) should be included in the counselling of incontinent women regarding treatment options.

1. **Regarding lifestyle interventions**, studies to date have reported associations and only a relatively small number of randomized trials have been carried out to assess the effect of a specific lifestyle on incontinence. However, there is evidence that:

- Obesity is an independent risk factor for the prevalence of urinary incontinence and weight loss would appear to be an acceptable treatment option for morbidly obese women. At this time, there is scant information on whether weight loss resolves incontinence in women who are moderately obese.

- Chronic straining may also be risk factor for the development of urinary incontinence, however, there have been no intervention trials that have examined the effect of resolving constipation on incontinence.

- The data on caffeine intake and incontinence are conflicting with a large cross sectional survey indicate no association, while smaller clinical trials have suggested that decreasing caffeine intake improves continence.

- The data relating to the association of smoking and incontinence is conflicting. Smokers may have a different mechanism causing their incontinence than non smokers. No data has been reported examining whether smoking cessation resolves incontinence.

- Strenuous exercise is likely to unmask the symptom of stress incontinence during the provocation. There is no evidence that strenuous exercise causes the condition of incontinence. In a small number of women without other known risk factors, extreme provocation, such as parachute jumping, may cause incontinence. There is scant uncontrolled data that suggests that women engaged in occupations with heavy lifting may be predisposed to genital prolapse and/or incontinence. The data is, however, insufficient to draw any firm conclusions.

- Apart from postural changes, there is no scientific evidence about whether other lifestyle changes affects either the treatment of or the prevention of urinary incontinence.

2. Regarding physical therapies

- There is Level 1 evidence to suggest that in women with the range of urinary incontinence symptoms (stress, mixed, urge), pelvic floor muscle training (PFMT) is better than no treatment and should be offered as therapy to women with those complaints. For those women with mixed and urge incontinence, it may be appropriate to offer PFMT in combination with bladder retraining.

- There is marked lack of consistency in PFMT programmes. On the basis of extrapolation from the exercise science literature, PFMT protocols should include 3 sets of 8 to 12 slow velocity maximal contractions sustained for 6 to 8 seconds each, performed 3 to 4 times a week and continued for at least 15 to 20 weeks. Prior to PFMT, a person with skills in the assessment and training of pelvic floor muscles should assess each woman to ensure that a correct voluntary pelvic floor muscle contraction is being performed and to determine what facilitation, techniques or adaptions, if any, are required to the recommended training programme to ensure an appropriate training intensity.

- In view of the failure of most studies to separately report self reported cure and improvement, it is difficult to estimate the size of the treatment effect. However, it seems that improvement is a more common outcome than cure. In a meta-analysis of trials comparing PFMT with no treatment, women in the PFMT groups were 7.25 times more likely to report cure than women in no treatment groups (RR7.25, 95% CI 1.99, 26.49) and this increased to 23.04 times for combined cure/improvement (RR23.04, 95% CI7.56, 70.22).

- Due to the lack of consistency in the trials evidence of effectiveness of PFMT versus ES for (urodynamic) stress incontinence is not clear, although three of the five trials show greater benefit of PFMT. On the basis of the limited evidence currently available there is no apparent difference in the effectiveness of PFMT with or without biofeedback, or intravaginal resistance devices, although clinicians may find occasions when these would be useful adjuncts to treatment for the purposes of teaching, motivation and compliance.

- There is insufficient evidence to determine whether electrical stimulation (ES) is better than no treatment for women with stress, mixed or urge incontinence.

- To date, the results of ES versus placebo ES in women with urodynamic stress incontinence are contradictory. There is a notable lack of consistency in ES types and parameters used to treat incontinence in women with detrusor overactivity/overactivity. There is a trend in favour of ES, but the trials are small and not easily comparable.

- For comparisons of ES with PFMT versus PFMT alone, the reporting was very poor in three of the four trials in women with stress incontinence, and only a single trial was found for women with detrusor overactivity. At present, it seems that there is no extra benefit in adding electrical stimulation to PFMT.

- The committee recommends that future trials of electrical stimulation place particular emphasis on identifying particular subgroups of the incontinent population that are likely to benefit most.

- Treatment with vaginal cones may be better than control treatment, however, it seems that it may be no better or worse than ES or PFMT. The addition of vaginal cones to a PFMT programme may add no further benefit over PFMT alone.

- Many of the factors traditionally supposed to effect the outcomes of physical therapy interventions (e.g. severity of incontinence) maybe less crucial than previously thought. The single factor that is consistently associated with positive outcome is greater motivation and/or compliance with the intervention. At present, there is no convincing evidence of the need for urodynamic evaluation to confirm diagnosis prior to the initiation of physical therapies.

- There is lack of evidence about the effectiveness of PFMT or other PF rehabilitation programmes (e.g. PFMT with electrical stimulation) for the prevention of urinary incontinence.

3. Regarding bladder retraining

- There is Level 1 evidence to suggest that for women with urge, stress and mixed urinary incontinence, bladder retraining is more effective than no treatment. Evidence is inconsistent about expected cure rates, which maybe dependent on when and how the outcome was measured or reflect differences in the bladder retraining protocol.

- There is a lack of consistency in bladder retraining programmes. On the basis of extrapolation from the bladder retraining literature, a retraining protocol should include an initial voiding interval typically beginning at 1 hour during waking hours only, which is increased by 15-30 minutes per week depending upon tolerance of the schedule until a 2-3 hour voiding interval is achieved. A shorter initial voiding interval, i.e. 30 minutes or less, may be necessary for women whose baseline voiding diaries reveal an average voiding interval of less than 1 hour. Education should be provided about normal bladder control and methods to control urgency such as distraction and relaxation techniques and pelvic floor muscle contraction. Self-monitoring of voiding behaviour using a voiding diary or treatment log should be included in order to determine adherence to the schedule, evaluate progress, and determine whether the voiding interval should be changed. Clinicians should monitor progress, determine adjustments to the voiding interval, and provide positive reinforcement to women undergoing bladder retraining at least weekly during the training period. If there is no reduction in incontinent episodes after three weeks of bladder retraining, the patient should be re-evaluated and other treatment options considered.

- One RCT has indicated that bladder retraining and pelvic floor muscle training have similar efficacy in women with urge, stress and mixed incontinence and this finding requires further investigation.

- The effectiveness of bladder retraining in combination with pelvic floor muscle training in comparison to bladder retraining alone is unclear and further investigation is also warranted.

- Bladder retraining appears to have similar benefits as drug therapy available prior to 1996 and may have greater long term benefit. The additional benefit of combining drug therapy with bladder retraining and vice versa was not consistently noted and further investigation is warranted.

- There is no convincing evidence of the need of urodynamic evaluation to confirm diagnosis prior to the initiation of bladder retraining.

4. Regarding anti-incontinence devices

- Although several classes of devices have demonstrated efficacy and tolerability in clinical studies, physician and patient acceptance have not been sufficient for commercial success. A lack of patient acceptance has been associated with a lack of knowledge and comfort with genital anatomy, limited manual dexterity in inserting and removing these devices, physical discomfort, or cost. There are no studies which characterize caregiver attitudes, although a commitment to patient training may be a barrier.

- There are currently no adequate external collection devices for the ambulatory female population.

- There are no RCT's on the utilization of pessaries for urinary incontinence. Pessaries are the most commonly prescribed devices for vaginal prolapse, but there are no studies to define those patients who will respond, or those patients in whom support of the prolapse will exacerbate urinary leakage.

- Bladder neck support prostheses, designed as a modification of a pessary, as an intravaginal insert, or as a modification of a tampon have shown efficacy in selected patients without significant prolapse or a history of vaginal surgery, but require patient acceptance and a degree of manual dexterity for use.

- External patch or cup devices, placed over the urethral meatus, and held in place by an adhesive or mild suction have demonstrated efficacy with minimal morbidity.

- Intraurethral devices have demonstrated the highest efficacy, but have been associated with higher incidence of urethral irritation, hematuria, and urinary tract infection. Device migration into the bladder, requiring cystoscopic removal, has also been reported.

- Incontinence devices may be considered as an adjunct to other forms of conservative therapy and may be considered as an alternative to surgery, in selected patients.

VII. RECOMMENDATIONS FOR FUTURE RESEARCH

1. LIFESTYLE INTERVENTIONS

- Further research is needed to evaluate the effect of several currently recommended lifestyle interventions on incontinence and whether their cessation can alleviate or prevent this condition. These include: weight loss, heavy exertion/exercise, smoking, caffeine intake, fluid intake, constipation on incontinence.

2. PHYSICAL THERAPIES

High quality RCTs with long term follow up are required to investigate:

- the effectiveness of PFMT in comparison to other interventions and to compare the effectiveness of different PFMT programmes in the management of urinary incontinence.
- the effectiveness of PFMT with other adjuncts in comparison to PFMT alone and effectiveness of different biofeedback protocols.
- all aspects of the use of electrical stimulation in the treatment of urinary incontinence.
- the effectiveness of physical therapies to prevent incontinence in women at risk or in the general female population.
- the subgroups of patients who would derive the greatest benefit from physical therapies.

3. BLADDER RETRAINING

- High quality RCTs with long term follow up are required to compare bladder retraining alone and in combination with lifestyle interventions, physical therapies and drug therapies in the management of stress, urge and mixed incontinence.
- Research is needed to determine the subgroups of patients who will derive the greatest benefit from bladder retraining along or in combination with physical therapies or drug therapy and also to determine the long term efficacy of bladder retraining.

4. DEVICES

- High quality RCT's with long term follow up are needed. However, it is acknowledged that device protocols may not easily employ a non-treatment group, cannot easily employ a 'placebo' model, and are usually designed as open longitudinal studies, utilizing the patients' baseline data as the control. Specifically within the field of device investigation, intention to treat and the inclusion of dropouts as treatment failures should be considered when evaluating efficacy, safety and satisfaction of outcomes. Similarly, studies to determine the subgroups of patients, who will derive the greatest benefit, should be performed.
- Studies on the effectiveness of devices following long term usage are needed. Long term data should consider: a) the degree and persistence of efficacy, b) the possibility of additional morbidity over time, c) the persistence of benefit following device discontinuation, which may result from a training effect, and d) the potential for loss of baseline function over time, resulting from tissue damage or an anti-rehabilitative effect.
- Device effectiveness and morbidity should be examined alone, in crossover studies with other devices, and in combination with other therapies.
- Devices should be compared with other devices and other interventions for efficacy, safety and cost effectiveness.

APPENDIX 1

1. SEARCH STRATEGIES

a) Lifestyle Interventions

Reports on lifestyle interventions were obtained by searching MEDLINE (languages English, Scandinavian, German) from 1976 to December 2000 using the following keywords which were linked to urinary incontinence: lifestyle interventions, weight, obesity, weight loss, exercise, work, physical activity, smoking, tobacco, coffee, caffeine, posture, constipation, bowel function, fluids, fluid restriction, timed voiding, clothing, pulmonary status, cough, and diet.

Anecdotal recommendations made in the literature unaccompanied by data of any sort are not reported.

b) Physical Therapies

• Systematic reviews

Reports of systematic reviews evaluating the effectiveness of physical therapies for prevention and treatment of female stress, urge and mixed incontinence were obtained by searching MEDLINE, EMBASE, CINAHL and The Cochrane Library. Key search terms were systematic review, meta-analysis, and incontinence. The date of the most recent search was November 2000. In addition the authors of this section on physical therapies had contributed to Cochrane systematic reviews of physical therapies for incontinence that were in press at the time of writing this chapter. The evidence from both these reviews (pelvic floor muscle training for female urinary incontinence, physical therapies for prevention of incontinence) was therefore available for inclusion.

• **Electrical stimulation**

The Trials Search Co-ordinator of the Cochrane Incontinence Group obtained reports of RCTs evaluating the effect of electrical stimulation for stress, urge and mixed incontinence from a search of the Specialised Trials Register of the Cochrane Incontinence Group. The Register contains trials identified from MEDLINE, CINAHL, The Cochrane Controlled Trials Register and handsearching of journals and conference proceedings. The date of the last search was November 2000.

c) Bladder Retraining

Reports of bladder retraining were obtained by searching MEDLINE and CINAHL from February 1966 to December 2000 using the following keywords which were linked to urinary incontinence and female: bladder, bladder training, behavior therapy, toileting, rehabilitation, therapy. In addition, the reference lists from Bladder Training for Urinary Incontinence in Adults ([149]Roe et al., 2000) published by the Cochrane Database of Systematic Reviews and those from review articles [146],[147], [148] and retrieved manuscripts were cross-referenced.

Inclusion/exclusion criteria

To be considered for inclusion, studies had to meet the following criteria:

1. Prospective research design: randomized controlled or nonrandomized controlled trials.
2. Types of participants: noninstitutionalized women with stress, urge, and mixed incontinence without mental or physical impairments
3. Type of intervention: Bladder retraining used in the management of urinary incontinence
4. Publication type: full published reports in English

d) Anti-Incontinence devices

Reports on anti-incontinence devices were obtained by searching MEDLINE 1980 to December 2000, and two abstracts from Cochrane as they were RCT's. A small number of descriptive studies performed on small groups of patients utilising devices which are not currently available, were included for historical value. Devices which are currently employed in clinical practice for the management of incontinence after being adopted from the standard usage, such as contraceptive diaphragms or pessaries, are reported in the subsection which is consistent with their presumed mode of action. Prospective trials of devices have generally not been randomised or parallel controlled, as these studies utilise the patient as their own control and derive outcome data based on change from baseline. There is only one abstract which compares one device to another. Two abstracts have been included, based on the use of comparative data and are noted as such in the references and text.

2. ACKNOWLEDGEMENTS

We would like to acknowledge the secretarial assistance of Maria Treloar and Christine Cooper in the coordination and preparation of this Chapter.

REFERENCES

1 Subak, L.L., Johnson, C., Whitcomb, E., Boban, D., Saxton, J. And Brown, J.S. Does weight loss improve incontinence in moderately obese women? Submitted for publication 2001.

2 Bump, R.C., Sugerman, J.H., Fantl, A. And McClish, D.M. Obesity and lower urinary tract function in women: effect of surgically induced weight loss. American journal of obstetrics & gynecology. 167 (2): 392-398, 1992.

3 Deitel, M., Stone, E., Kassam, H.A., Wilk, E.J. And Sutherland, D.J.A. Gynecologic-Obstetric changes after loss of massive excess weight following bariatric surgery. Journal of the American College of Nutrition. 7 (2): 147-153, 1988.

4 Kolbl, H. And Riss, P. Obesity and genuine stress incontinence: significance of indices of relative weight. Urologia internationalis. 43: 7-10, 1988.

5 Brown, J.S., Grady, D., Ouslander, J.G., Herzog, A.R., Varner, R.D. And Posner, S.F. Prevalence of urinary incontinence and associated risk factors in postmenopausal women. Obstetric gynecology. 94: 66-70, 1999.

6 Rasmussen, K.L., Krue, S., Johansson, L.E., Knudsen, J.H.H. And Agger, A.O. Obesity as a predictor of postpartum urinary symptoms. Acta Obstetrica Gynecologica Scandinavica. 76: 359-362, 1997.

7 Wilson, P.D., Herbison, G.P., Glazener, C.M.A., Lang, G., Gee, H. And MacArthur, C. Postnatal incontinence: a multicentre, randomised controlled trial of conservative treatment (Abstract 5). Neururology & Urodynamics. 16 (5): 349-350, 1997.

8 Mommsen, S. And Foldspang, A. Body mass index and adult female urinary incontinence. World journal of urology. 12: 319-322, 1994.

9 Dwyer, P.L., Lee, E.T.C. And Hay, D.M. Obesity and urinary incontinence in women. British Journal of Obstetrics and Gynaecology. 95: 91-96, 1988.

10 Yarnell, J.W.G., Voyle, G.J., Sweetnam, P.M. And Milbank, J. Factors associated with urinary incontinence in women. Journal of epidemiology and community health. 36: 58-63, 1982.

11 Brown, J.S., Seeley, D.G., Fong, J., Black, D.M., Ensrud, K.E. And Grady, D. Urinary incontinence in older women: who is at risk? Obstetric gynecology. 87 (5): 715-721, 1996.

12 Thom, D.H., Van Den Eeden, S.K. And Brown, J.S. Evaluation of parturition and other reproductive variables as risk factors for urinary incontinence in later life. Obstetrics & Gynecology. 90: 983-999, 1997.

13 Foldspang, A. And Mommsen, S. Overweight and urinary incontinence in women. Ugeskrift for Laeger. 157: 5848-5851, 1995.

14 Samsioe, G., Heraib, F., Lidfeldt, J., Nerbrand, C., Lindhom, L.,

Agardh, C. And Scherstein, B. Urogenital symptoms in women aged 50-59 years. Gynecological endocrinology. 13: 113-117, 1999.

15 Jörgensen, S., Hein, H.O. And Gyntelberg, F. Heavy lifting at work and risk of genital prolapse and herniated lumbur disc in assistant nurses. Occupational Medicine (Oxford, England). (44): 47-49, 1994.

16 Bø, K., Stein, R., Kulseng-Hanssen, S. And Kristofferson, M. Clinical and urodynamic assessment of nulliparous young women with and without stress incontinence symptoms: a case-control study. Obstetrics and gynecology. 84 (6): 1028-1032, 1994.

17 Bø, K., Mæhlum, S., Oseid, S. And Larsen, S. Prevalence of genuine stress incontinence among physically active and sedentary female students. Scandanavian Journal of Sports Sciences. 11 (3): 113-116, 1989.

18 Nygaard, I.E., Thompson, F.L., Svengalis, S.L. And Albright, J.P. Urinary incontinence in elite nulliparous athletes. Obstetrics & Gynecology. 84 (2): 183-187, 1994.

19 Davis, G.D. And Goodman, M. Genuine stress incontinence in nulliparous female soldiers in airborne infantry training. Journal of Pelvic Surgery. 2 (2): 68-71, 1996.

20 Bø, K. And Borgen, J.S. Prevalence of stress and urge urinary incontinence in elite athletes and controls. Medicine and Science in Sports and Exercise. In press: 2001.

21 Nygaard, I.E., Delancey, J.O., Arnsdorf And Murphy, E. Exercise and Incontinence. Obstetrics & Gynecology. 75 (5): 848-851, 1990.

22 Nygaard, I.E. Does prolonged high-impact activity contribute to later urinary incontinence? A retrospective cohort study of female Olympians. Obstetrics & Gynecology. 90 (5): 718-722, 1997.

23 Bump, R.C. And McClish, D.M. Cigarette smoking and pure *urodynamic* stress incontinence of urine: a comparison of risk factors and determinants between smokers and nonsmokers. American journal of obstetrics & gynecology. 170 (2): 579-582, 1994.

24 Tampakoudis, P., Tantanassis, T., Grimbizis, G., Papeletsos, M. And Mantalenakis, S. Cigarette smoking and urinary incontinence in women - a new calculative method of estimating the exposure to smoke. European Journal of Obstetrics, gynecology and reproductive biology. 63: 17-30, 1995.

25 Van Geelen, J.M., Van De Weijer, P.H.M. And Arnolds, H.T.H. Urogenital symptoms and resulting discomfort in non-institutionalised Dutch women aged 50-75 years. International Urogynecology Journal. 11: 9-14, 2000.

26 Hojberg, K.-E., Salvig, J.D., Winslow, N.A., Lose, G. And Secher, N.J. Urinary incontinence: prevalence and risk factors at 16 weeks of gestation. British Journal of Obstetrics and Gynaecology. 106: 842-850, 1999.

27 Hisayama, T., Shinkai, M., Takaynagi, I. And Toyoda, T. Mechanism of action of nicotine in isolated bladder of guinea-pig. British Journal of Pharmacology. 95: 465-472, 1988.

28 Milson, I., Arvidsson, L., Ekelund, P., Molander, U. And Eriksson, O. Factors influencing vaginal cytology, pH and bacterial flora in elderly women. Acta Obstetrica Gynecologica Scandinavica. 72: 286-291, 1993.

29 Bryant, C.M., Dowell, C.J. And Fairbrother, G. A randomized trial of the effects of caffeine upon frequency, urgency and urge incontinence. Neurourology and Urodynamics. 19: 501-502, 2000.

30 Creighton, S.M. And Stanton, S.L. Caffeine: does it affect your bladder? British journal of urology. 66: 613-614, 1990.

31 Ayra, L.A., Myers, D.L. And Jackson, N.D. Dietary caffeine intake and the risk for detrusor instability: a case-control study. Obstetrics and gynecology. 96: 85-89, 2000.

32 Tomlinson, B.U., Dougherty, M.C., Pendergast, J.F., Boyington, A.R. And Coffman, M.A. Dietary caffeine, fluid intake and urinary incontinence in older rural women. International Urogynecology Journal and Pelvic Floor Dysfunction. 10: 22-28, 1999.

33 Griffiths, D.J., McCracken, P.N., Harrison, G.M. And Gormley, E.A. Relationship of fluid intake to voluntary micturition and urinary incontinence in geriatric patients. Neurourology & Urodynamics. 12: 1-7, 1993.

34 Wyman, J.F., Elswick, R.K., Wilson, M.S. And Fantl, J.A. Relationship of fluid intake to voluntary micturitions and urinary incontinence in women. Neurourology & Urodynamics.: 463-473, 1991.

35 Roe, B. And Doll, H. Lifestyle factors and continence status: comparison of self-reported data from a postal survey in England. Journal of Wound, Ostomy & Continence Nursing. 26: 312-319, 1999.

36 Dowd, T.T., Campbell, J.M. And Jones, J.A. Fluid intake and urinary incontinence in older community-dwelling women. Journal of Community Health Nursing. 13: 179-186, 1996.

37 Diokno, A.C., Brock, B.M., M. Herzog, A.R. And Bromberg, J. Medical correlates of urinary incontinence in the elderly. Urology. 36: 129-138, 1990.

38 Moller, L.A., Lose, G. And Jorgensen, T. Risk factors for lower urinary trct symptoms in women 40 to 60 years of age. ObstetricS & Gynaecology. 96: 446-451, 2000.

39 Spence-Jones, C., Kamm, M.A., Henry, M.M. And Hudson, C.N. Bowel dysfunction: a pathogenic factor in uterovaginal prolapse and genuine stress incontinence. British Journal of Obstetrics & Gynaecology. 101: 147-152, 1994.

40 Jorge, J.M.N., Wexner, S.D., Ehrenpreis, E.D., Norgueras, J.J. And Jagelman, D.G. Does perineal descent correlate with pudendal neuropathy? Diseases of the Colon and Rectum. 36 (5): 475-483, 1993.

41 Lubowski, D.Z., Swash, M., Nicholls, R.J. And Henry, M.M. Increase in pudendal nerve terminal motor latency with defaecation straining. British Journal of Surgery. 75: 1095-1097, 1988.

42 Norton, P. And Baker, J. Randomized prospective trial of vaginal cones vs Kegel exercises in postpartum primiparous women. Proceedings of The 20th Annual Meeting International Continence Society, 1990, 9, 434-435.

43 Noble, E. Essential exercises for the childbearing year. 1988. Boston, Houghton Mifflin Company,

44 Polden, M. And Mantle, J. Physiotherapy in Obstetrics & Gynaecology. 1990. Oxford, Butterworth Heinemann,

45 Kegel, A.H. Progressive resistance exercise in the functional restoration of the perineal muscles. American Journal of Obstetrics & Gynaecology. 56: 238-249, 1948.

46 Delancey, J.O.L. Structural aspects of urethrovesical function in the female. Neururology & Urodynamics. 7: 509-518, 1988a.

47 Delancey, J.O.L. Anatomy and mechanics of structures around the vesical neck: How vesical neck position might affect its closure. Neururology & Urodynamics. 7: 161-162, 1988b.

48 Bo, K. Pelvic floor muscle exercise for the treatment of genuine stress incontinence: an exercise physiology perspective. International Urogynecology Journal. 6: 282-291, 1995a.

49 Constantinou, C.E. And Govan, D.E. Contribution and timing of transmitted and generated pressure components in the female urethra. In: Female Incontinence. 1981. Allan R Liss Inc, New York.

50 Miller, J.M., Ashton-Miller, J.A. And Delancey, J.O.L. A pelvic muscle precontraction can reduce cough-related urine loss in selected women with mild SUI. Journal of American Geriatrics Society. 46 (7): 870-874, 1998.

51 Plevnik, S., Janez, J., Vrtacnik, P., Trsinar, B. And Vodusek, B. Short-term electrical stimulation: Home treatment for urinary incontinence. World Journal of Urology. 4: 24-26, 1986.

52 Dinubile, N.A. Strength training. Clinics in Sports Medicine. 10: 33-62, 1991.

53 Godec, C., Cass, A.S. And Ayala, G.F. Bladder inhibition with functional electrical stimulation. Urology. 6: 663-666, 1975.

54 De Groat, W.C. A neurologic basis for the overactive bladder. Urology. 50 (Suppl 6A): 36-52, 1997.

55 Morrison, J. The excitability of the micturition reflex. Scandinavia Journal of Urology and Nephrology. 29 (Supp. 175): 21-25, 1993.

56 Berghmans, L.C.M., Van Waalwijk, Van Doorn, E.S.C., Nieman, F., De Bie, R.A., Smeets, L.W.H. And Ten Haaf, H.E.A. Efficacy of extramural physical therapy modalities in women with proven bladder overactivity: a randomized clinical trial. Neururology Urodynamics. 19 (4): 496-497, 2000.

57 Bouchard, D., Shephard, R.J. And Stephens, T. Physical activity, fitness, and health. International proceedings and consensus statement.: 1994.

58 Haskel, W. Dose-response issues from a biologial perspective. In: Bouchard, C., Shphard, R.J., Stephens, T. 1994. Champaing, I.L.: Human Kinetics Publishers, cl1994,

59 Fedorkow, D.M. Nonsurgical management of genuine stress incontinence. Journal of. 15 (6): 695-705, 1993.

60 Bo, K. Physiotherapy to treat genuine stress incontinence. 6: 2-8, 1996.

61 Berghmans, L.C., Hendriks, H.J., Bo, K., Hay-Smith, E.J., De Bie, R.A., Waalwijk, V. And Van Doorn, E.S. Conservative treatment of genuine stress incontinence in women: a systematic review of randomized clinical trials. British Journal of Urology. 82 (2): 181-191, 1998.

62 Hay-Smith, E.J., Herbison, P. And Morkved, S. Physical therapies for prevention of incontinence in adults (Cochrane Protocol). 2001. Update Software, Oxford.

63 Bo, K., Hagen, R.H., Kvarstein, B., Jorgensen, J. And Larson, S. Pelvic floor muscle exercise for treatment of female genuine stress incontinence: III effects of two different degrees of pelvic floor muscle exercises. Neururology & Urodynamics. 9: 489-502, 1990.

64 Bo, K., Talseth, T. And Holme, I. Single blind, randomised controlled trial of pelvic floor exercises, electrical stimulation, vaginal cones, and no treatment in management of genuine stress incontinence in women. British Medical Journal. 318 (7182): 487-493, 1999.

65 Cammu, H. And Van Nylen, M. Pelvic floor exercises versus vaginal weight cones in genuine stress incontinence. European Journal of Obstetrics & Gynecology, & Reproductive Biology. 77 (1): 89-93, 1998.

66 Wilson, P.D. And Herbison, G.P. A randomized controlled trial of pelvic floor muscle exercises to treat postnatal urinary incontinence. International Urogynecology Journal & Pelvic Floor Dysfunction. 9 (5): 257-264, 1998.

67 Gallo, M.L. And Staskin, D.R. Cues to action: pelvic floor muscle exercise compliance in women with genuine stress incontinence. Neururology & Urodynamics. 16 (3): 167-177, 1997.

68 Lagro-Janssen, A.L.M., Debruyne, F.M.J., Smits, A.J.A. And Van Weel, C. The effects of treatment of urinary incontinence in general practice. Family Practice. 9: 284-289, 1992.

69 Ramsay, I.N. And Thou, M.A. A randomised, double blind, placebo controlled trial of pelvic floor exercises in the treatment of genuine stress incontinence (Abstract 95). Neururology & Urodynamics. 9 (4): 398-399, 1990.

70 Burgio, K.L., Locher, J.L., Goode, P.S., Hardin, J.M., McDowell, B.J., Dombrowski, M. And Al., E. Behavioral vs drug treatment for urge urinary incontinence in older women. A randomized controlled trial. Journal of American Medical Association. 280 (23): 1995-2000, 1998.

71 Burns, P.A., Pranikoff, K., Nochajski, T.H., Hadley, E.C., Levy, K.J. And Ory, M.G. A comparison of effectiveness of biofeedback and pelvic muscle exercise treatment of stress incontinence in older community-dwelling women. Journal of Gerontology. 48 (4): M167-174, 1993.

72 Nygaard, I.E., Kreder, K.J., Lepic, M.M., Fountain, K.A. And Rhomberg, A.T. Efficacy of pelvic floor muscle exercises in women with stress, urge, and mixed urinary incontinence. American Journal of Obstetrics & Gynecology. 174 ((1 part 1)): 120-125, 1996.

73 O'Brien, J., Austin, M., Sethi, P. And O'Boyle, P. Urinary incontinence: prevalence, need for treatment, and effectiveness of intervention by nurse. British Medical Journal. 303 (6813): 1308-1312, 1991.

74 Laycock, J. and Jerwood, D. Does pre-modulated interferential therapy cure genuine stress incontinence? Physiotherapy. 79: 553-560, 1993.

75 Wyman, J.F., Fantl, J.A., McClish, D.K. And Bump, R.C. Comparative efficacy of behavioral interventions in the management of female urinary incontinence. Continence Program for Women Research Group. American Journal of Obstetrics & Gynecology. 179 (4): 999-1007, 1998.

76 Wells, T.J., Brink, C.A., Diokno, A.C., Wolfe, R. And Gillis, G.L. Pelvic muscle exercise for genuine stress incontinence in elderly women. Journal of the American Geriatrics Society. 39 (8): 785-791, 1991.

77 Haken, J., Benness, C., Cardozo, L. And Cutner, A. A randomised trial of vaginal cones and pelvic floor exercises in the management of genuine stress incontinence (Abstract 76). Neururology & Urodynamics. 10 (4): 393-394, 1991.

78 Henalla, S.M., Hutchins, C.J., Robinson, P. And Macvicar, J. Non-operative methods in the treatment of female genuine stress incontinence of urine. Journal of Obstetrics & Gynaecology. 9 (3): 222-225, 1989.

79 Klarskov, P., Belving, D., Bischoff, N., Dorph, S., Gerstenberg, T., Okholm, B. And Al., E. Pelvic floor exercise versus surgery for female genuine stress incontinence. Urologia Internationalis. 41 (2): 129-132, 1986.

80 Laycock, J., Brown, J.S., Cusack, C., Green, S., Jerwood, D., Mann, K. And Al., E. A multicentre, prospective, randomised controlled, group comparative study of the efficacy of vaginal cones and PFX (Abstract 47). Neururology & Urodynamics. 18 (4): 301-302, 1999.

81 Terry, P.B. And Whyte, S.M. Randomised trial comparing Enhance with physiotherapy for the treatment of GSI (Read by title abstract 242). Proceedings of The 26th Annual Meeting of the International Continence Society, Athens, Greece, 1996, 248-249.

82 Wong, K.S., Fung, B.K.Y., Fung, L.C.W. And Ma, S. Pelvic floor exercises in the treatment of genuine stress incontinence in Hong Kong Chinese women (Read by titles abstract 134). Proceedings of The 27th Annual Meeting of the International Continence Society, Yokohama, Japan, 1997b,

83 Hahn, I., Sommar, S. And Fall, M. A comparative study of pelvic floor training and electrical stimulation for the treatment of genuine female urinary incontinence. Neururology & Urodynamics. 10 (6): 545-554, 1991.

84 Henalla, S.M., Millar, D.R. And Wallace, K.J. Surgical versus conservative management for post-menopausal genuine stress incontinence of urine (Abstract 87). Neururology & Urodynamics. 9 (4): 436-437, 1990.

85 Hofbauer, J., Preisinger, F. And Nurnberger, N. Der stellenwert

der physikotherapie bei der weiblichen genuinen streb-inkontinenz. Zeitschrift Fur urologie Und Nephrologie. 83 (5): 249-254, 1990.

86 Smith, J.J.R. Intravaginal stimulation randomized trial. Journal of Urology. 155 (1): 127-130, 1996.

87 Lagro-Janssen, T. And Van Weel, C. Long-term effect of treatment of female incontinence in general practice. British Journal of General Practice. 48: 1735-1738, 1998.

88 Bo, K., Anders, K., Hextall, A., Tooz-Hobson, P. And Cardozo, L. Randomized trial of Reliance versus Femassist devices in the management of genuine stress incontinence. Neurourology & Urodynamics. 17 (4): 455-456, 1998.

89 Benevenuti, F., Caputo, G.M., Bandinelli, S., Mayer, F., Biagini, C. And Somavilla, A. Re-educative treatment of female genuine stress incontinence. American Journal of Physical Medicine. 66 (4): 155-168, 1987.

90 Sapsford, R., Hodges, P., Richardson, C., Cooper, D., Markwell, S. And Jull, G. Co-activation of the abdominal and pelvic floor muscle during voluntary exercises. Neururology Urodynamics. 20: 31-42, 2001.

91 Glavind, K., Nohr, S.B. And Walter, S. Biofeedback and physiotherapy versus physiotherapy alone in the treatment of genuine stress incontinence. International Urogynecology Journal and Pelvic Floor Dysfunction. 7 (6): 339-343, 1996.

92 Wilmore, J.H. And Costill, L.C. Physiology of sport and exercise. 1994. Champaign, I.L.: Human Kinetics, cl1994,

93 Astrand, P.O. And Rodahl, K. Textbook of work physiology: Physiological basis of exercise. 1986. McGraw Hill Company,

94 Ramsay, I.N., Ali, H.M., Hunter, M., Stark, D., McKenzie, S. And Al., E. A prospective, randomized controlled trial of inpatient versus outpatient continence programs in the treatment of urinary incontinence in the female. International Urogynecology Journal. 7: 260-263, 1996.

95 Laycock, J. Interferential therapy in the treatment of genuine stress incontinence (Abstract 74). Neururology & Urodynamics. 7 (3): 268-269, 1988.

96 Wise, B.G., Haken, J., Cardozo, L. And Plevnik, S. A comparative study of vaginal cone therapy, cones and Kegel exercises, and maximal electrical stimulation in the treatment of female genuine stress incontinence (Abstract 76). Neururology & Urodynamics. 12 (4): 436-437, 1993.

97 Peattie, A.B. And Plevnik, S. Cones versus physiotherapy as conservative management of genuine stress incontinence (Abstract 72). Neururology & Urodynamics. 7 (3): 255-256, 1988.

98 Tapp, A.J.S., Hills, B. And Cardozo, L.D. Randomised study comparing pelvic floor physiotherapy with the Burch colposuspension (Abstract 44). Neururology & Urodynamics. 8 (4): 356-357, 1989.

99 Elia, G. And Bergman, A. Pelvic muscle exercises: When do they work? Obstetrics & Gynecology. 81 (283-286): 1993.

100 Bo, K. And Talseth, T. Long-term effect of pelvic floor muscle exercise 5 years after cessation of organized training. Obstetrics & Gynecology. 87 (2): 261-265, 1996.

101 De Kruif, Y.P. And Van Wegen, E.E. Pelvic floor muscle exercise therapy with myofeedback for women with genuine stress incontinence: A meta-analysis. Physiotherapy. 82 (2): 107-113, 1996.

102 Berghmans, L.C., Frederiks, C.M., De Bie, R.A., Weil, E.H.J., Smeets, L.W.H., Van Waalwijk Van Doorn, E.S.C. And Al., E. Efficacy of biofeedback, when included with pelvic floor muscle exercise treatment, for genuine stress incontinence. Neurourology & Urodynamics. 15 (1): 37-52, 1996.

103 Aukee, P., Immonen, P., Penttinen, J. And Airaksinen, O. A prospective randomised study comparing Femiscan TM Home Trainer and pelvic floor muscle training alone (Abstract). Proceedings of The 30th Annual Meeting of the International Continence Association, Tampere, Finland, 2000,

104 Castleden, C.M., Duffin, H.M. And Mitchell, E.P. The effect physiotherapy on stress incontinence. Age & Ageing. 13 (4): 235-237, 1984.

105 Ferguson, K.L., McKey, P.L., Bishop, K.R., Kloen, P., Verheul, J.B. And Dougherty, M.C. Genuine stress incontinence: effect of pelvic muscle exercise. Obstetrics & Gynecology. 75 (4): 671-675, 1990.

106 Klingler, H.C., Madersbacher, S., Uher, E.M. And Schmidbauer, C.P. Pelvic floor exercise and Endotrainer for treatment of female genuine stress incontinence (Read by title abstract 122). Proceedings of The 24th Annual Meeting of the International Continence Society, Sydney, Australia, 1995,

107 Shepherd, A.M., Montgomery, E. And Aderson, R.S. Treatment of genuine stress incontinence with a new perineometer. Physiotherapy. 69 (4): 113, 1983.

108 Sherman, R.A., Davis, G.D. And Wong, M.F. Behavioral treatment of exercise-induced urinary incontinence amongst female soldiers. Military Medicine. 162 (10): 690-694, 1997.

109 Taylor, K. And Henderson, J. Effects of biofeedback and genuine stress incontinence in older women. Journal of Gerontological Nursing. 12 (9): 25-30, 1986.

110 Wong, K.S., Fung, B.K.Y., Fung, E.S.M., Fung, L.C.W. And Tang, L.C.H. Randomized prospective study of the effectiveness of pelvic floor training using biofeedback in the treatment of genuine stress incontinence in Chinese population. 1997a. Yokohama, Japan. 23-26 September 1997.

111 Shepherd, A.M., Tribe, E. And Bainton, D. Maximum perineal stimulation: A controlled study. British Journal of Urology. 56: 644-646, 1984.

112 Knight, S., Laycock, J. And Naylor, D. Evaluation of neuromuscular electrical stimulation in the treatment of genuine stress incontinence. Physiotherapy. 84 (2): 61-71, 1998.

113 Weil, E.H.J., Eerdmans, P. And Janknegt, R.A. A new randomized study of neuromodulation versus conventional treatment for incontinence or dysfunctional voiding patterns: A preliminary report. Neururology & Urodynamics. 15 (4): 284-285, 1996.

114 Yamanishi, T., Yasuda, K., Sakakibara, R., Hattori, T., Ito, H. And Murakami, S. Pelvic floor electrical stimulation in the treatment of stress incontinence: An investigational study and a placebo controlled double-blind trial. Journal of urology. 158: 2127-2131, 1997.

115 Blowman, C., Pickles, C., Emery, S., Creates, V., Towell, L. And Al., E. Prospective double blind controlled trial of intensive physiotherapy with and without stimulation of the pelvic floor in the treatment of genuine stress incontinence. Physiotherapy. 77: 661-664, 1991.

116 Luber, K.M. And Wolde-Tsadik, G. Efficacy of functional electrical stimulation in treating genuine stress incontinence: A randomized clinical trial. Neururology & Urodynamics. 16: 543-551, 1997.

117 Sand, P.K., Richardson, D.A., Staskin, D.R., Swift, S.E., Appel, R.A. And Al., E. Pelvic floor electrical stimulation in the treatment of genuine stress incontinence: A multicenter placebo-controlled trial. American Journal of Obstetrics & Gynecology. 173: 72-79, 1995.

118 Bower, W.F., Moore, K.H. And Adams, R.D. Randomised sham-controlled trial of two surface neuromodulation sites in women with detrusor instability. Neururology & Urodynamics. 16 (5): 428-429, 1997.

119 Yamanishi, T., Yasuda, K., Sakakibara, R., Hattori, T. And Suda, S. Randomized, double-blind study of electrical stimulation for urinary incontinence due to detrusor overactivity. Urology. 55: 353-357, 2000.

120 Brubaker, L., Benson, T., Bent, A., Clark, A. And Shott, S. Transvaginal electrical stimulation for female urinary incontinence. American Journal of Obstetrics & Gynaecology. 177: 536-540, 1997.

121 Tapp, A.J.S., Williams, S., Hills, B. And Cardozo, L.D. The role of phyisotherapy in the treatment of genuine stress incontinence (Read by title abstract). Proceedings of The 17th Annual Meeting of the International Continence Society, Bristol, UK, 1987, 204-205.

122 Lobel, R.W., Sasso, K.M. And Sand, P.K. Prospective randomized trial of maximal electrical stimulation for treatment of detrusor instability (Abstract). Proceedings of The 28th Annual Meeting of the International Continence Society, Jerusalem, Israel, 1998,

123 Abel, I., Ottesen, B., Fischer-Rasmussen, W. And Lose, G. Maximal electrical stimulation of the pelvic floor in the treatment of urge incontinence: A placebo controlled study. Proceedings of The 26th Annual Meeting International Continence Society, 1996, 15, 283-284.

124 Bidmead, J., Lose, G., Thyssen, H., Dwyer, P., Moller, L.A., Bek, K. And Cardozo, L. A new intravaginal device for stress incontinence in women. 2000. Aug 2000. ICS 2000 abstract.

125 Rosier, P.F.W.M., Meuleman, E.J.H. And Debruyne, F.M.J. Quality of life of patients with lower urinary tract dysfunction, after treatment with sacral neuromodulation. Neururology & Urodynamics. 16 (5): 483-484, 1997.

126 Plevnik, S. New method for testing aned strengthening of pelvic floor muscles. Proceedings of The 15th Annual Meeting, International Continence Society, 1985, 267-268.

127 Bo, K. Vaginal weight cones. Theoretical framework, effect on pelvic floor muscle strength and female genuine stress incontinence. Acta obstetrica et gynecvologica Scandinavica. 74: 87-92, 1995b.

128 Herbison, P., Plevnik, S. And Mantle, J. Weighted vaginal cones for urinary incontinence. 2001.

129 Olah, K.S., Bridges, N., Denning, J. And Farrar, D.J. The conservative management of patients with symptoms of stress incontinence: a randomized, prospective study comparing weighted vaginal cones and interferential therapy. American Journal of Obstetrics & Gynecology. 162 (1): 87-92, 1990.

130 Pieber, D., Zivkovic, F., Tamussino, K., Ralph, G., Lippitt, G. And Fauland, B. Pelvic floor exercise alone or with vaginal cones for the treatment of mild to moderate genuine stress incontinence in premenopausal women. International Urogynecology Journal and Pelvic Floor Dysfunction. 6 (1): 14-17, 1995.

131 Prashar, S., Simons, A., Bryant, C., Dowell, C. And Moore, K.H. Attitudes to vaginal/urethral touching device placement in women with urinary incontinence. Urogynecology Journal of Pelvic floor dysfunction. 11 (1): 4-8, 2000.

132 Bo, K. And Larsen, S. Pelvic floor muscle exercise for the treatment of female genuine stress incontinence: Classification and characterization of responders. Neururology & Urodynamics. 11 (5): 497-507, 1992.

133 Elser, D.M., Wyman, J.F., McClish, D.M., Robinson, D., Fantl, J.A. And Bump, R.C. The effect of bladder training, pelvic floor muscle training, or combination training on urodynamic parameters in women with urinary incontinence. Continence Program for Women Research Group. Neururology & Urodynamics. 18 (5): 427-436, 1999.

134 Ramsay, I., Hassan, A., Hunter, M. And Donaldson, K. A randomised controlled trial of urodynamic investigations prior to conservative treatment of urinary incontinence in the female. Proceedings of The 24th Annual Meeting International Continence Society, 1994, 13, 455-456.

135 Delancey, J.O.L. Genuine stress incontinence: Where are we now, where should we go? American Journal of Obstetrics & Gynecology. 175: 311-319, 1996.

136 Dougherty, M.C., Bishop, K.R., Abrams, R.M., Batich, C.D. And Gimotty, P.A. The effect of exercise on the circumvaginal muscles in postpartum women. Journal of Nurse-Midwifery. 34: 8-14, 1989.

137 Jonasson, A., Larsson, B. And Pschera, H. Testing and training of the pelvic floor muscles after childbirth. Acta obstetrica et gynecologica Scandinavica. 68: 301-304, 1989.

138 Jonasson, A., Fianus, S. And Larsson, B. Vagitrim - nyatt, enkelt, hjalpmedel for effectiv traning av backenbottenmuskulatur. Lakartioningen. 89 (38): 2820, 1992.

139 Meyer, S., Hohlfield, P., Achtari, C. And De Grandi, P. Pelvic floor education after vaginal delivery. Obstetrics & Gynecology. 97: 673-677, 2001.

140 Nielsen, C.A., Sigsgaard, I., Olsen, M., Tolstrup, M., Danneskiold-Samsoee, B. And Bock, J.E. Trainability of the pelvic floor. Acta obstetrica et gynecologica Scandinavica. 67: 437-440, 1988.

141 Reilly, E.T.C., Pedler, F., Steggles, P., Waterfield, A.E. And Freeman, R.M. Prevention of postpartum stress incontinence in at risk primigravide (Abstract). Proceedings of The 24h Annual Meeting of the International Urogynecology Association, Denver, U.S.A, 1999,

142 Sampselle, C.M., Miller, J.M., Mims, B.L., Delancey, J.O.L., Ashton-Miller, J.A. And Antonakos, C.L. Effect of pelvic muscle exercise on transient incontinence during pregnancy and after birth. Obstetrics & Gynecology. 91: 406-412, 1998.

143 Sleep, J. And Grant, A. Pelvic floor exercises in postnatal care. Midwifery. 3: 158-164, 1987.

144 Thorp, J.M., Stephenson, H., Jones, L.H. And Cooper, G. Pelvic floor (Kegel) exercises - a pilot study in nulliparous women. International Urogynecology Journal. 5: 86-89, 1994.

145 Porru, D., Campus, G., Caria, A., Madeddu, G., Cucchi, A., Roverto, B., Scarpa, R., Pili, P. And Usai, E. Impact of early pelvic floor rehabilitation after transurethral resection of the prostate. Neurourology & Urodynamics. 20: 53-59, 2001.

146 Hadley, E.C. Bladder training and related therapies for urinary incontinence in older people. Journal of American Medical Association. 256: 372-379, 1986.

147 Fantl, J.A., Wyman, J.F., McClish, D.K., Harkins, S.W., Elswick, R.K., Taylor, J.R. And Hadley, E.C. Efficacy of bladder training in older women with urinary incontinence. Journal of American Medical Association. 265: 609-613, 1991.

148 Fantl, J.A. Behavioural intervention for community-dwelling individuals with urinary incontinence. Urology. 51(2A Suppl): 30-34, 1998.

149 Roe, B., Williams, K. And Palmer, M. Bladder training for urinary incontinence in adults. The Cochhrane Database of Systematic reviews. 4: 1-22, 2000.

150 Jeffcoate, T.N.A., Francis, W.J. Urgency incontinence in the female. American Journal of Obstetrics & Gynecology. 94: 604-618, 1966.

151 Frewen, W.K. Urgency incontinence: review of 100 cases. Journal of Obstetrics & Gynecology of the British Commonwealth. 79: 77-79, 1972.

152 Frewen, W.K. An objective assessment of the unstable bladder of psychosomatic origin. British Journal of Urology. 50: 246-249, 1978.

153 Frewen, W.K. The management of urgency and frequency of

micturition. British Journal of Urology. 52: 367-369, 1980.

154 Frewen, W.K. A reassessment of bladder training in detrusor dysfunction in the female. British Journal of Urology. 54: 372-373, 1982.

155 Fantl, J.A., Newman, D.K. and Colling, J., Et Al Urinary Incontinence in Adults: Acute and Chronic Management. Rockville, MD: U.S. Department of Health and Human Services. Public Health Service. Agency for Health Care Policy and Research.1996.

156 Wyman, J.F. And Fantl, J.A. Bladder training in the ambulatory care management of urinary incontinence. Urological Nursing. 11 (3): 11-17, 1991.

157 Visco, A.G., Weidner, A.C., Cundiff, G.W. And Bump, R.C. Observed patient compliance with a structured outpatient bladder retraining programme. American Journal of Obstetrics & Gynecology. 18: 1392-1394, 1999.

158 Davies, J.A., Hosker, G., Lord, J. And Smith, A.R.B. An evaluation of the efficacy of in-patient bladder retraining. International Urogynecology Journal. 11: 272-276, 2000.

159 Jarvis, G.J., Millar, D.R. Controlled trial of bladder drill for detrusor instability. British Medical Journal. 281: 1322-1323, 1980.

160 Jarvis, G.J. A controlled trial of bladder drill and drug therapy in the mangement of detrusor instability. British Journal of Urology. 53: 565-566, 1981.

161 Columbo, M., Zanetta, G. And Scalambrino, S.E.A. Oxybutynin and bladder training in the management of female urinary urge incontinence: A randomized study. International Urogynecology Journal. 6: 63-67, 1995.

162 McClish, D.K., Fantl, J.A., Wyman, J.F., Pisani, G. And Bump, R.C. Bladder training in older women with urinary incontinence: Relationship between outcome and changes in urodynamic observations. Obstetric Gynecology. 77: 281-286, 1991.

163 Wyman, J.F., Fantl, J.A., McClish, D.K. And Al, E. Effect of bladder training on quality of life of older women with urinary incontinence. International Urogynecology Journal. 8: 223-229, 1997.

164 Macauley, A.J., Stern, R.S., Homes, D.M. And Stanton, S.L. Micturition and the mind: psychological factors in the aetiology and treatment of urinary symptoms in women. British Medical Journal. 294: 540-543, 1987.

165 Wiseman, P.A., Malone-Lee, J. And Rai, G.S. Terodiline with bladder retraining for treating detrusor instability in elderly people. British Medical Journal. 302: 994-996, 1991.

166 Szonyi, G., Collas, D.M. And Ding, Y.Y., Et All Oxybuynin with bladder retraining for detrusor instability in elderly people: A randomized controlled trial. Age Ageing. 24: 287-291, 1995.

167 Klarskov, P., Gerstenberg, T.C. And Hald, T. Bladder training and terodiline in females with idopathic urge incontinence and stable detrusor function. Scandanavian Journal of Urology Nephrology. 20: 41-46, 1986.

168 Nativ, O., Moskowitz, B., Issaq, E., Condrea, A., Kastin, A., Halachmi, S., Burbara, J. And Beyar, M. A new intraurethral sphincter prosthesis with a self contained urinary pump. ASAIO Journal 43 (3): 197-203, 1997.

169 Edwards, L. Objective and subjective results. British journal of urology.: 211-225, 1971.

170 Bonnar Silicone vaginal applicance for control of stress incontinence. Lancet.: 1161, 1977.

171 Cardozo, L. Evaluation of female urinary incontinence device. Urology. 13 (4): 398-401, 1979.

172 Nygaard, I. Prevention of Excercise Incontinence with mechanical devices. Journal of Reproductive Medicine. 40: 89-94, 1995.

173 Realini, J.B. and Walters, M.D. Vaginal diaphragm rings in the treatment of stress incontinence. Journal of the American Board of Family Practice. 2: 99-103, 1990.

174 Suarez, G. Use of a standard contraceptive diaphragm in management of genuine stress incontinence. Urology. 37 (2): 119-122, 1991.

175 Bhatia, N.N., Bergman, A. And Gunning, J.E. Urodynamic effects of a vaginal pessary in women with stress incontinence. American Journal of Obstetrics & Gynaecology. 147 (8): 876-884, 1983.

176 Bhatia, N.N. And Bergman, A. Pessary test in women with urinary incontinence. Obstetrics & Gynaecology. 65: 220-226, 1985.

177 Biswas, N.C. A silastic vaginal device for the treatment of genuine stress incontinence. Neurourology & Urodynamics. 7: 271-272, 1988.

178 Davila, G.W., Neal, D., Horbach, N., Peacher, J., Doughtie, J.D. And Karram, M. A bladder-neck support prosthesis for women with stress and mixed incontinence. Obstetrics & Gynaecology. 93 (6): 938-942, 1999.

179 Davila, G.W. And Osterman, K.V. The bladder neck support prosthesis: a nonsurgical approach to stress incontinence in adult women. 171. 1 (206-211): 1991.

180 Moore, K.H., Foote, A., Siva, S., King, J. And Burton, G. The use of the bladder neck support prosthesis in combined genuine stress incontinence and detrusor instability. Australian New Zealand Journal of Obstetrics & Gynaecology. 37: 440-445, 1997.

181 Moore, K.H., Foote, A.J., Burton, G. And King, J. An open study of the bladder neck support prosthesis in genuine stress incontinence. British Journal of Obstetrics & Gynaecology. 106: 42-49, 1999.

182 Kondo, A., Yokoyama, E., Koshiba, K., Gotoh, M., Yoshikawa, Y., Yamada, T. And Takei, M. Bladder neck support prosthesis: a non operative treatment for stress or mixed urinary incontinence. Journal of Urology. 157: 824-827, 1997.

183 Thyssen, H. New disposable vaginal device (continence guard) in the treatment of female stress incontinence: design, effical and short term safety. Acta Obstetricia et Gynecologica Scandinavica. 75: 170-173, 1996.

184 Thyssen, H., Lose, G. And Andersen, J.T. Effect of a vaginal device on quality of life with genuine stress incontinence. Obstetrics & Gynecology. 93 (3): 407-411, 1999.

185 Hahn, I. And Milson, I. Treatment of female genuine stress incontinence with a new anatomically shaped vaginal device (Conveen Continence Guard). British Journal of Urology. 77 (5): 711-715, 1996.

186 Glavind, K. Use of a vaginal sponge during aerobic exercises in patients with genuine stress incontinence. International Urogynecology Journal of Pelvic Floor Dysfunction. 8: 351-353, 1997.

187 Eckford, S.D., Jackson, S.R., Lewis, P.A. And Abrams, P. The continence control pad - a new external urethral occlusion device in the management of stress incontinence. British Journal of Urology. 77: 538-540, 1996.

188 Brubaker, L., Harris, T., Gleason, D., Newman, D. And North, B. The external urethral barrier for stress incontinence: a multicenter trial of safety and efficacy. Miniguard Investigators Group. Obstetrics & Gynecology. 93 (6): 932-937, 1999.

189 Versi, E., Griffiths, D.J. And Harvey, M.A. A new external urethral occlusive device for female urinary incontinence. Obstetrics & Gynecology. 2: 286-291, 1998.

190 Tincello, D.G., Bolderson, J. And Richmond, D.H. Preliminary experience with a urinary control device in the management of women with genuine stress incontinence. British Journal of Urology. 80: 752-756, 1997.

191 Tincello, D.G., Adams, E.J., Bolderson, J. And Richmond, D.H. A urinary control device for management of female stress incontinence. Obstetrics & Gynecology. 95 (3): 417-420, 2000.

192 Bellin, P., Smith, J., Poll, W., Bogojavlensky, S., Knoll, D., Childs, S., Tuttle, J., Barada, J. And Dann, J. Results of a multicentre trial of the CapSure continence shield on women with genuine stress incontinence. Urology. 51 (5): 697-706, 1998.

193 Versi, E. And Harvey, M.A. Efficacy of an external urethral device in women with genuine genuine stress incontinence. International Urogynecology Journal Pelvic Floor Dysfunction. 9 (5): 271-274, 1998.

194 Moore, K.H., Simons, A., Dowell, C., Bryant, C. And Prashar, S. Efficacy and user acceptability of the urethral occlusive device in women with urinary incontinence. Journal of Urology. 162 (2): 464-468, 1999.

195 Neilsen, K.K., Walter, S., Maeffaard, E. And Kromann-Andersen, B. The urethral plug II: an alternative treatment in women with genuine stress incontinence. British Journal of Urology. 72 (4): 428-432, 1993.

196 Peschers, U., Zen Ruffinen, F., Schaer, G.N. And Schussler, B. The VIVA urethral plug: a sensible expansion of the spectrum for conservative therapy of genuine stress incontinence? Geburtshilfe Frauenheilkd. 56 (3): 118-123, 1996.

197 Staskin, D.R., Bavendam, T., Miller, J., Davila, G.W., Diokno, A., Knapp, P., Rappaport, S., Sand, P., Sant, G. And Tutrone, R. Effectiveness of a urinary control insert in the management of genuine stress incontinence: early results of a multicenter study. Urology. 47 (5): 629-636, 1996.

198 Miller, J.L. And Bavendam, T. Treatment with the reliance urinary control insert: one-year experience. Journal of Endourology. 10 (3): 287-292, 1996.

199 Sand, P.K., Staskin, D., Miller, J., Diokno, A., Sant, G.R., Davila, G.W., Knapp, P., Rappaport, S. And Tutrone, R. Effect of a urinary control insert on quality of life in incontinent women. International Urogynecology Journal Pelvic Floor Dysfunction. 10 (2): 100-105, 1999.

200 Boos, K., Anders, K., Hextall A, Tooz-Hobson, P., Cardozo, L. Randomised trial of Reliance versus Femassist devices in the management of genuine stress incontinence. Neurourology Urodynamics. 17 (4): (abstract 113), 455-456, 1998.

201 Dunn, M., Brandt, D., Nygaard, I. Treatment of exercise incontinence with a urethral insert: a pilot study. The Physician and Sportsmedicine.: In press 2001.

Committee 10 D

Urinary Incontinence and Bladder Dysfunction in Older Persons

Chairman

D. Fonda (Australia)

Members

F. Benvenuti (Italy),

A. Cottenden (UK),

C. DuBeau (USA),

R. Kirshner-Hermanns (Germany),

K. Miller (USA),

M. Palmer (USA),

N. Resnick (USA)

CONTENTS

Urinary Incontinence and Bladder Dysfunction in Older Persons

D. FONDA,

F. BENVENUTI, A. COTTENDEN, C. DUBEAU, R.KIRSHNER-HERMANNS, K. MILLER, M. PALMER, N. RESNICK

I. INTRODUCTION

Incontinence is a very common condition that increases markedly with advancing age (See chapter 3 «Epidemiology»). This, together with ageing of communities throughout the world, means that we will be facing significantly increased numbers of older people who will be suffering from incontinence. This "demographic imperative" will impose increasing demands on limited health resources, especially in developing countries, and older people with incontinence may well find themselves with little opportunity for assessment or treatment.

A significant difference between young and older people is that usually in the former there is a single cause for the incontinence whilst in older people there are frequently co-morbid conditions, either related or unrelated to the lower urinary tract. The latter has particular importance as treatment directed to these causes may lead to modest or significant improvement in the incontinence even without attention to the lower urinary tract factors (which of course should also be attended to). Moreover, not to address these co-morbid conditions in frail older patients will likely limit the success of interventions limited to just the urogenital system.

Sound data for older and frail populations have been lacking because of difficulty in designing and performing good research studies. Reasons for this include:

- the heterogeneity of this population resulting in difficulty in designing studies that account for comorbidity, drug use, intercurrent illness, and shorter life expectancy;
- lack of standardized terminology to define and measure cure and improvement, and quality of life;
- lack of validated research tools to measure baseline and outcome variables in the frail older population;
- lack of long term follow-up to gauge impact, durability and applicability of the intervention;
- lack of information of the natural history of incontinence in this group.

To date there is a lack of specific data regarding conservative and surgical interventions in fit older people, even though they are often included in adult studies. Many of the studies cited throughout this book include older persons but few stratify the results by age. Furthermore, it has not been a requirement of this consultation for the respective committees to analyse or stratify data by age. Therefore it is difficult to extrapolate such interventions in older, and particularly frail, older people. The existence of co-morbid conditions makes such analyses most important and therefore reflects a major shortcoming of current research.

Despite the absence of clear scientific data management of incontinence in healthy older people is generally similar to the approach taken in younger individuals, except that greater caution should be taken when pharmacological or surgical intervention is contemplated because of the susceptibility of older people to adverse events. This chapter will focus on lower urinary tract dysfunction in older patients and particularly those who are frail and disabled. Specific reference or caution will be highlighted where current standard treatments that apply in other adult populations may have an impact on "frailer and disabled older people".

There is no agreed standard definition of frailty at this time but one useful one is "a state of reduced physiological reserve associated with increased susceptibility to disability [1]. In this chapter we will particularly focus on such frail older people as well as those sufficiently disabled that they require the assistance of others to perform some or all of the more basic activities of daily living (ADLs) including bathing, dressing, toileting and ambulating. Such people may be housebound, suffer from dementia or be living in a residential care facility. It is not surprising that results of interventions in younger or fit older populations cannot be extrapolated to the frail and disabled older population. Figure 1 shows the relationship between fit, frail and disabled older people. The potential reversibility of these conditions (as reflected by the two way arrows) emphasises the importance of focussing attention also away from the LUT.

The general approach to managing incontinence in

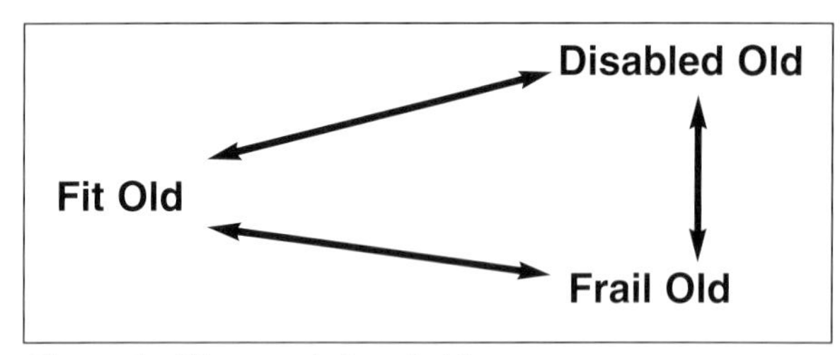

Figure 1 : Characteristics of older persons

patients with neurological conditions such as stroke, paraplegia or Parkinson's disease are covered in Chapter 10e «Conservative Treatment in Neuropathic». When frailty or significant disability is superimposed, as for example occurs in advanced Parkinson's, severe stroke or moderate to severe dementia, then the approaches in this chapter become more relevant. For these populations there is no validated research showing long term efficacy of treatment for urinary incontinence for the specific neurological condition. Good care can still be provided following comprehensive assessment and an integrated holistic management approach as will be outlined in this chapter.

During the International Consultation on Incontinence in 1998, the literature and Levels of Evidence were extensively reviewed and Grades of Recommendation were made. Unfortunately, in the area related to frail and disabled older people, evidence was generally found to be lacking. Nonetheless, based on Expert Opinion, the ICI team concluded that incontinence in the majority of older adults is amenable to improvement, and often cure, irrespective of the underlying condition.

However, such success demands appropriate assessment, investigation and management, informed by knowledge of the changes and morbidity that occur with aging and the multiple medications that such patients generally use.

By definition, 100% of these patients are wet at presentation and the goal is to achieve a 100% dry state (see figure 2). Ideally, improvement would be to the level of full, independent continence but the terms dependent continence and social continence were added and are defined further later in this chapter Figure 3 illustrates these relationships which shows that a patient can achieve a dry state by a combination of these strategies as will be outlined throughout this chapter [2].

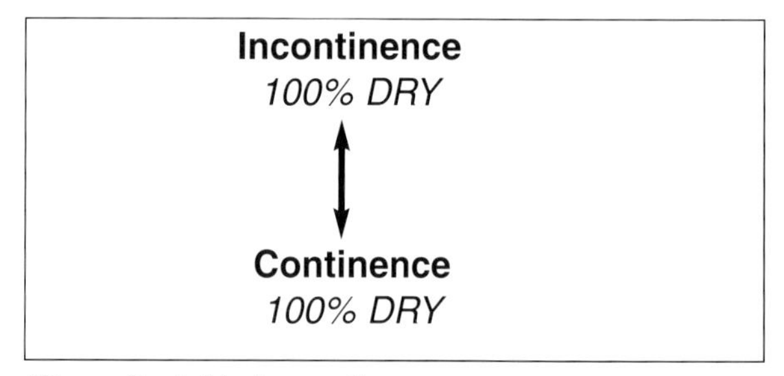

Figure 2 : Achieving continence

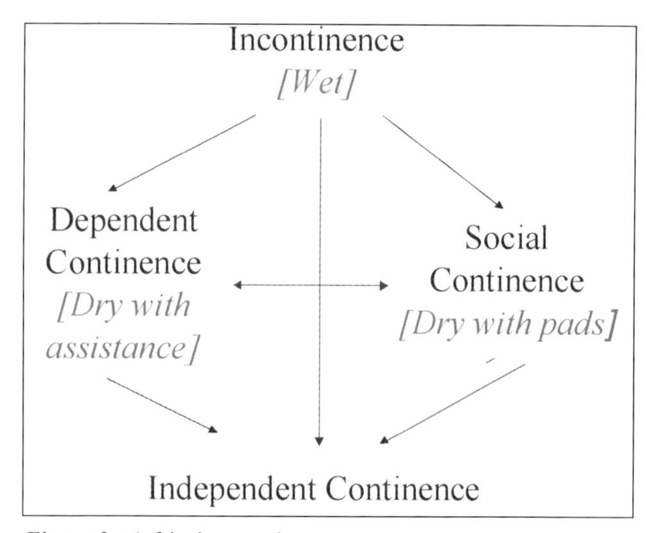

Figure 3 : Achieving continence

II. IDENTIFICATION OF URINARY INCONTINENCE

Incontinence increases markedly with age and frailty. Detailed prevalence data and the extent of under reporting are provided in chapter 2 «Basic Neurophysiology and Neuropharmacology» and will not be reported in this section.

Given the high prevalence of incontinence amongst older and frail populations it is important to seek any potential modifiable or reversible factors that could lead to a reduction in the severity of the incontinence or at least some amelioration of the symptoms. However, the significant under reporting of urinary incontinence compromises such.

Urinary incontinence usually comes to a health care professional's notice only when the patient complains of specific symptoms. However, research indicates that fewer than half of the older patients who suffer from urinary incontinence seek help for this problem [1-4]. Older people may think incontinence is part of the normal aging process [2,5-8] and health care professionals may dismiss incontinence as not worthy of investigation and treatment [8].

One of the problems with a number of the definitions used in the literature e.g. any leakage more than once a month, is that they turn up a great number of mild cases which does not define the prevalence of need. The latter may be much more important in frail, older people and residents of nursing homes. Furthermore, the relationship between severity and perceived impact is complex. There is a need to examine the effect of other urinary tract symptoms as these may be more bothersome than incontinence to the patient.

Older people without cognitive impairments should be always questioned about their continence status [9,10]. For patients who are cognitively impaired, family members are frequently helpful given the unpleasant experience of finding soiled clothes, wet beds, or detecting odor. In hospital and nursing homes, observation of voiding behaviour and wet episodes should be routinely performed.

In nursing homes reports of incontinence by nursing staff are not always reliable and valid [11]. To address this problem, in the USA, the Resident Assessment Instrument, which includes Minimum Data Set (MDS) and Resident Assessment Protocols, was devised to improve the quality of care for nursing home residents through maintenance and restoration of function. It was developed by the US Health Care Financing Administration [12] and is presently used in at least 18 different Countries. Identification of incontinence by the Minimum Data Set is mandated within 14 days of admission and every three months thereafter [13]. When a patient is incontinent or wears an indwelling catheter nurses and physicians are guided by the urinary incontinence Resident Assessment Protocol through the evaluation process to ascertain the cause, duration, and type of urinary incontinence or catheter. The interrater reliability of the 13 items of MDS related to incontinence was verified in nursing home residents of both genders by Resnick et al [14]. Use of the MDS has disclosed that, at least in the US, a substantial proportion of elderly incontinent institutionalized residents suffer from conditions that may be contributing to UI, are potentially remediable, and yet remain unaddressed [15].

RECOMMENDATIONS

- Strategies to increase recognition and reporting of UI are required and especially the perception that it is an inevitable consequence of ageing for which little or nothing can be done.

III. PHYSIOLOGIC AND PATHOLOGIC CHANGES RELEVANT TO INCONTINENCE IN OLDER ADULTS

This section builds on the general anatomy, physiology, and pathophysiology covered in chapters 1,2,4 «Anatomy, Cellular and Gross», «Basic Neurophysiology and Neuropharmacology», «Pathophysiology» and focuses on the specific issues related to older adults.

Aging affects the lower urinary tract in a number of ways, but it does not cause incontinence. Although data from continent elderly are sparse and longitudinal data virtually non-existent, it appears that bladder capacity and the ability to postpone voiding decline in both sexes, while urethral length and maximum closure pressure—as well as striated muscle cells in the rhabdosphincter—decline with age in women [1-4]. The prostate enlarges in most men, and it appears to cause urodynamic obstruction in approximately half [3, 5].

In both sexes, the post-voiding residual volume (PVR) probably increases, albeit to no more than 50-100 mls [1-3]. Increased PVR is found even in the absence of concurrent or prior obstruction, and it appears to reflect an age-related impairment in detrusor contractility [3]. Detrusor muscle biopsies from such individuals are characterized by an ultrastructural "dense band pattern" consisting of dense sarcolemmal bands with depleted caveolae [6-7]. Because caveolae are involved in ion transport (especially calcium), this change in detrusor architecture may mediate the observed decline in contractility.

Detrusor overactivity becomes more prevalent with age, even among continent individuals [1-3]. Although detrusor overactivity is rarely observed during standard urodynamic testing in continent younger adults, it can be documented in more than one-third of older people, even among those who are robustly healthy and who lack traditionally-impugned causes, such as neurological lesions or urethral abnormalities [3]. Detrusor biopsies from such individuals reveal a "complete dysjunction pattern" of smooth muscle. This pattern is characterized by a decrease in the number of normal smooth muscle junctions (adherens junctions) and emergence of a different type of junction known as "protrusion junction" or "ultraclose abutment." In this type of junction, cell-cell contacts occur via a much narrower intercellular space, with neither an interposed basement membrane nor the sub-sarcolemmal specialized structures that characterize the adherens junction. The complete dysjunction pattern differs from the "incomplete dysjunction pattern" found in age-matched older adults who do not have detrusor overactivity. In these individuals, normal adherens junctions are much more prominent, and any altered junctions that are present are sparse and do not connect multiple cells together in chains [7, 8].

The presence of DO in many continent elderly individuals suggests that the relationship between DO and urge incontinence is less straightforward in older adults than in younger individuals. A recent study suggests that in older patients, characteristics of the involuntary contraction, detrusor contractility, and urethral sphincter integrity, among other factors, all influence the severity of urge incontinence [9] and may affect the likelihood of becoming incontinent as well.

In addition, age-related changes in the secretion of

vasopressin and atrial natriuretic hormone result in older adults often excreting most of their fluid intake at night, even in the absence of venous insufficiency, renal disease, heart failure, or prostate obstruction [10, 11]. These changes, coupled with an age-associated increase in sleep disorders, leads to 1-2 episodes of nocturia in the majority of healthy elderly [1].

Because each of these changes was found in continent elderly, none of them causes incontinence. But they do predispose to it. This predisposition, combined with the increased likelihood that an older person will encounter an additional pathologic, physiologic, or pharmacologic insult, explains why the elderly are so likely to become incontinent. The implications are equally important. The onset or exacerbation of incontinence in an older person is likely to be due to precipitant(s) ***outside*** the lower urinary tract, which are amenable to medical intervention. Furthermore, ***treatment of the precipitant(s) alone may be sufficient to restore continence, even if there is coexistent urinary tract dysfunction.*** For instance, flare of hip arthritis in a woman with age-related detrusor overactivity may be sufficient to convert her urinary urgency into incontinence. Treatment of the arthritis—rather than the involuntary detrusor contractions—will not only restore continence but also lessen pain and improve mobility. These principles, depicted in Figures 4 and 5, [12,13] provide the rationale in the older patient for adding to the established lower urinary tract causes of incontinence a set of transient causes as well.

SUMMARY

Multiple changes of the lower urinary tract, which would be considered pathological in younger adults, are found commonly in continent elderly individuals and appear to have an ultrastructural basis. Thus, the relationship between lower urinary tract dysfunction and continence in older adults is more complex than in younger individuals. Further research is required to clarify this relationship.

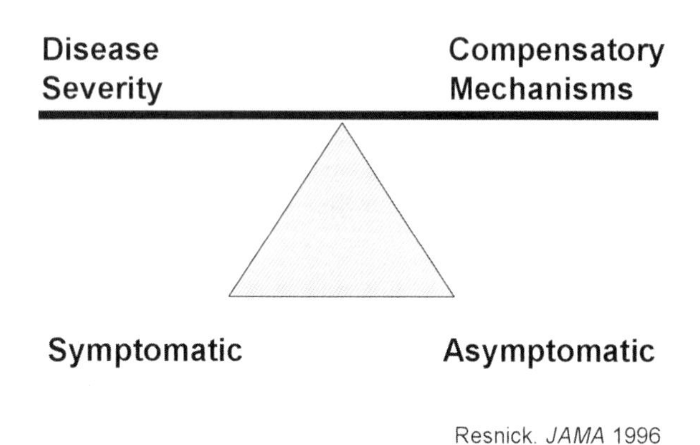

Figure 4 : Incontinence results when the ability to compensate for bladder dysfunction is inadequate. For instance, in the intact older person, detrusor overactivity or sphincter weakness may not cause leakage if the patient is more attuned to bladder fullness, drinks less, voids more often, eliminates precipitants such as coughing, and stays close to a toilet. This may explain how older patients remain continent despite such abnormalities and also suggests alternate therapeutic approaches independent of the urinary tract. (Modified from: Resnick NM, JAMA 1996: 276: 1832-1840)

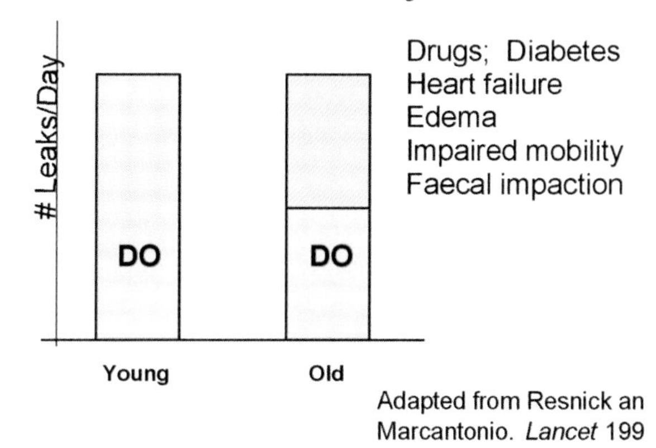

Figure 5 : This cartoon shows why treatment of UI in older adults has to differ and is often easier to treat than in younger adults. Both of these patients with detrusor overactivity (DO) have the same frequency of leakage. However, in the younger patient with intact compensatory mechanisms, such leakage reflects solely the contribution of the DO. In the older adult, other comorbid conditions make it more difficult to appreciate bladder fullness, adjust fluid output, and reach the bathroom. Such conditions magnify the impact of DO and will be unaffected by bladder relaxant therapy. But addressing them will result in a marked improvement in the UI even without treatment of the DO and will make bladder relaxant therapy—if still required—more effective. (Modified from Resnick NM, Marcantonio ER. Lancet 1997; 350: 1157-1158).

IV. NOCTURIA

Nocturia, waking more than once during the night to void, is an extremely common and bothersome global complaint. It affects all ages, increasing significantly with age from 50 years onwards. The pathophysiology is difficult to pinpoint, and to date there is no accurate reproducible method of diagnosis. Nocturia is commonly defined as the necessity to rise from bed more than once after one has retired there with the intention of sleeping until morning. Other definitions have been proposed and include; nighttime urine production greater than 33% of diurnal urine [1] and nighttime urine production of more than 0.9 ml/min [2]. Nocturia has long been considered a normal part of aging, yet its impact on quality of life (nocturnal incontinence, disrupted sleep, daytime sleepiness, risk of falling) calls for closer analysis of the parameters of normal and abnormal nocturnal urine production.

This section will deal only with nocturia in older people and not nocturnal incontinence as little specific data is available on the later.

1. Clinical evaluation

a) Background

There is more to nocturia than lower urinary tract dysfunction and the symptom alone does not suggest any one diagnosis. The main causes of nocturia are: *nocturnal frequency*, due to bladder pathology usually as a result of reduced bladder capacity; *nocturnal polyuria*, where there is nocturnal diuresis or overproduction of urine; or combinations of the above. Also awakening due to disturbed sleep or sleep apnoea can lead to nocturia. In these situations it may or may not be related to other LUTS of urinary incontinence, urinary frequency and urgency [3].

Bladder problems leading to nocturnal frequency include; age associated reduced bladder capacity, low compliant bladder, detrusor overactivity, and chronic retention of urine with overflow. Increased nocturnal urine production (noctunal polyuria) may be due to increased urine production both by day and night as occurs with diabetes insipidus or diabetes mellitus , or it may just be due to factors that create this problem at night. The later include congestive cardiac failure, hypoalbuminaemia, venous insufficiency and renal disease. Excessive intake of fluids, alcohol and caffeine especially later in the day, or use of a long-acting diuretic may also precipitate a nocturnal diuresis. Changes in posture from day to night can cause nocturia following reabsorption of peripheral fluid. Nocturnal polyuria may also be due to reduced nocturnal production of arginine vasopression (AVP) as is seen in some older people, so that urine production is increased at night and may exceed that produced in the day

It is generally agreed that in an older person the need to get up once at night should be accepted as normal and not treated. When a patient presents with the complaint of nocturia, the history taking is of paramount importance, covering the above mentioned conditions and with attention to sleep related problems. The later should include the time of going to bed and arising in the morning. Confirmation with a 48-hour frequency/volume continence chart is required, which provides information about the working capacity of the bladder, the diurnal volumes of urine, incontinent episodes (if any), and fluid intake.

b) Quality of Data

It is commonly understood that nocturia affects both sexes equally [4, 5, 6] and that its prevalence increases with age [7]. However, the lack of a formal definition and consequently public awareness and reporting makes the prevalence of nocturia difficult to ascertain. Prevalence figures are gleaned using different analytical methods and definitions of nocturia, but nonetheless gives a strong indication of the extent of the problem. Much research carried out on the mechanism of nocturia has been investigated in elderly men in conjunction with other lower urinary tract symptoms suggestive of bladder outlet obstruction. Since nocturia persists in 19-33% of men after prostectamy, pathophysiology other than obstruction is a contributing factor in the development of nocturia [1]. These mechanisms are yet to be clearly determined in persons not suffering from the above-mentioned predisposing conditions.

c) Results

Various studies have indicated the prevalence range to be 10% of the general population (older than 20 years), 16% in the fourth decade, 29% to 66% in the fifth decade, to rise to 55% in men aged over 70, reaching 70%-91% for those aged 80+ years [8]. Nocturia is particularly prevalent in residents of nursing homes be they male or female where the time spent in bed overnight is prolonged (8-14 hours). One investigation reported a high prevalence rate but found that 63% of men and 59% of women who were affected by their nocturia did not seek medical help [9], despite the findings that two-thirds of men and women with nocturia report it as bothersome [10]. Another study has shown a difference in reporting according to country of origin; more than 50% of the symptomatic patients in the United States and Germany were likely to consult a physician compared with 22% in Sweden and 24% in France [11].

The amount of time a patient is in bed may contribute to nocturia as it is common for older people to spend more time in bed but without requiring increased sleep. Hence the likelihood of nocturia increases especially as bladder capacity is frequently reduced in this population.

Those causes that wake the patient such as insomnia, sleep apnoea or pronounced snoring can be wrongly interpreted as a desire for micturition. In one sleep study, 65% of consecutive patients for evaluation of a suspected sleep disorder explained their awakenings the next morning as pressure to urinate. However, objective findings from a polysomnograph showed that 76% of these selected patients had awoken because of apnoea, hypopnoea or snoring [12]. The number of nocturnal voidings was also higher in a group of men referred for voiding disorders with habitual snoring compared to the non-snorers [13]. Sleep disordered breathing is very common in the older population [14]. Treatment of obstructive sleep apnoea with nasal continuous positive airway pressure reduces venous atrial natriuretic peptide concentrations and nocturnal voiding [15]. There is sufficient evidence therefore to suggest that a medical history including snoring habits and potential obstructive apnoeic events should be obtained from patients who complain of nocturnal urinary symptoms.

d) Summary

Nocturia is a bothersome, pathological symptom, affecting a person's quality of life.

The pathophysiology is thought to reside in bladder dysfunction and/or nocturnal diuresis, with or without a setting of other clinical conditions.

Accurate history taking of urinary symptoms and other active health problems is essential in the evaluation of a person with nocturia.

Prevalence is high and rises with age. Lack of public awareness makes exact figures difficult to determine.

e) Research priorities

- Consensus for a clinical definition and evaluation pathway for nocturia
- Public awareness
- Accurate appraisal of the underlying mechanisms

2. Conservative management

a) Background

Insight into the mechanisms of nocturia has provided direction for treatment and the potential for clinical improvement. First line treatment is always correction of any underlying conditions, biochemical abnormalities, with attention to medications. In patients with peripheral oedema and/or congestive cardiac failure, fluid accumulates in the lower limbs in the day and returns to the circulation at night. Appropriate management can prevent excessive variation of nocturnal intravascular volume, allowing the kidneys to excrete proportionally more fluid in the waking hours.

b) Quality of data

There are no studies on the effectiveness of conservative management strategies in older people, management relies on expert advice and common sense.

c) Summary

Fluid restriction, especially at night, has not been shown to effect symptoms unless there is obvious excessive intake or taken late at night [16]. It is reasonable to restrict caffeine and alcohol in the evening because of their effect on urine production and normal sleep. Compressive devices may prevent third-spacing of fluid. Late afternoon or evening elevation of oedematous legs for several hours stimulates a natural diuresis and limits the amount of oedema present at bedtime [17]. Making the patient aware of the consequences of prolonged time in bed may lead to nocturia may lead to simple possible strategies.

There are a number of suggested first-line clinical approaches to managing nocturia which may be useful in the management of nocturia, despite the lack of proof. These include modification of fluids, compressive stockings and elevation of the feet (Level of evidence 4).

d) Recommendations

- Conservative management of nocturia, whilst lacking hard data appear nonetheless to be effective or helpful in many patients. (Grade of Recommendation D)

e) Research priorities

- Further research into conservative management is warranted.
- Affect of strategies directed at sleep disturbance or sleep disorders.
- Association between snoring and nocturia.

3. Diuretic treatment

a) Background

Diuretics are a reasonable approach for patients with fluid retention, and there is anecdotal evidence that they might be given with more affect in the afternoon [18,19]. In the nursing home setting diuretics administered at varying times may reduce nocturia [20]. In older people with nocturia who do not have perioheral oedema, diuretics may still be of some value.

b) Quality of data

There are limited studies on this treatment in the community-dwelling older person with nocturia. The two randomised control trials to date have small sample sizes, and only one includes women.

c) Results

Reynard et al conducted a randomised double-blind placebo-controlled trial of 49 men older than 50 years who suffered from nocturia [18]. There was a significant reduction in night-time frequency when treated with 40mg of frusemide in the afternoon. Seven of 19 on the active treatment had a reduction in frequency by one, and four by two episodes, compared with only one of 20 experiencing a reduction on the placebo. Daytime voided volume increased, with a small but insignificant decrease (120ml) in nighttime volume. It is unclear as to what medications the subjects in both groups were taking, which could have interfered with the results. The other is a randomised double-blind cross-over study of bumetanide taken 4-6 hours before bed [19]. Twenty-eight patients (13 women, 15 men) of age ranging from 58-78 years (mean 66.5) completed the study, three were excluded due to adverse effects. The weekly number of nocturia episodes was reduced from 13.8 during placebo period to 10 on 1mg bumetanide. This statistically significant group effect was not seen in all patients.

d) Summary

Frusemide was shown to have a marked effect on some patients, without correlation between its effect and the severity of nocturia (Level of Evidence 3b).

Bumetanide had no benefit for the 10 men with a history of prostatic hyperplasia, and should not be used for those patients (Level of Evidence 3b).

Loop diuretics may alleviate nocturia, although each patient must be evaluated on a risk-benefit basis.

e) Recommendations

- Loop diuretic therapy could be considered for further therapeutic trial since it is a simple and effective treatment in some patients, provided they are screened and monitored for postural hypotension and electrolyte disturbance (Grade of Recommendation B).

f) Research priorities

- Role of daytime diuretics to reduce nocturia.

4. Desmopressin (DDAVP)

a) Background

The altered diurnal rhythm of AVP release and renal tubular sensitivity to AVP in older persons with nocturia, is thought to be corrected by a synthetic form of the hormone. Treatment of nocturnal polyuria with DDAVP has been explored in selected patients for a reduction in nocturnal diuresis and nocturnal frequency, and for longer term improvement of nocturia.

b) Quality of data

A tabulated summary is included of the ten notable therapeutic studies of intra-nasal and more recently, oral DDAVP in older people since 1980 (Table 1, 2). The randomised controlled trials are small, short-term studies with a marked male gender predominance. Sample size is limited by significant exclusion criteria of patients with any signs or symptoms, or receiving treatment for: heart disease, hypertension, liver disease, renal disease, Crohn's disease, neurological problems, primary polydipsia, diabetes insipidus, UTI, and those with medications that could create interactions or alter fluid and electrolye metabolism [1, 2]. Interpretation and generalisation of findings therefore to older patients is made difficult because of the frequency of co-existing conditions.

c) Results

- Nocturnal Diuresis

Cannon et al [1] selected a community-residing group of men with nocturia, defined as producing more than 33% of the 24 hour urine volume overnight. Intra-nasal DDAVP was given at bedtime for two weeks each at 20ug and 40ug in a double-blind, cross-over controlled study. Mean nocturnal volume as a percentage of 24-hour volume decreased from 47.3% at run-in, to 39.2% after two weeks of 20ug desmopressin, with some further but statistically insignificant decrease on the 40ug dose. Asplund et al conducted a dose-titration study of oral desmopression, the decrease in nocturnal diuresis in seventeen men and six women when administered 10, 20 and 40ug dosages was observed. It was found that the baseline nocturnal diuresis of 1.6ml/min decreased to 1.1ml/min after administration of the 10ug dose. Further decrease of nocturnal urine flow to 0.9ml/min with the 20ug dose, with no further decrease with the 40ug dose. Reduction occured almost exclusively in the group with a high nocturnal urinary output of ≥1.3ml/min. Diuresis returned to pre-treatment levels one week after treatment.

- Nocturnal frequency:

In the Cannon et al study, nocturnal frequency was only significantly reduced after the highest dose of 40ug DDAVP. The dose-titration study led Asplund et al to conduct a double-blind randomised control trial of oral desmopressin for the management of nocturnal polyuria in elderly subjects. The optimal dose (the dose which gave the best reduction in nocturnal diuresis without significant adverse effects [2]) of desmopressin for each patient was administered. Four patients received 10ug, 10 received 20ug, and 3 received 40ug.

Table 1 : Role of desmopressin in elderly people with nocturia

	Sex	Age	No.	Type	Definition of Nocturia	Dose DDAVP	Nocturnal Diuresis	Nocturnal frequency (n/night) pre-Rx	post-Rx	Level of Evidence
Cannon [1] (Intra-nasal)	M	52-80	20	DBCS Placebo	>33% of 24hr diuresis	20µg 40µg	↓15.4% ↓26.4%	3.0	2.3	3b
Asplund [22] (Oral)	M/F 12/5	60-74	17	RDBCS Placebo	>0.9ml/min at night	10µg - 40µg	↓37.5%	1.7	1.1	2b
Chancellor [24]	M	elderly	12	Case Series				3.6+/-0.5	1.8+/-1.1	4
Asplund [21] (Oral)	M/F 17/6	60-74	23	Dose-titration	>0.9ml/min at night	10µg 20µg 40µg	↓31.25% ↓43.75% no further ↓			3b

Table 2 : Role of desmopressin in elderly people with nocturia

	sex	Age (mean)	No.	Type	Dose DDAVP	Nocturnal Diuresis	Nocturnal frequency (n/night) pre-Rx	post-Rx	Level of Evidence
Obara [27]	M/F	44-77 (64)	8				4.6	2.5	4
Asplund [2]	M/F	(73)	19	2-month open	40µg	↓37.5%			3b
Asplund [16]	F	(71)	20	short term	20µg	↓29%+/-19%			3b
Seiler [28]	M/F	73-90	9	open	10µg 20µg 40µg	↓33% ↓10% ↓50%			4
Hilton [29]	F	Adult	25	DBCS	20µg	↓40%	3.2	1.9 (cf 2.9 with placebo)	3b
Mansson [30]	M	Adult	21	open	20µg	↓25%			3b

Results show fewer episodes of nocturia when on desmopressin compared with placebo, with reduction being related to the level of original nocturnal diuresis. Chancellor et al found that three months after intra-nasal therapy, ten of the twelve male patients had maintained a decreased nocturnal frequency. In a study of women with nocturia, the number of nocturnal voiding episodes was unchanged [16].

• ADVERSE EFFECTS

Three patients in the intra-nasal study [1], experienced effects of fluid retention, which led the authors to recommend extreme caution in the prescription of desmopressin. Oral DDAVP was not shown to affect body weight, and no serious adverse effects were found [21].

d) Summary

Overall there is still a lack of information on the use, dosage and safety of desmopressin in older people, particularly since cardiovascular disease and hypertension is very common in this age group.

The response to desmopressin is promising in patients with nocturnal polyuria, in whom other causes are excluded (Level of Evidence 2b-4; see Table 1 for details).

Desmopressin reduces nocturnal diuresis without affecting the 24 hour diuresis, however its efficacy in reducing nocturnal frequency and its continued efficacy is not clear in older people.

Intra-nasal administration of DDAVP may be associated with more adverse effects of water retention and hyponatraemia than oral DDAVP.

However some authors have concluded that any DDAVP therapy is dangerous with the risk of causing water retention in older patients [11].

e) Recommendations

- Until further information is available use of DDAVP should not be a routine treatment, although it may have beneficial effects , but only in healthy older patients. (Grade of Recommendation B). Close monitoring for side effects is important especially serium sodium and fluid balance status.. There is no data to support its use in frail older patients.

f) Research priorities

Role of antidiuretic hormone in managing nocturia in the old and frail older person.

5. Hormone Replacement Therapy (HRT)

a) Background

Post-menopausal women commonly experience a spectrum of urinary symptoms, including nocturia. The use of continuous or combined HRT is a possible treatment strategy for older women with nocturia. Chapter 10c provides a detailed analysis of HRT in management of incontinence in women.

b) Quality of data

There have been scant randomised control trials of HRT specifically as a therapy for nocturia. A recent prospective study showed promising results, however the conclusions were made by self-reporting questionnaire. Other studies have incorporated nocturia as well as other urinary symptoms. To illustrate the inconsistency of data just two studies are cited below and readers are referred to chapter 10c for more detailed review of the role of oestrogen therapy.

c) Results

In the prospective study, women took six months of estradiol (2mg) with different levels of dydrogesterone (2.5,5,10, or 15mg). A disappearance of nocturia in 65.4% of the 95 subjects, irrespective of the dose was reported. An earlier randomised placebo-controlled, double blind study of estrogen supplementation in 83 hypo-estrogenic women showed contrasting results. Women were given estrogen (0.625mg) and meroxyprogesterone (10mg) cyclically for 3 months after which no significant difference for nocturnal micturition, nor subjective improvement were reported.

d) Summary

There are mixed results for HRT in treating nocturia, with one study showing a positive effect (Level of evidence 3b), and another showing no effect (Level of evidence 1b).

e) Recommendations

- The disparity in results suggests a need for further studies on the effect of hormone replacement therapy for the treatment of nocturia in older women (Grade of Recommendation C).

f) Research conclusion

- Nocturia is a common condition which increases with age and fraility which may respond to conservative management

g) Other research priorites for the future.

- High quality studies on pharmacological management
- Comparison of DDAVP with diuretic therapy
- Role of anticholinergics in reducing nocturia.
- Specific research is needed on management of nocturnal incontinence.

V. CAUSES OF TRANSIENT INCONTINENCE

1. Background

Transient causes probably account for one-third of incontinent cases among community-dwelling older people, up to one-half of cases among acutely-hospitalized older people, and a significant proportion of cases among nursing home residents [1-3].

Most causes of transient incontinence in the older population lie outside the lower urinary tract but two points are worth emphasizing. First, the risk of transient incontinence is increased if, in addition to physiologic changes of the lower urinary tract, the older person also suffers from pathologic changes. Chronic retention of urine with overflow incontinence is more likely to result from an anticholinergic agent in a person with a weak or obstructed bladder, just as urge incontinence is more likely to result from a loop diuretic in someone with detrusor overactivity and/or impaired mobility [4,5]. This fact explains why some controversy persists regarding some causes of transient incontinence. It also emphasizes that continence depends on the integrity of multiple domains—mentation, mobility, manual dexterity, medical factors, and motivation, as well as lower urinary tract function. Although in younger individuals incontinence usually results from lower urinary tract dysfunction alone, incontinence in older patients often results from deficits in multiple domains that together result in incontinence [6]. Attention to any one or more of these risk factors can restore continence or at least improve it. Second, although termed "transient," these causes of incontinence may persist if left untreated, and so they cannot be dismissed merely because the incontinence is of long duration.

2. Quality of data

In frail older people, continence status is often not absolute. Infrequent leakage of small amounts may appear and disappear, and reporting accuracy varies as well [7]. Furthermore, ethical constraints and methodological issues preclude robust investigations of the conditions commonly impugned as causes of transient incontinence. Thus, it is not surprising that evidence supporting the association between these conditions and transient incontinence consists predominantly of case reports and case series.

3. Results of literature review

Transient causes of incontinence in older people are shown on the accompanying table and can be recalled using the mnemonic DIAPPERS [8] ("Diapers" misspelled with an extra "p." See Table 3).

"D" is for delirium, a confusional state characterized by fluctuating inattentiveness and disorientation. Its onset occurs over hours to days, as contrasted with dementia which develops over years. Delirium can result from almost any medication and from virtually any acute illness, including congestive heart failure, deep vein thrombosis, or infection. Many of these conditions may present atypically in older patients, and if the patient becomes confused because of them, incontinence may be the first abnormality detected [9]. Delirium leads the list because, if unrecognized, it is associated with significant mortality. Thus, in this case, meticulous medical evaluation—not cystometry—is crucial.

"I" is for infection. Symptomatic urinary tract infection is another cause of incontinence, although it is an uncommon one [1]. However, asymptomatic bacteruria and urinary tract infection, which is much more common in older people, is not a cause of incontinence [10, 11].

Table 3: Causes of Transient Incontinence in Older People

D	Delirium
I	Infection (UTI, symptomatic)
A	Atrophic urethritis/vaginitis (Women)
P	Psychological (e.g. severe depression, neurosis)
P	Pharmacologic
E	Excess fluid intake or output
R	Restricted mobility and environmental
S	Stool impaction (constipation)

"A" is for atrophic vaginitis is frequently a source of lower urinary tract symptoms in women. This occasionally includes incontinence. As many as 80% of older women attending an incontinence clinic are reported to have physical evidence of atrophic vaginitis, characterized by vaginal mucosal atrophy, friability, erosions, and punctate hemorrhages [12]. Incontinence associated with this entity usually is associated with urgency and occasionally a sense of "scalding" or pain on micturition, but both symptoms may be relatively unimpressive. The importance of recognizing atrophic vaginitis is that it will respond to low-dose topical or systemic estrogen. Moreover, like each of these conditions, treatment has other benefits as well: amelioration of dyspareunia and possibly reduction in the frequency of recurrent cystitis [13].

"P" is for pharmaceuticals which are one of the most common causes of incontinence in older people, with several categories of drugs commonly implicated [1]. (See table 4 and 5). Of note, many of these agents also are used in the treatment of incontinence, underscoring the fact that most medications used by older people are "double-edged swords." The first category of relevant drugs is the long-acting sedative/hypnotics, such as diazepam and flurazepam, which can cloud an older patient's sensorium. "Loop" diuretics, such as furosemide or bumetanide, by inducing a brisk diuresis, can also provoke leakage. Drugs with anticholinergic side effects are a particular problem and include major tranquilizers, antidepressants, anti-parkinsonian agents (e.g., benztropine mesylate or trihexyphenidyl), first generation (sedating) antihistamines, anti-arrhythmics (disopyramide), antispasmodics, and opiates. By decreasing detrusor contractility, they can cause urinary retention with overflow incontinence. They also can cause confusion. Anticholinergic agents are particularly important to ask about for two reasons. First, older patients often take more than one of them at a time. Second, they are contained in many nonprescription preparations that older people frequently take without consulting a physician.

Adrenergically-active agents have also been associated with incontinence. Many alpha-adrenoreceptor antagonists (used mainly for treatment of hypertension) block receptors at the bladder neck and may induce stress incontinence in women [14]. Older women are particularly at risk because their urethral length and closure pressure normally decline with age. Thus, prior to considering other interventions for stress incontinence in a woman taking such a drug, substitution of an alternative agent should be tried and the incontinence reevaluated. Calcium channel blockers can cause incontinence. As smooth muscle relaxants, they can increase residual volume. The increased residual urine may occasionally lead to stress incontinence in women with

Table 4 : Important anticholinergic drugs and drug side effects in the elderly

Drugs	Anticholinergic Effects
Antipsychotics	Dry mouth
Tricyclic Antidepressants (not SSRI's)	Constipation
Anti-parkinsonian agents	Confusion
First generation (sedating) antihistamines	Drowsiness, fatigue
Anti-arrhythmics (disopyramide)	Tachycardia
Antispasmodics	Inhibition of detrusor
contractility	
Opiates	Urinary retention Blurred vision Increased ocular pressure

Table 5 : Other Drug-Induced Causes of Incontinence

Alpha adrenergic antagonists	Decreased urethral resistance (esp in women)
Opiates	Constipation
Anticonvulsants	Confusion, ataxia
Antihypertensives resulting in poor mobility	Postural hypotension
Anti-parkinsonian agents	Confusion, postural hypotension
H_2 antagonists	Confusion
Potent ("loop") diuretics	Frequency, urgency
Sedative/Hypnotics	Excessive sedation
Spinal anesthetics	Detrusor paralysis
Calcium antagonist	Constipation, urinary retention
Angiotensin converting enzyme inhibitor	Cough
Others (alcohol, caffeine)	Polyuria causing frequency, urgency

a weak urethral sphincter, or to retention of urine with overflow incontinence in men with concurrent urethral obstruction and detrusor weakness. Finally, angiotensin converting enzyme inhibitors, by inducing cough (the risk of which is age-related), may precipitate stress incontinence in older women whose urethra has shortened and whose sphincter has weakened with age.

"P" is also for psychological factors such as depression, and anxiety states.

"E" is for excess fluid intake or urinary output which can cause incontinence, especially in individuals with impaired mobility, mentation, or motivation, particularly if they also have detrusor overactivity. Causes of excess output include excess intake, diuretics (including theophylline-containing fluids and alcohol), and metabolic abnormalities (e.g., hyperglycemia and hypercalcemia). Nocturnal incontinence can be caused or exacerbated by disorders associated with excess nocturnal excretion, such as congestive heart failure, peripheral venous insufficiency, hypoalbuminemia (especially in malnourished older people), and drug-induced peripheral edema associated with NSAIDs or some calcium channel blockers (e.g., dihydropyridines such as nifedipine, isradipine, and nicardipine). The role of caffeine and timing of drinking fluids (e.g. in the evening or before bedtime) is still not clear, but should nonetheless be considered a possible contributing cause for nocturia and nocturnal incontinence.

"R" is for restricted mobility which is an easily understood but frequently overlooked cause of incontinence. In addition to obvious causes, restricted mobility may be associated with orthostatic or postprandial hypotension, poorly-fitting shoes, physical deconditioning, or fear of falling, all of which are common geriatric conditions.

Finally; "S" is for stool as fecal impaction has been implicated as the cause of incontinence in up to 10% of older patients seen in acute hospitals [9] or geriatric incontinence clinics [1]. A clue to the presence of fecal impaction is the onset of both urinary and fecal incontinence, usually associated with oozing of loose stool around the impaction.

4. Summary

Aside from re-challenge data for alpha adrenergic agents (Level of Evidence = 2), it is not known how often treatment of these transient conditions results in improvement or continence, but the committee's experience suggests that improvement is common. Moreover, such causes are important to address in every incontinent older person because the risk is low and treatment has benefits even beyond the urinary tract; addressing some, such as delirium may even reduce mortality. (Level of Evidence = 4)

5. Recommendations

- Despite the current lack of compelling clinical trial data, these eight "transient" causes of urinary incontinence should be aggressively searched for in all older incontinent patients ***before embarking on complex assessment and management.*** Their prevalence is high and the "payoff" is great, not only in terms of improving or curing incontinence but also in terms of improving patients' overall function and quality of life. (Grade of recommendation C)

6. RESEARCH PRIORITIES

- Further research should be performed on the mechanisms, prevalence, incidence, and remission rates of each of the known causes of transient incontinence, and possible additional causes should be identified as well.
- Since frail older people are heterogeneous, studies should be conducted among several subgroups, including independent and homebound community-dwelling older people, bedfast and non-bedfast institutionalized older people, and acutely hospitalized older people.

VI. ESTABLISHED INCONTINENCE

Established urinary incontinence refers to incontinence that is unrelated to a comorbid illness and persists over time. There is a general consensus among experts that the identification of persistent incontinence is critically important for planning individually tailored treatment programs [1-6]. Three types of established urinary incontinence have been identified: urge, stress, and associated with impaired bladder emptying. They result from one or more basic abnormalities in lower urinary tract function:

1) failure to store urine, caused by an overactive bladder or by diminished outflow resistance;

2) failure to empty bladder, caused by poorly contractile bladder or by increased outlet resistance. For a detailed description of the pathophysiologic mechanisms of the different types of established incontinence see Chapter 4. In this section only the results of studies specifically designed for frail elderly will be reported.

• ***Urge incontinence*** is the most frequent type of established incontinence in elderly patients [7-14]. A distinction is usually made between detrusor overactivity that is associated with a central nervous system lesion (neurogenic detrusor overactivity) and that which is not (idiopathic detrusor overactivity) [15] but in elderly patients this distinction is often unclear [4, 5]. Detrusor overactivity in elderly patients exists in two subsets: one in which the contractile function is preserved and one in which contractile function is impaired. The latter is called "detrusor hyperactivity with impaired contractility" (DHIC) [9, 16] and is the most common form in frail elderly patients [9, 17]. The recognition of DHIC is important because an elevated post-voiding residual must be differentiated from other causes of urinary retention. Although patients with DHIC have symptoms of urge incontinence, they may also have symptoms of obstruction, stress or retention of urine with overflow incontinence. Anticholinergic therapy which is commonly used in this condition may increase the residual urine and cause urinary retention.

Local irritating factors (bladder tumors, stones, diverticuli, and cystitis) also cause urge symptoms but usually no incontinence. In these cases where urinary incontinence develops it is thought that sensory input overwhelms the central inhibitory influence on the brainstem micturition center and detrusor contraction occurs.

• ***Stress incontinence*** is common among elderly women in ambulatory clinic settings [18-20] and in nursing homes [10]. The most frequent cause is hypermobility of the proximal urethra due to weakness of pelvic floor musculature and/or derangement of bladder neck suspension mechanisms. Intrinsic urethral sphincter deficiency [21] is also frequently observed. It can be due to previous surgical procedures, radiation therapy, hypoestrogenism, or pelvic denervation. A rare cause of stress incontinence in elderly women is urethral instability in which the sphincter paradoxically relaxes in the absence of detrusor contraction [22, 23], however, most elderly women thought to have this condition may actually have DHIC [17]. Stress incontinence is rare in men in whom the most frequent cause is damage of the distal sphincterial mechanisms during prostatectomy.

Incontinence may be associated ***with impaired bladder emptying*** caused by an underactive or acontractile detrusor, bladder outlet or urethral obstruction, or both conditions together. In the most severe conditions with overdistension of the bladder retention of urine with ***overflow incontinence*** occurs. In elderly men the commonest cause is prostatic obstruction due to hyperplasia [24], and less frequently prostatic carcinoma, or urethral strictures. In women it is much less frequent. The most frequent causes are bladder outlet obstruction secondary to anti-incontinence surgery and severe genital prolapse. In both genders, fecal impaction is a frequent cause as well as underactive or acontractile bladder due to drugs (e.g. drugs with anticholinergic properties), or to autonomic neuropathy (e.g. diabetic cystopathy).

There is frequent overlap among the different types of incontinence in frail elderly. As many as one third of the female patients with idiopathic detrusor overactivity instability may have sphincter incompetence and vice versa (***mixed incontinence***)[25-27]. A substantial number of male patients with detrusor overactivity may have concomitant outlet obstruction [28, 29].

• ***Functional incontinence*** is also cited as a distinct type of geriatric incontinence and attributed to factors outside the lower urinary tract such as impairment of physical or cognitive functioning or both. This concept is problematic for several reasons. Functional incontinence implies that urinary tract function is normal, but studies of both institutionalized and ambulatory elderly reveal that normal urinary tract function is the exception even in continent subjects and rarely is observed in incontinent patients [9, 27]. Incontinence is not inevitable with either dementia or immobility [4, 30]. Functionally impaired individuals are the most likely to suffer from factors causing transient incontinence [7, 31-35] and therefore a diagnosis of functional incontinence may result in failure to detect reversible causes of incontinence. Finally, functionally impaired individuals still may have obstruction or stress incontinence and benefit from targeted therapy [8, 9, 27]. Nonetheless, the importance of functional impairments as a factor contributing to incontinence should not be underestimated because continence is also affected by environmental demands, mentation, mobility, manual dexterity medical factors and motivation.

VII. CLINICAL EVALUATION

Most of the characteristics of the components of basic evaluation (history, physical examination, urinalysis, and measurement of post void residual) and of further evaluation in older adults are similar to those described for younger adults (see Chapter 8 «Other Investigations»). Therefore, this section will deal only with studies specifically designed for frail older adults on algorithmic assessment strategies and on specific aspects of clinical and instrumental assessment.

1. Clinical algorithms

a) Background

Given the high prevalence of UI in the elderly population, limiting the evaluation and the management to specialist doctors is not feasible. Therefore, primary health care providers are encouraged to initiate evaluation of UI basing their judgment on the results of clinical non-instrumental approach. However, only few studies have evaluated diagnostic accuracy of non-specialist evaluation strategies of UI in frail older persons.

b) Quality of data

Diagnostic and therapeutic accuracy of clinical algorithms was investigated mainly in women by using different study designs and settings and comparing the clinical conclusions with those obtained from urological/urodynamic evaluation (Table 6).

c) Results

Results are summarized in Table 7.

d) Summary

Studies of algorithmic assessment strategies indicate that characterization of symptoms, when combined with other aspects of clinical evaluation can help plan management in most female frail older patients (level of evidence 2). On the other hand, very little evidence is available for males.

e) Recommendations

- In women algorithmic assessment strategies lead to an appropriate categorization of UI and initial treatment plan in most of the cases (grade of recommendation B). These strategies may be useful in specific settings (e.g. nursing homes) or where physical and financial costs of instrumental evaluation may outweigh those of empiric therapy (grade of recommendation D).

2. Clinical evaluation

a) Background

The aims of evaluation of UI in older persons are similar to those of younger adults, i.e. identifying reversible causes, associated serious conditions, and type of established UI in order to set up individually tailored treatment plans (see Chapter 8 «Other Investigations»). However, evaluation of UI in frail older persons differs from that in younger adults for several reasons. UI is frequently associated with deficits outside the urinary tract that affect mobility, mentation, manual dexterity and motivation, which impair the capacity of toileting independently. Lack of social support and environmental factors may worsen or precipitate UI. The coexistence of one to several pathological conditions of other organs and systems (comorbidity) may make less effective or even contraindicate treatment options directed at correcting lower urinary tract function.

It should be noted that in the evaluation of UI in frail older persons a greater deal of attention is paid to the identification not only of serious conditions (e.g. cancer) but also of the so called transient causes. Such transient causes (e.g., delirium, urinary tract infections, poliuria, drug side effects, volume overload) may be serious medical conditions which may lead to further mobidity or mortality. Restricted mobility prevents the possibility to live independently in the community. Nocturia is associated with an increased rate of falls and fractures. Therefore, it seems most appropriate to emphasize that identifying and evaluating frail older adults with UI is not only that to cure or ameliorate UI. Identifying and treating the transient conditions is essential in order to improve function and quality of life, and prevent potentially serious and expensive consequences of not identifying treatable conditions [1, 2].

The purpose here is to examine critically the available published methods for evaluation of UI. We will first review some aspects of history and physical examination with special attention to mental, functional, and social status since their alterations, highly prevalent in advanced age, contribute to incontinence and influence treatment/management approach. Subsequently some

Table 6 : Characteristics of studies on clinical algorithms.

Study	Number gender	Age (years)	Study design	Functional and cognitive status	Study setting	Clinical evaluation	Urologic and urodynamic evaluation
Hilton and Stanton [1]	100 F	Range 65-93 Mean 75	Retrospective	Not reported	Urodynamic unit referral	History, physical examination, PRV (manual palpation),urinalysis and urine culture	Uroflowmetry, subtracted water cystometry with patient supine and during postural change (selected cases), videocystourethrography (selected cases), urethtal closure pressure profilometry (selected cases), Urilos nappy test [2] (selected case).
Eastwood and Warrell [3]	65 F	Range 68-94 Mean 82	Prospective	Not reported	Geriatric outpatient clinic	History, physical examination, urinalysis and urine culture, PRV (manual palpation)	Simple cystometrogram and fluid bridge flow test [4]
Ouslander et al. [5]	205 F 59 M (136 F and 32 M underwent both clinical and urologic/ urodynamic evaluation)	Range 65-100 Mean 80	Prospective	Dependent in toileting 59% Dependent in transfer 50% MMSE score <20 26%	75% outpatient clinic 25% nursing home	History, physical examination, urinalysis and urine culture, PRV (catheterization), "Simple cistometry", CST, referral criteria	Urologic and urodynamic evaluation: history, physical examination, uroflowmetry, multichannel supine cystometrogram, static and dynamic urethral profilometry (selected cases), sphincter electromyography (selected cases), pressure-flow study (selected cases), stress and voiding cysto- urethrogram (selected cases), cystourethroscopy.
Resnick et al. [6]	102 F (complete data from 82 patients)	Mean 85	Prospective	Dependent in toileting 64% Dependent in transfer 67% MMSE score (mean) 17	Nursing home	History, functional assessment, physical examination, CST, urinalysis and urine culture, PRV (catheterization). Two algorhythms were tested one originally designed for men and women and one just for women.	Multichannel videourodynamics [7, 8]

F = female, M = male, PVR = post void residual volume, MMSE = Mini Mental State Evaluation9, CST = cough stress test.

Table 7 : Accuracy, sensitivity and specificity of clinical algorithms.

Study	Accuracy (%)	Sensitivity (%)	Specificity (%)	Comments
Hilton and Stanton [1]	Diagnostic 83 Therapeutic 95	DO 100 SI 97 Mixed 100 VD 71	DO= 76 SI 100 Mixed 100 VD 100	60% of invasive urodynamic testing could be avoided by using the proposed algorithmic method with minimal loss of diagnostic accuracy.
Eastwood and Warrell [3]	Diagnostic 71 Therapeutic 75	DO 93 SI 100 Mixed 100 VD 8	DO 50 SI 95 Mixed 91 VD 100	20% patients with urethral stenosis or acontractile bladder might have been harmed by the treatment inaccurately suggested by the algorithm. Since simple cystometry was used as "gold standard", detrusor hyperactivity with impaired contractility may have been misdiagnosed as outlet obstruction or stress incontinence.
Ouslander et al. [5]	Diagnostic 88 Therapeutic 88	DO 74 SI 75 VD 73	DO 86 SI 86 VD 94	50% met at least one criterion for further evaluation but only 25% of them did not require surgical intervention, and did not benefit from urologic and urodynamic evaluation. The urological and urodynamic evaluation changed the initial treatment plan in only ten (12%) of the 84 who did not meet any criteria for referral. The risks associated with the treatment plan based on the clinical assessment in these patients were relatively small.
Resnick et al. [6]	Diagnostic 70a Diagnostic 84b	DO 76 SI 76	DO 71 SI 97 UD 100 BOO 80	Serious misclassifications, which could lead to harmful therapy, were not observed with use of either algorithm. Misclassification errors were observed when stress test was performed at inadequate volume, for those with DHIC when the stress test was >200 ml, for women with normal urodynamic evaluation.

DO = detrusor overactivity, SI = stress incontinence, Mixed = DO and SI, VD = voiding difficulty, UD = underactive detrusor; BOO = bladder outlet obstruction, DHIC = detrusor hyperactivity with impaired contractility. aFor an algorithm designed for both genders; bfor an algorithm designed just for women.

specific aspects of basic and further evaluation of UI will be considered which will include voiding records, estimation of post-void residual volume, urinalysis, simplified bedside cystometry and complex urodynamic studies.

Voiding record is the initial noninvasive step in defining the severity and type of UI. Different types are available according to the mental and functional status of the patients. In a first type patients, ambulatory and with a good cognitive status, record (urinary diaries) the time and volume of all continent voidings or a qualitative estimate of incontinence episodes along with associated events and the hours of sleep. In the second type of record (wet checks) patients, generally inpatients or nursing home residents, are visually checked at regular intervals to determine wet episodes. However, problems have been identified with their use including difficulty to correctly identify wetness when newer absorbent products are used which "wick" away the moisture. Pad weighting (pad test) offers the potential for overcoming this limit and for quantifying the severity of incontinence.

Post-void residual volume provides data on voiding efficiency. It is frequently observed in elderly population [3, 4]. It can be measured by in-and-out catheterization or ultrasound in frail elderly. A dedicated portable ultrasound unit has also been developed for this purpose. There is no evidence in the published literature on the maximum normal and minimum abnormal post-void residual in an older population. However, According to experts' opinion [5-7], residuals <50 ml are considered to reflect adequate bladder emptying, while values >200 ml abnormal. Clinical judgment and other diagnostic tests are required to interpret the significance in the intermediate range. More information is needed to establish the association between the amount of post-void residual and urinary tract infection and renal failure.

The urinalysis screens for infection, hematuria and glycosuria. However, a clean mid-stream urine sample may be difficult to collect in frail incontinent patients and the use of in-and-out catheters may be necessary. Thus, attention has been paid to alternative non-invasive methods to collect urine samples suitable for analysis which use a sterile condom catheter in male patients [8], a disinfected collection pan [9], or disposable diapers [10].

A major part of the workload of the bacteriology departments is the processing of urine samples. This workload could be reduced if there was an effective ward screening test for bacteriuria. Only urine samples which were likely to be positive would be sent to the laboratory. The laboratory would then identify the casual organisms and determine its sensitivity to antibiotics. In this connection dipstick methods could reduce the number of urine samples submitted to laboratory for processing.

Urodynamic testing is not readily available in many communities and long-term care settings in which incontinence and other disorders of the urinary tract are especially prevalent. Thus, simple bedside cystometry has been advocated as a useful screening test because it does not require specialized equipment except for a catheter and open 50 ml syringe. Bladder capacity and stability is determined by incremental bladder filling by gravity. It could also provide an opportunity to measure post-void residual volume and to perform a stress test at a known volume. Finally, published literature on urodynamic studies will be reviewed. Urodynamic studies are considered fundamental for the definition of lower urinary tract disorders also in frail elderly persons although no study has specifically addressed the reproducibility, safety, feasibility and efficacy of these investigations in this age group.

b) Quality of data

• History and physical examination

All conclusions were based on experts'opinion [7, 11-22].

• Documentation of UI

Validity and reliability of urinary diaries have been investigated in two prospective studies of elderly community-dwelling persons without mental or physical disabilities [23, 24]. Sample size was 50 [24] and 200 [23]. The age of the patients ranged 55-90 (mean 68) [23] and 55-86 (mean 64) [24] years. Both studies included only women and compared urinary diary results with findings from urodynamic studies.

Wet checks reliability was investigated in nursing home residents by Hu et al. [25] in a clinical trial on behavioral therapy and by Ouslander et al. [26] in a quasiexperimental, nonequivalent control group design. Sample size were 26 [26] and 133 [25].

Four prospective studies investigated pad test in patients admitted in hospital geriatric wards [27-29] and in the community [30]. Sample size varied: 34 [30], 64 [27], 50 [28], 100 [29]. Three studies included patients of both genders [27, 28, 29] and one only women [30].

• Post-void residual volume

Prospective studies on the accuracy of ultrasound methods versus in-and-out catheterization for measuring post-void residual have been carried out in hospital patients [29] and nursing home residents [31]. Reproducibility of measures was prospectively investigated in hospital patients [29, 32, 33].

One study investigated only men [33] while five included patients of both genders [29, 31, 32]. Sample size was 30 [33], 100 [29], 201 [31], 14 [32].

• Urinalysis

Reliability of sampling urine by different methods were evaluated in cross sectional comparisons in nursing home residents [9, 34] and geriatric wards [10]. Reliability of different screening tests for bacteriuria was investigated in older patients in geriatric wards. Sample size was 26 [34], 101[9], 52 [10], 418 [35]. One study included patients of both genders [35], one only males [34] and two only females [9, 10].

• Simple bedside cystometry

Two studies compared simple cystometry with a continuous water filling multichannel cystometrogram in patients referred for persistent UI at out-patient clinics [36, 37] and long term care facilities [36]. Sample size was 171 (139 women and 32 men) [36] and 83 (49 women and 34 men) [37]. Furthermore, considerations on the limitations of this procedure were based on experts'opinion [7, 38, 39].

• Urodynamics

All conclusions were based or incidental observations in studies designed for other purposes [2, 17, 36, 37, 40-52].

c) Results

• History and physical examination

In patients with cognitive disorders a reliable history may be difficult to obtain. Information can be supplemented where necessary by data derived from caregivers and supplemented by medical records or data collection instruments, in particular for nursing home residents. It is important for decision-making to evaluate the bothersomeness of symptoms and their correlation with other clinical data [7, 11]. In community-dwelling disabled patients, the bothersomeness of symptoms to the primary caregiver is often critical. UI is stressful for caregivers and seems to play an important role in the decision to institutionalize an older person [11-15]. Often, caregivers of older person are older themselves or they may have their personal time and social activities restricted. Odor, physically demanding activities for transfers or necessity to get up at night to assist the consort or relative to pass urine may be the main complaints.

Direct observation of urinary leakage should always be attempted in female patients since it provides valuable information for defining the type of UI. A stress test is recommended, in which the patient coughs with a full bladder (at least 200 ml) [16]. A stress test can be performed in patients with dementia, but the staff performing the test requires special training [17, 18]. It is also important in men with post prostatectomy UI.

Psychological and social factors should be investigated [19, 20]. UI can cause a patient to withdraw from friends and family and isolate himself. Inattention to bladder cues and further UI may accompany depression. Chair or homebound older people may not have people around when help is needed. In nursing homes and hospitals (often crowded and understaffed), anger and hostility may lead to manipulative behavior.

The assessment of cognitive and functional status is necessary to evaluate patients' toileting capacity and is critical to realistically target diagnostic and therapeutic strategies. Tests of cognitive function, such as the Mini Mental State Evaluation [53] (MMSE), can be used for this determination. An informal evaluation of mobility and dexterity may be performed by observing the capacity of the patient to walk around, get up from a chair, undress and dress himself. Instruments such as the Barthel Index [54] and Katz scale [55] can be used to evaluate functional status.

There are no standardized tools for evaluating home setting [21]. Distance to the bathroom, environmental barriers such as stairs, position and height of the bed, lighting of the way to the bathroom at night, size of doors and bathroom which allows the use of walking aids or wheel chairs, height of the toilet seat, and clothing should be considered. Simple modification of home environment or clothing, adaptive equipment (hand rails, raised toilet seats), or toilet substitutes may allow self-toileting and help continence in the most disabled. However, self-adaptation to one's environment is such that patients should be evaluated in their own home before prescribing costly modifications. Home visits by nurses or occupational therapists are therefore extremely valuable to obtain this information and for planning intervention.

Fonda [22] proposed the classification of patients' toileting capacity, which may be helpful to realistically target the treatment/management options and defining the endpoints of intervention (Figure 3). He defined "independent continence" - that of persons not being wet and being able to void independently (without being reminded or physically assisted in any way) during the day and night; "dependent continence" - that of persons with mental or physical disabilities who can be dry because of assistance given; and "social continence" - that of persons who are incontinent but the problem is well contained with appropriate aids such that personal dignity and caregiver morale are improved.

• DOCUMENTATION OF UI

Wyman et al. [24], investigated the use of a one-week urinary diary in the evaluation of incontinent community-dwelling older women. All subjects kept a urinary diary for two consecutive weeks. Diurnal and nocturnal micturition frequency, and number of incontinent episodes were highly reproducible and consistent with urodynamic diagnosis. Test-retest correlation were highest with diurnal micturition frequency ($r = 0.89$) and incontinent episodes ($r = 0.91$). Lower correlation was observed with nocturnal micturition frequency ($r = 0.86$). Although weak, significant agreements between weekly diurnal and nocturnal frequencies and number of UI episodes collected by history and diary were found, but there were significant differences between different urodynamic diagnostic groups (those with detrusor overactivity had lower agreement rate). Diokno et al. [23] compared cystometric bladder capacity to self-reported voided urine volumes measured by the patient at home for a minimum of four 24-hour periods. The mean smallest and largest daily voided volumes, and the daily mean of all voided volumes were determined from the diary. Comparison of the cystometric bladder capacity with the daily voided volumes showed a significant positive correlation between cystometric bladder capacity and the largest voided volume. Comparison of the mean daily and mean largest daily void, and the cystometric capacity with the different urodynamic diagnoses using analysis of variance revealed a statistical significance among the groups.

Hu et al. [25] used 1-hour wet checks from 7 a.m. to 9 p.m. as the major outcome measure in a study to evaluate the efficacy of prompted voiding in female nursing home incontinent residents. The data collection was monitored by the research team during the first 3 weeks of the trial and then randomly by hired nursing students to ensure data accuracy. Of 2305 random observations the reliability of data collection was 94%. Ouslander et al. [26] compared different versions of UI monitoring records, one using black and white symbols and the other using colored circles in three nursing homes. The bladder record already in use in each facility served as control record. They found that recordings were made more frequently and interrater reliability was highest with the color version of the bladder diary.

Walsh and Mills [27] achieved complete collection of all urine, leakages in 220 (94%) of 234 incontinent episodes in patients from three long-term care wards. The attendant's subjective assessment of "wetness" was shown to be an extremely crude indicator of UI severity: the weight-gain in pads judged subjectively "wet" ranged from 0.7 to 341 g and there was considerable overlap between the weights of pads judged to be "dry", "damp", or "wet". Ekelund et al [30] investigated the ability of older women to perform a 48-h pad test in their home environment. 9% patients had poor vision, gait disorders or dementia and completed the test by involving a relative in the test procedure. The mean involuntary urinary loss was 80±88g (range 2-411 g) in the 48 hours. There was a good correlation between the patients own weighing of the pads and control weightings at the clinic performed on a precision weight scale. Griffiths et al [28] compared subjective (visual inspection) and objective methods (1-h and 24-h pad test) in older patients with established UI (62% had urge UI). Many patients had cognitive impairments (MMSE [53] median score 23/30) and limited mobility, although none was bedridden (activities of daily living median score [55] 3/8). The 24-hour in-patient monitoring of urine leakage was the most sensitive method of demonstrating UI (90%), with videourodynamic testing almost as good (78%). In comparison, the sensitivity of the 1-h pad test was poor (<50%). Visual inspection during physical examination seldom demonstrated leakage (20%). For quantitative assessment of severity, 24-h monitoring gave the most reproducible results; it was also able to reveal significant changes in severity in response to pharmaceutical treatment. A 1-h pad test was less reproducible and correlated poorly with 24-h monitoring. The subjective responses of the patients poorly correlated with changes in the severity of UI after treatment. Twenty-four hour monitoring thus stands out as a superior method of demonstrating and assessing UI. Finally, the high sensitivity (88%) of a 24-h pad test in frail older persons was also proved by a second study of Griffiths et al. [29]. Reproducibility of measurements was also investigated in the 31 patients who did not receive treatment (oxybutinin or prostatic surgery) by comparing 24-hour recordings at 2- to 6-week time intervals. They found fair reproducibility for 24 hour urine loss (r = 0.57), wettest pad weight (r = 0.54) and nocturnal weight loss (r = 0.61).

• Post-void residual volume

Post-void residual can be accurately measured by ultrasound in frail older persons as demonstrated by comparisons with in-and-out catheter determinations [29]. The correlation coefficient between the two sets of results was 0.97. Accuracy of measures with a portable ultrasound in frail older persons have been proved by Ouslander et al. [31]. They found that, in the 20-500 ml range of post void residual, similar values were obtained using ultrasound and catheterization (r = 0.86).

Birch et al. [33] studied thirty older men with prostatic hypertrophy by ultrasound in three occasions on the day before TURP. 66% of these patients had residual volumes that varied significantly on the same day. Griffiths et al. [29] estimated post-void residual urine three times by ultrasound techniques in the early afternoon, the evening, the early morning. They found diurnal variations: residuals were significantly larger in the early morning. In another study Griffiths et al. [32] measured residual urine by ultrasound at three different times of day on each of two visits separated by 2-4 weeks in 14 geriatric patients. Mean residual urine was 154 ml. Between-patient variability was large (standard deviation 246 ml). There was no significant difference between values in men and women, nor between visits. Within-patient variability was large because of a large systematic variation with time of day (standard deviation 128 ml), with greatest volumes in the early morning. The inherent, random variability of the measurement was much smaller (SD 44 ml). They suggested that if the physiological factors causing the temporal variation could be controlled, more reproducible measurements would be possible.

• Urinalysis

Ouslander et al. [34] compared urine cultures collected by a simple standardized technique from male nursing home residents wearing external catheters with culture results obtained by sterile in-and-out catheterization. The culture results were the same in 85% of the matched specimens. Specimens collected by the standardized technique were 100% sensitive and 94% specific in detecting significant growth of pathogenic organisms. In contrast, 57% of specimens collected from patients with external catheters by the nursing home staff using their routine technique yielded three or more organisms and were considered contaminated. Ouslander et al [9] compared cultures and dipstick screening test results from paired urine specimens, one collected by a clean catch technique using a disinfected collection pan, and the other collected by sterile in-and-out catheterization, in 101 incontinent female nursing home residents. Using the catheter specimen as gold standard, clean catch had sensitivity 90%, specificity 92%, positive predictive value 81%, and negative predictive value 95%. Finally, Belmin et al. [10] assessed the reliability for biochemical and microbiological analysis of urine collection from disposable diapers in older women with severe UI in a geriatric hospital ward. Urine was sampled by pressing a diaper which the patient had worn for 3 hours. Just after this collection, another sample was obtained by retrograde catheterization. Both samples were analyzed for sodium, potassium, chloride, proteins, urea, creatinine, calcium, phosphate, cell counts, bacteria, and bacteria culture. For all the biochemical parameters, the urinary concentrations obtained by the two methods were strongly and significantly correlated. For diagnosis of urinary tract infection, agreement between the two methods was good (kappa = 0.84), and bacteriological agreement was obtained in 89% of the cases. However, for diagnosis of microscopic hematuria, agreement was poor (kappa = 0.50), probably due to the overestimation of the true urinary red cell count in the samples collected by catheterization.

Flanagan et al. [35] compared four screening tests for bacteriuria with urine culture in 698 samples collected from 418 elderly patients in geriatric wards by a "clean catch" method with a standardized procedure. The screening tests were visual appearance, microscopy, and two dipstick methods. One dipstick method had ten reagent pads for glucose, bilirubin, ketones, blood, protein, urobilinogen, specific gravity, pH, nitrite and leucocyte esterase. The other had three reagent pads one for nitrite and two with dehydrated culture media for the growth of bacteria (one for both gram-positive and gram-negative organisms and the other for gram-negative organisms only). The sensitivity of the tests varied from 85.6% to 98.3% and the specificity from 18.4% to 82.9%. A combination of visual appearance and dipstick testing for nitrite and leucocyte esterase gave a sensitivity of 96.1% and a specificity of 50.6%.

• Simple bedside cystometry

Ouslander et al. [36] compared bladder capacity and stability determined by incremental bladder filling by gravity with the results of a continuous water filling multichannel cystometrogram in patients with persistent UI. They included patients with severe disability: 26% had MMSE score <20, 26% required walking aids, and 20% were not ambulatory. Bladder capacities measured by both methods were correlated significantly by simple linear regression (r=0.75) and they were not significantly different by paired t tests. DHIC was present on the multichannel cystometrogram in 64% patients, while simple cystometry had a sensitivity of 75%, specificity of 79%, and positive predictive value of 85% for this finding. Fonda et al. [37] also compared simple cystometry with multichannel cystometry. They also included patients with severe dementia (32%) or requiring walking assistance (9%) or walking aids (36%). They found a specificity of 75% and a sensitivity of 88% for the diagnosis of detrusor instability.

A number of considerations limit the utility of bedside simple cystometry in frail older patients [7, 36, 38, 39]. The accuracy for other conditions (stress incontinence, outlet obstruction, underactive detrusor, sensory urge detrusor-sphincter dyssynergia) was not assessed. Straining may be difficult to detect or misinterpreted as an involuntary bladder contraction. DHIC is easily missed. Furthermore, the involuntary detrusor contractions detected may be physiological because of age, pathological but unrelated to the leakage, or secondary to either obstruction or stress incontinence.

• Urodynamics

No study has specifically investigated reliability and validity of complex urodynamic testing in older persons. However, multichannel urodynamic and videourodynamic investigations have been successfully used in a number of studies (see e.g. references [2, 17, 36, 37, 40-52] to assist the accurate diagnosis of retentionof urine with overflow incontinence, DHIC and help clarify the cause of stress UI in frail older persons.

d) Summary

• History and physical examination

History and physical examination are similar to those in younger adults but greater attention is paid to comorbid conditions and to emotional, cognitive, functional, social and environmental status (level of evidence 5).

• Documentation of UI

Bladder diaries provide information on diurnal micturition frequency, nocturnal micturition frequency, and number of incontinent episodes (level of evidence 2). Further voided urine volumes give a measure of functional bladder capacity and maximum average bladder volume (level of evidence 2). However, reliability of bladder diaries when completed by community-dwelling frail older or their "untrained" carers has not been investigated.

In severely cognitively or functionally impaired patients living in institutions wet checks appear to be a reliable means of documenting UI (level of evidence 2). However, problems have been identified with their use including difficulty getting ward staff to reliably check and record wetness (level of evidence 2).

Pad weighting (pad test) is more reliable than visual inspection for identifying UI episodes and useful for quantifying the severity of UI (level of evidence 2). The 24-hour pad test is more sensitive than the 1-hour pad test for demonstrating UI (level of evidence 2).

• Post-void residual volume

Post-void residual volume is reliably estimated by in-and-out catheterization or ultrasound (level of evidence 2). In older persons post-void residual volume is very variable (level of evidence 2).

• Urinalysis

When a clean mid-stream urine sample is difficult to collect in frail incontinent patients, a condom catheter, a disinfected collection pan, or urine collection from a disposable diaper can be an alternative to the use of an in-and-out catheter to obtain urine for analyses and culture (level of evidence 2). A clean specimen can also be obtained by in-and-out catheters. Clinically significant bacteriuria is an unlikely finding in a dipstick-negative urine (level of evidence 2).

• Simple bedside cystometry

Simple bedside cystometry findings correlates with those derived from multichannel cystometrogram (level of evidence 2). However, further studies are needed to elucidate the test's optimum utility (level of evidence 5).

• Urodynamics

Urodynamic investigation is fundamental to understand pathophysiologic mechanisms underlying UI even in very frail older patients (level of evidence 5).

e) Recommendations

- Identification of comorbid conditions and evaluation of emotional, cognitive, functional, social and environmental status are fundamental for planning individually tailored treatment/management strategies (grade of recommendation D)
- Bladder diaries provide valuable information on severity and bladder capacity in older persons without disability in the community (grade of recommendation B). In severely cognitively or functionally impaired patients living in institutions wet checks performed by trained nursing staff provide information on frequency and severity of UI when bladder diaries are not feasible (grade of recommendation B). Pad weighting provides valid assessment of UI frequency and severity both in women living in the community and institutions (grade of recommendation B).
- Post-void residual can be accurately measured by catheterization or ultrasound in frail older persons (grade of recommendation B). In severely incontinent patients, post-void residual can be performed in association with frequent wet checks (grade of recommendation D). Ultrasound method is a safe method in patients in male with prostate obstruction while catheterization may cause urinary tract infection and, therefore, should be performed only with clear indications (grade of recommendation D). Given the intra-individual variability of residual urine volume repeated determinations are recommended; in these latter cases ultrasonography may be especially valuable (grade of recommendation D).
- Urinalysis should always be performed to evaluate the presence of conditions associated with UI in frail older patients (grade of recommendation D). Dipstick methods are useful in frail older patients to reduce the number of urine samples submitted to laboratory for processing; however, urine culture should be obtained when dipstick tests suggest infection (grade of recommendation B).
- Simple cystometry is of limited value for assessment and management of UI in a institutionalized frail older population and its use is not recommended (grade of recommendation D).
- Even in frail elderly, multichannel urodynamic evaluation is warranted when diagnostic uncertainty may affect therapy (grade of recommendation D).

f) Research priorities

- Validation of practical and useful clinical algorithms.
- Determine the normative range for post void residual volume in older patients.
- Determine when urodynamics should be used to benefit frail older patients.
- Understanding the barriers to improved continence care in institutional settings and piloting strategies to improve these.
- Identify patient characteristics that act as triggers for specific interventions.

VIII. MEASURING OUTCOME OF MANAGEMENT OF LOWER URINARY TRACT DYSFUNCTION IN FRAIL AND OLDER PEOPLE

1. Background

The ICS Working Party on Outcome Measures has indicated that outcome measures for fit and active older people should be the same as their middle aged counterparts. ***The broad principles of research methodology and measuring outcome is covered in Chapter 16 «Research and Outcomes».*** However, specific considerations are required for disabled and frail older people as outlined below [1,2].

2. Quality of data

To determine the effect of an intervention, accurate, valid, and meaningful outcome variables are needed. It is most important to define the major endpoints prior to commencing studies. Baseline diagnostic data should be gathered in order to characterise the patients' condition and to document the severity of incontinence. The selection of an outcome variable depends on the nature of the intervention being studied eg. pharmacological, surgical, behavioural, use of pads or appliances. Successful short term interventions should wherever possible have long term follow-up provided (at least 12 months) in order to gauge more accurately their impact, durability and relevance in this frail population.

Factors which can affect outcome of incontinence intervention should, wherever possible be addressed and reported at the time of follow-up. This includes:

- type and nature of data provided by patient or caregivers;
- level of compliance (by patients, staff or caregivers) such as compliance to exercise programs, toileting protocols, or drug use;
- type of bladder training or toileting programs (if used);
- changes in patient's physical, emotional and cognitive status;
- other intercurrent treatment not directly related to bladder function that might impact on outcome;
- medication which might impact on incontinence/continence;
- quality of life measures
- socio-economic data including impact of the intervention on the patient;
- changes in caregiver or staff status or numbers;
- cost of the treatment;
- cost-benefit data;
- acceptance of patient and/or caregiver with intervention, and satisfaction with the intervention;
- risk-benefit data;
- if part of an intervention study, number and reason for dropouts and deaths (ie were they trial related);
- lack of appropriate identifications of desired or appropriate outcomes hinder the evaluation of the effectiveness of an intervention.

3. Results

The ICS has defined Outcome measurements under five domains (see Table 8 «ICS recommendations for outcome measurements for frail older patients and their current status»). Because of the complexity of measuring and documenting incontinence, compliance and psychological factors, it is recommended, wherever possible, to document information in all of these domains, rather than in a single domain. A global single score is impractical and not useful. Table 8 summarises the findings of the ICS committee following review of the literature as it relates to frail and older people related to the current status of outcome measures. The current status of these measures is also listed in Table 8. More specific information can be found in the section on 'Evaluation' above.

4. Summary

Research methodology for studying incontinence in the frail and housebound older person is fraught with pitfalls. This has compromised the usefulness of past research. There is a great need for basic research to validate practical and useful outcome measures that will allow meaningful results to be obtained. In addition, an understanding is required of the importance of defining clinical rather than statistical significance. What the older incontinent person wants or needs should be strongly influencing all interventions.

5. Recommendations

- All studies involving intervention for incontinence should use sound research methodology, outcome measures and reporting practices.

IX. CONSERVATIVE MANAGEMENT

The previous men's and woman's chapters have provided overviews and detailed recommendations of various conservative strategies. Readers are referred to these chapters for more details. Unfortunately, there is no age stratification of most data to adequately understand, know or predict the impact of these strategies in older people. Therefore, in the absence of data to the contrary, it is assumed that pelvic floor muscle training, bladder retraining, biofeedback and electrostimulation should be offered to older, competent and motivated older people also.

The following sections will focus on additional information related to frail older patients.

X. BIOFEEDBACK AND ELECTRICAL STIMULATION

1. Introduction

Device-based conservative therapies for urinary incontinence have been studied very little in older persons, particularly in those who are frail. Functional, anatomical, and attitudinal barriers are more common in frail elderly than young persons. Many studies of biofeedback-assisted pelvic muscle exercises and electrical stimulation for stress, urge, and mixed urinary inconti-

Table 8 : ICS recommendations for outcome measurements for frail older patients and their current status

ICS outcome measure [2]	Comment and grade of Recommendation
Patient Observations and Symptoms	
Purely subjective. To be supplemented, where appropriate, by data derived from care-givers	
Practitioner Measures	
Bladder diaries, records or chart	Reliable and valid means in home bound hospitalised and institutionalised older people. (Grade of Rec B)
Pad weighing tests	Valid means in hospital setting and in elderly ambulant at home. (Grade of Rec B)
Wet checks	Reliable amongst research workers working with nursing home residents. (Grade of Rec B)
Anatomical and Functional measurements	
'Simple' cystometry	Validity not established. (Grade of Rec D)
Multichannel urodynamics	Validity not established in frail, older patients but is still the gold standard probably (Grade of Rec A)
Pelvic muscle strength	Validity not established
Ultrasound for residual urine	Convenient non-invasive tool to evaluate interventions which may affect bladder emptying. (Grade of Rec A)
Quality -of-life measurements	
	Continue to develop and validate in these diverse groups generic, condition specific and intervention specific instruments.
Socio-economic Measurements	Need to develop instruments to evaluate cost, cost-benefit and cost-effectiveness of interventions.

nence include young-elderly and some middle-elderly subjects. These studies are included in the review of biofeedback and related techniques in Chapter 10c «Surgical Treatment in Women». Most studies show a benefit, but do not specify whether age affects outcome. This section will discuss studies using electronically based biofeedback-assisted pelvic floor muscle training and electrical stimulation of the pelvic floor in frail elderly, and studies that noted whether or not age was a factor in success.

2. Biofeedback

a) Background

Biofeedback is not a treatment by itself, but is a method of learning pelvic floor muscle contractions. This section discusses the use of electronic biofeedback devices, but it should be kept in mind that the term "biofeedback" can be understood in a much broader sense, including office examination and education. Although biofeedback uses external and internal devices similar to those employed in electrical stimulation of the pelvic floor, they are fundamentally different techniques because of the necessity of patient participation and learning involved in biofeedback. Because pelvic floor muscle training (PFMT) with biofeedback requires active participation of the patient, cognitive status and motivation are important selection factors. Although there are no specific studies determining cognitive capabilities for use of this modality, Burns et al used a Folstein's Mini Mental State Examination score (MMSE) of 23 as the lowest mental status for inclusion in a biofeedback program [1]. McDowell et al used a score of >=24 [2]. Bear at al used a score of >25 on Issac and Akhtar's Set Test [3]. A willing and knowledgeable caregiver is a second requisite to instituting biofeedback in frail older people, since their understanding of the process and goals will also be critical to the success of the treatment.

b) Quality of studies included

Two prospective randomized controlled trials, one with cross-over design, both with unspecified urinary incontinence, inform the use of biofeedback in frail/impaired elderly. One compared stepped "behavioral management" with a control group in frail women over age 55 years, in a study stated by the authors to be a quasi-experimental design [3]. Frail, dependent women with at least two UI episodes per week, confirmed by voiding record, were recruited from a small county in Florida, USA. Cognitively or functionally impaired subjects required a participating caregiver. After initial screening, clinical evaluation, bladder diary and pad test were completed and reviewed over two visits. The patients were then randomly assigned to treatment or control. The control group received only one more follow-up visit, and "suggestions for UI management" were given if requested. The treatment arm consisted of three techniques: self-monitoring, scheduled toileting, or PFMT with biofeedback. Patients started one of these three management plans depending on symptoms and capabilities, and progressed to the next modality if insufficient progress had been made, up to six months. Treatments were not uniform in the treatment arm of this study. Although this precludes investigation of any specific treatment modality, it does approximate to an appropriately aggressive clinical approach to patients, and therefore informs about what one might expect in a clinical setting. Outcomes were based on voiding records and pad tests.

McDowell et al studied 105 homebound, cognitively intact (MMSE >23) adults age 60 and over with at least two UI episodes per week, as identified by nurses from two large Medicare-approved home health agencies [2]. Inclusion criteria included meeting Health Care Financing Administration criteria for being homebound (i.e., need assistance to leave home, have a medical condition that contraindicates leaving home, and generally, leaving home only for short period and for medical reasons); PVR <100 ml; toileting independently. Potentially correctible causes (hyperglycemia, UTI, constipation, and environmental barriers) were treated prior to randomization. Following initial evaluation, including voiding records, patients were randomized to control or treatment. Control subjects were visited for 35 minutes every one to two weeks (attention control). Treatment subjects received eight weekly 40-60 minute visits by skilled nurse practitioners with urge and stress strategies, bladder retraining, and biofeedback-assisted PFMT using surface EMG's. The PFMT protocol between visits consisted of 10-15 exercises three times a day. Voiding records were completed during and two weeks following the treatment period. Follow-up for one year was attempted. The thorough description of methods indicates much attention was given to quality of recruitment, protocol, and analysis.

In addition to these studies, seven prospective uncontrolled studies [4-10] and one post-treatment questionnaire of nonsurgical therapies including biofeedback and electrical stimulation [11] evaluated the effect of age on response. Shinopulos et al reported quality of life and pad test results from 42 subjects age 60 ±15 (range 21-78) referred for computerized EMG biofeedback therapy to evaluate the ability of a questionnaire (Health Promotion Lifestyle Profile II) to predict response [5]. The treatments, ranging from one to six in number, were not described. Smith et al evaluated women aged 25-81 years using a 16-week self-directed home biofeedback program [4]. Henderson et al reported results of weekly clinic biofeedback sessions in 9 women over age 55 and 5 younger women [9]. Baigis-Smith et al treated 54 patients over age 60 with PFMT augmented by biofeedback, habit training, and relaxation techniques [8]. They had biweekly sessions until improvement, then were followed for one year. Burgio et al evaluated a toileting regimen plus one to eight biofeedback sessions in 48 patient volunteers age 60-86 with stress, urge, and mixed UI [10]. Stein et al studied six sessions over three weeks of a 15 minute electrical stimulation session followed by 15 minutes of biofeedback-assisted PFMT in 26 women and 2 men, mean age 60, referred for stress, urge, or mixed incontinence [7]. "Quantifiable" outcomes of pad use, UI frequency, urinary frequency, and nocturia were assessed, but method of assessment is not defined. Susset et al reported semi-weekly 20 minute treatments of biofeedback alternating with electrical stimulation through vaginal probe for 6 weeks in 64 women ages 34-88 years [6]. Thirteen 13 subjects were over age 70. Clinical and urodynamic subject characteristics were reported. Compliance and pad tests were assessed. Weinstein et al evaluated subjective long-term outcomes by questionnaire of many nonsurgical treatments, including PFMT, bladder retraining, estrogen replacement, biofeedback, functional electrical stimulation, and pharmacologic therapy [11]. Subjects were over age 60, mean age 76, followed a mean of 21 months (range 12-45).

c) Results

Stepped "behavioral management" in 24 mostly functionally intact elders, mean age 68, resulted in a 33% reduction in incontinence episodes and volume lost, compared to 25% increases in the control group (p-value not specified) [3]. 6/12 treatment and 9/12 control subjects remained in the study for the entire 6 month duration. Of particular note is that only three elder-caregiver pairs entered the study. One was assigned to control; the other 2 did not complete the study due to the treatment regimens demands. It was found that recruitment, retention, and compliance were all difficult challenges in this population.

Of the 105 homebound adults treated for 8 weeks, the mean age was 77 +/- 7 years, (range 60-97) [2]. Eighty-five completed treatment. Urge accidents decreased by a median of 82% (mean 56%), and stress accidents by a median of 100% (mean 50%), compared to 6% median reduction in the control group ($p<0.001$). These favorable results were achieved despite high levels of co-morbidity and functional impairment. Exercise adherence was the best predictor of response.

Male sex and use of an assistive device for ambulation were negatively associated with reduction in incontinence. The influence of age on outcome was not evaluated.

In uncontrolled studies, age was inversely associated with therapeutic success in three biofeedback studies (4-5,9), in one study using both biofeedback and electrical stimulation [6], and in the long-term follow-up questionnaire of non-surgical UI management [11]. However, improvement was equal in older and younger subjects in two biofeedback studies [8, 10] and in one study using both biofeedback and electrical stimulation [7].

d) Summary

The only large study of biofeedback-assisted PFMT in impaired (homebound but cognitively intact) older persons found a very favorable response (Level of Evidence 1).

It is not clear whether advanced age diminishes response to this modality (Level of Evidence 5). No data exist to judge whether biofeedback improves response to PFMT in frail elderly.

e) Recommendations

- Biofeedback-assisted pelvic floor muscle training can effect dramatic continence improvements in cognitively intact but frail elderly. (Grade of Recommendation B)
- Although response in older persons can be good, it is not clear whether age is still a factor affecting response to biofeedback-assisted pelvic muscle exercises.

f) Research priorities

- Detailed analysis of baseline pelvic floor strength and function with multivariable analysis of biofeedback-related improvement is needed to better define the effects of age.
- Benefits and methods of application of external devices compared to internal devices in older persons need to be understood.

3. Electrical stimulation

a) Background

Unlike biofeedback-assisted PFMT, which requires active participation of the patient to be successful, electrostimulation is a passive exercise of the pelvic floor musculature. Issues that may complicate its use in frail or impaired elderly include cooperativeness, informed consent, and determination of the patient's level of comfort.

b) Quality of included studies

One prospective, uncontrolled study included 12 cognitively impaired long term care women residents, MMSE <14/30, with apparent urge urinary incontinence [12]. Patients identified by the nursing staff as incontinent of urine were recruited into the study. Functional and mental status assessment, rectal examination, simple cystometry, and urinalysis were performed initially. Urinary tract infections were treated. It is not stated whether any bowel management occurred based on rectal examination findings. Incontinence episodes were recorded for 48 hours by checks every two hours prior to treatment and at four and eight weeks of therapy. Patients were treated with electrical stimulation delivered by rectal probe 15 minutes twice weekly for 8 weeks, using 20 Hz and a maximum of 20 milliamps (mean 12 ±5).

All other published studies of electrical stimulation have included only independent, community dwelling elderly. Two studies reported on results of combined electrical stimulation and biofeedback-assisted PFMT (*vide supra*) [6,7]. Two studies of patients with overactive bladder symptoms reported subanalyses of those older and younger than age 60 [13-14]. In a double-blind randomized trial, Yamanishi et al studied electrical stimulation compared to a sham device in 68 patients with urge UI due to detrusor overactivity [13]. Patient recruitment was not well explained. Three women (of 39) had mild stress incontinence. Outcomes included frequency, incontinence episodes and pad changes as assessed by voiding records; subjective urgency; and urodynamic parameters. Electrical stimulation was delivered by surface, anal, or vaginal electrodes 15 minutes twice daily for 4 weeks, using 10 Hz and a maximum output current of 60 milliamps. Zöllner-Nielsen et al gave maximal electrical stimulation to 38 consecutive women patients with frequency, urgency, or urge UI, median age 70 years, range 35-90 [14]. Nine had simultaneous stress UI. Five to 15 treatments were given for 20 minutes twice weekly, using 5-10 Hz to a maximum of 100 milliamps. Outcomes were subjective improvement and voiding record volumes and frequencies.

Other studies with a mean age above 60 years failed to report whether age influenced outcomes [15-18].

c) Results

In the uncontrolled study of long term care residents, mean age was 82 years ±9 [12]. Therapy was well tolerated, but 2 hour wet checks increased from 11.8 to 14.1 per 24 hours. For the six subjects with documented detrusor overactivity , the volume at which involuntary contractions occurred increased by 50 ml. Mean age was 70 years ±11 in one study that compared improvement in those older and younger than age 60 [13]. In the other study, median age was 70 years (range 35-90) [14]. These 2 studies found equivalent improvement in older and younger subjects. As stated above, of the 2 studies using both electrical stimulation and biofeedback-assisted PFMT, one found that older subjects responded more poorly [6], and one found equal improvement in older and younger subjects [7].

d) Summary

Older persons may respond to electrical stimulation of the pelvic floor as well as younger persons. (Level of Evidence 4). The only published small study of electrical stimulation of the pelvic floor in cognitively impaired elderly found no benefit. However, there are too few studies with a very limited number of subjects in frail elderly to draw even preliminary conclusions. (Level of Evidence 5)

e) Recommendations

- Cognitively intact older persons respond well to electrical stimulation of the pelvic floor. (Grade of Recommendation C)
- Electrical stimulation of the pelvic floor may have equal benefit in older and younger persons. However, the evidence for this may reflect publication bias, because most studies do not report the effects of age. (Grade of Recommendation C)

f) Research priorities

- All aspects of electrical stimulation of the pelvic floor need further study in impaired populations, particularly noninvasive techniques.

4. Biofeedback-Assisted Pelvic Muslce Exercises and Electrical Stimulation for Post-Prostatectomy Incontinence

See chapter 10b on conservative Treatment in men for detailed discussion on this topic.

XI. OTHER BEHAVIORAL INTERVENTIONS

1. Background

Behavioral interventions have been especially designed for frail older people with cognitive and physical impairments that may affect the person's ability to learn new behaviors or to actively participate in self-care activities. These interventions evolved from classical behavioral change theory, using antecedent, consequent, or a combination of both stimuli to shape desired behavior. These interventions include habit training and prompted voiding. The need for these interventions is obvious for the many frail older persons who are dependent on the action of others to have access to toilet facilities. Nursing home admission criteria result in residents having high dependency needs whether cognitive, physical, or both. A survey of long-term care residents revealed that they preferred interventions designed to reduce urinary incontinence over other interventions designed to reduce loneliness, improve sleep or improve physical functioning [1].

2. Prompted voiding

b) Quality of data

The prompted voiding literature includes no recent (i.e., 1996 to early 2001) research articles on habit training in frail older people. (See Table 9). Several limitations exist in the papers reviewed. Some studies used small samples resulting in low powered studies [3-5]. Terminology and operational definitions also differed, making generalizations across studies difficult.

One study suffered from a high attrition rate (51%) threatening its internal validity [6]. Few men were included in the studies and sample characteristics reveal that most subjects were elderly white females [2, 4, 5, 7-9]. No replication studies using diverse populations were located. Neither was any long-term follow up studies located.

Most studies included exclusion criteria; thus many nursing home residents were excluded from the study due to the presence of physical or cognitive conditions [6,9], language ability [5], and/or other factors. Few studies employed random assignment. Some studies used delayed treatment [10], subjects serving as their own control [3] and repeated measures [9]. Ethical consideration for human subjects prohibits withholding treatment; therefore true "control" groups were nearly impossible to create. The dose of the intervention varied as well; some researchers offered the intervention hourly [8, 10] while others were offered every two hours [3, 5, 7, 9, 11] on a 12-hour [3, 7], 14-hour [5] or 24-hour schedule [9].

Few randomized controlled trials or quasi-experimental studies for behavioral interventions in frail older persons have been conducted in recent years limiting the applicability of the findings from earlier studies for current long-term care residents.

Findings vary in terms of the characteristics of the patients who respond to behavioral interventions. Lekan Rutledge [5] reported that residents with high

Table 9 : Other behavioural interventions for older people

Intervention	Authors	Study Design	Sample	Methods	Results
Prompted Voiding					
Prompted voiding	Creason et al[7]	Quasi-experimental	N=85, incontinent nursing home residents, average age 87 yrs, 20% fairly independent in functioning, 65% were at lowest level of cognitive functioning. Only 19% were in the normal range of cognitive functioning.	30 assigned to PV, 27 assigned to socialization, 28 were control. PV delivered, socialization consisted of 2-3 minute hourly contacts of social nature. Control got routine care.	PV group shifted from being equivalent to the control but different from the socialization group to being distinct from the control but not from the socialization group.
Hourly checking and prompting to toilet	Hu et al[8]	Randomized controlled experimental	N=133, female residents, age 65 yrs or older, ability to recognize her own name. Average age 85 yrs. Average MMSE 12.7	Hourly checking and prompting implemented 14 hours/day, 13-week treatment period with 22-week follow-up period. Outcome variable: frequency of incontinence/ day before, during and after program. Patients checked hourly and research staff monitored data collection for 1st 3 weeks of program.	By 6 wks, change in wetness was statistically significant in treatment (tx) group. During wks 7-9, 22% improvement, wks 10-12, 26% improvement. At 6 mo follow-up, improvement at 0.5 episodes/day. Those with high frequency of UI improve more than those with less, higher MMSE had better chance to improve, normal bladder capacity responded better to tx, and totally dependent benefited more than less dependent.
Prompted voiding	Schnelle[10]	Controlled experimental	N=101, nursing home residents average age 82 yrs, average length of time in facility 2.4 yrs. Average MMSE 7.9, average UI frequency per 12-hour day 4.5	Baseline phase consisted of checking patients for wetness, Phase 2 randomly assigned to immediate or delayed treatment groups, immediate group received PV.	No differences in groups at baseline, statistically significant in groups during phase 1 and no difference when delayed group received tx. Pts can be categorized into 3 groups: high dry, high change group, and no response group. Can reduce severity in 75% of NH residents.
Prompted voiding	Palmer et al[16]	Quasi-experimental	N=16, nursing home residents, median age was 80 years, average baseline level of dryness was 45%	Baseline level of dryness calculated for 5 days. Subjects served as their own controls. Prompted voiding intervention lasted 12-weeks at 2-hour intervals from 8am-8pm. Staff feedback was provided to supervisors and to individual staff members.	By end of first week, dryness was significantly increased to 64% and this increase was maintained to 12 weeks (66%)

Table 9 : Other behavioural interventions for older people (Ctd)

Intervention	Authors	Study Design	Sample	Methods	Results
Prompted voiding	Adkins & Mathews[3]	Case study	N=2, 68-year-old man living with wife at home, probable Alzheimer's Disease and UI 2 years prior to study. 63-year-old female living with husband, probable Alzheimer's Disease and UI for 4 years prior to study.	At baseline, caregivers asked to place soiled undergarments in plastic bag and mark bag with time and date. Researchers visited weekly and weighed undergarments. Prompted voiding was implemented and caregiver was taught how to conduct a dryness check on a regular schedule. If patient was wet, the caregiver changed wet clothing, bagged wet garments, and toileted person. After 6 days of 2 hour voiding schedule, it was converted to every hour schedule	For 68-year old man, 22% reduction during 2-hour PV and 69% reduction during 1-hour PV. Protocol was discontinued when caregiver became ill. For 63-year-old woman 55% reduction during 1-hour PV. Protocol was still in place 3 and 6 months after implementation.
Prompted voiding	Engberg et al[4]	Randomized controlled trial	N=14, cognitively impaired elderly women (average age 83 years) living at home with a full-time caregiver, mean number of accidents at baseline was 3.4	8-week long prompted voiding intervention performed every 2-hours.	Variable response to the prompted voiding intervention reported.
Prompted voiding	Lekan-Rutledge[5]	Quasi-experimental	N=9, residents of 120-bed long term care facility in 1991-1992 selected by the nursing staff. Average MMSE 10. Nursing staff sample consisted of RN, LPN. and CAN staff.	Residents received comprehensive UI assessment; PV based on Schnelle protocol, quality monitoring tool, and quality assurance nursing rounds. Formation of a continence team.	Overall dryness rate increased from 71% to 80% at 6-wks, 78% at 3-mos, 85% at 6-mos. Staff performance at 1-wk, 93% at 6-wks, 94% at 3-mos, and 81%, and 85% at 6-mos.
Prompted voiding	Eustice et al[14]	Systematic review	355 elderly persons mostly women.	5 randomized or quasi-experimental studies included in the review. Two reviewers evaluated studies for methodological quality; third reviewer proof read the review.	Appears prompted voiding increased self initiated voidings and decreased incontinent episodes in the short-term. One study used Oxybutinin and suggests short-term effect of reducing incontinent episodes.
Patterned Urge-Response Toileting					
Patterned urge-response toileting	Colling et al[9]	Experimental	N=113, residents of 4 non-profit nursing homes: 63 experimental group and 50	Nursing staff received 4 hr in-service UI education. Pre and post-tests of knowledge were	88 completed the study. Over 80% had involuntary contractions on cystometry. Impaired cognitive and mobility status was

Table 9 : Other behavioural interventions for older people (Ctd)

Intervention	Authors	Study Design	Sample	Methods	Results
			in the control group. Average age in experi-mental group 84.5 yrs and 85.4 in control group. Gender: experi-mental group female 74%, control group 92%, urge UI in experimental group 75% and 70% in control group	conducted. Facilities were reimbursed for participating in the study. 12-wk treatment period. Project staff collected daily voiding records and constructed weekly graphs of toileting results for staff. Project staff used verbal encouragement to staff who complied with PURT procedure. PURT consisted of toileting the patient 30 minutes prior to the meantime of voids within an hour's block of time (during 3 days of monitoring). Outcome measures: frequency and volume of all continent and incontinent voids for 14 24-hr data collection periods spaced at 2 wk intervals.	thought to have contributed to most subjects' UI. Subjects voided at PURT program 61% of time. Treatment most effective by wk 6 of inter-vention. Reduction of UI was .9 episodes per day per person. Improved con-tinence in 86% of experimental group (to some degree) and .33 of residents experi-enced 20% re-duction in UI. Staff knowledge and attitudes did not undergo significant changes. NAs did not benefit from toileting UI residents, especially immobile ones. It was hard for staff to change their routine; 70% compliance to protocol reported.
Functional Incidenctal Training and Prompted Voiding					
Functional Incidental Training and Prompted Voiding	Schnelle et al[6]	Randomized control group design	Residents who were UI, could pass a cognitive screen were eligible. 272 potential subjects identified and 155 consented, 99 completed 4-wk PV assessment, 36 completed FIT and 40 completed PV	FIT incorporated into toileting procedures average time 13.2 minutes. PV average time 7.7 minutes. Pts were randomly assigned to FIT.	Significant improvement in exercise tolerance in FIT group. Both groups had large and similar decreases in UI. High attrition (51%) during study.
General					
Self-care	Blair et al[15]	Repeated measures one-between subjects and one-within subjects factor	15 volunteers from nursing home residents with 42 beds in USA.	Staff received training over a 2-wk period in principles of behavioral management. Residents and staff were randomly assigned to 1 of 3 groups. Condition 1 staff met with residents and planned care. Staff prompted residents to do ADLs and reinforced behavior. Condition 2 staff met with residents and planned care, infrequently	Differences existed in scores of subjects under Condition and those of subjects in Condition 2 and 3. Group means were not helpful in understanding changes in individual behaviors. Majority of change scores for subjects in Condition 1 exceeded the expected.

Table 9 : Other behavioural interventions for older people (Ctd)

Intervention	Authors	Study Design	Sample	Methods	Results
				encouraged residents to do care. Condition 3 staff planned care and infrequently provided encouragement to do ADLs.	
Staff Intervention					
Formal staff behavioral management	Stevens et al[28]	Quasi-experimental	Nursing assistants (N=18) in one LTC facility on day and evening shifts, primarily black and female. Nursing assistants and resident dyads were observed.	Behavioral training 5-hour and subsequent on-the-job training. Formal staff management (FSM) included description of tasks, supervisory monitoring, supervisory performance feedback and praise, and incentives for NAs who achieve task criteria. Data were collected at baseline, intervention, 4-weeks post-intervention and approximately every 4 weeks for 12 months.	On-the-job training (OJT) facilitates use of skills taught during in-services. NA self monitoring and LPN feedback can be used effectively evaluate performance of management skills.
Staff compliance to PV	Remsberg et al[19]	Survey	88 nursing staff members participated.	Staff members were asked to rate perceptions regarding improvement of continence status of residents on a PV protocol.	52% thought residents were better on PV, 43% perceived no change. Staff thought compliance to PV was 80-90% when unobtrusive observations by research staff revealed it was 70%.
Pelvic Muscle Exercise					
PME with or without biofeedback, E-stim	Berghmans et al[21]	2000	RCTs between 1980-1999 on tx of UUI	Literature search, selection criteria: design, results in women with UUI, tx consisted of: bladder training, PME, or ES, reliable and clinically relevant outcomes	81 publications identified; 15 met inclusion criteria. Main methodological shortcomings were: small sample size, lack of prestratification on prognostic determinants, lack of description of random allocation procedure and suboptimal blinding. Weak evidence that bladder retraining is better than no tx. and that it is better than drug therapy. Insufficient evidence for PME exercises, exercises alone, toilet training, and ES for women with UUI.

Table 9 : Other behavioural interventions for older people (Ctd)

Intervention	Authors	Study Design	Sample	Methods	Results
Behavioral and drug	Burgio et al[22]	1998	197 women from ages 55-92 yrs formed a volunteer sample.	Randomized to 4 sessions of biofeedback assisted behavioral, drug (oxybutynin in range of doses), and placebo. Patients kept bladder diaries and reported perceptions of improvement and comfort and satisfaction with tx	All tx groups had reduction of UI in early stage of tx. Behavioral had most reduction, more so than drug and behavioral and drug more so than placebo. Patients reported most improvement with behavioral, only 14% in behavioral group wanted to change to another tx as compared to 75.5% in each of the other groups.
Combined behavioral and drug	Burgio et al[23]	2000	Same sample as above study with 8 (12.7%) women crossed from behavioral tx alone to combined tx (behavioral and drug) and 27 (41.5%) in drug alone to combined tx.	As above with a total of 35 subjects crossing to combined tx for 8 additional weeks after first 8 weeks of tx. Patients who were not completely dry or not completely satisfied with offered additional tx.	Women in the combined group (who added drug to behavioral) experienced additional improvement from average 57.5% reduction (with behavioral alone) to average 88.5% reduction of UI. Women in combined group (who added behavioral to drug) experienced additional improvement from average 72.7% reduction (with drug alone) to 84.3%.
Nonsurgical tx, PME, bladder retraining, estrogen replacement, biofeedback, ES, and pharmacological	Weinberger et[24]	1999	Community-dwelling women over age 60 who received treatment from April 1991-January 1994. GSUI in 18, detrusor overactivity in 14 and mixed in 13.	Mailed questionnaire at least one year after their final visit. Questions about persistent UI, pad use, treatment efficacy, characterization of UI severity and quality of life.	53/81 basis of analyses. PME, bladder retraining and estrogen replacement most frequently prescribed tx. Pt. Report of greater UI reduction with PME, bladder retraining, and caffeine restriction than with pharmacological tx, estrogen replacement, management of constipation, ES, and biofeedback.

baseline wetness rates, small voided volumes, and unsuccessful toileting attempts were not responsive to toileting regimes. Ouslander and his colleagues reported on the best predictors of responsiveness for prompted voiding programs in nursing home residents [12].

Those who could ambulate independently, had appropriate toileting rates (that is the number of times the resident voided into the toilet divided by the total number of voids) of 66 percent or higher, or achieved a wet rate of 20 percent or less in the initial days of the program were considered responders. The wet rate was the number of times the resident was wet when physically checked. In contrast, Hu and his colleagues [8] found that residents with a high rate of incontinence in baseline were responders to habit training with prompting intervention. The authors suggested that improvement was due to patient initiated requests to void. Residents who were cognitively intact and had normal bladder capacity were also more likely to respond than those without these attributes.

Cultural aspects of urinary incontinence are largely ignored in the research literature. One pilot study was located and it indicated that cultural differences do exist among women. Jewish and Muslim women with incontinence in this pilot study reported greater restriction on prayer than women of other religions, because of their religious requirement that they be in a state of cleanliness while at prayer and in a house of worship. Muslim and Hindu women discussed incontinence with close female friends and relatives, but not with male relatives. All 34 women in this study reported not feeling free to discuss urinary incontinence with outsiders for fear of appearing "unclean"[13].

Evidence exists then that socio-cultural factors for both the frail older person and the caregiver need to be taken into account as behavioral interventions are employed to improve continence. More research, however, is needed to understand the quality of life issues and interventions that may improve self-care activities in frail older persons.

b) Results

Evidence exists that prompted voiding is effective in the short-term for improving dryness (that is, improved continence) in nursing home residents and in some home care clients [4, 5, 7, 8, 10, 14]. Colling and colleagues reported that patterned urge response toileting (PURT), i.e., toileting residents at times when they most likely needed to empty their bladders, improved continence levels of nursing home residents [9]. Other research findings from a quasi-experimental study revealed that deconditioned and frail nursing home residents responded to an exercise intervention, Functional Incidental Training (FIT), with both increased mobility endurance and physical activity [6]. Although the evidence is modest, these findings support earlier reports that nursing home residents respond to behavioral and rehabilitative interventions and prefer interventions to help them control or manage urinary incontinence rather than interventions designed to reduce loneliness, improve sleep, or increase physical functioning. Blair and colleagues found the use of operant behavioral strategies effective in increasing self-care behavior in long-term care residents [15]. The underlying principle of these strategies is that behavior is modified by its consequences [16]. In this study, residents who performed self-care activities were verbally rewarded and received individual attention from staff members, thus reinforcing the desired behavior. Although this study did not discuss continence needs, it provides further evidence that frail older persons respond to stimuli that encourages and supports self-care activities.

c) Summary

Prompted voiding is an effective treatment in the short-term for nursing home residents and home-care clients, if staff members comply with the protocol (Level 1B).

d) Recommendations

- Prompted voiding should be offered to nursing home residents to decrease incontinence (grade A), and efforts made to increase and maintain staff compliance with prompted voiding programs (grade A).

e) Research priorities

Research is needed to determine:

- long-term effects of prompted voiding in nursing home residents and home care patients
- consumer preference for prompted voiding as treatment for urinary incontinence as compared to other treatments
- the effect of prompted voiding on the quality of life of frail older persons
- social and cultural influences on the effectiveness of prompted voiding in culturally diverse populations

3. Interventions with long term care staff

a) Background

Several authors of published studies acknowledged the difficulty of conducting research in the long-term care setting [2,7,9]. Factors such as staffing ratios and changes in administrative policies are beyond the researchers' control. Because most behavioral interventions in long-term care use a caregiver delivery system, several studies focused on the staff members' compliance to protocols. Evidence is available that a two-prong intervention, one geared towards the resident and the other geared towards the staff members, is necessary [2, 5, 7, 9]. In 1998 Schnelle and his colleagues noted that the direct care providers will be unlikely to implement programs unless long-term care residents and their families advocate for them [17].

b) Quality of data

Prompted voiding interventions are totally dependent on staff members' adherence to the protocol in order for the intervention to be effective. Several researchers reported that staff compliance was less than total. Creason and colleagues [7] experienced problems with staff training. For instance, several staff members did not attend group-training sessions and needed one-on-one training. Other staff members did not perform the protocol or document its use, especially when staffing levels were low. Hu and his colleagues noted that nursing assistants play a key role in the success of a behavioral program. They noted that organizational schemes need to be devised to create incentives for nursing assistants to make and keep residents continent [8].

b) Results

Colling and her colleagues also found an average of 70 percent of toiletings were completed and that staff knowledge and attitudes remained unchanged after inservice classes on urinary incontinence [9]. These researchers also noted that staff members believed that it was "not worthwhile toileting" some residents.

A staff survey revealed that nursing assistants' believed prompted voiding was very helpful to residents, that is, it reduces the frequency and volume of incontinent voids [18]. Perceptions of barriers to prompted voiding programs included inadequate staffing, workload, and turnover/absenteeism of staff. They believed that increased number of staff, improved communication, ongoing education, and alternative modes of care delivery were necessary to facilitate the implementation of prompted voiding programs. In sum, these authors found that the staff members believed the program improved the quality of life but the realities of long-term care (i.e., inadequate staffing, workload and absenteeism and turnover of staff) made it difficult to carry out the protocol.

Remsburg and colleagues compared staff perceptions regarding completed toiletings to research staff observed toiletings and found that staff over-inflated the percent of toiletings they completed believing 80-90 percent were completed when in actuality 70 percent were completed [19]. The staff members also believed that residents were happier while on a prompted voiding program but only 52 percent thought residents' continence status was improved due to the program.

c) Summary

Interventions designed to maintain implementation of patient-focused behavioral interventions by long-term care staff are helpful in promoting continence care (Level 2B).

d) Recommendations

- Long-term care institutions should implement staff development programs to increase knowledge and skills about continence care and the efficacy of behavioral methods (grade A)

e) Research priorities

Research is needed to determine:

- mechanisms of behavioral change in staff in both the short and long-term.
- the long-term effects of staff education and on-the-job training on patient outcomes, specifically urinary incontinence.

4. Pelvic Floor Muscle Exercises (PFME)

a) Background

Readers are referred to chapter 10c on Conservative Management in Women for a review of the role of PFME in women. These studies have included many older women but invariably have not stratified for age effects.

Little evidence exists to support the use of pelvic muscle exercise in nursing home residents. No randomized clinical trials were located. One major problem may be the high prevalence of cognitive impairment in this population that precludes its effective use. Pelvic muscle exercise has been used in the ambulatory or outpatient setting. Muscle hypertrophy is postulated as the primary mechanism for pelvic muscle exercise effectiveness in women with stress urinary incontinence (SUI) [20]. It is also probable that improvement in neuromuscular coordination (i.e. timing and intensity of contraction during intervals of increased abdominal pressure) are more important than pelvic muscle alone [20].

b) Quality of data

Small sample size and inadequate description of methodology hinder quality of several studies [21]. Women with different types of urinary incontinence (e.g. stress urinary incontinence, urge urinary incontinence, and mixed incontinence) have been included in studies [23,24] hindering interpretation of results. There is conflicting evidence regarding the effectiveness of pelvic muscle exercise as treatment for urge urinary incontinence in women [21, 22, 23]. Patient self-report of efficacy of treatment after at least one-year since treatment has also been used [24].

c) Results

Pelvic muscle exercise appears effective in combination with oxybutynin chloride in reducing incontinent episodes in older non-demented women with predominantly urge incontinence. Pelvic muscle exercise also appears effective one-year after treatment by patient report [24] and women appear to choose to behavioral therapy rather than drug therapy, as medication side-effects are troublesome [23].

d) Summary

Pelvic floor muscle exercise alone and in combination with medication is an effective treatment in older healthy women with urge urinary incontinence and in women with stress urinary incontinence and should be recommended to women who are able to perform the exercises correctly alone or in combination with medication

XII. PHARMACOLOGICAL MANAGEMENT

1. BACKGROUND

Several controlled trials that establish the benefit of pharmacologic agents for incontinence have included some fit elderly, but specific effects of age in these studies are not commonly delineated. For a more detailed discussion regarding results of drug intervention, please refer to Chapter 9 «Pharmacologic Treatment». This section focuses on the few published studies that are controlled and deal with the efficacy of pharmacologic agents for the treatment of urge incontinence in frail older patients; as noted below, adequate data for other types of incontinence could not be identified. Most of these studies were conducted in long-term care facilities [1-7], but one investigated frail community-dwelling older persons [8] and two included some independent older persons [9, 10].

Several points warrant emphasis.

- Caution is required when prescribing any medication to frail elderly because of increased susceptibility to potential side effects, including ones not commonly encountered in younger patients (Table 4, 5).
- Since many drugs have been associated with causing or contributing to incontinence, all current medications should be reviewed before initiating a new one.
- It is important when prescribing for older patients to start with a low dose and to increase it slowly, as necessary and as tolerated.
- Elderly patients are much more likely to respond to pharmacotherapy when all factors outside the lower urinary tract that could potentially contribute to incontinence have been treated first and after other lower urinary tract dysfunction, such as a weak urethral sphincter, has been addressed.
- In most cases, UI management in frail older persons should not consist of pharmacologic treatment alone, but should include behavioral therapy as well.

The available controlled studies in frail older persons all focus on treatment of detrusor overactivity. Although estrogens, alpha-adrenergic agonist and alpha-antagonist drugs have been used, respectively, for stress and mixed UI as well as for benign prostatic obstruction-related urge UI, we did not find any published controlled study regarding the efficacy of these drugs in frail older patients. No studies in frail older persons evaluated bladder relaxants for DHIC.

2. QUALITY OF DATA

We located 9 randomized controlled trials of treatment for urge UI [1-4, 6-10], six of which were also double blinded and placebo-controlled [2 ,6-10], and one non-randomized study [5]. Three studies of subjects with urge UI [5-6,10], and one with unspecified UI [3] compared drug efficacy when added to toileting assistance programs. Studies generally were small; of the 10 studies, three had fewer than 20 patients, and four others had fewer than 50. In most studies, the diagnosis was clinical alone, but in 5 studies [4-6,9-10] the diagnosis was made or supplemented by urodynamic evaluation. Many investigators included some information regarding patients' functional and cognitive status, as well as a list of comorbid conditions, but none addressed these issues adequately in the analyses. Study subjects were heterogeneous. Three studies excluded patients with detrusor underactivity , as defined by an elevated PVR [4-6], but none of these studies accounted for the spuriously low PVR that is found among women with a weak bladder when they strain during voiding; the remaining studies did not address bladder contractility. In six studies, investigators treated subjects with urinary tract infections before initiating bladder relaxant therapy [1, 3-7], and one study excluded such subjects [8]. In one study, investigators treated atrophic vaginitis prior to pharmacotherapy [3]. No other reversible causes were addressed prior to entry or randomization.

3. RESULTS

Ouslander et al found that oxybutynin, when added to

bladder training, did not affect the frequency of incontinence episodes in 15 nursing home residents [5]. These results differ somewhat from those of a subsequent and larger study by Ouslander et al [7]. In this study of institutionalized subjects who had failed prompted voiding alone, the addition of titrated oxybutynin resulted in a significantly greater reduction in wetness than did the addition of placebo. Improvement for the group was modest; the absolute frequency of UI decreased from 27% of checks at baseline to 24% on placebo and 20% on active drug, leading the authors to conclude that the improvement was statistically but not clinically significant. However, before beginning the study, the authors had decided that clinically significant improvement would consist of having one or fewer episodes of incontinence during the daytime hours. This status was achieved by 40% of patients on oxybutynin but by only 18% of patients on placebo ($p<0.05$); the dose generally associated with such improvement was 2.5 mg three times daily. In another controlled study of UI in institutionalized residents, Zorzitto et al found little effect of immediate release oxybutynin, but all of the residents were also toileted 10 times daily; the drug was given for only 8 days; and the dosing regimen was 5 mg twice daily, which may have been too high a dose given too infrequently [6]. In a two month, dose titration study of frail community-dwelling elderly, Szonyi et al found that the combination of oxybutynin and bladder training was subjectively and objectively superior to bladder training alone in improving urinary frequency (95% C.I. of 6 to 27 fewer voids per 2 weeks) but not in improving incontinence [8].

Other agents have also been evaluated, but with less impressive results. Robinson and Brocklehurst studied 20 patients seen in a continence clinic, only 14 of whom completed a trial of emepronium bromide; they reported an increase in PVR, but no significant change in incontinence episodes or cystometric detrusor overactivity after 2 weeks of treatment [9]. Williams et al found that emepronium bromide had no significant effect on daytime or nocturnal urinary incontinence among patients suffering from chronic organic brain syndrome or chronic functional psychiatric illness [2]. Similar results were reported by Zorzitto et al who treated institutionalized residents for only four days with 15 mg of propantheline given four times daily; when the dose was increased to 30 mg four times daily the useful clinical effects were overwhelmed by anticholinergic side effects in about half of the patients [4]. In addition, as in their oxybutynin study cited earlier, patients were likely to be toileted every two hours. Tobin and Brocklehurst found that institutionalized subjects who were toileted every 2 hours experienced more improvement in nocturia while on flavoxate four times daily plus propantheline three times daily than did those on placebo, but the effect on daytime incontinence was not significant [3]. Castleden et al administered titrated imipramine or placebo to 34 ambulatory patients, half of whom were elderly and also received habit training [10]. Although the proportion of patients who achieved complete continence was markedly better among those on imipramine (78% vs. 43%), it did not achieve statistical significance and the rate of UI at baseline was worse among the placebo group than among the imipramine group.

4. Summary

Pharmacologic suppression of overactive bladder symptoms appears to add to the effectiveness of behavioral therapy alone in frail and/or institutionalized older persons. This is an important point because trials in younger patients have generally not included a placebo group that was undergoing active behavioral intervention. Since such concurrent therapy would likely have attenuated the differences observed between the drug and placebo-treated groups, the results of these trials in frail elderly cannot be compared directly with those conducted in younger individuals.

The best outcomes reported to date have occurred in studies using-immediate-release oxybutynin (Level of Evidence 2), but trials of earlier agents suffered from more design flaws, and trials of newer agents in this population are not yet available. The characteristics of patients likely to respond to pharmacotherapy have not been well delineated. Therefore, at present it is reasonable to consider the use of drug therapy in a wide range of patients as an adjunct to other conservative measures. (Level of Evidence 4)

5. Recommendations

- Oxybutynin and potentially other bladder relaxants can improve the effectiveness of behavioral therapies in frail older persons. (Grade of Recommendation B)
- Before initiating drug therapy in frail older patients, all other currently prescribed medications that could be directly or indirectly contributing to incontinence should be reviewed and modified if possible. (Grade of Recommendation D)
- Because older persons frequently have multiple and complex medical and physical conditions that impair their capacity to toilet independently, pharmacological therapy should be used as an adjunct to other management programs (e.g., bladder retraining or prompted voiding). (Grade of Recommendation D).
- When drug treatment is necessary, it is important to start with low dosage, increasing it slowly while

reviewing the outcome and searching for side effects. (Grade of Recommendation D)

- Some agents that have proved effective in younger populations are associated with the potential for inducing serious side effects in older adults. These agents include vasopressin, tricyclic antidepressants (e.g., imipramine, desipramine, and amitriptyline), propantheline, and ephedrine. Because other agents are available, in whom the efficacy and toxicity have been established for this population, we believe that the agents just mentioned should not be used as first-line therapy for frail elderly. (Grade of Recommendation D)
- Data from frail elderly are not available regarding the efficacy and risks of treating types other than urge incontinence.

6. RESEARCH PRIORITIES

- Evaluation of the utility of pharmacologic agents in frail older persons. Studies should be conducted that include adequate numbers of patients, employ appropriate diagnostic methods, and adjust for comorbidity and concurrent LUT dysfunction (e.g., DHIC, sphincter incompetence).
- Definition of the benefit of pharmacological therapy in addition to behavioral therapy in frail and institutionalized older persons.
- Delineation of characteristics of frail or institutionalized older persons who are likely to respond to pharmacologic therapies.
- Determination of the beneficial or adverse effects of bladder relaxant use in subjects taking cholinergic agents for the treatment of Alzheimer's disease.
- Studies including outcome measures relevant in geriatric care, such as a modest improvement in incontinence, increased socialization, or decreased caregiver burden.
- Determination of the value of "PRN" rather than continuously scheduled bladder relaxant therapy in older persons.

XIII. SURGICAL INTERVENTION IN WOMEN

1. BACKGROUND

Eleven percent of women in the United States will undergo at least one operation for urinary incontinence or pelvic organ prolapse by age 80 [1]. Healthy elderly are managed similarly to younger patients, and surgical management in these populations is addressed in Chapter 11c «Surgical Treatment in Women». However, there are no published studies specifically addressing procedures for urinary incontinence in frail elderly women. This section discusses special considerations in the operative care of frail elderly, and data regarding the impact of age on response to surgery. Although particular attention must be paid to frail elderly, it must be noted because of the age-related but variable decrease in physiological reserve, all older persons are potentially more vulnerable to complications as discussed here. Even healthy older persons should be evaluated preoperatively and followed closely postoperatively for potential complications.

a) Preoperative Evaluation

The first decision to be made in surgical management of frail elderly is not whether the patient can survive the procedure, but whether the procedure will improve the patient's quality of life or enhance the patient's ability to function. Thus, a functional evaluation should ideally precede a medical evaluation. Every aspect of functional status and social support is important to plan the perioperative management and help the patient recover. Special considerations include the patient=s risk for postoperative delirium and for debilitation leading to dependence upon discharge. During the medical evaluation, special attention should be given to the cardiovascular system, both clinical and subclinical disease, because cardiovascular events cause the majority of serious morbidity and mortality. The patient should be evaluated for other risks that increase with age, including those of postoperative delirium, thromboembolic disease, renal failure, and pressure ulcerations.

The goals of identifying these risks are

- optimization of conditions, such as cardiopulmonary status, nutrition and mobility.
- prevention of complications, such as deconditioning, delirium, or renal failure.
- early recognition of complications that do occur, such as electrolyte imbalance or delirium.
- appropriate counseling about individual risks.

Standards for informed consent vary in different countries. If the patient is cognitively impaired, it is usually straightforward to obtain legal consent from appropriate family members.

Symptoms do not explicitly predict lower urinary tract pathology, and even less so in the elderly [2-3]. Complex urodynamic studies are universally recommended prior to incontinence surgery in elderly women, both because of the inaccuracy of symptoms, and also because of an increased prevalence in the elderly of low pressure urethra, detrusor overactivity, and voiding dysfunction, all of which might complicate surgical outcomes. However, abnormal urodynamic findings are common even in continent, asymptomatic older persons, and may not be the cause of the patient's bothersome symptoms. Thus, urodynamics cannot fully direct surgical therapy. As stated above, the surgeon must consider symptoms and urodynamic findings, together with the patient's functional ability and quality of life, to arrive at appropriate surgical management. There are no studies comparing surgical outcomes of older subjects who did and did not have preoperative urodynamic testing.

Preoperative estrogen therapy is considered beneficial for patients with urogenital atrophy, but has been studied very little. There are no studies of the effect of preoperative estrogen on surgical outcomes in frail elderly, nor on how long one might prescribe estrogen. Fecal incontinence is common in older women, and is particularly prevalent in those with urinary incontinence (>20%) [4-5]. This symptom should be specifically queried prior to any urinary incontinence procedure, to further evaluate and plan management for pelvic floor dysfunction.

b) Surgical choices

Choice of surgical procedure is essentially the same for a given urodynamic diagnosis in an elderly women as in a younger one, once the decision has been made to operate. Lower overall success rates would be expected in the frail or very old, because of the multifactorial nature of urinary incontinence. However, most published studies including elderly women find either no correlation of age with outcome or do not mention any evaluation of age effects. Thus, although some evidence exists to the contrary, one can expect the same success for a given surgical procedure in younger and older women. It may be prudent to perform a lesser procedure with less immediate morbidity but a lower long-term cure rate, such as anterior colporrhaphy or needle procedures, in frail elderly women. Because immediate quality of life is the paramount concern, the surgical success beyond 2 to 4 years will be irrelevant to many frail elderly.

c) Safety of surgery

The risk of major morbidity or mortality from continence procedures in older persons is extremely low. Sultana et al reviewed Medicare data on 66,478 patients over age 64 undergoing continence procedures from 1984 to 1991, mean age 72, median age 71 [6]. The 30-day mortality was 0.33%. Mortality increased linearly with age, from 0.2% at age 65 to 74, to 1.6% in those over age 84. It was concluded that incontinence surgery was safe in the «young elderly» woman, but that patients over 80 years old should be counseled about increased risks. However, the age-specific mortality rates were not adjusted for comorbid conditions. Patients who died had higher rates of diabetes and heart failure. It is unknown whether the increased morbidity was related to age or to comorbid conditions, as has been found in other studies [7].

2. Quality of data

Most publications about older women include primarily the «young old» and some «middle old». No studies have been conducted in frail elderly. Most retrospectively review a single surgical technique with a variable length of follow-up and without a control group. Selection bias is difficult to account for, whilst definitions and outcome measures are inconsistent. Variable definitions and statistical methods were used in the few studies that evaluated the effect of age on outcome. Most studies showing no correlation of age with outcome were not adequately powered to confirm the null hypothesis. In older women, more studies have been published about collagen injections than about any other procedure, followed by needle procedure studies.

3. Results

a) Needle procedures

Of six studies limited to or including elderly, one reported better results in older than younger women [8], three found that age did not correlate negatively with outcome [9-11], and two did not mention any analysis of age and outcomes [12-13]. Objective cures range from 39% [12] to 76% [8], with cured-or-improved rates as high as 88% [9].

b) Sling procedures

Of two pubovaginal sling studies, one found age not to be associated with outcome [14] and one did not analyze the effect of age on outcome [15]. Two studies of vaginal wall slings [16-17] and one of the vaginal wall island [18] did not evaluate the effect of age on outcome, nor did a study comparing sling with colposuspension [19].

c) Colposuspension

Two studies of colposuspension in women over age 65 found cure rates of 74-90%, but did not mention any specific evaluation of age as a factor [20-21]. One large retrospective evaluation of 289 colpourethropexies, including 50 women over age 65, found a non-significant trend toward less success in older patients (10% failure) compared to younger women (3% failure) [22]. This study did not state whether a greater percentage of the older patients had had previous anti-incontinence procedures. A study of colposuspension for persistent or recurrent stress urinary incontinence following previous surgery found a higher mean age (68 years) in those whose surgeries were unsuccessful compared to those with good results (mean age 57), but no statistical analyses were undertaken [23].

d) Other

A study of 12 patients, mean age 66, who received tension-free vaginal mesh for stress urinary incontinence and anterior vaginal wall prolapse reported 100% cure of incontinence in a short follow-up period [24].

e) Periurethral bulking agents

Three studies of collagen as a periurethral bulking agent found age not to be associated with outcomes [25-27]. Studies limited to women over age 65 found results ranging from favorable to poor [28-30]. Winters et al found that in 58 women, mean age 73 (range 65-86), 80% achieved at least social continence by subjective criteria, but 41% of these experienced recurrent incontinence, which was more difficult to treat [28]. Stanton and Monga found cure or improvement at 2 years 69% subjectively and 54% objectively [29]. Faerber found objective cure in 83% at an average of 10 months [30]. One study found that subjects who failed collagen were older, but the results were not further analyzed [31]. Three collagen studies including only women over age 65 [28,30,32] and 6 studies including both older and younger women [33-38], as well as one study of silicone micro-implants in older and younger women [39] did not evaluate whether age correlated with outcome. Results of collagen injection in these studies ranged from 83% objectively cured at 10 months [30] to 26% subjectively improved at 5 years [27]. A study of small volume periurethral polytetrafluoroethylene found no effect of age on outcome, with 72% dry or improved [40].

4. Summary

Elderly women probably have long-term results from incontinence surgery similar to those in younger women. (Level of Evidence 2) Advanced age *may*, however, correlate with worse outcome, as is found in one or 2 studies in each procedure group (needle procedures, sling procedures, colposuspension, periurethral bulking agents). (Level of Evidence 4) Data are lacking about the effects of age in most studies. No surgical trials or retrospective reviews have been done specifically in frail elderly, in whom surgical therapy is chosen less often. Since urge incontinence is much more prevalent than bothersome stress incontinence in frail elderly, particular efforts should be made to detect and treat this prior to any decision to operate (Level of Evidence 5).

5. Recommendations

- Robust older persons respond well to surgery and should be treated essentially the same as younger individuals, with the caveats that they are at increased risk for perioperative complications because of decreased physiological reserve. (Grade of Recommendation C)
- Frail older persons benefit in select cases from surgical intervention, and should not be denied consideration for this. (Grade of Recommendation D)
- Because urinary incontinence is more complex in frail elderly, the preoperative evaluation is of critical importance, including quality of life and functional assessment, as well as medical risk factors. (Grade of Recommendation D
- The increased complexity of lower urinary tract pathology in older persons necessitates full urodynamic evaluation prior to a surgical procedure. (Grade of Recommendation D)

6. Research priorities

- The functional response of frail elderly to incontinence surgery should be studied, including patients discharged to rehabilitation or long term care facilities, and how many gained an improvement in activities of daily living.
- The effect of surgery on quality of life in frail and robust elderly should be studied.
- Future studies should, at a minimum, define functional characteristics of elderly patients, as well as report success in subgroups of older persons, so that meta-analyses might be facilitated.

XIV. SURGICAL INTERVENTIONS IN OLDER MEN

1. Background

Although most men can be treated conservatively it is important to notice that age itself is no contraindication for surgical treatment in older men. The major indications are

incontinence after radical prostatectomy resulting in sphincter damage, radiation of the pelvis or other surgical procedures of the prostate, and retention of urine due to bladder outlet obstruction. Therapy of bladder outlet obstruction is covered extensively in chapter 11b

«Surgical Treatment in Men» and the ICI BPH Book [1] and will not be covered here.

Due to growing numbers of elderly men with localized prostate cancer undergoing radical prostatectomy or radiation therapy, the numbers of men with iatrogenic incontinence are increasing in spite of improved therapeutically methods. The introduction of new methods of anesthesia, effective prophylaxis against deep venous thrombosis, and sophisticated perioperative monitoring technology have contributed to lower surgical mortality for older adults [2]. In the last few decades economic pressures and technological advances have resulted in less invasive procedures allowing the patient to return quickly to their usual environment and functional status and thus help to reduce complications so commonly related to medications and immobilization associated with hospitalization. Especially in elderly with an increased risk for perioperative complication every indication for a surgical procedure must be weighed carefully against possible risks, expected benefit and the patient's and in some also the caregiver's wishes. Indices, which have been developed to estimate the perioperative risk, may help to find a suitable decision for the individual [3].

2. Quality of data

The main surgical procedures for iatrogenic stress incontinence are implantation of an artificial sphincter, injection of bulking agents and sling procedures. These surgical approaches are investigated in case series with a heterogeneous group of older persons focusing on cure rate and complication rate, but not stratifying the results by age or comorbidity [4-16]. Especially data about different techniques of sling procedures come from small case series including 10 to 30 patients of different ages. There are no data on augmentation cystoplasty or sacral implants-stimulators in older persons.

3. Results

All authors demonstrate that artificial urinary sphincter implantation provide good objective results [4-10] (see chapter 11b «Surgical Treatment in Men»). Martins [5] and Perez [10] demonstrate that patients older than 70, with previous radiotherapy or residual tumor may have good long-term outcome regardless of the underlying condition. Reported incontinence rate lie between 60 and 80% depending on the author's definition of incontinence [5-10]. Due to improved surgical methods in the newer series reoperation rates decreased to about 20% [9,10]. Surgical interventions were mainly due to infection and erosion. Haab et al conclude in a retrospective long-term study a positive impact of the artificial urinary sphincter on quality of life [9].

Injection of bulking agents are easy to perform and have a low morbidity but success rates are low and not durable [15,16]. Results are not stratified by age and data on comorbidity are quite sparse. Smith [15] reports in a series of 62 men that after a follow up of two years only 43 % were 'socially continent' (dry or minimal leakage) Success rates after radical prostatectomy was lower than after transurethral prostatectomy and patients with mild incontinence seem to respond better [16]. When recommending this procedure to older patients one has to keep in mind that often multiple injection procedures are required [16].

Different surgical approaches like fascial sling procedures [11,12], rectus fascial sling with needle suspension [13] or bone anchored sling [14] are presented as preliminary data and further experiences are needed to establish these procedures as treatment for incontinence due to sphincter incompetence.

Especially implantation of an artificial urethral sphincter provides cure of incontinence in a substantial number of patients. Complications and high rate of reoperation limit its use to a selected group of patients especially in the very old.

4. Summary

The surgical management of urinary incontinence due to sphincter incompetence in men is still a challenging issue for urologists to date. The best-investigated method is the implantation of an artificial urinary sphincter, which can provide fairly good continence rates. High reoperation rates because of mechanical failure, infection or erosion limit its use in elderly men. (Level of evidence 4)

Injection of bulking agent are have a low morbidity but cure rate and lack of durability limit its use in older men. (Level of evidence 4)

Different techniques for sling procedures in men with sphincter incompetence are published and although first results are quite promising further comparative studies are warranted. (Level of evidence 4)

5. Recommendations

- Implantation of an artificial sphincter is the most efficacious treatment currently available for significant male urinary incontinence due to sphincter incompetence, but the patient has to be informed that reintervention rates even in the hands of experts are about 20%. (Grade of recommendation C)

6. Research priorities

- Data on different surgical procedures should be stratified by age and whenever possible by comorbidity to enable the surgeons to better advise their patients.

XV. PADS AND APPLIANCES

Incontinence products come in relatively few fundamentally different design categories. However, a given category usually comprises a bewildering array of somewhat similar variants and, since robust clinical evaluations are available on virtually none of them, purchasers seeking to make informed choices face major difficulties. Choosing is especially difficult if manufacturers modify their designs frequently (as with disposable pads, for example) or if optimal product selection rests heavily on the details of the residual functions of the user(s) and/or their particular priorities and preferences (as with handheld urinals, for example). Indeed, no evaluation has ever found that one product best meets the needs of all testers. The generalisability of evaluation data is improved if the number of different products under test is increased but the multiple comparisons problem imposes constraints [1]. As the number of products (n) increases, the number of product pairs to be compared ((n2-n)/2) rises rapidly demanding ever bigger test panels to maintain a given study power, with concomitant increases in cost and delay to publication.

These difficulties do not justify the poor methodology that characterises much published work but they do underline the futility of seeking to provide purchasers with reliable data on all the products on the market, for all user categories. Following such a strategy would be immensely expensive and usually generate data doomed to fall out of date rapidly. There is little point in lamenting the fact that good quality data is not available on many products: it never will be. Pragmatically, many millions of incontinent people worldwide rely on pads and appliances to manage their incontinence and so the challenge is to glean from the literature the best advice possible.

1. Absorbent products

• Background and quality of data

Absorbent products account for the majority of expenditure on incontinence aids and appliances. They may be classified into four broad categories. There are bedpads (underpads) and bodyworn products, each available as disposable (single use) items and reusable (washable) variants designed to be laundered and reused many times.

Many comparative evaluations of absorbent products have been published. Some workers have sought to extend the usefulness of their data by generalizing results from sample products to whole product categories, for example, comparing a representative disposable bodyworn pad with a representative reusable bedpad. This is an attractive but dangerous approach as the diversity of product performance within categories may be as great as that between them and so generalizations can be meaningless and misleading. However, such evaluations can provide valuable insights into the nature of generic problems like those associated with laundering reusable products or discarding disposables. For this reason, meta-analysis of data from studies involving products which are very different from one another apart from one feature they have in common (eg the presence of superabsorber) is likely to reach spurious conclusions.

Comparisons within product categories are safer but still difficult: for example, comparing a disposable pad containing superabsorbent polymer and one without. But numerous design elements and material properties combine synergistically to determine performance and commercial products will invariably differ from one another in too many ways for it to be possible to isolate the impact of any particular feature or combination of features. The safest strategy is to evaluate experimental products engineered to differ from one another in limited, well-defined ways. Even then the synergy between product features may limit extrapolation of results. For example, a coverstock material (the surface layer next to the skin) which gives the best wet comfort when used in combination with a particular absorbent core may not provide the best wet comfort with all absorbent cores.

A completely different approach to product evaluation is to develop standard laboratory tests capable of predicting some aspects of clinical performance and several such tests are available. However, establishing tests of this kind is time-consuming as correlation with clinical data has to be proven for a good diversity of products. Also, it does not provide a permanent solution since new product designs and materials may not conform to the assumed correlation. But such tests are much easier to run than clinical evaluations and enable large numbers of products to be characterized rapidly and relatively inexpensively.

2. Disposable bodyworn absorbent products

a) Background

Disposable bodyworn absorbent products can be divided into several classes.

Inserts (sometimes called liners or, in the case of small pads, shields) are held in place by close-fitting underwear or stretch mesh briefs. They may have an adhesive strip on the back to help secure them; an indicator that changes colour when wet to signal the need for a pad change; and longitudinal, elasticated cuffsof hydrophobic material intended to impede lateral leakage of urine and faeces. They are sometimes rectangular but are often shaped to fit the body more snugly. Elastication at the legs may also be used to enhance fit.

Briefs are adult-sized diapers. They usually have elasticated waist and legs and self-adhesive tabs (usually resealable), and often a wetness indicator and standing gathers.

Pull-ups are similar in construction to trainer pants for toddlers. The absorbent material is built into a pull-up pant which is elasticated to give a close fit.

Male guards (sometimes called shields or pouches) are for lightly incontinent men and are designed to fit around the penis and sometimes the scrotum too. All are worn with close-fitting underwear or stretch mesh briefs. An adhesive strip is often provided.

All disposable products – except those used with water-proof pants – comprise three main layers: an absorbent core sandwiched between a water-proof polyethylene backing beneath and a water-permeable coverstock (sometimes called the topsheet) next to the wearer's skin. The main component in absorbent cores is invariably some kind of fluffed wood pulp fibres but most also contain some powdered superabsorber (sometimes referred to as SAP (superabsorbent polymer) or AGM (absorbent gelling material)), which is often concentrated in the crotch region. Superabsorbers hold much more urine – weight for weight – than fluff pulp and retain it far more tenaciously under pressure. They are usually based on cross-linked salts of polyacrylic acid whose chemistry can be varied according to the balance of properties such as absorption capacity and absorption speed desired. Some thermoplastic fibres are also sometimes included in absorbent cores to reduce core break up and the collapse of the structure when wet. It is increasingly common for absorbent cores to comprise two or more layers, each designed to perform a different function. For example, an inner layer might comprise low absorbency fibres selected to receive and distribute urine efficiently and maintain a dry layer next to the skin, while outer layers provide absorption capacity.

b) Quality of data

A large number of comparative evaluations of disposable bodyworn pads have been published but many of them have been poorly controlled and/or lacked statistical power. Nevertheless, some have found significant differences between products - especially regarding leakage performance, comfort, impact on skin health and discretion (invisibility beneath clothing). Unfortunately, none of the products described is still available in the variant evaluated and compared products almost always differed from one another in too many ways to yield reliable generic conclusions on the efficacy of different materials and design features. However, taken together these studies enable the key performance parameters to be identified and some broad conclusions to help product selectors can be drawn. Other studies have compared specially made experimental products that differed from one another in carefully controlled ways enabling more specific questions to be addressed robustly. In addition, a number of laboratory tests for predicting the leakage performance of pads have been clinically-validated in multi-centre trials

Drawing on the published literature, the International Standards Organisation has published guidelines on conducting user evaluations of bodyworn pads [2].

Considerable work has been done on measuring the impact of diaper materials on skin but most of it has used a normal adult volar forearm model and little work has been done on diaper-area skin.

c) Results

In a double-blind cross-over study involving 45 heavily incontinent adults (38 women, 7 men; mean age 82y, sd 7.6y) Clancy and Malone-Lee [3] compared the leakage performance of four different variants (each available in three sizes) of a large, shaped bodyworn pad. The results were complex but, in general, the variant with two layers of fluff pulp leaked significantly less than that with one layer while adding some superasborber to the lower pulp layer produced a further significant improvement. Increasing the quantity of superabsorber yielded no clear advantage. It was also found that pads were more likely to leak if they were not held in place by any pants ($p < 0.0001$) and that, if there was any leakage from a pad, this tended to be less severe if the supplied mesh pants were worn than if normal pants were worn ($p < 0.05$).

Thornburn et al. [4] compared three variants of a small shaped disposable pad by asking twenty lightly incontinent women living in the community (age range 37-89y) to evaluate each in turn for a week in random order. Women then blind tested a random sequence of 42 pads (14 of each variant) scoring the performance of each individual pad. One variant was engineered to have high absorbency and good wetback (resistance to allowing fluid to escape back on to the wearer's skin) by using a hydrophobic coverstock and including a substantial quantity of superabsorber in the core. A second variant had a hydrophilic coverstock and no superabsorber, chosen to give low absorbency and poor wetback. The third variant had intermediate properties. Whenever differences in wet comfort, absorbency or overall performance were found they were in the expected order but differences were small and few reached statistical significance.

The impact of wet pads on skin health has received particular attention. Brown [5] found that 33% of 166 incontinent elderly adult pad wearers from acute medical wards (80 women, 86 men; mean age 74.5y, sd 12y) had mild to severe dermatitis while Lyder et al. [6] found a prevalence of 23-25% in a very small sample (n=15) of elderly patients (of unspecified sex and age) in a geriatric psychiatry unit. Several studies have sought to measure the impact of different pad materials on skin, mostly through experiments on the volar forearm of adult volunteers. Orsmark et al. [7] have validated this model for infant perineal skin (most work has related to baby diapers) but there has been no validation for adult perineal skin. Zimmerer et al. [8] showed that normal adult forearm skin (age and sex of subjects not specified) that had been in contact with a patch of wet diaper for two hours had a significantly higher coefficient of friction than dry skin ($p < 0.05$) and was significantly more susceptible to damage by abrasion ($p < 0.02$). However, varying the level of fluid loading in the test patch had no significant effect on either parameter.

Wilson and Dallas [9] used the same adult normal volar forearm skin model to compare patches taken from 16 different infant diapers. They found that disposable diapers containing superabsorber left the skin significantly drier than washable diapers and disposable diapers without superabsorber ($p < 0.01$). Disposable diapers without superabsorber did not differ significantly from reusable diapers and there were no significant differences between products within any of the three groupings. However, in a subsequent study involving 20 disposable and washable adult incontinence pads incorporating a similar range of materials to the baby diaper study Dallas and Wilson [10] found significant differences between products within each of the three product groupings but not between groupings. Grove et al. [11] used a similar approach to compare three infant diapers and found a significant difference in skin wetness between two that contained similar quantities of superabsorber ($p < 0.001$). The one in which the superabsorber was in a layer near the water-proof backing kept the skin dryer than that in which it was near the coverstock. The third diaper – which had a microporous (breathable) backing kept the skin significantly dryer than each of the other two ($p < 0.001$).

Starting from an interest in infant skin health, Berg et al. [12] have examined the role of urine in the aetiology of "diaper dermatitis" using a hairless mouse model. They found that the irritant potential of urine by itself was minimal over short periods (48 hours) but after continuous exposure (10 days) skin damage became apparent. The researchers also measured skin permeability and found that continuous exposure to urine greatly increased skin permeability (more than 15 fold) compared to occluded skin or skin exposed only to water.

Using a similar mouse model Buckingham and Berg [13] examined the role of faeces in the aetiology of "diaper dermatitis". They identified proteases and lipases as the major irritants in the faeces of infants. They also noted that these faecal enzymes not only irritated the skin directly but also increased the susceptibility of the skin to other irritants such as bile salts. However, the combination of urine and faeces caused significantly higher levels of irritation than urine or faeces alone. The authors concluded that the presence of faecal urease results in the break down of urinary urea causing an increase in pH which increases the activities of faecal proteases and lipases leading to skin irritation. There is no published work specifically examining the impact on adult skin of exposure to faeces.

Because clinical evaluations are expensive and time-consuming, laboratory evaluation procedures are in widespread use. Few have been clinically validated but there are some clinically-validated International Standards relating to leakage performance. ISO 11948-1 [14] concerns large pads for heavy incontinence. It describes a method for measuring the absorption capacity of pads in the laboratory that was shown to correlate well with the leakage performance of 18 different products evaluated in an international multi-centre project involving 112 heavily incontinent adults [15]. The strength of the correlation between technical and clinical data depended on the exact parameters being compared but typically, $r = 0.9$. This method is in widespread use for product evaluation but needs to be revalidated with modern products that are more complex in structure than those used in 1990 for the original work.

ISO 11948-2 [16] relates to small pads for lightly incontinent women. It describes a method for measuring in the laboratory how much fluid wet pads release under pressure and the results have been shown to correlate well with the leakage performance of nine different products evaluated in an international multi-centre project involving 113 women [17]. The strength of the correlation between technical and clinical data depended on the exact parameters being compared but typically, $r = 0.85$.

Manufacturers often quote pad absorption capacities in sales literature but such numbers should be interpreted with caution. Firstly, different manufacturers base their values on different tests and so comparisons can be misleading. Secondly, the concept of a pad having a simple absorption capacity is flawed. There is no urine weight below which it can be guaranteed not to leak; rather, the more urine, the greater the probability of leakage [15, 17].

d) Summary

Although numerous studies have demonstrated significant differences in various aspects of performance between nominally similar products, none of the products evaluated is still on the market. Furthermore, compared products almost always differed from one another in too many ways for the efficacy of particular design features or materials to be established.

Insert pads leak significantly less if they are held in place by mesh pants than by ordinary pants, and using no pants at all is associated with significantly more leakage than if either kind of pant is worn (Level of evidence 2b). There is evidence that pads containing superabsorber leak less, are more comfortable, and keep the skin drier than those without (Level of evidence 2b). Wet skin is more susceptible to abrasion damage than dry (Level of evidence 2b).

The leakage performance of insert pads for light incontinence, and inserts and briefs for heavy incontinence can be predicted with reasonable precision using international standard laboratory tests (Level of evidence 2b).

e) Recommendations

Although published studies provide virtually no direct information on current commercial products they do consistently identify certain aspects of pad performance which should be considered in selecting products. They are summarized in an ISO guidance document [18] and below, along with guidelines where possible.

- *Individuality:* No study has ever identified one product that worked best for all testers: needs and priorities vary. Accordingly, users are advised to try a variety of products when possible (Grade B).
- *Freedom from leakage*: Where possible, international standard laboratory tests should be used to rank the likely leakage performance of different pads for heavy [14] and light [15] incontinence (Grade B). In general, pads containing superabsorber should be selected in preference to those without (Grade B). Nobody wants their pad to leak but compromises have to be made: the pad needed to contain a person's most severe accident may be substantially more bulky and expensive than is needed most of the time. Some users choose to tolerate a higher risk of pad leakage in exchange for being able to use cheaper, smaller (more discrete) pads. The balance of priorities for a given user should be investigated in making product selections (Grade D).
- *Comfort and skin health:* In general, pads containing superabsorber should be selected in preference to those without (Grade B). Shaped pads should usually be selected in preference to unshaped (Grade C).
- *Staying in place:* No product is effective if it slips from position. Inserts should be used with pants, preferably mesh pants (Grade B). Shaped pads are preferable to rectangular (Grade C).
- *Ease of putting on and taking off:* The ease of putting pads on and taking them off should be considered, especially for caregivers and for incontinent users with reduced mobility or dexterity (Grade C).
- *Aesthetics and discretion:* A possible preference for small, more discrete pads (even if they are more likely to leak) should be considered, especially for those wishing to wear close fitting clothing (Grade C). The possibility of plastic backing materials rustling noisily should be considered (Grade C).
- *Independence and lifestyle:* The ability of a user to change his/her own pad should be considered (Grade C): those able to change their own pad can often manage with a smaller (less absorbent) one than those reliant on a caregiver. Users who travel should consider in their choice of product(s) the practicalities of carrying a supply of pads, disposing of used ones, and dealing with laundry (Grade D).
- *Costs:* Cost issues should be approached with caution (Grade D). Expensive pads do not necessarily work better than cheaper ones. Cheaper pads do not necessarily save money. If pads leak more they may have to be changed more frequently and/or lead to higher laundry costs. More pad changes will mean increased caregiver workload. However, more absorbent pads will not necessarily reduce pad consumption rates: pads are often changed according to ward or personal routine.

3. Disposable absorbent bedpads

a) Background

The use of disposable bedpads has declined markedly over the last 25 years with the advent of increasingly effective bodyworn products. However, they still find widespread use for occasional light incontinence, or as back up to bodyworn products. They are square or rectangular and contain similar materials to bodyworn disposables.

b) Quality of data

Published trials comparing different disposable bedpads are few [19, 20, 21] and it is not possible to draw firm conclusions from them on the effectiveness of different product design features and materials. Some useful work has been done to highlight the risks of infection from disposable bedpads and to validate clinically some laboratory tests to assist with product selection by predicting pad leakage performance.

c) Results

Bedpads are generally supplied as non-sterile items and Bradbury [22] has drawn attention to the risk of infection, particularly from products containing recycled paper. Leigh and Petch [23] and Sprott et al. [24] have conducted microbiological tests on a range of products. Both studies identified low levels of bacterial contamination but concluded that the risk to patients was minimal unless they were immunocompromised in some way. More recently, Stansfield and Caudle [25] reported an outbreak of wound colonization on a surgical orthopaedic hospital ward which they attributed to the use of disposable underpads containing virgin wood pulp.

Due to the paucity of published clinical data many technical tests have been devised to evaluate products in the laboratory. The only tests with published clinical validations are described by Cottenden et al. [26] who subjected six different bedpads to a variety of laboratory tests and to a multi-centre clinical evaluation in which 95 incontinent subjects tested each product in turn for a week, in random order. A combination of two laboratory tests (one to measure the absorption capacity and the other the absorption time of bedpads) gave a strong correlation with the percentage of subjects finding the leakage performance of a product acceptable when used as their sole protection ($r = 0.94$) and predicted the acceptability scores of all six products accurate to within $\pm$ eight percentage points. A different absorption capacity test produced a strong correlation for the leakage performance of bedpads used as back-up to bodyworn products ($r = 0.96$) and predicted the acceptability scores of all six products to within $\pm$ five percentage points.

d) Summary

No robust data are available on the effectiveness of current disposable bedpads or of their various design features or constituent materials. There is a risk of infection from bedpads made from recycled paper for immunocompromised users (Level of evidence 2c). The leakage performance of bedpads (used alone or as back up to bodyworn pads) can be predicted with reasonable precision using clinically-validated laboratory tests (Level of evidence 2c).

e) Recommendations

- Immunocompromised people should not use bedpads made from recycled paper because of the risk of infection (Grade B). Where possible, clinically-validated laboratory tests [26] should be used to rank the likely leakage performance of different products (Grade B).

4. Reusable absorbent bodyworn products

a) Background

Reusable briefs (usually secured using snaps or VelcroTM); inserts and male guards all have geometries similar to their disposable counterparts. In addition, pants with integral pad comprise pants – often of normal exterior appearance – with an absorbent panel sewn into the crotch. Variants exist for light and moderate incontinence. Like disposables, reusable bodyworns usually have three layers: an absorbent core between a water-proof backing below, and a topsheet next to the skin. Topsheets are usually made from either cotton – which is hydrophilic and said to have good dry comfort – or polyester – which is hydrophobic and said to have good wet comfort. Absorbent cores are usually made from a needlefelt or knitted fabric comprising rayon and/or polyester fibres. A variety of polymers are used for the water-proofing. In general, the thicker, stiffer materials are more durable (the durability of the plastic backing often determines the lifetime of the product) but less comfortable.

b) Quality of data

There has been one robust clinical evaluation comparing the performance of different reusable pants with integral pad for lightly incontinent women [27]. No robust clinical evaluations have been published on reusable insert pads for lightly incontinent women; any reusable pad category for lightly incontinent men; or any category of reusable bodyworns for heavily incontinent users of either sex.

c) Results

In the only robust clinical evaluation of reusable absorbent bodyworn products published to date, Pettersson et al. [27] used a multi-centre evaluation to compare the performance of all ten pants with integral pad for lightly incontinent women on the UK market in 1999. Each of 72 subjects was offered each product to test for a week, in random order. The leakage performance of the products was disappointing with few significant differences ($p < 0.05$) between products. Based on plots of probability of leakage against urine weight, the best product leaked 31% and 50% of the time when confronted with 10 g and 20 g of urine, respectively. The greatest differences between products related to their appearance, discretion (invisibility beneath clothing), fit and comfort. Some products performed well in these respects and others poorly. Many significant differences ($p < 0.05$) were found (Level of evidence 2b).

Although there have been no robust evaluations of reusable bodyworn products for heavy incontinence, observational studies indicate that current products are commonly perceived to be unattractive and leaky.

d) Recommendations

- Particular attention should be paid to the appearance, discretion, fit and comfort of different reusable pants with integral pad for lightly incontinent women when choosing between products (Grade B). Reusable products for heavy incontinence should be considered with caution since, on balance, the literature suggests that they will not usually be as effective as disposables (Grade D).

5. Reusable absorbent bedpads

a) Background

Most reusable absorbent bedpads comprise three rectangular layers of material sewn together at the edges: a water-proof backing; an absorbent core; and a topsheet which goes next to the skin.

The choices of material for the three layers are similar to those for bodyworn products. Some designs have a high-friction plastic backing or tuck in flaps at the sides to impede them from slipping out of place. Sometimes the water-proof backing comes as a separate sheet.

b) Quality of data

There have been very few well-designed comparative evaluations of different reusable bedpads. One robust study addresses the risks of cross-infection between different users of bedpds.

c) Results

Cottenden [28] has reviewed comparative evaluations of different reusable bedpads up to about 1990. Leiby and Shanahan [29] have since published a study. Some evaluations have found significant differences between products relating, for example, to leakage performance and impact on skin health but none of the products evaluated is still available in the variant tested. In addition, compared products always differed from one another in many respects making it impossible to draw reliable generic conclusions relating to the products now available. However, the choice of topsheet material and the presence or absence of features like tuck-in flaps and integral water-proofing appear to be, primarily, matters of personal preference.

In institutional settings reusable bedpads are commonly used by multiple patients and questions are often asked about the risk of cross-infection. Cottenden et al. [30] assessed the risk by determining the microbial content of 145 bedpads of five different designs after a night's use by incontinent adults, followed by laundering using a standard foul wash procedure which included heat disinfection at 71oC for three minutes. Laundering destroyed all known pathogenic organisms, although some commensal flora were isolated in small numbers. It was concluded that foul wash laundry had left bedpads safe for multiple patient reuse with no demonstrable risk of cross-infection.

d) Summary

The literature contains insufficient robust data on which to base guidelines for choosing between reusable bedpads. Choice of topsheet material and the presence/absence of design features like tuck-in flaps and integral/separate water-proof backing appear to be, primarily, matters of personal preference (Level of evidence 4). Provided an approved foul wash procedure is used, the risk of cross-infection between different users of a bedpads is very low (Level of evidence 2c).

e) Recommendations

- Personal preferences of users with regard to topsheet material, tuck-in flaps and integral waterproofing should be considered in making product selections (Grade D). Provided an adequate foul laundry wash cycle is used, the risk of cross-infection between successive users of reusable bedpads is low and not a contra-indication for their use (Grade B).

6. Reusable versus disposable products

a) Background

The relative merits of disposable and reusable absorbent products have been debated for many years, focusing on a variety of issues. Currently in the western world, escalating bills for disposable bodyworn pads associated with the growing incontinent population have fueled a search for cost-saving strategies and so claims that reusable products can be cheaper have fallen on receptive ears. Reusability has acquired an image of environmental respectability and disposables usually suffer adverse press coverage when environmental issues come to the fore, as they did in the early 1990s. A valid environmental audit of either category of product should take a "cradle to grave" approach so that the energy, materials and environmental costs of manufacture, reuse (washing and drying) and disposal are taken into account. It has yet to be established in independent studies that either category is superior to the other on this basis. Currently, there is great demand for evidence that reusables can save money relative to disposables without compromising quality of care.

b) Quality of data

The quality of studies comparing disposable and reusable absorbent products is generally poor. Many studies have involved comparing a crude reusable product in established use with a modern disposable product, or *vice versa*. Furthermore, authors have sometimes made ill-justified generalisations from their results on a particular disposable and a particular reusable to all reusables and all disposables.

c) Results

Cottenden [28] has reviewed comparative evaluations of reusable and disposable absorbent products up to about 1990 since when studies have been published by McKibben [31], Gallo and Staskin [32], Brown [21, 33], Gibb and Wong [34] and Harper et al. [35]. These evaluations provide examples of cost-savings and performance improvements that have accompanied a change from a disposable product to a reusable or *vice versa*.

d) Summary

The literature provides no basis for declaring reusables superior to disposables or *vice versa*. It is clear that there are more and less effective products in each category and that local needs, priorities, motivations, laundry facilities and cost structures can be as important as product performance in determining the optimal solution in a given situation (Level of evidence 2c). The key issues are summarized below.

e) Recommendations

- ***Laundry issues:*** Access to good, reliable washing and drying facilities should be checked before reusable products are introduced (Grade B). Laundry – especially of bedpads – can be heavy work, beyond the capability of frail incontinent people or their caregivers. The number of reusable products needed per user depends on laundry turn-around times. Drying times for reusables can be long and expensive, especially for bodyworns for heavy incontinence and for bedpads.
- ***Personal preferences:*** Personal preferences (of both users and caregivers) with regard to choosing between reusable and disposable products should be taken into account carefully (Grade C). Some users prefer the chore of laundering reusables to anxiety over whether their next consignment of disposables will be delivered on time. Reusables generally require less storage space than disposables. Discreet disposal of disposables can be a challenge. The possibility of using a mix of disposable and reusable products should be considered (Grade C). Some users who choose disposables when at home prefer reusables when traveling because of the space that disposables occupy in luggage and the possible inconvenience of disposal. Others use reusables at home and disposables when away as they see the balance of disadvantages and advantages differently.
- ***Personalisation of products:*** In institutions, the chore of personalizing reusable products and sorting them after each laundry cycle should be considered before they are introduced (Grade D). Reusable bedpads are often personalised to particular users. In institutions this means marking products with users' names and sorting them after laundry, an extra task for caregivers. Reusable bedpads are not usually personalised.
- ***Staining:*** Reusable products should not usually be used by those with faecal incontinence – beyond occasional light smearing – because of staining (Grade C). Skin sprays and ointments may stain reusables too.
- ***Costs:*** Cost comparisons between reusable and disposable products should be made with caution (Grade C). Key factors are: local arrangements (mostly laundry and transport costs); the durability of the products (which depends on how carefully they are used and the criteria for deciding when they should be replaced); the costs of ordering, transporting and disposing of disposables; and product purchase costs. Much of the cost of reusables is encountered with the initial capital outlay for stock. This also represents a commitment to use the products for an extended period and so expensive mistakes can be made if it transpires that a better product was/has become available. It will usually be wise to experiment with samples of a variety of alternative products before committing to major purchases.
- Every effort should be made to get manufacturers to test new products against standardised local or universal standards.

5. Research priorities for Absorbent products

- Absorbent products which leak less, are more comfortable, less bulky and less damaging to the skin need to be developed, across all product categories
- The relative performances of disposable and reusable absorbent products (especially for heavy incontinence) need to be established to identify the strengths and limitations of different product subcategories for different user groups.
- The strengths and limitations of the different major sub-groups of disposable products for heavy incontinence (especially, briefs, inserts and pull-ups) need to be established for different user groups

- Given that manufacturers modify their absorbent products frequently, product evaluations should be designed so that data can be analysed to yield ***generic*** conclusions relating to the efficacy of specific product features and materials, rather than just determining the efficacy of the products tested. Such conclusions will outlive the (short-lived) products on which they are based.
- Predictive models which relate the clinical performance of pads (especially their ability to absorb urine without leaking) to their design and the properties of their constituent materials should be developed to facilitate the systematic development of improved designs.
- The impact of absorbent products on diaper-area skin needs to be studied to establish the mechanisms of skin damage and to identify/develop materials which minimise skin damage.

6. Catheters in older patients

a) Background

A full review of catheters – indwelling urethral, suprapubic, and intermittent – can be found in the chapter on the neurogenic bladder (Chapter 10 e). Discussion here focuses on catheter use by older patients.

Indwelling catheters are devices for carrying urine from the bladder to outside the body.

Bladder drainage in frail older persons with difficulty emptying their bladder may be unavoidable when there is complete failure of bladder emptying, the underlying cause is not treatable, surgical treatment is not wanted by the patient, or there is patient preference for catheterization. Table 10 lists the guidelines for long-term indwelling catheter use suggested by the Agency for Health Care Policy and Research of the U.S. Department of Health and Human Services [36].

Table 10 : AHCPR Guidelines for Long-Term Indwelling Catheter Use

1. For patients whose incontinence is caused by obstruction and no other intervention is feasible
2. For terminally ill, incontinent patients
3. Short term treatment for patients with pressure ulcers
4. For severely impaired individuals in whom alternative interventions are not an option
5. For patients who live alone and do not have a caregiver to provide other supportive measures

Morbidity associated with long term bladder catheterization has been evaluated in several prospective and retrospective studies and is well documented in several review articles [37-42]. Complications include: polymicrobial bacteriuria (universal by 30 days), febrile episodes (1 per 100 patient days), nephrolithiasis, bladder stones, epididymitis, and chronic renal inflammation and pyelonephritis (present, respectively, in 43% and 10% of patients catheterized over 90 days). Long-term catheterization morbidity is mainly related to symptomatic urinary tract infections, mechanical trauma to the urethra, catheter blockage, stone formation, bypass of urine around the catheter, and haematuria.

b) Quality of data

There are few randomised trials of long term transurethral catheterization in frail older persons [43, 44]. Existing data is predominantly expert opinion and reviews [45, 46] and case series or cohort studies [47-55].

c) Results

• *Choice of catheter*

In aged nursing home patients the indwelling catheter was the most commonly used device [53]. In women where few other options were available 93% were using urethral catheters, most men with devices were using urethral catheters (43%), condoms (39%), or suprapubic catheters (15%). The role of institutional factors in the choice of method for urine collection needs further investigation [53].

Especially in men, a suprapubic catheter is preferable to avoid urethritis, orchidoepidydimitis and prostatitis. However, there are no good studies in the literature comparing the complications of suprapubic versus urethral catheterization.in frail elderly people. Most studies look at suprapubic catheterization after surgical repair [56, 57] or in acute urinary retention [58]. Only one author compares suprapubic catheters with transurethral catheterization in aged nursing home patients [58]. In a prospectively conducted RCT with 25 patients with a transurethral catheter and 25 patients with a suprapubical catheter, the difference in pain and discomfort did not achieve statistical significance [44]. The authors - Vandoni et al. - concluded that suprapubic catheterization is preferable to the alternative using the urethral route in terms of improving urine sterility. Similar to Vandoni's findings, Horgan et al [58] found that the use of suprapubic catheters for acute urinary retention in men significantly reduced the risk of urinary tract infection and urethral stricture formation. A further advantage of the suprapubic catheter - especially when placed after acute retention - is that a voiding trial can be performed without removal of the catheter. The only complication that was repeatedly associated with suprapubic catheter was dislodgement (23%) [58]. None of the authors reported complications placing the suprapubic catheter such as misplacement and bleeding. There are no data concerning the possible advantages of suprapubic catherization in older women.

There have been no well-designed comparisons between intermittent catheterization and long-term indwelling catheterization in frail elderly. Retrospective analyses have shown that clean intermittent catheterization is seldom used in aged patients [53, 59]. Clean intermittent catheterization can still be an alternative for willing patients with sufficient dexterity. Strict sterility is not necessary, although good hand washing and regular decontamination of the catheters is needed. Bacteriuria can be minimized by a frequency of catheterization that keeps bladder volume <400 ml. Stiffer catheters are more acceptable because of easier insertion.

There appear to be no studies on frail elderly people which compare the quality of life achieved using indwelling transurethral catheters, suprapubic catheters and condoms.

• *Complications:*

Once a urethral catheter is inserted, even with the best of care, bacteriuria occurs at an incidence of 3% to 10% per day [39, 60]. In a prospective study of elderly patients in a nursing home Kunin et al. [50] found that although 74% of catheterized patients developed bacteremia, fewer than 2% had temperatures higher than 38°C. Ouslander et al. [51] found that none of the clinical factors they prospectively examined - including age, nutritional status, stool incontinence, diabetes mellitus, episodes of catheter blockage and the use of chronic suppressant antimicrobial therapy - were associated with the development of symptomatic infection. Zimakoff et al [52] looked at staff awareness of written guidelines for various aspects of catheter care. They found that only 25-68% of staff in hospitals, 27-45% in nursing homes and 7-17% in home care were aware of existing guidelines.

d) Summary

Long-term urethral catheterization has been well studied and is associated with universal bacteruria and with a number of complications like mechanical trauma to the urethra, catheter blockage, stone formation, bypass of urine around the catheter and haematuria. Several guidelines and reviews have been written with the aim of reducing catheter-associated complications [36, 37, 61, 62].

Although most studies have collected data from a very heterogeneous group of patients - including basically all patients with long-term use of indwelling catheters - these findings can still help in the care of frail elderly people. In frail elderly people the main goal may not be cure of a disease but improving quality of life of the individual.

Avoiding long term catheterization reduces the incidence of infection and other complications in frail elderly people. If, however, they are considered the best option for an individual, they should be placed cautiously and looked after diligently. (Level of evidence 1a)

The advantages of suprapubic catheters after surgery or when there is acute retention are well documented and it is known that suprapubical catheterization reduces epidydimitis and urethral strictures in men (Level of evidence 2b). Data on the benefit of suprapubic catheters for frail elderly people are sparse.

Intermittent self catheterization has a limited application with frail elderly people who often lack the necessary dexterity. But it should be considered in selected motivated patients who have chronic urinary retention or elevated post-void residual urine.

e) Recommendations

- Several general principles have been identified to enable safe and effective catheter care and these are described in the chapter on the neurogenic bladder (Chapter 10d). As with all catheter patients, bacteriuria is universal in elderly catheterized patients and it should not be treated unless there are clear symptomatic episodes (with fever, anorexia, or delirium), or if bacteriuria persists after catheter removal (Grade A).
- Data for suprapubic catheterization for frail elderly are sparse. After surgery or if there is acute retention the suprapubic route helps to decrease urethral injuries and infection, especially in men (Grade B).
- Clean intermittent catheterization is suitable for very few frail elderly patients and no recommendations can be given so far.

f) Research priorities

- Guidelines need to be established for helping caregivers find the best device for the individual. They should not only cover the medical status of the patient but also the patient's and the caregiver's perspectives. The quality of life of both the patient and the caregiver need to be covered, as well as economic issues.

7. Catheter valves

Catheters are usually connected to a drainage bag but they may also be used with a catheter valve which enables urine to be stored in the bladder until emptied. In the only robust comparative evaluation to date of different catheter valves Fader et al. [63] evaluated the seven different catheter valves on the UK market in 1996 using a two-part study. First, they ran a multicentre clinical evaluation in which each of 46 cognitively unimpaired, manually dexterous users of indwelling catheters (29 urethral, 17 suprapubic; 7 women, 39 men; age range 24-85y; mean age 65y) was invited to try each catheter valve for a week in turn. Second, they ran a single-centre ergonomic study of the same valves tested by 33 people with impaired manual dexterity (17 men, 16 women; age range 24-101y; mean age 70y; mostly catheter users). Substantial differences were found between valves and it was concluded that, to be successful, a valve needs to be easy to manipulate, leak-free, comfortable, and inconspicuous beneath clothing (Level of evidence 2c).

a) Recommendations

- In choosing between catheter valves, ease of manipulation, freedom from leakage, comfort and discretion beneath clothing should receive particular attention (Grade B). Compromises may need to be made, especially between ease of manipulation (which favours larger valves) and discretion (which favours smaller ones). The visual acuity and manual dexterity of the user and whether (s)he has the use of one or both hands will be vital considerations (Grade D).

b) Research priorities

The major challenge is to develop catheter valves which are easy to manipulate and leak-free while being discreet and reasonably priced.

8. Bodyworn urine collection devices

a) Background

Close-fitting penile sheaths (sometimes called condoms or external catheters) are the most commonly used male incontinence devices, and they may be considered provided a man has no trouble emptying his bladder, leaving little or no post void residual [47]. They are often unsuitable for elderly men, however, due to inadequate penile length and/or diameter for secure condom attachment.

Early products were made from latex and relied on friction between sheath and skin to stay in place, sometimes aided by an elastic strip or tape applied to the outside of the sheath. Almost all modern products use a skin adhesive which may be applied to the penis as a separate strip onto which the sheath is unrolled. Increasingly, however, the adhesive is integral to the inside of the sheath. Many sheaths continue to be made from latex but some are now made from silicone rubber to avoid possible problems with latex allergy. Some sheaths are supplied with an applicator intended to make them easier to apply and to reduce direct patient contact if they are applied by a caregiver.

b) Quality of data

There have been no major systematic studies of sheath use but the problems encountered by a number of patient series have been reported. Some data are available from comparative evaluations of different sheaths but there are no data relating to bulkier products like pubic pressure urinals, and very few on female collection devices.

c) Results

Although many men use sheaths successfully, problems have been reported in the literature. Saint et al. [55] showed that both patients and nursing staff prefer condoms to indwelling catheters for patient comfort, but recognised that dislodgment and leaking are major drawbacks of condoms. In a study on (an unspecified number of) spinal cord injured men, Golji [64] found that 15% experienced side effects or complications when using sheaths. These were irritative, allergic or compressive in nature. Jayachadran et al. [54] reported similar experiences with six incontinent men of widely varying aetiology and highlighted the importance of ensuring that the sheath does not become twisted near the distal end to avoid stagnation of urine and the risk of UTI. They also stressed the importance of good genital hygiene to avoid problems with infections. In a study of 94 men on medical/ surgical wards, Hirsh et al. [65] found that none of the 79 who were judged as co-operative and able to manage their sheaths properly developed UTI (mean period of use, 21.2 days). By contrast, eight of 15 patients who tended to tug and kink the drainage tube attached to their sheath developed UTI within a mean of 9.6 days. In a retrospective study, Johnson compared the frequency of UTI in users (mean period of use, 35 months) and non-users of sheaths amongst 64 elderly men on an extended care unit. He found that 63% of users but only 14% of non-users developed UTI. No difference was found between men who did and did not tug and kink their tubing. Ouslander et al. [47] reported that 40% of 30 nursing home sheath users (mean period of use, 35.9 months) developed at least one UTI.

Few comparative evaluations of different sheaths involving reasonable numbers of subjects are available. In a multi-centre study involving 35 men (age range 22-87y; mean age, 54y; 34 living in their own homes), the UK Medical Devices Agency [66] compared four latex sheaths: two with integral adhesive; and two in which the adhesive was supplied as a separate strip. They found the products with integral adhesive to be more successful in both overall performance and ease of application. Fader et al. [67] conducted al. a multi-centre study to compare all six sheaths with integral adhesive on the UK market in 1998. Five were made from latex, one from silicone rubber. Four were supplied with an applicator, two without. Fifty-eight men (age range 26-88y; mean age 53y) were given the opportunity to try each sheath in turn for one week. The silicone rubber sheath was found to be significantly better than four of the other sheaths in overall performance ($p<0.01$). The ease with which a sheath could be put on was found to be the best predictor of overall performance. Surprisingly, a significantly higher proportion of subjects found sheaths with an applicator to be unacceptable than those without ($p<0.0001$). Subjects found that the silicone sheath fell off/blew off significantly less frequently than two of the other products ($p<0.01$).

There are no published evaluations of the bulkier male bodyworn urine collection appliances (such as pubic pressure urinals) which rely on belts and straps to stay in place.

Pieper [68] has reviewed the many attempts to design bodyworn urine collection devices for women. None has found widespread success. The major challenge is in achieving a comfortable and aesthetically acceptable leak-proof seal with the body. The few devices for women that have been tested tend to leak frequently and are not recommended in frail elderly [68, 69].

d) Summary

For male non-obstructed patients the use of condom drainage can present a good alternative, but especially in frail elderly one should be aware of an increased risk for complications such as local skin breakdown, bacteriuria and infection. Also, there is the risk of urinary retention if the condom twists or the external band is too tight, leading to poor drainage to the urine bag (Level of evidence 2b). Sheaths with integral adhesive are more popular with users and easier to apply than those with separate adhesive strip (Level of evidence 4). The ease with which a sheath can be put on is the best indicator of its overall performance (Level of evidence 2b). Sheath applicators are often ineffective and unpopular (Level of evidence 2b).

e) Recommendations

- Condom drainage can be a suitable alternative for some elderly men who can empty their bladder sufficiently. It is viewed as comfortable by nurses and patients but dislodgment and leaking as well as some major potential complications limit their use in frail elderly (Grade of recommendation C).
- In general, sheaths with integral adhesive should be selected rather than those in which the adhesive is supplied separately (Grade C). Since the ease with which a sheath can be put on is the major predictor of the overall performance of a sheath, users should experiment with applying a range of products before making choices (Grade B). It should not be assumed that a sheath applicator makes sheath application easier: often it does not (Grade B).

f) Research priorities

- The need remains for condoms which are better than existing products in terms of ease of application, retaining a leak-free seal, protecting penile skin from damage and resisting twisting and kinking.

9. Urine drainage bags

a) Background

Urine drainage bags are used in conjunction with sheaths and indwelling catheters. Those for daytime use generally have a capacity of 350-750 ml and are secured to the wearer by means of straps or a "holster" suspended from the waist. Most have a drainage tap; those without are intended to be discarded once full. Some bags have urine sampling ports. Higher capacity bags (typically 2000 ml) are available for night time use. They may be connected directly to the sheath or catheter or to the (open) drainage tap of the day bag if repeated connection/disconnection between day bag and sheath/catheter is to be avoided, with its presumed increased risk of introducing infection. Floor stands to support night drainage bags are available. Most but not all bags are supplied sterile.

b) Quality of data

Several controlled comparative evaluations of urine drainage bags have been performed from which the key issues to be considered in choosing between different products can be identified.

c) Results

Kennedy et al. [70] tested the performance of ten different drainage bags in a simulation study involving 40 subjects (mostly health-care staff) which focused particularly on taps. Significant differences ($p<0.05$) were found between many pairs of bags with regard to each of the performance aspects studied: ease of tap opening and closing, ability to empty the bag without urine wetting fingers; and how easy the tap mechanism was to understand. Taps comprising caps or bungs were found to be particularly fiddly and messy to use.

In a study which focused primarily on the cross-infection risks associated with leg bags, Wilson and Coates [71] evaluated four leg bags. Each of ten long-term catheterised patients was invited to try each bag for a week in turn. The authors concluded that no one bag suited every patient; rather, each was liked by some. The popularity (or otherwise) of many features was a matter of personal preference. Adverse comments mostly related to the tap (difficult to operate; opened accidentally, causing leakage) and the straps.

The UK Medical Devices Agency [72] evaluated all 14 sterile 500 ml leg bags on the UK market in 1995 in a multi-centre study involving 83 test subjects (58 men, 25 women). About half (44) lived in their own homes and almost all the rest in nursing/residential homes. Subjects were divided into pairs matched for sex, mobility, manual dexterity and dependency and each pair was offered each of the 14 bags (seven each) to try for a week in turn. Preferences varied but the main concerns of users consistently focused on taps (many subjects found many taps difficult to operate), straps (discomfort was common) and the minimisation of leakage (through faults in bags and/or connectors; onto the fingers when emptying; or by the tap accidentally opening in use). The most popular bags tended to perform well in these three respects.

In a multi-centre study involving 34 men (age range 27-84y; mean age 55; all sheath users) Fader et al. [73] evaluated all seven non-sterile 500-700 ml leg bags on the UK market in 1997. Twenty five lived in their own homes and the rest in residential/nursing homes or long stay wards. Conclusions were substantially similar to those for the earlier MDA study.

The cross-infection risks of leg bags (particularly via the tap or sampling port) have been studied by Glenister [74] and by Wilson and Coates [71] Cross-infection is an important concern in hospitals and residential settings, particularly where indwelling catheters are in use. In community settings where patients manage their own leg bag the risks are considerably reduced. In her study Glenister [74] concluded that designs in which the tap and outlet spouts were most widely separated were most effective at preventing contamination of the hands with urine. Wilson and Coates [71] studied sampling ports and contamination of leg bag spouts. They suggested that the night connector tubing attached to the taps on the four leg bags in their study made decontamination difficult.

d) Summary

Taken together, published studies agree that the main factors to consider in selecting legbags are the ease of tap operation, the comfort of the straps and the minimisation of leakage (Level of evidence 2b). Bags in which the tap and outlet spout are widely separated are most likely to be effective at preventing contamination of the hands with urine and cross-infection (Level of evidence 4).

e) Recommendations

- In making legbag selections particular attention should be focused the ability of the user to operate the tap, the comfort of the straps and freedom from leakage, especially from and around the tap (Grade B).

f) Research priorities

- Improved urine drainage bags are needed which incorporate better taps (easy to operate, leak-free and discrete) and more comfortable straps (or other mode of support).

10. Occlusive and constrictive devices

Occlusive and constrictive devices are intended to prevent leakage from the bladder. They are not in widespread use and relatively few variants are available. Female devices are discussed in Chapter 10c «Conservative Treatment in Women».

The most common device for men in this category is the Cunningham clamp. It comprises an adjustable clamp lined with cushioning foam and, if adequate force is exerted, urinary incontinence is prevented by occluding the distal part of the urethra. It has the advantages of low cost and simplicity but wearing it for too long or applying too high a force can lead to skin necrosis, urethral erosion or peri-urethral abscess. Accordingly, it is vital that users have good sensation, manual dexterity and mental acuity (especially memory). In the case of detrusor overactivity upper urinary tract deterioration may occur.

Recommendations

- Penile clamps should not be considered unless alternative forms of management – especially, absorbent pads, sheaths or indwelling catheters – have failed or been judged inappropriate (Grade D)

11. Handheld urinals

Hand held urinals are designed to enable people to empty their bladders while not on the toilet and are therefore potentially useful in preventing incontinence. Most products for men are somewhat similar, involving a narrowed neck opening into which the penis is placed. Some products come with a detachable non-spill adaptor containing a flutter valve to impede back-flow of urine from the urinal. There are no published trials comparing different products.

A much greater diversity of products have been designed to meet the more challenging demands of the female anatomy. In the most comprehensive evaluation to date Fader et al. [75] ran a multi-centre study in which each of 37 community based women (age range 33-89y; mean age 61y) was invited to evaluate all 13 products on the UK market in 1997. No product suited everybody but each was successful for at least some subjects. The key requirements for success were that the user should be able to position the urinal easily and feel confident that it would catch her urine without spilling (Level of evidence 2c). Many products were successful when used in the standing/crouching position or when sitting on the edge of a chair/bed/wheelchair. Fewer worked well for users sitting in a chair/wheelchair. Only one worked even reasonably well when users were lying/semi-lying. In general, subjects with higher levels of dependency found fewer urinals to be suitable for their needs.

a) Recommendations

- Since the ability of female users to position a urinal depends on many factors – especially the postures they can adopt, their ability to abduct their hips, and their manual dexterity, as well as the geometry of the urinal – users should experiment with a range of products before making a selection (Grade B).

b) Research priorities

- Female handheld urinals which are effective for supine users and those unable to move to the edge of a chair should be developed.

12. General research priorities across all categories of FADS and appliances

- Since evaluation data on specific products invariably goes out of date quickly, studies should be designed so that, where ever possible, they yield generic conclusions on product categories, design features and materials which will apply to future products.
- Strategies/algorithms/guidelines which help product selectors to make the best informed choices possible given incomplete information should be developed.
- Tools should be developed for comparing the impact on quality of life (for users and caregivers) of using different products, and for measuring their cost-effectiveness, in order to help with product selection.
- More effective methods for dealing with incontinence-related odour should be developed.
- Products for the more effective containment of faeces should be developed.

XVI. PREVENTION OF INCONTINENCE

1. Background

Prevention strategies for urinary incontinence take the form of primary, secondary and tertiary strategies [1]. Prevention of urinary incontinence is receiving more attention from healthcare providers and policy makers due to its prevalence, economic costs, and impact on quality of life of affected older people and their caregivers [2-4].

Primary prevention strategies are focused towards continent individuals. Their primary purpose is to prevent urinary incontinence from occurring. Therefore identification of continent individuals who have the potential for becoming incontinent is an important primary prevention activity. Secondary prevention strategies are designed for incontinent people. Their prime objective is to improve or reverse incontinence. Finally, tertiary prevention interventions are designed to prevent complications and preserve the quality of life of the incontinent individual. With tertiary strategies the individual exhibits no rehabilitative potential of urinary elimination function [5].

No randomized clinical trials were located with primary prevention of urinary incontinence as an outcome. Few longitudinal studies within the past decade (1990-2001) investigating changes in continence status in older adults were located. Urinary continence appears to be a dynamic state [6], therefore longitudinal studies to investigate not only the incidence but the remission of urinary incontinence are needed in diverse populations and in a variety of settings, i.e. community, acute-care, long-term care, and outpatient.

There has been, however, research that addresses risk factors for urinary incontinence in the older population, see Table 11. Risk factors that lead to transient incontinence are addressed earlier in this chapter. Secondary prevention strategies include most of the interventions covered in this chapter including behavioral, pharmacological, and surgical interventions that aim to improve or reverse incontinence. Tertiary strategies such as devices and equipment are also addressed elsewhere in this chapter.

To date, no evidence exists that primary prevention strategies work, or do not work, in older populations. Using the information gleaned from epidemiological research on risk factors, longitudinal studies with groups known to be at risk for developing incontinence are needed. Widespread screening programs are also needed. Older people seldom report incontinence, especially those less bothered by incontinence than others, to their health care providers [7-9].

Using multi-media technology may help older people gain access to necessary information to improve and maintain bladder health. This type of intervention has proven effective in older people with urinary incontinence in changing both level of knowledge and behavior [10].

Efforts should continue in the identification of risk factors of urinary incontinence in culturally diverse groups. Johnson and his colleagues [11] found that the relationship between urinary incontinence and self-reported health differed between white and non-white subjects, suggesting that groups may use different frames of reference in rating health.

Longitudinal studies investigating the effectiveness of interventions designed to prevent urinary incontinence need to be undertaken. Education of health care providers must continue as evidence exists that physicians often do not screen older people for urinary incontinence [7].

2. Risk factor – Mobility impairment

a) Background

Mobility impairment and functional dependence has long been associated with urinary incontinence [3,12].

b) Quality of data

Few prospective longitudinal studies investigating the incidence of and risk factors for urinary incontinence in frail older adults were located. The continence status of 434 nursing home residents over their first year of admission was studied. Data were collected from staff members at 2 weeks, 2 months and one year after admission1 [13]. A large cross-sectional prospective study (N=7949) investigating osteoportic fractures in women from 69-101 years also collected information about their continence status [14]. Because of the large sample size the investigators were able to control for potential confounders.

Other cross-sectional studies show increase risk of urinary incontinence in the presence of functional dependence in community-dwelling older persons , N=927 [15] and limitations of activities of daily living of nursing home residents, N= 2014 [16] and community-dwelling older persons, N=3,809 [17].

c) Results

Mobility impairment at 2 months after nursing home placement increased the cumulative risk of being incontinent at one year post admission to 117% [13]. Community dwelling women with a faster gait speed were at decreased risk of incontinence OR 0.8 per 0.2 units, 95%CI 0.6-1.0) [14] (Brown et al). In older persons with sensory, affective, upper extremity and lower extremity impairments, the relative risk for urinary incontinence was 4.2 [15]. Activity of daily living impairment in nursing home residents was strongly correlated with urinary incontinence $p < 0.001$ [16]. Community-dwelling older men reported more difficulty in controlling urination than women with the same degree of functional impairment, but overall, more women reported functional impairment [17].

d) Summary

There is strong evidence that impaired mobility, functional dependence and limitations in activities of daily living increase risk for urinary incontinence for institutionalized and community-dwelling older adults, Level 2.

e) Recommendations

- Mobility impairments, functional dependence and limitations of activities of daily living should be considered significant risk factors for urinary incontinence, (Grade B).

f) Research priorities

- Research is needed to determine if : Interventions that improve or restore mobility and functional ability will decrease incidence of urinary incontinence.

2. Risk factor – Dementia

a) Background

Dementia, a highly prevalent condition in the frail older population, is associated with increased prevalence of urinary incontinence [18,19] and is discussed elsewhere in this chapter.

b) Quality of data

Some of the previously identified studies also investigated dementia or cognitive impairment as a risk factor for urinary incontinence. A prospective study with 100 hospitalized older adults being surgically treated for hip fracture repair was also located [20]. In an intervention study, older adults and their caregiver at home were randomly assigned to a program of individualized scheduled toileting (N=118 dyads) [21].

c) Results

Dementia increased risk of urinary incontinence in nursing home residents, cumulative risk 122% [13]. It was also found that urinary incontinence was independently associated with dementia in this same population, OR 2.3 95%CI 1.8-3.0) [16]. Dementia was found to be an independent risk factor for both men and women hip fracture patients. The risk of incontinence was similar between men (45%) and women (55%), $p > 0.05$ [20]. Cognitive ability was the best predictor of success in an

Table 11: Summary of risk factors prevention research

FIRST AUTHOR	Year	Design	Sample	Findings
Palmer[13]	1991	Longitudinal descriptive study measures taken at 2 weeks, 2 months, and 1-year post admission.	434 men and women over 64 years were enrolled; 196 remained in the nursing homes remained at one year.	Prevalence of UI increased from 37% at 2-weeks to 43.8% at 1-year. Incidence at 1 year 27%. Risk factors included male gender, Incontinence at 2 weeks, poor behavioral adjustment to nursing homes, impaired mobility at 2 months and impaired cognition at 2 months.
Wetle[17]	1995	Population survey of all residents aged 65 years and over in East Boston in 1982.	3809 (62% women), 28% had difficulty holding urine at least some of the time and 8% had difficulty most or all the time.	Difficulty holding urine was associated with depression, stroke, chronic cough, night awakening, fecal incontinence, problems with activities of daily living.
Brown[14]	1996	Cross-sectional study	7949 women aged 65 years and over	Prevalence of UI 41% with 14% reporting daily UI. Risks of daily incontinence increased with increasing age (OR=1.3), prior hysterectomy (OR=1.4), higher body mass index (OR=1.6), history of stroke (OR=1.9), diabetes (OR=1.7), chronic obstructive pulmonary disease (OR=1.4), poor overall health (OR=1.6).
Nygaard[6]	1996	Longitudinal cohort study	2025 women aged 65 years and over.	Baseline prevalence of urge UI 36.3% and stress UI 40.3%. 3-year incidence (between 3 and 6 years) was 28.6%. Only significant factor related to changed in incontinence status was age (with increased urge UI).
Brandeis[16]	1997	Secondary analyses of dataset constructed by Health Care Financing Administration for nursing home residents' information.	Minimum Data Set information for 2175 residents in 270 nursing homes in 10 states.	49% were incontinent, 84% managed by pads/briefs. UI was independently associated with impairment in ADLs (OR=4.2) dementia (OR=2.3), restraints-trunk (OR=1.7), bedrails (OR=1.3), and use of antianxiety/hypnotic medications (OR=.7).
Nakayama[28]	1997	Urinary incontinence (UI) and fecal incontinence (FI) subscores evaluated during hospitalization and at 6 months.	935 admissions to hospital for stroke over 19 months, average age 74 years with 56% female.	Risk factors for UI and FI were age, severity of stroke, diabetes, and comorbidity of other disabling diseases.
Palmer[20]	1997	Medical record from 2 hospitals were review of hospitalized patients over 55 years reviewed	100 consecutive admissions average age 78 years, majority were women (69%).	Prevalence of UI pre-operatively was 20% and increased to 43% post-operative. Incidence in men was 48% and 24% in women. Risk factors were gender and cognitive impairment. Risk similar for cognitively impaired similar for men and women (60% versus 55%).

Table 11: Summary of risk factors prevention research ((ctd)

FIRST AUTHOR	Year	Design	Sample	Findings
Hunskaar[19]	1998	Population based multi centre survey with stratified random sampling in Canada, sub-sample underwent clinical assessment..	N-8949, institutional sub-sample (n=1255) individuals aged 65 years and over.	16.9% women and 8.0% men reported UI, daily UI 7.0% and 5.2% respectively. UI associated with age, severity of dementia and decreasing ambulatory functioning.
Johnson[11]	1998	Cross-sectional analysis using multivariate logistic regression.	N=3485, community-dwelling subjects from the 1990-1991 National Survey of Self-Care and Aging	UI is independently and positively associated with poor self-rated health after adjusting for age, comorbidity, and frailty.
Koskimaki[24]	1998	Population based mailed questionnaire to men who were 50, 60 or 70 years old.	N=3,143 surveyed, 2,198 responded with 2, 128 included in the analyses.	Age adjusted RR of lower urinary tract (LUTS) symptoms significantly increased in former and current smokers compared to non-smokers. Risk of LUTS decreased in former smokers as years after smoking cessation increased. In current smokers risk of LUTS highest in men who had smoked 20 years or less.
Roberts[4]	1998	Community based cross sectional	2 cohorts, one of men and women (N=778, and N=762) and men (N=2150) living in Olmstead County, MN	Prevalence of UI in cohort I men was 24% and 49% in women and prevalence in cohort II was 17.3%. In cohort I moderate or severe UI was associated with care seeking for urinary symptoms in men and women. Urinary incontinence was associated with reduced quality of life.
Tomlinson[29]	1999	Descriptive study of caffeine consumption and fluid intake of subjects enrolled in the first phase of an interventional study.	N=218 women aged 55 years and over living in their own homes.	Relationship between a decrease in amount of dietary caffeine consumed and fewer daytime UI episodes p=0.0744
Brown[22]	2000	Systematic review of research articles on hysterectomy and urinary incontinence	12 articles met selection criteria	UI increased by 60% for women aged 60 years and older who had hysterectomy

Table 11: Summary of risk factors prevention research ((ctd)

FIRST AUTHOR	Year	Design	Sample	Findings
Dugan[8]	2000	Randomized controlled trial to determine the effects of AHCR Guideline implementation on primary care provider attitudes, beliefs, and beliefs and on geriatric patients UI, health status, quality of life, and satisfaction with care.	668 adults aged 60 years or older who completed endpoint survey and who made at least one visit to their primary care provider. Average age was 72.8 years.	Gender was not a significant predictor of depressive symptoms among incontinent people. Having higher odds of more depressive symptoms was related to UI status, poorer physical health, poorer mental health, and female gender.
Johnson[9]	2000	Cross-sectional analysis of national probability sample	N=787 from 1993-1994 National Follow Up Survey on Self-Care and Aging	Three self-care practices employed most frequently were limiting fluids, limiting trips and using disposable pads. Broken hip, coronary heart disease were independently and positively associated with contacting a physician about UI after adjusting for age, gender, instrumental activities of daily living, basic activities of daily living, and disposable pad usage.
Jirovec[21]	2001	2x2 mixed design analysis of variance to determine effectiveness of individualized scheduled toileting effectiveness Dyads randomly assigned to experimental and control groups.	118 dyads of caregiver and elder living at home were followed to 6 months: 36 men and 82 women elders with 39 men and 79 female caregivers.	Cognitive ability was best predictor of success with moderately impaired incontinent elders benefiting most. Mobility was a meaningful variable with walking speed correctly identifying 72.1% of those whose continence would improve with the intervention.

individualized scheduled toileting program with moderately impaired older adults benefiting the most [21].

d) Summary

Dementia creates risk of urinary incontinence in frail older adults, Level 2.

e) Recommendations

- Dementia should be considered a significant risk factor for urinary incontinence, (Grade B).

f) Research priorities

- Research is needed to determine:
- The efficacy of interventions designed to improve cognitive functioning in reducing the incidence of urinary incontinence in the frail older population
- The underlying mechanism for urinary development due to dementia.

3. Risk factor – Hyesterectomy

a) Background

A systematic review of research articles reporting on the association of history of hysterectomy and urinary incontinence was located [22].

b) Quality of data

Twelve papers (six studies were clinic-based and six were population-based) reporting on eight cross-sectional studies, two prospective cohort studies, and one case-control study were included in the review. Women ages ranged from 23-101 years. The main method urinary incontinence diagnosis was self-report.

c) Results

Summary odds ratio for urinary incontinence in women who had had a hysterectomy over the age of 60 years was increased by 60 percent, level 1B.

d) Summary

Evidence exists that hysterectomy significantly increases the risk of urinary incontinence in older women, grade A.

e) Recommendations

- Hysterectomy should be considered a significant risk factor for urinary incontinence in older women, (Grade A).

f) Research priorities

- Research is needed to determine the nature of the underlying mechanism that leads to the increase risk.

4. Risk factor – Smoking

a) Background

Chronic cough have been associated with urinary incontinence, especially in women [17] but there is conflicting evidence of the association between smoking and urinary incontinence in women [23].

b) Quality of data

A population-based study in Finland was conducted with men born in the years, 1924, 1934, and 1944 (N=3,143) [24]. Men answered questions about urinary symptoms and their history of smoking.

c) Results

Smoking was associated with lower urinary tract symptoms and after controlling for confounders (i.e. body mass index, alcohol consumption, previous prostate surgery, pelvic surgery, prostate cancer and bladder cancer), the increase in relative risks for current and former smokers remained significant. After smoking cessation, risk of lower urinary tract symptoms decreased with time, disappearing after 40 years.

d) Summary

Evidence exists that smoking is a significant risk factor for lower urinary tract symptoms (including urge incontinence) in older men, level 2.

e) Recommendations

- Smoking should be considered a risk factor for lower urinary tract symptoms in older men, (Grade B).

f) Research priorities

- Research should be replicated in other cultures and with older women.

5. Risk factor – Stroke

a) Background

Urinary incontinence has been associated with stroke [25] but study populations have been small [25, 26, 27].

b) Quality of data

Three recent studies with large samples were located. One study studied 935 acute stroke patients admitted to a hospital during a 19-month period [28]. Another study was a large cross-sectional prospective community-based study (N=7949) investigating osteoportic fractures in women from 69-101 years and the third study was a population-based cross-sectional study with 3,809 older adults.

c) Results

Logistic regression revealed the following risk factors

for urinary incontinence: age, stroke lesion diameter, diabetes mellitus, hypertension, other disabling diseases and initial Scandanavian Stroke Scale score. A 10-year increase in age, increased risk 1.7 times, 10mm increase in lesion diameter increased risk 1.2 times, diabetes mellitus increased risk 3.4 times, other disabling diseases increased risk 2.4 times. A 10-point increase in the Scandanavian Stroke Scale score decreased the risk by a third and hypertension descreased the risk by half [28]. For older women in the community, the odds ratio for stroke was 1.9 [95%CI1.3-2.7]. Stroke predicted severe difficulty in controlling urine in women, OR 2.93 but not in men [17].

d) Summary

Stroke is a significant risk factor for urinary incontinence immediately after the stroke in men and women and in the long-term for women, Level 2.

e) Recommendations

- Recent stroke and history of stroke should be considered as a significant risk factor for urinary incontinence in older persons, (Grade B).

6. RISK FACTOR – CAFFEINE

a) Background

Large population-based studies investigating caffeine as a risk for older men and women were not located. Two studies with older female subjects were located.

b) Quality of data

A case-control study of 259 women investigated risk of detrusor instability from dietary caffeine intake [23]. Women completed a voiding diary that contained information about their daily caffeine intake. Women who were randomally assigned to a Behavioral Management for Continence program (N=41) were instructed to reduce their consumption of caffeinated beverages in the first phase of the study [29].

c) Results

Caffeine intake was associated with detrusor instability and women with high caffeine intake had significantly higher odds for detrusor instability than did women with minimal caffeine intake, OR 2.7, 95%CI 1.2-5.8 [23]. The relationship between the decrease in consumption of caffeine and number of daytime involuntary urine loss approached significance p =0.0744 in women enrolled in a Behavioral Management for Continence study [29].

d) Summary

Some evidence exists that there may be a relationship between dietary caffeine consumption and detrusor instability in women, level 3.

e) Recommendations

- Caffeine may play a role in detrusor instability in women. More research is needed to elucidate this relationship, (Grade C).

f) Research priorities

Research is needed to determine :

- If a causal relationship exists between caffeine intake and urinary incontinence in women
- The relationship between caffeine intake and urinary incontinence in men.
- If reduction in caffeine intake reduces the incidence of urinary incontinence in older persons

7. RISK FACTOR - AGE

a) Background

Age is often cited as being associated with urinary incontinence [3,7,11,14] although no causal relation has been found [30].

b) Quality of data

Population based studies reported above also used age as a factor in the analyses of risk factors.

c) Results

In a study with stroke patients [28], age was found to be a risk factor for urinary incontinence. The authors reported for each 10-year increase in age, the incontinence risk increased 1.7 times. Brown and her colleagues [14] found in community based women that age increased the odds of urinary incontinence 1.3 per 5 years 95% CI1.2-1.5. In terms of changes in continence status in women, age was associated with an increased risk of urge incontinence OR 1.11 95%CI 1.019-1.20 3[6]. In a community-based population, Wetle and her colleagues [17] found that age and gender were associated with difficulty in controlling urination and therefore controlled for both variables in subsequent analyses, creating age-gender strata.

They concluded that increasing prevalence of urinary incontinence with increasing age may be due to the increased in prevalence of correlates of aging (such as age-specific changes in the urinary tract) rather than age itself. Age-adjusted prevalence of both urinary and fecal incontinence was reported in a community-based population study [31] with men having greater age-related effects, that is they had a higher prevalence of combined urine and faecal incontinence compared to women. In another study, age was not an important confounder of urinary incontinence and sef-rated health [11].

d) Summary

Age plays a role, yet elucidated, in the development of urinary incontinence, level 2.

e) Recommendations

- Age should be further explored in risk factor research, (Grade B).

f) Research priorities

- Longitudinal studies investigating changes in continence status are needed to explore the relation of age in the development or remission of urinary incontinence.

g) Conclusion

Whilst causal relationships exist for incontinence in frail and older patients, the efficacy of primary and secondary preventive interventions is lacking. Notwithstanding, it is recommended that clinicians use the information known about risk factors and associations by incorporating strategies into their care plans.

XVII. GENERAL RECOMMENDATIONS

1. Screening for incontinence especially in older and frail patients is important because its prevalence is high, its recognition is low, its consequences are great, it is frequently inappropriately or under investigated, and the probability of successful management is high.
2. Although there are age related changes to the LUT, incontinence is not an inevitable consequence of ageing. It is important to identify other non-lower urinary tract conditions that may be partly or fully reversible that can exacerbate or precipitate incontinence such as impaired cognition, mobility, dexterity, environment, concomitant factors (eg, immobility, heart failure, medications)and motivation.
3. Older people can be either fit, disabled or frail. With appropriate attention to their various co-morbid conditions they may become more independent or less frail. Awareness of this can lead to more successful outcome.
4. Health care providers should be able to initiate evaluation and treatment of UI basing their judgement on the results of history, physical examination, post-voiding residual and urinalysis (Grade of Recommendation B for women, D for men).
5. The baseline assessment for incontinence in frail and disabled older people should also include assessment of cognition, neurological and physical state, activities of daily living (ADL), and social and environmental factors (Grade of Recommendation D).
6. The extent of investigation and management in frail and/or disabled older people should take into account :

- degree of bother to the patient and / or their carer.
- patient motivation and level of co-operation
- patient/caregiver preferences
- patient's comorbidities, prognosis and life expectancy
- if more definitive procedures would lead to a change in management.

7. The needs for urodynamic, endoscopic and imaging tests should be considered when treatment based on a clinical diagnosis might be harmful if the patient is misdiagnosed, empiric therapy has failed and further treatments need to be tried, or if surgery is being considered (Grade of Recommendation D).
8. The management options for fit older people are similar to younger adults. However, in choosing these, special considerations must be given to the potential vulnerability of older people to drug and surgical interventions.
9. Nocturia and nocturnal enuresis is a major source of disability with multiple etiologies not usually limited to the bladder – hence its evaluation should involve identification of non LUT factors . Adjustment of fluids and diuretics may assist (Grade of Recommendation C) whilst cautious use of DDAVP in highly selected older patients may reduce nocturia (Grade of Recommendation B).
10. If PVR is small, treatment for either urge or stress UI can be safely initiated without invasive investigation, using conservative/ behavioral therapies +/- medications.
11. All conservative management options used in younger adults can be used in selected frail, older, motivated people. This includes :

- bladder retraining (grade of recommendation B)
- pelvic muscle exercises including biofeedback and /or electro-stimulation (grade of recommendation B)

12. Prompted voiding or habit training can be successful in frail and/or disabled patients (Grade of Recommendation A).
13. Before prescribing drugs to treat UI in frail, older people:

- modify/delete all other medications that could be contributing to UI
- consider drug use only as an adjunct to other conservative management strategies
- when possible, avoid using some drugs because of increased risk of side effects eg propantheline,amitriptyline,imipramine, vasopressin, ephedrine
- start with low dosage and titrate slowly, but continue until full effect realized
- review regularly outcome and side effects
- consider occasional (PRN) use of a drug

14. Age per se is not a contraindication to surgery for incontinence. However, in older people and especially frail or disabled older people :

- address non-LUT conditions prior to surgery
- whenever possible adequate trial of conservative treatment should be offered prior to surgery. The need for surgery should be reassessed following this.
- pre-op urodynamic assessment is valuable because clinical diagnosis may be inaccurate
- preoperative assessment and perioperative care is essential to minimize complications such as delirium, infection, dehydration and falls

15. Every person should be given the opportunity to become dry irrespective of their frailty or disability. This can be :

- 'independent continence'
- 'dependent continence' – dry with the assistance or reminder of carer
- 'social continence' – dry with the use of appropriate pads and appliances.
- Often a patient can achieve a dry state by combinations of the above

16. Selecting an appropriate pad or appliance to achieve social continence requires patient-centred consideration of: effective containment of urine/faeces, ease of use, comfort, skin health, aesthetics and discretion, disposability, laundry facilities and cost.
17. Where a catheter is used, it is important to determine the reason why it was introduced and to consider alternative management strategies. If the catheter is to remain in place the patient should have an appropriate indication for its chronic use.
18. Whilst evidence is lacking for successful interventions to prevent incontinence there is an increasing recognition of 'at risk' conditions associated with incontinence in older people. These conditions should be sought for and addressed.
19. Research methodology should be improved, particularly for frail older people, to account for population heterogeneity. Validated research tools are needed to reliably measure baseline and outcome measures including patient-defined clinical impact, side effects and quality of life. The durability of treatments should be reported.
20. Future drug studies impacting on older patients should compare the efficacy and tolerability of the drug against conservative interventions.
21. It should be emphasised that statistical significance in intervention studies in a frail elderly population may not equate to clinical or quality of life significance.
22. Practical and useful algorithms need to be created and validated to assist clinicians/caregivers in identifying the best treatment/management strategy for an individual.
23. There is a pressing need for all future research that includes older adults to stratify results by age in order to better understand the responsiveness of the elderly to various treatments.
24. Since older persons constitute the majority of UI patients, future consultations should seek to provide a more integrated approach to understanding the impact of age on physiology, evaluation and treatment.

XVIII. ALGORITHM *(see page 1104)*

REFERENCES

1. INTRODUCTION

1 Buchner DM and Wagner EH, Preventing frail health, Clin Ceriatr Med 1992;8: 1-17

2 Fonda, D, et al. Improving management of urinary incontinence in geriatric centres and nursing homes. Aust Clin Rev 1990;10:66-71

2. IDENTIFICATION AND PREVALENCE

1 Herzog A.R., Diokno A.C., Fultz N.H. Urinary incontinence: medical and psychosocial aspects. Annu Rev Gerontol Geriatr 1989;9:74-119

2 Branch L.G., Walker L.A., Wetle T.T., DuBeau C.E., Resnick N.M. Urinary incontinence knowledge among community-dwelling people 65 years of age and older. J Am Geriatr Soc 1994;42:1257-1262

3 Burgio K.L., Ives D.G., Locher J.L., Arena V.C., Kuller L.H. Treatment seeking for urinary incontinence in older adults. J Am Geriatr Soc 1994;42:208-212

4 Wyman J.F., Harkins S.W., Fantl J.A. Psychosocial impact of urinary incontinence in the community dwelling population. J Am Geriatr Soc 1990;38:282-288

5 Thomas T.M., Plymat K.R., Blannin J., Meade T.W. Prevalence of urinary incontinence. Br Med J 1980;281:1243-1245

6 Vetter N.J., Jones D.A., Victor C.R. Urinary incontinence in the elderly at home. Lancet 1981;2(8258):1275-1277

7 Mitteness L.S. Knowledge and beliefs about urinary incontinence in adulthood and old age. J Am Geriatr Soc 1990;38:374-378

8 McDowell B.J., Silverman M., Martin D., Musa D., Keane C. Identification and intervention for urinary incontinence by community physicians and geriatric assessment teams. J Am Geriatr Soc 1994;42:501-505

9 Diokno AC, Brown MB, Brock BM, Herzog AR, Normolle DP. Clinical and cystometric characteristics of continent and incontinent noninstitutionalized elderly. J Urol 1988;140:567-71

10 Maly RC, Hirsch SH, Reuben DB. The performance of simple instruments in detecting geriatric conditions and selecting community-dwelling older people for geriatric assessment. Age and Ageing 1997;26:223-31

11 Ouslander JG, Palmer MH, Rovner BW, German PS. Urinary incontinence in nursing homes: incidence, remission and associated factors. J Am Geriatr Soc 1993;41:1083-9

12 Resnick NM, Baumann MM. Urinary incontinence and indwelling catheter. In: Administration HCF. Long term care facility Resident Assessment Instrument (RAI) user's manual for use with version 2.0 of the Health Care Financing Administration's Minimum Data Set, Resident Assessment Protocols, and Utilization Guidelines. Baltimore (MD): Health care Financing Administration, 1995

13 Morris JN, Hawes C, Colling J, et al. Resident assessment instrument training manual and resource guide. Massachessetts: Elliot Press, 1991

14 Resnick NM, Brandeis GH, Baumann MM, Morris JN. Evaluating a national assessment strategy for urinary incontinence in nursing home residents: reliability of the minimum data set and validity of the resident assessment protocol. Neurourol Urodyn 1996;15:583-98

15 Brandeis GH, Baumann MM, Hossain M, Morris JN, Resnick NM. The prevalence of potentially remediable urinary incontinence in frail older people: a study using the Minimum Data Set. J Am Geriatr Soc 1997; 45: 179-184.

3. PHYSIOLOGIC AND PATHOLOGIC CHANGES RELEVANT TO INCONTINENCE

1 Resnick NM. Voiding dysfunction in the elderly. In: Yalla SV, McGuire EJ, Elbadawi A, Blaivas JG, eds. Neurourology and Urodynamics: Principles and Practice. New York: MacMillan Publishing Co., 1988:303-330.

2 Diokno AC, Brown MB, Brock BM, Herzog AR, Normolle DP. Clinical and cystometric characteristics of continent and incontinent noninstitutionalized elderly. J Urol 1988; 140: 567-571.

3 Resnick NM, Elbadawi A, Yalla SV. Age and the lower urinary tract: What is normal? Neurourol Urodyn 1995; 14: 577-579.

4 Strasser H, Tiefenthaler M, Steinlechner M, Bartsch G, Konwalinka G. Urinary incontinence in the elderly and age-dependent apoptosis of rhabdosphincter cells. Lancet 1999; 354: 918-919.

5 Botker-Rasmussen I, Bagi P, Jorgensen JB. Is bladder outlet obstruction normal in elderly men without lower urinary tract symptoms? Neurourol Urodyn 1999; 18; 545-542.

6 Elbadawi A, Yalla SV, Resnick NM. Structural basis of geriatric voiding dysfunction. II. Aging detrusor: normal vs. impaired contractility. J Urol 1993; 150:1657-67.

7 Elbadawi A, Yalla SV, Hailemariam S, Resnick NM. Structural basis of geriatric voiding dysfunction. VI. Validation and update of diagnostic criteria in 71 detrusor biopsies. J Urol 1997; 157; 1802-1813.

8 Hailemariam S, Elbadawi A, Yalla SV, Resnick NM. Structural basis of geriatric voiding dysfunction. V. Standardized protocols for routine ultrastructural study and diagnosis of endoscopic detrusor biopsies. J Urol 1997; 157: 1783-1801.

9 Miller KL, DuBeau CE, Griffiths DJ, Resnick NM. Quest for a detrusor overactivity index. J Urol 2001; 165 (Suppl): 297.

10 Miller M. Nocturnal polyuria in older people: Pathophysiology and clinical implications. J Am Geriatr Soc 2000; 48: 1321-1329.

11 Morgan K, Bergmann M, Kiely D, DuBeau CE, Resnick NM. Voiding pattern in normal elders (abstract). J Urol 2000: 163 (Supplement); 228

12 Resnick NM. Clinical Crossroads: Urinary incontinence in an 89 year old woman. JAMA 1996; 276:1832-1840.

13 Resnick NM, Marcantonio ER. How should clinical care of the aged differ? Lancet 1997; 350:1157-1158.

4. NOCTURIA

1. Cannon A, Carter OG, McConnell AA, Abrams P. Desmopressin in the treatment of nocturnal polyuria in the male. Br. J. Urol. 1999;84:20-24.

2. Asplund R, Sunberg B, Bengtsson P. Desmopressin for the treatment of nocturnal polyuria in the elderly: a dose titration study. Br. J. Urol. 1993a;72:38-41.

3. Perry, S, Shaw C, Assassa P, Dallosso H, Williams K et al. An epidemiological study to establish the prevalence of urinary symptoms and felt need in the community: the Leicestershire MRC incontinence study. Jour. Pub. Heal. Med. 2000;22:427-34.

4. Middlekoop HA, Smilde Van Den Doel DA, Kamphuisen HA, Springer CP. Subjective sleep characteristics of 1485 males and females aged 50-93: effects of sex and age, and factors related to self-evaluated quality of sleep. J Gerontol A biol Sci Med Sci. 1996;51:108-115.

5. Samuelsson E, Victor A, Tibblin G. A population study of urinary incontinence and nocturia among women aged 20-59 years. Prevalence, well being and wish for treatment. Acta Obstet Gynecol Scand. 1997;76:74-80.

6. Hale WE, Perkins LL, May FE, Marks RG, Stewart RB. Symptom prevalence in the elderly. An evaluation of age, sex, disease and medication use. J Am Ger Soc. 1986 ;34:333-340.

7. Malmsten UG, Milsom I, Molander U, Norlen LJ. Urinary incontinence and lower urinary tract symptoms: an epidemiological study of men aged 45 to 99 years. J Urol. 1997;158:1733-1737.

8. Blanker MH, Bohnen AM, Groeneveld FP. Normal voiding patterns and determinant of increased diurnal and nocturnal voiding frequency in elderly men. J. Urol. 2000;164:1201-5

9. Pinnock CB, Marshall VR. Troublesome lower urinary tract symptoms in the community: a prevalence study. Med J. Aust. 1997;167:72-75.

10. Schatzl G, Temml C, Schmidbauer J, Dolezal B, Haidinger G, Madersbacher S. Cross-sectional study of nocturia in both sexes: analysis of a voluntary health screening project. Urology. 2000;56:71-5.

11. Rembratt A, Mattiasson A. The prevalence of nocturia in the general population. ICS abstracts. 1998;201-202.

12. Pressman MR, Figueroa WG, Kenrick-Mohammed J, Greenspon LW, Peterson DD. Nocturia: a rarely recognised symptom of sleep apnoea and other occult sleep disorder. Arc. Int. Med. 1996;156:545.

13. Dahlstrand C, Hedner J, Wang WH, Pettersson S. Snoring: a common cause of voiding disturbance in elderly men. Lancet. 1996; 347 :270.

14. Young T, Palta M, Dempsey J, Skutrud J, Webber S and Badr S. The occurrence of sleep disorientated breathing among middle aged adults. New Eng. J. Med 1993;328:1230.

15. Krieger J, Laks L, Wilcox I et al. Atrial natriuretic peptide release during sleep in patients with obstructive sleep apnoea before and during treatment with nasal continuous positive airway pressure. Clin. Sci; 1989;77:407.

16. Asplund R, Aberg H. Desmopressin in elderly women with increased nocturnal diuresis. A short term study. Br. J. Urol. 1993b;72:42.

17. O'Donnell PD, Beck C, Walls RC. Serial incontinence assessment in elderly inpatient men. J. Rehab. Res. Dev. 1990;37:432-6.

18. Reynard JM, Cannon A, Yang Q, Abrams P. A novel therapy for nocturnal polyuria: a double blind randomised trial of frusemide against placebo. Br. J. Urol. 1998;81:215-8.

19. Pederson PA, Johansen PB. Prophylactic treatment of adult nocturia with bumetanide. Br. J. Urol. 1988;62:145-7.

20. Ouslander JG, Schnelle J, Simmons S, Bates-Jenson B, Zeitlin M. The dark side of incontinence in nursing home residents. J. Am. Geriatr. Soc. 1993;41:1083-9.

21. Asplund R, Sundberg B, Bengtsson P. Desmopressin for the treatment of nocturnal polyuria in the elderly: a dose titration study. Br. J. Urol. 1998;82:642-6

22. Asplund R, Sundberg B, Bengtsson P. Oral desmopressin for nocturnal polyuria in elderly subjects: a double-blind, placebo-controlled randomized exploratory study. Br. J. Urol 1999;83:591-595.

23. Chancellor MB, Atan A, Rivas D, Watanabe T, Tai HL, Kumon H. Beneficial effect of intranasal desmopressin for men with benign prostatic hyperplasia and nocturia: preliminary results. Techniques in Urology. 1999;5: 191-4.

24. Miller M. Nocturnal Polyuria in older people: pathophysiology and clinical implications. JAGS. 2000;48:1321-1329.

25. Kok ALM, Burger CW, Van De Weijer PHM, et al. Micturition complaints in postmenopausal women treated with continously combined hormone replacement therapy: a prospective study. Maturitas. 1999;31:143-9.

26. Fantl J, Bump, R, Robinson D, McClish,D, Wyman J. Efficacy of estrogen supplementation in the treatment of urinary incontinence. Obs & Gyn. 1996;88:745-749.

27. Obara K, Takahashi M, Sato S. The effect of desmopressin (DDAVP) in patients complaining of nocturia. Jap. J. Urol. 1993;84:2131-6.

28. Seiler WO, Stahelin HB, Hefti U. Desmopressin reduces night urine volume in geriatric patients: Iplications for treatment of the nocturnal incontinence. Clin. Invest. 1992;70:619.

29. Hilton P, Stanton SL. The use of desmppressin (DDAVP) in nocturnal urinary frequency in the female. Br. J. Urol. 1982; 54:252-5.

30. Mansson W, Swindin T, Gullberg B. Evaluation of a synthetic vasopressin analogue for treatment of nocturia in benign prostatic hyperplasia. Scand. J. Urol. Nephrol. 1980;14:139-41.

5. CAUSES OF TRANSIENT INCONTINENCE

1 Resnick NM. Voiding dysfunction in the elderly. In: Yalla SV, McGuire EJ, Elbadawi A, Blaivas JG, eds. Neurourology and Urodynamics: Principles and Practice. New York: MacMillan Publishing Co., 303-330, 1988.

2 Ouslander JG, Palmer MH, Rovner BW, German PS. Urinary incontinence in nursing homes: Incidence, remission and associated factors. J Am Geriatr Soc 1993; 41: 1083-1089.

3 Brandeis GB, Baumann MM, Hossain M, Morris JN, Resnick NM. The prevalence of potentially remediable urinary incontinence in frail elderly people: A study using the Minimum Data Set. J Am Geriatr Soc *1997*; 45: 179-184.

4 Diokno AC, Brown MB, Herzog AR. Relationship between use of diuretics and continence status in the elderly. Urol 1991; 38: 39-42.

5 Fantl JA, Wyman JF, Wilson M, Elswick RK, Bump RC, Wein AJ. Diuretics and urinary incontinence in community-dwelling women. Neurourol Urodyn. 1990; 9: 25-34,.

6 Resnick NM, Baumann M, Scott M, Laurino E, Yalla SV. Risk factors for incontinence in the nursing home: A multivariate study. Neurourol Urodyn 1988; 7:274-276.

7 Resnick NM, Beckett LA, Branch LG, Scherr PA, Wetle T. Short-term variability of self report of incontinence in older persons. J Am Geriatr Soc 1994; 42: 202-207.

8 Resnick NM. Urinary incontinence in the elderly. Medical Grand Rounds 1984; 3:281-290.

9 Resnick NM, Paillard M. Natural history of nosocomial incontinence. Gerontologist 1984; 24: 212A.

10 Boscia JA, Kobasa WD, Abrutyn E, Levinson ME, Kaplan AM, Kaye D. Lack of association between bacteriuria and symptoms in the elderly. Am J Med 1986; 81:979-982.

11 Ouslander JG, Schnelle JF. Incontinence in the nursing home. Ann Int Med 1995; 122:438- 449.

12 Robinson JM. Evaluation of methods for assessment of bladder and urethral function. In: Urology in the Elderly. In: JC Brocklehurst (ed.). New York: Churchill Livingstone, 19-54, 1984.

13 Raz R, Stamm WE. A controlled trial of intravaginal estriol in postmenopausal women with recurrent urinary tract infections. N Engl J Med 329: 753-6.

14 Marshall HJ, Beevers DG. α-adrenoceptor blocking drugs and female urinary incontinence: prevalence and reversibility. Brit J Clin Pharmacol 1996; 42: 507-509.

15 Hellstrom PM, Sjoqvist A. Involvement of opioid and nicotinic receptors in rectal and anal reflex inhibition of urinary bladder motility in cats. Acta Physiol Scand 1988; 133:559-562.

6. ESTABLISHED INCONTINENCE

1. Resnick NM, Yalla SV. Management of urinary incontinence in the elderly. N Engl J Med 1985; 313:800-5.
2. Hadley EC. Bladder training and related therapies for urinary incontinence in older people. JAMA 1986; 256:372-9.
3. Resnick NM. Geriatric incontinence. Urol Clin North Am 1996; 23:55-74.
4. Resnick NM. Urinary incontinence. Lancet 1995; 346:94-9.
5. Ouslander JG, Schnelle JF. Incontinence in the nursing home. Ann Intern Med 1995; 122:438-49.
6. Fantl JA, Newman DK, Colling Jea. Urinary incontinence in adults: acute and chronic management. Clinical Practice Guideline No.2, 1996 update. Rockville, MD: U.S. Department of Health and Human Services. Public Health Service, Agency for Health Care Policy and Research. AHCPR Publication No. 96-0682., 1996.
7. Ouslander JG, Uman GC, Urman HN, Rubenstein LZ. Incontinence among nursing home patients: clinical and functional correlates. J Am Geriatr Soc 1987; 35:324-30.
8. Ouslander J, Leach G, Staskin D, Abelson S, Blaustein J, Morishita L, Raz S. Prospective evaluation of an assessment strategy for geriatric urinary incontinence. J Am Geriatr Soc 1989; 37:715-24.
9. Resnick NM, Yalla SV, Laurino E. The pathophysiology of urinary incontinence among institutionalized elderly persons. N Engl J Med 1989; 320:1-7.
10. Resnick NM, Brandeis GH, Baumann MM, Morris JN. Evaluating a national assessment strategy for urinary incontinence in nursing home residents: reliability of the minimum data set and validity of the resident assessment protocol. Neurourol Urodyn 1996; 15:583-98.
11. McGrother C, Resnick M, Yalla SV, Kirschner-Hermanns R, Broseta E, Muller C, Welz-Barth A, Fischer GC, Mattelaer J, McGuire EJ. Epidemiology and etiology of urinary incontinence in the elderly. World J Urol 1998; 16:S3-9.
12. Rutchik SD, Resnick MI. The epidemiology of incontinence in the elderly. Br J Urol 1998; 82 Suppl 1:1-4.
13. DuBeau CE, Resnick NM. Evaluation of the causes and severity of geriatric incontinence. A critical appraisal. Urol Clin North Am 1991; 18:243-56.
14. O'Donnell PD. Special considerations in elderly individuals with urinary incontinence. Urology 1998; 51:20-3.
15. Blaivas JG, Appell RA, Fantl JA, Leach G, McGuire EJ, Resnick NM, Raz S, Wein AJ. Definition and classification of urinary incontinence: recommendations of the Urodynamic Society. Neurourol Urodyn 1997; 16:149-51.
16. Resnick NM, Yalla SV. Detrusor hyperactivity with impaired contractile function. An unrecognized but common cause of incontinence in elderly patients. JAMA 1987; 257:3076-81.
17. Resnick NM, Brandeis GH, Baumann MM, DuBeau CE, Yalla SV. Misdiagnosis of urinary incontinence in nursing home women: prevalence and a proposed solution. Neurourol Urodyn 1996; 15:599-613.
18. Diokno AC, Wells TJ, Brink CA. Urinary incontinence in elderly women: urodynamic evaluation. J Am Geriatr Soc 1987; 35:940-6.
19. Diokno AC, Brown MB, Brock BM, Herzog AR, Normolle DP. Clinical and cystometric characteristics of continent and incontinent noninstitutionalized elderly. J Urol 1988; 140:567-71.
20. Wells TJ, Brink CA, Diokno AC. Urinary incontinence in elderly women: clinical findings. J Am Geriatr Soc 1987; 35:933-9.
21. Blaivas JG, Olsson CA. Stress incontinence: classification and surgical approach. J Urol 1988; 139:727-31.
22. Ulmsten U, Henriksson L, Iosif S. The unstable female urethra. Am J Obstet Gynecol 1982; 144:93-7.
23. Low JA, Armstrong JB, Mauger GM. The unstable urethra in the female. Obstet Gynecol 1989; 74:69-74.
24. Diokno AC, Brock BM, Brown MB, Herzog AR. Prevalence of urinary incontinence and other urological symptoms in the noninstitutionalized elderly. J Urol 1986; 136:1022-5.
25. Hilton P, Stanton SL. Algorithmic method for assessing urinary incontinence in elderly women. Br Med J (Clin Res Ed) 1981; 282:940-2.
26. Eastwood HD, Warrell R. Urinary incontinence in the elderly female: prediction in diagnosis and outcome of management. Age Ageing 1984; 13:230-4.
27. Ouslander JG, Hepps K, Raz S, Su HL. Genitourinary dysfunction in a geriatric outpatient population. J Am Geriatr Soc 1986; 34:507-14.
28. Andersen JT, Nordling J, Walter S. Prostatism. I. The correlation between symptoms, cystometric and urodynamic findings. Scand J Urol Nephrol 1979; 13:229-36.
29. DuBeau CE. Urinary retention in the elderly. J Am Geriatr Soc 1993; 41:1372-3.
30. Skelly J, Flint AJ. Urinary incontinence associated with dementia. J Am Geriatr Soc 1995; 43:286-94.
31. Ouslander JG, Kane RL, Abrass IB. Urinary incontinence in elderly nursing home patients. Jama 1982; 248:1194-8.
32. Ouslander JG, Palmer MH, Rovner BW, German PS. Urinary incontinence in nursing homes: incidence, remission and associated factors. J Am Geriatr Soc 1993; 41:1083-9.
33. Brandeis GH, Baumann MM, Hossain M, Morris JN, Resnick NM. The prevalence of potentially remediable urinary incontinence in frail older people: a study using the Minimum Data Set. J Am Geriatr Soc 1997; 45:179-84.
34. Diokno AC, Brock BM, Herzog AR, Bromberg J. Medical correlates of urinary incontinence in the elderly. Urology 1990; 36:129-38.
35. Brown JS, Vittinghoff E, Wyman JF, Stone KL, Nevitt MC, Ensrud KE, Grady D, for the Study of Osteoporotic Fractures Research Group. Urinary incontinence: does it increase risk for falls and fractures? J Am Geriatr Soc 2000; 48:721-5.

7. CLINCAL EVALUATION

1. NIH Consensus Development Conference. Urinary incontinence in adults. J Am Geriatr Soc 1990; 38:265-72.
2. Resnick NM. Initial evaluation of the incontinent patient. J Am Geriatr Soc 1990; 38:311-6.
3. Bonde HV, Sejr T, Erdmann L, Meyhoff HH, Lendorf A, Rosenkilde P, Bodker A, Nielsen MB. Residual urine in 75-year-old men and women. A normative population study. Scand J Urol Nephrol 1996; 30:89-91.
4. Grosshans C, Passadori Y, Peter B. Urinary retention in the elderly: a study of 100 hospitalized patients. J Am Geriatr Soc 1993; 41:633-8.
5. Fantl JA, Newman DK, Colling Jea. Urinary incontinence in adults: acute and chronic management. Clinical Practice Guideline No.2, 1996 update. Rockville, MD: U.S. Department of Health and Human Services. Public Health Service, Agency for Health Care Policy and Research. AHCPR Publication No. 96-0682., 1996.
6. Kane RL, Ouslander JG, Abrass IB. Essentials of clinical geriatrics. Chapter 6: Incontinence. New York: McGraw Hill, 1993:146-96.
7. Resnick NM. Geriatric incontinence. Urol Clin North Am 1996; 23:55-74.

8. Ouslander JG, Greengold B, Chen S. External catheter use and urinary tract infections among incontinent male nursing home patients. J Am Geriatr Soc 1987; 35:1063-70.
9. Ouslander JG, Schapira M, Schnelle JF. Urine specimen collection from incontinent female nursing home residents. J Am Geriatr Soc 1995; 43:279-81.
10. Belmin J, Hervias Y, Avellano E, Oudart O, Durand I. Reliability of sampling urine from disposable diapers in elderly incontinent women. J Am Geriatr Soc 1993; 41:1182-6.
11. Mohide EA. The prevalence and scope of urinary incontinence. Clin Geriatr Med 1986; 2:639-55.
12. Noelker LS. Incontinence in elderly cared for by family. Gerontologist 1987; 27:194-200.
13. Nygaard HA. Strain on caregivers of demented elderly people living at home. Scand J Prim Health Care 1988; 6:33-7.
14. Ouslander JG, Zarit SH, Orr NK, Muira SA. Incontinence among elderly community-dwelling dementia patients. Characteristics, management, and impact on caregivers. J Am Geriatr Soc 1990; 38:440-5.
15. Markson EW. Functional, social, and psychological disability as causes of loss of weight and independence in older community-living people. Clin Geriatr Med 1997; 13:639-52.
16. Kadar N. The value of bladder filling in the clinical detection of urine loss and selection of patients for urodynamic testing. Br J Obstet Gynaecol 1988; 95:698-704.
17. Resnick NM, Yalla SV, Laurino E. The pathophysiology of urinary incontinence among institutionalized elderly persons. N Engl J Med 1989; 320:1-7.
18. Resnick NM, Brandeis GH, Baumann MM, Morris JN. Evaluating a national assessment strategy for urinary incontinence in nursing home residents: reliability of the minimum data set and validity of the resident assessment protocol. Neurourol Urodyn 1996; 15:583-98.
19. Wells TJ. Social and psychological implications of incontinence. In: Broklehurst JC, ed. Urology in the elderly. New York: Churchill Ligingstone, 1984:107-126.
20. Mitteness LS, Barker JC. Stigmatizing a "normal" condition: urinary incontinence in late life. Med Anthropol Q 1995; 9:188-210.
21. Steel K, Musliner M, Berg K. Assessment of home environment. In: Rubenstein LZ, Wieland D, Bernabei R, eds. Geriatric assessment technology: the state of art. Milan: Kurtis Editrice, 1995:135-45.
22. Fonda D. Improving management of urinary incontinence in geriatric centres and nursing homes. Victorian Geriatricians Peer Review Group. Aust Clin Rev 1990; 10:66-71.
23. Diokno AC, Wells TJ, Brink CA. Comparison of self-reported voided volume with cystometric bladder capacity. J Urol 1987; 137:698-700.
24. Wyman JF, Choi SC, Harkins SW, Wilson MS, Fantl JA. The urinary diary in evaluation of incontinent women: a test-retest analysis. Obstet Gynecol 1988; 71:812-7.
25. Hu TW, Igou JF, Kaltreider DL, Yu LC, Rohner TJ, Dennis PJ, Craighead WE, Hadley EC, Ory MG. A clinical trial of a behavioral therapy to reduce urinary incontinence in nursing homes. Outcome and implications [see comments]. JAMA 1989; 261:2656-62.
26. Ouslander JG, Urman HN, Uman GC. Development and testing of an incontinence monitoring record. J Am Geriatr Soc 1986; 34:83-90.
27. Walsh JB, Mills GL. Measurement of urinary loss in elderly incontinent patients. A simple and accurate method. Lancet 1981; 1:1130-1.
28. Griffiths DJ, McCracken PN, Harrison GM. Incontinence in the elderly: objective demonstration and quantitative assessment. Br J Urol 1991; 67:467-71.
29. Griffiths DJ, McCracken PN, Harrison GM, Gormley EA. Characteristics of urinary incontinence in elderly patients studied by 24-hour monitoring and urodynamic testing. Age Ageing 1992; 21:195-201.
30. Ekelund P, Bergstrom H, Milsom I, Norlen L, Rignell S. Quantification of urinary incontinence in elderly women with the 48-hour pad test. Arch Gerontol Geriatr 1988; 7:281-7.
31. Ouslander JG, Simmons S, Tuico E, Nigam JG, Fingold S, Bates-Jensen B, Schnelle JF. Use of a portable ultrasound device to measure post-void residual volume among incontinent nursing home residents. J Am Geriatr Soc 1994; 42:1189-92.
32. Griffiths DJ, Harrison G, Moore K, McCracken P. Variability of post-void residual urine volume in the elderly. Urol Res 1996; 24:23-6.
33. Birch NC, Hurst G, Doyle PT. Serial residual volumes in men with prostatic hypertrophy. Br J Urol 1988; 62:571-5.
34. Ouslander JG, Greengold BA, Silverblatt FJ, Garcia JP. An accurate method to obtain urine for culture in men with external catheters. Arch Intern Med 1987; 147:286-8.
35. Flanagan PG, Rooney PG, Davies EA, Stout RW. Evaluation of four screening tests for bacteriuria in elderly people. Lancet 1989; 1:1117-9.
36. Ouslander J, Leach G, Abelson S, Staskin D, Blaustein J, Raz S. Simple versus multichannel cystometry in the evaluation of bladder function in an incontinent geriatric population. J Urol 1988; 140:1482-6.
37. Fonda D, Brimage PJ, D'Astoli M. Simple screening for urinary incontinence in the elderly: comparison of simple and multichannel cystometry. Urology 1993; 42:536-40.
38. DuBeau CE, Resnick NM. Evaluation of the causes and severity of geriatric incontinence. A critical appraisal. Urol Clin North Am 1991; 18:243-56.
39. Ouslander JG, Schnelle JF. Incontinence in the nursing home. Ann Intern Med 1995; 122:438-49.
40. Diokno AC, Normolle DP, Brown MB, Herzog AR. Urodynamic tests for female geriatric urinary incontinence. Urology 1990; 36:431-9.
41. Diokno AC, Wells TJ, Brink CA. Urinary incontinence in elderly women: urodynamic evaluation. J Am Geriatr Soc 1987; 35:940-6.
42. Djavan B, Madersbacher S, Klingler C, Marberger M. Urodynamic assessment of patients with acute urinary retention: is treatment failure after prostatectomy predictable? J Urol 1997; 158:1829-33.
43. Elbadawi A, Hailemariam S, Yalla SV, Resnick NM. Structural basis of geriatric voiding dysfunction. VII. Prospective ultrastructural/urodynamic evaluation of its natural evolution. J Urol 1997; 157:1814-22.
44. Sakakibara R, Hattori T, Uchiyama T, Yamanishi T. Urinary function in elderly people with and without leukoaraiosis: relation to cognitive and gait function. J Neurol Neurosurg Psychiatry 1999; 67:658-60.
45. Resnick NM, Brandeis GH, Baumann MM, DuBeau CE, Yalla SV. Misdiagnosis of urinary incontinence in nursing home women: prevalence and a proposed solution. Neurourol Urodyn 1996; 15:599-613.
46. Leach GE, Yip CM, Donovan BJ. Post-prostatectomy incontinence: the influence of bladder dysfunction. J Urol 1987; 138:574-8.
47. Dennis PJ, Rohner TJ, Jr., Hu TW, Igou JF, Yu LC, Kaltreider DL. Simple urodynamic evaluation of incontinent elderly female nursing home patients. A descriptive analysis. Urology 1991; 37:173-9.
48. Resnick NM, Yalla SV. Detrusor hyperactivity with impaired

contractile function. An unrecognized but common cause of incontinence in elderly patients. JAMA 1987; 257:3076-81.

49. Elbadawi A, Yalla SV, Resnick NM. Structural basis of geriatric voiding dysfunction. IV. Bladder outlet obstruction. J Urol 1993; 150:1681-95.

50. Elbadawi A, Yalla SV, Resnick NM. Structural basis of geriatric voiding dysfunction. III. Detrusor overactivity. J Urol 1993; 150:1668-80.

51. Elbadawi A, Yalla SV, Resnick NM. Structural basis of geriatric voiding dysfunction. II. Aging detrusor: normal versus impaired contractility. J Urol 1993; 150:1657-67.

52. Elbadawi A, Yalla SV, Resnick NM. Structural basis of geriatric voiding dysfunction. I. Methods of a prospective ultrastructural/urodynamic study and an overview of the findings. J Urol 1993; 150:1650-6.

53. Folstein MF, Folstein SE, McHugh PR. Mini-mental state. A practical method for grading the cognitive state of patients for the clinician. J Psychiatr Res 1975; 12:189-98.

54. Mahoney RI, Barthel DW. Functional evaluation: the Barthel Index. Md State Med J 1965; 14:61-65.

55. Katz S, Ford AB, Moskowitz RW, Jackson BA, Jaffee MW. Studies of illness in the aged. The Index of ADL: a standardized measure of biological and psychological function. JAMA 1963; 185:914-19.

8. MEASURING OUTCOMES

1. Mattiasson A, Djurhuus JC, Fonda, D, Lose G, Nordling J, Stohrer M. Standardization of Outcome Studies in Patients with Lower Urinary Tract Dysfunction: A report on General Principles from the Standardisation Committee of the International Continence Society. Neurourol Urodyn. 17:249-253.1998

2. Fonda D, Resnick NM, Colling J, Burgio K, Ouslander JG, Norton C, Ekelund P, Versi E, Mattiasson A. Outcome Measures for Research of Lower Urinary Tract Dysfunction in Frail Older People. Neurourol Urodyn. 17:273-281. 1998

10. BIOFEEDBACK AND ELECTRICAL STIMULATION

1. Burns PA, Pranikoff K, Nochajski TH, et al. A comparison of effectiveness of biofeedback and pelvic floor exercise treatment of stress incontinence in older community dwelling women. J Gerontol 1993; 48:167-174.

2. McDowell J, Engbert S, Sereika S, Donovan N, Jubeck ME, Weber E, Engbert R. Effectivenessof behaviorial therapy to treat incontinence in homebound older adults. J Am Geriatr Soc 1999; 47:309-18.

3. Bear M, Dwyer JW, Benveneste D, Jett K, Dougherty M. Home-based management of urinary incontinence: A pilot study with both frail and independent elders. J Wound Ostomy Continence Nurs 1997; 24(3):163-71.

4. Smith DB, Boileau MA, Baun LD. A self-directed home biofeedback system for women with symptoms of stress, urge, and mixed incontinence. J Wound Ostomy Continence Nurs 2000; 27(4):240-46.

5. Shinopulos NM, Jacobson J. Relationship between health promotion lifesytle profiles and patient outcomes of biofeedback therapy for urinary incontinence. Urol Nurs 1999; 19(4):249-53.

6. Susset J, Galea G, Manbeck K, Susset A. A predictive score index for the outcome of associated biofeedback and vaginal electrical stimulation in the treatment of female incontinence. J Urol 1995; 153:146-66.

7. Stein M, Discippio W, Davia M, Taub H. Biofeedback for the treatment of stress and urge incontinence. J Urol 1995; 153:641-43.

8. Baigis-Smith J, Smith DAJ, Rose M, Newman DK. Managing urinary incontinence in community-residing elderly persons. Gerontologist 1989; 29(2):229-33.

9. Henderson JS, Taylor KH. Age as a variable in an exercise program for the treatment of simple urinary stress incontinence. J Obstet Gynecol Neonatal Nurs 1987; 44(4):266-72.

10. Burgio KL, Whitehead WE, Engel BT. Urinary incontinence in the elderly. Ann Intern Med 1985; 104:507-15.

11. Weinberger MW, Goodman BM, Carnes M. Long-term efficacy of nonsurgical urinary incontinence treatment in elder women. J Gerontol 1999;54A(3):M117-21.

12. Lamhut P, Jackson TW, Wall LL. The treatment of urinary incontinence with electrical stimulation in nursing home patients: A pilot study. J Am Geriatr Soc 1992; 40:48-52.

13. Yamanishi T, Yasuda K, Sakakibra R, Hattori T, Suda S. Randomized, double-blind study of electrical stimulation for urinary incontinence due to detrusor overactivity. Urology 2000; 55:353-357.

14. Zollner-Nielsen M, Samuelsson SM. Maximal electrical stimulation of patients with frequency, urgency or urge incontinence. Acta Obstet Gynecol Scand 1992; 71:629-631.

15. Bratt H, Salvesen KA, Eriksen BC, Kulseng-Hanssen S. Long-term effects ten years after maximal electrostimulation of the pelvic floor in women with unstable detrusor and urge incontinence. Acta Obstet Gynecol Scand 1998; supplement 168:77:22-24.

16. Kulseng-Hanssen S, Kristoffersen M, Larsen E. Evaluation of the subjective and objective effect of maximal electrical stimulation in patients complaining of urge incontinence. Acta Obstet Gynecol Scand 1998; supplement 168:77:12-15.

17. Geirsson G, Fall M. Maximal functional electrical stimulation in routine practice. Neurourol Urodyn 1997; 16:559-565.

18. Yamanishi T, Yasuda K, Sakakibara R, Hattori T, Ito H, Murakami S. Pelvic floor electrical stimulation in the treatment of stress incontinence: An investigational study and a placebo controlled double-blind trial. J Urol 1997; 158:2127-2131.

11. OTHER BEHAVIORAL INTERVENTIONS

1. Hays R, Siu A, Keeler E, Marshall G, Kaplan R, Simmons S, Mouchi D, Schnelle J. Long-term care residents' preferences for health states on the quality of well-being scale. Medical Decision Making, 16(3), 254-260, 1996.

2. Palmer MH, German PS, Ouslander JG, Rovner, E. Risk factors for urinary incontinence one year after nursing home admission. Research in Nursing and Health, 14, 405-412, 1992.

3. Adkins V, Mathews M. Prompted voiding to reduce incontinence in community-dwelling older adults. Journal of Applied Behavior Analysis, 30(1), 153-156, 1999.

4. E ngberg S, McDowell J, Donovan N, Brodak I., Weber E. Treatment of urinary incontinence in homebound older adults' interface between research and practice. Ostomy/Wound Management, 43(10), 18-26, 1997.

5. Lekan-Rutledge D. Diffusion of innovation. a model for implementation of prompted voiding in long-term care settings. Journal of Gerontological Nursing, 26(4), 25-33, 2000.

6. Schnelle J, Macrae P, Ouslander J, Simmons S, Nitta M. Functional incidental training, mobility performance, and incontinence care with nursing home residents. Journal of the American Geriatrics Society, 43(12), 1356-1362, 1995.

7. Creason NS Grybowski JA, Burgner S, Whippo C, Yeo SA, Richardson B. Prompted voiding therapy for urinary incontinence in aged female nursing home residents. Journal of Advanced Nursing. 14: 120-126. 1989.

8. Hu TW, Igou JF, Kaltreider DL, Yu LC, Rohner TJ, Dennis PJ, Craighead WE, Hadley EC, Ory M. A Clinical Trial of a behavioral therapy to reduce urinary incontinence in nursing homes.

Journal of the American Medical Association, 261(18), 2656-2662, 1989.

9. Colling J, Ouslander J, Hadley BJ, Eisch J, Campbell E. The effects of patterned urge-response toileting (PUR) on urinary incontinence among nursing home residents. Journal of the American Geriatrics Society 40: 135-141, 1992.

10. Schnelle JF. Treatment of urinary incontinence in nursing home patients by prompted voiding. Journal of the American Geriatrics Society, 38(3), 356-360, 1990.

11. McCormick KA, Cella M, Scheve A, Engel BT. Cost-effectiveness of treatment incontinence in severely mobility-impaired long-term care residents. Quality Review Bulletin, 16(12), 438-443, 1990.

12. Ouslander J, Schnelle J, Uman G, Fingold S, Nigam J, Tuico E, Bates-Jensen B. Predictors of successful prompted voiding among incontinent nursing home residents. Journal of the American Medical Association, 273(17), 1366- 1370, 1995.

13. Chaliha C, Stanton S. The ethnic cultural and social aspects of incontinence – a pilot study. International Urogynecology Journal, 10, 196-170, 1999.

14. Eustice S, Roe B, Paterson J. Prompted voiding for the management of urinary incontinence in adults. (Cochrane Review). In: The Cochrane Library, 1, 2001, Oxford: Update Software, 2001.

15. Blair C, Lewis R, Vieweg V, Tucker R. Group and single-subject evaluation of a programme to promote self-care in elderly nursing home residents. Journal of Advanced Nursing, 24, 1207-1213, 1996.

16. Baldwin J, Baldwin J. Behavioral Principles In Everyday Life, Second Edition. Prentice-Hall Co: Englewood Cliff, NJ, 1986.

17. Schnelle JF, Cruise PA, Rahman A, Ouslander JG. Developing rehabilitative behavioral interventions for long-term care: Technology transfer, acceptance, and maintenance issues. Geronotologist, 46(6), 771-777, 1998.

18. Lekan-Rutledge D, Palmer MH, Belyea M. In their own words: Nursing assistants' perceptions of barriers to implementation of prompted voiding in long- term care. Gerontologist, 38(3), 370-378, 1998.

19. Remsberg R, Palmer MH, Langford A, Mendelson G. Staff compliance with and ratings of effectiveness of a prompted voiding program in a long-term care facility. Journal of Wound, Ostomy and Continence Nursing 26(5), 261-269, 1999.

20. Dougherty, M. Current status of research on pelvic muscle exercise. Journal of Wound, Ostomy and Continence Nursing, 25(2), 75-83, 1998.

21. Berghmans, LC, Henriks, HJ, DeBie, RA, Van Doorn, ES, Bo, K & Van Kerrbroeck, PE Conservative Treatment of Urge Urinary Incontinence in Women: A Systemic Review of Randomized Clinical Trials. BJU International, 85(3), 254-263, 2000.

22. Burgio, KL, Locher, JL, Goode, PS, Hardin, JM., McDowell, BJ., Dombrowski, M. & Candib, D. Behavioral vs Drug Treatment for Urge Urinary Incontinence in Older Women: A Randomized Controlled Trial. Journal of the American Medical Association. 280(23), 1995-2000.

23. Burgio, KL, Locher, J. & Goode, P. Combined behavioral and drug therapy for urge incontinence in older women. Journal of the American Geriatrics Society, 48(4), 370-374.

24. Weinberger, MW, Goodman, BM, Carnes, M. Long-term efficacy of nonsurgical urinary incontinence in elderly women. Journals of Gerontology. Series A, Biological Sciences & Medical Sciences. 54(3): M117-M121, 1999.

25. Palmer, MH. A new framework for urinary outcomes in long-term care. Urologic Nursing, 16(4), 146-151, 1996.

26. Sloss, E., Solomon, D., Shekelle, P., Young, R., Saliba, D., MacLean, C., Rubenstein, L., Schnelle, J., Kamberg, C., Wenger, N. Selecting target conditions for quality of care improvement in vulnerable older adults. Journal of the American Geriatrics Society, 48(4), 363-369, 2000.

27. Silverman M, McDowell J, Musa D, Rodriguez E, Martin D. To treat or not to treat: Issues in decisions not to treat older persons with cognitive impairment, depression, and incontinence. Journal of the American Geriatrics Society, 48(4), 363-369, 1997.

28. Berstrom K, Carlsson C, Lindholm C, Widengren R. Improvement of urge-and mixed-typed incontinence after acupuncture treatment among elderly women a pilot study. Journal of Autonomic Nervous System, 79, 173-180, 2000.

29. Kutner N, Schechtman K, Ory M, Baker D, and the FICSIT group. Older adults' perceptions of their health and functioning in relation to sleep disturbances, falling, and urinary incontinence. Journal of the American Geriatrics Society, 42(7), 757-762, 1994.

30. Johnson T, Kincaide J, Bernard S, Busby-Whitehead J, De Friese G. Self-care practices used by older men and women to manage urinary incontinence: Results from the national follow-up survey on self-care and aging. Journal of the American Geriatrics Society, 48(8), 894-902, 2000.

31. Stevens A, Burgio L, Bailey E, Burgio K, Paul P, Capilouto E, Nicovich P, Hale G. Teaching and maintaining behavior management skills with nursing assistants in a nursing home. Gerontologist, 38(3), 379-384, 1998.

32. Kayser-Jones, J, Schell E, Porter C, Barbaccia J, Shaw H. Factors contributing to dehydration in nursing homes: Inadequate staffing and lack of professional supervision. Journal of the American Geriatrics Society, 47(10), 1187-1194, 1999.

33. Schnelle JF, Newman D, White M, Abbey J, Wallston KA, Fogarty T, Ory MG. Maintaining continence in nursing home residents through the application of industrial quality control. Gerontologist, 33(1), 114-121, 1993.

34. Dowd T, Campbell J. Fluid intake and urinary incontinence in older community-dwelling women. Journal of Community Health Nursing, 13(3), 179- 186, 1996.

12. PHARMACOLOGICAL MANAGEMENT

1. Dequeker J. Drug treatment of urinary incontinence in the elderly. Controlled trial with vasopressin and propantheline bromide. Gerontol Clin 1965; 7:311-317

2. Williams A.J., Prematalake J.K., Palmer R.L. A trial of emepronium bromide for the treatment of urinary incontinence in the elderly mentally ill. Pharmatherapeutica 1981; 2(8).539-542

3. Tobin GW, Brocklehurst JC. The management of urinary incontinence in local authority residential homes for the elderly. Age Ageing 1986; 15(5):292-298

4. Zorzitto ML, Jewett MA, Fernie GR, Holliday PJ, Bartlett S. Effectiveness of propantheline bromide in the treatment of geriatric patients with detrusor instability. Neurourol Urodyn 1986; 5:133-140

5. Ouslander JG, Blaustein J, Connor A, Pitt A. Habit training and oxybutynin for incontinence in nursing home patients: a placebo-controlled trial. J Am Geriatr Soc 1988; 36(1):40-46

6. Zorzitto ML, Holliday PJ, Jewett MA, Herschorn S, Fernie G. Oxybutynin chloride for geriatric urinary dysfunction: a double-blind placebo-controlled study. Age Ageing 1989;8:195-200

7. Ouslander JG, Schnelle JF, Uman G, Fingold S, Nigam JG, Tuico E, Jensen BB. Does oxybutynin add to the effectiveness of prompted voiding for urinary incontinence among nursing home residents? A placebo-controlled trial. J Am Geriatr Soc 1995; 43(6):610-617

8. Szonyi G, Collas DM, Ding YY, Malone-Lee JG. Oxybutynin with bladder retraining for detrusor instability in elderly people: a randomized controlled trial. Age Ageing 1995; 24:287-291

9. Robinson JM, Brocklehurst JC. Emepronium bromide and flavoxate hydrochloride in the treatment of urinary incontinence associated with detrusor instability in elderly women. Br J Urol 1983; 55:371-376

10. Castleden CM, Duffin HM, Gulati RS. Double-blind study of

imipramine and placebo for incontinence due to bladder instability. Age Ageing 1986; 15(5):299-303

13. SURGICAL INTERVENTIONS IN OLDER WOMEN

1. Olsen AL, Smith VJ, Bergstrom JO, Colling JC, Clark AL. Epidemiology of surgically managed pelvic organ prolapse and urinary incontinence. Obstet Gynecol 1997; 89(4):501-6.
2. Castleden CM, Duffin HM, Asher MJ. Clinical and urodynamic studies in 100 elderly incontinent patients. Br Med J (Clin Res Ed) 1981;282(6270):1103-1105.
3. Kirschner-Hermanns R, Scherr PA, Branch LG, Wetle T, Resnick NM. Accuracy of survey questions for geriatric urinary incontinence. J Urol 1998;159:1903-1908.
4. Roberts RO, Jabosen SJ, Reilly WT, Pemberton JH, Lieber MM, Talley NJ. Prevalence of combined fecal and urinary incontinence: a community-based study. J Am Geriatr Soc 1999;47(7):837-841.
5. Chassagne P, Landrin I, Neveu C, Czernichow P, Bouaniche M, Doucet J, Denis P, Bercoff E. Fecal incontinence in the instutionalized elderly: incidence, risk factors, and prognosis. Am J Med 1999;106(2):185-190.
6. Sultana CJ, Campbell JW, Pisanelli WS, Sivinski L, Rimm, AA. Morbidity and mortality of incontinence surgery in elderly women: An analysis of Medicare data. Am J Obstet Gynecol 1997;176(2):344-48.
7. Tiret L, Desmonts JM, Hatton F, Vourc'h G. Complications associated with anaesthesia – a prospective survey in France. Can Anaesth Soc J 1986;33(3):336-344.
8. Hilton P, Mayne CJ. The Stamey endoscopic bladder neck suspension: a clinical and urodynamic investigation, including actuarial follow-up over four years. Br J Obstet Gynaecol 1991;98:1141-49.
9. Nitti VW, Bregg KJ, Sussman EM, Raz Shlomo. The Raz bladder neck suspension in patients 65 yeasr old and older. J Urol 1993;149:802-7.
10. Golomb J, Goldwasser B, Mashiach S. Raz bladder neck suspension in women younger than sixty-five years compared with elderly women: three years' experience. Urology 1994;43(1):40-43.
11. Groutz A, Gordon D, Wolman I, Jaffa AJ, Kupferminc MJ, David MP, Lessing JB. The use of prophylactic stamey bladder neck susbension to prevent post-operative stress urinary incontinence in clinically continent women undergoing genitourinary prolapse repair. Neurourol Urodynam 2000;19:671-676.
12. Peattie AB, Stanton SL. The Stamey operation for correction of genuine stress incontinence in the elderly woman. Br J Obstet Gynaecol 1989;96:983-986.
13. Griffith-Jones MD, Abrams PH. The Stamey endoscopic bladder neck suspension in the elderly. Br J Urol 1990;65:170-72.
14. Carr LK, Walsh PJ, Abraham VE, Webster GD. Favorable outcome of pubovaginal slings for geriatric women with stress incontinence. J Urol 1997;157:125-28.
15. Chaikin DC, Groutz A, Blaivas JG. Predicting the need for anti-incontinence surgery in continent women undergoing repair of severe urogenital prolapse. J Urol 2000;163:531-34.
16. Couillard DR, Deckard-Janatpour KA, Stone AR. The vaginal wall sling: a compressive suspension procedure for recurrent incontinence in elderly patients. Urology 1994;43(2):203-8.
17. Kaplan SA, Te AE, Young GPH, Andrade A, Cabelin MA, Ikeguchi EF. Prospective analysis of 373 consecutive women with stress urinary incontinence treated with a vaginal wall sling: The Columbia-Cornell University experience. J Urol 2000;164:1623-27.
18. Ghoniem GM, Hassouna ME. Bladder neck prop using vaginal wall island for intrinsic sphincteric deficiency in elderly patients: A new technique. Urology 1998;52(4):668-72.
19. Sand PK, Winkler H, Blackhurst DW, Culligan PJ. A prospective randomized study comparing modified Burch retropubic urethropexy and suburethral sling for treatment of genuine stress incontinence with low-pressure urethra. Am J Obstet Gynecol 2000;182(1):30-34.
20. Stanton SL, Cardozo LD. Surgical treatment of incontinence in elderly women. Surg Gynecol Obstet 1980; 150:555-57.
21. Gillon G, Stanton SL. Long-term follow-up of surgery for urinary incontinence in elderly women. Br J Urol 1984;56:478-81.
22. Baker KR, Drutz HP. Age as a risk factor in major genitourinary surgery. Can J Surg 1992; 35(2):188-91.
23. Nitahara KS, Aboseif S, Tanagho EA. Long-term results of colpocystourethropexy for persistent or recurrent stress urinary incontinence. J Urol 1999;162:138-41.
24. Migliari R, Angelis D, Madeddu G, Verdacchi T. Tension-free vaginal mesh repair for anterior vaginal wall prolapse. Eur Urol 2000;38(2):151-55.
25. Herschorn S, Steele DJ, Radomski SB. Followup of intraurethral collagen for female stress urinary incontinence. J Urol 1996;156:1305-1309.
26. Herschorn S and Radomski SB. Collagen injections for genuine stress urinary incontinence: Patient selection and durability. Int Urogynecol J 1997;8:18-24.
27. Gorton E, Stanton S, Monga A, Wiskind AK, Lentz GM, Bland DR. Periurethral collagen injection: a long-term follow-up study. BJU Int 1999;44:966-971.
28. Winters JC, Chiverton A, Scarpero HM, Prats LJ, Jr. Collagen injection therapy in elderly women: Long-term results and patient satisfaction. Urology 2000;55(6):856-861.
29. Stanton SL, Monga AK. Incontinence in elderly women: is periurethral collagen an advance? Br J Obstet Gynaecol 1997;104:154-157.
30. Faerber GJ. Endoscopic collagen injection therapy in elderly women with type I stress urinary incontinence. J Urol 1996;155:512-514.
31. Monga AK, Stanton SL. Urodynamics: prediction, outcome and analysis of mechanism for cure of stress incontinence by periurethral collagen. Br J Obstet Gynaecol 1997;104:158-162.
32. Khullar V, Cardozo LD, Abbott D, Anders K. GAX collagen in the treatment of urinary incontinence in elderly women: a two year follow up. Br J Obstet Gynaecol 1997;104:96-99.
33. Monga AK, Robinson D, Stanton SL. Periurethral collagen injections for genuine stress incontinence: a 2-year follow-up. Br J Urol 1995;76:156-160.
34. Richardson TD, Dennelly MJ, Gaerber GJ. Endoscopic injection of glutaraldehyde cross-linked collagen for the treatment of intrinsic sphincter deficiency in women. Urology 1995;46:378-381.
35. O'Connell HE, McGuier EJ, Aboseif S, Usui A. Transurethral collagen therapy in women. J Urol 1995;154:1463-1475.
36. Elersgany R, Elgamasy A-N, Ghoneim GM. Transurethral collagen injection for female stress incontinence. Int Urogynecol J 1998;9:13-18.
37. Steele AC, Kohli N, Karram MM. Periurethral collagen injection for stress incontinence with and without hypermobility. Obstet Gynecol 2000;95(3):327-331.
38. Groutz A, Blaivas JG, Kesler SS, Weiss JP, and Chaikin DC. Outcome results of transurethral collagen injection for female stress incontinence: Assessment by urinary incontinence score. J Urol 2000;164:2006-2009.
39. Barranger E, Xavier F, Kadoch O, Liou Y, Pigné A. Results of transurethral injection of silicone microimplants for females with intrinsic sphincter deficiency. J Urol 2000;164:1619-1622.

40. Herschorn S and Glazer AA. Early experience with small volume periurethral polytetrafluoroethylene for female stress urinary incontinence. J Urol 2000;163:1838-1842.

14. SURGICAL INTERVENTIONS IN OLDER MEN

1. Chatelain et al (Eds). Benign Prostatic Hyperplasia. 5th International Consulation on Benign Prostatic Hyperplasia (BPH). Health Publication Ltd, Plymouth UK, 2001.
2 Palmber S, Hirsjavi E. Mortality in geriatric surgery. Gerontology 1979;25:103-112
3 Goldman L. Multifactorial index of cardiac risk in noncardiac surgery: ten-year status report. J Cardiothoracic Anesth 1987; 1:237-244.
4 Venn SN; Greenwell TJ; Mundy AR The long-term outcome of artificial urinary sphincters. J Urol 2000 Sep;164(3 Pt 1): p702-6; discussion 706-7.4.
5. Martins FE, Boyd SD. Artificial urinary sphincter in patients following major pelvic surgery and/or radiotherapy: are they less favorable candidates? [see comments]. J.Urol. 1995; 153:1188-1193.
6. Klijn AJ, Hop WC, Mickisch G, Schroder FH, Bosch JL. The artificial urinary sphincter in men incontinent after radical prostatectomy: 5 year actuarial adequate function rates. Br.J.Urol. 1998; 82:530-533.
7. Singh G, Thomas DG. Artificial urinary sphincter for post-prostatectomy incontinence. Br.J.Urol. 1996; 77:248-251.
8. Mottet N, Boyer C, Chartier-Kastler E, Ben NK, Richard F, Costa P. Artificial urinary sphincter AMS 800 for urinary incontinence after radical prostatectomy: the French experience. Urol.Int. 1998; 60 Suppl 2:25-29.
9. Haab F, Trockman BA, Zimmern PE, Leach GE. Quality of life and continence assessment of the artificial urinary sphincter in men with minimum 3.5 years of followup. J.Urol. 1997; 158:435-439.
10. Perez LM, Webster GD: Sucessful outcome of artificial urinary sphincter in men with post-prostatectomy urinary incontinence despite adverse implantation features. J.Urol. 1992; 148:1166-1170
11. Jorion JL. Rectus fascial sling suspension of the vesicourethral anastomosis after radical prostatectomy. J.Urol. 1997; 157:926-928.
12. Kakizaki H, Shibata T, Shinno Y, Kobayashi S, Matsumura K, Koyanagi T. Fascial sling for the management of urinary incontinence due to sphincter incompetence [see comments]. J.Urol. 1995; 153:644-647.
13. Shoukry MS, el-Salmy S. Urethral needle suspension for male urinary incontinence. Scand.J.Urol.Nephrol. 1997; 31:267-270.
14. Madjar S, Jacoby K, Giberti C, Wald M, Halachmi S, Issaq E, et al. Bone anchored sling for the treatment of post-prostatectomy incontinence. J.Urol.2001.Jan. 165:72-76.
15. Smith DN; Appell RA; Rackley RR; Winters JC Collagen injection therapy for post-prostatectomy incontinence. J Urol 1998 Aug;160(2): p364-7
16. Cummings JM; Boullier JA; Parra RO Transurethral collagen injections in the therapy of post-radical prostatectomy stress incontinence. J Urol 1996 Mar;155(3): p1011-3

15. PADS AND APPLIANCES

1. Fader MJ, Cottenden AM, Brooks RD. The CPE Network: creating an evidence base for continence product selection. Journal Wound Ostomy and Continence Nursing 28(2): 106-112; 2001.
2. International Standards Organisation. Basic principles for evaluation of single use adult incontinence absorbing aids from the perspective of users and caregivers. ISO 16021; 2000.
3. Clancy B, Malone-Lee J. Reducing the leakage of body-worn incontinence pads. Journal of Advanced Nursing 16:187-193; 1991.
4. Thornburn P, Fader M, Dean G, Brooks, Cottenden A. Improving the performance of small incontinence pads: a study of wet comfort. Journal of Wound Ostomy and Continence Nursing 24(4): 219-225; 1997.
5. Brown DS. Diapers and underpads, Part 1: skin integrity outcomes. Ostomy Wound-Manage 40(9): 20-28; 1994.
6. Lyder CH, Clemes-Lowrance C, Davis A, Sullivan L, Zucker A. structured skin care regimen to prevent perineal dermatitis in the elderly. Journal of Enterostomal Therapy 19(1): 12-16; 1992.
7. Orsmark K, Wilson D, Maibach H. In vitro transepidermal water loss and epidermal occlusive hydration in newborn infants: anatomical region variation. Acta Derm Venereol (Stockholm) 67: 403-407; 1980.
8. Zimmerer RE, Lawson KD, Calvert CJ. The effects of wearing diapers on skin. Pediatric Dermatology 3(2): 95-101; 1986.
9. Wilson PA, Dallas MJ. Diaper performance: maintenance of healthy skin. Pediatric Dermatology 7(3): 179-184; 1990.
10. Dallas MJ, Wilson PA. Adult incontinence products: performance evaluation on healthy skin. INDA Journal of Nonwovens Research 4(2): 26-32; 1992.
11. Grove GL, Lemmen JT, Garafalo M, Akin FJ. Assessment of skin hydration caused by diapers and incontinence articles. Current Problems in Dermatology 26: 183-195; 1998.
12. Berg RW, Buckingham KW, Stewart RL. Etiologic factors in diaper dermatitis: the role of urine. Paediatric Dermatology; 3(2): 18-20; 1986.
13. Buckingham KW, Berg RW. Etiologic factors in diaper dermatitis: the role of faeces. Paediatric Dermatology, 3 (2): 107-12; 1986.
14. International Standards Organisation. Urine absorbing aids – Part 1: Whole product testing; ISO 11948-1; 1996.
15. Cottenden AM, Ledger DJ. Predicting the leakage performance of bodyworn disposable pads using laboratory tests. Journal of Biomedical Engineering 15: 212-220; 1993.
16. International Standards Organisation. Urine absorbing aids – Part 2: Determination of short-time liquid release (leakage) under conditions of light incontinence and low pressure; ISO 11948-2; 1998.
17. Cottenden AM, Dean GE, Brooks RJ. Predicting the leakage performance of small disposable bodyworn incontinence pads using laboratory tests. Medical Engineering and Physics 19(6): 556-571; 1997.
18. International Standards Organisation. Urine absorbing aids – General guidance on evaluation. ISO 15621; 1999.
19. Henderson DJ, Rogers WF. Hospital trials of incontinence underpads. Nursing Times 4 Feb: 141-142; 1971.
20. Thornburn PH, Cottenden AM, Ledger DJ. Undercover trials. Nursing Times 88(13): 72-78; 1992.
21. Brown DS. Diapers and underpads, part 1: skin integrity outcomes. Ostomy/Wound Management 40(9): 20-32; 1994.
22. Bradbury SM. Incontinence pads and clostridium infection (letter). Journal of Hospital Infection 6(1): 115; 1985.
23. Leigh DA, Petch VJ. Sterility of incontinence pads and sheets (letter). Journal of Hospital Infection, 9: 91-93; 1987.
24. Sprott MS, Kearns AM, Keenlyside D. A microbiological study of absorbent pads. Journal of Hospital Infection 12: 125-129; 1988.
25. Stansfield R, Caudle S. Bacillus cereus and orthopaedic surgical wound infection associated with incontinence pads manufactured from virgin wood pulp. Journal of Hospital Infection 37(4): 336-338; 1997.
26. Cottenden AM, Dean GE, Brooks RJ, Haines-Nutt F, Rothwell JG, Penfold PH. Disposable bedpads for incontinence: predicting

their clinical leakage properties using laboratory tests. Medical Engineering and Physics 20: 347-359; 1998.

27. Pettersson L, Clarke-O'Neill S, Fader M, Brooks R, Cottenden A. Reusable pants with integral pad for light incontinence: an evaluation. Medical Devices Agency (London, England), September 2001.
28. Cottenden AM. Aids and appliances for incontinence. In Roe BH (ed): Clinical Nursing Practice: The promotion and management of continence, Prentice Hall, 1992.
29. Leiby DM, Shanahan N. Clinical study: assessing the performance and skin environments of two reusable underpads. Ostomy/Wound Management: 48(8): 30-37; 1994.
30. Cotteneden AM, Moore KN, Fader MJ, Cremer AWF. Is there a risk of cross-infection from laundered reusable bedpads? Bristish Journal of Nusring 8(17): 1161-1163; 1999.
31. McKibben E. Pad use in perspective. Nursing Times 91(24): 60-62; 1995.
32. Gallo M, Staskin DR. Patient satisfaction with a reusable undergarment for urinary incontinence. Journal of Wound/Ostomy and Continence Nursing 24(4): 226-236; 1997.
33. Brown DS. Diapers and underpads, part 2: cost outcomes. Ostomy/Wound Management 40(9): 34-40; 1994.
34. Gibb H, Wong G. How to choose: nurses' judgment of the effectiveness of a range of currently marketed continence aids. Journal of Clinical Nursing 3: 77-86; 1994.
35. Harper DW, O'Hara PA, Lareau J, Cass J, Black EK, Stewart A, Sigouin J. Reusable versus disposable incontinent briefs: a multiperspective crossover clinical trial. Journal of Applied Gerontology 14(4): 391-407; 1995.
36. Washington (DC): US Department of Health and Human Service. Agency for Health Care and Research. Clinical practice guidelines - managing acute and chronic urinary incontinence. Agency for Health Care and Research ;1996.
37. Falkiner FR. The insertion and management of indwelling urethral catheters-minimizing the risk of infection. J. Hosp. Infect. 25: 79-90; 1993.
38. Kunin CM, McCormack RC. Prevention of catheter-induced urinary-tract infections by sterile closed drainage. N. Engl. J. Med. 274: 1155-1161; 1966.
39. Kunin CM. Prevention of catheter-associated infections. In: Kunin CM, editor. Urinary tract infections. Detection, Prevention and Management. Baltimore: Williams and Wilkins, 245-278; 1997.
40. Warren JW. Catheter-associated urinary tract infections. Infect. Dis. Clin. North Am. 1: 823-854; 1987.
41. Newman DK. Managing indwelling urethral catheters. Ostomy. Wound. Manage. 44: 26-8, 30, 32; 1988.
42. Wilde MH. Long-term indwelling urinary catheter care: conceptualizing the research base. J. Adv. Nurs. 25: 1252-1261; 1997.
43. Ichsan J, Hunt DR. Suprapubic catheters: a comparison of suprapubic versus urethral catheters in the treatment of acute urinary retention. Aust. N.Z. J. Surg. 57: 33-36; 1987.
44. Vandoni RE, Lironi A, Tschantz P. Bacteriuria during urinary tract catheterization: suprapubic versus urethral route: a prospective randomized trial. Acta Chir. Belg. 94: 12-16; 1984.
45. Nicolle LE. Prevention and treatment of urinary catheter-related infections in older patients. Drugs Aging 4: 379-391; 1994.
46. Evans E. Indwelling catheter care: dispelling the misconceptions. Geriatr. Nurs. 20: 85-88; 1999.
47. Ouslander JG, Greengold B, Chen S. External catheter use and urinary tract infections among incontinent male nursing home patients. Journal American Geriatrics Society. 35: 1063-1070; 1987.
48. Bregenzer T, Frei R, Widmer AF, Seiler W, Probst W, Mattarelli G, et al. Low risk of bacteremia during catheter replacement in patients with long-term urinary catheters. Arch. Intern. Med. 57: 521-525; 1997.
49. Hedelin H, Bratt CG, Eckerdal G, Lincoln K. Relationship between urease-producing bacteria, urinary pH and encrustation on indwelling urinary catheters. Br. J. Urol. 67: 527-531; 1991.
50. Kunin CM, Chin QF, Chambers S. Morbidity and mortality associated with indwelling urinary catheters in elderly patients in a nursing home—confounding due to the presence of associated diseases. J. Am. Geriatr. Soc. 35: 1001-1006; 1987.
51. Ouslander JG, Greengold B, Chen S. Complications of chronic indwelling urinary catheters among male nursing home patients: a prospective study. J. Urol. 138: 1191-1195; 1987.
52. Zimakoff JD, Pontoppidan B, Larsen SO, Poulsen KB, Stickler DJ. The management of urinary catheters: compliance of practice in Danish hospitals, nursing homes and home care to national guidelines. Scand. J. Urol. Nephrol. 29: 299-309; 1995.
53. Hebel JR, Warren JW. The use of urethral, condom, and suprapubic catheters in aged nursing home patients. J. Am. Geriatr. Soc. 38: 777-784; 1990.
54 Jayachandran MD, Moopan UMM, Kim H. Complications from external (condom) urinary drainage devices. Urology 25(1): 31-34; 1985.55.
55 Saint S, Lipsky BA, Baker PD, McDonald LL, Ossenkop K. Urinary catheters: what type do men and their nurses prefer? J. Am. Geriatr. Soc. 47: 1453-1457; 1999.
56. Schiotz HA, Malme PA, Tanbo TG. Urinary tract infections and asymptomatic bacteriuria after vaginal plastic surgery. A comparison of suprapubic and transurethral catheters. Acta Obstet.Gynecol.Scand. 68: 453-455; 1989.
57. O'Kelly TJ, Mathew A, Ross S, Munro A. Optimum method for urinary drainage in major abdominal surgery: a prospective randomized trial of suprapubic versus urethral catheterization. Br. J. Surg. 82: 1367-1368; 1995.
58. Horgan AF, Prasad B, Waldron DJ, O'Sullivan DC. Acute urinary retention. Comparison of suprapubic and urethral catheterisation. Br. J. Urol. 70: 149-151; 1992.
59. Bakke A, Brun OH, Hoisaeter PA. Clinical background of patients treated with clean intermittent catheterization in Norway. Scand. J. Urol. Nephrol. 26: 211-217; 1992.
60. Garibaldi RA, Burke JP, Dickman ML, Smith CB. Factors predisposing to bacteriuria during indwelling urethral catheterization. N. Engl. J. Med. 291: 215-219; 1974.
61. Yoshikawa TT, Nicolle LE, Norman DC. Management of complicated urinary tract infection in older patients. J. Am. Geriatr. Soc. 44: 1235-1241; 1996.
62. Hardyck C, Petrinovich L. Reducing urinary tract infections in catheterized patients. Ostomy. Wound. Manage. 44: 36-3; 1998.
63. Fader M, Pettersson L, Brooks R, Dean G, Wells M, Cottenden A, Malone-Lee J. A multicentre comparative evaluation of catheter valves. British Journal of Nursing 6(7): 359-367; 1997.
64. Golji H. Complications of external condom drainage. Paraplegia 19: 189-197; 1981.
65. Hirsh DD, Fainstein V, Musher DM. Do condom catheter collecting systems cause urinary tract infection? JAMA 242(4): 340-341; 1979.
66. Medical Devices Agency (UK). Penile sheaths: a comparative evaluation. 1995.
67. Fader M, Pettersson L, Dean G, Brooks R, Cottenden A, Malone-Lee J. Sheaths for urinary incontinence: a randomized crossover trial. BJU International 87: 367-372; 2001.
68. Pieper B. Inventing urine incontinence devices for women. Journal of Nursing Scholarship 21(4): 205-209; 1989.
69. Johnson DE, Muncie HL, O'Reilly JL, Warren JW. An external

urine collection device for incontinent women. Evaluation of long-term use. J.Am.Geriatr.Soc. 1990; 38:1016-1022.

70. Kennedy AP, Brocklehurst JC, Faragher B. A comparison of 10 urinary drainage bags. Nursing Times, August 17, 1983: 56-60.

71. Wilson M, Coates D. Infection control and urine drainage bag design. Professional Nurse 11(4): 245-252; 1996.

72. Medical Devices Agency (UK). Sterile 500 ml leg bags for urine drainage. 1996.

73. Fader M, Pettersson L, Brooks R, Cottenden A. Selecting leg bags for sheath users: evaluation results. British Journal Community Nursing 4(7): 312-327; 1999.

74. Glenister H. The passage of infection. Nursing Times 83(22): 6873; 1987.

75. Fader M, Pettersson L, Dean G, Brooks R, Cottenden A. The selection of female urinals: results of a multicentre evaluation. British Journal Nursing 8(14): 918-925; 1999.

16. PREVENTION

1. Palmer, M, Interdisciplinary approaches to the treatment of urinary incontinence in older adults. Topics in Geriatric Rehabilitation, 16(1), 1-9, 2000.

2. Melchiro, H., Kumar, V., Muller, N., Van Maannen & NortonN C. National public health policies for prevention and care in urinary incontinence in the elderly. World Journal of Urology, 16[Suppl 1], S71-S72, 1998.

3. Fonda, D., Resnick, N. & Kirschner-Hermanns, R. Prevention of urinary incontinence in older people. British Journal of Urology, 82(Suppl 1), 5-10, 1998.

4. Roberts, RO., Jacobsen, SJ., Rhodes, T., Reilly, WT., Girman, CJ., Talley, NJ. & Lieber, MM. Urinary Incontinence in a Community-Based Cohort: Prevalence and Healthcare-Seeking. Journal of the American Geriatrics Society, 46(4), 467-472, 1998.

5. Palmer, M. A new framework for urinary continence outcomes in long-term care. Urologic Nursing, 16(4), 146-151, 1996.

6. Nygaard, IE. & Lemke, JH. Urinary Incontinence in Rural Older Women: Prevalence, Incidence and Remission. Journal of the American Geriatrics Society, 44(9), 1049-1054, 1996.

7. Cohen, S., Robinson, D., Dugan, E., Howard, G., Suggs, P., Pearce, K., Carroll, D., McGann, P. & Preisser, J. Communication between older adults and their physicians about urinary incontinence. Journal of Gerontology: MEDICAL SCIENCES, 54A(1), M34-M37, 1999.

8. Dugan, E., Roberts, C., Cohen, S., Preisser, J., Davis, C., Bland, D. & Albertson, E. Why older community-dwelling adults do not discuss urinary incontinence with their primary care physicians. Journal of the American Geriatrics Society, 9(4), 462-465, 2001.

9. Johnson, TM., Kincaide, JE., Bernard, SL, Busby-Whitehead, J., & DeFriese, GH. Self-Care Practices Used by Older Men and Women to Manage Urinary Incontinence: Results from the National Follow-Up Survey on Self-Care and Aging. Journal of the American Geriatrics Society, 48(8), 894-902, 2000.

10. Niewijk, A. & Weijts, W. Effects of a multi-media course on urinary incontinence. Patient education and counseling, 30, 95-103, 1997.

11. Johnson, T., Kincaide, J., Bernard, S., Busby-Whitehead, J., Hertz-Piccioto, I. & Defriese, G. The association of urinary incontinence with poor self-rated health. Journal of the American Geriatrics Society, 46(6), 693-699, 1998.

12. Ouslander, J. Uman, G., Urman, H. & Rubenstein, L. Incontinence among nursing home patients: Clinical and functional correlates. Journal of the American Geriatrics Society, 35(4), 324-330, 1987.

13. Palmer, M., German, P. & Ouslander, J. Risk factors for urinary incontinence one year after nursing home admission. Research in Nursing and Health, 14, 405-412, 1991.

14. Brown, J., Seeley, D. Fong, J., Black, D., Ensrud, K., Grady, D. For the study of osteoporotic fractures research group. Urinary incontinence in older women: Who is at risk? Obstetrics & Gynecology, 87(5 Part 1), 715-721, 1996.

15. Tinetti, M., Inouye, S., Gill, T. & Doucette, J. Shared risk factors for falls, incontinence, and functional dependence. Journal of the American Medical Association, 273(17), 1348-1353, 1995.

16. Brandeis, G. The Prevalence of Potentially Remediable Urinary Incontinence in Frail Older People: A Study Using the Minimum Data Set. Journal of the American Geriatrics Society, 45(2), 179-184, 1997.

17. Wetle, T., Scherr, P., Branch, LG., Resnick, NM., Harris, T., Evans, D. & Taylor, JO. Difficulty with Holding Urine Among Older Persons in a Geographically Defined Community: Prevalence and Correlates. Journal of the American Geriatrics Society, 43(4), 349-355, 1995.

18. Skelley, J. & Flint, A. Urinary incontinence associated with dementia. Journal of the American Geriatrics Society, 43(3), 286-294, 1995.

19. Hunskaar, S., Ostbye, T. & Borrie, M. The Prevalence of Urinary Incontinence in Elderly Canadians and its Association with Dementia, Ambulatory Function, and Institutionalization. Norwegian Journal of Epidemiology, 8(2), 177-182, 1998.

20. Palmer, M., Myers, A. & Fedenko, K. Urinary continence changes after hip fracture repair. Clinical Nursing Research, 6(1), 8-24, 1997.

21. Jirovec, MM. & Templin, T. Predicting Success Using Individualized Scheduled Toileting for Memory-Impaired Elders at Home. Research in Nursing & Health, volume number, 1-8, 2001.

22. Brown, J., Sawaya, G. Thom, D. & Grady, D. Hysterectomy and urinary incontinence: a systemic review. The Lancet, 356, 535-539, 2000.

23. Arya, L., Myers, D., & Jackson, N. Dietary caffeine intake and risk for detrusor instability: A case-control study. Obstetrics & Gynecology, 96(1), 85-89, 2000.

24. Koskimaki, J., Hakama, M., Huhtala, H. & Tammela, T. Association of Smoking with Lower Urinary Tract Symptoms. The Journal of Urology, 159, 1580-1582, 1998.

25. Brocklehurst, J., Andrews, K., Richards, B. & Laycock, P. Incidence and correlates of incontinence in stroke patients. Journal of the American Geriatrics Society, 33(8), 540-542, 1985.

26. Barer, D. Continence after stroke: Useful predictor or goal of therapy? Age and Ageing, 18, 183-191, 1989.

27. Borrie, M., Campbell, A., Caradoc-Davies & Spears, G. Urinary incontinence after stroke: A prospective study. Age and Ageing, 15, 177-181, 1986.

28. Nakayama, H., Jorgensen, HS., Pedersen, PM., Raaschou, HO. & Olsen, TS. Prevalence and Risk Factors of Incontinence After Stroke. Stroke, 28(1), 58-62, 1997.

29. Tomlinson, BU., Dougherty, MC., Pendergast, JF., Boyington, AR., Coffman, MA. & Pickens, SM. Dietary Caffeine, Fluid Intake and Urinary Incontinence in Older Rural Women. International Urogynecology Journal 10, 22-28, 1999.

30. Agency for Health Care Policy and Research. Urinary Incontinence in Adults: Acute and Chronic Management. Clinical Practice Guideline, Number 2, Update. US Department of Health and Human Services. AHCRP Publication No.96-0682, 1996.

31. Roberts, R., Jacobsen, S., Reilly, W., Pemberton, J., Lieber, M. & Talley, N. Prevalence of combined fecal and urinary incontinence: A community-based study. Journal of the American Geriatrics Society, 47(7), 837-841, 1999.

Committee 10 E

Conservative Management in Neuropathic Urinary Incontinence

Chairman

H. Madersbacher (Austria)

Vice-Chairmen

J.J. Wyndaele (Belgium),

Y. Igawa (Japan)

Members

M. Chancellor (USA),

E. Chartier-Kastler (France),

A. Kovindha (Thailand)

CONTENTS

Conservative Management in Neuropathic Urinary Incontinence

H. Madersbacher,

J.J. Wyndaele, Y. Igawa,

M. Chancellor, E. Chartier-Kastler, A. Kovindha

A. INTRODUCTION

This chapter deals with the conservative treatment of urinary incontinence due to neurological pathology, which can be caused by (a) suprapontine, (b) spinal cord and (c) subsacral (cauda equina and peripheral nerves) lesions (Figure1).

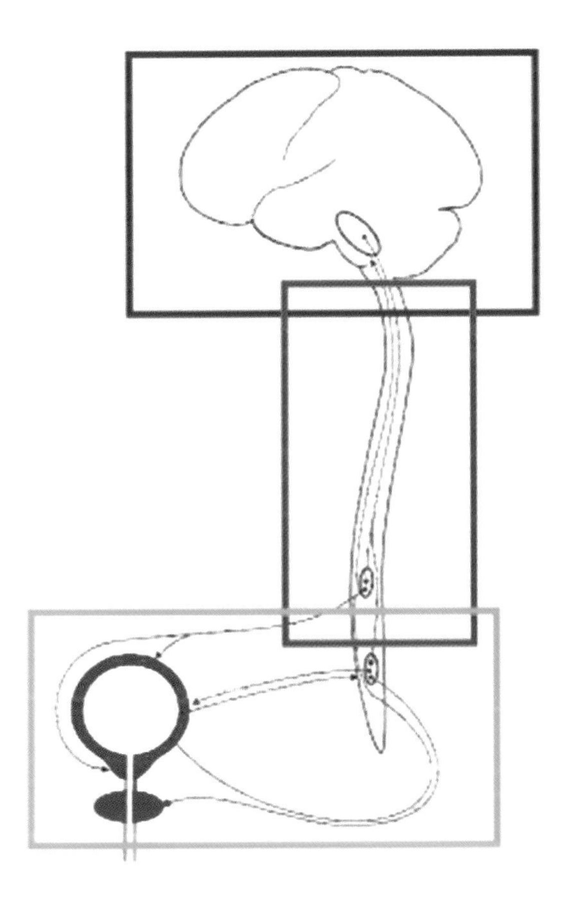

Figure 1 : Nervous control of continence and micturition is organised on a cerebral, spinal and peripheral level. All three are cross-linked, the circuiting is complex and contentious.

I. SUPRAPONTINE LESIONS

In suprapontine lesions urinary incontinence results from uninhibited detrusor contractions [Brocklehurst et al 1985]. This detrusor hyperreflexia is caused by damage to the cerebral inhibitory centers. Patients with lesions above the level of the pons characteristically demonstrate synergetic activity of the detrusor and the external sphincter [Tsuchida et al 1983]. Patients with suprapontine lesions may, however, purposely increase sphincteric activity during an uninhibited detrusor contraction to avoid urge incontinence. This guarding reflex or pseudo-dyssynergia may be confused with true dyssynergia by those less familiar with the interpretation of urodynamic studies [Siroky et al 1982].

In the absence of other urinary disease, such as outflow obstruction, as long as external sphincter activity remains coordinated with detrusor contraction, intravesical pressure should remain physiologic and therefore preserve the function of the urinary tracts. Residual urine may either be due to a coexisting morphologic infravesical obstruction, rigidity and spasticity of the pelvic floor (e.g. Parkinsons Disease) or due to a voluntary contraction of the external sphincter to control unhibitable detrusor contractions, a phenomenon, which has already become a reflex pattern in some patients.

A frequent reason for supraspinal detrusor hyperreflexia, causing reflex incontinence, are cerebrovascular accidents. A significant number of new stroke patients develop urinary retention for several weeks before detrusor hyperreflexia occurs. This phase of detrusor areflexia may be named "cerebral shock" much alike the classic "spinal shock" phase immediately after a spinal cord injury. Parkinsons Disease is one of the most common neurological entities causing voiding dysfunction, classically resulting in detrusor hyperreflexia, detrusor bradykinesia and an impairment of relaxation of the striated sphincter. According to Holliger et al (2001, in press), detrusor overactivity increases with progress and severeness of the disease and can then be found in up to 90 % of patients [Berger et al 1987]. Another reason for supraspinal reflex incontinence is dementia. The defect in cognitive function is responsible for the lack of social continence in these patients. In brain neoplasms alterations in lower urinary tract function tend to relate directly to the area of the brain affected.

Shy and Drager described a neurological syndrome characterized by autonomic dysfunction consisting of orthostatic hypotension, anhydrosis, impotence, extrapyramidal symptoms and poor urinary and fecal control [Wulfsohn et al 1981], however, the term mutiple system atrophy nowadays involves various syndroms, resulting in degeneration of neurons and associated fibers of motor and extrapyramidal systems including the cerebellum and brain stem. The urinary symptoms of incontinence are primarily caused by detrusor hyperreflexia although some element of external sphincter weakness may be present, with an open bladder neck during cystography indicating peripheral sympathetic dysfunction. The combination of detrusor dysfunction and sphincter denervation contraindicates the surgical management of symptoms [Beck et al 1994].

II. SPINAL CORD LESIONS

The degree of dysfunction is related to the disease process itself, the area of the spinal cord affected by the disease, and the severity of neurological impairment. Neurological injury, which can involve parasympathetic, sympathetic, and somatic nerve fibers, can result in a complex combination of signs and symptoms. The urodynamic investigation of those with neurological impairment can provide objective information regarding the nature and extent of the effect on lower urinary tract function. For this reason, urodynamic testing should be an integral part in the evaluation of all patients with complete and incomplete spinal cord dysfunction. In spinal cord injury (SCI) nearly 55% of patients develop tetraplegia, while 45% become paraplegic, neurologically incomplete injuries are slightly more common (53.8%) than complete injuries (46.2%) [Watanabe et al 1996].

Neurogenic lower urinary tract dysfunction resulting from SCI is an excellent model for the understanding of neuro-urological dysfunction (see below).

In multiple sclerosis voiding dysfunction is mainly due to spinal lesions, although cerebral lesions may contribute. Impairment of neurological function results from demyelinating plaques of the white matter of the brain and spinal cord, especially the posterior and lateral columns of the cervical cord, which serve as pathways for neurologic control over vesical and urethral function [Nathan & Smith 1982]. Symptoms of voiding dysfunction are appreciated by 90% of patients having the disease more than 10 years. These include not only frequency, urgency, and urge incontinence, but also urinary hesitancy, intermittency, and poor urinary stream.

Urodynamically, the most common pattern seen is detrusor hyperreflexia (in about 70%), 50% accompanied by detrusor-external sphincter dyssynergia [Goldstein et al 1982; Weinstein et al 1988; Sirls et al 1994]. Detrusor areflexia, associated with lower cord and cauda equina plaques, is seen in 20% to 30% of cases, and these patients usually strained to void [Gonor et al 1985]. The latter symptoms are caused by plaque formation in the sacral cord, impairing motor outflow to the detrusor.

Beside these most important reasons many other neurological lesions, affecting the spinal cord, may cause storage and emptying problems, e.g. transverse myelitis or the tethered cord syndrom, caused by a short filum terminale, intraspinal lipoma or fibres adhesions resulting from the surgical repair of spinal dysraphism [Al-Mefty et al 1979]. Detrusor areflexia has been reported to occur in 60% of the patients.

III. SUBSACRAL (CAUDA EQUINA AND PERIPHERAL NERVES) LESIONS

These lesions may affect the cauda equina including the sacral roots and the peripheral nerves. According to neurological classifications lesions of the conus, causing dysfunction of the peripheral neuron, are classified as peripheral lesions. For practical reasons these lesions, named for decades as lower motor neuron lesions of the spinal cord, are subsummarized under spinal lesions.

Pelvic plexus injury, common with abdominal perineal resection and hysterectomy, contains both parasympathetic and sympathetic fibers in a branching array, parasagittally adjacent to the rectum. Disruption of the pelvic plexus function may occur with traumatic pelvic fracture. Injury to the hypogastric, pelvic and sometimes also pudendal nerves results in damage to sympathetic, parasympathetic and somatic nerve fibers and, consequently, lower urinary tract dysfunction. Decreased parasympathetic innervation generally results in decreased detrusor contractility and potentially areflexia, while impaired sympathetic transmission results in incomplete bladder neck closure, internal sphincter dysfunction, and stress incontinence. Up to 80% of patients with voiding disturbances after significant pelvic procedures will resume normal voiding within 6 months [Blaivas, Chancellor 1995], if the urological management inbetween is adequate.

Another common medical condition, which causes neurogenic lower urinary tract dysfunction, is diabetes mellitus.

Deficits in bladder sensation occur initially, with insidious onset, usually associated with other sensory impairment. Classically, patients experience decreased urinary frequency, urinary hesitancy, and slowing of the urinary stream, symptoms which may progress even to urinary dribbling from overflow incontinence [Appel, Whiteside 1991]. Urodynamic studies commonly reveal impaired bladder sensation, increased cystometric bladder capacity, decreased detrusor contractility, an impaired uroflow, and an elevated post-void residual urine volume [Blaivas 1988]. One urodynamically controlled study showed detrusor hyperreflexia in 55%, while only 33% had either impaired contractility or areflexia [Kaplan et al 1995]. Diabetics with voiding symptoms are generally elderly people and subject to infection, outlet obstruction, and uninhibited detrusor contraction like others in this age group, which may contribute to these results.

Moreover, herpes zoster affecting the dorsal ganglion, Lyme disease with symptoms caused by encephalopathy, polyneuropathy and leukoencephalitis as well as Guillain-Barré syndrome, which represents an inflammatory demyelinating polyneuropathy affecting mainly the peripheral nervous system with a predilection to the nerve roots, may cause neurogenic voiding dysfunction with recovery depending on the course of the neurological disease.

Pattern of Lower Urinary Tract Dysfunction and Therapeutic Principles

Neurogenic urinary incontinence may be due to

1. **dysfunction of the detrusor,**
2. **dysfunction of the sphincter** and
3. **a combination of both.**

1. **Detrusor hyperreflexia leads to reflex-incontinence, detrusor areflexia to incontinence associated with poor bladder emptying** (previously and in the following named overflow-incontinence),

2. **an areflexic (incompetent) sphincter causes neurogenic stress-incontinence, a hyperreflexic (spastic) sphincter overflow-incontinence** and

3. quite often **detrusor and sphincter are affected simultaneously mostly from the same type** by the neurogenic lesions but also a dissociation may be possible, moreover, a normal functioning counterpart may be present with basically eight combinations, as shown in figure 2.

In most patients the storage problem, leading to incontinence, is associated with an emptying problem; therefore both aspects have to be considered at the same time.

Therapy of neurogenic incontinence is primarily a conservative one. Timed bladder emptying, by whatever means, controlled fluid-intake and avoidance of urinary tract infections are the prerequisites for successful treatment.

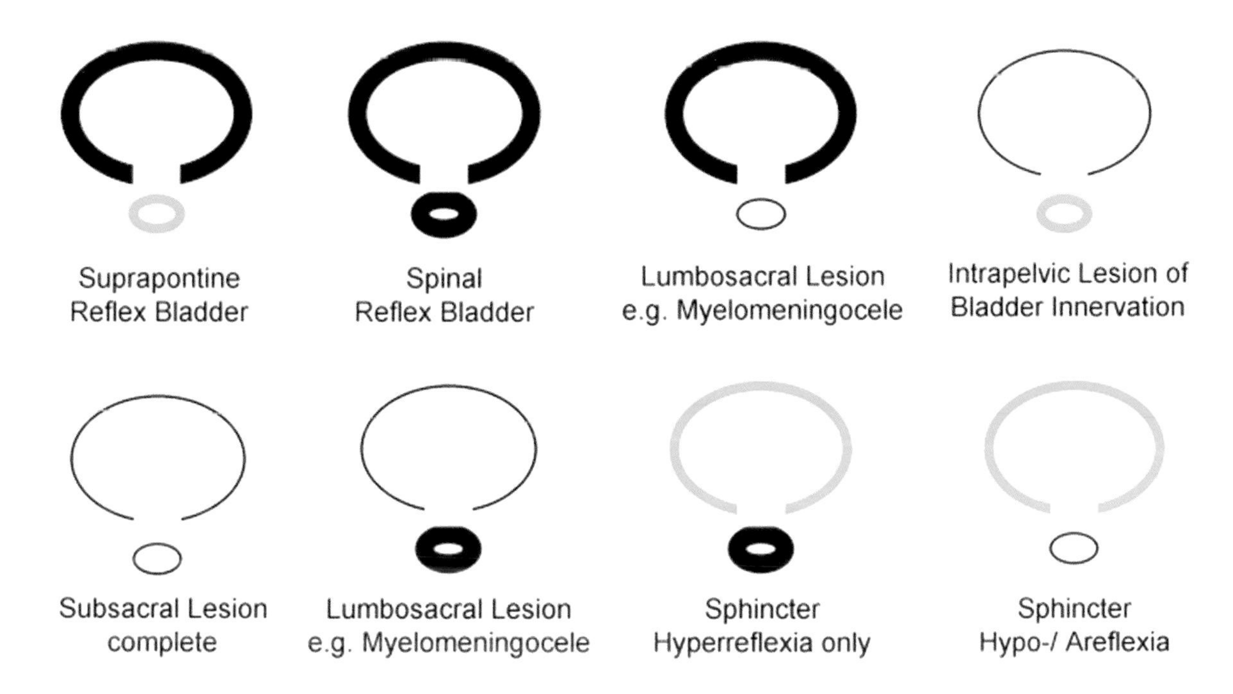

Figure 2 : Patterns of neurogenic detrusor-sphincter dysfunction Heavy lines symbolize hyperreflexia, thin lines hypo- or areflexia and green lines a normal innervation of the relevant structure, for further explanation see text.

In **I. Supraspinal lesions** detrusor hyperreflexia is mostly combined with normal sphincter function, reflex incontinence is the main symptom and anticholinergic therapy together with behavioural treatment, especially in patients with cognitive impairment, is the method of choice.

II. Spinal lesions mostly cause simultaneous dysfunction of the detrusor and the sphincter.

In **suprasacral lesions** the combination of a hyperreflexic detrusor with a hyperreflexic sphincter is characteristic for the spinal reflex bladder. Basically spontaneous reflex voiding is possible, however, it is uncontrolled, causing reflex-incontinence and is mostly unbalanced and basically unphysiologic. Detrusor contractions are mostly inadequate, and detrusor striated sphincter dyssynergia is present, both leading to unbalanced voiding with the possibility of a dangerous high pressure situation (Figure 3).

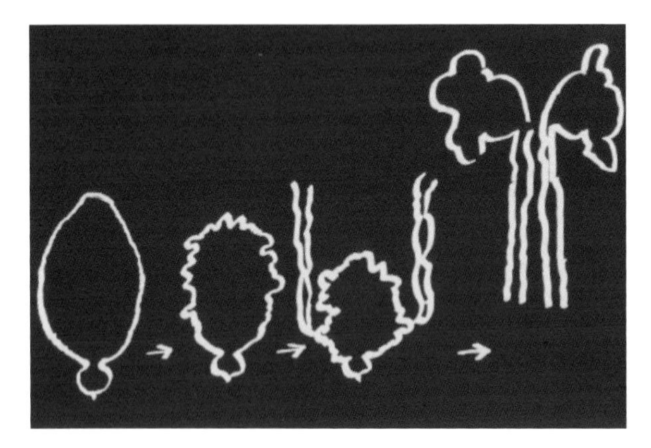

Figure 3 : Consequences of detrusor-sphincter dyssynergia: it creates a functional infravesical obstruction with the possible consequence of an intravesical high pressure situation, causing reflux, hydronephrosis and kidney-detoriation

Triggered reflex voiding is recommended only if it is urodynamically safe and reflex incontinence is manageable. The method of choice nowadays to empty an unbalanced reflex bladder and to manage reflex-incontinence is *intermittent (self-) catheterization*. However, to achieve the aims of therapy, - a low pressure situation and continence between catheterizations - additional *pharmacotherapy* may be necessary.

If bladder relaxing agents fail or are not tolerable, *electrotherapy* is an alternative in incomplete lesions: anogenital electrostimulation (penile, clitoral, vaginal and anal) can inhibit detrusor hyperreflexia by stimulating pudendal nerve afferents.

If none of the above mentioned treatment modalities is effective to control reflex incontinence and if operative procedures are not indicated/possible, appliances are the next choice, condom-catheters in males and pads in females.

The indwelling catheter – a suprapubic catheter is preferable to transurethral – remains the last resort for conservative therapy.

For complete **conus lesions**, also named lower motor neuron lesions, **areflexia of the detrusor with areflexia of the sphincter** is characteristic. Sphincter incompetence causes neurogenic urinary stress incontinence and may be combined with overflow-incontinence if adequate emptying is not achieved.

Basically, regular bladder emptying achieved by bladder expression, according to the individual bladder capacity, in combination with controlled fluid intake may decrease neurogenic urinary stress incontinence. However, continence is hard to achieve. *Bladder expression* is potentially dangerous. Pharmacotherapy is not helpful in this situation, appliances and condom catheters are therefore often necessary, continence can often be achieved only by operative therapy.

Areflexia of the detrusor combined with hyperreflexia of the sphincter may occur in lesions, comprising the conus and nearby areas above, however, this pattern may be also due to a decompensation of a hyperreflexic bladder after chronic urinary retention.

With this combination overflow incontinence can be controlled by intermittent catheterization mostly without additional pharmacotherapy. If intermittent catetherisation is not possible an indwelling catheter, preferable suprapubically, may be needed.

If **hyperreflexia of the detrusor is combined with areflexia of the sphincter**, a pattern sometimes found in epiconal lesions, especially in myelomeningoceles, reflex incontinence is combined with neurogenic stress incontinence. Bladder relaxant agents may abolish or deminish detrusor hyperreflexia. In incomplete lesions electrical stimulation of the pelvic floor musculature may improve sphincter function. Thus the combination of pharmacotherapy to treat reflex incontinence with electrotherapy of the pelvic floor muscle improves continence. However, with this type of neurogenic lower urinary tract dysfunction conservative treatment alone is generally unable to restore continence; therefore either appliances or operative treatment must be considered.

III. **Subsacral (cauda equina and peripheral nerves) lesion** are often incomplete lesions, hyporeflexia or areflexia of the detrusor may be combined with a normally functioning external striated sphincter, a combination which can be seen after intrapelvic surgery, when the pudendal nerve remaines intact. On the other side if the pudendal nerve is lesioned and the pelvic plexus remaines more or less intact, a combination of a normally functioning detrusor with a hypo- or areflexic external sphincter may be present. For a hyperreflexic detrusor, again, pharmacotherapy is the first choice. In the hyporeflexic detrusor cholinergics may increase the tone. If the lesions were incomplete, intravesical electrotherapy was reported to increase detrusor contractility. The chances for pharmacotherapy to improve external sphincter weakness as well as to decrease external sphincter spasticity are poor and operative therapy remains the therapy of choice.

B. BEHAVIOURAL THERAPY

I. TRIGGERED REFLEX VOIDING

1. Background

Following severe cord or cauda equina injury, the paralysed bladder behaves like an inert elastic bag and is unable to adapt itself to its contents or expel them. This areflexic phase is followed gradually by recovery of detrusor activity. The true automatic or reflex bladder occurs following recovery from spinal shock in spinal cord lesions not involving the conus or cauda equina. If the latters or the efferent branches of the pelvic nerve are involved, the reflex emptying is much less complete and considerable voluntary straining is required to empty the bladder to a satisfactory degree. It was just before World War II that Denny-Brown and Robertson (1933) did recognise this evolution of disturbance of micturition [Dick et al 1952].

With time concepts have been evolving and referring to Bors & Comarr (1971), stimulation of the sacral and lumbar dermatomes should be used to elicit reflex contractions of the detrusor in cases with upper motor neuron bladders and during treatment with intermittent or continuous catheterization, to evaluate if reflex voiding would be possible and an alternative.

The aims of regular triggered reflex voiding are to achieve balanced voiding [Corcos, Schick 1996], to decrease incontinence and/or to achieve continence [Wein et al 1984]. The prerequisites for this type of bladder emptying are: (1) the possibility of collecting the urine in a socially acceptable way and (2) the time needed for bladder emptying is adequate.

2. Objectives

To find evidence to answer the following questions:

1. How and when to do it?
2. Is it effective?
3. Is it safe?
4. Is it cost-effective?
5. Complications and how to treat them

3. Criteria for considering studies

The search was made from 1966 to 2000. Considering the historical aspect of this voiding management of bladder dysfunction, passed references are taken from books reporting on neurogenic bladder before 1970's [Bors, Comarr 1971].

Through Pubmed the following keywords were searched: Bladder, Neurogenic/etiology; Bladder, neurogenic/physiopathology. Case report. Child. Female. Human. Infant. Male. Urination disorders/congenital. Urination disorders/complications.

Qality of included studies. We did not find any prospective cohort study of patients using triggered voiding or any controlled or randomised study (Level evidence 4).

There are a few new references published within the last 3 years (1998- 2000) to be added to the previous report (1st ICI 1998).

4. Results

a) How and when to do it?

Referring to the ICS committee on standardisation of terminology [Andersen et al, 1992] bladder reflex triggering comprises various manoeuvres performed by patients in order to elicit reflex detrusor contractions by exteroceptive stimuli (Figure 4). The most commonly used manoeuvres are: suprapubic tapping, thigh scratching and anal/rectal manipulation. Frequency of use, intervals and duration have to be specified for each patient. Integrity of sacral reflex are requested for such voiding manoeuvres.

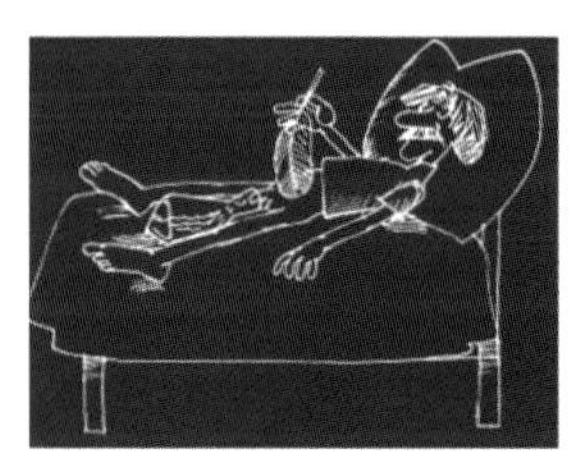

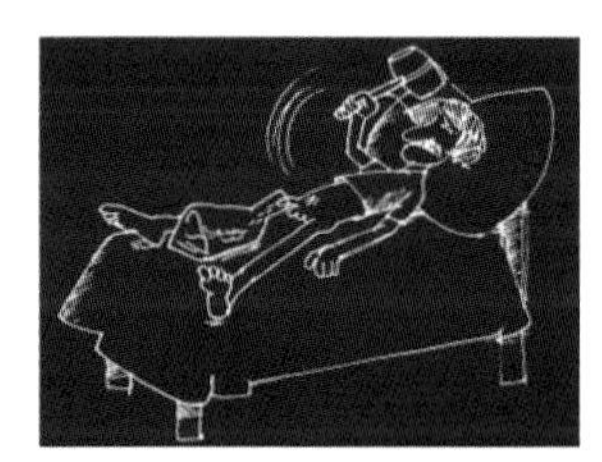

Figure 4 : Triggered reflex voiding comprises various techniques, the patient must find the best individual trigger zone and points (the technique on the left side is propably more effective than that on the right side ...)

Stimuli consist of [Bors, Comarr 1971; Wein et al 1984]:

- squeezing of glans penis or scrotal skin
- pulling on the pubic hair
- tapping the suprapubic areas
- stroking the skin of the thigh or the sole of the foot
- rectal digital stimulation

The latter has been described as the most effective stimuli for "triggered voiding" [Rossier, Bors 1964]. However the most popular and probably the most efficient and easy to do is inducing contractions with rhythmic suprapubic manual pressure. These manoeuvres are assumed to produce a summation effect on the tension receptors in the bladder wall, resulting in an afferent neural discharge, which activates the bladder reflex arc [Wein, Barret, 1988].

Today, learning of triggered voiding should not be done without taking care of:

1. Bladder outlet obstruction management;

2. Continence;

3. Appliances;

4. Gender; and

5. Level and type (complete or incomplete lesions). Literature cannot be seriously interpreted due to retrospective studies with none or poor specification of bladder outlet obstruction management associated with triggering reflex voiding.

There are two different steps in the management of reflex voiding in the neuropathic. Guidelines could be proposed as follows:

1. Period of recovery of bladder activity and type of drainage waiting for it: Use intermittent catheterization as soon as possible with voiding diary and do urodynamic study when signs of bladder wake-up are arriving (leakage, autonomic dysreflexia related to filling of the bladder, bladder sensation)
2. Period of full bladder activity: regular watching of bladder pressures, dyssynergia and upper tract deterioration (every six months).

Special attention must be taken to the problems of balance between continence and protection of upper tract, sex differences, level of the lesion and neurological handicap (para- vs tetraplegic patients).

There are few data comparing different types of voiding management. One is Bennett et al (1995) in female (Level of evidence 4). It shows that a definite trend as the management method of choice in contrast to reflex voiding and padding (or also indwelling catheter) is intermittent catheterization with anticholinergic therapy (statistically significant difference in long-term groups from 11 to 23 years). Some authors, Yokoyama et al, 1996 (Level of evidence 4) argue against triggered voiding because of high risk of upper tract deterioration during long periods with a full bladder.

The best choice of treatment for long-term use can be done with help of the analysis of 8 factors described by Maynard & Diokno (1982) (Level of evidence 4):

- Type of neurogenic bladder
- Prognosis of recovery
- Incontinence
- History of urethral trauma
- Decreased host resistance
- Dependence in catheterization
- Compliance (of patient)
- Patient preference (with informed choices)

One additional indication could be a tetraplegic patient who is unable to perform self-catheterization but able to do tapping or triggered voiding. They choose this option because it gives possible independence.

b) Is it effective?

The question of effectiveness of triggered voiding is separated as follows:

Is it an effective way of protecting upper urinary tract?

Is it an effective way of emptying the bladder?

Is it an effective way of ensuring a good quality of life for patients?

Is it an effective way of controlling incontinence?

So far no studies in the literature are able to give good answers to all these questions.

c) Is it safe?

This technique could be safe if patients are able to have adequate follow-up and monitored (see recommendations). As it is reported that complications occur more often in the first 15 years [Lamid 1988; van Kerrebroeck 1993; Gupta, Chawla 1994; Weld 2000] (Level of evidence 4), it is not recommended for patients who may fail to return for regular urological follow-up. Canupp et al (1997) reported reasons for poor compliance with regular follow-up: belief that follow-up was not necessary, cost of investigations, good local doctors, distance and transportation. These indicate a need to improve patient education.

According to Frankel et al (1998) reporting on a fifty year investigation in a spinal cord injury cohort, the risk of death related to a urological dysfunction is decreasing 50% each ten years. This was due to improvement of evaluation, indications, follow-up and urodynamics study. In addition the rate of patients using CISC was increasing and could be part of this success. Therefore it is not possible to give conclusion on the safety of triggered voiding (Level of evidence 4).

d) Is it cost-effective?

No studies on cost-effectiveness are available.

e) Complications

Complications such as clinically significant infections, upper urinary tract alteration/deterioration, autonomic dysreflexia have been reported in the past reports, levels of evidence 4 or lower. New publications did not report specifically on this topic [Weld 2000; Canupp et al 1997; Sekar 1997; McKinley 1999; MacDiarmid 2000; Yavuzer et al, 2000].

CONCLUSIONS

Reflex voiding is based on an unphysiological sacral reflex. It is potentially dangerous and has a limited role in managing the reflex bladder at present.

The long-term complication rate is not as high as with indwelling catheter, but enough to suggest a trend to avoid this triggered reflex voiding in detrusor hyperreflexia.

Costs of appliances and of adjuvant therapies (pharmacotherapy, surgery, urethral prosthesis etc) have to be evaluated.

Treatment of infralesional spasticity and co-morbidity should be taken into consideration.

5. Implications for practice

Before considering triggered reflex emptying, check if the bladder situation is urodynamically safe and if regular follow-up is guaranteed. The frequency of check-up is not validates, depends on risk factors, but should be between 6 months and 2 years.

Each patient has to find his best way of triggered reflex voiding. Adequate management of reflex incontinence is essential. Social continence may be achieved only by controlling fluid intake and regular bladder emptying according to each personal schedule.

Be sure that type of bladder emptying is socially (and sexually) acceptable to permit an adequate quality of life.

To improve emptying and control autonomic dysreflexia related to bladder filling and contraction, alpha-blockers should be tried before sphincterotomy and/or bladder neck incision is performed.

In a well-developed country, triggered voiding should not be recommended as the first line management of bladder hyperreflexia and micturition. Intermittent catheterization has become the gold standard to achieve continence, upper urinary tract protection and improvement of quality of life (see recommendations in the chapter of intermittent catheterization).

RECOMMENDATIONS

Triggered voiding could be recommended for patients whose situation has proven to be urodynamically safe and stable, and who can manage reflex incontinence. Moreover it is recommended for patients after sphincterotomy and/or bladder neck incision and/or alpha-blockers, in order to improve spontaneous reflex voiding.

Reflex voiding can only be recommended if an adequate follow-up is guaranteed. (Grande of recommendation C)

6. Implications for research

Due to lack of controlled studies and less patients using such bladder management nowadays, clinical research is recommended on the following issues:

- Alpha-blockers effect (see related chapter)

- Urodynamics pre- and post-sphincterotomy and/or bladder neck incision

- Long-term retrospective cohorts comparing triggered voiding with other types of management (e.g. CISC)

- Quality of life assessment

For future developments this topic should be analysed in accordance to sphincter status (sphincterotomy or not, alpha-blockers or not, bladder neck incision or not) and not as an isolated voiding management.

7. Acknowledgement

We would like to acknowledge the GENULF (French speaking neurourology study group) and its president (Jean-Jacques Labat, MD, Rehab. Phys., Nantes, France) who provided powerful information through its work.

8. Potential conflict of interest:

None

II. BLADDER EXPRESSION (CREDÉ AND VALSALVA)

1. Background

Bladder expression has been recommended since a long time for patients with so-called lower motor neuron lesions, resulting in a combination of an underactive detrusor with an underactive sphincter or with an incompetent urethral closure mechanism of other origin (e.g. after sphincterotomy).

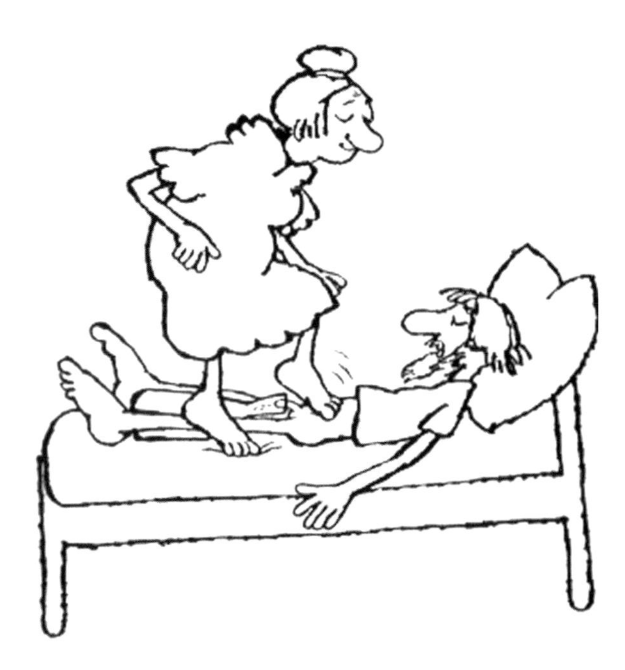

Figure 5 : Bladder expression comprises various manouvres, aimed at increasing intravesical pressure to enable / to facilitate bladder emptying.... (for details see text).

Difficulties in emptying the bladder by expression may be due to (1) an inability to open the bladder neck. However, especially in men, these techniques induce (2) a functional obstruction at the level of the striated external sphincter despite complete paralysis of the musculature of the pelvic floor. The pathophysiological mechanism of the bladder expression via Valsalva and Credé was evaluated by Madersbacher (1977) : voiding-cystourethrograms during these techniques show a typical bending, deformation and narrowing of the membranous urethra at the level of the pelvic floor. The interpretation of this phenomenon is, that during Valsalva and Credé, the bladder and its outlet are forced downwards and backwards, while the penile urethra is fixed via the Lig. suspensorium penis to the pubic symphysis. Thus the urethra becomes compressed by the musculature of the pelvic floor. Any further increase of the intraabdominal pressure increases the deformation of the membranous urethra and makes bladder emptying worse. This functional narrowing cannot be recognized by a retrograde urethrogram, nor felt by catheterization, nor it is visible endoscopically. However, through experience, some patients have learned that voiding can be improved by a manual counter pressing against the perineum.

Moreover, Clarke & Thomas (1981) studied static urethral pressure profiles in paraplegics with an acontractile bladder: (3) the urethral pressure in all flaccid male paraplegics investigated was much higher at the external sphincter than at the bladder neck. It was largely abolished by alpha-blockers. They conclude in flaccid male paraplegics the major component of urethral resistance is a constant, adrenergically innervated muscular resistance in the external sphincter region; however, this is still under discussion.

2. Objectives

To find evidence to answer the following questions:

1. How to do it?
2. Is it effective?
3. Is it safe?
4. Is it cost-effective?
5. How to treat complications?
6. Comparing between techniques
7. Long-term results and quality of life

3. Criteria for considering studies and searching strategy

All types of studies, adults and children only if necessary for understanding, dealing with Credé- and the Valsalva manoeuvre for emptying bladder in neurogenic lower urinary tract dysfunction were included.

Search from Medline through Pubmed 1966-2001/April and the list of publications used in the First International Consultation on Incontinence 1998.

Keywords: Credé, Credé voiding, Valsalva, Valsalva voiding in neurogenic bladder, in spina bifida, in spinal cord injury, in cauda equina syndromes, intervertebral disc protrusion, in lower urinary tract disorders, combined with anal stretch

All studies were considered in regards to efficacy, safety and cost-effectiveness (languages English, German).

Eleven studies (1 in Japanese languages, but with an abstract in English) were considered.

Quality of included studies. There were 7 case-series (level of evidence 4); 2 were case-reports, 1 of them with 1 patient and the other with 2 patients (level of evidence 5); 2 comprise basic research of bladder expression, one with operative therapy based also on a case-series.

4. Results

a) How to do it?

Bladder expression comprises various techniques aimed at increasing intravesical pressure in order to enable/to facilitate bladder emptying. The most commonly used are the Valsalva (abdominal straining) and the Credé (manual compression of the lower abdomen).

b) Is it effective?

There is no randomised controlled study on bladder expression, however, Barbalias et al (1983) prospectively evaluated the efficacy of Credé to promote voiding in 207 patients with a variety of lower urinary tract disorders using urodynamics, including urethral pressure measurement. They found an increase in urethral pressure during Credé manoeuvre while the vesical neck remained closed. Only 2% in this series the bladder neck opened and the external urethral sphincter relaxed. They concluded that Credé manoeuvre is an inefficient method of bladder empyting, in the majority of patients associated with a significant urethral obstruction.

Clinical experience shows that by straining and increasing abdominal pressure patients are able to empty their bladders, albeit mostly incompletely.

c) Is it safe?

With the development of urodynamics/videourodynamics, it could be demonstrated that despite high intravesical pressures created by these techniques, the urinary flow may be very poor and residual urine may also be present. This echoes Watkins' statement, 1936, that micturition by the Valsalva or Credé can be impeded despite flaccid paresis of the pelvic floor (see Background).

Reinberg et al (1984) reported a case of renal rupture with development of a large perinephrec urinoma and deterioration of renal function after the Credé technique in a girl with neurogenic bladder and detrusor sphincter dyssynergia (without vesico-ureteral reflux). Therefore bladder expression is not safe unless urodynamics have proved the contrast.

d) Is it cost-effective?

There are no data that evaluate the cost-effectiveness of bladder expression.

e) How to treat complications?

Complications with this method are caused by high intravesical pressure to overcome outflow resistance. Therefore complications with bladder expression can be treated either by lowering outflow resistance (see below) or by replacing bladder expression by CISC.

f) Comparing between techniques

Only Momose et al (1997) compared the clinical significance between Credé voiding (n=56, mean follow-up period 14.6 years) and Valsalva voiding (n=22, mean follow-up 13.7 years) in the urological management of spina bifida patients. **Although their findings suggest a possible superiority of Valsalva voiding over Credé voiding in the preservation of the urinary tract, the differences between the two groups were not statistically significant and they suggest further studies in neurogenic bladder patients.**

In other papers [Leroi et al 1994; Fanciullacci et al 1989; Sperling 1978] Credé and Valsalva are mentioned as part of the treatment without further judgement. Only Redman (1976) report on two cases with upper urinary tract improvement with Credé. Madersbacher (1977) as well as Clarke & Thomas (1981) documented a functional urethral obstruction at the level of the pelvic floor during bladder expression (as above-mentioned).

g) Long-term results and quality of life

Madersbacher (1977) demonstrated that with increasing time of using Valsalva and Credé techniques, more than 50% of patients showed demonstrable influx into the prostate and the seminal vesicles and other complications, e.g. epididymo-orchitis. Moreover, the high pressures cause reflux into the upper urinary tract with all known complications. The stress to the pelvic floor with these techniques several times a day also has a negative influence on existing minimal storage function of these structures and therefore makes incontinence worth, causing additional genital-rectal prolapse and haemorrhoides.

Adjunctive therapy to decrease outflow assistance includes alpha-blockers, if they are effective they usually cause or increase neurogenic urinary stress incontinence. Juraschek et al (1974) and Wyndaele (1998) advocated cystoprostatopexy to the abdominal wall to prevent kink of the urethra, however, no long-term results are available.

CONCLUSIONS

Bladder expression by Valsalva or Credé is potentially hazardous for the urinary tract due to functional obstruction at the level of the pelvic floor.

It is contraindicated if it creates a high intravesical pressure, or/and if prostatic reflux or/and a vesico-uretero-renal reflux are present. In addition, hernias, recto-genital prolapse and hemorrhoids as well as urethral pathology (stricture formation) and recurrent symptomatic UTIs are further contraindications.

It may have a negative influence on an existing minimal storage function of the flaccid pelvic floor and therefore incontinence may become worse.

Alpha-blockers may reduce the outflow resistance, and may also induce or increase urinary stress incontinence.

5. Implications for practice

Bladder expression is often recommended especially for patients with an underactive detrusor with an underactive / incompetent sphincter mechanism.

Expression of the bladder for voiding by Credé and Valsalva is effective. To empty the bladder, the pressures measured may be high and potentially dangerous for the upper urinary tract. **Bladder expression is not safe.**

According to the above-mentioned, it is clear that sphincter-hyperreflexia and detrusor-sphincter dyssynergia are contra-indications for bladder expression. However, there is one exception i.e., when used in the reflex bladder with the anal sphincter stretch described by Low & Donovan (1981). This method, by inserting one or two gloved fingers into the anal canal and then stretching the anal sphincter, does relax the external urethral sphincter; and voiding is then achieved by abdominal straining. Therefore, it can be used in those who have a reflex bladder with unbalanced voiding due to detrusor weakness and/or detrusor-sphincter dyssynergia. There is no evidence that Credé or Valsalva are superior or less dangerous as the other.

If complications, caused by high pressure during bladder emptying, occur, CIC is the alternative. Long-term results are good only if no contraindication exists or occurs over the years, urodynamic controlls are mandatory. If the situation remains safe and stable the method is cost-effective and guarantees an adequate quality of life. However if complications occur, patients have to be persuaded to change to CIC.

RECOMMENDATIONS

Before recommending bladder expression by Valsalva or Credé, it must be proved that the situation in the lower urinary tract is urodynamically safe. Basically the method is rather dangerous.

Exclude contraindications, such as a vesico-ureterorenal reflux, prostatic reflux, genito-rectal prolapse, hernias, urethra pathology and symptomatic UTIs before recommending this type of bladder emptying.

In general, bladder expression should be replaced by CIC in most patients with neuropathic bladder-sphincter dysfunction.

Alpha-blockers are not recommended as they may induce or increase urinary stress incontinence.

Valsalva and Credé only guarantee a good quality of life and are cost-effective in long term when the indication is proper and when the situation remains stabile throughout the years. (Grande of recommendation C)

6. Implications for research

A urodynamically controlled prospective study should be conducted to prove that Crede and/or Valsalva are really safe in patients with normal range intravesical pressure created by these techniques.

7. Acknowledgement:

None

8. Potential conflict of interest:

None

III. TOILETTING ASSISTANCE: TIMED VOIDING, HABIT RETRAINING, PROMPTED VOIDING

Bladder retraining and toiletting assistance aim to restore control over the urinary bladder. The different techniques have been reviewed especially in older persons with urinary incontinence, however, there are only few references directly related to neuropathic incontinence. Therefore in behalf of the bladder retraining and toiletting assistance see chapter on Incontinence in the Elderly. Randomised controlled studies are needed to get evidence also in patients with neuropathic incontinence.

C. CATHETERS

I. INTERMITTENT CATHETERIZATION [IC]

1. Background

The use of catheters for bladder emptying dates back to many thousands of years [Brosman 1965].

Intermittent catheterization (IC) and self-catheterization (ISC) have become properly introduced during the last 40 years [Guttmann, Frankel 1966; Lapides et al 1972].

The main aims of IC and ISC are to empty the bladder and to prevent bladder overdistension in order to avoid complications and to improve urological conditions. Many studies showed good results in continence with less complications leading to a better prognosis and a better quality of life in many with neurologic bladder [Maynard, Diokno 1982; Diokno et al 1983; Sutton et al 1991].

IC and ISC are nowadays considered as the methods of choice for the management of neurologic bladder dysfunction.

2. Objectives

To find evidence to answer the following questions:

1. *What is the best technique and what are the best materials for IC?*

2. *Is IC effective for treating neurogenic urinary incontinence and voiding dysfunction?*
3. *Is IC safe?*
4. *How to prevent complications?*
5. *How to treat complications?*
6. *Is IC preferable to other forms of bladder emptying/catheter drainage in the neuropathic patients?*
7. *What are the long-term results including the impact on quality of life?*
8. *What does IC cost?*

3. Criteria for considering studies and search strategy

All types of studies in adults dealing with IC and ISC in neurogenic bladder have been included in this search.

Medline through Pubmed from 1966-2000, and the list of publications used in First International Consultation Report if not included in the former list.

a) Keywords

Catheterization, catheterization, neurogenic, neurogenic bladder, bladder, urinary, intermittent catheterization, intermittent selfcatheterization

b) Method of review

All studies were considered in regards to outcome, efficacy, safety and cost effectiveness, in all languages. When written in Japanese the information in the English translation of the abstract was used.

c) Description of the review

477 studies were reviewed and 119 were in first instance selected because dealing with conservative treatment in adults with neurogenic bladder. Further analysis excluded 25 articles dealing with suprapubic or indwelling catheter. Fifty one articles were added to this list from a previous survey, bringing the total number to 145.

d) Methodological quality of the included studies

The articles withheld for evaluation are 9 randomized controlled trials, 23 propsective cohort studies, 12 retrospective case control studies, 87 case series, and 14 expert opinions.

4. Results

a) What is the best technique and what are the best materials for IC?

There exists not one best technique nor one best material as both depend greatly on patients' individual anatomic, social and economic possibilities.

Material and catheter type: Many types of catheters are used for IC and ISC, e.g. Nelaton, O'Neil, Tiemann and Foley. They are made of rubber, latex, plastic (PVC), silicon. They may be siliconized or of teflon coated rubber, glass or stainless steel. Some are packed in a sheet/bag [Wu et al 1981], others are reusable. A urethral introducer has been described which permits to bypass the colonized 1.5 cm of the distal urethra and which resulted in a significant lower infection rate in hospitalized men with spinal cord injury [Bennett et al 1997]. Most catheters need the use of some kind of lubricants, especially in men, e.g. jellies or aqueous solution but no studies were found comparing these. Lubricants are applied on the catheter or are instilled into the urethra [Burgdörfer et al 1997]. In developing countries, where resources are limited, patients sometimes use oil [Kovindha 1998] or just water [Orikasa et al 1976] as lubricant. For those with preserved urethral sensation, a local anesthetic jelly may be needed. Jellies would seem most effective when instilled into the urethra. This has been studied in endoscopy [Vogler 1980, Scholtmeijer, Dzoljic-Danilovic 1990] but can be accepted for catheterization too. The advantage is multiple: Lubricants injected into the urethra permit the catheter to glide in a film of jelly into the bladder; the desinfectant effect of jellies containing antiseptic substances is optimal; the local anesthetic effect, if one waits 5-10 min. after instillation, is fully developed. Many female patients do not use catheter lubrification. Some catheters have special properties such as a hydrophilic and self lubricated surface which can be activated with tap or sterile water. Regarding the size of the catheters, for adults 10–14 Fr for adult males and 14-16 Fr for adult females are mostly used but bigger size/lumen may be necessary for those with bladder augmentation. No studies on IC compared sizes in a randomized way.

Studies comparing materials in a randomized controlled way are scarce. Some recent studies evaluate the hydrophilic catheters. In an animal study in the rabbit, Lundgren et al (2000) found that osmolality of hydrophilic catheters is important in regards to removal friction and urethral trauma. To minimize the risk of urethral trauma high osmolality catheters are recommended especially when the catheterization times are a few minutes or more. Waller et al (1997) compared two different hydrophilic catheters in a crossover study of 14 male spinal cord injury patients, as to the maximum friction force during the removal of the catheters after bladder emptying. The catheter with the highest osmolality (approximately 900mOsm/kg) had much less sticking to the urethral epithelium and had a significantly lower friction force. Biering-Sorensen et al (1999) compared two types of hydrophilic catheters and found no difference regarding the number of urethral epithelial cells on the surface of the catheters after catheterization. Wyndaele et al (2000) evaluated the use of a hydrofilic catheter in 39 male patients with neurogenic bladder using conventional catheters for a long time. The hydrophilic catheter proved as easy to use but was better tolerated. Satisfaction was better especially in patients who experienced problems with conventional catheters. Some patients were unsatisfied for reasons of practical use or for economical reasons. Very recently Hedlund et al (2001) pleaded for a prospective, randomized longterm multicentre study in order to reach reliable conclusions. Studies comparing the use of hydrophilic catheters with the use of ordinary catheters and lubricant must take into account how this jelly is used: applied on the catheter or injected into the urethra.

Technique: Two main techniques have been adopted, a sterile IC (SIC) and a clean IC (CIC) (Figures 6, 7). The sterile non-touch technique advocated by Guttmann and Frankel implicates the use of sterile materials handled with sterile gloves and forceps. In an intensive care unit, some advocate wearing a mask and a sterile gown as well. In some centres, during a bladder training programme, SIC has been done only by a catheter team, which has proven to obtain a very low infection rate [Lindan, Bellomy 1971]. The sterile technique is used only during a restricted period of time and in a hospital setting. In the majority of cases a clean technique is used. Catheterization is done in many different positions: supine, sitting or standing. Female patients may use a mirror or a specially designed catheter to visualize the meatus [Bruijnen and Boer 1981]. After a while most women do not need these aids anymore. The catheter is introduced in a non-infecting and atraumatic way. The requirements for this have been described many times: non infecting means cleaning hands, using a non infected catheter and lubricant, cleaning the meatal region before catheter introduction. Here again different ways of application are used: the use of sterile components with the catheter introduced out of the sheath into the urethra as well as the use of resterilized catheters introduced by hand which have been washed before.

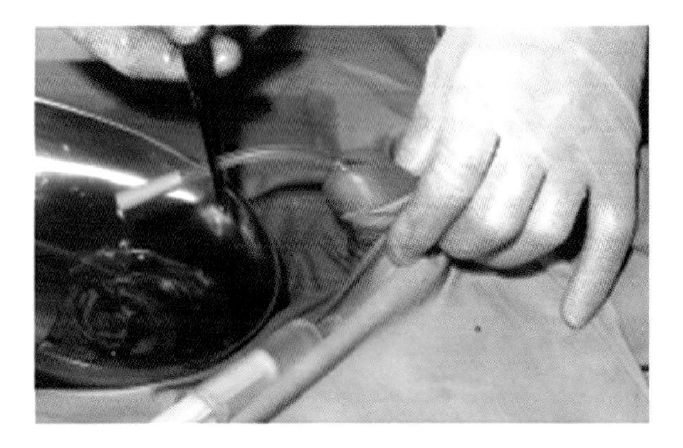

Figure 6 : Sterile non-touch technique of intermittent catheterization (Guttmann & Frankel, 1966)

Individual variation can be found in every patient group. Atraumatic requires a proper catheter size, sufficient lubrification, gentle introduction through the urethra, sphincter area and bladder neck [Wyndaele 1983, Corcos 1996]. The catheter has to be introduced until urine flows out. Urine can be drained directly in the toilet, in a urinal, a plastic bag or other reservoir. The catheter should be kept in place until urine flow stops. Then it should be pulled out slowly while gentle Valsalva or bladder expression is done in order to completely empty residual urine. When properly done the residual urine should be maximum 6 ml as demonstrated by Stribran and Fabian with fenolftalëine washing (1961). But routine can be different as shown by Jensen et al (1995). They measured residual urine repeatedly with ultrasonography and found rest urine in 70% of the catheterizations in their group of 12 patients with spinal cord lesion. The residual could exceed 50 ml and even 100 ml. Finally the end of the catheter should be blocked to prevent backflow of the urine or air into the bladder. Hydrophilic catheters can be left in place for a short time only to prevent suction by the urethral mucosa which may make removal difficult.

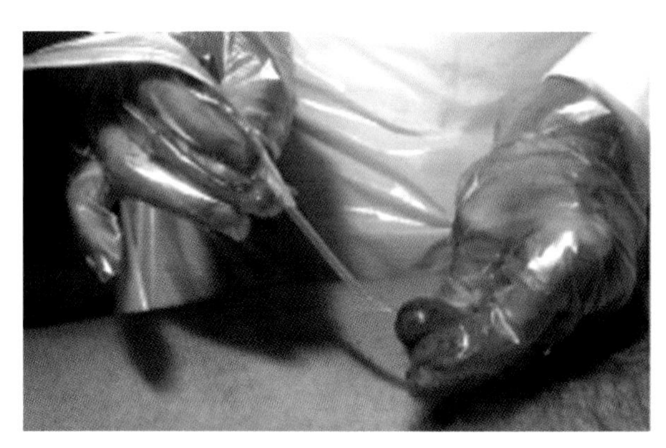

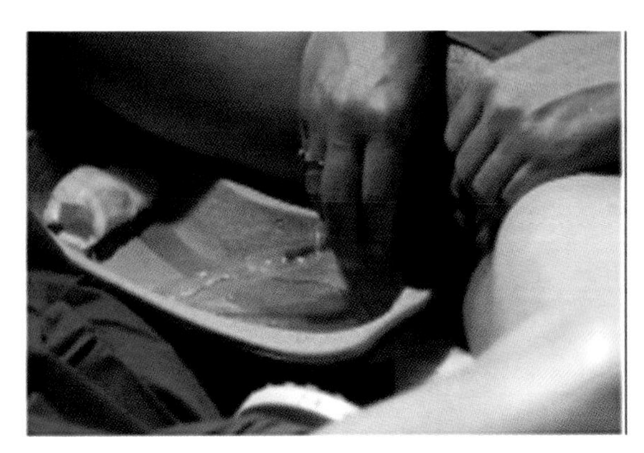

Figure 7 : Clean (self-) intermittent catheterization technique with catheterization out of the sheath.

During the rehabilitation phase clean ISC (CISC) can be taught to patients with good hand function fairly soon. Wyndaele and De Taeye compared the results of 25 paraplegic patients (23 men and 2 women) starting on CISC at a mean of 35 days (7 to 85+ days) post trauma with those of 48 paraplegic patients catheterized by nurses with a non touch technique. They found comparable results in final outcome of the bladder training and infection rate. Early self-catheterization permitted the patients to go home for weekends earlier and was considered positive by the majority of those participating. Champion (1976) found no bacteriological difference in urine specimens one year after 7 patients changed from sterile IC to CISC.

When resources are limited, catheters are reused many times, up to weeks and months. Some re-sterilise or clean them by soaking in an antiseptic solution or boiling water. Microwave to re- sterilise rubber catheters has been described by Silbar et al 1980. A silicone Japanese type self catheter has been reused for a long time [Igawa 1998, Kovindha 1998]. Van Hala et al (1997) used a questionnaire in 97 patients with pediatric onset neurogenic bladders to evaluate differences between IC with a sterile new catheter and IC with reused material. 98% used a clean technique. Their data suggest that reused supplies are not related to an increased likelihood of urinary tract infection. As only 2% used a sterile technique comparison between sterile and non sterile technique is not possible.

Frequency of catheterization: This depends on many factors as bladder volume, fluid intake, postvoid residual, urodynamic parameters (compliance, detrusor pressure). Usually it is recommended to catheterize 4 – 6 times a day during the acute stage after spinal cord lesion. Some will need to keep this frequency if IC is the only way of bladder emptying. Others will catheterize 1 – 3 times a day to check and evacuate residual urine after voiding or on a weekly basis during bladder retraining [Opitz 1976]. Clinical utility of a portable ultrasound device in IC has been evaluated in a randomized controlled trial by Anton et al (1998). The results show that the device reduces the number of required catheterizations and is associated with a high degree of patient satisfaction. De Ridder et al (1997) had used a similar device in multiple sclerosis patients and found some decrease in incontinence over 24 hours and one catheterization less needed a day in a small number of patients.

Adjunctive therapy: To overcome high detrusor pressure anticholinergic drugs or bladder relaxants can be indicated. As shown in the table 2 this is often needed in most series published. For those who develop a low compliance bladder, upper tract deterioration or severe incontinence, injection of Botuline toxin into bladder wall [Schurch et al 2000] or surgery as bladder augmentation may be necessary. Where a too high diuresis is noted during the night due to diurnal variation of antidiuretic hormone [Kilinc et al 1999], DDAVP can safely and effectively be used [Chancellor et al 1994]. In cases of catheterization difficulty at the striated sphincter, botulinum toxin injection in the sphincter can help [Wheeler et al 1998]. In individuals with tetraplegia reconstructive handsurgery is indicated [Kiyono et al 2000]. For those with poor handfunction or difficulty in reaching the meatus assistive devices might be needed [Bakke et al 1993].

Education: This is very important. Patients and caregivers must understand what is wrong with the bladder/sphincter, what the cause is and why IC is proposed for treatment. They have to learn how to catheterize properly. Teaching programmes have been successful in non-literate persons in developing countries [Parmar et al 1993] and in quadriplegic patients [Sutton et al 1991].

CONCLUSION

There is a wide variety of materials used and techniques applied for IC which does not seem to change the practical outcome much if the basic principles are applied: good education and training, clean and atraumatic technique, good patient compliance in the longterm.

b) Is IC effective for treating neurogenic urinary incontinence and voiding dysfunction?

In general, the purpose of catheterization is to empty the bladder and of IC is to resume normal bladder storage and regularly complete urine evacuation. With IC and ISC there is no need to leave the catheter in the lower urinary tract all the time, thus avoiding complications of indwelling catheterization (ID). Data on the results of continence in different neurological pathologies are given in table 1. It is striking that before the 1970's the articles on IC in neurogenic did not comment on continence specifically. Later the continence outcome was better reported. Some studies used bladder relaxants or surgery to obtain continence. (Table 1)

It is clear that IC can improve incontinence or make patients with neurogenic bladder continent if bladder capacity is sufficient, bladder pressure kept low, urethral resistance high enough, and if care is taken to balance between fluid intake, residual urine and frequency of catheterization.

c) Is IC safe? Several complications have been described

1. Urinary tract infection (UTI)

Prevalences of UTI vary widely in the literature. This is due to the various evaluation methods used, different techniques of IC, different frequencies of urine analy-

Table 1 : Outcome of continence

Authors	Number of patients	Follow-up	Adjunctive treatment	Result of continence
Lapides et al 1976	168	3 m – 5y	Anticholinergic + alfa-adrenergic	Majority dry
Madersbacher - Weissteiner 1977	12 women	2 – 4y		50% dry, other 50% some grade of incontinence
Wyndaele et al 1980	30 (18m,12f)	3m-30m	6 anticholinergic, 1 colocystoplasty	73% continent + 13% improvement
Iwatsubo et al 1984	60 spinal cord lesion (sci)		Overdistension during shockphase	100% continent
McGuire – Savastano 1986	22 f	2 – 11 y	Surgery 27%	Continent 73%
Kornhuber – Schultz 1990	197 multiple sclerosis			Continence improved with elimination of residual urine
Wyndaele –Maes 1990	75 (6 neurogenic)	1.5-12y	38 anticholinergics	47 dry, 22 seldom wet, 6 wet at least once a day
Kuhn et al 1991	22 sci	5 y	No	Continence did not change
Lindehall et al 1994	26 meningo-myelocoele	7.5 – 12 y		24/26 better
Waller et al 1995	30 sci	5 – 9 y	6 anticholinergics	22 dry, 8 incontinent
Vaidyanathan et al 1998	7 sci	14 – 30 m	Bladder relaxants intravesically	84 % dry, 3 dampness at awaking

sis, different criteria for infection, the administration or not of prophylaxis, the group of patients studied, et al. Some publications give the percentage of sterile urine: between 12% and 88% [Guttmann-Frankel 1966, Pearman 1971, Lapides et al 1974, Donovan et al 1978, Maynard et al 1984, Murray et al 1984, Wyndaele et al 1990]; others of asymptomatic: 11% [Sutton et al 1991] and others of symptomatic bacteriuria: 53% [Whitelaw et al 1987]. Bakke (1993) found in 407 patients, 206 men and 201 women, 252 with neurogenic bladder, during an observation period of one year, 24.5% with asymptomatic UTI, 58.6% with minor symptoms, 14.3% with more comprehensive or frequent symptoms while 2.6% claimed major symptoms. Also in other studies the prevalence of all types of UTI are given [Kass et al 1979, Webb et al 1990, Thirumavalavan et al 1992, Perrouin-Verbe et al 1995, Yadav et al 1993] with very different results. Biering-Sorensen et al (1999) studied 77 SCI patients on CIC after 5 years and found that 81% had been treated for at least one UTI, 22% had 2 – 3 UTI/year and 12% had 4 or more/year. Still it remains difficult from literature to get a proper estimate of the risk of infection when IC is done in a short- and in a longterm: the data differ so much that many factors must play a role in the prevalence of this complication.

In the acute stage of SCI with proper management urine can be kept sterile for 15-20 days without antibiotic prophylaxis and for 16-55 days if prophylaxis is given [Ott-Rossier 1971, Rhame -Perkash 1979, Anderson 1980]. Prieto-Fingerhut et al (1997) determined in a randomized controlled trial the effect of sterile and non sterile IC on the incidence of urinary tract infection in 29 patients after SCI. With urine analysis on a weekly basis they found in the group on sterile IC a 28.6% UTI incidence while in the nonsterile catheterization group 42.4% incidence was found. The cost of antibiotics for the sterile IC group was only 43 % of the cost for those on nonsterile IC. However the cost of the sterile IC kits was 371% of the cost of the kits used by the nonsterile IC group bringing the total cost of the sterile program on 277% of the other program. Rhame and Perkash (1979) published the results of UTI prevalence in 70 SCI patients in the initial rehabilitation hospitalization treated with sterile IC and a neomycin-polymixin irrigant. 54% developed an infection at an over-all rate of 10.3 infections per 1000 patient-days on IC. Bakke and Volset (1993) studied factors that may predict the occurence of bacteriuria and clinical UTI in 302 patients using CIC. Predictive factors of clinical infection were low age and high mean catheterization volume in women; low age, neurogenic bladder dysfunction and nonself-catheterization in men, in addition to urine leakage in patients with neurogenic dysfunction. Bacteriuria was a risk factor of future clinical infection. Risk factors for bacteriuria were present in men: low frequency of catheterization, high age and nonself-catheterization. If antibacterial prophylaxis was used fewer episodes of bacteriuria were noticed but significantly more clinical UTI. Shekelle et al (1999) made a systematic review of risk factors for UTI in adults with spinal cord dysfunction. In this review article they evaluated 22 studies from which many however had important methodological deficiencies. They found two studies that provide evidence supporting increased bladder residual volume as a risk factor. Patients on IC had fewer infections than those with ID. They found conflicting evidence over the value of sterile or "non touch" catheter techniques compared with CIC. They found insufficient evidence to assess risk due to psychological, behavioral and hygiene factors, sex, level of function and time since injury.

Schlager et al (1999) examined how frequently periurethral bacterial species produced bacteriuria in children followed longitudinally. Bacteriuria frequently occurs after inoculation of periurethral *E.coli* into the urine during CIC. Hull et al (1998) investigated virulence factors of *E. Coli* isolated from patients with symptomatic and asymptomatic bacteriuria and neuropathic bladders due to spinal cord and brain injuries. The results suggest that *E. Coli* isolated from patients who develop symptomatic UTI may be distinguished from bacteria recovered from patients who remain asymptomatic and possibly from normal fecal *E. Coli*. In order to diagnose UTI, Barnes et al (1992) found arguments that it should be recommended to obtain the urine by catheterization. The frequency of examining urine samples differs greatly between studies. Some advocate daily use of a dipslide technique during the acute phase after SCI, once a week during the subacute phase and monthly or a few times a year in longterm care [King et al 1992, Darouiche et al 1993, National Institute on disability and rehabilitation research consensus statement 1992]. If a urine culture reveals more than 10,000 cfu/ml, it indicates significant bacteriuria. Pyuria alone is not considered reliable in patients with neurogenic bladder [Gribble et al 1989, Menon -Tan 1992]. The bacteria found are *E. Coli, Proteus, Citrobacter, Pseudomonas, Klebsiella, Staphylococcus aureus* and *faecalis* in most short term cases while the same bacteria plus *Acinetobacter* and *Streptococcus faecalis* are found in the longterm IC patients [Noll et al 1988, Yadav et al 1993]. *E Coli* is considered the dominant species in several studies [Bakke 1993]. The detection of *E. Coli* on the periurethra corresponded in much higher percentage (93%) with bacteriuria than if other bacteria were present on the periurethra (80% or less) [Schlager et al, 1999]. Urinary sepsis is fortunately rare [McGuire et al 1977, Sperling 1978, Barkin et al 1983]. Previous treatment with an ID represented a special risk to develop sepsis in the series of Barkin et al (1983). In his thesis Wyndaele (1983) found sepsis in 21 of 115 patients with SCI during the in hospital rehabilitation. The prevalence of sepsis was highest in those treated beforehand with an ID. Factors of risk were the period of 24 hours to 3 days after changing from ID to IC drainage when UTI was present. The study of Wyndaele and Maes on 69 patients with neurogenic bladder and a literature survey till 1989 on CIC, found justification of several conclusions concerning the relationship between CIC and UTI: If catheterization is begun by patients with recurrent or chronic UTI and urinary retention, the incidence of infection decreases and patients may become totally free of infection. If symptomatic infections occur, improper CIC or misuse often can be found. Chronic infection persists if the cause of the chronicity remains.

2. Genitourinary complications: Urethritis and epididymo-orchitis have been reported in several case series (table 2). Again the prevalence figures vary widely. This is probably due to the many differences in technique, material used, primarily treatment and investigation method. Genital infections can lower fertility in SCI patients. In 1991 Allas reported on 14 paraplegics performing CIC. In each patient he performed two spermograms, one before and one after an episode of epididymitis (unilateral in 13). Azospermia increased from 7% to 50% when epididymitis occured. However if IC was used to empty the neurogenic bladder, slightly better sperm quality was seen. In a study by Ohl et al (1992) on 29 SCI men on electroejaculation, much better pregnancy rates than those patients using an alternative bladder management was the outcome. Also Rutkowski et al (1995) found in patients on IC a higher percentage of mobile sperms compared to those using ID.

Prostatitis, either acute or chronic is difficult to diagnose in patients with neurogenic bladder. Special tests have been developed [Kuhlemeier et al 1982; Wyndaele 1985]. The overall incidence was thought to be probably around 5% to 18% [Cukier et al 1976] but this may be underestimated. Perrouin-Verbe et al (1995) used the Meares-Steamy test and found a rate of 33%.

3. Other complications: Urethral bleeding is frequently seen in new patients and occurs regularly in one third on a long-term basis [Webb et al 1990]. Trauma of the urethra especially in men can cause false passage, meatal stenosis but the incidence is rare (table 2). The incidence of urethral strictures increases with a longer follow-up. Wyndaele and Maes followed 75 patients on CIC for a mean period of 7 years with a maximum of 12 years, the majority using CIC for neurogenic bladder. They found 11 urethral complications in 15 patients, mostly male, some of which were recurrent. Most events occurred after 5 years of CIC. Also Per-

Table 2 : Genitourinary complications (m=men)

Authors	Total no. of patients	Urethritis	Meatal stricture	Epididymitis	Urethral stricture
Lapides et al 1974	100(34m)	2 m	-	-	-
Lapides et al 1976	218 (90m)	2 m	-	2	
Orikasa et al 1976	26 (13m)			1	
Wyndaele et al 1980	30 (18m)	2 m		2	
Maynard,Diokno 1982	28 (m?)			4 (1 with infected penile prosthesis)	
Labat et al 1985	68 (48m)	9 m		3	
Maynard –Glass 1987	34 (m?)			3	2
Wyndaele-Maes 1990	75 (33m)		3	6	7
Webb et al 1990				2%	
Hellstrom et al 1991	41 (26m)			3	
Kuhn et al 1991	22 (11m)		1		1
Thirumavalan –Ransley 1992				12%	
Bakke 1993	407 (206m)	1%		1%	
Perkash –Giroux 1993	50 m			5	
Perrouin-Verbe et al 1995	159 (113m)			10% short-term, 28% long-term	5.3%
Waller et al 1995	30 SCI (26 m)			2	4

rouin-Verbe et al (1995) found that the risk of urethral stricture seems to increase with the number of years on CIC. These authors also showed that patients who developed strictures had a slightly higher catheterization rate than those who did not. Günther et al presented in 2000 their results in 230 men on IC and found urethral changes in 26.9% (3.7% strictures) when also in their history an ID had been used. In men with IC and no history of ID the prevalence was 16.9% urethral changes and no strictures. These results were compared with those in 311 men not on IC. In this last group with history of ID 25.4% urethral changes (2.5% strictures) and in those without history of ID 17.9% urethral changes (1.5%) strictures were found.

Urethral changes were also documented by Kovindha et al (2000) in 27 spinal cord injured men on CIC for an average of 5 years (between 1 to 14 years) and using one single re-usable silicone catheter for an average of 3 years (from 1 to 7 years). Urethrograms showed 70% normal, 11% minor abnormalities, 15% narrowed urethra and 4% with stricture (1 case) that needed operation.

The surface of the catheter is claimed to be an important factor with less stricture development when hydrophilic catheters are used. Vaidyanathan et all (1994) studied the degree of urethral inflammation by urethral cytology in two groups on CIC, one using ordinary catheters in PVC with lubricant, the other using hydrophilic catheters. The group using hydrophilic catheters had significantly less urethral inflammation. Waller et al (1995) found no extra stricture occuring in their patients using hydrophilic catheters after a mean follow-up of 7 years. Such data are suggestive for an advantage of using hydrophilic catheters to prevent stricture formation in the long-term but comparitive studies have not been published.

Other complications such as hydronephrosis, vesicoureteral reflux, bladder cancer seem to relate to infection, bladder trabeculation, detrusor pressure or neuropathy but not to CIC [Damanski 1965]. Bladder calculi caused by the introduction of pubic hair [Solomon et al 1980, Amendola et al 1983], loss of the catheter in the bladder [Morgan et al 1990], bladder perforation and bladder necrosis [Reisman, Preminger 1989] have been case reports on rare complications of CIC.

d) How to prevent complications?

To prevent UTI a non-infecting technique is needed. Barber et al (1999) evaluated the importance of nursing education and found this educational intervention by a clinic nurse to be a simple, cost-effective mean to decrease the risk of UTI's in SCI individuals on CIC who are at risk. Some other factors have been found to probably play a role in infection prevention: the frequency of IC is important as shown in several studies. Anderson (1980) found a fivefold incidence when IC is done 3 times a day compared to 6 times a day. In addition prevention of bladder overdistention is important [Lapides et al 1976, Shekelle et al 1999]. Cross infection is less if IC during hospitalization is done by a catheter team [Lindan, Bellomy 1971] or by the patients themselves [Wyndaele, De Taeye 1990]. As residual urine plays a role in infection, attention must be made to completely empty the bladder [Shekelle et al 1999].

Several studies have evaluated the infection rate during antibacterial prophylaxis. Randomized controlled trials are scarce. Pearman (1979) compared 2 groups of patients with acute SCI treated with non-touch IC: 22 had kanamycin colistin solution instilled into the bladder at the end of each catheterization and 25 patients were not given such instillations. Those with the instillation had only half the incidence of significant bacteriuria. The same effect could not be found in a comparison study by Haldorson et al (1978) with instillations of neomycin. Ascorbic acid has been used by several authors. It is considered only useful as adjuvant therapy together with other antibacterial drugs [Murphy et al 1965, Stover and Fleming 1980]. Johnson et al 1994 did a 3 months study of nitrofurantoin prophylaxis in 56 children with CIC. They found a reduction from 39% on placebo to 19% on single daily dose prophylaxis. Anderson (1980) in a randomized prospective study compared infection rate between control patients, patients treated with intravesical neomycin/polymyxin-B, with low dose of nitrofurantoin and with a combination of the intravesical and oral prophylaxis. There was a significant reduction in infection rates when oral and intravesical antibacterials were used.

Kevorkian et al (1984) evaluated the effect of methenamine mandelate with acidification in a randomized controlled trial with 17 and 22 patients. They found a statistically significant difference in infection rate between the group with methenamine and the group with placebo. Mohler et al (1987) on the other hand found no difference in infection rate in a controlled clinical trail in 46 patients comparing trimethoprim-sulfamethoxazole and placebo. Bakke (1993) found in 407 patients on CIC significant bacteriuria in 57.5% of those who used no prophylaxis while the corresponding figures in patients using methenamine hippurate and antibiotics were 42.5% and 37.5%. Cranberry juice has been evaluated recently. Schlager et al (1999) did a study in children on IC and found no effect on bacteriuria. Hofstetter (1987) showed a positive effect in vitro of chlorhexidine in the lubricant but no clinical data have evaluated this finding. But more studies are needed to permit a proper conclusion. Several studies have asked attention for the risk to develop dangerous resistance against antibiotics when either orally or by instillation prophylaxis is given [Dollfus, Molé 1969; Pearman 1971; Vivian, Bors 1974; Pearman et al 1991]. Galloway et al (1986) state that the threat of emergence of resistant organisms, the risk to patients for side effects of the antibiotics, the expense and the risk to other patients from cross infection with resistant organisms are strong arguments against prophylactic antibacterials.

To prevent urethal strictures gentle introduction of the catheter, lubrication of the catheter and perhaps the use of hydrophilic catheters can play a role. Forceful manipulation during catheter insertion and significant bleeding proved important contributory factors for the development of urethral strictures in patients on CIC studied by Mandal and Vaidyanathan (1993).

e) How to treat complications?

Treatment of UTI is necessary if the infection is symptomatic. Waites et al (1999) treated 25 men with SCI on IC to determine efficacy of ciprofloxacine 1 g per day for 10 days in to eradicate susceptible organisms from urine, urethra and perineum. Susceptible bacteria disappeared from urine in all and were significantly reduced in perineum and urethra. However they were replaced shortly after by resistant Gram-positive cocci. It is important to reserve the drug for symptomatic patients only and look closely into the antibiogram. This follows the conclusions of a study by Lewis et al (1984) on the significance of asymptomatic bacteriuria in neurogenic bladder disease: their results in 52 patients indicate the value of non-treatment for chronic non symptomatic bacteriuria throughout hospitalization.

In neurogenic patients on CIC, urethral trauma with false passages have been treated by Michielsen and Wyndaele (1999) with 6 weeks indwelling catheter and 5 days antibiotics. The false passages disappeared on cystoscopy and CIC could be restarted. Mandal and Vaidyanathan (1993) succesfully treated urethral strictures in 6 patients, with urethral dilatation in 4 and with optical internal urethrotomy in 2, followed by urethral stenting for 2 weeks.

f) Is IC preferable to other forms of bladder emptying/catheter drainage in the neuropathic patients including longterm results?

Almost all publications clearly state that IC is the preferable method for bladder drainage. It has less complications and give a better outcome. Most endorse this opinion by comparing the outcome with previous treatment methods. Wyndaele et al (1985) compared in a series of 115 SCI patients four different methods of bladder drainage used during spinal shock: suprapubic fine bore cystostomy, indwelling Foley catheter, IC and both ID and IC consecutively. The methods of bladder drainage used did not influence the number of patients becoming catheter-free but determined significantly the length of period before they acquired catheter-freedom. Patients on IC had the shortest time from injury to established micturition. Patients on IC and on cystostomy had few complications but the complication rate in the group treated with ID was high. McGuire and Savastano (1986) compared urological outcome in 35 women from 2 – 12 years after SCI and found that the 13 with ID had frequent and serious complications compared to those on IC. Bennett et al (1995) compared the outcome in 70 female SCI patients retrospectively after a mean follow-up of more than 15 years. The group on IC had significantly better outcome than those on reflex voiding and incontinence pads or the group on ID. Giannantoni et al (1998) compared the renal outcome in a small group of patients on IC with those on tapping, abdominal straining and Credé. The incidence of both urinary tract dilatation and vesicoureteral reflux was significantly lower in the IC group. The finding of upper tract complications also in patients on IC showing high intravesical pressures stresses the need of adding anticholinergic drugs. Weld et al (2000) compared the evolution in bladder compliance with time in association with the type of bladder management in 316 SCI patients. Logistic regression analysis revealed that IC and spontaneous voiding were associated more with normal compliance than Foley catheterization. This also explains why there are less upper tract complications in their IC group.

g) Reasons to stop IC.

Not all patients starting with IC continue this treatment. Reasons for this are given in several studies summarized in table 3.

Perrouin-Verbe et al 1995 found in their global population of 159 SCI patients that only 8 having practised CIC for at least 2 years stopped the technique. This indicates that in most SCI cases the definitive choice of voiding is made after 2 years post injury. A main reason to stop was continuing incontinence. The first factor of acceptance of the technique was continence. The second factor related to the patients' autonomy for practising IC. In a population of 50 patients Perkash and Giroux (1993) had also found that 4 out of 7 tetraplegics stopped IC because they needed to be catheterized by others. In addition 66% stopped IC mainly after surgery on sphincter and prostate or initiation of voiding.

Bakke and Malt (1993) found that among those who practiced IC independently 25.8% were sometimes and 6% always averse to IC. Young patients and females were more averse to CIC. In 30% aversion seemed to be related to a subjective evaluation of their situation, to an emotional status and above all to non-acceptance of their chronic disability. In a recent study [Yavuzer et al 2000] a retrospective analysis was made on the compliance with bladder management in SCI patients. Of 38 patients on CIC at discharge 52% discontinued the method and reverted to ID during follow-up. Dependence on caregivers, spasticity interfering with catheterization, incontinence despite anticholinergic agents and lack of availability of external collective devices for female patients were the main reasons for stopping CIC.

h) Is IC cost-effective?

There are no data about the cost and cost/efficacy available. In a study mentioned above Prieto-Fingerhut et al (1997) compared the cost of sterile and non-sterile IC and found that clean IC was less costly taking into account the price of sterile sets used for IC. Grundy et al (1983) compared the price of IC and suprapubic fine-bore catheterization after SCI and found the latter cheaper for material, average antibiotic cost and labour.

Table 3 : Reasons for stopping IC

Authors	Catheter-free	Incontinence	Inconvenient	Infection	Physical status	Choice of patient
Diokno et al 1983	17%	2%	2%		7%	
Maynard-Glass 1987	12%					6%
Whitelaw et al 1987	5%		5%		5%	5%
Webb et al 1990	9%		3%		2%	2%
Timoney-Shaw 1990		36%				
Sutton et al 1991		6%	6%	3%	3%	3%
Bakke et al 1993	10%		5%	4%	3%	
Hunt et al 1996	10 %					

Duffy et al (1995) evaluated cost-effectiveness in a population of male residents of VA nursing homes comparing CIC and SIC. In this randomized clinical trial they found similar outcome but less expenses if a clean technique was used.

5. Implication for practice

RECOMMENDATIONS

It should be recommended to use CIC as the first choice of treatment for those with inability to empty the bladder adequately and safely. It is a valuable tool for achieving continence in the neuropathic voiding dysfunction

Proper education and teaching are necessary to permit a good outcome

To prevent and reduce complications, a non-traumatizing technique with adequate frequency of catheterization and complete emptying should be strictly performed

Minimal requirements for regular follow-up are history taking, physical examination, imaging, laboratory results and urodynamic tests, in order to early detect risk factors and complications

There is still need for research in different parts of the world to determine the best catheter, the optimal technique and the best means to prevent and treat complications

Longterm results, cost and quality of life need to be further documented

CONCLUSIONS

CIC is effective and safe to treat the neuropathic bladder in the shortterm and in the longterm.

Complications such as UTI are regularely seen and seem to be related to both the catheterization itself and the existinglower urinary tract condition.

Urethral complication seem to be increase in the longterm.

In order to reduce and prevent complications, appropriate materials and correct techniques should be taught and performed

Adequate frequency of CIC, a non-traumatizing technique and suitable materials are the key factors for a successful outcome

So far, no study exists that proves that one catheter, one lubricant, or one special technique is significantly superior to another

5. Conflict of interest

None

6. Acknowledgement:

None

II. INDWELLING URETHRAL CATHETERS –TRANSURETHRALLY/ SUPRAPUBICALLY

1. Background

In early 19th century, a urinary catheter with a balloon bag (Foley cathether) was developed. After the World War I, majority of spinal cord injured (SCI) as well as other neuropathic patients were treated with *indwelling urethral cathetherization (ID)* or *suprapubic catheterization (SC)* due to difficulty in voiding or urinary incontinence. Nowadays, *intermittent catheterization (IC)* is recommended for neuropathic patients. Nevertheless many chose ID as a mean of treating urinary incontinence due to difficulty in performing IC or persistant leakage between catheterizations. In developing countries ID is still the method of choice for those with urinary retention or incontinence.

Studies have shown that ID caused and were associated with various complications such as urethral trauma and bleeding, urethritis, fistula due to pressure effect caused by improper size of the urethral catheters and improper technique of securing the catheters, bladder and renal stones, cystitis, acute and chronic urinary tract infection (UTI), bladder neck incompetence and urethral sphincter erosion, and bladder carcinoma. Many of these complications were related to long-term usage. Therefore instead of ID many experts advocate removal of the urethral catheter as soon as possible, use other methods such as IC or SC to decrease urethral complications. However nowadays these complications are much less due to better materials, using smaller size catheters and proper technique of securing the catheter.

2. Criteria for considering studies and search strategy

Types of studies: all types of studies.

Types of participants: mainly adults with spinal cord injuries/lesions (myelodysplasia), stroke, MS; animals and laboratories

Types of outcome measures: efficiency, safety, and quality of life

Search: Medline from 1966 to 2001

Keywords: neurogenic bladder, urethral catheter, indwelling catheteris(z)ation

Description of studies: randomised control trials (RCT); clinical trials, conhort studies, retrospective case-controlled studies, case series / case studies and reviews

Over all: there were 50 paper sorted and reviewed.

3. Results

a) Technique and Care of ID

Quality of included studies:

5 RCTs: Bull et al 1991; Liedberg, Lundeberg 1990; Liedberg et al 1990; Talja et al 1990; Priefer et al 1982. (Level of evidence 1)

5 clinical trials: Sugarman 1982; Cox et al 1989; Kunin et al 1987; Morris, Stickler 1998; Morris et al 1997. (Level of evidence 2/3)

1 case-controlled study: Burr et al 1993. (Level of evidence 3)

3 case series/case report: Warren et al 1982; Feneley 1983; Cuttino, Clark 1987. (Level of evidence 4)

3 experts'opinions: Kunin 1997; Wong 1983; Burgdoerfer et al 1997 (Level of evidence 5)

Transurethral ID needs a lot of meticulous skill and care. Materials used should be sterile and handled properly by a well-trained person such as a physician, a nurse, a patient or a carer. In some centers, a well-trained catheter team has proved to lessen complications related to catheterizations.

The following are procedures of urethral catheterization and catheter care recommended by Kunin (1997). First, cleanse the urethral meatus/perineum with antiseptic solution before catheterization. Followed by lubricating the catheter, using (non-touch) aseptic technique (either with sterile gloves or forceps). Then, gently insert the catheter into the meatus. Make sure to insert the catheter 1 inch beyond the balloon to provide enough room for inflation. In males fix the catheter and the penis to the abdomen (Figure 8), in females fix the catheter to the thigh. Wong (1983) also suggests maintaining aseptic closed drainage system according to the guidelines for catheter care developed by the Center of Disease Control. Besides, proper catheters and frequency of changing the catheter are also important in preventing complications related to the transurethral ID (Table 4).

• Materials

Nowadays there are various materials used for catheters e.g. rubber, latex, silicone, siliconised latex, taflon coated latex, silver coated latex, hydrogel coating catheter etc. Sugarman (1982) investigated different catheter materials to determine the extent of and differences among them in regards to bacterial adherance. He found that the adherence was significant less to siliconised rubber than to pure latex or teflon coated rubber. Generally, taflon coated rubber values exhibited intermediate and latex rubber the highest adherence.

Cox et al (1989) studied infection of catheterised patients by electron microscopy. Fifty catheters, of all-silicone or silicone elastomer-coated latex construction, studied were from long-stay geriatric patients. The duration of each catheter used was not mentioned. They found that bacteria had colonised the surfaces of nearly

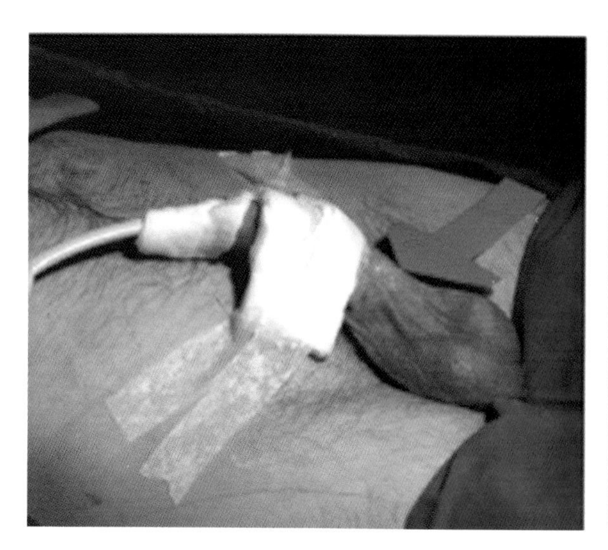

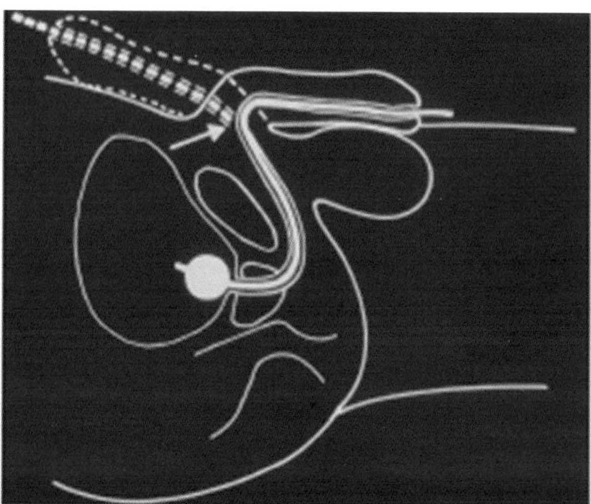

Figure 8 : In males the catheter should be fixed to the abdomen, expecially in spinal cord injured patients in order to avoid a pressure sore of the urethra with the possibility to develop abscess, fistula and diverticulum; when the penis is fixed to the lower abdomen this punctual pressure to the urethra can be avoided.

Table 4 : Shows studies of different materials used for transurethral indwelling catheterisation

Authors	Study	Results
Sugarman B (1982)	Bacteria adherence to catheters	Significant less adherence to siliconised rubber than to others; taflon coated rubber values exhibited intermediate and latex rubber the highest adherence
Cox AJ et al (1989)	Biofilm on catheter's surface by electron microscope	Bacteria had colonised the surfaces of nearly all the catheters examined (all-silicone or silicone elastomer-coated latex catheters)
Liedberg H. Lundeberg T. (1990)	RCT: Catheter-associated bacteruria after 6 days of catheterisation	Much less in the silver-coated catheters than in the taflon-coated latex catheters
Liedberg H, Lundeberg T, Ekman P. (1990)	RCT: Rate of bacteriuria after 5 days of catheterisation	Significant difference between a silver alloy and hydrogel-coated Foley catheter (SHC) and a non-coated (NC) catheter. No significant difference between the SHC catheter and a hydrogel-coated (HC) catheter, between the HC catheter and the NC catheter.
Talja M et al (1990)	RCT: Encrustation and degree of urethral inflammation	Hydrogel-coating catheter effectively prevented encrustation, siliconised latex catheters were the least resistant to encrustation. Full silicone catheters induced the mildest degree of inflammation.
Morris NS et al (1997)	Encrustation	None of the 18 types of catheter tested, including those coated with hydrogel or silver, were capable of resisting encrustation by P.mirabilis biofilm

all the catheters examined. This thick layer of bacteria (biofilm) appears not only to precede mineral deposition but also to bind the crystrals together as encrustation proceeds.

In *1990* Liedberg & Lundeberg did an RCT to study catheter-associated bacteruria in hospitalised patients. Sixty patients had a Foley catheter coated with silver alloy and 60 others used a taflonised latex catheter. After 6 days' catheterization, there was a statistically significant difference in the incidence of catheter-associated bacteriuria in the 2 groups, much less in the silver-coated catheters group and in 1989 they showed that *Pseudomonas auruginosa* cells did not grow on silver-coated. In addition, Liedberg et al (1990) did another RCT study. They found the significant difference in the rate of bacteriuria after 5 days of catheterization between a silver alloy and hydrogel-coated Foley catheter (SHC) and a non-coated (NC) catheter (p less than 0.002). However there was no significant difference between the SHC catheter and a hydrogel-coated (HC) catheter, nor was there a significant difference between the HC catheter and the NC catheter.

Besides, Talja et al (1990) did an RCT study and found that the full silicone catheters induced the mildest degree of inflammation in the urethra. Moreover, the hydrogel-coating catheter effectively prevented encrustation, while siliconised latex catheters were the least resistant to encrustation.

Morris et al (1997) studied different ID catheters and found that none of the 18 types of catheter tested, including those coated with hydrogel or silver, were capable of resisting encrustation by *P. mirabilis* biofilm.

- **Frequency of catheter change**

An optimal interval between catheter changes remains controversial. Some changes the catheters only when obstruction occurs, others propose routine weekly to monthly changes. Warren et al (1982) showed a high incidence (98%) of bacteriuria in SCI patients with a long-term ID (i.e. > 28 days).

According to a randomised study done in elderly patients by Priefer et al (1982), it showed that the practice of monthly catheter change had fewer symptomatic urinary tract infection (UTI) than those who changed the catheters when obstruction or infection had already occurred. However the number of patients in this study were small and done in elderly male patients, not in neuropathic patients; and types of catheters used were not mentioned.

Regarding elderly persons, Kunin et al (1987) reported the results of a clinical trial in which encrustation of siliconised rubber catheters was significantly less than that of teflon-coated latex or latex catheters. Bull et al (1991) addressed the relative performance of hydrogel-coated(HC)latex and silicone rubber coated (SC) latex catheters in a RCT involving 69 long-term catheter users (elderly patients), about half of whom evaluated each catheter. The HC latex catheters had to be changed less frequently than those of SC rubber catheters (mean times between changes of 89.6 and 56.7 days, respectively; $p < 0.0014$). Over the 16 weeks of the study, the HC and the SC rubber catheters required 17 and 39 changes, respectively, and the main causes were bypassing (6% and 41% of changes) and encrustation (77% and 13% of changes).

The time it takes for encrustation to block a catheter will be affected by the lumen size as well as the rate of deposition of encrusting material. Morris & Stickler (1998) have shown in experiments using a simulated laboratory bladder containing real urine that the time to blockage is proportional to lumen diameter for catheters made from a range of different materials. This suggests that, for example, the tendency of silicone rubber catheters to block less quickly than those made from latex has more to do with the larger lumen in silicone rubber catheters than to differences in material properties.

• Size of the catheters and the ballons

According to size of the Foley catheters for neuropathic paitnes, Burgdoerfer et al (1997) recommended smaller size such as 12-14F for men and 14-16F for women to reduce the pressure effect to the urethral surface and to minimise obstruction of the urethral glands in males. It should be noticed that full-silicone catheters size of 12-14F have bigger lumens than taflon-coated or siliconised catheters especially (Burr et al 1993).

Feneley (1983) studied 24 female with neuropathic bladder with incontinence. Six patients had a patulous and shortened urethra due to the use of large diameter urethral catheters and the instillation of increasing volumes of fluid into the self-retaining balloon. In addition, Cuttino & Clark (1987) reported a case that a 30 ml Foley balloon obstructed the ureteral orifices in a neuropathic patient with a contracted bladder and caused obstructive nephropathy. After partial deflation of the balloon by withdrawing 20 ml of fluid, the patient's creatinine fell from 1.8 on admission to 0.7 two days later.

CONCLUSIONS

Whenever transurethral catheter is applied, full silicone or hydrogel-coated catheters are preferable.

Catheters size 12-16F with as large a lumen as possible and smaller (5-10 ml) self-retaining balloons are recommended for adults to minimise the pressure effect on the bladder neck and to maximise time to blockage by encrustation.

Use sterile materials and aseptic technique followed by the routine catheter care to maintain aseptic closed drainage system.

Catheters should be changed regularly, if possible, before obstruction or infection occurs. Frequency of change depends on materials and size of catheter lumen e.g., every 1-2 weeks for siliconised latex catheters, every 2-4 weeks or longer for silicone or hydrogel-coated catheters.

In developing countries, siliconised catheters widely available and costing less may be used with more frequent change.

b) Effectiveness in controlling urinary incontinence

Quality of included studies as mentioned in 5.1 and

2 case series/case report: Stickler et al 1993; McGuire & Savastano 1986 (Level of evidence 4/5)

According to the above mentioned, ID with the Foley catheter does control urinary incontinence as long as there is no outflow obstruction or bladder neck or urethral erosion due to the self-retaining balloon or the strong bladder uninhibited contractions.

McGuire & Savastano (1986) studied SCI women, 13 with ID and 22 with IC. Incontinence occurred in 92% of those with ID, and 54% suffered urethral erosion or a totally incompetent or patulous urethra 2-4 years after ID. These were caused by pressure necrosis of the self-retaining balloon or by spontaneuos extrusion that occur during bladder spasm.

Stickler et al (1993) reported an old woman whose indwelling urethral catheter became blocked regularly due to 'worm-like' structures found either in the catheter, completely occluding the lumen, or in the drainage tube thereby blocking the valve of the drainage bag. These structures were composed of bacteria e.g., Pseudomonas aeruginosa, Escherichia coli, Enterococcus faecalis and Proteus mirabilis.

CONCLUSIONS

To control urinary incontinence, ID is effective if there is no blockade or urethral/bladder neck erosion.

c) Safety for a short-term user

Quality of included studies

2 case-controlled studies: Jacobs & Kaufman 1978; Lloyd et al 1986 (Level of evidence 3)

According to the study of Jacobs & Kaufman (1978) the group of SCI patients who had a short-term ID during the acute phase had the least complication rate (0.11) compared to other groups with intermediate (0.26) and long-term (0.25) ID. They were those of bladder, genital and renal but not urethral complications. No bladder cancers were found in the short-term ID group.

Lloyd et al (1986) studied initial bladder management in 204 SCI patients during acute and rehabilitation phases. Data showed no significant differences in regard to fever and chill, urinary tract infection, upper tract changes, and pyelocaliectasis between those with ID and those with IC or SC. Moreover, after one-year follow-up, they found that the duration of the initial period of ID was not the major determinant accounting for the high infection rate.

CONCLUSIONS

A short-term ID during the acute phase is still a safe method for neuropathic patients.

d) Long-term Results and Complications

Quality of included studies

1 Cohort studies: Chen et al 2000 (Level of evidence 2)

4 case-controlled studies: Jacobs, Kaufman 1987; Chao et al 1993; Jackson, DeVivo 1992; Burr 1993.(Level of evidence 3)

9 case series/case reports: West et al 1999; Chancellor et al 1994; Shenot et al 1994; Trop, Bennett 1992; Hall et al 1989; Andrews et al 1988; Lamid S 1988; Lindan et al 1987; Feneley 1983. (Level of evidence 4)

• Urethral trauma

Andrews et al (1988) reported 16 SCI men with iatrogenic hypospadias cuased by the downward pressure of an indwelling urethral catheter. The majority of such patients find the penile appearance unacceptable.

• Urine leakage

In neuropathic women with long-term ID, one major complication seen is leakage around the Foley catheters. Frequently this is due to urethra and sphincter erosion following ID with large urethral catheters and large balloons. In addition, Lindan et al (1987) and Feneley (1983) showed that the balloons provokes detrusor contractions and sometimes the contractions are strong enough to expel the catheter balloon and rupture the urethra.

In addition catheter blockage leads to urinary leakage. Burr et al (1993) studies factors related to the blockage of ID. They found that patients with frequent catheter blockage had significantly elevated urinary pH and ammonium and calcium concentration, and could be avoided by adequate fluide intake and proper diet.

Chancellor et al (1994) reported a series of 14 female with neurological disease and a patulous and non-functioning urethra. The duration of ID ranged from 2 to 17 years. Half of them had bladder capacity less than 100 ml. Trop & Bennett (1992) reviewed 48 neurologically compromised women treated primarily with ID. They found that patulous urethra expelling catheter and urinary incontinence were seen more over years.

• Renal function

In 1978 Jacobs & Kaufman reviewed the effect of permanent bladder catheter drainage on the course of 59 long-term SCI patients. Those with long-term use (> 10 years, average 20 years), had the lowest creatinine clearance (CCr) and also had a significantly higher complication rate (0.25 per year) than those short-term ID (0.11 per year). This means that a SCI patient with a long-term ID should expect 1 major urinary tract complication every 4 years, compared to 9 years for patients who are free of ID. Among major complications, bladder cancer was found more in the long-term ID group.

Jackson & DeVivo (1992), did a prospective long-term follow-up of renal function in SCI women with ID and compared to SCI men with condom catheter (CC). They found that renal function appears to be equally reduced for both women and men with SCI. Regardless of methods of bladder management, SCI women seem to have a slightly lower risk for post-injury urological complications than men do. This is supported by the retrospective study of Chao et al (1993) done in 81 SCI persons with more than 20 years post-injury. There were no significant difference in either renal function or upper tract images/complications except of a higher prevalence of scarring and calicectasis in the ID/SC group compared to the spontaneous group (with balanced bladder or IC). In the latter group a mean total bladder capacity was 350 ml with a mean maximum voiding pressure of 55 cm H_2O and a mean residual urine of 85 ml. However there were no urodynamic data of the ID and SC group and they did not mention whether an adjunctive therapy such as bladder relaxants were used in such group to prevent bladder contracture and involuntary detrusor contractions.

• Reflux

According to the study of 32 SCI patients by Lamid (1988), free drainage such as a Foley catheter did not prevent reflux formation. It was not effective in reflux treatment because in the long run it did not prevent progression of vesico-ureteral reflux (VUR) and did not protect the refluxing kidney from damage. Moreover, incidence of VUR was higher in those with an upper motor neuron lesion.

• Bladder cancer

Chao et al (1993) 6 patients developed bladder cancer: 3 were in the ID/SC group, 2 in the spontaneous voiding (SV) group and 1 had ileal conduit. The average time from injury to bladder cancer development was 25.7 years (range 9 to 34 years). West et al (1999) reported a large retrospective study on SCI patients with chronic ID. They found that 0.39% (130 out of 33,565 patients) had bladder cancer. An average age at diagnosis was 57.3 years. The histologic finding was transitional cell carcinoma in 23 (55%), squamous cell carcinoma in 14 (33%), and adenocarcinoma in 4 (10%). Bladder management of these patients was an transurethral ID in 18 (43%), SC in 8(19%), CIC in 8 (19%) and CC in 6. Squamous cell carcinoma was common in those with ID/SC than those without chronic catheterization.

• Stones

In the study of Trop & Bennett (1992), 22 out of 48 patients (46%) of long-term ID had bladder stones, and only 6 (12%) had renal stones. Hall et al (1989) reported higher incidence of 53% of bladder stones and 36% of renal stones.

Chen et al (2000) did a multi-center longitudinal study estimating the current trend in the incidence of first kidney stone among persons with SCI and delineating the potential contributing factors. They showed that bladder management played a stronger role during year 2 and later. Those with catheter-free at discharge less than 2% were estimated to get stones within 5 years, while 7% in those with ID, 5% in CC, 5% in IC and 3% in SC group.

• Allergy

Besides, urethral catheters induced latex allergy leading to a life-threatening reaction. Shenot et al (1994) reported a SCI woman with chronic ID who underwent bladder augmentation surgery. Intraoperatively, she developed cardiovascular collapse. Subsequent skin testing to a purified latex antigen revealed latex hypersensitivity.

CONCLUSIONS

Transurethral ID is not a safe method for a long-term use in neuropathic patients.

Bladder screening for bladder cancer is mandatory especially those with ID/SC more than 5-10 years. (Level of evidence 4)

4. Prevention and Management of Complications

Quality of included studies

3 RCTs: Garibaldi et al 1980, Muncie et al 1989; Classen et al 1991; (Level of evidence 1)

6 case series/case study: Stickler et al 1985; Kunin et al 1985, Elliot et al 1989; Trop & Bennett 1992; McGuire, Savastano 1986; Feneley 1983.(Level of evidence 4)

2 reviews: Galloway 1997, Wong, Hooton 1981. (Level of evidence 4/5)

A proper catheter protocol is essential in order to control and prevent complications. Wong & Hooton (1981) gave strong recommendations for prevention of catheter-associated UTI as follows: educate personnel in correct techniques of catheter insertion and care, catheterize only when necessary, use antiseptic technique and sterile equipment, secure catheter properly, maintain closed sterile drainage.

Galloway (1997) did an extensive review of prevention and management of urinary tract infection in SCI patients. He proposed 4 essential strategies: choice of drainage system, i.e. ID should be used for as short a time as possible in the early stage; treatment of complicating factors e.g., outflow obstruction and stones; infection control by hygiene catheter care, staff and patient education; and urological follow-up.

• Meatal care

Regarding catheter care, some suggest routine cleansing of external meatus, proper fixation of the catheter, bladder irrigation etc. Garibaldi et al (1980) showed evidence that the mucous sheath between the catheter and urethra is the major pathway for entry of bacteria into the bladder when closed drainage is used and that colonisation of the urethral meatus with potentially pathogenic bacteria is a major risk factor for subsequent bacteriuria. However in RCT done in 17 adult patients, a routine meatal care with providone-iodine twice a day or with soap and water did not prove to be better than non-treated group.

• Bladder irrigation

According to the study on infected Foley catheters of Stickler et al (1985) and other study of Kunin et al (1985) external agents such as antibiotics have difficulty penetrating the encrustation and effecting bacteria present on the catheter surface. In addition, bladder irrigation increased risk of infection from frequently breaking the closed drainage system, bacterial resistance and chemical cystitis. Elliot et al (1989) showed that bladder irrigation causes mechanical damage to the bladder and may lead to bacterial invasion into deeper mucosal layers.

Muncie et al (1989) performed a randomized crossover trial comparing ten weeks of once-daily normal saline irrigation with ten weeks of no irrigation in 32 long-term catheterized women. They concluded that it is a time-consuming and costly procedure that is unlikely to have an impact on the morbidity associated with such catheters.

• **Combined measures**

Classen et al (1991) conducted an RCT to assess the prevention of bacteriuria, using a three-way system including a hydrophilic polymer-coated and pre-connected sealed catheter system, daily catheter care, and disinfection of the outflow tube of the drainage bag with povidone-iodine. They concluded that the use of several simultaneous measures to prevent catheter-associated urinary infections is no more effective than the use of pre-connected catheters with junction seals alone and is clearly more expensive.

CONCLUSIONS

Use less irritating catheters and closed drainage system to minimise complications.

Bladder irrigation and antibiotic prophylaxis are not recommended as a routine infection-control measure.

Patient education on daily cleanliness and hygiene care and a thoroughly urological check-up are mandatory.

5. Suprapubic catheterization – special aspects

An alternative to indwelling urethral catheterization is an indwelling catheter placed in the lower abdomen into the dome of the bladder. This is most commonly called the suprapubic catheter (SC).

Overall the benefit and risks of the SC is very similar to the indwelling urethral catheter including the risk for urinary tract infection, stone formation, bladder cancer, and maintenance cost of catheter and bag. However, there are several benefits for the SC and one key disadvantage. Its advantages include: (1) minimized risk of urethra trauma in men and women, (2) minimized the risk of the urethral destruction that can sometime be seen in neurologically impaired women with even relatively short-term indwelling urethral catheters, and (3) minimized urethral pain. The key disadvantage is that it requires a minor surgical procedure to insert the supra SC with potential to injury adjacent structures to the bladder especially the large intestine. There are a large number of techniques described for the insertion of the SC. The preferred technique appears to be quite variable by region and country. There is no evidence that there is one best way to insert the SC.

Long-term management of the neurogenic bladder with the SC is a controversial topic in neurourology. The issue of controversy is that some rehabilitation centers across the world highly favor the suprapubic catheter as a safe and effective long-term management of the neuropathic bladder. On the other hand, a large number of experts have personal experience with suprapubic tube complications during its long-term use.

a) Description of studies and their results

The literature on suprapubic catheterization is small and most of them are 20 years or older. There are no prospective studies and no RCT on suprapubic catheterization. The bias of favorable single center case series is that the follow-up is short with a worrisome large number of patients who are lost to follow-up. It is concerned that patients lost to follow-up may have developed complications and have died or were treated with alternative bladder management at a different hospital.

There are 11 reports that discuss the management of the neurogenic bladder with the suprapubic catheter. There are no prospective randomized studies. All the studies are also limited by short follow-up time frame. It is well established that the risk of urological complications, especially urethral destruction and bladder cancer occurs most commonly beyond after 5-10 years. Therefore a favorable report of SC after two years is relatively meaningless [Grundy et al 1983; Barnes et al 1993] (Level of evidence 3-4). There are evidence that the complications associated with SC is similar to ID and both higher than IC in the long-term management of SCI patients [Weld & Dmochowski 2000] (Level of evidence 3-4).

Complications of the SC have been reported in seven case reports (Level of evidence 4). The unique complication associated with the suprapubic tube that non-urologists who takes care of neurologically impaired patients may not be aware of is bowel perforation during the insertion of the suprapubic catheter [Farina & Palou 1992]. Bowel injection would present with acute peritonitis and warrants emergency care [Browning 1977].

There are eight reports of short-term use of suprapubic catheter as adjunct management of abdominal or pelvic operations (Level of evidence 3). The consensus is that in the short-term in none neurogenic bladder patients the suprapubic tube appears to be better than indwelling urethral catheter. However, the risk of urinary tract infection appears to be the same [Horgan et al 1992].

CONCLUSIONS

Suprapubic catheter is a reasonable alternative to indwelling urethral catheter but both are clearly inferior to intermittent catheterization.

It is a safe and effective short-term management of urinary retention.

It is not recommended for the routine use for the long-term management of the neurogenic bladder.

6. Comparison between ID and SC

Quality of included studies

6 case series/case study: MacDiarmid et al 1995; Barnes et al 1993; Lloyd et al 1986; McGuire & Savastano 1986; Feneley 1983; Hackler 1982.(Level of evidence 4)

Regarding female incontinence after long-term ID, Feneley (1983) managed by SC with urethral closure and 19 out of 24 patients had satisfactory results. McGuire & Savastano (1986) suggests that SC may have advantage over ID with less urethral complications.

According to a comparison study between long-term SC and ID or external drainage, Hackler (1982) evaluated 31 SCI patients maintaining on SC for a least 5 years (average 8 years) by intravenous urography (IVU) and cystourethrography (CUG). Results showed that only 39% of 62 renal units were normal, 33% had evidence of chronic pyelonephritis, 18% with stones and 10% with hydronephrosis and hydroureters. He then compared this study with his previous studies on SCI patients with long-term (20 years) external appliance or ID. The renal units remained normal in 66% (128/195) of those with external appliance drainage, in 51% (77/152) of those with ID but in only 39% of those with SC. The incidence of VUR was significantly higher in the SC patients but the incidence of hydronephrosis was higher in the ID patients. He concluded that five years with SC might cause as much renal damage as 20 years with ID. However, only 6 were on anticholinergic therapy.

Lloyd et al (1986) did a study on initial bladder management in 204 SCI patients. Twenty-one patients were initially treated with fine bore SC but there was only 1 with such drainage one year after discharge. When compared those with SC to those with ID or IC, there were no difference in rate of UTI, bladder calculi and upper tract changes during acute and rehabilitation phases.

In addition, Barnes et al (1993) studied 40 neuropathic patients managed by SC. All received anticholinergics and daily clamped the catheter. Catheter-related problem reduced and 84% of the patients accepted it and it did not accelerated renal deteriotation during the 2-year follow-up.

MacDiarmid et al (1995) reported a case series of 44 SCI patients with SC for a mean duration of 58 months. They used latex Foley catheters and weekly irrigation with 500 ml to 1,000 ml of normal saline or 1:5,000 chlorhexidine solution; and changed the catheter every 2 weeks. In addition, after discharge the patients had routine urological check-up with cystometry and renal ultrasound every 6 months or annually. None of their patients had renal deterioration, vesicoureteral reflux (VUR) or bladder carcinoma. Uncomplicated infection (43%), bladder calculi (41%), catheter blockage (36%) and incontinence (11%) were reported.

CONCLUSIONS

Due to less urethral complications, SC is an alternative for a short-term management for neuropathic patients.

Adjuctive anticholinergic therapy, to minimise leakage and the development of bladder and renal abnormalities, is necessary especially in those with detrusor hyperreflexia.

7. Long-term Quality of Life

Quality of included studies

2 Case-control studies: Dewire et al 1992; Watanabe et al 1996

Dewire et al (1992) did a retrospective study of 57 tetraplegic SCI patients who were followed for a minimum of 10 years and compared urological complications between those with ID and without ID. They found no difference between these 2 groups. They suggest that the decision to manage tetraplegics with or without an ID should not be based on relative risk of complications or renal deterioration. The decision to avoid ID in these patients should reflect patient comfort, convenience and quality of life.

Watanabe et al (1996) investigated the changes in sexuality and quality of life in 18 neurologically impaired women treated with ID who underwent bladder reconstruction. All patients were followed 6 to 40 months (mean 18) after reconstructive surgery using a 9-part questionnaire to score numerically the effect of surgical reconstruction on sexuality and quality of life issues. In 4 of the 15 women who were sexually active preoperatively the frequency of sexual intercourse doubled from a mean of 3 to 6 times per month, respectively, and all 4 women reported improved sexual satisfaction.

RECOMMENDATIONS

Transurethral ID and suprapubic catheter are not recommended as a safe method for long term use in the neuropathic patients. *(Grade of recommendation C)*

Nowadays with less irritating catheter materials, improved closed drainage systems and regular urological check-up long term complications can be decreased, nevertheless ID/SC is still the last resource also in neuropathic women when other methods fail or are not applicable or are not accepted by the patient. *(Grade of recommendation C)*

One should consider patient comfort, convenience, sexuality and quality of life before prescribe ID as a long-term management for neuropathic patients. *(Grade of recommendation C)*

IMPLICATIONS FOR PRACTICE (Grade of recommendation B-C)

A silicone catheter with a smaller balloon of 5-10 ml is preferable.

For developing countries, use a siliconised catheter, change every 1-2 weeks or earlier, if possible, before obstruction or infection occurs.

Long-term ID may be safe only if a careful check-up of urodynamic, renal function, and upper and lower tract imaging are performed regularly at least yearly.

Annual cystoscopy and biopsy may be necessary for those after 10 years of ID and those with an episode of gross hematuria, chronic symptomatic UTI rafractory to therapy.

IMPLICATIONS FOR RESEARCH

More research to improve material used in the catheter's construction.

RCT on a proper duration of use of each type of catheters.

More research on impacts of ID on quality of life.

III. CONDOM CATHETER AND EXTERNAL APPLIANCES

1. BACKGROUND

Patients with neurogenic bladder and urinary incontinence usually need some kinds of urinary drainage system. In male, a condom catheter (CC) has been one of the choices (Figure 9). All CCs are connected to a urine or leg bag to collect the urine. Till now, there have been many variety of CCs available such as a simple thin latex or plastic or silicone CC or condom sheath, a rubber condom urinal which is a non-collapsable condom with funnel weld at the end, a CC with a double row of convolutions near the catheter tip to prevent kink with a unique inner flap to prevent backflow of the urine to the shaft of the penic and inner wall coated with a self-adhesive [deHoll JD et al, 1992], a special condom with a passage for catheterization without removal of the condom [personal communication].

2. OBJECTIVES

To find evidence to answer the following questions:

1. How to apply the condom catheter?

2. Is it effective?

3. Is it safe?

4. Is it cost-effective?

5. How to prevent complications?

6. Comparison between different types of CCs

7.Long term results and quality of life

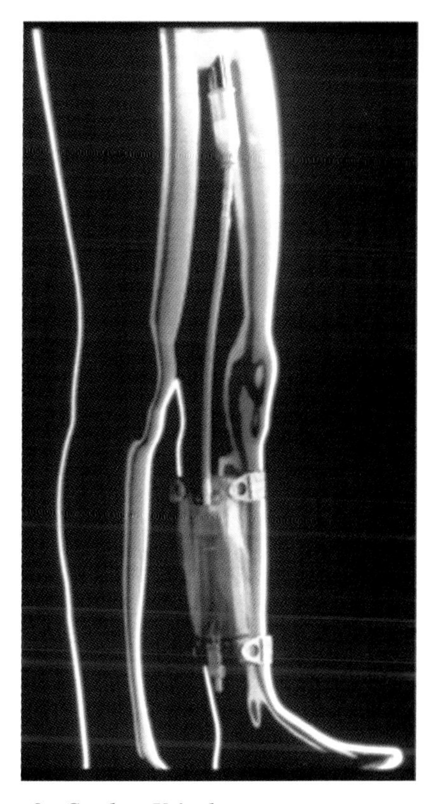

Figure 9 : Condom Urinal

3. Criteria for considering studies search strategy

Type of studies: all types of studies including experts' opinions

Type of participants: adult men

Type of outcome measure: efficiency, tolerability, safety and cost-effectiveness

Search from Medline (Pubmed) from 1966-2000:

With the keywords of 'condom catheter' and 'urinary continence' there were 37 papers sorted and only 15 papers were selected.

With the keywords of 'condom cathether' and 'neurogenic bladder' there were 18 papers sorted and only 10 were selected.

With the keywords of 'condom drainage' and ' neurogenic bladder' there were 12 papers sorted and only 6 papers were selected.

With the keywords of condom sheath' and 'urinary incontinence' only 1 paper was searched.

Overall 26 papers were reviewed.

4. Results

a) How to apply the condom catheter?

Quality of included studies:

1 Clinical trial: Peifer, Hanover 1997.

4 Case series and case reports: Brooks 1981; Pearman, Shah 1973; Smith et al 1980; Namiki 1984.

In the past, most of the CCs need devices to secure or fasten them to the penis to prevent slipping or detachment. They are as follows: an elastic tape/a fastener [Brooks 1981]; a non-elastic tape, an adhesive band or a strip; a supporting apparatus i.e., a proximal part of a conventional rubber urinal (Stoke Mandeville type) with straps and buckles [Pearman & Shah 1973]; skin adhesives etc.

Nowadays many commercial CCs with self-adhesives allowing easier application are available in developed countries. Peifer & Hanover (1997) did a clinical study comparing between a new 'easy-flow catheter' and other CCs. All except one of the 20 subjects found the new CC easier to apply and also easiest to remove. Moreover, it increased daytime and nighttime dryness in half of the studied group.

However they are some who have difficulty in applying CCs. They are those with overweight and/or some degree of penile atrophy. Smith et al (1980) successfully implanted penile prostheses to 10 patients who had neurogenic bladder and wore CCs. All indicated that the penile prosthesis helped keep the CC in place. Namiki (1984) reported a technique of teflon paste injection in the subdermal area directly below the glans penis to make a stopper to help maintain a secure position of the CC on th penic of a SCI patient.

In addition, to prevent the pubic hair to become trapped under the CC and to allow easy removal of the CC, the pubic hair should be removed.

b) Is it effective in preventing leakage?

Quality of included studies

1 Clinical trial: Peifer, Hanover 1997.

1 Case series: Saint et al 1999.

Saint et al (1999) did a questionnaire study in male patients and nursing staff. A major drawback of the CC is leaking and a more secure CC is needed to improve the management of male incontinence. Peifer & Hanover (1997) evaluated a new CC, the Easy-Flow External Condom Catheter in 20 subjects who were experienced user of CC. They found that the new CC reduced frequency of changing the CC, and increased daytime and nighttime dryness. Without an anatomical abnormality of the penis or overweight, cooperative neuropathic patients successfully apply CC and have no urine leakage.

c) Is it safe?

Quality of included studies

2 Case-controlled studies: Hirsch et al 1979; Kovindha & Wachirarat 1998.

7 Case series and case reports: Newman & Price 1985; de Holl et al 1992; Nanninga & Rosen 1975; Bang 1994; Pidde & Little 1994; Shenot et al 1994; Harmon et al 1995.

Hirsch et al (1979) studied urinary tract infection (UTI) among neuropathic patients with incontinence and using CCs. They found that 53.3% of those who were not cooperative had UTI while cooperative ones did not have UTI during the study. Newman & Price (1985) reported hazards and complications in 60 SCI men using CCs. Over 50% of patients in this study had positive urine cultures and 56% of patients with positive cultures had evidence of tissue invasion by bacteria. Many of these patients had numerous deficiencies in voiding habits causing incomplete bladder emptying, high residual urine and bladder overdistension. Stasis of urine within the CCs due to twisting of the CCs or kink of the drainage system was found especially when using a simple condom sheath. To overcome the twisting, those in developing countries an simple device e.g., a fixator, easily made by patients themselves may be added to the CC drainage system [Kovindha et al 1988] or those in developed countries non-collapsable CCs may be used [de Holl et al 1992].

Nanninga & Rosen (1975) reported penetrating or non-penetration lesions due to compressive effects of the condom fasteners or the proximal hard roller ring of the condom causing. Bang (1994) reported a neurogenic patient who continuously used the CC. He developed localised chronic edema on the dorsum of the penis and urethral fistula on the ventral surface. Pidde & Little (1994) reported a SCI patient with bilateral hydronephrosis due to CC retention strap. The hydronephrosis resolved when the strap was eliminated.

Other complications such as irritative or allergic reactions to latex CCs, to skin adhesives and to urine were also reported. Shenot et al (1994) reported 2 patients of allergic reaction to the latex CCs. The first one was paraplegic with 14 years managing with CC until the development of chronic penile dermatitis. Because of the morbidity associated with the latex CCs, he underwent cystectomy and ileal conduit diversion. Immediately after entering the peritoneal cavity, he became acutely hypotensive with evidence of bronchospasm. Last he was diagnosed with latex allergy using RAST and latex antigen skin testing. The other was also a paraplegic with 4 years managing with CCs. He presented with sever dermatitis and breakdown of the phallic skin. Subsequent skin testing to the latex antigen confirmed latex hypersensitivity. He then used a silicone CC resulting in the prompt resolution of the pathologic skin changes. Harmon et al (1995) also reported a patient after 25 years of wearing CCs, recurrent blister and sloughing of the penile shaft developed. He was found to have hypersensitivities to several allergenic components of the CCs. The condition improved after switching to a silicone CC and topical application of steroids.

d) Is it cost-effectiveness?

There have been no studies of cost-effectiveness of CCs.

e) How to prevent complications?

Quality of included studies

1 Clinical trial: Edlich et al 2000.

4 Case series and case reports: Zoller et al 1988; Hirsch et al 1979; Sotolongo & Koleitat 1990; Waites et al 1993.

If a condom catheter is the choice of treatment, proper size, type, material and application should be stressed to the patients to prevent the above-mentioned complications.

Edlich et al (2000) did a pilot clinical study of latex external condom catheters (ECCs) and silicone ECCs. It demonstrated the superior performance of the silicone ECC over that of the latex ECC. Moreover, the silicone ECC has a self-adhesive that binds more securely to human skin than the self-adhesive of the latex ECC. The moisture vapour transmission through silicone is significantly greater than through latex. Therefore silicone CCs which are now available should be used for those having allergic reaction to latex or those who need long-term CC usage to minimize a chance to develop such allergic reaction.

Zoller at al (1988) evaluated the prevalence of sensitization to natural latex in 50 children with congenital neurogenic bladder. They found that elevated latex-specific IGE values were statistically correlated with the number of past operations and a history of atopic or allergic reactions. They suggested serological examinations of latex-specific IGE in addition to patient history to better identify patient at risk.

Continuous use of the CC should be avoided. If used, silicone CC with self-adhesive is preferable to lesser both compressive and irritative effects.

Although bacteriuria is commonly found in those on CCs, it might not cause serious damage to the urinary tract. Hirsch et al (1979) found that no UTI developed in 79 episodes of CC use in patients who were cooperative or not be able to manipulate the CC drainage system. Sotolongo & Koleitat (1990) did a prospective study of 56 male SCI patients on CCs within 5 months of the injuries for 5 years. All had low bladder pressures (filling maximum 35 cm water and voiding maximum of 70 cm water) ascertained by video urodynamics. And all patients had colonized urine (asymptomatic) during the entire study period. However no patient sustained deterioration of the urinary tract on imagine or by serum creatinine. Therefore with low bladder pressure, aymptomatic bacteriuria is of no consequence to the integrity of the upper urinary tract.

Waites et al (1993) did a prospective study of 64 catheter-free SCI patients. They found that bladder management technique (IC programme, ICP or CC) was not associated with increased risk of UTI. The only factors correlated with increased risk were black ethnicity, less than excellent personal hygiene, and less than dailty change of CCs.

f) How to treat complications?

Quality of included studies

2 Case series and case reports: Nanninga & Rosen 1975; Harmon et al 1995.

If there is a skin lesion, a CC should be removed and the patient may have to resume IC or wear an ID until the skin is dry or healed sufficiently to reapply the CC. An additional surgical debridement may be necessary if the lesion is ulcerated or necrotic [Nanninga & Rosen 1975]. Those with allergic dermatitis, the latex CC should be removed and topical steroid should be applied [Harmon et al 1995].

g) Comparing between different types of CCs

Quality of included studies

2 Clinical trials: Edlich et al 2000; Peifer & Hanover 1997.

Edlich et al (2000) conducted a study comparing between a silicone CC with self adhesive and a latex CC. The silicone CC is much better than the latex CC in many ways. Peifer & Hanover (1997) found the new CC easier to apply and also easiest to remove when compared to previous CCs used. It also increased daytime and nighttime dryness in half of the studied group. (As mentioned above)

h) Long-term results related to quality of life

Quality of included studies

1 Case-controlled study: Sekar et al 1997.

Sekar et al (1997) did a comparison study of long-term renal function after SCI using different urinary management methods. They used effective renal plasma flow (ERPF) to evaluate renal function and found that renal function was adequately preserved in the great majority of persons and did not appear to be influenced to any great extent by method of bladder management. Although at discharge 33% of 913 patients used IC, they found that the percentage of men using CCs increased with advancing time post-injury while the percentage using IC decreased. The majority of men used CC in each time period while the majority of women used ID.

CONCLUSIONS ***(Level of evidence 4)***

CC still has a role in control urinary incontinence in neuropathic male patients.

Long-term use may cause bacteriuria but it does not increase the risk of UTI when compared to other methods of bladder management.

Complications may be less if apply it properly with good hygiene care, frequently change the CC and maintain low bladder pressures.

RECOMMENDATIONS
(Level of recommendation B-C)

To have better control of leakage, a more secure CC should be used and patients should be educated and cooperative.

To prevent latex allergy, a silicone CC should be used and serological examinations of latex-specific IGE is recommended in addition to patient history to better identify patient at risk.

To prevent compressive effects, choose proper size CC with self- adhesive.

To prevent infection, a CC should be changed at least daily.

To prevent bladder and upper tract damage, regular bladder emptying with low bladder pressures and low PVR should be persued.

D. PHARMACOTHERAPY

I. BACKGROUND

Pharmacological treatment of urinary incontinence is overviewed in the Chapter on the Pharmacological Treatment. Therefore, this section focuses on special aspects in regards to its indication and efficacy in patients with neuropathic bladder/urethral dysfunction. The principal causes of urinary incontinence in this subpopulation are detrusor hyperreflexia (DH) and/or incompetence of urethral closing function. Thus, to improve urinary incontinence the treatment should aim at decreasing detrusor activity, increasing bladder capacity and/or increasing bladder outlet resistance. Pharmacologic therapy has been particularly helpful in patients with relatively mild degrees of neurogenic bladder dysfunction. Patients with more profound neurogenic bladder disturbances may require pharmacologic treatment to augment other forms of management such as intermittent catheterization (IC).

Although the two most commonly used classes of agents are anticholinergics and alpha-adrenergic blockers, the drugs used for treating neuropathic bladder/urethral dysfunction should be classified as follows:

a) Drugs for incontinence due to detrusor hyperreflexia and/or low compliant detrusor

1. Bladder relaxant drugs

a) Oxybutynin

b) Propiverine

c) Trospium

d) Tolterodine

e) Propantheline

f) Oxyphencyclimine

g) Flavoxate

h) Tricyclic Antidepressants

2. Drugs for blocking nerves innervating the bladder

a) Vanilloids

1) Capsaicin

2) Resiniferatoxin

b) Botulinum toxin

b) Drugs for incontinence due to neurogenic sphincter deficiency

1. Alpha-adrenergic agonists

2. Estrogens

3. Beta-adrenergic agonists

4. Tricyclic antidepressants

c) Drugs for facilitating bladder emptying

1. Alpha adrenergic blockers

2. Cholinergics

II. OBJECTIVES

1. Is each of the drugs listed above effective for treating neurogenic urinary incontinence ?
2. Is the drug safe?
3. How to prevent complications?
4. Is the treatment cost-effective?
5. What are the long-term results including the impact on quality of life?

III. CRITERIA FOR CONSIDERING STUDIES AND SEARCHING STRATEGY

All types of publications dealing with pharmacotherapy in adult patients with neurogenic bladder/urethral dysfunction have been included in this search.

1. Medline through Pubmed from 1966-2000, and the list of publications used in first International Consultation Report if not included in the former list.
2. Keywords: Pharmacotherapy, urinary incontinence, neurogenic bladder, and the drug names listed above.
3. Method of review: all publications in adults (>=19 years old), humans were considered in regards to outcome, efficacy, safety and cost-effectiveness, in all languages.
4. Description of the review: There are 688 articles found by searching with the keywords-combination of "pharmacotherapy" & "urinary incontinence", and 319 articles with "pharmacotheray" & "neurogenic bladder". The number of the reviewed studies dealing with each of the drugs listed above is described separately in each section on the corresponding subtopics. Methodological quality of the included studies is indicated separately based on the subtopics dealling with each of the drugs listed above in each section on the corresponding subtopics.

IV. RESULTS/CONCLUSIONS

1. Drugs for incontinence due to DH and/or low compliant detrusor

a) Bladder relaxant drugs

Anticholinergic agents are by far the most useful pharmacologic agents in the management of neurogenic bladder. Anticholinergic agents are employed to suppress DH. Although there is an abundance of drugs available for the treatment of DH, for many of them, efficacy is estimated based on preliminary open studies rather than on controlled clinical trials [Andersson 1988]. However, drug effect in individual patients may be practically important. In developing countries, most of the bladder relaxant drugs listed below are not available mainly due to economical reasons, which makes the pharmacological treatment of DH in these countries difficult.

General indications of pharmacological treatment in DH are (1) to improve or eliminate reflex incontinence, (2) to eliminate/to prevent a high intravesical pressure situation and (3) to enhance the efficacy of intermittent catheterization (IC), triggered voiding and indwelling catheters (ID). Spinal DH is mostly associated with a functional outflow obstruction due to detrusor-sphincter-dyssynergia (DSD). For the most part, pharmacotherapy is used to suppress reflex detrusor activity completely and facilitate IC. On the other hand bladder relaxant drugs decrease detrusor-contractility also during voiding. With this situation residual urine increases and must then be assisted or accomplished by IC (Figure 10).

1. Oxybutynin (total 178 articles reviewed, including 36 articles searched in combination with the keyword

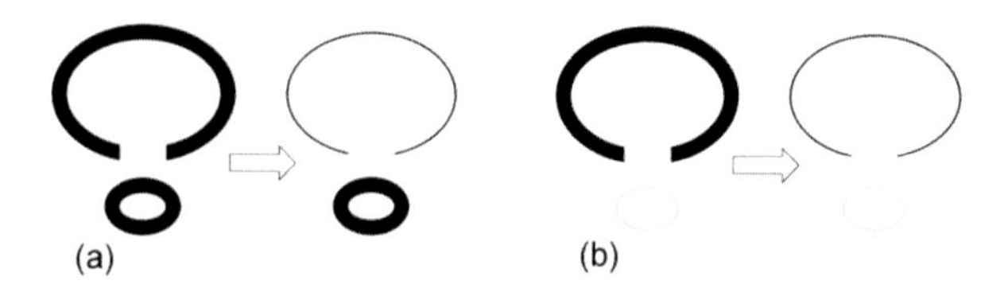

Figure 10 : The effect of bladder relaxant drugs on the hyperreflexic detrusor (schematic drawing). Aims of treatment are to change a hyperreflexic into a hyporeflexic detrusor. In the spinal reflex bladder (a) voiding may become unbalanced, as the spastic striated sphincter muscle remains unaffected; this problem does not occur in the suprapontine reflex bladder (b), as the sphincter mostly remains normally functioning)

of neurogenic bladder, 16 clinical trials (CTs) and 2 randomized controlled trials (RCTs), and 89 articles with the keyword of urinary incontinence, 35 CTs and 20 CRTs).

Oxybutynin hydrochloride is a moderately potent antimuscarinic agent with a pronounced muscle relaxant activity and local anesthetic activity as well [Andersson 1988; Anderson & Fredericks 1972; Yarker et al 1995; Wein 1997].

- Oral Administration

Several double-blind controlled studies have shown its efficacy for DH (Level of evidence 1) [Thompson & Lauvetz 1976; Hehir & Fitzpatrick 1985; Gajewski & Awad 1986; Koyanagi et al 1986; Zeegers et al 1987; Thüroff et al 1991]. The overall rates of good results (more than 50% symptomatic improvement) are 47 % with 3 mg t.i.d. and 61-86% with 5 mg t.i.d. Side effects were noted in all studies and severity increased with dosage. The overall incidence of possible side effects is 24.5% for 3 mg t.i.d. and 12.5% to 68% for 5 mg t.i.d. Most of them are related to antimuscarinic action with dry mouth as the most common complaint (incidence of 12.2% with 9 mg/day and between *12.5% to 47.6% with 15 mg/day).*

A once-a-day controlled-release formulation of oxybutynin, oxybutynin XL (Ditropan XL®) was recently developed. Parallel-group, randomized, controlled clinical trials comparing the efficacy and safety of cotrolled –release oxybutynin, oxybutynin XL with conventional, immediate-release oxybutynin in patients with overactive bladder demostrate that the urge urinary incontinence episodes declined log-linearly, and no significant difference was observed between the two formulations (Level of evidence 1) [Anderson et al 1999; Birns et al 2000; Versi et al 2000]. However, there was a trend toward higher efficacy with oxybutynin XL than with immediate-release oxybutynin at the same dose in one study. Dose-dry mouth analysis showed that the probability of dry mouth with an increasing dose was significantly lower with oxybutynin XL than with immediate-release oxybutynin [Gupta et al 1999]. However, no studies have been published on the efficacy and safety of oxybutynin XL dealing especially with neuropathic subgroup of patients.

Despite its adverse effects, oxybutynin (2.5-5 mg taken twice or three-times daily), especially Oxybutynin XL, a once-a-day controlled-release formulation of oxybutynin, is recommended for the treatment of overactive bladder (Grade of recommendation A). Further studies, however, are necessary to determine whether its controlled–release formulation has better tolerability also in neuropathic subpopulation. Clinical practice should aim at individual titration of drug dosage for a maximum therapeutic effect with minimal side effects [Yarker et al 1995; Wein 1997, Thüroff et al 1991].

- Intravesical application

Intravesical instillation of oxybutynin has been demonstrated its efficacy in patients with DH in whom oral oxybutynin failed or was not tolerated (Level of evidence 4) [Brendleret al 1989; Madersbacher & Jilg 1991; Greenfield & Fera 1991; Weese et al 1993; Prasad & Vaidyanathan 1993; Kasabian et al 1994; Mizunaga et al 1994; Connor et al 1994; Buyse et al 1995; Kaplinsky et al 1996; Painter et al 1996; Palmer et al 1997; Saito et al 2000; Pannek et al 2000], although no randomized controlled study has been reported. The rate of symptomatic improvement ranged from 55% to 90%. No antimuscarinic systemic side effects have been reported in early short-term follow-up studies. In recent relatively long-term studies [Madersbacher & Jilg 1991; Kasabian et al 1994; Buyse et al 1995], however, the incidence of side effects was 25-55%, and treatment was discontinued in 25-65 % mainly due to inconvenience and also due to side effects.

Intravesical instillation of oxybutynin is recommended for selected patients, who are already on IC but still incontinent between, due to persistent DH, if oral medication is not successful or not tolerated [Yarker et al 1995; Madersbacher & Jilg 1991] (Grade of recommendation C). The usual dose is a 5 mg pill dissolved in 10-30 ml saline or water. The solution is instilled intravesically twice daily and retained for at least 30 minutes. There has been no commercial preparation of this medication for direct instillation into the bladder.

2. PROPIVERINE (total 22 articles reviewed, including 14 CTs and 4 RCTs , 4 CTs and 2 RCTs searched in combination with the keyword of neurogenic bladder).

Propiverine hydrochloride is a benzylic acid derivative with musculotropic (calcium antagonistic) activity and moderate antimuscarinic effects [Tokuno et al 1993]. Several randomized double-blind, controlled clinical studies of this drug in patients with DH have been reported [Stöhrer et al 1999; Takayasu et al 1990; Madersbacher et al 1999]. In a placebo-controlled, double-blind, randomized, prospective, multicentric trial, Stöhrer et al (1999) evaluated the efficacy and tolerability of propiverine (15 mg t.i.d. for 14 days) as compared to placebo in 113 patients suffering from DH caused by spinal cord injury. The majority of patients practised intermittent catheterization for bladder emptying. The maximum cystometric bladder capacity increased significantly in the propiverine group, on average by 104 ml. Sixty-three % of the patients expressed a subjective improvement of their symptoms under propiverine in comparison to only 23% of the placebo group. Takayasu et al (1990) conducted a double-blind, placebo-controlled multicentric study in 70 neurogenic patients. During a treatment period of 14 days, 20 mg propiverine once daily or placebo were administered. An increase of maximum bladder capacity, a decrease of maximum detrusor pressure and an increase of residual urine were also obtained in this Japanese study, all statistically significant compared to placebo. Madersbacher et al (1999) in a placebo-controlled, multicentre study demostrated that propiverine is a safe and effective drug in the treatment of DH; it is as effective as oxybutynin, but the incidence of dry mouth and its severity is less with propiverine (15 mg, three times daily) than with oxybutynin (5 mg twice daily).

Propiverine has a documented beneficial effect in the treatment of DH, and seems to have an acceptable adverse effect profile (Level of evidence 1). The drug is recommended in the treatment of DH (Grade of recommendation A). The standard oral adult dose is 10-15 mg two or three times daily.

3. TROSPIUM (total 6 articles refer to the topic reviewed, including 6 CTs and 5 RCTs , and 3 RCTs searched in combination with the keyword of neurogenic bladder).

Trospium is a quaternary ammonium derivative with mainly antimuscarinic actions. In a placebo controlled, double-blind study in 61 patients with spinal DH, significant improvements in maximum cystometric capacity and maximal detrusor pressure were demonstrated with 20 mg b.i.d for 3 weeks compared with placebo [Stöhrer et al 1991]. Few side-effects were noted, comparable with placebo. Madersbacher et al (1995) compared the clinical efficacy and tolerance of trospium (20 mg b.i.d.) and oxybutynin (5 mg t.i.d.) in a randomized, double-blind, urodynamically controlled, multicentre trial in 95 patients with spinal cord injuries and DH. They found that the two drugs are equal in their effects on DH (increase of the cystometric bladder capacity by 30% and decrease of the maximum detrusor pressure by 30%), but trospium has fewer severe side effects (incidence of severe dry mouth 5% with trospium vs. 25 % with oxybutynin) [Madersbacher et al 1995].

Trospium has a documented effect on DH (Level of evidence 1). The drug is recommended to use for DH (Grade of recommendation A).

4. TOLTERODINE (total 28 articles refer to the topic reviewed, including 15 CTs and 8 RCTs , and 4 CTs and 2 RCTs searched in combination with the keyword of neurogenic bladder)

Tolterodine is a new competitive muscarinic receptor antagonist [Nilvebrant et al 1997a; 1997b]. Recently, several randomized, double-blind controlled studies in patients with overactive bladder have demonstrated its beneficial effect [Jonas et al 1997; Appel et al 1997; Rentzhog et al 1998; Abrams et al 1998; Van Kerrebroeck et al 1998; Goessl et al 2000; Malone-Lee et al 2001; Van Kerrebroeck et al 2001; Appel et al 2001] (Level of evidence 1). Jonas et al (1997) reported on a randomized, double-blind, placebo-controlled study of tolterodine including urodynamic analysis in a total of 242 patients. Two mg b.i.d. was significantly more effective than placebo in increasing maximum cystometric bladder capacity and volume at first contraction after 4 weeks treatment. However, there are no published reports on the specific effect on DH. The better tolerability profile of tolterodine compared to oxybutynin has been confirmed in an another randomized studies on detrusor overactivity [Abrams et al 1998]. Tolterodine (2 mg b.i.d.) appears to be as effective as oxybutynin (5 mg t.i.d.), but is much better tolerated, especially in regards to dry mouth. In a meta-analysis of 4 multicenter prospective trial of 1,120 patients, moderate to severe dry mouth was reported in 6% of the placebo, 4% of the 1 mg bid tolterodine, 17% of the 2 mg b.i.d. tolterodine and 60% of those patients receiving conventional 5 mg t.i.d. oxybutynin [Appel et al 1997]. An another randomized controlled trial by Malone-Lee et al (2001) demostrated superior tolerability than and comparable efficacy to oxybutinin in individuals 50 year old or older with overactive bladder.

Van Kerrebroeck et al (2001) reported a comparative study of the efficacy and safety of tolterodine extended release (ER; 4 mg once daily), tolterodine immediate release (IR; 2 mg twice daily), as well as placebo in 1,529 adult patients with overactive bladder. The primary efficacy variable was the change in mean number of incontinence episodes per week, which decreased 53% from baseline in the tolterodine ER group, 45% with tolterodine IR, and 28% in the placebo group. Tolterodine ER and IR provided a similar significant reduction in incontinence episodes versus placebo. Post hoc analysis of the data using median values, based on rational of skewed data distribution, demonstrated improved efficacy of tolterodine ER versus IR. Dry mouth was significantly lower with tolterodine ER than tolterodine IR (23% tolterodine ER 31% tolterodine IR, and 8% placebo). The incidence of other side effects was similar to placebo in the tolterodine ER and tolterodine IR groups.

A comparative study between controlled release oxybutynin (oxybutynin XL) and immediate release tolterodine (tolterodine IR), was recently published [Appel et al 2001]. Three hundred seventy-eight patients were randomized to receive either oxybutynin XL 10 mg. (n=185) or tolterodine IR 4 mg. (2 mg. b.i.d.) (n=193). The populations were evenly matched with respect to demographics. Oxybutynin XL reduced the number of weekly episodes of urge incontinence from 25.6 to 6.1 instances. Tolterodine IR decreased the number of weekly episodes from 24.1 to 7.8 instances. Oxybutynin XL demonstrated better efficacy (P=0.03) compared to tolterodine IR. Dry mouth and central nervous system side effects were similar between oxybutynin XL and tolterodine IR.

Although tolterodine has a documented effect on overactive bladder (Level of evidence 1), futher studies on the effect of the drug on DH in the neuropathic population are neccesary. Comparative studies of tolterodine ER with propiverine, trospium or oxybutynin XL, especially in regards to tolerability, could be useful to evaluate its position amongst other bladder relaxant drugs beside conventional oxybutynin or tolterodine IR.

5. Propantheline (total 8 articles searched in combination with the keyword of neurogenic bladder) including 2 CTs. No RCT was found.)

Propantheline bromide was the classically described oral antimuscarinic drug. Despite its success in uncontrolled case series [Andersson 1988; Blaivas et al 1980; Level of evidence 5], no adequate controlled study of this drug for DH is available. The usual adult oral dosage is 7.5 to 30 mg three to four times daily, although higher doses are often necessary [Wein 1997].

6. Oxyphencyclimine (total 1 CT refer to the topic reviewed)

Oxyphencyclimine is a cheap antimuscarinic that is usually used for treatment of peptic ulcer.

Kitisomprayoonkul and Kovindha (2000) reported their experience in 10 complete SCI patients who had urinary incontinence, treated with oxyphencyclimine HCl (15-20 mg/day) for 1-2 weeks.

All patients had clinical improvement even though some reported dry mouth and constipation that were tolerable. Significant improvement was observed regarding the mean frequency of incontinence per day, mean catheterization volume, mean maximum detrusor pressure, mean volume at the initial detrusor contraction and the cystometric capacity at the first leaking point (Level of evidence 4).

Due to its availability and very low cost, oxyphencyclimine may be an alternative bladder relaxant for SCI patients in developing countries where other potent bladder relaxant drugs are not available or too expensive (Grade of recommendation D).

7. Flavoxate (total 18 articles refer to the topic reviewed, including 11 CTs and 4 RCTs)

Flavoxate hydrochloride has a direct inhibitory action on detrusor smooth muscle in vitro. Early clinical trials with flavoxate have shown favorable effects in patients with DH [Kohler & Morales 1968; Pedersen et al 1972]. Several randomized controlled studies have shown that the drug has essentially no effects on detrusor overactivity (Level of evidence 1) [Zeegers et al 1987; Robinson & Brocklehurst 1972; Chapple et al 1990].

8. Tricyclic Antidepressants (total 20 articles refer to the topic reviewed with the keyword of imipramine, including 3 CTs and 0 RCTs, and no CTs searched in combination with the keyword of neurogenic bladder)

Many clinicians have found tricyclic antidepressants, particularly imipramine hydrochloride, to be useful agents for facilitating urine storage, both by decreasing bladder contractility and by increasing outlet resistance [Wein 1997; Barrett & Wein 1991]. However, no sufficiently controlled trials of tricyclic antidepressants in terms of DH in neuropathics have been reported. Nevertheless in some developing countries tricyclic antidepressants are the only bladder relaxant substances which people can afford. The down side with tricyclic antidepressants is the narrow safety profile and side effects. The potential hazard of serious cardiovascular toxic effect should be taken into consideration [Andersson 1988]. Combination therapy using antimascarinics and imipramine may have synergistic benefits (Level of evidence 5).

b) Drugs for blocking nerves innervating the bladder

1. Vanilloids

The vanilloids, capsaicin and resiniferatoxin, activate nociceptive sensory nerve fibers through an ion channel, recently discovered by Caterina et al (1997), known as vanilloid receptor subtype 1 (VR1). This receptor is a nonselective cation channel, and is activated by increases in temperature to within the noxious range and by protons, suggesting that it functions as a transducer of painful thermal stimuli and acidity *in vivo*. When activated the channel opens, allowing an influx of calcium and sodium ions that depolarizes the nociceptive afferent terminals, initiating a nerve impulse that travels through the dorsal root ganglion into the central nervous system. Noxious temperature uses the same elements, which explains why the mouth feels hot when eating chili peppers [Clapham 1997]. Previously called the capsaicin receptor, VR1 has been localized in the spinal cord, dorsal root ganglia and visceral organs, including the bladder, urethra and colon. Activation of VR1 results in spike-like currents [Liu & Simon 1996], and selectively excites and subsequently desensitizes C-fibers. Capsaicin-desensitization is defined as long lasting, reversible suppression of sensory neuron activity [Craft et al 1995]. How fast and for how long the desensitization develops is related to the dose and time of exposure to capsaicin, and the interval between consecutive dosing [Szolcsányi et al 1975; Maggi et al 1988]. The transient increase in intracellular concentration of calcium ions also leads to activation of intracelllar enzymes, peptide transmitter release and neuronal degeneration [Szallasi & Blumberg 1990a; Kawatani et al 1989].

1) Capsaicin (total 24 articles refer to the topic reviewed, including 3 RCTs and 8 CTs)

Recently, capsaicin, the "gold standard" in the vanilloid class of drugs, has been tried as an intravesical drug with limited success. If overactive bladder is due to sensitization and/or recruitment of C-fibers resulting in an overall increase in the C-fiber contribution to mechanoreception, then functional desensitization of C-fiber afferent neurons may decrease detrusor overactivity (Figure 11). However, capsaicin causes initial stimulation of the unmyelinated C-fibers, resulting in severe discomfort or pain, along with release of the neurotransmitters substance P and/or neurokinin A in the bladder. The use of capsaicin is still largely experimental, and includes patients with DH, however some trials are ongoing with the use of capsaicin for detrusor instability, especially when the patient has failed other forms of treatment. In a capsaicin study of DH, 44% of patients had satisfactory continence, 36% were improved and only 20% failed treatment [De Ridder et al 1997].

• Clinical results of intravesical capsaicin

Detailed descriptions of the key clinical report of intravesical capsaicin for treatment of detrusor hyperreflexia can be seen in a recently published article by Chancellor and de Groat (1999) (Level of evidence 4]. Most of the clinical studies report that intravesical capsaicin achieved over 60% urodynamic improvement 1-2 months after capsaicin instillation. The maximum cystometric capacity increased from 27% to 220%. The effect of capsaicin on clinical and urodynamic parameters was long lasting, exceeding one year in some patients. A meta-analysis of the six series on a total of 131 patients, mean pretreatment bladder capacity was 144 ml (range 72-195 ml). The mean post-capsaicin cystometric capacity, although at different time points, was 267 ml (range 185-321 ml). Mean symptomatic improvement was 72% (range 40-100%).

Wiart et al (1998) reported on 12 paraplegic patients treated either with 1 mM capsaicin in 30% alcohol or placebo (30% alcohol alone). One hundred ml of either

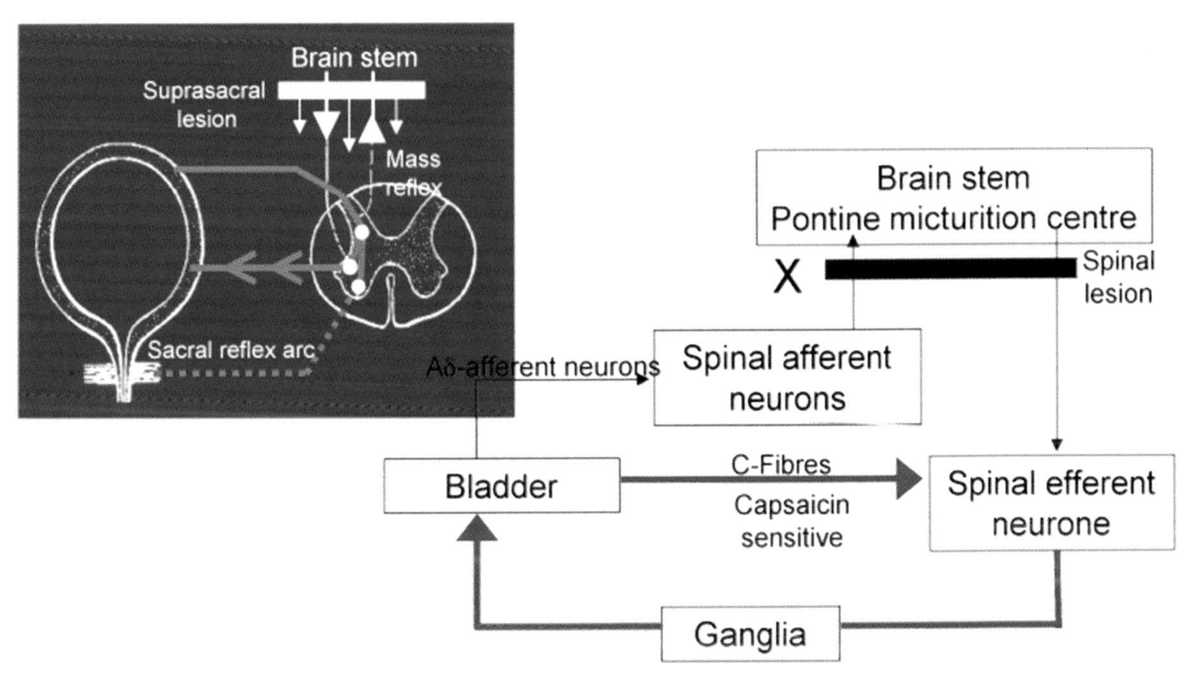

Figure 11 : With spinal cord injury, at least in the animal experiment, afferent stimuli are conducted in unmyelinated C-fibres (and not as normal, in myelinated aδ -fibres); vanilloids block the C-fibre reflexes in chronic spinal cat.

capsaicin or alcohol placebo was instilled for 30 minutes using outpatient procedures without anesthesia. Urodynamic studies and bladder diaries were compared before therapy and 30 days later. All of the capsaicin patients reported clinical improvement with significant regression of urine leakage episodes ($p=0.002$), and sensory urgency ($p=0.01$). Only one placebo subject had subjective improvement. This double-blind, placebo-controlled trial confirmed the efficacy of intravesical capsaicin for detrusor hyperreflexia (Level of evidence 2).

2) Resiniferatoxin (total 4 articles refer to the topic reviewed, including 1 CTs and 3 case series)

Resiniferatoxin (RTX) is a much more potent sensory antagonist than capsaicin. It is approximately 1,000 times more potent than capsaicin, based on the Scoville Heat Scale [Lewis 1998]. Like capsaicin, it possesses vanilloid receptor agonist activity, resulting in desensitization. However, RTX acts without the potent neuronal excitatory effect of capsaicin, and therefore elicits less discomfort. The use of this vanilloid promises an alternative to capsaicin that would be potentially therapeutic for overactive bladder and DH. However, formal controlled trials still have to be performed to determine the precise use and dosage for this agent. The key advantage of RTX is that it is at least as effective as capsaicin, without much of the local side effects, such as pain and inflammatory neuropeptide release.

RTX is the principal active ingredient in the classic drug Euphorbium, the air-dried latex (resin) of the cactus-like plant *Euphorbia resinifera* Berg [Hergenhahn et al 1975]. In 1990, RTX was recognized as an ultrapotent analogue of capsaicin [Szallasi & Blumberg 1990a]. At the same time, however, it was also realized that although RTX mimics most capsaicin actions, it also has unique pharmacological effects [Szallasi & Blumberg 1990b], such as the desensitization without prior excitation of the pulmonary chemoreflex pathway [Szolcsányi 1990]. The mechanisms underlying the differences between RTX and capsaicin actions are just beginning to be understood. RTX induces slowly activating, persistent currents in dorsal root ganglion neurons as measured under patch-clamp conditions [Liu & Simon 1994; 1996; Oh et al 1996]. These sustained currents prefer desensitization to excitation (the change in membrane potential is not sufficient to cause action potential formation, although the rising intracellular calcium levels can activate biochemical pathways leading to desensitization), which is in accord with the general pharmacological profile of RTX.

Cruz et al[Cruz et al 1997a; 1997b] instilled 50-100 nM RTX, dissolved in 100 ml solution of 10% alcohol, for 30 minutes in seven neurologically impaired patients with detrusor hyperreflexia. Itching or mild discomfort were the only symptoms evoked in four patients during the first minutes of the treatment. In five of the seven patients, urinary frequency decreased by 33-58%, and this effect was detected as soon as the first day after treatment. Three patients, who prior to treatment were incontinent, became dry most days following treatment. Improvement was sustained for up to 3 months. Four patients had urodynamic improvement with a rise in maximum cystometric capacity increasing from 50-900% of pretreatment measures. Lazzeri et al (1997) reported using intravesical RTX (10 microM) in eight normal patients, and seven patients with overactive bladder. RTX did not decrease the volume required to elicit the first desire to void and did not produce warm or burning sensations at the suprapubic or urethral level during instillation in normal subjects. However, in patients with overactive bladder, mean capacity increased from 175 ± 36 to 281 ± 93 ml ($p<0.01$) immediately after instillation, but was not significantly increased after four weeks (217 ± 87 ml).

RTX has also been reported to be helpful in patients who did not improve after capsaicin. Lazzeri et al (1998) presented data on 7 SCI patients with DH treated with RTX. These patients were reported to have failed intravesical capsaicin therapy. All nine patients received 30 ml of 10 microM RTX for 30 minutes. Fifteen days after RTX, mean cystometric capacity significantly increased from 188 ± 21 ml to 399 ± 120 ml ($p<0.01$) and remained increased four weeks later (402 ± 71 ml, $p<0.01$).

A recently completed North American multicenter RTX clinical trial was designed as a prospective, dose escalating, single-blind, placebo-controlled study comparing the effects of seven concentrations of RTX (0.005, 0.025, 0.05, 0.1, 0.2, 0.5, 1.0 microM of RTX 10% ethanol in saline) and placebo (10% ethanol) for treatment of neurogenic bladder [Rivas et al 1999]. Each patient received a single dose. Safety, tolerance and bladder function assessments were made at screen, immediately following dosing and at weeks 1, 3, 6, and 12 and quarterly thereafter, until a return to baseline bladder function was obtained. The final analysis of the results of this study is being complied a few trends can be seen. First, there were no significant differences between control and RTX at the lowest doses of 0.005-0.01 microM. Second, in patients with decreased bladder capacity, the mean change in cystometric capacity was markedly greater than for the placebo dose group. Third, the mean number of incontinence episodes from pretreatment of patients treated with 0.05 microM, 0.5 microM and 1.0 mM decreased by 1 to 2 fewer episodes compared to placebo. Adverse events, considered to be related to RTX, were generally mild to moderate and transient. One patient discontinued from study due to autonomic dysreflexia. In a patient population involving many SCI patients, the occurrence of autonomic dysreflexia is an expected event especially during urologic studies. Cystoscopic evaluation revealed no adverse treatment effect due to RTX. No signs of areflexia or urinary retention were noted. Clinically significant changes in laboratory abnormalities did not occur.

RTX seems to have a beneficial effect on spinal DH (Level of evidence 4). Ramdomized controlled studies need to determine its place in the treatment of DH.

2. Botulinum toxin A (total 13 articles refer to the topic reviewed, including 7 CTs)

Botulinum toxin A first isolated by van Ermengem in 1897, is the most potent biological toxin known to man [Van Ermengem 1897]. Through basic research, clinicians have been able to transform this lethal toxin into a health benefit. Clinicians have safely and successfully used this agent for the treatment of focal dystonias, muscle spasm and spasticity [Grazko et al, 1995; Jankovic et al 1990]. The toxin acts by inhibiting acetylcholine release at the presynaptic cholinergic junction (Figure 12). Inhibited acetylcholine release results in regionally decreased muscle contractility and muscle atrophy at the site of injection [Duchen 1970]. The chemical denervation that results in a reversible process as axons resprout in approximately 3-6 months [Borodic et al 1990].

Clinically, the urologic community has utilized botulinum toxin A to treat spinal cord injured patients who suffer from detrusor external sphincter dyssynergia (DESD) [Dykstra et al 1988; 1990; Schurch et al 1996; Petit et al 1998; Phelan et al 2001].

The toxin acts at the neuromuscular junction of the external sphincter to block vesicle transport of acetylcholine; in essence, producing a chemical denervation, a reversible chemical "sphincterotomy", which avoids a major surgical procedure (external sphincterotomy) with its attendant risks (bleeding, stricture, fistula). The clinical effects begin within 3-5 days and are reversible as terminal nerve sprouting occurs within 3-6 months [Phelan et al 2001]. Phelan et al (2001) have expanded the role of urethral injections to include patients with urinary retention secondary to pelvic floor spasticity and have even treated a female patient with MS and an acontractile bladder who wished to void by Valsalva.

More recently, Schurch et al (2001) reported successful treatment of spinal cord injured patients with DH using intravesical injections of botulinum toxin A. Under cystoscopic control a total of 200 to 300 units of botulinum toxin A (Botox®) were injected into the detrusor muscle at 20 to 30 sites (10 units per ml. per site), sparing the trigone. The authors demonstrated a significant increase in mean maximum bladder capacity (296ml to 480ml, $p<0.016$) and a significant decrease in mean maximum detrusor voiding pressure (65 to 35cm H_2O, $p<0.016$) in patients injected with the toxin when evaluated at 6 weeks after the injections. At the 6-week follow-up complete continence was restored in 17 of the 19 patients examineed after the treatment. Ongoing improvement in urodynamic parameters and incontinence was already present in all 11 patients reevaluated at 36 weeks after treatment.

Intravesical injection of botulinum toxin A into the detrusor muscle is promising therapy for spinal DH (Level of evidence 4) and this treatment may be recommended when standard pharmacotherapy using bladder relaxant drugs fails (Grade of recommendation C). Fur-

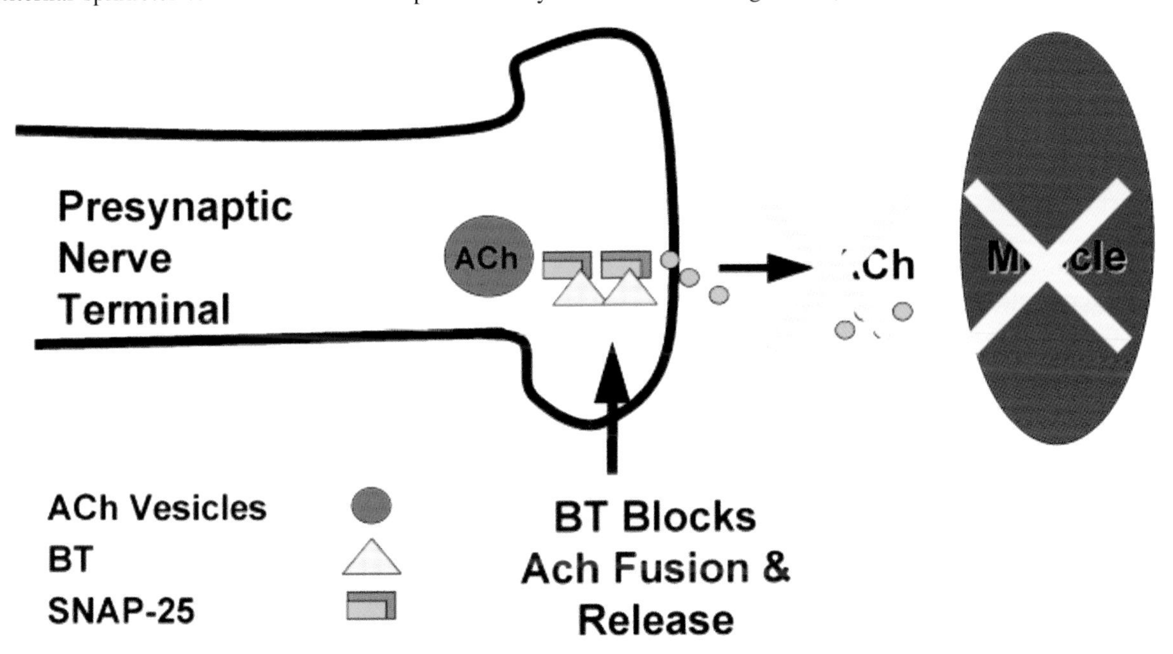

Figure 12 : Botulinum Toxine acts by inhibiting acetylcholine release at the presynaptic cholinergic junction

ther studies, however, are nessesary to confirm the efficacy of this treatment and to determine the duration of the therapeutic effect.

2. Drugs for incontinence due to neurogenic sphincter deficiency

Several drugs, including alpha-adrenergic agonists [Diokno & Taub 1975; Raezer et al 1977; Awad et al 1978; Ek et al 1978, Stewart et al 1976; Bauer 1994], estrogens [Beisland et al 1981], beta-adrenergic agonists [Gleason et al 1974] and tricyclic antidepressants [Gilja et al 1984], have been used to increase outlet resistance (Level of evidence 4). No adequately designed controlled studies of any of these drugs for treating neuropathic sphincter deficiency have been published. In certain selected cases of mild to moderate stress incontinence a beneficial effect may be obtained [Andersson 1988; Grade of recommendation D].

3. Drugs for facilitating bladder emptying

a) Alpha adrenergic blockers (total 61 articles refer to the topic searched in combination with the keyword of neurogenic bladder, including 13 CTs and 3 RCTs)

Alpha-adrenoceptors have been reported to be predominantly present in the bladder base, posterior urethra and prostate. Alpha-blochers have been reported to be useful in neurogenic bladder by decreasing urethral resistance during voiding. Recently, a multicenter placebo-controlled, double-blind trials of urapidil, an alpha-blocker on neurogenic bladder dysfunction [Yasuda et al 1996; Yamanishi et al 1999] by means of pressure/flow study demonstrated significant improvement of straining and of the sum of urinary symptom scores, which was associated with significant improvement of urodynamic parameters (decreases in the pressure at maximum flow rate and the minimum urethral resistance) over the placebo (Level of evidence 1).

Alpha adrenergic blockade also helps to prevent excess sweating secondary to spinal cord autonomic dysreflexia. Sweat glands, primarily responsible for thermoregulatory factors, are innervated by postganglionic cholinergic neurons of the sympathetic system. alpha receptor blockade inhibits this postsynaptic neuronal uptake of norepinephrine and reduces neurologic sweating [Chancellor et al 1994].

b) Cholinergics (total 1 CT refer to the topic searched in combination with the keyword of neurogenic bladder).

In general, bethanechol chloride seems to be of limited benefit for detrusor areflexia and for elevated residual urine volume. Elevated residual volume is often due to sphincter dyssynergia. It would be inappropriate to potentially increase detrusor pressure when concurrent DSD [Chancellor et al 1993].

CONCLUSIONS

Bladder relaxant drugs, including oxybutynin, propiverine, trospium and tolterodine have a documented suppressive effect on incontinence by controlling overactive bladder, thereby improving storage function (Level of evidence 1).

However, all of these drugs presently available have considerably high incidence of side effects (dry mouth, constipation, urinary retention, etc.), which limits their usage. Tolterodine, propiverine, trospium and controlled-release oxybutynin have significantly less side effects compared to immediate-release oxybutynin (Level of evidence 1).

Although the oral application is the usual way, intravesical instillation (oxybutynin) may be an alternative (Level of evidence 4).

Intravesical instillation of capsaicin/resiniferatoxin has been reported to improve spinal reflex incontinence for several months after instillation (presumably blocking sensory input) (Level of evidence 4).

Botulinum toxin injections into the detrusor muscle was reported to improve incontinence and increase functional bladder capacity in spinal cord injured patients with DH (Level of evidence 4).

There is no adequately designed controlled study of any of drugs for neuropathic sphincter deficiency.

RECOMMENDATIONS FOR PRACTICE

Bladder relaxant agents should be recommended for the treatment of reflex incontinence, in patients, in whom IC alone is unable to control it (Grade of recommendation A).

Titration of the dosage of these drugs individually should be done to achieve maximum therapeutic effect and minimal side effect. If one drug is not tolerated, try another drug as it may have less side effects (Grade of recommendation D).

In most of the developing countries bladder relaxant drugs are not available or only at costs people are unable to afford. Therefore the pharmaceutical industry must be encouraged to provide cheaper drugs (Grade of recommendation D).

Intravesical RTX and botulinum toxin injections may be an alternative for DH if conventional therapy fails (Grade of recommendation C).

Further attempts for the treatment of DH should be undertaken to develop the ideal drug in terms of good efficacy, tolerability and safety (Grade of recommendation D).

For neurogenic sphincter deficiency no effective drugs are available up to now; further research is needed (Grade of recommendation D).

4. Implications for research

During the past few years research in neurourology has stimulated the development of new therapeutic approaches for incontinence, including the intravesical administration of afferent neurotoxins, such as capsaicin and resiniferatoxin. What are the research priorities for the future? It will be important to focus on the development of neuropharmacologic agents that can suppress the unique components of abnormal bladder reflex mechanisms and thereby act selectively diminish symptoms without altering normal voiding function. To end this part we would like to speculate on a few areas of research that we feel may payoff within the next 5 years with new and better treatment of neuropathic urinary incontinence:

1. Bladder specific K channel openers. Can truly bladder smooth muscle or afferent neuron specific potassium channel openers be developed? This treatment may alleviate the overactive and sensitive bladder without any dry mouth.
2. Intravesical vanilloid treatment. Can the clinical utility of intravesical resiniferatoxin be perfected so that the preferred therapy for neurogenic bladder is a simple outpatient 30 minutes instillation of 30 ml resiniferatoxin that will last 3 months without system side effects?
3. Can pharmaceutical companies develop a truly bladder specific and effective anticholingeric drug with no dry mouth?
4. Tachykinin antagonists are appealing in that it may be effective without increasing residual urine volumes. Can clinically useful and safe NK antagonists be developed?
5. Urethral smooth and/or skeletal muscle specific alpha agonist or 5-HT reuptake inhibitor that may treat stress urinary incontinence. We need an effective drug for stress incontinence.

Beyond the horizon of near term advancement, we predict a brave new paradigm in neurourology. What has already started are the evolution of unstoppable forces of change in medicine that include pharmacogenomics, tissue engineering and gene therapy. These will change how we practice urology and gynecology:

1. Pharmacogenomics: Medicine will be tailored to the genetic make up of each individual. Through microarray gene chip technology we will know how a patient metabolizes medication, her receptors profile and allergy risk. These factors can be screen against a list of medications prior to therapy. A physician will then be able to always prescribe the best drug for each patient without the risk of allergic reaction.
2. Tissue Engineering: Rapid advances are being made in tissue and organ reconstruction using autologous tissue and stem cells feasible. We envision a day, in the not too distant future, where stress incontinence is cured not with a cadaver ligament and metal screws into the bones but rather minimally invasive injection of stem cells that will not only bulk up the deficient sphincter but actually improve the sphincter's contractility and function.
3. Gene Therapy: Diabetic neurogenic bladder and visceral pain maybe cured with one or more injection of a gene vector that the physician will inject into the bladder or urethra. Injection of nerve growth factor via a herpes virus vector into the bladder of a diabetic bladder may restore bladder sensation and innervation. Can the introduction of a virus that express the production of endorphin for site and nerve specific help alleviate pelvic visceral pain, regardless of the cause?

5. Acknowledgement:

None

6. Potential conflict of interest:

None

E. ELECTROSTIMULATION

I. ELECTRICAL NEUROMODULATION

1. Background

In the last decade sacral nerve neuromodulation [Schmidt RA 1988] has been confirmed as a valuable treatment option to treat patients with symptoms of the overactive bladder. The success with sacral neuromodulation has increased the interest in other neuromodulation techniques.

To find evidence to answer the following questions:

2. Objectives

a) How to do it?

The current techniques of neuromodulation for treating the overactive bladder – which includes per definition also detrusor hyperreflexia as detrusor overactivity of neurogenic origin - are (a) anogenital electrical stimulation, (b) transcutaneous electrical nerve stimulation (TENS), (c) sacral nerve neuromodulation, (d) percutaneous posterior tibial nerve stimulation (Stoller afferent nerve stimulation, SANS) and (e) magnetic stimulation.

b) How does it work, is it effective?

It is not really known how neuromodulation works, however, there is strong evidence that neuromodulation works at a spinal and at a supraspinal level [Bemelmans et al 1999].

The most important spinal inhibitory mechanisms of the micturition reflex [Fall & Lindström 1991] are (1) the guarding reflex: increased activity of the striated urethral sphincter in response to bladder filling, reflexively reducing detrusor contraction; (2) Edvardsen´s reflex: increased activity of the sympathetic nervous system in response to bladder filling; (3) anal dilation (afferent pathway: anorectal branches of the pelvic nerve, prevents voiding during defecation), (4) gentle mechanical stimulation of the genital region (afferent pathway: dorsal clitoral or penile branches of the pudendal nerve; prevents voiding during intercourse) and (5) physical activity (afferent pathway, muscle afferents from the limbs prevents voiding during fighting or fleeing).

At least two potential mechanisms are possible (1) activation of efferent fibres to the striated urethral sphincter reflexively cause detrusor relaxation and (2) activation of afferent fibres cause inhibition at a spinal and a supraspinal level.

Interesting studies supporting the second theory are those in which the dorsal or dorsal penile nerve, purely afferent branches of the pudendal nerve, were electrically stimulated: this induced a strong inhibition of the micturition reflex and of detrusor hyperreflexia [Vodusek et al 1986; Craggs et al 1998; Shah et al 1998].

Fowler et al [2000] measured the latency of the anal sphincter contraction during a peripheral nerve evaluation (PNE) and concluded that this response was mediated by a polysynaptic reflex. Experimental work in spinalized rats showed that neuromodulation reduced the degree of hyperreflexia as well as the expression of the c-fos after bladder instillation with acetic acid [Wang & Hassouna 2000]. This result shows that inhibition of afferent C fibre activity may be one of the underlying mechanism of neuromodulation. However, it does not explain the beneficial effects of neuromodulation in patients with idiopathic detrusor instability or urgency. However, stimulation of afferent pathways seems to play the crucial role.

As this chapter deals with conservative therapy sacral nerve stimulation (S3), which has been proved to be effective in refractory neurogenic urge incontinence, will not be discussed in this chapter.

c) Is it safe?

Neuromodulation has almost no complications, the methods must be regarded as safe.

d) Is neuromodulation cost-effective?

Comparing with the costs for anticholinergic therapy after one year of treatment the costs for pharmacotherapy and for neuromodulation including stimulator are equally, after one year electrical neuromodulation becomes cheaper.

e) How to prevent / to treat complications?

There are almost no complications with this type of therapy. According to the underlying working concept, which implies that the treshold for effectiveness is below the pain treshold even pains should not occur, therefore pains and skin irritation at the site of electrode placement are not found with a correct technique.

f) Comparing between techniques

There are no randomised controlled studies comparing one technique with the other.

g) Long term results and quality of life

Although there is a certain carry over effect with these methods about 75% of the patients in the neurogenic group need to continue the treatment on an individual schedule; if the patient accepts the manipulation involved with these techniques the quality of life is good because there are almost no side effects, which is in contrast to pharmacotherapy.

3. Criteria for considering studies and search strategies

Search strategies include all types of studies with adults treated with one of the techniques of electrical neuromodulation mentioned above.

From Medline through Pub.Med. 1966-2001/IV

Key words: Neurogenic bladder (4625) and urinary incontinence (13392) combined with electrical neuromodulation

Three studies were found which report on the effect of non-invasive electrical neuromodulation for detrusor hyperreflexia (Level of evidence 4)

4. Results

Only three papers report on results of non-invasive electromodulation techniques for detrusor hyperreflexia. Anogenital electrical stimulation (vaginal/anal) was used by Primus et al (1996), he found that the symptomatic and urodynamic results were the same in a group of patients with detrusor instability and a group

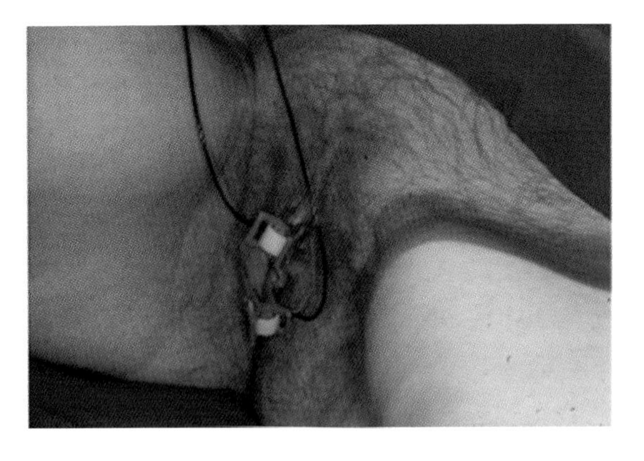

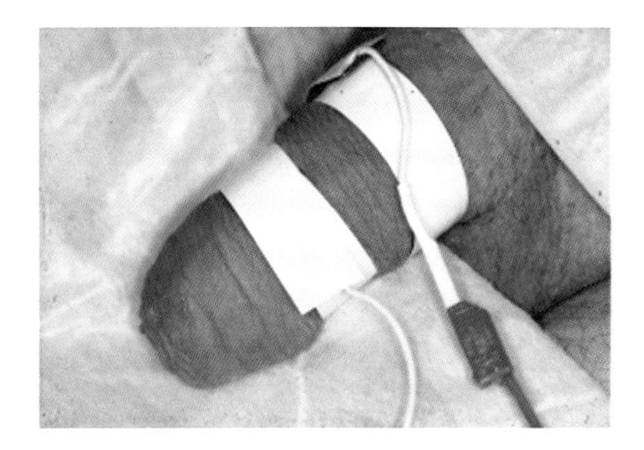

Figure 13 : For electrostimulation of the dorsal clitoral nerve clip-electrodes and of the dorsal penile nerve strip electrodes are used. Advantages: pure sensory nerves are stimulated with electrodes close to them.

of patients with multiple sclerosis. Madersbacher, Kiss & Mair (1995), by using dorsal clitoral and dorsal penile nerve stimulation (Figure 13) found even better results in the neurogenic group (detrusor hyperreflexia) than in the non-neurogenic group (detrusor instability) in regards to the increase of maximum cystometric bladder capacity and decrease of detrusor contractility. To maintain the results, however, 75% of the patients in the neurogenic group needed to continue the treatment on an individual schedule (however only 50% of the patients in the non-neurogenic group).

In contrast to these favourable results Prévinaire et al (1998) found no benefit in 6 patients with detrusor hyperreflexia due to suprasacral spinal cord injury by using continuous electrical stimulation of the penis or of the clitoris via bipolar surface electrodes and daily stimulation periods of 20 min. One possible reason for this discrepancy is the fact that in the two studies in which a beneficial effect was found, patients suffered from incomplete neurogenic lesions, however, the patients without success had complete suprasacral cord lesions. This may further support that effects of neuromodulation are mediated not only on a spinal, but, maybe even more important on a supraspinal level. In regards to percutaneous posterior tibial nerve stimulation and magnetic stimulation no reports refer to patients with neurogenic bladder dysfunction.

CONCLUSIONS

Electrical neuromodulation mostly is not the first line treatment for detrusor hyperreflexia, however it is indicated and beneficial in whom pharmacotherapy does not work or is not tolerated.

Non-invasive eletrical neuromodulation should always be applied and tested before invasive electrical neuromodulation (sacral nerve stimulation of S3) is considered.

5. Implications for Practice

Electrical neuromodulation is a valuable treatment option for patients with an overactive bladder, the non-surgical techniques can be applied as an alternative to standard conservative therapy or may be tried if such treatment fails. Experimental studies documented the effect of electrical stimulation of pudendal nerve afferents to inhibit detrusor hyperreflexia, however, only 3 published studies, using non-invasive techniques report on the effects on detrusor hyperreflexia: patients with detrusor hyperreflexia due to complete supraspinal cord lesions did not respond, patients with incomplete lesions did. Beneficial effects of invasive sacral neuromodulation (S3) are reported in the chapter of the surgical treatment of neuropathic urinary incontinence.

RECOMMENDATIONS

If pharmacotherapy fails to relax the hyperreflexic detrusor electrical neuromodulation is an alternative in patients with incomplete lesions and non-invasive electrical neuromodulation may be the first choice.(Grade of recommendation C/D)

Non-invasive electrical neuromodulation should always be applied before invasive electrical neuromodulation (sacral nerve stimulation of S3) is considered. (Grade of recommendation C)

6. Implications for Research

There are no sham-controlled studies with electrical neuromodulation in patients with detrusor hyperreflexia (although some studies exist for detrusor instability), therefore randomised sham-controlled studies should be undertaken in order to prove the efficacy of this method.

7. ACKNOWLEDGEMENT:

None

8. POTENTIAL CONFLICT OF INTEREST:

None

II. ELECTRICAL STIMULATION OF THE PELVIC FLOOR MUSCULATURE

1. BACKGROUND

The aim of electrical stimulation in patients with neurogenic urinary stress incontinence is to improve the function, that is strengh and/or timing of the pelvic floor muscle contraction.

2. OBJECTIVES

To find evidence to answer the following questions:

a) How to do it?

Electrical stimulation is provided nowadays mostly by portable battery powered stimulation. It offers a seemingly infinite combination of wave forms, frequencies, intensities, electrode placements etc.

b) Is it effective?

The nomenclature used to describe electrical stimulation has been inconsistent. Strength training theories suggest that near maximal contractions are the most significant factor in increasing strength and ideally, contraction need to be sustained for 6-8 seconds to recruit an increasing number of motor units and fast twitch fibres [Astrand & Rodahl 1986]. There is a fixed recruitment pattern during voluntary contraction: slow twitch (ST) fibres are recruited first, but with increasing resistance more and more fast twitch (FT) fibres are recruited. All types of muscle fibres will have hypertrophy in response to strength and training, but FT fibres have a greater potential for hypertrophy than ST fibres. According to Bazeed et al (1982) it was shown that in the animal experiment over months electrical stimulation is able to transform FT fibres into ST fibres, which basically should improve incontinence. As the strongest stimulation for strength increase is the intensity of the contraction (as close to maximum as possible), the main objective would be to recruit as many motor units as possible, regardless whether they are ST or FT fibres. To improve the potential for strength gains, also electrical stimulation should be conducted over sufficient time that both, neural adaptation and hypertrophy can occur. Thus, training periods of at least 20 weeks have been recommended [American College of Sports Medicine 1990].

c) Is it safe?

There are no complications reported with this type of therapy, if the technique is appropriate.

d) Is it cost-effective?

More studies are needed to evaluate this aspect. (see below)

e) How to prevent/treat complications?

There are no complications described

f) Comparing between techniques

There is a marked lack of consistancy in the electrical stimulation protocols used in clinical practice. Even in the group of women with urinary stress incontinence of obviously non-neurogenic origin due to the variation of stimulation protocols it is difficult to interpret the findings of trials comparing electrical stimulation with placebo stimulation.

f) Long term results and quality of life

There are no adequate data available.

3. CRITERIA FOR CONSIDERING STUDIES SEARCH STRATEGY

All studies dealing with adults suffering from neurogenic urinary stress incontinence

From Medline through Pub.Med 1966-2001/IV

Keywords: Neurogenic urinary stress incontinence, neurogenic sphincter weakness in combination of electrical neurostimulation, electrostimulation

All studies would have been considered in regards to efficacy, safety and cost-effectiveness (languages English, German).

No study was found dealing with electrical neurostimulation for neurogenic pelvic floor / striated sphincter weakness.

4. RESULTS

Although from the theoretical point of view and based on limited own clinical experience ***(Level of evidence 5)*** electrical stimulation via anal or vaginal plugs should be able to improve the strength of pelvic floor musculature including that of the striated sphincter muscle, there is no study published which deals with this matter. From our experience in selected patients with neurogenic urinary incontinence – patients being able to contract voluntarely pelvic floor musculature – electrical stimulation via anal or vaginal approach is able objectively, as assessed by perionometry, to improve the incontinence situation. In one of our patients the change after electrical stimulation over 4 months was as such that continence could be achieved even with sudden intraabdominal pressure rises.

5. Implications for practice

In patients with incomplete denervation of the pelvic floor muscle and the striated sphincter electrostimulation via anal or vaginal plugs performed over months, may improve pelvic floor function, thus improve incontinence. The incompleteness of the lesion should be as such that the patient is able to contract voluntary the pelvic floor, even if this is weak. ***(Grade of recommendation D)***

6. Implications for research

It would be worthwhile to assess in a prospective controlled study whether patient is likely to benefit or not, whether electrical stimulation can improve the situation. The amount of nerves damage to the pelvic floor muscle may also be crucial.

7. Acknowledgement:

None

8. Potential conflict of interest:

None

III. INTRAVESICAL ELECTRICAL STIMULATION (IVES)

1. Background

Already in 1887 the Danish surgeon Saxtorph described intravesical electrical stimulation for the "atonic bladder" by inserting a transurethral catheter with a metal stylet in it and with a neutral electrode on the lower abdomen. In 1899 two Viennese surgeons, Frankl-Hochwart and Zuckerkandl, stated that intravesical electrotherapy was more effective to induce detrusor contractions than external faradisation. In 1975 Katona introduced this method for the treatment of neurogenic bladder dysfunction. Ebner et al (1992) demonstrated in cat-experiments that intravesical electrostimulation activates the mechanoreceptors within the bladder wall.

Further basic research was undertaken by Jiang & Lindström (1991), who demonstrated that IVES at low frequencies (≥ 20 Hz) had a better modulatory effect than higher frequencies. Jiang (1998) proved in the animal experiment, that IVES induced modulation of the micturition reflex due an enhanced excitatatory synaptic transmission in the central micturition reflex pathway. The observed modulation may account for the clinical benefit of IVES treatment.

The afferent stimuli induced by IVES travel along afferent pathways from the lower urinary tract to the corresponding cerebral structures. This "vegetative afferention" [Katona 1975] results in the occurrence of sensation for bladder filling/urge to void, with subsequent enhancement of active contractions and possibly also in voluntary control over the detrusor (Figure 14).

A feedback training is mediated by enabling the patient to observe the change of the detrusor pressure on a water manometer, thus the patient is able to realise, when a detrusor contraction takes place. This also facilitates voluntary control (Figure 15).

2. Objectives

To find evidence to answer the following questions:

a) How to do IVES?

The technique involves a catheter with a stimulation electrode in it, introduced into the bladder and connected to the stimulator. Saline (0,9 %) is used as the current leading medium within the bladder. The neutral electrode is attached to the skin in an area with preserved sensation, usually in the lower upper abdomen. According to Ebner et al (1992) the following stimulation parameters have proved to be most effective in the animal experiment: pulse width 2 ms, frequency 20 Hz and current 1 to 10 mA. Each therapy session takes 90 minutes on a daily basis until the maximum response is achieved. For patients, who have never experienced the urge to void, e.g. children with myelomeningocele, or who have lost this ability, IVES is combined with a biofeedback training: on a water manometer attached to the system the patient is able to observe the change of the detrusor pressure. This way he is able to realize that the experienced sensation is caused by bladder contraction. This external feedback also facilitates achievement of voluntary control (see fig.4).

3. Criteria for considering studies and search strategies

All, clinical and experimental

from Medline 1966-2001

Intravesical electrostimulation, bladder stimulation, intravesical bladder stimulation, transurethral electrostimulation of the bladder; intravesical, transurethral bladder stimulation

30 studies were selected: 6 basic research papers (animal experiments and clinical research), only one randomised controlled trial ***(Level of evidence 1)***, 2 reviews within an editorial, one pro and contra IVES ***(Level of evidence 2)***, the rest were case series ***(Level of evidence 4).***

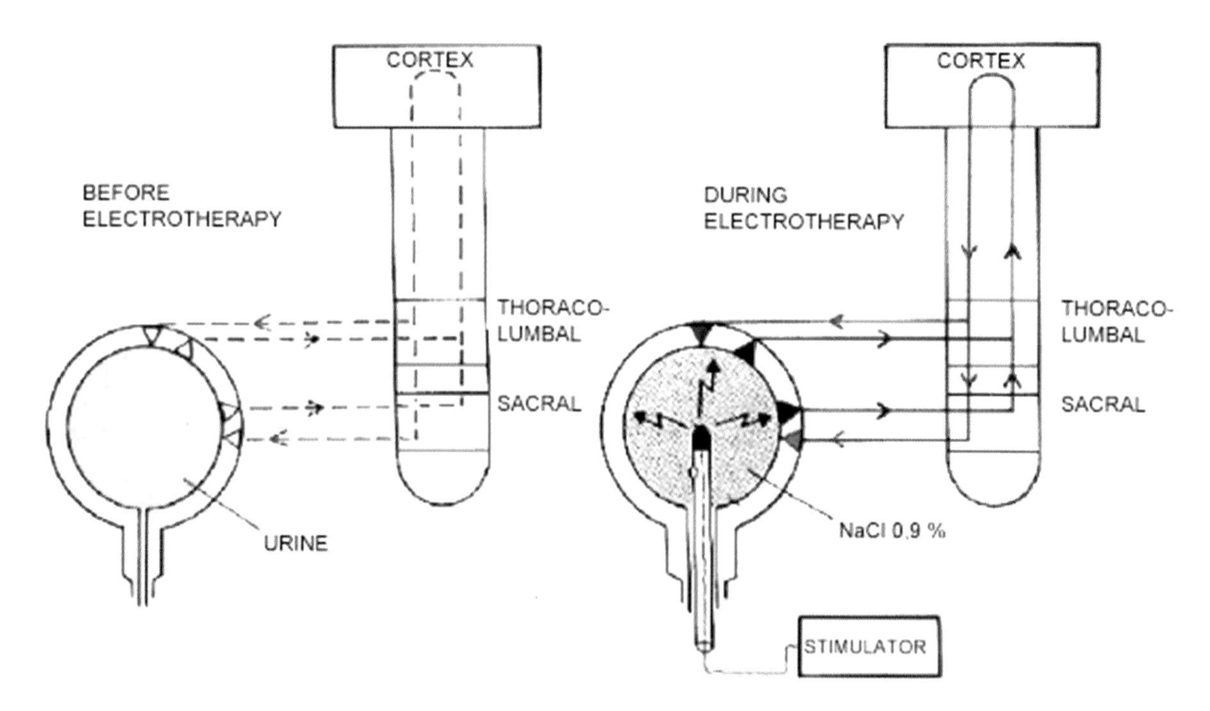

Figure 14 : Intravesical electrostimulation activates the mechanoreceptors within the bladder wall, thus increases the afferent and consequently the afferent input from and consequently also the efferent output to the bladder (Ebner et al., 1992)

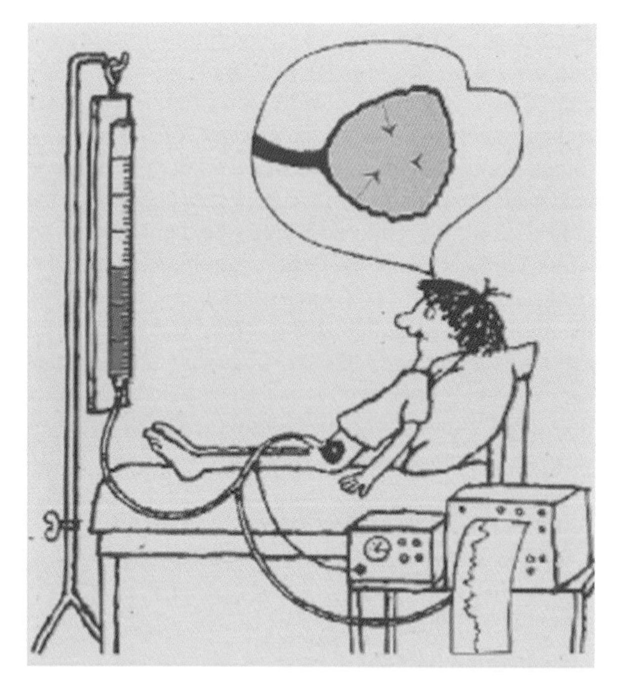

Figure 15 : With intravesical electrostimulation a feedback training is mediated by enabling the patient to observe the change of the detrusor pressure on a water manometer: the patient is able to realize when a detrusor contraction takes place.

4. Results

Intravesical electrical stimulation of the bladder (IVES) is still a controversial therapy for patients with neurogenic detrusor dysfunction, although basic research during the last decade has evidenced the mechanism of action and its efficacy [Ebner et al 1992; Jiang 1998]. At least in animal experiments optimal parameters have been determined [Ebner et al 1992; Buyle et al 1998]

Colombo et al (2000) demonstrated that intravesical electrostimulation also induces electrical changes on higher mictrution centres, measured by EEG. The evaluation of viscero-sensroy cortical evoked potentials after transurethral electrical stimulation of the bladder neck area has been proved to be useful in determine whether a patient is suitable for IVES or not [Kiss et al 1998].

This controversy about the value of IVES for detrusor (re-)habilitation is also reflected in an editorial recently published, in which Kaplan (2000) reported favourable results in 288 children, who received at least one series (20 outpatient sessions 90 minutes long):

87% have control and void or catheterize with sensation or have improved bladder compliance 18% have gained full control, they void synergistically and are continent, when before they were either voiding poorly and incontinent or used clean intermittent catherization and were more or less dry. Forty- four % void with sensation and are in biofeedback to try and gain control. Finally in 13 % the treatment failed, but the patients maintained their condition. Moreover, the results seen in an "early" group were followed up 10 years. As long as no intervening neurosurgical insult occurred, less than 3 % of cases needed to return for a tune up to maintain their "healthy bladder". The average number of daily session to achieve this results was 47.

In contrast the results reported by Decter (2000) were less favourable. In 25 patients during a 5 year period with all-together 938 sessions of stimulation, bladder capacity increased greater than 20% in regards to the age-adjusted and end-filling bladder pressure showed clinically significant decreases in 28% of patients. In response to a questionnaire, 56% of parents commented a subjective improvement in their childrens bladder function. However, the urodynamic improvements achieved after IVES did not signifincantly alter the daily voiding routine in these children [Decter et al 1994].

The only randomised controlled prospective clinical trial [Boone et al 1992] could not find differences between active and sham treatment, however, only 15 sessions were performed at first and another 15 sessions of IVES were applied after a 3-months hiatus. Moreover, the inclusion criteria were not defined.

Other studies are either individual case-controlled studies (Level of evidence 3) or case series (Level of evidence 4). They cannot be compared due to different or non-defined inclusion criteria, different technique details (different time of electrostimulation, varying follow-ups) and some with only a small number of patients included, [Eckstein & Katona 1974 - pro; Nicholas & Eckstein 1975 - contra ; Denes 1975 – pro; Janneck 1976 – pro; Seiferth et al 1978 – pro; Seiferth et al 1978 – pro; Schwock & Tischer 1981 – pro; Madersbacher et al 1982 - pro; Kaplan & Richards 1988 - pro; Madersbacher H 1990 - pro; Lyne & Bellinger 1993 – pro; Kölle et al 1995 - pro; Cheng et al 1996 – pro; in one 7 patients, in a second study 568 patients; Primus & Trummer 1993 – pro; Kroll et al 1998 – pro; Pugach et al 2000 - contra].

None really focused particularly on the inclusion criteria. According to basic research, only those with some intact afferent fibres from the bladder to the cortex and those with spinal cord lesions with the presence of pain sensation in the sacral dermatoms S3 and S4 can benefit from IVES. (according to Nathan the pathways of the bladder proprioception and for pain are lying close together). The value of viscerosensoric cortical evoked potentials from the bladder neck was demonstrated by Kiss et al (1999). A precise indication seems to be one prerequisite for a good result. Regarding children with myelomeningocele, one must also take into account that myelomeningocele bladders at birth may have a threefold increase in connective tissue and significant decrease of cholinergic receptors compared to normal controls [Shapiro et al 1991]. According to clinical experience this tempers the enthusiasm for intravesical electrical stimulation in this particular group of patients.

CONCLUSIONS

Basic research during the last decade has proved the underlying working concept

The results reported in the literature are controversial, mainly because of different inclusion and exclusion criteria.

In the only sham-controlled study the treatment period is too short and the inclusion and exclusion criteria are not really defined.

The alternative may be either life long intermittent catheterization or bladder augmentation. In this regards IVES is **cost-effective**

It is worthwhile to apply intravesical electrostimulation, bearing in mind inclusion and exclusion criteria, especially trying to varify functioning afferent fibres between the bladder and the cortex.

5. IMPLICATIONS FOR PRACTICE

Basically intravesical electrotherapy is able to improve neurogenic bladder dysfunction, primarily by stimulating a-delta mechanoafferents inducing bladder sensation and the urge to void and consequently increasing the efferent output with improvement of micturition and conscious control. Therefore IVES is the only available option to induce/improve bladder sensation and to enhance the micturition reflex in incomplete central or peripheral nerve damage. However, proper indication is crucial and this type of therapy should only be applied in those with at least some intact afferent fibres between the bladder and the cortex if possible, proved by the evaluation of viscerosensoric cortical evoked potentials. If these premisses are respected, IVES **is effective**.

Intravesical electrical stimulation is **safe**, no side-effects have been reported, beyond an occassional urinary infection. The question of cost-effectiveness was raised by Kaplan, stating that the most commonly used alternative for these patients is bladder augmentation, which is "miles apart in terms of cost, discomfort and short- and long-term complications".

One benefit of IVES was noted by most of the authors: improved sensation documents satisfactory long term results. The patients with successful IVES get great satisfaction from knowing when their bladder is full and when it is time to catheterise or to void. Moreover, even without direct bowel stimulation patients noted significant improvement in the warning of bowel fullness and gained greater control for their bowel movements.

IVES can only be effective with certain prerequisites, the most important one are at least some afferent fibres between the bladder and the CNS being intact and the detrusor able to contract. The method is safe, there are no real complications reported.

RECOMMENDATIONS

Intravesical electrotherapy is able to improve neurogenic bladder dysfunction, primarily by stimulating a-delta mechano-receptor afferents inducing bladder sensation and the urge to void and consequently increases the efferent output with improvement of micturition and conscious control.

IVES is the only available option to induce/improve bladder sensation and to enhance the micturition reflex in patients with incomplete central or peripheral nerve damage.

Indication is crucial and IVES should only be applied if afferent fibres between the bladder and the cortex are still intact and if the detrusor muscle is still able to contract.

If these premises are respected, IVES is effective.

The ideal indication is the neuropathic hyposensitive and hypocontracile detrusor (Grade of recommendation C)

6. Implications for research

There is definitely a need for placebo-(sham-)controlled prospective studies with clear inclusion- and exclusion-criteria and clear definitions of the aims. Recently De Wachter & Wyndaele (J.Urology, accepted for publication) demonstrated in the animal experiment and models that the position of the stimulating electrode, as well as the amount of saline within the bladder may be crucial for the effect. Additional research is needed to clarify these aspects of IVES.

7. Acknowledgement:

None

8. Potential conflict of interest:

None

REFERENCES

A. INTRODUCTION

Al-Mefty O, Kandzari S, Fox JL. Neurogenic bladder and the tethered spinal cord syndrome. J Urol 179:112-115, 1979

Appel RA, Whiteside HV. Diabetes and other peripheral neuropathies affecting lower urinary tract function. In Krane RJ, Siroky MB(eds.): Clinical Neurourology second edition. Boston, Little, Brown and Company, pp 365-373, 1991

Beck RO, Betts CD, Fowler CJ. Genitourinary dysfunction in multiple system atrophy: clinical features and treatment in 62 cases. J Urol 151:1336-1341, 1994

Berger Y, Blaivas JG, DeLaRocha ER, Salinas J. Urodynamic findings on Parkinson's disease. J Urol 138:836-838, 1987

Blaivas JG, Chancellor MB. Cauda equina and pelvic plexus injury. In Practical Neurourology-Genitourinary Complications in Neurologic Disease. Boston, Butterworth-Heinemann, pp 155-163, 1995

Blaivas JG. Neurologic dysfunctions. In Yalla SV, McGuire EJ, El-Badawi A, Blaivas JG (eds): Neurourology and Urodynamics-Principles and Practice. New York, Macmillan Publishing Company, pp 343-357, 1988

Brocklehurst JC, Andrews K, Richards B, et al. Incidence and correlates of incontinence in stroke patients. J Am Geriatric Soc 33:540-542, 1985

Goldstein I, Siroky MB, Sax DS, Krane RJ. Neurourologic abnormalities in multiple sclerosis. J Urol 128:541-545, 1982

Gonor SE, Carroll DJ, Metcalfe JB. Vesical dysfunction in multiple sclerosis. Urology 25:429-431, 1985

Holliger St, Kiss G, Poewe W, H.Madersbacher, 2001, in press

Kaplan SA, Te AE, Blaivas JG. Urodynamic findings in patients with diabetic cystopathy. J Urol 153:342-343, 1995

Nathan PW, Smith NC. The centrifugal pathway for micturition with the spinal cord. J Neurol Neurosurg Psychiatry 21:177, 1958

Sirls LT, Zimmern PE, Leach GE. Role of limited evaluation and aggressive medical management in multiple sclerosis: A review of 113 patients. J Urol 151:946-950, 1994

Siroky MB, Krane RJ. Neurologic aspects of detrusor-sphincter dyssynergia, with reference to the guarding reflex. J Urol 127:953-957, 1982

Tsuchida S, Noto H, Yamaguchi O, Itoh M. Urodynamic studies on hemiplegic patients after cerebrovascular accident. Urology 21:315-318, 1983

Watanabe T, Rivas DA, Chancellor MB. Urodynamics of spinal cord injury. Urol Clin NA 23:459-473, 1996

Weinstein MS, Cardenas DD, O'Shaughnessy EJ, Catanzaro ML. Carbon dioxide cystometry and postural changes in patients with multiple sclerosis. Arch Phys Med Rehabil 69:923-927, 1988

Wulfsohn MA, Rubenstein A. The management of Shy-Drager syndrome with propantheline and intermittent self-catheterization: A case report. J Urol 126:122-123, 1981

B. BEHAVIOURAL THERAPY

I. TRIGGERED REFLEX VOIDING

Andersen J, Blaivas J, Cardozo L, Thüroff J. Lower urinary tract rehabilitation techniques: seventh report on the standardisation of terminology of lower urinary tract function: Neurourol Urodyn, 11:593, 1992

Bennet CJ, Young MN, Adkins RH, Diaz F. Comparison of bladder management complication outcomes in female spinal cord injury patients: J urol, 153:1458-1460, 1995

Bors E, Comarr A. Neurological urology. Physiology of micturition, its neurological disorders and sequelae, Karger, Basel, 1971

Canupp K, Waites KB, DeVivo MJ, Richards JS. Predicting compliance with annual follow-up evaluations in person with spinal cord injury: Spinal cord, 35:314, 1997

Corcos J, Schick E. Les vessies neurogènes de l'adulte, Masson, Paris, 1996

Frankel HL, Coll SW, Whiteneck GG, Gardner BP, Jamour MA, Krishnan KR, Nuseibeh I, Savic G, Sett P. Long-term survival in spinal cord injury: a fifty year investigation: Spinal Cord, 36:266, 1998

Gupta S, Chawla JC. Review of urinary tract abnormalities in 100 patients with spinal cord paralysis: Paraplegia, 32:531, 1994

Lamid S. Long-term follow-up of spinal cord injury patients with vesicoureteral reflux: Paraplegia, 26:27, 1988

MacDiarmid S. Monitoring of renal function in patients with spinal cord injury: BKU International, 85:1014, 2000

MacKinley W. Long term medical complications after traumatic spinal cord injury: a regional model systems analysis: Arch Med Phys Rehab, 80:1402, 1999

Maynard F, Diokno A. Clean intermittent catheterisation for spinal cord injury patients: J Urol, 128:477, 1982

Mc Guire E, Savastano J. Comparative urological outcome in women with spinal cord injury: J Urol, 135:730, 1986

Mitsui T, Minami K, Furuno T, Morita H, Koyanagi T. Is suprapubic cystostomy an optimal urinary management in high quadriplegics?: Eur Urol, 38:434, 2000

Rossier A, Bors E. Detrusor responses to perineal and rectal stimulation in patients with spinal cord injuries: Urol Int, 10: 181, 1964

Sekar P. Comparison of long term renal function after spinal cord injury using different urinary management methods: Arch Med Phys rehab, 78: 992, 1997

van Kerrebroeck P. The morbidity due to lower urinary tract function in spinal cord injury patients: Paraplegia, 31: 320, 1993

Wein A, Barrett D. Voiding function and dysfunction, a logical and practical approach. in Treatment of voiding dysfunction 199 Year Book Medical Publishers, 1988

Wein A, Van Ardsalen K, Reilly, N. Treatment of voiding dysfunction in spinal-cord injured patients: non surgical. in Controversies in neuro-urology eds. Barrett, D. & Wein, A. 453 Churchill Livingstone, Edinburg, 1984

Weld J.: Effect of bladder management on urological complications in spinal cord injuries patients: J Urol, 163: 768, 2000

Yavuzer G, Gök H, Tuncer S, Soygür T, Arikan N, Arasil T. Compliance with bladder management in spinal cord injury patients: Spinal Cord, 38: 762, 2000

Yokoyama O, Hasegawa T, Ishiura Y, Ohkawa M, Sugiyama Y, Izumida S. Morphological and functional factors predicting bladder deterioration after spinal cord injury: J urol, 155: 271, 1996

II. BLADDER EXPRESSION (CREDE AND VALSALVA MANOUVRE)

Barbalias GA, Klauber GT, Blaivas JG. Critical evaluation of the Crede manoeuver: a urodynamic study of 207 patients. J Urol Oct;130(4):720-723, 1983

Clarke SJ, Thomas, DG. Characteristics of the urethral pressure profile in flaccid male paraplegics; BJU 53:157-161, 1981

Fanciullacci F, Sandri S, Politi P, Zanollo A. Clinical urodynamic and neurophysiological findings in patients with neuropathic bladder due to a lumbar intervertebral disc protrusion; Paraplegia Oct;27(5):354-358, 1989

Juraschek F, Dollfus P, Mennecier A, Moustafa C. Problèmes posés par les paralysies flasques des muscles du périnée; Rapport au Congres díUrologie 298-302, Ed.Masson e Cre,Pans, 1974

Leroi AM, Berkelmans I, Rabehenoina C, Creissard P, Weber J. Results of therapeutic management of vesico-urethral and anorectal disorders in 20 patients with cauda equina syndrome; Neurochirurgie 40(5):301-306, 1994

Low AI, Donovan WD. The use and mechanism of anal sphincter stretch in the reflex bladder; BJU 53: 430-432, 1981

Madersbacher H. The neuropathic urethra: urethrogram and pathophysiologic aspects; Eur Urol 3,321-332, 1977

Momose H, Kashiwai H, Kawata Y, Hirayama A, Hirata N, Xamada K, Yamamoto M, Hirao Y. Difference between the clinical significance of Crede voiding and Valsalva voiding in the urological management of spina bifida patients; Hinyokika Kiyo Nov;43(11):771-775, 1997

Redman JF. Crede expression of the bladder: a sometimes useful maneuver; J Urol Dec;116(6)794-795, 1976

Reinberg Y, Fleming T, Gonzalez R. Renal rupture after the Crede maneuver; J Pediatr Feb;124(2):279-281, 1994

Sperling KB. Intermittent catheterization to obtain catheter-free bladder function in spinal cord injury; Arch Phys Med Rehabil Jan;59(1):4-8, 1978

Watkins KH. The bladder function in spinal injury; Brit J Surg 23:734-736, 1936

Wyndaele JJ. 1998; Personal communication

C. CATHETER

I. INTERMITTENT CATHETERIZATION

Allas T, Colleu D, Le Lannon D. Fonction génitale chez l'homme paraplégique. Aspects immunologiques. Presse Med 29:2119, 1986.

Amendola MA, Sonda LP, Diokno AC, Vidyasagar M. Bladder calculi complicating intermittent clean catheterization. A J Roentgenol 141: 751-3, 1983

Anderson RU. Prophylaxis of bacteriuria during intermittent catheterization of the acute neurogenic bladder. J Urol 123: 364-366, 1980

Anton HA, Chambers K, Clifton J, Tasaka J. Clinical utility of a portable ultrasound device in intermittent catheterization. Arch Phys Med Rehab 79:172-175, 1998

Bakke A. Clean intermittent catheterization-physical and psychological complications. Scan J Urol Nephrol Suppl 150: 1 – 69, 1993

Bakke A, Digranes A, Hoisaeter PA. Physical predictors of infection in patients treated with clean intermittent catheterization: a prospective 7-year study. BJU 79: 85-90, 1997

Bakke A, Malt UF. Psychological predictors of sumptoms of urinary tract infection and bacteriuria in patients treated with clean intermittent catheterization: a prospective 7 year study. Eur Urol 34: 30-36, 1998

Bakke A, Vollset SE. Risk factors for bacteriuria and clinical urinary tract infection in patients treated with clean intermittent catheterization. J Urol 149: 527-531, 1993

Barber DB, Woodard FL, Rogers SJ, Able AC. The efficacy of nursing education as an intervention in the treatment of recurrent urinary tract infections in individuals with spinal cord injury. SCI Nurs 16: 54-56, 1999

Barnes D, Timoney A, Moulas G, Shaw P, Sanderson P. Correlation of bacteriological flora of the urethra, glans and perineum with organisms causing urinary tract infection in the spinal injuries male patient. Paraplegia 30:851-854, 1992

Barkin M, Dolfin D, Herschorn S, Bharatwal N, Comisarow R.The urological care of the spinal cord injury patient. J Urol 129:335-339, 1983

Bennett CJ, Young MN, Razi SS, Adkins R, Diaz F, McCrary A. The effect of urethral introducer tip catheters on the incidence of urinary tract infection outcomes in spinal cord injured pateients. J Urol 158: 519-521, 1997

Biering-Sorensen F, Nielans HM, Dorflinger T, Sorensen B. Urological situation five years after spinal cord injury. Scand J Urol Nephrol 33: 157-161, 1999

Biering-Sorensen F, Nielsen K, Hansen HV. Urethral epithelial cells on the surface on hydrophilic catheters after intermittent catheterization: cross-over study with two catheters. Spinal Cord 37: 299-300, 1999.

Brosman SN. History of the urethral catheter. J Wadsworth Gen Hospital 8:93-98, 1965

Bruijnen CLAH, Boer PW.Intermittent self-catheterization: a new instrument.BJU 53:198, 1981

Burgdörfer H, Heidler H, Madersbacher H et al.Manual-Neuro-urology and Spinal Cord lesion. Edited by the working party on Urological rehabilitation of Spinal Cord Injury Patients of the German speaking area.

Champion VL clean technique for intermittent self –catheterization. Nurs Res 25: 13-18, 1976

Chan H. Bladder management in acute care of stroke patients: a quality improvement project. J Neurosci Nurs 29: 187-190, 1997

Chancellor MB, Rivas DA, Staas WEJr. DDAVP in the urological management of the difficult neurogenic bladder in spinal cord injury: preliminary report. J Am Paraplegia Soc 17: 165-167, 1994

Corcos J. Traitements non médicamenteux des vessies neurogènes. In: Les vessies neurogènes de l'adulte. Corcos J, Schick E(Esd) Masson paris pp 173-187, 1996.

Cukier J, Maury M, Vacant J, Mlle Lucet. L'infection de l'appareil urinaire chez le paraplégique adulte.Nouv Presse Med 24:1531-1532, 1976

Damanski M. Vesico-ureteric reflux in paraplegics.Br J Surg 52:168-177, 1965.

Darouiche R, Cadle R, Zenon G 3rd, Markowski J, Rodriguez M, Musher DM. Progression from asymptomatic to symptomatic urinary tract infection in patients with SCI: a preliminary study. J Am Parap Soc 16:219-224, 1993.

De Ridder D, Van Poppel H, Baert L, Binard J. From time dependent intermittent selfcatheterisation to volume dependent selfcatheterisation in multiple sclerosis using the PCI 5000 Bladdermanager. Spinal Cord 35:613-616, 1997

Diokno AC, Sonda LP, Hollander JB, Lapides J. Fate of patients started on clean intermittent self-catheterization 10 years ago. J Urol 129:1120-1122, 1983

Dollfus P, Molé P. The treatment of the paralused bladder after spinal cord injury in the accident unit of Colmar.Paraplegia 7:204-205, 1969

Donovan W, Stolov W, Clowers D, Clowers M. Bacteriuria during intermittent catheterization following spinal cord injury. Arch Phys Med Rehab 59: 351-357, 1978.

Donovan WH, Hull R, Rossi CD. Analysis of gram negative recolonization of the neuropathic bladder among patients with spinal cord injuries. Spinal Cord 34:587-891, 1996.

Duffy LM, Cleary J, Ahern S, Kuskowski MA, West M, Wheeler L, Mortimer JA. Clean intermittent catheterization: safe, cost-effective bladder management for male residents of VA nursing homes. J Am Geriatr Soc; 43: 865-870. 1995

Fujimoto Y, Ueno K, Yamada S, Isogai K, Komeda H, Ban Y. Clinical investigation of clean intermittent catheterization. Hinyokika Kiyo; 40: 309-313. 1994

Galien P, Nicolas B, Robineau S, Le-Bot MP, Durufle A, Brissot R. Influence of urinary management on urologic complications in a cohort of spinal cord injury patients. Arch Phys Med Rehab; 79: 1206-1209. 1998

Galloway A, Green HT, Windsor JJ, Menon KK, Gardner BP, Krishnan RR. Serial concentrations of Creactive protein as an indicator of urinary tract infection in patients with spinal injury. J Clin Pathol;39:851-855. 1986

Giannantoni A, Scivoletto G, Di-Stasi SM, Silecchia A, Finazzi-Agro E, Micali I, Castellano V. Clean intermittent catheterization and prevention of renal disease in spinal cord injury patients. Spinal Cord; 36: 29-32. 1998

Gribble MJ, Puterman ML, McCallum NM.Pyuria: its relationship tp bacteriuria in spinal cord injured patients on intermittent catheterization.Arch Phys Med Rehab;70:376-379. 1989

Grundy DJ, Fellows GS, Gillett AP, Nuseibeh I, Silver JR. A comparison of fine-bore suprapubic and an intermittent urethral catheterization regime after spinal cord injury. Paraplegia;21:227-232. 1983

Günther M, Löchner-Ernst D, Kramer G, Stöhrer M. Intermittent catheterization in male neurogenics: no harm to the urethra. Abstract poster 93. Annual scientific meeting of IMSOP Sydney Australia 2000.Abstractbook p112.

Guttmann L, Frankel H The value of intermittent catheterization in the early management of traumatic paraplegia and tetraplegia Paraplegia;4:63-83, 1966

Haferkamp A, Stachler G, Gerner HJ, Dorsam J. Dosage escalation of intravesical oxybutin i the treatment of neurogenic bladder patients. Spinal Cord; 38: 250-254. 2000

Haldorson AM, Keys TF, Maker MD, Opitz JL. Nonvalue of neomycin instillation after intermittent urinary catheterization. Antimicrobial agents and chemotherapy; 14: 368-370. 1978

Hedlund H, Hjelmas K, Jonsson O, Klarskov P, Talja M. Hydrophilic versus non-coated catheters for intermittent catheterization. Scand J Urol Nephrol; 35: 49-53. 2001

Hellstrom P, tammela T, Lukkarinen O, Kontturi M. Efficacy and safety of clean intermittent catheterization in adults. Eur Urol 1991; 20: 117-121.

Herr HW. Intermittent catheterization in neurogenic bladder dysfunction. J Urol; 113: 477-479. 1975

Hill VB, Davies WE. A swing to intermittent clean self-catheterisation as a preferred mode of management of the neuropathic bladder for the dextrous spinal cord patient.Paraplegia; 26: 405-412. 1988

Hirano A, Tanaka H, Kuroda S. Experience with non-aseptic intermittent selfcatheterization. Hinyokika Kiyo; 34: 1751-1756. 1988

Hofstetter A. Antimikrobielle Wirksamkeit von Gleitmitteln. Urologe;27:359-360. 1987

Hunt GM, Oakeshott P, Whitacker RH.Intermittent catheterization: simple, safe and effective but underused. BMJ;312:103-107. 1996

Hull RA, Rudy DC, Wieser IE, Donovan WH. Virulence factors of Escherichia coli isolates from patients with symptomatic and asymptomatic bacteriuria and neuropathic bladders due to spinal cord and brain injuries. J Clin Microbiol; 36: 115-117. 1998

Igawa, 1998, personal communication. Iwatsubo E, Iwakawa A, Koga H, Imamura A, Yamashita H, Komine S. Functional recovery of the bladder in patients with spinal cord injury-prognosticating programs of an aseptic intermittent catheterization.

Hinyokika Kiyo; 31: 775-783. 1985 Iwatsubo E, Komine S, yamashita H, Imamura A, Akatsu T. Over-distension therapy of the bladder in paraplegic patients using self-catheterisation: a preliminary study. Paraplegia; 22: 201-215. 1984

Jensen AE, Hjeltnes N, Berstad J, Stanghelle JK. Residual urine following intermittent catheterisation in patients with spinal cord injuries. Paraplegia; 33: 693-696. 1995

Johnson HW, Anderson JD, Chambers GK, Arnold WJ, Irwin BJ, Brinton JR. A short-term study of nitrofurantoin prophylaxis in children managed with clean intermittent catheterization. Pediatrics; 93: 752-755. 1994

Kevorkian CG, Merritt JL, Ilstrup DM. Methenamine mandelate with acidification: an effective urinary antseptic in patients with neurogenic bladder. Mayo Clin Proc; 59: 523-529. 1984

Khoury JM, Freeman JA. Transitional cell carcinoma of the bladder in a patient on clean intermittent catheterization. BJU Int; 84: 378-379. 1999

Kilinc S, Akman MN, Levendoglu F, Ozker R. Diurnal variation of antidiuretic hormone and urinary output in spinal cord injury. Spinal Cord; 37: 332-335. 1999

King RB, Carlson CE, Mervine J, Wu Y, Yarkony SM: Clean and sterile intermittent catherization methods in hospitalized patients with spined cord injury Arch. Plys. Med. Rehabis 1992 - 73: 709-802

Kiyono Y, Hashizume C, Ohtsuka K, Igawa Y. Improvement of urological-management abilities in individuals with tetraplegia by reconstructive hand surgery. Spinal cord; 38: 541-545. 2000

Kornhuber HH, Schutz A. Efficient treatment of neurogenic bladder disorders in multiple sclerosis with initial intermittent catheterization and ultrasound-controlled training. Eur Neurol; 30: 260-267. 1990

Kovindha, 1998, personal communication.

Kovindha A, Na W, Madersbacher H. Radiological abnormaliteis in spinal cord injured men using clean intermittent catheterization with a re-usable silicone catheter in developing country. Poster 86 presented during the Annual Scientific meeting of IMSOP Sydney 2000. Abstract book p112.

Kuhn W, Rist M, Zach GA. Intermittent urethral self-catheterisation: long term results (bacteriological evolution, continence, acceptance, complications). Paraplegia; 29: 222-232. 1991

Kuhlemeier KV, Lloyd LK, Stover SL. Localization of upper and lower urinary tract infections in patients with neurogenic bladders.SCIDigest; 336-342. 1982

Labat JJ, Perrouin-Verbe B, Lanoiselée JM, Mathé JF, Buzelin JM. L'autosondage intermittent propre dans la réeducation des blesses medullaires et de la queue de cheval II. Annales de Réadaptation et de Médicine Physique; 28: 125-136. 1985

Lapîdes J, Diokno A, Silber S, Lowe B. Clean intermittent selfcatheterization in the treatment of urinary tract disease. J Urol; 107: 458-461. 1972

Lapides J, Diokno AC, Gould Fr, Lowe BS. Further observations on self-catheterization. Trans Am Assoc Genitourin Surg; 67: 15-17. 1975

Lapides J, Diokno AC, Lowe BS, Kalish MD. Follow-up on unsterile intermittent self-catheterization. J Urol; 111: 184-187. 1974

Lapides J, Diokno AC, Gould FR, Lowe BS. Further observations on self-catheterization. J Urol;116:169-172. 1976

Lewis RI, Carrion HM, Lockhart JL, Politano VA. Significance of aymptomatic bacteriuria in neurogenic bladder disease. Urology; 23: 343-347. 1984

Lindan R, Bellomy V. The use of intermittent catheterization in a bladder training program, preliminary report. J Chron Dis;24:727-735. 1971

Lindan R, Bellomy V. Effect of delayed intermittent catheterization on kidney function in spinal cord injury patients-a long-term follow-up study. Paraplegia; 13: 49-55. 1975

Lindehall B, Moller A, Hjalmas K, Jodal U. Long term intermittent catheterization: the experience of teenagers and young adults with myelomeningocoele. J Urol; 152: 187-189. 1994

Lundgren J, Bengtsson O, Israelsson A, Jonsson AC, Lindh AS, Utas J. The importance of osmolality for intermittent catheterizatio of the urethra. Spinal Cord; 38: 45-50. 2000

Madersbacher H, Weissteiner G. Intermittent self-catheterization, an alternative in the treatment of neurogenic urinary incontinence in women. Eur Urol; 3: 82-84. 1977

Mandal AK, Vaidayanathan S. Management of urethral stricture in patients practising clean intermittent catheterization. Int Urol Nephrol; 25: 395-399. 1993

Maynard F, Diokno A. Urinary infection and complications during clean intermittent catheterization following spinal cord injury. J Urol; 132: 943-946. 1984

Maynard FM, Diokno A. Clean intermittent catheterization for spinal cord injured patients. J Urol;128:477-480. 1982

Maynard FM, Glass J. Management of the neuropathic bladder by clean intermittent catheterization: 5 year outcomes. Paraplegia;25:106-110. 1987

McGuire EJ, Diddel G, Wagner FJr. Balanced bladder function in spinal cord injury patients. J Urol;118:626-628. 1977

McGuire EJ, Savastano J. Comparative urological outcome in women with spinal cord injury. J Urol; 135: 730-731. 1986

Menon EB, Tan ES. Pyuria: index of infection in patients with spinal cord injureis. BJU;69:141-146. 1992

Michelsen D, Wyndaele JJ. Management of false passages in patients practising clean intermittent self catheterisation. Spinal Cord; 37: 201-203. 1999

Mohler JL, Cowen DL, Flanigan RC. Suppression and treatment of urinary tract infection in patients with an intermittently catheterized neurogenic bladder. J Urol; 138: 3369-340. 1987

Morgan JDT, Weston PMT. The disappearing catheter-a complication of intermittent self-catheterization.BJU;65:113-114. 1990

Murphy FJ, Zelman S, Mau W. Ascorbic acid as urinary acidifying agent.II:Its adjunctive role in chronic urinary infection. J Urol;94:300-303. 1965

Murray K, lewis P, Blannin J, Shepherd A. Clean intermittent self-catheterization in the management of adult lower urinary tract dysfunction. BJU; 56: 379-380. 1984

National Institute on Disability and rehabilitation Research Consensus Statement Jan 27-29,1992.The prevention and management of urinary tact infections among people with spinal cord injuries.J Am Parap Soc;15:194-204. 1992

Noll F, Russe O, Kling E, Botel U, Schreiter F. Intermittent catheterisation versus percutaneous suprapubic cystostomy in th early management of traumatic spinal cord lesions. Paraplegia; 26: 4 – 9. 1988

Ohl DA, Denil J, Fitzgerald-Shelton K, McCabe M, McGuire EJ, Menge AC, Randolph JF. Fertility of spinal cord injuried males: effect of genitourinary infection and bladder management on results of electroejaculation. J Am Paraplegia Soc;15: 53-59. 1992

Opitz JL. Bladder retraining: an organized program. Mayo Clin Proc;51:367-372. 1976

Orikasa S, Koyanagi T, Motomura M, Kudo T, Togashi M. Experience with non-sterile intermittent selfcatheterization. J Urol; 115: 141-142. 1976

Ott R, Rosier AB. The importance of intermittent catheterization in bladder re-education of acute spinal cord lesions. In: Proc Eighteent Vet Admi Spinal Cord injury Conf;18:139-148. 1971

Ottolini MC, Shaer CM, Rushton HG, Majd M, Gonzales EC, Patel KM. Relationship of asymptomatic bacteriuria and renal scarring in children with neuropathic bladders who are practicing clean intermittent catheterization. J Pediatr; 127:368-372. 1995

Parmar S, Baltej S, Vaidynanathn S. Teaching the procedure of clean intermittent catheterization. Paraplegia;31:298-302. 1993

Pearman JW. Prevention of urinary tract infection following spinal cord injury. Paraplegia;9:95-104. 1971

Pearman JW. The value of kanamycin-colistin bladder instillations in reducing bacteriuria during intermittent catheterization of patients with acute spinal cord injury. BJU; 51: 367-374. 1979

Pearman J, Bailey M, Riley L. Bladder instillations of trisdine compared with catheter introducer for reduction of bacteriuria during intermittent catheterization of patients with acute spinal cord trauma. BJU;67:483-490. 1991

Pelosof HV, David FR, Carter RE. Hydronephrosis: silent hazard of intermittent catheterization. J Urol; 110: 375-377. 1973

Perkash I, Giroux J. Clean intermittent catheterization in spinal cord injury patients: a followup study. J Urol; 149: 1068-1071. 1993

Perrouin-Verbe B, Labat JJ, Richard I, Mauduyt De La Greve I, Buzelin JM, Mathe JF. Clean intermittent catheterization from the acute period in spinal cord injury patients. Longterm evaluation of urethral and genital tolerance. Paraplegia;33:619-624. 1995

Prieto-Fingerhut T, Banovac K, Lynne CM. A study comparing sterile and nonsterile urethral catheterization in patients with spinal cord injury. Rehabil Nurs; 22: 299-302. 1997

Reisman EM, Preminger GM. Bladder perforation secondary to clean intermittent catheterization. J Urol; 142: 1316-1317. 1989

Rhame FS, Perkash I. Urinary tract infections occurring in recent spinal cord injury patients on intermittent catheterization. J Urol; 122: 669-673. 1979

Rutkowski SB, Middleton JW, Truman G, Hagen DL, Ryan JP. The influence of bladder management on fertility in spinal cord injured males. Paraplegia;33:263-266. 1995

Schlager TA, Anderson S, Trudell J,Hendley JO. Effect of cranberry juice on bacteriuria in children with neurogenic bladder receiving intermittent catheterization. J Pediat; 135: 698-702. 1999

Schlager TA, Hendley JO, Wilson RA, Simon V, Whittam TS. Correlation of periurethral bacterial flora with bacteriuria and urinary tract infection in children with neurogenic bladder receiving intermittent catheterization. Clin Infect Dis; 28: 346-350. 1999

Schnider P, Birner P, Gendo A, Ratheiser K, Auff E. Bladder volume determination: portable 3-D versus stationary2-D ultrasound device. Arch Phys Med Rehab;81:18-21. 2000

Schurch B, Stöhrer M, Kramer G, Schmid DM, Gaul G, Hauri D. Botulinum-A toxin for treating detrusor hyperreflexia in spinal cord injured patients: a new alternative to anticholinergic drugs? Preliminary results. J Urol; 164: 692-697. 2000

Sekar P, Wallaca DD, Waites KB, De Vivo MJ, Lloyd LK, Stover SL, Dubovsky EV. Comparison of long-term renal function after spinal cord injury using different urinary management methods. Arch Phys Med Rehabil; 78: 992-997. 1997

Shekelle PG, Morton SC, Clark KA, Pathak M, Vickrey BG. Systematic review of risk factors for urinary tract infection in adults, with spinal cord dysfunction. J Spinal Cord Med; 22:258-272. 1999

Shenot P, Rivas DA, Kalman DD, Staas WEJr, Chancellor MB. Latex allergy manifested in ruologiucal surgery and care of adult spinal cord inhjured patients. Arch Phys Med Rehabil; 75: 1263-1265. 1994

Silbar E, Cicmanec J, Burke B,Bracken RB. Microwave sterilization.Method for home sterilization of urinary catheter. J Urol;141:88-90. 1980

Solomon MH, Foff SA, Diokno AC. Bladder calculi complicating intermittent catheterization. J Urol;124:140-141. 1980

Sperling KB.Intermittent catheterization to obtain catheter-free bladder in spinal cord injury.Arch Phys Med Rehab;59:4-8. 1978

Stover SL, Fleming WC. Recurrent bacteriuria in complete spinal cord injury patients on external condom drainage. Arch Phys Med Rehab;61:178-181. 1980

Stribrna J, Fabian F. The problem of residual urine after catheterization. Acta Univ Carol Med; 7: 931-935. 1961

Sutton G, Shah S, Hill V. Clean intermittent self-catheterization for quadriplegic patients-a five year follow up. Paraplegia;29:542-549. 1991

Sylora JA, Gonzalez R, Vaughn M, Reinberg Y. Intermittent selfcatheterization by quadriplegic patients via a catheterizable Mitrofanoff channel. J Urol; 157: 48-50. 1997

Takechi S, Nishio S, Yokoyama M, Iwata H, Takeuchi M. Clean intermittent catheterization in neurogenic bladder patients with vesicoureteral reflux. Nippon Hinyokika gakkai Zasshi; 86: 1520-1524. 1995

Tomoney AG, Shaw PJ. Urological outcome in female patients with spinal cord injury: the effectiveness of intermittent catheterization. Paraplegia;28:556-563. 1990

Thirumavalan VS, Ransley PG. Eididymitis in children and adolescents on clean intermittent catheterization. Eur Urol;22:53-56. 1992

Vaidyanathan S, Krishnan KR, Soni BM, Fraser MH. Unusual complications of intermittent self-catheterisation in spinal cord injury patients. Spinal Cord;34:745-747. 1996

Vaidyanathan S, Soni BM, Brown E, Sett P, Krisnan KR, Bingley J, Markay S. Effect of intermittent uerthral catheterization and oxybutinen bladder instillation on urinary continence status and quality of life in a selected group of spinal cord injury patients with neuropathic bladder dysfunction. Spinal cord; 36: 409-414. 1998

Van Hala S, Nelson VS, Hurvitz EA, Panzi A, Bloom DA, Ward MJ. Bladder management in patients with pediatric onset neurogenic bladders. J Spinal Cord Med; 20: 410-415. 1997

Vivian JM, Bors E. Experience with intermittent catheterization in the southwest regional system for tretament of spinal injury. Paraplegia;12: 158-166. 1974

Vogler H. Untersuchungen zur desinfizierenden Wirkung von Gleitmitteln bei transurethralen Electroresektionen. Z Urol u Nephrol;73:401-405. 1980

Waites KB, Canupp KC, Brookings ES, DeVivo MJ. Effect of oral ciprofloxacin on bacterial flora of perineum, urethra, and lower urinary tract in men with spinal cord injury. J Spinal Cord Medicine; 22: 192-198. 1999

Waller L, Jonsson O, Norlén L,Sullivan L. Clean intermittent catheterization in spinal cord injury patients: long-term followup of a hydrophilic low friction technique. J Urol; 153: 345-348. 1995

Waller L, Telander M, Sullivan L. The importance of osmolality in hydrophilic urethral catheters a crossover study. Spinal cord; 36: 368-369. 1998

Webb R, Lawson A, Neal D. Clean intermittent self-catheterization in 172 adults. BJU;65:20-23. 1990

Weld KJ, Dmochowski RR. Effect of bladder management on urological complications in spinal cord injured patients. J Urol; 163: 768-772. 2000

Weld KJ,Graney MJ, Dmochowski RR. Differences in bladder compliance with time and associations of bladder management with compliance in spinal cord injured patients. J Urol; 163: 1228-1233. 2000

Wheeler JS Jr, Walter JS, Chintam RS, Rao S. Botulinum toxin injections for voiding dysfunction following sci. J Spinal Cord Med; 21: 227-229. 1998

Whitelaw S, Hamonds J, Tregallas R. Clean intermittent self-catheterization in the elderly. BJU;60:125-127. 1987

Wu Y, Hamilton BB, Boyink MA, Nannninga JB. Re-usable catheter for longterm intermittent catheterization. Arch Physic Med Rehab; 62: 39-42. 1981

Wyndaele JJ. Early urological treatment of patients with an acute spinal cord injury. Thesis Doctor in Biomedical Science. State University Ghent 1983.

Wyndaele JJ. Chronic prostatitis in spinal cord injury patients. Paraplegia;23:164-169. 1985

Wyndaele JJ. Clean intermittent self-cathetrization in the prevention of lower urinary tract infections In: Dysfunction of the lower urinary tract: present achievements and future perspectives,

Ph Van Kerrebroeck, F Debruyne (eds) Bussum: Medicom, pp187-195. 1990 Wyndaele JJ, De Ridder D, Everaert K, Heilporn A, Congard-Chassol B. Evaluation of the use of Urocath-Gel catheters for intermittent self-catheterization by male patients using conventional catheters for a long time. Spinal Cord;38:97-99. 2000

Wyndaele JJ, De Sy A, Claessens H. Evaluation of different methods of bladder drainage used in the early care of spinal cord injury patients. Paraplegia; 23: 18-26. 1985

Wyndaele JJ, De Taeye N. Early intermittent selfcatheterization after spinal cord injury. Paraplegia;28: 76-80. 1990

Wyndaele JJ, Maes D. Clean intermittent self-catheterization: a 12 year follow up. J Urol; 143: 906-908. 1990

Wyndaele JJ, Oosterlinck W, De Sy W. Clean intermittent self-catheterization in the chronical management of the neurogenic bladder. Eur Urol; 6: 107-110. 1980

Yadav A, Vaidyanathan S, Panigraphi D. Clean intermittent catheterization for the neuropathic bladder. Paraplegia; 31:380-380. 1993

Yavuzer G, Gok H, Tuncer S, Soyger T, Arikan N, Arasil T. Compliance with bladder management in spinal ord injury patients. Spinal Cord; 38: 762-765. 2000

Yokoyama O, Hasegawa T, Ishiura Y, Ohkawa M, Sugiyama Y, Izumida S. Morphological and functional factors predicting bladder deterioration after spinal cord injury. J Urol; 155: 275-276. 1996

II. INDWELLING CATHETERIZATION

Andrews HO, Shah PJ. Surgical management of urethral damage in neurologically impaired female patients with chronic indwelling catheters. Br J Urol; 82(6):820-824. 1998

Barnes DG, Shaw PJR, Timoney AG, Tsokos N: Management of the neuropathic bladder by suprapubic catheterizaiton. Br J Urol 1993, 72(2): 169-172.

Browning, D.J.: Potential hazard of suprapubic catheterization. Med J Aust; 22:580, 1977

Bull E, Chilton CP, Gould CAL, Sutton TM.Single-blind, randomised, parallel group study of the Bard-Biocatheter and a silicone elastomer coated catheter.Br J Urol; 68(4): 394-9. 1991

Burgdoerfer H, Heidler H, Madersbacher H et al. Manual neuro-urology and spinal cord lesion: guidelines for urological care of spinal cord injury patient. Koeln: Parco-Pharma Gmbh, 1997.

Burke JP, Garibaldi RA, Britt MR. Jacobson JA, Conti M. Prevention of catheter-associated urinary tract infection. Am J Med; 70: 655-8. 1981

Burr RG, Chen C, Nuseibeh IM. Blockade of indwelling urinary catheters: the roles of urinary composition, the catheter, medication and diet. Paraplegia; 31: 234-241. 1993

Chancellor MB, Erhard MJ, Kiilholma PJ, Karasick S, Rivas DA. Functional urethral closure with pubovaginal sling for destroyed female urethra after long-term urethral catheterization. Urology; 43(4): 499-505. 1994

Chao E, Clowers D and Mayo ME. Fate of upper urinary tracts in patients with indwelling catheters after spinal cord injury. Urology; 42(3): 259-62. 1993

Chen Y, DeVivo MJ, Roseman JM. Current trend and risk factors for kidney stones in persons with spinal cord injury: a longitudinal study. Spinal Cord; 38: 346-53. 2000

Classen DC, Larsen RA, Burke JP, Stevens LE. Prevention of catheter-associated bacteriuria: clinical trial of methods to block three known pathways of infection. Am J Infect Control;19(3):136-42.1991

Cox AJ, Hukins WL, Sutton TM. Infection of catheterised patients: bacterial colonisation of encrusted Foley catheters shown by scanning electron microscopy. Urol Res; 17: 349-52. 1989

Cuttino JT, Clark RL. Bilateral ureteral obstruction caused by a Foley balloon in a patient with a contracted bladder. Am J Roentgenol; 149(6): 1197-3. 1987

Dewire DM, Owens RS, Anderson GA, Gottlieb MS, Lepor H. A comparison of the urological complications associated with long-term management of quadriplegics with and without chronic indwelling urinary catheters. J Urol;147(4):1069-71. 1992

Farina LA, Palou J. Suprapubic catheterization and bowel injury. Br J Urol; 70: 212-213, 1992

Feneley RC. The management of female incontinence by suprapubic catherisation, with or without urehtral closer. Br J Urol; 55: 203-7. 1983

Galloway A. Prevention of urinary tract infection in patients with spinal cord injury – a microbiological review. Spinal Cord; 35. 198-204. 1997

Garibaldi RA, Burke JP, Britt MR, Miller WA, Smith CB. Meatal colonization and catheter-associated bacteruria. N Engl J Med; 303: 316. 1980

Grundy, B.J., Fellows, G.J., Gillett, A.P., Nuseiheth, I., Silver, J.R.: A comparison of fine-bore suprapubic and intermittent urethral catheterization regime after spinal cord injury. Paraplegia; 21: 227-232. 1983

Hackler RH. Long-term suprapubic cystostomy drainage in spinal cord injury patients. Br J Urol; 54: 120-1. 1982

Hall MK, Hackler RH, Zampier TA et al. Renal calculi in spinal cord-injured patient: association with reflux, bladder stones, and foley catheter drainage. Urology; 34: 126-8. 1989

Horgan AF, Prasad B, Waldro DJ, O'Sullivan DC. Acute urinary retention. Comparison of suprapubic and urethral catheterization. Br J Urol 70; 149-151, 1992

Jackson AB, DeVivo M. Urological long-term follow-up in women with spinal cord injuries. Arch Phys Med Rehabil;73(11): 1029-35. 1992

Jacobs SC, Kaufman JM. Complications of permanent bladder catheter drainage in spinal cord injury patients. J Urol; 119:740-1. 1978

Kunin CM, Chin QF, Chambers S. Formation of encrustation on indwelling urinary catheters in the elderly: a comparison of different types of catheter materials in "blockers" and "non-blockers". J Urol; 138: 899-902. 1987

Kunin CM, Steele C. Culture of the surfaces of urinary catheters to sample urethral flora and study the effect of antimicrobial therapy. J Clin Microbiol; 21: 902-8. 1985

Lamid S. Long-term follow-up of spinal cord injury patients with vesicoureteral reflux. Paraplegia; 26: 27-34. 1988

Liedberg H, Lundeberg T, Ekman P. Refinements in the coating of urethral catheters reduces the incidence of catheter-associated bacteriuria. An experimental and clinical study. Eur Urol;17(3): 236-40. 1990

Liedberg H, Lundeberg T. Silver alloy coated catheters reduce catheter-associated bacteriuria. Br J Urol;65(4):379-81. 1990

Liedberg H, Lundeberg T. Silver coating of urinary catheters prevent adherence and growth of Pseudomonas aeruginosa. Urol Res; 17: 357-8. 1989

Lindan R, Leffler EJ, Bodner D. Urological problems in the management of quadriplegic women. Paraplegia; 25: 381-5. 1987

Lloyd LK, Kuhlemeier KV, Fine PR, Stover SL. Initial bladder management in spinal cord injury: does it make a difference? J Urol; 135: 523-7. 1986

MacDiarmid SA, Arnold EP, Palmer NB, Anthony A. Management of spinal cord injured patients by indwelling suprapubic catheterization. J Urol; 154: 492-4. 1995

McGuire EJ, Savastano J. Comparative urological outcome in women with spinal cord injury. J Urol; 135:730-1. 1986

Morris NS, Stickler DJ, Winters C. Which indwelling urethral catheters resist encrustation by Proteus mirabilis biofilms? Br J Urol; 80(1):58-63. 1997

Morris NS, Stickler DJ. Encrustation of indwelling urethral catheters by Proteus mirabilis biofilms growing in human urine. J Hosp Infect; 39: 227-34. 1998

Muncie HL Jr, Hoopes JM, Damron DJ, Tenney JH, Warren JW. Once-daily irrigation of long-term urethral catheters with normal saline. Lack of benefit. Arch Intern Med;149(2):441-3. 1989

Priefer BA, Duthie EH, Gambert SR. Frequency of urinary catheter change and clinial urinary tract infection. Urol; 20(2): 141-2. 1982

Shenot P, Rivas DA, Kalman DD, Staas WE Jr, Chancellor MB. Latex allergy manifested in urological surgery and care of adult spinal cord injured patients. Arch Phys Med Rehabil; 75:1263-5. 1994

Stickler D, Nickel JC, Gristina AG, Costerton JW. Electron microscopic study of an infected Foley catheter. Can J Surg; 28: 50-2. 1985

Stickler DJ, King JB, Winters C, Morris SL. Blockage of urethral catheters by bacterial biofilms. J Infect; 27(2): 133-5. 1993

Sugarman B. Adherance of bacteria to urinary catheters. Urol Res; 10: 37-40. 1982

Talja M, Korpela A, Jarvi K. Comparison of urethral reaction to full silicone, hydrogen-coated and siliconised latex catheters. Br J Urol; 66(6):652-7. 1990

Trop CS, Bennett CJ. Complications from long-term indwelling Foley catheters in female patients with neurogenic bladder. Semin Urol; 10(2): 115-20. 1992

Warren JW, Tenney JH, Hoopes JM, Muncie HL, Anthony WC. A

prospective microbiologic study of bacteriuria in patients with chronic indwelling urethral catheters. J Infect Dis;146(6):719-23. 1982

Watanabe T, Rivas DA, Smith R, Staas WE Jr, Chancellor MB. The effect of urinary tract reconstruction on neurologically impaired women previously treated with an indwelling urethral catheter. J Urol; 156(6):1926-8. 1996

Weld KJ, Dmochowski PR. Effect of bladder management on urological complication s in spinal cord injured patients. J Urol, 163:768-772. 2000

West DA, Cummings JM, Longo WE, Virgo KS, Johnson FE, Parra RO. Role of chronic catheterization in the development of bladder cancer in patients with spinal cord injury. Urology; 53(2): 292-7. 1999

Wong ES, Hooton TM. Guidelines for prevention of catheter-associated urinary tract infection. Infect Control; 2: 125-30. 1981

Wong ES. Guidelines for prevention of catheter-associated urinary tract infection. Am J Infect Control; 11: 28-33. 1983

III. CONDOM CATHETER AND EXTERNAL APPLIANCES

Brooks ME. Spector R. A new device for fastening the condom sheath. Paraplegia;19: 187-188. 1981

Bransbury AJ. Allergy to rubber condom urinals and medical adhesives in male spinal injury patients. contact Dermatitis;5:317-323. 1979

de Holl JD, Williams LA, Steers WD, Rodeheaver GT, Clark MM, Edlich RF. Technical considerations in the use of external condom catheter systems. J Burn Care Rehail;13(6):664-72. 1992

Edlich RF, Bailey T, Pine SA, Williams R, Rodeheaver GT, Steers WD. Biomechanical performance of silicone and latex external condom catheers. J Lon Term Eff Med Implants; 10(4): 291-299. 2000

Gear ALL, Nguyen WD, Bealle MA, Edlich RF. Evaluation of a new external condom catheter system. Medical Progress through Technology; 21: 181-185. 1997

Golji H. Complications of external condom drainage. Paraplegia; 19: 189-197. 1981

Hirsch DD, Fainstein V, Musher DM. Do condom catheter collecting system cause urinary tract infection? JAMA; 242(4): 340-341. 1979

Harmon CB, Connolly SM, Larson TR. Condom-related allergic contact dermatitis. J Urol; 153(4): 1227-1228. 1995

Jayachandran S, Moopan UM, Kim H. Complications from external (condom) urinary drainage devices. Urology; 25(1): 31-34. 1985

Johnson ET. The condom catheter: urinary tract infection and other complications. South Med J; 76(5): 579-82. 1983

Kovindha A, Wachirarat N. Srikisai P, Soonya O. A fixator to prevent twisting of a condom. Chiang Mai Med Bull; 37(1-2): 31-4. 1998

Lawson SD, Cook JB. An ergonomic appraisal of the use and functional efficency of condom urinals in the male patient with spinal cord paralysis. Paraplegia; 16: 317-21. 1978

Pearman JW, Shah SK, A new adaptor which obviates problems associated with condom external urinary drainage of male patients. Paraplegia; 11: 25-29. 1973

Pidde TJ, Little JW. Hydronephrosis due to improper condom catheter use. J Am Paraplegia Soc; 17(4): 168-170. 1994

Namiki T. Application of Teflon paste for urinary incontinence-report of 2 cases. Urol Int; 39(5): 280-282. 1984

Nanninga JB, Rosen J. Problems associated with the use of external urinary collectors in the male paraplegic. Paraplegic;13:56-8. 1975

Newman E, Price M. External catheters: hazards and benefits of their use by men with spinal cord lesions. Arch Phys Med Rehabil; 66: 310-313.1985

Peifer DJ, Hanover RY. Clinical evaluation of the easy-flow catheter. J Rehabil Res Dev; 34(2): 215-219. 1997

Saint S, Lipsky BA, Baker PD, McDonald LL, Ossenkop K. Urinary catheters: what type do men and their nurses prefer? J Am Geriatr Soc; 47(12): 1453-1457. 1999

Sekar P, Wallace DD, Waites KB, DeVivo MJ, Lloyd LK, Stover SL, Dubovsky EV. Comparison of long-term renal function after spinal cord injury using different urinary management methods. Arch Phys Med Rehabil; 78: 992-997. 1997

Shenot P, Rivas DA, Kalman DD, Staas WE Jr, Chancellor MB. Latex allergy manifested in urological surgery and care of adult spinal cord injured patients. Arch Phys Med Rehabil; 75: 1263-1265. 1994

Smith AD, Sazama R, Lange PH. Penile prothesis: adjunct to treatment in patients with neurognic bladder. J Urol; 124(3): 363-364. 1980

Sotolongo JR, Koleilat N. Significance of aymptomatic bacteriuria in spinal cord injury patients on condom catheter. J Urol; 143: 979-980. 1990

Stelling JD, Hale AM. Protocol for changing condom catheters in males with spinal cord injury. SCI Neur; 13(1): 28-34. 1996

Steinhardt G, McRoberts W. Total distal penile necrosis caused by condom catheter. JAMA; 244(11): 1238. 1980

Waites KB, Canupp KC, DeVivo MJ. Epidemiology and risk factors for urinary tract infection following spinal cord injury. Arch Phys Med Rehabil; 74: 691-5. 1993

D. PHARMACOTHERAPY

Abrams P, Freeman R, Anderstrom C, Mattiasson A: Tolterodine, a new antimuscarinic agent: as effective but better tolerated than oxybutynin in patients with an overactive bladder. Br J Urol, 81:801,1998.

Anderson GF, Fredericks CM: Characteriza-tion of the oxybutynin antagonism of drug-induced spasms in detrusor. Pharmacology, 15: 31, 1972.

Anderson, RU, Mobley, D, Blank, B, Saltzstein, D, Susset, J, Brown, JS: Once a day controlled versus immediate release oxybutynin chloride for urge incontinence. J. Urol. 161:1809, 1999.

Andersson K-E: Current concepts in treatment of disorders of micturition. Drugs, 35: 477, 1988.

Appell RA: Clinical efficacy and safety of tolterodine in the treatment of overactive bladder: A pooled analysis. Urology ,50: 90.39,1997.

Appell RA, Sand P, Dmochowski R, Anderson R, Zinner N, Lama D, Roach M, Miklos J, Saltzstein D, Boone T, Staskin DR, Albrecht D: Prospective randomized controlled trial of extended-release oxybutynin chloride and tolterodine tartrate in the treatment of overactive bladder: results of the OBJECT Study. Mayo Clin Proc, 76:358. 2001.

Awad SA, Downie JW, Kiriluta HG: Alpha-adrenergic agents in urinary disorders of the proximal urethra, part I: sphincteric incontinence. Br J Urol, 50: 332, 1978.

Barrett D, Wein AJ: Voiding dysfunction Diagnosis, classification and management. In Gillenwater JY, Grayhack JT, Howards SS and Duckett JW, eds: Adult and pediatric Urology, 2nd ed. St Louis, Mosby-Year book medical Publishers, pp 1001-1099, 1991.

Bauer S: An approach to neurogenic bladder: An overview: Problems In Urology, 8: 441, 1994.

Beisland HO, Fossberg E, Sander S: On incompetent urethral closure mechanism: treatment with estriol and phenylpropanolamine. Scand J Urol Nephrol, 60 (Suppl): 67, 1981.

Birns J, Lukkari E, Malone-Lee JG: A randomized controlled trial comparing the efficacy of controlled-release oxybutynin tablets (10 mg once daily) with conventional oxybutynin tablets (5 mg twice daily) in patients whose symptoms were stabilized on 5 mg twice daily of oxybutynin. BJU Int

Blaivas JG, Labib KB, Michalik J, Zayed AAH: Cystometric response to propantheline in detrusor hyperreflexia: Therapeutic implications. J Urol, 124: 259, 1980.

Borodic, GE, Joseph, M, Fay, L, Cozzolino, D, Ferrante, RJ: Botulinum A toxin for the treatmnent of spasmodic torticollis: dysphagia and regional toxin spread. Head Neck, 12: 392,1990.

Brendler BCH, Radebaugh LC, Mohler JL: Topical oxybutynin chloride for relaxation of dysfunctional bladders. J Urol, 141: 1350, 1989.

Buyse G, Verpoorten C, Vereecken R , Casaer P: Treatment of neurogenic bladder dysfunction in infants and children with neurospinal dysraphism with clean intermittent (self-) catheterisation and optimized intraversical oxybutynin hydro-chloride therapy. Eur J Pediatr Surg, 5 Suppl 1: 31, 1995.

Caterina MJ, Schumacher MA, Tominaga M, Rosen TA, Levine JD, Julius D: The capsaicin receptor: A heat-activated ion channel in the pain pathway. Nature, 389: 816,1997.

Chancellor MB, DeGroat WC: Intravesical capsaicin and resiniferatoxin therapy; spicing up the ways that we treat the overactive bladder. J Urol, 162: 3, 1999.

Chancellor MB, Erhard MJ, Hirsch IH, Staas WE: Prospective evaluation of terazosin for the treatment of autonomic dysreflexia. J Urol, 151:111,1994.

Chancellor MB, Karasick S, Erhard MJ, Abdill CK, Liu J, Goldberg BB, Staas WE: Intraurethral wire mesh prosthesis placement in the external urinary sphincter of spinal cord injured men. Radiology ,187:551,1993.

Chapple CR, Parkhouse H, Gardener C and Milroy EJ: Double-blind, placebo-controlled, cross-overbstudy of flavoxate in the treatment of idiopathic detrusor instability. Br J Urol, 66: 491, 1990.

Clapham DE : Some like it hot: spicing up ion channels. Nature, 389: 783,1997.

Connor JP, Betrus G, Fleming P, Perlmutter AD, Reitelman C: Early cystometrograms can predict the response to intravesical instillation of oxybutynin chloride in myelomeningcele patients. J Urol, 151: 1045, 1994.

Craft RM, Cohen SM, Porreca F: Long-lasting desensitization of bladder afferents following intravesical resiniferatoxin and capsaicin in the rat. Pain, 61:317,1995.

Cruz F, Guimaraes M, Silva C, Reis M: Suppression of bladder hyperreflexia by intravesical resiniferatoxin [letter]. Lancet, 350: 640,1997a.

Cruz F, Guimaraes M, Silva C, Rio ME, Coimbra A, Reis M: Desen sitization of bladder sensory fibers by intravesical capsaicin has long lasting clinical and urodynamic effects in patients with hyperactive or hypersensitive bladder dysfunction. J.Urol, 157: 585,1997b.

De Ridder D, Chandiramani V, Dasgupta P, Van Poppel H, Baert L, Fowler CJ: Intravesical capsaicin as a treatment for refractory detrusor hyperreflexia: a dual center study with long-term followup. J Urol, 158: 2087,1997.

Diokno AC, Taub M: Ephedrine in treatment of urinary incontinence. Urology 5: 624, 1975.

Duchen, L.W: Changes in motor innervation and cholinesterase localization induced by botulinum toxin in skeletal muscle of mouse: differences between fast and slow muscles. J. Neurol. Neurosurg. Psychiatry, 33: 40,1970.

Dykstra, D.D., Sidi, A: Treatment of detrusor-sphincter dyssyngeria with botulinum A toxin: a double blind study. Arch. Phys. Med. Rehabil., 71:24,1990.

Dykstra, DD, Sidi, AA, Scott, AB, Pagel, JM, Goldish GD: Effects of botulinum A toxin on detrusor-sphincter dyssyngeria in spinal cord injury patients. J. Urol., 139: 919, 1988.

Ek A, Andersson K-E, Gullberg B, Ulmsten K: The effects of long-term treatment with norephedrine on stress incontinence and urethral closure pressure profile. Scand J Urol Nephrol, 12: 105, 1978.

Gajewski JB, Awad SA : Oxybutynin versus propantheline in patients with multiple sclerosis and detrusor hyperreflexia. J Urol, 966, 1986.

Gilja I, Radej M, Kovacic M, Parazajdes: Conservative treatment of female stress incontinence with imipramine. J Urol, 132: 909, 1984.

Gleason D, Reilly R, Bottaccini M, Pierce MJ: The urethral continence zone and its relation to stress incontinence. J Urol, 112: 81, 1974.

Goessl C, Sauter T, Michael T, Berge B, Staehler M, Miller K: Efficacy and tolerability of tolterodine in children with detrusor hyperreflexia.. Urology, 55:414,2000.

Grazko MA, Polo KB, Jabbari B: Botulinum toxin A for spasticity, muscle spasms, and rigidity. Neurology; 45: 712,1995.

Greenfield SP, Fera M: The use of intravesical oxybutynin chloride in children with neurogenic bladder. J Urol, 146: 532, 1991.

Gupta SK, Sathyan G, Lindemulder EA, Ho PL, Sheiner LB, Aarons L: Quantitative characterization of therapeutic index: application of mixed-effects modeling to evaluate oxybutynin dose-efficacy and dose-side effect relationships.Clin Pharmacol Ther 1999; 65:672.

Hehir M , Fitzpatrick JM: Oxybutynin and prevention of urinary incontinence in spina bifida. Eur Urol, 11: 254, 1985.

Hergenhahn M, Adolf W, Hecker E: Resiniferatoxin and other esters of novel polyfunctional diterpenes from Euphorbia resinifera and euspina. Tetra Lett, 19: 1595, 1975.

Jankovic J, Schwartz K, Donovan DT : Botulinum toxin in the treatment of cranial-cervical dystonias and hemifacial spasm. J. Neurol. Neurosurg. Psychiatry., 53:633,1990.

Jonas U, Hofner K, Madersbacher H, Holmdahl TH: Efficacy and safety of two doses of tolterodine versus placebo in patients with detrusor overactivity and symptoms of frequency, urge incontinence, and urgency: urodynamic evaluation. The International Study Group. World J Urol , 15:144,1997.

Kaplinsky R, Greenfield S, Wan J and Fera M: Expanded followup of intravesical oxybutynin chloride use in children with neurogenic bladder. J Urol, 156: 753, 1996.

Kasabian NG, Vlachiotis JD, Lais A, Klumpp B, Kelly MD, Siroky MB, Bauer SB: The use of intraversical oxybutynin chloride in patients with detrusor hypertonicity and detrusor hyperreflexia. J Urol, 151: 944, 1994.

Kawatani M, Whitney T, Booth AM, de Groat WC: Excitatory effect of substance P in parasympathetic ganglia of the cat urinary bladder. Am J Physiol, 257: R1450, 1989.

Kitisomprayoonkul W, Kovindha A: The efficacy of oxyphencyclimine hydrochloride in treatment of urinary incontinence in spinal cord injured patients with detrusor sphincter dyssynergia. J Thai Rehabil, 10.23, 2000.

Kohler FP, Morales PA: Cystometric evaluation of flavoxate hydrochloride in normal and neurogenic bladder. J Urol, 100: 729, 1968.

Koyanagi T, Maru A, et al: Clinical evaluation of oxybutynin hydrochloride (KL007 tablets) for the treatment of neurogenic bladder and unstable bladder : A parallel double-blind controlled study with placebo. Nishinihonhinyouki: 48: 1050, 1986 (in Japanese).

Lazzeri M, Spinelli M, Beneforti P, Zanollo A, Turini D: Intravesical resiniferatoxin for the treatment of detrusor hypereflexia refractory to capsaicin. Scand J Urol Nephrol, 32: 331,1998.

Lazzeri M, Beneforti P, Turini D: Urodynamic effects of intravesical resiniferatoxin in humans: Preliminary results in stable and unstable detrusor. J Urol, 158: 2093, 1997.

Lewis R: Why red-hot peppers are red-hot. Biophoto Int J, 50:40,1998.

Liu L, Simon SA: A rapid capsaicin-activated current in rat trigeminal ganglion neurons. Proc Nat Acad Sci USA, 91: 738, 1994.

Liu L, Simon SA: Capsaicin-induced currents with distinct desensitization and Ca2+ dependence in rat trigeminal ganglion cells. J Neurophys, 75: 1503,1996.

Madersbacher H, Halaska M, Voigt R, Alloussi S, Hofner K: A placebo-controlled, multicentre study comparing the tolerability and efficacy of propiverine and oxybutynin in patients with urgency and urge incontinence. BJU Int, 84:646,1999.

Madersbacher H, Jilg G: Control of detrusor hyperreflexia by the intravesical instillation of oxybutynine hydro-chloride. Paraplegia, 29: 84, 1991.

Madersbacher H, Stöhrer M, Richter R, Burgdörfer H, Hachen HJ and mürtz G: Trospium chloride versus oxybutynin: a randomized, double-blind, multicentre trial in the treatment of detrusor hyperreflexia. Br J Urol, 75: 452, 1995.

Maggi CA, Santicioli P, Patacchini R, Geppetti P, Giuliani S, Astolfi M, Baldi E, Parlani M : Theodorsson E, Fusco B, Meli A, Regional differences in the motor response to capsaicin in the guinea pig urinary bladder: Relative role of pre- and postjunctional factors related to neuropeptide-containing sensory nerves. Neuroscience, 27: 675,1988.

Malone-Lee J, Shaffu B, Anand C, Powell C: Tolterodine: superior tolerability than and comparable efficacy to oxybutynin in individuals 50 years old or older with overactive bladder: a randomized controlled trial. J Urol, 165:1452,2001.

Mizunaga M, Miyata M, Kaneko S, Yachiku S, Chiba K, Intravesical instillation of oxybutynin hydrochloride therapy for patients with a neurogenic bladder. Paraplegia, 32: 25, 1994.

Nilvebrant L, Andersson K-E, Gillberg P-G, Stahl M, Sparf B: Tolterodine - a new bladder selective antimuscarinic agent. Eur J Pharmacol, 327:195, 1997a.

Nilvebrant L, Hallen B, Larsson G.: Tolterodine - A new bladder selective muscarinic receptor antagonist: preclinical pharmacological and clinical data. Life Sci, 60:1129, 1997b.

Oh U, Hwang SW, Kim D: Capsaicin activates a nonselective cation channel in cultured neonatal rat dorsal root ganglion neurons. J Neurosci, 16: 1659, 1996.

Painter KA, Vates TS, Bukowski TP, Fleming P, Freedman AL, Smith CA, Gonzalez R, Perlmutter AD: Long-term intravesical oxybutinin chloride therapy in children with myelodysplasia. J Urol, 156: 1459, 1996.

Palmer LS, Zebold K, Firlit CF and Kaplan WE: Complications of intravesical oxybutynin chloride therapy in the pediatric myelomeningocele population. J Urol, 157: 638, 1997.

Pannek J, Sommerfeld HJ, Botel U, Senge T: Combined intravesical and oral oxybutynin chloride in adult patients with spinal cord injury. Urology ,55:358,2000.

Pedersen E, Bjarnason EV, Hansen P-H: The effect of flavoxate on neurogenic bladder dysfunction. Acta Neurol Scand, 48: 487, 1972.

Petit H, Wiart E, Gaujard E, LeBreton F, Ferriere JM, Lagueny A, Joseph PA, Barat M: Botulinum A toxin treatment for detrusor-sphincter dyssynergia in spinal cord disease. Spinal Cord, 36:91, 1998.

Phelan MW, Franks M, Somogyi GT, Yokoyama T, Fraser MO, Lavelle JP, Yoshimura N: Chancellor MB: Botulinum toxin urethral sphincter injection to restore bladder emptying in men and women with voiding dysfunction. J. Urol., 165: 1107, 2001.

Prasad KV, Vaidyanathan S: Intravesical oxybutynin chloride and clean intermittent catheterisation in patients with neurogenic vesical dysfunction and decreased bladder capacity. Br J Urol, 72: 519, 1993.

Raezer DM, Benson GS, Wein AJ, Duckett JR JW: The functional approach to the management of the pediatric neuropathic bladder: A clinical study. J Urol, 177: 649, 1977.

Rentzhog L, Stanton SL, Cardozo L, Nelson E, Fall M, Abrams P.: Efficacy and safety of t olterodine in patients with detrusor instability: a dose-ranging study. Br J Urol, 81:42,1998.

Rivas DA, Shenot P, Kim DY, Fraser MO, Erickson JR, de Groat WC: Chancellor MB, ntravesical resiniferatoxin (RTX) treatment of detrusor hyperreflexia; results of prospective double-blind multicenter trial. J Urol, 161: 276,1999.

Robinson JM, Brocklehurst JC: Emepronium bromide and flavoxate hydrochloride in the treatment of urinary incontinence associated with detrusor instability in elderly women. Br J Urol, 55: 371, 1983.

Saito M, Tabuchi F, Otsubo K, Miyagawa I: Treatment of overactive bladder with modified intravesical oxybutynin chloride. Neurourol Urodyn ,19:683,2000.

Schurch B, Stohrer M, Kramer G, Schmid DM, Gaul G, Hauri D: Botulinum-A toxin for treating detrusor hyperreflexia in spinal cord injured patients: A new alternative to anticholinergic drugs? Preliminary results. J Urol, 164: 692, 2000.

Schurch B, Hauri D, Rodic B, Curt A, Meyer M, Rossier AB: Botulinum A toxin as a treatment of detrusor-sphincter dyssyngeria; a prospective study in 24 spinal cord injury patients. J. Urol., 155:1023, 1996.

Stewart BH, Banowski LHW, Montague DK: Stress incontinence: conservative therapy with sympathmimetic drugs. J Urol, 115: 558, 1976.

Stöhrer M, Bauer P, Giannetti BM, Richter R, Burgödrfer H, Murtz G: Effects of trospium chloride on urodynamic parameters in patients with detrusor hyperreflexia due to spinal cord injuries. A multicentre placebo-controlled double-blind trial. Urol Int, 47: 138, 1991.

Stöhrer M, Madersbacher H, Richter R, Wehnert J, Dreikorn K: Efficacy and safety of propiverine in SCI-patients suffering from detrusor hyperreflexia—a double-blind, placebo-controlled clinical trial. Spinal Cord, 37:196,1999.

Szallasi A, Blumberg PM : Vanilloid receptors: new insights enhance potential as therapeutic target. Pain, 30: 571, 1990a

Szallasi A, Blumberg PM: Resiniferatoxin and its analogs provide novel insights into the pharmacology of the vanilloid (capsaicin) receptor. Life Sci, 47: 1399, 1990b.

Szolcsanyi J, Jancso-Gabor A, Joo F: Functional and fine structural characteristics of the sensory neuron blocking effect of capsaicin. Naunyn Schmied Arch Pharm, 287: 157,1975.

Szolcsanyi J : Effect of capsaicin, resiniferatoxin and piperine on ethanol-induced gastric ulcer of the rat. Acta Physiol Hung, 75 (Supp): 267,1990.

Szollar SM, Lee SM: Intravesical oxybutynin for spinal cord injury patients. Spinal cord, 34: 284, 1996.

Takayasu H, Ueno A, Tuchida S, Koiso K, Kurito T, Kawabe K, Hanaoka K: Clinical Effects of propiverine hydrochloride in the treatment of urinary frequency and incontinence associated with detrusor overctivity: A double-blind, parallel, placebo-controlled, multicenter study. Igaku no Ayumi, 153: 459, 1990 (in Japanese).

Thompson IM, Lauvetz R: Oxybutynin in bladder spasm, neurogenic bladder, and enuresis. Urology, 8: 452, 1976.

Thüroff JW, Bunke B, Ebner A, Faber P, Degeeter P, Hannappel J, Heidler H, Madersbacher H, et al: Ramdomized, double-blind, multicenter trial on treatment of frequency, urgency and urge incontinence related to detrusor hyperactivity: Oxybutynin versus propantheline versus placebo. J Urol, 145: 813, 1991.

Tokuno H, Chowdhury JU, Tomita T: Inhibitory effects of propiverine on rat and guinea-pig urinary bladder muscle. Naunyn-Schmiedeberg's Arch Pharmacol 348: 659, 1993.

Van Ermengem E: Ueber einen neuen anaeroben Bacillus and seine Beziehungen zum Botulisms. Ztsch Hyg Infekt, 26: 1, 1897.

Van Kerrebroeck P, Kreder K, Jonas U, Zinner N, Wein AJ: Tolterodine once-daily: superior efficacy and tolerability in the treatment of the overactive bladder. Urology, 57:414, 2001.

Van Kerrebroeck PE, Amarenco G, Thuroff JW, Madersbacher HG, Lock MT, Messelink EJ, Soler JM.: Dose-ranging study of tolterodine in patients with detrusor hyperreflexia. Neurourol Urodyn, 17:499,1998.

Versi E, Appell R, Mobley D, Patton W, Saltzstein D: Dry mouth with conventional and controlled-release oxybutynin in urinary incontinence. The Ditropan XL Study Group. Obstet Gynecol, 95:718, 2000.

Weese DL, Roskamp DA, Leach GE, Zimmern PE: Intravesical oxybutynin chloride: Experience with 42 patients. Urology, 41: 527, 1993.

Wein AJ: Neuromuscular dysfunction of the lower urinary tract and its treatment. In Walsh, Retik, Vaughan and Wein AJ Eds: Campbell's Urology, 7th ed. pp.953-1006, 1997.

Wiart L, Joseph PA, Petit H, Dosque JP, de Seze M, Brochet B, Deminiere C, Ferriere JM, Mazaux JM, N'Guyen P, Barat M: The effects of capsaicin on the neurogenic hyperreflexic detrusor. A double blind placebo controlled study in patients with spinal cord disease. Preliminary results. Spinal Cord, 36: 95,1998.

Yamanishi T, Yasuda K, Kawabe K, Ohshima H, Morita T: A multicenter placebo-controlled, double-blind trial of urapidil, an a-blocker, on neurogenic bladder dysfunction. Eur Urol, 35 : 45, 1999.

Yarker YE, Goa KL and Fitton A: Oxybutynin, Oxybutynin: A review of its pharmacodynamic and pharmacokinetic properties, and its therapeutic use in detrusor instability. Drugs and Aging, 6: 243, 1995.

Yasuda K, Yamanishi T, Homma Y, Kawabe K, Morita T: The effect of urapidil on neurogenic bladder : a placebo controlled double-blind study. J Urol, 156 : 1125, 1996.

Zeegers AGM, Kiesswetter H, Kramer AEJ and Jonas U: Conservative therapy of frequency, urgency and urge incontinence: a double-blind clinical trial of flavoxate hydrochloride, oxybutinin chloride, emepronium bromide and pracebo. World J Urol, 5: 57, 1987.

E. ELECTROSTIMULATION

I. ELECTRICAL NEUROMODULATION

Bemelmans BL, Mundy AR, Graggs MD. Neuromodulation by implant for treating lower urinary tract symptoms and dysfunction. Eur Urol; 36:81-91. 1999

Craggs M, Edhem I, Knight S, McFarlane J, Shah N. Suppression of normal human voiding reflexes by electrical stimulation of the dorsal penile nerve. Eur Urol; 33(Supp.1):60. 1998

Fall M, Lindström S. Electrical stimulation. A physiologic approach to the treatment of urinary incontinence. Urol Clin North Am; 18:393-407. 1991

Kiss G, Madersbacher H, Poewe W. Cortical evoked potentials of the vesicourethral junction – a predictor for the outcome of intravesical electrostimulation in patients with sensory and motor detrusor dysfunction. World J Urol.;16(5):308-312. 1998

Madersbacher H, Kiss G, Mair D. Transcuataneous electrical stimulation of the pudendal nerve for treatment of detrusor overactivity. J.Neurourol Urodyn; 14: 501-502. 1995

Prévinaire JG, Soler JM, Perigot M. Is there a place for pudendal nerve maximal electrical stimulation for the treatment of detrusor hyperreflexia in spinal cord injury patients? Spinal Cord;36:100-3. 1998

Primus G, Kramer G. Maximal external electrical stimulation for treatment of neurogenic or non-neurogenic urgency and/or urge incongtinence. Neurourol Urodynam; 15:187-94. 1996

Shah N, Edhem I, Knight S, Shah J, Craggs M. Acute suppression of provoked detrusor hyperreflexia by electrical stimulation of dorsal penile nerve. Eur Urol; 33(Suppl.1):60. 1998

Schmidt RA. Applications of neurostimulation in urology. NeuroUrol Urodyn; 7:585. 1988

Stoller ML. Afferent nerve stimulation for pelvic floor dysfunction. Eur Urol; 37 (Suppl.):33. 2000

Vodusek DB. Light JK, Libby JM. Detrusor inhibition induced by stimulation of pudendal nerve afferents. Neurourol Urodyn; 5:381-9. 1986

Wang Y, Hassouna MM. Neuromodulation reduces c-fos gene expression in spinalized rats: a double-blind randomized study. J Urol; 163:1966-70. 2000

II. ELECTRICAL STIMULATION OF THE PELVIC FLOOR MUSCULATURE

American College of Sports Medicine. The recommended quantity and quality of exercise for developing and maintaining cardiorespiratory and muscular fitness in healthy adults" Med Sci Sports Exerc. Apr;22(2):265-74. 1992

Astrand & Rodahl. Personal communication by K. Boe, 2001

DiNubile NA. Strenght training. Clin Sports Med Jan;10(1):33-62. 1991

Plevnik S, Vodusek DB, Vrtacnik P et al: Optimization of pulse duration for electrical stimulation in treatment of urinary incontnience. World J Urol;4:22-23. 1986

Bazeed MG, Thüroff JW, Schmidt RA, Wiggin DM, Tanagho EA. Effect of chronic electrostimulation of the sacral roots on the striated urethral sphincter. J Urol Dec;128(6):1357-62. 19982

III. INTRAVESICAL ELECTRICAL STIMULATION (IVES)

Boone TB, Roehrborn CG, Hurt G. Transurethral intravesical electrotherapy for neurogenic bladder dysfunction in children with myelodysplasia: a prospective, randomized clinical trial. J Urol;148:550-554. 1992

Buyle S, Wyndaele JJ, D´Hauwers K, Wuyts F, Sys S. Optimal parameters for transurethral intravesical electrostimulation determined in an experiment in the rat. Eur Urol.; 33(5):507-510. 1998

Cheng EY, Richards I, Balcom A, Steinhardt G, Diamond M, Rich M, Donovan JM, Carr MC, Reinberg Y, Hurt G, Chandra M, Bauer SB, Kaplan WE. Bladder stimulation therapy improves bladder compliance: results from a multi-institutional trial. J Urol; 156:761-764. 1996

Cheng EY, Richards I, Kaplan WE. Use of bladder stimulation in high risk patients. J Urol Aug;156:749-5. 1996

Colombo T, Wieselmann G, Pichler-Zalaudek K, Steinbrenner B, Jantscher M, Halbwedl I, Zapotoczky HG, Hubmer G. Central nervous system control of micturition in patients with bladder dysfunctions in comparison with healthy control probands. An electrophysiological study. Urologe A Mar;39(2):160-5. 2000

Decter RM, Snyder P, Laudermilch C. Transurethral electrical bladder stimulation : a follow-up report. J Urol;152:812-814. 1994

Decter RM, Snyder P, Rosvanis TK. Transurethral electrical bladder stimulation: initial results. J Urol;148:651-653. 1992

Decter RM. Intravesical electrical stimulation of the bladder:Contra. Editorial. Urology;56(1):2-4. 2000

Denes J, Leb J. Electrostimulation of the neuropathic bladder. J Pediatr SurgApr;10(2):245-247. 1975

Ebner A, Jiang CH, Lindström S. Intravesical electrical stimulation - An experimental analysis of the mechanism of action. J Urol; 148:920-924. 1992

Eckstein HG, Katona F. Treatment of neuropathic bladder by transurethral electrical stimulation. Lancet 1:780-781, 1974

Fall M, Lindström S. Electrical stimulation. A physiologic approach to the treatment of urinary incontinence. Urol Clin North Am; 18:393-407. 1991

Frankel vL & Zuckerkandl O. in Die Erkrankungen der Blase, p 101, Hrsg. H.Senator, Wien 1899, Alfred Höbler Verlag

Janneck C. Electric stimulation of the bladder and the anal sphincter – a new way to treat the neurogenic bladder. Prog Pediatr Surg;9:119-139. 1976

Jiang CH, Lindström S, Mazières L. Segmental inhibitory control of ascending sensory information from bladder mechanoreceptors in cat. Neurourol Urodynam; 10:286-288. 1991

Jiang CH. Modulation of the micturition reflex pathway by intravesical electrical stimulation: an experimental study in the rat. Neurourol Urodyn.; 17(5):543-53. 1998

Kaplan WE, Richards I. Intravesical bladder stimulation in myelodysplasia. J Urol;140:1282-1284. 1988

Kaplan WE. Intravesical electrical stimulationof the bladder:Pro. Editorial. UROLOGY;56(1):2-4. 2000

Katona F. Stages of vegetative afferentiation in reorganization of bladder control during electrotherapy. Urol Int; 30: 192-203. 1975

Kiss G, Madersbacher H, Poewe W. Cortical evoked potentials of the vesicourethral junction – a predictor for the outcome of intravesical electrostimulation in patients with sensory and motor detrusor dysfunction. Worl J Urol.;16(5):308-312. 1998

Kölle D, Madersbacher H, Kiss G, Mair D. Intravesical electrostimulation for treatment of bladder dysfunction. Initial Experience after gynecological operations. Gynakol Geburtshilfliche Rundsch.;35 (4):221-225. 1995

Kroll P, Jankowski A, Martynski M. Electrostimulation in treatment of neurogenic and non-neurogenic voiding dysfunction. Wiad

Lek.;51 Suppl 3:92-97. 1998

Lyne CJ, Bellinger MF. Early experience with transurethral electrical bladder stimulation. J Urol;150:697-699. 1993

Madersbacher H, Pauer W, Reiner E, Hetzel H, Spanudakis St. Rehabilitation of micturition in patients with incomplete spinal cord lesions by transurethral electrostimulation of the bladder. Eur Urol;8:111-116. 1982

Madersbacher H. Intravesical electrical stimulation for the rehabilitation of the neuropathic bladder. Paraplegia;28:349-352. 1990

Nicholas JL, Eckstein HB. Endovasical electrotherapy in treatment of urinary incontinence in spina bifida patients. Lancet 2:1276-1277, 1975

Primus G, Trummer H. Intravesical electrostimulation in detrusor hypocontractility. Wien Klin Wochensch;105(19):556-557. 1993

Pugach JL, Salvin L, Steinhardt GF. Intravesical electrostimulation in pediatric patients with spinal cord defects. J Urol Sep;164:965-968. 2000

Saxtorph MH. Stricture urethrae - Fistula perinee - Retentio urinae. Clinisk Chirurgi, Copenhagen: Gyldendalske Fortlag; 265-280. 1878

Schwock G, Tischer W. The influence of intravesical electrostimulation on the urinary bladder in animals. Z KinderchirFeb;32(2):161-166. 1981

Seiferth J, Heising J, Larkamp H. Intravesical electrostimulation of the neurogenic bladder in spina bifida children. Urol Int;33(5):279-284. 1978

Seiferth J, Larkamp H, heising J. Experiences with temporary intravesical electro-stimulation of the neurogenic bladder in spina bifida children. Urologe A Sep;17(5):353-354. 1978

Shapiro E, Becich MJ, Perlman E, Lepor H. Bladder wall abnormalities in myelodysplastic bladders: a computer assisted morphometric analysis. J Urol. May;145(5):1024-9. 1991

Committee 11 A

Surgical Treatment of Urinary Incontinence in Children

Chairmen

M.Mitchell (USA),

C.Woodhouse (UK)

Members

D. Bloom (USA),

H.M. Snyder (USA),

Consultant

M. Fisch (Germany)

CONTENTS

Surgical Treatment of Urinary Incontinence in Children

M.Mitchell, C.Woodhouse

D. Bloom, H.M. Snyder, M. Fisch

I. INTRODUCTION

Urinary incontinence in children is a priori an issue of great social and medical importance and therefore constitutes an issue of the highest priority. Unfortunately, the proof of efficacy of the surgical procedures to correct this problem falls to levels three, four and five. The rarity and complexity of the conditions associated with congenital incontinence in children at this point precludes the establishment of higher levels of evidence because of the rarity and spectrum of the pathology. The modalities of treatment are in a state of flux and results dependent on the skills of the individual surgeon. Therefore at this point graded recommendations for specific procedures cannot be meaningfully provided. This report provides a schematic for the surgical approach to children based on the committee's consensus. Referenced literature is limited to reports of individuals' and institutional experience (Level 3,4) and there are no randomized controlled trials (level 1 and 2 evidence).

Congenital anomalies and acquired diseases may cause incontinence by interfering with the function of the sphincter mechanisms, the storage function of the bladder or by bypassing normal sphincter mechanisms. (Figures 1,2,3,4) Surgical treatments are designed to address these problems. In many cases conservative treatments such as intermittent catheterization and drug therapy are needed in addition to surgery since most of the surgical procedures can achieve continence, but seldom restore normal voiding. In the following sections we review these procedures. Multiple mechanisms for incontinence often coexist in the same patient.

Patients with bladder neck incompetence pose a real challenge and require a different approach. All surgical procedures to "reconstruct" the bladder neck have one thing in common; an anatomical obstruction is created to enhance bladder outlet resistance. Even if successful, normal voiding with low pressures and no external help is no longer possible in most patients. If resistance is too low they leak, if it is too high they have to strain or perform CIC. In either case, this is not a physiological situation. Considering the long-term outcome, it may be better not to void spontaneously when bladder outlet resistance is increased because longstanding outlet resistance may cause secondary changes of the bladder wall (as in benign prostatic obstruction), severe dysfunctional voiding or detrusor sphincter dyssynergia.

1. Abnormalities of storage (Figures 1 and 2)

a) Bladder exstrophy: The incidence for bladder exstrophy is 1 per 30,000 live births. (male to female ratio 2:3.1-6.1); closure of the bladder is generally performed within the first days of life; pelvic osteotomies facilitate reconstruction of the abdominal wall and may improve ultimate continence [1,2]. Some children will develop more or less normal capacities, while other patients end up with a poorly compliant small bladder, requiring later bladder enhancement or diversion (ureterosigmoidostomy). Reconstruction of the bladder neck can either be done at the time of bladder closure or at a later stage [3]. Early reconstruction may facilitate normal bladder function, but should be attempted only at centers experienced with such surgery [1,4]. Continence rates vary from center to center and may range between 43 to 87% [5,6].

b) Cloacal exstrophy: The incidence of cloacal exstrophy is 1 per 200,000 live births. This is a much more complex deformity that requires an individual approach. Most of these children have anomalies of the nervous system, upper urinary tract and gastrointestinal tract that can adversely affect urinary tract reconstruction. Before reconstructive procedures are considered, an extensive evaluation has to be carried out.

c) Agenesis and duplication of the bladder are both extremely rare. Agenesis is rarely compatible with life. In bladder duplication other associated congenital ano-

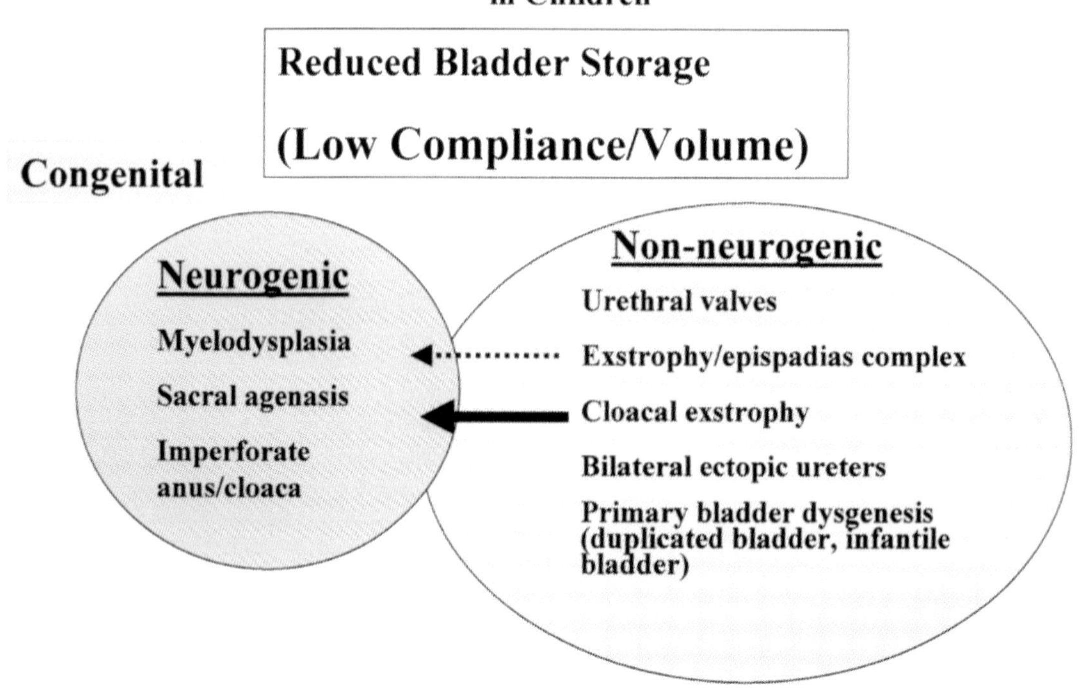

Figure 1 : Congenital diagnoses associated with urinary incontinence because of poor bladder compliance and /or reduced bladder volume.

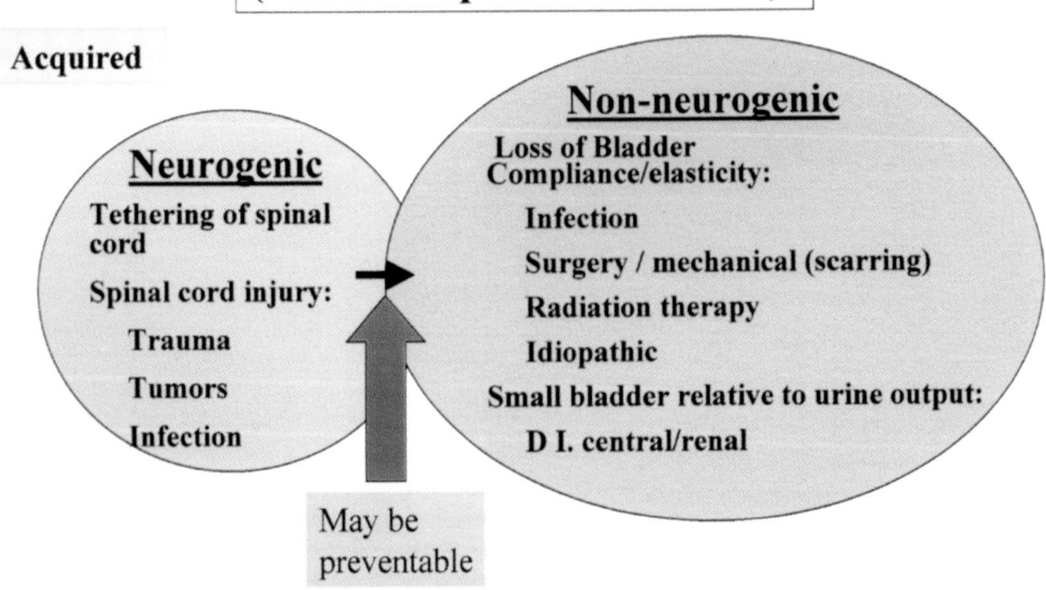

Figure 2 : Acquired diagnoses associated with urinary incontinence because of poor bladder compliance and /or reduced bladder volume.

malies are often observed such as duplication of external genitalia or lower gastrointestinal tract

d) Abnormal storage function in combination with other anomalies is usually caused by a neurologic deficit or is secondary to bladder outlet obstruction. Sacral anomalies are frequently seen with cloacal malformations and imperforate anus [8,9,10,11]. Posterior urethral valves may cause severe hypertrophy of the detrusor with a small poorly compliant bladder. Unfortunately, following valve ablation, particularly if not done soon after birth, these bladders may not return to normal function. Urinary incontinence is usually the result of detrusor overactivity. Some bladders become decompensated resulting in large residuals and overflow incontinence [12]. Different techniques will be described for enhancing bladder capacity.

2. Abnormalities of sphincteric function (Figures 3 and 4)

a) Epispadias: incidence 1 in 100,000 live births, male to female ratio: 3-5:1. All patients with bladder exstrophy also have complete epispadias. In patients with complete epispadias the sphincteric mechanism is deficient and causes complete incontinence. Reconstruction of the bladder neck is either performed at the time of epispadias repair or at a later stage [13,14]. The bladder function may or may not be normal in these patients.

b) Malformation of the Urogenital Sinus occurs exclusively in phenotypic females. The incidence is 1 in 50,000 live births. In patients with classical urogenital sinus or cloaca, the sphincteric mechanism is insufficient, and due to neurological abnormalities the bladder function may also be abnormal.

c) Ectopic ureteroceles protruding into the urethra may be responsible for a partial defect of the bladder neck. In these rare cases, sphincteric incontinence may be the result.

d) Sphincter Abnormalities secondary to spina bifida and other neurologic disorders are of particular importance. The sphincter may be overactive (like in detrusor sphincter dyssynergia) or incompetent. Overactivity of the sphincter causes secondary changes of the bladder wall (increased collagen type III with decreased elasticity and compliance). Continence is usually achieved with anticholinergic drug treatment or bladder augmentation (using the overactivity of the sphincter for continence). In cases of incompetence of the sphincter different types of surgical intervention are possible to enhance the sphincteric mechanism. In general all patients with a neurogenic bladder need Clean Intermittent Cauterization (CIC). In patients bound to a wheelchair a suprapubic channel can be created (Mitrofanoff) to facilitate CIC.

3. Bypass of sphincteric mechanisms (figures 3 and 4)

a)Ectopic Ureters occur more frequently in girls and are commonly part of a duplex system: in girls the ectopic orifice of the upper pole moiety drains into the urethra or vaginal vestibule, thus causing incontinence. When the ectopic ureter represents a single system, the trigone is usually asymmetrical and not well developed. These children may suffer from continuous incontinence as well as a deficient sphincteric mechanism: this is particularly true in bilateral ectopia of single systems. In these patients the trigone and bladder neck are functionally abnormal and treatment includes surgical reconstruction of the bladder neck. When the upper pole ureter opens in the mid or distal female urethra or outside the urinary tract (i.e. vulva or vagina) incontinence results [15]. Upper pole nephrectomy or ipsilateral uretero-ureterostomy solves the problem.

b) Urethral duplications. Most patients with urethral duplication will leak urine from the abnormal meatus during voiding. In rare cases, when the urethra bypasses the sphincteric mechanisms, continuous leakage may be present [16].

c) Vesicovaginal fistulas. Acquired fistulas may be traumatic or iatrogenic, following procedures on the bladder neck.

II. EVALUATION AND DIAGNOSIS *(Figure 5)*

1. History and Physical Examination

To understand and manage urinary incontinence in a child a clinician needs to become adept at the elimination interview. This interactive process requires practice and interpersonal skill far beyond a few simple questions such as "does your child wet his or her pants?." Just as a symptom of gross hematuria precipitates a targeted cascade of specific questions, any voiding dysfunction demands a well-tuned elimination interview and a careful search for physical clues [1].

The "Elimination History" should elucidate the following information; family history of genitourinary disorders; unexplained fevers in infancy, age of toilet training; evidence of urinary infections; previous or current voiding symptoms (dysuria, urgency, stranguria, stream abnormality, intermittency, retention episodes); number of voids per day; delay of first morning void (and, if so, for how long); nocturia; waking to drink (a hallmark of renal insufficiency). The present status of continence (diurnal, nocturnal, fecal) is carefully queried with quantitative analysis [2]. For

Diagnoses with potential Incontinence/wetting correlated to **Bladder** Function in Children

Reduced Bladder Storage

(Poor Sphincteric Function /Overflow/Bypass)

Congenital

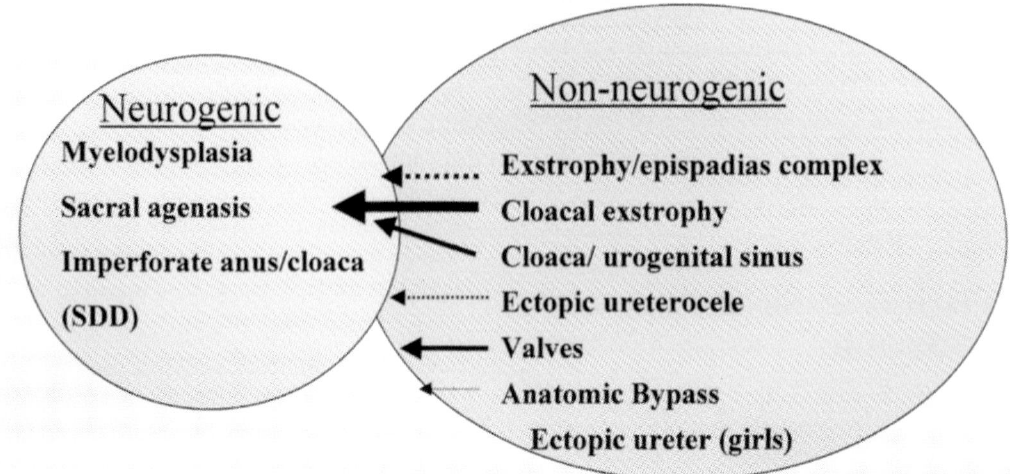

Figure 3 : Congenital diagnoses associated with urinary incontinence because of poor sphincteric function or anatomic bypass of the urinary sphincter.

Diagnoses with potential Incontinence/wetting correlated to **Bladder** Function in Children

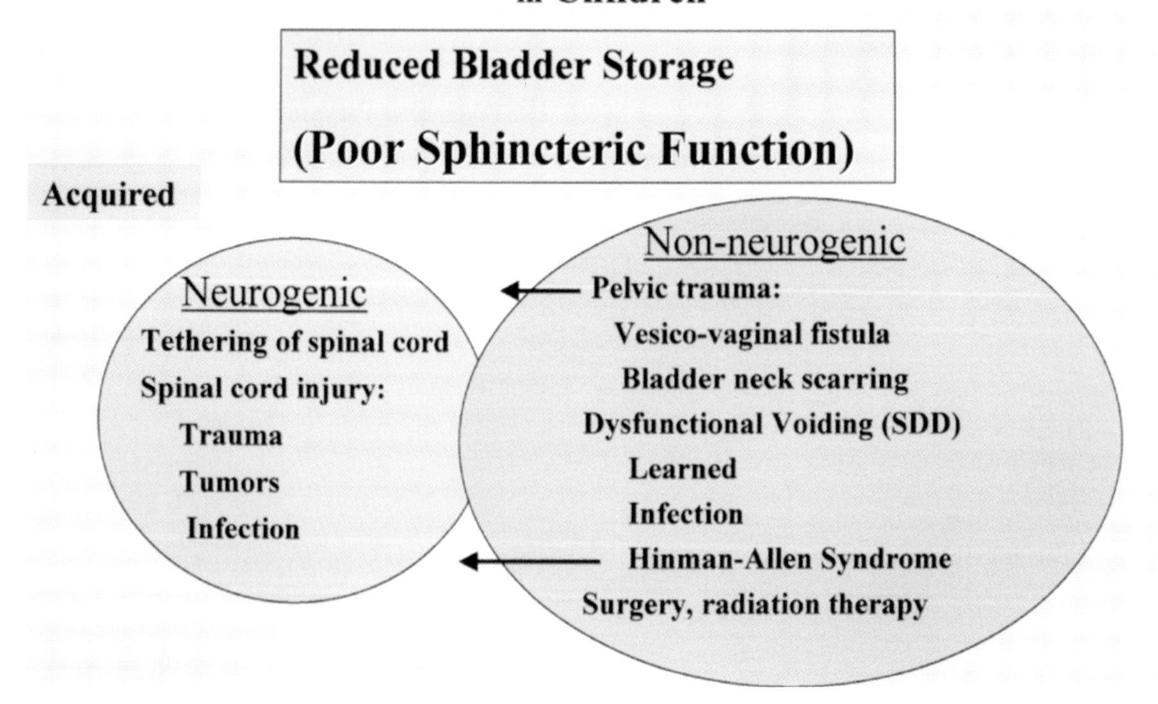

Figure 4 : Acquired diagnoses associated with urinary incontinence because of poor sphincteric function or anatomic bypass of the urinary sphincter.

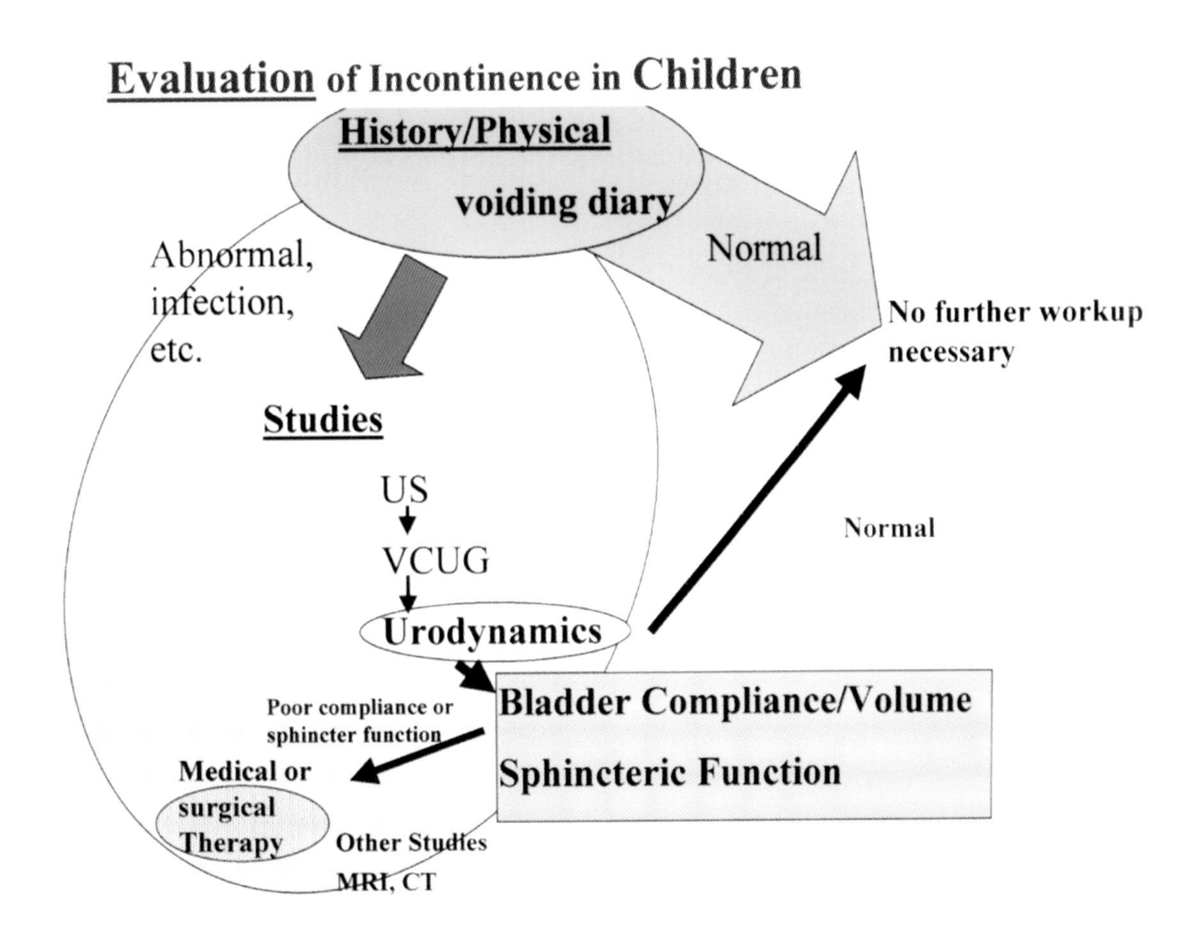

Figure 5 : Flow diagram for the evaluation of a child with urinary incontinence.

example, with diurnal incontinence ascertain the number of wet days (e.g. 2 per week), number of accidents on wet days, management of the accidents (e.g. number of pads, underwear or clothes changes/day). The pattern of incontinence is telling: does the child void normally but have continuous dribbling in between; are the accidents related to stress or physical activity; are the accidents related to large volumes and infrequent voiding; do the accidents occur just after voiding; are accidents only associated with giggling; are accidents random; are volumes usually large or small? Nocturnal incontinence is similarly probed; how many wet nights per week and accidents per night; how is the wet bed managed; does the accident waken the child; does the child wake to void on dry nights; what is the relationship of accidents to foods, stress, travels, menstrual periods; how has incontinence been managed thus far (medications, therapeutic programs, discipline)? An elimination diary is a very useful adjunct to the elimination interview. Bowel patterns are relevant [3].

Physical examination: Height and weight percentiles, blood pressure, and urine analysis are basic elements of the physical exam. Overall constitutional health, vigor and gait are assessed. Evidence for neglect or abuse is considered. The abdomen is inspected and palpated for organomegaly, particularly kidneys, bladder or masses. Genitalia are examined and described in terms of sexual maturity. Underwear and clothes are examined for dryness or stains. The penis is inspected for meatal stenosis, phimosis, hypospadias or epispadias. The introitus is examined for normal dimensions and landmarks. Absence of a distinct urethral orifice is a clue to a urogenital sinus anomaly. Failure of fusion of the labial folds anteriorly is a typical feature of female epispadias. Anal position and appearance are noted. We are reluctant to do routine rectal examination or intrusive pelvic examination in children unless a specific reason is present. The back and spine are examined and palpated for scoliosis, kyphosis, hemangiomas, lipoma, hair tufts, asymmetry, or dimples. The feet are inspected for asymmetry, arch disproportions, clubbing, and inversions. It is useful to observe the child's gait.

2. Imaging studies

Imaging studies are essential to define the anatomical abnormalities responsible for and associated with incontinence. Ultrasonography and a voiding cystourethrogram are the basic studies. Ultrasonography should assess not just the kidneys, but the entire abdomen including the bladder. Renal size is assessed by comparison to a nomogram for normal lengths. Parenchyma is described, hydronephrosis if present is graded and bladder wall is characterized. Stones, debris and foreign bodies are sought. In infants and small children sacral ultrasonography can demonstrate normal position and mobility of the spinal cord. The scout film of the contrast voiding cystourethrogram (VCUG) assesses the lower spine and sacrum, intersymphyseal distance, and fecal retention. The next images should be limited and collimated to minimize radiation. These films will show bladder configuration, presence of vesicoureteral reflux, incomplete voiding, bladder neck competence, urethral anatomy, and vaginal reflux. The amount of contrast instilled for the study is a useful parameter to record, in addition to initial catheter placement and postvoid residual. The VCUG is particularly important in patients with infection history or hydronephrosis. Occasionally, an intravenous urogram will provide the clearest assessment of the urinary tract. Rapid MRI and CT scanning can be helpful in defining spinal abnormalities as well as congenital abnormalities in the urinary tract.

3. Urodynamics

In addition to imaging studies, urodynamic studies, mainly cystometrography and when needed electromyography of the sphincters and urinary flow studies, are useful for all patients with neurogenic incontinence, and in some cases of bladder exstrophy and after posterior urethral valves are resected to help define the mechanism of incontinence. However in many patients much useful information on the function of the lower urinary tract can be obtained with very basic studies including ultrasound and cystometry.

Pediatric urodynamic assessment takes patience on the part of the pediatric specialist. These studies take time and care. They require experienced interpretation. The equipment may range from a simple water manometer with a 3-way stopcock in infants to a continuous recording device connected to a transducer, microtip transducer, or fiberoptic sensor. Concomitant electromyography with patch or needle electrodes is useful. The child should be emotionally prepared and put to ease. Catheterization affords another opportunity to examine the child. The filling curve will be essentially flat without significant pressure change, show low compliance, or evidence involuntary bladder contractions (detrusor overactivity). The absence of observable detrusor overactivity in the forced and artificial testing situation may not be representative of the day-to-day reality of bladder function for a child, and therefore does not necessarily rule out detrusor overactivity. Volume and pressure at the first sensation of fullness, first discomfort and the moment of voiding are critically important to note.

III INDICATIONS FOR SURGICAL PROCEDURES TO CORRECT INCONTINENCE IN CHILDHOOD *(Figure 6)*

1. Storage function

Reduced bladder capacity is the main indication for simple bladder augmentation. Reduced capacity can be congenital (bilateral single ectopic ureters, bladder exstrophy) or caused by previous surgery e.g. bladder neck reconstruction in exstrophy patients, where a part of the bladder is used to create an outlet resistance. Other indications are low functional bladder capacity as it may be present in neurogenic bladder (meningomyelocele) or bladder scarring from previous surgery or obstruction.

Bladder scarring from Bilharzia remains common in endemic areas and is increasingly common with immigration. In all such cases surgery is indicated when conservative treatment has failed.

2. Sphincter function

Most of the diseases in childhood requiring surgical repair for incontinence not only have an influence on bladder capacity but also on sphincter function. Conservative measures to improve sphincter function have limited value and surgery is required in many cases. There are different surgical options; either to increase outlet resistance or to create or implant a new sphincter mechanism. In neurologically normal patients such as classic exstrophy patients, early anatomic reconstruction may allow normal bladder and sphincter function.

Sling procedures are indicated when the residual sphincter function is not sufficient to avoid incontinence. This is the case in patients with neurogenic bladder disturbances and urethral incontinence. If there is no residual sphincter function or outlet resistance at all, an artificial sphincter may be required. Primary urinary diversion (rectal reservoirs/continent stoma) offers an alternative solution to this problem.

3 Procedures bypassing the sphincter

If bladder outlet surgery fails or urethral catheterization is not possible, a continent stoma may be constructed. Some patients prefer catheterizing through a continent stoma rather than through the sensate urethra. The continent stoma (Mitrofanoff principle) may be effectively combined with bladder augmentation and/or bladder neck closure. An alternative to such procedures would be the use of the anal sphincter for urinary continence.

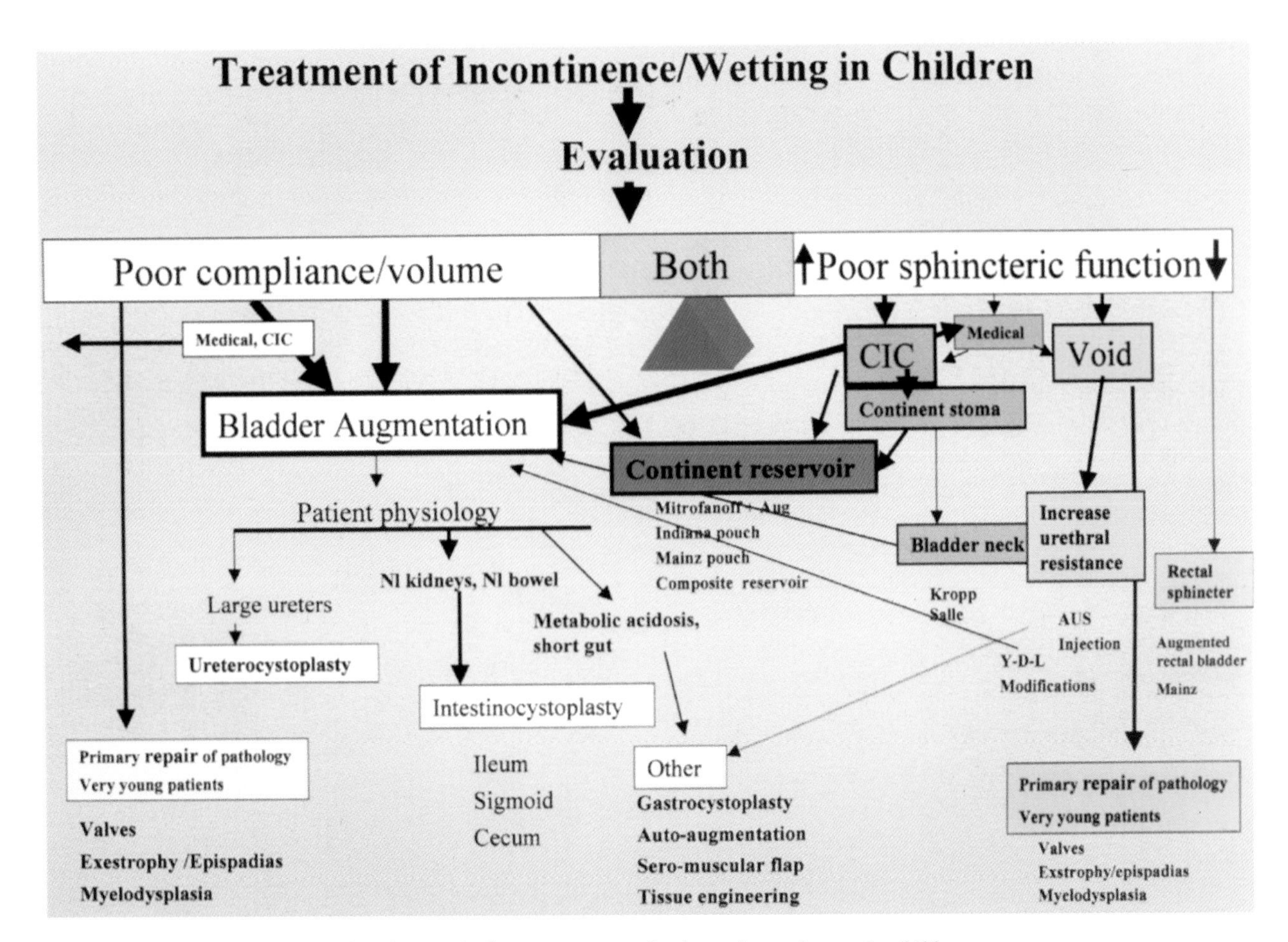

Figure 6 : Treatment schematic for the surgical management of urinary incontinence in children.

IV. BLADDER/RESERVOIR CONSTRUCTION

1. URETEROSIGMOIDOSTOMY/ THE SIGMA-RECTUM POUCH

This type of continent urinary reconstruction may be utilized in reconstruction for bladder exstrophy, an incontinent urogenital sinus or the traumatic loss of the urethral sphincter. As this reconstruction is totally dependent on the normal function of the anal sphincter, contraindications include incompetence of the anal sphincter, anal prolapse, previous anal surgery, and irradiation. Because of the potential for electrolyte resorption, renal insufficiency with creatinine greater than 2 mg/dl also is a contraindication. Furthermore, severely dilated and thick walled ureters are difficult to utilize for a direct ureterosigmoid anastomosis and may be a contraindication for this form of reconstruction in children.

Low pressure rectal reservoirs are superior to simple ureterosigmoidostomy because the augmented or reconfigured rectal bladder achieves lower pressure storage and accordingly, enhances continence. There are two techniques which have been utilized:

a) The Augmented rectal bladder (Figure 7). In which the rectosigmoid is opened on its antimesenteric border and augmented by an ileal segment [1]. The sigmoid may be invaginated to form a nipple valve, as shown in this figure, to avoid reflux of urine into the descending colon and thus to minimize metabolic complications.

b) The Sigma-rectum pouch (Figure 8). In which there is an antimesenteric opening of the recto-sigmoid and a side to side detubularization anastomosis. Ureteral reimplantation of normal sized ureters is by a standard submucosal tunnel (Goodwin, Leadbetter). If the ureter is dilated the technique utilizing a serosa lined extramural tunnel may be more appropriate.

As reported by Fisch et al. (1996) [2], the results of these low-pressure rectal reservoirs are excellent with day and night continence better than 90% and complications related to the surgical procedure range from 0-10% with the sigma-rectum pouch to 34% for the augmented rectal bladder. Late complications for the sigma-rectum pouch range from 6-12.5% and the late complications for the augmented rectal bladder are 17%. The complications are primarily pouch leakage early on, or late stenosis of the ureteral implantation into the bowel and pyelonephritis. Metabolic acidosis may also occur (Table 1).

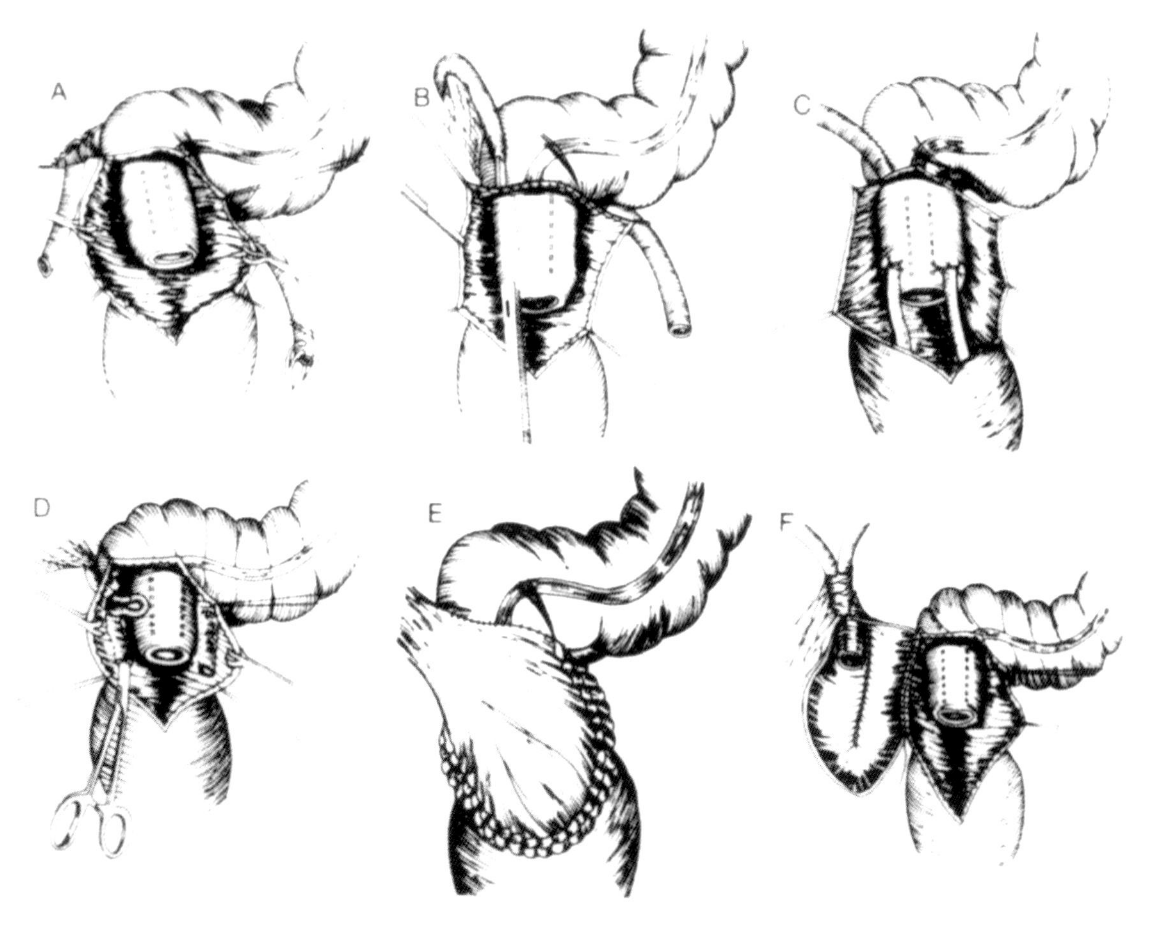

Figure 7 : Augmented rectal bladder

Table 1 : Mainz Pouch II

Author	# Of PTS	Mean age (Children)	Follow-up	Early Complication	Late Complication	Continence Day	Continence Night
El Damanhouri (Cairo)	38 (?)	53 15-17	8.5 mths	0	3%	100%	100%
Esen (Istanbul)	40 (?)	51.4 19-75	16.4 mths	2.5%	12.5%	1005	100%
Managadze (Tiblis)	21 (0)	36-69	?	0	5%	100%	100%
Orestano (Palermo)	40 (?)	?	3-31 mths	0	10%	?	?
Fisch (Mainz)	87 (18)	40.2 9 mths -73y	26.4 mths	6.9%	9.6%	93.8%	93.8%
Pansadoro (Rome)	47 (0)	64 38-74	15 mths	10%	6%	?	?

Abstract book Second International Meeting on Continent Urinary Reconstruction.June 28-30, 1995, Mainz, Germany

Augmented Rectal Bladder

Author	# Of PTS	Mean age (Children)	Follow-up	Early Complication	Late Complication	Continence Day	Continence Night
Dawaba Mansoura	18	8.1y 2-12y	5.2y	34%	17%	100%	100%

M.S. Dawaba et al. World J Urol 14:73-77, 1996.

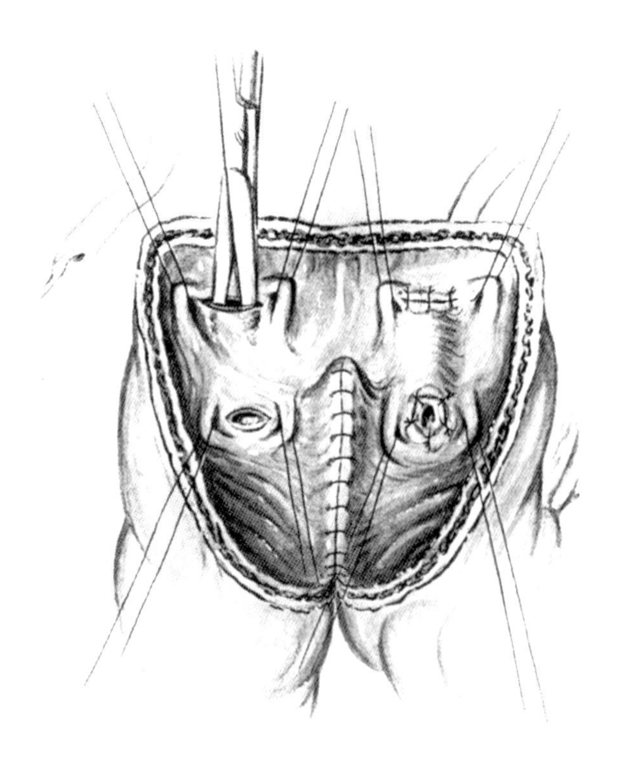

Figure 8 : Sigma-rectum pouch

2. Intestine: Bladder Augmentation, Bladder Replacement, Continent Urinary Diversion (Colon/Ileum/Stomach)

The indication for replacement of the bladder or a continent urinary diversion is either the morphological or functional loss of normal bladder function. A contraindication exists if the patient cannot be catheterized or there is an anticipation of poor patient compliance. When there is reduced renal function generally with a creatinine above 2 mg/dl or a creatinine clearance below 40 ml./min/1.73 m^2, there is a relative contraindication to the use of ileum or colon because of the anticipation of a metabolic acidosis secondary to reabsorption. The stomach with its excretion of acid may be used with a low creatinine clearance possibly in preparation for transplantation [3]. It is, however, not wise to use stomach with any questions of an incompetent bladder outlet because of the severe skin irritation that the acid urine may produce [4].

There are indications for different technical approaches to bladder augmentation or replacement that are dependent upon the clinical presentation of the patient:

• A simple bladder augmentation using intestine may be carried out if there is any bladder tissue, a competent sphincter and/or bladder neck, and a catheterizable urethra.

• An augmentation with additional bladder outlet procedures such as bladder neck reconstruction or other forms of urethral reconstruction are required when both the bladder and outlet are deficient. This occurs most commonly in bladder exstrophy. It must be appreciated that these procedures may complicate transurethral catheterization. Augmentation with surgical closure of the bladder neck may be required primarily, or as a secondary procedure in certain rare clinical situations. In this situation a continent stoma will be required.

• An augmentation with additional continent stoma is utilized primarily following failure of previous bladder outlet surgery. It is advisable also when it can be anticipated that there will be an inability to catheterize transurethrally. An abdominal wall continent stoma may be particularly beneficial to the wheelchair bound spina bifida patient who often can have difficulty with urethral catheterization. For continence with augmentation and an abdominal wall stoma, it is essential that there be an adequate bladder outlet mechanism to maintain continence.

• Total bladder replacement in anticipation of normal voiding in children is very rare, as there are infrequent indications for a total cystectomy, with preservation of the bladder outlet and a competent urethral sphincter. This type of bladder replacement is much more common in adult urologic reconstruction.

• A continent urinary intestinal reservoir with continent abdominal wall stoma is an alternative to procedures that depend on bladder neck reconstruction or compressive procedures for continence. It is also an alternative in patients who are not candidates for a reservoir dependent on anal sphincteric function [5,6,7].

a) Selection of Intestinal Segment to be Utilized (Figure 6)

• Stomach has limited indications primarily because of the complications that have been seen. It, however, is the only intestinal segment really suitable with significantly reduced renal function. Additionally, when no other bowel may be available, as after irradiation or there exists the physiology of a short bowel syndrome, as in cloacal exstrophy, this may be the only alternative remaining [4] (Table 2)

• Ileum/Colon

Clinically these two intestinal segments appear to be equally useful. In children, sigmoid colon is widely used except in those who have been treated for imperforate anus [8]. Use of the ileocecal region, however, can be associated with transient and sometimes prolonged diarrhea. This segment should be avoided in patients with a neurogenic bowel secondary to myelomeningocele or who have been subject to previous pelvic irradiation. If the ileocecal valve must be used, it

Table 2 : Gastric Pouches

Author	Technique	# Of PTS (Children)	Mean age	Follow-up	Early Complication	Late Complication	Continence Day	Continence Night	CIC
Bogaert 1994	Augmentation Artifi sphincter cont. stoma	28	9 (4-17)	2Y 5Mnths	0	18%	93%	93%	?
Ganesan Mitchell 1992 AUA	Augmentation replacement	73	14.1 (1.3-53)	26.5 mnths	6.8%	48%	86%	86%	?
Woodard 1995?	Continent diversion	22	11 (4-25)	24 mnths (6-38)	73%	73%	95.4%	95.4%	100%
Atala 1993	Gastrocystoplasty	43 20 follow	11 (1-23)	?	35%	35%	80%	80%	80%
Nguyen 1993	Augmentation total replacement	57	9.9 1.5-28	23.3 m (12-39)	Dysuria, hematuria 36%		?	?	?
Adams	Augmentation continent	13	6.4 (21m-14y)	13 m (6-23y)	0	23%	84.6%	85.6%	77%
Gosalbez 1993	Gastrocystoplasty continent stoma	30	9 (2.5-23)	14m (3-20)	6.7%	13.3%	81% 90%	81% 90%	92.3%
Ngan 1993	Gastrocystoplasty	1(0)	39.5 (30-84)	10y (4-16)	?	60%	100%	70%	0
Gonsalbez 1994	Continent stoma	15 (6)	15y 43y 12-60		0	46%	935	93%	100%

Stomach in combination with other intestinal segments

Author	Technique	# Of PTS (Children)	Mean age	Follow-up	Early Complication	Late Complication	Continence Day	Continence Night	CIC
McLaughlin 1995	Gastric+ileal	7	3-23y	13-59 m	85%		85.7%	85.7%	100%

may be reconstructed at the time of ileocolostomy. The ileum can be satisfactorily used for bladder augmentation: however because of its smaller diameter a longer segment of ileum is required to create a comparable colon reservoir [9]. Colon has greater flexibility for urethral implantation and construction of a continent. The colon is more frequently used for continent urinary reservoirs in children [6].

If the patient can be expected to void spontaneously, reconstructive surgery can be carried out at any age. If the child will be dependent on intermittent catheterization, either there must be a supportive parent or caregiver early in life or the procedure should be delayed until the child is sufficiently old enough to demonstrate a willingness to carry out self-catheterization. However, with bladder augmentation it is generally assumed that intermittent catheterization will be necessary.

There are several important principles for bladder augmentation and replacement that should be respected: (Grade C)

1. Use the minimal amount of bowel. Utilize hindgut segments or conduits if available.
2. A low-pressure large capacity reservoir is essential. This requires detubularization of any intestinal segment used.
3. For colonic reservoirs a sigmoid segment of 30 cm is generally satisfactory [10]. A slightly longer segment of ileum is wise. The length of the segments can be scaled down in smaller children. One should not utilize more than 60 cm of ileum in adolescents and comparable lengths in younger children because of reduction of the intestinal resorptive surface.
4. The jejunum is contraindicated in intestinal reconstruction of the urinary tract because of its metabolic consequences (hyponatremia, hyperkalemia, and acidosis) [11].
5. It is wise to strive to achieve an anti-reflux ureteral anastomosis to the reservoir to avoid potential for ascending infection.
6. A reliable continence mechanism (continent urinary outlet) must be assured.
7. Because of the risk of stone formation only resorbable sutures and staples should be used in bladder augmentation and reservoir construction.

b) Bladder Augmentation Techniques:

1. In gastric augmentation (Figure 9) A 10-15 cm wedge-shaped segment of stomach is resected. Most commonly this is based on the right gastroepiploic artery but can be based on the left as well. The segment is brought down to the bladder easily in the retroperitoneal space along the great vessels [4].

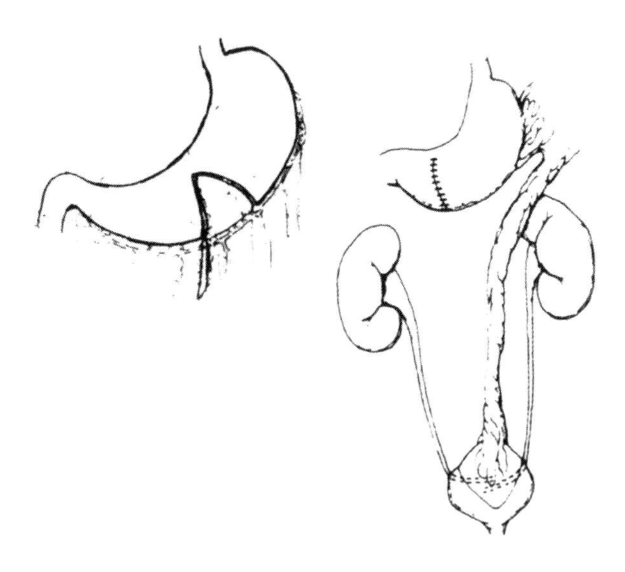

Figure 9 : Wedge-shaped segment of stomach is usually based upon right (or in this case the left) gastroepiploic artery and anastomosed to bladder remnant.

2. The technique for large and small bowel augmentation of the bladder is illustrated (Figure 10).: The bowel segment to be utilized is opened on the antimesenteric border and routinely detubularized prior to anastomosis to the bladder remnant. The anastomosis of the intestinal segment to the bladder remnant and to itself is usually carried out in one running layer of inverting semi-absorbable (polyglycolic acid or polyglactin) sutures. The procedures to create a competent bladder neck or to enhance bladder outlet continence have been reviewed elsewhere in this chapter.
3. The techniques for urinary diversion with continent stoma (Mainz pouch, Indiana pouch, Kock pouch) are all covered in the chapter on current urinary diversion in adults.

Currently, augmentation cystoplasty is the standard treatment for low capacity and/or low compliance bladders secondary to infectious, inflammatory, neurogenic and congenital disorders. Bladder augmentation using sigmoid or ileum has become popular world wide. However, due to the relatively high morbidity of such surgery there is renewed interest in alternative methods. These alternative techniques try to avoid the contact between the urine and intestinal mucosa. These innovative techniques include; gastrocystoplasty, bladder auto-augmentation, seromuscular augmentation, alloplastic or biodegradable scaffolds grafted with autologous urothelium developed in cell culture, and ureterocystoplasty [12].

3. Auto-augmentation

The principle of auto-augmentation procedure is the

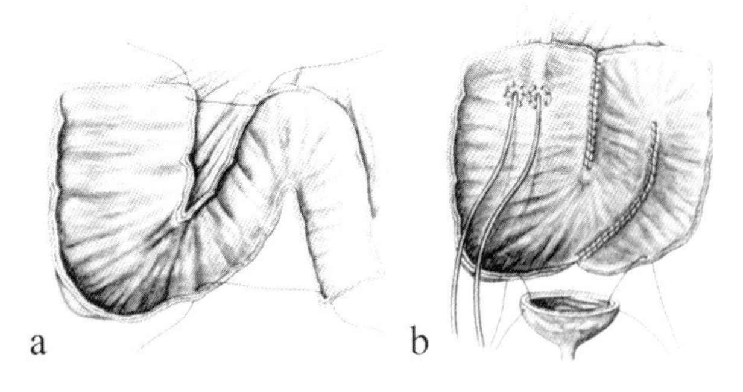

Figure 10 A, B : Bowel segment is isolated (here ileocecum) and opened and anastomosed to the bladder remnant. The ureters are tunneled into the cecum along the tinea.

excision or incision (myotomy) of a great portion of the bladder muscular layer whilst preserving the urothelium. Theoretically, this technique allows the creation of a large diverticulum able to store urine. This urine stored at a low pressure can be drained by intermittent catheterization. The theoretical advantages of this procedure are: the low complication rates of the surgery, reduced operative morbidity with shorter stay in the hospital; absence of urine salt resorption; minimal mucous in the urine and possibly absence of carcinogenic potential. Although some series showed good results with this procedure [13,14], most authors have been unable to achieve the reported success [15]. Twelve consecutive myelomeningocele patients were treated at the University of Sao Paulo by auto-augmentation in order to improve bladder capacity and/or compliance or to prevent deterioration of the upper urinary tract. Although some of them showed some improvement at the early postoperative period, 10 of them required ileal cystoplasty in order to obtain continence and/or to improve hydronephrosis. The inability of this procedure to achieve long-term good results may be due to the regeneration of nerve fibers divided during the surgery as well as the ischemic atrophy of the mucosa. More recently, some authors have proposed the laparoscopic auto-augmentation as a minimally invasive procedure for the treatment of low capacity/low compliance bladder [16]. Despite the indifferent results [17,18] some still suggest its consideration before a standard augmentation because of the reasons listed above. Although there are many potential advantages to this approach to a small poorly compliant bladder the inconsistency of success make it a less favorable option at this time. (Grade C)

4. Seromuscular patch

The first attempts at using intestinal segments free of mucosa to improve bladder capacity resulted in viable seromuscular segments covered with urothelial mucosa [19,20]. However, the intense inflammatory response and shrinkage observed in the intestinal segment discouraged its use in humans [21]. Further attempts consisted of using the association between demucosalized intestinal segments and auto-augmention in a procedure called: Urothelial lined colocystoplasty. In the initial model using sheep, the animals tolerated the demusculization procedure poorly, reflected by inflamed, hemorrhagic colonic segments in the animals sacrificed within one month. In addition, colonic mucosa regrowth occurred in one third of the animals [22]. Follow-up studies in a dog model with previously reduced bladder capacity suggested that the contraction of the intestinal patch in seromuscular enterocystoplasty can be avoided by the preservation of both the bladder urothelium and lamina propria, together with the submucosa and muscularis mucosa of the intestinal patch [23,24]. This form of bladder augmentation was shown to prevent absorption of toxic substances like ammonium chloride [25]. However, other authors using the same technique to line de-epithelialized gastric patches in the mini-pig model found it useless due to the fibrotic changes and decreased surface of the patch [26].

The initial experience in treating humans with colocystoplasty lined with urothelium involved 16 patients with a postoperative follow-up of 12 months. Bladder capacity increased an average of two to four-fold from a mean of 139 mL (+/-23 SEM) to 335 mL (+/- 38 SEM) in 14 patients ($p < 0.001$). In 13 patients submitted to postoperative urodynamics, bladder end filling pressures decreased from a mean of 51.6 cmH_2O (+/- 4.2 SEM) to 27.7 cm H_2O (+/- 2.4 SEM) ($p<0.001$). Of the 16 patients 10 underwent postoperative cystoscopy plus biopsy. Seven demonstrated urothelium covering the augmented portion of the bladder, two had regrowth of colonic mucosa and one showed a mixture of colonic mucosa and urothelium [27]. Another study analyzed 10 patients, nine of them with myelomeningoceles and one with posterior urethral valves using a similar technique [28]. Bladder capacity improved in all cases. However, larger series and longer follow-up are required before its wide application in patients with low capacity/low compliance bladder reservoirs. At this point, this procedure should remain as an experimental technique and should be performed only in regional or University centers until consistent data is obtained. (Grade C)

5. Ureteral bladder augmentation

Another alternative to avoid the morbidity of intestinal bladder augmentation is the use of ureteral segments to improve bladder capacity and/or compliance. Megaureters associated with poorly or nonfunctioning kidneys provide an excellent augmentation material with urothelium and muscular backing, free of potential electrolyte and acid base disturbance, and mucus production that plagues enterocystoplasty. In 16 patients augmentation cystoplasty using detubularized megaureter, with or without ipsilateral partial or total nephrectomy, was used to improve inadequate and dysfunctional bladders. Ten patients became completely continent with intermittent catheterization. Urodynamic evaluation performed in 13 patients showed good bladder capacity and compliance in 12 [29]. In another report three good results were observed in children with low bladder compliance secondary to urethral posterior valves and unilateral vesicoureteral reflux. [30] Another alternative in patients with ureteral dilation and good ipsilateral renal function, is to combine transureteroureterostomy with ureterocystoplasty [31]. Another alternative in bilateral dilated ureters with preserved renal function is bilateral reimplantation and the use of bilateral distal ends for detubularized bladder augmentation [32]. In another series of seven patients (six with neurogenic bladder and one with posterior urethral valves), two patients ultimately required augmentation with ileum [33]. No important complications were observed even in the two patients who required kidney transplantation. Bladder augmentation with ureter may be effective in a small sub group of patients with ureteral dilatation and poor bladder capacity but at this point is not generally applicable to most pediatric patients with surgical incontinence. (Grade B)

6. Experimental methods

The artificial bladder has been the topic of speculation and experiment that remains still outside the bounds of clinical application. Somewhat nearer to clinical use is the concept of tissue engineering using autologous urothelium and bladder muscle cells. These can be grown by tissue culture techniques on a degradable polymer scaffold and then implanted in animal models to fashion a bladder augmentation. Clinical trials with these methods are not far away [34,35,36,37,38].

The use of autologous urothelium could be very useful in many reconstructive urological procedures. Urothelial tissue grafts can be created using cultures of uroepithelial cells grown on appropriate synthetic substrate. A classic study was done using urothelial cell culture grown on a degradable polymer (acid polyglycolic), followed by implantation of the cell polymer scaffold in the mesentery, omentum, and retroperitoneum of athymic mice. It was demonstrated that the polymer degrades and viable urothelial cells layers of one to three cells in thickness remained 20 to 30 days after the implantation. The experiment shows that urothelial cells can be successfully harvested, survive in culture, and attach to artificial biodegradable polymers. These findings suggest that it may be possible to use autologous urothelium, reconfigured on a synthetic substrate, in reconstructive bladder surgery after implanting the urothelial-polymer scaffolds into host animals [34]. Follow-up experiments demonstrated the ability of human urothelial cells to produce monolayers up to 25 centimeters [35]. Later it was shown that human urothelial cells and bladder muscle cells, when implanted in polyglycolic acid fibers, form new urological structures in vivo composed of both cell types. The human cell-polymer xenografts can be recovered from host animals at extended time after implantation. These data suggest the feasibility of using polyglycolic acid polymers as substrates for the creation of human urothelial and muscle grafts for genitourinary reconstruction [36]. An additional contribution came when it was demonstrated that by combining collagen gel with a biodegradable mesh scaffold it was possible to create a surgically implantable cultured uroepithelial graft. This technique permits the use of cultured endothelium for reconstructive surgery [37]. In a recent study, uroepithelial cells were seeded onto de-epithelialized urothelial stroma. It was found that normal human urothelial cells retain the capacity to differentiate and reform a slow turnover stratified transitional epithelium.(38) Taken together, these studies and others not mentioned in this chapter, facilitate the potential use of urothelial artificial grafts for bladder substitution. Although this field of research may represent the future of bladder reconstructive surgery, currently only few experimental studies are available and it may be some time before all this knowledge can be used clinically. We strongly encourage further research in this field.

V. BLADDER OUTLET SURGERY

1. Native urethral enhancement

Procedures to increase urethral resistance, alone or in association with bladder augmentation should be considered when the evaluation of the incontinent child suggests that sphincteric incompetence is the only cause of incontinence or that it plays a mayor role in association with decreased bladder capacity or compliance. In this section, the indications, contraindications, advantages and disadvantages of some of these procedures will be discussed. We will review the published results and comment on our experience with three procedures commonly used to enhance urethral resistance, namely, the artificial urinary sphincter (AUS), urethral fascial slings and their variations, and periurethral injection therapy.

a) Injection procedures

The injection of bulking substances in the tissues around the urethra and bladder neck to increase outlet resistance in children dates back to at least 1985. However, concern about distant migration of the injected substance and risk of granuloma formation prevented this technique from gaining widespread acceptance [1] (Level 3).

The search for safer, biocompatible substances to create periurethral compression has led to the use of cross-linked bovine collagen. From the studies published it appears that satisfactory continence can be achieved in about 20-50% of children [2,3,4]. Although collagen injection appears to effectively improve urethral resistance, this does not always translate into satisfactory dryness. Also, the effect of the injection seems to be of short duration and repeated injections are often necessary [5]. However, complications are rare. Our experience in children with neurogenic incontinence has shown that collagen is only occasionally helpful. At present, given the cost and lack long term effectiveness, injection procedures for continence in children cannot be recommended as routine therapy. (Grade C).

b) Artificial urinary sphincter

In use since 1973, the AUS has undergone major transformations over the years [6]. The currently used model, AS800-T has been in use for almost 20 years. It consists of an inflatable cuff, a pressure regulating balloon and a unit containing a pump and control mechanisms. The inflatable cuff can only be implanted around the bladder neck in females and prepubertal males. In postpubertal males the bulbar urethral placement is possible but not recommended for wheelchair patients or those who perform intermittent catheterization.

Implantation of an AUS requires special training and difficulties may be encountered in the dissection of the space around the bladder neck in obese, post-pubertal males or in patients with a history of previous bladder neck procedures. The pressure-regulating balloon is positioned extra peritoneally to avoid risk of contamination or damage from intraperitoneal processes such as appendicitis. The pump is placed in the scrotum or labium major. A 61-70 cm H_2O pressure balloon is used exclusively when the cuff is around the bladder neck and a lower pressure balloon when it is around the bulbous urethra. Although high in cost the artificial sphincter remains the most effective means or increasing urethral resistance and preserving potential for voiding. (Level 3)

The ideal candidate for AUS implantation is a patient with pure sphincteric incompetence who voids spontaneously and has good bladder capacity and compliance. Unfortunately only a small proportion of children with sphincteric incontinence meet the criteria. However the AUS may also be used in patients dependent on clean intermittent catheterization. The compatibility of the AUS with intermittent catheterization and enterocystoplasty is well documented [7,8,9] (Level 3).

The ability to empty the bladder spontaneously or by Valsalva maneuver may be preserved after AUS implantation. In series reporting children with AUS, the majority having neurogenic incontinence, 25% void spontaneously [10]. When the AUS is implanted before puberty, the ability to void spontaneously may be lost after puberty. (Level 4)

Overall, 40 to 50% of neurogenic patients require a bladder augmentation concomitantly or subsequently to the AUS implantation [10,11] (Level 4). The continence rate ranges from 80 to 97% (Level 3).

The complications most commonly encountered in patients with AUS are mechanical failures [12,13]. Barring technical errors, the longevity of the present devices is expected to exceed 10 years. The second most common problem is the development of reduced bladder compliance with time. This may result from an error in the preoperative evaluation, the reaction of the detrusor to obstruction (a reaction noted in some patients with spina bifida). Or these changes can be seen after many years of follow-up [14,15]. The results of decreased capacity and compliance may be incontinence, upper tract deterioration, or the development of vesicoureteral reflux. Therefore long term follow-up with ultrasound (and, if indicated, urodynamics) is mandatory in all patients with an AUS. (Grade B).

Infection of the prosthesis should occur in no more than 15% of all cases. Erosions of the tissues in contact with the prosthesis are rather infrequent. Bladder neck erosions are practically non-existent when the sphincter is implanted around a "virgin" bladder neck. When the AUS is used as a salvage procedure following bladder neck reconstruction, the erosion rate may be as high as 30%. For this reason AUS implantation may be better considered as the initial treatment in selected cases.(16)

C. Fascial slings and variations

Fascial slings constructed with the aponeurosis of the anterior rectus muscle have been used to increase outlet resistance in incontinent children, particularly those with neurogenic dysfunction since 1982 [17°. The sling is used to elevate and compress the bladder neck and proximal urethra. From the technical point of view, the dissection around the urethra may be facilitated by a combined vaginal and abdominal approach, however, this option is limited to post-pubertal females [18]. (Grade C). Several technical variations of the sling have been reported. The fascial strip may be a graft or a flap based on the rectus sheath on one side. The fascial strip can be crossed anteriorly or wrapped around the bladder neck to enhance urethral compression. (Grade D)

Although the short-term success rate reported by most authors is encouraging, there are no series reporting detailed results at 5 years [19,20]. (Level 3) Most authors report a greater success when fascial slings are used in conjunction with bladder augmentation and success seems more likely in females than in males [21,22,23,24] (Level 3) In patients with neurogenic incontinence postoperative IC is recommended (Grade A).

Complications of sling procedures include difficulties with intermittent catheterization, erosion of the urethra and persistent incontinence. Overall, the increase in outlet resistance provided by slings seem less than that provided by the artificial sphincter. Experience with these procedures suggests an overall success of about 50% in females (Level 4).

From the data published it presently seems that the AUS provides more consistent results in boys and for girls capable of spontaneous voiding who have not had previous bladder neck surgery. Sling procedures are probably equally effective for girls dependant on intermittent catheterization and in conjunction with bladder augmentation. At present, given the cost and lack of effectiveness of injection procedures, their use does not appear justified in incontinent children. The cost of the AUS may restrict its use. (Grade C)

2. Bladder outlet reconstruction in children for continence and dryness

Surgical procedures to achieve urinary continence are dictated by functional and anatomic deficiencies and by the ultimate goal of either continence (with normal voiding) or dryness (dependent on intermittent catheterization).

Construction of a functional urethra for continence usually implies an anatomic defect without a neurogenic component (e.g. epispadias/exstrophy) and includes urethral and bladder neck narrowing (Young, 1922) and urethral lengthening [25,26,27,28,29]. Such procedures may initially require intermittent catheterization or occasional post voiding catheterization, but bladder empting by voiding is anticipated. (Level 3)

Urethral reconstruction for dryness, however, mandates intermittent catheterization. The goal in surgery to achieve dryness is to create a urethra suited to catheterization, which has closure such that intra-luminal pressures always exceed intravesical pressure. The most dependable procedures for dryness utilize a flap valve or tunnel to achieve urethral closure [30,31], although urethral slings, wraps and injections have also been used. (Grade C)

Reconstruction to achieve continence is based on the principle that proximal reduction of the caliber of the urethra supports the inherent proximal sphincteric mechanism of the bladder neck and proximal urethra. The narrowing must be dynamic to permit closure for continence and yet permit opening with funneling during voiding. Young [25] reported on the efficacy of this approach in patients with incontinence and epispadias. His procedure was actually a "double sphincter technique" that involved not only the excision of a wedge of tissue at the anterior bladder neck, but also removal of a wedge of tissue just proximal to the epispadiac meatus (external sphincter). Hendren [32] supported this approach in his report of six patients with epispadias. Dees [26] added the concept of lengthening the urethral tube to that of narrowing. In his procedure parallel incisions were made through the existing bladder neck area which created a posterior urethral plate from what had previously been the trigone of the bladder. This is tubularized to give added length to the proximal urethra. The added length provides increased potential for urethral closure and moves the bladder neck and urethra into the abdominal cavity. Leadbetter(27) modified the Young-Dees procedure by creating muscular flaps from the area of the bladder neck and proximal urethra which were used to wrap the newly created proximal tube (Figure 11). This procedure was popularized by Jeffs [33] who applied it to a staged repair of exstrophy. He supported a lengthened urethra by a suspension. They report their long term continence rate with this procedure as greater than 80%. Presently, this represents the gold standard for reconstruction for continence, however, modifications of the technique have reported similar or improved results [28,29] Most urethral lengthening procedures utilizing the posterior urethra and bladder neck also require ureteral reimplantation and preservation of the posterior urethral plate. The exception to this is the Tanagho procedure (Figure 12) which is based on a tube and formed from the anterior bladder wall after division of most proximal urethra. [34] Hendren [32] has promoted the concept of distal lengthening of the female urethra (urogenital sinus, cloaca, female hypospadias). (Level 4)

Bladder neck and urethral reconstruction for continence in patients who had previous attempts at repair has resulted in less success. Presumably this relates to tissue scarring with the loss of elasticity and contractility. Hendren also advocates a very persistent approach to reconstruction of a functional urethra for continence and maintains that several procedures may be necessary to secure continence or dryness in some patients, particularly in patients who have had previous surgeries. [35] However, if this reconstruction fails, "surgery for dryness (CIC)" or surgical closure of the bladder neck may be required. (Grade C)

Surgery for dryness is dependent on the effectiveness of intermittent catheterization and is usually reserved for patients with neurogenic dysfunction or multiple previous surgeries. Procedures to achieve dryness usually create a urethral closure pressure that exceeds bladder pressure. Usually this is achieved with the creation of a nipple valve or flap valve mechanism. A nipple valve is usually constructed when an intestinal segment used to construct an orthotopic urethra, as in the orthotopic Koch or Indiana Pouch.

A flap valve (Figure 13) can be constructed by using an anterior or posterior bladder flap (full thickness) to construct a tube that is placed in a submucosal tunnel [30,31,37] (Level 4) The major disadvantage of these procedures (flap valves) is that the valve will not allow leakage with high intravesical pressures, potentiating renal damage. (Level 1) Therefore, these procedures can be dangerous to the patient who is not totally committed to follow catheterization recommendations. (Grade A)

Unfortunately, the ideal procedure for surgical reconstruction of the bladder neck does not exist. The surgical approach to urinary incontinence in the child must be multifaceted because of the inherent complex and varied nature of the problem. (Grade A)

Recent data would support the concept that very early reconstruction in the exstrophy/epispadias group may result in physiologic bladder cycling which facilitates normal bladder and urethral development. This results in higher potential for continence without the need for bladder augmentation and bladder neck reconstruction (Level 3). More work and clinical experience in this area is strongly recommended. (Grade A)

3. Alternative continence channels

In the surgical treatment of incontinence in children every effort must be made to preserve the natural lower urinary tract. The bladder is the best urinary reservoir, the urethra the best outlet and the urethral sphincters the best control mechanism. If the bladder is partly or wholly unusable it may be augmented or replaced by a variety of techniques already described.

Urethral failure may occur either because the sphincters are incompetent or because it is overactive and does not allow spontaneous voiding. It would be preferable for the former to be treated by one of the techniques described above and the latter by intermittent catheterization (CIC). If all of these fail, continent supra pubic diversion is indicated.

a) The mitrofanoff principle

Mitrofanoff's name is given to the principle of burying a narrow tube within the wall of the bladder or urinary reservoir whose distal end is brought to the abdominal wall or perineum to form a catheterizable stoma sui-

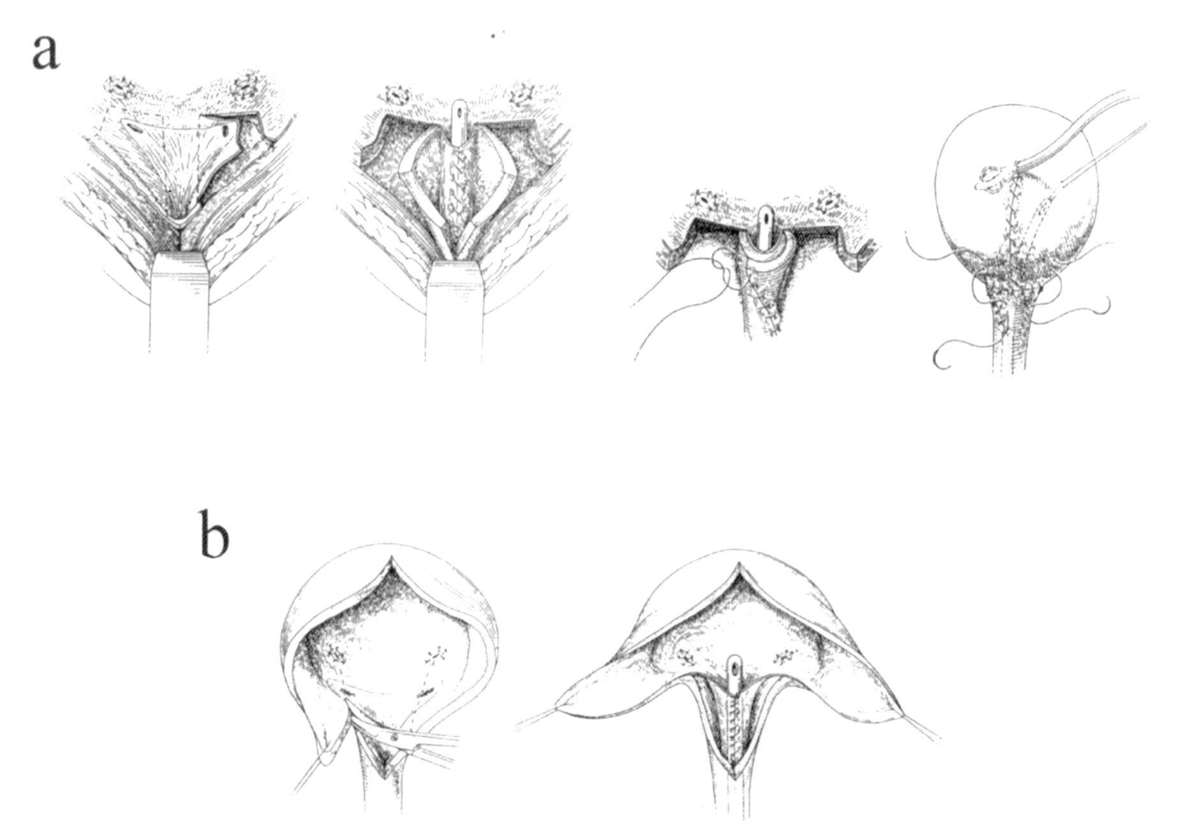

Figure 11 A, B : Extension of posterior urethra (useful in exstrophy) is a procedure for incontinence (potential for normal voiding). a) The Young-Dees-Leadbetter procedure is based on a proximal posterior urethral lengthening. The bladder and urethra are opened in the midline and parallel incisions made distally and extended proximally to the trigone through the mucosa. The ureters are reimplanted higher in the posterior bladder wall. The mucosa is tubularized and muscularis is closed in a vest-over pants technique. b) Variations include the Mollard technique the utilizes a muscular flap wrapped around the bladder neck. In the Mitchell technique the initial incisions are transverse across the distal urethra and then parallel incisions are made to define the urethral plate which extends to the trigone.

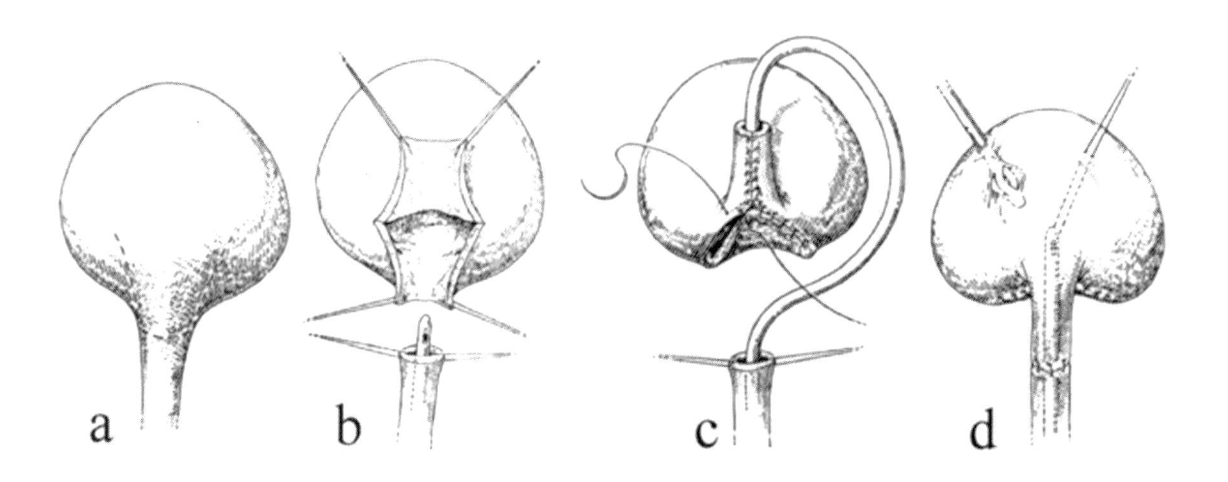

Figure 12 A-D : Extension of the urethra using an anterior bladder flap procedure for continence. In this Tanagho procedure the proximal urethra is divided and a full-thickness anterior bladder flap is tubularized to extend the proximal urethra.

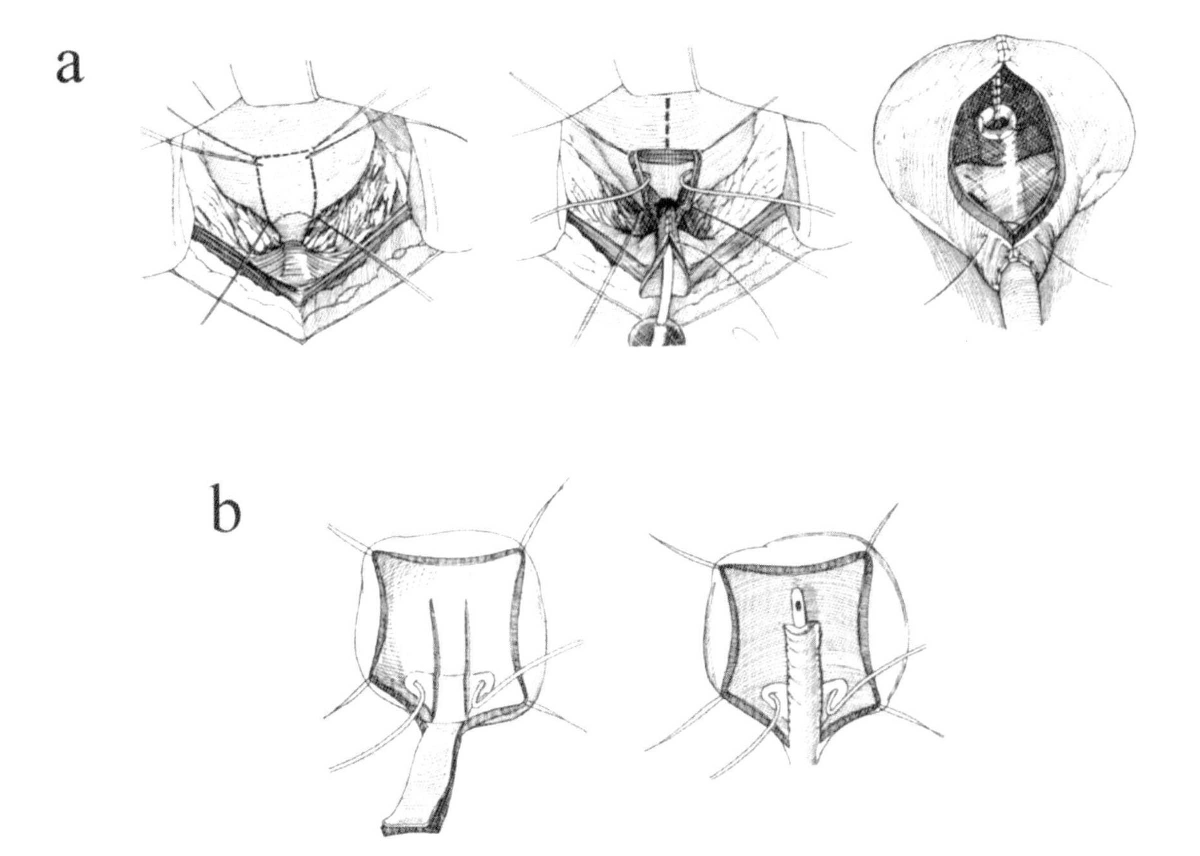

Figure 13 A, B : Procedures for dryness (useful in neurogenic bladder patients and patients with multiple previous surgeries) require intermittent clean catheterization. a) Kropp procedure which uses a full thickness bladder tube tunneled into the bladder wall. b) Salle procedure uses a flap tube made with anterior and posterior bladder wall.

table for intermittent catheterization [38]. The technique is simple and familiar to all urologists who are accustomed to re-implanting ureters. Furthermore, it is a procedure that is easily learned [39]. Several narrow tubes are available for the Mitrofanoff conduit. In the original description, the appendix was used. However, even if the appendix is still present, it may be unusable in 31% of patients [40]. (Level 4)

If no suitable tube is found, a good narrow tube can be formed by tailoring ileum. Ileum may be tailored longitudinally [41]. However, it has now been shown that it can be tailored transversely so that only 2-3cm of ileum can be made into a 7cm conduit. This very useful modification was originally described independently by Yang in humans and by Monti in experimental animals [42,43]. It is increasing used though great care must be taken in its construction to avoid an internal fistula [44] (Grade C)

The ureter may be used but there may be some difficulty in achieving sufficient caliber with a previously normal ureter. Earlier reports that the Fallopian tube could be used have not stood the test of time. (Level 5)

The Mitrofanoff system achieves reliable continence which is maintained in long term follow-up, for a high proportion of patients. (Grade C) The pressure generated within the lumen of the conduit is 2 to 3 times higher than that within the reservoir so that continence is preserved even when the intra abdominal pressure is raised by straining. Conversely, the pressure in the lumen of a Kock nipple is only slightly higher than that in the reservoir so that continence is less reliable [45,46] (Level 3).

The conduit may be buried either between the mucosal and muscle layers of the reservoir, or may be completely imbricated in the full thickness of the reservoir wall. Any well supported tunnel of about 5cm will suffice. The choice depends both on the nature of the reservoir and on the conduit [47] (Level 4)

Continence rates of 90-100% with the Mitrofanoff Principle are reported, regardless of diagnosis, reservoir or conduit type [48,41. Follow-up in small numbers of children for at least ten years has shown that the system is resilient [49] (Level 4)

Although perfect continence seems attractive, it may not be in the child's best interests. Studer has pointed out the need for a 'pop-off' valve if catheterization is impossible or forgotten [50].

b) The Ileocecal valve

The ileocecal valve is an obvious (and, indeed, the original) sphincter to combine with cecum and ascending colon as the reservoir and the terminal ileum as the conduit. The early continence rate of 94% was not sustained because of high pressures in the tubular reservoir and weakness of the valve [51,52] (Level 4)

The Indiana system is based on the competence of the ileocecal valve but with a detubularized reservoir [53] The valve itself is reinforced with non-absorbable plicating sutures and the terminal ileum which forms the conduit is tailored. The best reported continence rate is 96% with a 2% rate of catheterization difficulties [54] (Level 4)

In the complete Mainz I pouch a length of terminal ileum is intussuscepted through the ileocecal valve as a Kock nipple [55] (Thuroff et al 1988). It is impossible to say whether the nipple or the ileocecal valve (or both) produce the continence which is reported in 96% of patients. (Level 4)

Both these systems work well as complete reconstructions and are widely used as bladder replacements in children. The sacrifice of the ileocecal valve may cause gastro intestinal complications. (Grade C)

c) Kock pouch

The first workable continent diversion was the Kock pouch [56]. The reservoir is made from 40cm ileum reconfigured to reduce the intrinsic pressure. The continence mechanism is formed by intussusception of 12cm of ileum. In a complete form it requires 72cm of ileum which may be more than can be spared from the gastrointestinal tract. The stability of the nipple depends on three or four rows of staples, and fixation of the nipple to the wall of the reservoir [57]. To make it reliably continent, it is essential to pay attention to every detail. (Grade C)

It is the most commonly used continence system in adults by virtue of the large numbers reported by Skinner [58]. In Skinner's first 245 patients the continence rate was 77%; in the most recent 85 (of a total of 546) it was 89%. Although this improvement is encouraging, the high rate of leakage does illustrate the difficulty of making the Kock nipple work. For surgeons with a smaller practice, it may never be possible to achieve a complication rate as low as this. Although first described as a mechanism for a continent ileostomy in children the Kock Pouch is now not commonly used in children because of the problem with large amount of bowel needed, stone formation and mediocre success with dryness of the catheterizable stoma. (Grade D)

d) Artificial sphincter

As a last resort, the AUS may be considered to give continence to a reconstructed outlet. The cuff of an artificial sphincter is designed to encircle a normal urethra or bladder neck. Experimental evidence suggests that AUS cuffs can be placed safely around intestine providing the cuff pressure is low [59]. The AUS has been used successfully around large bowel, in three of four children with follow-up to 11 years [60] (Level 4)

e) Cutaneous stoma site

For most patients, the site of the cutaneous stoma should be chosen by cosmetic criteria. The umbilicus can be made into a very discrete stoma; the risk of stenosis is low and it is a readily identifiable landmark. Otherwise, the stoma should be as low on the abdominal wall as possible and certainly below the top of the underpants. However, many surgeons find the best results by placing the catheterizable stoma in the umbilicus. (Grade C)

In patients with spina bifida, particularly non-walkers, the site must be chosen with particular care. The natural tendency is for the spine to collapse with time so that the lower half of the abdomen becomes more pendulous and beyond the range of vision. A low site may seem appropriate in the child, but will become unusable in the adult. It is best to use a high, midline site, preferably hidden in the umbilicus. (Grade C)

The problem of stomal stenosis remains ever present. It can occur at any time so that only follow up of many years could determine whether any system of anastomosis to the skin is better than any other. The published rate of stomal stenosis is between 10 and 20%. The multi-flap V.Q.Z. stoma is claimed to have the lowest rate but follow up is short and it may well not pass the test of time [61].

VI. COMPLICATIONS OF CONTINENCE SURGERY IN CHILDREN (Table 3)

1. Storage and empting complications

In the short term, it has been shown that the continent diversions can store urine and can be emptied by clean intermittent catheterization (CIC). It is apparent that there is a constant need for review and surgical revision. This observation mirrors the late complications of augmentation cystoplasty for neuropathic bladder where the median time to revision surgery is as long as ten years [62]. (Level 4)

In general, once continent, they remain continent, although there are occasional reports of late development of incontinence. The problem lies more in difficulties with catheterization, particularly stenoses and false passages which may occur in up to 34% of patients [41] (Level 4)

The principal complications arise because the reservoir is usually made from intestine. Ideally, urothelium

Table 3 : Complications

AUTHOR	Bogaert, Kogan 1994	Ganesan, Mitchell 1992 AUA	Woodard	Atala 1990	Adams 1998
Complications	Bowel obstruction pouch fistula hematuria-dysuria hypochloremic alkalosis	Hematuria-dysuria 22% bowel obstruction bladder perforation hypochloremic alkalosis	Bowel obstruction hypochloremic Alkalosis Pouch fistula Abscess Pyelonephritis Fungyl sepsis Angulated outlet	Peptic cystitis Bleeding Bladder perforation Metabolic alkalosis	Hypochloremic Alkalosis Uretero-vesical Obstruction
AUTHOR	**Gosalbez**	**Ngan**	**Gosalbez**	**Ganesan**	
Complications	Ureterogastric stricture Abdomin. fluid collection Gastric hemorrhage Hypochloremic alkalosis	Ureteral stricture Gastrourethral stricture Renal stone	Stomal stenosis Traumatic performation Skin irritation Abscess Paracolic fluid collection	Ureterovesical stenosis Hematuria-dysuria Bladder perforation bowel obstruction	**Other complications described :** Peptic ulcer with subsequent perforation especially in the defunctionalized bladder

should be used. Although several ingenious systems have been devised that use urothelium. Detrusorectomy and preservation of the bladder epithelium gives fewer complications than enterocystoplasty [63] (Level 4)

Combinations of detrusorectomy and augmentation with demucosalized colon have given promising results in the short term. The surgery is difficult as the bladder epithelium must not be damaged and the intestinal mucosa must be cleared completely. When achieved there are no metabolic problems and many patients can void [64]. (Level 4)

When augmentation can be done with a dilated ureter, the results are good and the complication rate low even in children with compromised renal function or transplantation [65, 66]. (Level 4)

All intestinal reservoirs produce mucus. The amount is difficult to measure and most estimates are subjective. No regime has been shown to dependably reduce mucus production [67] (Level 4)

2. Reservoir rupture

The incidence of spontaneous rupture varies between different units. There may be delay in diagnosis although the history of sudden abdominal pain and diminished or absent urine drainage should make it obvious. The patient rapidly becomes very ill with symptoms of generalized peritonitis. 'Pouchogram' may not be sensitive enough to demonstrate a leak. Diagnosis is best made by history, physical examination, ultrasonography and CT cystogram. If diagnosed early, catheterization and broad spectrum antibiotics may sometimes lead to recovery. If the patient fails to respond within 12 hours on this regime or if the patient is ill, laparotomy should be performed at once. If there is any instability of the patient laparotomy should be considered as an immediate necessity as bladder rupture in this clinical situation can be lethal. (Grade A)

Figures are not available on the incidence of this complication in reservoirs made only of bowel but come from patients with intestinal segments in the urinary tract. Most papers report small numbers and the pool from which the population is drawn is uncertain. In a multicenter review from Scandinavia 'about' 1720 reconstructed patients were identified with a mean follow up of 53 months. The diagnoses were not given. There were 19 perforations in 17 patients giving an incidence of 1.5%. There were eight patients with neurogenic bladder which was said to be disproportionately high [68]. In a series of 264 children with any sort of bowel reservoir or enterocystoplasty 23 perforations occurred in 18 patients with one death [69]. Therefore, as this complication is more common in children it becomes a very important consideration. (Grade C)

Patients and their families should be warned of this possible complication and advised to return to hospital at once for any symptoms of acute abdomen, especially if the reservoir stops draining its usual volume of urine. All young patients with urinary reconstructions including intestinocystoplasty should carry suitable information to warn attending physicians of their urinary diversion in case of emergency. (Grade A)

3. METABOLIC COMPLICATIONS

Metabolic changes are common when urine is stored in intestinal reservoirs and must be carefully monitored. It is uncertain whether they are commoner in children or whether they just live longer and are more closely monitored. The near 60% serious complication rate in one series seems higher than most centers would recognize [70].

Nurse has made an experimental study of the handling of electrolytes instilled into intestinal reservoirs and subsequent arterial blood gas analysis. All patients were found to absorb sodium and potassium from the reservoirs but the extent was variable. A third of all patients (but 50% of those with an ileocecal reservoir) had hyperchloremia. All patients had abnormal blood gases, the majority having metabolic acidosis with respiratory compensation. The findings were unrelated to renal function or the time since the reservoir was constructed [71] (Level 3)

In 183 patients of all ages at St Peter's Hospitals who had any form of enterocystoplasty, hyperchloremic acidosis (HCA) was found in 25 (14%) and borderline HCA in 40 (22%). The incidence was lower in reservoirs with ileum as the only bowel segment compared to those containing some colon (9% v 16%). When arterial blood gases were measured in 29 of these children a consistent pattern was not found [72] (Level 4)

There are conflicting reports on the incidence of metabolic abnormalities from other units, though often with a smaller number of cases. For example, in a very careful study of 13 patients with colonic reservoirs, Koch et al did not find significant acid base changes compared to control patients with normal bladders [73]. In a series of 23 patients Ditonno et al found that 52% of patients with a reservoir of right colon had HCA.(74) In ileal reservoirs Poulsen et al found mild acidosis but no patients with bicarbonate results outside the reference range [75] (Level 4).

Many authors do not distinguish between patients with normal and abnormal renal function. All of 12 patients in one series with a pre-operative serum creatinine above 2.0mg% developed HCA within 6 months of enterocystoplasty [76]. It is prudent to monitor patients for metabolic abnormalities, especially HCA, and to treat them when found. (Level 4)

With increasing experience, it has become clear that there is a risk of developing vitamin B12 deficiency, sometimes after many years of follow up. It is likely that resection of ileum in children leads to an incomplete absorption defect. Stores of B12 may last for several years before the serum level becomes abnormal. At a mean follow up of six years, low levels of B12 have been found in 14% of children. There was a corresponding rise in the serum methyl malonic acid which is a metabolite that accumulates in B12 deficiency suggesting that the finding was clinically significant. Similarly, in adults, 18.7% have B12 deficiency at five years. In the adults the mean B12 level was significantly lower when the ileocecal segment as opposed to ileum alone had been used (413 ng/ml compared to 257 ng/ml) [77,78]. In order to avoid the serious neurological complications, regular monitoring of B12 levels is essential. (Grade B)

The stomach has had a checkered career as a urinary reservoir. Its non-absorptive role in the gastro intestinal tract has made it particularly useful in reconstruction of children with inadequate intestine, such as those with cloacal exstrophy. There is little effect on gastro intestinal function. Metabolically, the acid production leading to hypochloremic alkalosis may be positively beneficial in children with renal failure. It produces no mucus and the acidic urine is less easily infected and seldom grows stones. However bout a third of children have had serious long term complications, often multiple. The quite severe dysuria/hematuria and the skin complications from the acid urine, particularly, have limited its use [79,80] (Kurzrock et al, 1998; Mingin et al, 1999). (Grade C)

4. EFFECTS ON THE GASTROINTESTINAL TRACT

Little attention has been paid to the effects on gastro intestinal motility of removing segments of ileum or cecum for urinary reconstruction in children. When investigated in adults, disturbance of intestinal function has been found to be more frequent and more debilitating than might be expected. In a meticulous retrospective review of 71 patients with ileal conduits and 82 patients with reconstructions using ileum or the ileocecal segments, comparison was made between the bowel function that the patients remembered from the pre operative time (at least 30 months before) and their current status. In those with ileal conduits 17.5% had new symptoms persisting beyond the first year postoperatively but with minimal impact on quality of life. (Level 4)

The 28 patients having a clam cystoplasty for idiopathic detrusor overactivity fared the worst with 54% having new disturbance of bowel motility and function postoperatively. The negative effect on all aspects of quality of life was most marked in this group. (Level 4)

New symptoms were found in 26% of patients having a clam for neuropathic disease and in 14% of those having a reconstruction for non-neuropathic disease (mainly cancer and interstitial cystitis). The effect on quality of life was less marked in this group.

Disturbance of bowel habit does not mean diarrhea alone. It also includes urgency, leakage and nocturnal bowel actions. Although the study relies on the patients memory of bowel function in the pre operative period, it is clear that quality of life may be seriously undermined by changes in bowel habit [81] (Level 4)

It is known that the bowel has a considerable ability to adapt, especially in young animals, when parts are removed. Nonetheless, reconstruction should be undertaken with the smallest length of bowel possible. Particular care should be taken in children with neurologic abnormality in whom rectal control is already poor. Poorly controlled fecal incontinence may occur in a third of patients [82] (Level 4)

5. Renal function

In the follow-up so far available, undiversion or continent diversion seem not to have affected renal function. When function has improved after such surgery it is likely to be the result of eliminating obstruction or high bladder storage pressure.

In rats with 5/6ths nephrectomy the rate of progression of renal failure is no worse in those with ileocystoplasty compared to those with normal bladder [83]. This suggests, experimentally, that storage of urine in small intestine is not, on its own, harmful to renal function. (Level 5)

Clinically, in the longer term, the renal deterioration that has been found has been related to obstruction, reflux and stone formation. In one long-term study of Kock pouch patients, these complications occurred at the same rate as that found in patients with ileal conduits: 29% at five to 11 years [84]. Similarly, in a prospective follow up to a minimum of 10 years, it was found that the deterioration in glomerular filtration rate (GFR) that was found in 10 of 53 patients was due to a 'surgical' cause in all but one [85] (Level 2)

Although a complicated procedure, a renal transplant can be anastomosed to an intestinal reservoir with similar long term results as those using an ileal conduit. [86,87]. (Level 4)

6. Infection and stones

The incidence of reservoir stones is variously reported. In most series it lies between 12 and 25%, but the length of follow up is not always given. In an American series, the incidence was an extraordinary 52.5% at four years [88]. Renal stones are uncommon, occurring in about 1.6% of patients, an incidence which would be expected in a group with congenital urinary tract anomalies. (Level 4)

Stones are a particular problem in the Kock pouch where the nipple is fixed with metal staples. In Skinner's large series of adults the incidence was 17%. In those who had formed a stone, the recurrence rate was 22%. In a series comparing the Kock pouch with the Indiana (which does not have staples), 43.1% of 72 Kock reservoirs formed stones compared to 12.9% of 54 Indiana reservoirs. Furthermore, no patient with an Indiana formed a stone after 4 years, but patients with Kock pouches continued to do so at a steady rate up to eight years [89] (Level 4)

Apart from the presence of a foreign body, several factors have been blamed for the high stone risk. Almost all reservoir stones are triple phosphate on analysis, though Terai et al found carbonate apatite, urate and calcium oxalate in up to 50% of stones from patients with an Indiana pouch [90]. This suggests that infection is a key factor. Infection acts to form stones by rendering the urine alkaline. Thus organisms that produce urease and so split urea to form ammonia are the main culprits. The incidence of infection in reservoirs is high, 95% in one series [91] and yet the majority of patients do not form stones, suggesting that there are predisposing factors other than infection and the anatomical abnormality of the urine reservoirs. (Level 4)

It has been suggested that the immobility associated with spina bifida may be responsible, but this seems to have been in series with a predominance of such patients and was not confirmed in other studies [92].

The production of excess mucus has also been blamed. The problem is that the measurement of mucus is difficult. The production of excess mucus is, therefore, based on the patients statement and the doctors observation, neither of which are likely to be accurate. The finding of a spectrum of stone formation from mucus, through calcification to frank stone lends some support to this etiology. However, it could be a secondary event, with mucus becoming adherent to a stone that has already formed. Many surgeons encourage patients to wash out their reservoirs vigorously with water two or three times a week. It is difficult to monitor whether patients actually comply with this instruction, but there seem to be fewer stones in those that claim to practice regular washing. It is, of course, possible that washing only serves to clear 'dust' before a proper stone can be formed. In a prospective study a regime of weekly washouts did not improve the incidence of stones in 30 children compared to historical controls [93] (Level 4)

An interesting comparison has been made between children with a native bladder alone and those with an augmentation all of whom were emptying by self catheterization. There was no significant difference in the incidence of stones with or without an augmentation [94]. It was also found that catheterization through a urethra or a Mitrofanoff made no difference to either group. This would suggest that mucus was not a contributory factor though the authors are more circumspect, saying only that augmentation makes no difference to the risk of stone formation. (Level 4)

Stones are associated with inadequate drainage in the sense that CIC through the urethra, the most dependent possible drainage, has the lowest stone rate. Patients with the most 'up hill' drainage, that is with a Mitrofanoff entering the upper part of an orthotopic reservoir almost always form stones. Kronner et al made the observation, that the incidence of stones was statistically associated with abdominal wall stomas and a bladder outlet tightening procedure (21.1% compared to 6% in patients with augmentation alone) [91] (Level 4)

The universal acceptance that the stones are predominantly struvite would make a controlled trial of prophylactic antibiotics attractive. Unfortunately, clinical practice suggests that low dose antibiotics on their own do not reliably prevent symptomatic infections, though the incidence of stones might be reduced.

7. Growth

The suggestion that enterocystoplasty delayed growth in height seems to have been ill founded. In a group of 60 children reported in 1992 it was stated that 20% had delayed growth [95]. Current follow up of the same group has shown that all have caught up and achieved their final predicted height. Furthermore, measurements in a group of 123 children from the same unit have shown no significant delay in linear growth.(96) (Level 4)

Enterocystoplasty may have an effect on bone metabolism even if growth is not impaired. At least in rats with enterocystoplasty there is significant loss of bone mineral density especially in the cortical compartment where there is endosteal resorption. These changes are not associated with HCA and are lessened by continuous antibiotic administration [97,98].

8. Pregnancy

When reconstructing girls it is essential to have a future pregnancy in mind. The reservoir and pedicles should be fixed on one side to allow enlargement of the uterus on the other. (Grade D)

Pregnancy may be complicated and requires the joint care of obstetrician and urologist.(99) Particular problems include upper tract obstruction and changes in continence as the uterus enlarges.

Pregnancy with an orthotopic reconstruction appears to have a good outcome but chronic urinary infection is almost inevitable and occasionally an indwelling catheter is needed in the third trimester [100]. With a supra pubic diversion catheter drainage for incontinence or retention are usually needed in the third trimester [101]. Grade C

Except in patients with an artificial urethral sphincter, vaginal delivery is usual and caesarean section should generally be reserved for purely obstetric indications. The urologist should be present during Caesarean section to ensure protection for the reservoir and its pedicles.

9. Cancer

The possibility of cancer occurring as a complication of enterocystoplasty is a constant source of worry. It is known to be a frequent complication of ureterosigmoidostomy after 20 to 30 years of follow up. Experimental work suggests that there may be a risk in reservoirs with feces excluded [102]. Animal evidence suggests that fecal and urinary streams must be mixed in bowel for neoplasia to occur. However, if it is chronic mixed bacterial infection, rather than the feces per se, that is responsible, then all bowel urinary reservoirs may be at risk.

In patients with colonic and ileal cystoplasties high levels of nitrosamines have been found in the urine of most patients examined [103]. Clinically significant levels probably only occur in chronically infected reservoirs [104]. Biopsies of the ileal and colonic segments showed changes similar to those that have been found in ileal and colonic conduits and in ureterosigmoidostomies. More severe histological changes and higher levels of nitrosamines correlated with heavy mixed bacterial growth on urine culture [105] (Level 4)

In a review of the literature 14 cases of pouch neoplasm were identified [106]. Special features could be found in nearly all the cases. Ten patients had been reconstructed for tuberculosis; four tumors were not adenocarcinomas; one patient had a pre-existing carcinoma; six patients were over 50 years old. Cancer was found in bowel reservoirs at a mean of 18 years from formation. This is a few years earlier than the mean time at which malignant neoplasms are seen in ureterosigmoidostomies. Although the incidence of neoplasia is unknown, the risk in children cannot be ignored. (Grade D)

If cancer is going to be a common problem, there will be some difficulty in monitoring the patients at risk. Endoscopy with a small instrument through a stoma may not be sufficient. Ultra sound may not be able to distinguish between tumors and folds of mucosa. Three dimensional reconstruction of computerized tomography may be helpful, though the equipment is expensive and not widely available at present. Imaging takes about 45 minutes and the reconstruction about four to five hours [107].

10. Psychological consequences and quality of life

It would seem logical that continent urinary diversion would be better than a bag. This is not always the case. In adults the only sure advantage is cosmetic. Quality of life (QOL) surveys in children have not been done, primarily because of the lack of suitable instruments [108]. Our prejudice is that reconstruction does, indeed, improve the lives of children. Supporting evidence is very thin and based on experience in adults.

The main justification for performing a bladder reconstruction or continent diversion is to improve the individual's QOL. The ileal conduit has been a standard part of urological surgery for nearly 50 years, with hardly a change in surgical technique. It has well known complications but few would seriously suggest that they were more troublesome than those of the complex operations for bladder replacement. In an early investigation into quality of life issues, Boyd et al investigated 200 patients, half with an ileal conduit and half with a Kock pouch. It was shown that there was little difference between the groups except that those with a Kock pouch engaged in more physical and sexual contact. The only patients that were consistently 'happier' were those who had had a conduit and subsequently were converted to a Kock pouch [109]. (Level 4)

This observation is mirrored in every day practice. Many patients who have had life long cutaneous diversions ask for conversion to a continent diversion or bladder reconstruction. Few patients who, having apparently had a successful reconstruction, have been unhappy and requested a change back to an ileal conduit!

It is interesting to note that, in a recent QOL survey in adults, a wide range of complications were considered to be acceptable, although an ordinary urological clinic would be full of patients trying to get rid of such symptoms: mild incontinence (50%), nocturia (37%), bladder stones (12%), urinary infections (9%), hydronephrosis (5%). Nonetheless, their QOL was judged to good, primarily because 70% had experienced no adverse effect on their normal daily lives [110] (Level 4)

Quality of life does not mean absence of disease or a level of complications acceptable to the reviewing clinician. It is a difficult concept to measure because lack of validated instruments, difficulties in translating from one culture or language to another of the difficulties in selecting control groups and variations in clinical situations. Gerharz et al have constructed their own 102 item instrument and compared 61 patients with a continent diversion and 131 with an ileal conduit. The authors went to great lengths to validate the instrument and to remove bias in selection of patients. Patients with a continent diversion did better in all stoma related items indicating that containment of urine within the body and voluntary emptying is of major importance. In addition they had better physical strength, mental capacity, social competence and used their leisure time more actively. There was little difference in satisfaction with professional life, financial circumstances and in all interactions within the family including sexual activity [111] (Level 4)

V. CONSENSUS STATEMENT ON SURGICAL TREATMENT OF URINARY INCONTINENCE IN CHILDREN

Forms of urinary incontinence in children are widely diverse, however, a detailed history and physical and voiding diary obviate the need for further studies. These should identify that limited group that may require surgery. Many patients in this group will have obvious severe congenital abnormalities (Level 1).

Because of the spectrum of problems the specific treatment is usually dictated by the expertise and training of the treating physician. The rarity of many of these problems precludes the likelihood of any surgeon having expertise in all areas (resulting in recommendation Grades of C and D). Furthermore, nuances in surgical procedures develop gradually and often are tested without rigorous statistics (Level 4,5).

Nevertheless it may be that newer forms of very early aggressive surgical approach to severe complex anomalies such as exstrophy, myelodysplasia, and valves may provide a successful model for significant impact on the ultimate continence in such patients. Ultimately this may provide a basis for randomized studies to determine the most specific and effective mode of therapy.
The committee would encourage vigorous research in the molecular basis of bladder development and also support the development of surgical and treatment strategies which would utilize the natural ability of the bladder to transform in the early months of development and immediately after birth. Furthermore efforts to promote bladder healing, protecting and achieving normal bladder function should be supported. Such studies and research may lead to early and aggressive treatment of many of the complex anomalies now treated by the surgical procedures outlined in this report.

REFERENCES

I. INTRODUCTION SUMMARY OF CLINICAL PROBLEM

1. Ngan J, Carr M, Ansell J, Mitchell M: Factors contributing to urinary continence in classic exstrophy. J Urol 155:483A, 1996.
2. Stein R, Stockle M, Fisch M, Nakai H, Muller SC, Hohenfellner R: The fate of the adult exstrophy patient. J Urol 152:1413-1416, 1994.
3. Ben-Chaim J, Docimo SG, Jeffs RD, Gearhart JP: Bladder exstrophy from childhood into adult life. J R Soc Med 89:39P-46P, 1996.
4. Canning DA: Bladder exstrophy: The case for primary bladder reconstruction. Urology, 48:831-834, 1996.
5. Hollowell JG, Hill PD., Duffy PG, Ransley PG: Evaluation and treatment of incontinence after bladder neck reconstruction in exstrophy and epispadias. Br J Urol, 71:743-749, 1993.
6. Mollard P, Mouriquand PDE, Buttin,X : Urinary continence after reconstruction of classical bladder exstrophy (73 cases). Br J Urol 73:298-302, 1994.
7. Hohenfellner R, Stein R: Primary urinary diversion in patients with bladder exstrophy. Urology 48:828-830, 1996.
8. Sheldon CA, Gilbert A, Lewis AG, Aiken J, Ziegler MM: Surgical implications of genitourinary tract anomalies in patients with imperforate anus. J. Urol 152:196-199, 1994.
9. Boemers TML., Bax KMA, Rovekamp MH, Van Gool JD: The effect of posterior sagittal anorectoplasty and its variants on lower urinary tract function in children with anorectal malformations. J Urol 153:1919-1930, 1995.
10. Boemers TML, Van Gool JD, de Jong TPVM, Bax KMA: Urodynamic evaluation of children with caudal regression syndrome (caudal dysplasia sequence). J Urol, 151:1038-1042, 1994.
11. Sheldon C, Cormier, M, Crone K, Wacksman J: Occult neurovesical dysfunction in children with imperforate anus and its variants. J Pediatr Surg, 22:26:49-54, 1991.
12. Kim YH, Horowitz M, Combs AJ, Nitti vw, Borer J, Glassberg KI: Management of posterior urethral valves on the basis of urodynamic findings. J Urol 158:1011-1016, 1997.
13. Gearhart JP, Peppas DS, Jeffs RD: Complete genitourinary reconstruction in female epispadias. J Urol 149:1110-1113, 1993.
14. Ben-Chaim J, Peppas DS, Jeffs RD, Gearhart JP: Complete male epispadias: Genital reconstruction and achieving continence. J Urol 153:1665-1667, 1995.
15. Ahmed S, Morris LL, Byard RW: Ectopic ureter with complete ureteric duplication in the female child. J Pediatr Surg 27:1455-1460, 1992.
16. Psihramis KE, Colodny AH, Lebowitz RL, Retik AB, Bauer S: Complete duplication of the urethra. J Urol 139:63-67, 1986.

II. EVALUATION AND DIAGNOSIS DIAGNOSIS

1. Bloom DA, Faerber G, Bomalaski MD: Urinary incontinence in girls. Urol Clin North Am 22:521-538, 1995.
2. Bloom DA, Seeley WW, Ritchey ML, McGuire EJ: Toilet habits and continence in children: An opportunity sampling in search of normal parameters. J Urol 149:1087-1090, 1993.
3. Bloom DA, Pohl J, Norgaard JP: Comments on enuresis, particularly the nocturnal type. Scand J Urol Nephrol Suppl 163:7-13, 1994. Proceedings of First International Workshop. Editors: Norgaard, JP, Hjalmas, K, Djurhuus, JC, Jorgensen, TM.

IV. BLADDER/RESERVOIR CONSTRUCTION

1. Dawaba MS, Dawood A, Ghoneim MA: World J. Urol 14:73-77, 1996.
2. Fisch M, Wammack R, Hohenfellner R: The Sigma Rectum Pouch (Mainz pouch II). World J Urol 14:68-72, 1996.
3. Leong CH, Ong GB: Gastrocystoplasty in dogs. Aust NZ J Surg 41:272-279, 1972.
4. Nguyen D.H., Mitchell M.E.: Gastric bladder reconstruction. Urol clin North Am 18:649-657, 1991.
5. Kock NG, Nilson AE, Nilsson LO, Norlen LJ, Philipson BM: Urinary diversion via a continent ileal reservoir: Clinical results in 12 patients. J Urol 128:469, 1982.
6. Rowland RG, Mitchell ME, Bihrle R: The cecoileal continent urinary reservoir. World J Urol 3;185-190, 1985.
7. Thuroff JW, Alken P, Engelmann U, Riedmiller H, Jacobi GH, Hohenfellner R: The MAINZ pouch (mixed augmentation ileum and zoecum) for bladder augmentation and continent urinary diversion. Eur Urol 11:152-160, 1985.
8. Winter CC, Goodwin WE: Results of sigmoidocystoplasty. J Urol 80:467, 1958.
9. Goodwin WE, Turner RD, Winter CC: Results of ileocystoplasty. J Urol 8-:461, 1958.
10. Rowland RG: Complications of continent cutaneous reservoirs and neobladders – series using contemporary techniques. AUA Update Series, Vol XIV:25, 1995.
11. McDougal WS: Complications of urinary intestinal diversion. AUA Update Series Vol XI:37, 1992.
12. Duel BP, Ggonzales R, Barthold JS: Aalternative techniques for augmentation cystoplasty. J Urol 159:998-1005, 1998.
13. Kennely MJ, Gormley MA , McGuire EJ: Early clinical experience with adult auto-augmentation. J Urol 152:303-306, 1994.
14. Stoher M, Kramer A, Goepel M, Lochner, Ernst D, Kruse D, Rubben H: Bladder auto-augmentation – An alternative for enterocystoplasty: preliminary results. Urodyn 14(1) 11-23, 1995.
15. Usui A, Inoue K, Nakamoto T, Kadena H, Usui T: Usefulness of bladder auto-augmentation in neurogenic bladder: A case report. Nippon Nihyokika Gakkai Zasshi 87:802-805, 1996.
16. McDougall EM, Clayman RV, Figenshau RS, Pearl MS: Laparoscopic retropubic augmentation of the bladder. J Urol 153:123-126, 1995.
17. Poppas DP, Uzzo RG, Britanisky RG, Mininberg DT: Laparoscopic laser assisted auto-augmentation of the pediatric neurogenic bladder: Early experience with urodynamic follow-up. J Urol 155:1057-10601, 1996.
18. Gonzales R: Laparoscopic laser assisted auto-augmentation of the pediatric neurogenic bladder: Early experience with urodynamic follow-up. J Urol 156:1783, 1996.
19. Koontz WW, Jr, Prout GR, Jr., Mackler MA: Bladder regeneration following serosal colocystoplasty. Invest Urol 8(2):170-176, 1970.
20. DeBadiola F, Manivel JC, Gonzalez R: Seromuscular enterocystoplasty in rats. J Urol 146:559-562, 1991.
21. Salle JL, Fraga JC, Luvib A, Lampertz M, Jobim G, Putten A: Seromuscular enterocystoplasty in dogs. J Urol 144:454-456, 1990.
22. Dewan PA., Lorenz C, Stefanek W, Byard RW: Urothelial lined colocystoplasty in a sheep model. Eur Urol 26:240-246, 1994.
23. Buson H, Manivel JC, Dayanc M, Long R, Gonzales R: Seromuscular colocystoplasty lined with urothelium: Experimental study. Urology 44:743-748, 1994.

24. Garibay JT, Manivel JS, Gonzales R: Effect of seromuscular colocytoplasty lined with urothelium and partial detrusorectomy on a new canine model of reduced bladder capacity. J Urol 154:903-906, 1996.

25. Denes ED, Vates TS, Freedman AL, Gonzales R: Seromuscular colocystoplasty lined with urothelium protects dogs from acidosis during ammonium chloride loading. J urol 158:1075-1080, 1997.

26. Frey P, Lutz N, Leuba AL: Augmentation cystoplasty using pediicled and de-epithelialized gastric patches in the mini-pig model. J Urol 156:608-613, 1996.

27. Gonzales R, Buson H, Reid C, Reinberg Y: Seromuscular colocystoplasty lined with urothelium: Experience with 16 patients. Urology 45:124-19, 1995.

28. Lima SV, Araujo LA, Vilar FO, Kummer CL, Lima EC: Nosecretory sigmoid cystoplasty: Experimental and clinical results. J Urol 153:1651-1654, 1995.

29. Churchill BM, Aliabadi H, Landau EH, McLorie GA, Steckler RE, McKenna PH, Khoury AE: Ureteral bladder augmentation. J Urol 150:716-720, 1993.

30. Dewan PA, Nicholls EA, Goh DW: Ureterocystoplasty: An extraperitoneal, urothelial bladder autmentation technique. Eur Urol 26:85-89, 1994.

31. Gosalbez R, Jr, Kim CO, Jr: Ureterocystoplasty with preservation of ipsilateral renal function. J Ped Surg 31:970-975, 1996.

32. Ben-Chaim J, Partin AW, Jeffs RD: Ureteral bladder augmentation suign the lower pole ureter of a duplicated system. Urology 47:135-137, 1996.

33. Denes FT, Nahas WC, Borrelli M, Rocha FT, Mitre AI, Gianini PTR, Apexatto M, Arap S: Urererocistoplastia. J Bras Urol 23 (supl Espec):170-T590, 1997.

34. Atala A, Vacanti JP, Peters CA, Mandell J, Retik AB, Freeman MR: Formation of urothelial structures in vivo from dissociated cells attached to biodegradabel polymer scaffolds in vitro. J Urol 148:658-662, 1992.

35. Hutton KA: Trejdosiewicz LK, Thomas DF, Southgate J: Urothelial tissue culture for bladder reconstruction: An experimental study. J Urol 150:721-725,1993.

36. Atala A, Freeman MR, Vacanti JP, Shepard J, Retik AB: Implantation in vivo and retrieval of artificial structures consistingof rabbit and human urothelium and human bladder muscle. J Urol 150:608-612, 1993.

37. Hakim,S, Merguerian PA, Chavez D: Use of biodegradable mesh as a transport for a cultured uroepithelial graft: An improved method using collagen gel. Urology 44:139-142, 1994.

38. Scriven SD, Booth C, Thomas DF, Trejdosiewicz LK, Southgate J: Reconstruction of human urothelium from monloayers culture. J Urol 158:1147-1152, 1997.

V. BLADDER OUTLET SURGERY

1. Malizia AA, Jr., Reiman HM, Myers RP, Sande JR, Bahrman SS, Benson RC, Jr, Dewanjee MK, Utz WJ: Migration and granulomatous reaction after periurethral injection of polytef (Teflon). JAMA 251:3277-81, 1984.

2. Bomalski MD, Bloom DA, McGuire EJ, Panzi A: Glutaraldhyde cross-linked collagen in the treatment of urinary incontinence in children. J Urol 155:699-702,1996.

3. Chernoff A, Horowitz M, Combs A, Libretti D, Nitti V, Glassberg KL: Periurethral collagen injection for the treatment of urinary incontinence in children. J Urol 157:2303-5,1997.

4. Capozza N, Caione P, DeGennaro M, Nappo S, Patricola M: Endoscopic treatment of vesicoureteral reflux and urinary incontinence. Technical problems in the pediatric patient. Brit J Urol 75:538-42,1995.

5. Sundaram CP, Reinberg Y, Aliabadi HA: Failure to obtain durable results with collagen implantation in children with urinary incontinence. J Urol 157:2306-7,1997.

6. Scott FB, Bradley,WW, Timm GW: Treatment of urinary incontinence by implantable prosthetic sphincter. IV Urology 1:252-259, 1973.

7. Diokno AC, Sonda P: Compatibility of genitourinary prosthesis and intermittent self catheterization. J Urol 125:659-60,1981.

8. Gonzalez R, Nguyen,DH, Koilelat N, Sidi AA: Compatibity of enterocystoplasty and the artificial urinary sphincter. J. Urol 142:502-4, 1989.

9. Strawbridge LR, Kramer SA, Castillo OA, Barrett DM: Augmentation cystoplasty and the artificial genitourinary sphincter. J Urol 142:297-301, 1989.

10. Gonzalez R, Merino FG, Vaughn M: Long term results of the artificial urinary sphincter in male patients with neurogenic bladder. J Urol 154:769-70, 1995.

11. Levesque PE, Bauer SB, Atala A, Zurakowski D, Colodny, A, Peters, C, Retik, AB: Ten year experience with the artificial sphincter in children. J Urol 156:625-8, 1996.

12. Nurse DE, Mundy AR: One hundred artificial sphincters. Br J Urol 61:318-25, 1988.

13. Barrett DM, Parulkar BG, Kramer SA: Experience with AS800 artificial sphincter in pediatric and young adult patients. J Urol 42:431-6, 1993.

14. Singh G, Thomas DG: Artificial urinary sphincter in patients with neurogenic bladder dysfunction. Brit J Urol 77:252-5, 1996.

15. Simeoni J, et al: Artificial urinary sphincter for neurogenic bladder: A multi-institutional study in 107 children. Br J Urol 78:287-93, 1996.

16. Aliabadi H, Gonzalez R: Success of the artificial sphincter after failed surgery for incontinence. J Urol 143:987, 1996.

17. Woodside JR, BordenTA: Pubovaginal sling procedure or the management of urinary incontinence in a myelodysplastic girl. J Urol 78:808-9, 1986.

18. Gormley EA, Bloom DA, McGuire, EJ, Ritchey, M.: Pubovaginal slings for the management of urinary incontinence in female adolescents. J Urol 152:822-5,1994.

19. Kakizaki H, Shibata T, Kobayashi S, Matsumara K, Koyanagi T: Fascial sling for the management of incontinence due to sphincter incompetence. J Urol 153:644-7, 1995.

20. Elder JS: Periurethral and puboprostatic sling repair for incontinence in patients with myelodysplasia. J Urol 144:434-7, 1990.

21. Decter RM: Use of fascial sling for neurogenic incontinece: Lessons learned. J Urol 150:683-6, 1993.

22. Raz S, Ehrlich RM, Zeidman EJ, Alarcon A, McLaughlin S: Surgical treatment of the incontinent female patient with myelomeningocele. J Urol 139:524, 1988.

23. Bauer SB, Peters CA, Colodny AH, Mandell J, Retik AB: The use of rectus fascia to manage urinary incontinence. J Urol 142:516-9, 1989.

24. Perez LM, Smith EA, Broecker BH, Massad CA, Parrott TS, Woodard JR: Outcome of sling cystourethropexy in the pediatric population: A critical review. J Urol 156:642-6, 1996.

25. Young HH: An operation for incontinence associated with epispadias. J. Urol 7:1-32, 1922

26. Dees J: Congenital epispadias with incontinence. J. Urol 62:513-522, 1949.

27. Leadbetter GW: Surgical correction of total urinary incontinence. J. Urol 91:261-266, 1964.

28. Mollard P: Bladder reconstruction in exstrophy. J Urol 124(4) :525-529, 1980

29. Jones JA, Mitchell ME and Rink RC: Improved results using a modification of the Young-Dees-Leadbetter bladder neck repair. Br J Urol 71(5):555-561, 1993.

30. Kropp KA and Angwafo FF: Urethral lengthening and reimplantation for neurogenic incontinence in childrne. J. Urol 135(5):533-536, 1986.

31. Salle JL, et al: Urethral lengthening with anterior bladder wall flap (Pippi Salle procedure): Modifications and extended indications of the technique. J. Urol 158(2):586-590, 1997.

32. Hendren WH: Congenital female epispadias with incontinence. J Urol 125 (4)558-564, 1981.

33. Lepor H and Jeffs RD: Primary bladder closure and bladder neck reconstruction in classical bladder exstrophy. J Urol 123:1142-1145,1983.

34. Tanagho EA and Smith DR: Clinical evaluation of a surgical technique for the correction of complete urinary incontinence. J. Urol 107:402, 1972.

35. Mollard P, Mouriquand PD, et al: Urinary continence after reconstruction of classical bladder exstrophy (73 cases) (see comments). Br J Urol 73 (3):298-302, 1994.

36. Hendren WH: Construction of female urethra from vaginal wall and perineal flap. J Urol 123:657, 1980.

37. Snodgrass W: A simplified Kropp procedure for incontinence. J Urol 158:1049-1052, 1997.

38. Mitrofanoff P: Cystostomie continente trans-appendiculaire dans le traitement de vessies neurologique. Chirugae Paediatrica 1980;621:297-305.

39. Duckett JW, Snyder HM: Continent urinary diversion: variations on the Mitrofanoff principle. J.Urol 1986;136:58-62.

40. Leibovitch I, Avigad I, Nativ O, Goldwasser B: The frequency of histopathological abnormalities in incidental appendectomy in urological patients: the implications for incorporation of the appendix in urinary tract reconstructions. J.Urol 1992;148:41-3.

41. Woodhouse CRJ, MacNeilly AE: The Mitrofanoff principle: Expanding on a versatile theme. Brit J Urology 1994;74:447-53.

42. Yang WH: Yang needle tunnelling technique in creating antireflux and continence mechanisms. J.Urol 1993;150:830-4.

43. Monti PR, Lara RC, Dutra MA, Rezende de Carvalho R: New techniques for construction of efferent conduits based on the Mitrofanoff principle. Urology 1997;49:112-5.

44. Gerharz EW, Tassadaq T, Pickard RS, Shah PJR, Woodhouse CRJ: Transverse retubularised ileum: early clinical experience with a new second line Mitrofanoff tube. J Urol 1998;159:525-8.

45. Malone PR, d'Cruz VT, Worth PHL, Woodhouse CRJ: Why are continent diversions continent? J.Urol 1989;141:303-(A).

46. Riedmiller H, Burger R, Muller SC, Thuroff J, Hohenfellner R: Continent appendix stoma: a modification of the Mainz pouch technique. J.Urol 1990;143:1115-7.

47. Woodhouse CRJ: The Mitrofanoff principle for continent urinary diversion. World J Urol 1996;14:99-104.

48. Duckett JW, Lofti A-H: Appendicovesicostomy (and variations) in bladder reconstruction. J.Urol 1993;149:567-9.

49. Fishwick J, Gough DCS, O'Flynn KJ: The Mitrofanoff: Does it last? Br J Urol International 2000;85:496-7.

50. Studer UE: Editorial: continent urinary diversions. J.Urol 1994;151:341-2.

51. Gilchrist RK, Merricks JW, Hamlin HH, Rieger IT: Construction of substitute bladder and urethra. Surgery, Gynecology and Obstetrics 1950;90:752-60.

52. Harper JGM, Berman MH, Herzberg AD, Lerman F, Brendler H: Observations on the use of cecum as a substitute bladder. J.Urol 1954;71:600-2.

53. Rowland RG, Mitchell ME, Bihrle R, Kahnoski PJ, Piser JE: Indiana continent urinary reservoir. J.Urol 1987;137:1136-9.

54. Rowland RG, Webster G, Goldwasser B, editors: Urinary diversion. 1 ed. Oxford: Isis Medical Media; 1995; 22, Right colon reservoir using plicated tapered ileal outlet. p. 229-35.

55. Thuroff J, Alken P, Reidmiller H, Jakobi GH, Hohenfellner R: 100 cases of Mainz pouch: continuing experience and evolution. J.Urol 1988;140:283-8.

56. Kock NG, Nilson AE, Nilsson LO, Norlen L, Philipson BM: Urinary diversion via a continent ileal reservoir: Clinical results in 12 patients. J.Urol 1982;128:469-75.

57. Robertson GN, King L: Bladder substitution in children. Urol Clin of North Am 1986;13:333-44.

58. Skinner EC, Lieskovsky G, Boyd JD, et al. Hendry WF, editors: Recent advances in urology/andrology. 5 ed. Edinburgh: Churchill Livingstone; 1991; 9, Continent cutaneous diversion and total bladder replacement using the Kock principles. p. 135-48.

59. Engelmann UH, Felderman TP, Scott FB: The use of the AMS AS800 artificial sphincter for continent urinary diversion 1. investigations including pressure flow studies using rabbit intestinal loops. J.Urol 1985;134:-183

60. Light KK: Long term clinical results using the artificial sphincter around bowel. Brit J Urol 1989;64:56-60.

61. Mor Y, Quinn FMJ, Carr B, Mouriquand PD, Duffy PG, Ransley PG: Combined Mitrofanoff and antegrade continence enema procedures for urinary and fecal incontinence. J.Urol 1997;158:192-5.

62. Herschorn S, Hewitt RJ: Patient perspective of long term outcome of augmentation cystoplasty for neurogenic bladder. Urology 1998;52:672-8.

63. Leng WW, Balock HJ, Fredricksson WH, English SF, McGuire EG: Enterocystoplasty or detrusor myomectomy: comparison of indications and outcomes for bladder augmentation. J.Urol 1999;161:758-63.

64. Dayanc M, Kilciler M, Tan O, Gokalp A, Goktas S, Peker AF: A new approach to bladder augmentation in children: seromuscular enterocystoplasty. Br J Urol International 1999;84:103-7.

65. Landau EH, Jayanthi VR, Mclorie GA, Churchill BM, Khoury AE: Renal transplantation in children following augmentation ureterocystoplasty. Urology 1997;50:260-2.

66. Tekgul S, Oge O, Bal K, Erkan I, Bakkaloglu M: Ureterocystoplasty: an alternative reconstructive procedure to enterocystoplasty in suitable cases. Journal of Pediatric Surgery 2000;35:577-9.

67. N'Dow J, Robson CN, Matthews JNS, Neal DE, Pearson JP: Reducing mucus production after urinary reconstruction: prospective randomised trial. J Urol 2001;165:1433-40.

68. Mansson W, Bakke A, Bergman B: Perforation of continent urinary reservoirs. Scand J Urol and Nephrol 1997;31:529-32.

69. Rink RC, Hollensbe DW, Adams MC, Keating MA: Is sigmoid enterocystoplasty at greatest risk for perforation? Observations and etiology in 23 bladder perforations in 264 patients. Scand J Urol and Nephrol 1992;142(Supplement):179.

70. Bertschy C, Bawab F, Liard A, Valioulis I, Mitrofanoff P: Enterocystoplasty complications in children: A study of 30 cases. Eur J of Pediatr Surg 2000;10:30-4.

71. Nurse DE, Mundy AR: Metabolic complications of cystoplasty. Br J Urol 1989;63:165-70.

72. Wagstaff KE, Woodhouse CRJ, Rose GA, Duffy PG, Ransley PG: Blood and urine analysis in patients with intestinal bladders. Br J Urol 1991;68:311-6.

73. Koch MO, McDougal WS, Reddy PK, Lange PH: Metabolic alterations after continent urinary diversion through colonic segments. J.Urol 1991;145:270-3.

74. Ditonno P, Battaglia M, Ricapito V, Saracino GA, Selvaggi FP: Metabolic acidosis and urinary tract infections in ileocolic orthotopic reservoirs with an afferent ileal loop. Scand J Urol and Nephrol 1992;142:134-.

75. Poulsen AL, Thode J, Steven K: Acid base metabolism following urinary diversion with the ileal Kock reservoir. Scand J Urol and Nephrol 1992;142(Supplement):135-6.

76. Mitchell ME, Piser JA: Intestinocystoplasty and total bladder replacement in children and young adults: Follow up in 129 cases. J Urol 1987;138:579-84.

77. Kalloo NB, Jeffs RD, Gearhart JP: Long term nutritional consequences of bowel segment use for lower urinary tract reconstruction in pediatric patients. Urology 1997;50:967-71.

78. Racioppi M, D'Addessi A, Fanasca E: Vitamin B12 and folic acid plasma levels after ileocaecal and ileal neobladder reconstruction. Urology 1997;50:888-92.

79. Kurzrock EA, Baskin LS, Kogan BA: Gastrocystoplasty: Long term follow up. J Urol 1998;160:2182-6.

80. Mingin GC, Stock JA, Hanna MK: Gastrocystoplasty: Long term complications in 22 patients. J Urol 1999;162:1122-5.

81. N'Dow J, Leung HY, Marshall C, Neal DE: Bowel dysfunction after bladder reconstruction. J Urol 1998;159:1470-5.

82. Singh G, Thomas DG: Bowel problems after enterocystoplasty. Br J Urol 1997;79:328-32.

83. Vordemark JS, Irby PB, Shehata BM, Brown RF: The effects of ileocystoplasty on the development of renal failure in a rat model 5/6th nephrectomy. J Urol 1992;148:566-70.

84. Akerlund S, Delin K, Kock NG: Renal function and upper urinary tract configuration following urinary diversion to a continent ileal reservoir (Kock pouch): a prospective 5-11 year follow-up after reservoir construction. J Urol 1989;(142):-1193.

85. Fontaine E, Leaver R, Woodhouse CRJ: The effect of intestinal urinary reservoirs on renal function: a ten year follow up study. Br J Urol International 2000;86:195-8.

86. Crowe A, Cairns HS, Wood S, Rudge CR, Woodhouse CRJ, Neild GH: Renal transplantation following renal failure due to urological disorders. Nephrology, Dialysis and Transplantation 1998;13:2065-9.

87. Riedmiller H, Gerharz EW, Kohl U, Weingartner K: Continent urinary diversion in preparation for renal transplantation: a staged approach. Transplantation 2000;70:1713-7.

88. Palmer LS, Franco I, Kogan S, Reda E, Bhagwant G, Levitt S: Urolithiasis in children following augmentation cystoplasty. J.Urol 1993;150:726-9.

89. Ginsberg D, Huffman JL, Lieskovsky G, Boyd SD, Skinner DG: Urinary tract stones: a complication of the Kock pouch urinary diversion. J.Urol 1991;145:956-9.

90. Terai A, Ueda T, Kakehi Y, Terachi T, Arai Y, Okada Y, Yoshida O: Urinary calculi as a late complication of the Indiana continent urinary diversion: Comparison with the Kock pouch procedure. J.Urol 1996;155:66-8.

91. Kronner KM, Casale AJ, Cain MP, Zerin MJ, Keating MA, Rink RC: Bladder calculi in the pediatric augmented bladder. J.Urol 1998;160:1096-8.

92. Woodhouse CRJ, Lennon GN: Management and etiology of stones in intestinal urinary reservoirs in adolescents. Eur Urol 2001;39:253-9.

93. Brough RJ, O'Flynn KJ, Fishwick J, Gough DCS: Bladder washout and stone formation in paediatric enterocystoplasty. Eur Urol 1998;33:500-2.

94. Barrosso U, Jednak R, Fleming P, Barthold JS, Gonzalez R: Bladder calculi in children who perform clean intermittent catheterisation. Br J Urol International 2000;85:879-84.

95. Wagstaff KE, Woodhouse CRJ, Duffy PG, Ransley PG: Delayed linear growth in children after enterocystoplasty. Br J Urol 1992;69:314-7.

96. Gerharz EW, Woodhouse CRJ, Ransley PG: Growth failure revisited: a second look at the metabolic consequences of enterocystoplasty in childhood. J Urol 2001;165:106-.

97. McDougal WS, Koch MO, Shands C, Price RR: Boney demineralisation following urinary intestinal diversion. J Urol 1988;140:853-5.

98. Gerharz EW, Mosekilde L, Thomsen JS, Gasser J, Ransley PG, Reidmiller H, Woodhouse CRJ: Biomechanical consequences of bone loss following urinary diversion through intestinal segments. J Urol 1999;161:67

99. Hill DE, Kramer SA: Pregnancy after augmentation cystoplasty. J Urol 1989;144:457-9.

100. Creagh TA, McInerney PD, Thomas PJ, Mundy AR: Pregnancy after lower urinary tract reconstruction in women. J Urol 1995;154:1323-4.

101. Hatch TR, Steinberg RW, Davis LE: Successful term delivery by cesarean section in a patient with a continent ileocecal urinary reservoir. J.Urol 1991;146:1111-2.

102. Malone MJ, Izes JK, Hurley LJ: Carcinogenesis. Urologic Clinics of North Am 1997;24:723-8.

103. Groschel J, Riedasch G, Kalble T, Tricker AR: Nitrosamine excretion in patients with continent ileal reservoirs for urinary diversion. J Urol 1992;147:1013-6.

104. Creagh TA, Picramenos D, Smalley ET, Walters CL, Mundy AR: The source of nitrosamines in patients with enterocystoplasties. Br J Urol 1997;79:28-31.

105. Nurse DE, Mundy AR: Assessment of the malignant potential of cystoplasty. Br J Urol 1989;64:489-92.

106. Filmer RB, Bruce JR: Malignancies in bladder augmentations and intestinal conduits. J Urol 1990;143:671-8.

107. Stenzl A, Frank R, Eder R: 3-dimensional computerised tomography and virtual reality endoscopy of the reconstructed lower urinary tract. J.Urol 1998;159:741-6.

108. Eiser C: Need for a distinctive child quality of life measure. Dialogues in Pediatric Urology 1997;20:3-4.

109. Boyd SD, Feinberg SM, Skinner DG: Quality of life survey of urinary diversion patients. J Urol 1987;138:1386-9.

110. Sullivan LD, Chow VDW, Ko DSC, Wright JE, McLoughlin MG: An evaluation of quality of life in patients with continent urinary diversions after cystectomy. Br J Urol 1998;81:699-704.

111. Gerharz EW, Weingartner K, Dopatke T: Quality of life after cystectomy and urinary diversion: results of a retrospective interdisiplinary study. J.Urol 1998;158:778-85.

Committee 11 B

Surgical Treatment of Urinary Incontinence in Men

Chairman

S. HERSCHORN (CANADA)

Members

R.BOSCH (THE NETHERLANDS),

H.BRUSCHINI (BRAZIL),

T. HANUS (CZECH REPUBLIC),

A.LOW (AUSTRALIA),

E. SCHICK (CANADA)

Surgical Treatment of Urinary Incontinence in Men

S. Herschorn,

R.Bosch, H.Bruschini, T. Hanus, A.Low, E. Schick

INTRODUCTION AND SUMMARY

Surgery for male incontinence is an important aspect of treatment with the changing demographics of society and the global increase in surgery for prostate cancer.

Basic evaluation of the patient is similar to other areas of incontinence and includes primarily a clinical approach with history, voiding record, and physical examination. Since most of the surgeries apply to patients with incontinence after other operation or trauma, radiographic imaging of the lower urinary tract, cystoscopy, and urodynamic studies may provide invaluable information for the treating clinician.

Although prostatectomy for benign disease has become less frequent in many countries, the complication of incontinence is a rare but unfortunate occurrence that merits treatment. After a period of conservative therapy has been tried, surgical treatment, with implantation of the artificial urinary sphincter, has cured 75-80% of sufferers. Injection therapy with agents such as collagen has helped 40-50% of men.

Radical prostatectomy for prostate cancer, on the other hand, is performed far more frequently now than 10 years ago. Approximately 5-25% of patients will experience incontinence and of those a good number will require surgical treatment. The artificial sphincter has provided a satisfactory cure in most cases with a positive impact on quality of life. Other therapies such as collagen injections and sling procedures are being evaluated.

Incontinence following radiation therapy, cryosurgery, other pelvic operations and trauma is a particularly challenging problem because of tissue damage outside the lower urinary tract. The artificial sphincter implant is the most widely used surgical procedure but complications may be more likely than in other areas and other surgical approaches may be necessary. Unresolved problems from the pediatric age group and patients with refractory incontinence from overactive bladders may demand a variety of complex reconstructive surgical procedures. Other unique problems encountered are fistulae between the urethra and skin and the prostate and rectum. Surgical reconstructions in experienced hands are usually successful.

With extensive worldwide use of the artificial sphincter in the surgical management of male incontinence, its complications and their management are well known. Durability of the device is an important aspect that impacts on outcome and cost of treatment.

New surgical therapies such as slings are emerging. Although the literature is replete with well done cohort studies, there is a need for prospective randomized clinical trials.

• Materials and Methods

The committee was charged with the responsibility of assessing and reviewing the outcomes of surgical therapy that have been published since the first consultation [1] for non-neurogenic male incontinence. Articles from peer-reviewed journals, abstracts from scientific meetings, and literature searches by hand and electronically formed the basis of this review. The outcomes were analyzed, discussed among the members of the committee and included in the chapter.

In order to rationally discuss surgical therapy the incontinence problems were classified according to their etiology, i.e. either primarily sphincter or bladder related, and are listed in Table 1. Treatment of fistulae is covered separately.

Specific recommendations are made on the basis of published results and determined by the levels of evidence. Consensus of the committee determined the recommendations, which are found at the end of the chapter. New surgical modalities and recommendations for future research are also included.

Table 1 : Classification of surgically correctable problems

Sphincter related

Postoperative
- Post-prostatectomy for prostate cancer
- Post-prostatectomy for benign disease
- TURP and radiation for prostate cancer
- Post-cystectomy and neobladder for bladder cancer

Post-traumatic
- After prostato-membanous urethral reconstruction
- Pelvic floor trauma

Unresolved pediatric urologic incontinence
- Exstrophy and epispadias

Bladder related

Refractory urge incontinence due to detrusor overactivity

Small fibrotic bladder

Fistulae

Prostato-rectal

Urethrocutaneous

I. EVALUATION PRIOR TO SURGICAL THERAPY

Before surgical treatment of the incontinent male is undertaken, the following evaluations should be done. Basic evaluation includes history [2], physical examination (including neuro-urological examination: perineal sensation, anal tone, voluntary contraction and relaxation of the anal sphincter, bulbocavernosus reflex [3]) urinalysis, urine culture, and a frequency-volume chart [4] (indicating daytime and nighttime frequency of micturition, incontinence episodes, functional bladder capacity, 24-hour urinary output, etc.). No clear guidelines can be found in the literature indicating the minimum number of days necessary to furnish reliable data. According to Wyman et al. [5] the 7-day diary can be considered as the gold standard for voiding diaries. The pad test quantifies the severity of incontinence. The 24-hour home test is the pad test of choice for quantification and diagnosis of urinary incontinence because it is the most reproducible [6]. The 1-hour pad test is widely used, mainly because it is more easily done, and better standardized. Post-void residual urine is a good estimation of voiding efficiency [7,8]. Blood testing (BUN, creatinine, glucose) is recommended only if compromised renal function is suspected or if polyuria (in the absence of diuretics) is documented by the frequency-volume chart [9]. These basic investigations should be done in every incontinent male where surgical therapy, especially when eventual implantation of an artificial urinary sphincter is planned.

Further evaluation should be adapted to the particular patient. Cystourethroscopy is useful to verify integrity of the urethral wall (anterior aspect of the distal sphincteric mechanism in post-TURP incontinence [10], erosion by the cuff of the artificial sphincter, voluntary contraction of the pelvic floor, etc.) and the status of the bladder (trabeculation, stone, diverticula, etc).

Imaging techniques includes a plain abdominal X-ray in cases of incontinence following artificial sphincter implantation when, during the original procedure, the hydraulic system has been filled with contrast medium. Figure 1 illustrates the case of a young spina bifida patient in whom an artificial sphincter has been implanted with the cuff around the bladder neck. After more than 10 years, he became suddenly incontinent. Recent KUB compared to previous one clearly demonstrated fluid loss from the system. Cystography may demonstrate open bladder neck when bladder denervation is suspected [11] (e.g.: following abdominoperineal resection of the rectum). Cystourethrography is used to demonstrate fistula, stricture or urethral diverticulum following healing of the urethral wall erosion provoked by the cuff of the artificial urinary sphincter (Fig. 2). Ultrasound is widely used not only to evaluate the upper urinary tract, but also to evaluate post-void residual urine. The sensitivity of 66,7% and specificity of 96,5% when post-void residual is 100 ml or more is certainly adequate for routine clinical use [12]. It seems also to be cost-effective when compared to catheterization [13]. Other modalities (transurethral ultrasound [14], magnetic resonance imaging of the external sphincter, etc.) are still under development.

In the opinion of the Committee no incontinent male patient should be considered for surgical treatment without a thorough urodynamic evaluation to characterize the underlying pathophysiology. In patients with incontinence secondary to radical prostatectomy who developed bladder neck stenosis, the urethral catheter can create obstruction giving false values for Valsalva leak point pressure. Sphincter weakness can be documented by determining the Valsalva [15] or cough [16] abdominal leak point pressure. A recent study suggested that Valsalva leak point pressure is significantly lower than cough leak point pressure [17]. Its reproducibility has been studied almost exclusively in women. Catheter size seems to have a significant influence, but the correlation is extremely high between the test-retest leak point pressures when the same size of catheter is used [18,19]. In males, abdominal leak point pressure should be evaluated via a rectal catheter because a urethral catheter is much more likely to invalidate Valsalva leak point pressure measurements than it does in female [20].

It becomes more and more evident that bladder volume influences Valsalva leak point pressure, i.e. it decreases with bladder filling [21,22,23]. This observation, however, is not unanimous [24]. Unfortunately, no standardi-

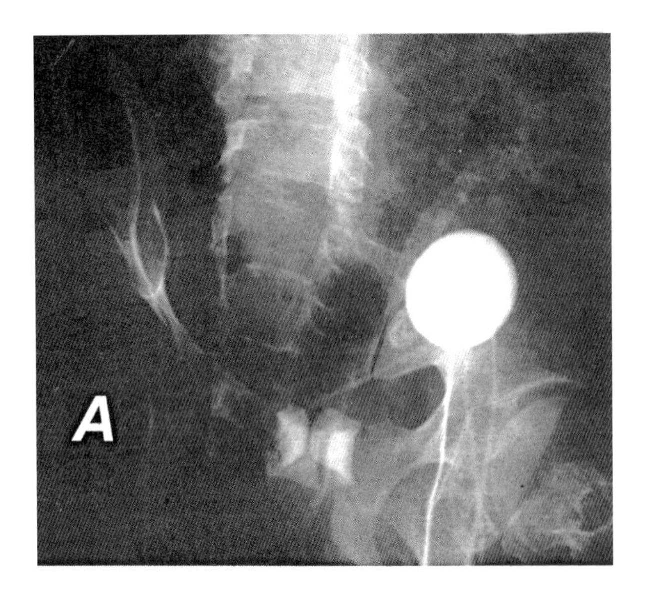

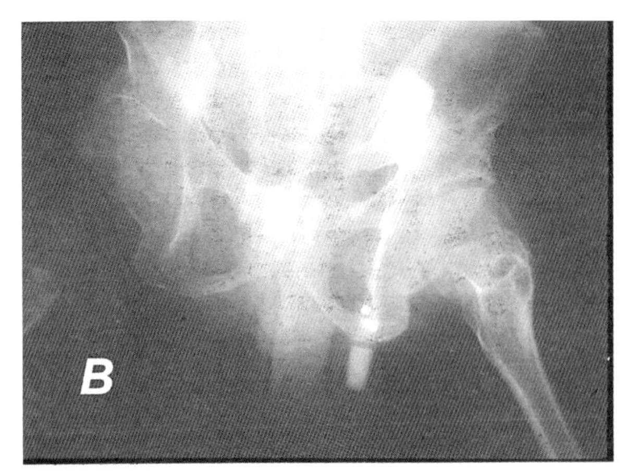

Figure 1 : Young spina bifida patient who had a bladder neck artificial sphincter implanted. After more than 10 years, he became incontinent. Early abdominal plain film, A, shows a full reservoir. After leakage started abdominal plain film, B, demonstrates loss of fluid from the reservoir.

zation of the technique and agreement upon it exists at the present time which somewhat limits its usefulness [25]. Measurement of leak point volume provides information on the functional capacity of the bladder [26]. Retrograde leak point pressure has been used to study incontinence following the placement of an artificial sphincter [27,28]. It correlates with the lowest abdominal leak point pressure [29]. The intraoperative use of this technique has been proposed as it allows early recognition of intraoperative urethral injury and mechanical malfunction [30]. Electrophysiological studies, mainly sphincter electromyography, may be useful to document denervation of the pelvic floor when nerve injury or neurological pathology is suspected [31].

Detrusor function is best evaluated by multichannel urodynamics, which is considered to be the gold standard today. Its main purpose is to detect detrusor overactivity and/or decreased bladder compliance. It can be coupled with fluoroscopic imaging (video-urodynamics). It has also been proposed by some that fluoroscopy be replaced with transrectal ultrasound [32,33]. It has even been suggested that ultrasound measurement of bladder wall thickness is a better predictor of bladder outlet obstruction such as an anastomotic stricture, than uroflowmetry [34]. Furthermore, non-invasive pressure-flow-like urodynamic evaluation based on Doppler ultrasound seems to have some definite potential for diagnosing bladder outlet obstruction [35].

However invasive, pressure-flow studies are still the gold standard in the incontinent male to rule out bladder outlet obstruction accompanied by detrusor overactivity [36], which in turn can cause incontinence.

The proposed evaluation of the incontinent male is summarized in Table 2.

Table 2 : Evaluation prior to surgical therapy

- **History**
- **Physical examination**
- **Urinalysis**
- **Urine culture**
- **Post-void residual (by ultrasound)**
- **Voiding diary (2-7 days)**
  - polyuria without diuretics: BUN, Creatinine, Glucose
- **Pad-test**
- **Cystourethroscopy**
- **Urodynamics :**
  - Valsalva leak-point pressure
  - Retrograde leak-point pressure
  - Multichannel urodynamics

II. INCONTINENCE AFTER RADICAL PROSTATECTOMY FOR PROSTATE CANCER

1. Incidence and risk factors

Urinary incontinence occurring after radical prostatectomy is a significant problem. The reported incidence of post-radical prostatectomy incontinence varies widely [37,38,39,40]. The main factors determining these reported percentages seem to be the definition of incontinence, the methodology used to determine the continence status of the patient, the duration of follow-up and the initial characteristics of the patient population. Whether or not a physiotherapist treated the patients after the operation may also have had an impact on these rates. Most authors reporting their continence rates do not give details on this subject although it seems likely that many men will have followed some program of pelvic floor exercises with or without the physician knowing about it. Incidence rates determined by telephone or face-to-face interview by the physician who treated the patient or his associates are presently considered to be invalid. Self-administered questionnaires or interviews by an independent party are more reliable; additionally, pad-testing can quantify urine loss more objectively. These tests will have to be done on the total population of treated patients to avoid selection bias.

The duration of follow-up is an important factor. Immediately after removal of the stenting urethral catheter more than 40-50% of the patients have serious difficulties with urinary control [38,39]. However, the percentage of incontinent patients decreases dramatically in the first one to one and a half years of follow-up [41].

Nerve sparing radical prostatectomy associated with a meticulous dissection of the apex of the prostate could theoretically lead to a lower incontinence rate. However, Steiner et al describing the Johns Hopkins experience in 593 patients have not found statistically significant differences in continence rates among patients with or without preservation of the neurovascular bundles [37]. Wei et al. recently reported improved continence rates in patients whose nerves were spared bilaterally whereas bladder neck preservation was not beneficial [42]. Advancing age was also a negative factor in that study. Other investigators have reported that patients who were more than 70 years old at the time of radical prostatectomy had a smaller chance of regaining continence [38,41]. Hautmann et al found that older patients regained continence less rapidly but eventually achieved continence rates comparable to the younger patients [39].

The major cause of post-radical prostatectomy incontinence is impaired function of the external urethral sphincter, although detrusor overactivity and/or decreased compliance seem to be an additional problem [43,44,45]. Conflicting data have been presented with regard to the percentage of patients with pure sphincteric weakness and detrusor overactivity, with or without decreased compliance, or a combination of these features [43,44,45]. The percentage of patients with post-radical prostatectomy incontinence, with sphincteric weakness as the only cause has varied between 8 and 57% [43,44,45]. The percentage of those with sphincteric weakness, in combination with other causes has varied between 39 and 52% [43,44,45]. All in all, sphincteric weakness is either the only cause or a major contributing cause in more than 80-85% of the patients.

The incidence of incontinence after radical prostatectomy as reported in papers published in 1997 and 1998 was reviewed for the First ICI. Most of these papers were from the USA. The percentage of incontinent patients, that is those wearing pads, varied between 9 and 48 %. In the National Medicare experience in the USA [40] it was found that 31% of patients "wear pads, diapers or a penile clamp" after a radical prostatectomy. European series have reported percentages of patients using incontinence pads after more than one year of follow-up in 18.8% [39] and 14.1% [38] of the men. In a recent paper from the USA, an incidence of 8% was reported [41]. Wei et al. found that "any leakage of urine" was reported by patients who underwent non-nerve sparing or nerve sparing radical prostatectomy in 35.4% and 25.8% respectively, after 24 months of follow-up [42].

2. Timing of surgical intervention

There are no clear data on timing of a surgical intervention for the treatment of post-radical prostatectomy incontinence. It seems that the largest percentage of patients who were incontinent after removal of the catheter regains continence during the first six months of follow-up [38,39,41]. Therefore, a certain period of watchful waiting supplemented with conservative measures, particularly pelvic floor physiotherapy, seems to be a reasonable option. This conservative management may be tried for periods of up to 6-12 months depending on whether there is any progress noted by the patient.

3. Surgical treatment options

a) Artificial sphincter

In the series of Leach et al [43], 54 out of 102 of patients incontinent after radical retropubic prostatectomy (53%) were eventually treated by implantation of the artificial urinary sphincter. In the Rotterdam series, 52% of the patients having to wear pads eventually underwent implantation of an artificial urinary sphincter [38]. Based on these figures one can tentatively postulate that about half of the patients with post-radical prostatectomy incontinence severe enough to necessitate the use of protective pads may be implanted with an artificial sphincter.

An overview of the results of the artificial urinary sphincter was reported previously: after an average of 3 years of follow-up, 75 to 87% are dry or require only one pad a day at most [1].

More recently some additional reports have been published and added (Table 3). Mottet et al. reported on 96 men treated with an AUS for post-radical prostatectomy incontinence in the period between 1995 and 1997 [50]. After a minimum follow-up of 1 year, 80% of the men were either dry or used 1 protective pad at most. The revision rate was 16.5%. Klijn et al. reported on 27 men treated with an AUS because of incontinence after radical prostatectomy [51]. The 5-year "primary adequate function rate" (P-AF) and the "additional procedure assisted adequate function rate" (APA-AF) based on Kaplan-Meier analysis, were 49% and 71% respectively. Although satisfactory continence in combination with a functioning AUS (without having had to exchange the complete AUS) was achieved in more than 70% at the 5-year follow-up mark, only about half of these patients did not need any operative revisions. If those patients who needed a complete exchange of the AUS were taken into account the satisfactory continence rate was more than 80%. Madjar et al. reviewed their experience with 131 AUS implants for post-radical prostatectomy incontinence [52]. Unfortunately, only 54% of the men were available for evaluation. The remaining men had an average follow-up of 7.7 years. Of these, 27% wear no pads and 32% one pad at most for a total of 59% being satisfactorily continent.

Table 3 : Results of the artificial urinary sphincter in post-radical prostatectomy incontinence

Author	No. pts.	years follow-up	0-1 pads/ day
Montague [46]	66	3.2	75%
Perez and Webster [47]	49	3.7	85%
Martins and Boyd [48]	28	2	85%
Fleshner and Herschorn [49]	30	3	87%
Mottet et al. [50]	96	1	86%
Madjar et al. [52]	71/131 followed	7.7	59%

A comparative study of the artificial urinary sphincter and collagen injections in men suffering from post-radical prostatectomy incontinence was reported by Kuznetsov et al. [53]. These authors conducted a retrospective comparative non-randomized study in in 85 men. Of these, 44 were treated with collagen and 41 with the AUS. The response rate to the quality of life and incontinence questionnaires was 93% in the collagen and 88% in the AUS group. 22% of the men in the AUS group were collagen failures. After an average follow-up of 19 months, 19% of the collagen patients versus 75% of the AUS patients used one pad or less. Quality of life based on the Incontinence Impact Questionnaire was better in the AUS patients.

Some patients who receive an AUS after a radical prostatectomy develop local recurrence and are candidates for external beam radiotherapy. Christie et al have demonstrated that irradiation of the device in a water bath with a dose of 400 Gy did not create any damage or malfunction [54]. A patient with an implanted AUS received a dose of 45 Gy without deleterious effects to the AUS.

b) Injectables

Periurethral injections using different substances either retrogradely or antegradely have achieved a variable improvement rate of 10-70% (first ICI) often with repeated injection sessions. Table 4 contains summarized results from different series of post-prostatectomy incontinence.

Recently, Klutke et al. followed 20 men who were antegradely injected with collagen for a mean of 28 months. Only 10% of the men were dry and an additional 35% were improved [69]. Bevan-Thomas reported on their experience with transurethral collagen injection and found that in a favorable group of post-radical prostatectomy incontinence patients who had normal bladder compliance and who had not needed dilatations or incisions of the neo-bladder neck, a continence rate of 21% could be achieved. An additional 28% were improved. These men had needed a mean of 3.8 injections with a mean total volume of 29 mL [70]. Kutznetsov et al. [53] reported a social continence rate of 19% (use of one pad or less per day) in patients treated with transurethral collagen injections. Only 2% were completely dry.

Summary

Based on these results it can be concluded that the AUS still is the preferred treatment option in properly selected men who are incontinent after radical prostatectomy.

III. INCONTINENCE AFTER PROSTATECTOMY FOR BENIGN DISEASE

1. Incidence and risk factors

The prevalence of urinary incontinence after prostatectomy for benign disease has been reviewed and described in the AHCPR Benign Prostatic Hyperplasia Clinical Practice Guidelines [71]. The following percentages for stress incontinence and total incontinence, respectively, were reported:

Open surgery (retropubic or transvesical prostatectomy): 1.9% and 0.5%.

TUIP (transurethral incision of the prostate): 1.8% and 0.1%.

TURP (transurethral resection of the prostate): 2.2% and 1.0%.

These figures were based on studies reported before 1990. Several other series were published after 1990. These series were reviewed for the 1st International Consultation on Incontinence [1]. A clear description of the method of follow-up and assessment of the continence status was indicated in only about one third of these studies. The incidence of incontinence after open surgery, TURP and TUIP was low but probably not as low as in the AHPCR review: The reported percentages ranged between 0 and 8.4%. Since the method of assessment of the continence status and the definition of incontinence is rarely stated it is actually not possible to make a distinction between simple stress incontinence and total incontinence. There is no clear indication that the incidence is affected by patient age or (resected) prostatic volume [1]. One comparative study of TURP and TUVP seems to indicate that the incontinence rate is somewhat higher after TUVP [72].

In summary, the prevalence of urinary incontinence after open surgery, transurethral resection of the prostate and transurethral incision of the prostate is low, but probably not as low as reported in the AHPCR review, which reported rates below 2%. The quality of reporting does not provide a distinction between total and lesser degrees of incontinence.

2. Timing of surgical intervention

There are no clear data on timing of a surgical intervention for the treatment of incontinence. Therefore, guidelines as to timing of the surgery cannot be formulated. A certain period of watchful waiting supplemented with conservative measures, particularly pelvic floor physiotherapy, seems to be a reasonable option. Thus, conservative management may be tried for periods of up to 6-12 months depending on whether there is any progress noted by the patient.

3. Surgical treatment options

a) Artificial sphincter

The literature on this subject was reviewed for the occasion of the 1st International Consultation on Incontinence [1]. Candidates for treatment with the artificial urinary sphincter (AUS) are patients with incontinence due to intrinsic sphincteric deficiency that have normal bladder compliance [73]. Detrusor overactivity is not an absolute contraindication but the response to medical treatment should be assessed before implantation of an AUS. The AUS has been placed around the bulbar urethra via a perineal route, around the bladder neck [74] and around the membranous urethra at the apex of the prostate via a retropubic route [75]. The above mentioned review of the results obtained with the AUS indicated that more than 70% of the men treated with the AUS for this indication are dry or almost dry after a follow-up of more than 2-3 years [1]. Unfortunately, most series on the AUS lump together post-prostatectomy incontinence after treatment for benign and malignant disease [1]. Placement of the AUS cuff around the bladder neck results in a slightly better continence rate than placement around the bulbar urethra [74].

Other surgical alternatives are mainly of historical interest, although bulbar urethral compression seems to be regaining some interest because of the availability of synthetic slings [76].

In summary, the AUS is a successful surgical treatment option for post-prostatectomy incontinence. The available literature seems to indicate that more than 70% of the men treated with the artificial urinary sphincter will be dry or almost dry. The artificial urinary sphincter is the treatment of choice in patients with incontinence after prostatectomy for benign disease, if the incontinence is due to intrinsic sphincteric deficiency and if the compliance of the bladder is normal.

b) Injectable agents

What has been said for the artificial sphincter is true for collagen injection as well: again most series lump together post-prostatectomy incontinence after treatment for benign and malignant disease (Table 4). A recent report on the use of transurethral collagen injections in men with intrinsic sphincter deficiency indicated that out of a total of 322 men only 14 were treated for incontinence after surgery for BPH [70]. There are no reports about the use of other types of injectables in this particular group of patients. The follow-up of patients treated with collagen ranged between 6 and 15 months. Based on the available data, the treatment fails in more than 50% of the patients and seems to lead to significant but short-term improvement in about 40% of the men or less.

In summary, bulking therapy fails in more than 50% of

Table 4 A : Results of transurethral collagen injection therapy for postprostatectomy incontinence

Investigators	No. Patients	Mean Follow-up (mo)	Mean No. Injections	Mean Volume (cc)	% Cured	% Improved	% Failed
Shortliffe et al [55]	14	19-23	1.6	28.4	21	36	43
Herschorn et al [56]	10	6	4.7	51.8	20	50	30
Bevan-Thomas et al [57]	257	28	4.4	36.6	20	39	41
Smith et al [58]	54	29	4	20	-	38	62
Cespedes et al [59]	110	7	4.2	28.4	53	9	38
Aboseif et al [60]	88	10	2.8	31	48	37	15
Martins et al [61]	46	26	2.8	31	24	46	30
Faerber and Richardson [62]	68	38	5	36	10	10	80
Griebling et al [63]	25	13.3	2.6	35.5	0	40	60
Cummings et al [64]	19	10.4	1.8	13.8	21	37	42
Elsergany and Ghoneim [65]	35	17.6	2	10	20	31	48
Tiguert et al [66]	21	12.5	2.9	18.2	5	57	38

Table 4 B : Results of antegrade injection collagen injection therapy for postprostatectomy incontinence

Investigators	No. Patients	Mean Follow-up (mo)	Mean No. Injections	Mean Volume (cc)	% Cured	% Improved	% Failed
Wainstein and Klutke [67]	48	8.5	-	14.5	25	45	30
Appell et al [68]	24	12	1	7.1	37.5	62.5	-
Klutke at al [69]	20	28	1	14.5	10	35	55

the men. Of those who are improved only a minority actually becomes dry with short-term follow-up. Therefore, bulking is of equivocal value in these men.

4. Problem of strictures in the sphincteric region

These should be treated actively if the patient is incontinent or if UTI, obstruction of the upper tracts or chronic retention are involved in the problem. Urethroplasty in combination with an AUS has been described by Mundy [77] with a relatively high chance on cuff erosion. Treatment of the stricture by incision followed by placement of a Wallstent and subsequent implantation of an AUS has been reported as well [78].

5. Summary of outcomes and recommendations

The data that were reviewed for this section were extracted from uncontrolled non-randomized observational studies only. RCT's in these patient groups are virtually non-existent. Based on the available literature on the subject more than 70% of the men treated with the artificial urinary sphincter will be dry or almost dry. Bulking therapy fails in more than 50% of the men. Of those who are improved only a minority seems to become dry with short-term follow-up.

The artificial urinary sphincter is the treatment of choice in appropriately selected cases with incontinence after prostatectomy for benign disease.

IV. INCONTINENCE AFTER EXTERNAL BEAM RADIOTHERAPY AND SURGERY FOR PROSTATE CANCER

The risk of incontinence after external beam radiotherapy for prostate cancer is low at 0-11%. Lawton et al. [79](1) reported a risk of urinary complications of 7.7% in more than 100 patients, proportional to dose. Perez et al. [80] (2) found incontinence in only 5 of 738 patients. Shipley et al. [81] (3) reviewed more than 2500 cases with an incontinence rate of 0.5%. Similar incidences have been reported in more recent series. Madalinska et al.[82] (4) reported an incidence of 6-7%. With three-dimensional conformal radiotherapy, Weil and colleagues [83] (5) reported no incontinence in 168 consecutive patients and Hanlon et al. [84] (6), in a series of 195 men, found that post treatment urinary symproms were no different than a control group without cancer.

Pre-radiotherapy transurethral prostatectomy appears to be a risk factor for incontinence. Jonler et al.[85] (7) reported an incontinence rate of 11% with pretreatment TURP. Green et al. [86] (8) and Lee at al. [87] (9) also reported a higher risk of incontinence with pretreatment TURP with 5.4% and 2% respectively. With conformal radiotherapy, Sandhu et al. [88] (10) reported a 9% incidence of stress incontinence in 110 patients. Very little data exist on treatment of incontinence following radiotherapy alone.

Adjuvant radiotherapy is frequently given after radical prostatectomy and may not increase the rate of incontinence, although little data have been published. Petrovich et al. [89] (11) reported no difference in incontinence in 2 cohorts of patients, one with and one without adjuvant radiation. On the other hand salvage radical prostatectomy following external beam radiotherapy has been generally reported to have a high incidence of urinary incontinence [90,91,92] (12,13,14) possibly because of radiation induced fibrosis of the external sphincter [92] (14).

1. Surgical treatment

Results of surgical treatment of incontinence in this setting are based on retrospective clinical series. The most commonly published treatment modality is the artificial urinary sphincter as therapy for sphincter damage. The series published contain both patients who had and had not received radiotherapy. Collagen injections have also been reported in retrospectively analysed case series.

There is a higher reported revision rate for the artificial sphincter following radiotherapy (Table 3) compared to low risk patients, 38% versus 22% [47,48,93,94,95]. This is due to a higher incidence of erosion and infection as well as urethral atrophy, possibly secondary to radiation induced vasculitis fibrosis of the urethra [48] (15). Good results are reported, however, and it is generally recommended that the cuff is placed outside the radiated field [97] (21).

Collagen injection has also been reported for incontinence after radical prostatectomy and adjuvant radiation [57,62-66] (22, 23, 24, 25, 26, 27) or after salvage radical prostatectomy following radiotherapy [98] (28). Continence results are poor when compared to those without radiation.

In summary, despite the higher incidence of complications of the artificial sphincter in patients after pelvic radiation, it has provided acceptable treatment benefits. Collagen injections have yielded poor results.

V. INCONTINENCE AFTER OTHER TREATMENT FOR PROSTATE CANCER AND NEOBLADDER FOR BLADDER CANCER

1. Brachytherapy is a form of radiation therapy in which radioactive materials are placed directly into the prostate gland. The incidence of incontinence following this modality is in Table 6. In a systematic review of brachytherapy series Crook et al.(108), reported the incidence of retention to be 1-14%. Many patients require prolonged or permanent alpha blocker or TURP. The main risk factor for incontinence after brachytherapy is TURP. Hu and Wallner [105] (35) reported on the incidence of urinary incontinence after TURP/TUIP following prostate brachytherapy for prostate cancer. Of the 10 patients who underwent an outlet relaxing procedure (TURP/TUIP) for refractory urinary obstruction, 7 developed some degree of permanent urinary incontinence. They surmised that the cause may be multifactorial and may include physical damage to the urinary sphincter and the radiation dose to the urethral region. Surgical therapy has included the artificial sphincter, when required [106] (36). Urethro-rectal fistula is another complication that has been reported in 1.8% of patients in a large U.S. medicare retrospective review [106] (36).

2. Cryosurgical ablation of the prostate is used for clinically localized prostate cancer as primary treatment or after unsuccessful external beam radiation therapy. The frequency of the main lower urinary tract complications are listed in Table 7. The artificial sphincter has been mentioned as one of the treatments for incontinence [120] (50). However, cryotherapy is an adverse factor for collagen injections. Urethrorectal fistulae can also occur in up to 5% of treated patients after cryosurgery. Severe incontinence and fistulae that occasionally result may have to be treated with extirpative surgery and diversion [121] (51).

3. Incontinence after Neobladder Construction

The incidence of incontinence after neobladder construction following radical cystectomy for bladder cancer ranges from 90 to 100% during the day and 55 to 94% at night (Table 8). Most patients achieve daytime continence after one year and nightime continence is reported after 2 years. Most of the published reports do not comment on specific surgical management and imipramine is mentioned as treatment in only the occasional paper. Martins and Boyd [48] (15) reported on 8 patients treated with the AUS. Six of these underwent revisions, 3 for infection and/or erosion and 3 for inadequate cuff compression. They cautioned against the use of the AUS and suggested alternatives such as intermittent catheterization at night. Collagen has been reported in women following neobladder construction [133] (63).

In summary there are not enough data upon which to recommend definitive surgical therapy although the artificial sphincter is probably the most commonly used method.

Table 5 : The artificial sphincter for incontinence after radiotherapy

Study	Pts. with Radiation Total number	Revision rate after radiotherapy	Continence
Martins and Boyd [48]	34/81	38% for whole group	88%
Wang and Hadley [93]	16	25% (Infection and Erosion - 12.5%)	87%
Perez and Webster [47]	11/75	55%	63%
Gundian et al. [94]	15/56	22%	90%
Elliott and Barrett [95]	46/313	22%	-
Manunta et al. [96]	15/72	53% (Infection and Erosion – 20%)	73%

Table 6 : Incontinence after brachytherapy for prostate cancer

Author	% Incontinence	% Post TURP	% No TURP
Beyer et al. [99]	1	-	-
Blasko et al. [100]	6	17	0
Stock et al. [101]	0	-	-
Wallner et al. [102]	0	-	-
Kaye et al. [103]*	4	11	1
Blasko et al. [104]	13	0	-
Hu and Wallner [105]	6	70	-
Benoit et al. [106]	6.6	-	-
Merrick et al. [107]	0	-	-
Crook et al. [108]	5.6	13	-

* Implant plus external beam radiation

Table 7 : Lower urinary tract complications after cryosurgery for prostate cancer

Author	N	% Incontinent	% Bladder outlet obstruction
Shinohara et al. [109]	102	15	23
Bahn et al. [110]	210	3	9
Cox and Crawford [111]	63	27	29
Wieder et al. [112]	83	2.5	13
Cohen et al. [113]	239	4	2.2
Coogan and McKiel [114]	95	3.5	6
Sosa et al. [115]	1467	11	6.8
Long et al. [116]	145	83/2.0*	17.2
Pisters et al. [117]	150	60	43
Derakhshani et al. [118]	48	10.4	22.9
Long et al. [119]	975	7.5	13
De la Taille et al. [120]	43	9	4

*Previously radiated/not previously radiated

Table 8 : Continence after neobladder construction for bladder cancer

Author	Number of patients	Follow-up (mo)	Continence (%) Day	Night
Alcini et al. [122]	34	12	100	83
Cancrini et al. [123]	89	24	97 (22% with SUI)	83
Elmajian et al. [124]	266	24	85	85
Studer et al. [125]	100	24	92	80
Benson et al. [126]	32	25	94	74
Abol-Enein and Ghoneim [127]	60	24	90	80
Rogers and Scardino [128]	20	24	90	55
Hautmann et al. [129]	211	36	85	85
Hautmann et al. [130]	363	57	95	95
Steven and Poulsen [131]	166	32.4	100 (After 5 years)	100
Abol-Enein and Ghoneim [132]	353	38	93.3	80

VI. TRAUMATIC INJURIES OF THE URETHRA AND PELVIC FLOOR

Incontinence following posterior urethral injuries occurs in 0-20% of patients [133,134] (64,65) and is thought to be due to the extent of injury rather than to the method of management.

The data on surgical treatment are all retrospective case series and the most commonly published surgical therapy is the AUS. The series published contain both patients with and without traumatic injuries. Perez and Webster [47] (17) reported on 27 patients after urethral or bladder neck strictures. The revision rate was 41% and the continence rate was 85%. In Montague's [46] (66) (series 22 out of 166 patients had incontinence after trauma. He did not separate the results of this group from those of the other patients. Martins and Boyd [48] reported on only one patient out of 81 with a traumatic urethral injury. This patient was dry and required no revisions. Venn at el. [97] (21) reported on 2 with pelvic trauma out of a total of 70.

Bladder neck reconstruction by excising the scar and narrowing the calibre was reported by Iselin and Webster [136] (67) in 6 patients who had incontinence with an open bladder neck on cystourethrography, following urethroplasty for traumatic strictures. Bladder neck closure with a Mitrofanoff catheterizable abdominal stoma has also been reported as treatment following severe urethral or bladder trauma, [137] (68).

For patients with severe bladder neck strictures and incontinence after radical prostatectomy Meulen et al. [138] (69) and Elliot and Boone [139] (70) reported on the use of a Urolume stent with a bulbar artificial sphincter.

In summary, while other treatments are possible the AUS provides a reasonable outcome in appropriate cases.

VII. UNRESOLVED PAEDIATRIC PROBLEMS: THE EXSTROPHY-EPISPADIAS COMPLEX

Despite a surprising number of publications on the exstrophy-epispadias complex over the last three years, there have been no major changes in management. Some new innovations have emerged both in primary treatment and in the management of persisting incontinence (as outlined below), and reports of good results from major centres continue. [140, 141, 142, 143, 144, 145]. A significant rate of incontinence persists across the board although it depends to some extent on how continence is defined [140,145]. Controversy continues regarding its management [140,145,146,147].

Deficiencies persist in the areas of long-term follow-up, the use of urodynamic assessment, the absence of clinical trials, and the continuing need for patients with exstrophy-epispadias complex to be managed in centres of excellence [146,147,148]. Recommendations regarding these issues are made.

1. New innovations

a) Initial management of exstrophy-epispadias complex

Several authors have advocated a reduction in the number of procedures in the standard staged surgical management of exstrophy-epispadias complex (early closure, repair of epispadias and bladder neck reconstruction) though this regime of three separate operations remains the backbone of treatment in most centres. The importance of careful selection of such patients is emphasized by Gearhart and Mathew [143], and the short time of follow-up in most series where a one-stage primary repair is used makes the long-term results uncertain [141,149,150,151]. Improvements in surgical techniques and experience justify continuation of these efforts in selected 'centres of excellence' along with the mandatory reporting of long-term outcomes [152]. The pivotal importance of the initial operation on a successful outcome is reinforced by several papers [140, 142, 144,148].

b) Management of persisting incontinence

While there appears to be a general acceptance that initial treatment with primary closure and (co-incident or separate) repair of epispadias is the basis of initial management in exstrophy-epispadias complex [142, 144,153] (with the notable exception of the Mainz group [145]), considerable differences of opinion remain regarding the management of persisting incontinence or failed primary repair [140,145,146,147]. Various options are shown in Table 9.

The Johns Hopkins group and others continue to champion the use of the 'native' bladder, with augmentation reserved for those whose capacity is decreased or bladder activity is increased that makes this necessary to achieve continence [142,143,144,146]. Their main arguments supporting this approach are the good continence that can be achieved in the hands of experienced surgeons, and the potential risks associated with the use of bowel reservoirs including malignancy, urolithiasis [154], deterioration of the upper tracts [155] and

Table 9 : Options for management of incontinence after unsuccessful exstrophy-epispadias surgery

Revision of bladder neck reconstruction

Augmentation enterocystoplasty
- Stomach
- Ileum
- Colon

Continent stoma
- with augmentation
- bladder neck transection and closure

Bladder replacement

Artificial urinary sphincter

Transurethral injections

Urinary diversion
- conduit
- continent reservoir
  • colon
  • ileal-cecal
  • rectal reservoir

decreased linear growth [156]. Others headed by those from Mainz, believe that all, but especially those who have 'failed' previous treatment, are best served by conversion to a rectal reservoir or ileocaecal pouch with a catheterizable stoma [140]. This belief is based on the excellent continence achieved compared with the incidence of 'complete' control with bladder neck reconstruction [145], the stability of the upper tracts and the likelihood of not needing any further surgery. The solution to this dilemma is the use of matched, comparative, quality of life trials between the differing centres of excellence [147]. For the patients involved, a full reassessment including upper tract studies and urodynamics is mandatory to allow individualization of treatment to optimize the chance of a successful outcome [148, 152, 157,158].

The armamentarium available for treatment of continuing incontinence is largely unchanged as set out in the original manuscript [1], though gastrocystoplasty has been advocated, particularly in cloacal exstrophy with its short bowel syndrome. The risk of complications of this procedure, such as the hematuria-dysuria syndrome, particularly with longer-term follow-up, was emphasized by several authors [159,160,161], though Plaire et al. believed it to be a good option in selected patients [162]. A possible solution to this problem may be the gastrointestinal composite urinary reservoir [163]. The problem of persisting nocturnal incontinence can be helped by desmopressin [164]. Finally, it has been shown that the presence of any neurological abnormality greatly reduces the chance of continence with standard reconstruction, even with augmentation, in cloacal exstrophy [158].

2. Deficiencies

a) Definition of continence

Most authors take a daytime three-hour voiding (or catheterization) interval without loss of urine at night as signifying continence, though even this is not universally accepted [141]. Even this achievement often requires the use of pads or other incontinence devices, and Hohenfellner quotes Jeffs as saying that only 20% of 5-10 year olds are completely dry [145].

There are still no apparent attempts to quantify the degree of wetness eg., pad tests. This assessment continues to rely on the history given by the patient or parents.

b) Lack of long-term follow-up

Many studies only quote relatively short periods of follow-up, and even those with longer median time intervals often contain a significant number who are excluded from assessment of continence because they are awaiting the attainment of an adequate bladder volume or a further procedure [141, 143,148,149,150]. Given the risks of urodynamic deterioration with bladder neck reconstruction (vide infra), and the potential problems with the use of bowel (vide supra), long-term (preferably life long) follow-up reports are essential.

c) Lack of urodynamic assessment

There is a dearth of urodynamic studies in exstrophy-epispadias complex patients even though many abnormalities are reported [141,152,157,160,165,166]. Its usefulness in making treatment decisions for those with persisting incontinence is commonly accepted, but even in those patients apparently doing well, urodynamic monitoring may be very helpful in detecting problems at an earlier stage [165,166]. Whether these patients ever void normally is uncertain, with bladder neck reconstruction being a delicate balance between preventing incontinence while avoiding obstruction [157,166,167].

d) Absence of trials

All the published material consists of reports of experience at various centres, and many of these are retrospective reviews. While even major institutions struggle to have large enough series to mount controlled trials, it should be possible to at least arrange comparative trials, including quality of life measurements, to assess different forms of treatment [147]. Until this happens we will be left with level 3 & 4 evidence at best and be no closer to establishing the best way to treat individual patients with this major disability.

RECOMMENDATIONS

- Patients with exstrophy-epispadias complex should be dealt with in centres of excellence
- The standard definition of incontinence and its assessment should be applied
- Life long follow-up including urodynamics should be undertaken
- Persisting incontinence should be fully investigated and its treatment tailored to the individual
- Comparative studies, including quality of life, should be established between units.

VIII. DETRUSOR OVERACTIVITY AND REDUCED BLADDER CAPACITY

1. REFRACTORY URGE INCONTINENCE AND IDIOPATHIC DETRUSOR OVERACTIVITY

According to the recent ***Terminology report of the International Continence Society*** the overactive bladder syndrome refers to the symptoms of urgency, with or without urge incontinence, usually with frequency and nocturia [168]. *Detrusor overactivity* has also been redefined to indicate a urodynamic observation characterized by involuntary detrusor contractions during the filling phase that may be spontaneous or provoked. *Idiopathic Detrusor Overactivity* exists when there is no defined cause. This term replaces "detrusor instability". *Neurogenic Detrusor Overactivity* is seen when there is a relevant neurological condition. This term replaces the term "detrusor hyperreflexia". Although the old terms will eventually be replaced they are still in common usage.

Idiopathic detrusor overactivity is a normal situation early in life. Children have urge incontinence as a stage in acquiring bladder control. The incidence of detrusor overactivity during the middle years (20 to 60) has been estimated as 10% [169]. In the asymptomatic elderly, detrusor overactivity once again becomes common, occurring in 50% of men over 70 [170]. In the symptomatic elderly, over 75 years old, it can reach 90% in men [171]. Detrusor overactivity may be a cause of severe storage symptoms such as frequency, nocturia, urgency and urge incontinence. Conservative treatment of these symptoms such as bladder training and pharmacotherapy is discussed in other sections. For symptoms that are refractory two interventional treatments have been reported: neuromodulation and bladder augmentation.

a) Electrical stimulation and neuromodulation

Electrical stimulation of the genital area was first used to control incontinence due to detrusor overactivity on an empirical basis [172], for different etiologies. Later, it was suggested that reflex sphincteric contraction induced by electrical stimulation can promote an inhibitory effect on detrusor activity, thus suppressing detrusor overactivity [173]. Many studies on external electrical stimulation for bladder inhibition on idiopathic urge incontinence have been published, mainly in female patients [174-179,182,183]. The results vary from 45 % to 85 % of success, with a mean of 38 %, and 26% improved. Electrodes implanted in the pelvic floor, did not yield good results [179].

Neuromodulation of sacral nerves has been reported as an alternative therapy for incontinence, urinary retention and chronic pelvic pain. Good results have been published in treating neurogenic bladder dysfunction [180,181]. Its use in refractory idiopathic urge incontinence has been limited to few patients, mostly women. Bosch and Groen [184] presented results of chronic implantation in 15 women and 3 men, with an average age of 46 years. Significant improvements in voiding frequency, average voided volume, number of incontinence episodes, and number of pads used were found, with no deterioration in response to stimulation with time. However, with subsequent experience in 14 men only 2 patients had a partial response [185]. Shaker and Hassouna [186] implanted 18 patients with refractory urinary urge incontinence, but only 2 were in men. Other studies are not clear about the etiology of the detrusor overactivity, neurogenic and non-neurogenic causes are grouped together [187,188]. Table 10 shows some recent prospective studies.

b) Surgical treatment by bladder myectomy and augmentation

Previous treatments by means of surgical bladder denervation, open bladder transection, cystolysis, endoscopic phenol injections, hydrostatic bladder distention did not produce good results.

Bladder autoaugmentation or myectomy has been reported as an alternative to augmentation in neurogenic and non-neurogenic dysfunction. Table 11 presents recent results of this treatment in patients with non-neurogenic detrusor overactivity. Additional and longer-term experience is still required to properly assess this modality.

Enterocystoplasty results are in Table 12, which includes male and female patients. Good results vary from 58% to 88%, with an average of 77%. A minimum of 10% of patients requires intermittent catheterization for bladder emptying. Ileum was the most frequently used bowel segment followed by sigmoid colon,

Table 10 : Neuromodulation for treatment of refractory urge incontinence due to detrusor overactivity (males and females)

Author	N	success (dry)	improved	control group	
Schmidt et al. [189]	34	47%	29%	42	prospective randomized
Weil et al. [190]	21	56%	19%	23	prospective randomized
Bosch et al. [191]	34 (females) 6 (males)	38% 16%	21% 16%	-	prospective longitudinal

Table 11 : Detrusor myectomy for treatment of refractory urge incontinence due to detrusor overactivity (both sexes)

Author	Detrusor overactivity N	Good results N
Swami et al. [192]	17	12
Leng et al. [193]	8	7
Total	**25**	**19 (76%)**

Table 12 : Enterocystoplasty for treatment of refractory urge incontinence due to detrusor overactivity (males and females)

Authors	Detrusor overactivity	Good or moderate result	Bowel segment
Hasan et al. [194]	33	19	46 ileum 2 colon
McInerney et al. [195]	50	44	
Bramble [196]	15	13	3 colon 2 ileum
Sethia et al. [197]	11	9	ileum
Mundy and Stephenson [198]	40	30	ileum, clam
Leng et al. [193]	2	2	
Total	**151**	**117 (77 %)**	

although no scientific reason for use of any particular segment was given. The surgery, as reported in other sections, has a significant complication rate and should be evaluated carefully when applying it to these patients.

c) Reduced bladder capacity

Fibrosis of the wall produces a low-volume low-compliant bladder, leading to diminished functional capacity. Symptoms of frequency and urgency occur with progressive decreases in volume but urinary incontinence may also be a consequence of a very small capacity, especially if accompanied by urethral weakness. The diagnosis can be suggested by the micturition chart and confirmed by cystogram and or urodynamics. The causes can be congenital or acquired. Acquired causes include multiple surgeries, inflammatory processes (chronic cystitis, interstitial cystitis, tuberculosis, schistosomiasis, chemical cystitis) or post radiation. Bilharzial contracted bladder is a problem that is primarily limited to endemic areas in Africa and the Middle East. Schistosoma haematobium migrates to the veins of the vesical and pelvic plexuses, where the female begins to lay eggs, promoting an initial inflammatory response. As a result, granulomatous lesions form in the lamina propria. Mucosal reactions vary from hyperplasia to polypoid cystitis. A contracted bladder occurs in 2% of cases [199]. Bladder augmentation seems to offer a reasonable result in these cases. Similarly small fibrotic bladders of other etiologies, can be treated successfully with enterocystoplasty. The results of this surgery are presented in Table 13.

These results are similar in all etiologies except radiation cystitis. The poorer results after radiation may be due to other tissue damage in the surgical area. New conformal techniques for radiotherapy may improve in the future, such that the need for and, the results of, augmentation improve.

Almost all of these studies do not distinguish bowel segments or separate males from females in reporting results. Therefore, it is not possible to correlate any particular aspect with the chance of success or failure. However, overall the results seem to be reasonable good with the exception of radiation.

Table 13 : Enterocystoplasty results for reduced bladder capacity

Authors	Bilharziasis cystitis		Tuberculous cystitis		Radiation cystitis		Unknown cause	
	TOTAL	SUCCESS	TOTAL	SUCCESS	TOTAL	SUCCESS	TOTAL	SUCCESS
Smith et al. [200]	-	-	7	4	9	3	12	7
Kerr et al. [201]	-	-	12	12	-	-	-	-
Zinman and Libertino [202]	-	-	2	2	1	?	1	1
Dounis et al. [203]	-	-	31	27	-	-	1	1
Lunghi et al. [204]	-	-	15	15	4	4	3	3
Shawket and Muhsen [205]	8	8	-	-	-	-	-	-
Whitmore and Gittes [206]	-	-	7	7	-	-	2	1
Chan et al. [207]	-	-	-	-	-	-	10	9
Shirley et al. [208]	-	-	10	10	4	2	-	-
Goodwin et al. [209]	-	-	3	2	-	-	3	3
Winter and Goodwin [210]	-	-	1	1	3	1	-	-
Fall and Nilsson [211]	-	-	1	1	-	-	1	1
Goldwasser and Webster [212]	-	-	-	-	-	-	7	7
Weinberg et al. [213]	-	-	2	2	1	1	1	1
Novak [214]	-	-	11	11	-	-	-	-
Sayegh and Dimmette [215]	2	0	-	-	-	-	-	-
Beduk et al. [216]	-	-	-	-	-	-	1	1
Kuo [217]	-	-	-	-	1	1	-	-
Kawamura et al. [218]	-	-	-	-	-	-	1	1
Hradec [219]	-	-	-	-	27	23	-	-
Lima et al. [220]	-	-	1	1	-	-	-	-
El Otmany et al. [221]	-	-	1	1	-	-	-	-
Yamada et al. [222]	-	-	1	1	-	-	-	-
Total	**10**	**8 (80%)**	**105**	**97 (92%)**	**50**	**35 (70%)**	**43**	**36 (84%)**

IX. URETHRO-CUTANEOUS AND RECTO-URETHRAL FISTULAE

Urethrocutaneous or rectourethral fistula may have congenital, inflammatory, neoplastic or traumatic origin. It is important to recognize this diversity of etiology because each type requires a different surgical strategy. All reports are still only retrospective case series.

1. Urethrocutaneous fistula (UCF)

a) Congenital

Sharma et al reported a case of congenital urethral fistula with an intact glandular urethra without chordee which was repaired in one-stage [224]. Harjai et al. managed the congenital urethral fistula in a 3-year-old male child with a life-long history of passing urine from the undersurface of penis and the meatus. A fistula was present on the ventral midshaft of penis through which a catheter could be passed [224]. Caldamone et al. reported a case of congenital anterior urethrocutaneous fistula. This is a rare anomaly that may present in an isolated fashion or in association with other penile abnormalities, such as chordee or hypospadias. To our knowledge the embryological events that cause anterior urethrocutaneous fistula are unclear but are likely to result from a defective urethral plate or an abnormality of the infolding of the urethral groove. There have been 18 cases of congenital anterior urethrocutaneous fistula reported in the literature. He treated 14 additional cases of congenital anterior urethrocutaneous fistula of whom 9 were uncircumcised at presentation. Two patients had evidence of chordee and 4 had distal hypospadias. The type of repair was determined by the anatomic variations of this anomaly. All cases were corrected electively by various techniques based on the degree of the defect, including primary closure via a Thiersch-Duplay urethroplasty, pedicle flap urethroplasty, hinged flap urethroplasty and interpositioned island pedicle tube, or onlay urethroplasty [225]

b) Acquired UCF

Hidden foreign bodies have been described as a rare cause of both strangulation of the glans penis and urethrocutaneous fistula. Tash and Eid [226] presented the case of a 30-year-old man who developed a urethrocutaneous fistula and penile shaft necrosis after a condom broke during intercourse. Neither the patient nor several physicians could identify the retained ring of condom, which had been buried under newly epithelialized skin. He underwent removal of the foreign body under general anaesthesia, followed 5 months later by a formal urethrocutaneous fistula repair.

Urethroperineal fistula, as a complication of open perineal prostate cryosurgery, occurs as an immediate perioperative complication in 10.7 % [227]. Thomas et al. retrospectively evaluated 250 patients after radical perineal prostatectomy and revealed only 1 (0.4%) urethroperineal fistula [228]. Fahal et al. [229] published an unusual complication of ***mycetoma***. The patient had an infection with Actinomadura madurae that involved abdominal wall, perineum and urethra. This resulted in urinary extravasation with a urethrocutaneous fistula.

c) Management of UCF

The diagnosis of UCF is made by physical examinations and retrograde urethrography, urethroscopy, fistulography, urethral ultrasound or color Doppler imaging. Urethral sonography provides additional information about an involvement of the surrounding tissue, location of vessels and associated abnormalities such as a periurethral abscess [230].

Treatment of UCF usually requires urethroplasty techniques with modifications involving fistula excision and multiple layer closure [231].

2. Rectourethral fistulas (RUF)

Culp and Calhoon described five basic groups of RUF according to the etiology [232]:

congenital, iatrogenic, traumatic, neoplastic, and inflammatory.

a) Congenital RUF

Endo et al. [233] described the results of the Japanese Study Group of Anorectal Anomalies (JSGA) to determine the relative incidence of specific types of these anomalies in Japan. They included discussion of RUF regarding the relationship between the fistula levels and blind end of the rectum, low type deformity, rare types, and associated anomalies. A total of 1,992 patients (1,183 boys and 809 girls) registered from 1976 to 1995 were analysed according to the pathogenesis of anorectal malformation in the field of molecular genetics. They reported that more than 20% of RUF should be categorized as intermediate or low deformity from the position of the rectal pouch. A significant preponderance of Down's syndrome in the deformities without fistulae suggests that investigation of associated anomalies and congenital diseases may provide further insights.

The purpose of Rintala´s study was to compare the long-term outcome of sacroperineal-sacroabdominoperineal pull-through (SP-SAP) to that of posterior sagittal anorectoplasty (PSARP). In boys with high anorectal anomalies, PSARP was superior to SP-SAP pull-through in terms of long-term bowel function and faecal continence [234].

b) Acquired RUF

In 1972 Smith and Venema [235] reported their 20-year experience with 160 patients undergoing radical retropubic prostatectomy (RRP) with the incidence of 15 rectal injuries. Only 4 fistulas developed in this group.

The most common single cause of RUF in the series of 23 male patients published by Tiptaft et al. [236] was a fracture of the pelvis and iatrogenic causes (two cases after transurethral prostatic surgery, two cases after open prostatectomy, and three cases after urethral instrumentation. Noldus et al. [237] reported 23 (3.9%) rectal injuries during 589 RRP and cystoprostatectomy. Eastham and Scardino [238] summarized the incidence of rectal injury during RRP in 3834 patients with an average of 0.7% (range 0.2-2.9%). The incidence of RUF, as an immediate perioperative complication of open perineal prostate surgery, is 1.4 %.

Nyam et al. [239] reviewed records of all patients who were diagnosed with rectourethral fistula between January 1981 and December 1995 and 16 males were identified. All patients were interviewed by telephone to establish follow-up. The mean age was 68 years and the mean follow-up was 80 months. Adenocarcinoma of the prostate in 15 patients and recurrent transitional cell carcinoma of the bladder in one patient were the underlying malignant diseases. Nine patients had had a RRP with 2 after radiation, 2 after brachytherapy, and 3 after a combination of radiation and brachytherapy. One patient formed a fistula after cystectomy and dilation of a stricture. This heterogenous group of patients received multiple therapies including initial colostomy (7 patients), transanal repair (2 patients), parasacral repair (2 patients), transperineal repair (2 patients), coloanal anastomosis (3 patients), and muscle transposition (3 patients). Four of the patients required a permanent stoma.

Zippe [240] reviewed preliminary results of prostate cryosurgery and reported a 2-5% incidence of RUF. Porter [227] found a 2.5% rate of RUF in 210 patients after TRUS-guided prostate cryosurgery and no urethroperineal fistulae.

Montorsi et al. [241] reported one complication of prostatorectal fistula after transrectal prostatic hyperthermia (43 degree C) in patients with advanced prostatic cancer after multiple treatment sessions. The fistula was cured after a urethral catheter was left in place for one month.

Kleinberg et al. [242] summarized results of 31 patients with stage T1 or T2 prostatic carcinoma following CT-guided transperineal (125) I implants and reported that only one patient developed a prostatorectal fistula managed with an ileal conduit.

Fengler and Abcarian [243] published their experience of eight patients with recto-urinary fistulae in the course of treatment of prostate cancer (3 fistulae after radiation therapy alone, 3 after prostatectomy and 2 after both surgery and radiation therapy).

Chang et al. [244] published a case of prostatic malakoplakia masquerading as a rectal tumor due to formation of a fistulous tract to the rectal muscular layers. Cools et al. [245] reported a very uncommon type of fistula between the large bowel and the prostatic urethra due to Crohn's disease. Felipetto et al. [246] described a prostato-cutaneous fistula as a complication of pseudomonas prostatitis.

c) Diagnosis of RUF

RUF may be strongly suspected from the patient's history (fecaluria, abnormal urethral discharge, pneumaturia, leakage of urine from the rectum during micturition). Rectal examination, proctoscopy, careful urethroscopy, intraurethral injection of methylene blue dye, radiopaque contrast agent placed into the bladder and then voided usually appears in the rectum on X-ray, are the most important diagnostic steps [230,247].

d) Therapy of RUF

Small fistulae may resolve "spontaneously" with urinary and/or fecal diversion. Therefore, an initial trial of conservative therapy is reasonable. Selected patients with chronic fistulas who are poor surgical candidates may also be managed conservatively with antiobiotics, pads and symptomatic care. Timing of repair is often individualized, mainly according to the etiology, delay in diagnosis, size of fistula, whether it is the first or subsequent repairs, and the general condition of patient. Diversion of urine (suprapubic cystostomy) is generally recommended as well as correction of any urethral stricture distal to the fistula. Fecal diversion, with colostomy is used by some as a mandatory part of double diversion or selectively by others. Gibbons [248] stressed the need for a diverting colostomy for 3-4 months.

However, as surgeons obtained more experience, bowel preparations became standardized, and effective antibiotics were developed, the enthusiasm for colostomy diminished. Currently, colostomy is recommended in circumstances where antibiotics alone cannot control the inflammation and infection associated with the fistula or when the fistula involves radiated tissue. Low residue diet is also useful for healing. Suitable drainage (perineal and urethral splinting) is stressed. Two-layer closure of the urethra and rectum with suture lines at right angles and with interposition of soft tissue (eg. omentum [249], gracilis muscle [250], or scrotal flap [251]) has been described. Surgical approaches include transabdominal, transvesical, direct exposure of RUF through a transperineal incision, transanal, transrectal with a transsphincteric approach or a flap technique with an intact anal sphincter [252,253], or the Latzko procedure [254]. The approaches to RUF repair are listed in Table 14.

Table 14 : Surgical approaches to Rectourethral fistula repair

Perineal	References
Posterior-sagittal	255-257
- Posterior (parasacrococcygeal) - transsphincteric	258
Transanal	236, 237, 247, 262
Anterior transanorectal	263
Endoscopic	264, 265
Other	246, 266

e) Surgical Approaches

1. Perineal

In 1926, Young [255] dissected the rectum away from sphincters, divided the fistula, closed the urethra, and mobilized the rectum further cephalad in such a fashion as to pull the affected rectum caudally out of the anus where it was then transected and discarded, suturing the proximal rectum to the anal skin. Subsequently Lewis, in 1947 [256], described suturing the levator muscle fibers together in the anterior midline when possible. Goodwin et al. [257] reported a series of 22 RUF approached perineally. They extensively mobilized the rectum posteriorly and the bladder anteriorly through wide perineal exposure allowing interposition of the levator ani muscles between the urinary tract and rectum.

2. Posterior sagittal

Kraske in 1885 described a posterior midline incision extending to the left paramedian aspect of the coccyx and sacrum that involved partial removal of the sacrum in addition to coccygectomy. His method did not involve division of the sphincters, but rather sweeping the rectum laterally to ultimately facilitate resection and reanastomosis of a tumour-bearing rectal segment, thereby preserving fecal continence. In 1962, Kilpatrick and Thompson [258] used this approach when the rectum was completely mobilized circumferentially proximal and distal to the fistula. The RUF was then divided, sparing as much as possible on the urethral aspect. The rectal opening was excised and closed in two layers, and the urethra was repaired and stented with a catheter.

3. Posterior (parasacrococcygeal) transsphincteric

In 1969 Kilpatrick and Mason [258] updated this method and advocated a more radical method of dividing the rectal sphincters to give direct access to the RUF. The procedure (the York-Mason approach) is simpler than some complicated transabdominal or transperineal approaches to RUF. It is still used because it allows direct visualization of the fistula via parasacrococcygeal (transsphincteric) incision especially to fistulae in the mid to lower rectum [259]. After the skin incision the mucocutaneous junction is marked with sutures and internal sphincter is exposed. Division of the sphincter mechanism and posterior rectal wall allows exposure of the fistula. Each sphincter muscle is tagged with color-coded sutures. The next step of this procedure is the incision around fistula, followed by excision of the fistulous tract exposing the catheter in prostatic urethra. The undermining of rectal wall allows sufficient mobilization. After closure of prostatic urethra it is recommended to close the full-thickness rectal wall flaps in a "vest over pants" technique. It is important to note that the suture lines do not overlie each other. The procedure is completed by suture of rectal wall and approximating the sphincter muscles (Figure 2). Fengler et al. [259] reported healing of RUF in all of 8 patients with the York-Mason approach. Bukowski et al. [260] managed 7 acquired recurrent RUF (3 after prostatectomy, 3 after trauma and 1 after perineal abscess) using York-Mason technique and similar experience was described by Fournier et al. [261] in the management of a case of the urethro-prostato-rectal fistula after a gunshot wound.

4. Transanal

Parks and Motson [262] popularized the addition of a full thickness local flap of anterior rectal wall as an adjunct to fistula repair through the intact anal canal (Figure 3). They modified the transanal technique by

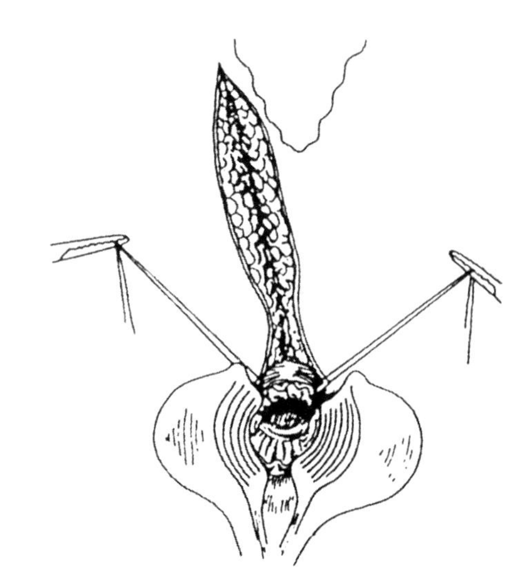

Figure 2 : York-Mason approach to a rectourethral fistula via a parasacrococcygeal (transsphincteric) incision. Sutures are used to mark the sphincters The speculum has been placed at the bottom of the incision and the anterior rectal wall is visible.

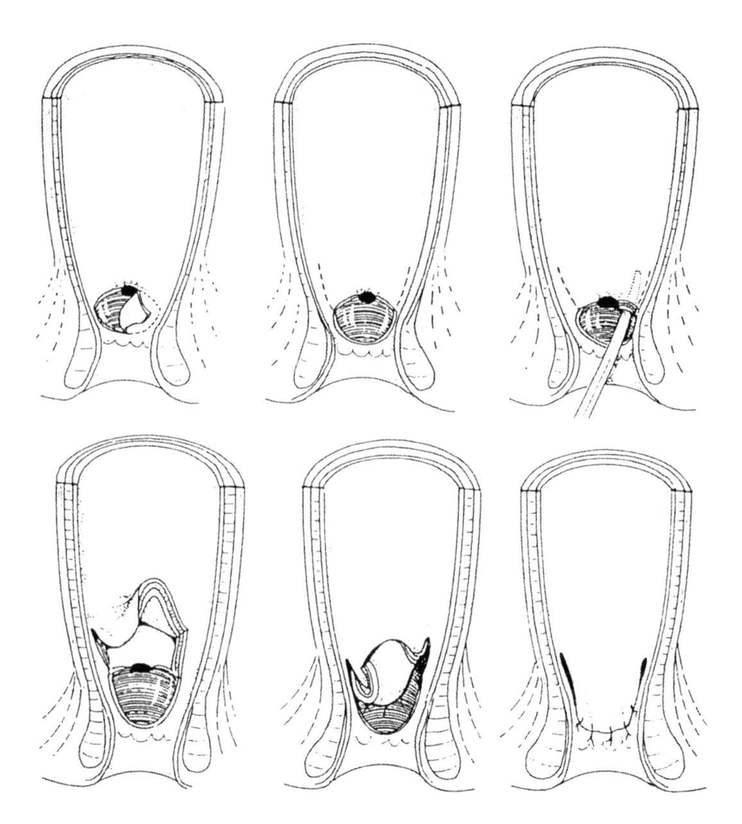

Figure 3 : Rectourethral fistula repair. Full thickness rectal wall is mobilized to close in a "vest over pants" technique to close the fistula.

denuding the rectal mucosa lateral and distal to the fistula, and mobilized the rectal wall away from Denonvilliers' fascia proximal to the fistula for four centimeters. Tiptaft et al. [236] also used a special anal retractor for this surgery.

With the Latzko procedure the RUF is closed in three layers with absorbable suture. A transurethral catheter is placed for 3 weeks. Noldus et al. [237] reported 23 patients (3.9%) with rectal injury during 589 RRP and cystoprostatectomy. Of these 23 patients, 12 developed a RUF. Seven fistulas closed spontaneously with prolonged catheter drainage. The remaining 5 fistulas were all successfully closed with the transanal Latzko procedure.

Al-Ali et al. [247] treated 30 men with RUF caused by war wounds. He used the method of posterior transsphincteric_anterior rectal wall advancement as the treatment of choice. Double diversion (end sigmoid colostomy and suprapubic cystostomy) for one month was performed in all patients. Double diversion alone resulted in "spontaneous" RUF healing in 47% of patients but 53% required reconstruction. Early repair was recommended for large fibrous fistulas. Undiversion was done after two months when the urethra and anorectal canals were normal.

5. Anterior transanorectal

In 1973 Gecelter [263] performed a midline perineal incision to gain access to the urinary tract after placing the patient in exaggerated lithotomy position. The sphincter was incised anteriorly, tag sutures carefully placed, and the rectal incision was carried to the fistulous tract, which was excised and repaired in multiple layers with transposition of tissue as available.

6. Endoscopic

Wilbert et al. [264] reported two patients with RUF who were repaired endoscopically transanally. The patients were positioned prone and the rectoscope mounted to the operating table was inserted into the rectum .The fistula was visualized and the opening excised to the level of the perirectal tissues with cautery. The rectal wall was mobilized full thickness with scissors and closed primarily in two layers with a microscope. The patient was then placed in lithotomy position and the urethral side of the fistula was coagulated and injected with fibrin.

Recently Bardari et al. [265] used biological glue (Glubran,) to close one prostato-perineal fistula complicating an abdominoperineal resection of rectum and one persistent neobladder-ileal fistula. The biologic sealant was administrated endoscopically through an open-end 6F ureteral catheter.

7. Other Modifications

Youssef et al. [266] successfully treated 12 male patients who presented with urethrorectal fistula from

1990 to 1997 using the perineal subcutaneous dartos flap procedure. Urethrorectal fistulas resulted from crush pelvic injury in 6 cases, gunshot wounds in 2, and post prostatectomy in 4. The fistula was associated with a urethral stricture in 4 cases. A perineal approach was used and combined with a transsymphyseal approach in the 4 patients with posterior urethral stricture. They interposed a subcutaneous dartos flap as a tissue flap between the repaired rectum and urethra. No leakage or perineal collection developed and there was no fistula recurrence. Follow-up ranged from 9 to 42 months. This technique of a perineal subcutaneous dartos flap may fulfill the principles for successful repair of urethrorectal fistulas.

Felipetto et al. [246] closed a prostato-cutaneous fistula (as a complication of pseudomonas prostatitis) with human fibrin sealant (Tissucol®). Venkatesh and Ramanujam [267] prospectively studied the efficacy of autologous fibrin glue application for closure of recurrent anorectal fistulas. Overall success rate was 60 percent however patients with fistulas associated with acquired immunodeficiency syndrome and the urinary tract failed to respond.

f) Summary

A review of recent literature shows an increasing number of papers describing treatment. All available studies are retrospective cases and case series. There are many causes of these fistulas described in the literature but there is a lack of valid epidemiologic data about the incidence of UCF and RUF. The diagnostic algorithm has not changed in many years. The aim of the surgical approach is the closure of all types of fistulas. While spontaneous closure and success with a one-stage procedure has been reported most cases to date involve 3 stages (double diversion, closure technique, undiversion). An endoscopic approach using biological sealants is promising. Only a few urologists and general surgeons have gained wide experience in the management of UCF or RUF. No single procedure has yet proved to be best or universally applicable.

X. THE ARTIFICIAL URINARY SPHINCTER (AUS)

A series of photographs depicting the artificial urinary sphincter (AUS) implant technique is shown in Figure 4.

1. Complications

Complications following implantation of the AUS can be divided into the broad categories of incontinence, erosion and/or infection.

a) Incontinence

Incontinence following implantation of an AUS can result from (1) alteration in bladder function, (2) atrophy of the urethra, or (3) mechanical failure of the device. These causes may co-exist.

1. Alteration in bladder function

This situation has been reported principally in patients with neurogenic bladder dysfunction, especially in children [268-273]. These changes include, de novo involuntary detrusor contractions, decrease in bladder compliance, and the development of a high pressure system, causing incontinence, hydronephrosis and ultimately renal failure. Modifications in detrusor behavior (including its consequences on the upper urinary tract) occur in up to 57% of cases [268-279]. It should be pointed out, however, that there has never been a published report of hydronephrosis following implantation of an artificial sphincter for incontinence after prostatectomy [280]. The best candidates for sphincter implantation are those with a low pressure, relaxed, and compliant bladder but an incompetent urethral sphincter [277].

2. Atrophy of the urethra

This occurs at the cuff site secondary to long-term mechanical compression of the periurethral and urethral tissues. It is not often reported and some authors do not even mention it as a possible cause of AUS failure [97,280,281]. About 4 months following implantation, cuff efficiency diminishes, presumably because pressure atrophy occurs in every patient to some extent [282]. The incidence of urethral atrophy leading to revision varies from 3% to 9.3% [46,278,283-287].

3. Mechanical failure

This includes perforation of one of the components with loss of fluid from the system, air bubbles or organic debris within the system causing inadequate function of the pump, kinking of the tubes, or disconnection of the tubes. The incidence of these complications varies widely with ranges from 0% [283] to 52.5% [288] with the longest follow-up. In this latter study, the cuff seemed to be the most vulnerable part of the system (22 cuff failures in 18 patients, most of them occurring during the first 2 or 3 years following implantation), followed by pump failure (6 times in 4 patients). Blockage is an exceptional event, occurring only once in 61 patients followed for 10 to 15 years [288]. An unusual mechanical complication has been reported recently. The locking tab became displaced distally into the cycling portion of the cuff preventing the fluid from flowing into the cuff surrounding the urethra [289].

b) Erosion and/or infection

Erosion and infection are two major complications that almost invariably necessitate removal of the prosthesis.

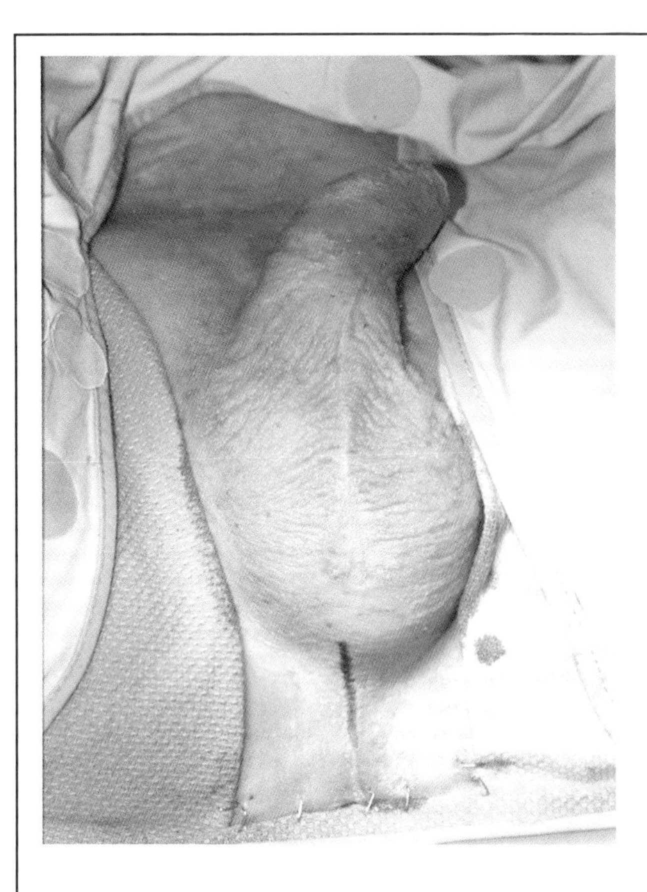

Figure 4 a : With the patient in lithotomy position, a perineal incision is made behind the scrotum to expose the bulbar urethra

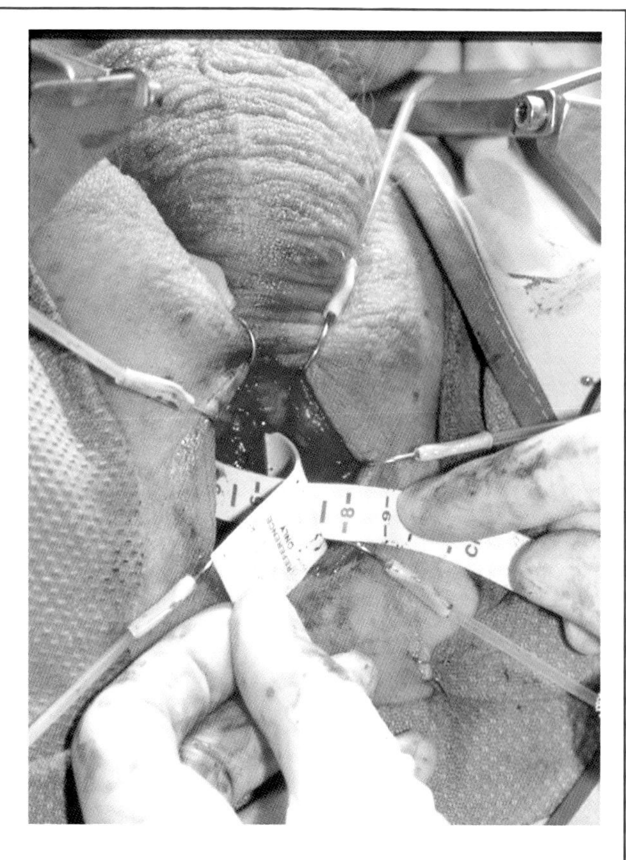

Figure 4 b: The urethra is mobilized circumferentially within the bulbospongiosus muscle and the measuring tape is used to obtain the cuff size.

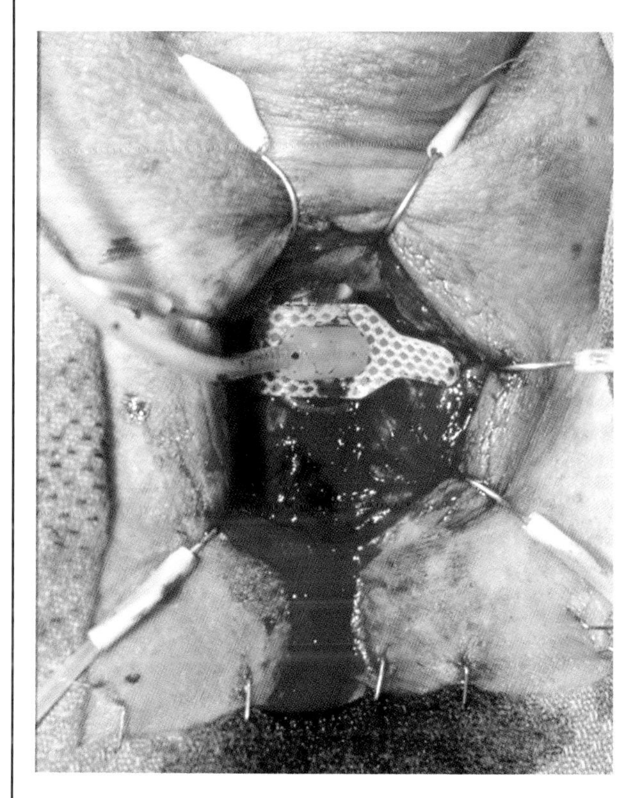

Figure 4 c : The belt-like cuff is positioned around the urethra.

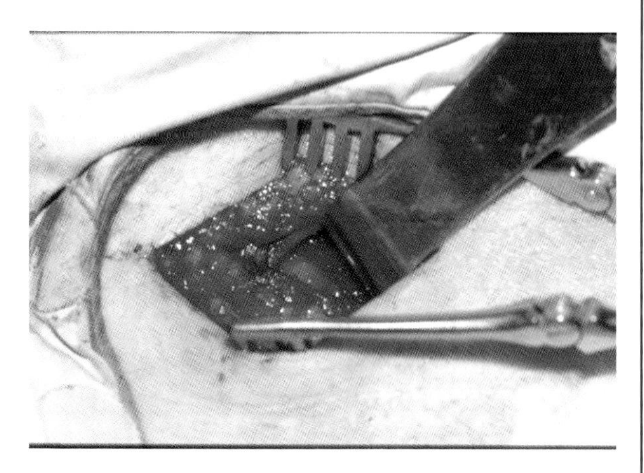

Figure 4 d : A right lower quadrant (RLQ) abdominal incision is made and the extraperitoneal space is entered lateral to the rectus muscle for insertion of the reservoir.

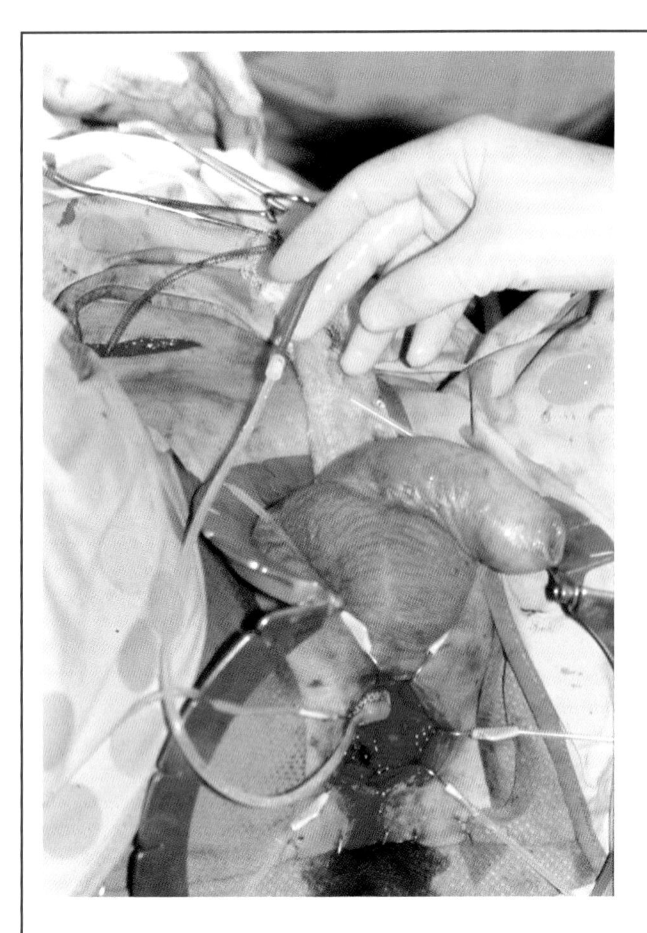

Figure 4 e : After reservoir insertion the cuff is pressurized with fluid

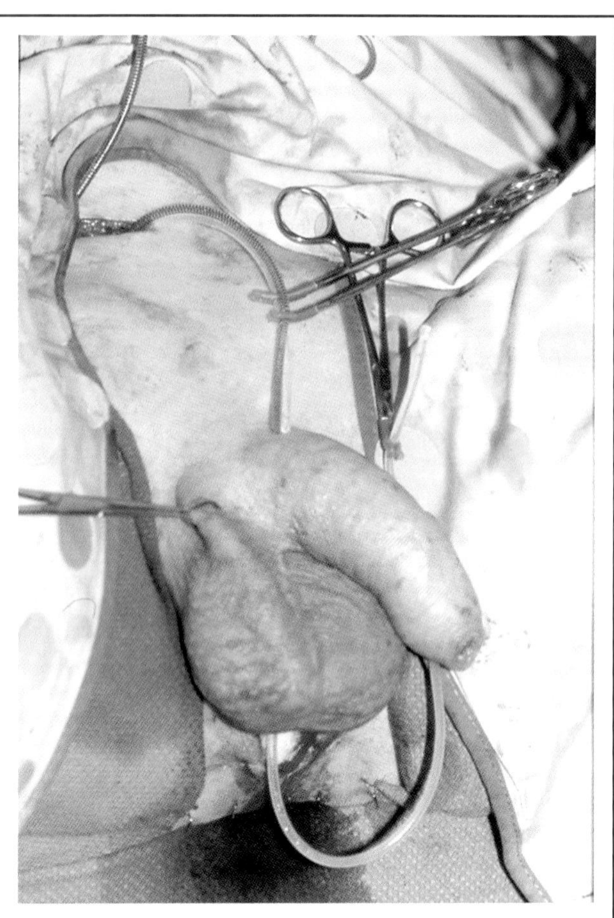

Figure 4 f : A scrotal space is created under the dartos and the pump is inserted (held with a Babcock clamp).

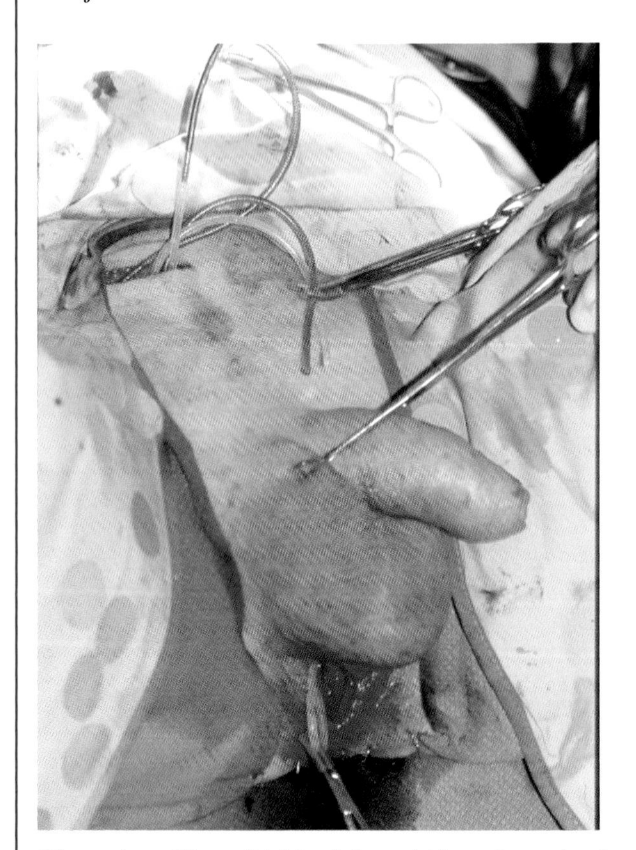

Figure 4 g : The cuff tubing is brought from the perineal incision to the RLQ incision with a tubing passer.

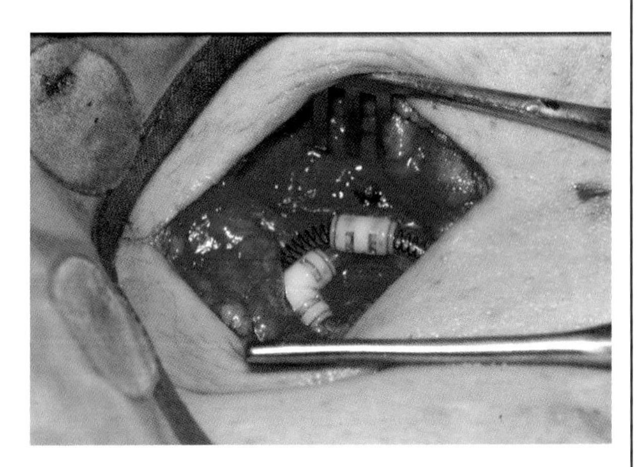

Figure 4 h : Connectors are placed to join the tubes from the cuff and reservoir to the corresponding tubes from the pump in the RLQ incision.

Their incidence is usually reported as a single complication.

The incidence of this complication varies from 0% to 24.6% [46,97,271,277,278,283,284,286,287,290,291]. As would be expected, the highest incidence has been reported with the longest follow-up (10 to 15 years) [283]. Two-thirds of the erosions occurred during the first year. Previous surgery [292] at the site of cuff placement increases the risk of erosion. This, however, can be decreased by delayed activation [293]. Some authors, however, did not find an increased incidence of complications when a new cuff was implanted at the site where several months previously a cuff was removed for infection or erosion [294]. Other risk factors include urethral catheterization and urethral endoscopic manipulations with an activated sphincter in place [295]. Whether or not previous radiation therapy constitutes a risk factor is still controversial although there is some compelling evidence [48,93,96,281].

The number of procedures done in a given center does not seem to be a determining risk factor. Comparable erosion/infection rates have been reported from centres with fewer than 50 or more than 100 cases [1]. This suggests that erosion and infection are more closely related to the physiological state of the host rather than the experience of the surgical team, provided that standard precautions are strictly applied.

2. Durability of AUS components

When defining durability of one of the components or the AUS as a whole, one should distinguish between explantation of the device due to device malfunction (e.g. leak in one of the components) or complications caused by an otherwise properly functioning sphincter unit (e.g. erosion by the cuff, infection at the site of implantation, etc.). This distinction is rarely made in the literature. Durability of a device is defined as time elapsed during which no mechanical problem alters the normal function of the device. This should exclude the second group from further analysis.

There are very few references in the literature pertaining to the length of time a device functioned normally before its removal due to mechanical failure. In a recently published multicenter trial, for neurogenic bladders, conducted in France [278], the authors mention that the "mean operational life" of the sphincter was 56 months (range 3-118 months). Haab et al [289] analyzed 68 patients and noted that the mechanical failure rate dropped from 44.4% to 12.4% since modifications were made to the device, mainly the cuff component. Survival time of these components was not provided. Similar conclusions can be drawn from a recent series from the Mayo Clinic [95] where the modification of the cuff design (narrower back) resulted in a significant drop of the reoperation rate at 5 years. In the narrow backing group 17% (31/184) required a first reoperation. Mean time to the first reoperation was 26.2 months (mean 2 to 68 months). Using Kaplan-Meier statistical analysis for this group of patients, the overall 5 year expected product survival was 75%.

In a recent review Venn et al [97] analysed the outcome of 100 patients in whom an artificial urinary sphincter was implanted more than 10 years before. Thirty-six percent of them still had the original sphincter and were continent at a median follow-up of 11 years. The bulbar cuff, as compared to the bladder neck cuff provided a slightly better continence rate at 10 years, 92% and 84%, respectively. The lowest erosion rate occurred with the bulbar cuff. Device survival rate at 10 years was 66% in this series.

It might be useful to consider patients with "primary adequate function" (PAF) when no revision is necessary to achieve continence separately from those with "additional procedure-assisted adequate function" (APA-AF), where one or more revisions are necessary to obtain favorable outcome. Applying Kaplan-Meier curves to this concept, Klijn et al [51] showed that in their series the median time to failure for the PAF group was 48 months, the mean time to the first failure following the initial implant was 14 months (range: 0-48 months).

In the APA-AF group at 72 months, the median time to definite failure could not yet be established while the mean time to a second failure after a revision was 15 months (range: 0-61 months).

3. Diagnostic procedures related to sphincter failure

The diagnostic evaluation of urinary incontinence after the placement of the AUS is critical for the management of these patients and represents a challenging problem for the urologist. Several diagnostic and management algorithms have been proposed, some relatively simple, others more complex [1, 27, 28, 96, 279, 296, 297]. Figure 5 shows a simple algorithm to investigate and treat the male patient with previously functioning AUS and who became incontinent.

Physical examination should exclude infection at the site of the cuff or the scrotal/labial pump. Difficulty compressing the pump suggests tube kinking, fluid loss or an obstructed system.

Cystometrogram or complete urodynamic study will demonstrate changes in bladder behavior following insertion of the AUS as described above.

Plain X-rays of the abdomen or pelvis may show fluid loss, if the system is filled with radio-opaque solution [298, 299] (Figure 1).

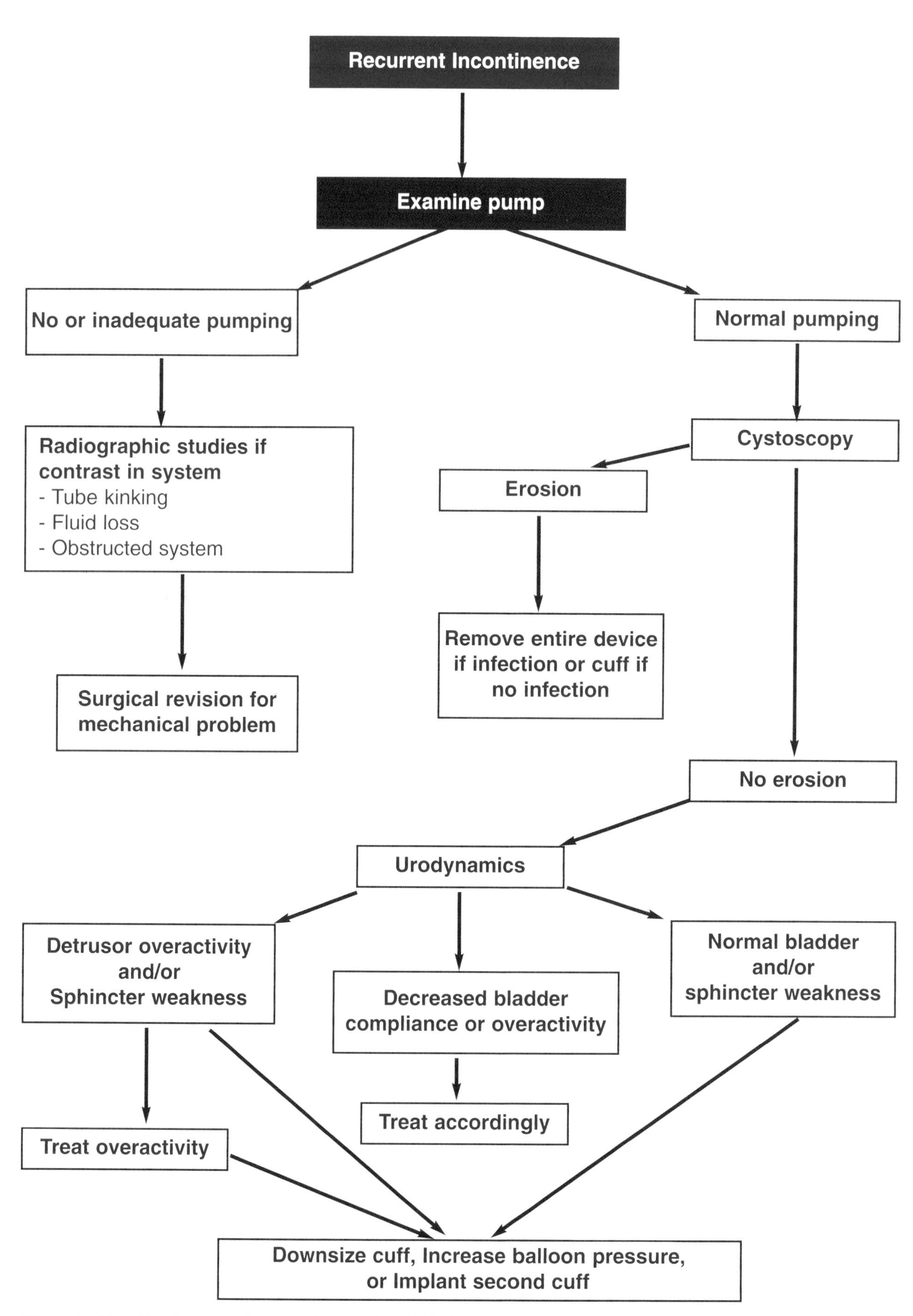

Figure 5 : Algorithm for managing incontinence after AUS placement

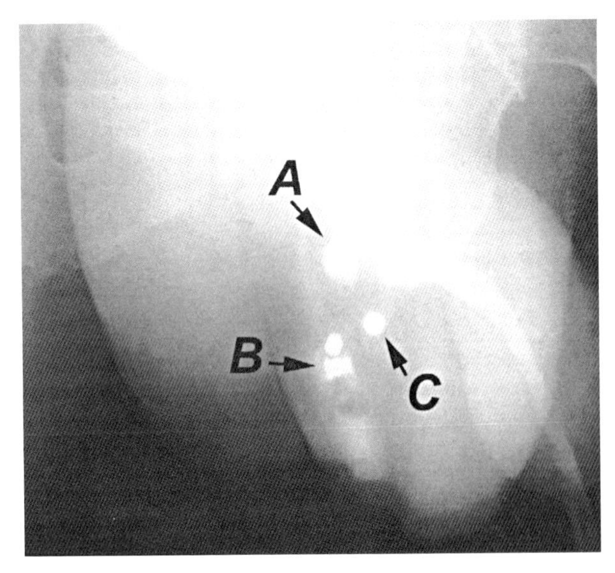

Figure 6 : Urethrogram of patient who underwent cuff removal for erosion into the urethra. A. Site of urethral diverticulum. B. scrotal pump. C. Tubing plug over tube from pump

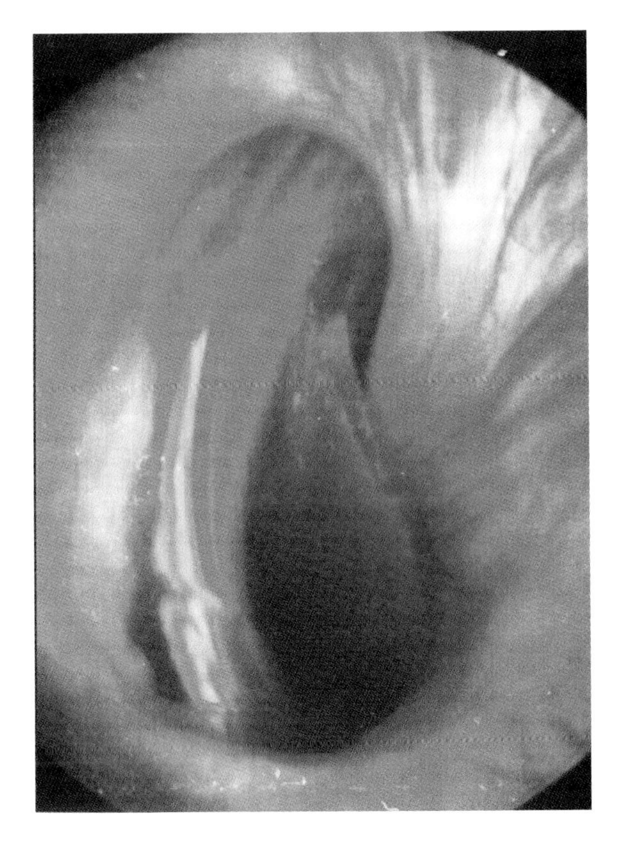

Figure 7 : Endoscopic view of AUS cuff erosion into the bulbar urethra. The patient had undergone radiation after radical prostatectomy.

Cystourethrography could eventually demonstrate a urethral diverticulum at the site of a previous cuff erosion (Figure 6).

Endoscopy will disclose any urethral erosion by the cuff (Figure 7).

Retrograde perfusion sphincterometry has been reported to diagnose the loss of compressive pressure in the urethral cuff [27]. This technique can also be used intraoperatively to detect urethral perforation or to adjust the pressure in the cuff [30]. This seems to be more useful than urethral pressure profile (UPP) [275].

Intraoperative electrical testing, using an ohmmeter [291,296] has been described to determine the site of fluid leakage from the system. This avoids the need to change the whole system, and allows replacement of the leaking part only.

4. TREATMENT OF COMPLICATIONS

As outlined above, complications directly related to the presence of an artificial urinary sphincter can be divided into categories: incontinence from alteration in bladder function, urethral atrophy, and/or mechanical failure, and infection/erosion. The treatment of each of these complications deserves comment, as no detailed reference can be found in the literature dealing with the treatment of these complications.

a) Alterations in bladder function

De novo (or pre-existing) detrusor overactivity can be treated with parasympatholytics. In a small proportion of patients systemic side effects will prevent the use of these drugs; there might also be some medical contraindications, or the drug may be ineffective. Other options such bladder autoaugmentation or enterocystoplasty may be considered. To date no report can be found where implantation of an artificial urinary sphincter resulted in a deterioration of the upper urinary tract in a post-prostatectomy or neurologically normal patient [280,300]. It has been reported that enterocystoplasty performed together with the placement of an AUS in the same operative session does not increase the morbidity of the procedure and does not affect the success rate [301]. However, in a recent review of 286 patients Furness et al. [302] demonstrated an infection rate of 14.5% and 6.8% with simultaneous and staged procedures, respectively. No clear urodynamic guidelines exist to select patients who need bladder augmentation in combination with an AUS [282].

b) Atrophy of the urethra

Several therapeutic options exist to increase cuff pressure around the atrophied urethral wall: changing the balloon reservoir for one generating a higher pressure, downsizing the cuff diameter initially by 0.5 cm [48,

303], or increasing the amount of fluid in the system. Some authors advocate the implantation of a second cuff around the urethra [304]. Others prefer the initial perineal implantation of a double-cuff AMS 800 in patients with total or severe incontinence [305]. It does not appear that morbidity increases with the double-cuff as compared to the single cuff system [305].

c) Mechanical failure

As with any device, mechanical failure can be expected with the AMS800 AUS. The treatment involves surgical replacement of the failed component and reconnecting the system.

d) Infection

With overt infection the accepted treatment option is removal of the entire device and appropriate antibiotics. A second system can be subsequently implanted with equally good results [293].

e) Erosion

In case of urethral erosion by the cuff, the "offending" cuff must be removed. No clear guidelines exist whether removal of the whole system is superior to removal of the cuff alone but it must be assessed for infection. If infection is present the whole device should be removed. Reservoir erosion into the bladder has been described following removal of an eroded cuff [306]. Furthermore, it is not known whether it is necessary to allow the urethra to heal over a catheter versus surgical repair. The former risks diverticulum formation (Figure 6) and the latter may increase the amount of periurethral fibrosis. This may compromise success of a new cuff. However, the new cuff should be positioned away from the erosion site. In case of erosion of one of the cuffs of a double cuff system removal of the eroded cuff can successfully convert a double-cuff system to a single cuff system [307].

5. Consensus protocol for follow-up of patients with AUS

As complications continue to be seen for years after implantation [308], it is helpful to have a structured follow-up plan. However, no standardized recommendations are available in the literature.

The consensus upon which the members of this subcommittee agreed and which is based on expert opinion (level of evidence 5) are as follows:

1. Antibiotics following implantation should be continued for 2 or 3 days, gram-negative enteric and Staphylococcus epidermidis being the most frequently encountered microorganisms in infected prostheses [295].
2. Hospital stay should be kept as short as possible to minimize the chances of nosocomial infections.
3. Urethral catheter should be withdrawn within 48 hours of surgery.
4. In general, the sphincter device should not be activated immediately postoperatively. In the initial period scrotal edema and pain prevent patients from manipulating the pump adequately. When this subsides after 6 to 8 weeks the device can be activated. Earlier activation may also be acceptable. Irradiated patients may benefit from a longer initial period of deactivation, up to 12 weeks [48]. Nocturnal deactivation should be considered in high-risk patients [46].
5. Patients are reviewed at 3 months after activation to ensure the device is working adequately, and to assess the continence status.
6. Long-term follow-up is different in the neurogenic and in the non-neurogenic patient. With time, alteration in bladder function can jeopardize renal function in the neurogenic patients. Periodic ultrasound evaluation of the upper urinary tract is advisable. If changes occur, urodynamic studies should be done to rule out detrusor overactivity. In non- neurogenic patients, periodic renal ultrasound may not be necessary.
7. When change in the continence status occurs diagnostic procedures related to sphincter failure (Figure 5) should be considered.

XI. NEW TECHNOLOGY - SLINGS

As a result of the cost of the AUS and the associated revisions non-prosthetic procedures are being evaluated. Shoukry and el-Salmy [309] used a rectus fascia sling to suspend the bulbar urethra to the abdominal wall in 12 men. After a mean of 13 months, 10 out of 11 patients were totally dry. One eroded sling had to be removed. Minowada et al. [310] described a sling procedure in one patient following an ileal neobladder. Elsharaby et al. [311] described an abdominal procedure for post-prostatectomy incontinence in which they lysed the pelvic urethra with preservation of the neurovascular bundles and suspended the prostatic capsule to the anterior abdominal wall in 21 men. After a mean of 19 months 17 patients were dry (81%). Kozizaki et al. [312] reported using a fascial sling around the bladder neck in 8 men and around the bulbar urethra in 2 of these men. Two males without neurogenic bladders were dry and voided normally after a mean of 36 months, while the remaining patients underwent augmentation cystoplasty and were dry or improved on intermittent catheterization.

Schaeffer et al, [313] reported a 75% success rate (67% cured, 8% improved) after a median of 18.1 months, with a bulbourethral sling suspended to the abdominal wall, in 64 men with post radical prostatectomy incontinence. The revision, erosion, and infection rates were 27, 6, and 3% respectively. Madjar et al. [314] described a bulbar sling suspended by bone anchor to the inferior pubic rami. After a mean of 12.2 months 12 of 14 patients with post radical prostatectomy incontinence were dry and 2 were improved.

XII. SUMMARY AND RECOMMENDATIONS

1. Evaluation

Prior to surgery a basic patient evaluation should consist of history and physical examination, urinalysis and postvoid residual urine. A voiding diary and pad test are very helpful. Blood testing (BUN, creatinine, glucose) is recommended if compromised renal function is suspected or if polyuria (in the absence of diuretics) is documented. Additional testing with cystoscopy and appropriate imaging of the urinary tract are also helpful in guiding therapy. Multichannel urodynamics are essential prior to invasive treatment for incontinence. A, B

2. Postprostatectomy incontinence

After a period of conservative treatment, which may be from 6 to 12 months, the artificial sphincter is the treatment of choice in appropriately selected patients with incontinence after prostatectomy for benign disease. Bulking agent therapy is of equivocal value. B, C

3. Postradical prostatectomy incontinence for prostate cancer

After a period of conservative treatment, which may also be from 6 to 12 months, the artificial sphincter is the preferred treatment for properly selected men who have stress incontinence after radical prostatectomy. Injectable agents are a less effective option for some men with mild to moderate incontinence. B, C

4. Incontinence following other treatments for prostate cancer

The artificial sphincter is most widely used but radiation may be a risk factor for an increase in complications. Injectable agents have not been successful in this setting. C

5. Incontinence following pelvic trauma

The artificial sphincter is most widely reported. Bladder neck reconstruction has also been reported on a limited basis. C

6. Incontinence in adult epispadias-exstrophy complex

Patients should be treated in centres of excellence. A patient-directed approach should be taken. The choices include further bladder neck reconstructive surgery (+/- AUS) or diversion with bowel. The data are insufficient for a specific recommendation. C, D

7. Refractory urge incontinence and detrusor overactivity

Neuromodulation is a treatment option with success reported in a limited number of patients. Detrusor myectomy has also been reported to be successful in a small number of patients. Augmentation cystoplasty is potentially successful in controlling symptoms but may be associated with unacceptable side effects. Urinary diversion is a final option. C, D

8. Reduced capacity bladder

Augmentation cystoplasty has been successful in most etiologies apart from radiation. C, D

9. Urethrocutaneous fistula and rectourethral fistula

Etiologic factors causing acquired urethrocutaneous fistulae are demonstrated by clinical, endoscopic and imaging studies. Surgical reconstruction is applied as required. Similar diagnostic maneuvers are applied to rectourethral fistulae. In those that do not close with or without temporary urinary and fecal diversion, surgical reconstruction may be carried out. Various techniques are available for closure and can be done in collaboration with colorectal surgeons. C, D

10. Management of AUS complications

Incontinence may result from alteration in bladder function, urethral atrophy, or mechanical malfunction. Infection and/or erosion of components demand surgical removal of all or part of the prosthesis. A treatment algorithm is presented to aid in management and in follow-up of patients. C, D

11. New technologies

Sub-urethral slings for postradical prostatectomy incontinence show early success. C, D

12. Recommendations for future research

- New technologies, bulking agents, sling materials, prosthetic devices should continue to be evaluated
- Clinical trial recommendations
  - Randomized trials
  - Standardized workup and outcome measures
  - Complete reporting of complications
  - Long-term results (>2 years)
  - Standardized reporting of durability

Take Home Messages

- Despite the significant revision and failure rate, the artificial sphincter is still the 'gold standard' for postprostatectomy incontinence.
- Bulking agents have an overall lower success rate than the artificial sphincter. Radiation, TURP, and cryotherapy negatively impact on the success of injectables.
- Treatment of complex incontinence problems, such as adult presentation of exstrophy epispadias complex and rectourethral fistulae, is difficult and has to be approached on an individual patient basis.
- The best surgical procedure for detrusor overactivity is still to be elucidated. Furthermore, the future of surgical treatment will depend on new developments in non-surgical therapy.
- New procedures and devices should only be introduced within the context of clinical trials.

REFERENCES

1. Herschorn S, Boccon-Gibod L, Bosch JLHR, et al.: Surgical treatment of urinary incontinence in men. In: Abrams P, Khoury S, Wein A, eds. Incontinence. Plymouth: Health publication Ltd, 1999: 691-729.
2. Mebust W, Rioso R, Schroeder F, Villers A. Correlations between pathology, clinical symptoms and the course of the disease. In A.T.K. Cockett et al., editors. Proceeding of the International Consultation on benign prostatic hyperplasia (BPH) – S.C.I., Paris – p. 53-62, 1991.
3. Blaivas JG, Zayed AAH, Labib KB. The bulbocavernosus reflex in urology: a prospective study of 299 patients. J Urol – 126:197-199,1981.
4. Griffiths DJ, McCracken PN, Harrison GM, Gormley EA. Relationship of fluid intake to voluntary micturition and urinary incontinence in geriatric patients. Neurourol Urodyn – 12:1-7, 1993.
5. Wyman JF, Choi SC, Harkins SW, Wilson MS, Fantl JA. The urinary diary in evaluation of incontinent women: a test-retest analysis. Obstet-Gynecol – 71:812-817, 1988.
6. Mouritsen L, Berild G, Hertz J. Comparison of different methods for quantification of urinary leakage in incontinent women. Neurourol Urodyn – 8:579-587, 1989.
7. S tarer P, Libow LS. The measurement of residual urine in the evaluation of incontinent nursing home residents. Arch Gerontol Geriatr – 7:75-81, 1988.
8. Diokno AC, Brown MB, Brock BM, Herzog AR, Normolle DP. Clinical and cystometric characteristics of continent and incontinent non-institutionalized elderly. J Urol – 140:567-571, 1988.
9. Fantl JA, Newman DK, Colling J et al. Urinary incontinence in adults: acute and chronic management. Clinical Practice Guideline, No 2, 1996 Update. Rockville, MD: U.S. Department of Health and Human Services. Public Health Service, Agency for Health Care Policy and Research, AHCPR Publication No 96-0682. March 1996.
10. Foote J, Yun S, Leach GE. Post-prostatectomy incontinence. Pathophysiology, evaluation and management. Urol Clin North Am – 18:229-241, 1991.
11. Leach GE, Yip CM. Urologic and urodynamic evaluation of the elderly population. Clin Geriatr Med – 2:731-755, 1986.
12. Goode PS, Locher JL, Bryant RL, Roth DL, Burgio KL. Measurement of postvoid residual urine with portable transabdominal bladder ultrasound scanner and urethral catheterization. Int Urogynecol J Pelvic Floor Dysfunct – 11:296-300, 2000.
13. Richter S, Hag'ag R, Shalev M, Nissenkorn I. Measuring residual urine by portable ultrasound scanner. Harefuah – 137:93-95, 176, 175;1999.
14. Strasser H, Frauscher F, Helweg G, Colleselli K, Reissigl A, Bartsch G. Transurethral ultrasound evaluation of anatomy and function of the rhabdosphincter of the male urethra. J Urol – 159:100-105, 1998.
15. McGuire EJ, Fitzpatrick CC, Wan J, Bloom D, Sanvordenker J, Ritchey M, Gormley EA. Clinical assessment of urethral sphincter function. J Urol – 150:1452-1454, 1993.
16. Schick E. The objective assessment of the resistance of the female urethra to stress: a scale to establish the degree of urethral incompetence. Urology – 26:518-526, 1985.
17. Peschers UM, Jundt K, Dimpfl T. Differences between cough and Valsalva leak-point pressure in stress incontinent women. Neurourol Urodyn – 19:677-681, 2000.
18. Bump RC, Elser DM, Theofrastous JP, McClish DK. Valsalva leak point pressure in women with genuine stress incontinence: reproducibility, effect of catheter size, and correlations with other measures of urethral resistance. Continence Program for Women Research Group. Am J Obstet Gynecol – 173:551-557, 1995.
19. Decter RM, Harpster L, Pitfalls in determination of leak point pressure. J Urol – 148:588-591, 1992.
20. Flood HD, Alevizatos C, Liou JL. Sex differences in the determination of abdominal leak point pressure in patients with intrinsic sphincter deficiency. J Urol – 156:1737-1740, 1996.
21. Faerber GJ, Vashi AR. Variations in Valsalva leak point pressure with increasing vesical volume. J Urol – 159:1909-1911, 1998.
22. Haab F, Dmochowski R, Zimmern P, Leach GE. Étude de la variabilité du seuil de pression de fuite à l'effort "Valsalva leak point pressure" en fonction du volume de remplissage de la vessie. Prog Urol – 7:422-425, 1997.
23. Theofrastous JP, Cundiff GW, Harris RL, Bump RC. The effect of vesical volume on Valsalva leak-point pressures in women with genuine stress incontinence. Obstet Gynecol – 87:711-714, 1996.

24. Petrou SP, Kollmorgen TA. Valsalva Leak point pressure and bladder volume. Neurourol Urodyn – 17:3-7, 1998.

25. Swift SE, Utrie JW. The need for standardization of the Valsalva leak-point pressure. Int Urogynecol J Pelvic Floor Dysfunct – 7:227-230, 1996.

26. McCormack M, Pike J, Kiruluta G. Leak point of incontinence: a measure of the interaction between outlet resistance and bladder capacity. J Urol – 150:162-164, 1993.

27. Leach GE. Incontinence after artificial urinary sphincter placement: the role of perfusion sphincterometry. J Urol – 138:529-532, 1987.

28. Wang Y, Hadley HR. Management of persistent or recurrent urinary incontinence after placement of artificial sphincters. J Urol – 1:1005-1006, 1991.

29. Comiter CV, Sullivan MP, Yalla SV. Retrograde leak point pressure for evaluating postradical prostatectomy incontinence. Urology 49:231-236, 1997.

30. Choe JM, Battino BS, Bell TE. Retrograde perfusion sphincterometry with a flexible cystoscope: method of troubleshooting the AMS 800. Urology – 56:317-319, 2000.

31. Beck R, Fowler CJ. Clinical neurophysiology in the investigation of genito-urinary tract dysfunction. In : Handbook of Neuro-Urology. Edited by D.N. Rushton. New York : Marcel Dekker, Inc. Ch. 6, p. 151-180, 1994.

32. Brown MC, Sutherst JR, Murray A, Richmond DH. Potential use of ultrasound in place of x-ray fluoroscopy in urodynamics. Br J Urol 57:88-90, 1985.

33. Bidair M, Tiechman JMH, Brodak PP, Juma S. Transrectal ultrasound urodynamics. Urology 42:640-645, 1993.

34. Manieri C, Carter SS, Romano G, Trucchi A, Valenti M, Tubaro A. The diagnosis of bladder outlet obstruction in men by ultrasound measurement of bladder wall thickness. J Urol 159:761-765, 1998.

35. Ozawa H, Chancellor MB, Ding YY, Nasu Y, Yokoyama T, Kumon H. Noninvasive urodynamic evaluation of bladder outlet obstruction using Doppler ultrasonography. Urology 56:408-412, 2000.

36. Abrams PH. Detrusor instability and bladder outlet obstruction. Neurourol Urodyn 4:317-328, 1985.

37. Steiner, M.S., Morton, R.A., Walsh, P.C.: Impact of anatomical radical prostatectomy on urinary continence. J.Urol., 145: 512, 1991.

38. Davidson, P.J.T., van den Ouden, D., Schröder, F.H.: Radical prostatectomy: Prospective assessment of mortality and morbidity. Eur.Urol., 29: 168, 1996.

39. Hautmann, R.E., Sauter, T.W., Wenderoth, U.K.: Radical retropubic prostatectomy: Morbidity and urinary continence in 418 consecutive cases. Urology, 43: suppl. Febr.: 47, 1994.

40. Fowler, F.J., Barry, M.J., Lu-Yao, G., Roman, A., Wasson, J., Wennberg, J.E.: Patient-reported complications and follow-up treatment after radical prostatectomy. The National Medicare experience: 1988-1990 (updated June 1993). Urology, 42: 622, 1993.

41. Catalona, W.J., Carvalhal, G.F., Mager, D.E., Smith, D.S.: Potency, continence, and complication rates in 1870 consecutive radical retropubic prostatectomies. J.Urol. 162: 433, 1999.

42. Wei, J.T., Dunn, R.L., Marcovich, R., Montie, J.E., Sanda, M.G.: Prospective assessment of patient reported urinary continence after radical prostatectomy. J. Urol. 164: 744, 2000.

43. Leach, G.E., Trockman, B., Wong, A., Hamilton, J., Haab, F., Zimmern, P.E.: Post-prostatectomy incontinence: urodynamic findings and treatment outcomes. J.Urol., 155: 1256, 1996.

44. Goluboff, E.T., Chang, D.T., Olsson, C.A., Kaplan, S.A.: Urodynamics and the etiology of post-prostatectomy urinary incontinence: The initial Columbia experience. J.Urol., 153: 1034, 1995.

45. Chao, R., Mayo, M.E.: Incontinence after radical prostatectomy: Detrusor or sphincter causes. J.Urol., 154: 16, 1995.

46. Montague DK: The artificial sphincter (AS800) experience in 166 consecutive patients. J Urol 147:302-304, 1992.

47. Perez LM, Webster GD: Successful outcome of artificial urinary sphincters in men with post-prostatectomy incontinence despite adverse implantation features. J Urol 148:1166-1170, 1992.

48. Martins FE, and Boyd SD: Artificial urinary sphincter in patients following major pelvic surgery and/or radiotherapy: are they less favorable candidates? J Urol 153: 1188-1193, 1995.

49. Fleshner N, Herschorn S: The artificial sphincter for postradical prostatectomy incontinence. Imapct on urinary symptoms and quality of life. J Urol 155:1201-4, 1996.

50. Mottet N, Boyer C, Chartier-Kastler E, Ben Naoum K, Richard F, Costa P.: Artificial urinary sphincter AMS 800 for urinary incontinence after radical prostatectomy: the French experience. Urol Int. 60: 25, 1998.

51. Klijn AJ, Hop WCJ, Mickisch G, Schröder FH, Bosch JLHR. The artificial urinary sphincter in men incontinent after radical prostatectomy: 5 year actuarial adequate function rates. Br. J. Urol. 82:530, 1998.

52. Madjar, S., Gousse, A.E., Lambert, M., Fishman, I.J.: Artificial urinary sphincter implantation for post radical prostatectomy urinary incontinence: which factors influence patient satisfaction? BJU international 86 (Suppl.3): 121 (abstr. P3.4.21), 2000.

53. Kuznetsov, D.D., Kim, H.L., Patel, R.V., Steinberg, G.D., Bales, G.T.: Comparison of artificial urinary sphincter and collagen for the treatment of postprostatectomy incontinence. Urology 56: 600, 2000.

54. Christie D, Hulbert P. Artificial urinary sphincters are resistant to radiotherapy. Australasian Radiology 42: 172, 1998.

55. Shortliffe LMD, Freiha FS, Kessler R, Stamey TA, Constantinou CE. Treatment of urinary incontinence by the periurethral implantation of glutaraldehyde cross-linked collagen. J Urol 141:538-541,1989.

56. Herschorn S, Radomski S, Steele D: Early experience with intraurethral collagen injections for urinary incontinence. J Urol 1992;148: 1797-1800.

57. Bevan-Thomas R, Wesley OL, Cespedes RD, et al: Long-term follow-up of periurethral collagen injections for male intrinsic deficiency. J Urol 1999; 161:257A

58. Smith DN, Appell RA, Rackley RR, Winters JC: Collagen injection therapy for post-prostatectomy incontinence. J Urol 1998; 160:364-367

59. Cespedes RD, O'Connell HE, McGuire EJ: Collagen injection therapy for the treatment of male urinary incontinence. J Rol 1996; 155:458A

60. Aboseif SR, O'Connell HE, Usui A, McGuire EJ: Collagen injection for intrinsic sphincteric deficiency in men. J Urol 1996; 155:10-13

61. Martins FE, Bennett CJ, Dunn M, Filho D, Keller T, Lieskovsky G: Adverse prognostic features of collagen injection therapy for urinary incontinence following radical retropubic prostatectomy. J Urol 1997; 158:1745-1749

62. Faerber GJ, Richardson TD: Long-term results of transurethral collagen injection in men with intrinsic sphincter deficiency. J Endourol 1997; 11:273-277

63. Griebling TL, Kreder KJ Jr, Williams RD: Transurethral collagen injection for treatment of postprostatectomy urinary incontinence in men. Urology 1997; 49:907-912

64. Cummings JM, Boullier JA, Parra RO: Transurethral collagen injection I the therapy of post-radical prostatectomy stress incontinence. J Urol 1996; 155:1011-1013

65. Elsergany R, Ghoniem GM: Collagen injection for intrinsic sphincteric deficiency in men: a reasonable option in selected patients. J Urol 1998; 159:1504-1506

66. Tiguert R, Gheller EL, Gudziak MR: Collagen injection in the management of post-radical prostatectomy intrinsic sphincter deficiency. Neurourol Urodyn 1999; 18:653-658.

67. Wainstein MA, Klutke CG: Antegrade techniques of collagen for post-prostatectomy stress urinary incontinence: indications, techniques, and results. World J Urol 1997; 15:306-309

68. Appell RA, Vasavada SP, Rackley RR Winter JC: Percutaneous antegrade collagen injection therapy for urinary incontinence following radical prostatectomy. Urology 1996; 48:769-772

69. Klutke, J.J., Subir, C., Andriole, G., Klutke, C.G.: Long-term results after antegrade collagen injection for stress urinary incontinence following radical retropubic prostatectomy. Urology 53: 974, 1999.

70. Bevan-Thomas, R., Westney, O.L., McGuire, E.J., Cespedes, R.D.: Long-term follow-up of transurethral collagen injections for male intrinsic sphincter deficiency. BJU International 86 (Suppl. 3): 121 (abstr. P3.4.19), 2000.

71. McConnell, J.D., Barry, M.J., Bruskewitz, R.C., Bueschen, A.J., Denton, S.E., Holtgrewe, H.L., Lange, J.L., McClennan, B.L., Mebust, W.K., Reilly, N.J., Roberts, R.G., Sacks, S.A., Wasson, J.H.: Benign prostatic hyperplasia: diagnosis and treatment. Clinical practice guidelines, No. 8. AHPCR Publication No.94-0582. Rockville, Maryland, Agency for Health Care Policy and Research, Public health service, US department of Health and Human Services, 1994.

72. Galluci, M., Puppo, P., Perachino, M. et al : Transurethral electrovaporization of the prostate vs. transurethral resection. Eur. Urol. 33: 359, 1998.

73. Scott, F.B.: The artificial urinary sphincter: experience in adults. Urol. Clin. N. Am., 16: 105, 1989.

74. Schreiter, F.: Operative Therapie der Harninkontinenz des Mannes. Urologe [A] 30: 223, 1991.

75. Singh, G., Thomas, D.G.: Artificial urinary sphincter for post-prostatectomy incontinence. Br.J.Urol. 77: 248, 1996.

76. Schaeffer AJ, Clemens JQ, Ferrari M, Stamey TA. The bulbourethral sling procedure for post-radical prostatectomy incontinence. J Urol 159: 1510, 1998.

77. Mundy, A.R.: The treatment of sphincter strictures. Br.J.Urol. 64: 626, 1989.

78. Zinman, L.N.: Rekonstruktion der hinteren Urethra. Urologe[A] 37: 31, 1998.

79. Lawton CA, Won M, Pilepich MV, Asbell S0, Shipley WU, Hanks GE, Cox ID, Perez CA, Sause WT, and Doggett SRL: Long-term treatment sequelae following external beam irradiation for adenocarcinoma of the prostate: analysis of RTOG studies 7506 and 7706. Int I Radiat Oncol Biol Phys 21:935-939, 1991.

80. Perez CA, Lee HK, Georgiou A, and Lockett MA: Technical factors affecting morbidity in definitive irradiation for localized carcinoma of the prostate. Int J Radiat Oncol Biol Phys 28: 811-819, 1994.

81. Shipley WU, Zietman AL, Hanks GE, Coen JJ, Caplan RI, Won M, Zagars GK, and Asbell SO: Treatment related sequelae following external beam radiation for prostate cancer: a review with an update in patients with Stages T1 and T2 tumor. J Urol 152: 1799-1805, 1994.

82. Madalinska JB, Essink-Bot ML, de Koning HJ, Kirkels WJ, van der Maas PJ, Schroder FH: Health-related quality-of-life effects of radical prostatectomy and primary radiotherapy for screen-detected or clinically diagnosed localized prostate. J Clin Oncol 19:1619-28, 2001.

83. Weil MD, Crawford ED, Cornish P, Dzingle W. Stuhr K. Pickett B. Roach M 3rd: Minimal toxicity with 3-FAT radiotherapy of prostate cancer. Seminars in Urologic Oncology. 18:127-32, 2000.

84. Hanlon AL, Watkins Bruner D, Peter R, Hanks GE: Quality of life study in prostate cancer patients treated with three-dimensional conformal radiation therapy: comparing late bowel and bladder quality of life symptoms to that of the normal population. Int J Rad Oncol, Biol, Phys. 49:51-9, 2001.

85. Jonler M, Ritter MA, Brinkmann R, Messing EM, Rhodes PR, and Bruskewitz RC: Sequelae of definitive radiation therapy for prostate cancer localized to the pelvis. Urology 44: 876-882, 1994.

86. Green N, Treible D, and Wallack H: Prostate cancer: postirradiation incontinence. J Urol 144: 307-309, 1990.

87. Lee WR, Schultheiss TE, Hanlon AL, Hanks GE: Urinary incontinence following external-beam radiotherapy for clinically localized prostate cancer. Urology 48:95-99, 1996.

88. Sandhu AS, Zelefsky MJ, Lee HJ, Lombardi D, Fuks Z, Leibel SA: Long-term urinary toxicity after 3-dimensional conformal radiotherapy for prostate cancer in patients with prior history of transurethral resection. Int J Rad Oncol Biol Phys 48:643-7, 2000.

89. Petrovich Z, Lieskovsky G, Langholz B, Bochner B, Formenti S, Streeter O, Skinner DG: Comparison of outcomes of radical prostatectomy with and without adjuvant pelvic irradiation in patients with pathologic stage C (T3N0) adenocarcinoma of the prostate. Am J Clin Oncol 22:323-31, 1999.

90. Tefilli MV, Gheiler EL, Tuguert R, Banerjee M, Forman J, Pontes JE, Wood DP Jr: Salvage surgery or salvage radiotherapy for locally recurrent prostate cancer. Urology 52:224-9, 1998.

91. Ornstein DK, Oh J, Herschman JD, Andriole GL: Evaluation and management of the man who has failed primary curative therapy for prostate cancer. Urol Clin N Amer 25:591-601, 1998.

92. Rogers E, Ohori M, Kassabian VS, et al: Salvage radical prostatectomy: outcome measured by serum prostate specifc antigen levels. J Urol 153:104-110, 1995.

93. Wang Y, and Hadley H R: Experiences with the artificial urinary sphincter in the irradiated patient. J Urol 147(3):612-3, 1992.

94. Gundian JC, Barrett DM, Parulkar BC: Mayo Clinic experience with the AS 800 artificial urinary sphincter for urinary incontinence after transurethral resection of the prostate or open prostatectomy. Urology 41:318-321, 1993.

95. Elliott DS, Barrett DM: Mayo Clinic long-term analysis of the functional durability of the AMS 800 artificial urinary sphincter a review of 323 cases. J Urol 159:1206-1208, 1999.

96. Manunta A, Guille F, Patard JJ, Lobel B: Artificial sphincter insertion after radiotherapy: is it worthwhile?. BJU Intl. 85:490-2, 2000.

97. Venn S, Greenwell TJ, Mundy AR: The long-term outcome of artificial urinary sphincters. J Urol 164:702-707, 2000.

98. Martins FE, Bennett CJ, Dunn M, Filho D, Keller T, Lieskovsky G: Adverse prognostic features of collagen injection therapy for urinary incontinence following radical retropubic prostatectomy. J Urol 158: 1745-9, 1997.

99. Beyer C Priestly JB: Biochemical disease-free survival following 1-125 prostate implantation [abstract]. Int J Radiat Oncol Biol Phys, 32: 254, 1995.

100. Blasko JC, Ragde H, Grimm PD: Transperineal ultrasound-guided implantation of the prostate: Morbidity and complications. Scand J Urol Nephrol Suppi, 137:113, 1991.

101. Stock RG, Stone NN, Dewyngaert JK: PSA findings and biopsy results following interactive ultrasound guided transperineal brachtherapy for early stage prostate cancer. In Proceedings of the American Radium Society 78th Annual Meeting, Paris,

France, 1995, p 58.

102. Wallner K, Roy J, Zelefsky M, Fuks Z, Harrison L: Fluoroscopic visualization of the prostatic urethra to guide transperineal prostate implantation. Int I Radiat Oncol Biol Phys, 29: 83-7, 1994.

103. Kaye KW, Olson DJ, Payne JT: Detailed preliminary analysis of 125-iodine implantation for localized prostate cancer using percutanous approach. J Urol, 53: 1020,1995.

104. Blasko JC, Ragde H, Luse RW, Sylvester JE, Cavanaugh W, Grimm PD: Should brachytherapy be considered a therapeutic option in localized prostate cancer? Urol Clin N Amer, 23: 633-650, 1996.

105. Hu K, Wallner K: Urinary incontinence in patients who have a TURP/TUIP following prostate brachytherapy. Int J Rad Oncol Biol Phys. 40:783-6, 1998.

106. Benoit RM, Naslund MJ, Cohen JK: Complications after prostate brachytherapy in the Medicare population. Urology. 55:91-6, 2000.

107. Merrick GS, Butler WM, Lief JH, Dorsey AT: Temporal resolution of urinary morbidity following prostate brachytherapy. Int J Rad Oncol Biol Phys 47:121-8, 2000.

108. Crook J, Lukka H, Klotz L, Bestic N, Johnston M, Genitourinary Cancer Disease Site Group of the Cancer: Systematic overview of the evidence for brachytherapy in clinically localized prostate cancer. Can Med Assn J 164:975-981, 2001.

109. Shinohara K, Connolly JA, Presti JC, Carroll PR: Cryosurgical treatment of localized prostate cancer (stages Tl to T4): preliminary results. J Urol, 156: 115, 1996.

110. Bahn DK, Lee F, Solomon MH, Gontina H, Klionsky DL, Lee FT: Prostate cancer: US-guided percutaneous cryoablation. Radiology, 190: 551, 1994.

111. Cox RL, Crawford ED: Complications of cryosurgical ablation of the prostate to treat localized adenocarcinoma of the prostate. Urology, 45: 170, 1994.

112. Wieder J, Schmidt JD, Casola G, Van Sonnemberg E, Stainken BF, Parsons CL: Transrectal ultrasound-guided transperineal cryoablation in the treatment of prostate carcinoma: preliminary results. J Urol, 154: 435, 1995.

113. Cohen JK, Miller RJ, Rooker GM, Shuman BA: Cryosurgical ablation of the prostate: two-year prostate-specific antigen and biopsy results. Urology, 7: 395, 1996.

114. Coogan CL, McKiel CF: Percutaneous cryoablation of the prostate: preliminary results after 95 procedures. J Urol, 154: 1813, 1995.

115. Sosa ER, Martin T, Lynn K: Cryosurgical treatment of prostate cancer: a multicenter review of compilations. J Urol, 155: 361, 1996.

116. Long JP, Fallick ML, Larock DR, Rand W: Preliminary outcomes following Cryosurgical ablation of the prostate in patients with clilnically localized prostate carcinoma. J Urol, 159: 477-484, 1998.

117. Pisters LL, von Eschenbach AC, Scott SM, et al: The efficacy and complications of salvage cryotherapy of the prostate. J Urol 157:921-925, 1997.

118. Derakhshani P, Neubauer S, Braun M, Zumbe J, Heidenreich A, Engelmann U: Cryoablation of localized prostate cancer. Experience in 48 cases, PSA and biopsy results. Eur Urol. 34:181-7, 1998.

119. Long JP, Bahn D, Lee F, Shinohar K, Chinn DO, Macaluso JN Jr: Five-year retrospective, multi-institutional pooled analysis of cancer-related outcomes after cryosurgical ablation of the prostate. Urology 57:518-523, 2001.

120. De la Taille A, Hayek O, Benson MC, Bagiella E, Olsson CA, Fatal M, Katz A: Salvage cryotherapy for recurrent prostate cancer after radiation therapy: the Columbia experience. Urology 55: 79-84, 2000.

121. Izawa JI, Ajam K, McGuire EJ, Scott S, von Eschenbach AC, Skibber J, Pisters LL: Major surgery to manage definitively severe complications of salvage cryotherapy for prostate cancer. J Urol 164:1978-1981, 2000.

122. Alcini E, Racioppi M, d'Addessi A, Menchinelli P, Grassetti F, Alcini A: Bladder replacement by detubularized ileal loop: 10 years experience using a personal technique. Brit J Urol 77: 688-93, 1996.

123. Cancrini A, De Carli P, Pompeo V, Fatthi H, Lamanna L, Giuseppi C, Cantiani R, Mainiero G, von Heland M: Lower urinary tract reconstruction following cystectomy: experience and results in 96 patients using the orthotopic ileal bladder substitution of Studer et al. European Urol 29: 204-9, 1996.

124. Elmajian DA, Stein JP, Skinner DG: Orthotopic urinary diversion: the Kock ileal neobladder. World J Urol 14: 40-6, 1996.

125. Studer UE, Danuser H, Hochreiter W, Springer JP, Turner WH, Zingg EJ: Summary of 10 years experience with an ileal low-pressure bladder substitute combined with an afferent tubular isoperistaltic segment. World J Urol 14: 29-39, 1996.

126. Benson MC, Seaman EK, Olsson CA: The ileal neobladder is associated with a high success and low complication rate. J Urol 155: 1585-8, 1996.

127. Abol-Enein H, Ghoneim MA: Further clinical experience with the ileal W-neobladder and a serous-lined extramural tunnel for orthotopic substitution. Brit J Urol 76: 558-64, 1995.

128. Rogers E and Scardino PT: A simple ileal substitute bladder after radical cystectomy: experience with a modification of the Studer pouch. J Urol 153: 1432-8, 1995.

129. Hautmann RE, Miller K, Steiner U, Wenderoth U: The ileal neobladder: 6 years experience with more than 200 patients. J Urol 150:40-5, 1993.

130. Hautmann RE, De Petriconi R, Gottfried HW, Kleinschmidt K, Mattes R, Paiss T, Thuroff JW: The ileal neobladder: complications and functional results in 363 patients after 11 years of followup, J Urol 161:142, 1999.

131. Steven K, Poulsen AL: The orthotopic Kock ileal neobladder: functional results, urodynamic features, complications, and survival in 166 men. J Urol 164:288-295, 2000.

132. Abol-Enein H, Ghoneim MA: Functional results of orthotopic ileal neobladder with serous–lined extramural ureteral reimplantation: experience with 450 patients. J Urol 165:1427-1432, 2001.

133. Tchetgen MB, Sanda MG, Montie JE, Faerber GJ, English S: Collagen injection for the treatment of incontinence after cystectomy and orthotopic neobladder reconstruction in women. J Urol 163:212, 2001.

134. Herschorn S, Thijssen A and Radomski SB: The value of immediate or early catheterization of the traumatized posterior urethra. J Urol 148:1428-31, 1992.

135. Kotkin L, Koch MO: Impotence and incontinence after immediate realignment of posterior urethral trauma: result of injury or management? J Urol 155: 1600-3, 1996.

136. Iselin CE, Webster GD: The significance of the open bladder neck associated with pelvic fracture urethral distraction defects. J Urol 162:347-51, 1999.

137. Jayanthi V R, Churchill BM, McLorie GA and Khoury AE: Concomitant bladder neck closure and Mitrofanoff diversion for the management of intractable urinary incontinence. J Urol 154 (Pt 2):886-8, 1995.

138. Meulen T, Zambon JV, Janknegt RA: Treatment of anastomotic strictures and urinary incontinence after radical prostatectomy with urolume wallstent and AMS 800 artificial sphincter. J Endourol 13:517, 1999.

139. Elliott DS, Boone TB: Combined stent and artificial urinary sphincter for management of severe recurrent bladder neck contracture and stress incontinence after radical prostatectomy: a long-term evaluation. J Urol 165:413-415, 2001.

140. Stein R, Fisch M, Black P, Hohenfellner R.: Strategies for reconstruction after unsuccessful or unsatisfactory primary treatment of patients with bladder exstrophy or incontinent epispadias. J Urol 161 : 1934-1941, 1999.

141. Grady WG, Mitchell ME: Complete primary repair of exstrophy. J Urol 162 : 1415-1420, 1999.

142. Gearhart JP. Editorial : The exstrophy-epispadias complex in the new millennium – science, practice & policy. J Urol 162 : 1421-1423, 1999.

143. Gearhart JP, Mathew R. Penile reconstruction combined with bladder closure in the management of classic bladder exstrophy : Illustration of technique. Urology 55 : 764-770, 2000.

144. Nicholls G, Duffy PG. Anatomical correction of the exstrophy-epispadias complex: Analysis of 34 patients. Br J Urol 82 : 865-869, 1998.

145. Hohenfellner R, Stein R. Primary bladder diversion in patients with bladder exstrophy (Editorial) Urology 48 : 828-830, 1996.

146. Canning DA. Bladder exstrophy : The case for primary bladder reconstruction (Editorial) Urology 48 : 831-834, 1996.

147. Gerharz WG, Riedmiller H, Woodhouse CR. Letter to the editor. RE : [1]. J Urol 162 : 1706-7, 1999.

148. Gearhart JP, Ben-Chaim J, Sciortino C, Sponseller PD, Jeffs RD. The multiple re-operative bladder exstrophy closure : What affects the potential of the bladder? Urology 47 : 240-243, 1996.

149. Kropp BP, Cheng EY. Total urogenital complex mobilisation in female patients with exstrophy. J Urol 164 : 1035-1039, 2000.

150. Caione P, Capozza N, Lais A, Matarazzo E. Periurethral muscle complex reassembly for exstrophy-epispadias repair. J Urol 164 : 2062-2066, 2000.

151. Kelley J. Vesical exstrophy : Repair using radical mobilisation of soft tissues. Paediatr Surg Int 10: 298-304, 1995.

152. Hollowell JG, Hill PD, Duffy PG, Ransley PG. Evaluation and treatment of incontinence after bladder neck reconstruction in exstrophy & epispadias. Br J Urol 71 : 743-749, 1993.

153. Surer I, Baker LA, Jeffs Rd, Gearhart JP. The modified Cantwell-Ransley repair for exstrophy & epispadias : 10 year experience. J Urol 164 : 1040-1043, 2000.

154. Silver RI, Gros D-Ac, Jeffs RD, Gearhart JP. Urolithiasis in the exstrophy-epispadias complex. J Urol 158 : 1322-1326, 1997.

155. Fontaine E, Leaver R, Woodhouse CRJ. The effect of intestinal reservoirs on renal function : A 10 year follow-up. Br J Urol Int 86 : 195-198, 2000.

156. Gros D-AC, Dodson JL, Lopatin UA, Gearhart JP, Silver RI, Docimo SG. Decreased linear growth associated with intestinal bladder augmentation in children with bladder exstrophy. J Urol 164 : 917-920, 2000.

157. Woodhouse CRJ, Redgrave NG. Late failure of the reconstructed exstrophy bladder. Br J Urol 77 : 590-592, 1996.

158. Husmann DA, Vandersteen DR, Mclorie GA, Churchill BM. Urinary incontinence after staged bladder reconstruction for cloacal exstrophy. The effect of co-existing neurological abnormalities on urinary continence. J Urol 161 : 1598-1602, 1999.

159. El-Ghoneimi A, Muller C, Guys JM, Coquet M, Monfort G. Functional outcome and specific complications of gastrocystoplasty for failed bladder exstrophy closure. J Urol 160 : 1186-1189, 1998.

160. Mingin GC, Stock JA, Hanna MK. Gastrocystoplasty : Long term complications in 22 patients. J Urol 162 : 1122-1125, 1999.

161. Leonard MP, Dharamsi N, Williot PE. Outcome of gastrocystoplasty in tertiary paediatric urology practice. J Urol 164 : 947-950, 2000.

162. Plaire JC, Snodgrass WT, Grady RW, Mitchell ME. Long-term follow-up of the haematuria-dysuria syndrome. J Urol 164 : 921-923, 2000.

163. Austin PF, Rink RC, Lockhart JL. The gastrointestinal composite urinary reservoir in patients with myelomeningocele and exstrophy : Long-term metabolic follow-up. J Urol 162 : 1126-1128, 1999.

164. Caione S, Nappo S, De Castro R, Prestipino M, Capozza N. Low-dose desmopressin in the treatment of nocturnal urinary incontinence in the exstrophy-epispadias complex. Br J Urol Int 84 : 329-334, 1999.

165. Yerkes EB, Adams MC, Rink RC, Pope JC, Brock JW. How well do patients with exstrophy actually void? J Urol 164 : 1044-1047, 2000.

166. Diamond DA, Bauer SB, Dinlenc C, Hendren WH, Peters CA, Atala A, Kelly M, Retik AB. Normal urodynamics in patients with bladder exstrophy : Are they achievable? J Urol 162 : 841-845, 1999.

167. Baker LA, Jeffs RD, Gearhart JP. Urethral obstruction after primary exstrophy closure: What is the fate of the genitourinary tract? J Urol 161 : 618-621, 1999

168. Terminology Report of the International Continence Society, Draft 7; 24.9.01.

169. Turner-Warwick R., Observations on the function and dysfunction of the sphincter and detrusor mechanisms. Urol Clin Norh Am 6:23, 1979.

170. Abrams PH, Bladder instability: concept, clinical association and treatment. Scand J Urol Nephrol Suppl 87:7, 1984

171. Malone-Lee JG, New data on urodynamics in the symptomatic elderly, Neurourol Urodyn 9:409, 1990

172. Godec, C, Cass, AS, Ayala, GF, Electrical stimulation for incontinence, Urology 7:388-397, 1976

173. Tanagho, E., Concepts of Neuromodulation, Neurourol Urodyn 12:487-488, 1993

174. Trsinar, B, Kraij, B, Maximal electrical stimulation in children with unstable bladder and nocturnal enuresis and or daytime incontinence : a controled study. Neurourol Urodyn 15 : 133-142, 1996

175. Primus, G, Kramer, G, Maximal External Electrical Stimulation for treatment of Neurogenic or Non-neurogenic Urgency and or Urge Incontinence, Neurourol Urodyn 15: 187-194, 1996

176. Fall, M, Does Electrostimulation cure urinary incontinence, J Urol, 131 : 664-667, 1984

177. McGuire, EJ, Shi-Chun, Z, Horwinski, ER, Lytton, B, Treatment of motor and sensory detrusor instability by electrical stimulation, J Urol 129 : 78-79, 1983

178. Siegel, SW, Richardson, DA, Miller, KL, Karram, MM, Blackwood, NS, Sand, PK, Staskin, DR, Tuttle, JP, Pelvic floor electrical stimulation for the treament of urge and mixed urinary incontinence in women, Urology 50 :934-940, 1997

179. Merril, DC, The treatment of detrusor incontinence by electrical stimulation, J Urol 122: 515-517, 1979

180. Dijkema, HE, Weil, EHJ, Mijs, PT, Janknegt, RA, Neuromodulation of Sacral Nerves for Incontinence and Voiding Dysfuncions, Eur Urol 24:72-76, 1993

181. Schmidt, RA, Treatment of Unstable bladder, Urology 37:28, 1991

182. Nakamura, M, Sakurai, T, Tsujimoto, Y, Tada, Y, Bladder inhibition by electrical stimulation of the perianal skin, Urol int 41 : 62-63, 1986

183. Nakamura, M, Sakurai, T, Suggao, H, Sonoda, T, Maximum electrical stimulation for urge incontinence, Urol int 42: 285-287, 1987

184. Bosch, JLHR, Groen, J: Sacral (S3) segmental nerve stimulation as a treatment for urge incontinence in patients with detrusor instability: results of chronic electrical stimulation using an implantable neural prosthesis. J Urol 154:504-507, 1995

185. Bosch, R, Groen, J: Disappointing results of neuromodulation in men with urge incontinence due to detrusor instability, Neurourol Urodyn, 16: 347-349, 1997

186. Shaker, HS, Hassouna, M, Sacral nerve root neuromodulation: an effective treatment for refractory urge incontinence, J Urol 159:1516-1519, 1998

187. Hassouna, M, Shaker, HS, Sacral nerve root neuromodulation: an effective treatment for refractory urge incontinence – J Urol 159:1516-1519, 1998.

188. Yamanishi, T, Yasuda, K, Sakakibara, R, Hattori, T, Suda, S, Randomized, double-blind study of electrical stimlation for urinary incontinence due to detrusor overactivity. – Urology 55:353-357, 2000.

189. Schmidt, RA, Jonas, U, Oleson, KA, Janknegt, RA, Hassouna, MM, Siegel, SW, Kerrebroeck, PEV, Sacral Nerve Stimulation for treatment of refractory urinary urge incontinece – J Urol 162:352-357, 1999.

190. Weil, EHJ, Ruiz-Cerdá, JL, Eerdmans, PHA, Janknegt, RA, Bemelmans, BLH, Kerrebroeck, PEV – Sacral root neuromodulation in the treatment of refractory urinary urge incontinence: a prospective randomized clinical trial – Eur Urol 37:161-171, 2000.

191. Bosch, JLHR, Groen, J, Sacral nerve neuromodulation in the treament of patients with refractory motor urge incontinence: long-term results of a prospective longitudinal study J Urol 163:1219-1222, 2000.

192. Swami, KS, Feneley, RCL, Hammonds, JC, Abrams, P, Detrusor myectomy for detrusor overactivity : a minimum 1-year follow-up, Br J Urol 81:68-72, 1998

193. Leng, WW, Blalock, HJ, Fredriksson, WH, English, SE, McGuire, EJ, Enterocystoplasty or detrusor myectomy ? Comparison of indications and outcomes for bladder augmentation – J Urol 161:758 763, 1999.

194. Hasan, ST, Marshall, C, Robson, WA, Neal, DE, Clinicial outcome and quality of life following enterocystoplasty for idiopathic detrusor instability and neurogenic bladder dysfunction, Br J Urol 76: 551-557, 1995

195. McInerney, PD, DeSouza, N, Thomas, PJ, Mundy, AR, The role of urodynamic studies in the evaluation of patients with augmentation cystoplasties, Br J Urol 76: 475-478, 1995

196. Bramble FJ: The treatment of adult enuresis and urge incontinence by enterocystoplasty, Br J Urol, 54: 693-696, 1982

197. Sethia, KK, Webb, RJ, Neal, DE, Urodynamic study of ileocystoplasty in the treatment of idiopathic detrusor instability, Br J Urol 67: 286-290, 1991

198. Mundy, AR, Stephenson, TP, " Clam" ileocystoplasty for the treatment of refractory urge incontinence, Br J Urol 57:641-646, 1985

199. Shokeir, AA, Ibrahim AD, Hamid MY et al : Urinary bilharziasis in Upper Egypt. I. A clinicopathological study. East Afr Med J 49:298-311, 1972

200. Smith, RB, Cangh, PV, Skinner, DG, Kaufman, JJ, Goodwin, WE, Augmentation enterocystoplasty: a critical review, J Urol 118: 35-39, 1977

201. Kerr, WK, Gale, GL, Peterson, KSS: Reconstructive surgery for genitourinary tuberculosis, J Urol 101:254-266, 1969

202. Zinman, L, Libertino, JA, Technique of augmentation cecocystoplasty. Surg Clin N Amer 60:703-710, 1980

203. Dounis, A, Abel, BJ, Gow, JG, Cecocystoplasty for bladder augmentation, J Urol 123:164-166, 1980

204. Lunghi, F, Nicita, G, Selli, C, Rizzo, M, Clinicial aspects of augmentation enterocystoplasties, Eur Urol 10:159-163, 1984

205. Shawket, TN, Muhsen, J, Treatment of bilharzial contracted bladder by ileocystoplasty or colocystoplasty, J Uro 97:285-287, 1967

206. Whitmore, WF, III, Gittes, RF, Reconstruction of the urinary tract by cecal and ileocecal cystoplasty : a review of a 15-year experience, J Urol 129:494, 1983

207. Chan, SL, Ankenman, GJ, Wright, JE, Mcloughlin, MG, Cecocystoplasty in the surgical management of the small contracted bladder, J Urol 124:338-340, 1980

208. Shirley, SW, Mirelman, S: Experiences with colocystoplasties, cecocystoplasties and ileocystoplasties in urologic surgery : 40 pacients, J Urol 120: 165, 1978

209. Goodwin, WE, Turner, RD, Winter, CC: Results of ileocystoplasty. J Urol 80:461, 1958

210. Winter, CC, Goodwin, WE: Results of sigmoidocystoplasty. 80:467, 1958

211. Fall, M, Nilsson, S: Volume of augmentation cystoplasty and persistent urgency, Scand J Urol Nephrol 16:125, 1982

212. Goldwasser, B, Webster, GD: Augmentation and substitution enterocystoplasty, J Urol 135:215224, 1986

213. Weinberg, AC, Boyd, SD, Lieskivsky, G, Ahlering, TE, Skinner, DG, The Hemi-Koch augmentation ileocystoplasty : a low pressure anti-refluxing system, J Urol 140 : 1380-1384, 1988

214. Novak, R, Surgical treatment of contracted tuberculous bladder, Tuberkuloza 2: 109-114, 1969

215. Sayegh, ES, Dimmette, RM, The fibrotic contracted urinary bladder associated with schistosomiasis and chronic ulceration : a clinicopathological study including treatment, J Urol 75:671-679, 1956

216. Beduk, Y, Anafarta, K, Baltaci, S, Adsan, O, Iskit, N, Urinary tract reconstruction in a patient with urethral stricture, contracted bladder and erectile impotence, Int Urol Nephrol 26:173-178, 1994

217. Kuo, HC, Clinical outcome and quality of life after enterocystoplasty for contracted bladders, Urol Int 58:160-165, 1997

218. Kawamura, S,Kumasaka, K, Noro, K, Aoki, H, Kubo, T, A case of replacement ileocystoplasty for contracted bladder. Hinyokika Kio 37: 1049-1052, 1991

219. Hradec, EA, Bladder substitution: indications and results in 114 operations, J Urol 94 : 406 - 47, 1965.

220. Lima, SVC, Araujo, LAP, Montoro, M, Maciel, A and Vilar, FO: The use of demucosalized bowel to augment small contracted bladders. Br J Urol 82:436-439, 1998

221. El Otmany, A, Hamada, H, Al Bouzidi, A, Oukheira, H, Boujida, M, Souadka, A, Amrani, M, Jahhid, A, Belabbas, M: Carcinome malpighien sur iléocystoplastie d´agrandissement pour vessie tuberculeusse. Progrès en Urologie 9:534-536, 1999.

222. Yamada, Y, Takenaka, A, Gotoh, K, Yamanaka, N: Augmentation ileocystoplasty and ileal ureter replacement for distal ureteral cancer in a patient with a contracted bladder. Int J Urol 6:475-478, 1999. 223.

223. Sharma A.K, Kothari S.K., Goel D., Chaturvedi V .: Pediatr.Surg.Int. 2000; 16(1-2): 142.

224. Harjai MM; Bal RK; Maudar KK Congenital urethral fistula. J.Indian Med Assoc 97: 500, 1999.

225. Caldamone-AA; Chen-SC; Elder-JS; Ritchey-ML; Diamond-DA; Koyle-MA Congenital anterior urethrocutaneous fistula. J-Urol. 1999 Oct; 162(4): 1430-2

226. Tash J.A ,Eid J.F.: Urethrocutaneous fistula due to a retained ring of condom. Urology 56: 508, 2000.

227. Porter A.T., Littrup P., Grignon D., Forman J., Montie J.E.: Radiotherapy and Cryotherapy for Prostate Cancer. In: Walsh PC, Retik AB, Vaughan Jr ED, Wein AJ, ed. Campbell's Urology, 7th Ed. Philadelphia,WB Saunders Company, pp 2605-2606, 1998.
228. Thomas R., Davis R., Ahuja S.: Toward out-patient radical prostatectomy: a cost effective cost management of patients with localized prostate cancer. BJU. (Suppl.) 80, 2, 261, 1997.
229. Fahal A.H., Sharfi A.R., Sheik H.E., el Hassan A.M., Mahgoub E.S.: Internal fistula formation: an unusual complication of mycetoma. Trans. R. Soc. Trop. Med. Hyg. 90(5), 550-2, 1996.
230. Chiou R.K., Anderson J.C., Tran R., Patterson R.H., Wobig R., Taylor R.J., McAninch J.W.: Evaluation of urethral strictures and associated abnormalities using resolution and color Doppler ultrasound. Urology 47:102,1996.
231. Blandy J.P., Singh M.: Fistulae involving the adult male urethra. Br. J. Urol. 44, 632, 1972.
232. Culp O.S., Calhoon H.W.: A variety of rectourethral fistulas: experiences with 20 cases. J. Urol. 91, 560, 1964.
233. Endo M., Hayashi A., Ishihara M., Maie M., Nagasaki A, Nishi T.,Saeki M.: Analysis of 1,992 patients with anorectal malformations over the past two decades in Japan. Steering Committee of Japanese Study Group of Anorectal Anomalies. J.Pediatr.Surg. 34: 435-41, 1999.
234. Rintala R.J.,Lindahl H.G.: Posterior sagittal anorectoplasty is superior to sacroperineal-sacroabdominoperineal pull-through: a long-term follow-up study in boys with high anorectal anomalies. J.Pediatr.Surg. 34: 334-7, 1999.
235. Smith A.M., Veenema R.J.: Management of rectal injury and rectourethral fistulas following radical retropubic prostatectomy. J. Urol. 108. 778, 1972.
236. Tiptaft R.C., Motson R.W., Costello A.J., Paris A.M.E., Blandy J.P.: Fistulae involving rectum and urethra: the place of Park's operations. Brit. J. Urol. 55, 711-715, 1983.
237. Noldus J., Graefen M., Huland H.: An "old technique" for a new approach for repair of rectourinary fistulas. J. Urol. (Suppl.) 157:1547, 1997.
238. Eastham J.A., Scardino P.T.: Radical prostatectomy. In: Walsh PC, Retik AB, Vaughan Jr ED, Wein AJ, ed. Campbell's Urology, 7th Ed. Philadelphia,WB Saunders Company, pp 2547-2564, 1997.
239. Nyam DC. Pemberton JH: Management of iatrogenic rectourethral fistula. Dis Colon & Rectum. 42:994-7, 1999.
240. Zippe C.D.: Cryosurgery of the prostate: technique and pitfalls. Urol. Clin. N. Am. 23, 147-163, 1996.
241. Montorsi F., Guazzoni G., Bergamaschi F., Galli L., Colombo R., Consonni P. Barbieri L., Rigatti P.: Transrectal prostatic hyperthermia and advanced prostatic cancer: Clinical results of one year follow up. Acta Urol. Ital. 6/Suppl. 6 (471-474), 1992.
242. Kleinberg L., Wallner K., Roy J., Zelefsky M., Arterbery V.E. Fuks Z., Harr J.K.: Treatment-related symptoms during the first year following transperineal (125) I prostate implantation. Int. J. Radiat. Oncol. Biol. Phys. 28/4 (985-990) 1994.
243. Fengler S.A., Abcarian H.: The York Mason approach to repair of iatrogenic rectourinary fistulae. Am. J. Surg. 173(3), 213-7, 1997.
244. Chang K.M., Lee R.C., Ciu A.W., Wang J.H., Chiang H.: Malakoplakia of the prostate forming a fistulous tract to rectum: a case report. Chung-Hua-I-Hsueh-Tsa-Chih-Taipei 58, 439-443, 1996.
245. Cools P., Vanderputte S., Van der Stighelen Y., Colemont L., Denis B.: Rectourethral fistula due to Crohn's disease. Acta Urol.Belg.64: 47-8, 1996.
246. Felipetto R., Vigano L., Cecchi M., Florentini L., Minervini R.: Use of fibrin sealant in the treatment of prostatic cutaneous fistula case of Pseudomonas prostatitis. Int. Urol. Nephrol. 27: 563-5, 1995.
247. Al-Ali M., Kashmoula D., Saoud I.J.: Experience with 30 posttraumatic rectourethral fistulas: presentation of posterior transsphincteric anterior rectal wall advancement. J. Urol. 158, 421-424, 1997.
248. Gibbons R.P.: Radical Perineal Prostatectomy. In: Campbell's Urology. Edited by P.C. Walsh, A.B. Retik, E.D. Vaughan, A.J. Wein. Philadelphia, Wiliam B. Saunders, 7, pp. 2589-2603, 1997.
249. Turner-Warwick R.: The use of the omental pedicle graft in urinary reconstruction. J. Urol. 116:341, 1976.
250. Ryan J.A. Jr., Beebe H.G., Gibbons R.P.: Gracilis muscle flap for closure of rectourethral fistula. J. Urol. 122:1242, 1979.
251. Venable D.D.: Modification of the anterior perineal transanorectal approach for complicated prostatic urethrorectal fistula repair. J. Urol. 142, 381-384, 1989.
252. Parks A.G., Motson R.W.: Peranal repair of rectoprostatic fistula. Brit. J. Surg. 70, 725, 1983.
253. Tiptaft R.C., Motson R.W., Costello A.J., Paris A.M.E., Blandy J.P.: Fistulae involving rectum and urethra: the place of Park's operations. Brit. J. Urol. 55:711-715, 1983.
254. Noldus J., Graefen M., Huland H.: An „old technique“ for a new approach for repair of rectourinary fistulas. J. Urol. (Suppl.) 157:1547, 1997.
255. Young HH: Repair of rectourethral fistula. In: Young's Practice of Urology, Edited by Young HH and Davis DM., Philadelphia, WB Saunders Co., vol. 2, p. 582, 1926.
256. Lewis LG: Repair of rectourethral fistulas. J Urol, 57:1173-1181, 1947.
257. Goodwin W.E., Turner R.D., Winter C.D.: Rectourinary fistula: principles of management and a technique of surgical closure. J. Urol. 80:246, 1958.
258. Kilpatrick F.R., Mason A.Y.: Postoperative recto-prostatic fistula. Brit.J.Urol.41:649-651, 1969.
259. Fengler S.A., Abcarian H.: The York Mason approach to repair of iatrogenic rectourinary fistulae. Am. J. Surg. 173:213-7, 1997.
260. Bukowski T.P., Chakrbarty A., Powell I.J., Frontera R., Perlmutter A.D., Montie J.E.: Acquired rectourethral fistula: Method of repair. J. Urol., 153:730, 1995.
261. Fournier R., Traxer O., Lande P., Tuech J.J., Vergos M.: Posterior trans-anal-sphincter approach in the management of urethro-prostate-rectal fistula. J. Urol. Paris,102:75-8, 1996.
262. Parks A.G., Motson R.W.: Peranal repair of rectoprostatic fistula. Brit. J. Surg. 70: 725, 1983.
263. Gecelter L: Transanorectal approach to the posterior urethra and bladder neck. J Urol. 109:1011-6, 1973.
264. Wilbert DM. Buess G. Bichler KH. Combined endoscopic closure of rectourethral fistula. J Urol 155:256-8, 1996.
265. Bardari F., D´Urso L., Leggero R., Coppola P., Muto G.: Conservative treatment of iatrogenic urinary fistulas: the value of a new synthetic biological glue (GLUBRAN). Eur.Urol 39, Suppl.5/1, 297, 2001.
266. Youssef A.H., Fath Alla M-. El-Kassaby A.W.: Perineal subcutaneous dartos pedicled flap as a new technique for repairing urethrorectal fistula. J.Urol. 161:1498-500, 1999.
267. Venkatesh K.S., Ramanujam P.: Fibrin glue application in the treatment of recurrent anorectal fistulas. Dis.Colon Rectum. 42:1136-9, 1999.
268. Murray KH, Nurse DE, Mundy AR. Detrusor behavior following implantation of the Brantley Scott artificial urinary sphincter for neuropathic incontinence. Br J Urol – 61:122-128, 1988.
269. Light JK, Pietro T. Alteration in detrusor behavior and the effect on renal function following insertion of the artificial urinary sphincter. J Urol – 136:632-635, 1986.
270. Bauer SB, Reda EF, Colodny AH, Retik AB. Detrusor instability: a delayed complication in association with the artificial sphincter. J Urol – 135:1212-1215, 1986.
271. Roth DR, Vyas PR, Kroovand RL, Perlmutter AD. Urinary tract deterioration associated with the artificial urinary sphincter. J Urol – 135:528-530, 1986.
272. Bitsch M, Nerstrom H, Nordling J, Hald T. Upper urinary tract deterioration after implantation of the artificial urinary sphincter. Scand J Urol Nephrol – 24:31-34, 1990.

273. Churchill BM, Gilmour RF, Khoury AE, McLorie GA. Biological response of bladders rendered continent by insertion of artificial sphincter. J Urol – 138:1116-1118, 1987.
274. Scott FB, Fishman IJ, Shabsigh R. The impact of the artificial urinary sphincter in the neurogenic bladder on the upper urinary tracts. J Urol – 136:636-642, 1986.
275. Warwick DJ, Abrams P. The perineal artificial sphincter for acquired incontinence – a cut and dried solution? Br J Urol – 66:495-499, 1990.
276. O'Flynn KJ, Thomas DG. Artificial urinary sphincter insertion in congenital neuropathic bladder. Br J Urol – 67:155-157, 1991.
277. Aprakian A, Berardinucci G, Pike J, Kiruluta G. Experience with the AS-800 artificial urinary sphincter in myelodysplastic children. Can J Surg – 35:396-400, 1992.
278. Simeoni J, Guys JM, Mollard P, Buzelin JM, Moscovici J, Bondonny JM, Melin Y, Lortat-Jacob S, Aubert D, Costa P, Galifer B, Debeugny P. Artificial urinary sphincter implantation for neurogenic bladder: a multi-institutional study in 107 children. Br J Urol – 78:287-293, 1996.
279. Ghoneim GM, Lapeyrolerie J, Sood OP, Thomas R. Tulane experience with management of urinary incontinence after placement of an artificial urinary sphincter. World J Urol – 12:333-336, 1994.
280. Montague DK, Angermeier KW. Postprostatectomy urinary incontinence: the case of artificial urinary sphincter implantation (Editorial). Urology 55:2-4, 2000.
281. Petrou SP, Elliott DS, Barrett DM. Artificial urethral sphincter for incontinence. Urology – 56:353-359, 2000.
282. Bosch JL. The contemporary role of the artificial urinary sphincter. Curr Opin Urol – 10:219-223, 2000.
283. Light JK, Reynolds JC. Impact of the new cuff design on reliability of the AS800 artificial urinary sphincter. J Urol – 147:609-611, 1992.
284. Leibovich BC, Barrett DM. Use of the artificial sphincter in men and women. World J Urol – 15:316-319, 1997.
285. Haab F, Trockman BA, Zimmern PE, Leach GE. Quality of life and continence assessment of the artificial urinary sphincter in men with minimum 3.5 years of follow-up. J Urol – 158:435-439, 1997.
286. Fishman IJ, Shabsigh R, Scott FB. Experience with the artificial urinary sphincter model AS800 in 148 patients. J Urol – 141:307-310, 1989.
287. Marks JL, Light JK. Management of urinary incontinence after prostatectomy with the artificial urinary sphincter. J Urol – 142:302-304, 1989.
288. Fulford SC, Sutton C, Bales G, Hickling M, Stephenson TP. The fate of the "modern" artificial sphincter with a follow-up of more than 10 years. Br J Urol – 79:713-716, 1997.
289. Smith DN, Fralick R, Appell RA. Incontinence after placement of a sphincter. Urology – 50:974, 1997.
290. Nurse DE, Mundy AR. One hundred artificial urinary sphincters. Br J Urol – 61:318-325, 1988.
291. Webster GD, Sihelnik SA. Troubleshooting the malfunctioning Scott artificial urinary sphincter. J Urol – 131:269-272, 1984.
292. Decter RM, Roth DR, Fishman IJ, Shabsigh R, Scott FB, Gonzales ET Jr. Use of the AS800 device in extrophy and epispadias. J Urol – 140:1202-1203, 1988.
293. Motley RC, Barrett DM. Artificial urinary sphincter cuff erosion. Experience with reimplantation in 38 patients. Urology – 35:215-218, 1990.
294. Frank I, Elliott DS, Barrett DM. Success of the novo reimplantation of the artificial genitourinary sphincter. J Urol – 163:1702-1703, 2000.
295. Martins FE, Boyd SD. Post-operative risk factors associated with artificial urinary sphincter infection-erosion. Br J Urol – 75:354-358, 1995.
296. Kreder KJ, Webster GD. Evaluation and management of incontinence after implantation of the artificial urinary sphincter. Urol Clin North Am – 18:375-381, 1991.
297. Wahle GR. Urinary incontinence after radical prostatectomy. Semin Urol Oncol – 18:66-70, 2000.
298. Taylor GA, Lebowitz RL. Artificial urinary sphincters in children: radiographic evaluation. Radiology – 155:91-97, 1985.
299. Lorentzen T, Dorph S, Hald T. Artificial urinary sphincters. Radiologic evaluation. Acta Radiol – 28:63-66, 1987.
300. Litwiller SE, Kim KB, Fone PD, de Vere White RW, Stone AR. Post-prostatectomy incontinence and the artificial urinary sphincter: a long-term study of patient satisfaction and criteria for success. J Urol – 156:1975-1980, 1996.
301. Gonzalez R, Nguyen DH, Koleilat N, Sidi AA. Compatibility of enterocystoplasty and the artificial urinary sphincter. J Urol – 142:502-504, 1989.
302. Furness PD 3rd, Franzoni DF, Decter RM. Bladder augmentation: does it predispose to prosthetic infection of simultaneously placed artificial genitourinary sphincters or in situ ventriculoperitoneal shunts? BJU Int – 84:25-29, 1999.
303. Barrett DM, Licht MR. Implantation of the artificial genitourinary sphincter in men and women. In : P.C. Walsh, A.B. Retik, E.D. Vaughan jr, A.J. Wein (Editors) : Campbell's Urology – 7th edition. Philadelphia: W.B. Saunders. Ch. 36, pp. 1121-1134, 1998.
304. Brito CG, Mulcahy JJ, Mitchell ME, Adams MC. Use of a double cuff AMS800 urinary sphincter for severe stress incontinence. J Urol – 149:283-285, 1993.
305. Kowalczyk JJ, Spicer DL, Mulcahy JJ. Erosion rate of the double cuff AMS800 artificial urinary sphincter: long-term follow-up. J Urol – 156:1300-1301, 1996.
306. Bartoletti R, Gacci M, Travaglini F, Sarti E, Selli C. Intravesical migration of AMS 800 artificial urinary sphincter and stone formation in a patient who underwent radical prostatectomy. Urol Int 64:167-168, 2000.
307. Bell BB, Mulcahy JJ. Management of cuff erosion of the double cuff artificial urinary sphincter. J Urol – 163:85-86, 2000.
308. Hajivassiliou CA. A review of the complications and results of implantation of the AMS artificial urinary sphincter. Eur Urol – 35:36-44, 1999.
309. Shoukry MS, el-Salmy S: Urethral needle suspension for male urinary incontinence. Scandinav J Urol Nephrol 31: 267 70, 1997.
310. Minowada S, Sasaki Y, Kano M, Okano Y: Sling operation for male urinary incontinence after ileal neobladder construction: a case report. Int J Urol 2: 132-4, 1995.
311. Elsharaby M, Abo-Farha O, Rasheed M, Omar A, Elgamasy OA, Ghoneim G: A new technique for treatment of simple post-prostatectomy urinary incontinence: preliminary experience. J Urol 156: 1972-4, 1996.
312. Kakizaki H, Shibata T, Shinno, Y, Kobayashi S, Matsumura K, Koyangi T: Fascial sling in the management of urinary incontinence due to sphincter incompetence. J Urol 153: 644-7, 1995.
313. Schaeffer AJ, Clemens JQ, Ferrari M, Stamey TA: The male bulbourethral sling procedure for post-radical prostatectomy incontinence. J Urol 159:1510-1515, 1998.
314. Madjar S, Jacoby K, Giberti C, Wald M, Halachmi S, Issaq E, Moskovitz B, Beyar M, Nativ O: Bone anchored sling for the treatment of post-prostatectomy incontinence. J Urol 165:72-6, 2001.

Committee 11 C

Surgical Treatment of Incontinence in Women

Chairman

A.R.B. Smith (U.K.)

Members

F. Daneshgari (USA),

R. Dmochowski (USA),

G. Ghoniem (USA),

G. Jarvis (U.K.),

V. Nitti (USA),

M. Paraiso (USA)

CONTENTS

Surgical Treatment of Incontinence in Women

T. Smith,

F. Daneshgari, R. Dmochowski, G. Ghoniem, G. Jarvis, V. Nitti, M. Paraiso

INTRODUCTION

The committee was asked to critically review the literature on the surgical treatment of incontinence in women. The literature on surgery for stress incontinence is large but has many shortfalls. These are detailed and the confounding variables which make it difficult to compare one paper or procedure with another are reviewed.

The remainder of the chapter includes surgery for urethral diverticulae, refractory detrusor instability and non-obstetric fistulae. This literature is almost entirely based on case series making critical review more limited. Whist not under-estimating the difficulty in conducting well constructed, prospective, randomised trials of surgical treatment the review highlights the need for such trials to be performed.

SURGERY FOR STRESS INCONTINENCE

1. Historical background

Surgery for stress incontinence of urine has been performed on women for over a century. The emphasis in the earlier reports focused predominantly on technical aspects of the surgery. In an attempt to address the problem of failure noted with vaginal continence surgery, (Bailey 1954) first classified types of stress incontinence according to the anatomical relationship between urethra and bladder, using radiographical studies. This classification was simplified by (Green 1973) and further modified by (McGuire 1976). However, by the early 70's the anterior vaginal repair was still the most popular primary procedure for stress incontinence. Failure or recurrence would be followed by a retropubic procedure. Over the last two decades this approach has been criticized because of the high recurrence rates reported for the vaginal repair and the more favourable and sustained results from retropubic surgery.

2. Literature shortfalls

The literature on surgery for stress incontinence is extensive. There are many deficiencies in the literature which make it difficult to compare the relative merits of the numerous procedures described. Case selection is varied and often not well described. Pre and post-operative assessment varies from full urodynamics including pad tests to symptoms review alone. The surgical technique and peri-operative complications are often ommitted. It has long been recognised that the risk of recurrence for any procedure is maximal in the first 2 years and continues with advancing age thereafter. Despite this, many reports include short-term follow up thereby producing an over-optimistic view of outcome.

Cure is defined in many different ways, both subjective and objective. The impact of complications from bladder neck surgery has only more recently been studied. What is the value of a procedure which cures stress incontinence but replaces it with urge incontinence or voiding dysfunction? Recent reports which include the social impact of stress incontinence surgery and the effect on Quality of Life help to address this question.

The inclusion of women whose symptoms have "significantly improved" with those who are cured is common. This group is often not well defined yet may greatly affect the apparent merit of a procedure. Research into the relationship between improvement of symptoms and objective parameters is needed.

The majority of surgical reports published, even in recent years, lack clarity in defining many of the variables that may influence outcome. In this chapter we have highlighted a number of confounding variables which might be expected to influence outcome. It is apparent that the level of evidence for most of these is such that no conclusions can be drawn about their level of impact or indeed whether they have any impact at all.

In order that the reader can evaluate the literature more clearly levels of evidence have been included for each of the surgical procedures described.

Ultimately, the role or value of a procedure will depend

on which outcome measure you choose to study. Some women regard absolute continence as the most important outcome. For them, a simple pad test would provide an adequate objective analysis of the chance of success from a procedure. Some women, whilst regarding continence as desirable, prefer to minimize the risk of complications such as voiding dysfunction. For them additional information on the risks is required. How much the complications of continence surgery impact on a woman's quality of life has not been fully studied. This needs to be addressed to determine whether surgery for stress incontinence should be offered on a one operation for all women basis or by selection of the procedure according to the outcome required. Currently most surgeons have a favourite procedure they use for women with stress incontinence. Some surgeons, particularly those with an interest in the field, will attempt to select the procedure according to pre-operative findings. The section on confounding variables highlights the difficulty in doing this accurately or at least on a scientific basis.

3. Review of procedures

a) Anterior colporrhaphy (Figure 1)

The anterior colporrhaphy procedure is perhaps better termed the anterior repair with bladder buttress when relating to the surgery for genuine stress incontinence. Anterior colporrhaphy and the Kelly type repair are also a part of pelvic reconstructive surgery for prolapse (vide infra).

Case report literature indicates a wide range of continence rates following this procedure, ranging between 31% and 100% continence (Jarvis 1994a). Meta-analyses of heterogenous studies suggest a continence rate of between 67.8 and 72.0% (Jarvis 1994a,b).

Randomised trials which include anterior colporrhaphy in one arm and generally suprapubic surgery in the other show a continence rate of 66% (Jarvis 1998). Only 257

women received anterior repair and were compared, in seven trials, with 454 comparable women randomised to another intervention.

The anterior colporrhaphy procedure remains in contemporaneous use largely because of the relatively low morbidity of the procedure. The 'serious complication rate' is in the region of 1%, the incidence of de novo detrusor instability is not greater than 6%, and compared with colposuspension there may be a shorter hospital stay and a 50% decrease in blood loss. The incidence of long-term voiding disorders following this procedure approaches zero (Jarvis 1994b, Beck 1991, Jarvis 1981, Loughlin 1982).

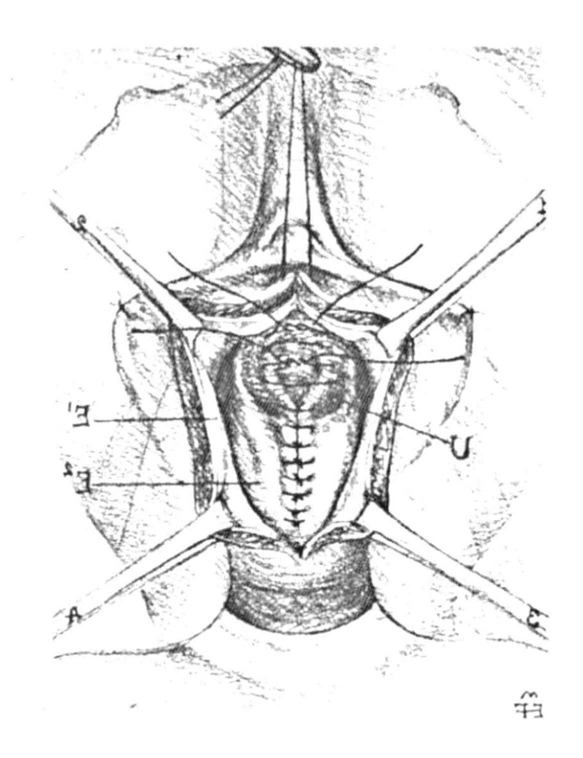

Figure 1 : The anterior repair is conventionally performed through a midline anterior vaginal wall incision. The diagram illustrates the creation of a layer of endopelvic fascia to provide additional support to the urethra.

Long-term results decrease with time such that a 63% cure rate at 1 year of follow up fell to 37% at 5 years of follow up (Bergman 1995). Long term follow up beyond the first year was only available in 3 randomised control trials (RCT). (Bergman 1989), (Liapis 1996), (Colombo 2000).

The view of the American Urological Association is that 'Anterior repairs are the least likely of the four major operative categories (anterior repair, suburethral sling, colposuspension, long needle suspension) to be efficacious in the long-term' (Leach 1997).

The literature regarding the anterior vaginal repair has also been reviewed fully by the Cochrane Library (Glazener 2000)

CONCLUSION

The view of the First International Consultation on Incontinence was 'Perhaps the major indication for bladder buttress in contemporary practice must be the patient who prefers to sacrifice some degree of chance of becoming continent for a reduced chance of complication' (Jarvis 1998)(Level 1). There is no scientific information which should lead to a revision of these opinions. (Recommendation Grade A)

b) Colposuspension (Figure 2)

Sixteen substantive articles were reviewed. Two of the studies are prospective randomised trials and 9 are prospective non-randomised studies. These articles report the treatment outcome on a total of 1363 women who underwent Burch colposuspension for stress urinary incontinence, mean age of 51 years. Among these women, 267 patients had had a previous anti-incontinence surgery. The mean cure rate (as defined by a combination of subjective and objective evidence) was 79% with an improvement rate of 90%. The follow up duration was 9 months to 16 years. The immediate and longer term results from colposuspension suggest that the procedure remains effective with time. There are two studies which report 5+ years cure rates of 82% (Alcalay 1995, Bergman 1989) Bergman (1995) reported a 90% continence rate at 8 years whilst Kjolhede (1994) reported only 55% cure at 10 years. Alcalay (1995) reported a gradual decline in success rate from 88% at 2 years to a plateau of 69% once 12 years or longer had been reached.

Voiding dysfunction has been reported in a mean of 10.3% of women after colposuspension (range 2-27%). De novo detrusor instability has been described in a mean of 17% women (range 8-27%). Genito-urinary prolapse (enterocoele, rectocoele or cystocoele has been reported in colposuspension follow up at 5 years in an average of 13.6% women (range 2.5 – 26.7%). This is reviewed later in the section under stress incontinence and prolapse. Other complications are reviewed in a separate section on complications. There was no reported mortality as a direct consequence of the procedure. The summary of the data is presented in table-1.

• **Marshall-Marchetti-Krantz**

The Marshall-Marchetti-Krantz (MMK) retropubic procedure was a common anti-incontinence procedure between 1950-90's. Krantz (Krantz 1980) described a personal series of 3861 cases with a follow up of up to 31 years and a 96% subjective cure rate. The success of MMK in treating SUI in women is reviewed in 58 articles that are predominantly retrospective studies between 1951-1998. The preoperative assessment was mainly with history and physical examination, with few studies reporting on other objective data such as urodynamic or pad test. These articles reported the treatment outcomes in a total of 3238 cases. The reported cure rate (mostly subjectively defined) was 88% (2850 patients). The improvement rate is reported as 91% (2946 patients). As a primary procedure in 1211 cases, the MMK had a success rate of 92%. In 1046 repeat cases, the success rate was 84%. The remaining 981 procedures could not be classified as primary or repeat. The mortality was 0.2%, with 22% overall complication rate. The one complication which would appear to limit the use of this procedure is osteitis pubis, a complication in 2.5% of these patients who undergo a MMK procedure (Mainprize 1988).

The longer term follow up data is limited. In the largest long term follow up series published, McDuffie reported a subjective continence rate of 89.7% at one year, 85.7% at 5 years and 75% at 15 years (McDuffie 1981)

CONCLUSION

Retropubic suspension can be expected, in primary or secondary surgery, to generate a mean cure rate of 79% and an improvement rate of 90% (Level 2). A decrease in continence rate is observed with time (Level 3).

c) Paravaginal repair

The concept of a paravaginal defect repair is, at least in theory, a logical one. It was first described by White in 1909 (White 1909) but the type of repair described by Kelly four years later (Kelly 1913) became more popluar. The Kelly type of anterior repair for genuine stress incontinence provides some central support but if there is deficiency in lateral support, then a central repair can only be of a limited benefit. It would be more logical to find the defect in the endopelvic fascia and repair it either in isolation or in combination with other procedures. Such defects in the fascia have been identified unilaterally and bilaterally, medially and laterally.

Individual cohort studies have suggested a subjective cure rate of 97% in patients undergoing a paravaginal repair (Schull 1989). However, there is as yet only a single published randomised comparison of colposuspension with paravaginal defect repair. In this study 36 patients were identified at the time of surgery when they were randomly allocated to treatment by either colposuspension or defect repair using non-absorbable suture material. At follow-up six months after surgery, there was an objective cure rate of 100% for those patients undergoing colposuspension but only 72% for those undergoing paravaginal repair (Colombo 1996).

CONCLUSION

Whilst there is some eveidence that repair of paravaginal defects may result in cure of stress incontinence (Level 2) there is also Level 1 evidence that paravaginal repair, performed abdominally, is less effective than colposuspension. Thus, at the current state of knowledge, the importance of recognition or repair of paravaginal defects is uncertain.

Table 1 : Summary of reported data on Retropubic suspension procedures for treatment of SUI in Women

Reference	Type of Op	No of Pts	Duration Follow up	Median age	Success criteria	Cure rate	Success rate
Alcalay M	Burch	109	13.8 yrs	46.6	Subjective -Objective clinically or on UD	70%	N/A
Bergman A 1989	Burch	101	1 yr	57	ICS criteria	87%	N/A
Bergman A 1995	Burch	33	5 yrs	55	UD and subjective cure	71%	N/A
Colombo M 1996	Burch	18	3 yrs	47.8	Subjective - Dry	100%	N/A
Feyereisi J 1994	Burch	87	5-10 yrs	49.9	Success of Fail – Dry or not	81.6%	N/A
Enzelberger H 1996	Burch	36		59.8	Dry	86%	N/A
Pentinen J) 1989	Burch	24		47	Dry, subjective satisfaction 9	6%	96%
Richmond D.H 1989	Burch	15		0	Dry	N/A	87%
Galloway N.T.M 1987	Burch	50		0	VUD	84%	N/A
van Geellen J.M 1988	Burch	34		46	Subjective satisfaction, VUD	75.8%	90%
Mutlu N 1997	Burch	98		0	Dry and Subjective	N/A	67%
Maher C1999	Burch	53		0	Women had no or occasional stress or urge incontinence	N/A	89%
Drouin J 1999	Burch	79		0	By Questionnaire Subjective	56%	81%
Akpinar H	Burch	50		0	Dry, subjective satisfaction	52%	82%
Maher C	Burch	50		0	No or occasional (<one episode per week)	72%	89%
Lee RA 1975	MMK	36		0	Dry	96%	N/A
Riggs JA 1986	MMK	490		0	Dry and Subjective	N/A	93%
Fatthy H	Lsc Burch	37 37	1.5 yrs				88% Lsc 85% Open
Summit RL	Lsc Burch	34 28	1 yr		Dry and Objective	93% Lsc 88% Open	
Su TH	Lsc Burch	46 46	1 yr			80% Lsc 96% Open	
Burton G	Lsc Burch	30 30	5 yrs		Urodynamic studies	57% Lsc 90% Open	
Persson J	Lsc Burch	83	1 yr		Pad test and subjective	83%	

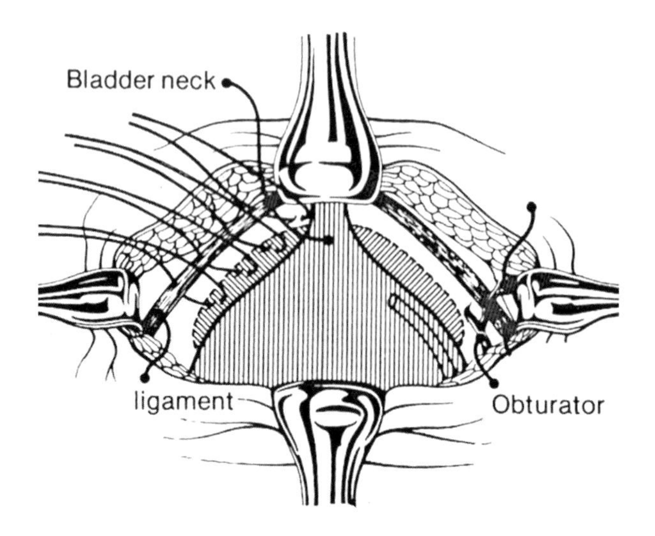

Figure 2 : The diagram illustrates the location of colposuspension sutures lateral to the urethra and bladder neck. A minimum of two sutures are normally placed bilaterally.

d) Laparoscopic colposuspension (Figure 3)

Although several case series and cohort studies show similar cure rates between laparoscopic and open Burch colposuspension, four prospective trials show similar or lower cure rates associated with laparoscopic Burch. Fatthy et al (Fatthy 200) and Summitt (2000) et al performed identical procedures by both routes and showed similar cure rates. The main criticisms of Burton's trial (Burton 1999) are that he had not gained sufficient experience with laparoscopic surgery prior to embarking on the study and that the suture used was absorbable with a small needle, which may have included insufficient thickness of tissue. Similarly, Su et al (1997) used three absorbable sutures in the open Burch compared to a single non absorbable suture in the laparoscopic procedure. Persson and Wolner Hanssen (Persson 2000) randomised patients to a one suture versus two suture laparoscopic colposuspension and found a significantly higher cure rate with the two stitch procedure at 1 year, 83% vs 58%. Unfortunately, Summitt et al (2000) and Burton's (1999) trials are published in abstract form only at present. In 2001 Morris et al (Morris et al 2001) reported on the 5 year follow up of a randomised, prospective study of 72 patients in which pre and post-operative subjective and objective assessment was performed. In this study laparoscopic colposuspension produced a cure rate of 77% at 5 years compared to a cure rate of only 48% for open colposuspension on objective testing. It is uncertain how much the experience of the surgeons influenced the results since the majority of the laparoscopic procedures were performed by a single surgeon whereas the open procedures were performed by a variety of surgeons. During the First International Symposium for Incontinence in Monte Carlo, Monaco, the laparoscopic Burch colposuspension was viewed with reservation because of lack of long-term follow up. The importance of avoiding compromise of the procedure by using tacks and mesh or placing fewer sutures because of technical difficulty of laparoscopic suturing must be stressed. Although quality of evidence is improving, more studies with long-term follow up are still required.

CONCLUSION

Although there are over 90 articles published on laparoscopic colposuspension the data is influenced by many confounding variables. A meta-analysis of the RCTs published by Fatthy, Summitt, Su and Burton show a continence rate of 80% for laparoscopic colposuspension compared with 90% for open colposuspension (Level 2). If the Glasgow study (Morris et al 2001) is included in the meta-analysis laparoscopic colposuspension is shown to be at least as effective. At this stage we must conclude that there is insufficient data available to determine the value of laparoscopic colposuspension.

e) Needle suspensions (Figure 4)

Multiple suspension procedures have been described in the past. The first procedure being described by Peyrera (1959). This was a standard needle type suspension. Numerous procedures have subsequently evolved from this including the Gittes procedure (an incision-less

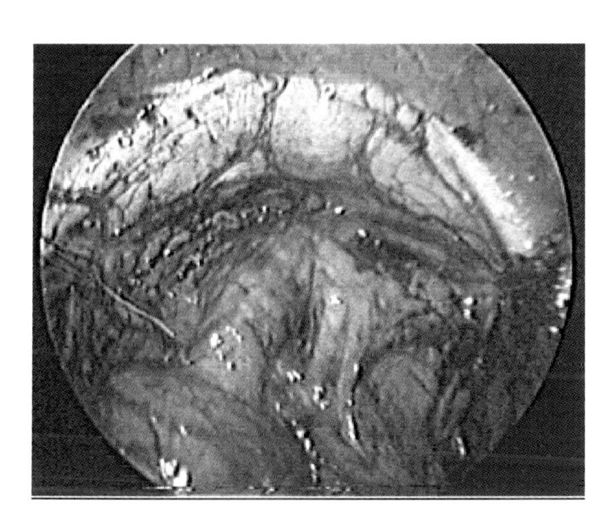

Figure 3 : The picture illustrates the view of the retropubic space seen through a laparoscope, after colposuspension has been performed

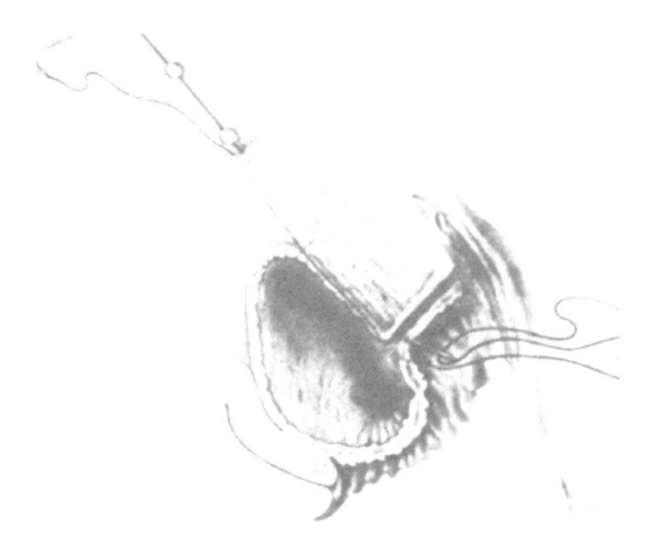

Figure 4 : The Stamey needle suspension is illustrated. The Stamey needle and suture is passed through the retropubic space from above and the suture is retrieved through a vaginal wound on each side of the urethra.

needle suspension procedure) and the Stamey procedure (Stamey 1973), utilizing suspending sutures and patch materials. Recently, procedures have evolved to the percutaneous bladder neck suspension utilizing bone anchors and a suspending system. The largest experience with these procedures was obtained by Raz (1992)

However, long-term follow up rates have recently been reported in two large group studies. Trockman et.al (1995) reported 77 patients at mean follow up of 9.8 years. These patients were surveyed by questionnaire means. At mean follow up only 20% of patients reported no incontinence of any type with 51% of patients reporting stress incontinence with or without urgency incontinence. 71% of patients reported significant improvement in incontinence and 73% were satisfied with the long-term success of the procedure.

Further long-term follow up of the percutaneous needle procedure specifically was reported by Tebyani et al (Tebyani), who reported 49 patients who underwent percutaneous bladder neck suspension, of whom 42 were available for interview. Mean follow up was 29 months (range 16 to 52 months). Only 5% of patients were cured of their stress incontinence with 12% significantly improved and 83% considering themselves a failure. In the only randomised controlled trial comparing Peyrera type suspension procedures and retropubic suspensions by Karram and Bhatia (Karram 1992), retropubic suspensions were found to be associated with a higher objective cure rate (98% versus 85% at minimum 1-year follow up). This study has been criticized because of alterations made in the type of suspending suture utilised in the Peyrera procedure performed in the inclusion criteria. Nonetheless, this does represent a randomised controlled trial, which was performed by the authors in an effort to compare these procedures directly.

CONCLUSIONS

The long term data indicates that the initial success rates reported with needle suspension procedures are not maintained with time.(Level 3) The risk of failure is higher than reported with retropubic suspension procedures (Level 1)

There would appear to be few, if any, indications to perform a needle suspension procedure. (Grade A recommendation)

f) Slings

Suburethral sling procedures were developed initially in 1888, by Schultze. Numerous authors have subsequently modified these procedures including Goebell and Stockell, who utilised pyramidalis muscle to form a muscular sheath beneath the urethra. This was subsequently modified by Frangheim to utilize strips of rectus fascia, which were left attached to the pyramidalis muscular group. Giordano also proposed utilization of muscle flaps and described the transposition of the gracilis muscle in a suburethral location. Martius utilised the bulbocavernosus muscle and associated fat to provide bulk around the urethra in a further modification of the procedure.

Miller (Miller 1947) utilised strips of rectus to elevate the bladder neck; and Price (Price 1933) used strips of fascia lata and fixed the two ends to the rectus muscles. In 1942 Aldridge (Aldridge1942) utilised rectus sheath strips and reported the technique in one patient and described the procedure as a salvage type operation for those women who had failed prior procedures (Figure 5).

The suburethral sling procedure has since been used predominantly as a treatment for patients who remain incontinent despite previous bladder neck surgery. Used in such an indication, the success rate recorded in the literature would appear to range between 64% and 100% with a mean cure rate in the region of 86% (Jarvis 1994 a, Jarvis 1994 b). The cohort literature relating to the use of a suburethral sling as a first procedure is

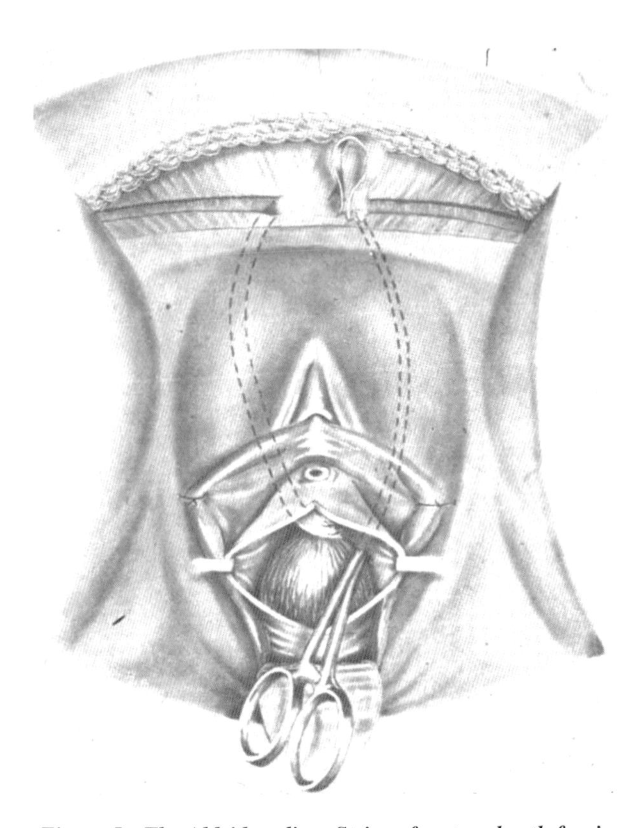

Figure 5 : The Aldridge sling. Strips of rectus sheath fascia are passed through the retro-pubic space and fixed under the urethra.

limited but a mean continence rate of 93.9% is quoted (Jarvis 1994 b).

Numerous materials are available for use in a suburethral sling. As a generalisation, autologous material is associated with a greater cure rate and fewer complications than either cadaveric material or synthetic materials (Bidmead 2000). Autologous rectus fascia and fascia lata are probably the commonest materials in use. Allogenic grafts harvested from a cadaveric donor are widely used. They do not seem to carry a risk of erosion and although the short-term results appear satisfactory, there appears to be a longer term material failure rate from fascia lata allografts in excess of 20% (Singla 2000, Fitzgerald 1999). The failure rate ascribed to cadaveric fascia lata is largely from the series reported by Fitzgerald et al (Fitzgerald 1999). This, however, was not replicated in data reported by Elliot and Boone (Elliot 2000), Amundsen et al (Admundson 2000)), Brown et al (Brown 2000), and Wright et al (Wright 1998). There seems to be wide variability in the quality of tissue; depending on its source and processing. Inconsistent fascia may lead to inconsistent results. The rationale for using allo and xenografts for suburethral slings is reinforcement of inherently weak endopelvic fascia. It remains to be seen whether this adds to the body's restorative processes of healing by fibrosis and granulation.

Long-term follow up at 48 months or greater (Morgan 2000) has revealed success rates that are persistent at greater than 90% with time. Morgan (Morgan 2000) reported a 10-year follow up of 247 women with type II and III incontinence. These patients were followed urodynamically, as well as with quality of life questionnaires. At a mean follow up of 51 months, continence rates were 88% overall with a 91% cure rate for type II and 84% for type III. Preoperative urge incontinence resolved in 81 of 109 (74%), while *de novo* urgency developed in 7% of women. Secondary procedures were necessitated in 14 patients for management of incontinence. 235 of the 247 women (95%) completed questionnaire data and 92% reported a high degree of satisfaction with resolution of symptoms.

Synthetic material tends to be associated with a risk of erosion and sinus formation (Duckett 2000). Modifications designed to achieve greater stabilisation, such as anchorage to the pubic bone, are associated with good results in the short-term but carry a longer term risk of osteomyelitis at the site of anchorage (Kovan 1997, Valley 1997).

The most extensive experience has been obtained utilizing Mersilene, which was initially described by Telind. Moir in 1968 (Moir 1968) reported an 83% cure or substantial improvement in incontinence with few complications. Other authors have reported success rates including the following: Nichols (Nichols 1973) reported 22 patients with a 1 to 2-year follow up with a 95% subjective cure rate without reported complications subjective. Herbertson (Herbertson 1993) reported 44 patients with follow up ranging from 3 to 11 years with a subjective success rate of 73% with 7 patients requiring sling revision for obstruction. Kersey (Kersey 1983) reported 100 patients with a 6-month to 5-year follow up with a 78% subjective cure rate with 2 suture exposures and approximately 23% persistent detrusor instability postoperatively. Recent studies include those of Guner (Guner 1994), who reported 24 patients with a 24-month follow up with a 96% subjective cure rate with a 4% persistent urge incontinence rate. Also, Young (Young 2001) reported 110 patients with a 13-month minimum follow up with 95% subjective and 93% objective cure rates. Two patients experienced vaginal erosions and one patient developed an inguinal sinus. These rates would imply fairly low rates of complications with this material.

Results using Gore-Tex have included Horbach (Horbach 1988) who reported 13 patients with 3 to 18-month follow up and an 85% subjective cure rate with 1 sling revision and 1 sling removal for sinus tract.

Silastic has been utilised by several authors. Chin (Chin 1995), who reported 30 patients with a 3 to12-month follow up and an 83% subjective cure rate, noted 4 sling removals for persistent retention and 1 patient with vesicovaginal fistula, and a 67% rate of de novo detrusor instability.

Overall, with all of these materials the risk of vaginal erosion ranges from zero to approximately 16%. Urethral erosion ranges from zero to 5%. De novo detrusor instability ranges from 3.7% to 66%, and procedures requiring sling revision or removal range from 1.8% to 35% of patients included in these studies.

When compared with colposuspension procedures, the suburethral sling carries a similar success rate (Jarvis 1998). This appears to be true even in patients with low maximal urethral closure pressure (Sand 2000). However, these studies involved small number of patients, short follow up and evaluated patients with a low-pressure urethra. This is not synonymous with intrinsic sphincter deficiency. In addition, the same author (Sand 1987) identified low-pressure-urethra as a risk factor for failure of colposuspension in a previous publication. (See section on urethral occlusive forces).

The intermediate and longer term results for suburethral slings suggest that the 10 year continence rate is not dissimilar from the 1 year continence rate (Jarvis 1988, Chaikin 1988).

Up to 10.8% of patients have some voiding disorder symptoms subsequent to the immediate post-operative period (Jarvis 1994b, Bidmead 2000). Long-term self-catheterisation has been reported in anywhere between 1.5 and 7.8% of patients, although a figure of 2% may be more realistic (Jarvis 1994 a, Bidmead 2000, Chaikim). De novo detrusor instability may arise in between 3 and 23% of patients and appears to be greater in patients who have urinary urgency but an apparently stable bladder pre-operatively (Jarvis 1994b, Leach 1997, Chaikin 1998).

The American Urological Association considered that 'Retropubic suspensions and slings are the most efficacious procedures for long-term success based upon cure/dry rate. However, in the panel's opinion, retropubic suspensions and sling procedures are associated with slightly higher complication rates, including post-operative voiding dysfunction and longer convalescence. In patients who are willing to accept a slightly higher complication rate for the sake of long-term cure, retropubic suspensions and slings are appropriate choices' (Leach 1997). The First International Consultation on Incontinence concluded that suburethral slings represented 'An effective procedure for genuine stress incontinence in the presence of previous failed surgery' (Jarvis 1998). A recent survey of North American Urological Surgeons showed a significant trend towards surgeons performing suburethral sling procedures in 1999 when they rarely performed such procedures in 1995 (O'Leary 2000). The Editor of the Journal of Urology considered 'Slings - an idea whose time has come' (Loughlin 2000).

CONCLUSION

Long term data suggests that sling procedures, using autologous or synthetic materials, produce a cure rate of approximately 80% and an improvement rate of 90% (Level 3). There is some data which shows that autologous material is associated with a higher cure rate and fewer complications than either cadaveric or synthetic material but there is a need to scientifically study whether the choice of material influences outcome.There is a need to address whether the choice of material influences the outcome. There is some evidence which suggests that placement of a sling without tension reduces the risk of post-operative voiding dysfunction (Level 3).

g) Tension-free vaginal tape (Figure 6)

The prolene tension-free vaginal tape (TVT) is a relatively new procedure although increasing numbers of cohort studies are being reported. The procedure is of particular importance in understanding the mechanisms by which surgery is effective, given that the suburethral sling is inserted without tension and the site of insertion is the mid urethra. The originator of the procedure reports that at 3 years 86% of women were 'completely cured', whilst a further 11% were 'significantly improved' (Ulmsten 1999). Others have reported comparable statistics; one series reporting that 80% of women were cured and a further 17.5% significantly improved, whilst a further series reported that 94% of treated women were either continent or significantly improved (Moran 2000, Nilsson 2001). The six month subjective and objective results of a randomised trial between TVT and colposuspension showed a similar cure rate from both procedures (Ward 2001). In this study, where TVT and colposuspension was employed as a primary procedure, the reporting of complete dryness in both groups was 38% and 40% respectively. Dryness with stress was reported in 66% and 68% of women. The 2 year follow up results of this study was reported in abstract form in December 2001. On the basis of a primary outcome measure of a negative cystometrogram and pad test 68% of TVT and 66% of colposuspension patients were cured. If pad test alone was used a cure rate of 75% was achieved in both groups. Over 60% of women were subjectively cured in both groups. This study highlights the difficulty with defining "cure". The only difference in outcomes at 2 years relates to voiding dysfunction and the need for surgery for utero-vaginal prolapse which appear to be more common in the colposuspension group.

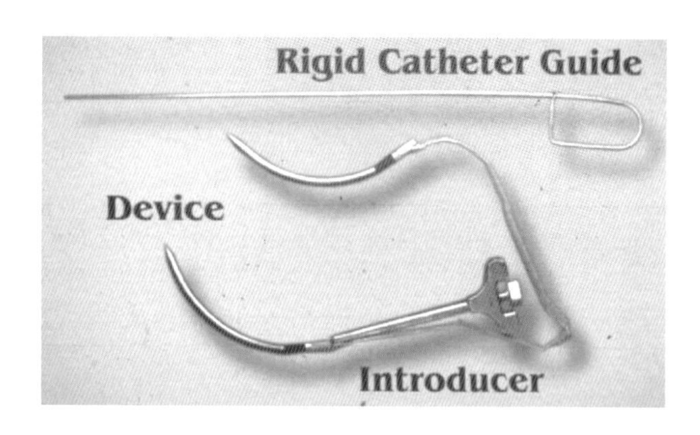

Figure 6 : The prolene mesh sling is inserted through a small vaginal incision under the mid-urethra. A needle with mesh attached is passed through the retropubic space on each side of the urethra and bladder and brought through the anterior abdominal wall.

The majority of patients are potentially treatable without general anaesthesia and on a day case basis (Ulmsten 1999). Somewhere between 3% and 15% of patients developed symptoms compatible with the onset of de novo detrusor instability (Moran 2000, Nilsson 2001). Short-term voiding disorder is described in 4.3% of women, although longer term voiding disorder does not appear to be a specific feature (Ulmsten 1999, Moran 2000, Nilsson 2001). Prolene mesh erosion has been reported 2 out of 137 women reviewed at 2 years.

In a multi-centre study, intra-operative bladder perforation was recognised in a mean of 9% of procedures (Ward 2001). A report from Finland (Kuuva 2000) on 1455 TVT procedures revealed 8 cases of significant bleeding, 3.8% chance of bladder perforation, and 2.3% chance of a voiding disorder. It was concluded from this evidence that the "TVT is a safe method for treatment of stress incontinence". There is a need for long-term results and randomised trials involving this procedure. Variations in technique and materials used need further evaluation.

CONCLUSIONS

Two year follow up data from a single RCT demonstrates a similar success rate to open colposuspension (Level 1). Large cohort analysis shows a cure rate of 80% and an improvement rate of 94% (Level 2).

h) Injectable agents

The cure rate, defined in 15 articles as completely dry, was 48%. The success rate (defined as dry and/or improved) was 76%. Only 8 studies defined intrinsic sphincter deficiency either as VLPP < 60 CM.H2O or through stress video urodynamics to assess bladder neck opening. Parity, BMI, uterovaginal prolapse and family history were not assessed as a potential influence on the outcome in the majority of the studies. Most of the studies include a small number of women and only short term follow up.

A number of bulking agents have been used for the treatment of SUI in women. The bulking agents (collagen, teflon, fat and recently Durasphere) are injected in a retrograde (more common) or antegrade fashion in the periurethral tissue around the bladder neck and proximal urethra. Among the eighteen larger published studies on bulking agents, fourteen are on Glutaraldedehyde Cross Linked Collagen. From the eighteen articles on bulking agents for the treatment of urinary incontinence in women (see Table 2), 8 are prospective non-randomised studies. A total 1221 patient were included, mean age 61 years. Follow up was between 3 months and 2 years, (mean of 12 months).

Macroplastique (Uroplasty bv.Geelan, The Netherlands) consist of solid polydimethylsiloxane (silicone) elastomer implants in a water-soluble hydrogel carrier suspension. Since its introduction in 1991, more than 20,000 patients with stress urinary incontinence and vesico-ureteral reflex were treated outside the United States.

Koelbl et al (998) found 75% and 60% objective success rates with it in the treatment of Type III stress urinary incontinence on a 6 and 12 month follow-up. Hennalla et al (2000), in a prospective multi-centre trial, reported success rates of 75% on a three month follow-up for treatment of genuine stress incontinence. Radley et al (2001) showed cure or improvement in 60% in a prospective chort of patients with recurrent stress urinary incontinence on a 19 month follow-up. Detrusor instability was an important cause of failures in this study.

Like collagen, it seems that efficacy deteriorate by time (Koelbl 1998) and (Sheriff 1997). Sherrif et al (1997) found success rate at 90% at one month, 75% at 3 months and 48% at 2 years. This raises the possibility of continuous sphincteric function deterioration versus absorption or degradation of the inected materials. RCTs are badly needed for bulking agents.

CONCLUSION

Bulking agents provide a relatively non-invasive method of treatment for stress incontinence. Short term data suggests a cure rate of 48% and an improvement rate of 76% (Level 3). Longer term results suggest a continued decline in success rate (greater than retropubic suspension procedures). It is not known whether the non-absorbable bulking agents last longer although in the short term there is no difference in results. This form of treatment may provide a more acceptable form of treatment for the women who wishes to avoid the complications associated with more invasive surgery.

The lack of morbidity associated with the bulking agents leads some people to believe that they should more meaningfully compared to conservative therapy such as pelvic floor physiotherapy.

j) Artificial sphincters

The literature related to the use of an artificial sphincter implanted around the proximal urethra is relatively difficult to interpret since most studies contain patients with a range of indications for surgery yet do not break down the result by indication.

There are, however, some studies in which the vast majority, or all, patients have undergone recurrent previous surgery for genuine stress incontinence. In such patients, and providing the detrusor remains stable, high levels of continence can be obtained, such as 92% (Webster 1992). These benefits must be balanced with the potential need for further surgery; in the above series 17% of patients required an average of two revisions each over an eight year follow up for either malfunction of the device or cuff erosion (Webster 1992, Richard 1996).

Table 2 : Summary of reported data on use of Bulking agents for treatment of SUI in Women

Reference	No of Pts	Median age	Bulking agent	Success criteria	Cure rate	Success rate
Eckford SD	25	52.3	Glutaraldedehyde CL Collagen	Cured- complete cessation Improved- reduction	64%	80%
Haab F	337	0	Glutaraldedehyde CL Collagen	N/A	N/A	N/A
Lopez A.E	45	63.3	FAT	0-100% subjective improvement	13%	64%
Lopez A.E	22	63.7	Glutaraldedehyde CL Collagen	success - dry 2	4%	62%
Smith D.N	74	54	Glutaraldedehyde CL Collagen	Cure – Completely Continent Success Minimal Pro	54%	76%
O'Connell H.E	94	67	Glutaraldedehyde CL Collagen	Cure - Continent Success Improved < 1 Pad 3	8.3%	67%
Herschon S	44	72	Glutaraldedehyde CL Collagen	cured- dry completely success - not > than 1 pad/	45%	63%
Shortliffe L/\. M.D	31	58	Glutaraldedehyde CL Collagen	Cured- dry completely success - not > than 2 pad/d	48%	90%
Stanton S.L	22	75	Glutaraldedehyde CL Collagen	Cured- dry completely success - not > than 1 pad/	N/A	86%
Winters J.C	160	0	Glutaraldedehyde CL Collagen	Cured- dry completely success - not > than 1 pad/	78%	78.4%
Winters J.C	50	0	Glutaraldedehyde CL Collagen	Cured- dry completely success - not > than 1 pad/	70%	48/50
Monga A.K	60	64	Glutaraldedehyde CL Collagen	Cured- dry completely 1 YR success - not > than 1	54%	40/60
Faerber G.J	12	76	Glutaraldedehyde CL Collagen	Subjective cure	83%	100%
Goldenberg S.L	190	0	Glutaraldedehyde CL Collagen	Cured- dry completely	30%	52%
Liu J	17	0	Glutaraldedehyde CL Collagen	Cured- dry completely	47%	82%
Stricker P	50 0		Glutaraldedehyde CL Collagen	Cured- dry completely	42%	82%
Corcos J	22	61	Glutaraldedehyde CL Collagen C	Cured- dry completely	40%	N/A
Henalla SM	10	0	Macroplastique	Subjective	N/A	74.3%

CONCLUSION

A cure rate of 80% and an improvement rate of 90% can be expected when an artificial sphincter is inserted as a primary procedure for stress incontinence (Level 3). Less favourable results are likely in women who have undergone multiple previous procedures (Level 3).

An attrition rate (revision, removal, non-function) of approximately 25% can be expected (Level 3).

SUMMARY OF CONCLUSIONS AND RECOMMENDATIONS

1. The major indication for anterior in contemporary practice must be the patient who prefers to sacrifice some degree of chance of becoming continent for a reduced chance of complication' (Level 1). The anterior repair should not normally be recommended as a procedure for the cure of stress incontinence. (Grade A Recommendation)

2. Retropubic suspension can be expected, in primary or secondary surgery, to generate a mean cure rate of 79% and an improvement rate of 90% (Level 2). A decrease in continence rate is observed with time (Level 3). The colposuspension can be recommended, on current evidence, as the procedure which produces the best chance of long lasting cure of stress incontinence.(Grade B Recommendation)

3. The long term data indicates that the initial success rates reported with needle suspension procedures are not maintained with time.(Level 3) The risk of failure is higher than reported with retropubic suspension procedures (Level 1)

   There would appear to be few, if any, indications to perform a needle suspension procedure. (Grade A recommendation).

   The results from small studies comparing laparoscopic and open colposuspension are conflicting. Until the data from larger studies are available no conclusions can be drawn about the value of this procedure. The evidence available suggests that the results are surgeon dependent.

4. Long term data suggests that sling procedures, using autologous or synthetic materials, produce a cure rate of approximately 80% and an improvement rate of 90% (Level 3). Sling procedures can be recommended as an effective treatment for stress incontinence (Grade C Recommendation).

5. 2 year data from a single RCT comparing open colposuspension and the TVT procedure demonstrates a similar success rate to open colposuspension (Level 1). Large cohort analysis with the TVT shows a cure rate of 80% and an improvement rate of 94% (Level 2). The short term results for this procedure are promising but it cannot be recommended for use before more data are available from long term studies. (Grade C Recommendation)

6. Short term data suggests that bulking agents produce a cure rate of 48% and an improvement rate of 76% (Level 3). Longer term results suggest a continued decline in success rate (greater than retropubic suspension procedures). (Level 3). The role of bulking agents is unclear but they may have a role as a non-invasive form of treatment with a lower chance of cure and a lower risk of complications. (Grade C Recommendation).

7. A cure rate of 80% and an improvement rate of 90% can be expected when an artificial sphincter is inserted as a primary procedure for stress incontinence (Level 3). Less favourable results are likely in women who have undergone multiple previous procedures (Level 3). The role of artificial sphincter should be limited to cases in whom previous attempts at surgical treatment have failed (Grade C Recommendation).

III. INCONTINENCE WITH PROLAPSE

Stress incontinence and prolapse of the anterior vaginal wall often co-exist. In addition prolapse of the uterus and posterior vaginal wall may be found in women with stress incontinence. Pelvic floor weakness is a common denominator to both conditions.

It has long been recognised that some women who are continent with stress prior to prolapse surgery develop stress incontinence after surgery. It has been suggested that if there is loss of support at the level of the bladder neck stress incontinence will occur. If the bladder neck is supported but the bladder base is not supported stress incontinence may not occur probably because of urethral kinking. Surgery which elevates the bladder base can then result in development of stress incontinence as urethral kinking is resolved.

Milani et al (Milani 1985) noted that the presence of vaginal prolapse pre-operatively led to a lower cure rate of stress incontinence with either the colposuspension or the MMK procedure; the greater the severity of the prolapse the greater the reduction in cure rate.

Urethro-vesical pressure dynamics have been studied by Richardson et al (Richardson 1983) and Bump et al (Bump 1988). In both studies elevation of the prolapse with a ring pessary led to development of stress incontinence in most cases. Richardson et al (Richardson 1983) demonstrated that women who did not demonstrate stress incontinence had a much higher urethral closure pressure with straining suggesting mechanical dysfunction of the urethra was preventing stress incontinence. Bump et al (Bump 1988) demonstrated a significant drop in pressure transmission and resting urethral closure pressure when the bladder base was supported in women with stress incontinence. These findings suggest that replacing or supporting the prolapse prior to surgery will reveal "latent incontinence" in women who are more likely to develop stress incontinence after prolapse surgery. This theory has not been tested by a rigorous prospective study.

Tanagho (Tanagho 1985) first suggested that prolapse surgery such as anterior repair damaged urethral innervation. Zivkovic et al (Zivkovic1996) found evidence of greater prolongation of nerve latencies in women whose bladder neck surgery had failed to cure their stress incontinence one year after follow up suggesting that surgery may increase denervation. The data on denervation and the role of surgery is not conclusive.

Burch recognised at an early stage that colposuspension led to the development of posterior vaginal wall prolapse in a significant number of women and recommended that a Moschovitz operation should be incorporated into the colposuspension procedure (Burch 1968). Despite introduction of this modification Burch found an 8% incidence of posterior vaginal wall prolapse after colposuspension. Wiskind et al (Wiskind 1992) demonstrated that 27% of women develop symptomatic prolapse within four years of a colposuspension and did not find that correction of prolapse at primary surgery prevented recurrence.

CONCLUSION

Surgery for stress incontinence may lead to the development of symptomatic prolapse in up to 27% women. (Level 3) Surgery for vaginal prolapse may lead to the development of stress incontinence (Level 3). The best way to predict or avoid this is not clear.

There is no evidence to support the view that surgery to prevent prolapse performed at the time of incontinence surgery prevents the development of prolapse in future. There is some evidence to suggest that prolapse, when present at the time of incontinence surgery, is associated with a poorer outcome for cure of stress incontinence(Level 3).

There is some evidence that surgery for stress incontinence may increase denervation of the striated muscle of the urethral sphincter (Level 3).

IV. COMPLICATIONS OF SURGERY

This topic has been comprehensively reviewed by Chaliha and Stanton (Chaliha1999). Complications can be conveniently divided into Immediate (0-24 hours); Short-term (24 hours to 6 weeks) and Long-term (6 weeks onwards).

1. Immediate complications

a) Haemorrhage

The perivesical/periurethral venous plexus can be a source of substantial haemorrhage during surgery for stress incontinence. The mean blood loss following anterior repair has been reported as 200 ml compared to 260 ml following a Burch colposuspension. (Van Geeland 1998).

Alcalay et all (Alcalay 1995) in a retrospective review of 109 Burch colposuspensions did not note any difference in blood loss between primary and secondary procedures but a blood loss of more than 1 litre was associated with a higher risk of failure to cure stress incontinence. Haematoma formation following bladder neck surgery may lead to the development of an abscess and possible wound breakdown. However, the relationship between haematoma formation and outcome from surgery has not been studied.

Needle suspension is associated with a lower blood loss (mean 53 ml) (Spencer 1987) and laparoscopic colposuspension is described by authors in cohort series as being associated with minimal blood loss (Liu 1993, Dorsey 1994).

Sling procedures which may involve more extensive dissection may be associated with haemorrhage requiring surgical drainage, Morgan et al (Morgan 2000) required drainage in 2.1% of cases. In a randomised prospective study comparing TVT and colposuspension blood loss was 50 ml and 135 ml respectively. (Ward 2000)

b) Urinary tract and visceral injuries

Bladder ureteric and urethral injuries have been reported during surgery for stress incontinence. Mainprize and Drutz (1988) reported 0.7% bladder injury in nearly 3,000 women undergoing an MMK procedure. Up to 6% of women may sustain injury to the bladder or ureter at open colposuspension. Reports on laparoscopic colposuspension note a risk of bladder injury in up to 10% cases (Smith 1998) In a randomised trail comparing open colposuspension with the TVT procedure an average of 9% bladder perforation was reported in the TVT group compared to 2% in the open colposuspension group (Ward 2000). Urethral injury during anterior repair appears to be uncommon but may follow the opening of an undetected urethral diverticulum.

Laparoscopic surgery when performed through a trans-peritoneal approach will also carry a risk of injury to intra-peritoneal viscera, particularly when previous surgery has been performed through the anterior abdominal wall. Suprapubic catheterisation, when performed blind, also carries a risk of bowel injury (Noller 1976, Louhglin 1990, Cundiff 1995).

Urinary tract infection is not uncommon following surgery for stress incontinence. Its frequency will increase with the duration of catheterisation at a rate of 6 to 7.5% per day (Foucher 1983). Anderson et al (Anderson 1985) compared suprapubic and transurethral catherisation in a randomised trial and reported a lower incidence of bactiuria on the 5th post-operative day following suprapubic catheterisation (21% versus 46%). A similar difference was reported by Bergman et al following a needle suspension procedure (Bergman 1987).

2. Short term complications

a) Infection

Wound infection appears to be uncommon or unrecognized following vaginal surgery. Vaginal hysterectomy however is associated with a vault haematoma in one in four women (Tincello 1998). There is no direct evidence that wound infection influences the cure rate for stress incontinent surgery, although infection in the presence of synthetic support materials may lead to removal. Mundy (Mundy 1983) removed 16% of Dacron Stamey buffers. Erosion rates of up to 21% have been reported with synthetic pubo-vaginal slings (Beck 1988, Bent 1993, Bryans 1979, Muznai 1992). Granuloma and abscess formation have been reported following peri-urethral injection (Politanoi 1974, Politano 1982, Lotenfoe 1993). Infection of artificial sphincters has been reported in up to 9.5% of cases (Appell 1988, Light 1988, Scott 1989).

Osteitis pubis is discussed within the section on MMK procedure but it has also been reported after needle suspension (Green 1986).

b) Voiding dysfunction

Voiding dysfunction is discussed under each of the operative procedures.and Section 6 on Post Surgical Outlet Obstruction Surgery.

c) Uro-genital fistulae

As described later in the Chapter, fistulae most commonly follow gynaecological surgery in the developed world. Fistulae may also develop following surgery for stress incontinence. Beck et al reviewed a series of over 500 women who underwent anterior repair and found two cases of urethro-vaginal fistula (Beck 1991). Fistulae have also been reported following needle suspension procedures (Guam 1984) MMK (Mainprize 1988) and sling (Kersey 1983).

Nerve injuries - No direct injuries have been reported to nerves following the anterior colporrhaphy but the abduction and flexion of the thigh in the lithotomy position may lead to femoral nerve injury. (Wang 1993). Denervation of the urethral sphincter may occur (see section on prolapse). Nerve injuries after needle suspension have been reported to the common perineal, sciatic, obturator, femoral, saphenous and ilio-inguinal nerves (Karram 1992). Seven cases of ilio-inguinal nerve entrapment were described following 402 needle suspension procedures. In three cases the suture was removed which led to resolution of the pain in two cases (Miyazaki 1992).

The 'post-colposuspension syndrome' has been described to include women who have pain in one or both ilio-inguinal regions following colposuspension (Galloway 1987).

3. Long term complications

Detrusor instability and uro-genital prolapse are discussed under the relevant procedures and also in the section for surgery for stress incontinence and prolapse.

Dyspareunia is seldom mentioned in reports on surgery for stress incontinence. It may be produced by the vaginal wound itself through scarring or vaginal narrowing. Erosion of synthetic material may also lead to dysparuenia in either partner. Alteration of the vaginal axis and the development of prolapse may lead to difficulty with intercourse. Dyspareunia has been reported in up to 40% of women after colposuspension. (Galloway 1987, Eriksen 1990), but less frequently after needle suspension 1.5% (Raz 1991).

a) Quality of life issues

There are only two studies in the literature which have looked at the quality of life after surgery for stress incontinence. Surgeons have tended to assume that the most significant outcome measure for surgery for stress incontinence is whether complete continence is achieved. This is despite evidence that patients may be satisified with the outcome without complete continence. Given that surgery for stress incontinence does not always produce continence and that this procedure can produce significant complications, it may be more relevant to consider the overall impact on the quality of life of the surgery rather than the single issue of continence. In the prospective cohort study of 442 women undergoing surgery for stress incontinence by various techniques, 68% of women declared themselves satisfied with the outcome of the surgery at one year follow up. However, 7% of women reported a deterioration in their general health by this time and 25% reported a deterioration in their mental health. Only 28% of these women achieved total continence. (Black 1997). Berglund et al (Berglund 1996) reported, in a prospective chohort study that, in addition to age and duration of symptoms, increased patient neurotiscism had a significant assocation with poorer outcome from surgery for stress incontinence.

It appears that clarification about most significant factors which influence satisfaction and improved quality of life after surgery for stress incontinence is required.

V. CONFOUNDING VARIABLES

The following variables which may impact on the outcome of surgery will be reviewed:

1. Age and activity
2. Race
3. Medical illness, psychiatric illness and drugs
4. Obesity
5. Parity
6. Previous history of continence surgery
7. Hysterectomy at the time of continence surgery
8. Severity and duration of symptoms
9. Detrusor instability
10. Urethral occlusive forces
11. Surgical factors

If the selection of a surgical procedure includes factors which may influence outcome, bias will be introduced. The degree of bias may be difficult to measure because the influence of factors such as age is not well defined. The influence of these confounding variables can be minimized by random allocation of treatment or structured non-randomised studies. Unfortunately there is a dearth of prospective randomised studies in incontinence surgery.

1. Age and activity

There is some evidence that advancing age is associated with a poorer outcome from surgery for stress incontinence (Berglund et al 1997). The chapter on treatment of incontinence in the elderly covers the influence of age on the outcome from incontinence surgery in detail.

There is no evidence that activity after surgery influences the cure rate following incontinence surgery. An early return to normal activity following surgery may have benefits such as reducing thrombo-embolic events but may also influence the strength of healing after surgery. Women are often advised to avoid high impact activity following incontinence surgery. There is no evidence to support this advice.

CONCLUSION

There is Level 3 evidence that advancing age is associated with a poorer outcome from surgery. There is no evidence that post-operative physical activity influences the outcome from surgery.

2. Race

There are no studies on the influence of race on the outcome of surgery for stress incontinence. A clinical and urodynamics study by Bump (Bump 1993) comparing black and white women in Virginia USA, demonstrated a different distribution of symptoms, different conditions causing incontinence and different risk profiles for their condition despite an equal prevalence of prolapse.

CONCLUSION

There is no evidence that race influences the outcome from surgery.

3. Medical illness, Psychiatric illness and Drugs

A patient with chronic obstructive airways disease might be expected to have a less favourable outcome from incontinence surgery. There is no data avilable about the influence of this or other medical illness on outcome from incontinence surgery.There is some evidence that the psych-neurotic state may influence the cure rate from continence surgery. A high degree of neuroticism, psychic anxiety and somatic anxiety was found in women who reported failure from their continence surgery (Berglund et al 1997). Obrink et al (1979) detected higher levels of neuroticism and depression in women who reported failure of their continence surgery at long term review even without objective evidence of stress incontinence. Some women have been found to have improved psychological status after successful surgery but a deterioration was found in women in whom the surgery was not successful. (Rozensweig et al 1991)

One might expect that some forms of drug therapy such as steroids might influence the outcome from surgery however there is no evidence on this issue.

CONCLUSION

There is Level 3 evidence that the psychiatric of the patient may influence the outcome from surgery. There is no data on the influence of other medical disease on surgical outcome.

4. Obesity

There are no studies reported which prospectively evaluate the influence of obesity on outcome from surgery for stress incontinence. Alcalay et al (Alcalay 1995) in a longitudinal retrospective study noted that women over 80 kg had a lower cure rate (46%) than women less than 80 kg (76%). The heavier women were also more likely to have had a hysterectomy and large blood loss at surgery which was also found to be associated with a lower success rate. Zirkovic et al (Zikovic 1999) performed a 5 year review on 198 women who were available for follow up. Obese women, defined as BMI>30 did not have a different cure rate than overweight (BMI 25-30) or normal women(BMI <25), although the authors assess that the statistical power was only 26% for the hypothesis that BMI does not influence surgical outcome. A record review of 16 women, classified as morbidly obese (200% or more than ideal weight) suggested that since there were only two surgical failures such women can undergo surgery with a good chance of success (Cummings 1998). Three needle suspension series (Varner 1990, O'Sullivan 1995, Bueger 1992) suggest that obesity is associated with a lower cure rate.

There are no studies which demonstrate a better cure rate in women who are overweight

CONCLUSION

There is conflicting evidence on the impact of obesity on outcome from surgery. There is no data on morbidity associated with surgery on obese patients.

5. Parity

There is evidence that the prevalence of incontinence increases with advancing parity. There is no direct evidence that parity influences the outcome from continence surgery although duration and severity of incontinence and age are related factors which may influence outcome.

CONCLUSION

There is no direct evidence that parity influences outcome from surgery but increased parity is associated with increased age, severity and duration of incontinence.

6. Previous history of incontinence surgery

It is widely believed that the first surgical procedure performed for stress incontinence is the most likely to be successful. Certainly most surgeons would prefer to operate in an area where no surgeon has previously been.

Hodgkinson (Hodgkinson 1978) notes "There is little doubt that the first operation for stress incontinence is the primary one and that every subsequent operation that fails lessens the chance of eventual success". However, in the final sentence of this paper he also writes "In the series of 205 patients with recurrent stress incontinence now under investigation, normal urinary control has been established in more than 90% control".

In 1978 Stanton et al (Stanton 1978) compared clinical and urodynamic features of 45 women whose stress incontinence was caused by colposuspension with 15 women in whom surgery had failed. A greater incidence of failure was found in the previous incontinence surgery group but detrusor instability was also more common in this group.

Stanton & Cardozo (Stanton 1979) reported on a 2 year follow up of colposuspension in 43 women. No difference in cure rate between women who had and had not undergone previous continence surgery was found.

Milani et al (Milani 1985) reviewed the outcome of 86 women who had undergone either a colposuspension or MMK procedure. Sixteen women had undergone a previous anterior repair which did not appear to influence the cure rate. Kjolhede et al (Kjolhede 1994) reviewed the 5 year cure rate of 236 women who underwent incontinence surgery and reported a 33% cure rate at 5 years in women who had undergone previous surgery compared to an overall cure rate of 68% . Jarvis, in a meta-analysis of surgery for stress incontinence demonstrated a trend towards lower cure rates with repeat surgery apart from when injectable agents are used (90% vs 83%). (Jarvis 1994).

CONCLUSION

The data available suggests a trend towards lower success rates with repeat surgery although the level of significance is in need of clarification.

7. Hysterectomy at the time of continence surgery

In a retrospective review of 147 women who underwent a MMK procedure with hysterectomy Green (Green 1975, Green 1978) noted an improved success rate compared to 47 women who underwent MMK alone. These series largely involved vaginal hysterectomy which may have produced a bias to women with uterine prolapse. Further retrospective reviews by Stanton and Cardozo (Stanton 1979) and Milani et al (Milani 1985) did not show any advantage to performing an abdominal hysterectomy at the same time as a colposuspension or MMK procedure. Langer et al (Langer 1988) demonstrated no advantage with respect to outcome of urinary symptoms when an abdominal hysterectomy was performed at the time of colposuspension in a prospective randomised control trial of 45 women. The women who underwent hysterectomy also had a Moschowitz procedure performed which appeared to offer some protection against enterocoele formation (three in the no Moschowitz group compared to none in Moschowitz group).

CONCLUSION

There is no evidence that hysterectomy performed at the time of incontinence surgery influences the outcome of the surgery.

8. Severity and duration of symptoms

A woman who experiences urinary incontinence over many years is likely to be older. Over time the incontinence is also more likely to have had an impact on her quality of life and may have impacted on her psychological state. Berglund et al (1996) demonstrated that older women who had experienced stress incontinence for a longer duration were less likely to have a favourable outcome from surgery. Hitchings et al (1998) in a prospective cohort study, demonstrated that women with more severe pre-operative incontinence have a greater liklihood of improvement in their ability to perform activities of daily living than women with mild pre-operative incontinence. Surgery in women with more severe stress incontinence pre-operatively was also found to have a more favourable impact on the woman's social activity. These findings highlight the fact that outcome depends on which measure you chose to study

CONCLUSION

There is Level 3 evidence that women with more severe incontinence of longer duration have a lower chance of cure from surgery. However, there is Level 2 evidence that women with more severe incontinence are more likely to gain benefit in terms of activities of daily living from surgery.

9. Detrusor instability

There are no prospective randomised trials which compare the outcome of colposuspension in women with and without detrusor instability. Colombo et al (Colombo 1996) performed a retrospective cohort study and compared 44 stress incontinent women with detrusor over-activity with a matched group of women with stress incontinence and a stable bladder. A cure rate of 95% in the stable group compared to 75% in the unstable group two years after surgery was reported. These results, although showing a less favourable outcome in women with stress incontinence with detrusor instability, show a more favourable outcome than cure rates of 24-43% shown in other series (Stanton 1978,Lose 1988, Milani 1995).

In a series of 46 women with urodynamically proved mixed incontinence Scotti et al (Scotti 1998) noted a significantly higher cure rate in women whose primary symptoms had been stress incontinence. A retrospective review of 36 women who underwent a sling procedure for stress incontinence and Valsalva induced detrusor instability revealed a cure rate of stress incontinence of 92% and urge incontinence of 75%.(Serels 2000). Pow-Sang et al (Pow-Sang1986) demonstrated in a retrospective study that high pressure detrusor instability is associated with a poorer outcome from bladder neck surgery. Further studies are required to clarify what type of detrusor over-activity is most likely to influence the surgical outcome. Since de novo detrusor instability is not uncommon after all forms of bladder neck surgery the relationship between pre and post-operative bladder function and pelvic surgery appears to merit further study.

CONCLUSION

There is Level 3 evidence that women who have detrusor instability pre-operatively are more likely to have a less favourable outcome from surgery.

10. Urethral occlusive forces

Several authors have reported a lower success rate for surgical treatment of stress incontinence in women with a maximum urethral closure pressure of < 20 cm (Sand 1987, Stanton 1979). Sand et al (Sand 1987) compared two similar groups of women who underwent colposuspension for stress incontinence. The group of women with a resting maximum urethral closure pressure (MUCP) of 20 cm water were less likely to be cures of stress incontinence if they were under 50 years of age but in women over 50 years the MUCP was not a discriminatior. All but three of the 86 women in this study had urethral hypermobility. McGuire et al (McGuire 1980) demonstrated that maximum urethral closure pressure measurement was not a reliable prediction of surgical outcome and more important was the identification of proximal urethral weakness by radiological studies. McGuire has suggested that such patients (classified as Type III incontinence) are best managed by a pubovaginal sling procedure. McGuire further reported (NcGuire 1993) no correlation between MUCP and clinical severity or the type of stress incontinence. In a series of 125 women with stress incontinence an inverse correlation between the abnormal pressure required to cause leakage and the grade and type of incontinence was demonstrated.

Bump et al (Bump 1997) studies urethral competence in 159 women with stress incontinence by measurement of maximum urethral closure pressure, Valsalva leak point pressure and straining urethral axis (urethral hypermobility). They found that a composite of a MUCP of < 20 cm water, a Valsalva leak point pressure (VLPP) of < 50 cm water and a stress urethral axis < 20 degrees was required to reliably diagnose intrinsic sphincter deficiency. Only low MUCP and VLPP had a significant association with the severity of incontinence.

Bump et al (1988) studied bladder to urethra pressure transmission ratios in addition to urethral pressure profilometry and demonstrated that an operative procedure producing a transmission ratio close to 100% was most likely to cure stress incontinence. This is consistent with other studies suggesting that stabilising urethral position is important for successful continence surgery (Hertogs1985, Bergland 1982 and Iosif 1982).

McGuire and Appell (McGuire 1994) reported that injection of a bulking agent improved the ability of the urethra to resist raised intra-abdominal pressure and therefore recommended such treatment for women who have intrinsic sphincter weakness with no urethral hypermobility. Kreden and Austin (Kreden 1996) demonstrated better cure rates with injectable agents in women without urethral hypermobility and concluded that injectable agents were only suitable for women with ISD in whom urethral support was satisfactory. Only 4 women were treated with ISD and urethral hypermobility for this study. Other groups have also used injectables on women with and without urethral hypermobility and found similar cure rates (O'Connell 1995 and Monga 1995)

CONCLUSION

Whilst there appears to be some growing consensus on the diagnosis and classification of types of incontinence in relation to urethral sphincter occlusive forces and urethral mobility there is conflicting data on whether this type of classification either influences outcome or should influence the type of surgical treatment.

11. Surgical factors

The seniority and experience of the surgeon is rarely mentioned in reports on continence surgery. It is therefore not known whether these factors are important in determining the outcome. Over the years many techniques have been described by their inventor which produce results that no other author manages to reproduce. The generalisability of a procedure is an important factor in assessing its value to the surgical community. There is some evidence in the literature on laparoscopic surgery that the learning process for this type of surgery may be longer and more difficult than open surgery. This is clearly of importance if a procedure is to be used by surgeons who have no familiarity with laparoscopic surgery.

The surgical technique and the materials used are little described in the literature. Burch used chromic catgut for his colposuspension in the series published in 1968 (Burch 1968) Only four suspension failures were described indicating that the suture material strength did not play an important role in the effectiveness of the procedure. It is difficult to evaluate the robustness of Burch's evaluation. Many surgeons now use non-absorbable sutures for colposuspension because they believe that the long-lasting support provided is important. There is no proven benefit of non-absorbable suture material and there is a potential risk of suture erosion.

Newer techniques such as testing for stress incontinence during the surgical procedure (and adjusting sling tension) need proper evaluation. It would be helpful to know whether local, regional or general anaesthesia influences the outcome of surgery. There are many techniques that have only anecdotal value and need proper evaluation.

CONCLUSION

There is no data to support the view that surgical technique or the experience of the surgeon influence the outcome from surgery or the associated morbidity.

VI. POST-SURGICAL OUTLET OBSTRUCTION SURGERY

The incidence of bladder outlet obstruction (BOO) and associated voiding dysfunction after anti-incontinence surgical procedures is not known but has been estimated to be between 2.5% and 24%. In table 3 the details of most recent six largest series reported in the English literature are summarized. As seen in this table, any of the retropubic, needle suspensions or pubovaginal sling procedures can cause BOO.

A newer cause of BOO is injection of Collagen. Since its introduction in late 1980s, glutaraldehyde cross-linked bovine dermal collagen has been used as a bulking agent for treatment of intrinsic sphincteric deficiency (ISD) in women with stress urinary incontinence.

Table 3 : BOO after previous anti-incontinence surgery

Author	No Pts	S/p surgery	Time interval	Diagnostic clue	Type of urethrolysis	Re-suspension	Results	Follow-up
Webster	15	6MMK 6 Stam. 2 Raz 1 Burch	2-24 7.6 mean	chronology of symptoms	Abd	Obturator shelf on all pts	93% success	N/A
Foster	48	Vaginal NS 19 sling 10 rpbns 17	2m-35 yr 11 months median	combination of sx, cysto and UDS	Vaginal	various types on 24 pts	65%	2-67 mean 17 m
McGuire	13	rpbns 6 vbns 4 sling 3	28 months	sx & UDS	Vaginal	various type in 4	77%	1-4 yrs
Zimmern	13	MMK 13	1-6 yr mean 3.5 yr	sx & UDS	vaginal	Raz in all	92%	12-44 m mean 20
Nitti	41	MMK 18 AP 7 Raz 7 Stamey 4 Burch 1	3-194 m mean 54 m	sx & UDS	vaginal	Raz in all	71%	3-78 m mean 21 m
Austin	18	average of 2.7/pt various procedures	at least 6 m	sx & UDS	vaginal	sling in 16	60% and 33%	N/A

Although its use has been reported to be safe with minimal or no complications, later reports have mentioned up to about 10% rate of urinary retention with subsequent urinary tract infection. The most recent report suggested 13% incidence of urgency with urge incontinence among 337 patients treated with collagen as early evidence of increased bladder outlet resistance·

According to Raz (Raz 1989) three distinct group of patients with BOO symptoms after previous anti-incontinence procedures exist. These groups are: 1) obstructed only- the patients who produce pdet>35 cm H2O without urinary flow. This group will benefit only from urethrolysis, 2) poor detrusor function- the patients who would continue to have problems post urethrolysis, and 3) obstructed and incontinent- the patient in whom an additional resuspension procedure seems appropriate. Many surgeons reserve urethrolysis for patients in whom intermittent self-catheterisation (ISC) is an unacceptable alternative. The use of ISC avoids the risk of return of the stress incontinence which can occur after urethrolysis.

1. Diagnosis

a) Symptoms

Women with BOO present with a variety of urinary symptoms. The most common of the presenting symptoms are frequency, urgency, urinary incontinence and nocturia. A similar constellation of symptoms in men has recently been termed as lower urinary tract symptoms (LUTS) with the underlying etiology ranging from simple benign prostatic hyperplasia (BPH) to severe bladder outlet obstruction. Classical symptoms of outflow obstruction such as poor urinary flow, hesitancy, abdominal straining or feeling of incomplete bladder emptying are less common. As a reaction to the obstructive mechanism, the detrusor muscle can become overactive and unstable resulting in frequency, urgency and urge incontinence, or even progress to the phase of detrusor decompensation heralded by urinary retention, recurrent urinary tract infections (UTIs) or overflow incontinence.

In table 4 the frequency of symptoms presented in women with BOO after anti-incontinence surgery is summarized.

In order to help reliably identify patients with voiding dysfunction use of questionnaires has increasingly become popular. Such a questionnaire is the Urogenital Distress Inventory developed by Uebersax and colleagues. With this questionnaire, a total score of >9 out of 18 usually points out to a underlying voiding dysfunction including BOO.

b) Voiding Diary

Urinary symptoms of women with suspected BOO could primarily be assessed through two methods:

Table 4 : Reported symptoms of BOO in women

Author	no of pts	frequency	urgency	nocturia	urge incontinence	new onset UI	inability to void	residual SUI
Webster	15	13	13	13	0	8	7	0
Foster	48	13	32	11	32	32	29	9
McGuire	13	N/A	N/A	N/A	N/A	N/A	5	N/A
Zimmern	13	4	4	N/A	N/A	N/A	2	3
Nitti	41	30	30	30	16	N/A	29	19
Austin	18	13	13	13	N/A	N/A	5	2

	pain	recurrent UTI	decreased force of stream	dysuria	post void dribbling	PVR	CIC
Webster	n/a	n/a	n/a	n/a	n/a		
Foster	10	8	6	6	6	63%	25%
McGuire	N/A	N/A	N/A	N/A	N/A	N/A	6/13
Zimmren	N/A	4	N/A	N/A	N/A	100%	2
Nitti	N/A	N/A	N/A	N/A	N/A	29	19
Austin	N/A	N/A	N/A	N/A	N/A	13	5

patient recall during history taking, and self-monitoring of voiding behavior using a diary. Although both methods have pitfalls in terms of providing reproducible information, voiding diary has been shown to be more accurate in demonstration of patient's symptoms. Seven-day diary does not provide any advantage over the three-day diary.

c) Physical examination

The physical examination of patients with suspected BOO should include: a general abdominal exam, a focused neurological exam including a back exam, and a detailed and a combined perineal/vaginal examination. During vaginal exam, careful investigation of possible anatomical causes for BOO including the urethrovesical angle should be performed. The entire length of urethra should be palpated carefully for any tender spot or mass. Periurethral scarring usually becomes apparent by a combination of observation and palpation of the urethra. In the case of excessive scarring, most of the urethra appears to be "cemented" in the anterior vaginal wall.

The value of urethral calibration in the management of BOO in women is difficult to assess. There is no agreement in the literature regarding the normal calibre of the adult female urethra, which ranges between 12 and 24 F. It has been determined however that restriction of the urethra to 10 F or less must be present to produce an obstructive urodynamic pattern (Tanagho et al 1971, Gleason et al 1969).

Partial or total urinary retention may be seen in women with bladder outlet obstruction. During the abdominal examination of a non-obese patient a minimal of 150 cc is needed in the bladder to make it palpable. In contrast to conventional thinking, urinary retention or large postvoid residuals in women more commonly are the result of a poor detrusor contractility rather than bladder outlet obstruction, although poor detrusor contractility does not rule out the presence of BOO in women. Incomplete bladder emptying is often associated with significant cystoceles.

d) Urodynamics

Interpretation of the results of urodynamic studies is the cornerstone of the diagnosis of BOO in women. Various elements of urodynamic studies can be used in the evaluation process depending on the guides received from history and physical examination.

e) Uroflowmetry

Despite its ease of use, wide availability and inexpensive nature, the uroflow information should be interpreted with caution. For an accurate interpretation of uroflowmetry data in men, the voided volume should be in excess of 150 ml. Although this data has never been replicated in women, it is commonly used in interpretation of uroflow data in them. Maximum flow rate (qmax), voiding time and the uroflow curve are other important elements in accurate interpretation of a noninvasive uroflow test. The caveat in uroflow interpretation is that it cannot distinguish between an obstructive process with a high-pressure detrusor contraction or impaired detrusor contractility as the cause of a weak stream. Following uroflowmetry, measurement of post voiding residual (PVR) is needed to determine the bladder capacity.

• **PRESSURE-FLOW STUDIES**

The simultaneous measurement of detrusor pressure and urine flow during voiding offers the best objective evidence for diagnosis of BOO in women. This is based on the physical principles that obstruction exists in a fluid-transporting system if an elevated pressure is required to transport the usual rate of flow through a relative narrowing. During the filling phase of the study, bladder compliance, presence or absence of detrusor overactivity/instability, and maximum bladder capacity are evaluated.

Filling and voiding cycles may be repeated twice to assure the persistency of the obtained values. Generally, the distinction between an unobstructed from an obstructed voiding pattern is made based on the following characteristics: a) the maximum flow rate (qmax) is lower; b) detrusor pressure at maximum flow (pdetqmax) is higher; c) the timing of void is longer and d) the slope/curve is of flattened or interrupted. In men, a number of pressure-flow plots have been created. These plots graphically show the changing pdet for each value of the flow rate as it rises and falls throughout a whole void. Based on this demonstration, patients voiding pattern is categorized to obstructed, unobstructed or equivocal.

Several groups have attempted to study obstruction in women on the basis of pressure flow analysis. Massey and Abrams defined the BOO when qmax of <12mL/s, pdetqmax of >50 cm H2O, urethral resistance (pdetqmax/qmax)>0.2 and "significant" residual urine. Farrar et al (Farrar 1975) used an arbitrary definition based on qmax of <15 mL/s and pdetqmax of >50 cm H2O. In order to establish the basis of a nomogram in women, Chassagne et al (Chassagne 1998) have recently proposed the pressure-flow cut off values for diagnosis of BOO in women. In a cohort of 35 clinically obstructed and 124 control women, different cutoff values were driven from receiver operator characteristic curves (ROC). Using cut off values of qmax of 15 mL/s or less and 12 mL/s or less, sensitivity of 85.7% and 71.4% and specificity of 78.2% and 90.3% was obtained. Also using cutoff values of pdetqmax of more than 25 and more than 30 cm H2O, sensitivity of 74.3% and 71.4% and specificity 79.8% and 88.7% was obtained. Based on these values, using a combined value of qmax of 15 mL/s or less and pdetqmax of more than 20 cm H2O with resultant sensitivity of 74.3% and specificity of 91.1% was proposed as the pressure-flow cutoff values for diagnosis of BOO in women.

• **URETHRAL PRESSURE PROFILE**

Urethral pressure profile can be performed as static or dynamic techniques. Its role in investigation of patients with stress urinary incontinence continues to be debated (see above). This test is technically challenging and is not currently recommended by most authors for investigation of patients with BOO. Moreover, some authors have found that UPP did not contribute to prediction of outcome after urethrolysis operation [1] in patients with BOO after a previous anti-incontinence surgery.

f) Cystourethroscopy

Using a flexible cystoscope with local anesthesia in the office, cystourethroscopy may be used to examine the likely cause of BOO. It is mostly useful in diagnosis of calculi and foreign bodies or suspension sutures in the bladder. However, the gross appearance of the urethra and bladder neck is usually inaccurate in diagnosis of obstruction in the absence of a defined pathology. Although the bladder trabeculation implies persistent detrusor damage, the significance of this finding is still unknown. Bladder trabeculation usually persist despite relief of obstructive process.

g) Voiding cystourethrogram

The voiding cystourethrogram (VCUG) is a reproducible method to evaluate the female lower urinary tract and may be used in the evaluation of patients presenting with BOO symptoms. The information gained includes angulation of the urethra, the position of urethrovesical junction, and the status of the bladder neck and proximal urethra during the voiding phase of micturition. Observation of post void residual contrast also confirms the incomplete emptying of the bladder.

SUMMARY

In summary, the combination of a) LUTS-like symptoms and continued incontinence in the presence of previous anti-incontinence surgery, b) physical finding of an overcorrected urethro-vesical junction or excessive scar on the urethral, and c) urodynamic confirmation of BOO as defined by high detrusor pressure with low flow rate during voiding phase constitute the foundation of diagnosis of post-surgical BOO in women. The value of imaging modalities has not been proven.

2. TREATMENT

The treatment options for BOO after anti-incontinence surgery in women primarily depends on the cause and the severity of the obstruction but the mainstay of treatment is:

a) Clean Intermittent Catheterization

Pioneering work of Lapides and colleagues has established clean intermittent catheterization (CIC) as an effective mean of bladder emptying when physiological voiding is not possible. The catheterization is ideally done by the patient herself or in certain cases by a care-worker or relative. Its ease, safety and low cost have made it a very attractive alternative for chronic bladder emptying. The recommended frequency varies depending on the patient's situation, but it has been suggested that catheterization volume be kept below 350 to 400 ml to prevent clinical infection.

b) Alternative treatment are

• **Anti-cholinergic medications**

In both clinical and animal models bladder/detrusor overactivity develops in response to BOO, and the main neurohumoral pathway of this physiologic response appears to be via acetylcholine-induced stimulation of the muscarinic receptors of the bladder smooth muscle. Anticholinergic agents thus can depress this physiologic response to BOO. The problem with the general muscarinic receptor anticholinergic agents is in their significant side effects on other systems such as salivary glands. The value of these drugs in BOO has not been formally evaluated.

• **Urethrolysis**

Surgical urethrolysis is an option for patients with BOO after a previous anti-incontinence surgery. The options for urethrolysis include retropubic, transvaginal and infra pubic approaches.

Series with either retropubic or transvaginal approaches have shown similar rates of success on the order of 80%. Although some authors have downgraded the importance of recurrent incontinence after urethrolysis and do not recommend resuspension (Foster and McGuire), most other authors do recommend resuspension. The choice of resuspension has varied from needle suspensions, pubovaginal slings, or obturator shelf repair in the case of abdominal approach to urethrolysis.

Several factors appear to have an impact on the outcome of urethrolysis in patients with BOO after an anti-incontinence surgery. A higher failure rate was seen when detrusor instability was demonstrated on the preoperative evaluation (McGuire et al 1989). In the group of patients reported by Nitti and Raz, preoperative postvoid residual was predictive of failure of urethrolysis. The presence or strength of the detrusor contraction preoperatively and pressure-flow analysis did not predict outcome in this report. Austin et al (Austin et al 1996) reported 60% success with urethrolysis and resuspension in 13 patients with highest mean maximal voiding pressure (MVP), and 33% for 5 patients with lowest MVP. Foster and McGuire have reported higher rate of success of transvaginal urethrolysis following needle suspension and retropubic urethropexy compared to patients with urethral obstruction secondary to pubovaginal sling.

• **Urethral incision**

Transurethral incision of the bladder neck (TUIBN) has been reported with good results in symptomatic patients with BOO after anti-incontinence surgery (Turner-Warwick 1976, Axelrod et al 1987 and Fenster 1990. Because of the vulnerability of the female urethra however, It has been suggested that TUIBN should only be used when a distinct anatomical obstruction exists. In animal studies, distinct differences between histological effects of urethrotomy and urethral dilation in female dogs were noted. The main difference was the prominence of sheared disruption of the musculature in the urethrotomy vs attenuation of circular striated and smooth muscles following dilatation

• **Urethral dilatation**

Dilatation of the female urethra has tradionally been used for a variety of lower urinary tract symptoms including BOO after anti-incontinence surgery. This is done by dilating the urethra up to 32 F using female urethral sounds, with or without anaesthesia. Due to lack of poor definition of indications and report of outcome, this option is rapidly falling out of favour. A recent survey by Lemack et al (Lemack et al 1999) showed that only 21% of urologists who have been trained more than ten years ago consider urethral dilatation as a viable option, whereas none of the urologists trained within the last decade consider it as a therapeutic option.

SUMMARY

Post-surgical incidence of BOO have been reported between 2.5-24%. All of the anti-incontinence procedures, including bulking agents can cause BOO in women. The diagnosis is made on the basis of symptoms, physical examinations and presence of high pressure voiding during pressure-flow studies. CIC is normally regarded as the mainstay of management but surgery may be required, particularly when there is marked over-elevation of the urethra and voiding dysfunction is severe.

VII. URETHRAL DIVERTICULAE

The diagnosis of female urethral diverticula is now being made with greater frequency due to awareness of the condition and its co-existence with incontinence. In a comprehensive videourodynamic study of 58 women with urethral diverticulum, Ganabathi et al (Ganabathi

1994) found that 53% had concomitant stress incontinence and 24% had detrusor instability (8 patients had both). In addition 2 patients (3%) had paradoxic incontinence (loss of urine associated with intermittent drainage of the diverticulum). Videourodynamics and voiding cystourethrography may be helpful to differentiate between true stress incontinence and paradoxic loss of urine (Figure 7).

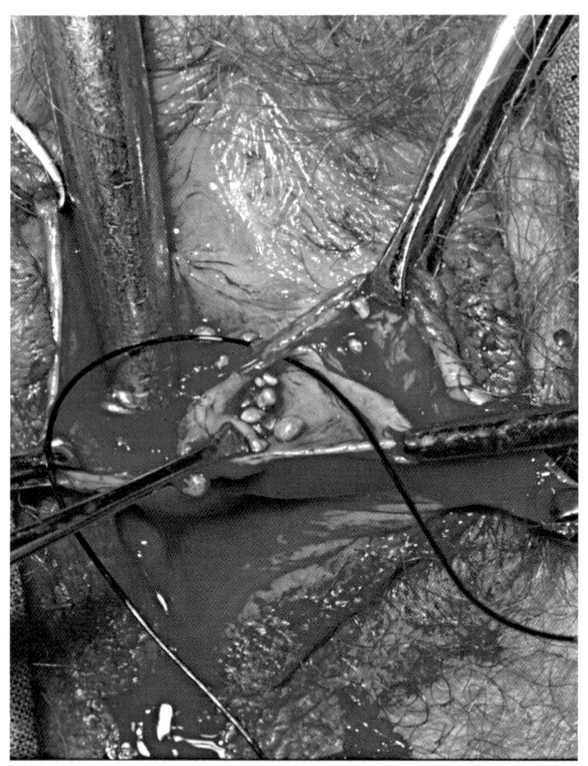

Figure 7 : A urethral diverticulum is illustrated. A dilator is placed in the urethra. The diverticulum contains small stones and a suture identifies the communication between the diverticulum and the urethral lumen.

Surgery for stress incontinence may be successfully performed along with urethral diverticulectomy (Table 5). Leach and Bavendam (Leach & Bavendam1987) described simultaneous needle bladder neck suspension in 22 women with stress incontinence. At a mean follow up of 20.5 months, 77% were totally continent and no significant complications were noted. Four of the five failures were secondary to ISD. In 1993, Swierzewski and McGuire (Swierzewski & McGiuire 1993) performed simultaneous autologous rectus fascia pubovaginal sling and urethral diverticulectomy in 14 women. All were cured of stress incontinence and one developed severe detrusor instability. A diverticulum recurred in 1 patient.

LEVELS OF EVIDENCE

All the evidence available is based on uncontrolled case series and therefore does not qualify for a more advanced level than 4.

VIII. SURGERY FOR REFRACTORY DETRUSOR INSTABILITY

Detrusor overactivity may be neurogenic (detrusor hyperreflexia) or non-neurogenic in origin. The underlying aetiology of the condition should be identified and appropriate medical therapy given for that aetiology. Surgical intervention for this condition is usually reserved for those patients who have failed conservative therapies, including pelvic floor exercises, bladder retraining, electrical stimulation of the pelvic floor, and pharmacologic treatment.

Surgery is a step of last resort and may be effective when detrusor overactivity is associated with involuntary contractions or diminished bladder compliance. In bladder disease the goal of surgical intervention is to prevent or modulate the development of intramural detrusor fibrosis (Sehn 1978). If it is initiated early enough within the natural history of the disease process poor compliance may be substantially decreased by early surgical intervention. However in patients with idiopathic detrusor instability, the aim is improved continence and preservation of upper urinary tract function.

A variety of surgical approaches have been tried for the management of the overactive bladder, including open and endoscopic approaches.

1. ENDOSCOPIC APPROACHES

Distension of the bladder utilizing hydrostatic pressure (cystodistension) has been used in the management of detrusor pathologies, including interstitial cystitis, urgency incontinence (Wang et al 1988) and even bladder tumours (Helmstein 1972). Overdistension is thought to reduce bladder dysfunction by causing degeneration of unmyelinated small sensory nerve fibers (c afferent). Success rates have varied from18% to 77%, with complications including hematuria, urinary retention, and bladder perforation in 5% to10% (Jorgenson et al 1985, Pengally et al 1978).

There are no long term studies on cystodistension. It may represent an intermediate step before considering more complicated surgical interventions. Although this method represents a very simple form of treatment, it may provoke interstitial fibrosis, leading to a contracted or non-distensible bladder. The proposed mechanism of activity is ischemic damage to sensory nerve endings reducing sensory input (Dunn1975). Initial supportive rates of 75% success have now not been upheld by more prolonged follow-up (Ramsden et all 1976, Delaere et al 1980).

A form of this technique is termed bladder "cycling," in which intermittent self-catheterization is used to increase bladder capacity periodically in an effort to improve

Table 5 : Complications of diverticulectomy from published series since 1956 in 872 women

Reference	No. Women	Follow up (mos)	No. Urethro-vaginal Fistula (%)	No. Recurrent Diverticulum (%)	No. Stress Incontinence (%)	No. Urethral Stricture (%)	No. Recurrent Urinary Tract Infections (%)
Wharton and Telinde	58	Not available	7		1.7	5.2	8.6
Davis and Telinde	84	Not available		11.9			13.1
MacKinnon et al	130	Not available	5.4	1.5	Several		10
Boatwright and Moore	48	Not available	8.3		4.2	2.1	
Hoffman and Adams	60	Not available	1.7		6.7	1.7	
Ward	24	Not available	8.3	29.2	12.5		
Davis and Robinson	98	Not available	4.1	1			
Pathak and House	42	Not available					
Benjamin et al	30	Not available	3.3	3.3	3.3		
Peters and Vaughan	32	24	6.3	25			10
Ginsburg and Genadry	52	12-240	1.9	25		1.9	
Rozsahegyi et al	50	Not available	2			2	
Lee RA	108	24-204	0.9	9.3	15	1.9	
Ganabathi et al	56	6 -136	1.8	3.6	16.1	0	0
Leng and McGuire	18	Not available	0	0	11	0	0

(Revised and reprinted from Leach GE, Trockman BA . Surgery for Vesicovaginal, and urethrovaginal fistula and urethral diverticulum. In Walsh PC, Retik AB, Vaughn ED, Wein A, eds:Campbell's Urology, 7th ed. Philadelphia, W.B. Saunders Company, 1997, pp1135 – 1153.)

overall bladder volumetric capacity. This technique has been described by Perlmutter for patients undergoing reconstruction of the lower urinary tract after revision of a urinary diversion and/or in transplant patients with a defunctionalized bladder. Although effective for the short-term management, this technique requires anaesthesia, and is usually only temporary in its overall symptomatic control. (Perlmutter 1980)

2. Open surgical interventions

a) Denervation

Denervation of the lower urinary tract can be accomplished at several levels:

1. in the bladder by injection of anesthetic or ablative chemicals or by hyperbaric bladder distention,

2. peripherally at the level of the pelvic nerves (immediately sub-trigonal, or more proximally at the anterior roots),

3. centrally at the level of sacral nerves,

Most of these procedures are associated with a high relapse rate of symptoms (or objective evidence of detrusor dysfunction) within 18 months after the procedure.

• ***Transvesical phenol injection:*** The utilization of dilute phenol (6%) injected through the base and trigone of the bladder has been described (Blackford et al 1982). Short term success followed by relapse rates approaching 100% within 18 months have been reported. Complications including vesicovaginal fistula have been reported (Chapple et al 1991, Nordling et al 1986).

• ***Ingelman-Sundberg Denervation:*** Initially described by Ingelman-Sundberg in 1950 (Ingelman Sundberg 1950), the procedure was utilized during radical hysterectomy for cervical carcinoma. It was subsequently modified as a transvaginal approach for the treatment of patients with refractory detrusor instability. Cespedes *et al.* utilized a modified technique composed of two steps. The first component was performed through a transvaginal approach to assess whether the patient would benefit from the procedure, utilizing a local anaesthetic block of the sub trigonal plexus. Subsequently, if successful, an open surgical neural ablation was carried out through an anterior vaginal wall dissection. 64% of patients (16) were cured at a mean of 14.8 months from surgery. A vaginal approach through which the terminal branches of the sensory pelvic nerves and postganglionic fibers are divided and/or are cauterised has been described. Cure rates of up to 70% of patients with documented motor instability have been reported, but is considered ineffective in sensory disorders such as interstitial cystitis (McGuire et al 1994).

• ***Cystolysis:*** Mundy (Mundy 1985) included a transection of the posterior and postero-lateral aspects of the bladder wall. This transection extended to a point approximately 1 cm above the ureteral orifices. In Mundy's study, 74% of patients were symptomatically cured, 12% failed, with 14% improvements at less than 12 months follow up. However, detrusor muscular atrophy occurred between two and five years, decreasing successful control of symptoms from a 65% to 16%. The transection technqiue has now been abandoned. This technique has given way to enterocystoplasty.

• ***Sacral bhizotomy:*** Sacral deafferentation of the bladder by dorsal sacral rhizotomy of the $S_{2\text{-}5}$ can be accomplished either peripherally or within the dura. A complete section of the anterior and posterior $S_{2\text{-}4}$ nerves results in permanent ablation of detrusor reflex function. Full rhizotomy, however, results in complete disruption of external anal and urethral sphincteric function, as well as loss of sexual function residing in erections and female lubrication, as well as sensation in the perineum and buttocks. The significant side effects of this technique have substantially limited its use.

Posterior sacral rhizotomy may be combined with anterior root stimulator implant, providing a means of voluntary stimulation of the motor efferents. This technique of deafferentiation and neurostimulation was developed by Brindley (Brindley 1982). Typically, an L4-L5 laminectomy is performed, the dura is opened, and the anterior and posterior sacral roots are identified and isolated using *in situ* stimulation. The posterior roots of S2, S3, and S4 are then transected, and a segment of the roots is removed. The anterior roots are then placed in an electrode "book", and the electrodes are connected to a Finetech-Brindley stimulator. The stimulator is driven by electromagnetic induction, and delivers intermittent bursts of stimulation to the anterior roots, timed in such a way as to offset the peaks of detrusor contraction and sphincter contraction, allowing the patient to void. The device can also facilitate defecation and erection. Egon et al (Egon et al 1998) recently reported a large series of patients with neurogenic bladder treated with posterior sacral rhizotomy and implantation of Brindley-Finetech sacral anterior root stimulators. Of 90 evaluable patients, 83 voided using their implants, and 82 were continent. Bladder capacity was significantly increased, and vesico-ureteral reflux disappeared. Re-operation was required in three patients with CSF leaks, and another two devices were explanted due to infection. In 1999, Weilink et al (Weilink 1999) demonstrated the potential for considerable health care cost savings in the long run, with positive effects on health status.

• ***Enterocystoplasty:*** The utilization of bowel segments to increase bladder capacity has been used for intractable detrusor instability. Some authors have also utilized this technique for interstitial cystitis. The goal of this procedure, like other procedures of this type, is to create a low-pressure, large-capacity reservoir with low-filling pressures (adequate compliance), which protects the upper urinary tract from pressure-related reflux and infection related to this reflux, as well as providing urinary continence. Augmentation enterocystoplasty is often utilized simultaneously with procedures to correct reflux or improve incompetent bladder outlets. Utilization of bowel to augment the bladder has been shown to decrease overall detrusor contractility and also to increase the volume at which the first detrusor contraction related to detrusor overactivity occurs. The bladder may be divided sagittally or transversely. There is still some argument regarding the appropriate configuration of the transected bladder and the type of bowel segment to be utilized. It is generally agreed that it is best to de-tubularize the intestine into a sphere, which will disrupt peristaltic contractions and increase overall bladder capacity. Herschorn and Hewitt (Herschorn and Hewett 1998) reported on 59 patients with neurogenic voiding dysfunction undergoing augmentation cystoplasty. In addition to showing improvement in urodynamic parameters (mean capacity increased from 220 ml to 523 ml and mean detrusor pressure at capacity decreased from 48.9 cmH2O to 15.8 cmH2O) continence improved, 67% demonstrating complete continence and 32% mild incontinence. They also reported patient satisfaction with a standardized questionnaire. Sixty-nine percent of patients were "delighted", 23% were "pleased" and 11% were "mostly satisfied " with the results of surgery. Complications specific to augmentation cystoplasty include: mucus production, which can cause either catheter or voiding obstruction, urinary tract infection, perforation resulting from incomplete or inadequate self-catheterization, and electrolyte abnormalities such as hyperchloremic acidosis. Perforation has been reported in 2-6% of patients in the long-term and surgical revision rates range from 15-36% (Herschorn and Hewitt 1998, Flood et al 1995). *N*-acetylcysteine instillation has been shown to be effective in decreasing mucus production in the bladder (Gillon et al 1989).

Ureterocystoplasty is another method utilizing native urothelium for bladder augmentation. Churchill *et al.* reviewed 16 patients, utilizing a catheterisation kidney ureter in 12 and a catheterisation duplex in 2. Fifteen patients required intermittent catheterisation and one voided spontaneously. This procedure has been modified to protect the distal blood supply with persistent improvements in compliance and capacity.

Gastrointestinal full-thickness segments may be utilized for augmentation or serial muscular graphs with de-epithelialized bowel segments may be used either alone or as a support for native urothelium. This was first proposed by Blandy in the early 1960s, and recently has attained new interest. Tissue engineering may provide further benefit in the future for augmentation indications. In Mundy's series (Mundy et al 1985), 37 of 190 patients experienced significant complications early in management, although 67 reported later urinary tract infections and later complications.

• ***Detrusor myomectomy:*** Detrusor myomectomy involves incising and removing the bladder muscle to allow bladder mucosa to form a pseudodiverticulum. The success of this procedure is incumbent upon removing large segments of muscle to prevent scarification of the muscle over the exposed mucosa.

From the recent literature, it appears that autoaugmentation is more successful in patients with idiopathic overactivity than those with neuropathic hyperreflexia, although success rates as high as 80% have been reported for this latter group (Swami, et al 1998). Seromuscular enterocystoplasty combines autoaugmentation with enterocystoplasty by laying a de-mucosalized detubularized segment of bowel over the exposed bladder mucosa following detrusor myectomy (Bunson, et al 1994). This theoretically avoids the complications associated with exposure of urine to gastrointestinal mucosa, and may prevent the loss in capacity seen over time with simple autoaugmentation. While recent literature cites encouraging results (Shekarriz et al, 2000), this technique remains limited to few centres, and long-term follow-up on significant numbers of patients is still pending.

• ***Urinary diversion:*** Urinary diversion is rarely needed, but may be useful in those patients with intractable detrusor instability with a very small reservoir. Diversion may be effective for helping the cause of pelvic pain that may be associated with detrusor overactivity. However, it represents a last-step intervention in the surgical management of incontinence resultant from detrusor overactivity.

CONCLUSIONS

1. Surgical therapy should only be considered when all conservative methods have failed.
2. Long-term results remain disappointing with surgical techniques for bladder overactivity.
3. Bladder augmentation appears to have supervened denervation procedures as being a reasonable intervention.
4. There is no evidence to support more extensive use of surgery.

LEVELS OF EVIDENCE

All the included studies in this section are non-randomized case series, usually with no cohort and only historical controls. The evidence available is therefore only Level 4 or 5.

IX. SURGERY FOR NON-OBSTETRIC FISTULAE

Extraurethral incontinence can be caused by an abnormal communication between the urinary tract, i.e bladder, urethra or ureter, and the vagina. Incontinence is often continuous, but can vary depending upon certain circumstances or patient position. Patients usually have "insensible incontinence" that is loss of urine without increase` in abdominal pressure or exertion or an` urge. Depending on the size of the fistula, incontinence can range from minimal to complete loss of all produced urine.

1. VESICO-VAGINAL FISTULAE

a) Aetiology

In developing countries birth trauma still accounts for the majority of fistulae. (Arrowsmith 1996). Prolonged labor induces tissue necrosis of the bladder base and urethra which results in tissue loss that can be substantial. Rarer causes include infectious disease (bilharziasis). In contradistinction, in developed countries, modern obstetric care has substantially limited the risk of vesicovaginal fistulae by reducing the duration of labour. In these areas fistulae are usually the consequence of complications of gynaecologic or other pelvic surgery. Regardless of the aetiology, fistulae can cause substantial life disruption for the patient and medical legal consequences for caring physicians. The most common cause of vesicovaginal fistula is abdominal or vaginal hysterectomy and approximately 75% of genitourinary fistulae are produced in this way. (Jonas 1984, Lee 1988; Symmonds 1984; Tancer 1992). Fistulae occurring after hysterectomy are thought to be due to tissue necrosis caused by inadvertent suture incorporation of vaginal tissue from the cuff closure into an unrecognised bladder wall injury. Tissue necrosis promotes fibrosis and induration, finally resulting in an epithelial or mucosal lining of the fistula tract (Kursh, 1988). In 1980 Goodwin reported 32 patients with fistulae as a direct result of gynaecologic surgery. Tancer (1992) noted a similar group of 151 patients and found that 91% (137) were post-surgical with 125 caused by gynaecologic surgery. The most common procedure accounting for fistula was hysterectomy in 73% (110) of cases (99 of which were performed transabdominally). Factors thought to contribute to the risk of fistula formation due to hysterectomy included prior cesarean section, intrinsic uterine disease (endometriosis) and the possibility of prior ablative treatment for carcinomas (pelvic radiation therapy). Similar risk factors were identified by Blandy et al. (1991) The incidence of fistula after hysterectomy is generally accepted to be 0.1 - 0.2%. (Harris, 1995) The influence of factors such as the grade/experience of the surgeon and the patient's habitus have not been studied. Other causes of fistulae include malignancy (Kottmeier, 1964), radiation (Cushing, 1968 , Stockbine 1970, and Villasanta, 1972), gastrointestinal surgery (low anterior resection) (Cross, 1993), inflammatory bowel disease and urinary tuberculosis (Ba-Thike et al, 1992). Symmonds' experience at the Mayo clinic revealed only 5% of 800 vesicovaginal fistulae to be due to obstetric causes (Symmonds1984). Rarely, foreign bodies such as pessaries, diaphragms, and intrauterine devices also may lead to fistula formations (Goldstein et al, 1990). Iatrogenic CO2 laser therapy for cervical disease has also resulted in bladder fistulae. (Colombel 1995) Autoimmune diseases such as Bechet's disease have also been recently implicated as causative for vesicovaginal fistulae due to extensive vasculitis related bladder wall necrosis. (Monteiro 1995)

b) Clinical features

The most common presenting symptom of an iatrogenic genitourinary fistula is continuous urinary drainage from the vagina after gynaecological or other pelvic surgery. A fistula may become apparent either immediately or much more commonly after a delay of several days to weeks after surgery. Patients may present while in the hospital with prolonged ileus, excessive pain, haematuria or loin pain (Kursh 1998). If the fistula tract is large enough a significant amount if not all urine drains through the vagina producing total incontinence. In other cases, fistula drainage may be minimal and intermittent and may be initially mistaken for stress incontinence occurring postoperatively. Patients with urethrovaginal fistulae arising from urethral catheter trauma may not develop symptoms until catheter removal has occurred. Incontinence arising from a urethrovaginal fistula may be intermittent unless the fistula extends across the bladder neck, in these cases severe and total incontinence is usually encountered.

c) Treatment

1. Conservative management

Most vesicovaginal fistulae are identified late after the initial surgical intervention. Regardless of the timing of presentation, a trial of conservative therapy may be implemented which uses continuous urethral / suprapubic catheter drainage supplemented with anticholinergics. This management technique is less likely to be successful in the woman with a mature tract (six weeks or longer after inciting event). Tancer et al (1992) reported 3 of 151 patients with spontaneous closure of fistula using this strategy.

Another possible conservative therapy utilizes electrocoagulation or fulguration of the lining of the fistulae tract (O'Connor 1980, Alonso 1985, Molina 1989, Stovsky 1994). In Stovsky's experience 11 of 17 (73%) of patients with small (less than 3mm) fistulae treated with electrofulguration and 2 weeks of catheter drainage resolved. This technique should not be used for large fistulous tracts. The magnitude of current intensity should be minimal. This technique is also not to be used for inflammatory, immature, or malignant fistulae. Another alternative, but similar strategy is the use of metallic objects to physically abrade the tract. The concept of this technique is physical disruption of the tract which instigates an inflammatory response leading to fistula closure. McKay (1997) recently described successful cystoscopically placed suture closure of a vesicovaginal fistula, with no secondary incision.

2. Surgical therapy

➡ *General concepts*

Optimal results for fistula closure are obtained when surgery is performed on a mature fistula tract. It is generally agreed that the first effort at surgical fistula closure is the most likely to succeed. Results approximating 90% are obtainable on the first operative intervention in woman who have not undergone radiation and do not have active carcinoma as the cause of the fistula. Multiple factors impact upon the success of fistula repair including the duration of fistula communication, the aetiology of the tract, the presence of necrotic tissues, surgical technique, and experience of the operating surgeon.

All suture lines should be watertight, tension-free, non-overlapping, and exist in an uninfected environment. If the repair is tenuous, interpositional graft materials may be helpful. (Wein 1980, Raz 1992, Raz 2000)

Previously, many authors have advocated a waiting period of at least 3 to 6 months before intervening with surgical therapy (O' Connor 1951, Wein 1980, Blandy 1991). More recently surgeons have advocated an individualized approach without an observational period. Several authors have reported superb results with early interventions (Persky, 1979, Goodwin 1980, Wang 1990, Raz 1992, Blaivas 1995, Raz 2000). Fistulae identified within the first 24 to 48 hours postoperatively can be safely repaired immediately. Those identified days to weeks after surgery require careful planning and selection. Wang and Hadley successfully managed 15 of 16 (94%) high lying (vaginal apical) fistulae through a transvaginal approach, with all 7 patients who were less than three months from initial surgery cured of fistula. (Wang 1990) Surgical judgment is needed since there are no prospective studies to determine the optimal technique for each aetiology.

➡ ***Surgical approaches***

Surgical approaches for vesicovaginal fistulae include: combined abdominal vaginal, vaginal, or abdominal approaches. The approach chosen is dependent upon several factors including location of fistula (position related to apex), quality and mobilty of tissue, the angle of the sub-pubic arch and the surgeon's experience. Vaginal surgery is usually quicker and results in less morbidity (avoiding an abdominal incision) and more rapid recovery. However, the vaginal route may be difficult in patients with a significant degree of fibrosis, pelvic immobility, or with large tracts with possible injury in close proximity to the ureteral orifices. The abdominal approach should be utilised for the poorly visualized tract , the narrow or immobile vagina, and those with close proximity to a ureteral orifice. All approaches should lend themselves to the possibility of interposition grafts. (see later).

➡ ***Vaginal approach***

The vaginal approach may utilize the creation of an anterior vaginal wall mucosal flap. Subsequently a tension free closure is performed utilizing a long acting (polyglycolic acid or polydioxanone) suture and non-overlapping multiple closure lines.

If the fistula repair is tenuous or there is concern regarding apposition of suture lines a Martius interpositional graft may be utilised. (see later on interpositional options) If this is not obtainable, alternative graft sources include peritoneal flap (Raz 2000) or interposition graft utilizing gracilis muscle tissue. The peritoneum can be freed from the posterior aspect of the bladder and easily advanced to cover the layers of the closure as well (Raz 1993).

Martius interposition utilizes the fibro- fatty tissues of the labia majora, which are well vascularised (Martius 1928, Raz 1992, Blaivas 1995, Blaivas 2000). The fat pad may be mobilized utilizing either a pudendal or epigastric based pedicle because of the constancy of blood supply.(Hoskins, 1984) After mobilization of the fat pad, the graft is tunnelled under the vaginal wall from labia to vaginal incision and is sutured in place over the fistula repair site with absorbable sutures. The vaginal mucosal flap is then closed over the site. A small Penrose drain is usually placed in the harvest site (the labia) to prevent haematoma accumulation. Several authors have used this graft as an adjunct to repair associated with complicated incontinence with excellent results. (Ghoniem 1995, Carr 1996)

In patients who are poor operative candidates, the Latzko (1942) technique of proximal vaginal fistula repair may also be attempted. This technique involves excision of the vaginal epithelium around the fistula site and colpocleisis with several layers of absorbable sutures from anterior to posterior wall obliterating the upper vagina. No actual excision of the fistula tract occurs during this procedure and therefore ureteral re-implantation should not be required (Raz 1992). Vaginal depth is compromised by this procedure but several authors (Raz 1992) have reported no impact on sexual function from this procedure.

The vast majority of vesicovaginal fistulae can be closed in one operation using a vaginal technique. Success rates range from 67-100%. Raz reported a success rate of 92% (64/69) for vesicovaginal fistulae, 2/3 of which had failed 1 to 3 prior repairs using this technique (Raz 1992).

a) Abdominal approach

All bladder fistulae (except those extending into the urethra) may be approached through the abdomen and this is the preferred approach in those patients requiring bladder augmentation or ureteral re-implantation. Experience in N America was reported by O'Conor (1951, 1973) for abdominal transvesical repair of vesicovaginal fistulae. Omentum may be interposed between the repaired bladder and vagina (Wein 1980;Turner-Warwick, 1976; Kiricuta, 1972). Reported success rates with the abdominal approach are approximately 85% - 90% (Marshall 1979, Wein 1980, Gil-Vernet

1989, Udeh 1985 ,Demirel 1993, Kristensen 1994, Blaivas 1995, Raz 2000). Table 6 summarizes a group published series for success rates and timing of repair. Recently, Nesrallah et al reported a 100% success rate using the O'Conor transabdominal supratrigonal technique in 29 patients. (Nesrallah 1999) Other authors have reported similar results (Table 6).

➨ *Interposition grafts*

Some authors feel that the routine interposition of healthy well vascularised tissue between the bladder and vagina is not necessary for uncomplicated fistula repairs, but rather should be reserved for complex cases such as failures, radiation, malignancy, compromised field, etc. Others place such grafts routinely. In a non-randomised retrospective review of transabdominal fistula repairs, where grafts were placed solely by surgeon's discretion, Evans et al reported a 100% success rate for benign fistulae repaired with an interposition flap, vs. 63% when a flap was not used. Similarly, fistula associated with malignancy success rates were 100% vs. 67%.

Reconstructive techniques have been described utilizing a variety of interpositional tissues including fibro-fatty labial interposition tissues, anterior/posterior bladder flaps (autografts), myocutaneous flaps including rectus, sartorius, gluteus, and gracilis muscle flaps as well as combined myocutaneous flaps (Garlock 1928, Byron 1969, Stirnemann 1969, Menchaca 1990, Blaivas 1991, Raz 1992, Candiani 1993, Tancer 1993, Brandt 1998, Raz 2000) as adjuncts to repair of the complex vesicovaginal fistula.

Table 6 : Results of fistula repairs, including timing of repair

Author (Date)	Number of patients	Success (%)	Fistula duration before surgery	Surgical technique
Collins (1960)	24	67	20 (<2 mth) 8 (> 4 mth)	24 vag
Eisen (1974)	29	90	29 (> 3 mths)	29 abd
Persky (1979)	7	86	7 (< 10 wks)	6 abd/1
vag Tancer (1980)	45	93	8 – 16 wks	43 vag / 1abd/ 1sp
Wein (1980)	34	88	> 3 mths	34 abd
Keetel (1982)	168	94	> 3 mths	156 vag/ 6 abd/ 6 com
Bisada(1983)	7	100	NS	7 abd
Cruikshank (1988)	11	100	< 1 mth	9 vag/ 1 abd / 1 comb
Lee (1988)	182	98	15 < 2 mths 167 > 2 mths	15 vag/ 130 vag/ 37 abd
Elkins (1990)	23	91	> 2 mths	23 vag
Wang (1990)	16	94	7 < 3 mths 9 > 3 mths	16 vag
Blandy(1991)	25	100	12 < 1.5 mths 13 > 1.5 mths	25 abd
O'Conor (1991)	77	91	> 2 mths	77 abd
Raz (1993)	19	84	>2 mths	19 vag
Demnirel (1993)	26	88	> 3 mths	8 vag /18 abd
Kristensen (1994)	18	94	>2 mths	18 Abd
Brandt (1998)	80	96	>1 mths	80 abd
Nesrallah (1999)	29	100	> 6 wks	29 abd

Vag = vaginal

Abd = Abdominal

Spon = spontaneous closure

Comb = combined abdominal and vaginal approach

2. URETHROVAGINAL FISTULAE

Urethrovaginal fistulae may be very small pinpoint fistulae demonstrated by vaginal voiding or may present as complete urethral and bladder neck loss with total urinary incontinence. This circumstance most commonly results from prior gynecologic surgery, with anterior repair and urethral diverticulectomy comprising the most common inciting procedures (Blaivas 1989, Raz 2000). Additionally, complete urethral loss due to trauma arising from prolonged urethral catheter malposition may occur.

Previously birth trauma was a cause of majority of urethral defects, however in developed nations this is now a rare cause of urethrovaginal fistulae. Prolonged obstructive labor, however remains a major cause of urethral injury in developing nations (Elkins 1994).

Techniques used for urethrovaginal fistula closure are very similar to those utilised for transvaginal vesicovaginal fistula repair (Webster 1984). Complete urethral loss is a more daunting surgical challenge and a multiplicity of techniques has been described for this (Blaivas 1989, Blaivas 1996, Hendren 1980 and 1998, Patil 1980). These techniques usually employ some type of flap utilizing either vaginal, bladder, or alternative tissue in an onlay versus tubularized reconstruction (Blaivas 1989). Simultaneous stress incontinence procedures should be performed to obviate the risk of postoperative incontinence (Blaivas 1990). Preoperative assessment of the degree of urethral loss as well as the function of the intrinsic urethral mechanism should be established prior to surgical intervention.

➡ *Urethral reconstruction*

Multiple procedures have been described for urethral reconstruction although many authors now prefer the transvaginal approach. Abdominal approaches previously described include posterior bladder flaps as described by Young and modified by Theiss as well as Ledbetter in 1964. Tanagho in 1981 also described an anterior bladder flap (Tanagho 1981). The abdominal approaches use omentum to reinforce the repair and also allow for simultaneous ureteral re-implantation.

The use of the vaginal approach has been well-described (Goodwin 1980, Blaivas 1991, Elkins 1992) and has been successfully used for all types of urethral bladder neck defects. Elkins also has described a transvaginal neoruethral reconstruction using the anterior bladder wall, however most investigators now use either vaginal flaps alone or in conjunction with Martius labial fascia interposition (Goodwin 1980, Webster 1984, Blaivas 1989 and 1991, Raz 1992, Bissada1997). Recently, utilization of rectus abdominis flaps for repair of recurrent urethrovaginal fistulae has been reported as a highly successful procedure. Bruce et al (2000) reported 100% success in 6 women with recurrent fistulae, 5 of whom were continent and able to void. Their technique used a combined abdominal-vaginal approach with rectus interposition. These authors recommended this flap as a salvage procedure after failed Martius graft. Another tissue alternative prior to bladder neck closure is the perineal based flap poineered by Hendren which provides an interpositional graft and also apparently conveys improved continence status possibly due to increased urethral length as compared to standard anterior bladder tube neourethral reconstructions (Hendren 1998).

In debilitated patients or patients with severe local tissue defects, bladder neck closure with a concomitant catheterisable stoma may be indicated (Ziedman 1989). Bladder neck closure should accomplish a tensionf ree circumferential closure of the remnant urethra at the bladder neck by complete disruption of the endopelvic fascia at the bladder neck, and layered inverting closure of the urethral stump.

Urethral incontinence after reconstruction may be a consequence of bladder and/or urethral factors as well as urethral fistula re-formation. Careful examination should help identify this consequence. Periurethral injections may be useful in selective cases (Lockhart 1988, Ganabathi 1994b) however, the quality of the surrounding tissues must be evaluated as the neo-urethral wall no longer has a well defined submucosa for injection. As with diverticulum repair, urethral strictures may result from a too narrow tubularization of the neo-urethra.

Blaivas (1996) reported on 49 women undergoing one stage vaginal flap reconstruction of urethra and/or bladder neck. Overall, 42 of 49 (87%) were continent, 6 of 7 failures were successful after a second procedure. Forty one patients underwent a sling and 5 a needle suspension (3 of whom subsequently required a sling). In 47 women a Martius was used and in one each a gracilis or anterior bladder tube functioned as the neourethra.

CONCLUSION

Surgical repair of non-obstetric vesico-vaginal fistulae may be performed abdominally or vaginally, the latter allowing a quicker post-operative recovery. (Level 4) Use of interpositional grafts may aid successful fistula repair (Level 3) There are no RCT's reported on the optimal method for fistula repair.

X. RESEARCH RECOMMENDATIONS

A. There is now a recognition that outcome from surgery for stress incontinence is not simply an issue of cure of stress incontinence. Research is required to understand:

1. What is the optimal measure of a good outcome? Is it cure of stress incontinence? Is it improved quality of life?
2. How do quality of life scores relate to objective measures of outcome?
3. How do symptom scores relate to objective measures of outcome?
4. Can improvement be defined in terms of symptom or QOL scores?

B. The Chapter has highlighted the large number of confounding variables which may influence outcome. Research is required to define the influence these variables may have on the outcome so that future research on surgical procedures can stratify for these variables if they are important.

C. Stress incontinence and prolapse commonly coexist. It appears that surgery for either condition commonly results in the development of the other. Research is needed into how to reduce the risk of prolapse developing after surgery for stress incontinence. The techniques used to try to predict "latent" incontinence need evaluation in order to prevent this unfortunate sequel to prolapse surgery.

D. It is evident from the literature that the risk of stress incontinence recurring after surgery increases with time. Some reports suggest that this risk evens out after approximately ten years. The risk of recurrence needs to be studied prospectively and the factors which influence the risk of recurrence over time should then become more fully understood.

E. Sling procedures are increasing in popularity. The optimal sling material needs to be determined. The advantages of using synthetic or cadaveric sling materials are obvious in avoiding the need for harvesting from the patient but the evidence to date illustrates the increased risks of infection and erosion. Large studies comparing slings with other retropubic procedures and different sling materials are required.

F. Pelvic floor physiotherapy is often tried before surgery in the treatment of stress incontinence. There is a need to determine whether pelvic floor physiotherapy *in conjunction with* surgery influences the outcome since the pelvic floor has both muscle and fascial components. Both components have a part to play in the normal continence mechanism.

G. It is to be hoped that pharmacotherapy will ultimately improve to the degree that surgery for detrusor instability will become obselete. In the meantime the procedures in current use need more rigorous evaluation than has been performed to date. This includes not only objective measures of continence but also evaluation of quality of life outcome. The magnitude and risks of these procedures is such that more objective analysis is required.

H. Women who develop a urinary fistula after gynaecological surgery suffer the misfortune of developing a more severe problem than at original presentation. The optimal management of a non-obstetric fistula, including which surgeon performs the repair, needs to be studied to reduce the risk of a chronic incontinence problem.

CONCLUSIONS

The medical press is still publishing case series of surgical procedures for stress incontinence that are scientifically flawed in many areas. This does not serve to inform and may mislead, often presenting an over-optimistic view of the outcome.

A minimum data set of information should be included in the assessment of any surgical procedure. Such a data set should include the following domains:

1. Anatomical / physiological- structured physical examination and urodynamics (POP-Q)

2. Symptoms (Validated questionnaire)

3. Urine loss (pad test)

4. Quality of Life (Validated questionnaire)

5. Full documentation of all confounding variables

6. Economic costs

It could be argued that, in complying with the type of scrutiny applied to new pharmacological agents, ethical approval should be sought before embarking on a study of any new procedure. Approval should only be then given if the study is designed in a manner which would have a reasonable chance of providing useful data.

In addition, when a new procedure becomes available for more widespread use, a central register, incorporating the same data set, could be employed to ensure that all the facts about the procedure could be learnt by the surgical community as soon as possible.

There is a recognition by the Research Funding Agencies that the literature on the surgical management of urinary incontinence needs to be improved by well constructed, multi-centre trials. It is up to the clinicians to present such trials for grant approval.

REFERENCES

Abrams PH, Griffiths DJ The assessment of prostatic obstruction from urodynamic measurements and from residual urine. Br J Urol 1979; 51: 129

Alcalay M. Monga A. Stanton S. Burch colposuspension: a 10-20 year follow up. British J. Obstet and Gynaecol. 1995, Vol. 102, 740-745.

Aldridge CW, Beaton, JH, Nanzig RP: A review of office urethroscopy and cystometry. Am J Obstet Gynecol 1978;131:432-435.

Alonso Gorrea M, Fernandez Zuaza J, Mompo Sanchis JF et al: Spontaneous healing of ureterovesicovaginal fistulas. Eur Urol 1985; 11:341 -344.

Amundsen CL, Visco AG, Ruiz H, Webster GD Outcome in 104 pubovaginal slings using freeze-dried allograFt fascia lata from a single tissue bank. Urology, 2000, 56 (soppl 6A) : 2-8

Anderson MJF: The incidence of diverticula in the female. J Urol 1967;98:96-98.

Anderson JT, Heisterberg S, Hebjorn S et al. Suprapubic versus transurethral bladder drainage after colposuspension/vaginal repair. Acta Obstet Gynecol Scand 1985; 64: 139-143

Andersson KE Current concepts in the treatment of disorders of micturition. Drugs 1988; 35: 477

Andersson KE Pharmacology of lower urinary tract smooth muscles and penile erectile tissue. Pharmacol Rev. 1993; 45: 253

Appel RA. Techniques and results in the implantation of the artifical urinary sphincter in women with type III stress urinary incontinence by the vaginal approach. Neurourol Urodyn. 1988; 7: 613-619

Appell R. A. Collagen Injection therapy for urinary incontinence. Urologic Clinics of North America, Vol. 21. Number 1, Feb 1994.

Appell RA Collagen injection therapy for urinary incontinence. Urol. Clin 1994; 21: 177

Appell RA Clinical efficacy and safety of Toterodine in the treatment of overactive bladder; a pooled analysis. Urology 1997; 50 (suppl 6A): 90-96

Aragona F, Mangano M, Artibani W, et al: Stone formation in female urethral diverticulum: Review of the literature. Int Urol Nephrol 1989;21:621-623.

Arrowsmith SD: Genitourinary reconstruction in obstetric fistulas. J Urol 1994;152:403-406.

Arrowsmith S, Hamlin EC, Wall LL: Obstructed labor injury complex: obstetric fistula formation and the multi-factorial morbidity of maternal birth trauma in the developing world. Obstet Gynecol Surv. 1996; 51: 568 –572.

Austin P, Spyropoulous E, LotenfoeR et al Urehtral obstruction after anti-incontinence surgery in women; evaluation, methodology and surgical results.

Axelrod SL, Blaivas JG Bladder neck obstruction in women. J Urol 1987; 137:497

Baert L, Willemen P, Oyen R: Endovaginal sonography: new diagnostic approach for urethral diverticula. J Urol 1992; 147: 464 -467.

Bailey K V A clinical investigation into uterine prolapse with stress incontinence treatment by modified Manchester colporrhaphy J Obstet Gynaec Brit Comm 1954 63 663-676

Bakke A, Vollset SE Risk factors for bacteremia and clinical urinary tract infectionin patients treated with clean intermittent self catheterisation. J. Urol 1993; 128:643

Ball TP: Editorial comment on Ginsberg et al: Posthysterectomy vaginal vault fistula : diagnosis and ma-nagement. Urol 1998; 52: 61 –65.

Ba-Thike K, Than-Aye, Nan-Oo: Tuberculous vesicovaginal fistula. Int J Gynecol Obstet 1992;37:127-130.

Beck RP, McCormick S, Nordstrom L. The fascia lata sling procedure for treating recurrent genuine stress incontinence of urine. Obstet Gynecol 1988; 72: 699-703

Beck R P, McCormick S and Nordstrom L. A 25-year experience with 519 anterior colporrhaphy procedures. Obstetrics and Gynecology, 1991, 78, 1011-18.

Benjamin J, Elliot L, Cooper J, et al: Urethral diverticulum in adult female: Clinical aspects, operative procedure, and pathology. Urology 1974; 3:1-7.

Bent AE, Ostergard DR, Zwick-Zaffuto M. Tissue reaction to expanded polytetrafluroethylene suburethral sling for urinary incontinence. Am J Obstet Gynecol 1993; 169: 1198-1204

Berglund AL, Eisemann M, Lalos A & Lalos O Predictive factors of the outcome of primary surgical treatment of stress incontinence in women. Scan J Urol Nephrol; 1997; 31: 49-55

Bergman A. Kooning P.P. Ballard A Primary stress incontinence and pelvic relaxation: prospective randomised comparison of three different operations. Am. J. Obstet Gynecol. And Gynaecol. 1989, Vol 161, Number 1, 97-101.

Bergman A, Matthews L, Ballard CA, Roy S. Suprapubic versus transurethral bladder drainage after surgery for stress urinary incontinence Obstet Gynecol 1987; 69: 546.

Bergman A, Ballard CA, Coonings PP Comparison of three different surgical procedures for genuine stress incontinence: prospective randomised study. Am. J. Obstet Gynacol. (1989); 160 (5 part 1): 1102-6

Bergman A. Elia G. Three surgical procedures for genuine stress incontinence: Five-year follow up of a prospective randomised study. Am. J. Obstet Gynecol. and Gynae, 1995, Vol. 173, Number 1, 66-71.

Berglung AJ, Eisemann M, Latos A, Lalos O. Prodictive factors of the outcome of primary surgical treatment of stress incontinence in women. Scan J Urol Nephrol. 1996; 31: 49-55

Bersland HO, Fossberg E, Sander S, Moer A Urodynamic studies before and after retropubic urethropexy for stress incontinence in females. Surg. Gynaecol. Obstet. (1982) 155: 133-6

Bidmead J and Cardozo L. Sling techniques in the treatment of genuine stress incontinence. Br. J. of Obstet. & Gynaecol. 2000; 107: 147-56

Bissada NK, McDonald D: Management of giant vesicovaginal and vesicourethrovaginal fistulas. J Urol 1983; 130: 1073 –1075.

Bissada NK, Morcos RR: Voiding patterns and urinary control after repair of giant vesicovaginal and vesicourethrovaginal fistulas and neourethral contruction. Neururol Urodyn 1986; 5: 321 –326.

Bissada SA, Bissada NK: Repair of active radiation induced vesicovaginal fistula using combined gastric and omental segments based on the gastroepiploic vessels. J Urol 1992; 147: 1368 –1369.

Bissada NK: Vesicovaginal fistulas. In Urinary Incontinence.

Blackford HN, Murray K, Stephenson TP, et al: Results of transvesical infiltration of the pelvic plexuses with phenol in 116 patients. Br J Urol 56: 647-649, 1982.

Blackford NN, Murray K, Stephenson TP et al. Transvesical infiltration of the pelvic plexuses with phenol. Br J Urol 1984; 56: 647-9

Blandy JP, Badenoch DF, Fowler CG et al: Early repair of iatrogenic injury to the ureter or bladder after gynecologic surgery. J Urol 1991; 146: 761 –765.

Blaivas JG, Apell RA, Fantl JA, Leach G, McGuire EJ, Resnick NM, Raz Shlomo, Wein AJ Standards of Efficacy for Evaluation of Treatment Outcomes in Urinary Incontinence: Recommendations of the Urodynamic Society (1997): Neurourology and Urodynamics. 16:145-147

Blaivas JG: Vaginal flap urethral reconstruction: An alternative to the bladder flap neourethra. J. Urol 1989;141:542-545.

Blaivas JG: Treatment of female incontinence secondary to urethral damage or loss. Urol Clin North AM 1991; 18:355-363.

Blaivas JG, Heritz, DM, Romanzi LI: Early versus late repair of vesicovaginal fistulas: Vaginal and abdominal approaches. J Urol 1995; 153:1110-1113.

Blaivas JG, Heritz DM: Vaginal flap reconstruction of the urethra and vesical neck in women: a report of 49 cases. J Urol 1996; 155: 1014 – 1017.

Blacklock ARE, Shaw RE, Geddes JR: Late presentation of ectopic ureter. Br J Urol 1982;54:106-110.

Boatwright DC, Moore V: Suburethral diverticula in the female. J Urol 1963;89:581.

Boyd SD, Raz S: Ectopic ureter presenting in midline urethral diverticulum. Urology 1993;41(6):571-574.

Brandt FT, Lorenzato FR, Albuquerque CD: Treatment of vesicovaginal fistula by bladder mucosa autograft technique. J Amer Coll Surg. 1998; 186: 645 - 650.

Brindley GS, Polkey CE, Rushton DN. Sacral anterior root stimulation for bladder control in paraplegia. Paraplegia 1982; 20: 363-81

Brown SL, Govier FE Cadaveric versus autologous fascia lata for the pubovaginal sling: surgical outcome and patient satisfaction. J. Urol, 2000; 164 : 1633-1637

Bruce RG, Rizk ES, El-Galley ES, Galloway NTM: Use of rectus abdominis muscle flap for the treatment of complex and refractory urethrovaginal fistulas. J Urol 2000; 163, 1212 – 1215.

Bryans FE. Marlex gauze hammock sling operation with Cooper's ligament attachment in the management of recurrent urinary stress incontinence. Am J Obstet Gynecol 1979; 133: 292-294.

Bueger G & Korden A The effect of obesity on the outcome of successful surgery for genuine stress incontinence Aust. New Zeal, J O&G 1992 32 71

Bump RC, Fantl JA,Hunt WG The mechanism of urinary incontinence in women with severe uterovaginal prolapse: results of barrier studiesObstet. Gynaecol 72 Sept 88 291-295

Bump RC Racial comparisons and contrasts in urinary incontinence and pelvic organ prolapse. Obstetrics & Gynaecology 1993 Vol 81 No 3 421-425

Bump RC, Coates JW, Cundiff GW, Harris RL & Weiner AC Diagnosing intrinsic sphincter deficiency: comparing urethral closure pressure, urethral axis and Valsalva leak point pressure. 1997.

Bump RC, Fantle JA, Hunt WG Dynamic urethral pressure profilometry pressure transmission ration determinations after continence surgery: understanding the mechanism of success, failure and complications. Obs & Gynae (1988) 72 No 6 : 870-874

Burch JC Coopers Ligament ureterovesical suspension for stress incontinence Am J O & G 1968 100 6: 764-774

Burton G. A five year prospective randomised urodynamic study comparing open and laparoscopic colposuspension. Neurourol and Urodyn 1999.

Bunson H, Manivel JC, Dayanc M, et al.: Seromuscular colocystoplasty lined with urothelium: Experimental study. Urology 44:773-748, 1994.

Buttyan R, Chen MW, Levin RM Animal models of bladder outlet obstruction; a molecular insight into the basis for dvelopment of bladder dysfunction. Act Neurol Scan. 1981; 64:175

Byron RL, Ostergard DR: Sartorius muscle interposition for the treatment of the radiation induced vaginal fistula. Am J Obstet Gynecol 1969; 104: 104 –107.

Cardozo L, Stanton SL, Williams JE Detrusor instability following surgery for genuine stress incontinence. Br J Urol , 1979; 51:204

Cespedes DR, Cross CA, McGuire Ej. Modified Ingelman-Sundberg bladder denervation procedure for intractable urge incontinence. J Urol 1996; 156: 1744-7

Chahliha C and Stanton SL Complications of surgery for genuine stress incontinence Br. J. Obstet. Gynaecol. 1999 Vol 106 pp 1238-1245

Chaikin DC, Rosenthal J and Blaivas JG Pubovaginal fascial sling for all types of stress urinary incontinence - long term analysis. J. of Urol. 1988 160: 1312-6

Chapple CR, Hampson SJ, Turner-Warwick RT, and Worth PH: Subtrigonal phenol injection: how safe and effective is it? Br J Urol 68: 483-486, 1991.

Chancellor MB, Blaivas JG, Kaplan SA et al Bladder outlet obstruction v impaired detrusor contractility; the role of uroflow. J. Urol 191; 145;810

Chassagne S, Bernier PA, Haab F, Roehrborn CG, Reich JS, Zimmern PE Proposed cut-off values to define bladder outlet obstruction in women. Urology 1998; 51: 408-411

Chin YK, Stanton SL. A follow up of silastic sling for genuine stress incontinence. Br J Ob Gynaecol. 1995; 102 (2): 143-147

Colombo M. Miliani R. Vitobello D. Maggioni A. Randomised comparison of Burch colposuspension abdominal paravaginal defect repair for female stress urinary incontinence. Am. J. Obstet Gynecol. And Gynaecol, 1996, Vol. 175, Number 1, 78-84.

Colombo M, Vitbello D, Proietti F, Milani R Randomised comparison of Burch colposuspension versus anterior colporrhaphy in women with stress urinary incontinence and anterior vaginal wall prolapse. Br. J. Obstet. Gynaecol (2000); 107 (4) : 544-551

Colombo M, Zanetta G, Vitobello D, Milani R. The Burch colposuspension for women with ? ? detrusor over-activity. Br J O&G March 1996 Vol 103 255-260

Concurrent genuine stress incontinence and detrusor instability Int. Urogynae J. 1990 1 128-131

Corcos J, Fournier C. Periurethral collagen injection for the treatment of female stress urinary incontinence: 4-year follow up results. Urology 1999 Nov;54(5):815-8

Cummings JM, Boullier JA & Parra RO Surgical correction of stress incontinence in morbidly obese women. J of Urology Vol 160 754-755 Sept 1998

Candiani P, Austoni E, Campiglio GL, et al: Repair of a recurrent urethrovaginal fistula with an island bulbocavernous musculocutaneous flap. Plast Reconstr Surg 1993;92:1393-1996.

Carr LK, Webster GD: Full-thickness cutaneous Martius flaps: a useful technique in female reconstructive urology. Urol 1996; 48: 461 –464.

Catalona S, Jones I: Transitional cell carcinoma in a urethral diverticulum. Aust N Z Obstet Gynecol 1992;32:85-86.

Chancellor MG, Liu JB, Rivas DA: Intraoperative endoluminal ultraosund evaluation of urethral diverticula. J Urol 1995; 153: 72 –75.

Clayton M, Siumi P, Guinan P: Urethral diverticular carcinoma. Cancer 1992;70:665-670.

Collins CG, Collins JH, Harrison BR et al: Early repair of vesicovaginal fistula. Am J Obstet Gynecol 1971;111: 524 –527.

Colombel M, Pedron P, Missirlu A et al: Vesicovaginal fistula after laser vaporization of vaginal condylomata. J Urol 1885; 154: 1860.

Cross SB, Copas PR: Colovaginal fistula secondary to diverticular disease. J Reprod Med 1993; 38: 905 -906

Cushing RM, Tovell HM, Leigner LM: Major urologic complications following radium and x-ray therapy for carcinoma of the cervix. Am J Obstet Gynecol 1968; 101: 750-755.

Dairiki Shortliffe L.M. Freiha F. S. Kessler R. Stamey A. Constantinou C. Treatment of urinary incontinence by the periurethral implantation of Glutaraldehyde cross-linked collagen. J. Urology, 1989, Vol. 141. 538-541.

Daneshgari F, Zimmern PE, Jacomides L: Magnetic resonance imaging detection of symptomatic noncommunicating intraurethral wall divertiucla in women. J Urol 1999; 161: 1259 –1262.

Davis BL, Robinson DG: Diverticula of the female urethra: Assay of 120 cases. J Urol 1970;104:850.

Davis HJ, Cian LG: Positive pressure urethrography: A new diagnostic method. J Urol 1956;75:753-757.

Davis HJ, Te Linde RW: Urethral diverticula: An assay of 121 cases. J Urol 1958;80:34-39.

Demirel A, Polat O, Bayraktar et al: Transvesical and transvaginal reparation in urinary vaginal fistulas. Int J Urol Nephrol, suppl, 1993; 25: 439 –443.

Derry DE: Notes on five pelves of women of the eleventh dynasty in Egypt. Brit J Obstet Gynecol 1935; 42:490 – 494.

Dmochowski RR, Ganabathi K, Zimmern PE, Leach GE: Benign female periurethral masses. J Urol 1994;152:1943-1951.

Dorsey JH, Cundiff G.Laparoscopic procedures for incontinence and prolapse. Curr Opin Obstet Gynaecol. 1994; 6: 223-230.

Drouin J, Tessier J, Bertrand PE, Schick E.. Burch colposuspension: long-term results and review of published reports. Urology 1999 Nov; 54(5):808-14

Duckett J.R.A. The use of periurethral injectables in the treatment of genuine stress incontinence. British. J. Urology, 1998, 105, 390-396.

Duckett JR and Constantine G. Complications of silicone sling insertion for stress urinary incontinence . J. Urology, 2000: 163: 1835-7

Eckford SD, Abrams P Para-urethral collagedn implantation for female stress incontinence. British J. Urology 1991; 68: 586-589.

Edwards, EA, Beebe RA: Diverticula of the female urethra. Obstet Gynecol 1955;5:729.

Egon G, Barat M, Colombel P, et al.: Implantation of anterior sacral root stimulators combined with posterior sacral rhizotomy in spinal injury patients. World J Urol 16:342-349, 1998.

Elkins TE: Surgery for the obstetric vesicovaginal fistula: A review of 100 operations in 82 patients. Am J Obstet Gynecol 1994; 170:1108-1120.

Elkins TE, Ghosh TS, Tagoe GA, Stocker R: Transvaginal mobilization and utilization of the anterior bladder wall to repair vesicovaginal fistulas involving the urethra. Obstet Gynecol 1992;79:455-460.

Ellik M: Diverticulum of the female urethra. A new method of ablation. J Urol 1957;77:234.

Elliot DS, Boone TB Is fascia lata allograft material trustworthy for pubovaginal sling repair? Urology 2000, 56: 772-776

Enzelsberger H. Helmer H. Schatten C. Comparison of Burch and Lyodura sling procedures for repair of unsuccessful surgery. Obstet. and Gynae. 1996, Vol. 88. NO 2, 251-256

Eriksen BC, Hagen B, Eik-Nes SH, Molne K, Mjolnerod D, Romslo I. Long term effectiveness of the Burch colposuspension in femail urinary stress incontinence. Acta Obstet Gynaecol Scand 1990; 69: 45-50.

Evans DH, Madjar S, Politano VA, Bejany DE, Lynne CM, Gousse AE. Interposition flaps in trandabdominal vesicovaginal fistula repairs: are they really necessary? Urology 57:670-674, 2001.

Faerber G.J. Endoscopic collagen therapy in the elderly women with type 1 stress urinary incontinence. J. Urology 1996,155,512.

Falk HC, Tancer ML: Vesicovaginal fistula: An historical survey. Obstet Gynecol 1954;3:337-341.

Farrar DJ, Whiteside CG, Osborne J et al A Urodynamic analysis of micturition symptoms in the female Surg Gynec Obstet 1975; 141:875

Fatthy H, El Hao M, Samaha I, Abdallah K. Modified Burch colposuspension: laparoscopy versus laparotomy. J Am Assoc Gynecol Laparosc 2001 Feb;8(1):99- 06.

Fenster HN Female bladder neck incision. Urology. 1990; 35 (2): 109-110

Feyereisl J. Dreher E. Haenggi W. Zikmund J. Schneider H. A. Long term results after Burch colposuspension. Am. J. Obstet Gynecol. And Gynaecol, 1994, Vol. 171, Number 3, 647-652.

Fitzgerald MP, Molenhauer J and Brubaker L. Failure of allograft suburethral slings. Br. J. of Urology, 1999; 84: 785-8

Flood HD, Malhotra SJ, O'Connell HE, Ritchey MJ, Bloom DA, McGuire EJ: Long-term results and complications using augmentation cystoplasty in reconstructive urology. Neurourol Urodynam 14:297-309, 1995.

Foster HE, McGuire EJ, Management of urethral obstruction with transvaginal urethrolysis. J. Urol 1993; 150: 1448-1451

Foucher JE, Marhsall V.Nosocomial catheter associated urinary tract infections. Infect Surg 1983; 2: 43

Galloway NTM, Davies N, Stephenson TP. The complications of colposuspension. Br J Urol 1987; 60: 122-124.

Ganabathi K, Leach GE, Zimmern, PE, Dmochowski RR: Experience with the management of urethral diverticulum in 63 women. J Urol 1994a;152:1445-1452.

Ganabathi K, Sirls L, Zimmern PE, Leach GE: Operative management of female urethral diverticulum. In McGuire E, ed: Advances in Urology. Chicago, CV, Mosby Company, 1994b, 199-228.

Garlock JH: The cure of an intractable vesicovaginal fistulas by the use of a pedicled muscle flap. Surg Gynecol Obstet 1928; 47: 255.

Guam L. Riccioti NA> Fair WR. Endoscopic bladder neck suspension for stress urinary incontinence. J. Urol 1984; 132: 1119-1121.

Ghoniem GM, Monga M: Modified pubovaginal sling and Martius graft for repair of the recurrent vesicovaginal fistula involving the internal urinary sphincter. Eur Urol 1995; 27: 241 –245.

Gillon G, and Mundy AR: The dissolution of urinary mucus after cystoplasty. Br J Urol 63: 372-374, 1989.

Gil-Vernet JM, Gil-Vernet A, Campos JA: A new surgical approach for treatment of complex vesicovaginal fistula. J Urol 1989;141:513-516.

Ginsberg DA, Rovner A, Raz S: Posthysterectomy vaginal cuff fistula: diagnosis and management of an unusual cause of incontinence Urol 1998; 52: 61 –64.

Ginsberg DS, Genadry R: Suburethral diverticulum in the female. Obstet Gynecol Surgery 1984;39:1-7.

Glazener CMA, Cooper K Anterior vaginal repair for urinary incontinence in women (Cochrane review) The Cochrane Library Issue 3 (2000). Oxford : Update Software.

Gleason DM, Bottaccini MR, Lattimer JK What does a bougie a boule calibrate? J. Urol 1969; 101:114

Goldenberg S.L. and Warkentin M.J. Periurethral collagen injections for patients with stress urinary incontinence. J.Urology 1994, 151,479A,abs. 1006

Goldstein I, Wise GJ, Tancer ML: A vesicovaginal fistula and intravesical foreign body: A rare case of the neglected pessary. Am J Obstet Gynecol 1990;163:589-591.

Goodwin WE, Scardino PT: Vesicovaginal and ureterovaginal fistulas: A summary of 25 years of experience. J Urol 1980;123:370-374.

Graham JB: Vaginal fistulas following radiotherapy. Surg Gynecol Obstet 1965;120:1019-1030.

Green TH Jnr Urinary stress incontinence: Differential diagnosis: Pathophysiology and management Am J Obstet Gynaecol 122 368 1975

Green TH Jnr Urinary stress incontinence, pathophysiology diagnosis and classification Gynaecologic & Obstetric Urology Ed by HS Buchsbaum, SB Schmidt Philadelphia ,W B Saunders 1978 162-188

Green DF, McGuire EJ, Lytton B. A comparison of endoscopic suspension of the vesical neck versus anterior urethropexy for the treatment of stress urinary incontinence. J. Urol 1986; 136: 1205-1207.

Gormley E.Ann . Editorial: Assessment of outcome and patient satisfaction in the treatment of stress incontinence-uses and problems. J. Urology, Vol. 157, 1287.

Green T H Jr Urinary stress incontinence: Differential diagnosis, pathophysiology and management Am J Obstet Gynaecol 1973 122 368-400

Griffth DJ Basics of pressure-flow studies. World J. Urol. 1995; 13: 30

Griffith DJ Pressure flow studies of micturition. Urol. Clinic. 1996; 23(2): 279.

Griifths D, Hofner K, van Mastricht R, Jan Rollema H, Spangberg A & Gleason D Standarisation of terminology of lower urinary tract function; pressure flow studies of voiding, urethral resistance and urethral obstruction. Neurourol Urody. 1998; 51: 408-411.

Guner H, Yildiz A, Erdem A, Tiftik M, Yildrim M. Syrgical treatment of urinary stress incontinence by a suburethral sling procedure using a Mersilene mesh graft. Gynecol Obstet Invest. 1994; 37(1): 52-55

Guner Haab F. Zimmern P. E. Leach G. E. Urinary stress incontinence due to intrinsic sphincteric deficiency: experience with fat and collagen periurethral injections. J. Urology 1997,Vol. 157. 1283-1286.

Hansen BJ, Horby J, Brynitz S, et al:Calculi in female urethral diverticulum. Int Urol Nephrol 1989;21:617-620.

Harris WJ: Early complications of abdominal and vaginal hysterectomy. Obstet Gynecol Survey 1995; 50: 795 – 805.

Helmstein K: Treatment of bladder carcinoma by a hydrostatic pressure technique. Report on 43 cases. Br J Urol 44: 434, 1972.

Hendren WH: Construction of female urethral from vaginal wall and a perineal flap. J Urol 1980;123:657-664.

Hendren WH: Construction of a female urethra using the vaginal wall and a buttock flap: experience with 40 cases. J Ped Surg. 1998; 33: 180 –187.

Hennalla SM, Hall V, Duckett JR, Link C, Usman F, Tromans PM, van Veggel L. A multicenter evaluation of a new surgical technique for urethral bulking in the treatment of genuine stress incontinence. BJOG 2000; 107(8):1035-9

Herbertsson G and Iosif CS Surgical results in urodynamics studies 10 years after retropubic colpourethropexy Acta Obstetrica and Gynaecologica Scandinavia. 1993; 72: 298-301

Herschorn S. Radomski S. B. Steele D. J. Early experience with intraurethral collagen injections for urinary incontinence. J. Urology, 1992, Vol. 148, 1797-.1800.

Herschorn S, Hewitt RJ: Patient perspective og long-term outcome of augmentation cystoplasty. Urology 52:672-678, 1998

Hilton P & Mayne CJThe Stamey endoscopic bladder neck suspension. Br. J. O&G 1991; 98 : 1141-9

Hirschorn RC: A new surgical technique for urethral diverticula in women. J Urol 1964;92:206-209.

Hitchings A, Griffiths J, and Black NA. Surgery for stress incontinence: factors associated with a successful outcome. Br J Urol 1998 82 634-641

Hoffman MJ, Adams WE: Recognition and repair of urethral diverticula: A report of 60 cases. Am J Obstet Gynecol 1965;92:106.

Horbach Hoskins WJ, Park RC, Long R et al: Repair of urinary fistulas with bulbocavernosus myocutaneous flaps. Obstet Gynecol 1984; 63: 588 –591.

Horbach NS, Blanco JS, Ostergard DR, Bent AE, Cornella JL. A suburethral sling procedure with polytetrafluorooethylene for the treatment of genuine stress incontinence in patients with low urethral closure profile. Obstet Gynecol 1988; 71(4): 648-652

Huffman AB: The detailed anatomy of the paraurethral ducts in the adult human female. Am J Obstet Gynecol 1948;55:86.

Hunner GL: Calculus formation in a urethral diverticulum in women.Urol Cut Rev 1938;42:336.

Hyams JA, Hyams MN: New operative procedures for treatment of diverticulum of female urethra. Urol Cut Rev 1939;43:573.

Ingelman-Sundberg A: Partial denervation of the bladder. A new operation for the treatment of urge incontinence and similar conditions in women. Acta Obstet Gynecol Scand 38: 487, 1959.

Iosif CS Comparative urodynamic studies of women with prolapse and stress incontinence before and after abdomino-vaginal sling urethroplasty.Int. J Gynaecol. Obstet. (19982) 20: 433-9

Jacoby K, Rowbothan RK: Double balloon positive pressure urethrography is a more sensitive test than voiding cystourethrography for diagnosing urethral diverticulum in women. J Urol 1999; 162: 2066-2069.

Jarvis G J . aIn Urodynamics (Ed Mundy, Stephenson and Wein), Stress incontinence, 1994, 299-326.

Jarvis G J. b.Surgery for bgenuine stress incontinence. British Journal of Obstetrics and Gynaecology, 1994, 101, 371-4.

Jarvis G J. In Incontinence (Ed Abrams, Khoury and Wein), Surgical treatment for incontinence in adult women, 1998, 637-68.

Jarvis G J.Detrusor instability, a complication of surgery. American Journal of Obstetrics and Gynecology, 1981, 319, 219.

Jensen D Jr. Pharmacological studies of the uninhibited neurogenic bladder. Acta Neurol Scan. 1981; 64: 175.

Jonas U, Petri E: Genitourinary fisulae. In Stanton SL, ed: Clinical Gynecologic Urology. St. Louis, CV, Mosby Company, 1984, 238-255.

Jorgensen L, Mortensen SO, Colstrup H, and Andersen JR: Bladder Distension in the management of detrusor instability. Scand J Urol Nephrol 19: 101-104, 1985.

Juma S, Serales L Aetiology of urinary retention after bladder neck suspension.J. Urol part 2, 1993; 149: 401A Abstract 752.

Karram MM, Angel O, Koonings P, Tabor B, Bergman A, Bhatia N.The modified Peryera procedure; a clinical and urodynamic review Br. J Obstet. Gynaecol 1992; 99; 655-658.

Keefe B, Warshauer DM, Tucker MS, Mittelstaedt CA: Diverticula of the female urethra: diagnosis by endovaginal and transperineal sonography. AJR 1991; 156: 1195 –1198.

Kelalis PPDistal urethral stenosis. (Editorial) Mayo Clinic Proc. 1979; 54: 690-692

Kersey J.The gauze hammock sling operation in the treatment of stress incontinence.Br. J Obstet. Gynaecol 1983; 90: 945-949

Khanna S: Posterior bladder flap plasty for repair of vesicourethrovaginal fistula. J Urol 1992; 147: 656 –657.

Khati NJ: MR imaging diagnosis of a urethral diverticulum.Radiographics 1998; 18: 517 –518.

Kjodhede P and Ryan GActa Obstetrica and Gynaecologica Scandinavia 1994; 73: 642-647

Kim B, Hricak H, Tanagho EA: Diagnosis of urethral diverticula in women: value of MR imaging. AJR 1993;161: 809 –812.

Kiricuta I, Goldstein AMB: The repair of extensive vesicovaginal fistulas with pedicled omentum: a review of 27 cases. J Urol 1972; 108: 724 –727.

Koelbl H, Saz V, Doerfler D, Haeusler G, Sam C, Hanzal E.Transurethral injection of silicone microimplants for intrinsic urethral sphincter deficiency. Obstet Gynecol 1998; 92: 332-6

Kottmeier HL: Complications following radiation therapy in carcinoma of the cervix and their treatment.AM J Obstet Gynecol 1964; 88: 854 – 858.

Kreden KJ and Austin JCTreatment of stress urinary incontinence in women with urethral hypermobility and intrinsic sphincter deficiency.J Urol (1996) 156: 1995-8

Kristensen JK, Lose G: Vesicovaginal fistulas: the transperitoneal repair revisited Scan J Urol Nephrol, syppl., 1994 ; 157: 101 –106.

Kovac SR and Cruikshank SRPubic bone suburethral stabilization sling for recurrent urinary incontinence. Obset. & Gynecol. 1997; 89: 624-7

Krantz KSurgery of female IncontinenceEd Stanton and Tanagho, Springer Verlag 1980 p54

Krieger JN: Vaginitis syndromes: a practical approach to diagnosis and teatment. AUA Update Series 1990; 9: 161 – 169.

Kursh ED, Morse RM, Resnik MI, Persky L: Prevention and development of a vesicovaginal fistula. Surg Gynecol Obstet 1988;166:409-412.

Kuuva and Nilsson Experience with TVT in FinlandNeurol Urodynam 2000, Vol 19, 364-365

Langer R, Ron-el R, Newman M, Herman A, Bukovsky I & Caspi EThe value of simultaneous hysterectomy during Burch colposuspension for urinary stress incontinenceObstet Gynecol 1988; 72: 6 866-869

Lapides J, Diokno AC, Silber EJ et al.Clean intermittent self-catheterisation in the treatment of urinary tract disease.J. Urol 1972; 107: 458

Lapides J: Transurethral treatment of urethral diverticulua in women. J Urol 1979;121:736-738.

Latzko W: Postoperative vesicovaginal fistulas: Genesis and therapy. Am J Surg 1942;58:211-228.

Lau TK, Wong WSF: Lymphatic vaginal fistula after Wertheim-Taussig hysterectomy: a case report. Gynecol Oncol 1994; 52: 411 –412.

Leach GE:Urethrovaginal fistula repair with Martius labial fat pad graft. Urol Clin North Am 1991;18:409-413.

Leach GE, Bavendam TG:Female urethral diverticula. Urology 1987;30:407-415.

Leach GE, Ganabathi K: Urethral diverticulectomy. Atlas Urol Clin North Am 1994;2:73-85.

Leach G E, Dmochowski R R, Appell R A et al. Female stress urinary incontinence clinical guidelines. Journal of Urology, 1997, 158, 875-80

Leach GE, Schmidbauer CP, Hadley HR, et al: Surgical treatment of female urethral diverticulum. Semin Urol 1986;4:33-42.

Leach GE, Sirls LT, Ganabathi K, et al: L N S C3; a proposed classification system for female urethral diverticulum. Neurourol Urodyn 1993;12:523-531.

Leach GE, Yip CM, Donovan BJ, Raz S: Tubovaginal leakage: An unusual cause of incontinence. J Urol 1987;137:287-288.

Lee AL, Symmonds RE, Williams TJ: Current status of genitourinary fistula. Obstet Gynecol 1988;72:313-319.

Lee RA, Symmonds RE. Repeat Marshall Marchetti procedure for recurrent stress urinary incontinence. Am J Obstet Gynecol 1975 May;122(2):219-29

Lee RA: Diverticulum of the urethra: Clinical presentation, diagnosis, and management. Clin Obstet Gynecol 1984;27:490.

Lee TG, Keller F: Urethral diverticulum: Diagnosis by ultrasound.AJR Am J Roentgeonol 1977;128:690-691.

Leng WW, McGuire EJ: Management of female urethral diverticula: a new classification. J Urol 1998; 160: 1297 – 1300.

Liapis AE, Asimiadis V, Loglis CD, Pyrgiotis E, Zourlas PA A randomised prospective study of three operative methods for genuine stress incontinence. J. Gynaec. Surg. (1996); 12 (1) : 7-14

Light JK.Abdominal approach for the implantation of the AS800 artifical urinary sphincter in females. Neurourol Urodyn. 1988; 7: 603-611.

Liu CY, Paek W.Laparoscopic retropubic colposuspension (Burch procedure).J. Am. Assoc. Gynecol. Laparosc. 1993; 1: 31-35.

Liu J. and Flood H.D.Selection of patients with intrinsic sphincter deficiency for treatment with collagen: can we do better? J. Urology, 1995, 153, 227A, abs. 818

Lockhart JL, Walker RD, Vorstman B, Politano VA: Periurethral polytetrafluoroethylene injection following urethral reconstruction in female patients with urinary incontinence. J Urol 1988;140:51-52.

Lotenfoe R, O'Kelly JK, Helal M, Lockhart JL.Periurethral polytetrafluorethylene paste injection in incontinent female subjects: surgical indications and improved surgical technique.J. Urol 1993; 149: 279-282.

Lopez A.E. Padron O. F. Patsias G. Politano V. A.Transurethral polyetrafluoroethylene injection in female patients with urinary continence.J. Urology, 1993, Vol. 150, 856-858.

Lose G, Jorgenson L, Johnson APredictive value of detrusor instability index in surgery for female urinary incontinenceNeurourol. Urodynam 1988 7 141-148

Loughlin K R, Gittes R F, Klein L A et al.The comparative costs of two major procedures available for the treatment of stress urinary incontinence. Journal of Urology, 1982, 127, 436-8.

Loughlin KR, Whitmore WF, Gittes RF, Richie JP. Review of an eight year experience with modifications of endoscopic suspension of the bladder neck for female stress urinary incontinence. J. Urol 1990; 143: 44-45

Loughlin KR Editorial. Slings – an idea whose time has come. J. of Urol. 2000; 163: 1843-4

Maher C, Dwyer P, Carey M, Gilmour D.The Burch colposuspension for recurrent urinary stress incontinence following retropubic continence surgery.Br J Obstet Gynaecol 1999 Jul;106(7):719-24

Maher C MacKinnon M, Pratt JH, Pool TL:Diverticulum of the female urethra. Surg Clin North Am 1959;39:953.

Mainprize TC, Drutz HP.The Marhsall-Marchetti-Krantz procedure: a clinical review.Obstet Gynecol Surv 1988; 43: 724-729

Marshall VF:Vesicovaginal fistulas on one urological service. J Urol 1979; 121: 25 –28.

Martius H: Die operative Wiedeherstellung der volkommen fehicnden Harn-rehre und des Schiessmuskels derselben.Zentfubl Gynak 1928;52:480.

Massey JA, Abrams PHObstructed voiding in the femaleBr J Urol 1988 Jan; 61(1):36-9

McDuffie RW, Littin RB & Blumdon KE Uretrovesical suspension.Am. J. Surgery 1981; 141 : 297-8

McGuire EJ, Lytton BPubovaginal sling procedures for stress incontinenceJ. Urol 1978; 119:82

McGulre EJ, Lytton B, Kohora EJ & Pepe V.The value of urodynamic testing in stress urinary incontinence.J. Urol (1980) 124 : 456.

McGuire EJ, letson W, Wang S Transvaginal urethrolysis after obstructive urethral suspension procedures.J. Urol 1989; 142: 1037.

McGuire EJ, Fitzpatrick CC, Wan J, Bloom D, Sondvordenker J, Ritchley M & Gormley EAClinical assessment of urethral sphincter function.J. Urol (1993) Vol 150 : 1452-1454

McGuire EJ and Appel RATransurethral collagen injection for urinary incontinence.Urology April 1994 Vol 43 No 4: 413-415

McGuire E J, Lytton B, Pope V and Kohorn E I Stress incontinenceObst Gynec 1976 47 255

McKay HA: Vesicovaginal and vesicocutaneous fistulas: transurethral suture cystorrhaphy as a new closure etchnique. J Urol 1997; 158: 1513 –1516.

McNally A:A Diverticula of the female urethra. Am J Surg 1935;28:177.

Meirowsky AM.Management of chronic interstitial cystitis by differential sacral neurectomy. J Neurosurg 1969; 30:604-7

Menchaca A, Akhyat M, Gleicher N, et al: Rectus abdominis muscle flap in a combined abdominovaginal repair of difficult vesicovaginal fistulae: A report of three cases. J Reprod Med 1990;35:565-568.

Milani R, Scalambrino S, Quadire G et alMMK procedure and Burch colposuspension in the surgical treatment of female urinary incontinenceBr. J. Obstet Gynaecol. 1985 92 1050

Miller NF: Treatment of vesicovaginal fistulas.Am J Obstet Gynecol 1935; 30: 675 –679.

Miyazaki F, Shook G.Ilio-inguinal nerve entrapment during needle suspension for stress incontinence.Obstet Gynecol 1992; 80: 246-248.

Mitchell ME, Hensle TW, Crooks KK: Urethral reconstruction in the young female using a perineal pedicle flap. J Ped Surg 1982;17:687-694..

Monteiro H, Nogueira R, Carvalho H:Bechet's syndrome and vesicovaginal fistula: an unusual complication. J Urol 1995; 153: 407 –408.

Moore TD: Diverticulum of the female urethra. An improved technique of surgical excision. J Urol 1952;68:611-616.

Moir JC The Gauze-Hammock operationThe J of Obstet Gynaecol Brit Commonw 1968; 75: 1

Monga A.K. Robinson D. Stanton S. LPeriurethral collagen injections for genuine stress incontinence: a 2-year follow up. British J. Urology, 1995, 76, 156-160.

Moran PA, Ward KL, Johnson D et al. Tension free vaginal tape for primary genuine stress incontinence. Br. J. of Urol. 2000; 86: 39-42

Morgan JE, Farrow GA, Stuart FE.The Marlex sling operation for the treatment of recurrent stress urinary incontinence:a sixteen year review. Am J Obstet Gynecol 1985; 151: 224-226

Morgan TO, Westney OL, McGuire EJ Pubovaginal sling: 4 year outcome analysis and quality of life assessment.J. Urology, 2000; 163: 1845-1848

Morris A R, Reilly E T C, Hassan A, Ramsey I N, Hawthorn R J S5-7 year follow up of a randomised trial comparing laparoscopic colposuspension and open colposuspension in the treatment of genuine stress incontinenceInt Urogynaecology Journal 2001 Vol 12 Suppl 3 S6 (Abstract)

Mundy AR. Long-term results of bladder transection for urge incontinence.Br J Urol 1983; 5: 642-4

Mundy AR.A trial comparing Stamey bladder neck suspension procedure with colposuspension for the treatment of stress incontinence. Br J Urol. 1983; 55: 687-690

Mundy AR, and Stephenson T: "Clam" ileocystoplasty for the management of the treatment of refractory urge incontinence. Br J Urol 57: 641-646, 1985.

Mutlu N, Kazado M, Culha M, Merder E, Baykal M, Canbazoglu N. Burch bladder neck colposuspension, comparison of early and late results. Mater Med Pol 1997 Jan-Dec;29(1-4):8-10.

Muznai D, Carrill E, Dubin C, Sliverman I. Retrobupic vaginopexy for the correction of urinary stress incontinence.Obstet Gynecol 1992; 59: 113-117.

Nataluk EA, Assimos DG, Kroovand RL Collagen injections for treatment of urinary incontinence secondary to intrinsic sphincter deficiency.J. Endourol. 1995; 9: 403.

Nel J: Diverticulum of female urethra. J Obstet Gynecol Br Commonw 1955;62:90.

Nesrallah LJ, Srougi M, Gittes RF: The O'Conor technique: the gold standard for the supratrigonal vesicovaginal fistual repair. J Urol 1999; 161: 566 –568.

Nichols DH. The mersilene mesh gauze hammock for severe stress urinary incontinence. Obstet Gynecol 1973; 41(1): 88-93

Niemic TR, Mercer LI, Stephens, JK, et al: Unusual urethral diverticulum lined with colonic epithelium with paneth cell metaplasia. Am J Obstet Bynecol 1989;160:186-188.

Nietlich JD, Foster HE, Glickman MG, Smith RC: Detection of urethral diverticula in women: comparison of high resolution fast spin echo technique with double balloon urethrography. J Urol 198; 159: 408 –412.

Nilsson CG and Kuuva N. The tension free vaginal tape procedure successful in the majority of women with indications for surgical treatment of urinary stress incontinence. Br. J. of Obstet. & Gynaecol. 2001; 108: 414-9

Nitti VW, Raz S. Obstruction following anti-incontinence procedures: Diagnosis and treatment with transvaginal urethrolysis. J. Urol 1994; 152: 93

Nitti VW, Raz S. Obstruction following incontinence procedures. Diagnosis and treatment with transvaginal urethrolysis. J. Urol 1994; 152: 93-98.

Nolan JF, Stillwell TJ, Bartelbort SW, Sands JP: Gracilis interposition in fistulas following radiotherapy for cervical cancer: A retrospective study. J Urol 1991;146:843-844.

Noller JI, Pratt JH, Symmonds HE. Bowel perforation with suprapubic cystostomy; report of two caes. Obstet Gynecol . 1976; 48: 675-695

Nordling J, Steven K, and Meyhoiff HH: ;Subtrigonal phenol injection: lack of effect in the treatment of detrusor instability. Neurourol Urodyn 5: 449, 1986.

Obrink A, Bunne G: Gracilis interposition in fistulas following radiotherapy for cervical cancer. Urol Int 1978;33:370-376.

Obrink A, Fedor-Freybruch P, Hjelmkvist M & Bunne GMental factors influencing recurrence of stress incontinence.Acta Obstet Gynecol Scan. 1979; 58: 91-94

O'Conor VJ JR: R Review of experience with vesicovaginal fistula repair. J Urol 1980;123:367-369.

O'Connell H. E. McGuire E. J. Aboseif S. Usui Transurethral collagen therapy in womenAm. J. Urology, Vol. 154, 1463-1465.

O'Conor VJ Jr, Kropp KA: Surgery of the female urethra. In Glenn JF, Boyce WH eds: Urologic Surgery. New York, Harper and Row, 1969.

O'Conor V, Sokol J: Vesicovaginal fistula from the standpoint of the urologists. J Urol 1951;66:367-369.

O'Conor VJ, Sokol JK, Bulkley GJ, Nanninga JB: Suprapubic closure of vesicovaginal fistula. J Urol 1973; 109: 51-53.

O'Donnell PD, Ed., Mosby, 1997O'Leary MP, Gee WF, Holtgrew L et al. American Urological Association Gallup Survey. J. of Urol. 2000; 164: 1311-6

Orikasa S, Metoki R, Ishikawa H, et al: Congenital urethral and vesical diverticula allied to blind ending ureters. Urology 1990;35:137-141.

O'Sullivan DC, Chilton CP & Munson KWShould Stamey colposuspension be our primary surgery for stress incontinence? Br. J Urology 1995 75 457

Palagiri A: Urethral diverticulum with endometriosis. Urology 1978;11:271.

Patanaphan V, Prempree T, Sewehand W, et al: Adenocarcinoma arising in female urethral diverticulum. Urology 1983;22:259-264.

Park G. S. Miller J Surgical treatment of stress urinary incontinence: a comparison of the Kelly plication, Marshall-Marchetti-Krantz, and Pereyra procedures. Obstet. And Gynaecol. \1988, Vol.71, NO 4, 575-579.

Parks J: Section of the urethral wall for correction of urethral vaginal fistula and urethral diverticula. Am J Obstet Gynecol 1965; 93:683.

Pathak UN, House MJ: Diverticulum of the female urethra. Obstet Gynecol 1970;36:789.

Patil U, Waterhouse K, Laungauni G: Management of 18 difficult vesicovaginal and urethrovaginal fistulas with modified Ingle-Sundberg and Martius operation. J Urol 1980;123:653-656.

Pengelly AW, Stephenson TP, and Milroy EJG: Results of prolonged bladder distension as treatment for detrusor instability. Br J Urol 50: 243-245, 1978.

Pentinen J. Kaar K . Kauppila A.Effect of suprapubic operation on urethral closure.British J. Urology, 1989,63, 389-391.

Perlmutter AD: Experiences with urinary undiversion in children with neurogenic bladder. J Urol 127: 402-406, 1980.

Persky L, Herman G, Guerner K: Nondelay in vesicovaginal fistula repair.Urology 1979;13:273-275.

Pereyra AJA simplified surgical procedure for the correction of stress urinary incontinence in women.Western Journal of Surgery Obstet and Gynecol. 1959; 67: 223-226

Persson J, Wolner-Hanssen P.Lapaorscopic Burech colposuspension for stress urinary incontinence: a randomised comparison of one or two sutures on each side of the urethra. Obstet Gynecol 2000 Jan;95 (1):151-5.

Peters WH, Vaughan ED Jr: Urethral diverticulum in the female. Obstet Gynecol 1976;47:549.

Politano VA, Small MP, Harper JM, Lynne CM.Periurethral Teflon injection for urinary incontinence.J. Urol 1974; 111: 180-183.

Politano VA.Periurethral polyterafluorethylene injection for urinary incontinence.J. Urol 1982; 127; 439-442

Pow-Sang J, Lochart JL, Suarez A, Lansman H & Politano VA Female urinary incontinence: pre-operative selection, surgical complications and results.J Urology 1986 136 831-833

Price B B Plastic operation for incontinence of urine and of faeces.Arch Surg 1933; 26: 1043-1053

Radley SC, Chapple CR, Mitsogiannis IC, Glass KS.Transurethral implantation of macroplastique for the treatment of female stress urinary incontinence secondary to urethral sphincter deficiency. Eur. Urol. 2001; 39: 383-89

Ramsden PD, Smith JC, Dunn M, and Ardan GM: Distension therapy for the unstable bladder. Later results including an assessment of repeat distension.Br J Urol 48: 623-629, 1976

Raz SEditorial .Comment.J. Urol 1989; 142: 1038-1039

Raz S, Brogg K, Nitti VW, Sussman E: Transvaginal repair of vesicovaginal fistula using a peritoneal flap. J Urol 1993;150:56-39.

Raz S, Little NA, Juma S: Female urology. In Walsh PC, Retik AB, Stamey TA, eds: Campbell's Urology, 6th ed. Philadelphia, WB Saunders Company, 1992, 2782-2828.

Raz S, Sussman EM, Ericksen DB, Bregg KJ, Nitti VW.The Raz bladder neck suspension; results in 206 patients.J. Urol 1992; 148: 845-850.

Redman J: Female urologic techniques. Urol Clin North Am 1990;17:5-8.

Richard F, Lefore TJM, Bitker NO et al. Female incontinence with primary sphincter deficiency – results of artificial urinary sphincter with long term follow up. J. of Urol. 1996; supplement 156A.

Richardson DA, Bent AE * Ostergard DRThe effect of uterovaginal prolapse on urethrovesical pressure dynamics Am J O&G 1983 146 No 8 901-905

Richmond D. H. Sutherst J. R.Burch colposuspension or sling for stress incontinence? A prospective study using transrectal ultrasound.British J. Urology, 1989, 64, 600-603

Riggs JA. Retropubic cystourethropexy: a review of two operative procedures with long-term follow-up.Obstet Gynecol 1986 Jul;68(1):98-105

Robertson JR: Genitourinary problems in women. Springfield, IL. Charles C. Thomas, 1978.

Roehrborn CG: Long-term follow up study of the marsupialization technique for urethral diverticula in women. Surg Gynecol Obstet 1988;167:191-195.

Rost A, Fiedler U, Fester CComparative analysis of the results of suspension-urethroplasty according to Marshall-Marchetti-Krantz and of urethrovesicopexy with adhesive.Urol. Into. 1979; 34: 167.

Routh A: Urethral diverticulum.Br Med J 1890;1:361.

Rozsahegyi J, Magasi P, Szule E: Diverticulum of the female urethra: A report of 50 cases. Act A Chir Hung 1981;25:33-38.

Rozensweig B, Hischke D, Thomas S, Nelson A & Bhatia N. Stress incontinence in women. Psychological status before and after treatment. J Reprod Med. 1991; 36: 835-838

Sand PK, Bowen LW, Panganiban R and Ostergard DR The low pressure urethral as a factor in failed retropubic urethropexy. Obs & Gynae (1987) 69 No 3 Pt 1 : 399-402

Sand 1997

Sand PK, Winkler H, Blackhurst DW et al. A prospective randomized study comparing modified Burch retropubic urethropexy and suburethral sling for the treatment of genuine stress incontinence with low pressure urethra. Am. J. of Obstet. & Gynecol. 2000; 182: 30-4

Schaffer W. Analysis of bladder out-let function with the linearized passive urethral resistance relation, lin PURR, and a disease-specific approach for grading obstruction – from complex to simple. World J. Urol 1995; 13: 47

Scott FB. The artificial urinary sphincter. Urol Clin N Am 1989; 16: 105-117.

Scotti RJ, Angell G, Flora R & Marjus Greston MT Obstet. & Gynaec. Vol 91 No 1 Jan 98

Seballos RM, Rich RR: Clear cell adenocarcinoma arising from a urethral diverticulum. J Urol 1995; 153: 1914-1915.

Sehn JR: Anatomic effect of distention therapy in unstable bladder: a new approach. Urology 11: 581-587, 1978.

Serels SR, Rackley RR & Appell Ra J of Urology March 2000 Vol 163 884-887

Sheriff MS, Foley S, McFarlane J, Nauth-Misir R & Shah PJR. Endoscopic correction of intractable stress incontinence with silicone micro-implants. European Urology, 1997, 32: 284-288.

Shekarriz B, Upadhyay J, Demirbilek S, et al.: Surgical complications of bladder augmentation: comparison between various enterocystoplasties in 133 patients. Urology 55:123-8, 2000.

Shull BL and Baden WF. A six year experience with paravaginal defect repair for stress urinary incontinence.Am.J. of O&G (1989): 161 43-240

Siegel CL, Middleton WD, Teefey SA et al: Sonography of the female urethra. AJR 1998; 170: 1269 –1274.

Sims JM: On the treatment of vesico-vaginal fistulas. Am J Med Sci 1852; 23: 59.

Silk MR, Lebowitz JM: Anterior urethral diverticulum. J Urol 1969;101:66.

Singla AK The use of cadaveric fascia lata in the treatment of stress urinary incontinence in women.Br. J. of Urology, 2000; 85: 264-9

Smith ARB and Stanton SLLaporoscopic colposuspension Br. J Obstet. Gynaecol 1998, 105: 383-4

Smith D. N. Appell R. A. Winters J. C. Rackley R. R. Collagen injection therapy for female intrinsic sphincteric deficiency. J. Urology, 1997, Vol. 157, 1275-1278.

Spence HM, Duckett JW: Diverticulum of the female urethral: Clinical aspects and presentation of a simple operative technique for cure. J Urol 1970;104:432-437.

Spencer WF, Stream SB: Diverticula of the female urethra roof managed endoscopically. J Urol 1987; 138: 147-148.

Spencer JR, O'Connor j, Schaeffer AJ.A comparison of endoscopic suspension of the vesical neck with suprapubic vesicoutrehtropexy for treatment of stress urinary incontinence. J. Urol 1987; 137: 411-515

Stamey TA. Endoscopic suspension of the vesical neck for urinary incontinence. Surgery Gynecol and Obstet 1973; 136: 547-554

StantonStanton SL, Cardozo L, Williams JE, Ritchie D & Allan V.Clinical and urodynamics features of failed incontnence surgery in the femal Obstet Gynaecol. 1978 51 515-520

Stanton SL, Cardozo LDResults of the colposuspension operation for incontinence and prolapse.Br. J Obstet Gynaecol 1979 86 693

Stanton S. Monga A. K.Incontinence in elderly women: is periurethral collagen an advance?British J. Obstet and Gynaecol, 1997, Vol. 104, 154-157.

Stirnemann H : Treatment of recurrent recto-vaginal fistula by interposition of a gluteus maximus muscle flap. AM J Proctol 1969; 20: 52 –55.

Stockbine MF, Hancock JE, Fletcher GH: Complications in 831 patients with squamous cell carcinoma of the intact uterine cervix treated with 3,00 rads or more whole pelvis radiation. AJR 1970;108:239-304.

Stothers L. Goldenburg S. L. Leone E.FComplications of periurethral collagen injection for stress incontinence. J. Urology, 1998, Vol. 159, 806-807.

Stovsky MD, Ignaroff JM, Blum MD, et al: Use of electrocoagulation in the treatment of vesicovaginal fistulas. J Urol 1994;152:1443-1444.

Stricker P, Haylen B. Injectable collagen for type 3 female stress incontinence: the first 50 Australian patients. Med J Aust 1993 Jan 18;158(2):89-91.

Summitt RL Jr., Lucente V, Karram M, Shull B, Bent A Laparoscopic versus open Burch colposuspension: a randomised clinical trial. Obstet Gynecol 2000.

Su Th, Wang KG, Hsu CY, Wei H, Hong BK Prospective comparison of laparoscopic and traditional colposuspensions in the treatment of genuine stress incontinence. Acta Obstet Gynecol 1997;76:576-82.

Sundberg I. Partial denervation of the bladder. A new operation for the treatment of urge incontinence and similar conditions in women. Acta Obst Gynec Scand 1959; 38: 487-91

Swami SK, Abrams P, Hammonds JC, et al: Treatment of detrusor overactivity with detrusor myomectomy (bladder autoaugmentation). Presented at the Twenty-Third Congress of the Societie Internationale d'Urologie, 1994; abstr 580.

Swami KS, Feneley RCL, Hammonds JC, et al.: Detrusor myectomy for detrusor overactivity: a minimum 1 year follow-up. Brit J Urol 81:68-72, 1998.

Swierzewski JJ III, McGuire EJ: Pubovaginal sling for treatment of female stress urinary incontinence complicated by urethral diverticulum. J Urol 1993;149:1012-1014.

Symmonds RE: Incontinence: Vesical and urethral fistulas. Obstet Gynecol 1984;27:499-514.

Tanagho EA: Bladder neck reconstruction for total urinary incontinence: 10 years of experience. J Urol 1981;125:321-326.

Tanagho EAEffect of hysterectomy and peri-urethral surgery on urethrovesical functionInt Gynaecologic Urology and Urodynamics Balitmore: Withams and Wilkins; 1985 537-544

Tanagho EA, McCurry E Pressure and flow rate as related to lumen calibre and entrance configuration. J. Urol 1971; 106: 583

Tancer ML: The post-total hysterectomy vesicovaginal fistula. J Urol 1980;123: 839 – 841.

Tancer ML: Observation on prevention and management of vesicovaginal fistula after total hysterectomy. Surg Gynecol Obstet 1992;175:501-506.

Tancer ML: A report of thirty-four instances of urethrovaginal and bladder neck fistulas. Surg Gynecol Obstete 1993;177:77-80.

Thomas RB, Maguire B: Adenocarcinoma in a female urethral diverticulum. Aust NZ J Obstet Gynecol 1991;869-871.

Tincello DGUltrasound detection of vault haematoma following vaginal hysterectomy Br J Obstet Gynaecol 1998 105(12) 1336-7

Torres S, Quartlebaum R: Carcinoma in urethral diverticulum. South Med J 1972;65:1374-1376.

Trockman BA, Leach GE, Hamilton J et al Journal of Urology 1995; 154: 1841-1847

Turner-Warwick R: The use of the omental pedicle graft in urinary tract reconstruction.J Urol 1976; 116: 341-344.

Turner-Warwick R.Impaired voiding efficiency and retention in Stanton SL (Ed): Clinics in Obstetrics & Gynecology, Philadelphia. WB Saunders Co. 1978; Vol.5; p138.

Turner WH, Brading AF.Smooth muscle of the bladder in the normal and the diseased state; pathophysiology, diagnosis and treatment Pharmacol. Ther., 1997; 75 (2); 77-110

Udeh FN: Simple management of difficult vesicovaginal fistulas by anterior transvesical approach. J Urol 1985;133:591-593.

Uebersax JS, Wyman JF, Schmake WA et al Short forms to assess life quality and symptom distress for urinary incontinence in women: the incontience impact questionnaire and the urogenital distress inventory. Neururol. and Urody. 1995; 14: 131-139.

Ulmsten U, Johnson P and Rezapour M. A 3 year follow up of tension free vaginal tape for surgical treatment of female stress urinary incontinence. Br. J. of Obstet. & Gynaecol. 1999; 106: 345-50

Valley MTPubic bone suburethral stabilization sling for recurrent urinary incontinence. Obstet. & Gynecol. 1997; 90: 481-2

Van Geelen J.M. Theeuwes A.G.M. Eskes T.K.A.B. Martin jr. C.B. The clinical and urodynamic effect of anterior vaginal repair and Burch colposuspension. Am. J. Obstet Gynecol. and Gynae, 1988, Vol. 159, Number 1, 137-144.

Varner ER Retropubic long needle suspension procedures for stress urinary incontinence Am J O&G1990 163 551

Villasanta V: Complications of radiotherapy for carcinoma of the uterine cervix. Am J Obstet Gynecol 1972; 114: 717- 720.

Wang SC, McGuire EJ, and Bloom DA: A bladder pressure management system for myelodysplasia—clinical out-come. J Urol 140: 1499-1502, 1988.

Wang Yu, Hadley R: Nondelayed transvaginal repair of high-lying vesicovaginal fistula. J Urol 1990;144:34-36.

Wang Y, Hadley R: The use of rotated vascularized pedicle flaps for complex transvaginal procedures. J Urol 1993; 149: 590 –592.

Wang Y, Mitchell D, Hadley R. The anatomical basis for femoral neuropathy due to procedures performed in the modified lithotomy postion. Int Urogynecol J 1993; 4: 390.

Ward KL, Hilton P and Browning J. A randomised trial of colposuspension amd tension free vaginal tape for primary genuine stress incontinence. Neuro-urology and Urodynamics. 2000; 19: 386-8

Ward KL and Hilton P A randomised trial of colposuspension and TVT for primary genuine stress Incontinence – 2 year follow up Presented to IUGA Melbourne 6th December 2001

Ward JN: Technique to visualize the urethra in female patients. Surg Gynecol Obstet 1989;168-278.

Wear JB: Urethral diverticulectomy in females. Urol Times 1976;4:2-3.

Webster GD, Sihelnik SA, Stone AR: Urethrovaginal fistula: A review of the surgical management. J Urol 1984;132:460-462.

Webster GD, Kreder KJ,. Voiding dysfunction following cystourethropexy; it's evaluation and management. J. Urol 1990; 147: 670-73

Webster SD, Perez LM, Khoury JM et al Management of stress urinary incontinence using artifical urinary sphincter. Urology 1992; 39: 499-503

Wein AJ, Malloy TR, Greenberg SH, et al: Omental transposition as an aid in genitourinary reconstructive procedures. J Urol 1980b;20:473-477.

Wharton LR Jr., Telinde RW: Urethral diverticulum. Obstet Gynecol 1956;7:503.

Wishard WN, Nourse NH, Mertz JHO: Carcinoma in diverticulum of the female urethra. J Urol 1963;89:431.

Weilink G, Essink-Bot ML, van Kerrebroeck PEV, Rutten FFH: Sacral Rhizotomies and electrical bladder stimulation in spinal cord injury. Eur Urol 31:441-446, 1999.

Wheeler JR, Culkin DJ, Walter JS et al Female urinary retention. 1990; 35: 428/

Winters J. C. Appell R. Periurethral injection of collagen in the treatment of intrinsic sphincteric deficiency in the female patient. Urologic Clinics of North America, Vol. 22. Number 3, Aug. 1995.

Wiskind AK, Creighton SM & Stanton SL The incidence of genital prolapse after colposuspension Am J O&G 1992 Vol 167 No.2 399-405

Wilson PD, Al Samarrai MT, Brown ADG. Quantifying female incontinence with particular reference to the Urillos system. Urol. Int. 1980; 35: 298.

Wright EJ, Iselin CE, Carr LK, Webster GD. Pubovaginal sling using cadaveric allograft fascia for the treatment of instrinsic sphincter deficiency. J. Urology, 1998; 160: 759-762

Wyman JF, Choi SC, Harkins SW, Wilson MS, Fantl A. The urinary diary in evaluation of incontinent women. A test-restest analysis. Obstet & Gynecol. 1988; 71: 812.

Young Young HH: An operation for the cure of incontinence associated with epispadias. J Urol 1922;7:1.

Young HH: Treatment of urethral diverticulum. South Med J 1938;31:1043-1047.

Youg SB, Howard AE, Baker SP. Mersilene mesh sling: short and long term clinical and urodynamic outcomes. Am J Obstet Gynecol 2001; 185: 32-40

Zacharin RE: Obstetric Fistula. New York, Springer-Verlag, 1988.

Zeidman EJ, Chiang H, Alarcon A, Raz S: Suprapubic cystotomy using Lowsley retractor. Urology 1988; 23: 54-55.

Zimmern PE, Hadley HR, Leach GE, Raz S. Female urethral obstruction after Marshall-Marchetti-Krantz operation. J. Urol 1987; 38: 517-520.

Zimmern PE The role of voiding cystourethropgraphy in the evaluation of the female lower urinary tract. Problems in Urology. 1991; 5(1): 23-41.

Zimmern PE, Ganabathi K, Leach GE: Vesicovaginal fistula repair. Atlas Urol Clin North Am 1994;2:87-99.

Zivkovic F, Tamussino K, Ralph G, Schied G, Auer-Grunbach M Long term effects of vaginal dissection on the innervation of the striated urethral sphincter. Obstet & Gynecol. 1996 87: 257-260

Zivkovic F, Tamusssino K, Pieber D & Haas J Body mass index and outcome of surgery Ostetrics & Gynaecology Vol 93, No 5 Part 1, May 1999

Committee 11 D

Surgery for the Neuropathic Patient

Chairman

D. CASTRO-DIAZ (SPAIN),

Members

D. BARRETT (USA),

P. GRISE (FRANCE),

I. PERKASH USA),

M. STÖHRER (GERMANY),

A. STONE (USA),

P. VALE (PORTUGAL)

CONSULTANTS

H. MADERSBACHER (AUSTRIA),

A. MUNDY

CONTENTS

Surgery for the Neuropathic Patient

D. CASTRO-DIAZ,

D. BARRETT, P. GRISE, I. PERKASH, M. STÖHRER, A. STONE, P. VALE

H. MADERSBACHER, A. MUNDY

INTRODUCTION

Incontinence is commonly associated with (a condition which may be secondary to) several types of neurological disease or injury. The neurological problem may primarily affect the sphincter, the detrusor, or both the sphincter and the detrusor. Surgery may correct the incontinence in many patients but is usually indicated only after all conservative therapies have been attempted and failed or have proved to be ineffective. In many cases, lessons learned from this conservative therapy, such as intermittent catheterisation, may enhance the changes achieved by surgery, allowing the patient to become more socially flexible and further improve quality of life.

As with all surgery on the urinary tract, certain principals must be adhered to in establishing the appropriateness of any procedure. These are: 1) preservation of renal function and 2) control of incontinence. In addition, for patients with neuropathic bladder, other issues need to be considered, namely:1) social circumstances, 2) degree of disability, 3) cost effectiveness, 4) technical difficulty and 5) complications.

The following chapter is a critical overview of the surgical procedures available to manage the various forms of neuropathic bladder.

A. FAILURE TO EMPTY

I. SURGERY TO ENHANCE DETRUSOR CONTRACTILITY

Restoration of the bladder's reservoir function in combination with the ability for complete voluntary evacuation has been the aim of the urinary bladder stimulation over the past decades. Various approaches have been reported to protect the upper urinary tracts and to prevent urinary incontinence in neurogenic bladder dysfunction.

A variety of implants have been used in patients with spinal cord injury or disease, with electrodes on the bladder wall, the splanchnic pelvic nerves, the conus medularis, the mixed sacral nerve or the sacral anterior roots.

Direct bladder stimulation has produced poor results and has been abandoned. Splanchnic pelvic nerves stimulation has also been abandoned due to a difficulties encountered with surgical access and because these nerves also include sympathetic fibers to the bladder neck and afferent fibers. Stimulation at the conus medularis level has been reported, with electrodes implanted directly into the gray matter in this section of the cord. Results have only been reported in one publication and the authors abandoned this work more than 15 years ago [1-2].

Intravesical electrical stimulation has been proposed as a method to improve the bladder function in conditions with weak detrusor contractility. The method is based on activation of the bladder mechanoreceptors, which initiate the normal micturition reflex. The results seem encouraging specially if there is residual detrusor contractility [3]. (Refer to chapter on Conservative Therapy for details)

1. SACRAL ANTERIOR ROOT STIMULATION TO CONTROL DETRUSOR CONTRACTION

Brindley, in London, started animal experiments in order to develop a system for intradural sacral anterior root stimulation in the 70's. The first successful sacral anterior root stimulator in a human subject with traumatic paraplegia, was implanted in 1978 [4]. Since then more than 3000 patients have been implanted worldwide. The technique of intradural sacral anterior root stimulation consists of the combination of complete posterior rhizotomies (S2, S3, S4) and simultaneous implantation of the Finetech-Brindley electrodes on the intact anterior roots. Posterior rhizotomy promotes detrusor arreflexia and normal compliance, thus avoiding reflex incontinence. With this technique more than 80% of the patients were able to achieve sufficient intravesical pressure to produce efficient voiding. Several attempts, since then, have been made to improve this technique. The principal purpose of the Finetech-Brindley bladder controller is to achieve bladder emptying. Stimulation of the anterior sacral roots, mainly S3 and S4, results in bladder contraction with simultaneous activation of the urethral sphincter and pelvic floor. The nerve roots contain a mixed population of somatic fibers innervating leg musculature, pelvic floor muscles, urethral and anal sphincters and pre-ganglionic parasympathetic fibers innervating the detrusor muscle. The somatic nerve fibers supplying the urethral sphincter have a larger calibre than the parasympathetic fibers; since large diameter fibers need a lesser stimulus for activation than the smaller ones, activation of the smaller diameter fibers is always accompanied by activation of the larger ones. The result is simultaneous activation of the detrusor and the urethral closure mechanism. The striated muscle of the sphincter relaxes more rapidly than the smooth muscle of the detrusor, which continues to contract after the cessation of the stimulation. Intermittent stimulation with bursts of impulses produces a rapid contraction of the urethral sphincter and a slow but more sustained contraction of the detrusor. Micturition occurs during the gap at the end of each burst of impulses, whilst the bladder is still contracted with the urethra relaxed (Figures 1-6). Electrical micturition occurs at physiologic pressures in 4 to 8 spurts, within one minute in most patients. The bladder then remains arreflexic until the next micturition sequence [5, 6, 7, 8] *LEVEL OF EVIDENCE 4.*

Several additional methods have been investigated to obtain a more physiological voiding pattern. These include surgical interruption of the somatic fibers, blockage of pudendal nerve transmission, fatiguing of the urethral sphincter, and selective small fiber activation. Some work has been done on the selective activation of the small diameter parasympathetic fibers on the anterior sacral nerve roots, using a selective anodal block. The principle of this technique is based on the observation that close to an anodal contact, the propagation of an action potential can be blocked by hyperpolarization of the fiber membrane. If the membrane is sufficiently hyperpolarized, action potentials cannot pass this zone and are wiped out. As large diameters fibers need a smaller stimulus for blocking than do the smaller fibers, a selective blockage of the large fibers is possible. Thus, selective small fibers activation can be obtained by a combination of excitation of both large and small diameter fibers and by blockage distal to the excitation point of the propagation of the induced action potentials in the larger fibers. This can be achieved with rectangular pulses or by the application of multichannel-generated quasitrapesoidal pulses in an anodal block stimulation technique. These studies have shown feasibility in animals but have not been applied to human subjects [9].

More recently attempts have been made to avoid the posterior rhizotomy, and obtain the same result, using selective urethral sphincter blockade and reversible deafferentation using cryotherapy. If these results can be reproduced in chronic trials and during intra operative evaluation, this technique may play some role in clinical practice [10].

Another technique recently described by Craggs et al is that of combining sacral anterior root stimulation for electromicturition with electrostimulation of the posterior sacral roots to suppress the neurogenic detrusor overactivity (SPARSI). Thus also achieving efficient emptying avoiding the rhizotomy.

2. Muscle augmentation to increase bladder contractility

Though neurostimulation, especially of the anterior sacral roots, is effective in inducing contraction in spinal cord lesions above the sacral micturition centre, it has no role to play in the flaccid neurogenic bladder due to lesions at or below the sacral micturition centre. The treatment of choice for detrusor underactivity is clean intermittent catheterisation. However, in an attempt to eliminate catheter related morbidity and improve quality of life for patients with acontractil detrusor, the restoration of bladder contractility may be desirable. The use of a striated muscle flap that can be electrically stimulated, to augment bladder contractility, is an attractive idea. Some authors have evaluated the use of the latissimus dorsi muscle wrapped around an artificial reservoir or wrapped around the acontractil bladder, after division of its motor supply and its reanastomosis to an active nerve [11, 12, 13]. Others have tried to use the rectus abdominus because of its proximity to the urinary bladder [14].

A pedicled latissimus dorsi muscle flap has been used as a myocardial substitute in patients with heart failure due to cardiomyopathy. Latissimus dorsi bladder myoplasty is more challenging and more complex. It involves latissimus transposition with microsurgical anastomosis of its blood supply as well as its innervation in order to be placed in the pelvis. This revascularization and reinnervation, though challenging, is achievable. It has been shown that the latissimus dorsi wrapped around the bladder is able to generate enough intravesical pressure to promote voiding. Although initial experience is promising [15, 16] more studies are needed in order to confirm the clinical applicability of these techniques.

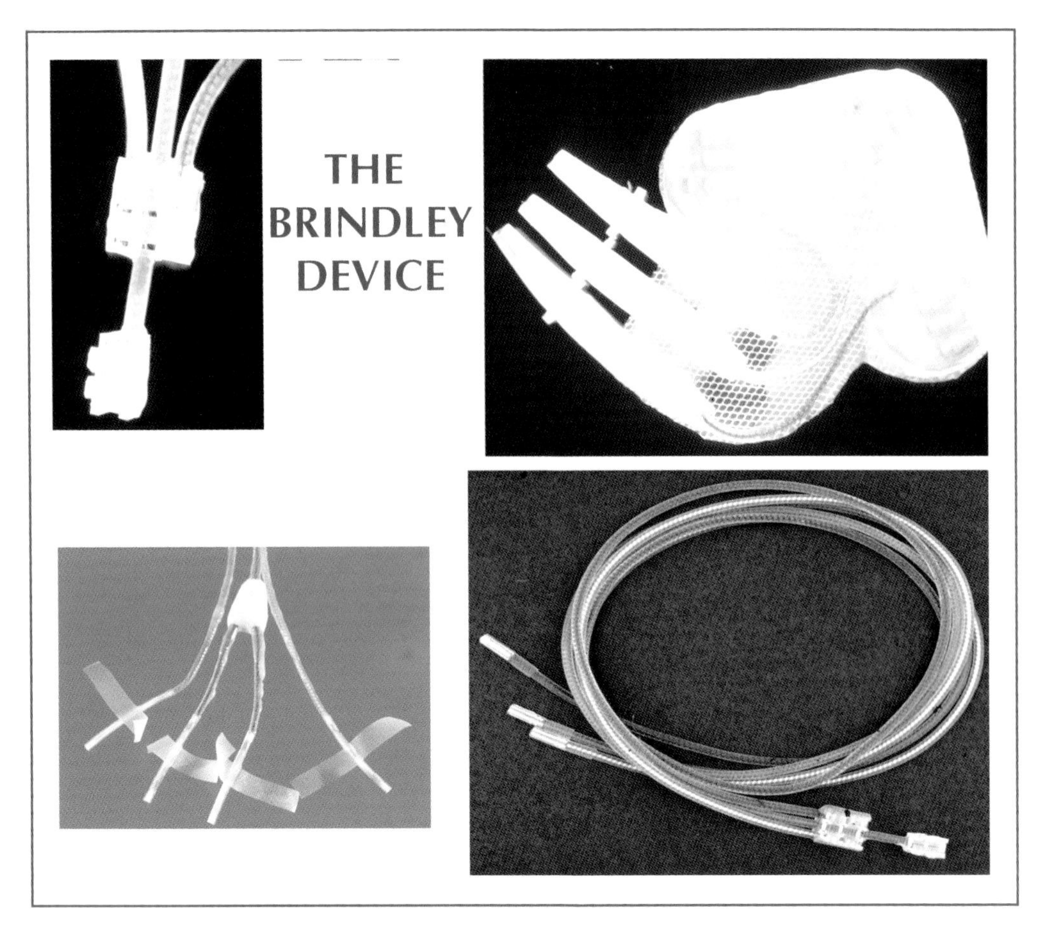

Figure 1 : Sacral Posterior Root Rhizotomy and Sacral Anterior Root Stimulation with the Brindley Device.

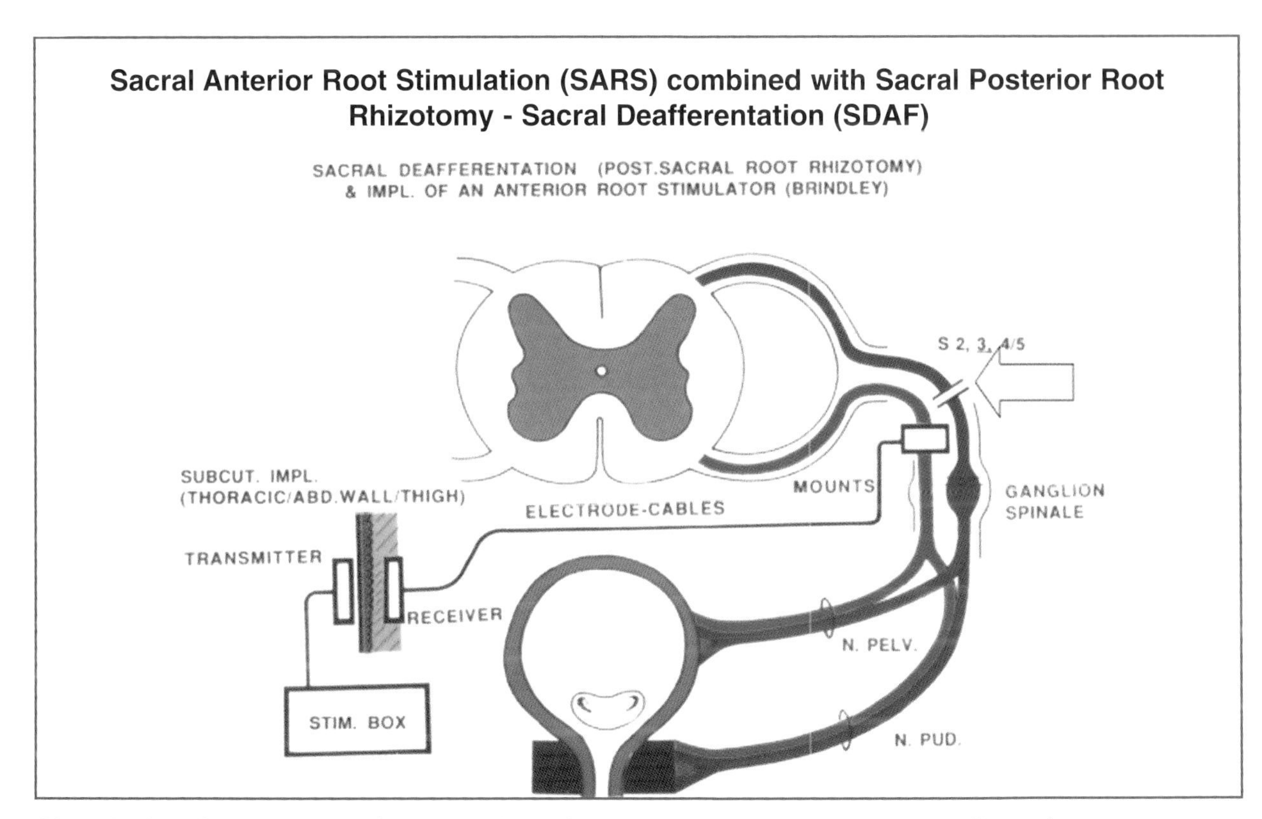

Figure 2 : Sacral Posterior Root Rhizotomy and Sacral Anterior Root Stimulation with the Brindley Device.

Blasensteuergerät
Ausgang zum Steuergerät
Akku geladen
Ladung
Laßegerät

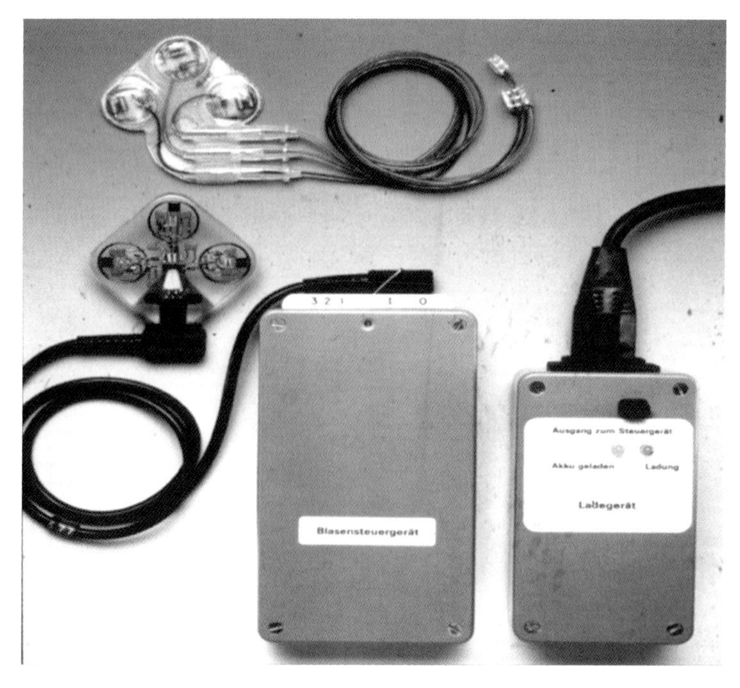

Figure 3 : Sacral Posterior Root Rhizotomy and Sacral Anterior Root Stimulation with the Brindley Device.

Sacral anterior root stimulation
SACRAL DEAFFERENTATION (POST.SACRAL ROOT RHIZOTOMY) & IMPL. OF AN ANTERIOR ROOT STIMULATOR (BRINDLEY)
S 2, 3, 4/5
SUBCUT. IMPL. (THORACIC/ABD.WALL/THIGH)
MOUNTS
GANGLION SPINALE
ELECTRODE-CABLES
TRANSMITTER
RECEIVER
N. PELV.
STIM. BOX
N. PUD.
Stim.
Bladder pressure
Sphincter pressure
Urine flow rate
Diagrammatic
1 sec.

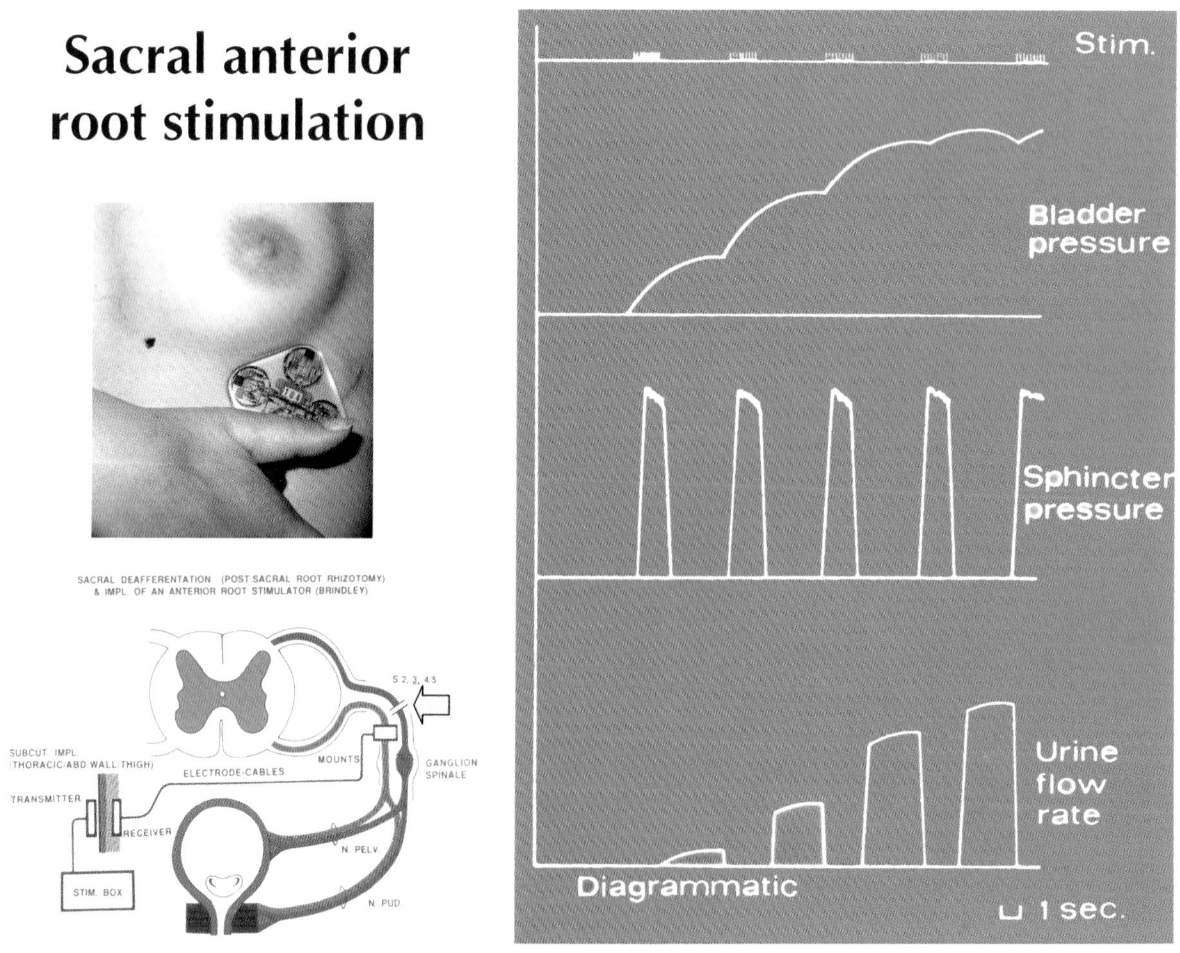

Figure 4 : Sacral Posterior Root Rhizotomy and Sacral Anterior Root Stimulation with the Brindley Device.

Electrostimulation Sacral Anterior Root Stimulation (SARS)

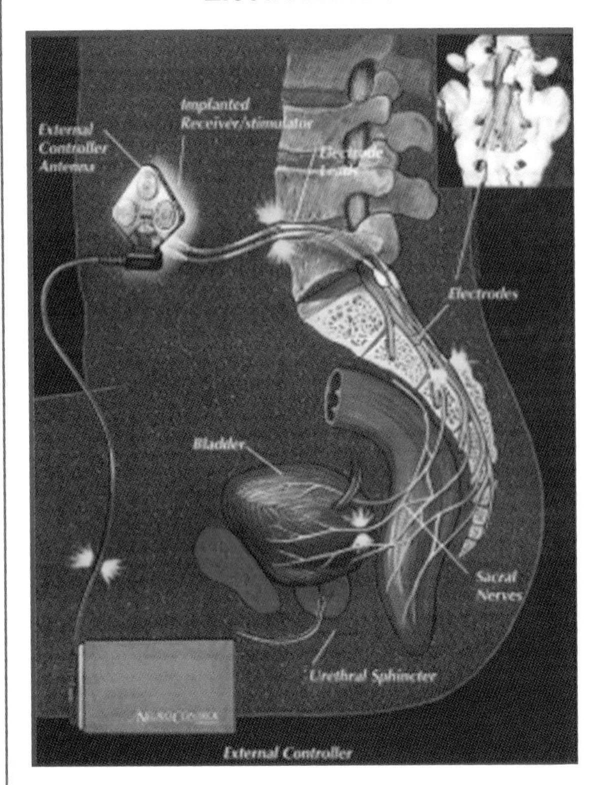

Prerequisite:
suprasacral lesion with intact efferent neurons and a detrusor able to contract

Technique:

- SARS to stimulate bladder contraction
- SDAF to abolish reflex voiding

Advantage: efficient voiding continence

Disadvantage: loss of reflex erections

Figure 5 : Sacral Posterior Root Rhizotomy and Sacral Anterior Root Stimulation with the Brindley Device.

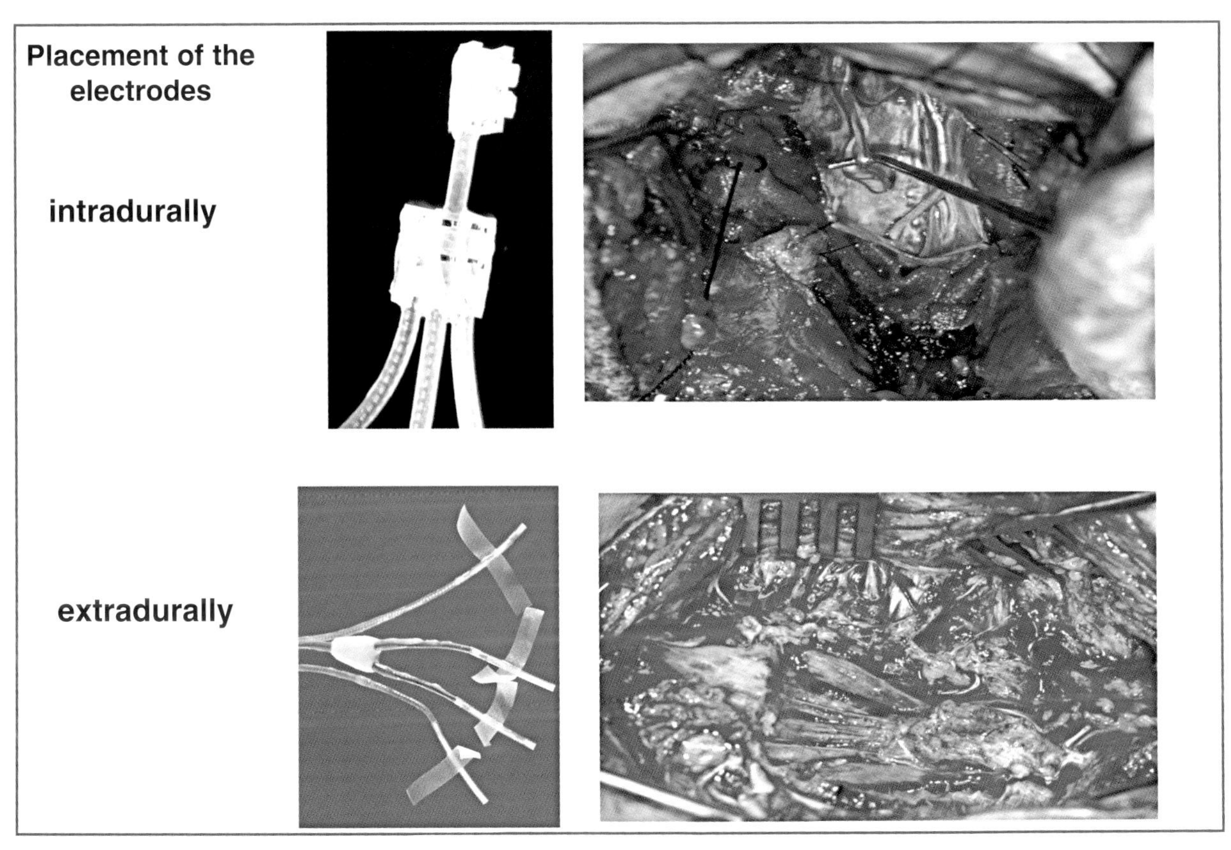

Figure 6 : Sacral Posterior Root Rhizotomy and Sacral Anterior Root Stimulation with the Brindley Device.

II. SURGERY TO DECREASE OUTLET RESISTANCE

1. SPHINCTEROTOMY

Transurethral incision of the external urinary sphincter (TUIS) is a reasonable option to promote bladder emptying and prevent urologic complications in the male spinal cord injured patient (or myelopathic disorders in male).

This procedure helps to decrease urinary outlet resistance due to detrusor-sphincter dyssynergia (DSN). The goal is to reduce the intravesical voiding pressure mediated by detrusor contractions against a dyssynergically contracted external urethral sphincter. The primary indication for sphincterotomy is in those individuals who have elevated residual urine volumes in the presence of good but involuntary detrusor contraction and who have failed conservative management. Other indications are repeated episodes of autonomic dysreflexia (17, 18) typically in a tetraplegic patient with poor hand function, whose bladder drainage through intermittent catheterisation (IC) is cumbersome and difficult to maintain 24 hours/day, repeated urinary tract infections, difficult catheterisations due to urethral false passages (19), and/or secondary bladder neck obstruction due to a "ledge" formation [20]. Inadequate bladder drainage resulting in upper tract changes, reduction of renal function, vesico-ureteric reflux, stone disease and prostate-ejaculatory reflux, with associated epididymo-orchitis, may also be considered for TUIS.

The goals of sphincterotomy are: stabilization or improvement in renal function, prevention of urosepsis, lowering the detrusor leak point pressure, stabilization or elimination of vesicoureteric reflux and eliminating the need for chronic indwelling catheterisation. Following successful sphincterotomy, improvement in bladder emptying and stabilization of the upper urinary tract function can be reasonably expected in 70-90% of patients (21).

Transurethral external sphincterotomy can be performed with either a knife electrode or using a resection loop at the l2 o'clock position [22]. Following electrosurgical TUIS significant intraoperative and postoperative bleeding may occur with subsequent clot retention requiring prolonged drainage with a large diameter catheter. In addition, urethral strictures, impotence and need for reoperation have been reported in 30 to 60% [23, 24] of patients. In some initial TUIS failures an additional bladder neck incision or a TURP is required [24]. Other failures reported are due to inadequate surgery, post TUIS bulbous urethral strictures and poor detrusor contractility. In order to improve these shincterotomy results using both contact and beam lasers have been applied through standard cystoscopes [25]. The laser energy is delivered fiberoptically either through a reusable contact laser probe screwed on to the tip of a rigid fiber or through the direct contact of fiber for the delivery of the Holmium laser (Figure 7). Free beam laser leads to coagulative necrosis, and therefore is not suitable for TUIS. Sphincterotomy with contact

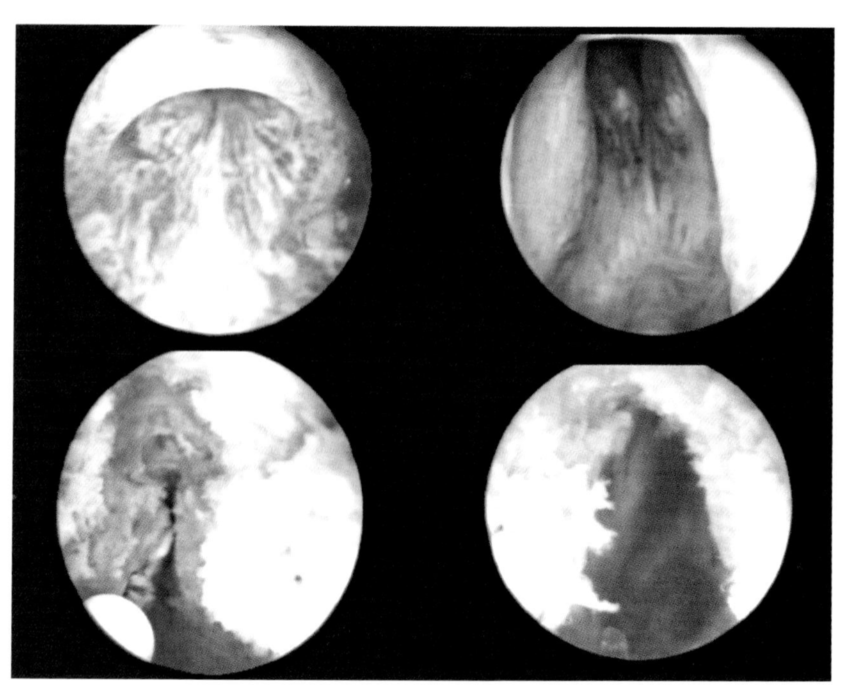

Figure 7 : Sphinterotomy with Holmium laser incision at 0´clock position

laser requires repeated passes to cut and vaporize all urethral tissue, stopped just short of the spongiosum to prevent perforation of the urethra [24, 25]. Results following the use of contact laser have been encouraging with significantly reduced incidence of operative and perioperative bleeding and reduced need for repeat sphincterotomy: 7% to 15% versus over 30% in reported series following conventional electrocautery TUIS [24, 25]. Detrusor leak point pressure below 40 cm water seems to be a useful urodynamic parameter for the successful outcome of TUIS [23, 26].

Following TUIS, some patients may have difficulty keeping the external condom in place. Although such patients have been helped in the past by placement of a semi rigid penile implant [27, 28], the incidence of infection, erosion and implant failure in this patient population has been significant compared to non paralyzed patients. Thus this procedure is now reserved for a very selected group. With adequate control of urinary tract infection, penile implant failure rate has been reduced in some series to 8% [27]. *(LEVEL OF EVIDENCE IV)*

2. Botulinum-A toxin to reduce outlet resistance

Botulinum-A toxin [150 I.U.] injected into the sphincter endoscopically as an alternative to conventional sphincterotomy, has been shown to be effective by some authors [29,30]. Schurch and co-workers reported that in 21 of 24 patients with detrusor-sphincter dyssynergia, urethral pressures were significantly reduced with a concomitant decrease in postvoid residual volumes in 38% patients. Botulinum-A toxin effects lasted 2 to 3 months making reinjections necessary. They concluded that, although costly, botulinum-A toxin injections, which aim at suppressing detrusor-sphincter dyssynergia but not bladder neck dyssynergia, appear to be a valid alternative for patients who do not desire surgery or who are unable to perform self-catheterisation [30]. *(LEVEL OF EVIDENCE IV)*

3. Implantable stents as an alternative to surgical sphincterotomy

The hope of neurological recovery or improvement is an important psychosocial issue for many SCI patients. They often refuse any procedure, medically indicated or not, if the procedure is destructive and irreversible. The sphincter stent gives the patient a treatment option that is potentially reversible. The UroLume prosthesis is made of a superalloy mesh that expands and shortens, similar to a Chinese finger toy when deployed from the insertion tool. This facilitates the device insertion and removal. The geometry, elastic property, and the radial force of the stent material allow it to maintain its position to continuously prevent obstruction by the external urethral sphincter. The large lumen (42 Fr) created by the prosthesis permits catheterisation and cystoscopy after epithelialization. In 153 patients at 15 centres, sphincter prosthesis placement has documented clinical success with up to two years of follow-up. The simplicity of placement and minimal associated morbidity makes the sphincter prosthesis an attractive modality to treat external sphincter dyssynergia and also in patients with failed previous external sphincterotomy. A prospective randomised study between the UroLume stent versus sphincterotomy at three model SCI centres has just been completed. Patient demographics for sphincterotomy patients (N=26) and UroLume patients (N=31) were statistically similar. Preoperative cystometric capacity, maximal voiding pressure, and residual urine were equivalent between the two groups. The decrease of voiding pressure was significant for both sphincterotomy and stent patients. No significant change in bladder capacity occurred after either sphincterotomy or stent placement. Residual urine decreased in both sphincterotomy and stent patients. The mean length of hospitalisation and operation were significantly shorter for stent patients rather than sphincterotomy [31]. Long-term results confirming the initial results have also been reported [32] *(LEVEL OF EVIDENCE II)*. However there have been several non randomised studies on the use of different stents for the treatment of detrusor sphincter dyssinergia showing disappointing results. The main reported complications are migration of the stent, persisting urinary tract and prostatic infection leading to autonomic dysreflexia, calculus formation, encrustation, tissue growth in addition to pain and irritative symptoms [33-36]

B. FAILURE TO STORE

I. SURGERY TO DECREASE DETRUSOR CONTRACTILITY

Patients with neurologic lesions above the sacral micturition centre will frequently exhibit detrusor overactivity [37-40]. This phenomenon is responsible for the majority of associated incontinence and may contribute to the development of upper tract deterioration. This latter problem may be exacerbated by the inability to generate a volitional detrusor contraction and the coexistence of detrusor sphincter dyssynergia. Dyssynergia can be predicted if the pontine micturition centre is cut off from bladder innervation [41-43]. Poor or absent volitional voiding function will increase residual urine. This will also occur in the presence of detrusor sphincter dyssynergia. More significantly detrusor pressures generated either volitionally or during storage due to the hyperreflexia, may be unphysiologically high, contributing significantly to the development of deleterious upper tract changes. In addition, these changes may be accompanied by the bladder exhibiting low compliance, further contributing to the abnormal bladdder pressures generated.

With these pathophysiologic changes in mind, management of detrusor overactivity will be directed at restoring storage function to as close to normal as possible, reducing the associated incontinence and possibility of upper tract changes. This management cannot be carried out in isolation as the patient's ability to empty may be compromised by the lesion itself or the therapy for the detrusor overactivity and must therefore also be considered [44, 45].

Surgery to decrease detrusor overactivity by altering the sacral reflex arc has historically been unsuccessful. Mainly because of this, enterocystoplasty and its alternatives have achieved a 'gold standard' position in the management algorithm of these cases. Continued concern regarding long-term complications of these procedures has prompted several alternatives to enterocystoplasty to be developed. These include gastrocystoplasty, autoaugmentation, ureterocystoplasty and the use of demucosalised bowel segments. This has also prompted a 'resurgence' of methods to peripherally denervate the bladder and the development of techniques to modulate the sacral reflexes. All these techniques will be discussed in the following sections.

1. Enterocystoplasty

It has been accepted practise for many years that patients with intractable neurogenic detrusor overactivity and or low compliance, with associated incontinence and/or upper tract deterioration, can be managed successfully by enterocystoplasty. This assumes that the patient can empty the bladder appropriately, the neurologic disease is not rapidly advancing and that all conservative measures have been exhausted. Despite this, the levels of evidence to support this in the literature are relatively poor. There are multiple series of studies describing retrospective results of this procedure. The results are uniformly good in terms of continence and improvement or stabilization of upper tracts. Many studies also confirm the associated enhancement of urodynamic storage characteristics [10-12].

As a general criticism, these papers vary greatly in number of patients studied. They are retrospective in nature and very often refer to a heterogeneous group of patients, not all of whom have a neurological etiology. Techniques, including choice of bowel segment, vary from series to series and many patients require additional surgery (outlet enhancement, reflux prevention, catheterizable stomas etc.) to achieve success. In addition results are not generally evaluated in any standardized fashion, such that there is significant physician bias in the interpretation of results, and attempts to compare series is compromised. Follow up is often too short to be truly meaningful [49, 50].

A universal theme found in all, is that complications are common. These include recurrent infection, stones, recurrent incontinence, bowel obstruction, and perforation. More remote complications included malignancy and metabolic abnormalities. The complication rate in some series reached more than 40%. Re-operation rates were similarly high, and intervention was needed both in short and long term follow up (>10 years).

Despite these observations, all authors refer to the overall success of this procedure. However, they do generally qualify this, in their conclusions, by commenting that careful patient selection is required along with life time follow up *(LEVEL OF EVIDENCE IV).*

2. Alternatives to enterocystoplasty

a) Gastrocystoplasty

Gastrocystoplasty was popularised as a more suitable segment for augmentation in the pediatric neurogenic population. The absence of metabolic acidosis and thinner mucus were some of its advantageous characteristics. There are very few meaningful studies on the use of gastrocystoplasty in the adult neuropath, so discussion of this will be dealt with in the pediatric section.

b) Ureterocystoplasty

Similarly, there are very few papers on the use of this technique in adults.

c) Detrusor myectomy (auto-augmentation)

Detrusor auto-augmentation therapy was introduced in 1989 by two separate research teams, one concentrating on children, and the other on adults. The treatment is intended to allow the bladder to enlarge when the functional capacity is reduced by detrusor overactivity in patients with neurological disease who are refractory to anticholinergic medication, mainly because of adverse effects. Follow-up times of up to ten years have now been published. Pre- and post-operative urodynamic evaluations are available and, because of the neuropathic conditions of these patients, these will be repeated every 1-2 years [52, 53]. A large part of the detrusor muscle is dissected, leaving the mucosa intact and thereby creating an "artificial diverticulum". This will expand and dissipate the pressure caused by the detrusor contraction and thus allow low-pressure storage. As a result the voiding contraction is reduced as well, and thus patients often need to empty their bladders by intermittent catheterisation after this procedure.

This surgery is generally performed under general anaesthesia. After introduction of a urethral catheter, the bladder is exposed extraperitoneally and filled to anatomical capacity. The peritoneum is dissected from the superior and superior-posterior of the detrusor the urachus, by blunt dissection from the bladder serosa. In trabeculated bladders it may be hard to remove every single muscle fibre, but this will not impair the therapeutic result.

The development of the bladder enlargement is a relatively slow process. It may take about 1-2 years before the final condition of low-pressure storage and eradication of the detrusor overactivity is achieved. During this period medical treatment with anticholinergics (mostly in a much lower dose than before surgery) may be beneficial [54].

In most studies the efficacy of this procedure has been documented by video-urodynamics, pre- and post-operatively. Outcome parameters are: improvement of incontinence, bladder compliance, maximum detrusor pressure during voiding, cystometric capacity, reduced use of anticholinergics, and patient satisfaction [55-58].

The maximum detrusor pressures during voiding decrease and the urine residual increases. The cystometric capacity and the bladder compliance both increase. Occasionally, late reduction of capacity, caused by fibrosis, has been reported. In these reports, the surgeons used tissue such as omentum, to cover the serosal side of the mucosa after the detrusor miectomy. However, in the reports from the two groups with the longest experience, this manoeuvre is not supported.

Motivation is extremely important when selecting patients for this procedure. Case reports exist on patients who were changed to intestinal augmentation within 6-12 months of auto-augmentation. Also, patients who will not perform intermittent catheterisation as their mode of voiding are not candidates for this procedure.

A study on 52 adult patients with various neurological (about 75% traumatic spinal cord injury) and a minimum follow-up of 4 years was published recently. The average follow-up was 6.4 years. The only complication noted was per-operative mucosal perforation in one third of the patients. This was easily closed and mostly had no late sequel. The results are encouraging: most patients did not use any anticholinergics, in the others drug use was reduced significantly. The cystometric capacity increased from 132 to 359 ml, bladder compliance from 9 to 25 ml/cm H_2O. The maximum voiding pressure decreased from 95 to 48 cm H_2O, and the residual volume increased from 45 to 163 ml (Figures 8-10). All these changes were statistically significant [58]. Reflux in four out of five patients, was ameliorated, but in one case, de novo reflux was observed. Sixteen failures were reported: nine patients were lost from follow-up and were conservatively counted as failures, four patients were submitted to other procedures, one had a fibrotic bladder, and one required indwelling catheterisation —, and three patients had low capacity after the surgery — one with recurrent infections and the other two had extensive mucosal perforations perioperatively.

In those patients who responded well to auto-augmentation, most were satisfied with their urinary condition, in particular they reported a much better quality of life [58].

In conclusion, detrusor myectomy is a valuable therapy in this difficult patient group, with approximately two thirds of patients responding favourably in the long term. *(LEVEL OF EVIDENCE IV)*. As these patients might otherwise be subjected to intestinal augmentation or sacral neuromodulation therapy, it is worthwhile having this relatively less invasive procedure available. Auto-augmentation does not preclude the use of these other modalities. Although the outcome is generally positive in the long term, a major drawback is the long delay between the procedure and the final result on the lower urinary tract function. This problem may be solved by combining this surgery with botulinum toxin injections into the detrusor. The bladder paralysis caused by botulinum toxin will immediately eliminate the detrusor overactivity and last for about one year.

3. DENERVATION TECHNIQUES FOR DETRUSOR OVERACTIVITY

Historically many techniques have been used and described in the literature to try and convert the overactive neuropathic bladder (upper motor neuron lesion) to an underactive bladder (LMN lesion). These methods will be briefly described. In general they are rarely used now because of poor long-term results, and significant complications.

a) Bladder distention (Helmstein's technique): although successful outcome was initially reported, long term results and the occasional reports of bladder rupture have discouraged the establishment of this technique.

b) Cystolysis: mostly used for the treatment of interstitial cystitis and other sensory conditions, with a few series including patients with neurogenic detrusor overactivity. Short-term results reported as good, but no long-term results available. The late complication of bladder contracture in 10% has precluded its further use.

c) Inglemann Sundberg procedure: transvaginal

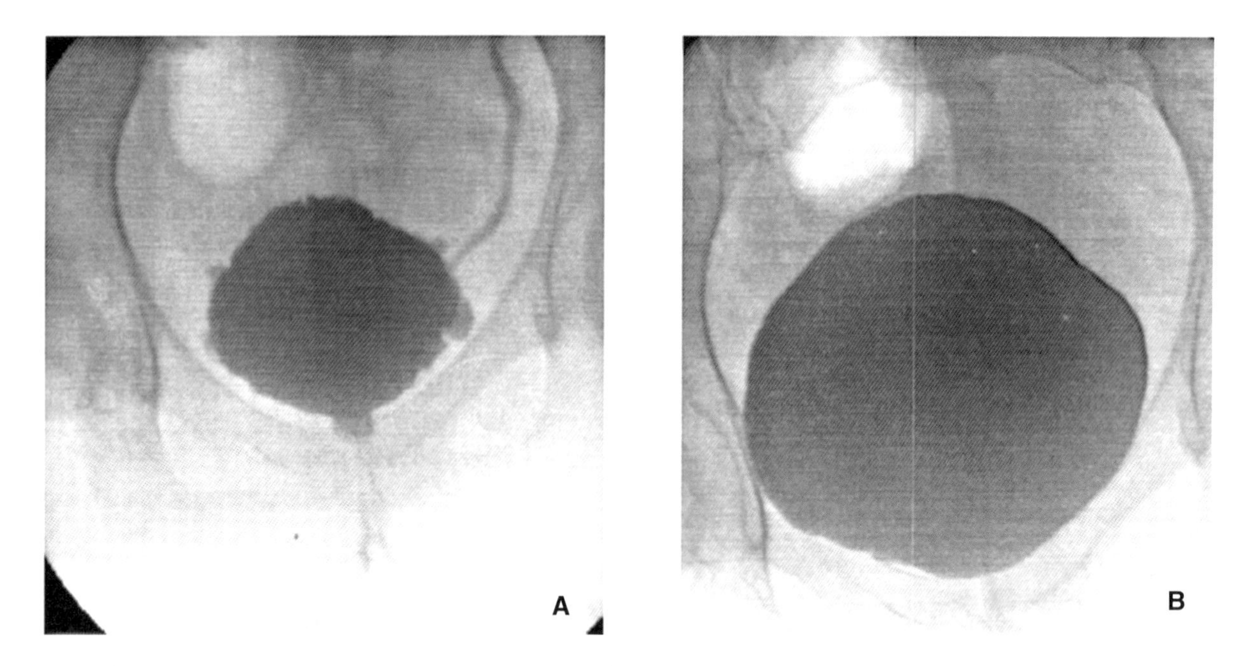

Figures 8 a-b : Cystography before and after autoaugmentation (Detrusor Myectomy)

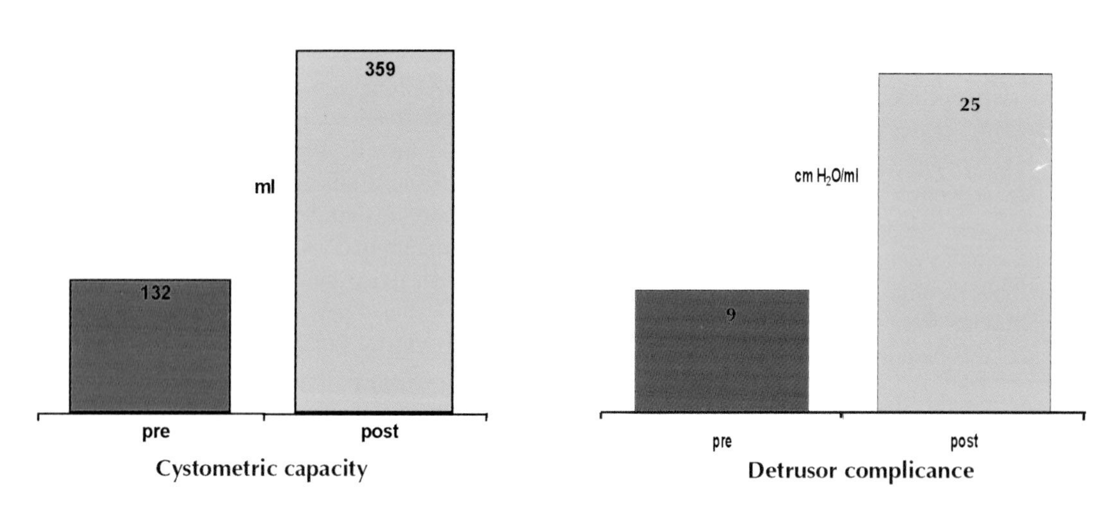

Figures 9 : Bladder capacity and compliance before and after autoaugmentation

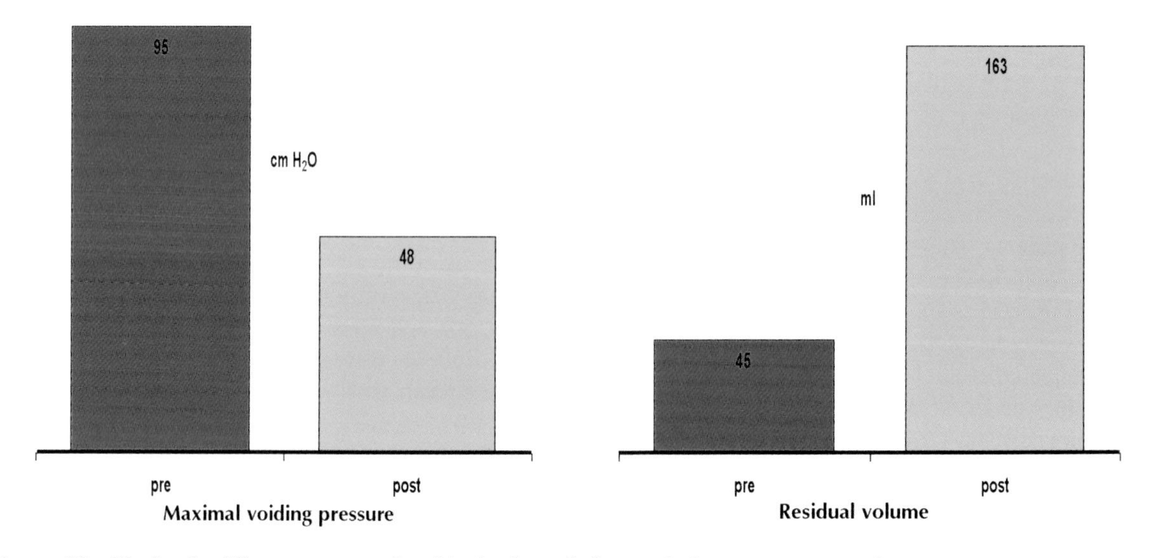

Figures 10 : Maximal voiding pressure and residual volume before and after autoaugmentation

denervation has been used in patients with detrusor overactivity with some short-term success. Series are all relatively small and there is no experience of this technique in the neurological population.

d) Bladder transection: various techniques have been described ranging from circumferential incision to an endoscopic supratrigonal technique. Patients in these small series were generally suffering from idiopathic detrusor overactivity or had sensory disorders (interstitial cystitis). Studies suffer from short follow up.

e) Subtrigonal injection: the logical extension of the above was the use of phenol or alcohol injected transtrigonally to effect a denervation of the bladder. Little experience is reported in neurological patients and effects were usually short lived. The occasional complication of fistula formation has further doomed these procedures to the 'history' books.

f) Sacral rhizotomy: Of all the techniques used to denervate the overactive detrusor, sacral rhizotomy has achieved the best success. In most series, presently, it is combined with implantation of sacral anterior root stimulator. In this way the overactivity is significantly reduced and functional bladder capacity is increased [4, 5, 7, 8]. The stimulator allows the patient to empty the bladder without resorting to catheterisation. The rhizotomy also reduces the development of sphincter dysynnergia during anterior root stimulation.

Rhizotomy is conventionally performed via a limited sacral laminectomy to expose S2-S4 nerve roots bilaterally. Visual magnification and continuous cystometry aid identification of the appropriate nerve roots. The nerves that evoke an adequate detrusor contraction when stimulated, are selected and severed.

Reported complications include fecal incontinence and erectile dysfunction. The later may be overcome by using the anterior root stimulator for this purpose. Fecal incontinence is rarely reported in published series [5, 6, 8]. *(LEVEL OF EVIDENCE IV)*

Recent developments focus on techniques to reversibly block the posterior roots during stimulation so that formal rhizotomy could be avoided. A technique using cryotherapy to produce a reversible nerve block has recently been described [10].

4. Sacral nerve stimulation / neuromodulation

Suppressing detrusor overactivity using a neuromodulation approach has been in the development stage for many years. Presently several clinical studies are available to demonstrates the efficacy of this technology. Unfortunately there are no good studies on its use in the neurogenic bladder patient. The exact mechanism, by which sacral nerve stimulation inhibits detrusor contraction, is not fully understood. However it is thought that sacral nerve stimulation induces reflex mediated inhibitory effects on the detrusor through afferent and or efferent stimulation of the sacral nerves. In addition activation of the pelvic floor muscles may occur via stimulation of the somatic fibers of the nerves, causing further detrusor inhibition [59].

The technique of initial percutaneous nerve stimulation to assess efficacy, followed by surgical implantation of the sacral nerve stimulator is well known.

Several reasonable clinical studies are available showing significant reduction in incontinence episodes etc. Unfortunately, as stated, the majority of patients in these studies, suffered from refractory urge incontinence and those with neurological conditions were specifically excluded. Complications of the technique included pain at implant site, infection, change in bowel habit and technical problems including lead migration [59].

This technique is certainly a promising development in a difficult group of patients. Technical details still need to be improved and although initial reports are encouraging [60, 61] it remains to be seen if this will be appropriate for neuropathic patients.

In general, surgical intervention to decrease detrusor contractility should still only be used when all conservative measures have failed. Choice of intervention at present will depend on many factors including the underlying pathogenesis of the condition, its natural history, the patients mobility, motivation, age and home support, to name the most significant. Although augmentation cystoplasty gives the most reproducible results its complication rate is still relatively high. Of the alternatives to cystoplasty, only autoaugmentation has some merit but will have to be carefully evaluated in the long term. Neuromodulation and denervation techniques such as rhizotomy have less morbidity than cystoplasty and their role will continue to evolve. The most pressing need in this field is to develop standardised methods of evaluating results. It is too much to ask for controlled trials for these surgical techniques, but a uniform method of assessing results would be extremely helpful.

5. Botulinum A toxin injections in the detrusor

This new therapy was used for the first time in 1998 and published in 1999. Subsequently, several clinical studies have been published including pre- and postoperative urodynamic evaluation and a follow-up time of up to three years. Patients with detrusor overactivity, refractory to anticholinergic medication, are suitable for this therapy [62-66].

The botulinum toxin blocks the local intramuscular nerve endings. This causes a flaccid paralysis of the detrusor that persists for several months. All patients must be established on intermittent catheterisation before embarking on this therapy. The combination of both these modalities leads to low pressure storage without upper tract damage and continence [62-66].

Botox® 300 IE or Dysport® 900 IE are approximately equivalent doses of botulinum A toxin. The agent is dissolved in 15 ml saline and injected in 0.5 ml aliquots over the whole of the detrusor using a standard endoscopic injection needle. The injections are performed preferably in visible muscular structures. The trigone and the ureteric orifices are spared, as is the bladder neck, in theory, preventing the development of post-injection stress incontinence.

The effects of Botox can be demonstrated within 7-14 days after the application. Over 100 patients have been treated in two centres (Murnau and Zurich). The majority of these patients had traumatic spinal cord lesions, but smaller groups with multiple sclerosis and myelomeningocele have also been treated. Patients with low bladder compliance secondary to neurological disease, caused by changes in the detrusor wall are excluded from this treatment. Patients at risk from autonomic dysreflexia are treated under local or general anesthesia.

In the published studies efficacy was documented by video-urodynamics, pre-operatively and at 6, 16, and 36 weeks after treatment. The outcome parameters were continence, functional reflex volume, bladder compliance, maximum detrusor pressure during voiding, cystometric capacity, reduced use of anticholinergics, and patient satisfaction [62-66].

In the vast majority of cases it was found that the detrusor overactivity was reduced, the functional reflex volume and cystometric capacity had increased, and the patients were continent.

The maximum detrusor pressures during voiding had decreased. The urine residual was almost always equal to the cystometric capacity. An improvement in autonomic dysreflexia was noted. About 5% of the patients did not respond to this therapy for unknown reasons. The authors suggest that these patients might have been in contact with the toxin earlier in their lives, and had developed antibodies. A single injection session offers therapeutic benefit for up to14 months, with most patients averaging between 10 and 12 months. Presently, 15 patients with a minimum follow-up of three years have received three injections, apparently without loss of efficacy [65,66].

This therapy is very well tolerated by patients, two thirds of them are completely continent, with some individuals reporting consistent bladder capacities of up to 800 ml.

In October 2000 an interim analysis was carried out on 43 patients. Forty patients had six weeks follow-up, and 24 had 16 weeks follow-up. The number of patients with 36 weeks follow-up was too small for evaluation. In this analysis, continence had improved and the detrusor overactivity had ameliorated significantly (Figure 11). The functional reflex volume increased from 178 to 412 and to 366 ml, the cystometric capacity from 284 to 487 and to 478 ml, the maximum voiding pressure decreased from 74 to 33 and to 24 cm H_2O, and the residual volume increased from 237 to 501 and to 508 ml. All these changes were statistically significant. The compliance increased non-significantly, probably because abnormally low compliance was excluded. It was noted that existing autonomic dysreflexia was also ameliorated.

Responders to this therapy (about 90%) will be completely continent and are able to stop or reduce the use of using anticholinergics. Both products seem to be equally effective. The detrusor paralysis lasts at least 10 months. This treatment is a safe and an impressive alternative when other methods for reducind detrusor overactivity have failed. This method is suitable for patients with neurogenic lower urinary tract dysfunction and detrusor overactivity, who can perform intermittent catheterisation. No adverse events have been reported up till now. This therapy may be combined with auto-augmentation, improving the development of low-pressure storage. [64-66] *(LEVEL OF EVIDENCE IV).*

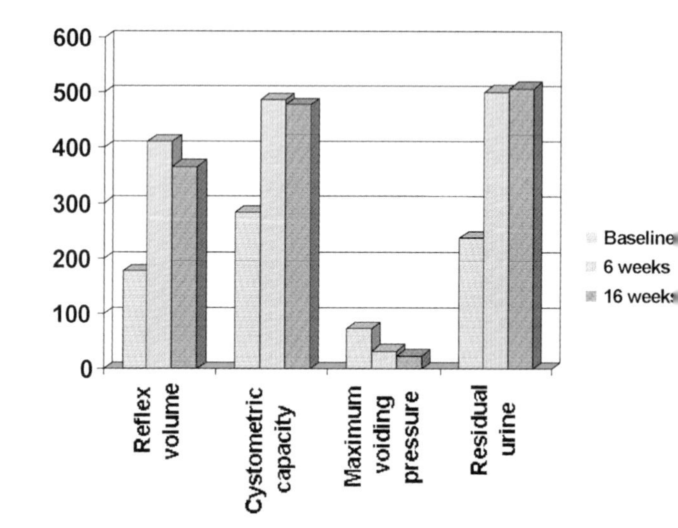

Figure 11 : Reflex volume, bladder capacity, maximum voiding pressure and residual urine at the baseline, 6 and 12 weeks after the inyection of Botulinum-A toxin at the detrusor.

II. SURGERY TO INCREASE SPHINCTERIC RESISTANCE

Patients with sphincteric incontinence due to neurologic disease or injury are candidates for surgical procedures to increase urethral resistance, assuming that associated bladder compliance and detrusor overactivity abnormalities can be satisfactorily managed. As all procedures to increase urethral resistance in neuropathic patients produce compression, urinary retention is not uncommon after the surgery.

Patient selection and preoperative evaluation play a critical role in the process of increasing urethral resistance. The work-up should include history and physical examination, urine culture, cystourethroscopy, upper urinary tract imaging and urodynamics.

The minimal conditions that a neurological patient should meet in order to be considered as a candidate for any of these procedures are:

- incontinence primarily due to intrinsic sphincter deficiency
- an acontractile detrusor or controllable detrusor overactivity
- a healthy, well-vascularized bulbar urethra or bladder neck
- absence of significant vesicoureteric reflux.

In addition the patient should have sufficient intelligence, motivation, compliance and manual dexterity and must be established on intermittent catheterisation. The neurological disease should be stable. Thus patients who have a progressive disease such as multiple sclerosis, are generally poor candidates.

There are several surgical options to increase urethral resistance in neuropathic patients. These include artificial urinary sphincter, sphincteric muscle augmentation, implantable valves and bulking agents. The rational for procedure selection depends on a number of patient's factors and the surgeon's preference and experience.

1. Artificial urinary sphincter

Although the artificial urinary sphincter (AUS) has been recommended for the treatment of sphincteric incontinence, and it is commonly used in patients with congenital neurological disease, there has not been a significant degree of popularity or success in the adult neurogenic population. In most of the reported series, the difference between the number of patients initially implanted and the number of patients using the device at the end of follow-up is unclear. Success rates reported range from 70% to 95% with a revision rate varying between 16% and 180% [67-77]. In a recent review on long-term outcome (more than 10 years) of 100 patients treated with the artificial urinary sphincter it has been shown that, in spite of the high revision rate, the artificial urinary sphincter is an effective long-term treatment for incontinence in male patients. In female patients the risk of erosion is high, although overall long-term continence is satisfactory [78] *(LEVEL OF EVIDENCE IV).*

Changes in bladder compliance leading to upper urinary tract deterioration may occur with any procedure to increase outlet resistance without bladder augmentation. This problem has been most frequently associated with the artificial urinary sphincter. The mechanism of these changes in bladder function is not fully understood but clearly the myelodysplasic population is most at risk [79]. Changes in compliance after artificial sphincter implantation are not documented in the adult incontinent population without myelodisplasia. It has been suggested that these changes might be associated with an increase of the alpha-adrenergic innervation [80], but could also be related to detrusor behaviour, not identified preoperatively. When post-treatment urodynamics reveals detrusor overactivity not demonstrated preoperatively, anticholinergic therapy is needed. If maximal doses of anticholinergic drugs do not control the detrusor overactivity, bladder augmentation may be necessary. Timing of the augmentation procedure in these patients, simultaneously or subsequently, is controversial alternatively. This procedure may be carried out as a first stage, prior to the sphincter implantation. It may be performed simultaneously, or as a secondary procedure if abnormal bladder behaviour is unmasked. Some authors advocate a staged approach, fearing sphincter infection if implanted at the same time as the cystoplasty [79]. Conversely other authors have not found a higher complication rate using the synchronous technique (Figure 12) [69, 74].

2. Sphincteric muscle augmentation

a) Dynamic myoplasty

Attempts have been made to correct intrinsic sphincter deficiency using a stimulated Gracilis muscle flap (dynamic myoplasty). First reported by Janknegt et al [81], initial experience has been gained in men and women with neurologically impaired sphincter function. Its use is based on the transposition of this muscle to the bladder neck [82] or to the urethral area [83]. The skeletal muscle is then converted into a functional sphincter by electrical stimulation. During an increasing stimulation protocol the fatigable type 2 fibres, the main fibres in skeletal muscle, are replaced by type 1 fibres, which can sustain long lasting contractions. A

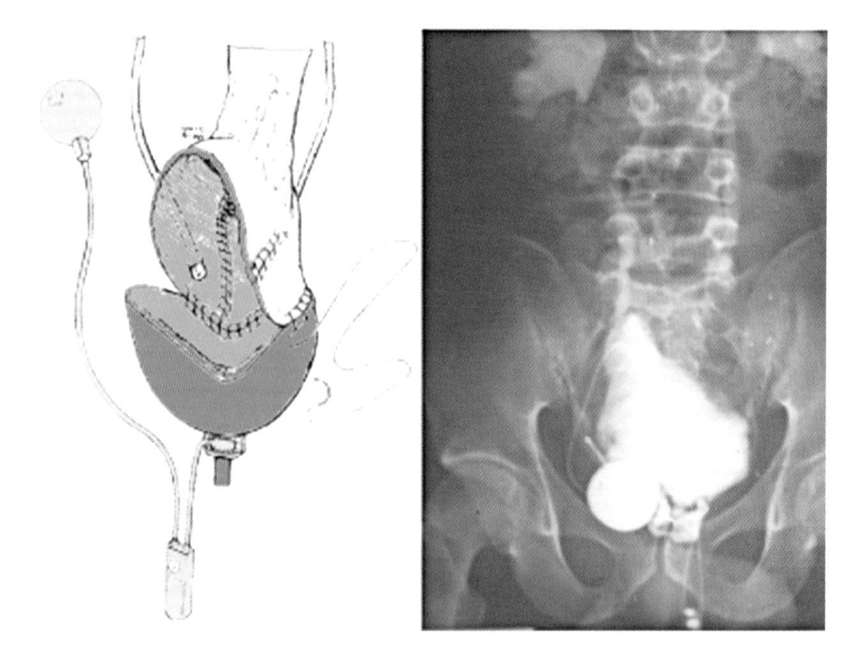

Figure 12 : Simultaneous bladder augmentation and artificial urinary sphincter implantation

subcutaneously placed pulse generator provides continuous low current electrical stimulation via electrodes, enabling the maintenance of constant sphincter tone. Urination is achieved by temporary termination of the neuromuscular stimulation. There have been very few reports on the dynamic graciloplasty for the treatment of urinary incontinence although results are encouraging with few complications. Presently, this technique could be applicable in incontinent patients with severe sphincteric intrinsic deficiency who are not candidates for conventional treatment, including the artificial urinary sphincter, or in whom such treatment has failed [84].

b) Slings

There have been many reports on the success of pubovaginal slings (PVS) for the treatment of intrinsic sphincteric deficiency in the neurogenic population in both children and adults. The procedure is established in the neurological female patient as an alternative to the artificial urinary sphincter. It should be assumed that following PVS, patients will have to empty their bladders by intermittent catheterisation [85]. The reported continence rate is generally high [86-88], with few complications, including difficulty with catheterisation, ventral hernia at the graft harvest site, bladder calculus and detrusor overactivity [89]. There have been a few reports using slings to correct male neurogenic urinary incontinence. Although some authors recommend its use in these patients, it is a procedure that has not gained widespread acceptance. The number of male patients in each series is small and there is a lack of long-term outcome [88, 90, 91, 92]. Walker et al have reported their results in a series of 15 patients with a 3-year followed-up who underwent a rectus fascial wrap. They found continence rates comparable to that of other bladder neck sling procedures in patients with spina bifida [93].

Recent reports suggest that the bulbourethral sling procedure for male incontinence, achieves continence by increasing urethral resistance in a dynamic fashion when intra-abdominal pressure increases, similarly to the pubovaginal sling used to treat female stress urinary incontinence [94] *(LEVEL OF EVIDENCE IV).*

c) Bulking agents

Periurethral injection of materials to provide bulk for urethral closure and continence has applicability for patients with neurogenic vesico-urethral dysfunction, although this has not gained much popularity. The reported continence rates achieved with the use of bulking agents in children ranges from 30% to 80% in the short term and 30% to 40% in the long-term [95-100]; At present there are no studies reporting the use of bulking agents in the adult neurogenic population.

3. Implantable valve/cath

During the last few years several intraurethral implantable devices for the treatment of intrinsic sphincteric incontinence in women have been introduced. The reported success varies in between 72 % and 94% [104,105]. High withdrawal rates have been observed in most studies as well as a significant number of complications. These include device migration, leakage around the catheter or through its lumen, blockage of the valve by sediment or stone formation, urinary tract infection, urethral/meatal bladder irritation, device malfunction and hematuria [106,107].

A remote controlled intraurethral insert has been used

for artificial voiding. In 49% of the patients the device had to be removed due to local discomfort or urinary leakage around the insert, rendering the results unsatisfactory [106,107].

In summary, there are several alternatives to surgically manage urinary incontinence due to neurogenic sphincteric incompetence. Increasing urethral resistance is possible only in those patients who have a good bladder capacity and accommodation or pharmacologically controlled detrusor overactivity. Otherwise when planning to increase the urethral resistance in these patients, bladder augmentation procedure should be considered. The implantation of an artificial urinary sphincter is the technique which has gained most popularity and which has passed the test of the time. As an alternative to the artificial sphincter a sling procedure might be use, assuming that the patient can perform intermittent catheterisation. Dynamic myoplasty appears promising although a cost-efficacy analysis needs to be done. Intraurethral valves need to be evaluated with longer follow up before they can be accepted. Bulking substances may play a limited role in the treatment of neurogenic sphincter deficiency.

III. BLADDER REPLACEMENT SURGERY

1. Orthotopic bladder

This technique aims to create a low-pressure reservoir in patients with severely damaged bladder wall by a partial cystectomy replaced by a substitution cystoplasty [108-110]. A severely thick and fibrotic bladder wall can result from supra sacral neurogenic bladder often complicated with recurrent infection or stones. Urodynamics usually shows detrusor overactivity associated with high intravesical pressure, severe low compliance and reduced bladder capacity. Failure of conservative treatment is an indication for bladder surgery. In these cases, conventional augmentation cystoplasty cannot be used and the majority of the diseased bladder wall needs to be excised. The cystectomy in these cases is supratrigonal, leaving the bladder neck and the trigone intact. The ureters are left in place or reimplanted in the intestinal segment if high-grade reflux or an abnormal urethrovesical orifice is identified.

Numerous factors must be taken into consideration. Urethral stricture or other outlet abnormality must be excluded. The patient must be able to carry out intermittent catheterisation (often this non-contractile reservoir and persistent dysynergia require catheterisation to empty); the patient's must be taught to perform catheterisation before surgery. Urethral sphincter deficiency can be treated by a sling [111] or implantation of an artificial sphincter [112]. These may be performed simultaneously or be held in reserve if it is anticipated that the reduction in bladder pressure by the orthotopic bladder reconstruction alone will be sufficient for continence.

The choice of bowel segment and configuration of that segment may differ but most authors agree that the segment should be detubularized in order to achieve a large capacity and a low-pressure reservoir according to Laplace's law. The segment of bowel used is often a 40 cm length of terminal ileum reconfigured in an S or W shape. Resection of a longer segment of ileum may be associated with diarrhea; due to the increased amount of bile acids reaching the colon [113]. This risk is increased in myelomeningocele patients and in those with short or diseased intestine. The diarrhea often resolves with diet and medication. The use of the caecum with the adjacent terminal ileal has been advocated, but ileocecal valve resection aggravates the risk of digestive disturbance due to reduction in transit time compared to ileum alone. The true incidence of diarrhea after the resection of ileum, ileocecal valve or colon is not known [113]. Absorption of urinary components, particularly chlorides can lead to metabolic acidosis when large resection or proximal ileum resection is associated with renal insufficiency, but in limited ileal resection and normal renal function patients do not develop acidosis [114]. In time, villous atrophy reduces the bowels absorptive properties as well as mucus secretion [115]. Incomplete emptying and mucus stagnation can lead to bladder calculi. Although bladder stones can develop in all types of neuropathic bladder, the main risk is intermittent catheterisation. However, the incidence of stones does not seem to be influenced by enterocystoplasty [116]. In a few cases, spontaneous overdistension leading to perforation has been reported [110]. The precise risk of malignancy in intestinal segments used for urinary reconstruction [117] is unknown. The incidence of adenocarcinoma of the ileum is far less than that of the colon. There is no consensus on cancer surveillance in these patients, but abnormal symptoms and hematuria should be investigated.

Ureteral reflux on pre-operative cystography is corrected by an antireflux procedure, as part of the reconstructive surgery. Severely dilated ureters can be reimplanted into the pouch using either an extramural tunnel, or a mucosal sulcus (Le Duc/Camay) or long afferent loop of bowel (Studer). Severe impairment of renal function is a contraindication, but this surgery can be considered if renal transplantation is planned. Low urine output after reconstruction, will require bladder irrigations in order to prevent mucus retention and pyocystitis. *(LEVEL OF EVIDENCE IV).*

2. Continent diversion

Continent cutaneous urinary diversion provides an alternative bladder outlet associated with a valve for urinary continence, which is catheterised to empty. The urinary reservoir must have low pressure and good capacity. The continent catheterisable stoma can either be implanted into the native bladder or into an intestinal neo-reservoir. In most cases of supra sacral neurogenic lesions and myelomeningocele, a bladder augmentation is carried out at the same procedure. In some cases the native bladder outlet needs to be closed to achieve continence. This is a difficult procedure, with recanalization observed in up to 25% [118]. In men a secondary closure may be particularly difficult but in women a secondary closure can be carried out transvaginally. If the bladder outlet is suitable, it may be preserved, maintaining continence with either a sling or endoscopic transurethral injections [119], or just left as access to the bladder and as a pop-off mechanism [120].

Indications for a continent catheterisable stoma are: inability to perform self-catheterisation through the normal urethral route. This may be due to severe urethral stricture, severe outlet lesions i.e. erosions related to permanent indwelling catheter, urethral pain, non accessible meatus (obesity or upper limb neurogenic partial deficit or spinal abnormalities, transfer difficulties or psychological factors). An additional factor is intractable incontinence particularly in women and in men with condom problems.

If patients are to be managed safely with long term indwelling catheters, they must adhere to a strict care guidelines to avoid complications. Thus altering management to a continent stoma, may be a better prospect. In addition, in some tetraplegic patients, a continent abdominal stoma is much more accessible and requires less dexterity than catheterising the native urethra [121].

In some patients a continent reconstruction may be performed in conjunction with orthopedic procedures. In other patients, the continent stoma provides easier bladder access for the patient's attendants. Finally, a continent stoma provides better self-image than an external appliance, thus further improving quality of life.

The continent conduit is constructed using the appendix or a segment of ileum, although the ureter or fallopian tube has been used occasionally [122]. If the conduit is as narrow as to admit a 14 Ch catheter, it can be implanted in a submucosal tunnel in the bladder or neo-reservoir. The Mitrofanoff procedure uses the appendix [123-125] and the Montie procedure [126-127] uses a short ileal or colonic segment sutured transversally. A narrow continent conduit can also be constructed by tapering the terminal ileum segment if it is combined with a right colon pouch (Indiana etc.). The continence mechanism in this case is the ileocecal reinforced by ileocecal plication [128-130]. Other techniques that have been used in conjunction with ileal reservoirs are the intussuscepted ileal nipple (Kock) [131], or the Benchekroun hydraulic valve [132]. Whichever mechanism is used, continence rates of more than 80% in short term has been reported. Unfortunately complications are relatively frequent, especially with longer tubes and with intussuscepted valves (dessusception, parastomal hernia, fistulae) [133] compared to narrow tube techniques [134]. These small bore-outlets (Mitrofanoff, Yang-Montie) are currently the commonest techniques used. They are however not without their own problems, with stoma stenosis being reported in 12 to 30% of cases. Liard [135] reported on 23 Mitrofanoffs continent with a minimum of 15 years follow-up. Complications that require surgical revision were: stomal stenosis or persistent leakage in 11 cases. Stenosis, particularly at skin level can be simply dilated or a V flap advancement used if necessary. The umbilical site for the stoma is popular and has cosmetic advantages, but may have a higher risk of stenosis [136]. Bladder stones can be treated endoscopically through the conduit or through a percutaneous route [137]. If the urethra is closed, patients should be advised to perform frequent and regular catheterisations and also to perform bladder irrigation through a catheter of minimum size, in order to evacuate the mucus. Metabolic disorders can occur in association with these reservoirs. A 20% rate of hyperchloremia has been reported without significant acidosis (Lockhart 128). Vitamin B12 deficiency and cholelithiasis have been reported but occur very rarely [113] *(LEVEL OF EVIDENCE IV).*

3. Conduit diversion

The indications for conduit (non-continent) supravesical diversion have been reduced significantly since the introduction of appropriate management, such as intermittent catheterisation, in these patients however this procedure may be considered in the case of intractable incontinence in bed bound patients, the devasted lower urinary tract following multiple failed surgery or where the use of long bowel segments for reconstruction is contraindicated (short bowel syndrome), It may also be considered in patients who do not accept the potential complications of a continent diversion, who are not able to perform catheterisation, or where the upper urinary tract is severely compromised. Proper location of the stoma must be determined before surgery by stomatherapist and urologist. This location is especially important in patients who are chair bound or who have specific deformities, such as patients with severe kyphoscoliosis or a small abdomen. The most common technique is to use a short ileal segment with the ureters anastomosed directly end to side. There is no evidence that an antireflux procedure is required and this may in fact increase the risk of implantation stenosis. Patients should be followed up indefinitely as stomal stenosis and or ureteric anastomotic stricture can occur years after surgery. Large bowel segments can be used when patients have a severe renal insufficiency in order to prevent metabolic disorders [138]. In the long term, complications will occur, namely pyelonephritis and calculi. Renal impairment has been estimated to occur in 16.5% to 50% of patients with 10 years or more follow-up [138-140]. *(LEVEL OF EVIDENCE IV)*

4. UNDIVERSION

Conversion from a conduit to a continent diversion or to the reconstructed bladder, may be indicated in few cases. Such patients will usually have been diverted many years ago when the newer technologies described above were not generally available. This will usually be considered in younger patients who have a strong desire to improve their body image by avoiding the use of an external appliance [110, 141, 142]. These young adults must be carefully counselled and must be compliant in following the medical instructions. The conduit can be anastomosed to the reconstructed bladder or to a continent self-cauterised pouch [128]. In some cases it can be anastomosed to the rectum [141-143]. The latter is an internal diversion that requires normal faecal continence and an efficient ureteral antireflux mechanism. It must be remembered that it does expose the patient to a greater risk of renal deterioration than external diversion *(LEVEL OF EVIDENCE IV)*.

C. THE FUTURE BLADDER

1. ESSENTIAL DESIGN CHARACTERISTICS

The need for bladder replacement because of malignancy or voiding dysfunction is a significant clinical problem. Numerous cystectomies and/or diversions are performed worldwide annually as a method of treating these maladies.

If an effective prosthetic bladder were available, it could be used in all of the above patients. It could also be used in a large proportion of the unquantified number of patients who are considered unsuitable for cystectomy and diversion because of unsuitable bowel or infirmity. Many patients who are being treated primarily with radiotherapy for bladder carcinoma might also receive primary surgery if prosthesis were available [144,145]. The proposed advantages of an alloplastic bladder, over methods of bladder substitution, are listed in Table 1. The characteristics required of the ideal prosthetic bladder are outlined in Table 2.

Table 1 : Advantages of prosthetic bladder

* Decreased peri-operative morbidity and mortality due to reduced operating time
* Availability of a device for all patients
* Postoperative complications related to the use of intestine, such as metabolic acidosis, anastomotic leaks, stoma problems, bowel obstruction, polyuria and cancer risk, would be avoided
* Complications related to inherent deficiencies of homologous tissue such as infection, mucous production and effects of prior irradiation would be avoided
* The ability to irradiate the pelvis without risk to the urinary reservoir.

Table 2 : Characteristics of an ideal prosthetic bladder

* Preservation of renal function
* Continent collection and adequate storage of urine
* Voluntary voiding without residual
* Easy to construct, insert and repair
* Biocompatible and does not degrade or shrink with time
* Does not interfere with the function or other organs.

2. DEVELOPING A PROSTHETIC BLADDER

The bladder has a number of complex features which are different to recreate, so much research is needed to develop a prosthetic bladder which can effectively substitute for these functions. The rate of progress in developing such a prosthesis will depend on

the interest of urological surgeons in the subject and on the amount of energy and enthusiasm with which the idea is promoted to the biomedical industry and healthcare providers. The degree of interest shown by the biomedical industry will also depend on the future need for a prosthesis, which is directly related to the potential bladder augmentation and cystectomy rates. In the recent past, there have not been any dramatic changes in the indications for these procedures. There has been some movement away from radiotherapy as first-line curative treatment in those countries where it is used, so a rise in cystectomy rates may well follow this trend particularly for patients with localized tumours. If effective chemotherapy is found for the treatment of transitional cell carcinoma, the number of patients who require cystectomy may well be reduced. On the other hand, chemotherapy could also make some patients, who are now thought to be inoperable because of locally extensive cancers, suitable for cystectomy by reducing the tumour mass to a resectable size. Patients with impaired renal function, who are not suitable for ileal conduits or bladder substitution with bowel and may be denied a cystectomy, would benefit from the availability of a prosthesis. Increasing numbers of patients are having intestinal augmentation or substitution of the bladder for functional disorders of the bladder. These patients would also benefit from an effective prosthesis. The numbers requiring such treatment for functional disorders will probably decrease again in the future as advances are made in electrostimulation of the pelvic nerves [146,147].

3. Protection of renal function

One of the primary objectives of a prosthetic bladder is to preserve renal function. In future work, this function will have to be studied more carefully than it has been in the past. Development of hydronephrosis on an intravenous urogram is not a sensitive enough method of following changes in renal function [148-156]. Monitoring changes in serum creatinine is also too vague to be of value in assessment of changes in the function of a prosthesis as it is delayed reaction and does not clearly identify what deficiencies in a design model are interfering with renal function. Direct measurement of renal function is required. Similarly, awaiting the development of complete obstruction or the results of postmortem examination of the specimens are not acceptable modes of determining how well a prosthesis is functioning [148-156]. Future models will have to incorporate in their structure, methods for recurrent, or preferably continuous, monitoring of pressure [157,158] urine flow rates and even urine constituents. Ideally, these should take the form of telemetric monitoring to avoid any external leads or connectors. These features will be essential, in future prototype bladders, so that definitive data can be collected on the effects of alterations in flow rates and pressures on renal function rather than depending on the intuitive approach used to date. In reality, most of the pressure and flow work can be done by bench studies in the laboratory.

The main cause of renal failure in most prosthetic bladder studies, when luminal occlusion and leakage are excluded, has been adynamic obstruction due to the large mass of fluid sitting in a passive prosthesis against which the kidney and native ureter have been expected to excrete more urine. If renal function is to be protected, some method of ensuring that urine drains into the bladder without either occlusive or non-occlusive resistance will have to be included in future prosthetic designs. This can be ensured by having a negative pressure draw the urine down, as in the Mayo [151,158, 159] and Aachen [148] models, or a positive-pressure mechanism which pumps urine down the ureter into the bladder. The latter would probably be more difficult to achieve as it would require continuous movement in the pumping mechanism and thus be more prone to mechanical failure. It would also require a continuous source of energy while the negative-pressure principle only requires a pumping action during bladder emptying and then the energy is stored, e.g. in a compressed spring, for use during the filling phase. A spring mechanism could conceivably be used to provide continuous energy, as used in clockwork mechanisms. Transcutaneous magnetic energy coupling is a mechanism which enables electrical power to be induced intracorporeally, with the use of magnets, without the need for internal batteries or percutaneous wires. It could be used to provide energy to create continuous positive or negative pressures but this would mean that the patient would have to wear a sizable battery pack continuously. Transcorporeal energy coupling would be very useful when an intermittent energy source is needed, such as during bladder emptying.

4. Filling, voiding and continence with the prosthetic bladder

From the research that has been done to date, there appears to be two directions for creating the actual structure of the artificial bladder. The first is to have a rigid outer shell which protects the bladder from any external compressive forces. A mechanism which allows outflow of urine during emptying is also necessary. In the Mayo bladder, this takes the form of a 300 ml reservoir but with modifications to the model this could be reduced to 20 ml. These rigid bladders will be placed in an extraperitoneal position, either subcutaneously or subfascially, to avoid the problem of fibrous capsule formation, bowel adhesion and ascites. A pump mechanism will be necessary to evacuate urine. This pump could be manually operated or be driven by a transcutaneous magnetic coupling device. The second approach, to the replacement of the storage and evacuation functions of the bladder, is to design a prosthesis with a semi-rigid shell. It would have to be stiff enough to resist the compressive forces of body tissues, and would have to be placed subcutaneously so that it could be emptied by manual compression. This is a simpler design concept but it would require a significant design effort to find an effective model which would be cosmetically acceptable and would have the capacity to manage urine production rates in the human. The surface of either design should be roughened to reduce the degree of tissue reaction. It would even be better to cover the shell with a bonded ingrowth material such as Dacron or Proplast to reduce movement and tissue reaction [148, 149, 155].

Advances in material research may allow a swing back from the rigid bladders to the collapsible bag idea. This system could possibly work if formation of a fibrous capsule around the bladder, which prevents its expansion, could be avoided. To do this, the surface which would be in contact with the intra-abdominal contents would have to be made from , or coated in, a material which would not induce an inflammatory reaction in the surrounding tissues. Hydrogels go some of the way to fulfilling this function, as they provide a moist lubricated surface, but further advances are still necessary. Ideally, this material should also allow gradual ingrowth of peritoneum without fibrosis enabling the prosthesis to be isolated from future intra-abdominal problems. The surface of the collapsible bladder, in contact with the back of the abdominal wall and the raw area are left after cystectomy, would be covered with an ingrowth material. It would be essential that adhesions could not form between this coating and bowel. Dense fixation of the bladder would reduce mobility and lessen tissue irritation. It if could be made to work effectively, the collapsible bladder would be the simplest, and thus most reliable, prosthesis available.

Mechanical reliability is an essential requirement for many prosthesis. This has been a problem with all bladder prostheses particularly the more complex designs [149, 157, 158]. This has nearly always been due to failure of the parts of the prosthesis and not to the implantation itself. Any future designs should be extensively bench tested before any in vivo studies are performed. Reliability of the parts and completed models should be ensured, before considering implantation, by extensive repeated testing on the bench under much wider ranges of pressures, fluid flow, moisture and temperature than could ever be experienced within the body. Short-term in vivo studies, of a few weeks, provide little added information over bench work because any functioning, non-infected prosthesis will have minimal negative effects on the laboratory animal and, conversely, the laboratory animal's system will not develop the reactions which can damage or interfere with the functioning of the prosthesis. The methods of preventing early failure of a prosthesis because of leakage or obstruction have been identified and do not need to be rediscovered. Thus, only long term in vivo studies should be required from now on.

Future models will have to provide excellent continence. This could be done by providing some feedback so that the patient can tell when the bladder is near to capacity rather than having to wait for the first few drops of overflow before he/she knows that the bladder is full. Sensors could monitor the volume or the pressure in the bladder. The patient could be alerted by an auditory signal, or by a mild subcutaneous electrical current. If, in future models, a satisfactory anastomosis can be made directly to the urethral sphincter, then the patient could be warned by a signal directed to the sphincter area giving the patient a natural feeling of having to pass urine. The external sphincter would then be relaxed voluntarily. If the neural control of the sphincter were damaged then the electrical signal could be used to actively control the sphincter.

While intraluminal access, through a stoma or subcutaneous injection port, would have the benefits of being able to monitor pressures directly, to perform contrast studies, and allow cleaning of the prosthesis, the risks of infection are too great to allow this feature to be included in future bladders. Further advances are needed in material research to find a substance which has the ability to prevent infection on a long-term basis.

The urethra will, however, always be the weak point of any alloplastic bladder because it is a connection to the outside world which provides a point of entry for infection. The urethra, although only a small part, is probably the area on which most future research and development will have to be performed if a viable prosthesis is to become a reality.

If development of an effective prosthesis is to advance the desire for short-term gain, an early publication of results must be resisted and long-term research and investment must be instituted.

RECOMMENDATIONS OF THE COMMITTEE

As with all surgery on the urinary tract, certain principals must be adhered to in establishing the appropriateness of any procedure. These are: 1) preservation of renal function and 2) control of incontinence. In addition, for patients with neuropathic bladder, other issues need to be considered, namely:1) social circumstances, 2) degree of disability, 3) cost effectiveness, 4) technical difficulty and 5) complications.

Surgical treatment for the neuropathic patient is actually focused to enhance detrusor contractility, to decrease outlet resistance, to decrease detrusor contractility, to increase sphincteric resistance or to circumvent the bladder.

A. Surgery to enhance detrusor contractility

Sacral anterior root stimulation combined with sacral posterior rhizotomy is a valuable method to restore bladder function in selected spinal cord injury patients suffering from hyperreflexia refractory to medical therapy *(LEVEL OF EVIDENCE IV).*

B. Surgery to decrease outlet resistance

Transurethral incision of the external sphincter is a reasonable option to adequately drain the bladder and prevent urologic complications in the spinal cord injury male patients *(LEVEL OF EVIDENCE IV)*. Intraurethral stents are showing promise as shown in prospective randomised clinical trials *(LEVEL OF EVIDENCE II)*.

C. Surgery to decrease detrusor contractility

Although there is a lack on prospective randomised studies, enterocystoplasty has passed the test of time in order to achieve a low pressure reservoir *(LEVEL OF EVIDENCE IV)*. As alternatives to this procedure it has been proposed the autoaugmentation and the injection of Botulinum-A toxin at the detrusor level *(LEVEL OF EVIDENCE IV)*.

D. Surgery to increase sphincteric resistance

Although there is a high revision rate Artificial urinary sphincter implantation remains a good option for the treatment of sphincteric incompetence in selected cases *(LEVEL OF EVIDENCE IV)*. In spite of a lack of long-term follow-up, sling procedures are an alternative to the artificial urinary sphincter implantation *(LEVEL OF EVIDENCE IV)*.

Resorbable or non-resorbable bulking agents might play some role in the treatment of neurogenic urinary incontinence *(LEVEL OF EVIDENCE IV)*.

E. Surgery to circumvent the bladder

Although less frequently used, after failure of more conservative treatment in patients with neurogenic bladder, continent or non continent urinary diversion represents an acceptable treatment for selected cases of neurogenic voiding dysfunction patients *(LEVEL OF EVIDENCE IV)*.

REFERENCES

1. Mersdorf , A. , Schmidt, R., Tanagho E.A.: Topographic-anatomical basis of sacral neurostimulation:neuroanatomical variations. J.Urol 149:345-349, 1993.
2. Rijkhoff, N.J.M., Wijkstra, H., Van Kerrebroeck, P, Debruyne, F. Selective detrusor activation by electrical sacral nerve root stimulation in spinal cord injury. J Urol (1997) 157:1504-1508
3. Kaplan, W.E. and Richards I. Intravesical transurethral electrotherapy for the neurogenic bladder. J. Urol 136,243-246, 1988
4. Brindley,G.S., Craggs,M.D.: A technique for anodally blocking large nerve fibres through chronically implanted electrodes. J. Neurol Neursurg Psychiatry.43:1083-1090.1980.
5. Creasey, G.H. Electrical stimulation of sacral roots for micturition after spinal cord injury.Urological Clinics of North America vol 20, 3:505-515, 1993
6. Rijkhoff, N,, Wijkstra, H., Van Kerrebroeck, P., Debruyne, F.. Selective detrusor activation by sacral ventral nerve-root stimulation: results of intraoperative testing in humans during implantation of a Finetech-Brindley system.World J Urol16:337-341, 1998.
7. Egon, G., Barat, M., Colombel,.P., Visentin, C., Isambert, J., Guerin, J.. Implantation of anterior sacral root stimulation combined with posterior sacral rhizotomy in spinal cord injury patients. World J Urol 16:342-349, 1998.
8. Schurch, B., Rodic, B, Jeanmond D. Posterior sacral rhizotomy and intradural sacral root stimulation for treatment of the spastic bladder in spinal cord injury patients. J. Urol, 157,2:610-614, 1997.
9. Stieglitz , T., Schumacher , S., Seif, C., Bross, S., Junemann, K.P., Meyer , J.U. Selective activation of the bladder with quasi-trapezoidal pulses in sacral anterior root stimulation in the dog. Biomed. Tech (Berl):42, Suppl: 492-493. 1997.
10. Schumacher, S. Bross, S. Scheepe, J.R., Seif, C., Junemann K.P. and Alken, P. Extradural cold block for selective neurostimulation of the bladder:development of a new technique. J. Urol: 161:950-954, 1999.
11. V.Heyden B, Anthony P, Kaula N, Brock GB, Jakse G, Tanagho Ea: The Latissimus dorsi muscle for the detrusor assistance:functional recovery after nerve division and repair.J.Urol 151:1081-1087, 1994
12. Stenzl A., Ninkovic M, Willeit J, Hess M, Feichtinger H, Schwabegger, Colleselli K, Pavelka M, Anderl H and Bartsch G. Free neurovascular transfer of latissimus dorsi muscle to the bladder. I. Experimental studies. J. Urol 157, 1103-1108, 1997.
13. Von Heyden B, Anthony JP,Brock GB, Kaula N, Tanagho EA. The latissimus dorsi bladder myoplasty to assist detrusor function. Urol Res, 26(3);215-212, 1998
14. Van Savage JG, Perez.-Badia GP, Palanca LG, Bardoel JW, Harralson T, Slaughenhpout BL, PalacioMM,Tobin GR,Maldonado C and Barker JH. Electricaly stimulated detrusor myoplasty .J. Urol 164,969-972, 2000.
15. Stenz A, Ninkovic M, Kolle D, Knapp R, Anderl H, Bartsch G.Restoration of voluntary emptying of the bladder by transplantation of innervated free skeletal muscle. Lancet 16,351:1483-1485, 1998
16. Stenzl A. Ninkovic M, Hannes S, Radmayr C and Bartsch G. Latissimus dorsi detrusor myoplpasty (LDDM) and autoaugmentation for the treatment of congenital neurogenic bladder dysfunction. Eur Urol, 37, S2,157, 2000.
17. Barton, CH, Khonsari, F, Vaziri, ND, Byrne, C, Gordon, S, Friis, R.: The effect of modified transurethral sphincterotomyon autonomic dysreflexia. J. Urol. Jan; 135 (1) : 83-5, 1986.

18. Perkash, I.: Autonomic dysreflexia and detrusor-sphincter dyssynergia in spinal cord injury patients. J. Spinal Cord Med. Jul;20(3):365-70, 1997.

19. Perkash, I. and Friedland, GW.: Ultrasonographic detection of false passages arising from the posterior urethra in spinal cord injury patients. J. Urol. 137:701-702, April, 1987.

20. Perkash, I. and Friedland, GW.: Posterior ledge at the bladder neck: the crucial diagnostic role of ultrasonography, Urol. Rad., 8:175, 1986.

21. Wein, AJ, Raezer, DM, Benson, GS: Management of Neurogenic Bladder Dysfunction in the Adult. Urology 1976;8:432.

22. Madersbacher, H., Scott, FB: Twelve o'clock sphincterotomy. Urol. Int. 30:75, 1975.

23. Juma, S, Mostafavi, M, Joseph, A.: Sphincterotomy: long-term complications and warning signs. Neurourol. Urodyn. 14 (1):33-41, 1995.

24. Noll, F, Sauerwein, D, Stohrer, M.: Transurethral sphincterotomy in quadriplegic patients: long-term-follow-up. Neurourol. Urodyn., 14(4):351-8, 1995.

25. Perkash, I.: Contact laser sphincterotomy: further experience and longer follow-up. Spinal Cord, Apr;34 (4) : 227-33, 1996.

26. Kim, YH, Kattan, MW, Boone, TB.: Bladder leak point pressure: the measure for sphincterotomy success in spinal cord injured patients with external detrusor-sphincter dyssynergia. J. Urol. Feb;159(2):493-6;discussion 496-7, 1998. Review.

27. Perkash, I, Kabalin, JN, Lennon, S, Wolfe, V.: Use of penile prostheses to maintain external condom catheter drainage in spinal cord injury patients. Paraplegia, May; 30(5):327-32, 1992.

28. Rossier, AB, Fam, BA: Indication and results of semirigid penile prostheses in spinal cord injury patients: long-term followup. J. Urol. 131:59-62, 1984.

29. Petit, H, Wiart, L., Gaujard, E., Le Breton, F., Ferriere, JM, Lagueny, A., Joseph, PA, Barat, M.: Botulinum-A toxin treatment for detrusor-sphincter dyssynergia in spinal cord disease. Spinal Cord 36(2):91-4, Feb. 1998.

30. Schurch, B, Hauri, D, Rodic, B, Curt, A, Meyer, M, Rossier, AB.: Botulinum-A toxin as a treatment of detrusor-sphincter dyssynergia: A prospective study in 24 spinal cod injury patients. J. Urol. 155:1023-1029, 1996.

31. Chancellor ; N;Bennett C;Simoneau AR; Finocchiaro MV;Kline C; Bennet JK;Foote JE;Green BG; Mafrtin SH;Killoran RW;Crewalk JA;Rivas DA. Sphincteric stent versus external sphincterotomy in spinal cord injured men:prospective randomized multicenter trial. J. Urol 161 (6);1893-8,1999.

32. Chancellor MB; Gajewski JB;Ackman CF;Appell RA;Bennett J;Binard J;Boone TB;Chetner MP;Crewalk JA;Defalco A;Foote J;Green B; Juma SY;Linsenmeyer TA; Macmillan R; Mayo M; Ozawa H;Roehnborn CG; Shenot PJ; Stone A; Vazquez A;Killorin W; Rivas DA. Long-term followup of the North American muticenter UroLume trial for the treatment of external detrusor-sphincter dyssynergia-.J. Urol 161 (5):1545-50,1999.

33. Low AI; McRae PJ. Use of the Memokath for detrusor-sphincter dyssynergia after spinal cord injury -cautionary tale. Spinal Cord ;36(1):39-44,1998.

34. Chartier-Kastler EJ ; Thomas L; Bussel B; Chancellor MB; Richard F; Denys P. A urethral stent for the treatment of detrusor-striated sphincter dyssynergia. BJU Int: 86(1)52-57,2000.

35. Juan García FJ; Salvador S;Montoto A;Lion S; Balvis B;Rodríguez A; Fernández M;Sánchez J. Intraurethral stent prostheses in spinal cord injured patients with sphincter dyssynergia. Spinal Cord : 37(1):54-7,1999.

36. Corujo M;Badlani GH. Uncommon complications of permanent stents. J. Endourol: 12(4):385-8,1998.

37. Chalfin SA, Bradley WE., The etiology of detrusor hyperreflexia in patients with infravesical obstruction. J. Urol.: 127(5):938-42,1982.

38. Madersbacher H. The various types of neurogenic bladder dysfunction: an update of current therapeutic concepts. Paraplegia :28(4):217-29,1990.

39. Stohrer M. Alterations in the lower urinary tract after spinal cord injury--diagnosis, prevention and therapy of late sequelae. World J. of Urology : 7: 205-211.1990.

40. Cardenas DD, Mayo ME, Turner LR. Lower urinary changes over time in suprasacral spinal cord injury. Paraplegia 33: 326-329,1995.

41. Goldstein I, Siroky MB, Sax DS, Krane Neurourologic abnormalities in multiple sclerosis. J Urol. : 128(3):541-545,1982.

42. Siroky MB, Krane RJ. Neurologic aspects of detrusor-sphincter dyssynergia, with reference to the guarding reflex. J Urol. : 127(5):953-7,1982.

43. Nordling J, Meyhoff HH, Hald T. Neuromuscular dysfunction of the lower urinary tract with special reference to the influence of the sympathetic nervous system. Scand J Urol Nephrol.:15(1):7-19,1981.

44. Stone AR, Rentzepis M. Augmentation cystoplasty In O"Donnell PD, Urinary Incontinence Mosby - Year Book, Inc.,1997Chapter 51 375-383.

45. Madersbacher H. The various types of neurogenic bladder: an update of current therapeutic concepts. Paraplegia : 28: 217-229,1990

46. Hasan ST, Marshall C, Robson WA, Neal DE. Clinical outcome and quality of life following enterocystoplasty for idiopathic detrusor instability and neurogenic bladder dysfunction. Br J Urol. 76(5):551-7.1995.

47. Mast P, Hoebeke P, Wyndaele JJ, Oosterlinck W, Everaert K.Experience with augmentation cystoplasty. A review. Paraplegia.: 33(10):560-4. 1995.

48. Khoury JM, Webster GD. Evaluation of augmentation cystoplasty for severe neuropathic bladder using the hostility score. Dev Med Child Neurol.:34(5):441-7,1992.

49. Radomski SB, Herschorn S, Stone AR, Urodynamic comparison of ileum v. sigmoid in augmentation cystoplasty for neurogenic bladder dysfunction. Neurourol. Urodyn;14:231-237,1995.

50. Freedman ER, Singh G, Donnell SC, Rickwood AM, Thomas DG. Combined bladder neck suspension and

augmentation cystoplasty for neuropathic incontinence in female patients.Br J Urol.: 73(6):621-4,1994.

51. McInerney PD, DeSouza N, Thomas PJ, Mundy AR.The role of urodynamic studies in the evaluation of patients with augmentation cystoplasties. Br J Urol.:76(4):475-8,1995.

52. Cartwright PC, Snow BW: Bladder auto-augmentation: early clinical experience. J Urol 142: 505-508,1989

53. Cartwright PC, Snow BW: Bladder auto-augmentation: partial detrusor excision to augment the bladder without the use of bowel. J Urol : 142: 1050-1053,1989..

54. Stöhrer M, Kramer A, Goepel M, Löchner-Ernst D, Kruse D, Rübben H: Bladder auto-augmentation — an alternative for enterocystoplasty: preliminary results. Neurourol Urodyn : 14: 11-23, 1995..

55. Stöhrer M, Kramer G, Goepel M, Rübben H. Excision of detrusor muscle in patients with neurogenic bladder disease. In: McGuire EJ, Bloom D, Catalano WJ, Lipshultz LI (eds) Advances in Urology. Chicago: Mosby, 1997: 191-217.

56. Kennelly MJ, Gormley EA, McGuire EJ: Early clinical experience with adult bladder auto-augmentation. J Urol 152: 303-306,1994.

57. Stöhrer M, Kramer G, Goepel M, Löchner-Ernst D, Kruse D, Rübben H. Bladder autoaugmentation in adult patients with neurogenic voiding dysfunction. Spinal Cord :35: 456-462,1997.

58. Stöhrer M, Goepel M, Kramer G, Löchner-Ernst D, Rübben H. Die Detrusormyektomie (Autoaugmentation) in der Behandlung der hyperreflexiven Low-compliance Blase. Urologe A: 38: 30-37,1999.

59. Hohenffellner, M., Dahms, S.E.,.Matzel, K. and Thüroff J.W.. Sacral neuromodulation for treatment of lower urinary tract dysfunction. BJU International:85,Supp 3,10-19,2000.

60. Chartier-Kastler, E.J., Bosch, R., Perrigot ,M., Chancellor, M.B., Richard, F. and Denis P. Long-term results os sacral nerve stimulation (S3) for the treament of neurogenic refractory urge incontinence related to detrusor hyperreflexia. J. Urol.:164,1476-1480,2000.

61. Chartier-Kastler, Denis, P., Chancellor, M.B., Haerting, A., Bussel, B. and Richard, F. Urodynamic monitoring during percutaneous sacral nerve neurostimulation in patients with neurogenic detrusor hyperreflexia. Neurourology and Urodynamics 20:6170, 2001.

62. Schurch B, Schmid DM, Stohrer M. Treatment of neurogenic incontinence with botulinum toxin A. N Engl J Med.; 342: 665.2000.

63. Schurch B, Stöhrer M, Kramer G, Schmid DM, Gaul G, Hauri D. Botulinum A-toxin for treating detrusor hyperreflexia in spinal cord injured patients: A new alternative to anticholinergic drugs? Preliminary results. J Urol : 164: 692-697.2000.

64. Stöhrer M, Schurch B, Kramer G, Schmid DM, Gaul G, Grosse J, Hauri D. Detrusor injections of botulinum A-toxin for detrusor hyperreflexia. BJU Int : 86 Suppl. 3: 134.2000.

65. Stöhrer M, Schurch B, Kramer G, Schmid DM, Gaul G, Hauri D. Botulinum A-toxin detrusor injections in the treatment of detrusor hyperreflexia. J Urol : 163 Suppl.: 244.2000.

66. Stöhrer M, Schurch B, Kramer G, Schmid D, Gaul G, Hauri D. Botulinum-A toxin in the treatment of detrusor hyperreflexia in spinal cord injury: A new alternative to medical and surgical procedures? Neurourol Urodyn : 18, 401-402,1999..

67. Light K, Scott FB.. Use of the artificial urinary sphincter in spinal cord injury patients. J. Urol: 130: 1127. 1983.

68. Aprikan A; Berardinucci G; Pikr J; Kiruluta G. Experience with the AS-8OO artificial urinary sphincter in myelodysplastic children. Can J. Surg.: 35 (4):396.1992.

69. Fulford S.C.V., Sutton C., Bales G; Hickling M and Stephenson TP. The fate of the modern artificial urinary sphincter with a follow-up more than 10 years. Br. J. Urol.: 79:7 13,1997.

70. Levesque PE; Bauer SB; Atala A; Zurakowski D; Colodny A;Peters C and Retik AB; Ten-year experience with the artificial urinary sphincter in children. J. Urol; 156:625.1996.

71. Belloli G; Campobasso P; Mercurella A. Neuropatic urinary incontinence in pediatric patients: management with artificial urinary sphincter. J. Ped. Surg:27(11): 1461. 1992.

72. Barret DM; Parulkar BG. The artificial sphincter (AS 800). Experience in children and young adults. Urol Clin North Am; 16(1):1 19,1989.

73. Mouriquand PG, Mollard P. Management of urinary incontinence in neurogenic bladder. Scand Jurol Neph: Suppl 14 1:28, 1993..

74. Singh G and Thomas DG. Artificial urinary sphincter in patients with neurogenic bladder dysfunction. Br. J. Urol.: 77:252,1996.

75. Gonzalez R; Merino F.C. and Vaughn M.. Long term results of the artificial urinary sphincter in mate patients with neurogenic bladder. J. Urol , 154:769, 1995.

76. Jacobsen H and Hald T. Management of neurogenic urinary incontinence with AMS artificial urinary sphincter. Scand J Urol Nephrol : 20 (2):137,1986.

77. Elliot DS and Barret DM. Mayo Clinic Long term analysis of the functional durability of the AMS 800 Artificial Urinary sphincter. A review of 323 cases. J. Urol. : 159:1206,1998.

78. Venn SN; Greenwell TJ and Mundy AR. The long-term outcome of artificial urinary sphincters. J. Urol:164.702-707,2000.

79. Light JK; Lapin S and Vohra S. Combined use of bowel and the artificial urinary sphincter in reconstruction of the lower urinary tract: infectious complications. J. Urol. :153:331, 1995.

80. Light K and Pietro T. Alteration in detrusor behavior and the effect on renal function following insertion of the artificial urinary sphincter. J. Urol.; 336:632,1986.

81. Janknegt RA, Baeten CG, Weil EH and Spaans F: Electrically stimulated gracilis sphincter for treatment of bladder sphincter incontinence. Lancet. : 340: 1129, 1992.

82. Janknegt R.A., Heesakkers JPFA; Weil EH and Baeten CG. Electrically stimulated gracilis sphincter (dynamic graciloplasty) for treatment of intryinsic sphincter deficiency: a pilot study on feasibylity and side effects. J. Urol.: 154:1830, 1995.

83. Chancellor MB; Watanabe T; Rivas DA; Hong RD; Kumon H;Ozawa and Burgeois I. Gracilis urethral myoplasty: preliminary experience using an autoiogous urinary sphincter for post-prostatectomy incontinence. J. Urol. : 158:1372,1997.

84. Chancellor MB; Rivas DA; Shenot PJ; Crewalk JA;Figueroa E. Gracilis urethromyoplasty. The creation of new autologous urinary sphincter in neurologically impaired patients. J. Urol.:155 (Suppl) 591:A1:307, 1996.

85. McGuire EJ; Wang C; Usistalo H; Savastano J, Modified pubovaginal sling in gilrs with myelodysplasia. J.. Urol:135:94, 1986.

86. Gomley EA ; Bloom DA ; McGuire EJ; Ritchey MI.. Pubovaginal slings for the management of urnary incontinence in female adolesteces. J.. Urol.:152:822,1994

87. Raz S; Ehrlich RM; Zeidman EJ;Alarcon A and McLaughlin S. Surgical treatment of the incontyinent female patient with myelomeningocele. J. Urol : 139:524,1988.

88. Walker RD; Flack CE; Hawkins-Lee R;Lim DJ; Parramore H and Hackett RL. Rectus fascial wrap: early results of a modification of the rectus fascial sling. J. Urol.: 154:771-4, 1995.

89. Kakizaki H; Shibata T; Shino Y; Kobayasshi S; Matsumura K; Koyanagi T. Fascial sling for the management of urinary incontinence due to sphincter incompetence. J. Urol : 153: 644.1995.

90. Herschorn S; Radomski SB. Fascial sling and bladder neck tapering in the treatment of male neurogenic incontinence. J. Urol.:147(4):1073-5, 1992.

91. Kryger JV; Gonzalez R and Barthold JS. Surgical management of Urinary incontinence in children with neurogenic sphincteric incompetence. J. Urol.:163(1):256-63, 2000.

92. Austin PF; Westney OL;Wendy WL; McGuire EJ; Ritchey ML. Advantages of rectus fascial slings for urinary incontinence in children with neuropathic bladders. J. Urol :165:2369-2372, 2001.

93. Walker RD; Erhard M; Starling J. Longterm evaluation of rectus fascial wrap in patients with spina bifida. J. Urol. : 164:485-486,2000.

94. Clemens JQ; Bushman W; Shaeffer AJ; Golomb J; Madersbacher S. Urodynamic analysis of the bulbourethral sling procedure. J. Urol :162;1977-1985, 1999.

95. Kim YH; Katan M; Boone TB. Correlation of urodynamic results and urethral coaptation with success after transurethral collagen injection. Urology, 50, 941.1997.

96. Sundaram CP; Reiberg Y; Aliabadi HA. Failure to obtain durable results with collagen implantation in children with urinary incontinence. J.Urol. :157, 6, 2306,1997.

97. Silveri, M; Capitanicci M; Mosiello G; Endoscopic treatment for urinary incontinence in children with a congenital neuropathic bladder. Br. J. Urol. 82:694,1998.

98. Chernoff A, Horowitz M; Combs A. Periurethral collagen injection for the treatment of urinary incontinence in children. J. Urol. 157,157:2303, 1997.

99. Kassouf W; Capolicchio G; Berardinucci G;Corcos J. Collagen injection for the treatment of urinary incontinence in children. J. Urol.:165:1666-1668,2001.

100. Guys JM;Fakhro A; Louis-Borrione C; Prost J; Hautier A. Endoscopic treatment of urinary incontinence: longterm evaluation of the results. J. Urol :165:2389-2391,2001.

101. Nielsen K; Kromann-Andersen B;Jacobsen H. The urethral plug: a new treatment modality for genuine stress incontinence in women. J. Urol.;144:l,199, 1990.

102. Staskin D ;Sant G ; Rappaport S et all. One year experience with an expandable urinary control insert: multicenter clinical update. J.. Urol.: 155 (Suppl) 638-.A, 1996

103. Natif O; Moskowitz B; Condrea A; Halachami S; Burbura J; Madjar S and Beyar M.: A new intraurethral sphincter prosthesis with a self contained urinary pump. ASAIO-J: 43, 3, 197,1997.

104. Schurch B; Suter S; Dubs M. Intraurethral prostheses to treat hyporeflexic bladders in women:does it work?. BJU Int : 84(7):789-94,1999.

105. Sand PK; Staskin D; Miller J; Diokno A; Sant GR; Davila GW; Knapp P; Rappaport S; Tutrone R, Int Urogynecol J Pelvic Floor Dysfunction : 10(2):100-105,1999.

106. Madjar S; Sabo E; Halachmi S; Wald M; Issaq E; Moskovitz B; Beyar M, Nativ O. A remote controlled intraurethral insert for artificial voiding:a new concept for treating women with voiding dysfunction. J. Urol :161 (3);895-898, 1999.

107. Pannek J; Muller M; Haupt G. An unexpected complication of the remote-controlled intraurethral valve pump for urinary incontinence. Urol Int.: 61(4):235-236, 1998,

108. Chartier-Kastler EJ, Mongiat-Artus P, Bitker MO, Chancellor MB, Richard F, Denys P. Long-term results of augmentation cystoplasty in spinal cord injury patients. Spinal Cord:38:490-494,2000.

109. Woodhouse C.R. Reconstruction of the lower urinary tract for neurogenic bladder. Lessons from adolescent age group. Brit J Urol:69:589-593,1992.

110. Stein R., Fisch M., Ermert A., Schwarz M., Black P., Filipas D., Hohenfellner R. Urinary diversion and orthotopic bladder substitution in children and young adults with neurogenic bladder: a safe option for treatment? J Urol:163: 568-573,2000.

111. Fontaine E., Bendaya S., Desert J.F., Fakacs C., LeMouel M.A., Beurton D. Combined modified rectus fascial sling and augmentation ileoplasty for neurogenic incontinence in women. J Urol :157:109-112,1997.

112. Gonzales R., Merino F.G., Avughn M. Long-term results of the artificial urinary sphincter in male patients with neurogenic bladders. J Urol :154:769, 1995.

113. Steiner M.S., Morton R.A. Nutritional and gastrointestinal complications of the use of bowel segments in the lower urinary tract.Urol Clin North Am :18,4:743-752,1991.

114. Studer U.E., Gerber E., Springer J., Zing E.J. Bladder

reconstruction with bowel after radical cystectomy. World J Urol : 10:11-19,1992.

115. Nurse D.E., Mundy A.R. Metabolic complications of cystoplasty. Brit J Urol:63:165-170,1989,

116. Barroso U., Jednack R., Fleming P. Bladder calculi in children who perform clean intermittent catheterisation. Birt J Urol Int :148:575,2000.

117. Treiger BFG, Marshall FF. Carcinogenesis and the use of intestinal segments in the urinary tract. Urol Clin North Am :18:737-742,1991.

118. Mollard P. Long-term results of incontinence surgery in neuropathic bladder. In Long-term outcome in padiatric surgery and urology. Ed M. Stringer, K. Oldham, E. Howard. London: W.B.Saunders, 1998

119. Guys J.M., Simeoni-Alias J., Fakhro A. Use of polydimethylsiloxane for endoscopic treatment of neurogenic urinary incontinence in children. J Urol : 162: 2133, 1999.

120. Kaefer M., Retik A. B. The Mitofanoff principle in continent urinary reconstruction. Urol Clin North Am: 24: 795,1997.

121. Moreno J.G., Chancellor M.B., Karasick S., King S., Abdill C., Rivas D. Improved quality of life and sexuality with continent urinary diversion in quadriplegic women with umbilical stoma. Arch Phys Med Rehabil: 76:758-762,1995.

122. DuckettJ.W., Lofti A.H. Appendicovesicostomy (and variations) in bladder reconstruction J Urol :149 :567-569,1993.

123. Mitrofanoff P. Cystostomie continente transappendiculaire dans le traitement des vessies neurologiques Chir Pediatr :21:297-305, 1980.

124. Sylora JA, Gonzales R, Vaughn R, ReinbergY. Intermittent sef-cathterisation by quadriplegic patients via catherizable Mitrofanoff channel. J Urol :157:48-50,1997.

125. Cain M.P., Casale A.J., King S.J.,Rink R.C. Appendicovesicostomy and newer alternatives for the Mitrofanoff procedure: results in the last 100 patients at Riley Children's Hospital. J Urol:162:1749-1752,1999.

126. Monti PR., Lara RC, Dutra MA, Rezende de Carvalho J. New technique for construction of efferent conduits based on the Mitrofanoff principles. Urology :49 :112-115,1997.

127. Atan A., Konety B.R., Nangia A, Chancellor M.B.Advantages and risks of ileovesicostomy for the proper management of neuropathic bladder. Urology.: 54(4):636-640, 1999.

128. Lockhart JL, Pow-Sang J, Persky L, Kahn P, Helal M, Sanford E. A continent colonic urinary reservoir: the Florida pouch. J Urol :144:864-867,1990.

129. Plancke HR, Delaere KP, Pons C. Indiana pouch in female patients with spinal cord injury. Spinal Cord:37 (3):208-210,1999.

130. Goldwasser B., Ben-Chaim J., Golomb J., Leibovitch I., Mor Y., Avigad I. Bladder neck closure with an Indiana stoma outlet as a technique for continent vesicostomy. Surg Gynecol Obstet :177:448-450, 1993.

131. Skinner DG. Intussuscepted ileal niple valve-development and present status. In Colleen S, Manson W (eds) Proceedings of Continent Urinary Reconstruction. First International Meeting. Scand J Urol Nephrol : 142 (suppl) : 63-65,1992.

132. Benchekroun A., Essakalli N, Faif M., Marzouk M., Hachimi M., Abbakka T. Continent urostomy with hydraulic ileal valve in 136 patients: 13 years of experience J. Urol:142:46-51, 1989.

133. Arai Y., Kawakita M., Terachi T., Oishi K., Okada Y., Takeuchi H. Long-term follow up of the Kock and Indiana procedures J Urol :150:51-55, 1993.

134. Helal M., Austin P., Spyropoulos E., Pow-sang J., Persky L., Lockhart J. Evaluation and management of parastomial hernia in association with continent urinary diversion J Urol:157 :1630-1632, 1997.

135. Liard A., Seguier-Liepszyc E., Mathiot A., Mitrofanoff P. The Mitrofanoff procedure: 20 years later. J Urol: 165: 2394-2398,2001.

136. Van Savage J., Khoury A., Mac Lorie G. Outcome analysis of Mitrofanoff principle applications using the appendix and ureter to umbilical and lower quadrant stomal sites. J Urol:156:1794-1797,1996.

137. Roth S., Van Halen H., Semjonow A. Percutaneous pouch lithotripsy in continent conduit diversions with narrowed Mitrofanoff conduit. Brit J Urol :73:316-318, 1994.

138. Shapiro S.R., Lebowitz R., Colodny A.H. Fate of 90 chidren with ileal conduit urinary diversion a decade latter; analysis of complications, pyelography, renal function and bacteriology. J Urol :114:289-295,1975.

139. Cass A.S., Luxenberg M., Gleich P., Johnson C.F. A 22-year followup of ileal conduits in children with a neurogenic bladder. J Urol :132:529-531,1984.

140. Schwartz G.R., Jeffs R.D. Ileal conduit urinary diversion in children: computer analysis of follow up from 2 to 16 years J Urol : 114, 289-295,1975.

141. Hendren W. H. Nonrefluxing colon conduit for temporary or permanent urinary diversion in children. J Ped Surg: 10: 381-398, 1975.

142. Herschorn S., Rangaswamy S., Radomski S.B. Urinary undiversion in adults with mylodysplasia: long-term followup. J Urol :152:329-333, 1994.

143. Gonzales R., Sidi AA, Zhang G.. Urinary undiversion : indications, technique, and results in 50 cases. J Urol : 136: 13-16, 1986.

144. Boring, C.C., Squires, T.S. and Tong, T. Cancer Statistics CA-A Cancer J. Clin., 42 (1), 19-38, 1992.

145. Catalona, W.J. Bladder cancer. In: Gillenwater, J.Y., Howard, S.S. and Duckett, J.W. (eds) Adult and Pediatric Urology, Vol. 1, pp. 1000-1043. Year Book Medical Publishers, Chicago, 1987.

146. Barat, M., Egon, G., Daverat, P., Vcolombel, P., Guerin, J., Ritz, M., Marit, E. and Herlant, M.Electrostiumulation of anterior sacral nerve roots in the treatment of central neurogenic bladders. G.S. Brindley's technique. Results of the first 40 French cases. J. d'Urol., 99, 3-7, 1993.

147. Tanagho, E.A. Principles and indications of electrostimulation of the urinary bladder. Urologie (A), 29, 185-190, 1990..

148. Abbou, C. and Auvert, J. Prosthetic bladder replacement in dogs. In: Wagenknecht, L.V., Furlow, W.L. and Auvert, J. (eds) Reconstruction with Prostheses. Pp. 71-75. Georg Thieme Veriag, Stuttgart, 1981.

149. Lutzeyer, W., Gerlach, R., Hannappel, J., Heinreichs, B. and Gregoir, W. (1984) Development and animal experimental investigation of an artificial urinary bladder with sphincter. Presented at 95th Annual Meeting of the American Association of Genitourinary Surgeons, Boca Raton, Florida, 2-4 March, 1984.

150. Apoil, A., Granger, A., Sausse, A. and Stern, A.. Experimental and clinical studies of prosthetic bladder replacement. In: Wagenknecht, L.V., Furlow, L.V. and Auvert, J. (eds) Genitourinary Reconstruction with Prostheses pp.75-80. Georg Thieme Verlag, Stuttgart.1981.

151. Donovan, M.G. Testing of Biocompatibility of Alloplastic Materials in the Genitourinary Tract Suitable for use as Prosthetic Materials. Master in Surgery Thesis, National University of Ireland, Trinity College, Dublin, 1962.

152. Bordat, J.P. Erude experimentale d'une prosthese vesicale en elastomere de silicone. J. Urol. Nephrol., 88 (Suppl. 2). 498-505, 1976.

153. Kline, J., Eckstein, E., Block, N., Lyon, F., Kelly, R., Morgan, D. and Ehrlich, S. Development of a total prosthetic urinary bladder. Trans.Am. Soc. Artif. Int. Organs. 24,254-256, 1978.

154. Pentermann, E., Kammbic, H., Matsushita, M., Kay, R. and Nose, Y.Prerequisites for urinary bladder design. Trans. Am. Soc. Artif. Int. Organs. 31, 308-312, 1985.

155. Friedman, B., Smith, R. and Finkle, A. Prosthetic bladder of silicone rubber in dogs. Inves. Urol., 1, 323-338, 1964.

156. Belden, L., Kushner, G., Wascher, U., Naslund, M. and Mostwin, J. Design, fabrication, evaluation and iterations of tailored urinary bladder prosthesis. J. Urol., 143, Part 2 (888), 409A, 1990.

157. O'Sullivan, D.C. Design, Development and in vivo Testing of a Complete Active Alloplastic Urinary Bladder, Masters of Surgery Thesis, National University of Ireland, University College, Cork, 1992.

158. O'Sullivan, D.C. and Barrett, D.M. Prosthetic bladder: in vivo studies on an active negative pressure driven device. J. Urol., 151 (3), 776-780, 1994.

159. Barrett, D.M., O'Sullivan, D.C., Parulkar, B.G. and Donovan, M. Artificial bladder replacement: a new design concept. Mayo Clinic Proc., 67, 215-220, 1992.

Committee 12

Urinary Incontinence in the Developing World: The Obstetric Fistula

Chairman

L. L. WALL (USA),

Members

S.D. ARROWSMITH (USA),

N. D. BRIGGS (NIGERIA),

A. LASSEY (GHANA)

CONTENTS

Urinary Incontinence in the Developing World: The Obstetric Fistula

L. L. WALL

S.D. ARROWSMITH, N. D. BRIGGS, A. LASSEY[1]

«In vast areas of the world, in South East Asia, in Burma, in India, in parts of Central America, South America and Africa 50 million women will bring forth their children this year in sorrow, as in ancient Biblical times, and exposed to grave dangers. In consequence, today as ever in the past, uncounted hundreds of thousands of young mothers annually suffer childbirth injuries; injuries which reduce them to the ultimate state of human wretchedness.

Consider these young women. Belonging generally to the age group 15-23 years, and thus at the very beginning of their reproductive lives, they are more to be pitied even than the blind, for the blind can sometimes work and marry. Their desolation descends below that of the lepers, who though scarred, crippled and shunned, may still marry and find useful work to do. The blind, the crippled and the lepers, with lesions obvious to the eye and therefore appealing to the heart, are all remembered and cared for by great charitable bodies, national and international.

Constantly in pain, incontinent of urine or faeces, bearing a heavy burden of sadness in discovering their child stillborn, ashamed of a rank personal offensiveness, abandoned therefore by their husbands, outcasts of society, unemployable except in the fields, they live, they exist, without friends and without hope.

Because their injuries are pudendal, affecting those parts of the body which must be hidden from view and which a woman may not in modesty easily speak, they endure their injuries in silent shame. No charitable organization becomes aware of them. Their misery is utter, lonely, and complete.»

RHJ Hamlin and E. Catherine Nicholson, 1966

People in the developing and the industrialized worlds share a common humanity and with this comes a common susceptibility to the pathophysiological processes that can lead to urinary incontinence; however, there is one continence issue that is both unique to and particularly prevalent in developing countries: the obstetric fistula. Although once common in Western Europe and the United States, the obstetric fistula is virtually unknown in these regions today. The prevalence of this condition has also fallen precipitously in the more industrialized nations of Asia and Latin America; but fistulas nonetheless remain prevalent and problematic in Africa and in the less developed regions of Asia and Oceania. This fact alone requires special attention, all the moreso because the obstetric fistula is unique among the causes of urinary incontinence in that it can be completely and reliably prevented by the provision of appropriate health care. It is this lack of appropriate health care—-specifically the lack of appropriate health care for pregnant women in developing countries—-that is responsible for the widespread prevalence of this devastating condition in certain areas of the world today. Quite clearly, the obstetric fistula has vanished from industrialized nations due to the creation in those countries of efficient and effective systems of maternity care which provide prompt emergency obstetrical services to women when complications arise in labor. The problem of obstetric fistulas in the developing world will not be solved until similarly effective systems of maternal health care are created there. Unfortunately, "Safe Motherhood" has largely become an "orphan" initiative (Rosenfield and Maine 1985; Graham 1998, Weil and Fernandez 1999). In virtually no other area in which health statistics are commonly collected is the disparity between the industrialized and the developing worlds so great as in the area of maternal health (AbouZahr and Royston 1991). This situation remains one of the most glaring, and one of the most neglected, issues of international social injustice in the world today. For this reason, the committee has chosen

1. The committee would like to thank Dr. Jonathan Karshima and Dr. Gunter Rienhart, who served as consultants to the committee

to focus its discussion of incontinence in the developing world on the obstetric fistula as the first and most pressing continence priority, rather than attempt to recapitulate our understanding of all forms of incontinence within the particular context of non-industrialized countries.

This chapter provides an overview of the pathophysiology of obstetric fistula formation and discusses the relationship of this condition to the broader issue of maternal mortality with which it is intimately linked. This chapter also summarizes the most important issues in the treatment of obstetric fistulas, and suggests directions for much-needed future research in this area.

I. LEVELS OF EVIDENCE CONCERNING OBSTETRIC FISTULAS

Scientific data on the problem of obstetric fistulas, their prevalence and forms of treatment, are limited by unusual historical circumstances. Prior to the middle of the 19th Century, an obstetric vesicovaginal fistula was generally regarded as an incurable and hopeless condition. It was only after the work of the American surgeon J. Marion Sims and his colleague and successor Thomas Addis Emmett (Sims 1852, Emmett 1868, Harris 1950, Zacharin 1988) that surgical cure of this condition could be undertaken with confidence. As obstetrics developed as a scientific specialty in the first half of the 20th Century, maternal mortality underwent a precipitous decline throughout Europe, the United States, and other developed nations (Loudon 1992a, 1992b). This meant that the obstetric fistula vanished from the clinical and social experience of the West just as it was starting to become rigorously scientific. As a result of these historical circumstances, the Western medical literature on obstetric fistulas is old and generally uncritical by current scientific criteria. This literature consists almost entirely of anecdotes, case series (some quite large), and personal experiences reported by dedicated surgeons who have labored in remote corners of the world while facing enormous clinical challenges with scanty or absent resources at their disposal (Evidence Levels 4 and 5). The committee charged with producing this report was able to locate only a handful of articles, all quite recent, that rise to a higher level of evidence. For example, there appears to be only one prospective, randomized clinical trial in the literature on vesico-vaginal fistulas in the developing world (Tomlinson and Thornton 1998), and only one comparative study of surgical technique (Rangnekar et. al. 2000). This fact underlines how the entire problem of obstetric fistulas in developing countries has been neglected by the bioscientific medical community of the industrialized world. The paucity of well-designed studies makes it impossible to produce a sophisticated meta-analysis of hard scientific data on the fistula problem at this time. While acknowledging this difficulty, the members of the committee feel that it is still possible to arrive at a consensus view of the broad outlines of the fistula problem. This report is therefore a general summary of the current state of our knowledge regarding obstetric fistulas in the developing world and the challenges thus presented. It should be regarded as a point of departure for further work—-and further action—- while recognizing that many important issues remain unclear and urgently require more intensive scientific study.

II. THE RELATIONSHIP OF OBSTETRIC FISTULAS TO MATERNAL MORTALITY

The commonly accepted definition of a maternal death is «the death of a woman while pregnant or within 42 days of termination of pregnancy, irrespective of the duration and the site of the pregnancy, from any cause related to or aggravated by the pregnancy or its management but not from accidental or incidental causes» (Abour Zahr and Royston 1991). The most common measure of maternal mortality used for international comparative purposes is the maternal mortality ratio: the number of maternal deaths per 100,000 live births. The available statistics show huge discrepancies between the developed and the developing worlds (WHO 1996). The overall world maternal mortality ratio is estimated at 430 maternal deaths per 100,000 live births. In more developed regions of the world the ratio is 27 deaths per 100,000 live births, contrasted with 480 deaths per 100,000 live births in less developed regions. The numbers are substantially worse for Africa: 870 for the continent as a whole, 950 in middle Africa, 1,020 in West Africa, and 1,060 in East Africa. In northern Europe and North America there are 11 maternal deaths per 100,000 live births. There are many problems associated with the collection of maternal mortality statistics, especially in developing countries, and all such statistics are acknowledged to be underestimates to some (usually to a substantial) degree. For an individual woman, a more important statistic than the maternal mortality ratio is her lifetime risk of pregnancy-related death. This statistic is a function of the risk of dying in any particular pregnancy multiplied by the number of times she is likely to become pregnant. The risks are therefore highest in areas of high fertility where access to emergency obstetric care is poor. Overall, the global lifetime risk of maternal death is 1 in 60. In more developed regions, the risk is only 1 in 1800; in less developed regions the risk is 1 in 48. In North America or Northern Europe, a woman has a lifetime risk of pregnancy-related death of approximately 1 in 4,000; in Africa, the risk is 1 in 16, and in the poorest parts of Africa a woman's lifetime risk of dying as the result of pregnancy or childbirth is as high as 1 in 7. The currently accepted world maternal mortality statistics are summarized in Table 1 (WHO 1996).

The majority of maternal deaths are due to five principal causes: hemorrhage, sepsis, hypertensive disorders of pregnancy, unsafe abortion, and obstructed labor (AbouZahr and Royston 1991). The vast majority of fistulas are due to obstructed labor. Not surprisingly, obstetric fistulas are most prevalent in areas where maternal mortality is high and where obstructed labor is a major contributor to maternal deaths. These are areas where access to emergency obstetric care is poor; correspondingly, accurate epidemiological information is also poor in these regions—-a continuing point of difficulty in the evaluation of maternal mortality in general and in the evaluation of obstetric fistulas in particular.

The problem of obstetric fistula formation is linked directly to that of maternal mortality. Maternal mortality is embedded in a complex network of social issues that have to do with the social status of women, the distribution and availability of healthcare resources, perceptions about the nature and importance of maternal health problems, and the social, economic and political infrastructures of developing countries. Indeed, it is commonly said that obstetric fistulas result from the combination of «obstructed labor and obstructed transportation.» Thaddeus and Maine (1994) have articulated the concept of three «stages of delay» that result in maternal mortality: delay in deciding to seek care, delay in arriving at a health care facility, and delay in receiving adequate care once a woman arrives at such a facility. All of these factors are present in the formation of an obstetric fistula. Women in labor are often neglected in the hopes that «everything will come out all right» on its own. Other women refuse to seek care for fear they will be perceived as "weak" or "cowardly." Frequently the seriousness of the situation is not appreciated or help is not sought for fear of incurring high financial costs. Even if help is sought, poor roads and

Table 1 : Revised estimates of maternal mortality by United Nations regions (WHO 1996)

	Maternal Mortality Ratio (Maternal deaths per 100,000 live births)	Number of Maternal Deaths	Lifetime Risk of Maternal Death, 1 in:
World total	**430**	**585,000**	**60**
More developed regions*	27	4,000	1,800
Less developed regions	480	582,000	48
Africa	**870**	**235,000**	**16**
Eastern Africa	1,060	97,000	12
Middle Africa	950	31,000	14
Northern Africa	340	16,000	55
Southern Africa	260	3,600	75
Western Africa	1,020	87,000	12
Asia*	**390**	**323,000**	**65**
Eastern Asia	95	24,000	410
South-central Asia	560	227,000	35
South-eastern Asia	440	56,000	55
Western Asia	320	16,000	55
Europe	**36**	**3,200**	**1,400**
Eastern Europe	62	2,500	730
Northern Europe	11	140	4,000
Southern Europe	14	220	4,000
Western Europe	17	350	3200
Latin America & the Caribbean	**190**	**23,000**	**130**
Caribbean	400	3,200	75
Central America	140	4,700	170
South America	200	15,000	140
Northern America	**11**	**500**	**3,700**
Oceania*	**680**	**1,400**	**26**
Australia-New Zealand	10	40	3,600
Melanesia	810	1,400	21

*Australia, New Zealand and Japan have been excluded from the regional totals but are included in the total for developed countries. Figures may not add to total due to rounding.

inadequate public transportation often result in long delays in reaching a health care facility, and even if the laboring woman arrives at a hospital, inadequate facilities or untrained personnel may preclude the performance of an emergency cesarean section or meeting her other medical needs.

The three "stages of delay" keep women on what is sometimes termed the "road to maternal death." In similar fashion it seems that there is also a «road to obstetric fistula» that begins when young girls grow up in nutritionally marginal circumstances, are married around the age of menarche, become pregnant while still adolescents, and labor at home either alone or under the care of untrained birth attendants for prolonged periods of time and with inadequate access to emergency obstetrical care. In addition, many become victims of harmful traditional medical practices that further complicate matters. The obstetric fistula pathway is summarized in Figure 1.

III. EPIDEMIOLOGY OF THE OBSTETRIC FISTULA

In industrialized countries most vesico-vaginal fistulas (VVF) are the result of radiation therapy or surgery (Latzko 1942; Everett and Mattingly 1956; Counsellor and Haigler 1956; Radman 1961; Moir 1966; Massee et. al. 1964; Weed 1967; Taylor and Droegemueller 1967; Goodwin and Scardino 1980; Enzelsberger and Gitsch 1991; Langkilde et. al. 1999). In the developing world, on the other hand, most fistulas occur from the neglect of obstetric complications. As such, they occur under very different circumstances. As Gharoro and Abedi remarked in their short case series of fistulas from Benin City, Nigeria (1999), «Any pregnant patient could develop VVF from substandard care.»

To date there has never been a comprehensive worldwide survey designed to determine precisely where obstetric fistulas occur. Questions regarding the incidence and prevalence of obstetric fistulas have never been included on the standardized demographic and health surveys (DHS) that are carried out to evaluate population characteristics and overall health status in developing countries. Virtually no population-based surveys have been carried out in countries where there appears to be a high incidence and high prevalence of obstetric fistulas. Furthermore, the urinary and/or fecal incontinence that accompanies fistula formation makes its sufferers social outcasts, pushing them to the margins of society where they are ignored, further obscuring the true extent of the problem. There is a very real need for ongoing scientific research in this area. Until such work is forthcoming, we are left with only indirect means of describing the epidemic. In a short survey of available information on obstetric fistulas published by the World Health Organization in 1991 that encompassed a literature review and correspondence with over 250 individuals, institutions and organizations in developing countries, a map was created showing the distribution of countries where obstetric fistulas had been reported (Figure 2). The committee members, from personal experience and contact with other workers in the field, know that this map should include virtually all of Africa and south Asia, the less developed parts of Oceania, Latin America, and the Middle East; and, we suspect (though we cannot prove) the more remote regions of Central Asia and selected isolated areas of the former Soviet Union and Soviet-dominated eastern Europe.

The true magnitude of the fistula problem worldwide is unknown, but it is clearly enormous. The situation in Nigeria may be cited as an example. Arrowsmith (1994), writing from the plateau region of central Nigeria, noted that «the local popular press estimates that the region may harbor up to 150,000 victims of vesico-vaginal fistula.» Harrison, also writing from northern Nigeria, reported a vesico-vaginal fistula rate of 350 cases per 100,000 deliveries at a university teaching hospital (1985). Karshima, who has carried out village-based survey work on obstetric fistulas in the middle belt of Nigeria, suspects that there may be as many as 400,000 unrepaired fistulas in Nigeria (J. Karshima, personal communication, 2001), and the Nigerian Federal Minister for Women Affairs and Youth Development, Hajiya Aisha M.S. Ismail, has estimated the number of unrepaired vesico-vaginal fistulas in Nigeria at between 800,000 and 1,000,000 (personal communication, 2001).

The data on maternal morbidity (non-fatal obstetric complications) in developing countries are poor, but it is obvious that the number of serious morbid episodes or «near misses» greatly exceeds the number of maternal deaths in the developing nations (Prual et. al., 1998). In parts of the world where a woman's lifetime risk of maternal death is high, a woman's lifetime risk of suffering serious maternal morbidity (including obstetric fistula) may be extraordinarily high. In one of the few studies that has looked at the issue of maternal morbidity, Fortney and Smith calculated the ratios of serious morbidities to maternal mortalities in Indonesia, Bangladesh, India and Egypt. For each maternal death, they calculated that there were 149, 259, 300 and 591 serious morbidities in these respective countries, and 112, 114, 24, and 67 life-threatening morbidities respectively (Fortney and Smith, 1996). In the face of such sobering statistics, Danso and colleagues suggested that in regions of the world where obstructed labor is a major contributor to maternal mortality, the obstetric fistula rate may approach the maternal mortality rate

Figure 1 : The obstetric fistula pathway: Origins and consequences (©Worldwide Fund for Mothers Injured in Childbirth, used by permission).

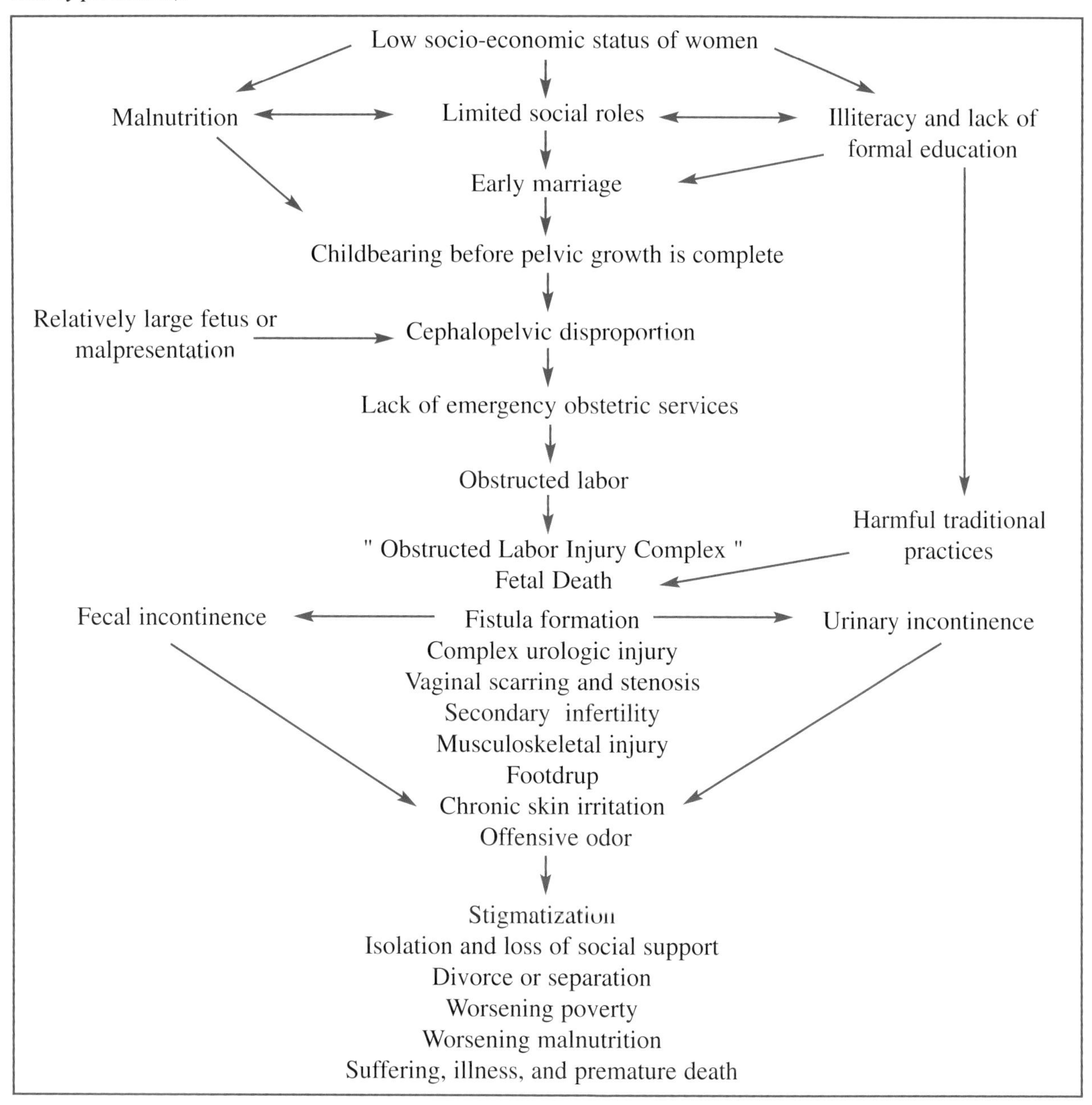

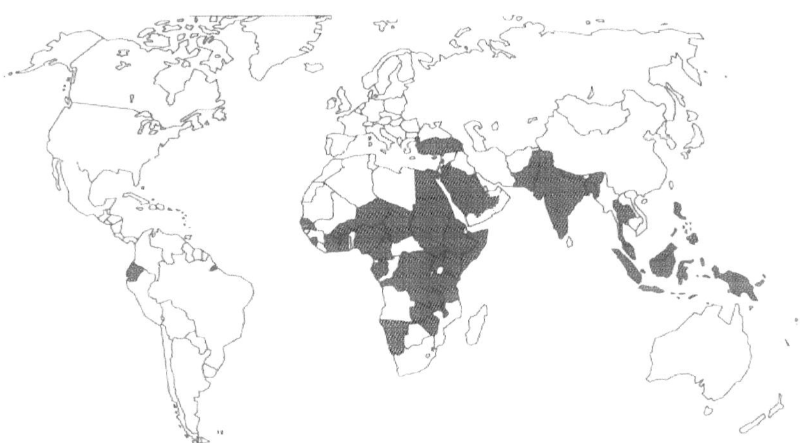

Figure 2 : Countries from which obstetric vesico-vaginal fistulas have been reported (WHO 1991). The prevalence is actually greater than this map indicates.

(Danso et. al., 1996). Other authors have reached similar conclusions (Hilton and Ward, 1998).

In the absence of good population-based epidemiological studies, most information on fistulas has come from large series of patients seen at teaching hospitals or at dedicated fistula centers. Just as there are reasons to be wary of hospital-based statistics in surveys of maternal mortality (AbouZahr and Royston 1991), there are reasons to be cautious about considering hospital-based surveys of fistula patients to be representative of the over-all population of women with fistulas from obstructed labor. Answers to the following questions appear to be crucial in delineating the true extent of the fistula problem worldwide:

- Where do fistula patients come from?
- What is their social background?
- What is their educational level?
- What is the age at marriage of women who develop fistulas?
- What is the distribution of fistulas by age and parity at the time of their occurrence?
- In which pregnancy do obstetric fistulas occur?
- What proportion of women who develop fistulas had access to obstetric care, and if such care was available, why was it not used in a timely fashion?
- Where do women who develop fistulas deliver and who attends those deliveries?
- How long are these women in labor before they recognize that labor is obstructed and seek help, and how long is the delay before effective help is obtained?
- What is their marital/social status at the time of labor?
- How long must women who develop fistulas wait before they undergo an attempt at surgical repair, and at what age do they present for repair?
- What is the social status of fistula victims after they develop this problem?
- Does this status change after fistula closure?
- What role do harmful traditional beliefs and practices play in the genesis of prolonged obstructed labor and fistula formation?

Although detailed answers to these questions await detailed population-based research, preliminary impressions can be obtained from surveys taken of fistula patients in hospital settings in several countries. The overall impression is that fistula patients come from poor rural areas where infrastructure development is rudimentary and access to health care—particularly access to basic midwifery and emergency obstetric services—is lacking. Fistula patients tend to be young women, many of whom married very early, of short stature, poorly educated, married to farmers or petty traders who themselves have little or no formal education. They typically have had little or no access to prenatal care, and even if they have had access to antenatal screening, they have often nonetheless delivered at home attended by family members or traditional midwives. If they have sought help from trained midwives or medical doctors, this often occurs late in labor after serious complications have already set in.

Several papers from Africa support this picture of the fistula patient. Kelly and Kwast (1993b) reviewed a 10% sample of fistula patients seen at the Addis Ababa Fistula hospital between 1983 and 1988, by reviewing the records of every tenth patient. The mean age of these women was 22.4 years (range 9 – 45 years); 42% were less than 20 years of age, and 65% were less than 25 years of age. Of the women surveyed, 52.3% had been deserted by their husbands and 21.5% had to live by begging for food. Nearly 30% had delivered alone, and the mean duration of labor was 3.9 days (range 1-6 days).

In one review of 150 fistulas from Ghana, 91.5% were the result of obstructed labor and 8.5% were the result of complications of difficult gynecological surgery (Danso et. al. 1996). Nearly 53% of the obstetric fistula patients were under the age of 25 and nearly 43% of patients were primigravid. Interestingly, nearly 25% of the patients had a parity of 5 or more, indicating that labor can become obstructed even in women who have previously delivered vaginally. This probably represents the tendency for birth weights to increase with successive pregnancies, as well as the effects of aging on changes in pelvic anatomy.

Information from several studies in northern Nigeria is similar. Tahzib reviewed records of 1,443 patients with vesico-vaginal fistulas seen in the clinics at Ahmadu Bello University in Zaria between 1969 and 1980. Delivery occurred at home in 64.4% of these women. Among women who developed fistulas, 54.8% were under the age of 20 and only 22.7% were older than 25 years. The majority of women developed a fistula in their first pregnancy (52%), and 21.5 % of fistula patients were parity 4 or greater. Two case control studies from northern Nigeria have found fistula patients to be shorter, to be of lower socioeconomic status, and to have less education than control patients without fistulas (Ampofo, Otu, and Uchebo 1990; Onolemhemhen and Ekwempu 1999).

Virtually every paper on vesico-vaginal fistulas from developing countries demonstrates that the most common cause of fistula formation by far is prolonged obstructed labor (Amr 1998; Arrowsmith 1994; Azia 1965; Bird 1967; Coetzee and Lithgow 1966; Gharoro and Abedi 1999; Goh 1998; Hilton and Ward 1998; Iloabachie 1992; Kelly 1992; Lavery 1955; Krishnan 1949; Lawson 1972; Mahfouz 1957; Mustafa and Rushwan 1971; Naidu 1962; Tahzib 1983; Tahzib 1985; Naidu 1962; Waaldijk 1989; Yenen and Babuna 1965) accounting for between 76% and 97% of fistulas in most large series. Additional important causes include injuries sustained during complicated gynecologic surgery performed under very difficult circumstances, accidents such as penetrating injuries to the vagina and bladder involving cattle horns or impalement by falling on a stick, infection (particularly lymphogranuloma venereum, but also diphtheria, measles, schistosomiasis, infected centipede bites, etc.), and cervical cancer. In their series of 309 urinary fistulas treated in Pietermaritzburg, Natal, South Africa between 1954 and 1963, Coetzee and Lithgow (1966) reported 248 as resulting from obstructed labor (80%), 9 (3%) from complications of pelvic surgery, and 52 (17%) from advanced carcinoma of the cervix. Particularly troubling are fistulas caused by sexual abuse, rape, or from attempts forcibly to enlarge the vaginal introitus of child brides so that sexual relations can commence (Tahzib 1985; Muleta and Williams 1999).

In some parts of the world, harmful traditional practices are also responsible for fistula formation. For example, in northern Nigeria, a harmful traditional practice called *gishiri*-cutting is responsible for fistula formation in 6 – 13% of cases (Ampofo, Otu and Uchebo 1990; Tahzib 1983, 1985). *Gishiri* is the Hausa word for «salt.» It is often used to refer to the encrustations of salt that occur on the outsides of porous water jars as their contents evaporate. *Gishiri* is an important ethnomedical condition in Hausa traditional medicine. The belief is that an imbalance of salty or sweet foodstuffs can cause a «film» to grow over the woman's vagina, causing a variety of gynecological complaints, the most important of these being difficult labor (Wall 1988). When this diagnosis is made, surgical treatment is often undertaken. A midwife or barber is summoned. A sharp object such as a knife, razor blade, or piece of broken glass is inserted into the vagina, and a series of random cuts is made to alleviate the postulated obstruction and «open the way» for the baby to come out. Serious infection, life-threatening hemorrhage, and fistulas frequently result from this practice. The *gishiri* fistula typically presents as a direct longitudinal slit in the bladder neck and urethra, occasionally presenting as a similar posterior injury affecting the rectum.

Another traditional practice that have been reported to produce fistulas is the insertion of caustic substances into the vagina, either as part of a traditional herbal remedy for a gynecologic condition (Lawson 1968) or as part of traditional puerperal practices to «help» the vagina return to its nulliparous state. The latter practice is a part of the traditional folk medicine of several Arab countries (Kingston 1957, El Guindi 1962, Frith 1960). The practice was summarized by Betty Underhill in her 1964 report of 65 such cases seen at the Bahrain Government Hospital between 1957 and 1963 thus:

«For hundreds of years it has been the custom of Arab women to pack the vagina with salt for the first week after delivery. This is popularly supposed to restore the vagina to its nulliparous state and to add to the husband's sexual pleasure. Since the practice has survived for so long it must be presumed that this desirable effect is sometimes achieved. It is certainly true, however, that in a great many cases the end results are devastating and it is these unhappy women who are driven to hospital for relief. ... The substance used is crude rock salt sold in the bazaar. A piece of salt roughly the size and shape of an egg is pushed into the vagina daily for 2 to 15 days after the delivery. An additional incentive to the use of salt is its supposed antiseptic property, and some women are said to employ it between pregnancies as a contraceptive.

The immediate effect of the pessary on the hyperaemic vagina is the production of severe inflammation which goes on to ulceration. Healing of the ulcers leads to a very severe fibrosis and the vagina becomes partly or completely occluded by a substance with an almost cartilaginous texture. The walls of the upper third of the vagina are held apart by the cervix and the lower third is constantly pulled upon by the levator ani muscle. The lax middle third is commonly the area affected by fibrosis and the patient is left with a tiny lower vagina 2 to 5 cm long, then a block or cord of fibrous tissue with an upper chamber indented by the cervix.»

The fibrosis that results is extensive enough to produce obstructed labor in many cases (Fahmy 1962). Fistulas may result from either obstructed labor (Fahmy 1962) or by direct chemical action. As Naim has written, «The method of salt packing determines the site and types of the fistulae that may develop. Thus in Kuwait, where the whole vagina is packed with rock salt, combined rectovaginal and vesicovaginal fistulae develop due to rock salt being in contact with both the anterior and posterior vaginal walls. In Saudi Arabia, where pieces of rock salt are inserted high in the vagina, rectovaginal fistulae only were met with.» In some cases the vagina is completely occluded, leading to the formation of a hematocolpos, dysmenorrhea, infertility and related gynecological conditions (Underhill 1964).

Much popular concern has focused on the problem of «female circumcision» («female genital mutilation») in recent years (for example, Abdalla 1982; Aziz 1980; Boddy 1982; El-Dareer 1982; Gruenbaum 2001; Toubia 1994; WHO 1998). While these practices should rightly be condemned by the medical community as being markedly injurious to the health of women and female children, there is absolutely no evidence in the world literature to suggest that practices of this type are the *major* cause of fistula formation in developing countries. Although fistulas are common in communities where various forms of female genital mutilation are practiced, the former are not usually caused directly by the latter. Rather, these two phenomena both reflect the low social status of women in these countries, which in turn is reflected by a striking underinvestment in women's reproductive health care in those countries, with a consequent lack of access to emergency obstetric care and poor gynecologic health.

Where female genital mutilation is practiced, it contributes to the genesis of fistulas in two ways. First, as in the case of *gishiri*-cutting among the Hausa, surgical attempts to modify the female genitalia in any fashion can cause direct injury to the bladder or urethra. When such procedures are carried out without anesthetic under unsterile conditions by unskilled practitioners who do not understand female pelvic anatomy, the risks of catastrophic complications are great. Fistula formation may occur in these cases through direct surgical trauma to the urinary tract. Secondly, in cases where large amounts of vulvar or vaginal tissue are removed, particularly in the case of infibulation («Pharaonic circumcision») where the vaginal introitus is sewn almost completely shut or where excessive vulvar scarring has occurred as a result of these practices, the vaginal outlet may become extremely narrow and constricted by dense scar tissue. This may prevent expulsion of the fetus at the end of the second stage of labor; indeed, an anterior episiotomy is usually required in order to effect vaginal delivery in such women. If the outlet cannot be opened sufficiently to allow passage of the fetus, obstructed labor may result and may end in fistula formation. However, obstructed labor from this cause would only occur at the end of labor.

The available evidence suggests that in the majority of cases in which fistulas occur, labor becomes obstructed in the mid-pelvis or at the pelvic brim, rather than at the pelvic outlet. Further evidence for the primary importance of obstetric factors in the development of vesicovaginal fistulas can be seen in the fact that the Hausa, who have one of the highest prevalences of obstetric fistula formation in the world, do not practice «female circumcision.» Comparative radiographic studies suggest that the Nigerian pelvis is considerably smaller than that of European (Welsh) women, particularly at the pelvic inlet, least significantly at the pelvic outlet (Kolawole, Adamu and Evans 1978). This suggests that there are anatomic differences that predispose African women to obstructed labor (Briggs 1983). Because sexual maturity and adult height are reached before growth of the pelvic dimensions has been completed, pregnancies that occur in early adolescence are more likely to be complicated by obstructed labor than those that occur in older women (Moerman 1982). Early marriage and accompanying early pregnancy are also linked to a relatively low social status of women, tying these factors together in one more way.

IV. THE «OBSTRUCTED LABOR INJURY COMPLEX»

Obstructed labor occurs when the presenting fetal part cannot pass through the maternal bony pelvis. The presenting part then becomes wedged against the maternal pelvic bones, compressing the soft tissues in between (Figure 3). The uterine contractions force the presenting part deeper into the pelvis, compressing the maternal soft tissues more forcibly. If this process is not relieved by surgical intervention, the blood supply to the entrapped soft tissues becomes compromised, ultimately resulting in tissue death and fistula formation.

The pathophysiology of obstructed labor was described clearly and succinctly by Mahfouz in 1930:

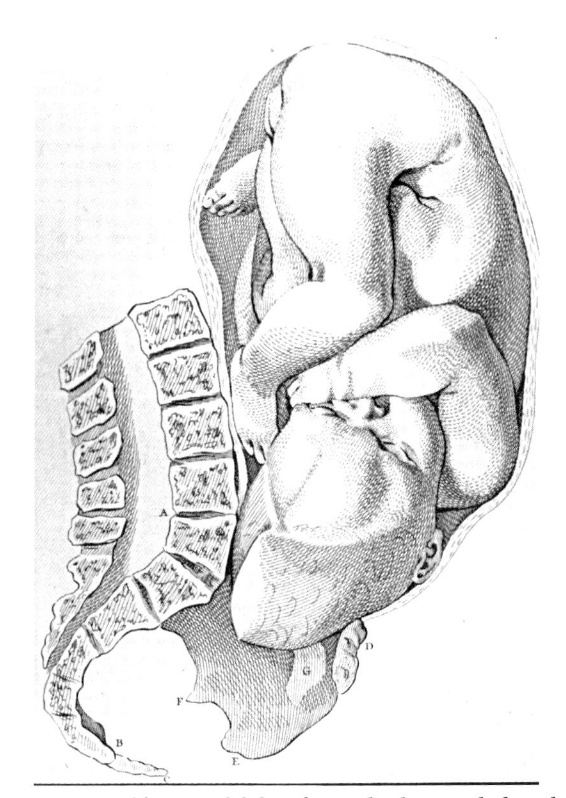

Figure 3 : Obstructed labor from absolute cephalo-pelvic disproportion, from William Smellie's Sett of Anatomical Tables with Explanations, and an Abridgment of the Practice of Midwifery. London, 1754

«The process by which a fistula develops after labour is the following. When labour becomes difficult, on account of disproportion between the pelvis and presenting part, or when the presentation is abnormal, the uterine contractions increase in strength and endeavour to force the presenting part through the brim. The membranes protrude unduly in the vagina, and premature rupture occurs. In consequence of early rupture and disproportion the full force of the uterine contractions is directly exerted upon the foetus and the presenting part is forced against the brim of the pelvis or gets tightly impacted therein. The vesico-vaginal septum, and the cervix if the latter is not dilated, will be tightly compressed against the back of the symphysis pubis. The uterus in such cases usually passes into a state of tonic contractions which prevents any remission in the pressure exerted on the soft parts. As a result of the continued pressure the tissues undergo necrosis and slough away. The duration of compression in such cases is usually very long, but I have seen cases in which a fistula developed after 3 hours of compression only. At about the fifth day of the puerperium the slough begins to separate and urine dribbles involuntarily into the vagina. ...

The slough that develops from this pressure necrosis most commonly results in a vesico-vaginal fistula (Figure 4). Once this has occurred, the unfortunate woman suffers from constant, unremitting loss of urine. She can attempt to stay this flow with the use of rags or cloth, but she can never get rid of it. J. Marion Sims, who first developed a consistently successful method of fistula closure, expressed well the situation of the patient with a fistula (1852):

«Its diagnosis is sufficiently easy. Incontinence of urine, following a tedious labour after a lapse of from one to fifteen days, will always prove its existence. But to determine the exact size, shape, and relative position of the artificial opening require some nicety of examination. The consequences of the involuntary discharge of urine are indeed painful. The vagina may become inflamed, ulcerated, encrusted with urinary calculi, and even contracted; while the vulva, nates, and thighs are more or less excoriated, being often covered with pustules having a great resemblance to those produced by tartar emetic. These pustules sometimes degenerate into sloughs, causing loss of substance, and requiring a long time to heal. The clothes and bedding of the unfortunate patient are constantly saturated with the discharge, thus exhaling a disagreeable effluvium, alike disgusting to herself and repulsive to others.

The accident, per se, is never fatal; but it may well be imagined that a lady of keen sensibilities so afflicted, and excluded from all social enjoyment, would prefer death. A case of this kind came under my observation a few years since, where the lady absolutely pined away and died, in consequence of her extreme mortification on ascertaining that she was hopelessly incurable.»

The location and nature of the maternal injury that results from prolonged obstructed labor is a function of the force and duration of the compression that occurs, as well as the level at which labor becomes obstructed (Figure 5). As Mahfouz remarked (1930): "The situation of the fistula depends to a great extent on the state of the cervix, when impaction and compression occur, and also on the plane of impaction. If pressure and compression occur before the cervix is pulled up over the head, the vault of the vagina and the cervical tissues may be involved in the slough. The resulting fistula will be vesico-cervico-vaginal, or uretero vaginal, as the case may be." The location of the fistula is often determined by the particular configuration of the woman's pelvis. Thus, John St. George noted (1969):

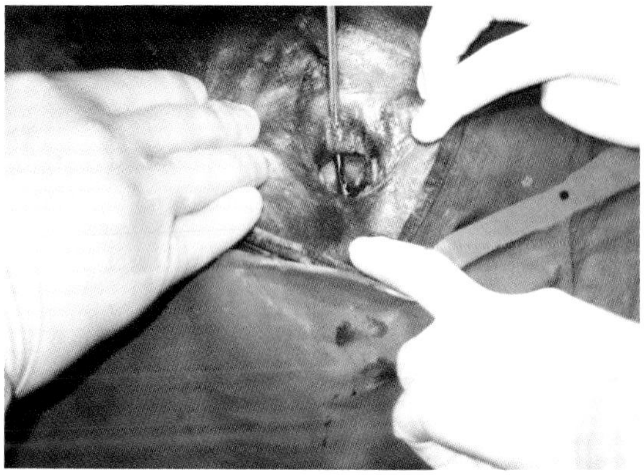

Figure 4 : Typical mid-vaginal vesico-vaginal fistula from obstructed labor. A metal sound passed through the urethra can clearly be seen inside the bladder. (©Worldwide Fund for Mothers Injured in Childbirth, used by permission).

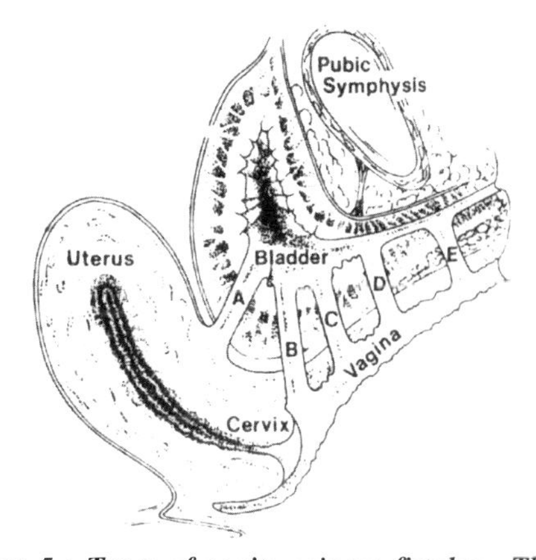

Figure 5 : Types of genito-urinary fistulas. The location depends on the point at which labor becomes obstructed. A. Utero-vesical fistula. B. Cervico-vesical fistula. C. Mid-vaginal vesico-vaginal fistula. D. Vesico-vaginal fistula involving the bladder neck. E. Urethro-vaginal fistula. From Elkins (1994).

«Vesico-vaginal fistulae occurred more often in primigravidae (often very young) than in multiparae. Deep transverse arrest of the fetal head was commoner in primiparae with an android type of pelvis, and therefore the site of the fistula was more often at the bladder neck or was juxta-urethral. Primiparae were also permitted longer labour by their folk because of their youth, and hence their fistulae were extensive. On the other hand, labour in multigravidae was often obstructed at the inlet because of a secondary flat pelvis; in these cases mid-vaginal or juxta-cervical fistulae, which were more amenable to surgery, were more common.»

Many women who develop an obstetric vesico-vaginal fistula have been delivered vaginally with the use of instruments or have had an abdominal delivery by Cesarean section. As early as the 19th Century, obstetricians were often blamed for creating fistulas through the injudicious use of operative techniques. Although incompetent surgical delivery is undoubtedly responsible for some fistulas, the vast majority of patients undergoing operative delivery have been in labor for a prolonged period of time and have already suffered the ischemic insult that ultimately leads to fistula formation. The mode of delivery is therefore often unrelated to the development of the fistula that subsequently occurs (Emmett 1879). As Das and Sengupta noted in their series from India (1969):

«Pressure necrosis is responsible to a great extent for the fistula. Most of the instrumental labour group were also prolonged labour cases and would probably have resulted in vesico-vaginal fistula even without instrumentation. Therefore, all cases were not caused by instrumental delivery as such but were due to pressure necrosis that had already existed.»

The prevalence of women who have had prolonged labors and then undergone operative delivery is in part a function of increasing access to obstetric care, even if that access is not timely enough to prevent the development of a fistula. In his review of vesico-vaginal fistulas in Jordan, M.F. Amr (1998) summarized the relationship between women's health care and fistula formation with these words: «The incidence of urinary fistula reflects the standard of obstetric and gynaecological care and its availability to the population. Most fistulae are due to obstetric causes such as prolonged and obstructed labour, difficult instrumental delivery and other obstetric manipulations, and ruptured uterus.»

The vast majority of women in non-industrialized countries who develop a vesico-vaginal fistula do so as the result of prolonged obstructed labor from cephalo-pelvic disproportion. The presenting fetal part is wedged into the pelvis, trapping the woman's soft tissues between two bony plates which effectively shut off the blood supply to the affected tissues. This results in extensive tissue necrosis which frequently destroys the vesico-vaginal septum and results in fistula formation; however, it is important to realize that obstructed labor produces a broad-spectrum "field injury" that may affect many parts of the pelvis. The damage that occurs is not limited to vesico-vaginal or recto-vaginal fistula formation alone. This fact is not generally appreciated by most Western doctors. Although the fistula that results is usually the dominant clinical injury, it is wrong to focus solely on the «hole in the bladder» to the exclusion of the other consequences of obstructed labor. Women who have sustained an obstetric fistula are usually injured in multiple ways, all of which impact their lives and well-being, and all of which must be considered in their care. Arrowsmith, Hamlin and Wall (1996) have called this spectrum of injury the «obstructed labor injury complex» (Table 2). The understanding that one must treat the "whole person" with a fistula—-and not just her injured bladder or rectum—-is the single most important concept in fistula care. Doing this effectively requires some understanding of the multi-system consequences of prolonged obstructed labor.

1. Urologic injury

Obstetric vesicovaginal fistulas are not caused by tearing or laceration of the bladder; rather they result from ischemic injury. Normal tissue perfusion is disrupted by compression of the soft tissues by the fetal head. This leads to ischemia, tissue death, subsequent necrosis, and fistula formation, along with varying degrees of injury to surrounding tissues which, although they have not died, nonetheless are often not completely healthy either, having suffering a non-fatal but debilitating ischemic vascular injury as well. This process has an impact at various levels throughout the urinary tract.

a) Bladder. The most familiar injury from obstructed labor is the vesicovaginal fistula. The loss of bladder tissue from pelvic ischemia during obstructed labor affects both the technique needed for, as well as the functional outcome of, fistula repair. Loss of bladder tissue is one of the main reasons why obstetric fistula repair is technically difficult. The surgeon must try to close large defects in the bladder often with only small remnants of residual bladder tissue. Although there are as yet no basic histologic studies of the tissue surrounding obstetric fistulas, it seems clear that these tissues have themselves sustained significant damage during obstructed labor. The fistula itself develops in an area which has sustained enough damage to become necrotic; the process by which this occurs also appears to affect another, variable zone surrounding the fistula in which the tissues have been damaged but not killed. In

Table 2 : Spectrum of Injuries Seen in the "Obstructed Labor Injury Complex"

Urologic Injury
Vesicovaginal fistula
Urethrovaginal fistula
Ureterovaginal fistula
Uterovesical fistula
Complex combinations of fistulas
Urethral damage, including complete urethral loss
Stress urinary incontinence
Secondary hydroureteronephrosis
Chronic pyelonephritis
Renal failure
Gynecologic Injury
Amenorrhea
Vaginal stenosis
Cervical damage, including complete cervical destruction
Secondary pelvic inflammatory disease
Secondary infertility
Gastrointestinal Injury
Rectovaginal fistula
Acquired rectal atresia
Anal sphincter incompetence
Musculoskeletal Injury
Osteitis pubis
Neurological Injury
Foot-drop
Complex neuropathic bladder dysfunction
Dermatological Injury
Chronic excoriation of skin from maceration in urine/feces
Fetal Injury
Approximately 95% fetal case mortality rate
Social Injury
Social isolation
Divorce
Worsening povery
Malnutrition
Depression, sometimes suicide

repairing obstetric fistulas, it is this unhealthy surrounding tissue that must be used to close the defect—-a problem that has led many fistula surgeons over the generations to the brink of despair (Figure 6).

In some cases pressure necrosis may destroy virtually the entire bladder, so that when the defect is finally closed the afflicted woman is left with a remarkably small (30 - 50 ml) bladder that remains virtually functionless. Because most of the innervation of the bladder runs through the base and trigone, ischemic injury to these areas probably also produces an element of neuropathic bladder dysfunction. Basic scientific studies confirming this hypothesis have yet to be undertaken. Clinical experience with fistula patients also suggests that bladder compliance may be altered by the extensive fibrotic changes that often take place. To date there has been only one urodynamic study of post-repair fistula patients (Schleicher et. al 1993), but compliance was not measured in this study and the number of patients

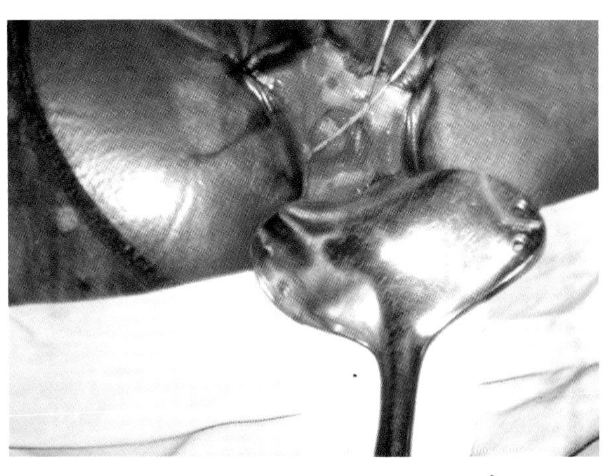

Figure 6 : Large mid-vaginal vesico-vaginal fistula with scarring. The ureters, which have been catheterized for better visualization, lie directly on the margins of the fistula. (©Worldwide Fund for Mothers Injured in Childbirth, used by permission).

evaluated (18) is too small to allow meaningful generalizations to be made. There is a great need for further investigation of these issues; unfortunately, those hospitals most likely to see large numbers of patients with obstetric fistulas lack the resources for such urologic investigation. The potential use of bladder augmentation operations to restore the functional bladder capacity of such patients remains largely uninvestigated. Although there are well-established surgical techniques for bladder augmentation that can be used in the health care systems of industrialized countries, for the most part those developing countries in which fistulas are most likely to be major problems are precisely those countries in which the capacity is lacking to perform such operations safely, competently, and successfully. At least for the present, complex bladder augmentation operations (cecocystoplasty, ileocystoplasty, gastrocystoplasty, etc.) do not appear to be feasible therapies for most women with contracted bladders after obstetric fistula repair. One possible solution to this problem may lie in the use of "auto-augmentation" operations in which a portion of the detrusor muscle is removed, permitting the underlying bladder mucosa to expand, in essence creating a large bladder diverticulum (Kennelly et. al. 1994; Snow and Cartwright 1996; Leng et. al. 1999). At present the potential of these techniques in the treatment of fistula patients with small fibrotic bladders remains completely unexplored within the context of the developing world.

b) Urethra. The ischemic changes produced by obstructed labor often have a devastating impact on urethral function. The great Egyptian fistula surgeon Naguib Mahfouz was well aware of this problem. As he wrote in 1930:

I have carefully examined 100 patients suffering from

what was termed vesico-vaginal fistula during the last 10 years. I found by careful examination and measurement of the urethra that the sloughing which ultimately led to the formation of the fistulae had in more than half the cases involved from one-third to half of the urethra. This is not to be wondered at, since in most cases of obstructed delivery in which the bladder is pulled up above the brim of the pelvis the urethra is pulled up with it. If the seat of obstruction happens to be at the brim of the pelvis, the neck of the bladder and a small portion of the upper third of the urethra seldom escapes compression.. In cases in which the presenting part is impacted in the cavity of the pelvis, or detained at the outlet, the entire urethral canal will be lying in the plane of compression. In some of these cases the urethra sloughs away completely.»

The finest centers in the world report fistula closure rates in excess of 90%, yet many patients who have had a successful fistula repair continue to have severe urinary incontinence. Although the bladder defect has been closed successfully, many patients have defective, injured urethras which are often foreshortened, fibrotic, functionless «drainpipes» densely bound in scar tissue. Patients with these findings may remain almost totally wet in spite of fistula closure, and perhaps as many as 30% of fistula patients have some element of persistent stress incontinence after repair (Hudson and Henrickse 1975; Hassim and Lucas 1974; Schleicher et. al. 1993). The development of successful techniques for dealing with this problem remains an unmet challenge in fistula surgery (Hilton et. al., 1998).

Loss of the urethra traditionally has been the most feared form of obstetric fistula. Complete urethral loss occurs in about 5% of fistula patients, with about 30% of fistula patients sustaining partial urethral injury. Mahfouz stated (1930) that fistulas «in which the whole urethra has sloughed» are «the most troublesome of all.» The experience of subsequent surgeons seems to bear this out. In a 1980 series based on 1,789 fistula patients, Sister Ann Ward reported that only 26 cases were inoperable; but in all 26 urethral loss was present. In urethral fistula repair, the surviving tissues must be reassembled not just as a tube, but as a supple, functional organ that serves both as a conduit for urine as well as a «gatekeeper» ensuring that the passage of urine occurs only at socially appropriate times and places. There are no comparative surgical studies that evaluate differing techniques of urethral reconstruction in patients with obstetric fistulas. Work of this kind is badly needed.

c) Ureters. Ureterovaginal fistulas from direct injury to the distal ureter during obstructed labor are uncommon, comprising only about 1% of fistula cases. Depending on the amount of tissue that is lost at the bladder base, the ureteral orifices can be found in bizarre locations, ranging from the lateral vaginal walls all the way up to the level of the vesicourethral junction and the pubic arch (Figure 6). Aberrant ureteral locations of this kind can easily be missed on clinical examination and are one cause of persistent incontinence after otherwise «successful» fistula closure. Standard urological tools such as ureteral stents are usually not available in hospitals in the developing world, and most of the surgeons who work in such hospitals are not trained in «urologic» techniques such as ureteral reimplantation (Waaldijk 1995).

d) Kidneys. The incidence of secondary injury to the upper urinary tract in fistula patients has received little study, but this phenomenon appears to be clinically important. Clinical experience suggests that renal failure is a common cause of death in women with obstetric fistulas. Upper tract damage could result from chronic ascending infection, obstruction from distal ureteral scarring, or even from reflux in very young patients. Lagundoye et al (1976) found that 49% of fistula patients had some abnormality of the kidneys when intravenous urograms were performed. Most of the pathology that was detected consisted of minor calyceal blunting, but 34% of patients had hydroureter, 9.7% had ureteral deviation, four patients had bladder stones, and 10 patients had a non-functioning kidney. In the developing world, hospitals typically have neither the laboratory capability to detect azotemia, nor the radiographic facilities to diagnose hydroureteronephrosis. It is clear, however, that injury to the kidneys is a common complication in patients with obstetric fistulas.

2. Gynecologic injury

a) Vagina. An impaction of the fetal head serious enough to cause ischemic injury to the bladder will also cause ischemic injury to the vagina, which is likewise trapped between the two bony surfaces. The necrotic areas that develop subsequently heal with varying degrees of scarring. A small sonographic study by Adetiloye and Dare (2000) detected fibrotic changes in 32% of fistula patients and minor vaginal wall fibrosis in another 36%. Vaginal injuries in fistula patients are arrayed along a spectrum the includes only small focal bands of scar tissue on one end all the way to virtual obliteration of the vaginal cavity on the other. Roughly 30% of fistula patients require some form of vaginoplasty at the time of fistula repair.

The degree of vaginal injury has several important implications. In the first instance, severe vaginal injury results in loss of substantial portions of the vagina. In many instances the scarring is such that vaginal intercourse is simply not possible. There is virtually no information available on the sexual functioning of fistula patients, yet this is obviously an important concern in healthy marital relationships and undoubtedly contributes to the high rates of separation and divorce that appear common among these women. Surgical repair of fistulas in women with extensive vaginal scarring often requires the use of flaps and tissue grafts in order to close the fistula. Little work has been done to assess whether or not sexual function normalizes in women who have had such operations. The presence of scarring that requires the use of plastic surgical techniques of this kind markedly reduces the effectiveness of surgical repair when fistula closure is attempted by surgeons who lack experience in reconstructive gynecologic surgery. Although several papers have described various techniques for vaginoplasty that may be required in fistula patients (Dick and Strover 1971; Hoskins et. al. 1984; Margolis et. al 1994), there is a pressing need to investigate the role of vaginal plastic surgery at the time of fistula repair and to evaluate subsequent sexual functioning in patients who require surgery of this kind.

Vaginal scarring impacts more than just sexual functioning. The presence of vaginal scarring appears to be an important prognostic factor in determining the likelihood both of successful fistula closure, and also for the development of debilitating urinary stress incontinence after otherwise successful fistula repair. In one unpublished series of 26 fistula patients with severe vaginal scarring, 57.7 percent suffered from stress incontinence after fistula repair and 23.5 percent had a persistent or recurrent fistula This would compare to an expected stress incontinence rate of around 26% and a failed fistula closure rate of about 7% in the overall population of fistula patients (Arrowsmith, personal communication). As Lawson Tait remarked in his book, *Diseases of Women* (1879): «One case, which I utterly failed to improve in any way, had the whole vagina destroyed by sloughing, so that the rectum, ureters, and uterus opened into a common cloaca about two inches deep, with walls of cartilaginous hardness. In such cases the damage is nearly always very extensive and very difficult to remedy.» Kelly and Kwast have also reported worsening surgical outcome in fistula patients who have vaginal scarring than in those without such findings (1993a).

Cervix, Uterus, and Future Reproductive Performance. Many patients sustain severe cervical damage as well as vaginal injury in the course of obstructed labor. When fistula patients are examined, a completely normal cervix is rarely seen. The presence of cervical injury would also help explain the apparently high prevalence of pelvic inflammatory disease encountered among these patients. In the worst cases, prolonged obstructed labor may result in complete cervical destruction, leaving the patient with no identifiable cervical tissue at all. Unfortunately, detailed descriptions of the condition of the cervix have not been included in the series of fistulas published to date. Since cervical competence is such an important factor in future reproductive performance, this is yet another clinical area that demands further study.

A review of the menstrual histories of 998 patients with obstetric fistulas in Ethiopia (Arrowsmith et. al. 1996) showed 63.1 percent were amenorrheic. Other studies have shown amenorrhea rates from 25% to 44% (Aimakhu 1974; Bieler and Schnabel 1976; Evoh and Akinla 1978). Many of these patients undoubtedly have hypothalamic or pituitary dysfunction (Bieler and Schnabel 1973). While the high incidence of amenorrhea in VVF patients is widely recognized, only one unpublished study has been done to look specifically at uterine pathology in the VVF population. Dosu Ojengbede of the University of Ibadan (personal communication) performed hysteroscopy on fistula patients in Nigeria and found that intrauterine scarring and Asherman's syndrome are common. The combination of widespread amenorrhea, vaginal scarring, and cervical destruction leads to a tremendous problem of secondary infertility among these patients. To date, there have been no serious scientific efforts to explore treatment of cervical and uterine damage in VVF patients.

Subsequent reproductive performance of women who have had an obstetric vesicovaginal fistula has been analyzed in a few articles (Naidu and Krishna 1963; Aimakhu 1974; Evoh and Akinla 1978; Emembolu 1992). Emembolu analyzed the subsequent reproductive performance of 155 fistula patients delivered at Ahmadu Bello University Teaching Hospital in Zaria, Nigeria, between January 1986 and December, 1990. This series included pregnancies in 75 women who became pregnant after successful fistula closure and 80 women who became pregnant while still afflicted with an unrepaired fistula that had occurred in a previous pregnancy. The data presented do not allow one to determine the subsequent fertility rates of women who develop a fistula, but clearly indicate that women can, and do, become pregnant after sustaining an obstetric fistula. The proportion of booked pregnancies receiving antenatal care was higher in the repaired group (73%) than in the unrepaired group (51%), and reproductive performance was better (but still dismal) in those patients who had had a fistula repair. Of the 69 patients whose fistulas had been repaired, there was a recurrence in 8 (11.6%), and among those undergoing a trial of vaginal delivery, the fistula recurrence rate was nearly 27%. In women with unrepaired fistulas who did not register for prenatal care, maternal mortality and morbidity in subsequent pregnancies was high and severe, and reflects the conditions that led to fistula formation in the first instance:

«Mrs. A.A., a 25-year-old unbooked para 1+0 (neonatal death) whose VVF was as yet unrepaired was admitted at 40 weeks gestation in the second stage of labor. She had been in labor at home for over 20 h before admission. Vaginal examination revealed that the vagina was markedly stenosed and the patient in advanced obstructed labor with an intrauterine fetal death. At cesarean section, the uterus was found to have ruptured. The macerated female fetus weighting 2800 g was delivered and the patient had a repair of the uterus with bilateral tubal ligation. She however died on the sixth post-operative day of persistent anemia and overwhelming infection due to Klebsiella species.

Mrs. M.A., a 28-year old unbooked para 1+0 (stillbirth) who had a residual vesico-vaginal fistula was admitted in labor at 34 weeks gestation. She had been in labor at home for about 19 h prior to admission in the second stage of labor. Vaginal examination revealed marked vaginal stenosis admitting only one finger. A diagnosis of advanced obstructed labor with fetal distress was made. At cesarean section, a severely asphyxiated female baby weighing 2200 g with Apgar score of 1 and 2 at 1 and 5 min was delivered. The baby died within 30 min of delivery. The mother subsequently developed post-partum eclampsia with septicemia from Staphylococcus aureus and died on the fourth post-operative day.

The commonest maternal morbidity, excluding recurrence of VVF, was hemorrhage requiring blood transfusion in 35 patients (27.3%). Others included ruptured uterus in 3 unbooked patients whose fistulae had not been repaired, bladder injury at cesarean section in 1.6% and acute renal failure in 0.8%. The maternal complication occurred more frequently in the patients whose fistulae had not been repaired and who were also unbooked.»

The largest series is that of Aimakhu, who analyzed subsequent reproductive performance in 246 women who underwent successful fistula closure at University College Hospital in Ibadan, Nigeria, between 1957 and 1966. Only 48 patients became pregnant following fistula repair with a total of 65 pregnancies. All but 6 of these were managed at University College Hospital. Five patients had aborted prior to the 16th week of gestation, leaving only 60 viable pregnancies. The plan was to perform elective Cesarean section on all patients who became pregnant after fistula surgery, but only 49 Cesarean operations were carried out. The results of the vaginal deliveries were not encouraging. Aimakhu summarized the results in this fashion (1974):

«Of the eight vaginal deliveries, six were our booked patients, and they were all admitted in the second stage of labor; one patient had in fact delivered the first of her twins before arrival. There were no maternal deaths among these six patients and there was no reopening of the fistulae after delivery. Five of the seven babies survived. The seventh patient with vaginal delivery had an instrumental vaginal delivery elsewhere. The baby was stillborn and the fistula recurred. At the beginning of the repair of the new fistula in our unit, this patient died from cardiac arrest. The eighth patient with vaginal delivery sustained her first fistula in her first delivery in 1952. This was successfully repaired elsewhere 4 years later. In 1962 she was allowed a vaginal delivery in another hospital. The baby was stillborn and the fistula recurred.. Following another successful repair of the fistula she became pregnant again. She defaulted from a cesarean section offered her in our unit. She delivered at home another stillborn baby and the fistula was again reopened.»

Patients who underwent cesarean delivery fared better. There were 49 fetuses delivered and 47 survived. There was no recurrent fistula among women previously repaired who became pregnant and had a subsequent cesarean section. There was one maternal death from pulmonary embolism in a woman who underwent a emergency delivery at 32 weeks gestation due to a prolapsed fetal umbilical cord.

3. The recto-vaginal fistula

Rectovaginal fistulas appear to be significantly less common than vesico-vaginal fistulas. In case series of patients presenting with vesico-vaginal fistulas, between 6% and 24%% have a combined recto-vaginal and vesico-vaginal fistula (Figure 7) (Arrowsmith 1994; Ashworth 1973; Aziz 1965; Bird 1967; Coetzee and Lithgow 1966; Emmett 1878; Hilton and Ward 1998; Mustafa and Rushwan 1971; Naidu 1962; Tahzib 1983, 1985; Waaldijk 1989). In most series, isolated recto-vaginal fistulas are less common than combined fistulas. Indeed, most series do not even mention isolated recto-vaginal fistulas as a clinical phenomenon. In a series of patients from Turkey reported by Yenen and Babuna (1965), 7.1% had recto-vaginal fistulas and 6.5% had «combined» fistulas. From the report it is not clear if this latter figure was comprised solely of recto-vaginal and vesico-vaginal fistulas, or if it included other combinations of urinary tract fistulas as well (vesico-cervico-vaginal, urethro-vaginal, etc.). Kelly and Kwast (1993), reporting data from the Addis Ababa Fistula Hospital, noted a 15.2% prevalence of combined fistulas, and a 6.8% prevalence of isolated rectovaginal fistulas in that population. Ethiopia appears to have one of the highest rates of recto-vaginal fistulas reported in the literature. Whether this relates to specific obstetric characteristics of the Ethiopian population or whether this relates to other social factors—-such as

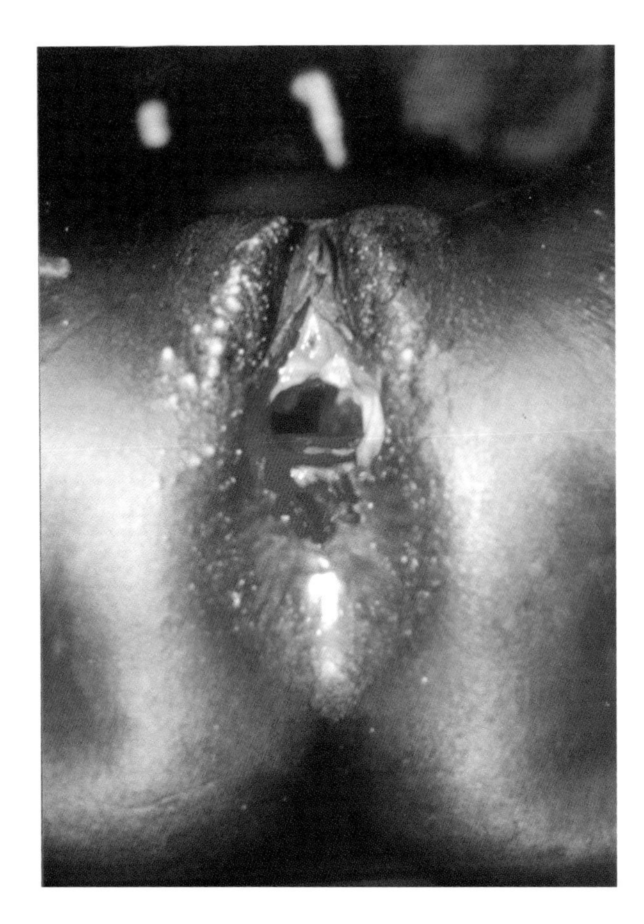

Figure 7 : Large combined vesicovaginal and rectovaginal fistula. (©Worldwide Fund for Mothers Injured in Childbirth, used by permission).

the cases of rape and sexual abuse of young Ethiopian girls reported by Muleta and Williams (1999)—is unclear.

Since the pubic symphysis poses an obstruction to delivery through the anterior pelvis, in normal birth mechanics the fetal head is normally forced posteriorly towards the rectum, anus, and perineum towards the end of the second stage of labor. In non-obstructed labor, direct laceration of the perineum is not uncommon, occasionally resulting in a complete perineal tear with complete disruption of the anal sphincter. If this is not repaired, a complete perineal tear with sphincter disruption can create a recto vaginal fistula at the anal outlet. This mechanism of fistula formation seems more likely to account for low recto-vaginal fistulas, whereas recto-vaginal fistulas higher in the pelvis would seem more likely to be caused by direct tissue compression from obstructed labor. As Mahfouz noted in 1938:

«The process by which faecal fistula forms after labour differs greatly from that which leads to the formation of a urinary fistula. Sloughing, due to pressure-necrosis produced by impaction of the presenting part, which accounts for the overwhelming majority of urinary fistulae, is seldom the cause of faecal fistula. It accounted for 2 case only in my series of 75. The majority of the remaining cases were the result of a complete tear of perineum which extended into the recto-vaginal septum. The lacerated edges of the perineum united spontaneously in the lower part where the tissues were fleshy, but remained ununited at the upper end where tissues were thin. This results in a permanent communication between the vagina and rectum at the upper end of the healed tear.»

In Das and Sengupta's series of 135 obstetric fistulas from India, there were 12 patients with recto-vaginal fistulas, 6 patients with complete perineal tears, 1 patient with both a recto-vaginal fistula and a complete perineal laceration, and 1 patient with a recto-vaginal fistula as well as a fistula-in-ano, giving a posterior fistula rate of 20/135 or 14.8%.

Because recto-vaginal fistulas appear to be less common than genito-urinary fistulas in the developing world, less attention has been paid to describing techniques for their repair in this setting. Mahfouz recommended different approaches to recto-vaginal fistulas, depending on their location (1938).

«The methods of treatment of faecal fistula differ according to their site. If the fistula is situated at the vaginal outlet, incorporated in or lying immediately above an incompletely healed perineal tear, the perineum should be cut through. In other words, the recto-vaginal fistula is converted into a complete tear of the perineum and is dealt with as such. The vaginal and rectal walls are next separated from one another by a transverse incision. This separation should be carried well above the upper edge of the fistula. The rent in the rectum is now carefully sutured with catgut. The sutures should not pierce the mucous membrane of the gut. The next step is to unite the levator ani muscles in the middle line so that a thick mass of tissue is interposed between the lines of sutures in the vagina and rectum respectively. The cut ends of the sphincter should now be very carefully brought together and the perineum reconstructed in the usual manner.

In dealing with rectal fistulae situated at a distance from the perineum the latter should not be cut through. These fistulae should be dealt with by a flap-splitting operation performed on the same principles employed in operating on urinary fistulae. The separation of the rectal from the vaginal wall should be carried until a point well beyond the upper and lower limits of the fistulae. In rectal fistulae this separation can be effected more easily, and much more widely, than separation of the bladder in urinary fistulae.»

These general principles still prevail. For example,

Arrowsmith (1994) recommended oral cathartics and cleansing enemas (where the fistulas were small enough to allow the patient to retain some enema fluid), followed by wide mobilization of the fistula, a two-layered rectal closure, with perineal reconstruction and the use of Martius bulbocavernosus fat flaps for large defects. These general principles have also been endorsed by Hudson (1970).

More problematic is the very high recto-vaginal fistula, where the fistula occurs in the upper vagina (Bentley 1973; Eden 1914; Lawson 1972; Mahfouz 1934). Such cases are particularly troublesome if the vagina is very stenotic or the fistula is fixed and tethered in such a manner as to prevent its being dissected free and brought down low enough so that a vaginal repair can be attempted. In these cases, the route of repair must be transabdominal. Before an abdominal attempt at recto-vaginal fistula repair, the patient should always have a temporary transverse colostomy performed prior to fistula repair and undergo as thorough a bowel preparation regimen as is possible. In Hudson's series of 88 high rectovaginal fistulas, successful closure was significantly more likely if a colostomy had been performed prior to attempted fistula closure (1970). Each abdominal repair operation is likely to be different, due to the comparative rarity of the high rectovaginal obstetric fistula and the variable severity and extent of the concurrent pathology that is likely to accompany it, but in general the surgeon should attempt to separate the vagina from the rectum, close the rectum in multiple layers, interpose a pedicled graft of omentum between the rectum and the vagina and, where possible, close the vagina separately (Bentley 1973).

Clinical experience suggests that «double fistulas» (combined vesico-vaginal and recto-vaginal fistulas) are more difficult to repair than solitary rectovaginal fistulas (Hudson 1970). In patients with double fistulas, the amount of normal tissue available for use as vaginal flaps is often very limited, and the reduction in vaginal space that occurs after successful closure of a double fistula can be formidable. The presence of a rectovaginal fistula also decreases the success rate for repairing the vesicovaginal fistula that is present.

Rectovaginal fistula repair presents special problems for the fistula surgeon, particularly in cases where the fistula is high or complex. Many gynecologic surgeons may not be comfortable performing a colostomy, let along more complex colon and rectal operations such as a colo-anal pull-through procedure. Colostomy surgery requires access to more sophisticated anesthesia capability than vaginal fistula repair, and in many cultures a colostomy is no more acceptable than a rectovaginal fistula, particularly as useable colostomy appliances are often difficult or impossible for most fistula patients to obtain. From a research perspective, the issue of anal sphincter function in obstetric fistula patients remains virtually unaddressed, both with regard to the presence of injuries in women who only have a vesico-vaginal fistula, as well as in patients who have had successful recto-vaginal fistula repair.

4. Orthopedic trauma

Ischemic injury from obstructed labor not only affects pelvic organs, but also the pelvis itself. These changes are most pronounced in the pubic symphysis. The normal radiography of the symphysis pubis has been described in detail by Vix and Ryu (1971). In obstructed labor, the pubic bones are often directly involved as one side of the bony vise in which the vulnerable soft tissues are trapped. In fistulas where large amounts of bladder tissue are lost, the periosteum of the pubic arch can often be palpated directly through the fistula defect. It is these cases in which ischemic damage to the pubic bones is most likely to be demonstrable. In a study of 312 Nigerian women with obstetric vesicovaginal fistulas Cockshott (1973) noted bony abnormalities in 32 percent on plain pelvic radiographs. The findings included bone resorption, marginal fractures and bone spurs, bony obliteration of the symphysis, and wide (>1 cm) symphyseal separation. Most of these changes appear to be the result of avascular necrosis of the pubic symphysis. Their long-term significance remains uncertain and further study is required.

5. Neurologic injury

Another tragic injury associated with obstetric fistula formation is foot-drop (Waaldjik and Elkins 1994). The relationship between difficult labor and neurological injury has been known for centuries, and the condition was traditionally called «obstetric palsy» (Sinclair 1952). Women with this condition have an inability to dorsiflex the foot and therefore walk with a serious limp, dragging their injured foot, and using a stick for support [Figure 8]. In Sinclair's paper on maternal obstetric palsy in South Africa (1952), he made the comment that «There are no records of this lesion associated with vaginal fistulae, where there has been prolonged pressure by the foetal skull in the lower part of the pelvis.» This statement is clearly wrong. In Waaldijk and Elkins' review of 947 fistula patients, nearly 65% of those studied prospectively had evidence of peroneal injury either by history or physical examination (1994). The prevalence of clinical footdrop among patients seen at the Addis Ababa Fistula Hospital is about 20% (Arrowsmith, Hamlin and Wall, 1996). Various theories have been proposed for the etiology of this condition. In general clinical series of peroneal nerve palsy, the most common etiologies appear to be direct trauma

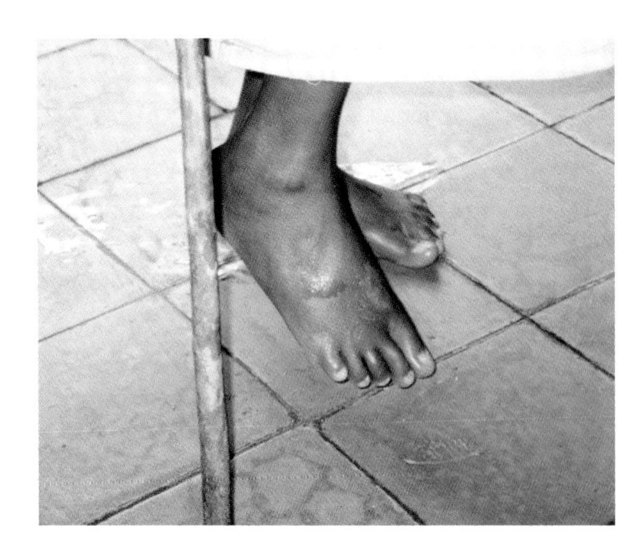

Figure 8 : Fistula patient with foot-drop, manifested by an inability to dorsiflex the foot. In particular note the trauma to the toes, as well as the constant puddle of urine in which she walks. (©Worldwide Fund for Mothers Injured in Childbirth, used by permission).

from ankle inversion, fractures of the hip, femur, fibula or tibia; knee injuries, alcoholic neuropathies, and a variety of miscellaneous or idiopathic causes. In obstetric patients the lesion most likely develops from one of three causes: prolapse of an intravertebral disk, pressure from the fetal head on the lumbo-sacral nerve trunk in the pelvis leading to direct compression of the peroneal nerve, or direct trauma to the peroneal nerve from prolonged squatting and pushing in the second stage of labor (Sinclair 1952; Colachis et. al. 1994, Reif 1988). Of the three possible etiologies, the last seems the most likely, however, to date no one has performed electromyographic studies of the lower extremities in fistula patients with foot-drop to evaluate the neurophysiological abnormalities that are present. Foot-drop has also been associated with trauma sustained in difficult forceps deliveries, particularly mid-pelvic rotations, but again, as others have emphasized «The peripheral nerve lesion following instrumental delivery may have developed in any case and forceps were but incidental or at the most a precipitating factor in border-line cases» (Sinclair 1952). The prognosis for recovery from this injury is unclear, as there are no proper prospective studies of women who have developed this condition. Waaldijk and Elkins suggest that most patients recover some or all of their nerve function spontaneously within two years of the injury (1994); however 13% showed persistent signs of nerve trauma. In some cases the affected women are almost completely crippled with bilateral lesions and suffer tremendously from the additional burden imposed by immobility on someone who already suffers from intractable urinary incontinence. Physiotherapy and the use of posterior splints improve the condition of some patients. Others may require surgical intervention: the use of posterior tibialis tendon transfer is a well-established procedure for patients with foot-drop from other causes (such as leprosy), and it may be that this method will be useful in treating women with unresponsive obstetric palsy as well (Hall 1977; Richard 1989).

6. Dermatologic injury

The condition of the skin, which is in constant, unremitting contact with a stream of urine or feces, is one of the most bothersome problems for the fistula patient [Figure 9]. The problems thus encountered have been eloquently described since the early days of fistula surgery. The great American gynecologist Thomas Addis Emmett summarized the clinical situation in 1868:

«Unless the greatest care has been given to cleanliness, the sufferer, in a few weeks after receiving the injury, becomes a most loathsome object. From the irritation of the urine, the external organs of generation become excoriated and oedematous, with the same condition extending over the buttocks and down the thighs. The labia are frequently the seat of deep ulcerations and occasionally of abscesses. The mucous membrane of the vagina is in part lost, and the abraded surface rapidly becomes covered at every point with a sabulous or offensive phosphate deposit from the urine. If the loss of tissue has been extensive, the inverted posterior wall of the bladder protrudes in a semi-strangulated condition, more or less incrusted with the same deposit, and bleeding readily. This deposit will frequently accumulate to such an extent in the vagina that the sufferer becomes unable to walk or even to stand upright, without the greatest agony.

The deposit must be carefully removed as far as possible by means of a soft sponge, and the raw surface brushed over with a weak solution of nitrate of silver. If, at any point, it cannot be at first removed without causing too much bleeding, the deposit itself must be treated in the same manner, or coated with the solid stick. Warm sitz-baths add greatly to the comfort of the sufferer. The vagina must be washed out several times a day with a large quantity of tepid water. After bathing, it is best for the patient to protect herself by freely anointing the outlet of the vagina and the neighboring parts with any simple ointment. She must be instructed to wash her napkins thoroughly when saturated with urine, and not simply to dry them for after-use. Time, and increased comfort of the patient, are gained by judicious attention to such details.

About every fifth day, the excoriated surfaces yet unhealed should be protected with the solution of nitrate of silver; and it is frequently necessary to pursue the same general course for many weeks, before the parts

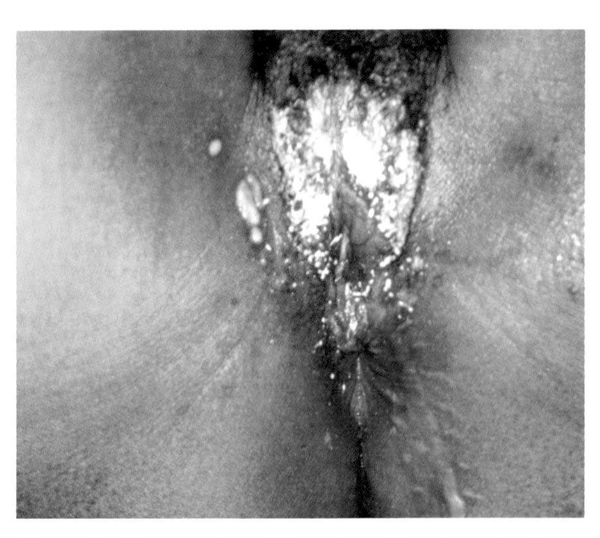

Figure 9 : Encrustation of the vulva with uric acid salts, as the result of the constant trickle of urine from the fistula. (©Worldwide Fund for Mothers Injured in Childbirth, used by permission).

can be brought into a perfectly healthy condition. This point is not reached until not only the vaginal wall, but also the hypertrophied and indurated edges of the fistula, have attained a natural color and density. This is the secret of success; but the necessity is rarely appreciated; without it, the most skillfully performed operation is almost certain to fail.

When the proper condition has been brought about, the surgeon may then be able to decide upon some definite plan of procedure for the closing of the fistula».

Further work remains to be done on determining the optimal regimen of skin care for patients with fistulas within the context of developing countries. It seems clear that efforts of this kind will produce marked improvements in the reduction of patient suffering, even before fistula closure is undertaken.

7. Social consequences of prolonged obstructed labor

Although physicians tend to think in terms of clinically definable injuries, much of the suffering that fistula patients endure is a result of the social consequences of their condition. It is vitally important to understand the social context in which these injuries occur (Wall 1998). Although there is no such thing as a monolithic «African culture», in many areas where fistulas are endemic there appear to be recurring patterns that allow for some general observations to be made regarding the position of women. In countries where there are high fistula rates, women generally have a lower social status than men. Often a woman's role in family life centers around a strong obligation to satisfy the sexual needs of her husband and to provide him with offspring (preferably male), and both men and women are dependent on their children for care when they become old. In many African societies, women are often called upon to perform heavy manual labor, tending the fields, carrying water and firewood. Religion—be it Islam, Christianity, or a traditional African religion—-also plays a more central role in day-to-day life than is common in Western countries. Each of these areas of human life is affected in a profoundly negative way by the injuries sustained in obstructed labor.

a) Marriage and family life

In societies where obstetric fistulas are still prevalent, a woman's role in life is defined almost exclusively in terms of marriage, childbearing, and the family life that results (Wall 1998). Because most women in these societies appear to accept this role at present, the inability to have children or to satisfy her husband's sexual needs may diminish her own sense of self worth. Vaginal injuries often make intercourse impossible, and the constant stream of urine makes it otherwise unpleasant. As members of agrarian societies, women are often expected to contribute long hours of hard labor working on the family farm. Foot drop and associated pelvic injuries may make the satisfactory performance of these tasks impossible. The woman, formerly a productive laborer, then becomes an economic burden as an invalid. The combination of all of these factors often leads to a gradual disintegration of the marriage over time, which then ends with complete rupture of the relationship. The existing data suggest that large numbers of fistula patients become divorced or separated from their husbands, particularly when it becomes evident that their condition is chronic, rather than transient. Unpublished data from Ethiopia suggest that almost 50 percent of VVF victims are divorced or separated (S.D. Arrowsmith, personal communication). Murphy's research documented similar findings in northern Nigeria (1981).

Infertility is a devastating problem to couples in any culture, but it is difficult to underestimate the importance of fertility in African societies. Large families are a source of pride and a symbol of affluence. Since the social, economic, and political lives of these societies are still dominated in many respects by ties of kinship, not having offspring is a disaster on many fronts. Furthermore, large families may be the only source of reliable (or affordable) farm labor, a critical economic factor in societies based on peasant agriculture. Because governmental social welfare programs are unreliable or non-existent in most African countries, children are the only hope one has for security in old age. The fetal mortality in obstructed labor is staggering, generally above 90%. Since obstructed labor is most commonly a complication of a woman's first labor, and since she is usually infertile thereafter, the majority of fistula victims (about 70%) have no living children. Not only is this a disaster for the affected woman, but from her husband's perspective, it puts his whole future in jeopardy as well. Faced with this prospect, many men find it easier to rid themselves of their damaged wives and seek other, fertile, spouses.

Although obstructed labor is most common as a complication of a first pregnancy, it can occur in any pregnancy if the baby is too large, presents wrong, or other complications arise. In a review of 121 obstetric fistulas from Kumasi, Ghana, Danso and colleagues found that 43% of patients had had three or more pregnancies, and that 25% had had five or more (Danso et. al. 1996). Similarly, at the Addis Ababa Fistula Hospital, nearly 25% of fistula patients have had three or more pregnancies, and 11 percent have had six or more children (Kelly and Kwast, 1993). What happens to the living children when their mother's life is ruined in this fashion? Important indirect health consequences of fistula formation such as this have been largely unexplored.

b) Religious and social implications

In some parts of the world, such as northern Nigeria, married women live under a system of «wife seclusion» in which their social contacts are severely restricted to their immediate family and female neighbors (Wall 1998). The offensive odor that accompanies total urinary and/or fecal incontinence usually curtails even this limited opportunity for social interaction. In order to deal with the never-ending problem of foul smells and omnipresent urine and fecal loss, the families of these patients may remove them from the main family dwelling into a peripheral hut, sometimes even forcing them to live outdoors. Not uncommonly, they are often forced out of the family compound altogether over time.

Because of the nature of her injury, a fistula patient simply cannot maintain normal hygiene, no matter how hard she tries. This fact has an enormous impact on all aspects of her life, including her participation in religious or spiritual life. Fistula women are generally regarded as both physically and ritually unclean. Many African religious groups, especially Muslims, require personal cleanliness as a prerequisite for worship. This often excludes them from participation in religious activities (often a central concern of African social life); this further diminishes their sense of self-worth and social connectedness.

The tragedy faced by these women was described very eloquently by Kelsey Harrison, who had extensive experience with their plight as a result of his long tenure as Professor of Obstetrics and Gynaecology at Ahmadu Bello University in Zaria, Nigeria (1983):

«Whether in hospital or outside, their own society goes to great lengths to ostracize these girls, an action disparaged by outsiders but considered reasonable by most local people including certain (male) health workers. Their point of view is straightforward enough. The safe delivery of a healthy baby is always an occasion for great rejoicing and at the naming ceremony held on the eighth day after birth, the whole family and local community celebrate. In the case of the girl with an obstetric fistula, the baby is usually stillborn and this together with the fact that her odour is offensive means that such celebrations cannot take place. Soon, her incontinence becomes confused with venereal disease, and the affected family feels a deep sense of shame. The consequences are devastating: the girl is initially kept hidden; subsequently, she finds it difficult to maintain decent standards of hygiene because water for washing is generally scarce; divorce becomes inevitable and destitution follows, the girl being forced to beg for her livelihood. So traumatic is this experience that even when cured, some girls never regain their self esteem."

In considering the overall impact of the fistula problem, one should consider the life-time burden of suffering that this condition presents. The vast majority of these women are young and develop their fistula in their first pregnancy. In a series of over 9,000 fistula victims in Ethiopia the average patient age was 19 yrs (Arrowsmith, Hamlin and Wall, 1996). Most of the injuries associated with prolonged obstructed labor cause permanent disability without causing early death. The members of the committee have seen patients presenting for surgery over 40 years after the initial injury: the wasted years of human life represented by such cases is mind-numbing.

Professor Abbo Hassan Abbo, Professor of Obstetrics and Gynaecology at the University of Khartoum in the Sudan, himself an international authority on fistulas, tells a powerfully poignant story of a group of Somali women with fistulas who, in despair, chained themselves together and jumped off the dock in Mogadishu in a mass suicide because their suffering had become unendurable. (A.H. Abbo, personal communication).

The social ramifications of having a fistula is a major co-morbidity that is easy to forget unless one has seen the patient in her own social setting. This is why the proper care of fistula victims must be based on a holistic approach that pays as much attention to healing the psycho-social wounds inflicted on these women as it does to curing their physical injuries. Programs for women with obstetric fistulas must encompass education, literacy training, the development of social networks, and the provision of skills with which to earn an adequate livelihood, if the social problems that these women face are to be overcome (Bangser 1999). Some women are so injured that they can never return to their home villages, and many have such serious medical problems that they linger around fistula centers and become permanent residents. At the Addis Ababa Fistula Hospital, many of these women become nursing aides, taking care of other fistula patients. In a unique social experiment, that institution is developing a permanent residential farm for the most severely injured of these women, in essence forming a new women's community based on shared experiences and the «sisterhood of suffering» that has resulted (E.C. Hamlin, personal communication).

V. THE CLASSIFICATION OF OBSTETRIC FISTULAS

At the present time, there is no generally accepted, standardized system for describing, classifying, or staging obstetric fistulas. The situation remains much the same as it was in 1951, when Bayard Carter and colleagues lamented, «It is difficult to interpret and to compare many of the reported series of fistulas. There is a real need for standard methods to describe the fistulas, the actual operations, and results.» McConnachie (1958) eloquently summed up the problems surrounding discussions of fistula repair in the following words:

«It is common to find that each author has either used his own form of classification based solely on the anatomical structures involved, or the size of the fistula, or even one of convenience. But no two writers seem to have reached any common grounds for agreement other than that a urinary fistula is present. This lack of agreement has prevented comparison between individual workers' material or results, based on a common scientific classification. Such classification needs to be full yet simple, workable in its details so that it will not be cumbersome, to be based on the three principal anatomical structures involved in urinary leakage [bladder, urethra, ureters], and to take into account the clinical aspects of site, size, accessibility and condition of the tissues involved in attempted repair.»

In describing their experience with fistula repair, many surgeons have put forth various systems or rationales for grouping cases together. The earliest such system was that of Sims (1852) who classified fistulas according to their location in the vagina: 1) urethro-vaginal fistulas, where the defect was confined to the urethra; 2) fistulas situated «at the bladder neck or root of the urethra, destroying the trigone;» 3) fistulas involving the body and floor of the bladder; and 4) utero-vesical fistulas where the opening of the fistula communicated with the uterine cavity or cervical canal. Succeeding authors have added to, modified, and re-grouped the categories of fistulas in a variety of ways (Emmett 1868, Mahfouz 1930; Thomas 1945; Krishnan 1949; Lawson 1968; McConnachie 1958; Moir 1961; Hamlin and Nicholson 1969; Hilton and Ward 1998; Waaldijk 1994, 1995). Mahfouz (1930) listed the main points to be considered in the evaluation of a fistula as follows:

- The situation, size, form and variety of the fistula
- The scarring of the vagina and its effect on the mobility of the fistula
- The attachment of the fistula to the pelvic walls
- The condition of the urethral sphincter and permeability of the internal orifice of the urethra (occasionally the urethra is completely occluded by fibrosis)
- The location of the ureteral orifices, and their relation to the edges of the fistula
- The presence of complications such as recto-vaginal fistula, inflammatory lesions of the pelvis, vagina, vulva or peritoneum
- The presence of more than one fistula

There is an urgent need to develop a standardized, generally-accepted system for describing and classifying fistulas, to aid communication between fistula centers and to facilitate research in this field. The committee has not taken upon itself the task of developing such as system, but recommends that the Standardization Committee of the International Continence Society make this a priority in the future. The committee feels that the following factors should be taken into account in the development of a standardized ICS Classification System:

- The system should provide a simple yet precise method of describing fistula location and size. Although the size of the fistula may be quite impressive in cases of prolonged obstructed labor, the actual size of the opening is probably less important in the overall prognosis than other factors. As John St. George noted in 1969, «This [size] is not very important as long as other factors are favourable. It has been found that an opening of 1 cm or less with unhealthy tissues, fixed to bone within a stenosed vagina, is worse than an opening of 5 cm or more with lax vaginal walls, no fixity and a wide vaginal introitus. Also, a small bladder neck fistula is found to be more difficult and less successful at repair than a large mid-vaginal fistula.»
- The system should make some attempt to assess the impact of the fistula on function; i.e. how does the fistula impact the bladder neck, urethra, ureters, or (in the case of rectovaginal fistulas) the anus and its sphincter mechanism?

- The presence, location, and degree of vaginal scarring should be quantified, as this appears to be directly related to the probability of successful fistula closure. Many authors have commented on the grim prognosis for fistulas complicated by vaginal scarring. Das and Sengupta noted (1969) «Massive scarring is frequently present and is definitely a great handicap for a successful vaginal operation. Annular constriction ring around the vagina, distal to the fistula, with fixity to the pubic bones with cartilagenous margins are very unfavourable signs. But, fortunately it is noted that once the neighbouring bands of adhesions are released, the bladder can be brought down easily and anatomic apposition made.»

Any classification system for fistulas should be based on criteria that correlate with the prognosis for successful surgical repair. This will require looking at the whole patient, rather than simply looking at just the fistula. In a comparative study of failed fistula repairs carried out in Addis Ababa, Kelly and Kwast (1993a) found a statistically significant association ($p < 0.001$) with failed fistula repair and a ruptured uterus, with a previous history of failed surgical repair (especially repairs carried out at other, non-specialist, institutions), with the presence of limb contractures, with the need for special preoperative feeding in order to become fit enough for surgery, and with the presence of a «complicated» fistula requiring more extensive and more complicated surgical intervention. These authors believed that these factors reflected a more extensive injury from prolonged obstructed labor. McConnachie (1958) suggested that failures in fistula surgery were due to previous failed repairs with increased scar tissue formation, differences in the grade and type of fistulas reported in various series, to inexperienced operators taking on cases beyond their surgical capabilities, and «residual urinary sepsis and alkalinity.» Further comparative studies are needed to ascertain if these factors are reliably associated with surgical failure, and to determine if other, as yet unascertained, factors are also related to a poorer surgical prognosis.

- There should be a standardized definition of «success» in fistula surgery. In his series of 303 fistulas, McConnachie (1958) refused to regard the patient as «cured» even though the fistula was «closed» unless «she also has complete urinary continence and control.» This principle reduced his overall success («closed and dry») rate from 79.5% to 65.1%. Perhaps as many as one third of women who undergo successful fistula *closure* still have significant incontinence due to the presence of sphincteric damage and/or other persistent alterations in bladder or anorectal function. To classify as a «success» a woman who has a closed fistula but continuous, debilitating stress incontinence from a non-functioning urethra is both dishonest and clinically unhelpful.

- In describing surgical success rates, the time at which this assessment is made must be clearly specified. Long-term outcome data on women who have undergone fistula repair surgery are almost entirely lacking in the literature. Given the difficult circumstances from which most fistula patients come, and the difficulties of travel and communication in rural Africa, this is not surprising. As a result of these problems, most «successes» are evaluated as such only at the time of discharge from hospital, with almost no further follow-up. This may well be misleading as to actual outcome. Coetzee and Lithgow (1966) defined «cure» of a patient with a vesicovaginal fistula as follows:

«For a 100% cure the following conditions must be fully satisfied: 1) The patient should have complete continence by day and by night, and to achieve this it has been found that the bladder should hold a minimum of 170 ml. 2) No stress incontinence should be present. 3) The vagina should allow normal coitus without dyspareunia. 4) Traumatic amenorrhea should not result. 5) The patient should be able to bear children.»

- Achieving standards this high in patients who have undergone extensive pelvic trauma from obstructed labor will not be easy, but honesty is the first prerequisite if progress is to be made with true scientific integrity.

- General agreement should be reached concerning what constitutes an «irreparable fistula»—that is, which women should be offered urinary and/or colonic diversion as their first surgical procedure, rather than undergo an attempt at fistula closure? The committee recommends that the term «irreparable fistula» be used in preference to the phrase «hopeless fistula,» which is sometimes encountered in these discussions.

- Any system for the classification or staging of obstetric fistulas must emphasize low-technology clinical assessment, since such a system will have to be used in areas of the world with extremely limited resources. Fistulas afflict the world's poorest women, not the affluent elites of industrialized economies.

- In view of the multi-system pathology produced by obstructed labor, any classification system should note the presence of associated conditions related to the primary pathophysiological process in obstructed labor, such as the presence of neurologic injury, damage to the pubic symphysis, the concurrent presence of a recto-vaginal fistula, the presence of chronic skin ulcers, nutritional state, etc.

- Because most of the suffering endured by fistula victims is the result of social isolation and abandonment and the subsequent loss of self-esteem and economic deprivation that results from this social isolation, the evaluation of women with obstetric fistulas should include information on these social «co-morbidities.» The fistula problem in the developing world is inextricably intertwined with its social milieu, and this must be openly acknowledged.

VI. EARLY CARE OF THE FISTULA PATIENT

Although many patients with vesico-vaginal fistulas appear for care many years after they have sustained their injury, others arrive at a medical facility in obstructed labor, or shortly after the fistula appears. The traditional teaching has been that an attempt at repair should be deferred for three months until the extent of the injury has fully manifested itself and any infection/inflammation in the injured tissues has resolved. However, it also appears to be true that some fistulas might be prevented by prompt treatment of women who arrive after obstructed labor, that some fistulas might close spontaneously if the bladder is drained for a prolonged period of time, and that a subset of fistulas might even be amenable to early closure. John St. George (1969) believed that prompt medical treatment of patients after obstructed labor could prevent post-partum sepsis and promote the healing of injured tissues, thus preventing some fistulas altogether, or at least minimize the extent of injury that developed. He advocated vigorous local care of the injured tissues and prompt antibiotic treatment as soon as such patients were seen. He described one particularly noteworthy case:

«The patient, who was aged 18, was brought to the hospital three days after delivery, following labour which lasted seven days. She was incontinent of urine and faeces. She was very pale (haemoglobin concentration 3.7 g per 100 ml), dehydrated, toxic and unable to walk. Vaginal examination revealed a gaping opening with offensive purulent lochia and discharge. The lateral walls of the vagina had sloughed, revealing both pubic rami and the right ischial tuberosity. The perineum was torn, leaving an indefinite anal sphincter. A large vesico-vaginal fistula and a small recto-vaginal fistula, both with infected edges, were seen. Apart from blood transfusions, parenteral antibiotics and high protein diet were given: the vagina was douched twice daily with warm Dettol solution; this was followed each time by insertion of layers of ofra tulle gauze. After three weeks, the local treatment was given only once daily for another three weeks. When the patient was examined under anesthesia ten weeks after admission, and before discharge from hospital, the vaginal walls had healed over and returned to normal; the perineum had healed, leaving only a wide vaginal introitus; the recto-vaginal fistula had healed and the vesico-vaginal fistula was reduced to 1 cm diameter with mobile surrounding edges. She returned for repair three months later, and this was successfully carried out. Prevention of sepsis was the chief factor in such a transformation as occurred in this case, as in many others, and repair would otherwise have failed.»

Further research on the effectiveness of immediate local care after fistula formation should be encouraged. Waaldijk (1994) found that 50 - 60% of smaller fistulas (< 2 cm) would heal spontaneously, if prompt prolonged bladder drainage was started within three months of the initial injury. If the fistula did not close with simple catheter management, he performed an early closure. Using this regimen, he reported a successful closure rate in 92% of cases, with continence in 94% of those in whom the fistula was closed successfully. These results are encouraging, but await replication at other centers.

VII. SURGICAL TECHNIQUE FOR FISTULA CLOSURE

In general, specific issues of surgical technique are among the least important issues in obstetric fistula repair today. In practiced hands, skilled fistula surgeons routinely achieve fistula closure rates of 80% or better. Multiple papers reporting large case series support this contention (Abbott 1950; Amr 1998; Arrowsmith 1994; Ashworth 1973; Aziz 1965; Bird 1967; Coetzee and Lithgow 1966; Ghароror and Abedi 1999; Goh 1998; Hamlin and Nicholson 1966, 1969; Hilton and Ward 1998; Iloabachie 1992; Kelly 1992; Krishnan 1949; Lavery 1955; Lawson 1972; Mahfouz 1929, 1930, 1938, 1957; Moir 1966; Mustafa and Rushwan 1971; Naidu 1962; Waaldijk 1989; Yenen and Babuna 1965). There is a fairly general consensus concerning the basic principles of fistula repair, which can be summarized as follows:

- The best chance for successful fistula closure is at the first operation. In their large series of 2,484 fistula patients, Hilton and Ward (1998) reported successful fistula closure in 82.8% of patients at the first attempt. Successful closure was achieved in only 65% of those patients who required two or more operations.
- The fistula should be widely mobilized from the surrounding tissues at the time of repair, so that fistula closure can be achieved without tension on the site of repair.

- The repair must be «water-tight» at the time of closure. If it is not, failure is virtually certain. The simplest way to test this is to instill a solution of colored water into the bladder at the time of fistula closure and make certain that no leakage can be demonstrated. If leakage occurs, the repair should be taken down and repeated or reinforced until no leakage can be demonstrated. As J. Marion Sims wrote in his original paper on fistula repair (1854), «if a single drop of urine finds its way through the fistulous orifice, it is sure to be followed by more, and thus a failure to some extent is almost inevitable.»
- The fistula should be closed in multiple layers, avoiding over-lapping lines of suture, whenever this can be achieved.
- After fistula repair, the bladder should be emptied by prolonged continuous catheter drainage in order to prevent distention of the bladder and increased tension on the suture lines. The traditional duration of bladder drainage is 14 days, but no comparative trials have been carried out to see if shorter duration of bladder drainage (for example, 7 or 10 days) is associated with increased risk of failed repair. Research on the optimal duration of bladder drainage is important, and has obvious consequences for fistula centers with large clinical volumes. If, for example, the duration of post-operative catheterization could be decreased from 14 days to 10 days without a significant increase in failure rates, the center could increase the number of fistula patients undergoing surgical repair by almost 30%.
- Especially in the case of fistulas due to prolonged obstructed labor where the injury is the result of prolonged ischemia and tissue necrosis, successful closure is enhanced by the use of tissue grafts (bulbocavernosus graft, gracilis muscle graft, etc.) which bring a new blood supply to the site of repair. There is one retrospective paper in the literature that evaluated the repair of comparable fistulas with and without the use of Martius bulbocavernosus flaps and demonstrated substantially higher rates of successful closure when such a graft was employed (Rangnekar et. al. 2000).

Each fistula is unique, and an ability to improvise in the face of unexpected findings or complications is a virtue that every fistula surgeon must strive to develop. It is clearly not possible to illustrate here every different type of fistula and all of the various techniques that may be employed to close them. However, a generally accepted technique—-based largely on the work of Drs. Reginald and Catherine Hamlin at the Addis Ababa Fistula Hospital in Ethiopia where nearly 20,000 obstetric fistulas have now been repaired— can be described and illustrated as follows [Figures 10 - 29]. The first prerequisite for successful fistula repair is meticulous attention to detail. As Abbot aptly (if somewhat quaintly) noted (1950), «There must be no attempt to operate on these cases with one eye on the clock and the other on the tea wagon. In fact, the operator upon vesico-vaginal fistulae should combine the traits of daintiness, gentleness, neatness and dexterity of the pekinese, with the tenacity and perseverance of the English bulldog.»

The position for fistula surgery depends upon the nature and location of the fistula to be repaired. For the vast majority of straightforward fistulas (especially for mid-vaginal fistulas) a high lithotomy position with the buttocks pulled well over the edge of the operating table, provides excellent exposure [Figure 10]. Surgery in this position is easy to perform under spinal anesthesia, which is the cheapest and easiest form of anesthesia for «low technology» settings in developing countries. To operate in the knee-chest position is relatively uncomfortable for patients and can compromise pulmonary function. Performing operations in the knee-chest position generally requires intubation of the patient, the use of general anesthesia, and continuous ventilation. Trans-abdominal surgery with the patient in the supine position is rarely needed, except for certain complex fistulas. An abdominal approach increases both the cost of surgery and the likelihood of complications, such as wound infections. When doing fistula surgery in the developing world, failure to use a trans-vaginal approach requires special justification, such as cases in which additional intra-abdominal pathology must be addressed.

The first requirement for successful fistula repair is adequate exposure of the operative field. Figure 11

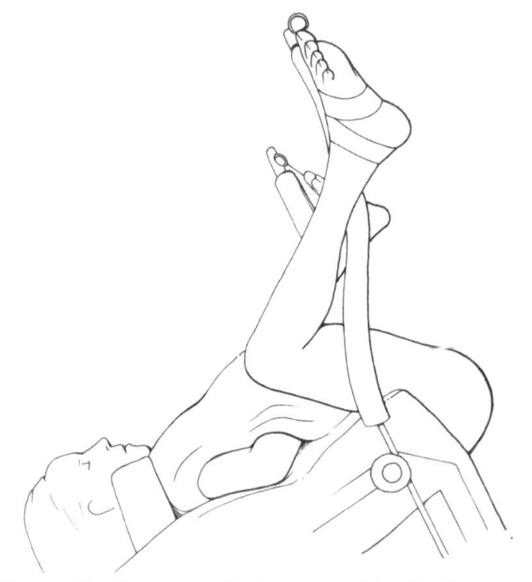

Figure 10 : Exaggerated lithotomy position for fistula repair. The patient is positioned at 35 - 45 degrees, head down position, with the use of shoulder supports and the buttocks pulled over the edge of the table. (©Worldwide Fund for Mothers Injured in Childbirth, used by permission).

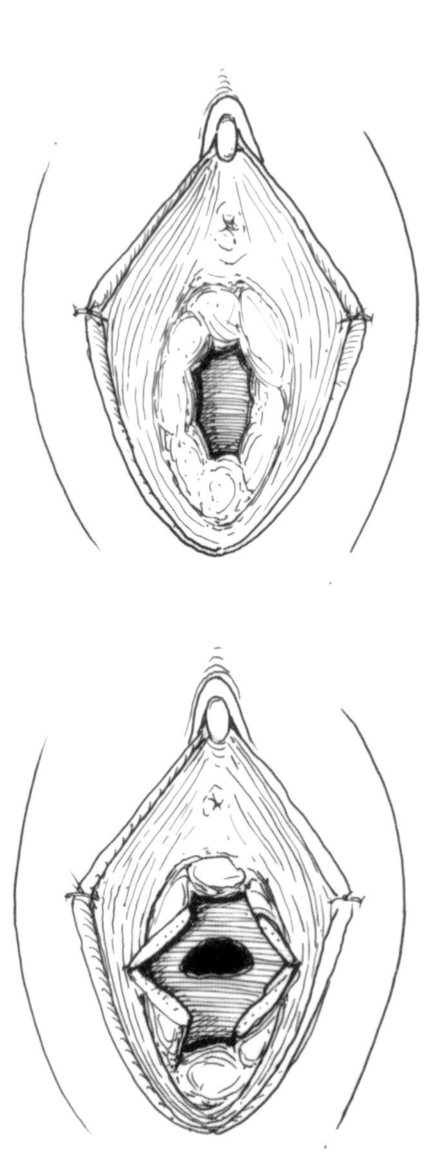

Figure 11 : Placement of labial stay sutures helps increase lateral exposure. Incisions through bands of scar tissue are often necessary to allow insertion of retractors. The upper illustration shows the vagina prior to relaxing incisions. The lower illustration shows enhanced exposure after relaxing incisions. (©Worldwide Fund for Mothers Injured in Childbirth, used by permission).

depicts a typically narrow, scarred vagina of the type that often develops after obstructed labor. The vesico-vaginal fistula is not clearly visible as it is obscured by scar tissue and a constriction ring. When this scar tissue is released by performing vaginal relaxing incisions, the fistula can be seen and repaired. The fistula depicted here is a straightforward mid-vaginal vesico-vaginal fistula.

It is generally preferable to identify and catheterize the ureters in most operations so that they are readily identifiable throughout the course of the operation. This can usually be done by passing catheters through the fistula into the ureters under direct vision [Figure 12]. The purpose of ureteral catheterization is ensure that the ureters are not inadvertently ligated during the fistula repair, with subsequent renal damage or death. (This was the cause of death in Sims' only operative fatality; unfortunately, it occurred in a very public demonstration of his technique for fistula closure in London at the Samaritan Hospital; see McKay 1922:518). Although some fistula surgeons prefer to leave ureteral catheters in place for up to 14 days after surgery, current Western urological practice would suggest that such catheters can be removed immediately at the end of the case, or within a day or two after surgery at most.

Once the fistula is exposed and the ureters are identified, it is important to mobilize the fistula fully so that it may be closed without tension. Figure 13 demonstrates the first move in mobilizing a mid-vaginal fistula. The posterior border of the fistula is incised and the incision is carried out laterally onto the vaginal sidewalls. The incision extends only through the vaginal epithelium, not into the bladder itself. Wide vaginal dissection will allow complete mobilization of the fistula.

Following the initial vaginal incision, the posterior vaginal flap is developed, always keeping the course of the ureters in mind [Figure 14].

Continued mobilization of the fistula is achieved by extending the incision circumferentially around the fistula, then anteriorly towards the urethra [Figure 15]. As before, the incision extends only through the vaginal epithelium, not into the bladder. When this portion of the operation has been completed, the bladder should be freed completely from the vagina. When this has been accomplished, the ureteral catheters can be passed through back into the bladder and brought out through the urethra to keep them out of the operative field.

The anterior vaginal flaps then are developed widely to mobilize the fistula more completely [Figure 16]. Due to the presence of scarring and tethering of the fistula, it is generally useful to carry the anterior dissection upwards behind the pubic symphysis, opening the retropubic Space of Retzius and detaching the bladder from its supports in this area. This allows full mobilization of the fistula [Figure 17]. The anterior vaginal flaps can be sutured out of the operative field using «stay sutures.»

Additional tension may be taken off the fistula at this point by performing a partial bladder suspension by passing sutures from the bladder up behind the pubic symphysis and anchoring the sutures in the symphyseal periosteum [Figure 18]. Persistent stress incontinence is relatively common in patients after otherwise successful fistula closure. It has been argued that suture placement of this type reduces the prevalence of this problem post-operatively (Hudson, Hendrickse, and Ward 1975;

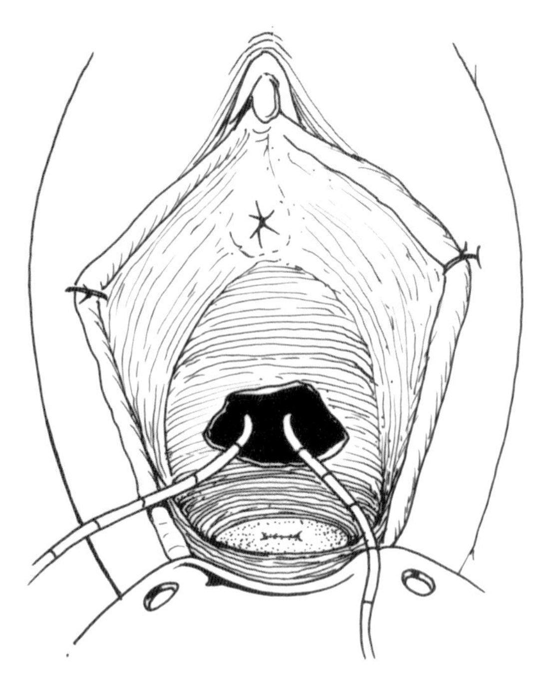

Figure 12 : Ureters are identified and cannulated, if possible. The use of intravenous diuretics and/or vital dyes can be used to improve ureteric localization, if needed. (©Worldwide Fund for Mothers Injured in Childbirth, used by permission).

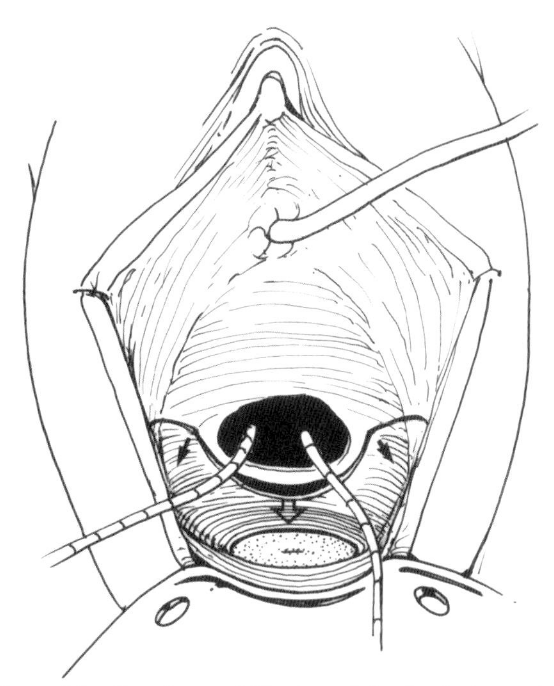

Figure 14 : Complete mobilization of the fistula is continued by raising posterior vaginal flaps. The mobilization is carried out to each vaginal sidewall as well as to the cervix (if one is still present). Special care must be taken at the 4 and 7 o'clock positions to avoid possible injury to the ureters. (©Worldwide Fund for Mothers Injured in Childbirth, used by permission).

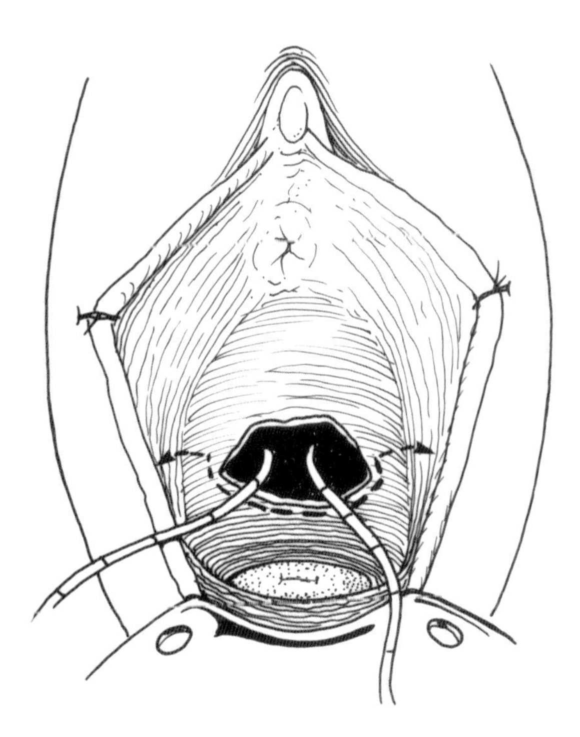

Figure 13 : Dissection of the fistula begins at its posterior margin by making an incision that runs from one vaginal sidewall to the other. Accentuation of tissue planes in some cases may be aided by local infiltration of saline or local anesthetic. (©Worldwide Fund for Mothers Injured in Childbirth, used by permission).

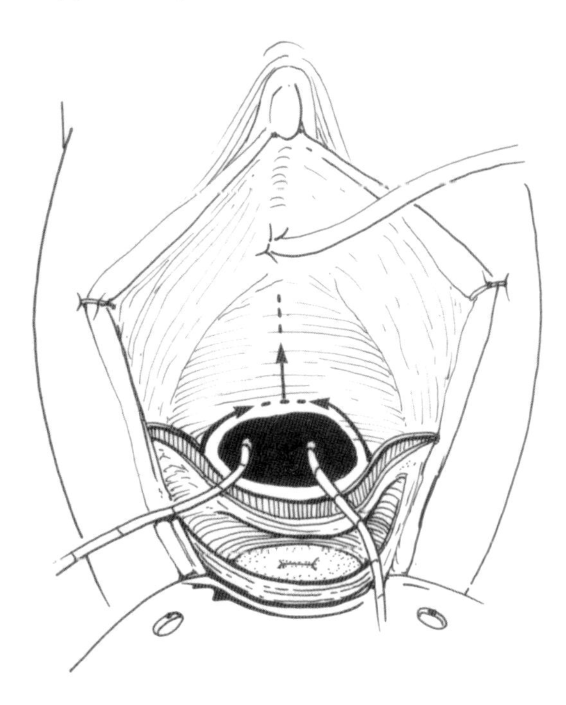

Figure 15 : The mobilizing incision is extended circumferentially around the fistula. When this is completed, an anterior midline incision is made in the vagina and extended up towards the external urethral meatus. (©Worldwide Fund for Mothers Injured in Childbirth, used by permission).

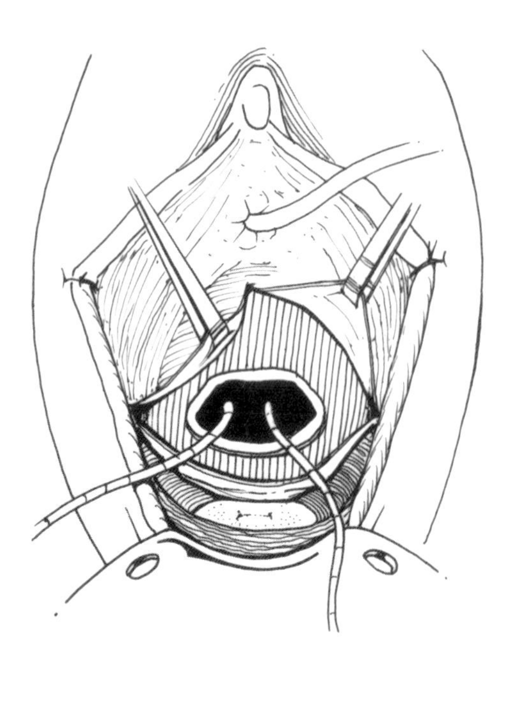

Figure 16 : The anterior vaginal flaps should be mobilized all the way from the edge of the fistula to the pubic arch. (©Worldwide Fund for Mothers Injured in Childbirth, used by permission).

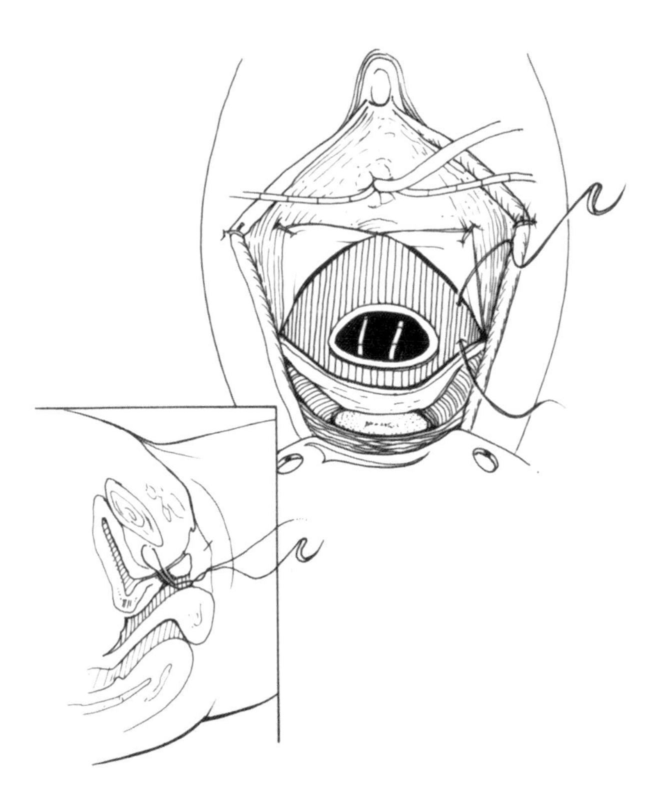

Figure 18 : Closure of the fistula begins by placing anchoring sutures lateral to the bladder defect and superiorly through the periosteum of the pubic arch. The sutures are designed to decreases tension across the line of bladder closure. (©Worldwide Fund for Mothers Injured in Childbirth, used by permission).

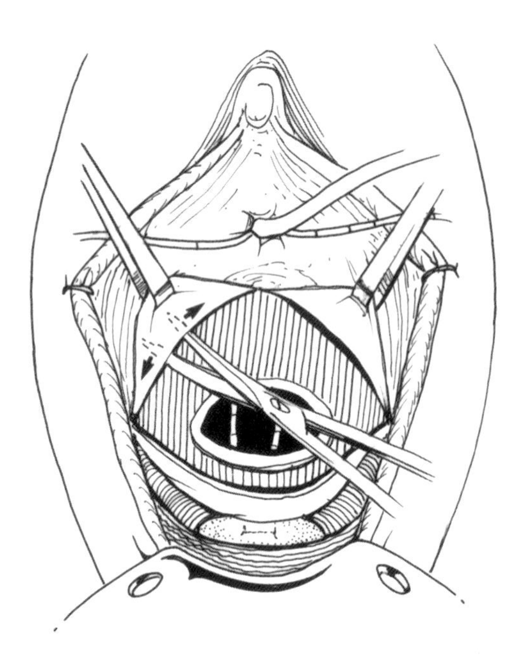

Figure 17 : Once the anterior flaps have been fully developed, the endopelvic fascia is perforated and the space of Retzius is entered, to complete the full mobilization of the fistula. This portion of the operation is often technically challenging. The apices of the anterior vaginal flaps can be retracted out of the operative field with stay sutures to improve visualization of the fistula. At this point, the bladder base and vagina should be completely separated from one another. It is generally not necessary (or advisable) to trim or "pare back" the edges of the fistula. This only increases the size of the defect and decreases the amount of remaining bladder tissue. (©Worldwide Fund for Mothers Injured in Childbirth, used by permission).

Hassim and Lucas 19740); however, no controlled studies have yet been carried out that document this assertion.

Once the fistula has been mobilized as fully as possible, fistula closure can begin. There are many different techniques by which this task may be accomplished. One proven technique is to close the first layer of the bladder with a continuous, running, interlocking stitch of an absorbable suture [Figure 19]. The initial suture bite should be placed beyond the lateral margin of the fistula and the last suture should be placed in a similar position on the opposite side of the fistula. Although Sims initially «pared back» the edges of the fistula in his closure technique, there seems to be no need to do this in the vast majority of obstetric fistulas: a better philosophy is to preserve as much bladder tissue as possible, particularly when attempting to close extensive fistulas.

After initial fistula closure has been completed, the primary suture line should be reinforced by a second layer of closure if at all possible. Ideally this should be done in such a fashion that the second row of sutures imbricates the initial closure, rolling more bladder tissue over the first line of closure in order to protect it [Figure 20]. When the second layer has been closed, the integrity of the repair should be checked by instilling 150 - 250 ml of water colored with indigo carmine, methylene blue, or another suitable dye. If there is no leakage of colored water, the fistula repair can be assumed to be «water tight,» and the operation can proceed. If leakage is observed, the repair should be taken down and repeated until no more leakage is observed.

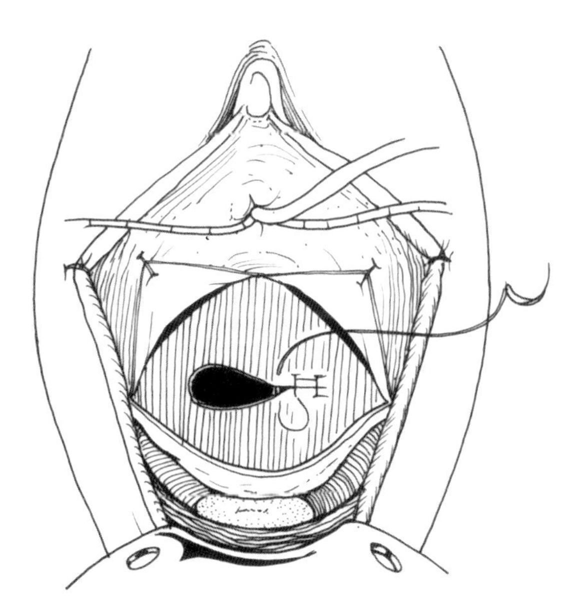

Figure 19 : Fistula closure. The bladder defect is closed in two layers using absorbable suture. If any tension is encountered during bladder closure, the initial dissection has been inadequate and should be revised. The first closure can be made with either interrupted sutures or a continuous running, interlocking, suture. (©Worldwide Fund for Mothers Injured in Childbirth, used by permission).

Extensive experience with fistula repairs has led many surgeons to believe that successful fistula closure is markedly enhanced by the use of a bulbocavernosus fat pad (Martius) graft (Hamlin and Nicholson 1969; Elkins et. al 1990; Baines et. al. 1976; Punekar et. al 1999; Rangnekar et. al. 2000; Given and Acosta 1989; Fitzpatrick and Elkins 1993; Zacharin 1980; Shaw 1949; Martius 1956). There is one small comparative surgical study that documents this finding (Rangnekar et. al. 2000).

Development of the fat pad graft should begin with a vertical midline skin incision on the left or right labium majus, extending from the base of the mons pubis to about the level of the middle of the vaginal introitus [Figure 21]. Sharp dissection with a surgical scissors is used to expose a central «cord» of labial fat, and this dissection is carried down to the deep fascial layer [Figure 22]. Even in thin, malnourished women, dissection of this fat is always possible. Once this «cord» of fat has been identified and dissected, it is cross-clamped superiorly with a single clamp and transected [Figure 23]. The superior stump is suture-ligated to achieve hemostasis.

Next, the superior aspect of the graft is grasped gently with an Allis forcep and the cord of fat is further mobilized down to its base. It is important to protect the base of the pedicle to insure that its blood supply remains intact [Figure 24]. At this point, surgical scissors are used to dissect a tunnel which extends from the base of the fat pad's pedicle into the vagina, traveling between the vaginal epithelium and the pubic arch [Figure 25]. The tunnel should be large enough to allow passage of the surgeon's finger from the labial defect down to the bladder base [Figure 26].

Prior to passing the graft through the tunnel, four anchoring stitches of absorbable suture should be placed into the muscularis of the bladder at the 2,4, 8, and 10 o'clock positions. This allows the Martius graft to be anchored into place securely against the repaired fistula, protecting it and bringing in a new blood supply to nourish the surgical site [Figure 27]. The graft is then passed through the tunnel to the bladder base and is anchored into position using the previously placed anchoring stitches. The fistula site should be completely covered at this point [Figure 28].

Finally, the stay sutures which had been holding the anterior vaginal flaps out of the surgical field are released and the vaginal defect is closed as an "inverted T» [Figure 29]. The ureteric catheters can now be removed and a vaginal pack placed, if desired.

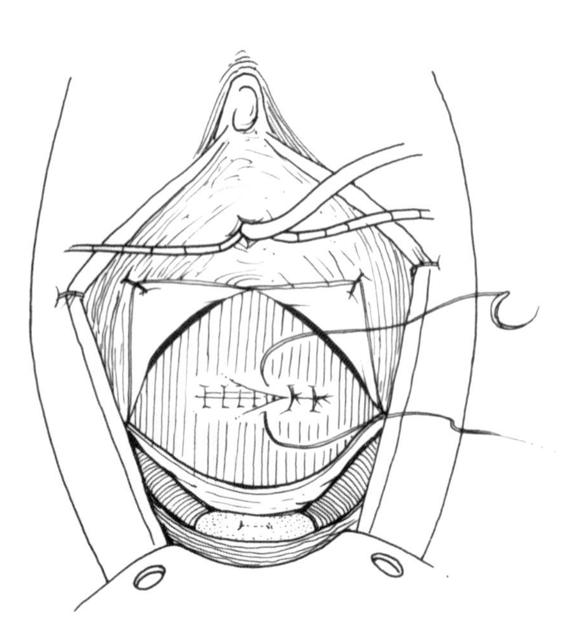

Figure 20 : Fistula closure. A second set of sutures is placed, imbricating the second suture line over the first. When this has been completed, «water tight» closure of the fistula should be confirmed by gentling filling the bladder with a solution of colored water or sterile infant feeding formula to check of leakage. If any leakage is noted, the repair should be taken down and reclosed until no leakage can be demonstrated. (©Worldwide Fund for Mothers Injured in Childbirth, used by permission).

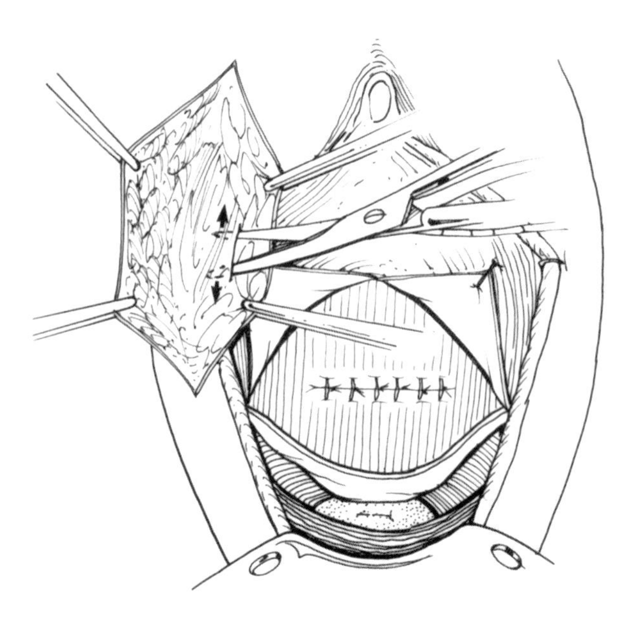

Figure 22 : Martius flap. Lateral and medial dissection of the bulbocavernosus fat is made down to the deep fascial layer, exposing a "cord" of labial fat. (©Worldwide Fund for Mothers Injured in Childbirth, used by permission).

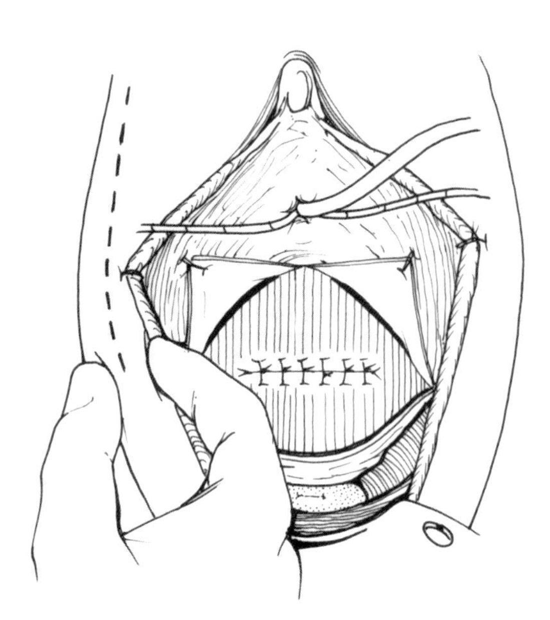

Figure 21 : Martius bulbocavernosus fat flap. A vertical skin incision is made in the labium majus from the base of the mons to the level of the middle of the vaginal introitus. (©Worldwide Fund for Mothers Injured in Childbirth, used by permission).

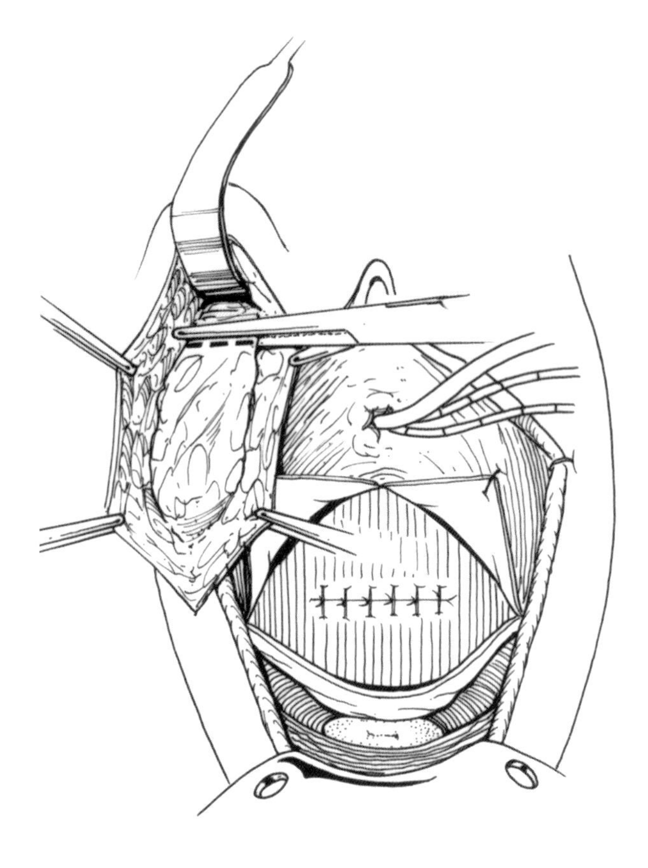

Figure 23 : Martius flap. Once the "cord" of fat has been identified and dissected, it is cross-clamped superiorly and divided. The superior stump is suture-ligated to insure hemostasis. (©Worldwide Fund for Mothers Injured in Childbirth, used by permission).

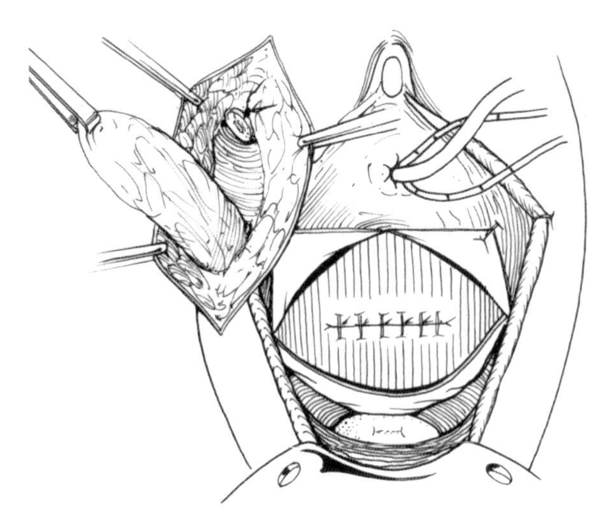

Figure 24 : Martius flap. The superior aspect of the graft is gently grasped with an Allis forcep and the labial fat is further mobilized down to its base, which is left intact to maintain its blood supply. (©Worldwide Fund for Mothers Injured in Childbirth, used by permission).

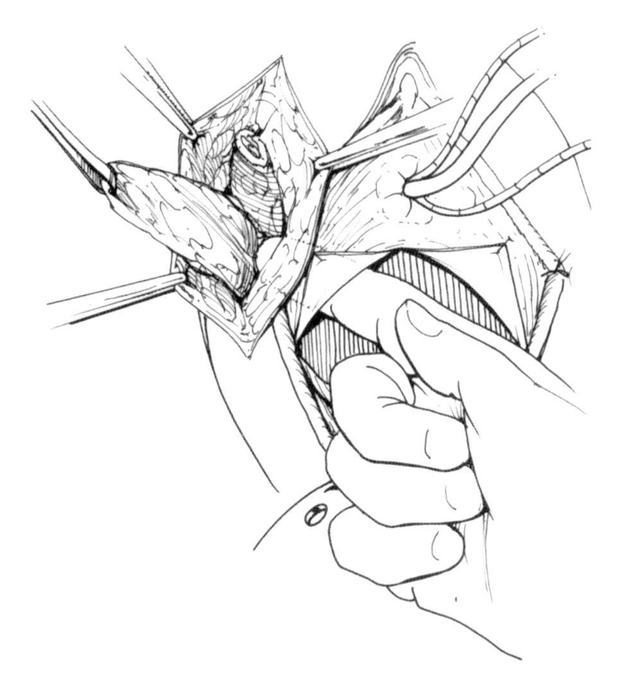

Figure 26 : Martius flap. The final caliber of the tunnel should be large enough to allow passage of the surgeon's finger from the labial defect down to the bladder base. (©Worldwide Fund for Mothers Injured in Childbirth, used by permission).

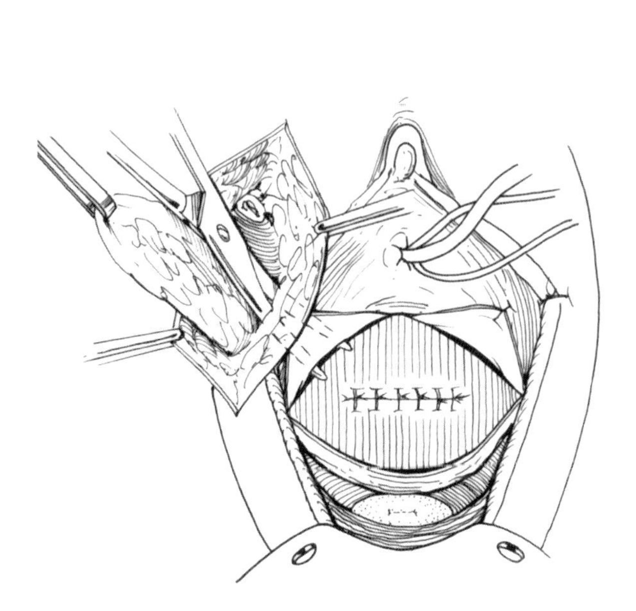

Figure 25 : Martius flap. A tunnel is dissected from the base of the labial fat graft into the vagina, running between the vaginal epithelium and the pubic arch.. (©Worldwide Fund for Mothers Injured in Childbirth, used by permission)..

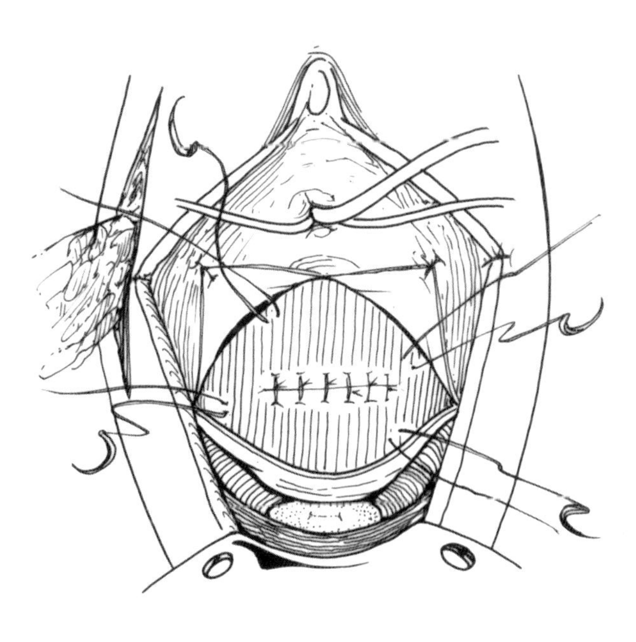

Figure 27 : Martius flap. Prior to passing the graft through the tunnel, four anchoring stitches of absorbable material are placed into the muscularis of the bladder at the 2, 4, 8, and 10 o'clock positions. (©Worldwide Fund for Mothers Injured in Childbirth, used by permission).

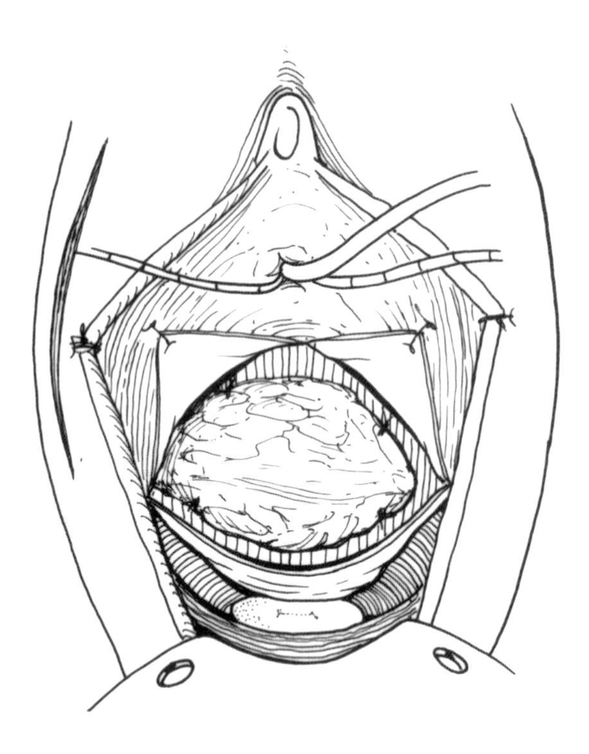

Figure 28 : Martius flap. The graft is then brought through the tunnel and anchored securely into place against the repaired fistula. The site of fistula repair should be completely covered at this point. (©Worldwide Fund for Mothers Injured in Childbirth, used by permission).

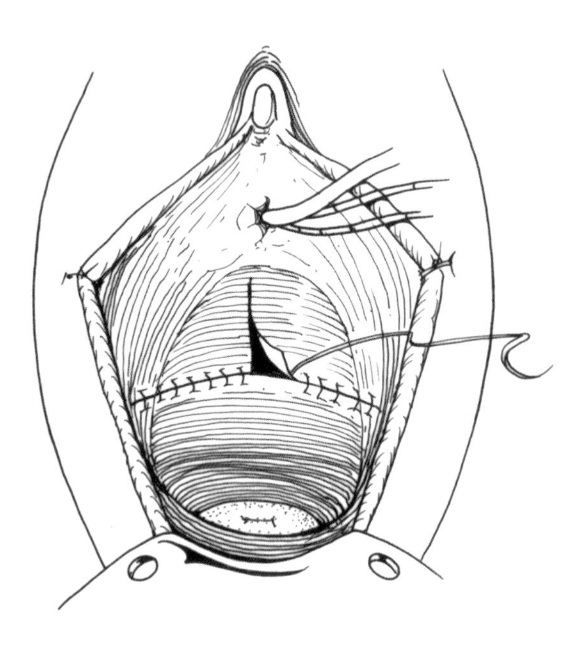

Figure 29 : Vaginal closure. The stay sutures holding the vaginal flaps are released and the vaginal defect is closed as an "inverted T" using absorbable sutures. (©Worldwide Fund for Mothers Injured in Childbirth, used by permission).

VIII. COMPLICATED CASES AND TECHNICAL SURGICAL QUESTIONS

1. The fistula complicated by urethral damage

Virtually all authors with extensive experience in the management of obstetric fistulas comment on the great difficulty in achieving post-operative continence in patients who have had extensive damage to the urethra, even if the fistula defect itself can be closed successfully. J. Chassar Moir, the great British gynecologist, referred (1965) to the worst of these cases as «circumferential» fistulas, which «involve a destruction of the bladder neck not only on the vaginal side but, in many instances, on the pubic side as well. The result is a circumferential sloughing with subsequent discontinuity of the urethra and bladder; the intervening tissue is merely the epithelium that has grown over, and become adherent to, the periosteum of the back of the pubic bone.» Fistulas involving this level of destruction are daunting, and are rarely seen in developed countries. According to Moir, the three great problems involved in dealing with this type of fistula are:

1. extremely difficult exposure;

2. technical difficulty in dissecting the tissue remnants from the pubic bone; and

3. difficulty in joining the bladder neck to the urethral remnant or stump, if, indeed, any portion of the urethra is still intact.

The basic principles of technique needed to deal with this type of injury are complete mobilization of the bladder so that it can be drawn down low enough to create a tension-free anastomosis with the urethral remnant. Freeing the urethral remnants from their adherence to the pubic bone may require a suprapubic incision with dissection from above in order to accomplish this. In such cases Moir took care to reinforce the bladder neck with buttressing sutures, and generally brought in a Martius' graft for better support and a renewed blood supply.

If only the posterior portion of the urethra had been sloughed and the anterior portion of the urethra was intact, Moir (1964) advocated a different technique for urethral reconstruction. In this technique, a thin catheter was stitched into position to serve as a splint for the new urethra. The margins of the urethral bed were freed from the vagina and were mobilized to allow them to be pulled together over the underlying catheter without tension. The vaginal incision was extended above the bladder neck and then reinforced with «inrolling stitches.» The repair was usually buttressed with a Martius bulbocavernosus fat graft, after which the vagina was closed over the repair with vertical mattress sutures to achieve a «broad apposition» of the vaginal wall. The bladder was then drained for 10 days and the vaginal sutures were removed after 21 days. Although he reported good success with this technique, with 23 of 34 women (67%) having «perfect or near perfect control» six months after surgery, 8 of 34 (24%) had persistent stress incontinence, and 9% had no improvement, reconfirming the view that persistent stress incontinence remains a significant problem for many women after successful fistula closure. Similar techniques with similar results have been reported by other authors (Noble 1901; Symmonds 1969; Symmonds and Hills 1978)

Various authors have described neourethral reconstruction using bladder flaps (Barnes and Wilson 1949; Flocks and Culp 1953; Su 1969; Quartey 1972; Tanagho and Smith 1972). All of these operations are based upon transabdominal techniques; however, a transvaginal approach to neourethral reconstruction using an anterior bladder flap technique was described by Elkins, Ghosh and co-workers (1992). In this technique, a neo-urethra is created by mobilizing a flap from the anterior bladder, which is then rolled into a tube. In this technique, the anterior and lateral edges of the fistula are freed up and the space of Retzius is entered transvaginally beneath the pubic bone. The anterior bladder is then pulled down into the vagina and mobilized. A 3 cm incision is made into the bladder and the anterior bladder wall is then rolled around a 16 Fr. Foley catheter to create a tube. After this is tacked down, a similar incision is made on the other side to complete mobilization of the tube. The anterior surface of the neourethra is then sutured in two layers and the posterior edge of the fistula is closed transversely, also in two layers. The neourethra is reattached to the posterior edge of the pubic symphysis, and a Martius graft is placed, before reapproximating the vaginal epithelium. This technique resulted in successful closure of the fistula in 18 of 20 cases, 4 of whom had severe stress incontinence post-operatively.

Based on their extensive experience with fistulas in Addis Ababa, Ethiopia, in 1969 Hamlin and Nicholson introduced the concept of the «difficult urinary fistula» to describe the complicated aspects of the problem touched on by Moir. According to them, the «difficult fistula»

«...is a complex of several grave injuries occurring together—-namely, a) total destruction of the urethra (all walls), the remaining tissue being merely fibrous connective tissue and squamous epithelium which has grown over and become adherent to the periosteum on the back of the pubic bones; b) an extensive sloughing of the bladder neck and trigone sometimes so large as to cause one or both ureteric orifices to open directly into the vagina; and c) fibrosis to an incredible degree which 1) narrows the vagina to the diameter of one fingerbreadth, and 2) binds the remains of the bladder high up to the descending pubic rami and to the pubic symphysis. In a word, no part of the patient's lower urinary tract has escaped some degree of damage. This is the fistula which daunts the hearts of most observers who see it for the first time. ... The gynaecologist bold enough to attempt the classical flap-splitting operation for a case like this soon discovers that he is operating in an area as confined and almost as inaccessible as the inside of the toe of a leather shoe. He will find himself freeing the bladder of scar and the lateral fixation of its torn edges by touch only. ... Within the vagina nothing exists ... except, almost quite literally, skin and bone.»

In such cases, Hamlin and Nicholson recommended constructing a new urethra by creating a new «inner» urethra using the skin and fibrous connective tissue covering the pubic bones and the inferior border of the pubic symphysis. In this technique, two lateral vertical incisions about 2 cm part are made in the skin, and left and right skin flaps were then created and reflected medially until their edges could be joined together without tension in the midline underneath the urinary catheter that had been placed in the bladder. When joined, these fragile skin flaps are rolled into a tube. At this point the neourethra is a fragile, untenable creation. As the authors noted, «Such a fragile neourethra, standing unsupported, would almost certainly necrose, and even if it survived would not restore any worthwhile degree of function.» The neourethra was then reinforced using a gracilis muscle flap taken from the thigh, preserving its neurovascular pedicle. The gracilis tendon is pulled through a tunnel in the thigh that crosses the ischiopubic ramus at the level of the urethra and is guided into the vagina, under the pubic symphysis, and is sutured to the anterior lip of the cervix, the lateral vaginal fascia, and the fibrous connective tissue covering the periosteum of the ischiopubic rami and the pubic symphysis. Once this has been accomplished, additional grafting is necessary using a Martius flap which is then covered with skin flaps.

Using this technique, the authors reported no deaths and only one «complete failure» in 50 operations, this case being due to failure of the blood supply to the gracilis muscle flap. In some cases small urethro-vaginal fistulas remained, which were repaired at a subsequent operation. Surprisingly, only 8 women (16%) developed «severe» stress incontinence after this reconstruction, four of whom regained «satisfactory» continence over time, and four of whom required an operation for stress incontinence. In the latter four patients, only two of these operations were completely successful. Six patients (12%) developed a urethral stricture, three of which were successfully treated by passage of a sound and three of which required surgical correction. The remaining 35 patients (70%) were discharged home within six weeks of surgery clinically cured or with mild residual stress incontinence which did not appear to be clinically bothersome for them.

Complete urethral loss from obstructed labor remains a daunting surgical challenge, to which an ideal solution has yet to be found.

2. Urinary diversion for the irreparable fistula

Although there is a general consensus in the literature that some fistulas simply cannot be repaired with restoration of full continence, there is no general agreement as to which fistulas should be treated initially by primary urinary diversion rather than an attempt at fistula closure. Similarly, there are no accepted criteria in failed cases to dictate when further attempts at closure should be abandoned and the patient should be offered some form of urinary diversion as a treatment. The dilemma has been summarized by Hodges (1999):

Many centres which perform VVF repairs have a small group of «problem» patients who have failed to gain continence despite often repeated attempts by different surgeons. Urinary diversion, with all its disadvantages, is seen as an admission of defeat by the VVF surgeon and so this decision is reached reluctantly. This reluctance is compounded by the concern of performing such a major procedure in often basic conditions. However, in the best interests of the patient, eventually the experienced VVF surgeon must admit when all attempts to gain continence have failed and consider urinary diversion.»

Because urinary diversion tends to be a «high technology» approach to fistula management, its use in countries that do not have a well-developed nursing infrastructure to support the ongoing care of such patients suggests that this technique should be used with extreme caution. For example, transplantation of the ureters into an ileal conduit requires the use of an external collecting device. The use of such appliances may well be unacceptable in the local culture and patients are likely to experience significant difficulty in obtaining suitable external appliances and may have trouble performing good stoma care. The result of such a policy could well be simply to transpose the fistula from the vagina to the abdomen! Likewise, if continent urinary diversions are performed with the creation of a catheterizable stoma, the problem of clean intermittent self-catheterization remains. This can be compounded by loss of the catheter or the development of stomal stenosis, with urinary retention, reservoir breakdown, sepsis, and death. Hodges (1999) has reported a series of seven patients with intractable fistulas who were treated in Uganda by continent urinary diversion using a Mitrofanoff procedure in which the appendix is mobilized as the catheterizable stoma. There was one death 6 days after surgery, apparently from coincidental complications rather than as a direct result of the operative technique. The other six patients were reported as doing well up to 14 months after surgery. Because of the possibility of the complications already alluded to, «patients are encouraged to remain near a hospital which can deal with any likely complications; five of the six patients have taken this advice. All patients carry spare catheters and a letter clearly explaining the nature of the procedure and the emergency treatment if there is a complication.» Whether these arrangements would be suitable for employment in different environments in other countries remains unknown.

The «traditional» operation for dealing with the irreparable fistula has usually been uretero-sigmoidostomy in which the ureters are transplanted into the sigmoid colon, which then functions as a reservoir for both urine and feces. The long-term consequences of this operation, such as anastomotic leakage with peritonitis, ureteral stenosis and hydronephrosis, acute and chronic pylonephritis, electrolyte imbalances, diarrhea, long-term renal failure, and the development of adenocarcinoma of the colon at the site of ureteral implantation, are well-known. These complications should give compassionate surgeons pause before recommending operations of this kind.

Several small series of fistula patients who have undergone ureterosigmoidostomy have been reported in the literature (Attah and Ozumba 1993, Humphries et. al. 1961, Thompson 1945, Foda 1959). These series are somewhat difficult to evaluate, as the numbers of patients reported are small and follow-up is often unsatisfactory. For example, Das and Sengupta (1969) resorted to urinary diversion and ureteral transplantation in 20 of 135 fistula patients that they reported in one series from India. Of these patients, two died of uremia after the surgery—one of the 9th and one on the 21st post-operative day after a stormy post-operative course. They did not know the follow-up of the other patients. Case fatality rates as high as 38.5% have been reported following these procedures in developing countries (Thompson 1945); although such grim statistics tend to come from the older surgical literature, the conditions of surgical practice and the facilities available for patient care may not have changed appreciably in those countries in which fistulas are still prevalent.

In recent years it has been discovered that many of the

disadvantages of «classical» ureterosigmoidostomy could be overcome by modifications of technique, the so-called «Mainz II» pouch (Fisch et. al 1993; Gerharz et. al. 1998). In this modification the anterior colon is opened 12 cm distal and proximal to the rectosigmoid junction, and a side-to-side anastomosis is made. This detubularization of the bowel reduces the force of colonic contractions and creates a «low pressure» system that does not appear to predispose such patients to the development of hydronephrosis. The bowel is attached to the sacral promontory for stabilization, and the ureters are mobilized bilaterally and transplanted into the colon through a 4-5 cm submucosal tunnel on each side. Aside from the continuing need to monitor such patients for the development of hyperchloremic metabolic acidosis and the possibility of the growth of malignant polyps at the uretro-colonic implantation site, patients undergoing the Mainz II procedure have done quite well, and almost all have had socially acceptable urinary continence and improved body image compared to patients undergoing urinary diversion using an ileal-conduit.

Good long-term follow-up studies of patients who have undergone urinary diversion of this type for irreparable fistulas in developing countries are virtually non-existent. If ureterosigmoidostomy is contemplated for a fistula patient, it is essential that she have normal anal sphincter control pre-operatively. This can be assessed by giving a large volume enema as a continence test to see how long she can retain it. It is also essential that patients be given enough time and counseling to understand the possible consequences of this type of surgery for their lives and future health. Treatment of intestinal parasites and a thorough bowel-prep prior to surgery are obvious essential components of this type of therapy. The optimal use of such techniques in fistula patients remains to be determined; however, it is clear that «salvage therapy» of this type will continue to have a place in the treatment of some patients with obstetric fistulas for many decades to come.

IX. PREVENTION OF OBSTETRIC FISTULAS

The ultimate strategy for dealing with obstetric fistulas should be to prevent them entirely. Indeed, this is precisely how the Western world solved the problem within its borders. Because obstetric fistulas are tied closely to overall maternal mortality, the best way to reduce fistula formation is to provide essential obstetric services at the community level with prompt access to emergency obstetric services at the first referral level. The success of this strategy has been amply demonstrated by Loudon (1992), by Maine (1991) and the essential elements of such obstetric care have been elaborated in some detail by the World Health Organization (1986). Figure 30 shows the historical trends in maternal mortality in the United States, England and Wales, and the Netherlands since 1920 (Loudon 1992a). At the beginning of the 20th Century, maternal mortality in Western Europe and North America was similar to that which currently exists in the developing world. The introduction of antibiotics, blood transfusion, safe Cesarean section, better transporation and improved access to care, along with the professionalization of obstetric care and midwifery services, led to a dramatic and continued decrease in maternal mortality in all these countries (Loudon 1992a, 1992b, 2000). During the same period the obstetric fistula virtually vanished from the experience of the industrialized world. Elimination of obstetric fistulas from the developing world will require that their health care systems undergo a similar transformation.

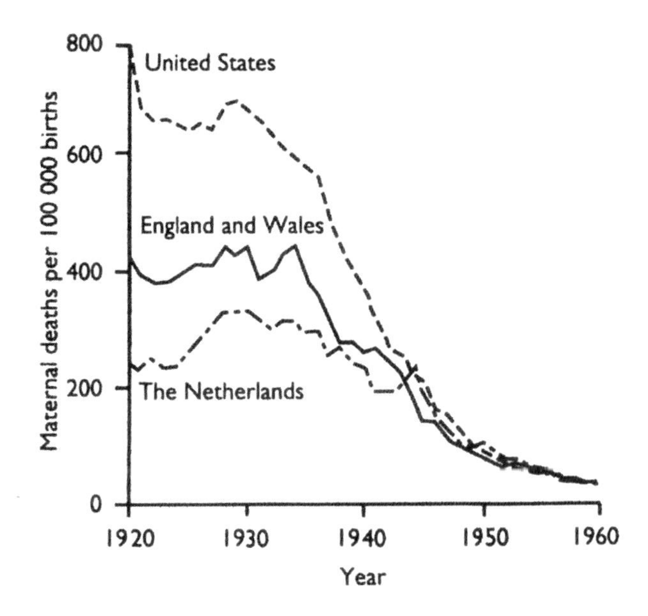

Figure 30 : Historical trends in maternal mortality in the United States, England and Wales, and the Netherlands, 1920 - 1960. (Loudon 1992a).

The committee believes that the fundamental components of such a program include the following:

- Promotion of breastfeeding and the elimination of childhood infections which hamper growth, such as gastroenteritis, respiratory infections, along with immunization against the six «killer diseases» of childhood: measles, diphtheria, tetanus, polio, pertussis, tuberculosis.
- Adequate childhood nutrition to allow young women to achieve full pelvic growth before childbearing begins

- Delay in childbearing until full pelvic growth is completed. There is substantial evidence to suggest that education is the best way to shelter girls from premature childbearing.
- Provision of family life education, education about women's health, sex education, and contraception to adolescent girls
- Elimination of traditional customs that promote early marriage. While respect for the principle of individual autonomy would argue for the elimination of early betrothal and arranged marriages, even in cases where such practices continue there should be a mutually-understood and agreed-upon delay in the consummation of such marriages until the young woman has reached full pelvic maturity. There is no advantage to any community in having early adolescent pregnancies.
- Supervision of the labor of every pregnant woman by a trained birth attendant. For developing countries this requires a commitment to developing culturally-acceptable community midwifery programs and an expansion of midwifery training services everywhere.
- Monitoring of every labor with the use of partograms to detect cephalo-pelvic disproportion early and to prevent the development of obstructed labor. There is overwhelming evidence that simple technology can accomplish this goal (Kwast 1994).
- Prompt, universal access to emergency obstetric care at the first referral level. This should be a fundamental goal of every health care system in the world. This will require removal of cultural and institutional, as well as physical, barriers (Prevention of Maternal Mortality Network 1995; Maine 1991; Thaddeus and Maine 1994)
- Universal basic education for women. There is substantial evidence that the education of women plays a major role in promoting maternal health, reducing maternal mortality, and eliminating obstetric fistulas (Harrison 1997). These goals appear to be achieved largely through better access to and utilization of life-saving health care services; however, it must be emphasized that for education to be effective in achieving these goals, effective health care services must first exist. Maternal mortality, and with it obstetric fistula formation, is largely a problem of the world's poor: the affluent countries of the world bear substantial responsibility for allowing this situation to continue when relatively low cost, low technology interventions exist that could prevent it (Rosenfield and Maine 1985; Weil and Fernandez 1999)
- Finally, education of men concerning the importance of women's reproductive health for their own families in particular and for the community at large. Because men control a disproportionate share of social resources in almost every developing country, they must understand that «women's health» is not «just a women's issue,» but is one in which they too must become intimately involved.

X. DEALING WITH THE BACKLOG OF SURGICAL CASES

The WHO Technical Working Group on the prevention and treatment of obstetric fistulas which met in Geneva from April 17-21, 1989 naively suggested that a plan could be put forth by which the backlog of existing fistula cases could be cleared up within five years (WHO 1989). Greater experience now suggests that solving the problem of cases awaiting surgery will require a generation or more. Not only is the backlog of unrepaired cases huge, but the absence of adequate maternal health care and emergency obstetrical services means that large numbers of new cases are continually occurring in those parts of the world where the fistula problem is greatest, thus adding continually to the burden of injury, which is not diminishing.

The special nature of the injuries produced by obstructed labor, the stigmatizing and socially isolating nature of the injury, and the long periods of rehabilitation needed before operation and the length of nursing care required after surgery, strongly argue in favor of the creation of specialized fistula centers in areas of the world where fistulas are highly prevalent. Ideally, each country or region in which this problem exists should have its own dedicated center, and centers in neighboring countries should be encouraged to collaborate in sharing information and establishing common protocols for research and training. There is an urgent need to create an international network of fistula centers in the developing world that can collaborate with one another in advancing the care of patients who have sustained an obstetric fistula.

Why are specialized fistula units needed? The first argument is the efficiencies obtained from «economies of scale.» A «focused factory» that does nothing except repair fistulas and take care of the related problems stemming from obstructed labor will develop special expertise in managing those problems. Such a center can deal with more cases more efficiently than a smaller service attached to a general hospital. Such a center also allows for the concentration of a sufficient volume of cases for meaningful training programs to be established through which additional fistula surgeons and fistula nurses can be developed for other centers in developing countries.

Second, the large volume of existing cases in developing countries justifies this approach in terms of the sheer numbers of patients involved. The Addis Ababa Fistula Hospital in Ethiopia, for example, has repaired approximately 20,000 cases to date, and still there is no shortage of women needing services.

Third, fistula units in general hospitals must compete for scarce resources with the needs of the general medical and surgical population. Since fistula repairs are rarely emergencies, it is difficult to book and keep scheduled operating theater time in the face of ongoing emergencies such a road traffic accidents, incarcerated hernia, intestinal perforations from typhoid or parasites, women in obstructed labor who need a surgical delivery, and so on. In settings where the health care system is already overwhelmed and where resources are scarce, scheduled fistula repairs are continually getting «bumped» from the operating schedule by more acute emergencies. While this is perfectly understandable, it augurs poorly for the development of an efficient fistula service in such a setting. Furthermore, because fistula patients traditionally have required two weeks of post-operative care for catheter drainage, they are more «bed intensive» than other surgical cases. In Lavery's (1955) series of 160 obstetric fistula cases from South Africa, the average duration of stay in hospital was 57.3 days, with a range of 11 to 264 days. In an environment with constant pressure to turn over hospital beds more quickly, fistula patients are likely to receive short shrift.

Fourth, fistula patients tend to integrate poorly into general hospital wards. By the time most such patients arrive for surgical treatment, they have been cast out and stigmatized by the society in which they live. They are psychologically and spiritually vulnerable, and they are socially offensive due to the odor that surrounds them. Many of these women are further stigmatized by unwarranted beliefs about why they developed a fistula in the first place: it is assumed by many to be a punishment for some offense against God (such as a pregnancy originating from an adulterous relationship) or as the result of a hideous venereal disease, which some consider contagious. Fear of the unknown breeds hostility towards these patients in the community at large.

Fifth, for reasons cited above, these patients do better in a communal environment. It is a great psychological relief to fistula patients to realize that they are not alone, to meet fellow sufferers with whom they can share experiences. A «sisterhood of suffering» develops in a dedicated fistula center that is immensely beneficial in restoring psychological health and hope to these women. At the Addis Ababa Fistula Hospital, most of the nursing care is provided by former fistula patients, who provide a level of empathetic nursing unequaled anywhere in the world.

It seems unlikely that large, dedicated fistula centers similar to that which exists in Addis Ababa will be developed in every country where there is great need within the foreseeable future. What then can be done? For the reasons enumerated above, it is important that facilities be created that are dedicated exclusively to the care of women with obstetric fistulas. Such facilities need not be identical everywhere; their capabilities could be stratified into those capable of dealing with «simple» cases, and those dealing with more complicated «high risk» fistulas (Elkins et. al., 1994).

Hamlin and Nicholson's concept of the «difficult» fistula has already been alluded to (1969). It is unrealistic to expect (and undesirable to encourage) a neophyte fistula surgeon to tackle cases of this complexity in a small, low volume fistula unit. However, the majority of obstetric fistulas seen in developing countries are not this complicated, and the size of the fistula has little bearing on the degree of urinary incontinence and resulting disability that the affected woman experiences: The same amount of urine runs out of an unscarred, freely mobile, 1 cm mid-vaginal fistula as runs out of a 5 cm fistula in which the bladder neck and proximal urethra have been destroyed, the vagina stenosed, and the fistula scarred against the pubic symphysis in dense bands of fibrosis. A relatively unskilled fistula surgeon could easily fix the former, thereby restoring continence and hope to the afflicted patient, whereas he or she would likely get into serious difficulties in an attempt to operate on the latter.

Elkins and Wall (1996) have demonstrated that trained obstetrician-gynecologists and general surgeons can quickly become proficient with the basic principles of fistula surgery if they are given appropriate training and supervision through an intensive «short course» in fistula repair: it does not take years of additional training to create capable fistula surgeons. Although such trainees may not be fully able to tackle difficult or «high risk» cases, they can certainly close the less complicated fistulas (Hamlin and Nicholson 1969; Elkins et. al. 1994). What is required in order to achieve this level of skill is an adequate volume of surgical cases that can be done under supervision while the basic techniques are mastered. Thus, it does seem feasible to create a «tiered» system of fistula centers within countries where that need exists. The key to making such programs work is trained, committed personnel who have adequate local resources. Small programs can be started with a few dedicated beds in a general hospital. If additional resources are provided, such programs can expand to occupy a dedicated ward at the same facility. Ultimately, the program can become transformed into an entirely separate facility dedicated exclusively to the care and rehabilitation of fistula patients.

The following recommendations can be made for the creation of specialized fistula centers in developing countries:

- For the reasons outlined above, the creation of dedicated fistula centers should be encouraged.
- Fistula centers should be located close to an all-weather road and good public transportation to facilitate access by patients. Wherever possible, such centers should be located in the geographic region in which fistulas are most prevalent, rather than in capital cities which have few fistulas and which therefore require patients to travel long distances to obtain care.
- Fistula centers should be located reasonably close to a general hospital so that emergency cases can be referred elsewhere, thus protecting the overall mission of the fistula program.
- Each fistula center should have a dedicated operating theater, ideally one in which two or more operations can be carried out simultaneously to maximize the turnover of cases.
- An in-patient ward of adequate size should be provided to deal with the expected number of cases. A ward of 40 or 50 beds should allow 500 to 1,000 operative cases to be treated each year.
- A «step-down unit» or hostel should be located at the fistula center to allow for pre-operative nutritional and educational support for fistula victims, and to allow better post-operative monitoring of non-acute patients.
- Care for fistula patients should be provided free of charge as a matter of principle. Fistula victims overwhelmingly tend to be young, poor, uneducated women, often deserted by husband and family, and from rural areas. There are many tragic stories of women who have suffered with fistulas for decades because they were unable to scrape together bus fare to a hospital or the cost of surgical supplies. Many studies of health care in developing countries have demonstrated that the institution of «user fees» dramatically reduces the utilization of services, often with worsening health outcomes (Ekwempu 1990; Prevention of Maternal Mortality Network 1995). The total cost of supplies and services for fistula repair is generally quite modest ($150 - $200). Although this still represents a large expenditure in developing countries, set against the value obtained from giving a woman back her life, it represents excellent cost-effective treatment. In order to bear these expenses, most fistula centers will probably require some degree of external funding through international medical aid; efforts in this direction should be encouraged. As the famous British surgeon Lawson Tait wrote in 1889, «I have already said that operations for vaginal fistulae are rarely paid for, except in gratitude, because the patients are nearly always poor. I must have operated on two or three hundred cases, and I have not yet been remunerated to an extent which would pay for the instruments I have bought for the purpose.»
- Fistula centers will require an on-site kitchen and laundry facilities. In African general hospitals, many of these services are typically provided by the family and relatives of the patient. The nature of the injury sustained by fistula victims means that many have been abandoned and lack this fundamental resource for coping with their condition. Fistula centers should therefore be prepared to provide the essentials of nutrition and laundry. Due to the vagaries of water and electric power in developing countries, fistula centers should have their own diesel generators and self-contained water supply, wherever feasible.
- Facilities and surgical care should be provided within a framework of «low technology» medicine. Almost all surgical procedures can be provided under simple spinal or ether anesthesia using standard surgical instruments, simple suture, and transurethral catheter drainage. Clinical laboratory requirements should be kept to a minimum. Cinder block construction, open wards, sheet metal roofing and simple architecture can be used to keep construction and operating costs to a minimum.
- Adequate housing for doctors and nursing staff should be provided, within the appropriate expectations of the local culture. If current and former patients are trained to work as nursing assistants, they can be housed acceptably in dormitory-style housing.

XI. CONCLUSIONS AND RECOMMENDATIONS

- The precise extent of the fistula problem in developing countries is unknown. The available evidence suggests that at a minimum, hundreds of thousands (if not several millions) of women are afflicted with this condition worldwide, most especially in sub-Saharan Africa. The enormous burden of suffering caused by fistulas is borne principally by young women living under conditions where their opportunities for education, economic prosperity, self-determination, and «the pursuit of happiness,» are limited by poverty, illiteracy, restricted social roles, the absence of adequate reproductive health services, and political disenfranchisement. Fistulas are primarily a condition that afflicts society's «have nots,» and the prevalence of obstetric fistulas closely tracks world maternal mortality statistics, especially in those areas where obstructed labor is a principal contributing cause of maternal death. The continued prevalence of obstetric fistulas represents a tragic waste of some of the most precious of the world's human resources: its young women.
- In theory, obstetric fistulas are completely preventable. When they do occur, they should be curable in over 90% of cases by the provision of appropriate, low-technology medical and surgical care.
- The fistula problem has been shamefully neglected by the governments of those countries in which they occur, by local health services, by non-governmental organizations, by international health organizations such as WHO, and by the foreign aid and international development agencies of the world's wealthy countries. The fistula problem has been almost uniformly neglected by the world's «Safe Motherhood» initiative, which itself has been largely ineffectual in reducing maternal death in developing countries. The fistula problem has been, and still is, an «orphan.» This situation is intolerable, and must be changed.
- There is a great need for village-based community studies of the incidence and prevalence of obstructed labor and fistula formation. It is clear that most fistulas arise from the combination of «obstructed labor and obstructed transportation,» but much more work is needed to understand the social context in which obstetric emergencies arise and how they are dealt with in developing countries. Nonetheless, the urgent needs of pregnant women should not be sacrificed on the altar of epidemiological research; rather, more attention should be paid to improving emergency treatment for obstetric complications at existing referral facilities, to upgrading peripheral facilities to provide essential life-saving obstetric care, to educating the community about the danger signs of obstetric complications, and to working with community leaders to improve access to emergency obstetric care in areas where maternal mortality and obstetric fistula rates are high.
- There is no standard classification system for obstetric fistulas. The committee recommends that the ICS take this task upon itself and that a sub-committee of the committee on the standardization of terminology be appointed to begin dealing with this task.
- Although the solution to the fistula problem will ultimately come from the provision of essential obstetric services for all the world's women, the current needs of those women who have already developed an obstetric fistula cannot be ignored. The committee recommends that specialized fistula centers should be created in all countries where obstetric fistulas are prevalent. Women with fistulas should have access to prompt, high quality surgical reconstruction which should be provided free of charge. Such facilities should serve as centers of compassionate excellence and should provide high quality patient care, medical and nursing education, and clinical research as part of their mandate for existence. It is unlikely that essential obstetric services will be available to all of the world's women within the foreseeable future; therefore, development of a sustainable clinical infrastructure to deal with the effects of maternal morbidity is likely to be an essential need in reproductive medicine for the rest of the 21st Century.
- Although current surgical techniques consistently result in fistula closure rates of 80% - 95% of cases, there has been almost no scientifically rigorous research carried out on most of the persistent technical surgical questions raised by fistulas. Urgent work is needed in this area. Among the issues that should be addressed are:

1. The problem of persistent stress incontinence after successful fistula closure;
2. The management of dramatically reduced bladder capacity in patients with large fistulas who have undergone successful closure;
3. The best technique for rectovaginal fistula repair;
4. The role of urinary diversion for the «incurable» fistula, usually involving some form of ureterosigmoidostomy;
5. The role of vaginoplasty in patients with vaginal atresia from obstructed labor;

6. The best method of caring for patients who present with a «fresh» fistula a few days or weeks after delivery, including the role of early repair in selected obstetric fistulas;
7. Future reproductive function in patients who have sustained an obstetric fistula;
8. The proper role and choice of flaps and grafts in fistula surgery;
9. The optimum duration of post-operative bladder drainage after fistula repair;
10. The role of nutritional support in improving the outcomes of patients with obstetric fistulas; and
11. The role of physical therapy and reconstructive orthopedic surgery in the management of women with obstetric foot-drop from prolonged obstructed labor.

REFERENCES

Abbott DH. 1950 The repair of vesico-vaginal fistulae. East African Medical Journal 27109-118.

Abdalla RHD. 1982 Sisters in Affliction: Circumcision and Infibulation of Women in Africa. London: Zed Press.

AbouZahr C, Royston E. 1991 Maternal Mortality: A Global Factbook. Geneva: World Health Organization.

AbouZahr C. 1998 Maternal mortality overview. Pp. 111-164 in: Murray CJL and Lopez AD (Eds), Health Dimension of Sex and Reproduction: The global burden of sexually transmitted diseases, HIV, maternal conditions, perinatal disorders, and congenital anomalies. Boston: Harvard University Press. Published by the Harvard School of Public Health on behalf of the World Health Organization and the World Bank

Aimakhu VE. 1974 Reproductive functions after the repair of obstetric vesicovaginal fistulae. Fertility and Sterility 25:586-591.

Ampofo K, Otu T, Uchebo G. 1990 Epidemiology of vesico-vaginal fistulae in northern Nigeria. West African Journal of Medicine 9:98-102.

Amr MF. 1998 Vesico-vaginal fistula in Jordan. European Journal of Obstetrics and Gynecology and Reproductive Biology 80:201-203.

Arrowsmith SD. 1994 Genitourinary reconstruction in obstetric fistulas. Journal of Urology 152:403-6.

Arrowsmith S, Hamlin EC, Wall LL. 1996 «Obstructed labor injury complex:» Obstetric fistula formation and the multifaceted morbidity of maternal birth trauma in the developing world. Obstetrical and Gynecological Survey 51:568-574.

Ashworth FL. 1973 Urinary vaginal fistulae: A series of 152 patients treated in a small hospital in Ghana. West African Medical Journal April:39-43.

Attah CA, Ozumba BC. 1993 Management of unrepairable urinary vaginal fistulae in a developing country. Australia New Zealand Journal of Surgery 63:217-220.

Aziz FA. 1965 Urinary fistulae from obstetrical trauma. Journal of Obstetrics and Gynaecology of the British Commonwealth 72:765-768.1980 Gynecologic and obstetric complications of female circumcision. International Journal of Gynaecology and Obstetrics 17:560-563.

Baines REM, Orford HJL, Theron JLL. 1976 The repair of vesicovaginal fistulae by means of omental slings and grafts. South African Medical Journal 50:959-961.

Bangser M, Gumodoka B, Berege Z. 1999 A comprehensive approach to vesico-vaginal fistula: A project in Mwanza, Tanzania, pp.157-165 in M Berer and TKS Ravindram (Eds); Safe Motherhood Initiatives: Critical Issues.. Oxford: Blackwell Science, for Reproductive Health Matters.

Barnes RW, Wilson WM. 1949 Reconstruction of the urethra with a tube from bladder flap. Urologic and Cutaneous Review 53:604-606.

Bentley RJ. 1973 Abdominal repair of high rectovaginal fistula. Journal of Obstetrics and Gynaecology of the British Commonwealth 80:364-367.

Bieler EU, Schnabel T. 1976 Pituitary and ovarian function in women with vesicovaginal fistulae after obstructed and prolonged labour. South African Medical Journal 50:257-266.

Bird GC. 1967 Obstetric vesico-vaginal and allied fistulae. Journal of Obstetrics and Gynaecology of the British Commonwealth 74:749-752.

Bland KG, Gelfand M. 1970 The influence of urinary bilharziasis on vesico-vaginal fistula in relation to causation and healing. Transactions of the Royal Society of Tropical Medicine and Hygiene 64:588-592.

Boddy J. 1982 Womb as oasis: The symbolic context of Pharaonic circumcision in rural northern Sudan. American Ethnologist 9:682-698.

Briggs ND. 1983 Occipito-Posterior Positions: Predictive Indices on the Outcome of Labor. M.D. Thesis, University of Lagos..

Carter B, Palumbo L, Creadick RN, Ross RA. 1952 Vesicovaginal fistulas. American Journal of Obstetrics and Gynecology 63:479-496.

Cockshott WP. 1973 Pubic changes associated with obstetric vesicovaginal fistulae. Clinical Radiology 24:241-247.

Coetzee T, Lithgow DM. 1966 Obstetric fistulae of the urinary tract. Journal of Obstetrics and Gynaecology of the British Commonwealth 73:837-844.

Colachis SC III, Pease WS, Johnson WE. 1994 A preventable cause of foot drop during childbirth. American Journal of Obstetrics and Gynecology 171:270-272.

Cottingham J, Royston E. 1991 Obstetric Fistulae: A Review of Available Information. Geneva: World Health Organization (WHO/ MCH/ MSM91.5)

Counsellor VS, Haigler FH. 1956 Management of urinary-vaginal fistula in 253 cases. American Journal of Obstetrics and Gynecology 72:367-376.

Danso KA, Martey JO, Wall LL, Elkins TE. 1996 The epidemiology of genitourinary fistulae in Kumasi, Ghana, 1977-1992. International Urogynecology Journal 7:117-120.

Das RK, Sengupta SK. 1969 Vesico-vaginal fistula of obstetric origin. Journal of Obstetrics and Gynaecology of India 19:383-389.

Dick JS, Strover RM. 1971 Vaginoplasty following vesicovaginal fistula repair: a preliminary report. South African Medical Journal 45:617-620.

Eden TW. 1914 A case of superior recto-vaginal fistula dealt with by the abdominal route after preliminary colostomy. Journal of Obstetrics and Gynaecology of the British Empire 26:175-185.

Ekwempu CC, Maine D, Olorukoba MB, Essien ES, Kisseka MN. 1990 Structural adjustment and health in Africa. Lancet 336:56-7..

El-Dareer A. 1982 Woman, Why Do You Weep? Circumcision and Its Consequences. London: Zed Press.

El-Guindi I. 1962 Vaginal atresia in Saudi Arabia. Journal of Obstetrics and Gynaecology of the British Commonwealth 69:996-998.

Elkins TE. 1994 Surgery for the obstetric vesicovaginal fistula: A review of 100 operations in 82 patients.. American Journal of Obstetrics and Gynecology 170:1108-1120.

Elkins TE, DeLancy JOL, McGuire EJ. 1990 The use of modified Martius graft as an adjunctive technique in vesicovaginal and rectovaginal fistula repair. Obstetrics and Gynecology 90:727-733.

Elkins TE, Ghosh TS, Tagoe GA, Stocker R. 1992 Transvaginal mobilization and utilization of the anterior bladder wall to repair vesicovaginal fistulas involving the urethra. Obstetrics and Gynecology 79:455-60.

Elkins TE, Mahama E, O'Donnell P, Fort D, Park RC. 1994 Recognition and management of patients with high-risk vesicovaginal fistulas: Implications for teaching and research. Internatiional Urogynecology Journal 5:183-187.

Elkins TE, Wall LL. 1996 Report of a pilot project on the rapid training of pelvic surgeons in techniques of obstetric vesico-vaginal fistula repair in Ghana and Nigeria. Journal of Pelvic Surgery 2:182-186.

Emembolu J.. 1992 The obstetric fistula: Factors associated with improved pregnancy outcome after a successful repair. International Journal of Gynecology and Obstetrics 39:205-212.

Emmet TA. 1868 Vesico-Vaginal Fistula from Parturition and Other Causes: With Cases of Recto-Vaginal Fistula. New York: William Wood.

1879 The necessity for early delivery, as demonstrated by the analysis of one hundred and sixty-one cases of vesico-vaginal fistula. Transactions of the American Gynecological Society 3:114-34.

Enzelsberger H, Gitsch E. 1991 Surgical management of vesicovaginal fistulas according to Chassar Moir's method. Surgery, Gynecology and Obstetrics 173;183-186.

Everett HS, Mattingly RF. 1956 Vesicovaginal fistula. American Journal of Obstetrics and Gynecology 72:712-724.

Evoh NJ, Akinla O. 1978 Reproductive performance after the repair of obstetric vesico-vaginal fistulae. Annals of Clinical Research 10:303-306.

Fahmy K. 1962 Cervical and vaginal atresia due to packing the vagina with salt after labor. American Journal of Obstetrics and Gynecology 84:1466-1469

Fisch M, Wammack R, Muller SC, Hohenfellner R. 1993 The Mainz Pouch II (sigma rectum pouch). Journal of Urology 149: 258- 263.

Fitzpatrick C, Elkins TE. 1993 Plastic surgical techniques in the repair of vesicovaginal fistulas: A review. International Urogynecology Journal 4:287-295.

Flocks RH, Culp DA. 1953 A modification of technique for anastomosing membranous urethra and bladder neck following total prostatectomy. Journal of Urology 69:411-415

Foda MS. 1959 Evaluation of methods of treatment of urinary fistulae in women: A report of 220 cases. Journal of Obstetrics and Gynaecology of the British Empire 66:372-381.

Fortney JA, Smith JB (Eds). 1996 The Base of the Iceberg: Prevalence and Perceptions of Maternal Morbidity in Four Developing Countries (The Maternal Morbidity Network). Research Triangle Park, NC: Family Health International.

Frith K. 1960 Vaginal atresia of Arabia. Journal of Obstetrics and Gynaecology of the British Empire 67:82-85

Gerharz EW, Kohl UN, Weingartner K, Kleinhans BJ, Melekos MD, Riedmiller H. 1998 Experience with the Mainz modification of ureterosigmoidostomy. British Journal of Surgery 85:1512-1516.

Gharoro EP, Abedi HO. 1999 Vesico-vaginal fistula in Benin City, Nigeria. International Journal of Gynecology and Obstetrics 64:313-314.

Given FT Jr, Acosta AA. 1989 The Martius procedure—bulbocavernosus fat flap: A review. Obstetrical and Gynecological Survey 45:34-40.

Goh JTW. 1998 Genital tract fistula repair on 116 women. Australia New Zealand Journal of Obstetrics and Gynaecology 38:158-161.

Goodwin WE, Scardino PT. 1980 Vesicovaginal and ureterovaginal fistulas: A summary of 25 years of experience. Journal of Urology 123:370-374.

Graham W. 1998 The scandal of the century. British Journal of Obstetrics and Gynaecology 105:375-6.

Gruenbaum E. 2001 The Female Circumcision Controversy: An Anthropological Perspective. Philadelphia: University of Pennsylvania Press.

Hall G. 1977 A review of drop-foot corrective surgery. Leprosy Review 48:184-192.

Hamlin RHJ, Nicholson EC. 1966 Experiences in the treatment of 600 vaginal fistulas and in the management of 80 labours which have followed the repair of these injuries. Ethiopian Medical Journal 4(5):189-192. 1969 Reconstruction of urethra totally destroyed in labour. British Medical Journal 1:147-1150

Harris, S. 1950 Woman's Surgeon: The Life Story of J. Marion Sims. New York: Macmillan.

Harrison KA. 1983 Obstetric fistula: one social calamity too many. British Journal of Obstetrics and Gynaecology 90:385-386.

1985 Child-bearing, health, and social priorities: A survey of 22,774 consecutive deliveries in Zaria, northern Nigeria. British Journal of Obstetrics and Gynaecology 92(Suppl 5):1-119.

Hassim AM, Lucas C. 1974 Reduction in the incidence of stress incontinence complicating fistula repair. British Journal of Surgery 61:461-465.

Hilton P, Ward A. 1998 Epidemiological and surgical aspects of urogenital fistulae: A review of 25 years' experience in southeast Nigeria. International Urogynecology Journal 9:189-194.

Hilton P, Ward A, Molloy M, Umana O. 1998 Periurethral injection of autologous fat for the treatment of post-fistula repair stress incontinence: A preliminary report. International Urogynecology Journal 9:118-121.

Hodges AM. 1999 The Mitrofanoff urinary diversion for complex vesicovaginal fistulae: experience from Uganda. BJU International 84:436-439.

Hoskins WJ, Park RC, Long R, Artman LE, McMahon EB. 1984 Repair of urinary tract fistulas with bulbocavernosus myocutaneous flaps. Obstetrics and Gynecology 63:588-593.

Hudson CN. 1970 Acquired fistulae between the intestine and the vagina. Annals of the Royal College of Surgeons of England 46:20-40.

Hudson CN, Henrickse JP, Ward A. 1975 An operation for restoration of urinary incontinence following total loss of the urethra. British Journal of Obstetrics and Gynaecology 82:501- 504.

Humphries SV. 1961 Transplantation of ureters for vesico-vaginal fistula. South African Medical Journal 35:643-646.

Iloabachie GC. 1992 260 cases of juxta cervical fistula. East African Medical Journal 69:188-190.

Kelly J. 1992 Vesico-vaginal and recto-vaginal fistulae. Journal of the Royal Society of Medicine 85:257-258.

Kelly J, Kwast BE 1993a Obstetric vesicovaginal fistulas: Evaluation of failed repairs. International Urogynecology Journal 4:271-3. 1993b Epidemiological study of vesicovaginal fistulas in Ethiopia. International Urogynecology Journal 4:278-281.

Kennelly MJ, Gormley EA, McGuire EJ. 1994 Early clinical experience with adult bladder auto-augmentation. Journal of Urology 152:303-306.

Kingston AE. 1957 The vaginal atresia of Arabia. Journal of Obstetrics and Gynaecology of the British Empire 64:836-839.

Kolawole TM, Adam SP, Evans KT. 1978 Comparative pelvimetric measurements in Nigerian and Welsh women. Clinical Radiology 29:85-90.

Krishnan RG. 1949 A review of a series of 100 cases of vesicovaginal fistulae. Journal of Obstetrics and Gynaecology of the British Empire 56:22-27.

Kwast BE. 1994 World Health Organization partograph in management of labour. Lancet 343:1399-1404

Lagundoye SB, Bell D, Gill G, Ogunbode O. 1976 Urinary tract changes in obstetric vesico-vaginal fistulae: A report of 216 cases studied by intravenous urography. Clinical Radiology 27:531-539.

Langkilde NC, Pless TK, Lundbeck F, Nerstrom B. 1999 Surgical repair of vesicovaginal fistulae: A ten-year retrospective study. Scandinavian Journal of Urology and Nephrology 33:100-103.

Latzko W. 1942 Postoperative vesicovaginal fistulas: Genesis and therapy. American Journal of Surgery 58:211-228.

Lavery DWP. 1955 Vesico-vaginal fistulae: A report on the vaginal repair of 160 cases. Journal of Obstetrics and Gynaecology of the British Empire 62:530-539.

Lawson JB. 1968 Birth-canal injuries. Proceedings of the Royal Society of Medicine 61:22-24. 1972a Rectovaginal fistulae following difficult labour. Proceedings of the Royal Society of Medicine 65:283-286. 1972b Vesical fistulae into the vaginal vault. British Journal of Urology 44:623-631.

Leng WW, Blalock J, Fredriksson WH, English SF, McGuire EJ. 1999 Enterocystoplasty or detrusor myectomy? Comparison of indications and outcomes for bladder augmentation. Journal of Urology 161:758-763.

Loudon I 1992a The transformation of maternal mortality. British Medical Journal 305:1557-1560. 1992b Death in Childbirth: An International Study of Maternal Care and Maternal Mortality, 1800-1950. Oxford: Clarendon Press. 2000 Maternal mortality in the past and its relevance to developing countries today. American Journal of Clinical Nutrition 2000;72(suppl)241S-246S.

McConnachie ELF. 1958 Fistulae of the urinary tract in the female: A proposed classification. South African Medical Journal 32:524-527.

McKay WJS. 1922 Lawson Tait: His Life and Work. New York: William Wood and Co.

Mahfouz N. 1929 Urinary and rectovaginal fistulae in women. Journal of Obstetrics and Gynaecology of the British Empire 36:581-589. 1930 Urinary fistulae in women. Journal of Obstetrics and Gynaecology of the British Empire 37:566-576. 1934 A new technique in dealing with superior recto-vaginal fistulae. Journal of Obstetrics and Gynaecology of the British Empire 41:579-587. 1938 Urinary and faecal fistulae. Journal of Obstetrics and Gynaecology of the British Empire 45:405-424. 1957 Urinary Fistulae in women. Journal of Obstetrics and Gynaecology of the British Empire 64:23-34.

Maine DM. 1991 Safe Motherhood Programs: Options and Issues. New York: Center for Population and Family Health, Columbia University School of Public Health.

Margolis T, Elkins TE, Seffah J, Oparo-Addo HS, and Fort D. 1994 Full-thickness Martius grafts to preserve vaginal depth as an adjunct in the repair of large obstetric fistulas. Obstetrics and Gynecology 84:148-152.

Martius HR. 1956 Martius Gynecological Operations, With Emphasis on Topographic Anatomy. Boston: Little, Brown, and Company.. Translated and edited by Milton L. McCall and Karl A. Bolten (from Die Gynakologischen Operationen und ihre Topographisch-Anatomischen Grundlagen, 7th ed).

Massee JS, Welch JS, Pratt JH, Symmonds RE. 1964 Management of urinary-vaginal fistula: Ten year survey. Journal of the American Medical Association 190:124-128.

Moerman ML. 1982 Growth of the birth canal in adolescent girls. American Journal of Obstetrics and Gynecology. 143:528-32

Moir JC. 1964 Reconstruction of the urethra. Journal of Obstetrics and Gynaecology of the British Commonwealth 71:349-359. 1965 The Sir Kendarnath Das Oration: The «circumferential» vesico-vaginal fistula. Journal of Obstetrics and Gynaecology of India 15:441-448. 1966 Vesicovaginal fistula: Thoughts on the treatment of 350 cases. Proceedings of the Royal Society of Medicine 59:1019-1022.

Muleta M, Williams G. 1999 Postcoital injuries treated at the Addis Ababa Fistula Hospital, 1991-1997. Lancet 354:2051-2052.

Murphy M. 1981 Social consequences of vesico-vaginal fistula in northern Nigeria. Journal of Biosocial Science 13:139-150.

Murphy M, Baba TM. 1981 Rural dwellers and health care in northern Nigeria. Social Science and Medicine 15A:265-271.

Mustafa AZ, Rushwan HME. 1971 Acquired genito-urinary fistulae in the Sudan.. Journal of Obstetrics and Gynaecology of the British Commonwealth 78:1039-1043.

Naidu PM. 1962 Vesico-vaginal fistulae: An experience with 208 cases. Journal of Obstetrics and Gynaecology of the British Commonwealth 69:311-316.

Naidu PM, Krishna S. 1963 Vesico-vaginal fistulae and certain obstetric problems arising subsequent to repair. Journal of Obstetrics and Gynaecology of the British Commonwealth 70:473-475.

Naim A. 1965 Vaginal fistulae complicating salt atresia in Arabia. Alexandria Medical Journal 11:218-226.

Noble CP. 1901 The new formation of the female urethra, with report of a case. American Journal of Obstetrics 43:170-178.

Onolemhemhen DO, Ekwempu CC. 1999 An investigation of sociomedical risk factors associated with vaginal fistula in northern Nigeria. Women and Health 28;103-116. Prevention of Maternal Mortality Network. 1995 Situation analyses of emergency obstetric care: Examples from eleven operations research projects in West Africa. Social Science and Medicine 40:657-667.

Prual A, Huguet D, Garbin O, Rabe G. 1998 Severe obstetric morbidity of the third trimester, delivery, and early puerperium in Niamey (Niger); African Journal of Reproductive Health 2:10-19.

Punekar SV, Buch DN, Soni AB, Swami G, Rao SR, Kinne JS, Karhadkar SS. 1999 Martius' labial fat pad interposition and its modification in complex lower urinary fistulae. Journal of Postgraduate Medicine 45:69-73.

Quartey JKM. 1972 Bladder rotation flap for repair of difficult vesicovaginal fistulas. Journal of Urology 107:60-62.

Radman HM. 1961 Vesicovaginal fistula. American Journal of Obstetrics and Gynecology 82:1238-1242..

Rangnekar NP. Imdad Ali N. Kaul SA. Pathak HR. 2000 Role of the Martius procedure in the management of urinary-vaginal fistulas. Journal of the American College of Surgeons 191:259-63.

Reif ME. 1988 Bilateral common peroneal nerve palsy secondary to prolonged squatting in natural childbirth. Birth 15:100-102.

Richard BM. 1989 Interosseous transfer of tibialis posterior for common peroneal nerve palsy. Journal of Bone and Joint Surgery – British Volume 71:834-7.

Rosenfeld A, Maine D. 1985 Maternal mortality—a neglected tragedy. Where is the 'M' in «MCH?' Lancet 2:83-85. St. George, J. 1969Factors in the prediction of successful vaginal repair of vesicovaginal fistulae. Journal of Obstetrics and Gynaecology of the British Commonwealth 76:741-745.

Schleicher DJ, Ojengbede OHA, Elkins TE. 1993 Urologic evaluation after closure of vesicovaginal fistulas. International Urogynecology Journal 4:262-265.

Shaw W. 1949 The Martius bulbo-cavernosus interposition operation. British Medical Journal 2:1261-1264.

Sims JM 1852 On the treatment of vesico-vaginal fistula. American Journal of the Medical Sciences (new series) 23:59-82.

Sinclair RSC. 1952 Maternal obstetric palsy. South African Medical Journal 26:708-714.

Snow BW, Cartwright PC. 1996 Bladder autoaugmentation. Urologic Clinics of North America 23:323- 331.

Su CT. 1969 A flap technique for repair of vesicovaginal fistula. Journal of Urology 102:56-59.

Symmonds RE. 1969 Loss of the urethral floor with total urinary incontinence: A technique for urethral reconstruction. American Journal of Obstetrics and Gynecology 103:665-678.

Symmonds RE, Hill LM. 1978 Loss of the urethra: A report on 50 patients. American Journal of Obstetrics and Gynecology 130:130-138.

Tahzib F 1983 Epidemiological determinants of vesico-vaginal fistulas. British Journal of Obstetrics and Gynaecology 90:387-391 1985 Vesicovaginal fistula in Nigerian children. Lancet 2:1291-3.

Tait L. 1879 Diseases of Women, second edition. New York: William Wood and Co. 1889 Diseases of Women and Abdominal Surgery. London.

Tanagho EA, Smith DR. 1972 Clinical evaluation of a surgical technique for the correction of complete urinary incontinence. Journal of Urology 107:402-411.

Taylor ES, Droegemueller W. 1967 Repair of urinary vaginal fistulas. Obstetrics and Gynecology 30:674-678.

Thaddeus S, Maine D. 1994 «Too far to walk:» maternal mortality in context. Social Science and Medicine 38:1091-1110.

Thompson DJ. 1945 Vesicovaginal fistula: A review of 42 cases treated by plastic repair or ureterosigmoidostomy. Journal of Obstetrics and Gynaecology of the British Empire 52:271-277.

Tomlinson AJ. Thornton JG. 1998 A randomised controlled trial of antibiotic prophylaxis for vesico-vaginal fistula repair. British Journal of Obstetrics and Gynaecology. 105:397-9.

Toubia N. 1994 Female circumcision as a public health issue. New England Journal of Medicine 331:712-716.

Underhill BML. 1964 Salt-induced vaginal stenosis of Arabia. Journal of Obstetrics and Gynaecology of the British Commonwealth 71:293-298.

Vix VA, Ryu CY. 1971 The adult symphysis pubic: normal and abnormal. American Journal of Roentgenology, Radium Therapy, and Nuclear Medicine 112:517-525.

Waaldijk K. 1989 The (surgical) management of bladder fistula in 775 women in Northern Nigeria. Thesis: University of Utrecht, Netherlands. 1994a Step-By-Step Surgery of Vesicovaginal Fistulas. Edinburgh: Campion Press. 1994b The immediate surgical management of fresh obstetric fistulas with catheter and/or early closure. International Journal of Gynecology and Obstetrics 45:11-16. 1995 Surgical classification of obstetric fistulas. International Journal of Gynecology and Obstetrics 49:161-163.

Waaldijk K, Elkins TE. 1994 The obstetric fistula and peroneal nerve injury: an analysis of 947 consecutive patients. International Urogynecology Journal 5:12-14

Walker AHC. 1954 The management of urinary fistulas in a primitive population. Surgery Gynecology and Obstetrics 99:301-309

Wall LL 1988 Hausa Medicine: Illness and Well-being in a West African Culture. Durham, NC: Duke University Press. 1998 Dead mothers and injured wives: the social context of maternal morbidity and mortality among the Hausa of northern Nigeria. Studies in Family Planning 29:341-359.

Ward A. 1980 Genito-urinary fistulae: a report on 1,789 cases. Proceedings of the 2nd International Congress on Obstetrics and Gynaecology, Lagos, Nigeria.

Weed JC. 1967 Management of vesicovaginal fistula: Experience with 75 cases. American Journal of Obstetrics and Gynecology 97:1071-1075.

Weil O, Fernandez H. 1999 Is safe motherhood an orphan initiative? Lancet 354:940-943.

World Health Organization. 1986 Essential Obstetric Functions at First Referral level to Reduce Maternal Mortality: Report of a Technical Working Group, June 23-27, 1986. Geneva: WHO. (FHE/86..4) 1989 The Prevention and Treatment of Obstetric Fistulae: Report of a Technical Working Group, Geneva, 17-21 April, 1989. Geneva: Division of Family Health, World Health Organization WHO/FHE/89.5 1998 Female Genital Mutilation: An Overview. Geneva: WHO, 1998.

World Health Organization and UNICEF. 1996 Revised 1990 Estimates of Maternal Mortality: A New Approach. Geneva: WHO.

Yenen E, Babuna C. 1965 Genital fistula: A study based on 197 consecutive cases. Obstetrics and Gynecology 26:219-224.

Zacharin RF. 1980 Grafting as a principle in the surgical management of vesicovaginal and rectovaginal fistulae. Australia New Zealand Journal of Obstetrics and Gynaecology 20:10-17. 1988 Obstetric Fistula. New York: Springer-Verlag.

Committee 13

Promotion, Education and Organization for Continence Care

Chairman

D. K. Newman (USA)

Members

L. Denis (Belgium),

C. B. Gartley (USA),

I. Gruenwald (Israel),

P.H.C. Lim (Singapore),

R. Millard (Australia),

R. Roberts (USA)

CONTENTS

Promotion, Education and Organization for Continence Care

D. K. Newman

L. Denis, C. B. Gartley, I. Gruenwald, P.H.C. Lim, R. Millard, R. Roberts

I. INTRODUCTION

Urinary incontinence (UI) is a most common problem, affecting over 200 million people worldwide. UI seriously affects both sufferers and caregivers and leads to major deterioration in quality of life (QOL). It is surrounded by taboos, misinformation and ignorance. Most sufferers fail to seek help despite safe and effective treatments that are available.

The chapters in this volume have outlined the tremendous advances over the past two decades in the understanding of the causes of UI, and in the ability to diagnose and treat those patients who present for help. However, this is of limited usefulness if:

1) The majority of incontinent people remain unaware and too embarrassed to seek professional help;

2) Health care professionals who provide primary care services are often unaware of the improvement in health status resulting from the active detection of UI.

3) Health care professionals' attitudes towards incontinence in general is faulty due to lack of basic knowledge of the effect of incontinence on QOL, on mental, social and economical aspects.

4) Many health care professionals generally lack basic knowledge in this field and are unaware of recent advances;

5) Those who provide specialist services are unaware of, or fail to liaise with, the services provided in primary care

6) Those responsible for funding health care often do not pay for continence services.

The Committee on *Promotion, Education and Organization for Continence Care* had a challenge, as there is little evidence available on these issues. Countries throughout the world continue to be at various stages of addressing the challenges posed by the following questions.

1) Given the millions of incontinent people worldwide, how can the message that help is possible be communicated?

2) And how can this be done in the best interests of patients?

3) How can countries without any current service for incontinent people most effectively initiate development of those services?

UI is such a common problem that in most healthcare systems it is unrealistic, and probably undesirable, to expect that every incontinent person will have access to a specialist center and a thorough evaluation as a first option. Indeed, for countries with less developed health services, treatment of UI will not be a priority compared to more basic services. It is only as countries become more affluent that the relative luxury of continence services can be afforded. In countries with existing services, these have largely grown up on an *ad hoc* basis with little coordinated planning. In most countries, the structure of the medical services payment system has directed access to UI evaluation and treatments, making direct comparisons difficult [1]. As other countries develop services, they will have the opportunity to consider the most efficient and effective use of scarce resources, and hopefully learn from what has happened elsewhere.

There is likely to be a shift in what is needed and what is affordable over time. For example, in the past maternal and infant mortality eclipsed all other issues surrounding pregnancy. In the developed world, incontinence and pelvic floor dysfunction are now being addressed as an issue in childbirth. Increasing the use of incontinence services will require a change in public and professional knowledge, attitudes and behaviors. There are some data to suggest that public awareness programs can impact knowledge and attitudes; there is scant evidence describing the best strategies for promoting the behavior changes needed to prevent, diagnose and treat urinary incontinence.

There has been very little work on how to monitor the success of continence promotion and public awareness, education of professionals, international organization initiatives and delivery of continence care and services. Education for the public and for professionals is simplistically assumed to be a good thing in its own right. However, there has been little debate on outcome criteria, and on what constitutes success or progress. It is vital that the ultimate goal of improving care and quality of life for incontinent people is kept to the forefront - none of these other activities makes sense except in that context.

This chapter attempts to summarize the current information available on promotion of continence awareness, professional education, and organization and delivery of services for urinary incontinence. Fecal incontinence has not been addressed in this chapter.

II. PROMOTION OF CONTINENCE AWARENESS

1. Background

The 1992 clinical practice guideline on Urinary Incontinence in Adults of the USA Agency for Health Care Policy and Research (AHCPR) added a section on public and professional education [2]. AHCPR is now known as the Agency for Healthcare Research and Quality (AHRQ). This panel of experts recommended:

- Increased efforts to inform and educate the public about incontinence
- The public should be aware that incontinence is not inevitable or shameful but is treatable or at least manageable.
- Patient education needs to be comprehensive and multidisciplinary so as to explain all management alternatives.
- Research to test the effectiveness of patient education is lacking and essential.

Taboos on mentioning disorders of the bladder generally and UI in particular are gradually lifting in some cultures. Two decades ago it was almost impossible to have incontinence discussed in the media. Now popular magazines, local and national papers, radio and television cover the subject in some countries regularly. Many countries have run national or local public awareness campaigns, usually spearheaded by a national continence organization. Many also have confidential help lines, which can be accessed anonymously. A list of international continence organizations is given in Appendix 1, and many are willing to share their experiences with others.

There is a need to evaluate the impact of public awareness campaigns. It cannot be assumed that everyone who has a continence problem would want or welcome information.

The World Wide Web provides a convenient source of health information for a minority of consumers. There are more than 10,000 health related sites, but all information may not be accurate and timely. Some believe that persons with incontinence might get valuable advice and comfort by using interactive services such as email [3].

2. Quality of Data *(Level of evidence-4)*

There is a great deal of published information on building public awareness of incontinence but very little to no information of the effectiveness in changing the public's attitudes and knowledge about the problem and health-seeking behavior.

3. Conclusions and Recommendations - *(Grade of recommendation D)*

1. Continence organizations are often pivotal in stimulating and maintaining awareness. Many countries, including many developed nations, have a very low level of public awareness of incontinence and have not had any public awareness activities. There has been great progress in some countries with active continence awareness program. There is growing knowledge about what works and what does not.

2. The goal should be to promote health-seeking behaviour using simple language and terminology (e.g. bladder health, bladder control, overactive bladder). Public awareness should convey the messages that:

- Healthy bladder habits may help to prevent problems
- Bladder control problems are common and affect all ages and both sexes
- A problem with bladder control is a medical condition that can be investigated and frequently improved or cured.
- Bladder control problems are not inevitable.

3. There is a need for research on the best route for the delivery of the message and on the appropriate vocabulary, message and format in different cultures. For many it will be more appropriate to refer to "bladder control" than "incontinence." There is also a need to identify routes for obtaining health information in each culture.

4. There is a need for research on the long-term consequences of ignoring incontinence.

5. There is a lack of evidence on translating awareness into behavior change and triggers for health-seeking behavior. Success of campaigns should be measured by behavioral changes, and ultimately by improved patient outcomes.

6. There can be conflict of interest issues with public awareness, particularly where the motivation for funding a campaign is product or practice promotion.

7. Evaluation and outcome measures should be built into all projects and their funding.

8. There is a need for research to substantiate the benefits of preventive strategies.

9. The potential role of peer educators in developing countries should be explored.

a) Primary Prevention of Incontinence

There has been very little work on the prevention of incontinence. There is a lack of epidemiological studies focusing on the identification of risk factors for developing incontinence. Primary prevention strategies should be focused towards preventing UI from occurring [4]. Any activity taken for primary prevention of incontinence serves the target of promotion and awareness. Therefore, primary prevention can be viewed as another means for promotion of awareness of continence.

Identification of continent individuals who have the potential for becoming incontinent is one important primary prevention activity. Some risk factors have been clearly identified (e.g. more than two vaginal deliveries for stress incontinence). Interventions recommended to prevent incontinence through the use of pelvic muscle rehabilitation or caesarean deliveries may prevent future stress incontinence. Prevention should include education about behavioural changes that increase the probability of continence, the normal functioning of the urinary tract, expected age related and developmental changes, and how to find the appropriate treatment providers.

Primary prevention should be the target of all healthcare professionals as it means taking an active part in preventing its appearance. All preventive measures require a high level of community awareness, public education and health professional education [5]. The process of storing and expelling urine is shaped by social rules for acceptable times and places for elimination. This may well be one of the main reasons why shame and denial of the problem are some of the main barriers for seeking medical attention.

From the literature and from previous survey results it is clear that there is a lack of public knowledge and awareness about the concept of incontinence as a medical problem that is common and has negative effects on quality of life, economics, social functions, etc [6]. The public is not aware that incontinence can often be cured with conservative, non-invasive or minimally invasive techniques.

Studies looking into risk factors for incontinence are scarce and sometimes conflicting. One study in older men showed an increased risk for urinary incontinence in post-prostatectomy and hip fracture patients [7]. In elderly women, risk factors were hysterectomy after the age of 60 years, age (odds ratio 1.3 per 5 years); higher body mass index (odds ratio 1.6 per 5 units), history of stroke (OR 1.9), diabetes (OR 1.7), chronic obstructive pulmonary disease (OR 1.4), and poor overall health (OR 1.6). In frail older persons in nursing homes, other risk factors included incontinence and poor adjustment to the nursing home at two weeks post admission, and both mobility and cognitive impairment at two months post admission [8]. In 100 hip fracture patients, men had a higher incidence of incontinence than women (48% versus 24%, $p < 0.03$). Individuals with cognitive impairment also had higher incidence of incontinence (56% versus 25%, $p < 0.03$) [9]. It has been reported that UI in Caucasian, community dwelling older persons is associated with reports of poor self-rated health, after adjustments for age, comorbidity and frailty [10]. Another report lists antecedents of UI including impaired mobility, impaired cognition, poor pelvic muscle tone, lack of access to bathroom, decreased fluid intake, medications, lack of knowledge regarding normal functioning, abrupt changes in cognition, functional status and physical health, depression and social withdrawal [11]. Primary prevention strategies should be addressed for these high-risk populations.

An expert consensus meeting on prevention of incontinence made the following recommendations on promoting prevention education to the public, although it was recognized that these have yet to be substantiated by research [12].

1. The general public should be informed about healthy bladder habits and when/how to seek help.

2. Parents should know about the possible effects of toilet training practices and attitudes.

3. Teachers and schools should be informed about the importance of healthy bladder habits and appropriate toilet environments.

4. People with neurological disease (and their doctors) should know that management is possible.

5. Relatives of people with existing incontinence might prove the most receptive and relevant audience to target with a prevention message.

6. More research is needed to determine the most effective delivery of continence health education.

The group felt that it was important to target the prevention message to government bodies (especially health departments, but also education and employment), health insurance companies and other health funders, national organizations and societies whose members may have continence risks (e.g., organizations of people with neurological diseases), health professional organizations and commercial companies producing continence-related products. Persons at the administrative and clinical level need to be educated about the basics of urinary health and precipitating factors for incontinence before attempting to impart a prevention message.

b) Educating the public about continence

There is little research investigating public education to promote continence. Building awareness among the general public is usually attempted via the media. Using the media to disseminate information in the form of Public Service Announcements (PSAs) has been used extensively in the USA to promote AIDS awareness and as anti-smoking campaigns. In 2001, National Association for Continence (NAFC) produced and disseminated television PSAs to 380 media markets in the USA for the purpose of promoting continence awareness

In many cultures, one of the best vehicles to reaching the public is through an informed journalist. Journalists often use a "media hook," an interesting story that will take priority over other news on the television, radio or newspaper. Having a spokesperson with the problem or finding a celebrity who is willing to speak for the cause can help. These individuals can act as "influence leaders."

A promotion program for raising awareness must consider several aspects:

- **Target population –** Population studies reveal that older women followed by younger women are most affected by incontinence. The prevalence of UI and the lack of knowledge about incontinence are sufficient enough to justify a health-promotion program without segmentation by age or gender [13].
- **Target issues -** A promotion program should identify the issues that warrant promotion effort as well as barriers to promotion. Issues such as lack of willingness or readiness to seek treatment prevent women from seeking help [14].
- **Content of promotional material** -Any type of advertisement that deals with incontinence, even advertising campaigns for absorbent products can have a positive impact on lessening taboos against talking about incontinence. This increased willingness to discuss UI can be followed by advice on effective methods of coping with incontinence followed by directing patients to more effective methods of coping with incontinence.
- **Channels of communication.** Health care professionals may launch campaigns to increase practice revenues. Commercial companies often fund public campaigns in order to sell their products. Regardless of motivation, care should be taken to avoid raising public expectations beyond what the products or services can deliver.
- **Outcome assessment.** Prior to implementing an UI awareness campaign it is important to identify outcome variables that will evaluate its effectiveness.

c) Funding public awareness

Raising money for public awareness is often difficult. In some countries there are numerous granting charities. However, like the general public, these foundations are seldom aware of the impact of incontinence. Therefore, before starting public awareness campaigns, groundwork is needed to educate potential grant-givers. One way to do this is to publish a newsletter and to personalize letters to all of the staff at these organizations. Another is to offer to be a grant reviewer in order to promote better understanding in funding priorities and to stimulate proposals for incontinence that meet those priorities.

In countries where provision of continence products is only by a government funded health service (e.g. UK), there tend to be poorly developed retail markets with little commercial advertising directly to the public. This may limit public awareness about incontinence. Many countries also prohibit public advertising of prescription medication, so companies are forced to create awareness of their product and demand for treatment through indirect public awareness campaigns.

There are many opportunities for collaboration between commercial companies and not-for profit organizations. Companies wish to expand their market and have more incontinent people or caregivers come forward for help. Organizations aim to build public awareness.

d) Examples of public education campaigns in the USA

In order to get correct information to the public, and to allow persons to get their questions answered by a professional, the "I Will Manage" program was developed by the Simon Foundation for Continence. This program was modeled after the American Cancer Society's program "I Can Cope" and was marketed to professionals as a tool to promote continence at the community level. The program was designed to be multidisciplinary and included lectures and a small group format [15]. However, this program was not widely used by professionals in the USA.

The Oklahoma State Health Department developed "Dry Anticipations," which was a community demonstration project that included a curriculum on UI for small groups of elderly women. [16] This project had three components: an educational intervention with physicians, an educational campaign for the general public and a test of behavioral treatments for older women. It was implemented by contracting with six sites in Oklahoma using a train-the-trainer model. A train-the-trainer approach, in which a project prepares a group of instructors to deliver an educational intervention to members of a target population, is a useful method when one wishes to introduce an intervention into existing agencies or ongoing social settings [17, 18].

In the last 5 years, promoting continence to the American public has exploded, primarily because of direct to consumer advertising that uses print, TV and radio marketing. This advertising is primarily developed and funded by pharmaceutical companies. Of course, in other countries such as the Netherlands, law bars the advertising and promotion of prescription drugs. In the USA each fall, a particular bladder condition is highlighted during "Bladder Health Week". Twice in the last ten years, UI has been the featured topic.

e) Other national campaigns

An interesting campaign has been New Zealand's "Dry Pants Day". In Auckland a continence product fashion show began with fully dressed models who then stripped down to their incontinence products to demonstrate how well the products fit and how easy to disguise they are. The narrator told the audience about price and absorbency. Throughout New Zealand, stickers were placed on the inside of public toilet doors encouraging people, in honor of Dry Pants Day, to do their pelvic muscle exercises. No outcomes were measured.

In 1998 the Commonwealth of Australia granted AU$15 million (Australian dollars) for improved continence management in elderly care, targeting those persons living at home. The Advisory Board to this grant included professionals, consumers, caregivers, and organization representatives. Projects are funded under four phases: public awareness, education and information, prevention and health promotion, quality of service, and research. National Continence Awareness Weeks will be held in both 2001 and 2002 but similar activity in each of the last 10 years has not has significant impact. Among the various consumer projects is the Public Toilet Map – a national mapping of toilets to assist travel for persons with incontinence that will show information about opening hours and disability access. Each funded project is independently evaluated or has inbuilt outcome measures.

In Belgium, patients, caregivers, and industry founded an interest group to coordinate activities. It was named "Ucontrol" indicating "you can be in control." The purpose of Ucontrol is to improve incontinence by giving information to patients and caregivers and by supporting and combining coordinated actions involving various government authorities. Ucontrol includes a permanent telephone line, information leaflets which can be obtained free of charge and posters for waiting rooms and hospitals. The organization has prepared a workbook for family doctors, which offers practical information on diagnosis and treatment of incontinence and when to refer for specialist investigation. Ucontrol has published articles in all major Belgian newspapers and magazines and has organized public talks for organizations of women and caregivers, schools and the general public. A scientific organization was formed to provide communication, quality control and continuous post- academic education for the different professionals who provide incontinence services.

f) Public awareness materials

The interventions that best reach the public and trigger the desired behavior seem to vary between countries and cultures. The Japan Continence Action Society held a "Toll Free Telephone Clinic" and callers were asked how they heard about the line. Sixty five percent replied from a newspaper; 26% from television and 8% from a poster. In a United Kingdom (UK) campaign it was found that newspapers were by far the most common source of information, followed by radio [19]. Television and newspapers work best in Singapore, with a cured patient bearing testimony to former suffering and its alleviation having the most impact. In the USA, television advertising targeting overactive bladder and funded primarily by pharmaceutical companies, has yielded a significant response. Nationwide TV reaches more people than the circulation of any single newspaper or the distribution of a booklet even through physician offices.

Experience from a toll-free help line in Australia suggests that television exposure produces a better response than radio, Sunday newspapers are better than dailies, tear-off reply slips are well-used and engaging a celebrity as a spokesperson is more effective than a doctor or nurse. The Australian toll-free help line started with a $A5,000 donation and ran for 18 months before attracting a major ($Australian 900,000) government grant. The Australian Continence Strategy grants have covered multiple projects including epidemiology of incontinence, outcome measure, toilet surveys and service delivery. The words "continence" or "incontinence" are poorly understood and simpler terms achieve greater public recognition in many languages and cultures. The use of overactive bladder in advertising has increased reporting of the condition to primary care professionals in the USA.

Little evaluation of the importance of leaflets or brochures has been undertaken. An information booklet has been found to improve patients' knowledge, acceptance and management of an indwelling catheter at home [20]. More evaluation of the impact of educational materials is needed.

g) Evaluating the effectiveness of public awareness campaigns

It is important to assess that all the efforts to educate the public have the desired effect, and to define the criteria by which to judge "success." Measures of success could include the number of media "impressions" through newspaper, television or radio, the number of people who sought help or the numbers who were actually helped. The message should be crafted to encourage and motivate the desired action. A questionnaire survey of callers three months after phoning the Continence Foundation UK help line during National Continence Week 1994 found that callers appreciated the information, but did not necessarily act on it [19].

A media campaign should use multiple channels to insure the broadest coverage [16]. An initial channel should include press and radio. A second channel would be specialized age and health publications. A third channel is the use of posters and brochures placed in physician's offices, hospitals, senior center, pharmacies and churches. A final channel is direct presentations to the public, such as at senior centers.

In France, the effect of health education was evaluated in a randomized study in sheltered accommodations for the elderly [21]. Twenty centers were randomized to a single one-hour health information meeting or control group. During a 30-minute talk a nurse encouraged people to visit a doctor if they had urinary problems. A questionnaire three months later found that the experimental group were much more likely to have had treatment if they were incontinent (41% vs. 13% controls) and 82% said that they had received some information about incontinence in the previous 3 months (compared to 22% controls).

A health promotion project called Dry Expectations was developed and implemented in six ethnically diverse, predominantly minority, and inner city senior centers in the USA. The program was designed to address an older population. The project consisted of three phases: orientation and training of key staff members/peer educators at the centers (train-the-trainer model); educating seniors through four one-hour weekly sessions involving visual aids and completion of bladder records and quizzes; and follow up sessions with senior staff/peer educators to reinforce the previous training. The program was very well received by the participants and roughly 80% felt they had more control over their bladder by the end of the last session [22].

This project was recently expanded to determine the health promotion needs of senior citizens concerning bladder control issues. Focus groups of older adults attending health seminars in an urban, community setting were conducted. The primary objective of the project was to determine the understanding of older adults in the areas of general health and their beliefs surrounding the problem of UI. The 81 participants were predominantly African-American women representing all socio-economic levels. Seniors expressed confusion when asked if "overactive bladder, bladder control issues and urinary incontinence" were the same condition. Most seniors said they felt comfortable about discussing bladder control issues but most admitted that their doctor had never asked them, nor had they raised the issue. However, they did discuss UI with family members and friends and they were aware that many persons with whom they socialize might have a problem with UI. The majority of seniors answered "no cure" when asked if treatments were successful [23].

A 1996 survey of community-based incontinent people by the National Association for Continence (NAFC) showed that on average women wait 3 years before seeking treatment while men wait only 6 months [24]. This survey also indicated that when women did tell their doctor or nurse about their problem many were told to "live with it". The most common reasons cited for failure to seek treatment are either that incontinence is not seen as abnormal or that there is a low expectation of benefit from treatment. A 1999 NAFC membership survey (mailed to 98,000 consumers with 2,000 surveys returned) indicated that 62.1% registered dissatisfaction with treatment outcome [25]. Only 3.3% of all respondents considered themselves "cured" following their most helpful treatment and only 6.8% overall explicitly expressed that they were "very pleased" with their outcomes. It appears that a gap continues to exist between outcome objectives of consumers and what is available among preferable treatment options.

h) Taboos and health-seeking behavior

Triggers for health-seeking behavior are complex and multifactorial. It is beyond the scope of this chapter to review these here. With a chronic problem like UI, it is important to understand what triggers the patient to consult. Many people also do not consider themselves "incontinent," as this has a negative connotation, or is not well understood. For this reason it may be better to use non-technical terms in most languages and cultures.

Incontinence and bodily functions remain taboo in many cultures. In a series of in-depth interviews with 28 young and middle aged women with urinary incontinence, it was found that incontinence was considered a taboo, making it difficult to seek professional help or even to focus on and think clearly about [26]. Some reacted with apathy; others were always on the brink of taking action. Some feel guilty or associated with despised groups. Many worked hard to maintain "normalcy," and hide the problem. For some there was defensive denial, or they subordinated the problem to other priorities.

One of the aims of a UK study was to explore why people with urinary symptoms (incontinence, urgency, frequency and nocturia) sought help, particularly to identify the triggers that caused them to seek help [27]. The most frequently cited reason for seeking help was raised awareness. The authors postulated that this suggests that health promotion campaigns could be effective and raise not only awareness but also demand on services.

i) Non-compliance: Guilt and Apathy

Pelvic muscle exercises are often recommended post partum. The evidence that these exercises can prevent incontinence is not conclusive but is promising [28]. Patients often do not comply with the advice. A study of in-depth interviews found some recurrent themes [29]. Women often felt guilty that they had not done the exercises, and were subsequently apathetic about the possibility of help for incontinence. Non-compliance with exercises was seen as a reason to expect no further help from doctors, made patients feel embarrassed and was a reason for inaction. Women have found these exercises difficult to remember and to do. If exercises had not been done this was seen as an irretrievable past error that must now be lived with. Consequently many women find themselves in a situation that they feel is their own fault - because exercises were not done, were not done correctly. This led to apathy and reluctance to seek help. Women have a perception that health professionals will blame them for their incontinence.

Self-interest may be a motivator for public education. Direct advertising raises public awareness to advance sales and to serve a commercial advantage. In Australia, medical entrepreneurs advertised widely in the press to promote urodynamic centers and in doing so stimulated the inception of the Australian Urodynamic Society. Such profit-motivated initiatives may also have the effect of raising the profile of incontinence as a health issue, to the benefit of all. It is unrealistic to expect industry to be totally altruistic. Continence organizations may consider partnering with industry to reach a wider, general public audience.

III. PROFESSIONAL EDUCATION

1. Background

A comprehensive service will only work well if those responsible for primary health care are educated about incontinence and know how to refer appropriately. However, professional education with reference to urinary and fecal incontinence remains only a small part (if any) of the basic training of medical practitioners, nurses or allied health professionals. An early survey in the UK found minimal attention given to incontinence in both medical and nurse training, and a key recommendation for improving continence care was an increase in quality and quantity of professional education [30].

There is a dilemma in most countries as to whether to educate the public or the health professional first. In some places it is felt unfair to raise false expectations among incontinent people by creating awareness without having knowledgeable professionals or services already in place. But it may be argued that it is necessary to stimulate professional interest by creation of public demand for help. Ideally, the two would develop together, but this is not always realistic in practice.

Survey results indicated that in most countries incontinence is covered little or not at all in undergraduate medical education and only selectively in postgraduate training [6].

2. Quality of data- *(Level of evidence - 4)*

There is a paucity of published work on professional education in the realm of urinary or fecal incontinence. Similarly there are few studies addressing the effectiveness of education either in improving the knowledge base of the learners, or in whether there are changes in the standard of care for patients, or the outcomes of their interventions.

3. Conclusions and Recommendations - *(Grade of Recommendation - D)*

1. There is a dilemma as to whether public or professional education should come first. In countries where continence has not been developed as a medical service, professional education will usually need to precede public awareness.

2. There should be compulsory inclusion of incontinence in undergraduate curriculum (doctors, nurses, physiotherapists, pharmacists, and others). Incontinence must be identified and planned and preferably delivered as a separate topic, not fragmented between different modules of the educational curriculum.

3. There must be specialist education programs, with relevant accreditation mechanisms (and planned periodic re-credentialing) to safeguard patient interests, for urologists, gynecologists, specialist nurses, physical therapists and others.

4. Funding of education needs to be addressed.

5. There is a need for research on translation of education and research into improved clinical practice and how to ensure that this happens.

6. There needs to be research into mechanisms for increasing professional motivation to acquire education and improve performance.

a) Medical professionals

Most physicians have received little education about incontinence, fail to screen for it and view the likelihood of successful treatment as low [31]. When most of today's professional leaders were undergraduates, UI had almost no part in the medical curriculum. Gynecologists in the course of taking a history occasionally mentioned the term incontinence, but there were no lectures on the subject. Many urologists had no interest or practice in the continence sphere and those that did regarded urinary incontinence as being a post-graduate rather than an undergraduate subject. Bladder and pelvic floor anatomy is poorly covered in preclinical schools and relevant physiology is not mentioned.

- **Medical Undergraduates**

Many undergraduate curricula include information about incontinence. Incontinence may appear in the geriatric medicine, gynecology or urological sections of the curriculum. While co-ordination between the disciplines is rare, some give joint seminars on urinary and fecal incontinence (University of New South Wales) and physiotherapists may have an input to the curriculum (University of Newcastle). Most students today learn about pad and bell alarms for enuresis training, but that is often the extent of their pediatric continence knowledge. In few medical schools are undergraduates exposed to more than five hours of lectures or tutorials on incontinence in the 5-year medical course. In a 1995 survey in UK, undergraduate medical students received an average of 3.3-hours on incontinence causes and treatment, compared with 4.2 hours for physiotherapists and 9.4 hours for pre-registration nurses [32].

It may not be realistic to expect more input than this, given the overburdened medical curriculum. In-depth education may be best given at the postgraduate level for those who will manage incontinence in clinical practice.

- **Family doctors**

The training of family doctors is extremely heterogeneous, varying between different regions and nations. In the UK, two-thirds of newly qualified family doctors received between 1 and 4 hours of training on incontinence; one third had no training at all [33]. Ninety-two percent of doctors in practice for over 5 years had received no training on incontinence and 80% of all doctors felt that their training on the subject was inadequate. Ninety-two percent expressed a desire for specific postgraduate education on incontinence. Knowledge about incontinence was found to be limited, with 76% having "no idea of its prevalence." Only 30% of family doctors felt confident diagnosing and managing incontinence.

There have been few concerted efforts to educate family doctors. However, in Australia in 1989 the New South Wales state government gave $A25, 000 (approx. US$ 18,000) for the development of an educational kit on incontinence [34]. The Australian Federal Government ultimately funded 15000 copies to be distributed to all family doctors in the country. The evaluation of that educational program showed a significant retention rate among 124 volunteers, 80 of who got the pack and were compared with 44 controls [35]. There was no difference in initial knowledge between the groups, but there was a significant difference in post-pack scores between the groups with no difference in scores on questions not in the pack. Sixty-three percent continued to use components of the kit later in clinical practice. However, the study also found a great lack of interest, in that only 16% of those initially selected randomly agreed to participate.

A similar study conducted in 2001, showed a similar initial lack of interest among family doctors. However, after using an educational flip chart and lectures over one evening, family doctors and their practice nurses, showed significant changes in their attitude, with 64% indicating that they would adopt a more pro-active role in the future. Only 10% remained disinterested after the educational intervention [36].

Family doctors can be effective in treating incontinence by conservative measures when educated and motivated [37, 38]. Typical cure or improvement rates range around 60 - 70%. Education can also increase referral rates to specialist practitioners [39]. However, the best format for education needs further delineation. It gas been found that videos are not necessarily the best format for use in primary care practices. It is not known whether commercially produced videos are more successful in reaching their target; some may be, especially when the company has a sales force actively promoting the videos. As the price of video reproduction has come down, many companies are now prepared to give them away free, even for individual patients.

The 1992 and 1996 USA AHCPR clinical practice guidelines were produced to help to standardize the assessment and management of urinary incontinence in adults [2, 40]. Aimed at health professionals the guidelines are widely quoted, but they failed to inform the practice of medical practitioners or their trainees [41]. The concept of using bladder diaries or checking post-void residual urine as part of basic assessment is still foreign to most urologists, gynecologists and family doctors not specializing in continence. Nurses seem to have taken up the AHCPR recommendations, incorporating them in curricula, evidence-based clinical practice and care pathways, whereas doctors have not [42, 43]. In a USA survey, 50% of physicians in the USA who treat bladder disorders (25% of which were family practice physicians) were not familiar with the AHCPR guidelines [44]. Although UI is prevalent it mainly goes underdectected and is inadequately managed. Physicians are inquiring about incontinence in only a minority of their at-risk patients.

Changing the current patterns of medical care with respect to detection and management of incontinence will not be easy [45]. Guidelines for medical practice can contribute to improved care only if they succeed in moving actual practice closer to the behaviors the guidelines recommend [46]. Unless there are other incentives or the removal of disincentives, guidelines are unlikely to effect rapid changes in actual practice. It is recognized that other tools or strategies are needed to augment and build on educational endeavours [47]. Strategies that aid in implementation of a guideline include reminder systems to remember when to implement guidelines, tracking systems to identify patients who need follow-up and continuous quality improvement monitoring and regulations. Educational programs alone may change knowledge and attitude but rarely change behaviors. Guidelines combined with continuing medical education programs may be more successful [48].

Even evidence-derived guidelines may not always result in better practice or outcomes. The implementation and evaluation of such a guideline in one family practice from which 1503 patients were selected randomly has been reported [42]. Thirty-five percent of women and 9.9% of men suffered from incontinence in the previous 2 months, but 61% had never sought help. Of those who did, 63% were referred on mostly to specialists. Only 53% had a urine test, only 1 in 4 women had a vaginal examination and only 4 of 206 persons with UI had done a frequency/volume chart. After implementing the guideline, two abdominal examinations and one new rectal examination were performed, but no new vaginal examinations were performed. Frequency/volume charts were given to three people. Two people used less drugs. The severity of incontinence was not changed following the intervention. Family doctors did not effectively implement the guideline. It remains to be tested whether, properly used, guidelines can improve incontinence in practice.

In a 1999 repeat of a 1996 survey, among 6481 patients (>50 yo), it was found that after numerous UI awareness and education campaigns, German physicians were even less likely to address incontinence [49]. The "don't ask, don't tell" attitude between physicians and patients, has fiscal implications for managed care. The consequence of not treating the condition may increase the annual cost of care by an estimated $3941 per individual [50]. Funding for conservative management of UI, or better-informed public demand, may stimulate more interest and improved performance among this pivotal group.

If family doctors are to be engaged in continence care, they need to be involved in the process and it's planning. As clinical encounter time is limited, there is a need for a validated assessment tool to aid in the assessment of a patient. The family doctors need effective, practical treatments relevant to their care setting.

- **Medical Specialist Training**

Specialist training in incontinence is not always adequate to their needs in subsequent clinical practice. A survey of urological trainees between 1988 and 1994 in Australia showed many felt their training in the management of incontinence (and infertility) had not been adequate[51].

Much the same can be said of continuing medical education for already-credentialed specialists who are erroneously assumed to know something about the subject from their training. The Colleges of Obstetrics and Gynecology in the United Kingdom and Australia and the American Board of Obstetrics and Gynecology have developed courses and credentialing of specially trained urogynaecologists with separate examinations. However, incontinence may be in danger of being seen as the province of an elite group of super-specialists who get further and further away from their colleagues.

A recent survey of 163 urodynamic services in the UK found that only 43% of doctors, nurses and others performing urodynamic investigations felt that training to do these studies had been adequate [52].

The plethora of meetings put on by medical specialist groups (International Continence Society, Pelvic Floor Society, Asian Society for Female Urology, International Urogynecology Association) and meetings of recently-formed national Continence Foundations in Thailand, the Philippines, Taiwan serve both as stimulants to trainees, and as continuing education for practicing clinicians.

b) Other medical professionals

Nurses have often been more closely involved in continence care and management than physicians or allied health professionals. Those dealing with the elderly at home (through domiciliary nursing services), in hostels, nursing homes or geriatric institutions are especially familiar with the problem. Only in the last 15 years has education really empowered nurses to intervene to change the continence status, rather than coping with its consequences.

Nurses called "Continence nurse advisers" were appointed in the UK throughout the 1980s with no central planning or direction. In 1983, there were only 17 continence advisers, [30] by 1998 there were over 420 [53] with nearly every purchasing authority having at least one in their area. Some cynics claim that the program was created to reduce spending on incontinence absorbent products, which have traditionally been provided, free of charge in the UK. Most continence nurses have developed a service in which individual patients are seen and assessed in hospital, at home or in community clinics, as well as offering professional advice and support to colleagues.

The Royal College of Nursing Continence Care Forum conducted a consensus exercise amongst continence advisers [54]. Recommendations were that the principal functions of the continence adviser should be education, management, clinical practice and research, and that each of these elements should be recognized as equally important. At present there is no research on the most appropriate mix of these functions, nor on the optimum caseload or number of continence advisers per population. Most areas seem to be moving towards a small team to cover a geographical area rather than a lone individual.

The UK Department of Health has commissioned a survey of continence nurses which found that most had both hospital and community responsibilities. Ninety percent were involved in clinical practice, advice and training, but fewer in management and research. Only 20% were involved in all 5 of these. There was a wide variation in the amount of time and the importance ascribed to different activities. Seventy-three percent carried a personal caseload. Eighty-five percent did home visits and 65% ran a clinic. Thirty-eight percent ran a telephone advisory service. Many had developed a link nurse network in each clinical unit to encourage liaison. Most worked as part of several different multidisciplinary teams. Gaps in the service were identified as children, people with disabilities and those with mental health problems. Few referrals were from ethnic minority groups. With time many had moved away from clinical work towards education and training, and towards developing a team of advisers [55].

Other countries, such as Australia, have adopted this model of a continence nurse specialist. Australia provides domiciliary continence services via the District nursing service or geriatric assessment teams. The Continence Foundation also runs centers in several state capitals. The Netherlands has a well-developed system of continence nurses, and Scandinavia has a university course requirement to practice as an "Urotherapist."

The specialist nurse role varies from independent nurse practitioner, continence consultant on call to other generalist domiciliary nurses, appliance specialist, assessor, trainer or therapist. Funding arrangements may determine whether and how a specialist nurse post can be developed. For example, in Singapore, most posts have started in large hospitals because that is the source of funding.

There are health care systems that make it very difficult to fund nurses working as independent practitioners across hospital and community boundaries. Elsewhere, the prevailing culture and philosophy within nursing does not favor the development of specialist roles. For example, historically in Denmark the system prepared highly trained generalist nurses and did not encourage clinical nurse specialists [56].

In Canada, a Nurse Continence Adviser collaborative database has been set up. Information gathered during patient assessments is recorded on a standard assessment data entry form. The system generates reports and consultation letters and can be updated at each visit. There is a care-mapping feature, which allows evaluation of each patient's progress against expected outcomes, facilitating audit and comparison between advisers. The system is reported to have reduced paperwork by 75% [57].

- **Specialist Nurses**

As has been previously noted, much of the change in the role of nurses has come about through the emergence of nurse continence advisers and to a lesser extent, special interest groups within stoma (enterostomy) therapy. Educational courses on incontinence are available for nurses are in the UK, USA, Europe and Australia and are beginning to appear in Asia, notably Hong Kong and Singapore. These courses vary from 2 to 4 weeks face to face didactic courses to distance learning courses lasting 4 - 6 months and leading to a post-basic nursing certificate. Australia has a graduate certificate course for continence nurses, as well as a variety of distance learning and certificated courses. A 1-year graduate certificate course is available at several university Schools of Nursing within Australia - in particular, Flinders University of South Australia, Univ. of Western Australia, University of Technology Sydney and Deakin University. At Flinders, the Certificate in Continence Management can be upgraded to a Master degree after 2 years of further study and research. Integral to some of these courses has been instruction in educational skills that enable the graduates to teach not only other nurses, but also patient and caregiver groups.

This accords with the needs in the community and the emerging role of the continence nurse practitioner (CNP). The English National Board has defined a role and an appropriate curriculum involving introduction, clinical practice, and health promotion and bowel dysfunction. The course evaluation was by controlled trial in which graduates were shown to improve knowledge scores from 18(38%) to 25 (53%) [58].

There is a need for properly validated courses as a prerequisite to practice as a nurse specialist. The University of Gothenburg has a well-established multidisciplinary course for the recognized qualification of "Urotherapist," of whom there are several hundred throughout Scandinavia. Most participants are nurses or physiotherapists, but there have also been some doctors who completed the training. In the USA, nurse practitioners are prepared at the graduate nursing level, but there are few nurse practitioners specializing in incontinence care [59]. In many other countries, recognized preparation is not in place, and any one can potentially claim to be a continence specialist.

The Japan Nurses Association has an accredited 6-month specialist course on wound care, ostomy and continence nursing, but the emphasis is on stoma nursing. The course costs $Y750, 000 (approximately American$ 5,500) and 90% of attendees pay their own tuition fees. The Japan Continence Action Society also provides 4-day primary and secondary courses. The Danish Nurses Organisation has a 220 hour course, divided into 5 modules [60].

In Canada, 38 nurses were trained in a 3-month program funded by the Ontario Ministry of Health in 1995. This was found to be expensive, so McMaster University, with local preceptors and a tutor available developed distance learning Nurse Continence Advisor education program by phone. Assignments are posted on-line. The students have 6-9 months to complete the course, which has so far enrolled 34 students, for the same cost, as training four students under the previous program. It is planned to offer this distance learning on a national basis in 1998 [61]. The same group has developed standards for management, clinical practice, education and research [62].

The funding of educational continence programs in incontinence by governments will inform both the need for CNPs and the types of service they provide. Non-surgical treatment remains under-recognized and poorly reimbursed in the USA, where the demands for CNPs is low, whereas in many other countries (e.g. UK, Europe, Australia) CNPs are not only funded, but also are highly regarded. The potential roles of CNP's as clinical providers, advisors, educators, researchers and managers, [55] and the relative need for each skill, will inform curricula of certificate courses in the future [63].

- **General Nurses**

Setting nursing standards of practice can help by requiring clinicians to acquire the skills to meet the standards. In Australia, for example, government funding to nursing homes is dependent upon their reaching certain standards in continence assessment and management. The standards set were those based on advice from the Continence Foundation, which was commissioned in 1991 to produce an educational resource for nurses working in elder care [64] which was distributed to 1400 nursing homes. Changing negative attitudes among health workers and low expectations amongst elderly people themselves are among the obstacles to such educational endeavours [65]. Nursing records, which are designed to extract and document continence status, may assist the nursing process [66].

The development of Continence Care Pathways has been tested and found that the use of care pathways ensured that generalist nurses identified reversible causes (e.g. UTI, drugs, fluid intake, constipation, dexterity and mobility issues), and addressed quality of life, bothersomeness and specific symptoms [67]. Patients could then be referred to CNPs for specific treatment beyond the scope of the generalist nurse, or when they failed to respond to first line therapy. The care pathway identified the needs of the patient, directed simple investigation and primary therapy, but also identified the resources needed by the nurses (e.g., urine testing dipsticks, lists of drugs, frequency/volume charts). The pathway could be modified according to the equipment and expertise locally available. Educating large numbers of general nurses to follow a simple pathway with basic continence-care competencies [68] may make better use of a CNPs time and specialized skills [69].

The level of knowledge within the general nursing community appears to be less than ideal in both the USA [68, 70] and Sweden [71]. Many non-specialist nurses desire, and have a need for, more education about what they can do to better manage incontinent individuals. Moreover, the quality of life of the incontinent nursing home resident is often more dependent upon the skill, education and attitude of the nursing aide than of the nursing unit manager.

In a detailed UK study of learner and qualified nurses' knowledge and the content of nurse education, only 12% of qualified nurses had received any education on incontinence in the previous 12 months, and for those who had, most was on products. Forty-four percent of charge nurses and 81% of staff nurses had received no additional training on incontinence since qualifying [72]. Further work on attitudes via a questionnaire to qualified student nurses on hospital wards found predominantly therapeutic, rehabilitative attitudes, but also a number of misconceptions. Twenty one percent thought their primary role with incontinent patients should be supplying products and 11% saw incontinence as an inevitable part of aging. Sixteen percent agreed that incontinence was often due to laziness and 28% thought that incontinence was more distressing for a younger than for an older adult [73]. In a further survey of trained student nurses, the author found that nurses still focus primarily on palliative rather than therapeutic care and lacked knowledge on which to base care [74]. However, nurses with a post-basic qualification or in-service education were more likely to have positive attitudes, although it was not clear whether this was as a result of the education, or whether these nurses already had a positive attitude and had therefore self-selected themselves to receive further education.

In the USA, although there are a growing number of nurses who are developing expertise caring for incontinent patients, there are no academic or clinical proficiency requirements to be considered a "continence nurse practitioner or specialist." In 1993, the Wound, Ostomy, and Continence Nurses Society (WOCN) developed the first certification program for continence care nurses in the USA. To date, the number of nurses certified through this process has not been significant probably because of views of specific requirements. The norm is that most nurses in the USA obtain their knowledge and skill through self-motivated activities. A survey of nurses attending a national nursing conference on UI asked about educational preparation related to this condition. Respondents reported that less than half (40%) received academic education including course work in accredited post-baccalaureate or graduate programs related to UI. However, most nurses (76%) obtained instruction at professional conferences, continence clinics supervised by nurse practitioners or physicians, "on-the-job" training, self-study, or in-service programs [63].

These findings were supported by a national survey of USA nursing school curriculum [75]. Schools of nursing agreed that incontinence is important and 90% of curricula included it specifically, but with an average of only 2.1 hours of lecture time in undergraduate nurse preparation. There was no commitment to requiring clinical experience in this area, there was a lack of awareness of available educational resources and there were few experts available to teach. The authors offer evidence that incontinence is not well managed in clinical practice, suggest that 2 hours is insufficient and make recommendations for improvements and research on which instructional methods are most effective. Because incontinence crosses so many boundaries, it is difficult to know where to fit it into a curriculum as a coherent whole rather than fragmented between different modules.

Nurses are not always positive towards continence education, with 20% in one study feeling that nurses in USA nursing homes would be apathetic or resistant to a program on incontinence [75].

It is not clear how the need can be met in a timely fashion, or who will pay for the time and expertise it will require. Governments, as chief funders of nursing home care have a vested interest in promoting continence where it is possible. It is believed that the continent nursing home resident requires less nursing time than an incontinent resident. Expert intervention also has the possibility to reduce the need for, and cost of incontinence devices and products [77]. It therefore falls to the funders to underwrite the education that is needed to promote continence. More emphasis on incontinence care and the nurses' role in continence promotion should be encompassed in basic nurse training courses. CNP's and nurse continence advisors are the best instructors to provide this education. Fundamental texts on incontinence should get onto the reading lists of basic training schools and colleges [78, 79, 80, 81, 82, 83].

A clinical handbook has been found to be a good method of disseminating research findings to nurses [84]. A significant improvement in reported clinical practice was found for 86% of variables in the experimental group compared to a 59% improvement in controls. However, only 54% of those approached agreed to enter the study, and only 29% of them attended the second session, suggesting a lack of interest and motivation generally. As with physicians, it is felt that improving nursing knowledge will not actually translate into improved clinical practice, or into the ultimate goal of improved patient outcomes. A review of ward policies and community nursing practice in an area with a well-established continence service and education program demonstrated very little evidence that education had tangible effect on practice. The authors conclude that nurse specialists are most usefully employed providing a clinical service to individual patients rather than spending their time educating other nurses. [85]

There is a lack of consensus or guidelines on what it is reasonable to expect different nursing groups to be taught at each educational level.

c) Allied Health Professionals

Physiotherapists or physical therapists (PT) have long

played a part in continence care and the management of incontinence. In some countries, patient self-referral to specializing physiotherapists has become commonplace. Physiotherapists' involvement in incontinence appears to be either on the basis of individual interest or through association with women's hospitals or obstetric departments, rather than as part of a general physiotherapy practice. As such they tend to be highly motivated and enthusiastic.

Post-basic PT education has largely been post-graduate through specialist courses run by specialists. In the UK, the University of East London has a degree level module run part-time over 15 months. Over 100 physiotherapists have completed this to date [86].

Pharmacists have a variety of roles to play in continence care. In Australia, they have been avid consumers of recent continence education programs. The public sees them as important and approachable sources of health information. Many retail pharmacies display health promotion literature on a range of subjects including incontinence. From such displays people can pick up the information they need without drawing attention to themselves. The pharmacist may also become the continence adviser on appropriate continence products. Liaison between continence organizations, continence advisers and medical practitioners may be an important avenue for promoting continence information into the community, often at no charge, or with the cost born either by the pharmacy chain or by sponsoring pharmaceutical houses. Educational seminars for pharmacists are generally well received.

There is also a need to address the training needs of unqualified nursing assistants and aides, particularly in the nursing home setting. In the USA of concern is the high turnover rate among first-line caregivers in institutionalized and in home care settings, making it economically difficult to maintain desired training levels. These individuals are nursing assistants who are the people providing incontinence care and who are the least trained.

Reimbursement schemes strongly affect who is the provider of intervention measures. In the Netherlands, for example, up to 14 visits to a physiotherapist are paid for by the government for incontinence (e.g., biofeedback therapy). Before 2001, there was little chance of getting coverage of biofeedback assisted pelvic muscle exercises in the USA.

d) Educational materials and funding

There is a range of teaching packs, videos, and books on the topic of UI available. The Continence Promotion Committee of the International Continence Society (ICS) publishes a directory of material available from national continence organizations. There have been many advances in the field of information technology and interactive and distance learning methods which are starting to be applied to continence.

One interesting innovation in delivering continence education was reported by Teleac, a Dutch broadcasting company, who offered sufferers training therapy consisting of pelvic floor muscle exercises, bladder training and advice on relaxation and posture. They reached an average of 140,000 viewers per broadcast; 51% of participants reported an improvement in their incontinence, and 83% were satisfied with the results of the course [87].

Education can be expensive, for courses or production of materials, and to replace personnel who are away from work. The first two specialist nurse courses in Australia cost AU$110,000 to train 20 nurses.

In practice much education and many materials are produced or sponsored by commercial companies marketing incontinence-related products. While some are highly ethical, and fund broadly based materials without product mention, others attempt to influence the content to market their product. A partnership between ethical companies and professionals can be mutually beneficial, but the boundary between education and marketing is not always clear.

e) Internet education resources

Many Internet sites now exist for the education of professionals and public. Providers have developed web sites and educational materials which are available in CDROM format (Japan) and as computerized decision pathways. In future, online real time video will be accessed through the Internet. The CONTInet, a site sponsored by the ICS, provides interchange between national continence organizations and the public. A number of sites now exist from trade and professional bodies providing up to date information about new products and operative interventions. Interactive educational sites have yet to appear. One study reported on the accuracy of web sites developed by organizations based in the USA that included information on UI [88]. A total of 265 web sites were located but only 15 sites met the inclusion criteria. The authors felt there is a rapid proliferation of information on the WWW and there is a need to critically evaluate new sites or updated information as it becomes available. A physician evaluated the Internet as a source of interactive information about UI by posing as a fictitious woman with symptoms of stress UI. He found that few sites provided comprehensive information, but most information was correct [3].

IV. ORGANIZATIONS

A. Delivery of Continence Care and Services

1. Background

The organization of incontinence services in each country will depend on the organization and structure of health services generally. It is difficult to make recommendations that will apply in such a variety of contexts. In addition, incontinence is so widespread and affects so many different types of people that they can present for help to literally any health care professional. This means that there will seldom be one portal of entry to a continence service. The challenge is to plan a service that ensures a systematic care pathway (i.e., that patients follow a step-wise progression of investigation and treatment, without overlaps or omissions) and the best use of scarce resources [89].

When new services are created there is a temptation to focus on the high technology investigation and medical treatment elements without considering the infrastructure needed to support that service. However, there has never been a comprehensive examination of an optimal service. It is not known whether a hospital-based specialist-led clinic will achieve better and more cost-effective results than primary care clinics, domiciliary services or any other model.

In some health systems incontinence traditionally has been seen solely as a nursing problem, with little interest or input from other members of a multidisciplinary medical team. Except for a few isolated areas, the main intervention has been trying to help the individual and caregivers cope with symptoms rather than attempting to cure the incontinence. For example, in the UK it is common for an elderly person presenting with incontinence to be referred directly to the district nurse "for assessment for pads and pants," with no physical examination or further investigation considered.

In fact, incontinence is often a complex and multi-faceted problem, particularly in frail or dependent individuals and it may require input from a wide variety of disciplines to tackle it effectively. While it may not be practical for all specialities to work in close proximity, there needs to be careful consideration of who does what, with protocols to guide appropriate referral and ensure good liaison. It is important that there are neither gaps nor overlaps in the service. In countries such as Australia, New Zealand and the UK, where there is a national network of CNPs, part of their job is to organise this liaison, integrate services, and guide individuals through the referral route most appropriate to their individual needs.

Although some might see multidisciplinary working as the ideal, the reality is not always smooth. In some situations, rivalries and competition between disciplines and medical specialities is evident. This may be because of competition for patients and income, or because of disputes over the demarcation of the scope of different disciplines (such as the boundary between urology and gynecology, or between nursing and physical therapy). In Israel, physical therapists are not permitted to perform any invasive procedure (e.g. insertion of vaginal and rectal sensors and pelvic examination procedures are considered invasive and physical therapists are not reimbursed). Only nurses and doctors perform these procedures and examinations.

2. Quality of the Data - *(Level of evidence - 4)*

There are no studies directly comparing the effectiveness of specific delivery systems for continence care. In certain cases, enthusiasts have conducted research. The results may not generalize to the wider setting. However, there are examples of models for service delivery in some countries. Others have combined the expertise of multidisciplinary to maximize service delivery.

3. Conclusions and Recommendations - *(Grade of Recommendations - D)*

1. World Health Organization recognition of continence as an important health issue will encourage those countries with no current provisions to plan a strategy for meeting continence needs.

2. Government support and co-operation is needed to develop services, and responsibility for this should be identified at a high level in each Health Ministry. Incontinence should be identified as a separate issue on the health care agenda. There is a need for funding as an independent service, not to be linked to any one patient group (e.g. elderly or disabled), and not an optional service.

3. No one model for Continence services will apply. In all health care systems much will depend on the local health care structure. Given the high prevalence of incontinence, there is a need for a stratified service. There should be a community based primary health care continence service (family doctor or continence nurse led) to assess each presenting individual and to implement conservative treatment when appropriate. Specialist consultation and modern investigations should generally be reserved for those patients where appropriate conservative options have failed, or for specified indications.

4. Continence services should be planned according to the needs and wishes of incontinent people and their caregivers. Consumers should be actively consulted

and involved in the planning process in order to empower consumers of services.

5. At present many clinical decisions are determined by reimbursement structures, which are not always in concordance with the results of scientific research or professionally developed guidelines.
6. While developing countries may have other pressing health priorities, there is a need to encourage future planning of continence services together with promoting awareness in anticipation of the aging population.
7. There is a need for research on outcomes, not just the process of service delivery. These outcomes must be patient-focused, and evaluate the outcomes of all comers to a service (not just specific treatments for specified groups). To do this, validated audit tools are needed as well as longitudinal studies of services (e.g., nursing home admission rates).
8. There is a need for cost-effectiveness studies of a whole service and evidence on whether high quality services save on costs.

a) The needs of service users

It is only recently that the desires or needs of people with incontinence themselves have been seriously considered. With an embarrassing problem like incontinence, many have been reluctant to report or to complain when they experienced symptoms. Many do not seek help anyway, and expect little when they do. In the UK, continence was one of a series of qualitative studies into users' views on health services. Responses were mixed [90]. Some people were appreciative of the compassionate treatment they had received, but others seemed bewildered by the intricacies of getting help. A series of 14 recommendations on making services accessible and acceptable were made.

It is important not to assume that all incontinent people want or need help, and this may vary considerably between different cultures. One community study found that only half of people who identified themselves as having incontinence of urine took up the offer of a local consultation [91]. In another study, a postal questionnaire asking about urinary symptoms found that nocturnal problems caused the most bother (69% were bothered by nocturnal enuresis, 63% by nocturia). Only 50% found stress incontinence a bother, 56% were bothered by urge incontinence [92].

A community interview study found that only 15% of severely incontinent women (daily incontinence requiring protective pads most of the time) were worried about it, and 15% felt that their activities were restricted. Most seemed able to cope. Overall, 78% were not worried by their incontinence and the authors concluded that their findings "do not support the hypothesis of severe psychological effects of hidden incontinence". They therefore suggested that services should be targeted towards the minority who do find it a problem [93].

In Japan it has been found that 55% of elderly incontinent people do not consider incontinence a bother, but 15% did not go out, 10% found it difficult to go out and 10% felt that they caused bother to family and neighbours [94]. A Japanese survey of over 1,000 caregivers of elderly incontinent people in the community found that more than 80% of caregivers are female and over half were more than 60 years old. (Kitagawa, 1997) The caregivers felt that incontinence caused problems with the home getting dirty (10%); extra laundry (9%); need to wake at night (7%) and not being able to go out because of incontinence (9%). When asked what kind of government service they wanted, caregivers replied "health training" (10%); "knowledge about incontinence" (10%); and "supply of a portable toilet" (3%). Only 6% wanted the government to send them professional caregivers and 4% desired referral to a specialist doctor.

Some people seemed to cope better than others with symptoms, and some had coping strategies which were easily undermined by any suggestion that professional help was required [95]. Few people seemed prepared to take action to prevent incontinence. In France, where the state will pay for women to have up to 10 sessions of pelvic floor rehabilitation after childbirth, only 30% take up this offer.

This can create a dilemma - should health professionals attempt to persuade people who do not see incontinence as a problem that it is an abnormal condition? Is lack of bother genuine, or simply a defence against having to tackle an unpleasant problem? Does early intervention prevent later deterioration in symptoms? Does delay in treatment mean that success rates are lowered? There is scant evidence on any of these issues, or on the most acceptable way of providing help.

In a USA survey, UI was seen in 53% of homebound patients and was a leading reason for caregivers to place a family member in a nursing home [96]. The relatives of 50 patients admitted to the hospital because caregivers could no longer cope were asked which factors, if alleviated, would have enabled coping. Micturition at night, fecal incontinence and incontinence in an opposite-gender parent who needed intimate care were among the least well-tolerated problems [97].

b) The United Kingdom Continence Care model

The UK continence services have grown up over the past 2 decades without, until recently, any central planning or guidance. Local needs, interests and often personalities have driven developments. Two main models have emerged. One is a service led by a hospital consultant doctor (urologist, gynecologist or geriatrician), often focused around an urodynamic unit providing medical or surgical treatment. The other model is a nurse continence adviser-led model. The continence nurses often work in both hospital and community, and the service is focused on primary care (particularly district nurse) assessment of patients and organization of free incontinence product delivery to the home. Only recently, except in a few notable situations, have truly multidisciplinary services emerged. It is unknown if these model are effective for addressing all needs of persons with incontinence.

The Royal College of Physicians set up a multidisciplinary working party, which made a number of recommendations on continence services [98] (See Table 1). The Department of Health has identified the key elements of a continence service and strongly advised Health Authorities to implement this [99]. It is a very complex job to integrate all elements into a coherent service. Some continence services or information are targeted to a specific segment of the population, such as a project to provide continence advice to the 23 % of women in the East End of London who were Bangladeshi [100].

Table 1 : Royal College of Physicians' Recommendations for a Continence Service

The structure required to achieve these aims might include: a designated manager, an expert advisory panel and a budget to provide staff, their training and support services, and containment materials and equipment.

A continence service should include:

- a defined method of entry for patients referred by family doctors, nurses, hospital staff and patients themselves
- access to appropriate diagnostic facilities, including urodynamics and anorectal investigations
- access to medical and surgical consultants with a special interest in incontinence
- integration of incontinence services for children with other paediatric services
- attention to the wishes of patients and caregivers
- access to nurses and physiotherapists with special training in treatment modalities for incontinence
- a role for one or more specialist continence advisors in the education of the public and professionals in continence maintenance
- a policy concerning the purchasing and supply of containment materials and equipment in the community, in residential and nursing homes and in hospitals
- well defined audit and quality assurance systems.

Source Royal College of Physicians, 1995

The Department of Health in the UK has commissioned an evaluation of different models of nursing services, with and without specialist continence advisers [101]. It was found that where there is a continence nurse, incontinent people are more likely to receive targeted referral to specialists such as an urologist, and are more likely to have had investigations and to receive more appropriate treatment and care for their incontinence. These patients were also more likely to report satisfaction with the service. In most areas the continence nurse is involved in individual patient assessment, to sort out the simple problems at the primary care level and implement conservative therapy where appropriate.

c) The Israeli model – starting an integrated service

In January 1994, a national center for geriatric incontinence was established in Israel. Previously, there were very limited services and it had previously been found that 20% of older people and 53-100% of those living in institutions had urinary incontinence. Only 2% had received proper evaluation and treatment [102].

A National Center for Continence was formed that included a team of professionals (two urologists, two geriatricians, two nurses skilled in geriatrics and in home care, a social worker, a co-ordinator and a secretary) from different institutions. This allowed promotion of interdisciplinary exchange as well as maximum co-operation between the Medical Centers and the community health services. After 6 months of training, the team was ready to address the goals of the Center. After trying various education and training programs an approach which fits the healthcare system was developed. A clinic was pre-selected to be trained according to certain criteria: it must be a large clinic with at least 3 family doctors and a service population of over 20% elderly patients. A local team composed of a physician and a nurse are also pre-selected to be in charge of promotion, detection and treatment of incontinence at the clinic. Questionnaires and evaluation sheets developed by the Center were to be used. The education program included training the entire staff of the clinic, and the team received supplementary training. A new position of regional continence advisor was created. The best physician and nurse among teams in a region received additional training to be in charge of incontinence in the whole region.

This system enables professionals to approach local or regional advisors as well as to contact the Center directly, and it gives the Center feedback on the activity and success of individual clinics. Centers staff make frequent visits to the clinics, maintain contact via telephone and by a quarterly newsletter. There is also an update program every 6 months for all professionals. The Center has developed a training program in nursing homes, where mostly nursing staff and aides provide treatment.

The outcomes of this program are constantly examined. Data on patients, detection, and success rates are collected each month from the clinics and nursing homes. Results have shown that this model of training combined with consultancy back up is beneficial. Detection rates are high, and there is an average of 70% success rate for patients treated at the clinics. In the nursing homes, in addition to a surprisingly high success rate, treatment of incontinence made family members more involved with the patients' progress, saved costs on diapers and added to the prestige of the nursing home.

The Center has also set up a central clinic equipped with advanced diagnostic tools (e.g., urodynamics), and a selection of treatment options including surgery. Other activities include the development and production of effective tools intended for professional staff, telephone advisory services to healthcare providers as well as to the public, production of information brochures and audiocassettes, and promotion of awareness through lectures in the community. The Center organised the first national meeting on incontinence and conducts clinical and epidemiological trials along with basic science research. Most recently, fecal incontinence management has been included in the Center's training program and a catalogue of all products available in Israel is being completed.

A countrywide program for establishing satellite centers is currently in progress. Plans for the near future are to establish a Hotline for the public, to promote education programs in nursing and medical schools, hospitals and nursing homes and to develop guidelines for diagnosis and management of incontinence by primary healthcare staff.

d) Community continence services – is there an ideal model?

The Israeli experience suggests that, where few services exist, it is feasible and effective to stimulate effective community management of incontinence, with limited specialist back- up. There are many factors that can persuade health care planners of the importance of adequate investment in community continence services: the prevalence and the number of incontinent people is likely to increase with an aging and increasingly dependent population; many frail, disabled or elderly people are incontinent for reasons extraneous to the urinary system (such as poor mobility, an inappropriate physical environment or lack of an individualised care regime). It is often best to provide a first assessment for such individuals in their usual surroundings and to reserve hospital or clinic referral for those who do not respond to simple measures such as treatment of constipation, modifying a diuretic medication or provision of accessible toilet facilities. A number of guidelines have suggested an algorithmic, step-wise approach to assessment and treatment of incontinent people and many conservative treatments have a good success rate in primary care [2, 40, 103].

Incontinence is an expensive problem. It is likely, but as yet unproven, that more investment in prevention and early detection could prevent progression of symptoms for some people and prevent them from eventually becoming major users of resources (such as needing a nursing home place because incontinence can no longer be coped with at home). However, it is recognised that in some health care systems, such as Japan, primary health care is not well developed. In such situations primary care continence services may not be realistic.

e) Family doctors and incontinence

Family doctors are often ideally placed to delivery UI services through early detection. For example, 87% of older Australians visit their family doctor at least once per year [104]. However, many family doctors lack the necessary training, time, self-assessment tools and effective primary care strategies, knowledge or confidence to manage UI successfully.

A New Zealand study of 600 family doctors found that most respondents provided continence care, and 2.6% offered special clinics for continence promotion [105]. Fewer than half felt confident to diagnose the causes of incontinence. Confidence in managing incontinence in children was consistently lower than for other childhood problems. There was no difference by sex in confidence, although female respondents were more likely to consider management of continence care as part of a practice nurse's role and to routinely ask well women about incontinence. Most respondents (71.9%) could not remember having had any formal training in the management of incontinence either at the undergraduate or postgraduate level. Recall of postgraduate education was associated with greater levels of confidence in management of continence problems.

In a questionnaire study in the UK replies were received from 560 family doctors. They were more likely to refer men than women and younger rather than older patients with UI to a specialist. Fifty-three percent had seen 3 or more incontinent patients in the past month. Twenty-nine percent routinely ask about incontinence at well man clinics, 54% do so at well women clinics, 6% do not ask at over 7 years of routine screenings. Eighty percent would always test the urine, 60% would always send a sample for microscopy. Women and older doctors were more likely to refer and felt that the most helpful people were the community nurse, gynecologist and urologist. Only two-thirds used geriatricians or continence nurses, half use physiotherapists. The author concluded that family doctors see a lot of incontinence, and vary in how they manage it [106].

Family doctors have been shown to be successful in treating incontinence. A UK study examined assessment and treatment of 65 women, who were treated according to their type of incontinence. Those with stress incontinence were treated by pelvic muscle exercise, those with urge incontinence by bladder training and medication, and those with mixed incontinence by both. Both stress and urge, but not mixed, improved compared to controls at 12 weeks [107]. A Dutch study of 110 women reporting UI to a family physician were randomly assigned to treatment or control. Treatment was pelvic muscle exercises for stress and bladder training for urge. Patients were interviewed at 3 and 12 months, with crossover at 3 months for controls. At 3 months, 60% were dry or only slightly incontinent. Mean wet episodes were down from 27 to 7 per week. Seventy-four percent felt improved or cured and there was further slight improvement at 1 year [38].

A study in a community clinic in Israel showed that after training, family doctors detected 100 patients with UI during a period of 19 months. Mean age was 71years (range 56-89), 94 females and 6 males. Most patients (53) were detected by the physicians on direct questioning, some by nurses (29) and only 18 by self-referral. After a mean follow up of 10 months, 35 were dry and 32 significantly improved. Cure or improvement was achieved at the clinic with no involvement of urologist or gynecologist [108].

f) Multidisciplinary care

Some countries are starting to tackle problems of coordinating continence services by consulting on and agreeing to referral criteria and pathways. Others have set up multidisciplinary clinics, such as a "Pelvic Floor Clinic" where gynecologist, urologist, colorectal surgeon, physiotherapist and continence nurse work together [109]. The issue of fecal incontinence services is not included in this chapter but consideration should be given to the desirability of close co-operation where the patient has double incontinence.

There is some evidence on the effectiveness of multidisciplinary clinics. A Canadian study looked at 184 women, with a mean age of 60. Eighty-eight patients were treated and seen weekly for 6 months. Ninety-four controls were also seen at 6 months. The main interventions were pelvic muscle exercises, bladder training, and advice on fluids and the reduction of weight and smoking. Thirty-four percent of the treatment group were cured and there was a significant improvement in the amount of leakage and bladder control compared to controls. The study did not report on the outcomes in the control group [110].

An Australian study took all community referrals of those who had been incontinent for at least two months and had at least one episode in past 2 weeks to a continence clinic. Patients were randomised to conservative treatment or control, with a crossover design. Patients were asked subjective questions about embarrassment, odor, depression, family relationships, isolation and laundry on a 4-point scale ranging from no effect to major effect upon life. The questionnaire was completed at the start, and at 2, 4, 8, and 12 months. Seventy-eight patients entered the study; 87% improved with treatment (41% controls also improved). Fifty-two percent were moderately or severely embarrassed at the start of the study period; only 17% were at 4 months. Depression decreased from 49% to 22% and isolation from 28% to 12%. Odor and extra laundry also decreased. All benefits were maintained at 12 months. Controls did not improve on these items until crossed over to active treatment, despite feeling better. The authors conclude that conservative treatment in a multidisciplinary community clinic improves continence and well being [111].

g) Other specialists practitioners

One study found that a nurse was competent to assess and manage community patients after 3 weeks of training [112]. Patients received 4 sessions of exercises and bladder training. Sixty-eight percent of women were subjectively cured or improved after nursing intervention, compared to 5% of controls. Only 22 of 86 men were suitable for treatment by the nurse, 17 were cured or improved (no controls improved). They concluded that many incontinent people could be effectively managed by a nurse with limited additional training, reserving specialist medical help for resistant cases. These results seem to be sustained in the long term. In a follow up study 89% were followed up 4 years later. 69% had maintained or improved their continence status. Improvement was strongly associated with continuing pelvic floor exercises for more than a year.

In a Canadian study, 421 subjects were assessed by a nurse and then randomised to treatment or control. The treatment group improved in voiding frequency and wet episodes as compared to the control group [37]. Another Canadian study found that interventions were effective in reducing incontinence and patients were satisfied and felt that they had received control over the problem [113].

In UK, a new mode of service delivery that was dependent on specially trained CNPs was shown to be effective in reducing urinary symptoms and led to high levels of patient satisfaction [114].

A recent study in the USA demonstrated significantly improved outcomes for three clinical problems; urinary incontinence, depression and pressure ulcers when advanced practice gerontological nurses (APNs) worked with nursing home (NH) staff to implement scientifically based protocols [115]. In addition to working with NHs to provide resident evaluation as physician extenders, this research indicates that APNs can be an effective link between current research based knowledge about clinical problems and NH staff. This study also showed that consistent educational efforts with staff and residents demonstrated that interventions could improve or stabilize the level of UI in many persons.

In some countries, physical therapists (PTs) have also developed a specialized practice with incontinent clients. In France all women are entitled to up to 10 sessions of pelvic floor rehabilitation physiotherapy, paid for by the government, after childbirth. In Australia, Scandinavia and the UK, research on pelvic floor exercise has been led by PTs. However, there is a lack of consensus as to best practice for incontinence. In a postal survey of British PTs found that many were providing a specialized service. Gynecologists were the most common source of referral. The majority said physiotherapy was first line of treatment. Pelvic floor muscle exercises and electrical stimulation were the most used modalities. However, there was little consensus about optimum treatment regimes and a wide variety in the details of therapies used [26, 29].

h) Childhood enuresis services

Very few countries have well-developed services for nocturnal enuresis in childhood. These are seldom well integrated with adult continence services, although some continence nurses do run enuresis clinics. Most clinics are the responsibility of pediatric, school health or psychology services.

i) Services in developing nations

Continence services are a relative luxury, to which countries with a low per capita income are unlikely to devote scarce resources until more "life and death" issues are addressed. For example, in Brazil, priorities for their health budget are childhood immunizations, AIDS/STDs, basic sanitation, healthy environment and literacy to help with the problem of street children. The Mission Statement of the Pan American Health Organization is "to promote the full development and utilization of human capabilities through health promotion activities and stronger intersectoral and community action to improve the living conditions of the most socially neglected groups." In such circumstances it is unrealistic to expect a major priority given to a subject such as UI. The one instance where UI has become a recognised problem in developing countries is incontinence secondary to obstetric fistula.

Ethiopia's Health Minister has stressed the need to develop rural health services to reduce the incidence of fistula and to have first time mothers examined by Traditional Birth Attendants (TBAs). It is planned that TBAs will be trained to identify high-risk women, and thereby divert expenditure from high cost doctors and urban health services to training community health workers and health education. Attitudes on female circumcision, contraception and women's health, which are often decided by their husbands, obviously have much wider implications than just continence care.

A demonstration project in northern Nigeria has reported training obstetric fistula patients to act as peer educators to help prevent vesico-vaginal fistula [116]. The concept of peer health educators has been used in many developing countries. Given local traditions of seclusion of women, only their peers may have access to women of childbearing years.

j) Financial issues and funding of services

It seems that the major share of expenditure goes toward additional hospital admissions, longer hospital stays, home care, and routine care expenses rather than toward therapeutic interventions. It is not known what impact might be made by diverting a portion of current expenditure to education of professionals or the public, or to investigation and cure.

There are always decisions to be made on how to allocate scarce resources, for instance between hospital and community services; high tech and conservative treatments; cure and products to support people with intractable incontinence in their own homes. Cure should always be the aim where this is feasible, and no continence service should merely manage the incontinence without individual assessment, care planning and an attempt to improve continence. Where there is one overall mechanism for planning the whole service, there is the potential for rational allocation of resources and a seamless service. Where the service is fragmented and the responsibility of several different agencies, there is the danger of competition for funds, or shifting responsibility between budgets without actually benefiting the patient or saving on costs.

Funding arrangements will also mould the configuration of a service. For instance, in France, where postnatal pelvic exercises are reimbursed, many PTs have developed a continence expertise; in the USA, where it is more difficult to be reimbursed, fewer PTs are expert in this area. In the USA in 2001, the Commission on Medicare and Medicaid Services (CMS), formerly the Health Care Financing Administration, which administers Medicare, the insurer of the disabled and elderly, recommended biofeedback assisted pelvic muscle exercises and pelvic floor electrical stimulation as a reimbursable service. It is important that professionals involved in continence care make funders aware of optimum clinical efficacy, and how funding arrangements can potentially distort clinical decisions.

k) Cost-effectiveness of continence services

It has sometimes been argued that good continence services may ultimately save on costs. The evidence for this is scant and difficult to measure. A survey of 49 homebound patients with indwelling catheters in Israel showed that one year after the intervention of a trained team, there was a significant reduction in emergency calls, hospitalisation rate and complication rate due to proper management [117].

Provision of a service can increase costs when many people who were not previously treated seek help. Whether the cost per case can be decreased by better management remains to be proven, as does the cost implication of prevention of symptom progression by early treatment. However, the ultimate aim of services should be to improve quality of life rather than simply minimize costs.

l) Protocols and guidelines

There have been several attempts to improve clinical practice by issuing centrally produced guidelines. The USA has done this on the largest scale [2, 40, 103, 118]. From the first Urinary Incontinence in Adults guideline issued in 1992, and the second completely re-worked edition in 1996, over 3.5 million copies of the three documents (detailed report, summary and patient guide) have been issued in English and Spanish, 58% to consumers. However, it is not clear that a paper guideline always reaches the intended target. Only 17% of physicians had seen or read the 1992 AHCPR guidelines [17]. A huge effort and expense may not result in a change in behaviour, and research on effective dissemination and implementation of research findings should be a priority. This effort is now being further developed by the USA National Institutes of Health (www.nih.gov) by way of computer-based patient assessment documentation linked to the guidelines. By linking in to a server, health practitioners can access on-line information relevant to the individual patient under assessment.

The USA has also attempted to influence and improve clinical practice in nursing homes by statutory regulation. The 1987 Omnibus Budget Reconciliation Act made it a statutory requirement that nursing homes maintain as normal a level of bladder function as possible. To ensure that this happens, the CMS issued a minimum data set (MDS) to be completed for all nursing home residents. The MDS includes items about bladder function, which, if positive, should trigger a more detailed assessment of bladder function.

The NAFC developed a Blueprint for Continence Care for Assisted Living Facilities (ALFs) in the USA. The Blueprint addresses gaps between intentions and practices and discusses assessment of residents, management of their conditions and training of caregivers [119].

The UK Department of Health has commissioned a multidisciplinary panel of experts to draw up recommendations on outcome indicators by which to measure the performance of continence services [120]. The effectiveness of the indicators has yet to be evaluated.

B. World Wide Organizations

1. Background

The International Continence Society, in setting up a Continence Promotion Committee, and in hosting this International Consultation of Incontinence (1998 & 2001), has recognised a broader responsibility than its former role as a forum for scientific research. Many in the scientific and medical community have also been active in developing national policies services and organizations, in teaching professionals and in public awareness activities. Although it may not be practical to develop global and uniform strategies for continence promotion and public awareness, much can be learned from the positive and negative experiences of other organizations in other countries.

Continence promotion is a most challenging endeavour. Although the ratio between affected patient populations and continence organizations funding has not been formally studied, anecdotal information suggests that fundraising for continence programs is among the most difficult of medical problems for which to obtain funding. In view of all these challenges, the proliferation of new continence organizations, especially in the Far East, is a validation of both the need for continence promotion and the dedication of those who have recognized and are addressing this need.

2. Quality of data *(Level of Evidence - 4)*

There is a paucity of published work on the formation of national organizations that target consumers or the general public. Appendix 1 gives the contact details for national continence organizations. A professional or medical organization is listed if there is no organization that targets the lay public in that country. The countries where there is an organization generally seem to have greater public and professional awareness about continence and more educational activity and materials available, although the direction for causation in this relationship is not always clear. The countries where there is more interest are more likely to develop an organization. A CD-ROM on how to set up a continence organization is available from the Society for Continence Singapore.

3. CONCLUSIONS - *(Grade of Recommendations - D)*

1. A worldwide association of continence organizations, under the auspices of the Continence Promotion Committee of the International Continence Society should be explored. This will create a central co-ordinating body for continence activity to be encouraged and should be a catalyst in countries where there has as yet been little development of services, education and awareness. This Worldwide collaboration must spearhead the formation of a "World Bladder Health Day".

2. Resources for promoting continence are scarce, especially in proportion to the magnitude of the problem. Unique, creative solutions must be found to maximize all available resources.

3. Free exchange of continence information and materials between countries should be encouraged. This can be co-ordinated via the Continence Promotion Committee (CPC) of the International Continence Society and the CONTInet Internet site. In order to accomplish this task, funding for an experienced executive director for the CPC should be a priority.

4. A "media bank" should be created. This "bank" would contain medical art, illustrations, and animations related to incontinence (a set for consumer education and a set for medical education), which could be used by any organization, eliminating the costs all organizations generate when creating educational materials.

5. A data bank should be established on the CONTInet Internet site and formatted for standardized reporting of program launches worldwide. This "experience bank" database would create an avenue for fast and efficient experience exchange.

6. "Information modules" with ICS-approved language should be created (and posted on CONTInet) to help organizations communicate clear, standardized information in their educational material for the general public.

7. Organizations must undertake market research to better understand the needs of people with incontinence, so as to set their own agenda and priorities rather than being led by the availability of funding.

8. Adequate funding will often involve commercial collaboration, but attention must be given to ethical considerations, in particular avoiding direct product endorsement.

• Summary of Current International Organizations

National organizations, which promote continence, are as diverse as the cultures they serve. They represent a wide diversity of models, including consumer-led, company sponsored, professionals only, and organizations which have deliberately set about trying to bring together all relevant stakeholders in a relatively democratic set-up. In every part of the world these organizations play a dynamic role in building both public and professional awareness of this under-served and under-reported condition. Most continence organizations are poorly capitalized, being either under or unfunded (i.e., run by volunteers) and are held together initially by either a dedicated patient advocate or an energized health professional. Yet, despite this limitation, these organizations often provide their country with the first wake-up call that incontinence is common.

Although the exact founding date of the first continence organization is not known, none have been in existence longer than three decades. Even so, the wealth of experience, the creativity of endeavours which have been tried, and the method in which older organizations are evolving into established foundations are all worth studying. However, the challenges of cross cultural communications, language barriers, and the costs of travelling to international meetings make information sharing a unique challenge.

Each of the organizations listed in Appendix 1 were sent a survey requesting general information about the organization. Organizations that primarily target the general public generally do not participate in educating professionals. Those countries where a consumer-based organization does not exist do engage in educating professionals as well as raising the awareness of incontinence to the population in general. Except for the USA, most countries responded that incontinence services are paid through national health insurance plans. The USA has a combination of government and private insurance. In those countries that have consumer-based Continence organizations, there are national public awareness campaigns about USA programs (e.g., has a designated "Bladder Health Week" every fall). Organizations were quizzed about the origin of funding or financial support. Most receive funding from members or charitable donations. Other sources included lottery funds (Great Britain) or corporations. It was generally felt that media coverage in these countries is inadequate. Only the USA indicated that there was a national organization that addresses fecal incontinence.

In 1994, the Singapore Continence Society set up "CONTInet", an electronic network on the World Wide Web [121]. This service will eventually develop an index system to facilitate rapid easy communication of information between organizations and individuals. The initial focus has been networking of continence organizations and internal International Continence

Society business, but there is also the facility for announcements of meetings, publication of abstracts, rapid sharing of resources and teaching materials and co-ordination of multi-centre research. The CONTInet can be found at: http://www.org.sg/continet/, or at: http://www.dpa.org.sg/continet.

While there is little data on the outcomes of the use of organizations to change consumers' views and awareness of incontinence, there is one model that indicates coordination of countries may be a more efficient use of resources and time. The Asia Pacific Continence Advisory Board (APCAB) was established with a mission to develop "Continence Promotion" programs that work together with healthcare providers and the general public to develop strategies to increase awareness and reduce the social burden of urinary incontinence in the Asia Pacific Rim. APCAB member countries are the following: Thailand, Korea, China, Hong Kong, Taiwan, Malaysia, Indonesia, India, Philippines, Singapore and Pakistan. APCAB's secretariat is under the administration of Society for Continence Singapore (SFCS) since its formation in 1998. APCAB conducted its first Asia-wide prevalence survey on "Overactive Bladder" to obtain epidemiological data in the respective countries [122]. The SFCS coordinated this project and successfully completed the study in six months. By the end of year 2000, SFCS helped nine out of these eleven countries to form their own continence organizations.

The Committee would like to thank Nancy Mueller, Executive Director, National Association for Continence and Carole Mertz for their review of this chapter.

REFERENCES

1. Fonda D, Ouslander JG, Norton C: Continence across the continents. [Review] [25 refs]. JAGS, 42:109-112, 1994
2. Agency for Health Care Policy and Research, Urinary Incontinence in Adults: Clinical Practice Guideline. AHCPR Pub. No. 92-0038. Rockville, MD, Public Health Service, U.S. Department of Health and Human Services, March, 1992.
3. Sandvik H. Health information and interaction on the Internet: a survey of female urinary incontinence BMJ, 319:29-32, 1999.
4. Palmer, MH. Urinary Continence: Prevention Focused Research in Swanson, E., Tripp-Reimer, T, Buckwalter, K. Eds Health Promotion and Disease Prevention in the Older Adult, Springer Publishing Co., NY: 127-145, 2000.
5. Palmer MH. A health promotion perspective of urinary continence. Nursing Outlook. 42(4):163-169, 1994.
6. World Health Organization's (1998) meeting and publication of the 1st Consultation on Urinary Incontinence. (Abrams, P, Khoury, S, Wein, A (Eds). Incontinence, Plymouth, UK: Health Publications, Ltd, 838-868, 1999.
7. Fonda D, Resnick NM, Kirschner-Hermanns R. Prevention of urinary incontinence in older people. British Journal of Urology, 82[Suppl 1]: 5-10, 1998.
8. Ouslander JG, Palmer MH, Rovner BW, German PS. Urinary incontinence in nursing homes: incidence, remission and associated factors. JAGS, 41:1083-1089, 1993.
9. Palmer M, Myers, A., & Fedenko, K Urinary continence changes after hip-fracture repair. Clinical Nursing Research. 6(1). 8-24, 1997.
10. Johnson, T., Kincaide, J., Bernard, S., Busby-Whitehead, J., Hertz-Picciotto, I. & Defriese, G. The association of urinary incontinence with poor self-rated health. JAGS, 46(6), 693-699, 1998.
11. Palmer, MH., German, P., Ouslander, J. Risk factors for urinary incontinence one year after nursing home admission. Research in Nursing and Health, 14, 405-412, 1991
12. Cottenden, A., Gartley, C. B., Norton, C., and Saltmarche, A. Consensus statement of the first international conference for the prevention of incontinence (Danesfield House). Conference Proceedings, 1997.
13. Melchior H, Kumar V, Muller N, Van Maanen H, Norton C. National public health policies for prevention and care in urinary incontinence in the elderly. World J Urol. Suppl I:S71-S73, 1998.
14. McFall SL & Yerkes AM: Targets, messages, and channels for educational intervention on urinary incontinence. J Applied Gerontology 17:403-418, 1998.
15. Haugen V, Moore A. "I will manage": promoting continence through community education JWOCN 22(6):291-295, 1995.
16. McFall SL, Yerkes AM, Belzer JA, et al: Urinary incontinence and quality of life in older women: a community demonstration in Oklahoma. Family & Community Health 17:64-75, 1994
17. McFall SL, Yerkes AM, Cowan, LD: Overcomes of a small group educational intervention for urinary incontinence, Health-related quality of life. J Aging and Health 12(3) August,:301-317, 2000.
18. McFall SL, Yerkes AM, Cowan, LD: Overcomes of a small group educational intervention for urinary incontinence, episodes of incontinence and other urinary symptoms. J Aging and Health 12(3) August, 250-267, 2000.
19. Norton C, Brown J, Thomas E: Continence: a phone call away. Nursing Standard 9:22-23, 1995.
20. Roe B: Study of the effects of education on the management of urine drainage systems by patients and carers. J Advanced Nursing 15:517-524, 1990.
21. Beguin AM, Combes T, Lutzler P, et al: Health education improves older subjects' attitudes toward urinary incontinence and access to care: a randomised study in sheltered accommodation centers for the aged (letter). JAGS, 45:391-392, 1997.
22. Newman DK, Wallace J, Blackwood N: Promoting healthy bladder habits for seniors. Ostomy Wound Management 42:18-28, 1996.
23. Newman, DK, Palmer, MH, O'Connor, MP, Flynn, L, Brown, D Health promotion needs of Older Adults concerning Bladder Control Issues, Abstract - Sixth Multi-Specialty Conference on Urinary Continence, New Orleans, LA, 2001.
24. National Association for Continence. Consumer Focus 96: A Survey of Community-dwelling Incontinent people. NAFC: Spartanburg, SC. 1996.
25. National Association for Continence. Consumer Focus 99: A Survey of Community-dwelling Incontinent people. NAFC: Spartanburg, SC. 1999.
26. Ashworth PD, Hagan MT: The meaning of incontinence: a qualitative study of non- geriatric urinary incontinence sufferers. J Advanced Nursing 18:1415-1423, 1993.
27. Brittain, KR, Perry, S, Williams, K. Help seeking and goal setting in people with urinary symptoms: an exploratory study. University of Leicester, 1999.

28. S ampselle, CM, Miller, JM, Mims, BL, Delancey, JOL et al. Effect of Pelvic muscle exercise on transient incontinence during pregnancy and after birth. Obstet & Gynecol, 91(3):406-412, 1998.
29. Ashworth PD, Hagan MT: Some social consequences of non-compliance with pelvic floor exercises. Physiotherapy 79:465-471, 1993.
30. Incontinence Action Group. Action on incontinence; report of a working group. Project Paper No 43. London, Kings Fund, 1983.
31. Resnick N, Improving treatment of urinary incontinence JAMA 1998, 280,2034-5.
32. Laycock J: Must do better. Nursing Times 91:64-64, 1995.
33. Jolleys JV, Wilson J: GPs lack confidence (Letter). British Medical Journal 306:1344-1344, 1993.
34. Continence Foundation of Australia. Tackling urinary incontinence in the community. Continence Foundation of Australia, 1989.
35. Szonyi G, Millard RJ: Controlled trial evaluation of a General Practitioner education package on incontinence: use of a mailed questionnaire. British Journal of Urology 73:615-620, 1994
36. Lazzarini RS Report on Continence Education in the Hunter Region. Australian Government Report, May 2001 – personal communication.
37. Borrie MJ, Bawden ME, Kartha AS, et al: A nurse/physician continence clinic triage approach for urinary incontinence: a 25 week randomised trial. Neurourology and Urodynamics 11:364-365, 1992.
38. Lagro-Janssen ALM, Debruyne FMJ, Smits AJA, et al: The effects of treatment of urinary incontinence in general practice. Family Practice 9:284-289, 1992.
39. Snape, J., Allardice, A. J., Lemberger, R. J., and Pickles, C. J. The continence roadshow: a method of educating primary health care workers about services available and management of urinary incontinence. Proceedings of the International Continence Society, Halifax, Nova Scotia. 284-284, 1992.
40. Fantl, JA, Newman, DK, Colling, J. et.al. Urinary Incontinence in Adults: Acute and Chronic Management Clinical Practice Guideline, No 2, Update, Rockville, MD: US Department of Health and Human Services. Public Health Service, Agency for Health Care Policy and Research, AHCPR Publication No. 96-0682. March. 1996
41 McFall S, Yerkes AM, Bernard M, Le Rud T. Evaluation and treatment of urinary incontinence. Report of a physician survey. Arch Fam Med., 6(2), 114-9, 1997.
42. Button D, Roe B, Webb C, Frith T, Colin-Thome D, Gardner L. Consensus guidelines for the promotion and management of continence by primary health care teams: development, implementation and evaluation. J Adv Nurs. 1998, 27, 91-99
43. Sampselle CM, Wyman JF, Thomas KK, Newman DK, Gray M, Douglas, Burns PA
42. Continence for Women: A test of AWHONN's evidence-based protocol in clinical practice. J Obstst Gyneol Neonatal Nurs, 29(1): 18-26, 2000.
44 Wein, AJ, Appell, R A., Blavias, JG, Bump, RC, Diokno, AC, Fantl, JA., Norton, P, Resnick, NM. Bladder Disorders Monitor – Bladder Disorders Clinical Practice Consensus Report. The Center for Bio-Medical Communications, Hackensack, NJ, 1998.
45. Cohen SJ, Robinson D, Dugan E, Howard G, Suggs PK, Pearce KF, Carroll DD, McGann P, Preisser J. Communication between older adults and their physicians about urinary incontinence J Gerontology 54A(2): M34-M37, 1999.
46. Lomas, J., Anderson, GM, Domnick-Pierre, K., Vayda, E., Enkin, MW., Hannah, WJ. Do practice guidelines guide practice? The effect of a consensus statement on the practice of physicians., N Eng J Med, Nov 9; 321(19):1306-11, 1989.
47. Woolf, SH. Changing physician practice behavior: the merits of a diagnostic approach. J Fam Pract. Feb, 49(2):126-9, 2000.
48. Davis, DA, Thomson, MA, Oxman, AD, Haynes, B. Changing physician performance: A systematic review of the effect of continuing medical education strategies. JAMA, September 6, 274(9):700-705, 1995.
49. Welz-Barth A, Fusgen I, Melchior HJ. A 1999 rerun of the 1996 German Urinary Incontinence Survey: will doctors ever ask? World J Urol, 18, 436-8, 2000.
50. Cochran A. Don't ask, don't tell: the incontinence conspiracy. Manag Care Q. 8(1). 44-52, 2000.
51. Nichol D, Ward J, McMullin R, et al: Urological training in Australasia: perceptions of recent fellows and current trainees. Australian and New Zealand Journal of Surgery 65:278-283, 1995.
52. Hosker GL, Kilcoyne PM, Lord JC, et al: Urodynamic services, personnel and training in the UK. British Journal of Urology 79:159-162, 1997.
53. Continence Foundation (UK). Index of continence advisory services. London, The Continence Foundation, 1998.
54. Royal College of Nursing Continence Care Forum. Role of the continence adviser. Royal College of Nursing, 1992.
55. Rhodes P, Parker G. The role of the continence adviser in England and Wales. Int J Nurs Stud, 32, 423-433, 1995.
56. Roe B: Promoting continence in Denmark and UK. Nursing Standard 7:28-30, 1993.
57. Skelly, J., Krouse Cutler, K., and Corradetti, P. Simplifying communication, quality assurance and research using the NCA database. P-22. Association for Continence Advice conference proceedings, Edinburgh, 1998.
58. Williams KS, Assassa RP, Smith NK, Shaw C, Carter E. Educational preparation: specialist practice in continence care. Br J Nursing. 8(18), 1198 – 1207, 1999.
59. Newman, D. K. Urinary incontinence management in the USA: the role of the nurse. Bri J Nursing 5(2),Jan-Feb:78,80,82-88, 1996.
60. Basse, K. Educational programme for nurses in healthcare for people with incontinence. P-12. Association for Continence Advice Conference Proceedings, Edinburgh, 1998.
61. Skelly, J. Nurse continence advisor distance education pilot programme. P-23, Edinburgh, Association for Continence Advice Conference proceedings, 1998.
62. Corradetti, P., Krouse Cutler, K., Putman, L., Pyatt, B., and Skelly, J. Developing standards of practice for continence advisors. P-24. Association for Continence Advice conference proceedings, Edinburgh, 1998.
63. Jacobs M, Wyman JF, Rowell P, Smith D. Continence nurses: A survey of who they are and what they do. Urologic Nursing, 18, 13-20, 1998.
64. Hunt, S. Promoting continence in the nursing home. Continence Foundation of Australia., 1993
65. Wellings C: Ageist attitudes promote urinary incontinence in older people and can lead to demoralisation of nursing staff. Australian Journal on Ageing 7,:6-8, 1988.
66. Palmer MH, McCormick KA, Langford A: Do nurses consistently document incontinence? Journal Gerontological Nursing. 15:11-16, 1989.
67. Bayliss V, Cherry M, Locke R, Salter E. Pathways for continence care: development of pathways Br J Nurs, 9(17), 1165-1172, 2000.
68. Jirovec MM, Wyman JF, Wells TJ Addressing urinary incontinence with educational continence-care competencies. Image J Nurs Sch. 30, 375-8, 1998.
69. Hall C, Castleden CM, Grove GJ Fifty six continence advisers, one peripatetic teacher. BMJ; 297:1181-2., 1988.

70. Connor PA, Kooker BM: Nurses knowledge, attitudes and practices in managing urinary incontinence in the acute care setting. Medsurg Nursing 5:87-92, 1996.

71. Mansson-Linstrom A, Dehlin O, Isacsson A: Urinary incontinence in primary health care: perceived knowledge and training among various categories of nursing personnel and care units. Scandinavian Journal of Primary Health Care 12:169-174, 1994.

72. Cheater, F. M. Urinary incontinence in hospital in-patients. A nursing perspective. University of Nottingham, UK, 1990.

73. Cheater FM: Attitudes towards urinary incontinence. Nursing Standard 5:23-27, 1991.

74. Cheater FM: Nurses' educational and knowledge concerning continence promotion. J Advanced Nursing 17:328-338, 1992.

75. Morishita L, Uman GC, Pierson CA: Education on adult urinary incontinence in nursing school curricula: can it be done in two hours? Nursing Outlook 42:123-129, 1994

76. Palmer MH: Nurses' knowledge and beliefs about continence interventions in long-term care. J Advanced Nursing 21:1065-1072, 1995.

77. Fonda, D., Woodward, M., D'Astoli, M., and Chin, W. F. Sustained subjective improvement of quality of life before and after treatment for incontinence. 286-286. Conference Proceedings of the International Continence Society, Halifax, Nova Scotia, 1992.

78. Norton C: Nursing for continence. Beaconsfield, Beaconsfield Publishers:1996

79. Doughty, D (Ed) Urinary and Fecal Incontinence: Nursing Management. Philadelphia: Mosby:325-383, 2000.

80 Getliffe, K, Dolman, M. Promoting Continence: A Clinical and Research Source, London: Bailliere Tindall and the Royal College of Nursing, 1997.

81. Newman, D.K. 2nd edition The Urinary Incontinence Sourcebook, California: Lowell House, 1999.

82. Palmer, M.H. Urinary Continence: Assessment and Promotion. Aspen: Gaithersburg, MD, 1996.

83. Roe, BH. Clinical Nursing Practice: The Promotion and Management of Continence UK: Prentice Hall International, 1992.

84. Williams KS, Crichton NJ, Roe B: Disseminating research evidence. A controlled trial in continence care. J Advanced Nursing 25:691-698, 1997.

85. Wells, A. and Malone-Lee, J. G. The assessment of a continence advisory service. 146-146. Rome, International Continence Society, 1993.

86. Mantle J, Versi E: Physiotherapy for stress incontinence: a national survey. British Medical Journal 302:753-755, 1991.

87. Neiwijk AH, Weijts WB Effects of a multi-media course on urinary incontinence Patient Educ Couns, 30, 95-103, 1997.

88. Diering C, Palmer MH. Professional information about urinary incontinence on the World Wide Web: Is it timely? Is it accurate? JWOCN 27(6): 1-9, 2001.

89. Clayton J, Smith K, Qureshi H, Ferguson B. Collecting patients' views and perceptions of continence services: the development of research instruments. J Advanced Nursing 28(2): 353-361, 1998.

90. NHS Management Executive. Incontinence. 1994. London, Citizens Charter & National Health Service Executive.

91. O'Brien J, Austin M, Sethi P: Urinary incontinence: prevalence, need for treatment and effectiveness of intervention by a nurse. British Medical Journal 303:1308-1312, 1991

92. Swithinbank, L. V., Donovan, J., Shepherd, A. M., and Abrams, P. Female urinary symptoms: just how much "bother" are they? Proceedings of the International Continence Society, Tokyo. 431-432. 1997.

93. Lagro-Janssen ALM, Smits AJA, Van Weel C: Women with urinary incontinence - self-perceived worries and general practitioner's knowledge of the problems. British Journal of General Practice 40:331-334, 1990.

94. Kitagawa, K. Annual report on Health and Welfare 1995-6. Tokyo, Ministry of Health & Welfare of Japan., 1997.

95. Talbot LA: Coping with urinary incontinence: a conceptualization of the process. Ostomy Wound Management 40:28-37, 1994

96. Noelker L. Incontinence in elderly cared for by family. The Gerontologist 27: 194-200, 1987.

97. Sander P, Mouritsen L, Andersen JT, Fischer-Rasmussen W. Evaluation of a simple, non-surgical concept for management of urinary incontinence (minimal care) in an open-access, interdisciplinary incontinence clinic. Neurourology and Urodynamics 19:9-17, 1999.

98. Royal College of Physicians: Incontinence. Causes, management and provision of services. A Working Party of the Royal College of Physicians. Journal of the Royal College of Physicians of London 29:272-274, 1995.

99. Department of Health. An agenda for action on continence services. ML(91)1. London, Department of Health, 1991.

100. Haggar V: Cultural challenge. Nursing Times 90:71-72, 1994

102. Gruenwald, I. The Center for Continence: A different concept for an old problem. JAGS 47:912-914, 1999.

103. Association of Women's Health, Obstetric and Neonatal Nurses; Evidence Based Clinical Practice Guideline: Continence for Women. Washington DC, AWHONN. 2000.

104. Gingold R: Prevention of health problems in later life. Medical Journal of Australia 159 :682-690, 1993

105. Dovey S, McNaughton T, Tilyard M: General Practitioner's opinions of continence care training. New Zealand Medical Journal 109:340-343, 1996

106. Grace J: Incontinence: your views. Geriatric Medicine March:52-57, 1993

107. Jolleys JV: Diagnosis and management of female urinary incontinence in general practice. J Royal College of General Practitioners 39:277-279, 1989

108 Aharoni, L., Gruenwald, I., Rosen, T., and Vardi, Y. Management of urinary incontinence for the old aged in the primary care clinic. Proceedings of the International Continence Society, Jerusalem, 1998.

109. Nijeholt, AAB. The Leiden pelvic floor center: a patient-oriented multidisciplinary diagnostic center. Proceedings of the International Continence Society, Jerusalem, 1998.

110 Bawden, M. E., Kartha, A. S., Kerr, P. S., Durko, N. A., Haslam, I. F., and Lytwynec, S. Treating women with stress incontinence in a multidisciplinary clinic: a randomised study. Proceedings of the International Continence Society, Halifax, Nova Scotia. 276-276. 1992.

111. Fonda D, Woodward M, D'Astoli M, et al: Effect of continence management programme on cost and useage of continence pads. Neurourology and Urodynamics 12:389-391, 1993.

112. O'Brien J, Long H: Urinary incontinence: long tern effectiveness of nursing intervention in primary care. British Medical Journal 311:12081995

113. Saltmarche, A., Reid, D. W., Harvey, R., and Linton, L. A community nurse continence service delivery model - a demonstration project. Proceedings of the International Continence Society meeting, Halifax, Nova Scotia. 274-274. 1992..

114. Williams KS, Assassa RP, Smith NKG, Jagger C, Perry S, Shaw C, Dallosso, H, McGrother, C., Clarke, M., Brittain, KR, Castleden, CM., Mayne, C. Development, implementation and evaluation of a new nurse-led continence service: a pilot study. J Clinical Nursing 9:566-573, 2000.

115. Ryden, MB, Snyder, M, Gross, CR, Savik, K., Pearson, V., Krichbaum, K., Mueller, C. Value-added outcomes: the use of advanced practice nurses in long-term facilities. The Gerontologist, 40(6):654-662, 2000.

116. Ojanuga D: Training obstetric patients to prevent vesico-vaginal fistula: a report of a demonstration project in northern Nigeria. Social Work and Social Sciences Review 5:236- 245.1994.

117. Gruenwald, I. A profile of indwelling catheter in the community. Israel Urology Society Annual Congress., 1997.

118 American Medical Directors Association, Urinary Incontinence Clinical Practice Guideline, AMDA, Maryland, 1996.

119. National Association for Continence Blueprint for Continence Care in an Assisted Living Setting, NAFC: Spartanburg, SC. 2000.

120 Brocklehurst, J. C. Chairman. Working Group on outcome indicators for urinary incontinence: report to the Department of Health. Oxford, Unit of Health Care Epidemiology, 1997.

121. Lim PHC, Fonda D. The ContiNet of the International Continence Society Neurourology and Urodynamics 16:609-616, 1997.

122. Lapitan, MC, Chye, PLH. The Epidemiology of overactive bladder among females in Asia: a questionnaire survey. Int Urogynecol J 12: in press, 2001.

APPENDIX 1

INTERNATIONAL CONTINENCE ORGANIZATIONS

Note: Only organizations, which have their major focus on continence for the consumer/general public, are included here. Professional organizations are listed if they are the only formal consumer/lay public based organization in a particular country.

AUSTRALIA

CONTINENCE FOUNDATION OF AUSTRALIA LTD
AMA House, 293 Royal Parade
Parkville, Victoria 3052
Tel: 61 3 93472522 Fax: 61 3 93472533
website: info@contfound.org.au

CANADA

The Canadian Continence Foundation
2100 Marlowe Ave, Suite 350
Montreal, Quebec H4A 3L5
Tel: (1) 514 488-8379 Fax: (1) 514 488-1379
Website: www.continence-fdn.ca

GERMANY

Gesellschaft fur Inkontinenzhilfe e.V. (GIH)
Friedrich-Ebert-Strasse 124
34119 Kassel
Tel: (49) 0561 780604 Fax: (49) 561 776770
Website: http://www.gih.de

HONG KONG

Hong Kong Continence Society
Room 214, 2/F Tung Ying Bldg
100 Nathan Road
Hong Kong
Tel: 852 2311 2218 Fax: 852 2311 2633
Email: kwokfook@netvigator.com

INDIA

INDIAN CONTINENCE FOUNDATION
c/o Bangalore Kidney Foundation
CA6, 11th Cross, 15th Main Padmanabhanagar
Bangalore 560 010
Tel: 91 80669 0084/6691145
Fax: 91 80669 2466
Website: www.indiancontinencefoundation.org

INDONESIA

INDONESIAN CONTINENCE SOCIETY
Unit Urology, University of Diponegoro
Dr Kariadi Hospital
Jl. Dr Sutomo No 16 Semarang
Indonesia
Tel: 62 24 310152
Email: drrudi@indosat.net.id

ISRAEL

National Center for Continence
Rambam Medical Centre, POB-9602 Haifa 31096
Tel: 972-4-8543197 Fax: 972-4-8542883
Email: ig054@hotmail.com

JAPAN

Japan Continence Action Society
Continence Centre
103 Juri Heim, 1-4-2 Zenpukuzi Suginami-Ku
Tokyo, 167 0041
Tel: 81 03 3301 3860 Fax: 81 03 3301 3587
Website: http://www.shodouka.com/

KOREA

Korea Continence Foundation
Department of Urology, Dong-A
University Hospital, 3 Ga-1
Dongdaeshin-dong, Seo-Gu
Pusan City 602-715
Tel: 82 51 240 5446 Fax: 82 51 253 0591
Email: hykwon@seunghak.donga.ac.kr

Hee Seon, Yu, RN
7-206, 3-GA, Shinheung-Dong
Jung-gu Inchon, 400-103
Korea
Tel: 82 32 890 2365 Fax: 82 32 890 2363
Email: forever@inha.com

Sun Yeon Hwang
Hyundae Apt 103-1701, Dadae 2 dong, Sahagu
Pusan, S-Korea
Tel: 80 051 240 5766 Fax: 80 051 255 9286
Email: HSY1701@damc.or.kr

MALAYSIA
Continence Foundation (Malaysia)
c/o University Hospital, Lembah Pantai
Kuala Lumpur 59100
Tele: 603 7956 4422 Fax: 603 758 6003
Email: lohcs@medicine.med.um.edu.my

NEW ZEALAND
New Zealand Continence Assn Inc
41 Pembroke Street
Hamilton, New Zealand
Tel: 64 7 834 3528 Fax: 64 7 834 3532
Website: www.continence.org.nz

NORWAY
NOFUS (Norwegian Society for Patients with Urologic Diseases)
Linjeveien 178, N-1400 Ski
Norway
Tel: 47 64 87 28 45 Fax: 47 64 87 42 08
Email siralf@sensewave.com

PHILIPPINES
Continence Foundation of the Philippines
319 M.O.L.B. Bldg
Katipunan Road
Loyola Hts
Quezon City, Philippines
Tel: (63)-2-4333602 Fax: (63)-2-4333602
Website: continence99@yahhoo.com

SINGAPORE
Society for Continence (Singapore)
c/o Department of Urology
Changi General Hospital
2 Simei Street 3
Singapore 529889
Tel: (65) 787 0337 Fax: (65) 5881723
Website: http://sfcs.org.sg

SWEDEN
Swedish Urotherapists
Nordensioldsgatan 10, S-418 04
Goteborg
Tel: 46 31 50 26 89 Fax: 46 31 53 68 32
Email: birgtha.lindehall@vgregion.se

TAIWAN
Taiwan Continence Society
Department of Urology
Taipei Medical College Hospital
(TMCH)
No. 250 Wu-Hsin St.,
Taipei, Taiwan
Tel: + 886 2 2737 5076 Fax: + 886 2 273 77470
Email: hansun@mail.tmc.edu.tw

UNITED KINGDOM
The Continence Foundation, UK
307 Hatton Square
16 Baldwin Gardens
London EC1 N 7RJ
Tel: (44) 207 404 6875 Fax: (44) 207 404 6876
http://www.continence.foundation@dial.pipex.com

Enuresis Resource and Information Centre (ERIC)
34 Old School House, Britannia Road
Kingswood, Bristol BS15 2DB
Tel: (44) 117 960 3060 Fax: (44) 117 960 0401
Website: www.eric.org.uk

***In*contact**
United House, North Road
London N79DP
Tel: (44) 207 700 7035 Fax: (44) 207 700 7045
Website: www.incontact.demon.co.uk/

UNITED STATES OF AMERICA
American Foundation for Urologic Disease
Bladder Health Council
1128 North Charles Street
Baltimore, Maryland 21201-5559
Tel: 410-468-1800 Fax: 410 468 1808
Website: www.afud.org

International Foundation for Functional Gastrointestinal Disorders
P O Box 170864
Milwaukee WI 53217-8076
Tel: 414 964 1799 Fax: 414 964 7176
Website: www.iffgd.org

National Association for Continence
P O Box 8306,
Spartanburg, SC 29305-8310
Tel: 864 579 7900 Fax: 864 579 7902
Website: www.nafc.org

Simon Foundation for Continence
P O Box 815
Wilmette Illinois 60091
Tel: (1) 847 864 3913 Fax: (1) 847 864 9758
Website: www.simonfoundation.org

Committee 14

Economics of Incontinence

Chairman

T.-w. Hu (USA)

Members

K. Moore (Australia),

L. Subak (USA),

E. Versi (USA),

T. Wagner (USA),

N. Zinner (USA)

Consultant

J. Ouslander

CONTENTS

Economics of Incontinence

T.-W. Hu

K. Moore, L. Subak, E. Versi, T. Wagner, N. Zinner

J. Ouslander

I. INTRODUCTION

1. WHAT ARE THE "ECONOMICS OF INCONTINENCE"?

Understanding the economic impact of urinary incontinence on society is important for evaluating competing demands for the use of scarce health care resources. Knowing the magnitude of the economic impact of incontinence is also essential for the medical community and for government entities to determine funding priorities. The cost of incontinence includes both the direct use of resources for the care or treatment of incontinence and indirect economic effects that result from incontinence, such as the loss of productivity, resulting from morbidity or disability.

The economic issues surrounding incontinence revolve around two main issues: efficiency and equity. Efficiency is the concept of delivering services in the least costly manner, and equity is the concept of distributing the burden of cost fairly. With regard to either of these topics, one must first know the costs associated with incontinence.

In the context of health or health care, cost is conceptually equivalent to the value of resources consumed or lost as a result of illness. Thus, the economic costs of incontinence are equivalent to the sum of the values of resources consumed or lost by patients, treatment providers, government entities, or other segments of society as a direct or indirect result of incontinence. Since resources that are used to care for patients vary from medical personnel to equipment, supplies, spaces, etc, it is much easier to estimate direct costs by defining types of treatment services, measuring units of these treatment services used and multiplying these by the cost per unit of services.

2. WHY EVALUATE COSTS OF INCONTINENCE?

Costs can be evaluated from four different perspectives: society, payer, provider and patient, all of which have different interests. Since the economic impact on society is significant, regardless of where the burden falls, it would be helpful for government policymakers to know the overall burden of incontinence on society. It is also useful to have a number for cost comparison of various types of illness within a country, as well as a comparison between countries for a given illness.

Public or private insurance (third party) payers often incur major financial expenses in caring for patients. Therefore, these payers are interested in costs and the financial impact of a disease so that future health care financial budgets or insurance premiums can be planned. In addition, many European countries would like to determine the transfer payment, such as sick leaves or disability times, which is to be paid by the purchaser.

Providers, such as hospitals, managed care plans, health maintenance organizations and nursing homes are interested in the costs associated with a particular illness, such as incontinence or dementia, so that they can be taken into account for their capitation rates, global budgeting and/or service fees.

Finally, depending on different insurance coverage, patients would also like to learn what their shares of copayment and out-of-pocket expenditures are. The coverage of surgery for incontinence and lack of coverage for incontinence supplies would have different cost implications for patients. Furthermore, there are loss of productivity and loss of wages costs that directly affect a patient's well being.

While the costs of incontinence vary depending on the perspective, it has been recommended that researchers first use a societal perspective [1–2]. Maintaining the societal perspective facilitates comparisons of costs of various illnesses within a country, as well as comparisons of costs between countries for a given illness. Tallying societal costs and then exploring the costs of incontinence from different perspectives provides a lens through which one can better understand incontinence and the competing incentives.

One useful example is the international comparison (Canada, France, Sweden, UK, US) of the proportion of client incontinence costs paid by third party payers and by patients. The analysis followed patients for three months; all had urge or mixed incontinence. Costs included an initial visit, drug treatment, pad costs, extra costs for laundry, and treatment for urinary tract infections. It can be seen from Figure 1 that the costs from the patients' perspective varied depending on the country's insurance coverage and treatment/care practices.

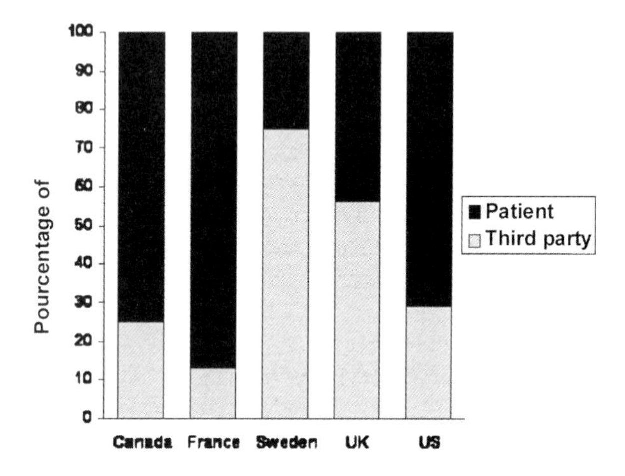

Figure 1 : Proportion of costs paid by health insurance and patients, 1997 [7].

3. Cost-effectiveness, cost-utility, and cost-benefit analyses

Estimating costs provides valuable information on the magnitude of the economic burden of an illness, which guides health policy decision-making. These data are also critical for comparing the costs and outcomes of medical interventions. In today's society, it is important to provide services that offer the most "value" for the least amount of money. To aid decision making, we often turn to cost and outcome analysis, which is a systematic method for comparing alternative medical interventions.

A medical intervention that yields better outcomes for less cost than an alternative intervention is considered dominant. Dominance is rare, since most new interventions yield better outcomes at an additional expense. In these situations, it is important to ask whether the value is worth the investment. The three most commonly used cost and outcome methods are:

1. Cost-Effectiveness Analysis (CEA),
2. Cost-Utility Analysis (CUA), and
3. Cost-Benefit Analysis (CBA).

In cost-effectiveness analysis, interventions are compared to alternatives by estimating a cost-effectiveness ratio (CER). The CER is the ratio of the marginal cost of the intervention to the marginal health effect of the intervention, compared to the next less costly alternative. In traditional CEA, the health effect is measured in units that are relevant to the illness (e.g. incontinence episodes). Although this may facilitate interpretation of the results among incontinence experts, these CERs cannot be compared with CERs from a heart failure medication, because the outcome measures are not the same. To permit this type of comparison, many researchers have turned to using a single outcome measure, such as life expectancy that is adjusted to account for quality of life.

Cost-utility analyses are useful for comparing the cost of treating different diseases. This type of analysis is particularly important for diseases that have a major impact on quality of life, such as incontinence. The primary difference between a CEA and a CUA is the choice of outcome measures. A CUA uses a global outcome measure (utilities) that allows the comparison of dissimilar interventions. For example, with a CUA, a researcher could compare a new incontinence treatment to a new heart disease treatment.

The quality adjusted life year (QALY) model is the preferred measure for estimating utilities [1]. QALYs are estimated by multiplying each life year gained with an intervention by a quality-weighting factor that reflects the individual's utility or preference in the health state for that year. This type of analysis, while often still referred to as a CEA, is also known as a CUA because the QALYs represent utilities. Utilities are measured on a scale from zero (death or the worst health imaginable) to one (perfect health), and can be used as quality-weighting factors. Utilities are typically gathered through direct assessment, such as standard gamble or time tradeoffs methods, or through indirect assessment, such as the Health Utilities Index (HUI) [3] or the EuroQol (EQ-5D) [4].

Cost-Benefit Analysis represents a deviation from CEA and CUA models in that it attempts to measure benefits in dollars. Theoretically, this holds some advantages over CEA and CUA in that it permits efficiency analysis [3]. An increasingly common way to measure benefit is to use a survey that considers patients' willingness to pay. This type of analysis accounts for the treatment outcome and the utility/preference, but is expressed by the patient's willingness to pay a given amount of money in return for a healthy status. Debate continues on the value of willingness to pay [4–5]. While researchers continue to explore better ways of developing the willingness to pay scenario [6], a CUA with QALYs still represents the most widely accepted cost and outcome method.

II. METHODS OF ECONOMIC ANALYSIS

Detailed discussions on methods of measurement and estimation of costs of illness and outcomes have already been presented in the previous consultation volume [7]. Therefore, this section will provide a very brief summary.

1. Definition and measurement of costs of illness

Costs of incontinence include direct costs and the value of lost productivity due to illness. Direct costs include diagnosis, treatment, routine care and consequence costs. Table 1 details the items associated with direct costs of incontinence. The value of productivity lost includes time lost due to incontinence. Since incontinence is not often associated with premature death, time loss in incontinence refers to work-related productivity loss. These values of productivity loss can be obtained from the amount of lost wages in different age/gender categories. Often, older adults are productive inside and outside the home in ways that are not reimbursed through wages (e.g. household work). These efforts can be valued by imputing estimates from national age-sex adjusted averages or by using minimum wage. It could be argued that productivity loss is a subset of indirect costs on the assumption that all patients are productive members of the workforce.

In estimating the cost of illness, it is important to first obtain the prevalence of incontinence. Differences in gender, community and institutions all impact the cost of illness associated with incontinence. Therefore, it is important to obtain accurate prevalence estimates for those sub-populations. There is a difference between disease prevalence and utilization rates for health services. In order to estimate direct costs for incontinence, it is necessary to evaluate the number and type of resources used in treatment (e.g. visits, tests, supplies, hospital days, medications, etc). At the same time, per unit costs of each service should be obtained from national surveys or statistics. Multiplying the quantity of the services by the unit cost of each service will yield the total costs of treatment.

Table 1 : Direct costs associated with urinary incontinence

Diagnostic costs	Laboratory tests Physician consultations Physical examinations Urodynamic evaluations
Treatment costs	Medication Surgery Behavioral Therapy Devices
Routine care costs	Incontinence pads and briefs Laundry, dry cleaning Hygiene and odor control products New clothing to replace those worn from frequent laundering Cleaning/replacing carpet and/or furniture Nursing time Disposable bed pads Indwelling urinary catheters
Consequence costs	Treatment for falls Treatment for skin infections due to incontinence Treatment of urinary tract infections Lengthened hospital stay Nursing home admission

2. Definition and measurement of outcome

Combining measures of effectiveness and costs provides a powerful tool to evaluate the cost per unit of effectiveness of a specific intervention. As urinary incontinence is a multidimensional syndrome and treatments often do not provide a cure but rather an alleviation of symptoms, it is not easy to define a single disease-specific effectiveness measure that is acceptable and meaningful to patients, physicians and purchasers.

A composite construct incorporating all the dimensions of the disease (physical, psychosocial, etc) is preferred in economic evaluations over objective clinical measures, which cannot be transformed easily into such a construct. Subjective outcome measures, however, can be incorporated into this construct and at present, they are considered more relevant for economic analysis. The most commonly used objective clinical outcomes in incontinence treatment are measures of improvement in symptom severity: for example, reduction in number of incontinent episodes, or clinical tests such as pad tests or urodynamic measurements. These are often obtained from voiding diaries, self-report or interview. Recently, a new method for measuring response to surgical treatment of incontinence was described [8]. Results obtained from patient questionnaires, 24 hour voiding diaries, and 24 hour pad tests were scored into five categories based on new criteria (cure, good response, fair response, poor response, failure), and scores were pooled to create a new response scoring system. The authors observed that this new tool was more accurate than previous methods (which evaluated each outcome separately using previously published criteria that assessed only cure, improvement, and failure).

Subjective quality of life measures should be responsive to treatment. Since the goal of treatment for incontinence is to improve the patient's quality of life, specific instruments more relevant and sensitive to measure incontinence outcomes have been developed. These include the Incontinence Impact Questionnaire [9], Urinary Distress Inventory, Incontinence Quality of Life [10] and Kings Health Questionnaire [11]. Since these disease-specific quality of life measures do not measure quality of life on a continuum anchored by perfect health and death, they cannot be used to quality adjust life expectancy. QALYs, which are the preferred measure for economic analysis in clinical trials, require patient preferences called utilities which are determined using a scale anchored by life and death. Utilities may be estimated through direct assessment, such as standard gamble or time tradeoffs methods, or through indirect assessment, such as the Health Utilities Index (HUI) or the EuroQol (EQ-5D). One of the primary limitations of utilities and QALYs, however, is that they are typically not responsive to treatment.

Other subjective measures that do not directly assess incontinence severity are rapidly emerging as important secondary outcomes [12]. Data regarding secondary outcome measures such as global assessment of patient satisfaction, symptom bothersomeness assessments, and anatomical and functional assessments can and should be collected using quantifiable criteria.

III. DATA SOURCES AND DATA INTERPRETATION

With increasing frequency, studies are assessing the costs associated with urinary incontinence. Recent examples include descriptive studies that identified the cost of urinary incontinence in the US [13], Italy [14] and Sweden [15]. There have also been a few comparative studies with cost analyses [16–19]. Nevertheless, the use of economic analysis in urinary incontinence studies remains rare.

1. Data sources

One obstacle to economic studies is the lack of available data. Most industrialized countries track the health of their citizens with complex surveys, such as the National Medical Care Expenditure survey in the USA, the National Health Survey in Australia, National Population Health Survey in Canada, and the National Health and Lifestyle Survey in Ireland [20]. However, the vast majority of national health surveys do not query respondents about bladder control problems or urinary incontinence.

Several countries are collecting data on urinary incontinence (Table 2). The majority of studies are national health surveys that have been amended to include questions on urinary incontinence. For example, questions on bladder problems were added to the Scottish Health Survey in 1998 and to the Nurses Health Study (USA) in 2001.

Most national surveys that include data on incontinence have been cross-sectional studies. Although this study design provides data on incontinence prevalence, the data may be confounded by unobserved factors. Additional limitations of cross-sectional data include the sensitivity and specificity of the questions to identify incontinence, misclassification of incontinence type or severity, and inability to establish a causal relationship (for example, incontinence causes nursing home admission).

Several longitudinal data sets, which hold some advantages over cross-sectional data, include questions on bladder control (Table 2). These data sets may be used to assess the consequences of urinary incontinence on outcomes including health care utilization, falls, urinary tract infections and institutionalization. While these studies may provide critical data to determine the probability that people will use specific health care resources, none of these data sets include information on costs. Therefore, if researchers are conducting a cost analysis, costs need to be estimated from different sources.

2. Data interpretation

Estimating costs can be difficult. Most items that we purchase daily have a readily observable cost. In markets with perfect competition, the cost is determined by market conditions. In these situations, the market self-regulates, requiring little or no outside regulation. However, health care markets involve uncertain heterogeneous goods where there are large information asymmetries. All of these factors contribute to market failure, resulting in some need for external regulation [21–23]. Although all countries regulate health care to some degree, they do so in very different ways. This has implications for estimating costs, and places an even greater burden on researchers to describe explicitly where, when and how the costs were calculated.

Regulations can have a large effect on costs. Health care providers, as a nation, province, or health plan, can set and regulate prices for health services. Alternatively, the health provider can limit the treatments for

Table 2 : Health surveys with information on urinary incontinence

Health Surveys	Year	Notes
AUSTRALIA		
Women's Health project	1998	Longitudinal study of 3 age cohorts
National Continence Management Strategy (NCMS)		
Survey of Disability, Ageing & Careers 1998 (ABS 1999a)	1998	Cross-sectional
National Women's Longitudinal Health Survey	1996	Cross-sectional
CANADA		
National Population Health Surveys	1994/95 1996/97	Cross-sectional
http://www.statcan.ca/english/survey/household/health/health.htm		
DENMARK		
Denmark Survey of Health and Illness	1994	Cross-sectional
http://www.dda.dk/gbcat/s2323gb.html		
UK		
Scottish Health Survey	1998	Cross-sectional
http://www.show.scot.nhs.uk/		
Household Survey of England	1995	Cross-sectional
http://qb.soc.surrey.ac.uk/surveys/hse/hsecontent95.htm		
US		
Hospital Discharge Data		Cross-sectional
National Nursing Home Survey		Cross-sectional
National Medical Care Expenditure		Cross-sectional
National Health Interview Survey		Cross-sectional
National Overactive BLadder Evaluation (NOBLE)	2000	Cross-sectional
Health and Retirement Survey	1993–present	Longitudinal

which it will pay. Pharmaceuticals are often regulated in this fashion, where many providers limit access to expensive patent drugs by using formularies.

Various forms of regulation result in the same service having very different "costs" across health care providers. Accounting systems are used to identify "costs." These estimates are usually in the form of charges that are highly (but not perfectly) correlated with economic costs, in the true economic sense. Therefore, different accounting systems can yield highly divergent cost estimates.

Most of the hospital accounting systems in the US focus on billing and payments. The charges listed on the bill usually overstate costs and are rarely paid in full by the purchaser. In the US, researchers have developed imperfect methods for adjusting the charges with a hospital specific ratio of costs to charges so that they have a better estimate of costs [24]. However, countries with nationalized health care systems often do not routinely generate bills. In these situations, researchers have developed methods for generating pseudo-bills and more detailed gross cost estimates [25–28]. In some instances, researchers rely on an average cost per encounter that is calculated by dividing the total annual cost by the number of inpatient days or the number of outpatient visits. Pseudo-bill methods tend to be more precise than average encounter costs. This is particularly true for inpatient care, where average daily rates make the untenable assumption that costs are solely a function of length of stay.

Another common problem with accounting systems is the distinction between professional services and facility costs. Systems in many countries have evolved to pay the physician separately from the facility. Therefore, it is important to identify both the facility costs and the professional fees. These costs are sometimes kept in different databases. For instance, the Medicare program keeps inpatient facility information in the Part A database, while the outpatient and provider fees are kept in the Part B database.

Another caveat with accounting systems is that they always report the health care payer's costs or charges. Society's costs are usually of interest [1–2], therefore it is important to distinguish between provider-incurred costs and patient-incurred costs. This distinction is important for urinary incontinence, since most providers do not pay for routine care (e.g. pads and protection). These costs are usually borne by individuals, and in 1995 the routine care costs represented approximately 45% of the total cost of urinary incontinence [13].

The word "cost" is often casually used, yet researchers should be careful and explicit when cost data are presented. It becomes difficult to compare costs if they are not put in context. As mentioned above, it is important to provide information on what the costs represent and how they were obtained in order to judge how much they can be generalized.

It is also important to consider when and where the costs were gathered. Costs are time-dependent and it is important for studies to identify the year for which the costs were calculated. Economic studies can collect costs over many years and make projections about the future. When this is done, the costs should be adjusted so that they reflect a single year. Future costs should be discounted to represent the present value. There is controversy over the appropriate discount rate and therefore there is no international standard [29–31]. Despite the lack of consensus, it is important to discount future costs to reflect time preferences [1–2]. Given the uncertainty surrounding the discount rates, a sensitivity analysis should be done with alternative discount rates.

Costs borne in past years should be expressed in the current year's dollars. In the US, past and future costs can be adjusted by the Consumer Price Index or other appropriate indices for all urban consumers (www.stats.bls.gov). In the UK, the Health Service Cost Index or the Retail Price Index, published by the NHS Executive, Leeds, UK, can be used to adjust the costs of health care services; other indices would be used to adjust other items, such as wages (www.statistics.uk.gov). Most counties track inflation, thereby providing a method for inflating past costs. The best method for inflating costs is not free from controversy, and again this should be varied in a sensitivity analysis. See the articles by Berndt [32] and Cleeton [33] for detailed discussions on price indices.

While the use of economic analysis in health services research is increasing, a sufficiently large number of published studies provide insufficient background information. This problem was evident in the early 1990s [34], and unfortunately continues to persist [35–36]. While we hope that the future will see more economic analyses for urinary incontinence, studies that follow generally accepted standards [1–2] will minimize confusion and may encourage others to follow suit [37].

IV. ECONOMIC ANALYSIS OF URINARY INCONTINENCE

1. Global cost of illness

Cost of illness analyses describe the economic impact of a disease. These studies are used to determine health policy or to make decisions about broad treatment guidelines, and are descriptive in nature. Cost of illness studies quantify costs incurred by a population over a defined time, ignoring outcome. Prevalence-based studies estimate the total cost to society due to a given disease by aggregating data on the average amount of health care resources used and the average cost of treatments, forming population estimates [38]. Total cost can either be calculated from national statistics when available (top-down approach), or by collecting detailed costs for a cohort of patients during a given time and combining them with prevalence estimates (bottom-up approach). Alternatively, in incidence-based analyses, lifetime costs are estimated for a cohort of patients (from the time they contract the disease to death), adjusting for incidence estimates.

Cost of illness for urinary incontinence has been addressed by several studies, most of which focus on a particular sub-population (gender, age, institutionalization status), type of incontinence (stress, urge, mixed, neurogenic), or cost type (direct, indirect) [13,39–46]. The most recent estimates of the annual direct costs of incontinence in all ages are approximately $16 billion: $11 billion in the community and $5 billion in nursing homes (1994 dollars) [47]. This cost estimate increased by 250% over 10 years, with previous estimates of $6.6 billion (1984 dollars) [38] and $10.3 billion (1987 dollars) [41]. This increase is greater than can be accounted for by medical inflation. Direct and indirect costs of care for the elderly alone were recently estimated to be $26 billion (1995 dollars) [13].

One recently recognized condition related to incontinence is overactive bladder (OAB), which includes urinary urgency, frequency and nocturia, with or without urge incontinence. The National Overactive BLadder Evaluation (NOBLE) program in the US surveyed approximately 5,000 adults. The prevalence of OAB was estimated to be 16.9% in females and 16.0% in males [48]. A follow-up survey collected detailed information on treatment costs of OAB (with and without urinary incontinence). The cost data include routine personal care, treatment, and health related consequences due to OAB. The estimated costs of OAB for community residents in the US in 2000 were around $9.14 billion. The estimated nursing home care costs (largely routine care costs such as pads, laundry, nursing aids, etc) were about $4.4 billion. The total costs of OAB in 2000 were $13.6 billion [49].

The US National Institutes of Health recently published disease-specific estimates of costs of illness comparing different diseases. The annual direct cost of urinary incontinence ($17.5 billion in 1995 dollars) was comparable to the direct costs of other common acute and chronic diseases in women: gynecological and breast cancers ($11.1 billion), osteoporosis ($13.8 billion), pneumonia and influenza ($15.8 billion) and arthritis

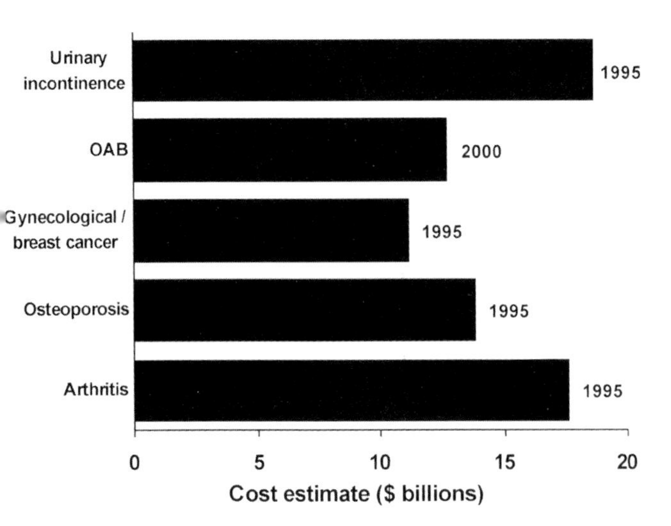

Figure 2 : Comparison of urinary incontinence direct costs with other illnesses in the US. Numbers beside each bar denote the year of the estimate [49–50].

($17.6 billion) [50]. While these illnesses vary in their effects on quality of life, daily functioning, indirect costs, and prevalence, this is a striking example of the large cost of illness of urinary incontinence. Figure 2 compares different cost estimates for selected illnesses in the US.

Several non-USA studies on the overall costs of urinary incontinence have recently been published. The total cost of illness can be calculated from national statistics (top-down approach) or by collecting detailed costs for a cohort of patients and combining them with prevalence estimates (bottom-up approach). By using the top-down approach, an Australian study [51] (based on [52] and extrapolated to longitudinal data from Women's Health Australia, as described in [53]) estimated the economic cost of urinary incontinence in community-dwelling Australian women in 1998. An estimated 1.83 million community-dwelling women over the age of 18 years in Australia had urinary incontinence. The total annual cost of this urinary incontinence is estimated at AU$710 million (US$378 million at the 2001 conversion rate), or AU$387 (US$208) per incontinent woman, comprising AU$339 million (US$182 million) in treatment costs or AU$372 million (US$200 million) in personal costs. An estimated 60% of women with incontinence in 1998 were aged 40 years and over. Assuming the prevalence of incontinence remains constant and allowing for inflation, the total annual cost in 20 years time will be AU$1268 million (US$682 million), 93% of which will constitute costs associated with women aged over 40 years. Urinary incontinence imposes a considerable burden on Australian health care resources.

An Italian study [14] shows that the annual treatment costs in 1997 were L351.85 billion (US$166 million at the 2001 conversion rate), considering only the costs of diapers and drugs. A 1995 French study [54] estimated that the annual direct costs associated with incontinence treatment in women, excluding diapers and sanitary towels, were about 3 billion French Francs (US$417 million). Table 3 provides a summary of the direct cost estimates in US dollar values for the four countries discussed above.

Cost-of-illness analyses of urinary incontinence have several limitations. There are limited data on incontinence prevalence, institutionalization due to incontinence, routine care costs, and the impact of incontinence on hospitalizations and outpatient medical management. In addition, estimating productivity loss and intangible costs for urinary incontinence is difficult and imprecise.

2. Direct costs

a) Routine care or "self-help"

Routine care costs include pads or other protective products such as disposable and reusable underpants, laundry, and miscellaneous items such as skin care, odor control products and extra dry cleaning. Incontinence-related laundry costs include cleaning linens, bed pads and clothing.

One of the features of incontinence is that patients need to take care of themselves on an ongoing basis by changing incontinence pads, bed pads, underwear and clothing, laundry and occasionally skin care. Among community residents, these activities are usually done by

Table 3. International comparison of urinary incontinence community treatment cost estimates

Country	Cost estimate		Year
	Local currency	US$ (millions)	
Australia [51]	AU$710 million	378	1998
France [54]	FF3 billion	417	1995
Italy [14]	L352 billion	166	1997
US [50]	US$17.5 billion	17,500	1995

the individual. If an individual is in a nursing home or has a disability, then they may have to be taken care of by aides. This type of care is no longer called self-help, although it is still considered a routine care cost. Because of the two different settings, community versus nursing home, the costs of routine care are different. Furthermore, the accuracy of data collection varies. It is much easier and more accurate to collect routine care costs in nursing homes than in the community. Costs in the community are largely self-reported and types of products used vary.

Since the last consultation on incontinence (1998), a number of refinements have been suggested for cost estimation. New studies have been carried out at the community level in the US and other countries. There has been a gap in understanding routine care costs at the community level and attempts have been made to address this. The cost of pad consumption is a major element in routine care costs. There have been four studies [14,52–53,55] in Australia and Italy, three studies in the US [56–58], and one on the international comparison of pad use in 12 countries [59].

A detailed residential survey [53] (based on the bottom-up cost approach) indicated that incontinent women in Australia spent a median AU$12.89 per week on direct incontinence costs (US$6.94 at the 2001 conversion rate), which comprised the personal costs of AU$5.61 or 43.5% of total costs. Within personal cost, 70% of personal costs are incontinence pad costs. It has been found, as expected, that the more severe the status of incontinence, the higher the personal costs. Laundry costs were 16% of personal costs, while protection costs (e.g. bath towels, tissues, toilet paper, bed pad, old sheets, etc) and miscellaneous costs accounted for 13%. In Australia, quite a few patients used non-commercial products because they could not afford commercial products or they preferred the home remedies. This was the first detailed non-US study on direct personal costs of routine care at community level. In Australia, a detailed laundry cost formula was also developed by taking into account electricity, water and washing powder.

An Italian study [14] on costs of incontinence collected data on the number of pads used for stress incontinence and other incontinence conditions (urge or mixed), as well as data on the frequency of incontinence. Stress incontinent patients used a mean of 34 pads a month, while patients with urge and other incontinence conditions used 59 pads a month. Those with one or more incontinent episode per day used 56 pads a month, while those who had less than one incontinence episode per day use 25 pads. Overall, the cost per patient for diapers was L240,000 (US$114 at the 2001 conversion rate). The annual costs of adult diapers and drugs for urinary incontinence was L352 billion (US$167 million). These costs represent out-of-pocket expenses for patients, with diapers comprising the bulk of the costs (94%).

A recent US study also compared types of pads used in community incontinent residents [58]. They divided the products into three groups:

1. mini pads, panty liners, toilet paper, tissue paper;

2. maxi-pads; and

3. incontinence products. They classified condition of incontinence as stress incontinence, detrusor instability, or both.

In this US study, it was found that 92% of patients used only commercial incontinence products and 8% used non-commercial. The daily usage was 1.7 pieces (mean) or 1.4 (at median). The median annual costs were $46 for all subjects or $76 for pad users (assuming the average costs per pad is around 10 cents). This study also confirms that costs and pad usage are significantly associated with number of incontinent episodes and quality of life.

Kornides & Moore [59] conducted an international comparison of incontinence pad use based on global commercial marketing data from Molnycke Corporation in Sweden in 1998. The per capita female use of heavy incontinence pads is highly associated with either per capita gross domestic product (high users such as the US and Canada, and low users such as Australia, Spain and Taiwan) or heavy government subsidies (Scandinavian countries), as shown in Figure 3.

These recent studies have provided additional refinement of costs of routine care in the community in all age groups, and have increased awareness of the economic importance of routine care around the world.

b) Treatment

Little is known about the costs and practice patterns for individuals with urinary incontinence patients in the managed care setting. Data from Day et al. [60] showed that within a health management organization, new prescriptions for urinary incontinence were filled at a continuous rate over the 3-year period. Although it would seem logical that the refill rate would also increase by the same proportion, the new prescription fill rate far exceeded that for refills, indicating that compliance with therapy was less than desirable. A similar study [61] indicated poor compliance in a study of 246 women with overactive bladder (OAB) from the UK, most of whom (83.5%) had been prescribed oxybutynin therapy for their symptoms. At 6 months, only 18.2% remained on therapy. Therefore, patient compliance with drug treatment is a key element for successful outcomes.

Both pharmacologic and non-pharmacologic treatments

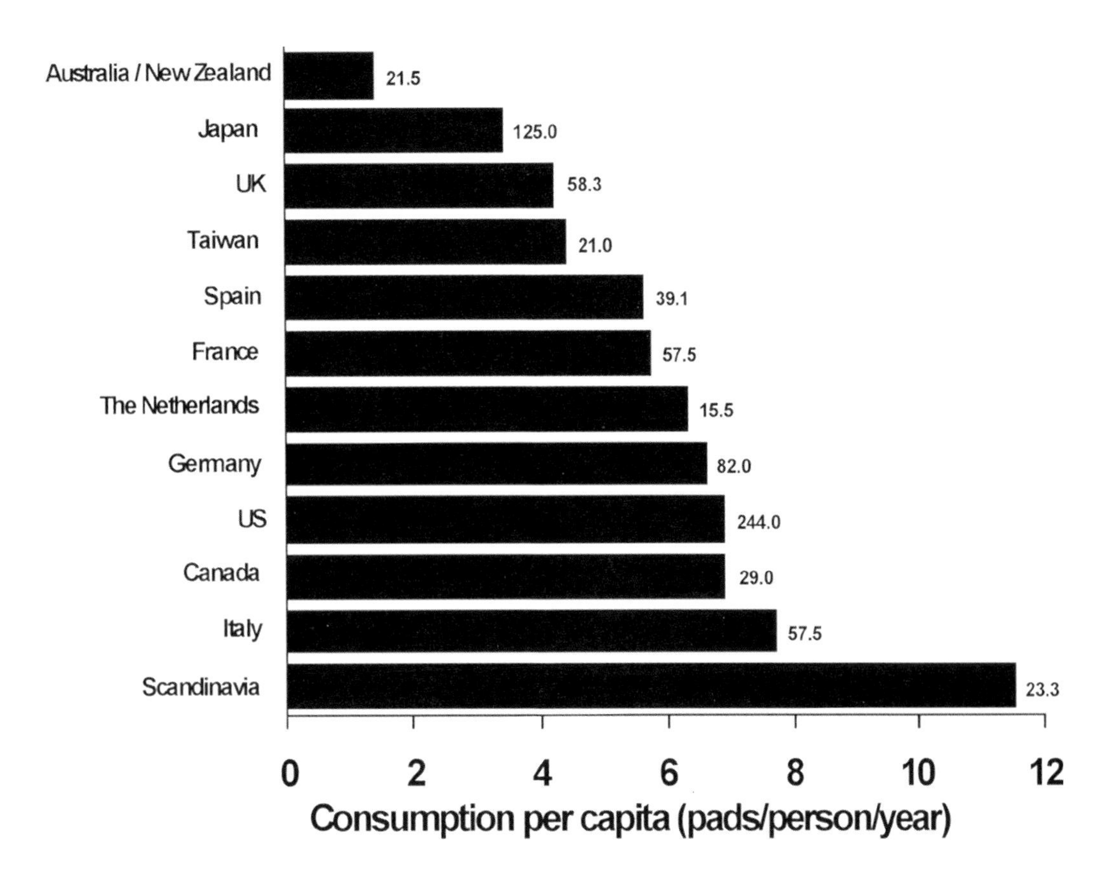

Figure 3 : Heavy incontinence pads used per capita, 1998. Numbers beside each bar denote population (millions) [59].

are available to patients who suffer from incontinence. Non-pharmacologic treatment (e.g. bladder retraining) can be successful, but has demonstrated only limited long-term efficacy because patients are often non-compliant with therapy. It has been suggested that treatment plans should combine drug therapy and behavioral modification, but such combinations have not been evaluated for their cost-effectiveness.

Patient compliance is critical to cost-effective treatment. Anticholinergic drugs, such as oxybutynin, are the drugs of choice for the treatment of incontinence. Although oxybutynin treatment is effective [62], it is frequently limited by poor acceptability, often due to adverse side effects, which in turn can lead to the discontinuation of treatment. To overcome the problems of intolerable side effects with immediate-release oxybutynin, extended-release formulations have been developed. However, not all studies have shown an improved rate of dry mouth rate [63–64].

New antimuscarinic compounds have been introduced for urge incontinence, because they have a greater selectivity for the bladder. Tolterodine was developed specifically for the treatment of OAB, of which a major component is urge incontinence. It has a greater selectivity for the bladder than other anticholinergic drugs, which may explain the lower incidence of dry mouth [62]. Only half as many patients taking immediate-release (IR) tolterodine report dry mouth compared to oxybutynin [65]. A new, long-acting formulation of tolterodine (extended-release; ER) was recently shown to be 18% better in controlling urge incontinence episodes than the IR formulation, producing a 71% overall decrease in incontinence [65]. Tolterodine ER also has a better side effect profile than immediate release tolterodine and oxybutynin. There was a 23% lower occurrence of dry mouth for patients taking tolterodine ER compared to patients taking tolterodine IR, and the overall occurrence of severe dry mouth was only 1.8% for tolterodine ER patients [66]. Tolterodine ER's improved efficacy and acceptability combined with convenient, once-daily dosing may result in improved compliance with therapy. This appears to translate into greater cost-effectiveness in that tolterodine ER has a lower cost per successfully treated patient than tolterodine IR or oxybutynin [67].

A large USA managed care organization (more than 3 million members) collected data on women seeking care for urinary incontinence and pelvic floor disorder (PFD) [68]. There was an age-related increase in the incidence of women seeking care for all PFD symptoms from June 1997 to May 1999, from 2 to 19 consults per 1000 woman-years in the 30-to-39 year old and 70-to-79 year old age groups, respectively. Applying data from the US Census Bureau, the authors estimated that there would be more than 620,000 consultations for PFD in the US in 2000, and that by 2030 there would be more than 1 million. According to these projections, there will be an 11% increase in women 30 to 59 years of age seeking care for PFD, which is consistent with the anticipated growth in the population. The greatest percentage increase in demand for services will occur among older women (60 to 89 years of age), where there is expected to be an 81% increase in demand for consultations. These are conservative estimates because they do account for changes in the characteristics of women or increased public awareness of PFD, two factors that are expected to increase the number of people seeking help for PFD.

A recent study [69] estimated the annual costs to society of pelvic organ prolapse (POP) operations in the US. The study estimated the number of POP surgeries identified in the 1997 National Hospital Discharge Survey, by direct medical costs to society estimated by national average Medicare reimbursement for physician services and hospitalizations. In 1997, the direct costs of POP surgery were $1 billion (95% confidence interval $775-1,251 million), including $499 million (49%) for vaginal hysterectomy, $279 million (28%) for cystocele/rectocele repair, and $2 million (2%) for abdominal hysterectomy. Physician services accounted for 29% ($298 million) of total costs and hospitalization accounted for 71% ($715 million). Twenty-one percent of POP surgeries included urinary incontinence surgery ($218 million). If all surgeries were reimbursed by non-Medicare sources, the annual estimated cost would increase by 52% to $1.5 billion. It was concluded that the annual direct costs of operations for POP are substantial and similar to other surgical interventions for women (breast cancer, gynecological cancer, urinary incontinence).

These recent studies have provided additional refinement of costs of routine care in the community in all age groups, and have increased awareness of the economic importance of routine care around the world.

c) Acute complication

Acute complication due to urinary incontinence usually refers to urinary tract infection (UTI), skin irritation, falls and fractures, and extended length of stay in hospitals. Recent studies have provided further firm evidence that urinary incontinent older women were significantly more likely to have hip fractures than the general population [70–71]. In multivariate analysis, incontinence was independently associated with falls and fractures; women with weekly urge incontinence had a 26% greater risk of sustaining a fall (Odds Ratio = 1.26, 95% Confidence Interval [CI] 1.14-1.40) and a 34% increase risk of fracture (Relative Hazard = 1.34; 95% CI 1.06-1.69), after adjusting for all other causes (e.g. age, frailty, poor overall health, and previous fall or fracture) [71]. More frequent incontinence was associated with increased risk, and women with daily urge incontinence had increased risks of 35% and 45% of sustaining falls and fractures, respectively. Previous studies have demonstrated that urge incontinence is associated with frequency/urgency and nocturia, suggesting that any OAB symptom, not just urge incontinence, has the potential to increase the risk of falls and fractures among elderly women. The NOBLE program [72] used multivariate analysis to estimate that individuals with OAB have more than twice the risk of being injured in a fall than those without OAB.

UTI and skin infection have also been associated with urinary incontinence. A 5% random sampling of the 1996-1997 California Medicaid Program (Medi-Cal) claims data showed that 22% and 8% of the OAB population received treatment for UTIs and skin infections, respectively. After OAB was diagnosed, the number of services received for UTIs and skin infection decreased by 40% and 60%, respectively, and was associated with potential cost savings [73]. Also, the NOBLE program used the multivariate analysis to estimate the association of OAB and UTI. It was estimated that an individual with OAB had more UTIs than individuals without OAB, after controlling for sociodemographic and other illness conditions [72].

Several recent studies [74–76] have suggested that there is a strong association between depressive symptoms and urge incontinence. Urge incontinence was classified as being idiopathic or neuropathic, depending on whether neurologic findings were absent or present. The results [74] were compared with those of continent controls. Depressive symptoms were highly prevalent among those with idiopathic urge incontinence, occurring in 60% of patients. In contrast, depressive symptoms were observed in only 14% of those with stress incontinence and 42% of those with mixed incontinence. Of all patients with incontinence, only those with idiopathic urge incontinence were significantly more likely than controls to have an elevated Beck Depression Inventory score or a history of depression.

d) Chronic complication – long-term care

Urinary incontinence has been considered one of the common factors contributing to decisions on admission to nursing homes [39,42,77]. Thom [77] found that in the US, the risk of nursing home admission was 2.0 times greater for incontinent women (95% CI 1.7-2.4) and 3.7 times greater for incontinent men (95% CI 2.7-3.8), after adjustment for age and co-morbid conditions. In addition, the risk of hospitalization was 30% higher in women following the diagnosis of incontinence (relative risk [RR] = 1.3, 95% CI 1.2-1.5) and 50% higher in men (RR = 1.5, 95% CI 1.3-1.6).

Once patients are admitted to an institution, nursing home staff consider urinary incontinence to be one of the most difficult conditions to manage, in terms of time, resources and stress. In Australia, 77% of Australian nursing home residents are affected by urinary incontinence and up to 25% of nursing staff time is spent on incontinence care. It was estimated that approximately AU$450 million a year in 1991 dollars [52].

Two US studies [78–79] have evaluated the time and motion studies of added costs of caring for incontinent nursing home residents. Shih et al. [79] estimated incremental labor, supply and laundry costs associated with incontinence care at more than $15 per resident per day, or more than $5,000 per resident annually. Costs varied according to frequency of incontinence, and ranged from $8.70 to $17.28 per resident per day in 1997. Frenchman [57] provided a detailed breakdown by supplies, labor and laundry with total costs of $17.21 per resident per day in 1999. Although these studies were carried out at different locations, cost results are quite comparable.

Finally, urinary incontinence has been associated with extended length of hospital stay or multiple admissions, independent of other co-morbid conditions [77]. Treating incontinence may prevent extended stays in hospitals or admission into nursing homes.

3. Indirect costs – productivity loss

Loss of productivity is usually due either to the individual's premature death or due to illness. Urinary incontinence rarely causes premature death [80], but it may often affect individual's lost work time or interfere with job performance.

Although limited in number and scope, reports of studies to investigate the impact of urinary incontinence on workers' productivity are beginning to appear [81–86]. While incontinence is more prevalent in the elderly, it can also affect younger people who are more likely to be employed in the workplace [87–89]. Most studies of productivity and incontinence focus on women, since incontinence among men of working age is less common.

Recent surveys of white-collar women [81–82], female and army service members [83–86], public school teachers [84] and athletes [90] demonstrate that a relatively high proportion – 21%-33% – suffer from incontinence, with the potential to significantly impact their work productivity. This impact includes loss of sleep leading to fatigue at work, loss of concentration, and interference with job performance. Women reported taking time from work for frequent urination to reduce incontinence episodes. Women also reduced fluid intake to minimize incontinent events, which may cause dehydration and a greater risk of UTI. Many women reported embarrassment, altered social interactions, loss of self-esteem, depression, and other factors that could impede work performance and reduce productivity. Incontinence is also associated with absence from work secondary to health care visits, shame, and the need to change clothing.

While it is probable that these factors contribute to lost productivity, to date no objective data have quantified the loss. Given the larger number of younger women in the work force and the relatively high prevalence of incontinence among this group [81,84–86], future efforts to objectively quantify the fiscal impact of their lost productivity is needed.

V. ECONOMIC ANALYSIS OF URINARY INCONTINENCE TREATMENT STRATEGIES

More studies on CEA and CUA have been published since the last consultation. Rather than evaluating just the cost of the disease, these studies focus on particular treatments or procedures and their effectiveness in treating particular incontinence conditions.

1. Cost-effectiveness analysis

There have been a number of international cost-effectiveness studies. A US study [91] examined the cost-effectiveness of preoperative urodynamic testing in women with prolapse and stress incontinence, using a theoretical decision-analytical model. This study evaluated the cost-effectiveness of basic office evaluation before surgery in women with prolapse and stress incontinence symptoms, and compared it with that of urodynamic testing. Costs were obtained from US government data; effectiveness of treatment for urinary incontinence was based on published literature. The strategies of basic office evaluation and urodynamic testing had the same cure rate of urinary incontinence (96%) after initial and secondary treatment. Under baseline assumptions, the incremental cost-effectiveness of urodynamic testing was $328,601 per case of urinary incontinence. According to sensitivity analyses, basic office evaluation was more cost-effective than urodynamic testing when the prevalence of pure detrusor instability was <8% or when the cost of urodynamic testing was >$103. It was concluded that urodynamic testing is not cost-effective before surgery for prolapse and stress urinary incontinence symptoms. However, it should be noted that the assumption about the prevalence of detrusor instability and the routine use of sling procedures for all genuine stress incontinence may limit the broad applicability of the study.

In Australia, the Dowell Bryant Incontinence Cost

Index (DBICI) was used as an outcome measure following non-surgical therapy, to determine whether the magnitude of leakage would correlate with the magnitude of reduced personal cost [55]. The commercial price for a simple urethral occlusive device was compared to reductions in the cost of incontinence. The severity of leakage was significantly reduced on all parameters and the median personal costs of incontinence fell from AU$6.52 per week (US$3.49 at the 2001 conversion rate; inter-quartile range [IQR] 1.50-10.59) to a median of AU$1.57 per week (US$0.84; IQR 0-4.89). A significant correlation was observed between reduction in personal costs and reduction in visual analog scale, pad test loss, and quality of life scores. The pad test showed a median reduction of 83%, but the personal costs fell by a median of 71%, because some women do not stop using pads as soon as they are cured. Thus it was concluded that measurement of the personal costs of incontinence as an outcome measure actually provides a different dimension of the patient's burden, in keeping with the recommendations of the ICS standardization committee that cost impact is an important, but separate, measurement of the burden of the disease.

The manufacturer's recommended price of AU$12.50 (US$6.70) for the urethral occlusive device, to be changed each week, was not supported by the median reduction of personal cost of AU$4.22 (US$2.26; 95% CI 3.00-5.63). However, pad testing of the patient sample revealed that most patients had only moderate leakage (median baseline loss of 22 ml/hr, IQR 6-83.5 ml). Therefore, that sensitivity analysis for a cohort of patients with severe leakage and high costs might have reached different conclusions.

The Dutch Study [92] on sacral anterior root stimulation evaluted the costs of this procedure versus "routine care" for 51 incontinent patients with spinal cord lesions. Costs were measured at baseline (mean duration 7.5 months), to form the comparison "routine care" data set. Patients then underwent sacral posterior rhizotomy and implantation of a Brindley sacral anterior root stimulator, requiring an average hospital stay of 15.6 days. Post-implantation costs were measured again for an average 14 months' follow up.

For the sacral anterior root stimulation group, incidence rates and survival rates for the total Dutch population were calculated (controlled for mean age and average duration of conventional care of the patient population). The baseline pre-implantation costs were NLG4,710 (US$1965 at the 2001 conversion rate) per patient per year. The implantation costs were high at NLG33,402 (US$13,933) over 2 years (50% due to hospital stay and implantation surgery). After implantation, direct routine care costs dropped to NLG1,421 (US$593) per patient per year. However, no significant overall changes in Nottingham Health Profile nor Karinovsky index were observed, although other scores related to impact of incontinence upon household work etc showed significant beneficial effects. Long-term effects of bladder cancer and renal failure over 30 years were NLG20,999 (US$8,760) for those with implanted stimulators and NLG33,723 (US$14,066) for those without stimulation, but the methods of calculation were not elaborated. The long-term cost model showed the stimulation implantation care program to be cheaper than routine care after 8 years.

An economic model was developed in the UK to estimate the comparative cost-effectiveness of treating unstable bladder with tolterodine IR, tolterodine ER and oxybutynin. The model employs the purchaser, patient and societal perspectives over a one-year timeframe. The treatment population was based on the percentage of patients seeking treatment in the UK, and the treatment population was divided into successfully treated patients (STPs) and patients failing treatment. The percentage of STPs was calculated from clinical efficacy and adjusted by annual persistency; the percentage of STPs and the number of patients seeking treatment were multiplied to calculate the number of STPs. The prevalence of sufferers in the UK was estimated to be 19% of people 40 years and over (approximately 5.15 million sufferers), with only 5.9% of those patients seeking treatment [93]. Efficacy was considered approximately equal for tolterodine IR and oxybutynin; however, tolterodine ER has an 18% greater efficacy than tolterodine IR [66]. Persistence on therapy (measured as the percentage of patients remaining on therapy at 12 weeks) was higher for tolterodine than for oxybutynin [65]. Therefore, effectiveness, defined as the percentage of STPs, was higher for tolterodine than for oxybutynin (42.00% for tolterodine IR, 54.67% for tolterodine ER and 9.50% for oxybutynin [67]. Cost per successfully treated patient was lower for tolterodine than oxybutynin, with the lowest cost per successfully treated patient being for tolterodine ER (US$1,473 for tolterodine ER, US$1,992 for tolterodine IR, US$5,729 for oxybutynin) [67].

2. Cost-utility analysis

Foote & Moore [94] measured changes in quality of life and calculated the cost per QALY gain for each of five treatments for incontinence shown in Figure 4. The York questionnaire was used because it provides a common yardstick to measure improvement in quality of life, and can also be employed to compare these treatments with any other medical treatment and to rank treatments overall in a league table.

The percentage improvement in quality of life on the York Questionnaire was similar for all five treatment groups varying from 1.21% (urogynecologist conservative treatment) to 2.09% (laparoscopic colposuspension). In contrast, there was a large difference between the costs, varying from $901/year (urogynecologist conservative treatment) to $6,124/year (open colposuspension). The most cost-effective treatment was the conservative treatment of urinary incontinence by the nurse continence advisor. However, confidence intervals were wide, as shown in Figure 4. These wide confidence intervals were due to loss of the York data when the quality of life gain was zero (making an infinite number with quality of life in the denominator for the cost/QALY), hence resulting in smaller numbers available for QALY calculation.

A review study on cost-effectiveness and cost-utility analysis of urinary incontinence surgical procedures was carried out [37]. The review identified 10 basic principles that should be incorporated in cost-effectiveness analyses (Table 4). These principles were derived by reviewing recommendations in publications describing standard methods for cost-effectiveness analysis of health care practices and comprise an appropriate minimum standard for performing and reporting cost-effectiveness analyses. This review of gynecologic surgical procedures suggests that much of the existing cost analysis literature does not adhere to basic recommended analytic guidelines. However, those authors who specifically planned to perform a CEA analysis met all or nearly all of the methodologic principles. Investigators who use CEA are strongly encouraged to use the many outstanding methodologic reviews of CEA. For example, Kung et al. [16] compared the cost per cure of stress urinary incontinence of laparoscopic Burch strategy and open Burch procedures. The probability of cure after each procedure was estimated from a retrospective cohort of 62 women with a mean follow up of 1.2 years for the laparoscopic Burch strategy and 2.7 years for the open Burch strategy. The authors found that the laparoscopic Burch dominated, with lower costs and a higher cure rate. However, the analysis would be more informative with a much longer follow-up, because most women who undergo an incontinence procedure have a life expectancy greater than 1–2 years.

3. COST-BENEFIT ANALYSIS

A willingness-to-pay survey [56], in which 411 Americans with urge incontinence were solicited via their membership of the National Association for Incontinence, found a mean willingness to pay US$87.74 per month for a 25% reduction in micturition and incontinence episodes. For a 50% reduction in symptoms, respondents were willing to pay a mean $244.54 per month (1997 dollars). Corresponding median reductions were $27.24 and $75.92, respectively. Using both mean and median results, willingness to pay increased

Table 4 : Principles for performing and reporting cost-effectiveness analysis [37]

1. RESEARCH QUESTION	• Explicitly stated • Interesting, feasible • Appropriate for CEA
2. TIME FRAME	• Explicitly stated Appropriate
3. PERSPECTIVE	• Explicitly stated • Appropriate • Costs and outcomes appropriate for perspective
4. ANALYTIC MODEL	• Explicit (spreadsheet, tree, Markov process) • Strategies, intermediate and terminal states described • Includes reasonable alternative strategies
5. PROBABILITIES	• Source of data • Quality of data
6. COSTS	• Appropriate measure (cost, charge; direct, indirect costs) • Source of data • Quality of data
7. OUTCOME MEASURE	• Explicitly stated • Appropriate • [Utility measure (source of data, appropriate methods)]
8. INCREMENTAL ANALYSIS	• Done • Appropriate "basecase" • Appropriate summary measure
9. SENSITIVITY ANALYSES	• Done • Appropriate range • Appropriate variables
10. DISCOUNTING (WHEN APPROPRIATE)	

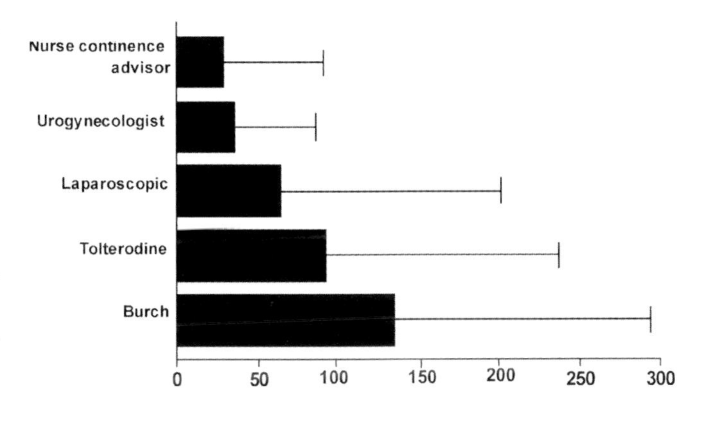

Figure 4 : Costs of QALYs gained with 5 different treatments for incontinence in female patients (means and standard errors) [95].

by a factor of 2.75 when the percentage reduction in symptoms doubled (from 25% to 50%).

In summary, selection of an effectiveness measure after surgical intervention is often difficult and controversial. For benign disease, life years or QALYs may not be sensitive to a reasonable safe intervention. In the short-term, utility may be negatively affected by surgery and recovery. In longer-term analyses, these effects will be diluted by time and may be negligible. Nevertheless, QALYs are the current gold standard [1, 2]. Researchers are encouraged to use QALYs, but they may find it very worthwhile to add other outcome measures, such as disease-specific quality of life measures that are more sensitive to treatment.

VI. SUMMARY

Urinary incontinence continues to be a costly illness that affects personal resources, medical treatment, and quality of life, as evidenced from quantitative estimates from middle to high-income counties. The magnitude of urinary incontinence costs is quite comparable to other illnesses afflicting the female population, such as breast cancer, osteoporosis and arthritis. Most studies focus on the direct costs of the illness, which are relatively easier to quantify than indirect costs, such as productivity loss. Among the direct costs, personal care (routine care costs) took an overwhelming share of total direct costs. It was found that there is a strong correlation between the economic status of the country and the amount of incontinence pads used.

In recent years, a special effort has been made to follow up treatment cost analysis, both in terms of the effect of new medication on the treatment of urge incontinence and procedures on treating stress incontinence. A number of studies have examined the patterns of treatment among the managed care system.

More quantitative analysis has been carried out to study health related cost consequences due to urinary incontinence. This is a more challenging task. Through direct survey and multivariate analysis, more reliable estimates are now available.

Finally, cost-effectiveness analyses and cost-utility analyses of alternative treatment protocols have been studied, but in limited quantity, and largely under quasi-experimental design. More studies are needed using randomized trials.

VII. FUTURE RESEARCH PRIORITIES

Since the last review, more studies have been published on the costs of urinary incontinence among community dwelling residents, the detailed costs estimate of routine care, cost consequences of urinary incontinence, and the costs of OAB (which overlaps the subset of urinary incontinence – urge and mixed condition). The estimation of costs of urinary incontinence has been expanded beyond the US in the last few years, and in countries such as Australia, France, Germany, The Netherlands, Italy and the UK urinary incontinence continues to be a significant illness affecting personal resource use in the health care system and quality of life. However, there is still a need to know more about these costs in low-income countries. One of the reasons for the paucity of these cost studies in low-income countries is that this topic has not been widely recognized either due to cultural differences or differences in economic status. In addition, most of the available data only exists from high-income countries. To encourage low-income countries to engage these cost estimates, it would be useful to explore findings for these types of study in the future.

We have identified the following priority areas for research on the economics of incontinence:

1. direct medical costs of urinary incontinence
2. productivity loss and indirect intangible costs of incontinence
3. routine care costs
4. effect of incontinence on institutionalization and hospitalization
5. costs of incontinence for the population under 65 years
6. cost variation by type of urinary incontinence
7. costs of treating incontinence in different health care systems
8. the sensitivity of utilities and willingness to pay in economic evaluations
9. national differences in the costs of incontinence and funding of care
10. cost implication of disease progression and remission in incontinence and OAB

To facilitate economic research, it is imperative to establish validated and accepted outcome measures of symptom severity as well as measures for symptom improvement following therapy. We need to define when a treatment works and what is a clinically significant change.

These research priority areas should not be viewed as mutually exclusive. For instance, there are costs associated with urinary incontinence whether or not a person is treated. If a person is treated and becomes continent, direct treatment costs are incurred but the cost consequences of indirect costs and intangible costs are avoided. In contrast, if a person does not seek medical attention, then the direct medical costs will be minimal but the indirect and intangible costs will be increased. In addition, such people will likely contribute to an underreporting of the prevalence of urinary incontinence. There has been no research on the different types of costs associated with urinary incontinence with respect to national and cultural differences. Clearly, it will depend on people's knowledge of incontinence and their willingness to seek medical advice for it based on severity and cultural conditioning. Understanding the costs and cost-effectiveness as well as effectiveness of intervention will help to guide health policy.

Another area that has not been explored is the effect of remission and recurrence in terms of the cost impact and how prevention programs may be cost-effective. For example, patients with OAB may be continent because they are using coping strategies to deal with their frequency and urgency, but if they decompensate then incontinence ensues. Hence, an understanding of costs related to prevention of decompensation would be of value.

Cost analyses are necessary to help health policy planners determine how to allocate resources. For such analyses to be meaningful, it is necessary to abstract data only from studies that are tightly focused, and to keep references to these data within the context of the original work. Generalizations or extrapolations that do not relate directly to each aspect of a survey will be misleading. To date, most analyses have not been so stringent because data are lacking. Such information is urgently needed to allow meaningful interpretation.

It should be emphasized that research on costs should be carried out in the developing world as well as in more developed countries outside of the US. Data from the US, such as they exist, will help to guide such endeavors.

This committee wishes to encourage inclusion of the following in future incontinence studies:

- Direct and indirect measurement of patient preferences (utilities)
- Economic evaluation preferably cost-effectiveness analysis (especially cost-utility analysis)

In order to facilitate economic studies regarding the cost of incontinence treatment, each country should gather data regarding the costs of the available treatments and investigations and publish average figures, which could be employed in economic studies. The actual cost of visits to each type of continence clinician should be obtained from the cost of doing business rather than relying on charges. Policy guidelines should be based not only on evidence-based medicine but also on cost-effectiveness.

REFERENCES

1. Gold MR, Siegel JE, Russell LB, Weinstein Mc, Eds. Cost-effectiveness in health and medicine. Oxford: Oxford University Press, 1996.
2. Drummond MF, O'brien B, Stoddart Gl, Torrance Gw. Methods for the economic evaluation of health care programmes. Second Ed. Oxford: Oxford University Press, 1997.
3. Feeny D, Furlong W, Boyle M, Torrance GW. Multi-attribute health status classification systems. Health Utilities Index. Pharmacoeconomics 1995;7:490--502.
4. The EUROQOL GROUP. EuroQol – a new facility for the measurement of health-related quality of life. Health Policy 1990;16:199–208.
5. Gafni A. Willingness to pay. What's in a name? Pharmacoeconomics 1998;14:465–70.
6. Donaldson C. Valuing the benefits of publicly-provided health care: does 'ability to pay' preclude the use of 'willingness to pay'? Social Science and Medicine 1999;49:551–63.
7. Versi E, Defever M, Hu T, et al. Socioeconomic considerations. In: Incontinence (Abrams P, Khoury S, Wein A, Eds). Plymouth: Health Publication Ltd, 1999, pp.869–91.
8. Groutz A, Blavias JG, Rosenthal JE. A simplified urinary incontinence score for the evaluation of treatment outcomes. Neurourol Urodyn 2000;19:127–35.
9. Shumaker SA, Wyman JF, Uebersax JS, Mcclish D, Fantl JA. Health-related quality of life measures for women with urinary incontinence: the Incontinence Impact Questionnaire and the Urogenital Distress Inventory. Continence Program in Women (CPW) Research Group. Qual Life Res 1994;3:291–306.
10. Wagner TH, Patrick Dl, Bavendam TG, Martin ML, Buesching Dp. Quality of life of persons with urinary incontinence: development of a new measure. Urology 1996;47:67–71.
11. Kelleher CJ, Cardozo LD, Kuhller V, Salvatore S. A new questionnaire to assess the quality of life of urinary incontinent women. Br J Obstet Gynaecol 1997;104:1374–9.
12. Blaivas JG. Outcome measures for urinary incontinence. Urology 1998;51(Suppl.2A):11–9.
13. Wagner T, Hu T. Economic costs of urinary incontinence in 1995. Urology 1998;51:355–61.
14. Tediosi F, Parazzini F, Bortolotti A, Garattini L. The cost of urinary incontinence in Italian women: a cross-sectional study. Pharmacoeconomics 2000;17:71-6.
15. Milsom I, Fall M, Ekelund P. Urinary incontinence – an expensive national disease. Lakartidningen 1992;89:1772–4.
16. Kung RC, Lie K, Lee P, Drutz HP. The cost-effectiveness of laparoscopic versus abdominal Burch procedures in women with urinary stress incontinence. J Am Assoc Gynecol Laparosc 1996;3:537–44.

17. Gomes CM, Broderick GA, Sanchez-Ortiz RF, Preate D Jr, Rovner Es, Wein Aj. Artificial urinary sphincter for post-prostatectomy incontinence: impact of prior collagen injection on cost and clinical outcome. J Urol 2000;163:87–90

18. Baker DI, Bice TW. The influence of urinary incontinence on publicly financed home care services to low-income elderly people. Gerontologist 1995;35:360–9.

19. Schnelle JF, Keeler E, Hays RD, Simmons S, Ouslander Jg, Siu Al. A cost and value analysis of two interventions with incontinent nursing home residents. J Am Geriatr Soc 1995;43:1112–7.

20. Van Doorslaer E, Wagstaff A, Van Der Burg H, Christiansen T, De Graeve D, Duchesne I, et al. Equity in the delivery of health care in Europe and the US. Journal Health Econ 2000;19:553–83.

21. Cutler DM. The cost and financing of health care. Am Econ Rev 1995;85:32–7.

22. Arrow K. Uncertainty and the welfare economics of medical care. Am Econ Rev 1963;53:941–73.

23. Feldstein M. The economics of health and health care: What have we learned? What have I learned? Am Econ Rev 1995;85:28–31.

24. Schwartz M, Young DW, Siegrist R. The ratio of costs to charges: how good a basis for estimating costs? Inquiry 1995;32:476–81.

25. Barnett PG. Research without billing data. Econometric estimation of patient- specific costs. Med Care 1997;35:553–63.

26. Miller ME, Welch WP. Analysis of Hospital Medical Staff Volume Performance Standards: Technical Report. Washington D.C.: The Urban Institute, 1993.

27. Wagner TH, Chen S, Yu W, Barnett PG. HERC's inpatient average cost dataset for VA care: fiscal years 1998 and 1999. HERC Working Paper #3 2001; Menlo Park, California.

28. Farley D, Goldman D, Carter G, Davis L, Carleton J, Cherry G, et al. Interim Report: Evaluation of the Medicare-DOD subvention demonstration. Santa Monica: RAND MR–1106.0–HFCA, 1999.

29. Krahn M, Gafni A. Discounting in the economic evaluation of health care interventions. Med Care 1993;31:403–18

30. Ganiats TG, Carson Rt, Hamm RM, Cantor SB, Sumner W, Spann Sj, et al. Population-based time preferences for future health outcomes. Med Decis Making 2000;20:263–70.

31. Olsen JA. On what basis should health be discounted? J Health Econ 1993;12:39–53.

32. Berndt ER, Busch SH, Frank RG. Price indexes for acute phase treatment of depression. NBER working paper 6799, 1998.

33. Cleeton Dl, Goepfrich VT, Weisbrod Ba. What does the Consumer Price Index for prescription drugs really measure? Health Care Financ Rev 1992;13:45–51.

34. Adams Me, Mccall Nt, Gray DT, Orza MJ, Chalmers TC. Economic analysis in randomized control trials. Med Care 1992;30:231–43.

35. Neumann Pj, Stone Pw, Chapman Rh, Sandberg Ea, Bell CM. The quality of reporting in published cost-utility analyses, 1976-1997. Ann Intern Med 2000;132:964–72.

36. Udvarhelyi Is, Colditz Ga, Rai A, Epstein AM. Cost-effectiveness and cost-benefit analyses in the medical literature. Are the methods being used correctly? Annals Intern Med 1992;116:238–44.

37. Subak Ll, Caughey AB. Measuring cost-effectiveness of surgical procedures. Clin Obstet Gynecol 2000;43:551–60.

38. Hu TW. The economic impact of urinary incontinence. Clin Geriatr Med 1986;2:673–87.

39. Ouslander J, Kane R. The cost of urinary incontinence in nursing homes. Med Care 1983;22:67–9.

40. Sowell V, Al A. A cost comparison of five methods of managing urinary incontinence. Qual Rev Bull. 1987;13:411–4.

41. Schnelle J, Sowell V, Hu T. Reduction of urinary incontinence in nursing homes: does it reduce or increase costs? J Am Geriatr Soc 1988;36:34–9.

42. Hu TW. Impact of urinary incontinence on health-care costs. J Am Geriatr Soc 1990;28:292–5.

43. Cella M. The nursing costs of urinary incontinence in a nursing home population. Nurs Clin North Am 1988;23:159–68.

44. Ramsey Sd, Wagner Th, Bavendam TG. Estimating costs of treating stress urinary incontinence in elderly women according to the AHCPR clinical practice guidelines. Am J Managed Care 1996;2:147–54.

45. Hu TW. The cost of Urinary Incontinence on Health Care Services. A paper prepared for the 1997 Clinical Practice Guideline Panel for Urinary Incontinence, Agency for Health Care Policy and Research, also presented at the National Multi-Specialty Nursing Conference on Urinary Incontinence, Phoenix, Arizona, June 1994.

46. Wilson L, Oark Ge, Luc Ko, Brown Js, Subak LL. Annual costs of urinary incontinence. Obstet Gynecol (in press).

47. Fantl J, Newman D, Colling J, Delancey J, Keeys C, Mcdowell B. Urinary incontinence in adults: acute and chronic management. Clinical Practice Guideline, No.2. Rockville, Maryland: AHCPR, 1996.

48. Stewart Wf, et al. Overactive bladder in the United States: what is the burden? ICS, Korea, 2001.

49. Hu T, Wagner T, Bentkover J, Leblanc K, Piacentini A, Stewart W, Corey R, Zhou Z, Hunt T. Economic costs of overactive bladder. Presented at the 2nd International Consultation on Incontinence, July 1–3, 2001, Paris.

50. National Institutes Of Health. Disease-Specific Estimates of Direct and Indirect Costs of Illness and NIH Report. US Public Health Services, 1997.

51. Doran Cm, Chiarelli P, Cockburn J. Economic costs of urinary incontinence in community-dwelling Australian women. Med J Aust 2001;174:456–8.

52. Moore KH. The costs of incontinence. Med J Aust 2001;174:436–7.

53. Dowell Cj, Bryant Cm, Moore Kh, Simons AM. Calculating the direct costs of urinary incontinence: a new test instrument. BJU Int 1999;83:596–606.

54. Ballanger Ph, Rischmann P. Incontinence urinaire de la femme: evaluation et traitment. Prog Urol 1995;5:739–63.

55. Simons Am, Dowell Cj, Bryant Cm, Prashar S, Moore KH. Use of the Dowell Bryant Incontinence Cost Index as a post-treatment outcome measure after non-surgical therapy. Neurourol Urodyn 2001;20:85–93.

56. O'conor Rm, Johannesson M, Hass Sl, Kobel-Nguyen G. Urge incontinence. Quality of life and patients' valuation of symptom reduction. Pharmacoeconomics 1998;14:531–9.

57. Frenchman IB. Cost of urinary incontinence in two skilled nursing facilities: a prospective study. Clin Geriatr 2001;9:49–52.

58. Mcclish Dk, Wyman Jf, Sale Pg, Camp J, Earle B. Use and costs of incontinence pads in female study volunteers. J Wound Ostomy Continence Nurs 1999;26:207–13.

59. Kornides M, Moore K. Per capita use of continence pads in 12 countries in relation to per capita gross domestic product. Aust Cont J 1999;5:36–7.

60. DAY PL. Findings of a three-year retrospective study to investigate prevalence and incidence of urinary incontinence and overactive bladder in a typical managed care setting. Pharm Pract Manag Q 2000;20:1–11.

61. Kelleher Cj, Cardozo L, Khullar V, Salvatore S. A medium-term analysis of the subjective efficacy of treatment for women with detrusor instability and low bladder compliance. Br J Obstst Gynaecol 1997;104:988–93.

62. Abrams P, Freeman R, Anderstrom C, Mattiasson A. Tolterodine, a new antimuscarinic agent: as effective but better tolerated than oxybutynin in patients with overactive bladder. Br J Urol 1998;81:807–8.

63. Anderson R, Mobley D, Blank B, Saltzstein D, Susset J, Brown J. Once daily controlled versus immediate release oxybutynin for urge urinary incontinence. J Urol 1999;161:1809–12.

64. Versi E, Appell R, Mobley D, Patton W, Saltzstein D. Dry mouth with conventional and controlled-release oxybutynin in urinary incontinence. Obstet Gynecol 2000;95:718–21.

65. Appell RA. Clinical efficacy and the safety of tolterodine in the treatment of overactive bladder: a pooled analysis. Urology 1997;50(Suppl.6A):90–6.

66. Van Kerrebroeck P, Kreder K, Jonas U, Zinner N, Wein A, on behalf of The Tolterodine Study Group. Tolterodine once-daily: superior efficacy and tolerability in the treatment of overactive bladder. Urology 2001;57:414–21.

67. Chapple C, Hill S, Corey R, Bentkover J, Kurth H. Tolterodine: The cost-effective choice for treating unstable bladder in the UK. Neurourol Urodynam 2001;20:424-6.

68. Ouslander Jg, Shih Y-Ct, Malone-Lee J, Luber KM. Overactive bladder: special considerations in the geriatric population. Am J Managed Care 2000;6:599–606.

69. Subak Ll, Waetjen Le, Van Den Eeden S, Thom Dh, Vittinghoff E, Brown J. The social cost of pelvic organ prolapse surgery in the U.S. Obstet Gynecol (in press).

70. Johansson C, Moldander U, Milsom I, Ekelund P. Association between urinary incontinence and urinary tract infections, and fractures in postmenopausal women. Maturitas 1996;23:265–71.

71. Brown J, Vittinghof E, Wyman J, Stone Kl, Nevitt Mc, Ensrud Ke, Grady D. Urinary incontinence: does it increase risk for falls and fractures? Study of Osteoporotic Fractures Research Group. J Am Geriatr Soc 2000;48:721–5.

72. Wagner T, Hu T, Bentkover J, Leblanc K, Piacentini A, Stewart W, Corey R, Zhou Z, Hunt T. Health-related consequences and costs of overactive bladder. Presented at the 2nd International Consultation on Incontinence, July 1–3, 2001, Paris.

73. Bailey Kl, Torigoe Y, Zhou S, Mo Ls, Flewelling SL. Overactive bladder cost of illness: analysis of Medi-Cal claims. Presented at the International Society for Pharmacoeconomics and Outcomes Research 5th Annual International Meeting, May 21–24, 2000, Arlington, Virginia.

74. Zorn Bh, Montgomery H, Pieper K, Gray M, Steers WD. Urinary incontinence and depression. J Urol 1999;102:82–4.

75. Brown Js, Grady D, Ouslander Jg, Herzog Ar, Varner Re, Posner SF, for the Heart and Estrogen/progestin Replacement (HERS) Research Group. Prevalence of urinary incontinence and associated risk factors in postmenopausal women. Obstet Gynecol 1999;94:66–70.

76. Bodden-Heidrichr, Beckmann Mw, Libera B, Rechenberger I, Bender HG. Psychsomatic aspects of urinary incontinence. Arch Gynecol Obstet 1999;262:151–8.

77. Thom D. Variation in estimates of urinary incontinence prevalence in the community: effects of differences in definition, population characteristics and study type. J Am Geriatr Soc 1998;46:473–80.

78. Ouslander Jg, Shih Yt, Malone-Lee J, Luber KM. Overactive bladder: special considerations in the geriatric population. Am J Managed Care 2000;6:S599.

79. Shih Yct, Hartzema Ag, Tolleson-Rinehart S, Gorospe Ja, Foldfarb SD. Costing the care for urinary incontinent patients in long-term care facilities. Presented at the 21st Annual Meeting of the Society for Medical Decision Making, October 5, 1999, Reno, Nevada.

80. Johnson Tm, Bernard Sl, Kincade Je, Defriese GH. Urinary incontinence and risk of death among community-living elderly people: results from the National Survey on Self-Care and Aging. J Aging Health 2000;12:25–46.

81. Fitzgerald St, Palmer Mh, Berry Sj, Hart K. Urinary incontinence. Impact on working women. AAOHN J. 2000;48:112–8.

82. Palmer Mh, Fitzgerald S, Berry Sj, Hart K. Urinary incontinence in working women: an exploratory study. Women Health. 1999;29:67–80.

83. Sherman Ra, Davis Gd, Wong MF. Behavioral treatment of exercise-induced urinary incontinence among female soldiers. Military Med 1997;162:690–4.

84. Nygaard Je, Linder M. Thirst at work - an occupational hazard? Int Urogynecol J Pelvic Floor Dysfunct 1997;8:340–3.

85. Linder M, Nygaard I. Void where prohibited: rest breaks and the right to urinate on company time. Ithaca, New York: ILR Press, 1998.

86. Davis G, Sherman R, Wong Mf, Mcclure G, Perez R, Hibbert M. Urinary incontinence among female soldiers. Military Med. 1999;164:182–7.

87. Turan C, Zorlu Cg, Ekin M, Hancerliogullari N, Saracoglu F. Urinary incontinence in women of reproductive age. Gynecol Obstet Invest 1996;41:132–4.

88. Samuelsson E, Victor A, Tibblin G. A population study of urinary incontinence and nocturia among women aged 29–59. Acta Obstet Gynecol Scand 1997;76:74–80.

89. Elving Lb, Foldspang A, Lam Gw, Mommsen S. Descriptive epidemiology of urinary incontinence in 3100 women age 30–59. Scand J Urol Nephrol Suppl 1989;125:37–43.

90. Nygaard Ie, Thompson Fl, Svengalis Bs, Albright JP. Urinary incontinence in elite nulliparous athletes. Obstet Gynecol 1994;84:183–7.

91. Weber Am, Walters MD. Cost-effectiveness of urodynamic testing before surgery for women with pelvic organ prolapse and stress urinary incontinence. Am J Obstet Gynecol 2000;183:1338–46.

92. Wielink G, Essink-Bot Ml, Van Kerrebroeck Ph, Rutten FF. Sacral rhizotomies and electrical bladder stimulation in spinal cord injury. Eur Urol 1997,31.441–6.

93. Milsom I, Abrams P, Cardozo L, Roberts Rg, Thuroff J, Wein AJ. How widespread are the symptoms of an overactive bladder and how do we manage them? A population-based prevalence study. BJU Int 2001;87:760–6.

94. Foote Aj, Moore KH. Comparative cost-utility analysis of 5 treatments for female urinary incontinence. Austr Continence J, 2001; 7 (in press).

Committee 15

Anal Incontinence

Co-Chairs

C. Norton (U.K.),

J. Christiansen (Denmark)

Members

U.Butler (U.K.),

D. Harari (U.K.),

R. L. Nelson (USA),

J. Pemberton (USA),

K. Price (U.K.),

E. Rovnor USA),

A. Sultan (U.K.),

CONTENTS

Anal Incontinence

C. Norton, J. Christiansen

U.Butler, D. Harari, R.L. Nelson, J. Pemberton, K. Price, E. Rovnor, A. Sultan

A. INTRODUCTION

Faecal incontinence has been a largely neglected topic in the world health care literature. Many patients with faecal incontinence become housebound because of the stigma associated with the condition. It is an embarrassing complaint that is socially disruptive.

I. DEFINITIONS

Faecal incontinence has been variously defined and there are no internationally accepted or accredited definitions available. The Royal College of Physicians has proposed "the involuntary or inappropriate passage of faeces"[1]. An international panel of experts has defined "functional faecal incontinence" as "recurrent uncontrolled passage of faecal material for at least one month, in an individual with a developmental age of at least four years...." [2]. Some authors also include inability to control passage of flatus, or an arbitrary frequency with which symptoms must occur to be included. The "objectively demonstrable" criteria specified by the International Continence Society for urinary incontinence is not practical in clinical practice for faecal incontinence. Therefore, clinicians must rely on patients' self-report of symptoms.

This chapter will adopt the widely accepted distinction between "anal incontinence" denoting any loss of stool or flatus per anus and "faecal incontinence" as denoting any loss of solid or liquid stool.

The literature is confusing on the subject of definitions. The term "idiopathic incontinence" is often used to denote incontinence not due to trauma, congenital defects or neurological disease. "Neurogenic incontinence" in the colorectal literature often denotes faecal incontinence presumed to be secondary to damage to the pudendal nerve during childbirth, rather than that associated with major neurological disease. It is recommended that this term should not be used since it in principal it is identical with idiopathic incontinence and may be confused with incontinence due to neurological disease which is quite distinct. "Sensory incontinence" is not an entity but should be a description added to incontinence of any aetiology when the patient has no defecation urge at all and does not feel the passage of stool. "Motor incontinence" is an ill defined term which mainly covers incontinence in connection with diarrhoea and irritable bowel syndrome. It is recommended that this term should not be used.

The committee proposed the definition **"Anal incontinence is the involuntary loss of flatus, liquid or solid stool that is a social or hygienic problem"** as a working definition for this review. This definition takes cognisance of the fact that people react very differently to the same objective situation. For example, loss of flatus which is hardly noticed by one person is experienced as socially incapacitating by another. We recognise the need for, and would welcome, further debate and refinement of this definition.

II. SERVICES FOR PEOPLE WITH FAECAL INCONTINENCE

In many settings there is a lack of designated services for people with faecal incontinence. Locally, a service may be provided by a colorectal surgeon, gastroenterologist, specialist nurse (e.g. in stoma care, colorectal practice or biofeedback practitioner), but more often there is no interested professional and absent investigation facilities.

People with faecal incontinence are reluctant to seek health care for their problem [3, 4]. It is not clear the relative importance played in this by embarrassment and social taboos, lack of awareness that treatment is possible, lack of services, or a genuine unconcern at the symptom.

III. PROFESSIONAL EDUCATION AND PUBLIC AWARENESS

The majority of health professionals receive little or no training on faecal incontinence and even those who might be supposed to have a special interest, such as continence nurse specialists or colorectal surgeons, often focus on other areas. Public awareness of the symptom is very poor and there have been very limited attempts to alter this as yet.

B. EPIDEMIOLOGY AND THE INCIDENCE OF ANAL INCONTINENCE; THE MAGNITUDE OF THE PROBLEM

Most discussions of the aetiology of anal incontinence (AI) have been based upon the assumption that women, particularly under the age of 65 years, are more at risk for AI than men. Obstetric injury to the pudendal nerve or sphincter muscle are described as the primary risk factors [5-7], irritable bowel syndrome as second [8] and other aetiologies such as diabetes as a distant third [9]. Yet each population based survey of AI prevalence has shown a surprisingly high prevalence in males [10-15]. Clearly other aetiologies than childbirth must be sought. In the most broadly based survey, it was apparent that factors that impact on an individual's general health or physical capabilities independently of age and gender place that individual at greater risk for anal incontinence than either age or gender [16].

Evidence in epidemiologic investigations comes principally from cohort and cross sectional surveys (level 2 – in which risk can be calculated and expressed as an odds ratio and 95% confidence intervals) in which the statistical significance of the associations can be assessed. Secondarily risk factors arise from case series (level 4) and insightful observation (level 5). Systematic reviews of epidemiologic observations have for the most part been difficult to perform, since different studies usually adjust for differing variables and individual patient data are needed to overcome this difficulty. Therefore level 1 evidence does not exist for any risk factor related to faecal incontinence. In the tables below, when odds ratios and confidence intervals are presented it can therefore be assumed that that evidence is level 2 and when only lists of associations are presented, the level is most usually 4, occasionally 5.

I. PREVALENCE

Most reports of AI prevalence have been from single institutions and the patients described therein subject to referral bias when demographics and aetiology are discussed. The accuracy of prevalence estimates of AI may also be diminished by difficulty in ascertainment. Underestimates of prevalence are common due to patients' reluctance to report symptoms of incontinence in strange settings or to seek support services [9, 17,4] (Table 1). It has been shown that women are more willing to report AI than men [16]. In addition, the character (incontinence to solid faeces, diarrhoea or flatus) and frequency (daily versus episodic) of AI varies greatly in each population. Prevalence depends on the definition of AI. The entry question quoted in one survey was written by a patient with faecal incontinence [16]. That individual regarded the inclusion of gas as critical. The same individual, and many others have said that one does not have to be incontinent all the time or only to solid stool to think that one is incontinent all the time and to be disabled by it.

Only seven population based estimates of prevalence in non-institutionalized individuals have been reported (Table 2). Prevalence has varied in these reports from 0.5% to 11%. The first report was restricted only to individuals over 65 years of age, both living at home and in institutions in New Zealand. The overall prevalence was 3.1%. FI was more prevalent in men, though further details of the population are not given [11]. The second, from Holland, was restricted to women over 60 years of age, and a non-representative sample of this group surveyed for prevalence by mail [12]. The prevalence varied with advancing age from 2.3% to 17.8%. These reports focused, as have most reports, on urinary incontinence. The third report was from Britain and compared prevalence obtained from a survey of community support services concerning individuals known to be incontinent in the region and a follow-up postal survey of all individuals living in the region. There was a marked disparity between those having sought help from community support services for faecal and double (urinary and faecal) incontinence and those reporting incontinence in the postal survey (Table 1). The difference was 8 fold for men below 65, four fold for women below 65 and roughly two fold for both genders over 65 years of age [10]. The total population prevalence of

Table 1 : Prevalence of anal or double incontinence in Middlesex, England [10]

	MEN 15-64 years	MEN > 64	WOMEN 15-64	WOMEN > 64
Community Services Reported	0.5%	4.9%	0.4%	8.8%
Postal Survey Reported	4.2%	10.9%	1.7%	13.3%

Table 2 : Anal incontinence; population based surveys

Country (ref)	Population	Prevalence
New Zealand [11]	> 65 years old	3.1%
Holland [12]	Women > 60 years	4.2% to 16.9 % with rising age
U.K. [10]	Community Service	1.9% (Table 1)
France [13]	All > 45 years	11%, 6% to faeces 60% women
U.S.A. [14]	Market mailing	7% soiling, 0.7% to faeces
U.S.A. [16]	Wisconsin Households	2.2%, 63% women
Australia [15]	Household survey	6.8% Men, 10.9% Women > 15 years old
U.S.A. [19]	Wisconsin Nursing Homes	47%

faecal or double incontinence of that British health region was 1.9% by survey of health service personnel and 4.3% by postal survey.

From France, a prevalence study has been reported limited to individuals over the age of 45 years [13]. FI prevalence was determined in a "Gallup poll" style telephone interview, as well as in the practices of several medical specialists. In the population based survey, an overall prevalence of 11% was reported, roughly half to gas only and half to solid or liquid stool. 60% were women and prevalence was increased independently of gender if subjects had urinary incontinence or neurological disorders. FI prevalence increased with age, with disability resulting in bed confinement, with dementia and with nursing home residence. From the United States, FI prevalence was determined through the addition of questions concerning functional bowel disorders to a commercial marketing survey mailing [14]. Because the means by which the addressees were chosen was proprietary information and was not made available to the investigators, there was great potential for selection bias in this population that cannot be accurately assessed. (Marketers may be more interested in "buyers" than obtaining a group representative of the general population). Response to the survey was also subject to many factors that affect the generalisability of the results. The survey encompassed 5430 respondents, which was 66% of the mailing. Faecal soiling was present in 7.4% of the males in the respondents and 6.9% of the females, with incontinence to solid stool in 0.5% of the males and 0.9% of the females.

The population of the State of Wisconsin was sampled in the 1993 Wisconsin Family Health Survey [16]. Subjects were identified by random digit dialing of Wisconsin residences with telephone interview. The individual within each household identified as most knowledgeable about the health status of all other members of the household was asked about the health status of each member of the household. Approximately 200 households were surveyed each month. The presence of anal incontinence to solid, liquid or gas within the past year, who suffered from it, the frequency of incontinence, and how that individual coped with it were assessed.

2570 Households comprising 6959 individuals were surveyed. 153 individuals were reported to have AI, representing 2.2% of the population (95% confidence interval (CI) = + 0.3%). 30% of the incontinent subjects were greater than 65 years of age; 63% were women. Of those with AI, 36% were incontinent to solid faeces, 54% to liquid and 60% to gas. In a multivariate analysis, independent associations of the following risk factors with AI were found in increasing order of importance: female gender, age, physical limitations and poor general health (Table 3).

From Australia, a population based household survey was reported encompassing 3010 interviews with individuals ranging in age from 15 to 97 years [15]. In face to face interviews, the prevalence of incontinence to either flatus or solid stool was found to be 6.8% and 2.3% in men, and 10.9% and 3.5% in women respectively. The male to female ratio is also very similar to the Wisconsin report, being 64% women for flatus incontinence and 60% for incontinence to solid stool.

II. ASSOCIATIONS

The most prominent association with faecal incontinence by far is nursing home residence. Whereas the prevalence of faecal (not just anal) incontinence is probably around 2% to 3%, and may rise in age with community dwelling individuals to greater than 10%, among nursing home residents the prevalence approaches 50% [19, 20]. Indeed it is one of the most common reasons for nursing home admission. In a survey of residents of Wisconsin nursing homes, risk factors for faecal incontinence, as directly observed by nursing home personnel, were sought [19]. Surprisingly, in this very old population (mean age 84 years), neither age, gender nor diabetes were found to be associated with FI. Positive associations included most prominently the loss of ability to perform the activities of daily living, followed by tube feedings, restraints, diarrhea, dementia, impaired vision, constipation and faecal impaction. Inverse associations were noted with body

Table 3 : Adjusted odds ratios for anal incontinence risk factors [16] (Level 2 evidence)

Risk Factor	Adjusted odds ratio*	95% Confidence interval
AGE @	1.01	1.01 - 1.02
FEMALE GENDER	1.51	1.10 - 2.11
PHYSICAL LIMITATIONS	1.82	1.20 - 2.74
POOR GENERAL HEALTH @	1.64	1.42 - 1.91

** Each factor adjusted for all other factors in the Table*
@ Age and health (using all five strata from excellent to poor) are continuous variables. The others are dichotomous.

weight, heart disease, arthritis and surprisingly, depression. This was a large survey encompassing over 18,000 residents (Table 4).

Pregnancy, though not the exclusive cause of anal incontinence, is certainly a prominent association [5-7]. Factors leading to incontinence both during [21] pregnancy, immediately after [15, 22, 23] and long after pregnancy [24] have been investigated. Irritable bowel syndrome has been an important correlate with post partum anal incontinence [23] (Table 5). Quantitative assessment of risk related to pregnancy, and various methods of delivery, has only recently been feasible in data presented from an Australian survey [15]. It is most interesting to note how similar risk is comparing caesarean section and vaginal delivery. However, these odds ratios are not adjusted for age or parity and it is not known which caesarean sections were done as an emergency versus electively (Table 6).

Several specific diseases have been associated with AI in case series and mechanisms investigated to explain the associations [25]. These include diabetes, multiple sclerosis, Parkinson's disease, spinal cord injury, systemic sclerosis, myotonic dystrophy and amyloidosis (Table 7). Many of these conditions directly affect a patient's mobility, their ability to perform activities of daily living, or cause diarrhoea or faecal impaction. In addition children with congenital anal anomalies, such as imperforate anus, despite anatomic correction of their deformity, often have life long problems with incomplete evacuation and soiling. A similar group are children born without anomalies, but who for a variety of reasons withhold stool at a point beyond which toilet training should be complete and develop faecal soiling and a megarectum (see section 8, below). Failure to retrain the child at an early age often leads to chronic impaction and AI.

Ttable 4 : Associations with faecal incontinence in wisconsin nursing homes. minimum data set reports from 1992 and 1993. Odds ratios and 95% confidence intervals; each variable adjusted for all other variables in the table

ASSOCIATION	1992	1993
Urinary Incontinence	12.6; 11.5-13.7	11.3; 10.3-12.4
Tube Feeding	7.6; 5.6-10.4	8.8; 6.3-12.3
Loss of ADLs	6.0; 4.7-7.7	7.3; 5.5-9.7
Diarrhea	3.3; 2.7-4.2	2.4; 1.9-3.1
Trunk Restraints	3.2; 4.7-7.7	3.0; 2.7-9.8
Pressure Ulcer	2.6; 2.2-3.0	2.3; 2.0-2.6
Dementia	1.5; 1.4-1.7	1.4; 1.3-1.5
Impaired Vision	1.5; 1.4-1.7	1.4; 1.3-1.5
Faecal Impaction	1.5; 1.1-2.1	2.1; 1.3-3.3
Constipation	1.4; 1.3-1.6	1.3; 1.2-1.4
Stroke	1.3; 1.2-1.5	1.2; 1.1-1.3
Male Gender	1.2; 1.1-1.3	1.3; 1.1-1.4
Non-white Race	**NS**	1.3; 1.0-1.7
Age	1.0; 1.0-1.01	1.0; 1.0-1.01
Body Mass Index	1.0; 1.0-1.3	1.0; 1.0-1.04
Diabetes	**NS**	**NS**
Heart Disease	0.9; 0.8-1.0	**NS**
Arthritis	0.9; 0.8-1.0	0.8; 0.7-0.9
Depression	**NS**	0.9; 0.8-1.0

2b evidence
ADLs; Activities of Daily Living
NS; Not statistically significant
Age and Body Mass Index are adjusted as continuous variables.

The importance of diarrhoea or liquid stool in AI cannot be overemphasized. One case series noted that 51% of individuals with chronic diarrhoea were incontinent [4]. In the Wisconsin Family Health Survey of AI, 41% of the 25 subjects with AI disclosed in April and May of 1993 lived in Milwaukee [16]. At this specific time there was a water-borne outbreak of cryptosporidium diarrhea in southern Milwaukee [26], reportedly the largest outbreak of water born disease in U.S. history. This is an important reminder that infectious sources of incontinence should be part of the diagnostic evaluation of AI when diarrhoea is present. Non-infectious causes of diarrhoea must also be considered, including those initiated by leisure activities such as running [27]. Additional aetiologies for anal incontinence that have been described include stroke [28] and hospitalisation for acute illness [29].

The surgeon is often concerned that he might be the originator of a patient's AI. On a population wide basis,

Table 5 : Events related to anal incontinence

Running
Pregnancy (That is, during pregnancy)
Vaginal Childbirth; Obstructed Labor;
Rectovaginal Fistula
Hospitalisation For An Acute Illness
Advancing Age
Tube Feedings
Patient Restraints
Faecal Impaction

Running and Hospitalisation are type 4 evidence risk factors. The others are all type 2.

Table 6 : The association of pregnancy and the method of delivery with incontinence to faeces and flatus. Unadjusted Odds Ratios and 95% Confidence Intervals; (level 2 evidence) [15]

Comparison	Faecal Incontinence	Flatus Incontinence
Vaginal Delivery vs. Nulliparous	2.93; 1.23 – 7.33	2.59; 1.58 – 4.28
Instrumented Delivery vs. Nullip.	2.46; 0.87 – 7.12	3.37; 1.93 – 5.91
Cesarean Section vs. Nulliparous	2.54; 0.61 – 9.88	1.76; 0.73 – 4.16
Vaginal Delivery vs. C Section	1.16; 0.38 – 3.94	1.47; 0.69 – 3.23

Table 7 : Diseases associated with anal incontinence (Level 4 Evidence)

Diabetes
Stroke
Multiple sclerosis
Parkinson's disease
Systemic sclerosis
Mytonic dystrophy
Amyloidosis
Spinal cord injury
Imperforate anus
Hirschsprung's disease
Retarded or interrupted toilet training
Procidentia
Any illness causing diarrhea (HIV, Inflammatory Bowel Disease, radiation, infection)
Irritable bowel syndrome

this would seem a fairly insignificant factor, since prior anal surgery has not been an apparent risk factor in the larger surveys. Yet much of a colorectal surgeon's training is directed towards avoidance of this disabling complication. Nevertheless, several operations performed frequently can result in AI (Table 8). The first of these is lateral internal sphincterotomy for fissure in ano. The risk of this procedure causing AI was thought to be insignificant when compared to midline sphincterotomy (which is the operation done most frequently for fistula in ano). A recent reappraisal of the outcome of this operation has shown an AI risk as high as 8% [30]. Similarly fistulotomy was thought to have a negligible risk of AI when compared to fistulectomy. However the risk of AI after fistulotomy has been reported to be as high as 18-52% [31]. New approaches to fissure and fistula have been recently developed specifically to lower this risk [31, 32]. Ileo-anal pouch reconstruction has enabled individuals afflicted with inflammatory bowel disease to live without a stoma, but at high risk of AI. A more proximal anal anastomosis is now commonly done in hopes of diminishing this risk. There is controversy as to whether a pouch should also be made for patients having an ileorectal anastomosis. Low anterior rectal resection has also made it possible for patients with mid-rectal cancer to avoid a permanent stoma, but the functional results, even in the absence of prior radiation, may be poor and new procedures have also been described to deal with this [33]. Lastly, mixing urine and stool has been found to have an adverse effect on anal sphincter control in patients having ureterosigmoidstomy after urinary bladder resection [34].

The development of incontinence in previously continent nursing home residents has also been studied. Significant associations have been found, as would be expected, with dementia, stroke and blindness. However the most prominent association is with the use of patient restraints, even when adjustment has been made for factors that might be associated with restraint, such as immobility and dementia (Table 9) (Nelson; submitted).

III. SUMMARY

Anal and urinary incontinence commonly co-exist, particularly in the elderly [2].

The prevalence of anal incontinence increases with age, but is present in all age groups and both genders varying from 1.5% in children to over 50% in nursing home residents [2].

Though pregnancy is a common association with anal incontinence, in younger and older populations, AI is more common in men [2].

As populations age, comorbid disease becomes a significant component of anal incontinence risk [2].

Table 8 : Operations associated with risk of anal incontinence . Level 4 Evidence

Midline internal sphincterotomy
Lateral internal sphincterotomy
Fistulectomy
Fistulotomy
Ileo-anal reservoir reconstruction
Low anterior rectal resection
Total abdominal colectomy
Ureterosigmoidostomy

IV. RECOMMENDATIONS

Epidemiologic investigations of AI and urinary incontinence should be performed jointly. (D)

The use of truncal restraints in nursing homes should be re-assessed. (D)

Table 9 : Adjusted Odds Ratios and 95% Confidence Limits Associated With Risk Factors for the Development of Incontinence of Urine, Faeces, and Both Urine and Faeces from 1992 to 1993 in Wisconsin Nursing Home Residents (Level 2 Evidence)*

	URINE **Incontinent of bladder=940, Not incontinent of bladder=3054,**	**FAECES** **Incontinent of bowel=609, Not incontinent of bowel=3386**	**BOTH** **Incontinent of both=470, Not incontinent of both =3535**
Trunk restraints	2.4 (1.7-3.3)	2.8 (2.0-4.0)	2.4 (1.7-3.6)
Dementia	1.5 (1.3-1.8)	1.6 (1.3-1.9	1.7 (1.4-2.1)
Impaired vision	NS	NS	NS
Stroke	1.2 (1.0-1.5)	NS	NS
Constipation	NS	NS	NS
Heart disease	NS	NS	NS
Arthritis	0.8 (0.7-1.0)	0.8 (0.6-1.0)	0.7 (0.6-0.9)
Diabetes	NS	NS	NS
Faecal impaction	NS	NS	NS
Race (NW = 1, W = 0)	NS	2.1 (1.3-3.5)	1.8 (1.0-3.0)
Age	1.03 (1.02-1.04)	1.02 (1.01-1.03)	1.02 (1.01-1.04)
Body mass index	NS	0.98 (0.97-1.0)	0.98 (0.96-1.00)
Depression	NS	NS	NS
Diarrhea	NS	NS	NS
Male gender	0.8 (0.6-0.9)	NS	NS
Pressure ulcer	NS	NS	NS
Tube feeding	NS	NS	NS

**Adjusted odds ratios were derived from multivariable logistic regression models with all risk factors included.*

C. BOWEL SYMPTOM QUESTIONNAIRES, INCONTINENCE GRADING AND SCORING AND QUALITY OF LIFE STUDIES

In order to better understand anal incontinence as a medical entity, reliable and validated questionnaires and instruments are essential. Although it is considered fundamental by experts in the field of outcomes research that a self administered questionnaire or other instrument must be psychometrically tested for validity and reliability to have scientific merit or value, this is often overlooked in the published literature. Not uncommonly, bowel symptom questionnaires, anal incontinence grading systems and quality of life scoring have relied on individual clinician's opinions and their subjective collection of only certain data elements that they felt salient. Uncontrolled studies using non-validated instruments to assess populations, measure outcomes and draw conclusions often prevent objective, scientific comparisons within and between many of the studies in the literature.

I. BOWEL SYMPTOM QUESTIONNAIRES

Due to inherent problems in investigating certain aspects of anal incontinence due to the attached social stigma [4], detailed, objective and pointed questioning is often necessary to delineate symptoms in patients with this condition.

There is a large amount of information that may be obtained and recorded on a suitably constructed bowel symptom questionnaire depending on the particular goals of the researcher in anal incontinence (Table 10). Accordingly, the material covered in the questionnaire may vary with the goal of developing the instrument. The goal of a self-report bowel symptom questionnaire may be multiple including:

1. measuring outcomes including quality of life from medical and surgical interventions
2. assessing individual symptoms and grading the severity of the problem
3. screening for the condition to determine a prevalence or incidence of the condition
4. providing a forum or template from which to begin physician-patient interactions
5. providing an organised basis for recording symptoms in order to better understand the underlying pathophysiology, facilitate diagnosis or improve the management of the condition
6. helping to identify patterns of disease or identifying risk factors.

Bowel symptom questionnaires, although not widely utilised clinically, have been developed and validated for a number of conditions including irritable bowel syndrome [36-39], and Crohn's disease [40-42]. These

Table 10 : Potential data recorded on a bowel symptom questionnaire*

Chief complaint	
Bowel pattern	
	Sensation of the urge to defaecate, number of movements per day, consistency: loose, soft, hard, hard pellets, faecal urgency or ability to defer defaecation , evacuation pattern: straining, anal or vaginal digitation
Continence of flatus	
Presence of passive soiling	
Pain, tenesmus, etc.	
Presence of blood or mucus	
Sensations of incomplete emptying, or prolapse	
Quantification of pad or incontinence pant use	
Fluid intake	
Toileting access	
Past medical/surgical/obstetric history, co-morbid conditions	
Medications	
Associated risk factors such as diet, smoking, and body weight	
Associated symptoms of bladder control	
Skin problems due to local irritation	
Quality of life assessment	

**Adapted from: Norton & Chelvanayagam [35].*

questionnaires were developed as general instruments for gastrointestinal disorders, and not specifically for investigating anal incontinence.

Very few anal incontinence specific self-administration questionnaires have been developed and validated. A 38-item questionnaire was tested in a small series of normal controls, patients with anal incontinence and patients with constipation [43]. This instrument performed well in the original patient population but has not been widely adapted or validated by others in the field.

Based on prior work assessing general gastrointestinal symptoms, another anal incontinence specific self-administered questionnaire, the Faecal Incontinence Questionnaire (FIQ), has been developed and validated. This instrument was designed to measure the prevalence of anal incontinence in the community and assess risk factors associated with the condition. When compared to the AUA Symptom Score, it performed favourably [44]. This instrument has subsequently been used to measure the prevalence of anal incontinence in selected populations including those with combined urinary and anal incontinence [45, 46]. Whether this instrument will be widely adopted for clinical and research purposes is unclear.

1. Summary

Objective and complete symptom assessment of anal incontinence is essential.

The information contained on a bowel symptom questionnaire may vary with the goal of the questionnaire both clinically and as a research tool.

At present, there are no widely utilised, validated anal incontinence specific bowel symptom questionnaires.

The FIQ, although lengthy may be a useful instrument in the initial assessment of the patient with AI.

2. Recommendations

- Future work should determine whether the Faecal Incontinence Questionnaire or other subsequently developed bowel symptom questionnaires are applicable, reliable and appropriately validated across all age groups, all languages, as well as all conditions including benign, malignant, acquired and congenital conditions resulting in anal incontinence.

II. ANAL INCONTINENCE GRADING AND SCORING

An anal incontinence scoring system is useful, not only for epidemiological purposes, but also in order to objectively grade the severity of anal incontinence as well as provide a basis for the comparison of outcomes of both surgical and non-surgical therapies for the condition. A universally agreed upon standard scoring/grading system does not exist.

The ideal scoring system should be reproducible, simple to use and include parameters such as frequency, quantity, and type of incontinence (solid, liquid or gas), descriptions of the circumstances under which anal incontinence occurs (e.g.: passive/active, awareness of urgency, etc.), quantify the use of adjunctive measures such as pads or plugs in an effort to control or manage the condition, as well as assess the effects of anal incontinence on quality of life (occupational, social, etc.). To some degree, classification of incontinence is linked to grading and scoring systems as authors have often devised their own systems in an effort to describe baseline patient symptomatology before and after interventions. These classification/grading/scoring systems are numerous and diverse. Many are not validated and have been used only by the author who devised the system. Therefore reproducibility across and between surgeons, patients, procedures and treatments remains unknown.

Many of the grading/scoring systems recorded in the current literature suffer from a variety of shortcomings including: a lack of objectivity, being primarily descriptive in nature [47, 48] mixing subjective and objective parameters [49], using objective parameters such as anal manometry [50, 51] or difficult to classify subjective parameters [52] which often do not correlate with clinical conditions, or do not account for frequency of the incontinent episodes in individual patients [53-56].

Several anal incontinence grading or scoring systems have been prospectively developed and tested. The Faecal Incontinence Severity Index (FISI) was developed and evaluated as a questionnaire for assessing the severity of anal incontinence [57]. Using a 20 cell matrix table, the researchers constructed the FISI by looking at both type (gas, mucus, liquid and solid) and frequency (5 categories) of incontinence episodes. This generated a graded numerical result. The FISI was administered to both physicians and patients for weighting and scoring, with surgeons and patients responses of severity correlating very well.

Perhaps one of the most widely used scales or grading systems is the Wexner score [59]. This was the first system to account for the use of pads, changes or alterations to lifestyle, consistency and frequency of incontinence. The Wexner Score is derived from numerical values assigned to the frequency of occurrence (scored 0-4) in each of several categories including type of incontinence (solid, liquid, gas), pad use, and lifestyle alteration. A minimum score of 0 indicates perfect continence, and a maximum score of 20 indicates complete incontinence (Table 11).

Table 11 : The Wexner score [59]

Type of incontinence	Never	Rarely	Frequency Some-times	Usually	Always
Solid	0	1	2	3	4
Liquid	0	1	2	3	4
Gas	0	1	2	3	4
Wears Pad	0	1	2	3	4
Lifestyle Alteration	0	1	2	3	4

Never: 0 Rarely: <1month
Sometimes: <1/week, ≥1/month Usually: <1/day, ≥1/week
Always: ≥1/day 0= perfect continence
20=complete incontinence

A modified version of the Wexner score was compared with the original version, a 28 day diary and several other scoring systems in 23 patients and then the results were correlated with an independent clinical assessment by two clinicians [60]. Ten patients were assessed before and after surgery.

The newly devised scale showed the best correlation although all the scales performed well. The modified scale included details regarding urgency, and the use of anti-diarrhoeal medications. Categories scored 0-4 (0=never, to 4=daily) included type of incontinence (solid, liquid, gas), and alteration in lifestyle. Scored separately were the need to wear a pad or plug (0=no, 2=yes), taking anti-diarrhoeal medications (0=no, 2=yes) and lack of ability to defer defecation (0=no, 4=yes). The maximum score in the modified Wexner scale was 24 implying complete incontinence.

1. Summary

Many of the existing grading/scoring scales are empirically derived, and are not prospectively validated.

There are no widely utilised, validated grading/scoring systems for AI.

2. Recommendations

- Faecal incontinence grading and scoring are an important part of the initial assessment of patients with AI. (D)
- Future work should be directed towards development, validation and widespread dissemination of a standardised faecal incontinence grading/scoring system.
- Interventional studies for anal incontinence should utilise a validated grading/scoring system at baseline and following intervention. (D)

III. QUALITY OF LIFE

Quality of Life (QOL) instruments are designed to measure the subjective perception of a given patient's health state including the emotional and social impact of a medical condition. When applied appropriately, this is a reliable outcome measure that can be objectively and scientifically quantified. The optimal methodology by which QOL is measured has been constantly evolving and is not yet ideal [61, 62]. Although the severity of a given condition may correlate with quality of life in some patients, QOL instruments measure different aspects of the health/disease continuum and should not be considered an indicator of disease severity. Both generic and disease-specific QOL instruments have been developed.

Several authors have utilised well-validated generic QOL instruments such as the SF-36 or MOS-36 [63, 64] to study anal incontinence in certain populations [65-67]. Numerous studies in the colorectal and anal incontinence literature have utilised some form of a QOL scale as an outcome measure, but these are for the most part unvalidated instruments. Disease specific QOL instruments have been developed for several gastrointestinal conditions including inflammatory bowel disease [68, 69] and are generally felt to have good reliability and validity [62]. However, with one exception, good quality disease specific QOL instruments for anal incontinence do not yet exist. The Faecal Incontinence Quality of Life Scale (FIQLS) is, however, a QOL instrument developed, tested and psychometrically evaluated for the assessment of patients with anal incontinence [70]. This instrument is a self-administered questionnaire containing 29 items covering 4 scales: Lifestyle, Coping/Behaviour, Depression/Self-perception and Embarrassment. Each of the 29 items are scored 1-5 and a mean score is obtained within each of the 4 scales. Due to unresolved issues regarding potential differential weighting of the 4 scales, it is unclear whether an overall score can be obtained by simply summing the 4 mean scores. In a study of 190 patients, the FIQLS discriminated well between those with anal incontinence and those with other gastrointestinal conditions and also correlated well with the MOS-36 [70]. As the process of validation continues, refinement of the weighting between the four scales are necessary to arrive at an overall score, as is further testing of this instrument in an interventional setting and in different countries, languages and cultures [71].

1. Summary

Patients with AI have a diminished QOL as measured by general QOL instruments [4].

The FIQLS may be a promising disease specific QOL instrument to study those with anal incontinence [4].

2. RECOMMENDATIONS

- A validated, disease specific QOL instrument is essential in the study of anal incontinence. (D)
- General and disease specific QOL instruments should be an integral part of the initial assessment of patients with AI and should be a standardised outcome measure when evaluating interventions. (D)
- Future work should be directed towards development, validation and widespread dissemination of a standardised disease specific QOL instrument. (D)

D. PATHOPHYSIOLOGY AND INVESTIGATION OF FAECAL INCONTINENCE IN ADULTS

I. INTRODUCTION

Normal defecation and faecal continence are the result of a complex interplay among a number of factors. Colonic transit, consistency and volume of stool, rectal compliance and capacity, anal sphincter function and anorectal sensation, and reflexes all play an important role. Faecal incontinence may be the result of abnormalities in any one or more of these functions. Progressive diminution loss of anal sphincter function occurs [72]. Eventually, there may be incontinence to solid stool. The purpose of this section is to describe the investigation of faecal incontinence with particular reference to the value of physiologic tests.

II. FAECAL CONTINENCE

Faecal continence is achieved by a combination of a competent, closed anal sphincter; normal anorectal sensation and sampling reflex; adequate rectal capacity and compliance; and conscious control. Continence is maintained as long as anal canal pressure is greater than rectal pressure [73]. The rectum is supported by the pelvic floor muscles, and the anal sphincter is augmented by the acute rectoanal angle maintained by the sling effect of the puborectal muscle. Reflexes quickly increase muscular activity in response to changes in intra-abdominal pressure to augment mechanical barriers to the aboral movement of rectal content.

Maintenance of faecal continence at times when the anal sphincter is under maximal strain, such as when the rectum is filled with liquid, is associated with marked electrical activity in the anal sphincter complex and puborectal muscle. Pressures measured within the rectal lumen are consistently lower than those recorded in the anal canal as long as continence is preserved. Support for this hypothesis comes from patients in whom a successful postanal repair has been carried out. This operation was originally described for faecal incontinence in the belief that correction of an obtuse anorectal angle would restore faecal continence. A successful operation is associated not with correction of the angle, which often remains unchanged, but rather with a rise in anal sphincter resting and squeeze pressures [74].

The significance of the external anal sphincter in maintaining continence is illustrated by the finding of faecal seepage or soiling in 50% of patients who have a simple defect in the muscle after obstetric tears [75].

The flap valve theory of faecal continence suggests that when intra-abdominal pressure is applied to the rectum, the anterior rectal wall is pressed down onto the upper anal canal and thereby prevents rectal content from gaining contact with the upper anal canal [76]. The anterior rectal wall acts as a plug. In support of this theory is the regular association of an obtuse anorectal angle, and presumably the inability of the anterior rectal wall to close off the upper anal canal, with faecal incontinence. In studies in which the anal sphincter was maximally stressed and the rectum visualised radiographically, however, no contact between rectal wall and anal canal was seen [77]. It is likely that the flap valve effect is effective only when the rectum is less distended. The relevance of the puborectal muscle to continence is illustrated by the high degree of continence in children with congenital absence of internal and external anal sphincters [78] and by the high incidence of incontinence in patients with constipation in whom division of the puborectal muscle has been carried out to relieve outlet obstruction [79].

The flutter valve theory suggests that intra-abdominal pressure applied to a high pressure zone within the lower rectum leads to the occlusion of this area and thereby prevents any rectal content from reaching the anal canal [80]. According to this theory, the anal sphincter serves to provide fine control. The idea is analogous to that observed about the lower oesophageal sphincter, in which a flutter valve mechanism has been proposed to explain control of gastroesophageal reflux. Manometric studies clearly demonstrate, however, that the high pressure zone lies in the mid-anal canal and that no such higher pressure zone is demonstrable in the lower rectum either in static studies or in ambulatory subjects [81].

1. Role of rectal compliance in maintaining faecal continence

The anorectum acts as a functional unit. The first sensation volume of rectal filling varies from 11 to 68 mL in published studies, whereas the mean maximum tolerated volume ranges from 220 to 510 mL [82]. Mean rectal compliance also shows a wide range (4 to 14 mL/cm H_2O). The compliance, and hence the capacitance, of the rectum is integral to this function. Reflex adaptation of the rectum in response to filling occurs in a manner analogous to that of the bladder. The rectum tolerates volumes up to about 300 mL without showing any marked change in intraluminal pressure. Beyond this, pressure waves become more pronounced until tolerance is approached and the feeling of urgency to defaecate develops [83]. Rectal compliance is reduced in patients in the presence of diseases such as Crohn's disease or radiation proctitis. Low compliance leads to increased frequency of bowel actions, urgency of defecation, and often faecal incontinence despite a normal pressure profile of the anal sphincter. In such cases, removal of the diseased rectum and replacement with a compliant neorectum, either an ileal pouch or healthy colon may restore continence [84, 85].

Contractility of the rectal wall increases in response to a meal [86]. The rectum is usually empty [87]. The main reservoir for faeces is located more proximally, and the transverse colon appears to be the principal region for storage and mixing of enteric contents [88, 89]. Solids and liquids are stored equally in the transverse colon [88]. Transit of ^{111}indium pellets through unprepared colon shows that although the ascending and transverse colon are sites of storage of solid residue, the descending and rectosigmoid act mainly as conduits [90]. If stool is emptied into the rectum from the sigmoid colon when the tone of the rectum is increased, a more marked increase in intraluminal rectal pressure occurs. This leads to a prompt urge to defecate. In constipated patients, rectal contractility is blunted such that the sensation of rectal filling appears to be less pronounced, and the usual prompt desire to defecate is not appreciated [91].

III. MECHANISM OF DEFAECATION

Events leading to defecation start when the volume of content in the sigmoid colon becomes large enough to initiate contractions, which empty the stool into the rectum. Conscious awareness of a full rectum is brought about by receptors in the rectal wall, pelvic floor, and upper anal canal by way of the rectoanal inhibitory reflex. Rectal filling is recognised at a volume of about 50mL. If the rectum continues to fill, a temporary sensation of an urge to defecate is elicited, followed by a constant urge and eventually pelvic discomfort—the maximal tolerable volume. The puborectal muscle is stretched by rectal pressure waves, and the amplitude of these waves increases [92] as the rectum distends. The urge to defecate is probably mediated by stretch receptors in the pelvic floor because tugging a small balloon against the puborectal muscle produces this feeling [93]. The precise influences of the rate of rectal filling and the nature of its content on conscious awareness are unknown. Distension of the rectum leads to relaxation of the internal anal sphincter and sampling of the contents. The external sphincter contracts. If it is socially convenient, the pressure within the rectum must be made to exceed that of the anal canal. This is largely achieved by increasing the intra-abdominal pressure by contraction of the diaphragm, abdominal muscles, and performance of the Valsalva manoeuvre.

Relaxation of the puborectal muscle allows the anorectal angle to become less acute, increasing from a mean of 92 degrees to a mean of 111 to 137 degrees [94], and this is helped if the individual adopts the squatting position, which increases the anorectal angle more than that achieved by flexion of the hips to 90 degrees [95]. Inhibition of pelvic floor activity allows descent of the pelvic floor by about 2 cm, which further straightens out this angle [96]. As the rectum evacuates, there is prolonged inhibition of the internal anal sphincter and external anal sphincter, and anal pressure falls. Whether physiologically important contractions of the rectal wall occur during defecation is unknown. Conversely, if it is not socially convenient, brief conscious contraction of the external sphincter allows the internal sphincter to recover and the rectal contents are propelled in an oral direction by forceful contraction of the puborectal muscle and the rest of the pelvic floor musculature. Internal anal sphincter tone then returns to normal and the urge to defaecate becomes less imperative.

Defaecation is influenced by the size and consistency of the stool. The time to expel a single solid sphere is inversely proportional to its diameter [97]. More effort is required to evacuate small, hard stools, and the ideal stool diameter is about 2 cm.

Straining at defaecation is associated with the co-contraction of laryngeal, respiratory, and abdominal muscles and the inhibition of anal sphincter muscles, and this patterned recruitment is closely linked to the extrapyramidal system. Paradoxical contraction of the puborectal muscle and the external anal sphincter during defecation is seen in patients with Parkinson's disease [98]. Higher control is needed for appropriate defaecatory responses as illustrated by patients with damage to the frontal lobes [99]. Defaecation occurs without any warning in these patients.

IV. CAUSES OF FAECAL INCONTINENCE

The cause of major incontinence, the total loss of control of solid stool, is poorly understood. Progressive loss of anal sphincter function occurs with no definite time of onset of symptoms. Initially, loss of control of flatus occurs followed by seepage of faecal material onto undergarments and then incontinence to solid stool. Finally, the call to stool is also lost.

Two types of history are typical in colorectal practice. Patients may have a history of prolonged or difficult childbirth with vaginal delivery, with occult sphincter damage [100] or there may be a history of several years' duration of forceful straining at defecation. Incontinence may be passive, in which there is leakage of faeces without the patient being aware, or motor, in which the patient is aware of an urge to defaecate but is unable to prevent the passage of faeces.

1. Dysfunction of the internal anal sphincter

Resting anal pressure is usually reduced in patients with faecal incontinence, often to a level similar to that recorded in the rectal lumen. Electrical activity in the internal sphincter as measured by electromyography (EMG) is reduced. Marked descent of the pelvic floor may be apparent, and this laxity may cause disruption of the sympathetic innervation. This denervation is evidenced by atrophy, fibrosis, and increased fibre density. Ultrastructural changes include disruption and loss of smooth muscle cells, increased deposition of collagen, and stretching of elastic tissue [101]. The internal sphincter may relax inappropriately in response to relatively low amounts of rectal distension. Continence then depends on external sphincter activity [102].

Internal sphincter relaxation in response to rectal distension occurs more frequently, is more pronounced, and lasts longer in incontinent patients compared with controls [103]. A subgroup of patients may show not only anal relaxation, but also failure of external sphincter contraction at the time of rectal distention [104]. Endoanal ultrasound has demonstrated that thinning of the internal anal sphincter occurs in patients with idiopathic faecal incontinence, and this correlates with reduced resting anal sphincter pressure [105]. Furthermore, the adrenergic response of the internal sphincter may be impaired [106]. The clinical significance of isolated internal sphincter dysfunction is unknown.

2. Dysfunction of the external anal sphincter and puborectal muscle

Persistent repeated traction on the pudendal nerve leads to denervation and weakness of the external anal sphincter. There is loss of myelinated and demyelinated nerves and fibrous replacement [107]. Chronic partial denervation of the striated nerves of the pelvic floor is also associated with prolonged vaginal delivery often associated with delivery of a large infant or use of forceps. This situation may result in prolonged stretch being applied to the pudendal nerve or traumatic injury to the sacral nerves by the foetal head. EMG studies before and after breech or forceps deliveries have shown increased fibre density in the external anal sphincter and prolonged pudendal nerve latency times [108]. Interestingly, while vaginal deliveries may result in cumulative injury, women who have undergone caesarean section also show evidence of denervation of the pelvic floor [109]. Partial denervation injury may occur with repeated straining, with denervation secondary to abnormal perineal descent. The pudendal nerve is stretched from its point of fixity in Alcock's canal. Anal sensation is also impaired in this group of patients [110].

3. Impaired rectal sensation and compliance

Repeated deferral or ignoring the call to stool may lead to faecal impaction. This is a common cause of overflow incontinence in elderly people. Impaired anorectal sensation may be associated with an abnormal response of the external anal sphincter to rectal distension and hence incontinence. Recruitment of external anal muscle activity is reduced [111].

The rectum, if damaged by radiation or Crohn's disease, becomes less complaint any may develop increased rectal pressures. Accommodation of stool is therefore reduced, and patients may complain of symptoms of urgency of defaecation and faecal incontinence.

V. INVESTIGATIONS

1. History and clinical examination

A careful, thorough history and full physical examination are essential and will identify the majority of causes of faecal incontinence. There may be a history of prolonged or difficult childbirth. A long history of forceful straining at defecation suggests denervation of the pelvic floor. Incontinence may be sensory in which there is leakage of faeces without the patient being aware or motor with patients being aware but unable to prevent the passage of faeces, or a mixture of both. True faecal incontinence must be differentiated from conditions that cause seepage such as grade 3 or 4 haemorrhoids, fistulas, low rectal or anal tumours, and poor perineal hygiene. Diagnostic administration of an enema may be useful in this respect; retention of the enema suggests that the patient does not have clinically significant faecal incontinence [112].

Severity of faecal incontinence can be classified as a minor if faecal seepage occurs less than once a month, moderate if there is incontinence to solids more than once a month or liquids more than once a week, and severe if there is loss of control of solids several times a week or liquids on a daily basis. An alternative classification grades continence as follows [113]:

Grade 1: Complete

Grade 2: Incontinence of flatus

Grade 3: Incontinence of flatus and liquid stools

Grade 4: Incontinence of flatus, liquid stools, and solid stools.

Physical examination should include inspection of underclothing for soiling and staining by stool, pus, or mucus. Perianal skin should be examined for irritation, fistulous tracks, and hygiene. Scars from previous episiotomies or obstetric tears should be noted. Abnormalities at the anal verge from previous surgery or a gaping anus suggestive of marked loss of function may be present. Digital rectal examination includes assessment of the tone of the anal sphincter (at rest and squeezing) and identification of faecal impaction or a rectal mass. Function of the puborectalis muscle (palpable at the anorectal junction) is assessed by asking the patient to squeeze the sphincter at which time the puborectalis should push the examiner's finger anteriorly. Anoscopy and rigid proctoscopy should be performed to exclude anorectal pathology. Procto-sigmoidoscopy and/or colonoscopy should be performed to exclude anorectal pathology such inflammatory bowel disease, neoplasm or radiation changes. Patients with complete rectal prolapse (Procidentia) often complain of faecal incontinence – examination of the patient while straining on the toilet facilitates determining the severity of the prolapse.

Physiologic and complimentary radiologic tests are used to confirm clinical suspicions and provide objective data on the function of the anorectum. Pelvic floor dysfunction is a complex problem and multiple tests may be needed [114]. An algorithm for the investigation of faecal incontinence is shown in Figure 1.

2. Anorectal manometry

Anal manometry provides a sphincter pressure profile and measures resting and maximum squeeze pressures, length of the anal canal and demonstrates the presence or absence of the anorectal inhibitory reflex [115]. The resting anal pressure reflects the functional status of the internal anal sphincter, the squeeze pressure reflects the functional status of the external sphincter and the anorectal inhibitory reflex demonstrates coordination between rectum and anal canal. The length of the anal canal can be the only detectable change in anorectal function tests after successful postanal repair or overlapping sphincteroplasty.

The data generated can be used to create a three-dimensional pressure map of the anal canal both at rest and during contraction. Several different catheters have been used, such as air- or water-filled microballoons, water-perfused catheters, sleeve catheters, or solid-state microtransducers. With water-perfused catheters, ports are arranged circumferentially around the catheter tip and generate a 360° pressure image along the length of the anal canal. Recorded pressures vary with type and size of probe used. A station pull-through technique is most commonly used, with resting and squeeze pressures being recorded at 0.5-cm intervals along the lower 6 cm of the anorectum. Directional manometry describes a pressure vector that can identify the site of a sphincter defect. Simple digital examination by an experienced clinician gives a very good estimation of anal sphincter pressures [116].

Unfortunately, there can be considerable overlap between the pressure profiles of normal and incontinent patients; patients with normal resting pressures but reduced squeeze pressures may be incontinent because of failure of the external anal sphincter to contribute to continence at critical times. A significant number of continent patients have impaired pressure profiles and some incontinent patients generate normal pressure profiles. Manometric studies of the anal canal do not always predict the patient's clinical status.

3. Anorectal sensation

To measure rectal sensation, a balloon is attached to the manometry catheter. The balloon is placed in the rectum and slowly inflated. The patient announces when the sensation of a faecal mass within the rectum is first noticed and filling of the balloon continues to the point at which the patient would wish to defecate. Both blunted and hyperacute rectal sensation can be detected from this test.

Sensation of the anal canal can be measured by means of small electrical probe inserted into the anal canal and connected to a constant current stimulator [110]. The amplitude of current is gradually increased until the patient experiences a tapping or pricking sensation. This threshold to electrostimulation is increased in patients with incontinence but the test is quite specialised and may be of limited value in clinical practice.

4. Electromyography of the pelvic floor and pudendal nerve latency

Electromyography (EMG) of the anal sphincter demonstrates electromuscular activity of the puborectalis and will identify re-innervation of the sphincter typi-

Figure 1 : Algorithm for assessment of adults

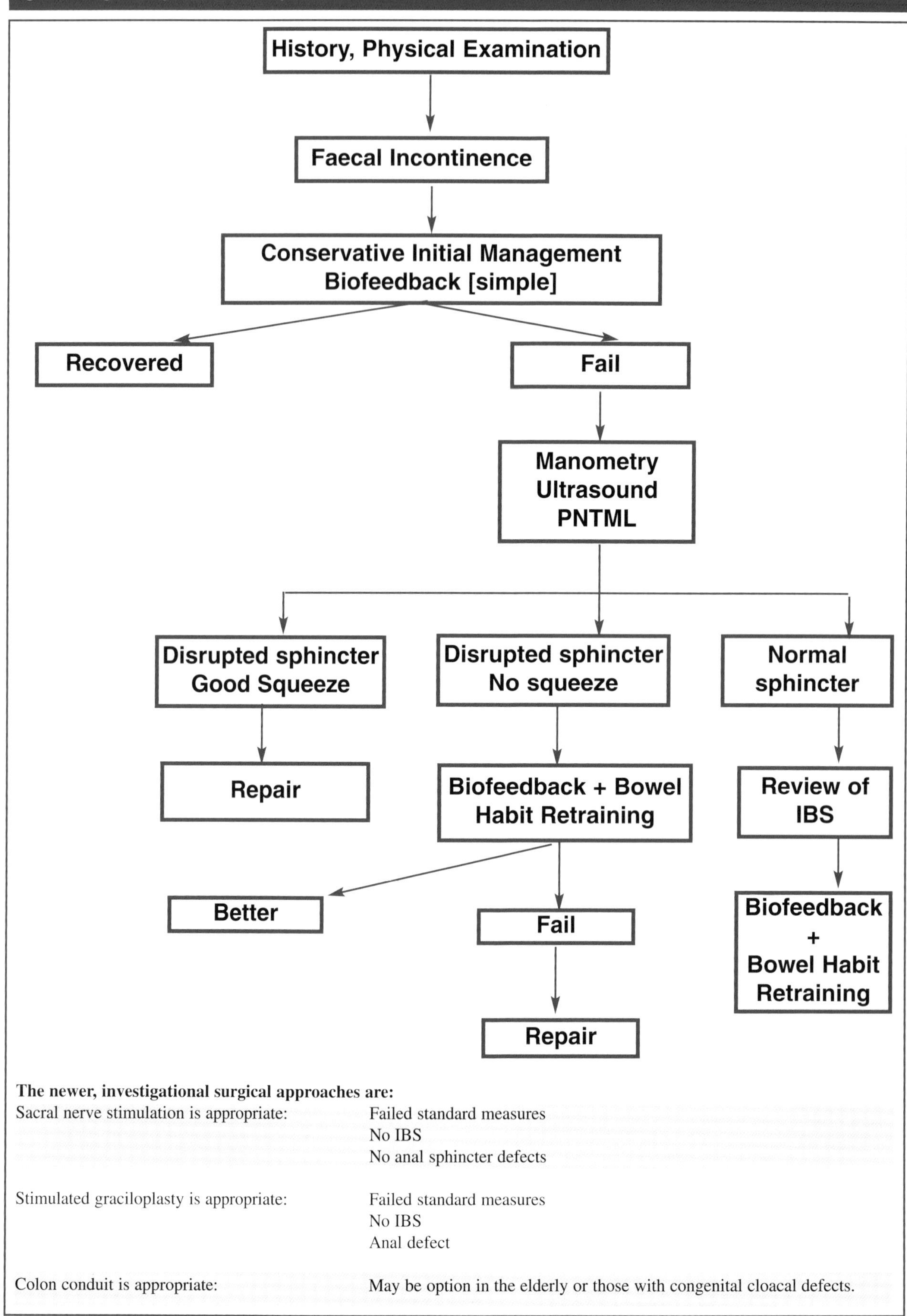
History, Physical Examination
Faecal Incontinence
Conservative Initial Management
Biofeedback [simple]
Recovered
Fail
Manometry
Ultrasound
PNTML
Disrupted sphincter
Good Squeeze
Disrupted sphincter
No squeeze
Normal
sphincter
Repair
Biofeedback + Bowel
Habit Retraining
Review of
IBS
Better
Fail
Biofeedback
+
Bowel Habit
Retraining
Repair
The newer, investigational surgical approaches are:
Sacral nerve stimulation is appropriate:
Failed standard measures
No IBS
No anal sphincter defects
Stimulated graciloplasty is appropriate:
Failed standard measures
No IBS
Anal defect
Colon conduit is appropriate:
May be option in the elderly or those with congenital cloacal defects.

cal of pelvic neuropathy. The test can be carried out with single-fibre or concentric needle techniques. Single-fibre electrodes detect potentials that originate from a single motor unit. Fibre density may be determined from the mean number of spikes recorded from the uptake area of a single-fibre EMG electrode sited in 20 different positions [117]. Increased fibre density, suggested by increased number of spike potentials detected by the single-fibre EMG electrode, implies denervation followed by re-innervation as axons sprout from intact neurons to re-innervate muscle fibres. Incontinent patients usually show smaller and prolonged motor unit potentials.

A needle electrode is inserted into either the puborectalis or, more commonly, the external anal sphincter to carry out concentric needle EMG. Electromyography is an uncomfortable investigation that is unpopular with patients and objective interpretation of concentric EMG can be very difficult. An alternative, less painful technique is to use a sponge EMG electrode, which is inserted into the anal canal. Two electrodes, placed 180 degrees apart, record electrical activity of the puborectalis at rest, squeezing, and pushing (which simulates defecation). Normally, the puborectalis generates the greatest signal during contraction and normal defaecation requires relaxation of the puborectalis to permit straightening of the anorectal angle. Incontinent patients may show diminished activity in all phases of activity. It should be noted that EMG of the EAS and pelvic floor is not performed for diagnostic purposes at this time.

Pudendal nerve terminal motor latencies are measured by placing a glove-mounted, stimulating electrode that is inserted through the anal canal onto the nerve as it crosses the ischial spine. A recording electrode, adjacent to the external sphincter, detects the evoked potential associated with muscle contraction [118]. The process is carried out for each pudendal nerve. The normal delay between stimulating and recording is 2.0 +/-0.5 (SD) ms). Increased delay suggests damage to the pudendal nerves.

Although no medical or surgical treatment has been shown to be effective for pudendal nerve damage at present, it is an important diagnosis to make. First, surgical intervention (such as overlapping sphincteroplasty) is usually less successful [119]. Second, if the surgeon is persuaded to attempt a procedure (such as postanal repair), then the surgeon can prepare the patient for the likelihood of failure. Third, some surgeons would argue that some form of neosphincter might be appropriate for this subgroup of incontinent patients.

5. Defaecating proctogram

Defaecography is a dynamic study of rectal emptying and the complex process of defaecation. The patient is positioned sitting upright upon a radiolucent commode and barium paste is instilled into the rectum and distal sigmoid. Lateral fluoroscopic images are taken as the patient squeezes the sphincter, while deferring defaecation, and while straining to defaecate. A number of interactive processes can be seen and assessed. A defaecating proctogram assesses the function of the puborectalis, efficiency of emptying length of the anal sphincter, movement of anorectal angle, and perineal descent [120]. Defaecating proctograms are, however, difficult to interpret as 50% of normal subjects will show some abnormality [121]. Occult or overt rectal intussusception may be seen, as well as the presence or absence of a rectocele, sigmoidocele, or enterocele. It should be noted that although a careful history and physical examination may lead to a diagnosis of a rectocele, its role in incontinence may be unclear until clarified by defaecography.

6. Ultrasound

Endoanal ultrasound has only recently been used for the investigation of patients with faecal incontinence. The morphology of the internal anal sphincter, part of the external anal sphincter, the puborectalis, and the rectovaginal septum can be seen remarkably well [122] (Figure 2). It is particularly useful if there is a history suggestive of a sphincter defect. Defects, evident as a break in the ring of the sphincter deep to the submucosa, may be identified and mapped. Endoanal ultrasound has shown that up to 85% of patients with incontinence of traumatic origin have external sphincter defects and 40% of these patients also have disruption of the inter-

Table 12 : Tests of anorectal function for the patient with faecal incontinence

A. Initial Evaluation	1. History of symptoms to include psychosocial history 2. Physical exam to include visual and digital exam (including examination while straining on the toilet)	
B. Prior to Surgical Intervention	1. Anorectal manometry to include compliance (P/V relationship) 2. Ultrasound of the anal canal 3. Visualise the colon (proctosigmoidoscopy, colonoscopy) 4. Abdominal X-ray	
C. Optional	1. Pudendal nerve terminal motor latency 2. Electromyography	
D. Research	1. Barostat 2. MRI 3. Vector manometry	
E. Levels of Evidence for:		
Anorectal Manometry	2—for accuracy	3—for outcomes
Ultrasound	2—for accuracy	3—for outcomes
PNTML	3	

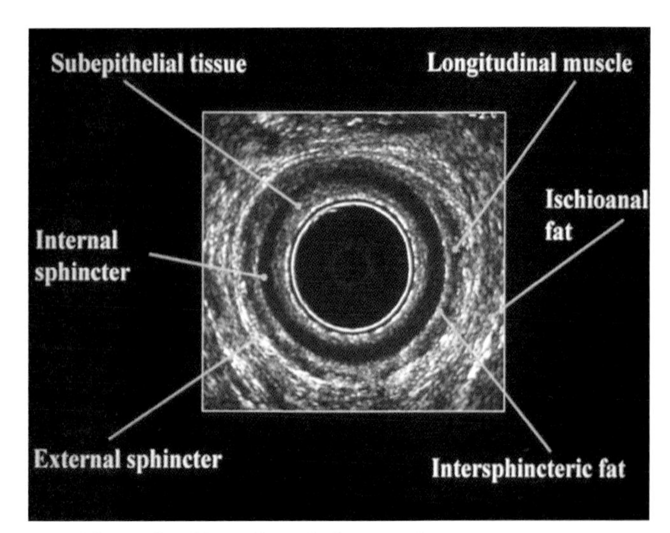

Figure 2 : Normal anal ultrasound

nal sphincter [105]. Such defects are often associated with a weak puborectalis sling that can be relatively inert on dynamic testing (when the patient is asked to squeeze the sphincter). It may reveal cryptoglandular infection as well as the relative bulk of the upper, middle, and lower parts of the anal sphincter. Incontinent patients with low resting anal pressures may have a thinner internal anal sphincter compared with controls. Endoanal ultrasound is superseding electromyography in the investigation of patients with faecal incontinence.

7. Magnetic resonance imaging (MRI)

MRI alone and in conjunction with intra-anal and intrarectal ultrasound may enhance our understanding of pelvic floor function as a whole and delineate abnormalities of function perhaps not seen with more standard tests [123]. Agreement between radiographers regarding the anatomy specifically delineated by MRI remains a problem, however [124].

VI. SUMMARY AND RECOMMENDATIONS

Anorectal incontinence is multifactorial in origin: it rarely presents as a single, easily identifiable abnormality in individual patients. An algorithmic approach (Figure 1) is needed for the evaluation, quantification of anorectal function, and finally, categorization of patients with faecal incontinence. In this way, appropriate conservative medical, aggressive non-surgical (biofeedback), and surgical modalities can be undertaken with an enhanced degree of long-term success.

E. CHILDBIRTH AND ANAL INCONTINENCE

I. INTRODUCTION

Pregnancy and childbirth have a significant impact on the emotional and physical wellbeing of a woman. It is reported that as many as 91% of women report at least one new symptom eight weeks post-partum [125]. A fall in maternal mortality accompanied by an increase in female life expectancy (80 years in the UK) has now shifted the focus of attention towards identification of factors that may minimise morbidity. Although pre-existing bowel symptoms may be aggravated during pregnancy and childbirth, the development of symptoms *de novo* is a more frequent occurrence. Obstetric trauma is the commonest precursor to faecal incontinence. However the onset of symptoms may occur many years after delivery with a peak incidence in the perimenopausal years. This may reflect the effect of contributory factors such as the process of ageing, the effect of the menopause or progression of neuropathy. This section focuses on the association between obstetric trauma and faecal incontinence. However to avoid confusion, the term anal incontinence is used to include incontinence to flatus, liquid and solids.

II. MECHANISM

The mechanism that maintains continence is complex and affected by various factors such as mental function, lack of a compliant rectal reservoir, enhanced colonic transit and changes in stool consistency and volume. However the most important factors are appear to be an anatomical intact anal sphincter complex and neurological function. In about 80% of women with presumed "idiopathic" anorectal incontinence there is histological evidence of denervation of the striated pelvic floor muscles, particularly the puborectalis and external sphincter [126]. This feature has also been demonstrated electro-physiologically by means of an increased fibre density in patients with idiopathic faecal incontinence indicating re-innervation following denervation [127]. Another finding in these patients is a conduction delay in pudendal nerves as measured by pudendal nerve terminal motor latency (PNTML) [128].

Although Hertz in 1909 suggested that pelvic floor damage may result from a normal vaginal delivery, objective scientific evidence for this was only produced in 1984 [129] and a follow-up of 14 patients 5 years later [130]. These authors studied 122 women, 71 after delivery with manometry, perineometry, PNTML and EMG, and 51 before and after delivery with EMG. This study demonstrated an increase in anal sphincter striated muscle fibre density in the vaginal delivery group at 2 months post-partum indicating evidence of re-innervation following denervation. The fibre density was not altered following elective caesarean section. Thirty three percent of primiparae and 50% of multiparae had prolonged PNTML within 48 hours of delivery. However by 2 months, the PNTML had returned to normal in 60% of these women, indicating that damage to pudendal nerve conduction is reversible. Multiparity, forceps delivery, increased duration of the second stage of labour, third degree perineal tears and high birth weight were important factors leading to pudendal nerve damage. In the 5 year follow-up study of 14 women, only multiparae who did not have a forceps delivery were selected; the denervating process was found to be progressive in the majority of women and 5 women suffered from stress incontinence of urine, 3 of whom were also incontinent to flatus.

In another prospective neurophysiological study, Allen et al [131] studied 96 nulliparous women with EMG, PNTML and vaginal pressure measurements during pelvic floor contraction. They found evidence of re-innervation in the pelvic floor muscles of 80% of primiparae 2 months after vaginal delivery. The only obstetric factors associated with re-innervation were a high birth weight and a longer active stage of labour. Forty five of the original 96 women were studied again 6 years later and they concluded that changes in pelvic floor neurophysiology occur with time and do not appear to be related to further childbearing [132].

A third prospective study [133] measured anal pressures, anal sensation and the perineal plane in 72 antenatal women and repeated 72 hours post-partum and in 41 women 2 months postpartum. Anal sensation was unchanged. Cornes et al [134] measured anal sensation in 96 primiparae within 10 days after delivery and measurements were repeated in 74 women 6 months after delivery. They found that at 6 months anal sensation had returned to normal. Anal sensation remained unchanged after caesarean section. In women who had a torn external sphincter, only impairment of sensation in the upper anal canal persisted at 6 months. More than half the women who admitted to persistent anal incontinence had normal anal sensation. Chaliha et al [135] measured anal electro-sensitivity before and after childbirth and found it unchanged. Anal sensation in isolation therefore probably plays a minor role in the development of obstetric related faecal incontinence.

1. Mechanical trauma

Until the recent advent of anal ultrasound, mechanical trauma to the anal sphincters was only suspected when there was a history of a difficult vaginal delivery, particularly a third or fourth degree tear. Consequently, when anal endosonography was first performed in patients believed to be suffering from "neurogenic" faecal incontinence, unsuspected internal and external sphincter defects were identified [105]. The sonographic appearance of external anal sphincter defects has been verified histologically to represent fibrosis [136] while the appearance of internal sphincter defects have been validated prospectively in patients undergoing lateral internal anal sphincterotomy [137]. Trauma identified by ultrasound may be occult or recognised (third/fourth degree tear).

a) Occult anal sphincter trauma

To date Sultan et al [100] have performed the only prospective study (before and after childbirth) to demonstrate both occult anal sphincter trauma (Figure 3) and pudendal nerve damage during childbirth in both primiparous and multiparous women (n=150). Thirty five percent of primiparous women and 44% of multiparous women developed anal sphincter defects during vaginal delivery. Thirteen percent and 23% respectively developed defaecatory symptoms (faecal urgency and/or anal incontinence) after delivery. Only 2 of the 150 women (both primiparous) had recognised tears of the anal sphincter at the time of delivery. A strong association was demonstrated between the presence of any defect and the development of symptoms. Only 4% of multiparous women sustained new sphincter damage following a subsequent delivery. The single independent factor associated with anal sphincter damage was forceps delivery. The 23 women delivered by caesarean section remained asymptomatic and none developed sphincter defects. No relationship was demonstrated between pudental latency measurements and defaecatory or urinary symptoms.

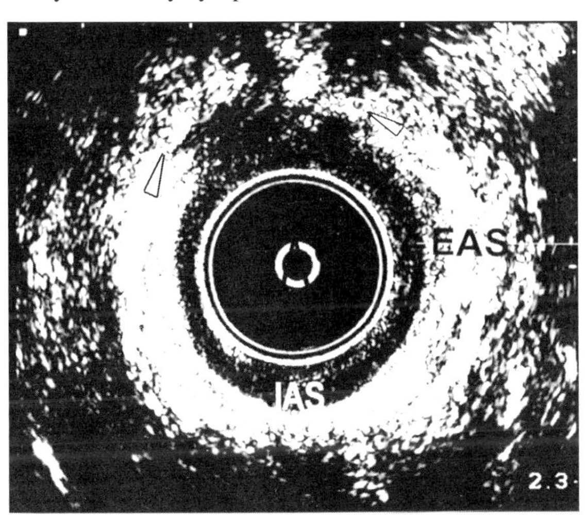

Figure 3 : Anal ultrasound image of the mid anal canal. EAS= external anal sphincter. IAS= internal anal sphincter. The area between the arrows at 10 and lo' clock represents an external anal sphincter defect.

Donnelly et al [22] interviewed 219 nulliparae regarding bowel habit in the third trimester and performed anal vector manometry. At 6 weeks postpartum 184 women returned and the same bowel symptom questionnaire was completed and anal vector manometry plus PNTML measurements were performed. Anal endosonography was performed in 81 women with altered faecal continence or abnormal physiology. Instrumental vaginal delivery and a passive second stage of labour prolonged by epidural analgesia were significantly associated with the greatest risk of anal sphincter trauma and impaired faecal continence. As instrumental delivery is a known risk factor (8 fold increased risk of sphincter trauma), early use of oxytocin was recommended to shorten the second stage. A continuation of the same study [138] reported that pudendal nerve latencies were prolonged and the squeeze pressure increment was reduced in those women who had a caesarean section in the late first stage (>8cm cervical dilatation) or second stage.

Chaliha et al [135] measured anal sensation and manometry in 286 nulliparae during the third trimester and repeated in 161 women postpartum when anal endosonography was also performed. Anal endosonography revealed sphincter defects in 38% of women and this was associated with a lowering of anal squeeze and resting pressures. Threshold anal electrosensitivity remained unchanged and bore no relationship to symptoms. Postpartum sphincter defects were associated with perineal laceration and vaginal delivery.

Abramowitz et al [139] performed a prospective study of 233 women who had anal endosonography performed before and 6 to 8 weeks after childbirth. Of the 233 women (118 primiparae), 202 had a vaginal delivery. Postpartum anal incontinence in the 233 women was reported by 13% of primiparae and 8.5% of multiparae and anal sphincter defects in 21% and 12% respectively. However, the prevalence of anal sphincter defects amongst those that had a vaginal delivery (n=202) was 26% and 13% respectively. Previous studies [140, 141] including others mentioned in Table 13 and 14 have shown that the first delivery is at greatest risk for anal

Table 13 : Prospective studies before and after vaginal delivery of "occult" anal sphincter injury and anal incontinence excluding faecal urgency

Study	Parity Numbers	Vaginal delivery postpartum	FU in weeks	Sphincter Defects	Anal incontinence
Sultan et al 93 [100]	Primi	79	6	35%	5%
	Multi	48	6	44%	19%
Donnelly et al 98 [22]*	Primi	168	6	35%	25%
Rieger et al 98 [144]	Primi	37	6	41%	8%
Zetterstrom et al 99 [145]	Primi	38	9	20%	18%
Fynes et al 99 [142]*	Multi	59	6-12	37%	17%
Abramowitz et al 00 [139]	Primi	202 including	8	26%	15%
	Multi	multi	13%	10%	
MEAN	**Primi**			**31%**	**14%**
	Multi			**31%**	**15%**

**modified continence score questionnaire used and may include urgency*

Table 14 : Studies of "occult" anal sphincter injury sustained during vaginal delivery and anal incontinence excluding faecal urgency only done postnatally

Study	Vaginal delivery	Parity	FU postpartum	Defects	Anal incontinence
Varma et al 99 (143)*	78	Primi	4 weeks	11.5%	0%
	31	Multi	4weeks	19%	0%
Damon 00 [146]	197	Primi	3 months	34%	6%
Faltin 00 [147]**	150	Primi	3 months	28%	15%

**Ultrasound performed < 1 week after delivery*

*** anal ultrasound performed immediately after delivery before perineal repair* sphincter trauma but this study is at variance as it claimed that secundiparous females have the same risk as primiparous women. However this finding remains unsubstantiated and is further disputed by a more recent prospective study [142].

Fynes et al [142] undertook a prospective study of 59 previously nulliparous women through 2 successive pregnancies and found that 34% had anal sphincter injury after their first delivery but only 2 new injuries occurred after the second delivery confirming the findings in Sultan's study [100]. An important finding in this study was that 42% of women (5 of 12) who had occult sphincter injury during their first delivery (squeeze pressure increment < 20mmHg or anal sphincter defect > one quadrant) developed anal incontinence after the second delivery.

In three further studies [143-145] anal ultrasound was performed only after delivery and defects were identified in 11.5 to 34% (Table 14). Varma et al [143] studied 159 postnatal women (105 primiparous and 54 secudiparous) and found occult anal sphincter defects in 11.5% of primiparous and 19% of secundiparous vaginal deliveries but 80% of forceps deliveries. None of their patients suffered faecal incontinence but only 72% of questionnaires were returned. However their cohort had a high caesarean section rate (25%) and a low forceps rate (4%).

b) Third/fourth degree obstetric tears

It is unclear as to whether the sonographic anal sphincter defects described above represent tears that have been missed at delivery or true "occult" defects that may not be visible to a trained doctor or midwife. Groom and Patterson [148] conducted a study in which they demonstrated that the rate of third degree tears rose to 15% when all "second degree tears" were examined by a second person confirming that at least some tears are being missed. This reflects inadequate training and was highlighted by Sultan et al [149] who reported that 91% of doctors who had done at least 6 months of training in obstetrics and 60% of midwives indicated inadequate training in perineal anatomy and 84% and 61% respectively reported inadequate training in identifying third degree tears. Another possible reason for under-diagnosis is that tears of the anal sphincter have been wrongly classified and therefore anal sphincter tears have been under-reported. Any involvement of the anal sphincter should be classified as third degree. However 41% of doctors and 16% of midwives classified a torn anal sphincter as a second degree tear [149]. Sultan and Thakar reviewed every relevant text book (n=65) in the library of the Royal College of Obstetricians and Gynaecologists (RCOG) and found that there was a lack of consistency in classification and in about 40% the classification was omitted or wrong [150]. Furthermore, previous classifications are incomplete because they do not incorporate depth of external sphincter rupture or involvement of the internal sphincter. This therefore has epidemiological, clinical and medicolegal implications. If a third degree tear is incorrectly classified as second degree, then inappropriate repair could result in sub-optimal outcome (see below). Sultan (151) has therefore proposed the following classification to be incorporated in the 29th RCOG green top guidelines:

First degree: laceration of the vaginal epithelium or perineal skin only.

Second degree: involvement of the perineal muscles but not the anal sphincter.

Third degree: disruption of the anal sphincter muscles and this should be further subdivided into:

3a: <50% thickness of external sphincter torn.

3b: >50% thickness of external sphincter torn.

3c: internal sphincter torn also.

Fourth degree: a third degree tear with disruption of the anal epithelium.

An isolated rectal tear without involvement of the anal sphincter is rare and should not be included in the above classification.

Primary sphincter repair of a third or fourth degree obstetric tear is usually performed by obstetricians using the end-to-end repair technique [152]. However as shown in Table 15, anal incontinence occurs in 15 to 59% and in addition, urgency can affect a further 6 [152, 153] to 28% [154]. Frank faecal incontinence affected 9% (range 2 [155] to 23% [156]. In five studies [152, 154, 157-159] anal endosonography was performed to demonstrate persistent anal sphincter defects following repair in 40 to 91% of women. Forceps delivery, first vaginal delivery, large baby, shoulder dystocia and a persistent occipito-posterior position have been identified as the main risk factors for the development of a third/fourth degree tear [139, 140, 152, 157].

The most popular method of repair of the external sphincter is the end-to-end technique but colorectal surgeons prefer the overlap technique for secondary repair because of better outcome [160]. It is now known that like other incontinence procedures outcome can deteriorate with time and one study has reported 50% continence at 5-year follow-up [161]. However some women in this study had more than one attempt at sphincter repair [161]. Sultan et al [160] were the first to describe the overlap technique for acute anal sphincter rupture and in addition advocated the separate identification and repair of the internal sphincter. Compared to matched historical controls [152] who had an end-to-

Table 15 : Prevalence of anal incontinence following primary repair of obstetric anal sphincter rupture

Authors	Year	Country	N	Follow-up Months	Anal incontinence
Sangalli et al [153]	2000	Switzerland	177	13 years	15%
Wood J et al [162]	1998	Australia	84	31	17%*
Walsh et al [163]	1996	UK	81	3	20%
Sander et al [164]	1999	Denmark	48	1	21%
Crawford et al [165]	1993	USA	35	12	23%
Sorensen et al [166]	1993	Denmark	38	3	24%
Nielsen et al [167]	1992	Denmark	24	12	29%
Go & Dunselman [168]	1988	Netherlands	20	6	30%
Uustal Fornell et al [169]	1996	Sweden	51	6	40%
Poen et al [157]	1998	Netherlands	117	56	40%
Sultan et al [152]	1994	UK	34	2	41%
Zetterstrom et al [155]	1999	Sweden	46	9	41%
Sorensen et al [170]	1988	Denmark	25	78	42%
Tetzschner et al [171]	1996	Denmark	72	24-48	42%
Kammerer-Doak et al [159]	1999	New Mexico	15	4	43%
Haadem et al [172]	1988	Sweden	62	3	44%
Bek & Laurberg [173]	1992	Denmark	121	?	50%
Fitzpatrick et al [154]	2000	Ireland	154	3	53%
Gjessing H et al [156]	1998	Norway	38	12-60	57%
Goffeng et al [158]	1998	Sweden	27	12	59%
MEAN					**37%**

* *Includes 2 with secondary sphincter repair*

end repair, anal incontinence could be reduced from 41% to 8% using the overlap technique and separate repair of the internal sphincter [156]. However as the two operators performing the repair had a specialised knowledge of the anal sphincter anatomy it could have biased their results and they therefore recommended a randomised trial. The only published randomised trial published to date is by Fitzpatrick et al in Dublin [154] who found no significant difference between the 2 methods of repair although there appeared to be trend towards more symptoms in the end-to-end group. There were methodological differences in that the torn internal sphincter was not identified and repaired separately and they used a constipating agent for 3 days after the repair. Nevertheless as the authors concur, a better outcome would be expected with both techniques as a consequence of focused education and training in anal sphincter repair. A longer-term follow-up is awaited and further randomised trials using the described technique [160] are currently in progress.

• **Management of subsequent pregnancy**

All women who have sustained a third/fourth degree tear should be assessed in hospital by a senior obstetrician 6 to 8 weeks after delivery. Some centres have established dedicated multidiscliplinary perineal clinics. It is important that a careful history is taken regarding bowel, bladder and sexual function. As these symptoms are embarrassing, a structured questionnaire may be useful. A careful vaginal and rectal examination should be performed to check for complete healing, scar tenderness and sphincter tone [174, 175]. We recommend that all women should have ano-rectal investigations (endosonography and manometry) but if such facilities are unavailable locally then at least symptomatic women should be referred for investigations (Figure 4) [150]. Mild incontinence (faecal urgency or flatus incontinence) may be controlled with dietary advice, constipating agents (loperamide or codeine phosphate), physiotherapy or biofeedback. However women who have severe incontinence should, in addition, be offered secondary sphincter repair by a colorectal surgeon. Asymptomatic women must be advised to return if symptoms develop.

There are no randomised studies to determine the most appropriate mode of a subsequent delivery. Women who have had a successful secondary sphincter repair for faecal incontinence should be delivered by caesarean section [176]. Some women with faecal incontinence may chose to complete their family prior to embarking on anal sphincter surgery. It remains to be established whether these women should be allowed a vaginal delivery as it could be argued that damage has already occurred and risk of further damage is minimal and possibly insignificant in terms of the outcome of surgery.

Very few text books discuss management of a subsequent pregnancy but some indicate that caesarean section should be considered particularly after a difficult primary repair [150]. It has been suggested that a caesarean section should be performed even after transient anal incontinence [171] but this has been questioned [177].

In order to counsel women with previous third/fourth degree tears appropriately, we find it useful to have a symptom questionnaire, anal ultrasound (Figure 2) and manometry results. If vaginal delivery is contemplated then these tests should be performed during the current pregnancy unless performed previously and found to be abnormal (Figure 4). Current evidence suggests that if a large sonographic defect (more than one quadrant) is present or if the squeeze pressure increment is less than 20 mmHg then the risk of impaired continence is increased to 42% after a subsequent delivery [142]. One policy is to counsel these women and offer a caesarean section especially especially to those who are symptomatic. Asymptomatic women who do not have compromised anal sphincter function can be allowed a normal delivery by an experienced accoucher. Although 11% of textbooks recommend a prophylactic episiotomy [150] there is no evidence that an elective episiotomy prevents subsequent anal sphincter disruption. Some studies have indicated that episiotomy may increase the prevalence of anal sphincter disruption. Preliminary results of a multicentre study (Sultan, unpublished data) do not support the practice of prophylactic episiotomy and therefore it should only be performed if clinically indicated.

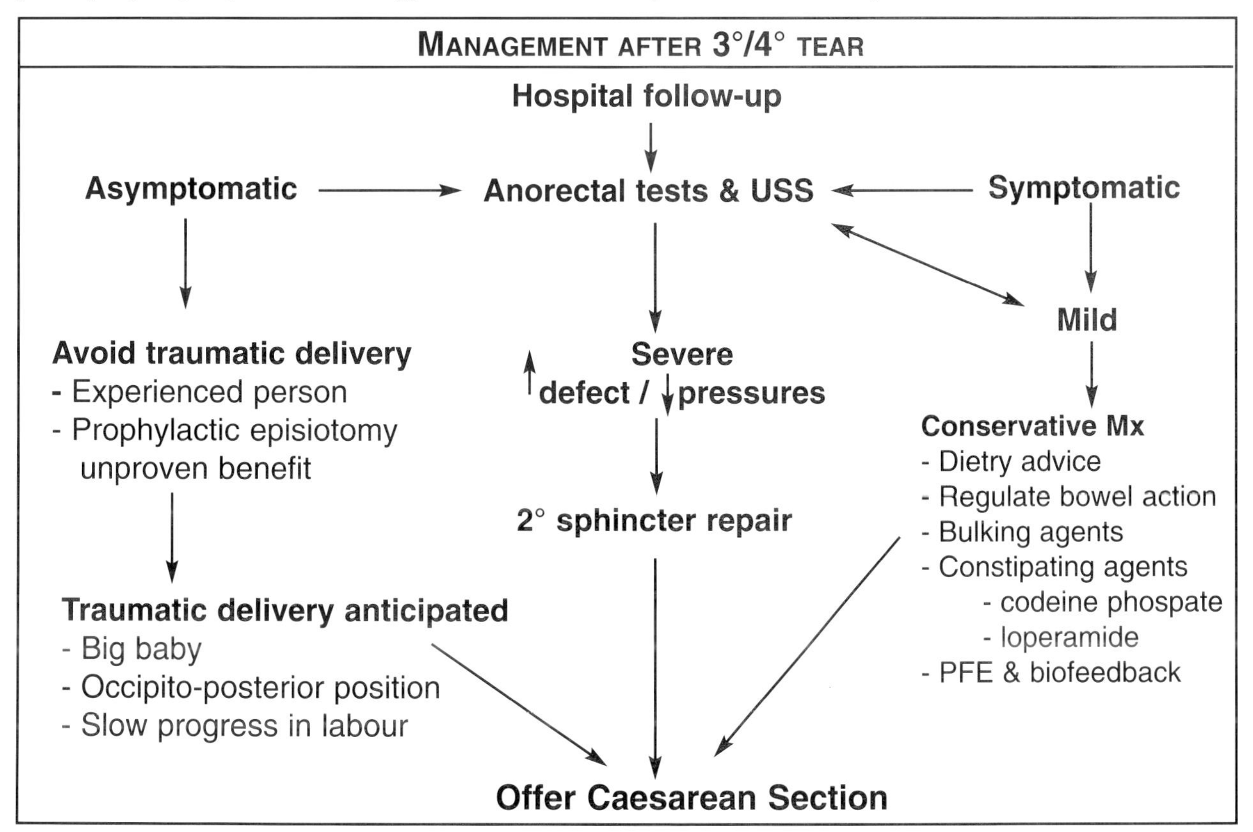

Figure 4 : Management of obstetric injury

III. EFFECTS OF INSTRUMENTAL VAGINAL DELIVERY

Although only 4% of women delivered by forceps sustain a third/fourth degree tear, up to 50% of those that do tear have an instrumental delivery [152]. Vacuum extraction is associated with fewer third/fourth tears than forceps and this view is supported by 2 large randomised studies [178, 179]. A UK study [178] where mediolateral episiotomy is practised reported severe vaginal lacerations in 17% of forceps compared to 11% of vacuum deliveries and a Canadian study [179] where midline episiotomy is practised reported third/fourth tears in 29% of forceps compared to 12% of vacuum deliveries. In a Cochrane review (ten trials) [181] use of the vacuum extractor instead of forceps was associated with significantly less maternal trauma (odds ratio 0.41, 95% confidence interval 0.33 to 0.50) and with less need for general and regional anaesthesia. There were more deliveries with vacuum extraction (odds ratio 1.69, 95% confidence interval 1.31 to 2.19) and fewer caesarean sections were carried out in the vacuum extractor group. However the vacuum extractor was associated with an increase in neonatal cephalhaematomata and retinal haemorrhages. Serious neonatal injury was uncommon with either instrument.

The reduction in cephalhaematoma and retinal haemorrhages seen with forceps may be a compensatory benefit. A 5 year follow-up of infants who participated in a randomised study of forceps and vacuum delivery has confirmed that there is no difference in terms of neurological development and visual acuity with use of either instrument [59]. Occult trauma to the anal sphincter has also been identified more frequently in forceps delivery occurring in up to 80 percent [100, 143, 182]. A small randomised study (n=44) confirmed this by identifying occult anal sphincter defects in 79% of forceps compared to 40% of vacuum deliveries [182]. Trauma occurs more frequently when a second instrument is used to attempt vaginal delivery [182] and therefore if delivery fails with the appropriate technique and vacuum cup, one should resort to a caesarean section. Metal cups appear to be more suitable for 'occipito-posterior', transverse and difficult 'occipito-anterior' position deliveries [183]. The soft cups seem to be appropriate for straightforward deliveries as they are significantly more likely to fail to achieve vaginal delivery (odds ratio 1.65, 95% confidence interval 1.19 to 2.29). Although they were associated with less scalp injury (odds ratio 0.45, 95% confidence interval 0.15 to 0.60), there was no difference between the two groups in terms of maternal injury. Farrell et al [184] performed a prospective study of 690 primigravid women and found that forceps delivery was associated with a higher incidence of flatal incontinence (RR 2.6) compared to vaginal delivery and both flatal (RR 2.6) and faecal (RR 3.6) incontinence compared to caesarean delivery. Vacuum delivery did not increase the risk of flatal incontinence. In another recently study MacArthur et al [185] performed the largest questionnaire based multicentre study to establish the prevalence of faecal incontinence at 3 months post-partum. They reported a prevalence of 9.2%, with 4.2% reporting it more often than rarely. Forceps delivery was associated with almost twice the risk of developing faecal incontinence whereas vacuum extraction was not associated with this risk. These studies support the recommendation by the U.K. Royal College of Obstetricians and Gynaecologists (RCOG) that the vacuum extractor should be the instrument of choice [186].

IV. EPISIOTOMY

There is now considerable observational data to indicate that a reduction in episiotomy rate is not associated with an increase in anal sphincter rupture [187]. The Cochrane database [188] shows that restricting the use of episiotomy is associated with less posterior vaginal trauma. Although anterior perineal trauma was increased it had no effect on the development of urinary incontinence. Henrikssen et al [189, 190] performed an observational study in which they noted that when midwives who previously had a high episiotomy rate reduced their rate, the prevalence of anal sphincter rupture also reduced. However this beneficial effect was abolished when midwives with a low rate of episiotomy attempted to reduce it even further. Based on this evidence, it was suggested that the ideal episiotomy rate should lie between 20 to 30% and no more. Midline episiotomies are more popular in North America as it is believed that they are more comfortable and recovery is less complicated. However Coats et al [191] performed a randomised study of 407 primiparae and found 12% of midline episiotomies extended into the anal sphincter compared to 2% of mediolateral episiotomies. Although the perineum was significantly less bruised in the midline group and sexual intercourse commenced earlier, pain and wound breakdown was similar in both groups.

V. DELIVERY TECHNIQUES

Pirhonen et al [192] compared the frequency of anal sphincter rupture in low risk deliveries between two Scandinavian countries (26,541 vaginal deliveries) and found the risk to be 13 times higher in Sweden (Malmo) *vs* Finland (Turku). They speculated that the only explanation for this was a difference in manual support given to the baby's head during crowning and pushing the perineum under the chin.

VI. TRAINING

There is evidence from one study [149] that perineal anatomy is poorly understood by midwives and trainee doctors, who perform the bulk of deliveries in the UK. In this study 41% of trainees and 16% of midwives incorrectly classified a partial or complete tear of the EAS as 'second degree'. Inconsistency in classification of tears would allow many injuries to pass unrecognised. Intensive and focused training in perineal anatomy and repair should therefore become an essential module in the programme for trainees.

VII. IRRITABLE BOWEL SYNDROME (IBS)

IBS affects 3-17% in selected populations and the cause remains unknown. Donnelly et al [23] recruited 312 primiparous women and reported that 11% of young primiparous women (n= 34 of 208) suffered from pre-existing IBS prior to their first pregnancy. Twenty four percent reported symptoms of impaired faecal continence in the puerperium but symptoms were found significantly more frequently in those with IBS compared to those with normal bowel habit (71% vs 18%). However women suffering from IBS are no more likely to incur mechanical or neurologic injury to the anal sphincter. Women with IBS delivered by caesarean section did not have altered continence postpartum. However 6 months postpartum there were no symptomatic differences between those with IBS and those without, but only 90 of the 107 women who had either impaired faecal continence or abnormal anal manometry were studied. Treatment is directed towards the predominant symptom and although antispasmodics such as hyoscine, mebeverine and dicyclomine are used widely to relax intestinal smooth muscle, they should be avoided during pregnancy.

VIII. RECOMMENDATIONS

a) Compared to forceps the vacuum extractor is associated with less perineal and anal sphincter trauma and should therefore be the instrument of choice. (Level 1)

b) Compared to midline episiotomy, mediolateral episiotomy is associated with a lower risk of anal sphincter rupture (12% vs 2%). (Level 1)

c) Liberal use of episiotomy is not beneficial (Level 1) and restricting the rate of episiotomy to about 30% may reduce the risk of trauma to the anal sphincter.(Level 4)

d) A prolonged active second stage of labour is associated with denervation of the pelvic floor and one study has suggested that this also occurs with a prolonged passive second stage of labour with epidural analgesia. In these circumstances, early use of oxytocics in the second stage of labour may be useful. (Level 4)

e) Selective use of caesarean section particularly in those who have evidence of compromised anal sphincter function and those who have had previous successful continence or prolapse surgery. (Level 5)

f) The value of antenatal pelvic floor exercises in the prevention of incontinence and prolapse could be of benefit but is currently being evaluated in randomised studies.

g) Modification in techniques of delivery of the baby may reduce anal sphincter injury and further research is needed (Level 5)

g) A more focused training program for doctors and midwives needs to implemented. There is a poor understanding of perineal and anal sphincter anatomy and hence identification of anal sphincter trauma, incorrect classification and poor outcome of repair (Level 5)

F. CONSERVATIVE MANAGEMENT OF FAECAL INCONTINENCE IN ADULTS

I. DRUG THERAPY

Patients who experience urge incontinence of faeces associated with loose stool, or who have a passive anal seepage of soft stool may benefit from low dose constipating medication [193]. Loperamide has been found to reduce faecal incontinence, improve stool consistency, and reduce stool weight compared to placebo. Continence to rectally infused saline improved on 4mg three times per day in 26 patients with chronic diarrhoea, and there was additionally a small increase in resting anal pressure [194]. Loperamide oxide has a similar effect [195] There is also some evidence that loperamide increases water absorption by slowing colonic transit and, in an animal model, that it decreases internal anal sphincter relaxation in response to rectal distension [196] and increases mucosal fluid uptake [197].

Codeine phosphate is a naturally occurring opiate which also acts to increase transit time. It is prescribed in in doses of 30 to 120mg daily in divided doses. The use of codeine is limited by the relatively high incidence of side-effects, principally drowsiness. Additionally, long term usage of codeine may be associated with tolerance and dependence. Despite these problems, codeine is a useful agent in the treatment of faecal incontinence [198] although formal evidence from trials is lacking. It may be given in addition to loperamide when maximal doses have failed to reduce symptoms.

Some patients may choose to effectively stop spontaneous evacuation by using these agents and then plan evacuation at a convenient time by using suppositories or a micro-enema. Although not ideal, this regime can at least give the patient an element of control and predictability to enable a reasonable quality of life. This has been found to be effective in a nursing home environment, even when staff compliance with prescribed regimes is not good [199].

One study has suggested some benefit from hormone replacement therapy (HRT) in post-menopausal women with faecal incontinence [200]. Resting and squeeze anal pressures were increased, as was the maximum volume tolerated in the rectum. The presence of an anal sphincter defect did not preclude symptomatic benefit. 90% of women reported some improvement and 25% became symptom-free. These results must be viewed with caution as it was a small (20 patient) uncontrolled study, and it has been suggested with urinary incontinence that subjective well-being rather than objective improvement may be the mode of action [201]. It is known that hormone replacement can increase collagen and elastic tissue in the pelvic floor, that there are oestrogen receptors in the external anal sphincter [202], and that anal pressures have a tendency to decrease with advancing age [203]. It is theoretically possible that HRT could decrease or even reverse this trend.

A more recent pharmacological approach has been to modulate anal sphincter activity. Alpha-stimulant medication has been found to increase anal resting tone in healthy volunteers [204] and to improve incontinence in patients after formation of an ileo-anal pouch [205]. However, initial results in patients with "idiopathic" incontinence have been disappointing [206].

II. BIOFEEDBACK

Biofeedback is a technique which gives the patient immediate feedback about normally subconscious body processes. Equipment is used to detect and amplify a physiologic response [207]. Biofeedback has been extensively used in clinical practice and has been advocated to be "the treatment of choice" for faecal incontinence [208]. Many different treatment modalities have been used in the name of "biofeedback". As described by the original authors, it was thought to be an operant conditioning therapy [209]. The aim was for the patient to learn to enhance the presumed reflex contraction of the external anal sphincter (EAS) in response to a reflex relaxation of the internal anal sphincter (IAS) induced by stimulating the recto-anal inhibitory reflex by distension of a rectal balloon [209]. It has subsequently become evident that the EAS response is mostly a voluntary (if usually subconscious) response [210]. Later authors have recognised this and have focused on training the patient to improve this voluntary response.

1. MODALITIES OF BIOFEEDBACK

Three main modalities, with many variations and many adjunctive measures, have been described, although there is a wide variety of methods used within each modality, and some studies give very little detail on equipment or training programme used. No two studies have described exactly the same treatment as "biofeedback".

The first method is the use of an intra-anal electro-myographic (EMG) sensor, anal manometric probe (measuring intra-anal pressure), or perianal surface EMG electrodes to teach the patient how to exercise the anal sphincter, usually as a variation of pelvic floor muscle or "Kegel" exercises more commonly used for treatment of urinary incontinence [211]. Some have used this simply to demonstrate correct isolation and use of an anal squeeze in response to rectal filling or an urge to defaecate. Others have devised a programme of home exercises and use the clinic biofeedback sessions to demonstrate correct technique and monitor progress in achievement. Early studies tended to focus on the peak muscle strength (squeeze increment) [212], while later workers have suggested that it is the overall muscle capacity (strength and endurance of the squeeze) that is important [213, 214].

The second modality is the use of a 3-balloon system to "train" the patient to correctly identify the stimulus of rectal distension and to respond without delay by immediate and forceful EAS contraction to counteract reflex inhibition of the internal anal sphincter. Some have felt that sensory delay is an important factor in faecal incontinence and that abolishing any delay in response to the sensation of distension is the crucial element in successful therapy [215, 216].

The third method is the use of a rectal balloon to "retrain" the rectal sensory threshold, usually with the aim of enabling the patient to discriminate (and thus respond to) smaller rectal volumes. However, tolerance of larger volumes by the use of progressive distension and urge resistance is also reported [217, 218].

One study has used anal ultrasound to show patients contraction of the anal sphincter on a screen [219].

Two studies have attempted to evaluate the different components of biofeedback in randomised controlled trials [216, 220]. Unfortunately, both had very complex designs which makes analysis of the different components impossible from the data presented, except that improving (lowering) the threshold for sensing rectal distension did seem to be beneficial in reducing symptoms [216].

2. Results of biofeedback

A systematic review found 46 studies in adults published in English, including a total of 1364 patients treated [221]. In all but four studies the majority of patients were female. Ages in the included studies ranged from 6-97 years (studies where the majority of participants were children were excluded). Most were mixed or unstated aetiology groups, but a few studies related to specific patients groups (e.g. obstetric [222, 223], or elderly [224]) or to those with a common surgical history (e.g. sphincter repair [225], or anterior resection of the rectum [226]). Two studies involved patients undergoing formation of an ileo-anal pouch and looked at the prophylactic rather than treatment effect of biofeedback; these patients initially had a covering stoma, so it was not known how many had the symptom of faecal incontinence [217, 227]. One study followed a cohort of women who had a repaired third degree obstetric tear, treating symptomatic women more intensively than those without symptoms [223].

Studies have used between one and twenty-eight sessions over 2 days to one year duration of therapy. A wide variety of outcome measures has been employed in studies of biofeedback. Most take reduction of episodes of faecal incontinence as their primary endpoint, although few explicitly stated that diaries or questionnaires were used to gather this information. Criteria for success varied from 90% [228, 229] to 50% [230] reduction in episodes of incontinence. Success rates ranged from 0% [231] to 100% [232]. Thirty four studies quoted an overall response rate (usually combined cure and improvement). Of these, only 3 had a response rate under 50%; 13 had a response rate of 50-75% and 19 studies had a response rate of 75% or greater (6 over 90%).

Of those studies which gave data on patients who were free of the symptom of faecal incontinence, 275 of 566 patients (48.6%) were said to have no incontinence at the end of the study or follow up period. Criteria for "responders" varied greatly, but overall, 617 of 861 patients were reported as responders (71.7%). Many did not specify a follow-up period. Some had no follow up and reported results at the end of the treatment period only [218, 222]. Of those that had longer follow up, most included a wide variation within a mean. Only 4 studies reported results at 2 or more years for all patients [216, 233-5]. One study reported immediate results and then at 3 years follow-up, with success deteriorating from 22 to 15 of 37 patients over time [235].

Adjunctive therapies have included the use of electrical stimulation [222, 223]. Others mention the use of medication (bulking agents or anti-diarrhoeals) and dietary modification. The majority of studies mention that patients were instructed to practice at home, but few specified in detail what instructions were given to the patients. Some instructed patients to squeeze whenever rectal distension was felt; other gave a structured exercise programme.

From these studies, there are few clear indicators of which patients are likely to benefit from biofeedback, and some of the evidence is contradictory. Few studies had the benefit of anal ultrasound to define sphincter structural defects. Two studies did not find that success correlated with defects [236, 237], while another obtained better results if the anal sphincters were structurally intact [218]. Pudendal nerve damage was the common factor in the only study to find no benefit at all from biofeedback [231], but others have found that success is independent of pudendal nerve function [236]. Although patients with pudendal neuropathy failed to increase their anal squeeze pressure, this did not preclude symptomatic improvement [236]. Pre-treatment manometry does not seem to predict success or failure [237-9], but sensitivity to balloon distension with air may be important, with some authors concluding that those with an initially insensitive rectum are less likely to respond [229], and others finding that decreasing sensory threshold is the single most important element of biofeedback [216]. Many studies have shown improvement in both resting and squeeze anal pressures, but improvement does not necessarily correlate with symptomatic relief. For example, one study found that pressures increased in both successes and failures [228]; another found that even those who failed to improve their pressures could improve their symptoms [236]. Two studies concluded that duration rather than strength of squeeze was the important element [213, 214].

A Cochrane review of controlled studies of biofeedback and exercises for faecal incontinence has concluded that " there is not enough evidence from trials to judge whether these treatments are helpful, nor which aspects of the treatment are the most helpful and which patients are the most likely to be helped" [240]. Four trials reported in published papers and one reported in abstract form met the inclusion criteria of a randomised or quasi-randomised controlled trial [216, 220, 222, 224, 241]. The total number of participants was 109. All included trials but one [222] presented with potential methodological bias. The quality of allocation concealment was judged to be adequate in one trial [222], unclear in three trials [220, 216, 241] and inadequate in one trial [224]. Only two of the included trials provided data in a form suitable for statistical analysis.

No two studies employed the same outcome measures and consequently a quantitative synthesis was not possible. Results from a single trial in this review suggest that anal biofeedback is superior to vaginal, and that electrical stimulation might enhance the results of exercises [222]. However, the trial focused on the use of electrical stimulation as an adjunct to biofeedback and compared two very different types of interventions (vaginal pelvic floor manometric pressure biofeedback and home exercise with anal EMG biofeedback and home exercises in combination with anal electrical stimulation) and did not just single out the effects of electrical stimulation or biofeedback. Moreover, it is difficult to know how much of this improvement is a consequence of the natural history of faecal incontinence following childbirth as a no-treatment group was not included.

It appears also that training to enhance rectal discrimination of sensation may be helpful in reducing faecal incontinence, at least in the short term [216]. It may be that adding this technique to the more commonly-available pelvic floor muscle training would enhance results, but this cannot be a strong recommendation in view of the small numbers and lack of follow-up data.

The evidence suggests that biofeedback and exercises have an effect in clinical practice and a role in the treatment of patients with faecal incontinence, with only one treatment study reporting no benefit at all and the majority improving at least 50% of patients at least to some degree. However, it cannot be claimed that "biofeedback" is the effective element in what is inevitably a complex package of care, including assessment and the opportunity to discuss these taboo symptoms, time and attention with an enthusiastic therapist, patient information and teaching, and often supplementary advice on diet, medication and lifestyle. It is not known whether these elements, exercises alone, or the biofeedback itself, are the determining factor in symptom improvement. Well-designed controlled trials are needed to clarify these issues.

a) Summary

It is not possible to draw definitive conclusions for practice from the currently available evidence. Research does not provide sufficient evidence on which to judge the effectiveness of sphincter exercises and or biofeedback therapy in the management of people with faecal incontinence. In particular there is not enough evidence on which to select patients suitable for anal sphincter exercises and/or biofeedback, nor to know which modality of biofeedback or exercises is optimal.

b) Recommendations

No study has reported adverse events from biofeedback and it seems unlikely that the treatment itself could cause worsening of symptoms. Given this, and the potential for adverse events from surgery [161], biofeedback may be considered as a first-line option in therapy for many patients with faecal incontinence which has not responded to simple dietary advice or medication, with surgery reserved for those with major structural abnormalities of the anal sphincter, severe symptoms and those who fail to respond to biofeedback (D). Although some results from the studies reviewed here are equivocal, the majority report at least some positive benefit.

III. ELECTRICAL STIMULATION

Electrical stimulation was first described for treatment of faecal incontinence nearly 40 years ago [242] and was described as efficacious in several uncontrolled studies over the subsequent decades [243-5]. Only one study has reported minimal clinical benefit, and this in patients with major pudendal neuropathy, who probably could not be expected to respond [246].

Stimulation has never been properly evaluated in a controlled manner. A recent review of controlled trials of electrical stimulation concluded "Only one eligible trial with 40 participants was identified. At present, there are insufficient data to allow reliable conclusions to be drawn on the effects of electrical stimulation in the management of faecal incontinence. There is a suggestion that electrical stimulation may have a therapeutic effect, but this is not certain" [247]. There are no controlled studies comparing different stimulation parameters or active with sham stimulation. There have been very few studies and most have been very small, with some using inappropriate stimulation parameters, particularly too low a frequency, for optimum muscle hypertrophy. Some have not even stated their stimulation parameters. Interferential therapy has been judged ineffective, in this and many other areas of physiotherapy [248]. Many have used very few treatments, or over a period of time too short to reasonably expect change. Some have used home exercise [244] and/or biofeedback [222] as well (often instructions not stated), so it is not possible to tell which has an effect. One controlled study has compared biofeedback and exercise with adjunctive electrical stimulation, but in this study different therapists were used to compare vaginal biofeedback with anal biofeedback plus electrical stimulation, and so electrical stimulation was not the only variable and the difference in outcome found could have been the effect of a different therapist or biofeedback method [222]. One attempted controlled study after repair of third degree tears during childbirth abandoned stimulation as it caused discomfort [223].

Most have used unselected patient groups and some have not had the benefit of any physiological investigations to ascertain the cause of incontinence. Few have had the benefit of endoanal ultrasound and so the structural status of the internal and external anal sphincters is unknown in most studies.

a) Recommendations

Given the reasonable success rates of treatment for urinary incontinence [211], and clinical observations of some therapeutic effect in clinical practice, this is a treatment modality which warrants proper investigation (D).

IV. BOWEL MANAGEMENT IN THE NEUROLOGICAL PATIENT

While there is a considerable literature on the prevalence and pathophysiology of bowel dysfunction in neurological disease or injury, there has been remarkably little work done on practical management. In particular, there are very few controlled trails of interventions, and many articles finish their review of causes with rather vague advice on the importance of a good fluid intake and balanced diet. Many patients with neurological problems will be treading a fine dividing line between constipation and faecal incontinence. Great care is needed that in treating one, the other is not precipitated [249, 250].

Many patients will prefer constipation to incontinence as being more socially acceptable, but care is needed that side-effects of constipation such as exacerbation of bladder symptoms [251] or limb spasticity [249] or faecal impaction with overflow diarrhoea do not in turn cause problems. In patients with high spinal lesions impaction can precipitate autonomic dysreflexia and so is potentially life-threatening [252]. Many patients with neurological problems will need to actively plan bowel evacuation rather than wait until problems develop.

The importance of a multidisciplinary assessment in order to identify and minimise impairments disabilities and handicaps related to bowel dysfunction, and in setting person-centred goals in line with desired post-rehabilitation lifestyle are often emphasised [253]. Any bowel schedule has to fit with other activities, of the patient and any carer involved.

Bowel control is often easier to manipulate than bladder control as, if complete evacuation can be achieved, the rectum is normally empty, mass movements are an infrequent event and stool consistency can be regulated by diet or medication. Most patients, with careful planning of a bowel regime, should be able to achieve bowel continence and adequate evacuation. Often this will involve a "package" of care rather than a single intervention - attention to diet, bowel habit, evacuation techniques, and in selected cases, use of medication or surgery.

1. MEDICATION IN NEUROLOGICAL PATIENTS

There are no data on the use of constipating agents in patients with neurological problems and faecal incontinence.

Dunn et al have compared "thervac" micro enemas (5ml stimulant enemas) to bisacodyl suppositories in spinal cord injury (SCI) patients and found that patients need over 45 minutes to respond to the suppositories. The micro enemas reduced both digital stimulation time and evacuation time, and could potentially reduce carer time by up to one hour per day, with obvious cost savings [254]. Another two randomised studies have found that the carrier is important for suppositories, with hydrogenated vegetable oil bisacodyl taking longer to work than polyethylene glycol based bisacodyl, assumed to be the result of sooner bioavailability as the former has to dissolve in body heat [255, 256].

2. BOWEL TRAINING IN NEUROLOGICAL PATIENTS

Many different interventions have been described as "bowel training" [257]. Most extol the virtues of a high fibre diet, adequate fluid intake, as much exercise as feasible, and a regular toileting regime to capitalise on the gastro-colic reflex. Where this fails to establish a habit, use of a suppository or digital stimulation is often advocated. In practice many patients resort to evacuation by Valsalva or straining. However, this can eventually lead to problems with haemorrhoids or even rectal prolapse.

Children with spina bifida have been found to respond to behaviour modification, a regular toilet habit and dietary manipulation, with laxative medication or evacuants as indicated [258]. Most programmes stress the importance of teaching the child to self-initiate toileting after each meal, rewarding successful defaecation and use of suppositories or an enema if there is no self-initiated bowel motion in 2 days.

A protocol of a step-wise programme for bowel management in spina bifida, has been developed [259]. In a prospective evaluation of this protocol 40 patients with spina bifida were entered, "social continence" (defined as one or less episodes of faecal incontinence per month) was increased from 13 to 60% of subjects. Success was associated with younger age at onset of the programme, compliance with the prescribed regime and presence of the anocutaneous reflex. Of those who had been previously incontinent and who complied, 79% achieved continence.

Patients following a CVA have been found to develop a consistent elimination pattern by a programme of daily digital rectal stimulation [260]. Daily stimulation was more effective than alternate day stimulation, with 24/25 patients achieving success.

The most developed protocols for bowel management are with SCI patients. Patients with an upper motor neurone lesion are usually taught to stimulate reflex bowel emptying every 1-3 days by gentle rotation of a gloved finger in the anus until the rectal wall is felt to relax, or flatus is passed and the stool comes down. In a survey of 424 members of the Danish Paraplegic Association it was found that 65% use digital stimulation [261]. Lower motor neurone lesion patients often need to manually evacuate the rectum once or more per day to stay continent.

In a nursing home population, frequency defaecation and number of continent stools was increased significantly in a trial of prompted voiding for urinary incontinence [262]. The authors suggest that this incidental finding may relate to increase opportunity to sit on the toilet, together with improved mobility and fluid intake. This suggests that dependent individuals may increase bowel frequency simply by being able to access a toilet more frequently. This has particular relevance for people with a urinary catheter who may seldom be offered use of the toilet.

3. Bowel washout regimes in neurological patients

There is limited research on optimal regimes and techniques, or on which fluids are the most effective. Shandling has developed a catheter incorporating an inflatable balloon and reported 100% success with 40% of 112 children with spina bifida, but did not make selection criteria clear or state length of follow-up [263] Others are more cautious in their appraisal. Thirty one children with spina bifida who were dissatisfied with current bowel management were started using the catheter, using saline at 20ml/kg body weight every 24 or 48 hours [264]. There were 6 immediate dropouts and a further 9 had stopped using the catheter, at 30 months. Of those who continued to use the catheter the percentage of continent stools rose from 28 to 94% and the percentage of constipated stools dropped from 55 to 15%.

One group report 83 of their 190 patients with spina bifida using irrigation daily or on alternate days via a cone in the anus, with good compliance [265]. Details of the technique are given by Scholler-Gyure and colleagues [266]. Of 41 patients with spina bifida who had failed other bowel management, 66% were continent at a mean follow up of 33 months, seven had monthly incontinence and 7 weekly incontinence; none had daily incontinence. Minor side effects included abdominal pain, headaches and poor appetite, but these were rare. Parental satisfaction was high in 63% and good in 37%. 66% of the children rated continence as the most important advantage, but half felt that it took up too much time and energy. Six found irrigation painful and 3 unpleasant; five were dependent on others to help.

Where a rectal washout is incomplete a catheterisable continent conduit may be surgically constructed to achieve antegrade colonic irrigation (see ACE procedure, section G, below).

4. Manual evacuation in neurological patients

There is a group of patients who have little or no reflex activity in the lower colon (and so cannot stimulate peristalsis), who have little alternative to planned manual evacuation either done by themselves or a carer or nurse. The majority of SCI patients need to use this regularly [267]. The UK Royal College of Nursing has reviewed manual evacuation and suggested a procedure and safety points [268].

V. GENERAL MEASURES AND ADVICE

Patients with bowel problems often need considerable psychological support, together with teaching and information on the normal working of the bowel. Knowledge about peristalsis, the gastro-colic reflex and the normal co-ordination of internal and external anal sphincters can enable planning and development of coping strategies. A few patients present following sexual abuse and may need intensive psychological support.

Fibre supplements have been found to contribute to faecal incontinence in frail immobile people [198, 269]. Softer stool is more difficult to hold during an urge to defaecate, and is also more likely to passively leak. There are no trials on the effect of fibre reduction on faecal continence, but clinically a lot of patients derive benefit from moderating their fibre intake [270]. People with faecal incontinence which is not secondary to severe constipation may find it helpful to keep the stool firm and formed by moderating the fibre content of their diet. Immobile people are often found to have a colon loaded with soft stool or coinstipation, which is more likely to leak than firm stool [198, 271]. Conversely, those with incontinence secondary to loose stool or constipation may benefit from additional fibre [272]. Fibre must be used with caution in immobile people as it has been found to increase the risk of faecal incontinence compared to placebo [269] and a soft impaction can be caused [271].

Caffeine seems to act as a gut stimulant for some people and clinically some patients with urgent defaecation benefit from caffeine reduction [270].

VI. MANAGING FAECAL INCONTINENCE

There are no perfect answers to the problem of coping with faecal incontinence. It is very difficult to find anything that reliably disguises bowel leakage and smell and very few products have been designed specifically for faecal leakage.

Most of the disposable pads used for urinary incontinence can be used for containment, but some people find them unnecessarily thick, bulky, and not exactly the right shape to contain anal leakage.

An anal plug has been developed to help people with faecal incontinence. It is designed to be worn inside the rectum to plug the entrance to the anus from the inside and is available in two sizes. Some people find an anal plug uncomfortable, or that it gives a constant feeling of needing to open the bowels. It has to be taken out before a bowel action, and so is not suitable for someone who needs to open the bowels very frequently Christiansen [273] found that 11 of 14 patients (71%), withdrew because of discomfort. In another evaluation [274], the majority of patients (14/20) could not tolerate the plug due to discomfort. Four patients (20%) wished to continue to use a plug on a regular basis after the study, and two others on an occasional basis. However, for this minority who could tolerate a plug, it was highly successful in controlling faecal incontinence. There was no association between comfort in using the plug and anorectal sensitivity as measured by electrophysiological tests. It was not possible to predict which patients would benefit from plug use.

G. SURGERY FOR FAECAL INCONTINENCE

Standard surgical treatment for faecal incontinence has been postanal repair for idiopathic incontinence and external sphincter repair for traumatic faecal incontinence.

Although idiopathic faecal incontinence should be defined as incontinence in subjects where neither trauma nor underlying disease are recognized as cause of the condition, the patients with idiopathic faecal incontinence treated by postanal repair are usually confined to middle-aged and older women. The introduction of intra-anal ultrasound has revealed that up to 60% of these patients have an overlooked obstetric lesion of the external sphincter [275] which means that the standard treatment should be sphincter reconstruction and not postanal repair. The recognition that a large fraction of the patients previously treated as idiopathic incontinence in fact has an external sphincter lesion may explain some of the conflicting results published.

I. POST-ANAL REPAIR

The post-anal repair was originally designed to improve continence by restoring an obtuse anorectal angle and to elongate the functional length of the anal canal [76]. The operation is carried out with the patient in the lithotomy or prone jack-knife position according to the surgeons preference. Bowel preparartion and peroperative antibiotic prophylaxis is used. The technique consists of a transverse post-anal incision and dissection of the intersphincteric space, opening of Waldeyers fascia and mobilisation of the rectum off the sacrum by finger dissection. The central pelvic floor muscles, i.e. the puborectalis, the ischiococcygeus and the pubococcygeus are sutured behind the rectum either by mass suture or by a layered suture. After the operation the patients should be instructed not to strain during defecation and a bulk laxative may be advisable. Pelvic floor exercises should be encouraged 3-4 weeks after the operation.

The initial results reported were encouraging, obtaining continence of faeces in 60 to 75% of the patients [276, 277] but later, critical assessment by independent observers could not confirm these results. In a study from St. Marks hospital where this technique was first described, only 26% of the patients were continent to faeces at a median follow-up of 6 years [278]. Similar results were reported by Jameson et al [279] where only 28% of the patients experienced a major improvement after a median follow-up of 2 years compared to 83% after 6 months. A recent study from United States reported satisfactory continence in 35% of the patients after an average follow-up of 3 years [280].

Hypothetically, the same effect on anal continence should be obtained whether the puborectalis sling is shortened by suturing the muscle posterior or anterior to the anal canal. This was eventually demonstrated [281-3] and it was furthermore shown that neither post-anal repair nor anterior perineoplasty decreased the anorectal angle [282, 283]. A randomised study comparing anterior and posterior pelvic floor repair with total pelvic floor repair (combined anterior and posterior repair) showed a significantly better results for the latter operation which also was the only of the three which increased the length of the anal canal [284]. This difference may partly be explained by the knowledge provided by intranal ultrasound examination that 60% or more of these patients may have had an anterior external sphincter defect which would be repaired by the anterior sphincteroplasty.

Persisting incontinence after rectopexy for complete rectal prolapse, a condition which manometrically resembles idiopathic faecal incontinence, has also been treated by post-anal repair with results which do not differ from those described above [285, 286].

In conclusion, the long term effect of postanal repair for idiopathic anal incontinence is poor and there are no predictors for a successfull outcome. It has been argued [280] that despite the low success rate, the absence of mortality and the low morbidity may justify its use in selected patients in whom conservative tratment has failed and who are not candidates for other surgical procedures.

II. ANAL SPHINCTER REPAIR

Traumatic lesion of the external anal sphincter, which in the large majority of patients is due to an obstetric tear, is treated by reconstruction of the external sphincter usually by an overlapping suture. The defect, which is diagnosed by intra-anal ultrasound, will in obstetric lesions always be located anteriorly whereas defects following anal fistula surgery are usually located in the posterior half of the external sphincter. Patients should go through conservative treatment including biofeedback training before sphincter reconstruction is performed. It is our experience, however, that patients with external sphincter lesion and severe incontinence (comparing to a Wexner score of 10 or more) usually will require surgery.

The procedure is carried out with the patient either in the lithotomy or prone jack-knife position and with bowel preparation and antibiotic prophylaxis. In patients with obstetric lesions an anterior curvilinear incision parallel to the anal verge is made. The length of the incision should be limited to approximately 180 degrees antero-laterally. The scar tissue is dissected from the posterior vaginal wall to the level of the anorectal ring and lateral dissection is continued until solid external sphincter muscle is reached. The ends of the external sphincter are mobilised and the repair is performed by placing 3 to 4 2-0 polyglycolic acid mattress sutures which overlap the cut ends of the muscle and finally another 3-4 sutures to complete the overlap repair. In patients without a total disruption of the muscle an imbrication without division of the muscle may be performed. In patients with a lax internal sphincter imbrication of this muscle should be done [287] and in patients with signs of perineal descent 2 or 3 anterior levator sutures may be added. Faecal diversion is unnecessary since it offers no benefit in terms of wound healing or functional outcome, and is a source of morbidity [288].

Early results of external sphincter repair for obstetric lesions have generally been favourable with satisfactory continence in approximately 75% of the patients [287-293] but after 3 to 5 years this figure has decreased to roughly 50% [293, 294, 161]. Furthermore, higher age seems to reduce the success rate with inferior results reported in women over 40 and 50 years [292, 295]. Whether the repair is performed as an overlapping suture or as a simple end to end suture seems of no importance [296].

Some of the poor results are due to an insufficient repair, whether insufficiently performed or due to post-operative dehiscence of the repair, which can be demonstrated by intra-anal ultrasound at follow-up. Dehiscence may be due to infection which occurs in up to 24% resulting in disruption in about 10% [297]. In a study of 10 consecutive patients who had undergone external anal sphincter reconstruction by overlapping suture for obstetric lesions and who had no infection or wound disruption, ultrasound revealed sphincter defects in 4 of 5 patients who were still incontinent [298]. In such patients, repeated external sphincter reconstruction may be performed successfully [299] indicating that intra-anal ultrasound should be part of the follow-up procedure in patients with persisting incontinence.

Damage to the pudendal nerve expressed by a prolonged pudendal nerve terminal motor latency has been claimed to be a predictor of poor outcome of sphincter repair for anal incontinence due to obstetric lesion [119]. Recent studies have, however, do not support this [292, 294].

In conclusion, external sphincter repair for traumatic,

mainly obstetric, lesions results in satisfactory long-term continence in approximately 50%. The principal predictors for a successful outcome are age and post-operative infection.

III. NOVEL SURGICAL APPROACHES

In patients with refractory end stage faecal incontinence who have failed or who are not candidates for sphincter repair or other standard therapy more advanced surgical procedures may be tried. These are dynamic graciloplasty, implantation of an artificial anal sphincter and sacral nerve stimulation.

1. DYNAMIC GRACILOPLASTY

Graciloplasty for faecal incontinence was originally developed for use in paediatric surgery [300]. It gained a certain use also for incontinence in adults [301, 302], but the functional results were too unreliable. Since striated muscles are composed of a mixture of fatigue-resistant type 1 fibres and fatigue-prone type 2 fibres they are usually not able to sustain contraction for more than a few minutes which means that it can only to a limited degree act as a sphincter. By electrical stimulation which replaces voluntary contraction, fatigue-prone fibres are converted to fatigue-resistant fibres which is the physiological basis for the use of a stimulated gracilis transplant. The anatomical basis for use of the gracilis muscle as an anal sphincter is the fact, that the muscle receives its vascular and nerve supply through one bundle at its proximal end which allows mobilisation of the full length of the muscle from its insertion at the tibial tuberosity.

The operation is carried out with the patient in the lithotomy position. The gracilis muscle is mobilized to its insertion in the tibial tuberosity through one long or two short incisions. Care must be taken not to damage the neurovascular bundle. The muscle is transposed around the anal canal in subcutaneous tunnels through two perianal incisions at 3 and 9 o´clock. The tendon of the muscle is usually fixed to the ischial spine, but may also be fixed to the skin. Intramuscular electrodes are implanted at the site of nerve entry and connected through a subcutaneous tunnel to a neurostimulator placed in a subcutaneous pocket in the abdominal wall. Prophylactic antibiotics are given from 1 to 3 days. Before continuous stimulation is applied the muscle is trained for 4 to 8 weeks according to a protocol. The amplitude, pulse width, rate and duty cycle can be programmed telemetrically.

Satisfactory continence has been reported in 50 to 73% of the patients [302-4].Complication rate is rather high and especially infectious complications which occur in up to 30% of the patients are followed by a high rate of therapy failure [304, 305]. The most serious of these complications are necrosis of the transplant and erosion through the anal canal. Impaired rectal emptying without sign of anatomical obstruction but with a severe impact on quality of life has been described in all series. A multicentre study showed a convincing relationship between volume of patients and success rate as well as rate of complications indicating that this therapy should only be carried out in specialist centres with a reasonably large number of patients [306].

Since impaired rectal emptying with severe impact on quality of life has occurred in a few patients in all series, a history of obstructed defecation should probably be a contraindication for this procedure.

2. ARTIFICIAL ANAL SPHINCTER

Implantation of an artificial anal sphincter was first reported in 1987 [308]. The sphincter used was originally designed for treatment of urinary incontinence but subsequently the device has been modified to meet the demands of a bowel sphincter, i.e. higher closing pressure and increased strength of the cuff. The system consists of an inflatable cuff placed around the upper anal canal, a pressure-regulating balloon to maintain closure of the cuff placed in the subperitoneal space lateral to the bladder and a control pump accessible to the patient to empty the cuff for defaecation placed in the scrotum or labium. There is a button on the pump which allows for deactivation and activation of the system. The cuff is available in lengths from 10 to 12 cm and in widths from 2 to 3.4 cm. In the reported series the size mostly used has been a length of 11 cm and a width of 2.9 cm. The pressure-regulating balloon contains 40 ml of fluid and is available in pressure ranges from 60 to 110 cm H_2O.

The patients should have a full bowel preparation and peri-operative antibiotic prophylaxis from 1 to 3 days. The procedure begins with implantation of the cuff around the anal canal. This is done either through two perianal incisions at 3 and 9 o´clock or through one transverse perineal incision. A tunnel is created around the anal canal preferably at the anorectal junction and posteriorly above the anococcygeal ligament. Through a suprapubic incision the pressure regulating balloon is placed in the laterovesical subperitoneal space. From this incision the pump can be placed in the scrotum or labium by blunt dissection and the components are connected by tubings through subcutaneous tunnels. The system is left deactivated for 4 to 6 weeks. No diverting stoma is used.

In the first published series of 12 patients the indication had mainly been faecal incontinence due to neuro-muscular disease, a condition where no other treatment was available [308]. Subsequent series have mainly included patients where sphincter repair for traumatic lesions has failed and patients with idiopathic incontinence and anal atresia [309-313].

All series are relatively small with 6 to 14 patients from each participating centre. Acceptable continence has been obtained in approximately 70% of the patients. One series with long-term follow up (more than 5 years) showed that 7 of 17 patients had the system removed due to infection, malfunction or obstructed defaecation. It should be emphasised, however, that the majority of these patients had an implant either with an unmodified urinary sphincter or with one of the earlier modifications of the sphincter; the patients available for follow-up all had good to acceptable continence [314].

Complication rate in most series has been relatively high with infection around the device being the most serious and responsible for removal in up to 23% of the patients [315]. Technical complications like rupture of the cuff which occurred frequently with the earlier modifications of the device are now rare. Obstructed defecation without anatomical stenosis as described for dynamic graciloplasty has also occurred in most series and has in some patients required explantation. Other complications leading to explantation have been erosion of the cuff through the skin or into the anal canal which emphasises the importance of placing the cuff as close to the anorectal junction as possible and not to overpressure the system. At present a total removal rate of 20-25% probably must be expected, an important fact to discuss with patients prior to the operation.

Implantation of the artificial anal sphincter may be done on the same indications as for dynamic graciloplasty except in patients with previous perianal infections or with a thin and scarred perineum where a muscle transplant is preferable. It should be emphasised that due to the relatively high risk of treatment failure and of complications requiring re-operation patient selection for both procedures should be very strict.

3. Sacral nerve stimulation

One of the newer modalities for faecal incontinence is stimulation of the sacral nerves through the foramina of the sacrum. The technique is at present under evaluation but in contrast to dynamic graciloplasty and the artificial sphincter it is not a sphincter replacement therapy and consequently requires an anal sphincter with some degree of function.

This means that its main indications probably will be incontinent patients with an intact anal sphincter, i.e. idiopathic incontinence, patients who are still incontinent after external sphincter repair for traumatic lesions, incontinence after spinal lesions and patients with persisting incontinence after surgery for rectal prolapse and possibly also patients with continence disturbances after low anterior resection for rectal cancer.

Unlike the two other operations this is a minimally invasive procedure which is usually performed in two steps. The operation is carried out with the patient in the prone position. The outline of the sacral bone is marked on the skin and the sacral foramina are located. Sheathed needles are inserted in the sacral foramen of S2, S3 and S4. After placement of the needles current is applied in graduated amplitude until a muscle response is obtained, monitored visually and by anal electomyography and pressure recording. Typically, S2 stimulation results in contraction of the perineum and usually also in an inward movement of the heel and contraction of the toes and foot, S3 stimulation results in a clamp-like contraction of the levator ani and plantar flexion of the great toe, and S4 stimulation in contraction of the levator ani but no leg or foot activity. The nerve that gives the most efficient contraction is chosen for temporary stimulation.

An incision is made over the sacrum with the needle left in place and when the foramen is identified the needle is replaced by a stimulating electrode which is fixed to the periosteum of the sacrum with two non-absorbable sutures. After having checked the efficiency of stimulation, the electrode is through a subcutaneous tunnel to the flank connected to a temporary pulse generator. The system is now tested for 2 to 3 weeks, and if the patient gains satisfactory continence a permanent pulse generator is implanted by the same technique as described for dynamic graciloplasty. The operation requires no bowel preparation but antibiotic prophylaxis from 1 to 3 days is recommended.

It is possible in some patients to replace the first step of the operation with an even less invasive test procedure simply by inserting temporary stimulating electrodes into the sacral foramina through the needles (percutaneous needle electrodes).

The first results with this technique was published by Matzel et al in 1995 [316] who described a successful outcome in three patients with traumatic incontinence in two and incontinence after rectopexy in one. Similar encouraging results both for short term and permanent stimulation have been reported from other centres [317, 318]. Satisfactory long-term continence has been described in a series of 6 patients with a follow up from 5 to 66 months [319].

4. Injectable biomaterial

Perianal injection of fat [320], glutaraldehyde cross-linked collagen [321] and silicone biomaterial [322] in patients with passive anal incontinence due to internal sphincter dysfunction or disruption have been sucessfully reported in small series.

IV. ANTEGRADE LAVAGE (ACE PROCEDURE)

An option which should be considered in patients unsuitable for the procedures described above is the antegrade colon lavage through an appendicostomy originally described for faecal incontinence in children [323]. A recent study where the technique was used for faecal incontinence in 10 adults showed that 6 gained satisfactory continence [324].

V. COLOSTOMY

A number of patients in whom the surgical procedures described above are inapplicable or do not lead to satisfactory bowel control should be offered a permanent colostomy. With the stoma appliances now available a colostomy offers the patient a far more social acceptable life than severe uncontrolled faecal incontinence. There are no published studies comparing quality of life in patients with anal incontinence with and without a colostomy.

VI. SUMMARY

There is a number of surgical options for the treatment of faecal incontinence.

Post anal repair is associated with poor long term results (4).

Overlapping anal sphincter repair achieves good long term results in about 50% of patients (4).

In patients where simple sphincter reconstruction fails or is unsuitable there is a number of newer options available. The role of these is as yet not well-established, nor are the long-term success rates. Some of these methods carry a considerable risk of side effects and consequently a careful patient selection is mandatory.

Sacral nerve stimulation for faecal incontinence is a promising therapy but indications and contraindications are still not clarified.

VII. RECOMMENDATIONS

Surgery should normally be reserved for patients who have failed conservative therapy, except in cases of severe sphincter disruption and symptoms (D).

Surgery is seldom, if ever, indicated for minor symptoms (D).

H. FAECAL INCONTINENCE IN CHILDREN

I. INTRODUCTION

Faecal incontinence during childhood may be a symptom of delayed acquisition of toileting skills or may reflect serious underlying organic or functional pathology. Whatever the cause, the social and psychological consequences for the child and their family are often profound. For management to be successful the physical and psychological components will need to be addressed.

There are considerable cultural differences in toilet training and across the world children acquire bowel control at anytime between 1 year and 4 years of age [325-7]. Children tend to be trained earlier when the carer is able to immediately respond to signals that the child is about to defaecate. The trend in Western cultures has changed in the past 30 years to allow a more child-oriented approach in which the behaviour of the child dictates when toilet training is introduced [328]. In the USA the average age at which bowel control is gained is 28 months and the vast majority of children will have acquired bowel control by 4 yrs of age [329].

The pattern of bowel actions changes during early life from an average of 3 stools per day in the neonate to 1.7 stools per day at 1 year of age. 97% of preschool children in the UK will pass stool within the range 3 times per day to alternate days [330].

Epidemiological data on faecal incontinence in the normal childhood population is variable. Bellman observed a prevalence of 1.5 % among 7 yr old Swedish children [331] and Rutter in the UK reported a similar prevalence in 10-11 year olds [332]. It accounts for 3% of referrals to a medical clinic in Boston [333] and 25% of referrals to specialist paediatric gastroenterology clinics.

II. DEFINITIONS

Differences in definition can lead to confusion when comparing literature. In the USA encopresis is defined as "involuntary faecal soiling in the presence of functional constipation, in a child over the age of 4 years". Within the UK and Australian literature this is usually called "soiling" with the term encopresis being reserved for those where there appears to be voluntary passage of stool into a socially unacceptable place, implying a large behavioural element. This is a far less common cause of incontinence.

A Multinational Consensus Document On Functional Gastrointestinal Disorders: Rome II [334] identifies functional faecal retention and functional non-retentive soiling as separate entities with the following descriptions:

"Functional faecal retention is the most common cause of constipation and faecal soiling in children. It consists of repetitive attempts to avoid defecation because of fears associated with defaecation. Consequently, a faecal mass accumulates in the rectum."

"Functional non-retentive soiling may be a manifestation of an emotional disturbance in a school-aged child. Soiling episodes may have a relationship to the presence of a specific person (e.g., a parent) or time of day, and may represent impulsive action triggered by unconscious anger."

III. CAUSES OF CONSTIPATION AND FAECAL INCONTINENCE IN CHILDHOOD

1. ORGANIC

Table 16 gives the most common organic causes of childhood bowel symptoms.

The first role of the paediatrician is to identify those few children with underlying organic disease such as Hirschsprung's Disease, anorectal anomaly and those with a neuropathic bowel. One in 5000 children is born with Hirschsprung's disease. Reports of faecal incontinence after surgery vary widely. Several studies show a prevalence of 10 – 20% [335, 336] but Catto-Smith and colleagues in Melbourne have described soiling in 80% of 60 patients followed up by questionnaire and interview [337].

Table 16 : Organic causes of constipation and faecal incontinence in childhood

Neuropathic – meningomyelocoele, spinal dysraphism, spinal tumour, sacral agenesis, Cerebral palsy, dystrophia myotonica

Anorectal anomaly – anal atresia, stenosis, ectopic anus

Acquired anal conditions - anal fissure, Group A streptococcal infection, lichen sclerosis et atrophicus, anal sexual abuse

Congenital bowel disorders – Hirschsprung's, neuronal intestinal dysplasia, chronic intestinal pseudo-obstruction

Miscellaneous medical conditions

Hypothyroidism
Hypercalcaemia
Cow's milk protein intolerance

Drugs
Opiate analgesia
Loperamide
Anticonvulsants
Oxybutynin

Ninety percent of those with meningomyelocoele will experience faecal incontinence of some degree [338]. It is important to identify children with less overt spinal abnormalities, such as spinal dysraphism and sacral agenesis as the majority in this group will also have a neuropathic bladder. Preservation of the upper renal tract from reflux and infection is a priority in order to protect future renal function.

2. FUNCTIONAL RETENTIVE SOILING

95% of children who soil have no inherent bowel or neurological abnormality but are incontinent as a result of functional constipation. There has been considerable debate as to the relative influences of psychological, behavioural and physical factors in the development of constipation but the cause of severe constipation is probably multifactorial.

In young children, stool holding is a common antecedent of constipation seen in 13% of 480 children followed through the toilet training process by Taubman [329]. Parents may describe manoeuvres and postures adopted by the child that almost certainly represent avoidance of defaecation. Such behaviour is reinforced by episodes of painful defaecation, as with anal fissure. In older children, reluctance to use toilet facilities at nursery and school may also precipitate stool holding and subsequent constipation (Ross and Price – personal communication).

The stool in overflow soiling may be loose and therefore interpreted as diarrhoea. 10-20% of children are thought by their parents not to be constipated [339, 333]. However in these children, the fact that they have little sensation of the passage of this stool should alert the paediatrician to the likelihood of constipation as the underlying cause of the soiling.

3. FUNCTIONAL NON-RETENTIVE SOILING

Children over four years who do not have underlying constipation and have no organic or anatomical abnormality are defined as having "non-retentive soiling". They often pass normal stools into clothing at normal stool frequencies. Day and night time enuresis is commonly associated.

Primary and involuntary soiling may be due to delayed toilet training. This may be associated with general developmental delay or with the group of interrelated conditions that includes developmental coordination disorder, autism, other language impairments and attentional difficulties such as Attention Deficit Hyperactivity Disorder

[340]. Functional constipation is also common in this group.

Secondary or voluntary soiling is more likely to have an underlying psychological cause especially when it is related to specific and identifiable triggers. Children with a history of abuse or neglect often have continence problems with soiling in 26% [341]. However chronic faecal retention needs to be excluded.

IV. SECONDARY EFFECTS

1. Psychological and behavioural

Whatever the cause of faecal incontinence, loss of bowel control is one of the most devastating symptoms a child can suffer. Soiling results in increased anxiety and loss of self-esteem. There are significant negative effects on relationships with family members and at school where bullying can become a serious problem. Children are often blamed for being "lazy" as it is not understood that they have little or no bowel control. Many children respond by denial and will hide soiled pants rather than admit to an accident. The whole family, not just the affected child, can experience guilt and failure with associated shame and secrecy leading to isolation [342]. Parents and other carers often give confusing messages by being cross and punitive at times but encouraging and forgiving at others. Continuing problems can lead to "learned helplessness" as all attempts to control the soiling fail [343-5]. Behaviour problems defined by parents are found in up to 40% of children with soiling (344, Butler, personal communication) but these are not generally as severe as in children referred to child mental health services [346]. Most of these behaviour difficulties resolve with successful treatment of soiling indicating they are likely to be secondary. However some children with severe behavioural difficulties associated with poor intra family relationships do not have good outcomes [347]. Breaking these negative cycles by engaging the child and family with appropriate explanations in a non-blaming fashion is vital. It should generate the motivation to cooperate with the management of the condition.

2. Educational

Although up to 40% of children will not have gained full bowel control by entry into nursery at 3 years of age, lack of adequate provision for these children can cause difficulties. In the UK, Department of Health guidance suggests that schools should "recognise the need for unrestricted access to non-threatening toilet facilities". However, school toilets are often unsatisfactory or viewed as such by children [348].

V. ASSESSMENT

The aim of assessment is to identify the cause of faecal soiling and especially identify those children where there may be an underlying organic condition. Other related problems need exploring and an appropriate management plan developed that takes into account the whole child and family.

1. History

A careful history is vital. The areas that should be covered are given in Table 17.

2. Examination

The soiling child should be examined as follows:

Growth and general overview to exclude failure to thrive and neglect.

Abdomen – distension, palpable faecal mass.

Anus and genitalia – careful inspection for abnormality.

Perianal sensation, inspect lower back, spine and buttocks, check lower limb reflexes to exclude any suggestion of neuropathy.

Rectal examination is not usually necessary and may cause distress to younger children.

3. Investigations

In functional constipation few investigations are indicated. Cow's milk protein intolerance may present as intractable constipation and should be considered in an atopic child [349].

Anal manometry and rectal biopsy are indicated if Hirschsprung's disease is a possibility. This should be suspected with a history of delayed passage of meconium or severe constipation starting shortly after birth. Endoanal sonography may provide information about external anal sphincter configuration.

Where there is doubt and perhaps when parents need convincing evidence a plain abdominal X ray can show significant faecal loading and gross rectal enlargement. A rectopelvic ratio greater than 0.61 has been suggested as demonstrating enlargement [350]. Scoring systems have been devised in an attempt to quantify faecal loading [351, 352]. Measurement of bowel transit time using radiological markers may contribute to the clinical picture [353].

- **Anal Manometry**

Anal manometry is an invasive investigation and is not regarded as routine. It may contribute useful information in children suspected of having a neuronal abnormality or where response to conventional treatment is poor.

Table 17 : History in childhood faecal incontinence

	Reason
Age of onset, any initiating factors. Primary or secondary	Constipating event?
Present stool habits – interval, size (any huge) and consistency	
Soiling – interval, amount, consistency, when and where.	
Coping strategies. Hiding soiled pants? School involved?	
Attitude of child, parent, school friends etc.	
Co existing conditions. Congenital or acquired disorders	Neuropathy?
Atopy	Cow's milk intolerance?
Medication (e.g. anticholinergics, anticonvulsants, opiates)	Constipating effect
Learning or attentional difficulties, language impairment.	Delayed toileting
Behavioural problems	1° or 2° to soiling?
Previous surgery – especially related to GI tract	Association
Previous GI symptoms	Constipation associated
Birth history – delay in passage of meconium, early constipation	Hirschsprung's
Family history of bowel related difficulties	Genetic or dietary
Social history, any past history of any type of abuse	Abuse associated
Toilet training history – delay, holding, toilet refusal.	Constipation
Age when could identify need to pass stool without prompting	1° or 2° soiling
Nocturnal enuresis, day wetting, frequency, urgency	Association
Diet (fibre content and balance)	Very low fibre, restricted
Fluid intake and type.	Poor total intake or milk in excess

Children with chronic constipation have significantly increased rectal volume [353] and rectal myohypertrophy [354]. 50% of 34 constipated children studied by Loening-Baucke had an abnormal increase in external sphincter activity during attempts to pass a balloon [354]. There is no evidence for any underlying abnormality in rectal sensation or rectal wall compliance in children with faecal impaction [350]. Anal manometry abnormalities have been shown to persist even after effective treatment of constipation and encopresis [354].

VI. MANAGEMENT

Most authors advocate a multidisciplinary approach in which psychosocial and biological issues are both addressed [356, 344]. Nolan and colleagues in a large randomised found a multimodal approach (disimpaction, maintenance laxatives and behaviour modification) and to be superior to behaviour therapy alone [357].

There are various components to a successful treatment plan (Figure 5):

1. Explanation / "demystification"

It is crucial that parents, carers and the child understand the reason why soiling is occurring. The child is likely to have little or no sensation of soiling episodes. Acknowledging this is a relief for children who previously have not been believed, although it may cause guilt for those parents.

2. Toileting program

Establishing a normal and regular pattern of bowel evacuation is central to eventual success for children with soiling from any cause. Star charts and reward systems can be used to reinforce this behaviour. Externalisation of the bowel problem by using ideas such as goal scoring charts or beating that "sneaky poo" can be helpful. Behavioural programmes like these on their own have been shown to be of benefit [358] but are even more successful when used in conjunction with appropriate laxative medication [357]. Continuing follow up and support to maintain motivation is important.

3. Diet and fluid intake

A well balanced diet with a reasonable fibre intake is likely to be helpful. Experimental studies have shown that increasing fibre results in shorter bowel transit times and stool with greater volume and water content [359]. Mean daily fibre intake in constipated children was statistically lower than that of controls in a series from Greece [360] but low fibre intake is not thought to be the only causative factor. Excessive consumption of milk or poor fluid intake probably contributes.

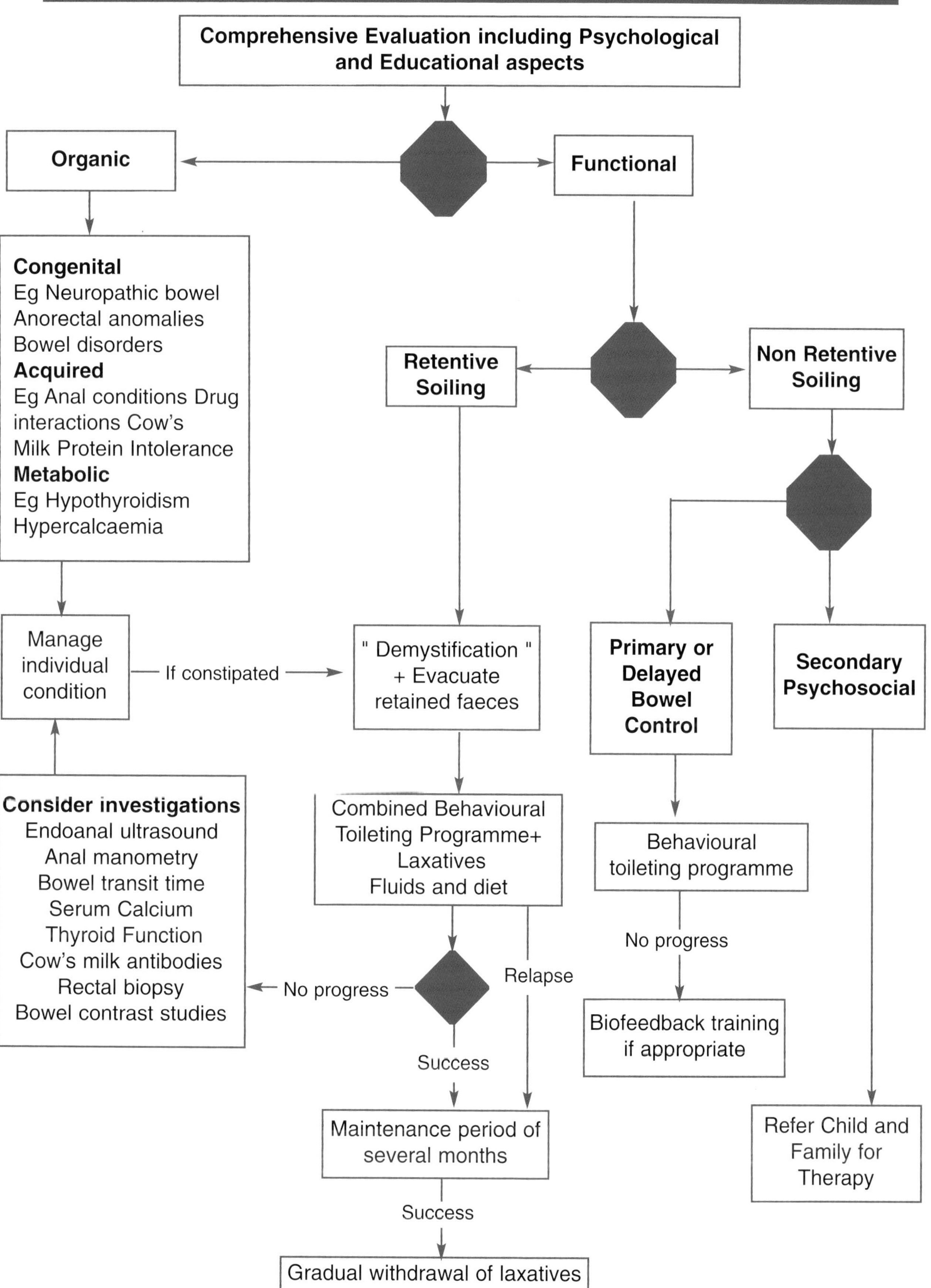

Figure 5 : Algorithmic approach to management of childhood soiling

4. Laxatives

There is general consensus that the child with constipation and overflow soiling requires laxative treatment with the aim of evacuating retained stool and maintaining regular bowel actions thereafter [343, 361, 362]. The evidence base to support the choice of laxatives is however small. Within the UK and Australia the common practise is to combine osmotic laxatives such as lactulose with stimulants such as senna, sodium picosulphate or sodium dioctyl. There are however very few relevant clinical trials and none which contribute significantly to the debate. Lubricants such as mineral oil provide the mainstay of treatment in USA often in combination with laxatives such as senna. Lipoid pneumonia has been described with mineral oil treatment and this should be used with caution in a child at risk of aspiration [363]. Faecal impaction can often be cleared with oral laxatives and lubricants in adequate doses, but in more resistant cases, enemas may be required. Many children find these distressing and effective evacuation of stool is often possible without resorting to rectally administered treatment [364]. Isotonic intestinal lavage with polyethylene glycol is effectively and clears retained faeces in severe refractory constipation [365, 366].

Once retained stool is cleared soiling will dramatically reduce. Various approaches have been used to maintain regular bowel actions – the mainstay being laxative treatment with behavioural approaches, designed to establish a regular toileting routine, enhance compliance and maintain motivation.

5. Biofeedback

Biofeedback training appears to have short term benefits [367, 368] but more recent controlled studies have not demonstrated that these are greater than the success following standard combined behavioural and laxative therapy with supportive follow up [369, 370]. There is some evidence it may be helpful in children who have nonretentive soiling [371].

6. Complementary therapies

Abdominal massage with or without aromatology, reflexology, homeopathy and acupuncture can all be helpful, sometimes in conjunction with standard management, where they assist in establishing a regular toileting routine. Evidence base for these therapies is poorly established.

7. General support

Faecal incontinence has socially isolating effects for the whole family. The network of support is generally less than for other chronic conditions but appropriate literature and advice can be very helpful. Within the UK, the charitable organisation ERIC, Enuresis Resource and Information Centre [372], has done much to raise the profile of this disabling childhood problem.

8. Specialist psychology and psychiatry Services

Children whose soiling is associated with complex family functioning difficulties may need the expertise of a child and family mental health team.

VII. ASSOCIATED DISABILITIES

In those with structural or neuropathic abnormalities the aim is to achieve social continence. The treatment approach, once corrective surgery is complete, is remarkably similar – namely to remove faecal impaction and maintain regular bowel actions. Laxatives and regular toileting plans (with physical aids for those with additional disabilities) may be sufficient but in those with inadequate bowel emptying additional techniques such as use of enemas or rectal washouts may be required to prevent overflow soiling. Malone in 1990 introduced the surgical technique of the antegrade colonic enema (ACE) whereby the large bowel is irrigated via a caecostomy tube or appendix stoma [373, 374]. By keeping the large bowel empty in this way overflow soiling can be largely abolished. This technique has also been used in severe intractable functional constipation with megacolon [375].

VIII. OUTCOME OF CHILDHOOD FAECAL INCONTINENCE

Several studies have demonstrated the chronicity of this condition. The prognosis seems better in those diagnosed before the age of 4 years with recovery in 63% of children followed up by Loening Baucke [376]. In older children approximately 50% will have discontinued laxatives at 12 month follow up, with a further 20% coming off laxatives in the next 2 years [377-9]. In Clayden's series of over 300 children with severe constipation, laxative treatment was required by 56% for over 12 months [343]. At a mean of 6.8 years after treatment nearly 70% of 43 constipated children reviewed by Sutphen were entirely asymptomatic. Mild constipation persisted in 13. Faecal incontinence persisted in 3 of the 17 children who first reported it [380].

IX. SUMMARY

Most children have gained bowel control by 4 years of age [2].

The prevalence of faecal incontinence is around 1.5% at 10 – 11 years of age (2).

Functional results of reconstruction of congenital anorectal anomalies (eg imperforate anus and Hirschsprung's disease) may be poor. These children require long term follow up (3).

The vast majority of soiling children have functional retentive soiling secondary to constipation with no underlying organic abnormality. Stool holding is a common antecedent of constipation (3).

Psychological and behavioural problems are common and are usually secondary to the soiling. These improve when the child becomes continent (3).

Functional non-retentive soiling is less common and may be due to delay in establishing bowel control or to significant psychological and behavioural problems associated with other family and relationship difficulties.

Biofeedback training has been found useful for some children with functional non-retentive soiling (3).

A multidisciplinary approach to the management of functional retentive soiling is more likely to be successful. Parents and children need a clear understanding of the reasons why soiling is occurring in order to prevent intolerance and encourage compliance with the programme. Behavioural issues need to be addressed in conjunction with a combined laxative and toileting programme (2).

Laxative therapy may be needed for many months to maintain regular bowel actions (2).

Outcome is generally better when the condition is diagnosed early (2).

Figure 5 gives an algorithm for management of soiling in children.

X. RECOMMENDATIONS

- A comprehensive and holistic assessment is necessary with consideration of family, psychological and educational issues (D).
- The few children with organic causes of faecal incontinence must be identified, investigated and managed appropriately. Children with a neuropathic bowel or congenital bowel anomalies should be managed within specialist paediatric units (D).
- There is often a considerable delay before children with FI present to knowledgeable health professionals indicating a need for general health promotion and professional training in this area.
- Levels of evidence and research into the most common cause of FI in children – functional retentive soiling - are generally poor although combined laxative and behavioural toileting programmes have been shown to be more effective than either alone (B).

I. ANAL INCONTINENCE IN THE OLDER ADULT

I. INTRODUCTION

Few medical symptoms are as distressing and social isolating for older people as anal incontinence (AI), a condition which places them at greater risk of morbidity, dependency, hospital admissions, and instutionalisation. Many older individuals with AI will not volunteer the problem to their general practitioner, and regrettably, doctors and nurses do not routinely enquire about the symptom. This 'hidden problem' therefore leads to social isolation and a downward spiral of psychological distress, dependency, and poor health. The condition takes its toll on carers also; anal incontinence surpasses even dementia as a leading reason for requesting nursing home placement.

• **Data sources**

A computer-assisted search of the English language literature using Medline (to present), Cochrane Library databases, reference lists from recent systematic reviews and book chapters.

II. EPIDEMIOLOGY OF ANAL INCONTINENCE IN OLDER PEOPLE – PREVALENCE AND RISK FACTORS

Details are presented in Section B (above); the following is a summary of current evidence. The studies reviewed include one prospective short-term cohort study [381]; all the others are cross-sectional surveys [45, 16, 382-6]. Risk factor analyses were unadjusted in several studies [383, 385], and retrospectively conducted in all but one [381].

1. Summary

The prevalence of AI increases with age, particularly in the 8th decade and beyond (2). The prevalence of AI also varies with the general health of the patient, and is therefore higher in the acute hospital and nursing home setting than in the community (2). The prevalence of AI in elderly people is equal or greater in men than women. Nursing home studies show great variablity in prevalence between institutions (2). AI is often combined with urinary incontinence in older individuals (2). Impaired mobility, dementia and loose stool are primary risk factors for AI in older people (2).

2. Recommendations

Bowel continence status should be identified by direct questionning and/or direct observation in nursing home residents, hospital inpatients aged 65 and over, people aged 80 and beyond living in the community, and older adults with impaired mobility and/or cognition (B).

The high prevalence of AI in older men (B) should prompt exploration of aetiologies other than childbirth in ageing adults.

Variability of AI prevalence between nursing homes (B) implies that different standards of care may impact the occurence of the condition.

Standardised definition of AI in older people would be useful in both clinical and research arenas.

Further epidemiological studies are required to further characterise AI in older people, particularly in the acute hospital and primary care settings. Such studies should include evaluation of unmet need for patients and carers.

III. ANAL INCONTINENCE IN OLDER ADULTS - THE 'HIDDEN' PROBLEM

In a British primary care study of patients aged 75 years and over, only half of those reporting AI (or their carers) had discussed the problem with a health care professional, and only one out of eight patients with daily AI had done so. The GP's involved in this study reported full knowledge of incontinence status in only 33% of patients with a continence problem [382].

In Australian survey of acutely hospitalised patients of all ages, only 1 in 6 of those reporting AI had the symptom documented by ward nursing staff [384].

A US nursing home study showed that nursing staff were aware of AI in only 53% of residents self-reporting the condition [387]. The kappa value for concordance between resident and nurse reporting of AI was only 0.34 (0.24-0.43 95% CI).

In an English nursing home study, only 4% of patients with long-standing AI had been referred to their general practitioner for further assessment of this problem [199].

1. Summary

Physicians and nurses have a low awareness of AI (2). Within the nursing home, there is a low rate of referral by nursing staff of residents to their primary care physicians for further assessment of AI (2), which may reflect a tendency toward conservative nursing managment (e.g. use of pads only without further evaluation).

2. Recommendations

General practioners, primary care nurses, hospital ward staff, and nursing home nursing staff should routinely enquire about bowel incontinence in older patients (B).

Older patients with AI should be further assessed for reversible causes, regardless of their institutionalisation status (B).

IV. THE AGEING LOWER BOWEL AND PATHOPHYSIOLOGY IN OLDER ADULTS WITH ANAL INCONTINENCE

1. Quality of data

The findings from physiological studies of the lower bowel in older adults tend to be variable due to a) a variety of different techniques used in measuring anorectal function, b) unclear definition of the normative range of manometric measures for older people, c) poor matching between cases and controls of clinical factors which may affect gut function (e.g. level of mobility), or inadequate clinical information [388, 389] and d) small subject numbers in some cases [389-91]. Studies reviewed are cohort case-control to evaluate age-effect [392-4], young-old healthy subject comparisons [390, 391], and age- and sex-matched case-control studies of continent versus incontinent patients [388, 389, 395].

- **Anorectal function in healthy older adults**

Studies of age effect in healthy volunteers have shown a linear reduction with ageing in squeeze pressures in women after the age of 70, and in men from the 9th decade onwards [392, 393]. Age beyond 70 years was associated with reduction in basal pressures in both genders, but to a greater degree in women [392, 393]. A study of healthy adults in early old age showed no differences in sphincter pressures when compared with healthy young people [391].

Rectal motility appears to be unaffected by healthy ageing [390], but an age-related increase in anorectal sensitivity thresholds has been observed, starting at an earlier age in women than men [394].

2. Anorectal function in older adults with faecal incontinence

Rasmussen et al found prolonged pudendal nerve terminal motor latency (>2.2ms) in 34% of women aged over 50 with AI, though no relationship was observed between pudendal neuropathy and basal or squeeze pressures [396]. Advancing age was however related to declining basal pressures. Vaccaro et al similarly found an age-related increase in pudendal neuropathy in incontinent women, again unrelated to squeeze pressures [397]. Single fibre EMG in incontinent patients aged over 70 years showed increased fibre density in the external anal sphincter muscles compared with continent subjects, indicating some local reinnervation of these muscles following neurogenic damage [389].

Barrett et al. examined anorectal function in elderly medically frail incontinent patients and continent age- and sex-matched controls [388]. Individuals with AI had reduced internal anal sphincter pressures, and a lower threshold for expulsion of a rectal balloon. Patients with AI and dementia were more likely to exhibit multiple rectal contractions in response to rectal distension, though the role of these 'uninhibited' contractions in causing incontinence was unclear [388, 398].

A similar matched case-control study showed that elderly patients with rectal impaction and soiling had impaired rectal sensation (needing a larger volume before feeling the presence of a rectal balloon and the urge to void), lower rectal pressures during rectal distension, and impaired anal and perianal sensation ('rectal dyschezia') [395]. Basal and squeeze pressures were however unimpaired in these patients, and the rectoanal inhibitory response was well-preserved. The authors concluded that overflow AI is primarily due to locally secreted mucus from around an irritative rectal faecal mass leaking out, despite well-preserved anal sphincter integrity.

a) Summary

Anorectal function in healthy older persons is characterised by a tendency towards an age-related reduction in internal anal tone (2), and a more definite decline in external anal sphincter tone, especially in older women (2). An age-related decline in anorectal sensitivity in women has been observed (3), but rectal motility is well-preserved (3). Ageing alone however, appears to have little impact on anorectal function until later old age – from the 7th decade upwards in women and even later in men (2).

Age-related internal anal sphincter dysfunction is an important factor in faecal incontinence in elderly people (2).

Although pudendal neuropathy is an age-related phenomenon in women with AI (2), its significance as a predisposing factor for incontinence is unclear.

Stool impaction predisposing to overflow is related to rectal dyschezia in frail older adults, a condition characterised by reduced tone, increased compliance and impaired sensation (3b). Overflow AI is due to mucus secretion from around a rectal faecal bolus, rather than to impaired sphincter function (3).

b) Recommendations

- Overall, the physiological data suggests that AI should not be considered an inevitable consequence of ageing (B).
- Older adults with AI should be evaluated for age-related reduction in internal and external sphincter function (B).
- Older patients with AI require a digital examination to identify rectal stool impaction causing overflow (B). Patients who are unaware of the presence of a large faecal bolus in the rectum may have rectal dyschezia, and should be considered at risk of recurrent impaction with overflow (B)

V. CAUSES OF FAECAL INCONTINENCE IN OLDER PEOPLE

1. Quality of data

Risk factor studies have been reviewed above, and there is little additional data on causes of AI in this population. The causes of AI in older people, unlike in younger adults, are often multifactorial. The aim of this section is to categorise AI in the older adult by primary cause in a clinically meaningful way, emphasising the identification of potentially reversible factors.

a) Overflow incontinence secondary to constipation and stool impaction

The prevalence of faecal impaction and overflow AI is high in nursing home patients, implying that insitutionalisation may place older individuals at greater risk of this condition. Tobin et al showed overflow to be the underlying problem in 52% of nursing home residents with long-standing AI [199], while Read reported that faecal impaction was the main reason for acute hospitalisation in 27% of nursing home residents admitted over the course of a year [395].

While there is virtually no published data on causes of impaction and overflow, there are several studies evaluating potentially modifiable risk factors for constipation in older adults. Only one of these was prospective; Robson et al looked at baseline characteristics predictive of new-onset constipation in elderly nursing home patients, using the US Minimum Data Set instrument. Seven percent (n=1,291) developed constipation over a 3-month period. Independent predictors were white race, decreased fluid intake, Parkinson's disease, decreased mobility, arthritis, greater than 5 medications and dementia [399]. In mainly retrospective studies, other researchers have identified the following causes of constipation in older people:

Immobility - Symptoms of constipation, and level of laxative use have been shown to be less in older people who are more physically active [400-402].

Medication side-effects - Drugs most implicated are iron supplements, calcium supplements, calcium channel blockers, opiates, and non-steroidal anti-inflammatory drugs [403, 404]. Another important group of drugs affecting the bowel are those with anticholinergic properties (e.g. antipsychotics, tricyclic antidepressants, oxybutynin) which may induce irreversible colonic laxity with long-term use [402].

Parkinson's disease patients may suffer greatly from constipation because of dual pathologies of primary degeneration of dopaminergic neurons in the enteric nervous system resulting in prolonged transit throughout the entire gut [405], and pelvic dyssynergia resulting in rectal outlet delay and prolonged straining (406)

Low dietary fibre intake is common in the elderly, and has been associated (through meta-analysis) with increased stool weight and decreased transit time in healthy and constipated adults [407].

Low fluid intake in older adults has been related to slow colonic transit [408], and in young male volunteers over a 1-week period has been shown to reduce stool output [409]. Elderly people are at greater risk of dehydration due to impaired thirst sensation, and less effective hormonal responses to hypertonicity, while those in nursing homes and hospitals may in addition have functional reasons for being unable to drink.

Dementia predisposes individuals to rectal dyschezia [395, 398], possibly partly through ignoring the urge to defecate; a study in which young men deliberately suppressed defecation resulted in a prolongation of transit through the rectosigmoid with a marked reduction in frequency of bowel movements [410].

2. Functional incontinence

Functional incontinence occurs in individuals who are unable to access the toilet in time due to impairments in mobility, dexterity, or vision. These patients may even have normal lower gut function. Epidemiological studies of nursing home residents (see above) have repeatedly shown that poor mobility is a strong risk factor for AI after adjustment for other variables [381, 16, 386].

3. Dementia-related incontinence

Patients with advanced dementia may have a neurologically disinhibited rectum, with a tendency to void formed stool once or twice daily following mass peristaltic movements. Tobin et al documented dementia as the primary cause of AI in 46% of nursing home residents [199]. These individuals are very commonly incontinent of urine also.

4. Comorbidity-related incontinence

The following diseases may cause AI, and are more common in older people:

Stroke - Immediately following a stroke 40% of individuals are incontinent, and 10% remain so 6 months after the acute event [29]. There is very little data examining the pathophysiological basis for AI following stroke. AI in 3-month stroke survivors was shown to be more strongly associated with potentially modifiable factors of anticholinergic medication use, and functional difficulties in getting to the toilet, than with stroke severity or location in a multivariate adjusted analysis [411].

Diabetes mellitus - AI may occur in people with diabetic neuropathy affecting the gut through the dual mechanisms of a) bacterial overgrowth resulting from severe prolongation of gut transit causing the characteristic nocturnal diarrhoea and b) multifactorial anorectal dysfunction [412]. Case-control studies show that diabetic patients with AI have reduced basal and squeeze pressures, spontaneous relaxation of the internal anal sphincter, reduced rectal compliance, and abnormal rectal sensation [412, 413].

Sacral cord dysfunction - The neuropathophysiology of rectal dyschezia [18] is compatible with diminished parasympathetic outflow from the sacral cord. Conditions in older persons that could impair sacral cord function are ischaemia and spinal stenosis.

5. Anorectal incontinence

Age-related anal sphincter dysfunction is likely to contribute to the increased prevalence of AI in men and women in their 80's and beyond (see above). Rectal prolapse is also a cause of AI which occurs more commonly in older adults [393].

6. Loose stools

Loose stool increases the risk of AI in normally continent older adults by overwhelming a functional but age-compromised sphincter mechanism. Forty-four percent of cases of AI in a prospective nursing home study had diarrhoea as a primary cause [386].

Potentially reversible causes of loose stools in older adults are:

Excessive use of laxatives - One-third of community-dwelling people aged 65 and over regularly take laxatives, far exceeding the prevalence of constipation in this population [414]. Laxative use has been linked to AI in nursing home residents, in particular 'Codanthramer' [385].

Lactose intolerance is an age-related phenomonon - Goulding et al. found a lactose malabsorption rate of 15% in healthy women aged 40-59 years as compared with 50% in those aged 60-79 [415].

Antibiotic-related diarrhoea – Among hospitalised patients, age, female gender and nursing home residency sigificantly increases the risk for Clostridium difficile-associated diarrhoea associated with antibiotic use [416].

7. Summary

Overflow incontinence secondary to stool impaction is a primary cause of AI in nursing home residents (3).

There are multiple potentially modifiable causes of constipation in older people (2)

Older people may be incontinent because they are unable to use the toilet for functional reasons (2)

Dementia-related AI is an important cause of AI in nursing home residents (2b)

AI is a common complication following stroke (2), but causes other than stroke status itself may also contribute to incontinence in stroke survivors (2).

Loose stools predispose elderly people to soiling (2), and have potentially reversible causes (2).

8. Recommendations

- Nursing home residents with AI should be evaluated for the presence of overflow and impaction (B)
- Older patients with constipation should be carefully assessed for potentially modifiable causes of immobility, medication side-effects, low fibre intake, and low fluid intake (B).
- Functional AI should be identified early on in the assessment process (B)
- Cognitive status should be assessed when evaluating causes of AI in older individuals (B)
- The symptom of loose stools should be elicited in older people, and reversible causes sought (B).

VI. ASSESSMENT AND DIAGNOSIS OF FAECAL INCONTINENCE IN OLDER ADULTS

Table 18 summarises the clinical evaluation of faecal incontinence in older people. The emphasis is on a structured comprehensive clinical approach. In most cases this approach will provide sufficient diagnositic information on which to base a feasible management plan without resorting to more specialised tests and assessments.

Table 18 : Assessment and diagnosis of faecal incontinence in older people

Emphasis in older people is on a *structured clinical approach* to identify all contributing factors for faecal incontinence

• *History*

Duration of faecal incontinence

Frequency of episodes

Type (soiling, small amounts, complete bowel movement)

Stool consistency Stool-stained mucus

Passive or urge AI

Constipation symptoms / current laxative use

Systemic illness (confusion, depression, weight loss, anemia)

Antibiotic use

• *General examination*

Abbreviated Mental Status Examination (score of 6 or less out of 10 suggests significant cognitive impairment)

Mood assessment (for depression)

Neurological profile (stroke, autonomic neuropathy, Parkinson's disease)

• *Toilet access*

Evaluate ability to use toilet based on muscle strength, coordination, vision, limb function, and cognition.

Place in context of current living environment.

• *Specific examination*

Abdominal inspection for distension and tenderness

Perineal inspection for skin breakdown, dermatitis, surgical scars

Observe for excessive downward motion of the pelvic floor when asking patient to bear down in the lateral lying position

Digital examination for stool impaction

Digital examination for evaluation of impaired sphincter tone

• Anal gaping, and/or easy insertion of finger (internal sphincter)

• Reduced squeeze pressure (external sphincter)

Ask patient to strain while sitting on commode and observe for rectal prolapse

• *Tests*

An abdominal Xray should be performed to look for stool impaction in the colon

In the case of diarrhoea – send stool sample for culture, including C.Difficile

Blood tests for full blood count, glucose, urea and electrolytes, calcium, thyroxine

There is however much room for improvement in this clinical area; current surveys indicate a lack of thoroughness by doctors and nurses in assessing faecal incontinence in older people in all settings (community, acute hospital, and nursing home), with failure to obtain an accurate symptom history or to perform rectal examinations. A recent UK survey of physcian practice in performing rectal examinations in acutely hospitalised elderly patients found that of the 5% (n=10) of patients with AI, only two had undergone a rectal exam [417].

• ***Data quality***

There are few quality data evaluating methods of assessing and diagnosing AI in older adults. The information presented below is largely derived from review articles, and non-age specific studies.

• ***Results***

Documentation of the *type of incontinence* is diagnostically helpful. Self-report of bowel symptoms relating to AI have been shown to be reliable and reproducible in older cohorts [43, 39]. Constant leakage of loose stool or stool-stained mucus is characteristic of overflow around an impaction, while patients with anal sphincter dysfunction tend to leak small amounts of stool. Engel et al. showed in younger adults that where external anal sphincter weakness predominates the patient often reports urgency prior to leaking (urge AI), while those with internal sphincter dysfunction tend to have unconscious leakage of stool (passive AI) [418] Patients with dementia-related incontinence often pass complete bowel movements, especially after meals in response to the gastrocolic reflex.

Evaluation of *toilet access* should be multidisciplinary, and include a broad functional assessment (e.g. Barthel Index), mobility test (e.g. 'up and go' test), visual acuity test (count fingers), upper limb dexterity assessment (undoing buttons), and cognitive measure (e.g. Abbreviated Mental Test Score). For community patients, the health care provider should be aware of the physical layout of the patients home, and in particular bathroom details (location, distance from main living area, width of doorway for accomodating walking aids, presence of grab rails or raised toilet seat). Low lighting levels, high degree of clutter and hard to manage clothing may also be relevant.

Digital examination can reasonably assess anal sphincter tone in the clinical setting. Easy finger insertion with gaping of the anus on finger removal indicates poor internal sphincter tone, while reduced squeeze pressure around the finger when asking the patient to 'squeeze and pull up' suggests external sphincter weakness. Hallan et al. found that digital assessment of squeeze and basal tone was as sensitive and specific as manometry in discriminating sphincter function between continent and incontinent patients aged over 50 [116].

A digital rectal examination is essential for identifying stool impaction, although an empty rectum does not exclude the diagnosis of constipation [400]. All incontinent patients without evidence of rectal stool impaction should ideally undergo a *plain abdominal radiograph* in order to a) establish or rule out the diagnosis of overflow, b) measure the extent and severity of faecal loading, c) evaluate the degree of bowel obstruction secondary to impaction, d) rule out acute complications of impaction such as sigmoid volvulus and stercoral perforation and e) identify colonic motility/dysmotility [419-21].

1. Summary

Current evidence suggests that assessment of AI in older adults is suboptimal (2).

Documentation of the type of incontinence by self-report, proxy report or observation is diagnostically helpful (2).

Evaluation of ability to access and use the toilet should be multidisciplinary.

Digital assessment of sphincter tone can accurately discriminate between continent and incontinent adults (3).

2. Recommendations

- Standardisation of assessment methods of older adults with AI in all health care settings is required
- The emphasis in older people is on a structured clinical approach to identify multiple causes of AI (D), including cognitive and functional assessments (B).
- A careful bowel symptom history and assessment of voiding pattern should form part of the assessment (B).
- Digital assessment of sphincter tone in older people should be a first-line approach (B), with anorectal manometry testing reserved for a minority in whom surgery or biofeedback seems feasible (D).
- Digital rectal examination is essential in assessing older patients with AI, but those without evidence of rectal stool impaction should undergo a plain abdominal radiograph to rule out higher impaction and other problems (C).

VII. TREATMENT OF FAECAL INCONTINENCE IN OLDER ADULTS (Figure 6)

Quality of data

There are very few published trials of treatment of AI in

older people, and no trials on prevention of AI. The studies reviewed suffer from small numbers [199, 224], poor methodology (e.g. not applying intent-to-treat rule, unclear reporting of drop-outs) [199, 422], and no blinding (all). Randomised controlled trials examining effective laxative treatment for constipation in older adults also largely lack power, and are therefore unlikely to detect effects of treatment [423].

1. Treatment of faecal impaction and overflow anal incontinence in older people

Tobin et al. evaluated a therapeutic intervention in 52 nursing home residents with AI, based on treatment recommendations to general practitioners [199]. Patients with rectal impaction and continuous faecal soiling were classed as having overflow and recommended treatment with enemas until no further response followed by lactulose - complete resolution of incontinence was achieved in 94% of those in whom full treatment compliance could be obtained.

A French nursing home study of 206 frail elderly nursing home residents found that treatment of constipation was only effective in improving overflow AI (incontinence at least once weekly associated with impaired rectal emptying) when long-lasting and complete rectal emptying (monitored by weekly rectal examinations) could be achieved using daily lactulose, daily suppostories and weekly tap-water enemas [422]. Patients randomised to the group receiving lactulose only showed no reduction in frequency of AI. The analysis was not performed on an intent-to-treat basis and there was no description of the high number of subjects lost to follow-up.

Over half of nursing home residents take laxatives at least once daily, prompting speculation that nonpharmacological approaches to optimise management of constipation may be under-utilised in this setting [385]. A recent systematic review of effective laxative treatment in elderly persons found that RCT's in this area are potentially flawed due to small numbers, but nevertheless commented that significant improvements in bowel movement frequency have been observed with cascara and lactulose, while bulk laxative psyllium and lactulose have been reported to improve stool consistency and related symptoms in placebo-controlled trials [423]. Observational studies of nursing home residents (i.e. those at risk of impaction with overflow) suggest that stimulant and osmotic laxatives (lactulose and polyethylene glycol) may be effective [423, 424].

Although enemas are considered useful in the clinical setting for acute disimpaction and treatment of overflow, there are no data examining effectiveness other than case-reports. Case-series suggest that phosphate enemas should be used with caution in people with renal failure (no more than once weekly) [425].

2. Treatment of dementia-related faecal incontinence

Ouslander et al showed that prompted voiding programmes significantly increased the number of continent bowel movements in an uncontrolled study of elderly nursing home residents with dementia-related incontinence over a period of a few weeks, but no impact was seen on frequency of AI [262].

Tobin et al evaluated a bowel programme in 25 nursing home residents with dementia-related AI, consisting of daily codeine phophate and twice weekly enemas; continence was achieved in 75% of those fully treated [199].

3. Treatment of AI in older adults due to anal sphincter weakness

Biofeedback treatment for AI in older people resulted in a 75% reduction in incontinent episodes short-term in one small study of a highly selected group of patients with no cognitive impairment, good motivation and intact anorectal sensation [224].

Loperamide is recommended for treatment of anorectal incontinence [193], though there are no data on its efficacy in older people. In one small placebo-drug crossover trial in older adults, loperamide oxide significantly reduced visual analogue scores for incontinence and urgency, and both prolonged colonic transit and increased basal tone [195].

a) Summary

There are too few data to determine what constitutes effective laxative treatment of faecal impaction with overflow AI (1) Although good quality data are lacking, stimulant and osmolar laxatives may be effective in treating constipation in older people at risk of overflow (2).

Treatment approaches to dementia-related AI (prompted toileting, controlled evacuation) may be helpful in the nursing home setting (3).

Biofeedback is unlikely to help more than a minority of older adults with AI (3).

Loperamide is a useful drug treatment for anorectal AI in the absence of constipation (4).

b) Recommendations

All underlying causes of AI in each older individual should be identified and treated (D).

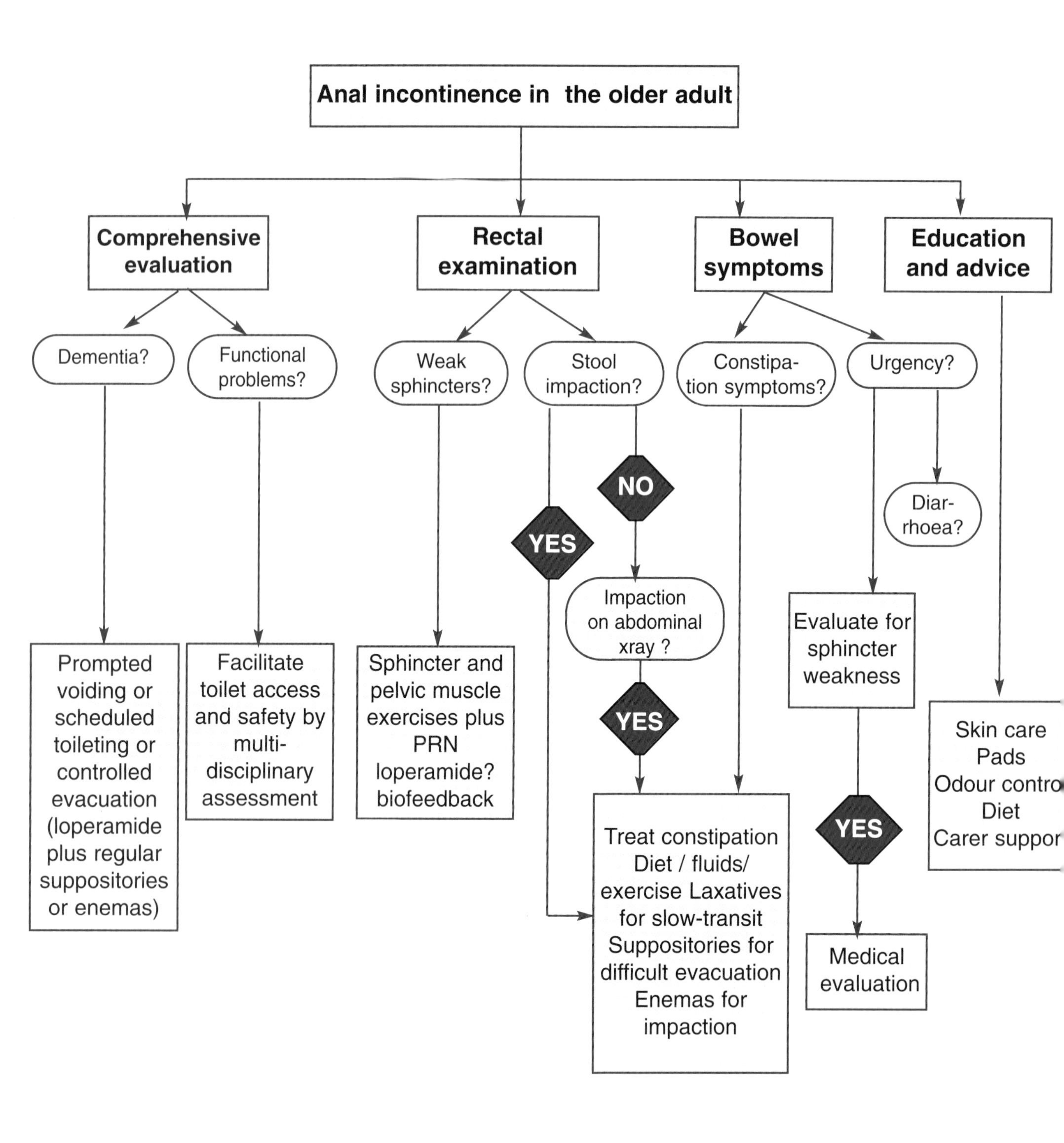

Figure 6 : Algorithmic approach to management of AI in older adults

As older adults with AI are not a homogenous group, a multicomponent research approach in the form of a randomised controlled trial evaluating a structured managment protocols versus usual care would be helpful. Such a study should be sufficiently large to permit subgroup analysis of targeted treament protocols are required.

RCT's of laxative and nonpharmacological treatment and prevention of faecal impaction in and overflow are needed to optimise standards of prescribing and care.

A multidisciplinary RCT assessing a step-wise approach to management of dementia-related AI in nursing home residents (prompted voiding in those with mild to moderate dementia, scheduled toileting plus suppositories next step, bowel programme of controlled evacuation in those with persistent incontinence) would be of great value.

Greater emphasis needs to be placed on systematic and effective management of faecal incontinence in older people backed up by sound communications between doctors and nurses, especially in the nursing home and acute hospital setting (D)

Patient and carer education should be undertaken to promote self-efficacy and other coping mechanisms, and where appropriate self-management (e.g. reducing risk of constipation and impaction through dietary and lifestyle measures, advice on how to take loperamide) (D). Advice on skin care, odour control, and continence aids is also important (D).

Figure 6 shows an algorithmic approach to management of AI in older adults.

REFERENCES

1. Royal College of Physicians. Incontinence. Causes, management and provision of services. A Working Party of the Royal College of Physicians. Journal of the Royal College of Physicians of London 29, 272-274. 1995.
2. Whitehead,W.E., Wald,A., Diamant,N.E., Enck,P., Pemberton,J.H. and Rao,S.S.C. Functional disorders of the anus and rectum. Gut 45, 1155-1159. 1999.
3. Johanson,J.F. and Lafferty,J. Epidemiology of fecal incontinence: the silent affliction. Am.J.Gastroenterol. 91, 33-36. 1996
4. Leigh,R.J. and Turnberg,L.A. Faecal incontinence: the unvoiced symptom. Lancet 1, 1349-1351. 1982.
5. Small KA and Wynne JM. Evaluating the pelvic floor in obstetric patients. Aust. New Zeal. Obstet. Gynecol., 30:41-45, 1990.
6. Madoff RD, Williams JG and Caushaj PF. Current Concepts; Fecal Incontinence. NEJM., 326:1002-7,1992.
7. Abou-Zahr C. Obstructed labour. In Murray CJL, Lopez AD. Health dimensions of sex and reproduction: the global burden of sexually transmitted diseases, HIV, maternal conditions, perinatal disorders and congenital anomalies. Cambridge. Harvard University Press, 1996.
8. Drossman DA. What can be done to control incontinence associated with the irritable bowel syndrome? Am. J. Gastroent., 84:355-57, 1989.
9. Schiller LR, Sanat Ana CA, Schmulen AC, Hendler RS, Harford WV and Fordtran JS. Pathogenesis of fecal incontinence in diabetes mellitus. NEJM., 307:1666-71, 1982.
10. Thomas TM, Egan M, Walgrove A and Meade TW. The prevalence of faecal and double incontinence. Comm. Med., 6:216-20, 1984.
11. Campbell AJ, Reinken J and McCosh L. Incontinence in the elderly: prevalence and prognosis. Age and Aging, 14:65-70, 1985.
12. Kok ALM, Voorhorst FJ, Burger CW, van Houten P, Kenemans P and Jansens J. Urinary and faecal incontinence in community-residing elderly women. Age & Aging, 21:211-15, 1992.
13. Denis P, Bercoff E, Bizien MF, Brocker P, Chassagne P, Lamouliatte H, Leroi AM, Perrigot M and Weber J. Etude de la prevalence de l'incontinence anale chez l'adulte. Gastroent. Clin Biol., 16:344-50, 1992.
14. DA, Li Z, Andruzzi E, Temple RD, Talley NJ, Thomp-son WG, Whitehead WE, Janssens J, Funch-Jensen P, Corazziari E, Richter JE and Koch GG. U.S. Householder survey of functional GI disorders: prevalences, sociodemography and health impact. Dig. Dis. & Sciences, 38:1569-80, 1993.
15. MacLennan AH, Taylor AW, Wilson DH, Wilson D. The prevalence of pelvic floor disorders and their relationship to gender, age, parity and mode of delivery. BJOG, 107:1460-1470, 2000
16. Nelson RL, Norton N, Cautley E and Furner S. Community based prevalence of anal incontinence. JAMA, 274:559-562, 1995.
17. Enck P, Bielefeld K, Rathmann W, PurrmannJ, Tschope D, Erkenbrecht JF. Epidemiology of faecal incontinence in selected patient groups. Int J Colorectal Dis., 6:143-146, 1991
18. Wisconsin Family Health Survey, Center for Health Statis-tics, Division of Health, Department of Health and Social Serv-ices, P.O. Box 309, Room 172, Madison Wisconsin 53701-0309, 1994.
19. Nelson RL, Furner S, Jesudason V. Fecal incontinence in Wisconsin nursing homes. Dis Colon & Rectum, 41:1226-1229, 1998
20. Borrie MJ, Davidson HA. Incontinence in institutions: costs and contributing factors. CMAJ, 147:322-328, 1992.
21. Hojberg KE, Salvig JD, Winslow NA, Bek KM, Laurberg S, Secher NJ. Flatus and faecal incontinence: prevelence and risk factors at 16 weeks of gestation. BJOG, 107:1097-1103, 2000.
22. Donnelly V, Fynes M, Campbell D, Johnson H, O'Connel PR, O'Herlihy C. Obstetric events leading to anal sphincter damage. Obstet Gynecol., 92:955-961, 1998.
23. Donnely VS, O'Herlihy C, Campbell DM, O'Connel PR. Postpartum fecal incontinence is more common in women with irritable bowel syndrome. Dis. Colon & Rectum, 41:586-589, 1998.
24. Nygaard IE, Rao SSC, Dawson JD. Anal incontinence after anal sphincter disruption: a 30 year perspective. Obstet. Gynec., 89:896-901, 1997.
25. Wald A. Systemic diseases causing disorders of defecation and continence. Sem Gastroint Dis., 6:194-202, 1995.
26. MacKenzie WR, Hoxie NJ, Proctor ME, Gradus MS, Blair KA, Petersen DE, Kazmierczak JJ, Addiss DG, Fox KR, Rose JB and Davis JP. A massive outbreak in Milwaukee of cryptosporidium infection transmitted through the public water supply. NEJM, 331:161-7, 1994.
27. Sullivan SN, Wong C. Runner's diarrhea. Different patterns and associated factors. J. Clin Gastroent., 14:101-104, 1992.

28. Bliss DZ, Johnson S, Savik K, Clabots CR, Gerding DN. Fecal incontinence in hospitalized patients who are acutely ill. Nursing Res., 49:101-108, 2000.

29. Nakayama H, Joergensen HS, Pedersen PM, Raaschou HO, Olsen TS. Prevelance and risk factors of incontinence after stroke: The Copenhagen stroke study. Stroke, 28:58-62, 1997

30. Pernikoff BJ, Eisenstat TE, Rubin RJ, et al. Reappraisal of partial lateral internal sphincterotomy. Dis. Colon & Rectum, 37;1291-5, 1994.

31. del Pino A, Nelson RL, Pearl RK, Abcarian H. Island flap ano plasty for treatment of transsphincteric fistula-in-ano. Dis. Colon & Rectum, 39;224-6, 1996.

32. Gorfine SR. Treatment of benign anal disease with topical nitroglycerin. Dis. Colon & Rectum, 38;453-7, 1995.

33. von Flue M, Harder F. A new technique for pouchanal reconstruction after total mesorectal excision. Dis. Colon & Rectum, 37:1160-2, 1994.

34. Ishigooka M, Hashimoto T, Izumiya K, Sasagawa I, Nakada T. Incidence of anal incontinence after long-term follow-up of patients treated by ureterosigmoidostomy. Int Urol Nephrol., 25:455-460, 1993.

35. Norton,C. and Chelvanayagam,S. A nursing assessment tool for adults with fecal incontinence. Journal of Wound, Ostomy, & Continence Nursing 27, 279-291, 2000.

36. Talley, N.J., Phillips, S.F., Melton, L.J., Wiltgen, C., Zinsmeister, A.R.,: A patient questionnaire to identify bowel disease. Ann Intern Med.111:671-4, 1989.

37. Talley, N.J., Phillips, S.F.Wiltgen, C.M., Zinsmeister, A.R., Melton, L.J.: Assessment of functional bowel disease: The bowel disease questionnaire. Mayo Clin. Proc. 65:1456-79, 1990.

38. Manning, A.P., Thompson, W.G., Heaton, K.W., Morris, A.F.,: Towards positive diagnosis of the irritable bowel. Br. Med. J. 2:653-4, 1978.

39. O'Keefe, E.A., Talley, N.J., Tanagalos, E.G. and Zinsmeister, A.R.: A bowel symptom questionnaire for the elderly. Journal of Gerontology. 47(4):M116-M1, 1992.

40. Best, W.R.,Becktel, J.M., Singleton, J.W., Kern, F.: Development of a Crohn's disease activity index: National Cooperative Crohn's Disease Study. Gastroenterology 70:439-44, 1976.

41. Harvey, R.F., Bradshaw, J.M.: A simple index of Crohn's disease activity. Lancet 1:514, 1980.

42. Van Hees, P.A.M., Van Elteren, P.H., Van Lier, H.J.J., Van Tongeren, J.H.M.: An index of inflammatory activity in patients with Crohn's disease. Gut 21:279-86, 1980.

43. Osterberg, A., Graf, W., Karlbom, Pahlman, L.: Evaluation of a questionnaire in the assessment of patients with faecal incontinence and constipation. Scand J. Gastroenterol. 31:575-580, 1996.

44. Reilly, W.T., Talley, N.J., Pemberton, J.H. and Zinsmeister, A.R.: Validation of a questionnaire to assess fecal incontinence and associated risk factors. Dis. Colon Rectum 43:146-154, 2000.

45. Roberts, R.O., Jacobsen, S.J., Reilly, W.T., Pemberton, J.H., Lieber, M.M. and Talley, N.J.: Prevalence of combined fecal and urinary incontinence: A community based study. J. Am. Geriatric Soc. 47:837-841, 1999.

46. Bishoff, J.T., Motley, G., Optenberg, S.A., Stein, C.R., Moon, K.A., Browning, S.M., Sabanegh, E., Foley, J.P. Thompson, I.M.: Incidence of fecal and urinary incontinence following radical perineal and retropubic prostatectomy in a national population. J Urol. 160:454-458, 1998.

47. Hiltunen, K.M., Matikainen, M., Auvinen, O., Hietanen, P.: Clinical and manometric evaluation of anal sphincter function in incontinent patients. Am J. Surg. 151:489-92, 1986.

48. Broden, G., Dolk, A., Holmstroem, B.: Recovery of the internal anal sphincter following rectopexy: a possible explanation for continence improvement. Int. J. Colorectal Des. 3:23-8, 1988.

49. Kelly, J.H.: Cineradiography in anorectal malformation. J. Pediatric Surg. 4:538, 1968 and Parks, A.G.: Anorectal incontinence. J. R. Soc. Med. 68:21-30, 1975.

50. Shelton, A., Madoff, R.: Defining anal incontinence: establishing a uniform continence scale. Semin. Colon Rectal Surg. 8:54-60, 1997.

51. Holschneider, A.M.: Treatment and functional results of anorectal continence in children with imperforated anus. Acta Chir Belg 3:191-204, 1983.

52. Keighley,M.R. and Fielding W.L.: Management of faecal incontinence and results of surgical treatment. Br. J. Surg 70:463-468, 1983.

53. Rudd, W.W.: The transanal anastomosis: a sphincter saving operation with improved continence. Dis. Colon Rectum 22:102-5, 1979.

54. Womack, N.R., Morrison, J.F., Williams, N.S.: Prospective study of the effects of post-anal repair in neurogenic fecal incontinence. Br. J. Surg. 75:48-52, 1988.

55. Corman, M.: Gracilis muscle transposition for anal incontinence. Late results. Br. J. Surg 72:S21-22, 1985.

56. Rainey, J.B., Donaldson, D.N., Thomson, J.P.: Post-anal repair: which patients derive most benefit? J.R. Coll Surg. Edinb 35:101-105, 1990.

57. Rockwood, T.H., Church, J.M., Fleshman, J.W., Kane, R.L., Mavrantonis, C., Thorson, A.G., Wexner, S.D., Bliss, D., and Lowry, A.C.: Patient and surgeon ranking of the severity of symptoms associated with fecal incontinence. The Fecal Incontinence Severity Index. Dis. Colon Rectum. 42:1525-1532, 1999.

58. Pescatori, M., Anastasio, G., Bottini, C., Mentasti, A.: New grading and scoring for anal incontinence. Dis. Colon Rectum 35:482-487, 1992.

59. Jorge, J.M.N., Wexner, S.D.: Etiology and management of fecal incontinence. Dis. Colon Rectum 36:77-97, 1993.

60. V aizey, D.J., Carapenti, E., Cahill, J.A. and Kamm, M.A.: Prospective comparison of faecal incontinence grading systems. Gut. 44:77-80, 1999.

61. Gill, T.M., Feinstein, A.R.: A critical appraisal of the quality of Quality of Life measurements. JAMA 272(8):619-626, 1994.

62. Maunder, R.G., Cohen, Z., McLeod, R.S., Greenberg, G.R.: Effect of intervention in inflammatory bowel disease on Health-Related Quality of Life: A critical review. Dis. Colon Rectum 38:1147-1161, 1995.

63. Stewart, A.L., Greenfield, S., Hays, R.D. et al: Functional status and well-being of patients with chronic conditions. Results from the Medical Outcomes Study. JAMA 262:907-912, 1989

64. Stewart, A.L., Hay R.D., Ware, J.E.: The MOS short form general health survey: reliability and validity in a patient population. Medical Care 26:724-35, 1988.

65. Hassink, A.A.M., Rieu, P.N.M.A,, Brugman, A.T.M., Festen, C: Quality of Life after operatively corrected high anorectal malformation: A long-term follow-up study of patients aged 18 years and older. Journal of Pediatric Surgery. 29:773-776, 1994.

66. Tiainen, J., Matikainen, M.: Health related quality of life after ileal J-pouch anal anastomosis for ulcerative colitis: Long term results. Scand J. Gastroenterol. 34:601-605, 1999.

67. Fazio, V.W., O'Riordain, Lavery, I.C., Church, J.M., Lau, P., Strong, S.A., Hull, T.: Long term functional outcome and quality of life after stapled restorative proctocolectomy. Annals of Surgery 230:575-586, 1999.

68. Guyant, G., Mitchell, A., Irvine, E.J. et al: A new measure of health status for clinical trials in inflammatory bowel disease. Gastroenterology. 96:804-810, 1989.

69. Drossman, D.A., Lesserman, J., Li, Z., Mitchell, C.M., Zagami, E.A., Patrick, D.L.: The rating form of IBD patient concerns: A new measure of health status. Psychosom Med. 53:701-12, 1991.

70. Rockwood, T.H., Church, J.M., Fleshman,J.W., Kane, R.L., Mavrantonis, C., Thorson, A.G., Wexner, S.D., Bliss, D., Lowry, A.C.: Fecal incontinence quality of life scale: Quality of life instrument for patients with fecal incontinence. Dis. Colon Rectum 43:9-17, 2000.

71. McLeod, R.S: Re: Fecal incontinence quality of life scale: Quality of life instrument for patients with fecal incontinence (editorial) Dis Colon Rectum 43:16-17, 2000.

72. McHugh SM, Diamant E: Effect of age, gender, and parity on anal canal pressures. Contribution of impaired anal sphincter function to fecal incontinence. Digestive Diseases & Sciences 32 (7): 726-36, 1987.

73. Ferrara A, Pemberton JH, Hanson RB: Preservation of continence after ileoanal anastomosis by the coordination of ileal pouch and anal canal motor activity. AM J Surg 163:83-89, 1992.

74. Womack NNR, Morrison JFB, Williams NS: Prospective study of the effects of post anal repair in neurogenic faecal incontinence. Br J Surg 75:48-52, 1988.

75. Parks AG, Porter NH, Melzak J: Experimental study of the reflex mechanism controlling the muscles of the pelvic floor. Dis Colon Rectum 5:407-414, 1962.

76. Parks AG: Anorectal incontinence. Proc Roy Soc Med 68:681-690, 1975.

77. Bartolo DCC, Roe AM, Locke-Edmonds JC: Flap valve theory of anorectal incontinence. Br J Surg 73:1012-1014, 1986.

78. Varma KK, Stephens D: Neuromuscular reflexes of rectal continence. Aust N Z J Med 41:263-272, 1972.

79. Barnes PR, Hawley PR, Preston DM, et al: Experience of posterior division of the puborectalis muscle in the management of chronic constipation. Br J Surg 72:475-477, 1985.

80. Phillips SF, Edwards DAW: Some aspects of anal continence and defecation. Gut 6:396-405, 1965.

81. Taylor BM, Beart RW, Jr., Phillips SF: Longitudinal and radial variations of pressure in the human anal sphincter. Gastroenterology, 86(4):693-7, 1984.

82. Rasmusson OO: Anorectal function. Dis Colon Rectum 37:386-403, 1994.

83. O'Connell PR, Pemberton JH, Kelly KA: Motor function of the ileal J pouch and its relation to clinical outcome after ileal pouch-anal anastomosis. World J Surg 11:735-741, 1987.

84. Pemberton JH, Kelly KA, Beart RW, Jr., Dozois RR, Wolff BG, Ilstrup DM: Ileal pouch-anal anastomosis for chronic ulcerative colitis. Long-term Results. Annals of Surgery, 206(4):504-13, 1987.

85. Beart RW, Jr., Dozois RR, Wolff BG, Pemberton JH: Mechanisms of rectal continence. Lessons from the ileoanal procedure. American Journal of Surgery, 149(1): 31-4, 1995.

86. Grotz RL, Pemberton JH, Levin KE, et al: Rectal wall contractility in healthy subjects and in patients with chronic severe constipation. Ann Surg 218:761-768, 1993.

87. McNeil NI, Rampton DS: Is the rectum usually empty? A quantitative study in subjects with and without diarrhea. Dis Colon Rectum 23:596-599, 1981.

88. Hammer J, Phillips SF: Fluid loading of the human colon: Effects on segmental transit and stool composition. Gastroenterology 105:988-998, 1993.

89. B, Malmud L, D'Ercole F, et al: Colonic transit scintigraphy: A physiologic approach to the quantitative measurement of colonic transit in human. Gastroenterology 91:1102-1112, 1986.

90. Proano M, Camilleri M, Phillips SF, et al: Transit of solids through the human colon: Regional quantification in the unprepared bowel. Am J Physiol 248:G856-862, 1990.

91. Ferrara A, Pemberton JH, Grotz RL, Hanson RB: Prolonged ambulatory recording of anorectal motility in patients with slow-transit constipation. American Journal of Surgery, 167(1):73-9, 1994 January.

92. Haynes WG, Read NW: Anorectal activity in man during rectal infusion of saline: A dynamic assessment of the anal continence mechanism. J Physiol 330:45-56, 1982.

93. Scarli AF, Kiesewetter WB: Defecation and continence. Dis Colon Rectum 13:81-107, 1970.

94. Womack NR, Williams NS, Holmfield JH, et al: New method for the dynamic assessment of anorectal function in constipation. Br J Surg 72:994-998, 1985.

95. Barkel DC, Pemberton JH, Pezim ME, Phillips SF, Kelly KA, Brown ML: Scintigraphic assessment of the anorectal angle in health and after ileal pouch-anal anastomosis. Annals of Surgery 208(1):42-9, 1988 July.

96. Womack NR, Williams NS, Holmfield JHM, et al: Anorectal function in the solitary rectal ulcer syndrome. Dis Colon Rectum 30:319-323, 1987.

97. Ambroze WL, Pemberton JH, Bell AM, et al: The effect of stool consistency on rectal and neorectal emptying. Dis Colon Rectum 34:1-7, 1991.

98. Christmas TJ, Kempster PA, Chapple CR: Role of subcutaneous apomorphine in Parkinsonian voiding dysfunction. Lancet 2:1451-1453, 1988.

99. Andrew J, Nathan P: Lesions of the anterior frontal lobes and disturbances of micturition and defaecation. Brain 87:233-262, 1964.

100. Sultan AH, Kamm MA, Hudson CN, et al: Anal sphincter disruption during vaginal delivery. N Engl J Med 329:1905-1911, 1993.

101. Swash M, Gray A, Lubowski DZ, et al: Ultrastructural changes in internal anal sphincter in neurogenic faecal incontinence. Gut 29:1692-1968, 1988.

102. Read NW, Bartolo DCC, Read MG: Differences in anal function in patients with incontinence to solids and in patients with incontinence to liquids. Br J Surg 71:29-42, 1984.

103. Sun WM, Read NW, Miner PB, et al: The role of transient sphincter relaxation in faecal incontinence. Int J Colorect Dis 5:31-36, 1990.

104. Bannister JJ, Read NW, Donnelly TC, et al: External and internal anal sphincter responses to rectal distension in normal subjects and in patients with idiopathic faecal incontinence. Br J Surg 76:617-621, 1989.

105. Law PJ, Kamm MA, Bartram CI: Anal endosonography in the investigation of faecal incontinence. Br J Surg 78:312-314, 1991.

106. Speakman CTM, Hoyle CHV, Kamm MA: Adreneregic control of the internal anal sphincter is abnormal in patients with idiopathic faecal incontinence. Br J Surg 77:1342-1344, 1990.

107. Parks AG, Swash M, Urich H: Sphincter denervation in anorectal incontinence and rectal prolapse. Gut 18:656-666, 1977.

108. Snooks SJ, Setchell M, Swash M: Injury to the innervation of the pelvic floor causing damage to the pelvic floor musculature in childbirth. Lancet 2:546-550, 1984.

109. Fynes M, Donnelly VS, O'Connell PR, O'Herlihy C: Cesarean delivery and anal sphincter injury. Obstetrics & Gynecology 92(4 Pt 1):496-500, 1998.

110. Miller R, Bartolo DCC, Cervero F, et al: Differences in anal sensation in continent and incontinent patient with perineal descent. Int J Colorectal Dis 4:45-49, 1989.

111. Read NW, Abouzekry L: Why do patients with faecal impaction have faecal incontinence? Gut 27:283-287, 1986.

112. Madoff RD, Williams JG, Caushaj PF: Fecal incontinence. N Engl J Med 326:1002-1007, 1992.

113. Fleshman JW, Dreznick Z, Fry RD, et al: Anal sphincter repair for obstetric injury: Manometric evaluation of functional results. Dis Colon Rectum 34:1061-1067, 1991.

114. Pemberton JH: Anorectal and pelvic disorders: Putting physiology into practice. J Gastroenterol Hepatol 5:127-143, 1990.

115. Barkel DC, Pemberton JH, Pezim ME, et al: Scintigraphic assessment of the anorectal angle in health and following ileal pouch-anal anastomosis. Ann Surg 208:42-49, 1988.

116. Hallan RI, Marzouk DEMM, Waldron DJ, et al: Comparison of digital and manometric assessment of anal sphincter function. Br J Surg 76:973-975, 1988.

117. Neill ME, Swash M: Increased motor unit fibre density in the external anal sphincter muscle in anorectal incontinence: a single fibre EMG study. J Neurol Neurosurg Psychiatry 43:343-347, 1980.

118. Snooks SJ, Barnes PRH, Swash M: Damage to the innervation of the pelvic floor musculature in chronic constipation. Gastroenterology 89:977-981, 1985.

119. Laurberg S, Swash M, Henry MM: Delayed external sphincter repair for obstetric tear. British Journal of Surgery 75(8):786-8, 1988.

120. Bartram GI, Turnbull GK, Lennard-Jones JE: Evacuation proctography: An investigation of rectal expulsion in 20 subjects without defecatory disturbance. Gastrointest Radiol 13:72-80, 1988.

121. Goie R: Anorectal function in patients with defaecation disorders and asymptomatic subjects. Radiology 174:121-123, 1990.

122. Law PJ, Kamm MA, Bartram CI: Anal endosonography: Technique and normal anatomy. Gastrointest Radiol 14:349-353, 1989.

123. Stoker J, Halligan S, Bartram CI: Pelvic floor imaging. Radiology 218(3):621-41, 2001 March

124. Malouf AJ, Halligan S, Williams AB, Bartram CI, Dhillon S, Kamm MA: Prospective assessment of interobserver agreement for endoanal MRI in fecal incontinence. Abdominal Imaging 26(1):76-8, 2001.

125. Glazener CMA, Abdalla M, Stroud P, Naji S, Templeton A, Russell IT. Postnatal maternal morbidity: extent, causes, prevention and treatment. Br J Obstet Gynaecol 102:282-87, 9195.

126. Beersiek F, Parks AG Swash M. Pathogenesis of anorectal incontinence: a histometric study of the anorectal musculature. J Neurol Sci 42:111-127, 1979.

127. Neill ME, Swash M. Increased motor unit fibre density in the external anal sphincter in ano-rectal incontinence: a single fibre EMG study. J Neurol Neurosurg Psychiatry 43:343-347, 1980.

128. Kiff ES and Swash M. Slowed conduction in the pudendal nerves in idiopathic (neurogenic) faecal incontinence. B J Surg 71:614-616, 1984.

129. Snooks SJ, Swash M, Setchell M, Henry MM. Injury to innervation of pelvic floor sphincter musculature in childbirth. Lancet 2:546-50, 1984.

130. Snooks SJ, Swash M, Mathers SE and Henry MM. Effect of vaginal delivery on the pelvic floor: a 5-year follow-up. Br J Surg 77:1358-60, 1990.

131. Allen RE, Hosker GL, Smith ARB, Warrell DW. Pelvic floor damage and childbirth: a neurophysiological study. Br J Obstet Gynaecol 97:770-779, 1990.

132. Mallett V, Hosker G, Smith ARB, Warrell D. Pelvic floor damage and childbirth: a neurophysiologic follow up study. Neurourol Urodyn 13:357-8, 1994.

133. Small KA, Wynne JM. Evaluating the pelvic floor in obstetric patients. Aust NZ J Obstet Gynaecol 30:41-5, 1990.

134. Cornes H, Bartolo DCC, Stirrat GM. Changes in anal canal sensation after childbirth. Br J Surg 78:74-7, 1991.

135. Chaliha C, Sultan AH, Kalia V, Monga AK, Stanton SL. Anal incontinence during pregnancy and following childbirth Am J Obstet Gynecol 2001, in press.

136. Sultan AH, Kamm MA, Talbot IC, Nicholls RJ, Bartram CI. Anal endosonography: Precision of identifying sphincter defects confirmed histologically. Br J Surg 81:466-9, 1994.

137. Sultan AH, Kamm MA, Nicholls RJ, Bartram CI. Internal anal sphincter division during lateral sphincterotomy. Prospective ultrasound study. Dis Colon Rectum 37:1031-33, 1994.

138. Fynes M, Donnelly VS, O'Connell PR, O'Herlihy C. Cesarean delivery and anal sphincter injury. Obstet Gynecol 92:496-500, 1988.

139. Abramowitz L, Sobhani I, Ganasia R, Vuagnat A, Benifla JL, Darai E, Madelenat P, Mignon M. Are sphincter defects the cause of anal incontinence after vaginal delivery? Results of a prospective study. Dis Colon Rectum 43:590-8, 2000.

140. DeLeeuw JW, Struijk PC, Vierhout ME, Wallenburg HCS. Risk factors for third degree perineal ruptures during delivery. Br J Obstet Gynaecol 108:383-7, 2001.

141. Buchhave P, Flatow L, Rydhystroem H, Thorbert G. Risk factors for rupture of the anal sphincter. Eur J Obstet Gynecol Reproduct Biol 87:129-32, 1999.

142. Fynes M, Donnelly V, Behan M, O'Connell PR, O'Herlihy C. Effect of second vaginal delivery on anorectal physiology and faecal incontinence: a prospective study. Lancet 354:983-6, 1999.

143. Varma A, Gunn J, Gardiner A, Lindow SW, Duthie GS. Obstetric anal sphincter injury. Prospective evaluation of incidence. Dis Colon Rectum 42:1537-43, 1999.

144. Rieger N, Schloithe A, Saccone G, Wattchow D. A prospective study of anal sphincter injury due to childbirth. Scand J Gastroenterol 33:950-5, 1998.

145. Zetterstrom J, Mellgren A, Jensen LJ, Wong WD, Kim DG, Lowry AC, Madoff RD, Congilosi SM. Effect of delivery on anal sphincter morphology and function. Dis Colon Rectum 42:1253-60, 1999.

146. Damon H, Henry L, Bretones S, Mellier G, Minaire Y, Mion F. Postdelivery anal function in primiparous females. Ultrasound and manometric study. Dis Colon Rectum 43:472-7, 2000.

147. Faltin DL, Boulvain M, Irion O, Bretones S. Stan C, Weil A. Diagnosis of anal sphincter tears by postpartum endosonography to predict fecal incontinence. Obstet Gynecol 95:643-7, 2000.

148. Groom KM, Paterson-Brown S. Third degree tears: are they clinically underdiagnosed? Gastroenterology International 13(2):76-7, 2000.

149. Sultan AH, Kamm MA, Hudson CN. Obstetric perineal tears: an audit of training. Journal of Obstetrics and Gynaecology 15:19-23, 1995.

150. Sultan AH, Thakar R. Lower genital tract and anal sphincter trauma. In: Baskett and Arulkumaran: Operative and Intrapartum Surgery. Bailliere's Best Practice & Research – Clinical Obstetrics and Gynaecology, 2002 in press.

151. Sultan AH. Editorial: Obstetric perineal injury and anal incontinence. Clinical Risk 5 (5):193-6, 1999.

152. Sultan AH, Kamm MA, Hudson CN, Bartram CI. Third degree obstetric anal sphincter tears: risk factors and outcome of primary repair. BMJ 308:887-91, 1994.

153. Sangalli MR, Floris L, Weil A. Anal incontinence in women with third or fourth degree perineal tears and subsequent vaginal deliveries. Aust N Z J Obstet Gynaecol 40:244-8, 2000.

154. Fitzpatrick M, Behan M, O'Connell R, O'Herlihy C. A randomized clinical trial comparing primary overlap with approximation repair of third degree obstetric tears. Am J Obstet Gynecol 183:1220-4, 2000.

155. Zetterstrom J, Lopez A, Anzen B, Norman M, Holmstrom B, Mellgren A. Anal sphincter tears at vaginal delivery: Risk factors and clinical outcome of primary repair. Obstet Gynecol 24:21-8, 1999.

156. Gjessing H, Backe B, Sahlin Y. Third degree obstetric tears; outcome after primary repair. Acta Obstet Gynecol Scand 77:736-40, 1998.

157. Poen AC, Felt-Bersma RJF, Strijers RLM, Dekkers GA, Cuesta MA, Meuwissen SGM. Third-degree obstetric perineal tear: long-term clinical and functional results after primary repair. Br J Surg 85:1433-8, 1998.

158. Goffeng AR, Andersch B, Berndtsson I, Hulten L, Oresland T. Objective methods cannot predict anal incontinence after primary repair of extensive anal tears. Acta Obstet Gynecol Scand 77: 439- 43, 1988.

159. Kammerer-Doak DN, Wesol AB, RogersRG, Dominguez, Dorin MH. A prospective cohort study of women after primary repair of obstetric anal sphincter laceration. Am J Obstet Gynecol.;181(6):1317-23, 1999

160. Sultan AH, Monga AK, Kumar D, Stanton SL. Primary repair of obstetric anal sphincter rupture using the overlap technique. Br J Obstet Gynaecol ;106:318-323, 1999.

161. Malouf AJ, Norton CS, Engel AF, Nicholls RJ, Kamm MA. Long term results of overlapping anterior anal-sphincter repair for obstetric trauma. Lancet ;355: 260-5, 2000.

162. Wood J, Amos L, Rieger N. Third degree anal sphincter tears: risk factors and outcome. Aust N Z J Obstet Gynaecol ;38:414-7, 1998

163. Walsh CJ, Mooney EF, Upton GJ, Motson RW. Incidence of third-degree perineal tears in labour and outcome after primary repair. Br J Surg ; 83:218-21, 1996.

164. Sander P, Bjarnesen L, Mouritsen A, Fuglsang-Frederiksen A. Anal incontinence after third- /fourth degree laceration. One-year follow-up after pelvic floor exercises. Int J Urogynecol.;10:177-81, 1999.

165. Crawford LA, Quint EH, Pearl ML, DeLancey JOL. Incontinence following rupture of the anal sphincter during delivery. Obstet Gynecol ;82:527-31, 1993.

166. Sorensen M, Tetzschner T, Rasmussen OO, Bjarnessen J, Christiansen J. Sphincter rupture in childbirth. Br J Surg ; 80:392-94, 1993.

167. Nielsen MB, Hauge C, Rasmussen OO, Pedersen JF, Christiansen J. Anal endosonographic findings in the follow-up of primarily sutured sphincteric ruptures. Br J Surg ; 79: 104-6, 1992.

168. Go PMNYH, Dunselman GAJ. Anatomic and functional results of surgical repair after total perineal rupture at delivery. Surg Gynecol Obstet ;166:121-4, 1988.

169. Uustal Fornell EK, Berg G, Hallbook O, Matthiesen LS, Sjodahl R. Clinical consequences of anal sphincter rupture during vaginal delivery. J AM Coll Surg ;183:553-8, 1996.

170. Sorensen SM, Bondesen H, Istre O, Vilmann P. Perineal rupture following vaginal delivery. Acta Obstet Gynecol Scand :67;315-8, 1988.

171. Tetzschner T, Sorensen M, Lose G, Christiansen J. Anal and urinary incontinence in women with obstetric anal sphincter rupture. Br J Obstet Gynaecol ;103:1034-40, 1996.

172. Haadem K, Ohrlander S, Lingman G. Long-term ailments due to anal sphincter rupture caused by delivery - a hidden problem. Eur J Obstet Gynecol Reprod Biol ; 27: 27-32, 1988.

173. Bek KM, Laurberg S. Risks of anal incontinence from subsequent vaginal delivery after a complete obstetric anal sphincter tear. Br J Obstet Gynaecol ;99:724-7, 1992.

174. Sultan AH, Abulafi MA. Anal incontinence – the role of the obstetrician and gynaecologist. In: Sturdee D, Olah K, Keane D (eds) The yearbook of obstetrics and gynaecology. Vol 9. London: RCOG press. :170-187, 2001.

175. Nichols DH. Gynecologic and Obstetric Surgery. Boston:Mosby. :1053-4, 1993.

176. Sultan AH, Stanton SL. Preserving the pelvic floor and perineum during childbirth - elective caesarean section? Br J Obstet Gynaecol ;103:731-4, 1996.

177. Sultan AH, Monga AK. Anal and urinary incontinence in women with obstetric anal sphincter rupture. British Journal of Obstetrics and Gynaecology ; 104: 753-4, 1997.

178. Johanson RB, Rice C, Doyle M et al. A randomised prospective study comparing the new vacuum extractor policy with forceps delivery. Br J Obstet Gynaecol ;100: 524- 30, 1993.

179. Bofill JA, Rust OA, Schorr SJ et al. A randomized prospective trial of the obstetric forceps versus the M-cup vacuum extractor. Am J Obstet Gynecol ;175:1325-30, 1996.

180. Johanson RB, Menon BKV. Vacuum extraction versus forceps for assisted vaginal delivery (Cochrane Review). In: The Cochrane Library, Issue 2. Oxford: Update Software 2001

181. Johanson RB, Heycock E, Carter J, Sultan AH, Walklate K, Jones PW. Maternal and child health after assisted vaginal delivery: five-year follow up of a randomised controlled study comparing forceps and ventouse. Br J Obstet Gynaecol ;106:544-9, 1999.

182. Sultan AH, Johanson RB, Carter JE. Occult anal sphincter trauma following randomized forceps and vacuum delivery. Int J Gynecol Obstet ; 61:113-9, 1998.

183. Johanson RB, Menon BKV. Soft versus rigid vacuum extractor cups for assisted vaginal delivery; Vacuum extraction versus forceps for assisted vaginal delivery. In: The Cochrane Library, Issue 1. Oxford: Update Software 2001.

184. Farrell SA, Allen VM, Baskett TF. Anal incontinence in primaparas. J Soc Obstet Gynaecol Can ; 23(4):321-6, 2001.

185. MacArthur C, Glazener CMA, Wilson PD, Herbison GP, Gee H, Lang GD, Lancashire R. Obstetric practice and faecal incontinence three months after delivery. Br J Obstet Gynaecol;108:678-83, 2001.

186. RCOG Audit Committee. Effective procedures in obstetrics suitable for audit. Manchester: RCOG Medical Audit Unit, 1993.

187. Woolley RJ. Benefits and risks of episiotomy: A review of the English language literature since 1980. Obstet Gynecol Surv;50:806-35, 1995.

188. Carroli G, Belizan J. Episiotomy for vaginal birth (Cochrane Review). In: The Cochrane Library, Issue 2. Oxford: Update Software, 2001

189. Henriksen TB, Bek KM, Hedegaard M, Secher NJ Methods and consequences of changes in use of episiotomy. BMJ ;309:1255-8, 1994.

190. Henriksen TB, Bek KM, Hedegaard M, Secher NJ. Episiotomy and perineal lesions in spontaneous vaginal deliveries. Br J Obstet Gynaecol ; 99:950-4, 1992.

191. Coats PM, Chan KK, Wilkins M, Beard RJ. A comparison between midline and mediolateral episiotomies. Br J Obstet Gynaecol ; 87: 408-12, 1980.

192. Pirhonen JP, Grenman SE, Haadem K, Gudmundsson S, Lindqvist P, Sihola S, Erkkola RU, Marsal K. Frequency of anal sphincter rupture at delivery in Sweden and Finland – result of

difference in manual help to the baby's head. Acta Obstet Gynecol Scand ;77:974-7, 1998.

193. Kamm MA. Faecal incontinence: clinical review. British Medical Journal ; 316: 528-532, 1998.

194. Read M, Read NW, Barber DC, Duthie HL. Effects of loperamide on anal sphincter function in patients complaining of chronic diarrhoea with faecal incontinence and urgency. Digestive Diseases and Sciences ; 27: 807-814, 1982.

195. Sun WM, Read NW, Verlinden M. Effects of loperamide oxide in gastrointestinal transit time and anorectal function in patients with chronic diarrhoea and faecal incontinence. Scandinavian Journal of Gastroenterology ; 32: 34-38, 1997.

196. Rattan S, Culver PJ. Influence of loperamide on the internal anal sphincter in the opossum. Gastroenterology ; 93: 121-128, 1987.

197. Kamm MA. Functional disorders of the colon and anorectum. Current Opinion in Gastroenterology ; 11: 9-15, 1987.

198. Barrett JA. Faecal incontinence and related problems in the older adult. London: Edward Arnold, 1993.

199. Tobin GW, Brocklehurst JC. Faecal incontinence in residential Homes for the elderly: prevalence, aetiology and management. Age and Ageing ; 15: 41-46, 1986.

200. Donnelly V, O'Connell PR, O'Herlihy C. The influence of oestrogen replacement on faecal incontinence in postmenopausal women. British Journal of Obstetrics & Gynaecology ; 104: 311-315, 1997.

201. Fantl JA, Cardozo L, McClish D. Estrogen therapy in the management of urinary incontinence in postmenopausal women: a meta-analysis. First report of the hormones and urogenital therapy committee. Obstetrics & Gynecology ; 83: 12-18, 1994.

202. Haadem K, Ling L, Ferno M, Graffner H. Oestrogen receptors in the external anal sphincter. American Journal of Obstetrics & Gynecology , 164: 609-610, 1991.

203. Laurberg S, Swash M. Effects of aging on the anorectal sphincters and their innervation. Dis.Colon Rectum ; 32: 737-742, 1989.

204. Carapeti EA, Kamm MA, Evans BK, Phillips RK. Topical phenylephrine increases anal sphincter resting pressure. British Journal of Surgery ; 86: 267-270, 1999.

205. Carapeti EA, Kamm MA, Nicholls RJ, Phillips RKS. Randomized, controlled trial of topical phenylepherine for fecal incontinence in patients after ileoanal pouch construction. Dis.Colon Rectum ; 43: 1059-1063, 2000.

206. Carapeti EA, Kamm MA, Phillips RKS. Randomized controlled trial of topical phenylepherine in the treatment of faecal incontinence. British Journal of Surgery ; 87: 38-42, 2000.

207. Burgio KL, Engel BT. Biofeedback-assisted behavioral training for elderly men and women. Journal of the American Geriatrics Society ; 38: 338-340, 1990.

208. Whitehead WE, Drossman DA. Biofeedback for disorders of elimination: fecal incontinence and pelvic floor dyssynergia. Professional Psychology: Research and Practice ; 27: 234-240, 1996.

209. Engel BT, Nikoomanesh P, Schuster MM. Operant conditioning of rectosphincteric responses in the treatment of faecal incontinence. New England Journal of Medicine ; 290: 646-649, 1974.

210. Whitehead WE, Orr WC, Engel BT, Schuster MM. External anal sphincter response to rectal distension: learned response or reflex. Psychophysiology ; 19: 57-62, 1981

211. Schussler B, Laycock J, Norton P, Stanton S. Pelvic floor re-education: principles and practice. London: Springer-Verlag, 1994.

212. MacLeod JH. Management of anal incontinence by biofeedback. Gastroenterology ; 93: 291-294, 1987.

213. Chiarioni G, Scattolini C, Bonfante F, Vantini I. Liquid stool incontinence with severe urgency: anorectal function and effective biofeedback treatment. Gut ; 34: 1576-1580, 1993.

214. Patankar SK, Ferrara A, Larach SW, et al. Electromyographic assessment of biofeedback training for faecal incontinence and chronic constipation. Dis.Colon Rectum ; 40: 907-911, 1997.

215. Buser WD, Miner PB. Delayed rectal sensation with faecal incontinence. Successful treatment using anorectal manometry. Gastroenterology ; 91: 1186-1191, 1986.

216. Miner PB, Donnelly TC, Read NW. Investigation of the mode of action of biofeedback in the treatment of faecal incontinence. Digestive Diseases & Sciences ; 35: 1291-1298, 1990.

217. Oresland T, Fasth S, Nordgren S, Swenson L, Akervall S. Does balloon dilatation and anal sphincter training improve ileo- anal pouch function? International Journal of Colorectal Disaese ; 3: 153-157, 1988.

218. Norton C, Kamm MA. Outcome of biofeedback for faecal incontinence. British Journal of Surgery; 86: 1159-1163, 1999.

219. Solomon MJ, Rex J, Eyers AA, Stewart P, Roberts R. Biofeedback for fecal incontinence using transanal ultrasonography: novel approach. Dis.Colon Rectum ; 43: 788-792, 2000.

220. Latimer PR, Campbell D, Kasperski J. A components analysis of biofeedback in the treatment of faecal incontinence. Biofeedback and Self-Regulation ; 9: 311-324, 1984.

221. Norton C, Kamm MA. Anal sphincter biofeedback and pelvic floor exercises for faecal incontinence in adults - a systematic review. Alimentary Pharmacology & Therapeutics ; 15: 1147-1154, 2001.

222. Fynes MM, Marshall K, Cassidy M, et al. A prospective, randomized study comparing the effect of augmented biofeedback with sensory biofeedback alone on fecal incontinence after obstetric trauma. Dis.Colon Rectum ; 42: 753-758, 1999.

223. Sander P, Bjarnesen J, Mouritsen L, Fuglsang-Frederiksen A. Anal incontinence after obstetric third- /fourth-degree laceration. One-year follow-up after pelvic floor exercises. International Urogynecology Journal & Pelvic Floor Dysfunction ; 10: 177-181, 1999.

224. Whitehead WE, Burgio KL, Engel BT. Biofeedback treatment of faecal incontinence in geriatric patients. Journal of the American Geriatrics Society ; 33: 320-324, 1985.

225. Jensen LL, Lowry AC. Biofeedback improves functional outcome after sphincteroplasty. Dis.Colon Rectum ; 40: 197-200, 1997.

226. Ho YH, Chiang JM, Tan M, Low JY. Biofeedback therapy for excessive stool frequency and incontinence following anterior resection or total colectomy. Dis.Colon Rectum ; 39: 1289-1292, 1996.

227. Jorge JM, Wexner SD, Morgado PJ, James K, Nogueras JJ, Jagelman DG. Optimization of sphincter function after the ileoanal reservoir procedure. Dis.Colon Rectum ; 37: 419-423, 1994.

228. Berti Riboli E, Frascio M, Pitto G, Reboa G, Zanolla R. Biofeedback conditioning for faecal incontinence. Archives of Physical & Medical Rehabilitation ; 69: 29-31, 1988.

229. Cerulli MA, Nikoomanesh P, Schuster MM. Progress in biofeedback conditioning for faecal incontinence. Gastroenterology ; 76: 742-746, 1979.

230. McHugh S, Kersey K, Diamant NE. Biofeedback training for faecal incontinence: outcome according to physiological parameters. Gastroenterology 94: A295, 1988.

231. van Tets WF, Kuijpers JH, Bleijenberg G. Biofeedback treatment is ineffective in neurogenic fecal incontinence. Dis.Colon Rectum ; 39: 992-994, 1996.

232. Magrini P, Pallotta L, Koch M, Capurso L. Manometric biofeedback in the management of faecal incontinence and pelvic floor dyssynergia. International Journal of the Proctological and Perineal Diseases ; 1: 269-270, 1997.

233. Enck P, Daublin G, Lubke HJ, Strohmeyer G. Long-term efficacy of biofeedback training for faecal incontinence. Dis.Colon Rectum ; 37: 997-1001, 1994.

234. Guillemot F, Bouche B, Gower-Rousseau C, et al. Biofeedback for the treatment of fecal incontinence. Long-term clinical results. Dis.Colon Rectum , 38: 393-397, 1995.

235. Ryn A-K, Morren GL, Hallbook O, Sjodahl R. Long-term results of electromyographic biofeedback training for faecal incontinence. Dis.Colon Rectum ; 43: 1262-1266, 2000.

236. Leroi AM, Dorival MP, Lecouturier MF, et al. Pudendal neuropathy and severity of incontinence but not presence of an anal sphincter defect may determine the response to biofeedback therapy in fecal incontinence. Dis.Colon Rectum ; 42: 762-769, 1999.

237. Rieger NA, Wattchow DA, Sarre RG, et al. Prospective trial of pelvic floor retraining in patients with faecal incontinence. Dis.Colon Rectum ; 40: 821-826, 1997.

238. Ko CY, Tong J, Lehman RE, Shelton AA, Schrock TR, Welton ML. Biofeedback is effective therapy for fecal incontinence and constipation. Arch.Surg. 132: 829-833, 1997.

239. Wald A. Biofeedback therapy for faecal incontinence. Annals of Internal Medicine ; 95: 146-149, 1981.

240. Norton C, Hosker G, Brazzelli M. Effectiveness of biofeedback and/or sphincter exercises for the treatment of faecal incontinence in adults. Cochrane electronic library 2000.

241. McHugh S, Walma K, Diamant NE. Faecal incontinence: a controlled trial of biofeedback. Gastroenterology ; 90: 1545-1545, 1986.

242. Caldwell KPS. The electrical control of sphincter incompetence. Lancet ; ii: 174-175, 1963.

243. Mills PM, Deakin M, Kiff ES. Percutaneous electrical stimulation for ano-rectal incontinence. Physiotherapy ; 76: 433-438, 1990.

244. Pescatori M, Pavesio R, Anastasio G, Daini S. Transanal electrostimulation for faecal incontinence: clinical, psychologic and manometric prospective study. Dis.Colon Rectum ; 34: 540-545, 1991.

245. Jost WH. Electrostimulation in fecal incontinence: relevance of the sphincteric compound muscle action potential. Diseases of the Colon & Rectum ; 41: 590-592, 1998.

246. Scheuer M, Kuijpers HC, Bleijenberg G. Effect of electrostimulation on sphincter function in neurogenic fecal continence. Dis.Colon Rectum ; 37: 590-593, 1994.

247. Hosker G, Norton C, Brazzelli M. Effectiveness of electrical stimulation for faecal incontinence in adults. Cochrane electronic library 2000.

248. Sylvester KL, Keilty SEJ. A pilot study to investigate the use of interferential in the treatment of ano-rectal incontinence. Physiotherapy ; 73: 207-208, 1987.

249. Hinds JP, Wald A. Colonic and anorectal dysfunction associated with multiple sclerosis. Am.J.Gastroenterol. ; 84: 587-595, 1989.

250. Wald A. Systemic diseases causing disorders of defaecation and continence. Seminars in Gastrointestinal Disease ; 6: 194-202, 1995.

251. O'Regan S, Yazbeck S, Schick E. Constipation, bladder instability, urinary tract infection syndrome. Clin Nephrol ; 23: 153-154, 1985.

252. Banwell JG, Creasey GH, Aggarwal AM, Mortimer JT. Management of the neurogenic bowel in patients with spinal cord injury. Urologic Clinics of North America ; 20: 517-526, 1993.

253. Stiens SA, Bergman SB, Goetz LL. Neurogenic bowel dysfunction after spinal cord injury: clinical evaluation and rehabilitation management. Archives of Physical Medicine & Rehabilitation ; 78: S-86-S-104, 1997

254. Dunn KL, Galka ML. A comparison of the effectiveness of Therevac SB and bisacodyl suppositories in SCI patients' bowel programs. Rehabilitation Nursing ; 19 : 334-338, 1994.

255. Glen House J, Stiens SA. Pharmacologically initiated defaecation for persons with spinal cord injury: effectiveness of three agents. Archives of Physical Medicine & Rehabilitation ; 78: 1062-1065, 1997.

256. Stiens SA. Reduction in bowel programme duration with polyethylene glycol based bisacodyl suppositories. Archives of Physical Medicine & Rehabilitation ; 76: 674-677, 1995.

257. Doughty D. A physiologic approach to bowel training. Journal of Wound, Ostomy, & Continence Nursing ; 23: 46-56, 1996.

258. Younoszai MK. Stooling problems in patients with myelomeningocele. Southern Medical Journal ; 85: 718-724, 1992.

259. King JC, Currie DM, Wright E. Bowel training in spina bifida: importance of education, patient compliance, age, and anal reflexes. Archives of Physical Medicine & Rehabilitation ; 75: 243-247, 1994.

260. Munchiando JF, Kendall K. Comparison of the effectiveness of two bowel programs for CVA patients. Rehabilitation Nursing ; 18: 168-172, 1993.

261. Krogh K, Nielsen J, Djurhuus JC, Mosdal C, Sabroe S, Laurberg S. Colorectal function in patients with spinal cord lesions. Dis.Colon Rectum ; 40: 1233-1239, 1997.

262. Ouslander JG, Simmons S, Schnelle J, Uman G, Fingold S. Effects of prompted voiding on fecal continence among nursing home residents. Journal of the American Geriatrics Society ; 44: 424-428, 1996.

263. Shandling B, Gilmour RF. The enema continence catheter in spina bifida: successful bowel management. J.Pediatr.Surg. ; 22: 271-273, 1987.

264. Lipak GS, Revell GM. Management of bowel dysfunction in children with spinal cord disease or injury by means of the enema continence catheter. Journal of Pediatrics ; 120: 190-194, 1992.

265. De Kort LMO, Nesselaar CH, Van Gool JD, De Jong TPVM. The influence of colonic enema irrigation on urodynamic findings in patients with neurogenic bladder dysfunction. Br.J.Urol. ; 80: 731-733, 1997.

266. Scholler-Gyure M, Nesselaar CH, van Wieringen H, Van Gool JD. Treatment of defaecation disorders by colonic enemas in children with spina bifida. European Journal of Pediatric Surgery ; 6: 32-34, 1996.

267. Glickman S, Kamm MA. Bowel dysfunction in spinal-cord-injury patients. Lancet ; 347: 1651-1653, 1996.

268. Addison, R. Digital rectal examination and manual removal of faeces. London, Royal College of Nursing, 1995.

269. Ardron ME, Main ANH. Management of constipation. British Medical Journal ; 300: 1400, 1990.

270. Norton C, Kamm MA. Bowel control - information and practical advice. Beaconsfield: Beaconsfield Publishers, 1999.

271. Barrett JA. Effects of wheat bran on stool size. British Medical Journal ; 296: 1127-1128, 1988.

272. Bliss,D.Z., Jung,H., Lowry,A.C., Savik,K., Jensen,L., LeMoine,M. and Werner,C. Effects of dietary fiber therapy for fecal incontinence. Gerontologist ; 325-325, 1997.

273. Christiansen J, Roed-Petersen K. Clinical assessment of the anal continence plug. Dis.Colon Rectum ; 36: 740-742, 1993.

274. Norton C, Kamm MA. Anal plug for faecal incontinence. Colorectal Disease ; 3: 323-327, 2001.

275. Rasmussen OØ,Christiansen J,Tetzschner T, Sørensen M. Pudendal nerve function in idiopathic fecal incontinence. Dis Colon Rectum ;43:633-635, 2000.

276. Browning GGP, Parks AG. Postanal repair for neuropathic fae-

cal incontinence: correlation of clinical results and anal canal pressures. Brit J Surg ;70:101-104, 1983.

277. Keighley MRB.Postanal repair. Int J Colorectal Dis ;2:236-239, 1987.

278. Carraro PS,Kamm MA, Nicholls RJ.Br J Surg ;81:140144, 1994.

279. Jameson JS,Speakman CTM,Darzi A,Chia YW,Henry MM. Audit of postanal repair in the treatment of fecal incontinence.Dis Colon Rectum ;37:369-372, 1994.

280. Matsuoka H,Mavrantonis C,Wexner SD,Oliveira L,Gilliland R,Pikarsky A. Postanal repair for fecal incontinence-is it worthwhile?. Dis Colon Rectum ;43:1561-1567, 2000.

281. Christiansen J, Skomorowska E. Persisting incontinence after postanal repair treated by anterior perineoplasty.Int J Colorect Dis 7;2:9-11, 2000.

282. Miller R,Orrom WJ,Cornes H,Duthie G,Bartolo DCC. Anterior sphincter plication and levatorplasty in the treatment of faecal incontinence. Br J Surg ;76:1058-1060, 1989.

283. Orrom WJ,Miller R,Cornes H,Duthie G,Mortensen NJM, Bartolo DCC. Comparison of anterior sphincteroplasty and postanal repair in the treatment of idiopathic fecal incontinence. Dis Colon Rectum ;34:305-310, 1991.

284. Deen KI,Oya M, Ortiz J,Keighley MRB. Randomized trial comparing three forms of pelvic floor repair for neuropathic faecal incontinence. Br J Surg ; 80:794-798, 1991.

285. Keighley MRB, Williams NS. Surgery of the Anus Rectum and Colon. Saunders. London 1993 p.548.

286. Carraro PS,Nicholls RJ. Postanal repair for faecal incontinence persisting after rectopexy. Br J Surg ;81:305-307, 1994.

287. Wexner SD,Marchetti F,Jagelman DG. The role of sphincteroplasty for fecal incontinence reevaluated: a prospective physioogical and functional review.Dis Colon Rectum ;34:22-30, 1991.

288. Hasagawa H,Yoshioka K,Keighley MR. Randomized trial of fecal diversion for sphincter repair.Dis Colon Rectum ; 43:961-964, 2000.

289. Sitzler PJ,Thompson JP. Overlap repair of damaged anal sphincter. A single surgeons series. Dis Colon Rectum ;39:1356-1360, 1996.

290. Engel AF,Kamm MA,Sultan AH,Bartram CI,Nicholls RJ. Anterior sphincter repair in patients with obstetric trauma. Br J Surg; 81:1231-1234, 1994.

291. Jacobs PP,Scheuer M, Kuijpers JH Vingerhoets MH. Obstetric fecal incontinence.Role of pelvic floor denervation and results of delayed sphincter repair. Dis Colon Rectum ; 3:494-497, 1990.

292. Rasmussen OØ,Puggaard L,Chistiansen J. Anal sphincter repair in patients wit obstetric trauma. Dis Colon Rectum; 42:193-195, 1999.

293. Karoui S,Leroi AM,Koning E,Menard JF,Michot F, Denis P.Results of sphincteroplasty in 86 patients with anal incontinence.Dis Colon Rectum ;43:813-820, 2000.

294. Morren GL, Hallböök O,Nyström PO, Baeten CGM,Sjödahl R. Audit of anal-sphincter repair Colorectal Dis ; 3:17-22, 2001.

295. Nikiteas N,Korsgen S, Kumar D, Keighley MRB. Audit of sphincter repair. Factor associated with poor outcome.Dis Colon Rectum ;39:1164-1170, 1996.

296. Arnaud A, Sarles JC, Sielezneff I, Orsoni P, Joly A. Sphincter repair without overlapping for fecal incontinence.Dis Colon Rectum ;34: 744-747, 1991.

297. Cook TA, Mortensen NJM. Management of faecal incontinence following obstetric injury. Br J Surg ;85:293-299, 1998.

298. Nielsen MB, Dammegaard L,Pedersen JF. Endosonographic assessment of the anal sphincter after surgical reconstruction. Dis Colon Rectum ; 37:434-438, 1994.

299. Engel AF, Brummelkamp WH. Secondary surgery after failed postanal or anterior sphincter repair. Int J Colorect Dis ; 9:187-190, 1994.

300. Pickrell K,Georglade N, Maguire C,Crawford H. Gracilis muscle transplant for rectal incontinence.Surgery ;40:349-363, 1956.

301. Corman ML. Follow-up evaluation of gracilis muscle transposition for fecal incontinence.Dis Colon Rectum ;23:552-555, 1980.

302. Christiansen J,Rasmussen OØ,Lindorff-Larsen K. Dynamic graciloplasty for severe anal incontinence.Br J Surg ; 85:88-91, 1998.

303. Baeten CGMI,Geerdes BP,Adang EMM,Heineman E, Konsten J,Engel GL,Kester ADM,Spaans F,Soeters PB. Anal dynamic graciloplasty in the treatment of intractable fecal incontinence. N Engl J Med ;332:1600-1605, 1995.

304. Madoff,RD,Rosen HR,Baeten CG,LaFontaine LJ,Cavina E,Devesa M,Rouanet PR,Christiansen J,Faucheron J-L,Isbister W,Köhler L,Guelinckx J,Påhlman L. Safety and efficacy of dynamic muscle transplant for anal incontinence:lessons from a prospective multicenter trial. Gatroenterology ;116:649-556, 1999.

305. Geerdes BP,Heineman E,Konsten J,Soeters PB,Baeten CGMI. Dynamic graciloplasty. Complications and management. Dis Colon Rectum ;39:912-917, 1996.

306. Baeten CGM and the Dynamic Graciloplasty Study Group.Dis Colon Rectum ;43:743-751, 2000.

307. Christiansen J,Lorenzen M. Implantation of artificial sphincter for anal incontinence. Lancet ; 1:244-245, 1987.

308. Christiansen J, Sparsø B. Treatment of anal incontinence by an implantable prosthetic anal sphincter. Ann Surg;215:383-386, 1992.

309. Wong DW,Jensen LR,Bartolo DCC,Rothenberger DA. Artificial anal sphincter. Dis Colon Rectum ;39:1345-1351, 1996.

310. Lehur P-A, Michot F, Denis P,Grise P, Leborgne J, Teniere P,Buzelin J-M. Results of artificial sphincter in severe anal incontinence.Dis Colon Rectum ;39:1352-1355, 1996.

311. Lehur P-A, Glemain P, Bruley des Varannes S, Buzelin JM,Leborgne J. Outcome of patients with an implantable artificial anal sphincter for severe anal incontinence. Int J Colorect Dis ;13:88-92, 1998.

312. Vaizey CJ,Kamm MA,Gold DM,Bartram CI, HalliganS, Nicholls RJ. Clinical,physiological, and radiological study of a new purpose-designed artificial bowel sphincter.Lancet;352:105-109, 1998.

313. Dodi G,Melega E, Masin A, Infantino A, Cavallari F, Lise M. Artificial bowel sphincter (ABS) for severe faecal incontinence: a clinical and manometric study. Colorect Dis ;2:207-211, 2000.

314. Christiansen J, Rasmussen OØ, Lindorff-Larsen K. Long-term results of artificial anal sphincter implantation for severe anal incontinence. Ann Surg ;230:45-48, 1999.

315. Spencer M, Wong W,Congilosi S. Artificial anal sphincter:preliminary results of a multicenter prospective trial. Dis Colon Rectum ;41: A15, 1998.

316. Matzel KE, Stadelmaier U, Hohenfellner M, Gall FP. Electrical stimulation of sacral spinal nerves for treatment of faecal incontinence.Lancet ;346:1124-1126, 1995.

317. Vaizey,CJ,Kamm MA,Turner IC,Nicholls RJ,Woloszko J.Effects of short term sacral nerve stimulation on anal and rectal function in patients with anal incontinence.GUT ;44:407-412, 1999.

318. Malouf AJ, Vaizey CJ, Nicholls RJ,Kamm MA.Permanent sacral nerve stimulation for fecal incontinence. Ann Surg; 232:143-148, 2000.

319. Matzel KE,Stadelmaier U,Hohenfellner M,Hohenberger W. Chronic sacral spinal nerve stimulation for fecal

incontinence:long-term results with foramen and cuff electrodes. Dis Colon Rectum ; 44:59-66, 2001.

320. Shafik A. Perianal injection of autologous fat for treatment of sphincteris incontinence. Dis Colon Rectum ;38:583-87, 1995.

321. Kumar D. Benson M. Glutaraldehyde cross-linked collagen in the treatment of faecal incontinence. Br J Surg ; 85:978-79, 1998.

322. Malouf AJ,Vaizey CJ,Norton CS,Kamm MA. Internal anal sphincter augmentation for fecal incontinence using injectable silicone biomaterial. Dis Colon Rectum ;44: in press 2001.

323. Griffiths DM, Malone PS. The Malone antegrade continence enema. J Pediatric Surg ;30:68-71, 1995.

324. Krogh K,Laurberg S. Malone antegrade continence enema for faecal incontinence an constipation in adults. Brit J Surg; 85:974-977, 1998.

325. Vries MW,de Vries MR Cultural relativity of toilet training readiness: a perspective from East Africa. Pediatrics, 60(2):170-7, 1977.

326. Largo RH, StutzleW. Longitudinal study of bowel and bladder control by day and at night in the first six years of life. I: Epidemiology and interrelations between bowel and bladder control. Developmental Medicine and Child Neurology, 19(5):598-606, 1977.

327. Largo RH, StutzleW. Longitudinal study of bowel and bladder control by day and at night in the first six years of life. II: The role of potty training and the child's initiative. Developmental Medicine and Child Neurology, 19(5): 607-613, 1977

328. Brazelton TB: A child oriented approach to toilet training. Pediatrics, 29: 121, 1962.

329. Taubman B Toilet training and toileting refusal for stool only: a prospective study. Pediatrics, 99(1): 54-8, 1997.

330. Weaver LT, Steiner H. The bowel habit of young children. Arch. Dis. Child, 59: 694-652, 1984.

331. Bellman M. Studies on encopresis. Acta Paediatr Scand Suppl:170: 1-151, 1966.

332. Rutter M. Helping Troubled Children. Harmons-Worth, England, Penguin Education 1995.

333. Levine MD.Children with encopresis: a descriptive analysis. Pediatrics, 56(3):412-416, 1975.

334. Rasquin-Weber A, Hyman PE et al. Childhood functional gastrointestinal disorders. Gut, 45 Supp II 60-68, 1999.

335. Marty T et al. Gastrointestinal function after surgical correction of Hirschprung's disease: Long term follow up in 135 patients. J Pediatr Surg, 30:655 – 658, 1995.

336. Moore et al. Clinical outcome and Long term quality of life after surgical correction of Hirschprung's disease. J Pediatr Surg, 31(11): 1496 – 1502, 1996.

337. Catto-Smith Ag, Coffey CM, Nolan TM, Hutson JM. Fecal incontinence after surgical treatment of Hirschprung disease. J Pediatr, 127:954-957, 1995.

338. Loening-Baucke VA, Desch L Wolraich M Biofeedback training for patients with meningomyelocoele and fecal incontinence. Dev Med Child Neurol, 30; 78-90, 1998.

339. Davidson M,Kugler MM, Bauer CH. Diagnosis and management in children with severe and protracted constipation and obstipation. J Pediatr, 62:261, 1963.

340. Johnston BD, Wright JA. Attentional dysfunction in children with encopresis. J. Dev & Beh. Ped, 14; 381-385, 1993.

341. Gohlke BC, Khadilkar VV, Skuse D, Stanhope R. Recognition of children with psychosocial short stature: a spectrum of presentation. J Ped Endocrinology & Metabolism, 11: 509 – 517, 1998.

342. Levine MD. Encopresis: its potentiation, evaluation and alleviation. Pediatr. Clin. North Am, 29(2): 315-30, 1982.

343. Clayden GS. Management of chronic constipation. Arch Dis Child, 67:340, 1992.

344. Buchanon A. Children who Soil. Wiley. Chichester ISBN 0-471-93479-8, 1992.

345. Slukin A. Behavioural social work with encopretic children, their families and the school. Child Care, Health & Dev, 7: 67-80, 1981.

346. Gabel S, et al. prevalence of behavior problems and mental health utilisation among encopretic children: Implications for behavioral pediatrics. J. Dev & Beh Ped, 7(5) 293-297, 1986.

347. Young M, Brennen L, Baker R, Baker S. Functional encopresis: Symptom reduction and behavioral improvement. J Dev & Beh Ped, 16(4) 226-232, 1995.

348. Jewkes RK, O' Connor . Crisis in our schools: survey of sanitation facilities in schools in Bloomsbury health district. BMJ, 301(6760):1085-7, 1990.

349. Iacono G, Cavataio F, Montalto G, et al. Intolerance of cow's milk and chronic constipation in children. N Engl J Med, 339:1100-1104, 1998.

350. van der Plas RN, Benninga MA et al. Megarectum in constipation. Arch Dis Child, 83(1): 52-58, 2000.

351. Blethyn AJ, Verrier Jones K, Newcombe R, Roberts GM, Jenkins HR. Radiological assessment of constipation. Arch Dis Child, 73:532-533, 1995.

352. Leech SC, McHugh K, Sullivan PB. Evaluation of a method of assessing faecal loading on plain abdominal radiographs of children. Pediatr Radiol, 29(4): 255-8, 1999.

353. Papadopoulou A, Clayden GS, Booth IW. The clinical value of solid marker transit studies in childhood constipation and soiling. Eur J Pediatr, 153;560-564, 1994.

354. Loening-Baucke V. Abnormal rectoanal function in children recovered from chronic constipation and encopresis. Gastroenterology, 87:1299, 1984.

355. Clayden GS, Lawson JON. Investigation and management of long-standing chronic constipation in childhood. Arch Dis Child, 51: 918-923, 1976.

356. Poenaru D, Roblin N, Bird M, Duce S et al. The pediatric bowel management clinic: initial results of a multidisciplinary approach to functional constipation in children. J Pediatr Surg, 32(6) 843-848, 1997.

357. Nolan T, Debelle G, Oberklaid F, Coffey C. Randomised trail of laxatives in treatment of childhood encopresis. Lancet, 338;523-527, 1991.

358. Taitz LS, Wales JKW, Urwin OM et al . Factors associated with outcome in management of defaecation disorders. Arch Dis Child, 61:472, 1986.

359. Graham YD, Moser ES, Estes KM. The effect of bran on bowel function in constipation. Am J Gastroenterol, 77: 599 – 603, 1982.

360. Roma E, Adamidis D et al. Diet and chronic constipation in children: The role of fibre. J Ped Gastro & Nutr, 28(2): 168-174, 1999.

361. Loening-Baucke V. Encopresis and Soiling. Ped Clin of N Am, 43 (1) 279-298, 1996.

362. Drug and Therapeutics Bulletin. Managing Constipation in Children, 38(8): 57-60, 2000.

363. Bandla HP, Davis SH, Hopkins NE . Lipoid pneumonia: a silent complication of mineral oil aspiration. Pediatrics, 103(2): E19, 1999.

364. Gleghorn EE, Heyman MB, Rudolph CD: No enema treatment for idiopathic constipation and encopresis. Clin Pediatr, 30:669-672,1991.

365. Ingebo KB , Heyman MB. Polyethylene glycol-electrolyte solu-

tion for intestinal clearance in children with refractory encopresis. AJDC, 142:340-342, 1988.

366. Sondheimer JM , Sokol RJ, Taylor SF, Silverman A, Zelasney B . Safety, efficacy and tolerance of intestinal lavage in pediatric patients undergoing diagnostic colonoscopy. J Pediatr, 119:148-52, 1991.

367. Loening-Baucke V. Modulation of abnormal defaecation dynamics by biofeedback treatment in chronically constipated children with encopresis. J Pediatr; 116:214, 1990.

368. Benninga MA, Büller HA, Taminiau JAJM. Biofeedback training in chronic constipation. Arch. Dis Child, 68: 126-129, 1993.

369. van der Plas RN, Benninga MA, Buller HA et al. Biofeedback training in treatment of childhood constipation: a randomised controlled study. Lancet, 348 (9030):776-80, 1996.

370. Loening-Bauke V. Biofeedback treatment for chronic constipation and encopresis in childhood: long-term outcome. Pediatrics, 96: 105-110, 1995.

371. van Ginkel R, Benninga MA et al. Lack of benefit of laxatives as adjunctive therapy for functional nonretentive fecal soiling in children. J Pediatr, 137:808-813, 2000.

372. ERIC (Enuresis resource and Information Centre, Bristol, UK) Helpline +44 117 960 3060. www.enuresis.org.uk

373. Malone PS, Ransley PG, Keily EM. Preliminary report; the antegrade continence enema. Lancet, 336:1217-1218, 1990.

374. Griffiths DM, Malone PS. The Malone antegrade continence enema. J Pediatr Surg, 30 68-71, 1995.

375. Vos A, Cuesta M, Meuwissen S . Antegrade colonic enema (ACE): a new therapeutic approach to chronic constipation. Acta Gastroenterol Latinoam 26(4):225-6, 1996.

376. Loening-Baucke V. Constipation in early childhood: patient characteristics, treatment and long term followup. Am Fam Physician, 49:397, 1994.

377. Loening-Baucke V. Factors determining outcome in children with chronic constipation and fecal soiling. Gut, 30:999,1989.

378. Loening-Baucke V. Factors responsible for persistence of childhood constipation. J Pediatr Gastroenterol Nutr, 6:915, 1987

379. Rockney R, McQuade, W et al. Encopresis treatment outcome: Long-term follow-up of 45 cases. J Dev & Beh Ped. 17(6): 380-385, 1996.

380. Sutphen JL,Borowitz SM, Hutchinson RL, Cox DJ. Long-term follow-up of medically treated childhood constipation. Clin Pediatr (phila) 34(11);576-80, 1995.

381. Chassagne P, Landrin I, Neveu C, Czernichow P, Bouaniche M, Doucet J, Denis P, Bercoff E. Fecal incontinence in the institutionalized elderly: incidence, risk factors, and prognosis. Am J Med106(2):185-190 1999;1999.

382. Prosser S, Dobbs F. Case-finding incontinence in the over-75's. Br J Gen Pract ; 47:498-500, 1997.

383. Peet SM, Castleden CM, McGrother CW. Prevalence of urinary and fecal incontinence in hospitals and residential and nursing homes for older people. Br Med J ;311:1063-4, 1995.

384. Schultz A, Dickey G, Skoner M. Urologic Nursing ;17:23-8, 1997.

385. Brocklehurst J, Dickinson E, Windsor J. Laxatives and faecal incontinence in long-term care. Nursing Standard ;52:32-36, 1999.

386. Johanson JF, Irizarry F, Doughty A. Risk factors for fecal incontinence in a nursing home population. J Clin Gastroenterol ; 24:156-60, 1997.

387. Harari, D, Gurwitz JH, Choodnovskiy I, Avorn J, Minaker KL. Constipation: Assessment and management in an institutionalised population. J Am Geriatr Soc ;4 2:1-6, 1994.

388. Barrett JA, Brocklehurst JC, Kiff ES, Ferguson G, Faragher EB. Rectal motility studies in faecally incontinent geriatric patients. Age and Ageing ;19:311-317, 1990.

389. Percy JP, Neill ME, Kandiah TK et al. A neurogenic factor in faecal incontinence in the elderly. Age Ageing ;11;175-179, 1982.

390. Loening-Baucke V, Anuras S. Sigmoidal and rectal motility in healthy elderly. J Am Geriatr Soc ;32:887-891, 1984.

391. Loening-Baucke V, Anuras S: Effects of age and sex on anorectal manometry. Am J Gastroenterol ;80(1):50-53, 1985.

392. McHugh SM, Diamant NE. Effect of age, gender, and parity on anal canal pressures. Dig Dis Sci ;32(7):726-736, 1987.

393. Matheson DM, Keighley MRB: Manometric evaluation of rectal prolapse and faecal incontinence. Gut ;22:126-129, 1981

394. Ryhammer AM, Laurberg S, Bek KM. Age and anorectal sensibility in normal women. Scand J Gastroenterol ;32:278-84, 1997

395. Read NW, Abouzekry L, Read MG, Howell P, Ottewell D, Donnelly TC. Anorectal function in elderly patients with fecal impaction. Gastroenterology ;89:959-966, 1985

396. Rasmussen OO, Christiansen J, Tetzschner T, Sorensen M. Pudendal nerve function in idiopathic fecal incontinence. Dis Colon Rectum 43:633-6, 2000;

397. Vaccaro CA, Cheong DM, Wexner SD, Nogueras JJ, Salanga VD, Hanson MR, Phillips RC. Pudendal neuropathy in evacuatory disorders. Dis Colon Rectum ;38:166-71, 1995

398. Barrett JA, Brocklehurst JC, Kiff ES et al. Anal function in geriatric patients with fecal incontinence. Gut ;30:1244-1251, 1989

399. Robson KM, Kiely DK, LemboT. Development of constipation in nursing home residents. Dis Colon Rectum ;43:940-3, 2000

400. Donald IP, Smith RG, Cruikshank JG, Elton RA, Stoddart ME. A study of constipation in the elderly living at home. Gerontology ;31:112-8, 1985.

401. Kinnunen O. Study of constipation in a geriatric hospital, day hospital, old people's home and at home. Aging ;3:161-170, 1991.

402. Harari, D, Gurwitz JH, Choodnovskiy I, Avorn J, Minaker KL. Correlates of regular laxative use in frail elderly persons. Am J Med :99(4);513-8, 1995.

403. Harari D, Gurwitz JH, Minaker KL. Constipation in the elderly. J Am Geriatr Soc 41(10):1130-1140, 1993.

404. Jones RH, Tait CL. Gastrointestinal side-effects of NSAIDs in the community. Br J Clin Pract ;49:67-70, 1995.

405. Singaram C, Ashraf W, Gaumnitz EA et al. Dopaminergic defect of enteric nervous system in Parkinson's disease patients with chronic constipation. Lancet ;346:861-64, 1995.

406. Bassotti G, Maggio D, Battaglia E et al. Manometric investigation of anorectal function in early and late stage Parkinson's disease. J Neurol Neurosurg Psychiatry :68:768-770, 2000.

407. Muller-Lissner SA: Effect of wheat bran on the weight of stool and gastrointestinal transit time: a meta analysis. Br Med J 296:615-617, 1988.

408. Towers AL, Burgio KL, Locher JL, Merkel IS, Safaeian M, Wald A. Constipation in the elderly: Influence of dietary, psychological, and physiological factors. J Am Geriatr Soc ;42:701-6, 1994.

409. Klauser AG, Schindlbeck NE, Muller-Lissner SA: Low fluid intake lowers stool output in healthy male volunteers. Z Gastoenterol 28(11):606-609, 1990.

410. Klauser AG, Voderholzer WA, Heinrich CA, Schindlbeck NE, Muller-Lissner SA. Behavioural modification of colonic function: can constipation be learned? Dig Dis Sci ;35:1271-5, 1990.

411. Harari D, Patel M, Rudd SG, Wolfe CDA. Prevalence, corre-

lates, and impact of new-onset faecal incontinence following stroke. J Cerebrovascular Dis (in press).

412. Wald A, Tunuguntla AK. Anorectal sensorimotor dysfunction in fecal incontinence and diabetes mellitus. NEJM ;310:1282-7, 1984.

413. Sun WM, Katsinelos P, Horowitz M, Read NW. Disturbances in anorectal function in patients with diabetes mellitus and faecal incontinence. Euro J Gastroenterol Hepatology ; 8:1007-12, 1996.

414. Harari D, Gurwitz JH, Avorn J, Bohn R, Minaker KL. Bowel habits in relation to age and gender: Findings from the National Health Interview Survey and clinical implications. Arch Int Med;156:315-320, 1996.

415. Goulding A, Taylor RW, Keil D, Gold E, Lewis-Barned NJ, Williams SM. Lactose malabsorption and rate of bone loss in older women. Age and Ageing ; 28:175-180, 1999.

416. Al-Eidan FA, McElnay JC, Scott MG, Kearney MP. Clostridium difficile-associated diarrhoea in hospitalised patients. J Clin Pharm Therapeutics ;25:101-9, 2000.

417. Morgan R, Spencer B, King D. Rectal examinations in elderly subjects: attitudes of patients and doctors. Age and Aging; 27:353-6, 1998.

418. Engel AF, Kamm MA, Bartram CI, Nicholls RJ. Relationship of symptoms in faecal incontinence to specific sphincter abnormalities. Int J Colorect Dis ;10:152-5, 1995.

419. Harari D, Minaker KL. Megacolon in patients with chronic spinal cord injury. Spinal Cord ;38:331-339, 2000.

420. McKay LF, Smith RG, Eastwood MA et al: An investigation of colonic function in the elderly. Age Ageing 12:105-110, 1983.

421. Starrveld JS, Pols JS, Van Wijk MA et al: The plain abdominal radiograph the assessment of constipation. Z Gastroenterol 28:335-338, 1990.

422. Chassagne P, Jego A, Gloc P et al. Does treatment of constipation improve faecal incontinence in institutionalized patients. Age Ageing :29:159-164, 2000.

423. Petticrew M, Watt I, Sheldon T. Systematic review of the effectiveness of laxatives in the elderly. Health Technology Assessment ;1(13):i-iv,1-52, 1997.

424. Puxty JA, Fox RA. Golytely: a new approach to faeçal impaction in old age. Age Ageing ;15(3):182-184, 1986.

425. Korzets A, Dicker D, Chaimoff C, Zevin D. Life-threatening hyperphosphatemia and hypocalcemic tetany following the use of Fleet enemas. J Am Geriatr Soc 40:620-1, 1992.

Committee 16

Research Methodology in Urinary Incontinence

Chairman

C. Payne (USA),

P. Van Kerrebroeck (The Netherlands),

Members

J. Blaivas (USA),

D. Chaikin (USA),

H. Herrera (USA),

U. Jonas (Germany),

L. Kusek (USA),

A. Mattiasson (Sweden),

L. Nyberg (USA),

T. Peters (U.K)

M-A Stothers (Canada),

A. Webers (USA)

CONTENTS

Research Methodology in Urinary Incontinence

C. PAYNE, P. VAN KERREBROECK,

J. BLAIVAS, H. HERRERA, D. CHAIKIN, U. JONAS, L. KUSEK, A. MATTIASSON, L. NYBERG, T. PETERS, M-A STOTHERS, A. WEBERS

I. INTRODUCTION

Lower urinary tract dysfunction comprises a group of common diseases, and we need far more knowledge of their origin, diagnosis, treatment, and ultimately prevention than we have today. Clinical research is a precondition for any progress in these areas. The task for the present committee is to provide recommendations for good research practice, including principles of trial design and correct statistical methodology. In addition, the aim is to give recommendations, when possible, on current concepts and outcome measurements, as well as to provide specific recommendations for various methods and their application in different groups of patients. Other ICI committees report on the etiology, epidemiology, pathophysiology, prevention, and economics of lower urinary tract dysfunction. This committee only covers these areas briefly, when appropriate.

Methodology and terminology in incontinence research should comply with standards established by the International Continence Society (ICS) [1-15]. The ICS Standardization Committee describes the "now-state" (how to do things right using present knowledge) with regard to interventions in patients by a number of "Outcome Groups" [12,13,14,15] while the future "desired state" (to do the right things in order to develop the area) is processed by a number of work groups with the collective name "Clinical Research Assessment". The recommendations from the ICS Standardization Committee on "General Outcomes" [12] and subcommittee recommendations [13,14,15] lower urinary tract dysfunction in women, men, frail older people, children, and neurogenic disorders are integrated into this chapter. Recommendations from national working groups have also been included when appropriate, for example, the Urodynamic Society's recommendations for outcome research [16,17,18].

The aim of clinical research is clear – namely, to offer freedom or relief from symptoms, and eventually to prevent the origin of disease. The need for high quality research is similarly evident. The prevalence and impact of genitourinary disease has been underestimated in the past, impairing research efforts. Many factors, including embarrassment and ignorance keep patients from seeking care and contribute toward making incontinence a silent disease. A gradually increasing degree of openness in society means that patients feel less guilty about urinary incontinence and other lower urinary tract symptoms. When these factors are coupled with the marked demographic trend toward an older society it produces an explosive increase in demand for incontinence therapy. At the same time, our knowledge of the etiology of incontinence, optimal treatment strategies, and prevention is greatly inadequate. In order to meet this need effectively, we need to intensify research. Proper choice and use of methods decides whether or not we will be successful in our efforts. The quality of research is not only important immediately (to improve treatment) but in a larger sense that research funding is severely limited in relation to need. There is great competition for government funding and other resources. While there is ample evidence that urinary incontinence is a greatly troublesome disease creating a major impact on patient's quality of life, priority for funding research may be compared against heart disease, cancer, infections, as well as in relation to other non-life-threatening diseases. We must therefore constantly strive to produce the highest quality work so as to make the best use of each research dollar and to encourage future competitive funding. We must also acknowledge the wide spectrum of interest in incontinence research. While clinicians are primarily interested in specific disease outcomes, government bodies may require more generalized assessment of global impact on quality and quantity of life.

There are many goals of research—foremost to improve care of patients, but also to promote understanding of the disease process. We need a broad spectrum of information if we are to not only understand which treatments work but also how and why they work (or don't). The ultimate goal is to produce credible research. When research is inherently credible due to strong study design the impact is maximized. The clinical application of the research will be hastened and other investigators will be energized to use the information in their own quest for knowledge. The recommendations given in this document have less the character of definitive standards than of guidelines and options, although on occasion the current state of evidence is such that standards are available. We have tried to keep a discursive style, but also give firm and practical advice when possible and appropriate.

II. GENERAL RECOMMENDATIONS FOR CLINICAL RESEARCH IN INCONTINENCE

1. THE PLANNING PHASE OF A CLINICAL STUDY ON INCONTINENCE

Meticulous planning is essential in all clinical research. The work done before initiating a research protocol does not in itself guarantee success but it is the obligatory first step in that direction. At the same time, inadequate planning can doom even carefully conducted protocols. Both prospective and retrospective studies require the same deliberate approach in the planning stage. The background and rationale for the study as well as the study objectives and/or hypotheses must be clearly elucidated and documented. There are many mistakes that should be avoided in the planning and conduct of a clinical study. A detailed list of common pitfalls in preparing and writing protocols has been taken from Spilker [19] to illustrate many avoidable errors (Table 1).

The first step of the planning phase involves reviewing previous and, if possible, ongoing work in the field. A study may be well performed but clinically irrelevant. A thorough knowledge of related clinical work is the cornerstone of protocol development. Fortunately, in urinary incontinence the work of the Cochrane Collaboration (www.cochrane.org) and its Cochrane Incontinence Group (www.otago.ac.nz/cure/) provide a tremendous asset to the potential investigator. The Cochrane reviewers have registered over 1300 trials in the field and produced 16 reviews (with others in progress) that cover most issues in conservative therapy as well as many other topics. This concentrated collection of data allows researchers to hone in on key questions

Table 1: Common pitfalls in preparing and writing protocols (from Spilker 1984)

A. Study objectives

1. Expressed too generally to allow a specific study design to be constituted
2. Ambiguous or vague
3. Not achievable with the current study design. The study may be too complex or there may be inadequate resources to conduct the study

B. Study design

1. Insufficient statistical planning—the design will not adequately address study objectives
2. The design chosen is beyond current state of the art
3. Inadequate validation of outcome measures
4. Inadequate statistical power. The chosen sample size is too small to detect clinically meaningful differences
5. Inappropriate use of active or inactive controls
6. Lack of placebo or double blind when one or both should be incorporated
7. Dose regimen too restrictive (e.g., range of allowed doses, alterations of dosing for adverse reactions)
8. Failure to consult with statistician regarding randomization process

C. Inclusion/exclusion criteria

1. Too stringent to allow adequate numbers of subjects to be enrolled. Overly stringent criteria also reduce the generalizability and thus the impact of research
2. Too broad to create homogenous groups.

D. Screen/baseline/treatment

1. Time periods for data collection are either too long or too short for optimal conduct of the study
2. Too few or too many measurements are requested
3. Subjects may be inappropriately entered into the study before complete screening
4. Excessive blood volume removed for testing or an excessive period of fasting is required. This is especially common in pharmacokinetic studies

E. Drug packaging/dispensing

1. Drug packaging that does not permit all options allowed by protocol to be followed

F. Study blind

1. Study blind easily broken because of "obvious" characteristics (e.g., adverse reactions, changes in laboratory parameters, drug odor) that are difficult or impossible to adequately mask
2. Study blind easily broken by observation of drug interactions or other situations by the investigator (e.g. marked improvement in study group or changes in blood levels of concomitant drugs)
3. Study blind inappropriate

G. Data collection and analysis

1. Poorly designed data collection forms
2. Incorrect statistical methods used to analyze data, including baseline comparisons
3. Failure to make the primary research question the main focus of the analysis
4. Reliance on within group rather than between group comparisons in parallel group trials
5. Overreliance on p-values without presenting confidence intervals

H. Overall

1. Ambiguous language that allows different interpretations
2. Too many comparisons requested. Five of every 100 independent comparisons will be statistically significant by chance alone, when alpha is 5% and there are no true differences between the comparison groups.
3. Lack of internal consistency in the protocol
4. Discretionary judgments allowed by the investigator. This may seriously affect the quality and quantity of data obtained
5. Presentation/reporting fails to accord with CONSORT guidelines

and focus their research. Recommendations of the group help to assure that future studies will be interpretable in the context of past work. This is an appropriate starting point for any literature search.

A rule of thumb for all research is that one should seek the least complex approach to adequately answer or address a given problem, hypothesis or question. The project must provide a convincing answer to the question in an efficient manner. At the same time, the committee has struggled with the desire to gain more from clinical research than an answer to treatment efficacy. We still need to understand how our treatments work. It may be helpful to think of the dilemma as a balance between breadth and depth [19]. While it is important to remember that only a limited number of questions should be posed in one study protocol it is still relevant to record as many observations as possible without jeopardizing subject recruitment or retention with onerous demands.

2. Study design: types of clinical trials

Discussion of the various types of studies and other aspects of study design can be described as the framework by which the study objectives will be met. Different considerations might be made for etiological, epidemiological and pathophysiological studies on the one hand, and for clinical trials on the other. Ideally, clinical research should be prospective, controlled and randomized. However, some studies can only be performed retrospectively and good clinical research methodology does not always mean controlled or blinded studies. Sometimes open and uncontrolled studies are accepted, as in a phase I study when a new pharmacological agent is tested for the first time in humans, and in pilot studies where a new surgical technique is being developed.

The following definitions of Phase I-IV studies have been constructed from Senn [20].

- ***Phase I studies:*** The first studies with the actual drug in humans. Often, but not exclusively carried out in healthy volunteers. Pharmacokinetics and tolerance information are obtained in these studies.
- ***Phase II studies:*** The first attempts to prove efficacy of a treatment. These are often the first studies in patients. Dose finding is a common objective of such studies.
- ***Phase III studies:*** Large-scale "definitive" studies carried out once probable effective and tolerated doses of the drug have been established with the object of proving that the drug is suitable for registration.
- ***Phase IV studies:*** Studies undertaken either during or after registration with the purpose of discovering more about the drug safety and efficacy in different populations. Such studies are often larger and simpler than regulatory studies and may lack a control group.

Randomized Controlled Trials (RCTs) are the most important method for demonstrating the effectiveness of treatments. Phase III studies are usually RCT in format, using the regimen indicated from phase II, in comparison with placebo and/or a comparator, such as equivalent drug or other therapy. Parallel groups are recommended as the first choice, while the crossover design is best suited for intra-individual comparisons (see below).

a) Types of trials

- ***Parallel Designs:*** *Parallel clinical trial* designs offer subjects only one treatment during the study. In a placebo-controlled trial, the patient is assigned to receive placebo or the active drug according to the study protocol, with the predetermined outcome measure obtained at the time of the study follow-up. During a drug trial, the dosage of drug may be held steady or, in a variable dose trial, the dosage may be increased to maximize clinical benefit or decreased if side effects occur.
- ***Crossover trials***: An alternative to the parallel groups design is the *crossover trial*, in which patients experience both arms of the study [21,22,23]. Like parallel designs, randomization is important in the limitation of bias; in crossover trials, patients are randomly allocated to receive the treatments in one order or the other. Crossover trials allow for within subject comparisons, which may provide a more precise measure of treatment effectiveness. The effect of variance between subjects is removed, unlike in parallel group designs. Crossover studies are particularly well suited for small study groups with chronic stable disease states in which the primary objective is to measure a short-term response in symptoms. The treatment itself should not have a long lasting result once it is stopped. The duration of treatment is important in this design. If the duration of treatment is too short, the treatment may not show its effect or make too small an effect to be adequately measured. If the duration of treatment is too long, compliance may be poor or the disease may not remain stable. *Crossover effects* may occur, where the results of the first treatment linger and affect the second treatment. To avoid crossover effects, a *washout period* is planned where subjects receive either no treatment or placebo. To ensure adequate disease stability before the start of the study, a *run-in period* of monitoring relevant signs or symptoms can be undertaken. Those with transitory or labile disease can then be excluded.

- ***Equivalence trials:*** The primary objective of an equivalence trial is to demonstrate that two treatments are similar in outcome or that there is no difference between treatment and controls. This can be of relevance when one treatment is significantly more cost-effective, offers a better quality of life, or is less toxic or time consuming for the patient when similar clinical outcome can be achieved. In this scenario, it is the primary objective to demonstrate that a more conservative therapy is no different than the standard by a degree of measure that the investigator feels would make the two treatments equivalent. It should be emphasized that this type of trial is not the same as failing to find a difference between two groups. In contrast, this is a powerful design when appropriately employed. The goal is to demonstrate that the observed difference between two treatments is small with a narrow confidence interval. Specific statistical methods are needed to ensure adequate power to find a difference between the groups if one truly exists.

The magnitude of clinically unimportant differences may be quite small, which is one reason why equivalence trials often need large sample sizes [20,24]. Equivalence trials need to be designed and conducted with particular care. Unlike the other approaches, equivalence trials aim to demonstrate that the trial arms are equivalent or, at least, are not particularly different. For a conclusion of this kind to be valid, researchers should be especially vigilant that failure to demonstrate a difference is not merely a consequence of poor study design and procedures.

3. Study conduct and statistical considerations

Research must be planned early, and planned often. All issues should be addressed at the start of the planning process, and many will need to be re-addressed at suitable times throughout the project. Many of these issues are statistical; indeed, the major statistical input to a study should be at the design stage, including planning the data analysis in advance to follow the design of the study. Leaving this until the end of a study will almost always lead to difficulties that cannot be resolved, resulting in a study which is at best inefficient, and at worst inconclusive.

The issues covered here relate to: study design; sampling strategies; randomization and stratification; primary and secondary outcomes; inclusion and exclusion criteria; blinding and effects on validity; control of bias; sample size considerations; pragmatic and explanatory trials; data analysis; and reporting of randomized controlled trials (RCTs). Only the principal features of study design and analysis will be covered here; extensive coverage is available elsewhere [24]. Regarding presentation, the Consolidated Standards of Reporting Trials (CONSORT) statement provides guidelines for reporting the design, detailed methods, and results of RCTs [25]. The original statement [26,27] has recently been revised with the aim of improving clarity and, where appropriate, increasing flexibility [28-31]. Many of the points discussed here relate to those guidelines.

a) Study design

The most fundamental planning issue is whether the study is observational or experimental. Observational studies include a variety of designs, from cross-sectional descriptive studies (where the primary purpose is estimation of the prevalence of incontinence in a defined population) to case-control designs and long-term prospective or retrospective cohort studies. Observational studies may be purely descriptive, or they may be analytic when designed with a control or comparison group. The limitation that all comparisons based on observational data have in common, however, is that it is not possible to ensure that one is comparing like with like. In particular, the bias that results from differential selection effects (both patient and clinician induced) cannot be eliminated, even by the use of advanced statistical methods.

Properly planned and executed, the RCT is the optimal approach to limiting selection bias [32] RCTs compare outcomes in groups of subjects with the allocation of treatment determined by chance. In this way, the treatment groups will not differ in any systematic fashion, and comparisons between them will be unbiased [21]. Subject assignment must be concealed during enrollment (e.g., by separating allocation from the process of recruiting subjects, and by using sealed envelopes or, preferably, telephone randomization). In addition, treatment allocation must be concealed during the trial (e.g., through blinding with or without use of placebo). In some studies, blinding of subjects and health care providers may be impossible or undesirable. This can occur with some surgical trials, or with studies of health care delivery. In all cases, however, those personnel collecting outcome data should be blinded to the subjects' treatment allocation.

RCTs provide the optimum level of evidence about the clinical effectiveness of different interventions [28]. Observational studies can contribute useful information on many aspects of health care [33], and may be necessary pre-cursors to a randomized trial, but the central position of the RCT in terms of influencing patient care should and will continue. The classical (two) parallel groups RCT is not the only option within the experimental paradigm; complex randomized designs such as factorial and cross-over designs may overcome some of the limitations of and objections to the standard approach [23].

The type of study design for a clinical trial is dependent upon the *primary research question*. In particular, the primary question is critical in determining the *sample size* needed for the study. Obtaining adequate numbers of patients to address the primary research question is crucial to avoid the problem of an underpowered study and insufficiently precise estimates of the comparisons between the treatments (for details see below). A sufficient *power* (probability of detecting a difference if it exists) is required to minimize the risk of a Type II or *beta error* – that is, failing to find a difference between the treatment groups even when one exists.

Secondary factors that influence the choice of a study design may be related to the natural history of the disease, the treatment itself or patient endpoints. Patient-related endpoints may be short term such as changes in signs or symptoms or may be more long term such as increased survival. Once the sample size required for the primary research question has been calculated it is usually obvious if the study can be performed in a *single institution* or if a *multicenter* study is required. Single institution studies have the benefit of being less complicated since all personnel are on site and study coordination is less difficult. However, if a large sample size is required a single institution may take years to accrue the required number of patients. While multicenter trials are more complex from an administrative point of view and are generally more expensive, they provide larger numbers of patients in a shorter period of time, and have benefits in terms of the generalizability of the research findings.

b) Strategies

Whether a study is descriptive or analytical, the first practical issue to resolve is the selection of participants. Some studies require a sample that is representative of the community overall. In principle, this is achieved by taking a simple random sample from a known population. In practice, a list of all eligible and consenting individuals is obtained and then a sample is drawn by a method in which each member of the population has an equal probability of selection ('epsem'). Even in ideal circumstances, however, some sophistication on this basic method is usually desirable or necessary. For example, in *stratified sampling*, subjects are arranged into subgroups and the sampling is performed within each subgroup separately. This ensures that the sample is representative of the population in terms of these subgroup characteristics. In *multi-stage random sampling*, the population is first divided into 'primary sampling units' (such as hospital, health center, or surgeon), and a sample of primary units is selected. The 'secondary sampling units' (usually individual subjects) are then selected just within the primary sampling units that have been selected. A special case of multi-stage random sampling is *cluster sampling* where all individuals within each primary unit are included. Standard procedures for sampling should be followed [34].

It is important to note that, while the technicalities of random selection of subjects for a study are closely related to the random allocation of patients in a clinical trial (and indeed there are similar issues in trials relating to stratification and clustering [35]), there is an important distinction in the objectives of the two procedures. First, the (ideally random) *selection* from the population of eligible subjects concerns the *external validity* or generalizability of the study findings (RCT or otherwise). Independent of this, the random *allocation* of subjects in an RCT is concerned with the *internal validity* or comparability of the trial groups.

In principle, sampling should involve random selection. In practice, however, this ideal is rarely met outside of large-scale epidemiological studies. Rather, a consecutive series of patients at a particular health care setting over a specified period of time often forms the basis of recruitment to a study. Where this is the case, it is crucial to provide descriptive information about the study sample, so that broad representativeness can be judged. This is as important for trials as for observational studies. Guidelines for reporting of RCTs include requirements to state the study population, give details of inclusion and exclusion criteria, and present clearly the numbers of eligible subjects who were not randomized and the reasons [28,29,36] Nevertheless, "the basic logic of clinical trials is comparative and not representative" [20]. In other words, the principal benefit of conducting a randomized trial is to provide groups that allow valid comparisons to be made.

c) Randomization and stratification

Randomization is the process of allocating subjects to groups by chance [21,32]. Neither the subject nor the clinical staff responsible for recruitment to the trial should be able to predict to which group the subject will be assigned. Randomization removes treatment selection from the hands of the clinician thereby removing selection bias.

In order to minimize bias, the randomization process must be concealed from those recruiting subjects to the trial [28,36]. This can be achieved most effectively for multicenter trials by the use of central telephone randomization. Sealed opaque envelopes can be used for studies performed at a single institution. In drug studies, a pharmacy can maintain identical treatment drug and placebo already randomly allocated into individual subject portions. These are distributed consecutively as subjects are enrolled in the study.

• ***Simple randomization*** can use computer-generated random numbers, either prepared specifically for the trial or using existing tables of random numbers where the digits of 0-9 appear with equal likelihood in each entry. Treatments are assigned to odd or even numbers. As the total number of subjects in the trial increases, the balance of numbers and characteristics of subjects between the groups improves. In small trials, however, balance is not assured by simple randomization. Appreciable imbalances in subjects per group may be particularly important in a multicenter study where imbalances in assignment can occur within individual institutions.

• ***Block randomization*** is one method used to prevent imbalances in subject numbers assigned to each group, particularly when the number of subjects in the trial is small. With block randomization, the total sample size is divided into blocks of a given size. Within each block, the group is assigned so that there are equal numbers allocated to each group. To prevent investigators from learning the block size and being able to guess order of assignment, the block size can be varied, usually at random from a small number of alternatives.

Most disease states have factors known to influence the outcome of treatment. A form of randomization that accounts for such factors is called *stratified randomization* [21,32]. Stratified randomization ensures equal distribution of subjects with a particular characteristic in each group. Stratification is usually restricted to a small number of factors, in particular those most likely to influence outcome. Despite its complexity, stratified randomization is usually helpful in a multicenter trial, so that both the numbers of subjects in each group and the important factors influencing the outcome can be balanced within each site. An alternative method exists to cater for more factors at once, known as *minimization,* where the characteristics of individuals already randomized alter in a systematic manner the chances of a given subject being allocated to the different trial groups, so as to maximize the resulting balance of these factors [21,32].

d) Primary and secondary outcomes

Specific discussions of the most appropriate outcome measures for particular studies of incontinence will be dealt with elsewhere in this book; the purpose here is to define the general concepts of primary and secondary outcomes in the context of RCTs, which are relevant to both sample size determination and data analysis. The distinction between these two sets of outcomes depends on the context of the trial, and should be decided at the planning stage of the study. Primary and secondary outcomes should not be confused with the distinction between primary and secondary analyses of trial data, which will be discussed later. Primary outcomes are those viewed by the researchers to be of central interest. Trial results that lead to major changes in patient care will be based on primary outcomes.

The number of primary outcomes in a particular trial will depend on the nature of the interventions and the number of independent domains. The number of primary outcomes is usually limited to three, and rarely will there be reasonable justification for more than six. Sample size calculation is based on the primary outcomes and is unlikely to be based on more than two outcome measures. The number and nature of outcome domains in a particular study will vary depending on the study's perspective (e.g., those of patients, clinicians, regulatory bodies, and health care purchasers). In almost all situations, the outcome set should include a dimension representing the viewpoint of the patient (such as a questionnaire relating to symptoms and impact on quality of life) as well as an appropriate clinical outcome measure.

Secondary outcomes are the remaining outcome measures and could be relatively large in number. They are not the focus of the main study objectives and are rarely used directly in sample size estimation. Secondary outcomes are often subject to the dangers of multiple hypothesis testing, for which suitable corrections should be considered as described below. Analyses of secondary outcomes are often best viewed as exploratory, i.e., as hypothesis-generating exercises for which independent confirmation is essential.

e) Inclusion and exclusion criteria

Inclusion and exclusion criteria should provide a relevant population to address the study question, and together define the heterogeneity or homogeneity of the study population. Broadening the inclusion criteria can make a study more generalizable and facilitate recruitment. Making the entry criteria too broad, however, may dilute the effect being sought in the most suitable patients. If the study population is defined too narrowly with many exclusion criteria, applicability of the results may be limited and subject recruitment may be difficult.

Inclusion criteria govern what patient characteristics are required for eligibility to enter the study. Some exclusion criteria such as age, weight and gender are determined implicitly by corresponding inclusion parameters. Issues of patient safety determine other exclusion parameters (e.g., avoiding nephrotoxic drugs in patients with renal insufficiency). All parameters should be precise enough to allow the study to be reproduced by other groups of researchers.

The most important inclusion criterion is how the disease in question is defined. Eligibility criteria are critical to both the interpretation of the study and its reproducibility. If possible, established international criteria for the presence and severity of disease should be used. Inclusion criteria should screen for patients who are known 'non-responders' to the treatment being studied.

Including these patients can result in false negative clinical trial results since they do not have a reasonable expectation of improvement.

f) Informed consent

Peer review of protocols by a multidisciplinary team may include members of the scientific community, clinicians, pharmacists, the public, the legal profession and religious representatives. Each member of this team reviews the protocol from their particular type of expertise and in doing so aids in safeguarding patient health and well-being.

Informed patient consent is required for participation. The length and depth of detail in consent forms vary widely between institutions. In the most extreme, they involve exhaustive pages of information, which explain every alternative treatment and its pros and cons in detail. A general list of requirements for a consent form includes: name of the investigators and contact numbers, a detailed description of the new treatment and its known side effects, rationale for why the new therapy may be better compared to standard therapy. A summary table of the results of previous studies using the drug can be helpful in some circumstances. A statement that the patient may decline to be in the study with no subsequent consequence to their ongoing medical care is generally provided and whether or not remuneration is expected. An understanding that the patient will be randomly assigned to treatment should be included.

A review committee should be established prior to initiation of the trial. In addition to reviewing results of the study for safety monitoring they may conduct an interim analysis to ensure that a treatment is not producing unacceptable levels of side effects. Rules for stopping the study in this case are agreed upon usually prior to the start of the trial. Emergency procedures for unblinding a patient are put in place in the case of a severe side effect or concomitant serious illness.

g) Bias, blinding, and effects on validity

All human players in a clinical trial can introduce bias (systematic error), which can result in erroneous conclusions regarding treatment effects. Bias can occur in every aspect of a clinical trial from the process of randomization to observation of the outcome variables and the statistical analysis itself. Bias occurs because of previously conceived ideas held by those involved, which unconsciously affect their actions and observations. In addition to *observer bias*, an amount of *observer error* is inherent in outcome measures that require clinical interpretation. To avoid or limit bias, blinding should be employed whenever possible, with concealment of allocation and blinding of outcome assessors being the most important. *Blinding* is the process by which key elements of knowledge are withheld that can otherwise lead to bias. Blinding should not be confused with *concealment of allocation*, referring to withholding knowledge of assignment in advance, which is a prerequisite for the validity of any trial (Moher, Schulz et al, 2001; Altman et al, 2001) [28,36].

Unblinded trials are conducted in an open manner where both subjects and clinicians are aware of which treatment has been assigned. While certain types of therapy may require investigation in this manner (e.g., some surgical trials), there remains considerable opportunity for bias. Both subjects and clinicians may have preconceived ideas regarding the benefits of a particular treatment that can influence the reporting of symptoms and/or their outcome.

In a ***single blind*** trial, the subject is blinded to group assignment. It may be advantageous for the clinical staff to be aware of the assignment to allow them to monitor the health and safety of individuals, since the potential effects of the treatment (side effects) will often be known in advance. Single blinding ameliorates biased reporting of symptoms and/or side effects by subjects. However, clinical staff can influence data collection and change other aspects of subjects' care when they know which study treatment subjects are receiving. Moreover, particularly when a placebo is used in a trial, clinicians can systematically introduce co-interventions (or even the treatment under study itself) to the placebo group, thereby potentially diluting any differences between the trial arms.

In ***double blind*** trials, both parties who could influence outcome are unaware of group assignment. Often this is just the subjects and the clinical team responsible for their care. More generally, the term *double blind* relates to subjects and research personnel responsible for the measurement and assessment of outcome [21,28]. While this reduces potential sources of bias considerably compared with unblinded or single blind trials, it does introduce other levels of complexity. For example, safety monitoring must be performed by a third party.

Triple blind trials include blinding of subjects, outcome assessors, and those involved in data analysis. If the same persons carry out data analysis and safety monitoring, it can be difficult to ensure proper monitoring of complications and outcome. It might be argued that subject safety may not be properly ensured unless the monitoring committee knows which arm of the study is the treatment and which is the control (placebo). For the same reasons, clinical staff may not feel comfortable participating in such a study.

If investigators are aware of the results of interim analyses, this may cause bias by influencing how vigorously any given patient is recruited into the study. Another opportunity for bias occurs if an appreciable number of subjects drop out or withdraw during a study, and fail to provide outcome data. This can be particularly problematic if withdrawal is related to group assignment and if it unequally affects one arm of a parallel group design. In this scenario, both the monitoring team and the trial data analyst must carefully consider the reasons for subject withdrawals.

h) Sample size considerations

Sample size should be calculated in the planning stage of all studies. There are many formal equations to assist in this process, details of which will not be given here [21,37,38,39]. Rather, the emphasis for this discussion is on the concepts involved and the information required for the calculations to proceed. Determination of sample size is not an exact science. Many decisions about design and analysis are interrelated with specifications for sample size, and the process does not have a single solution. This is no reason to abandon the exercise, but reinforces the need to include someone with appropriate statistical expertise in the research team.

There are three fundamental approaches to sample size calculation. One is based on the required precision of an estimate. The second requires that the study have adequate probability (power) of detecting a given (target) magnitude of effect. The third aims to demonstrate equivalence between treatment groups. In all cases, appropriate adjustment for attrition (loss to follow-up) should be performed.

The first of these approaches is relevant to both descriptive and analytical investigations. The basic issue is one of precision (measured by the standard error, SE) or margin of error (which depends on the SE but is more specifically defined as half the width of the 95% confidence interval [CI] around the estimate). The higher the level of precision specified in advance (i.e., the smaller the SE and the narrower the CI), the larger the sample size will need to be. However, the margin of error depends on the nature of the primary outcome variable, i.e., whether it is a continuous variable (such as maximum urinary flow rate) or a binary variable (such as the presence or absence of self-reported urge incontinence). For a continuous variable, the variability (standard deviation) of the measure must be estimated for relevant patients; this may be derived from some combination of clinical experience, the literature, or a pilot study. The larger the variability, the larger the sample size required. For a binary variable, its prevalence must be estimated in the population to be studied, since the SE for such variables depends on their prevalence.

The second approach, based on power, is the most commonly used. It requires similar prior information, including estimates of the variability for continuous measures and the magnitude of proportions for binary variables. In addition, it requires specification of three other quantities: the *significance level*, the *power*, and the *target difference*. The *significance level*, termed alpha, is conventionally, though not necessarily, set at 5%. *Power* is defined as the probability that the study will detect (as statistically significant at the alpha level specified) a given target difference between the groups, if such a difference exists. Power is commonly specified in the range of 80% to 90%, which implies a risk of not detecting the target difference of between 20% and 10%, respectively. For a trial involving anything other than minor risks and expenditure, a power closer to 90% than 80% would seem preferable [24], which leads to a larger sample size (as does a stricter alpha level of, say, 1%). This is most pertinent when a lack of statistical significance is obtained in a small trial, particularly when the sample size was not planned using a power calculation [21]. This is the basis for the adage that "the absence of evidence is not evidence of absence" [20]. A planned unequal allocation to the trial groups also requires an inflation of the sample size [21], as does interim analyses. By multiplying the number of significance tests performed, studies with interim analyses generally require stricter significance levels at each analytical point [20,37].

The *target difference* is the last, and arguably the most important, quantity that must be specified for the power-based approach to sample size calculation. The target difference is defined as the minimum difference needed for clinical significance. Clinical significance is an entirely different concept from statistical significance. Investigators must estimate the clinical significance as the magnitude of difference (in means or proportions) that would lead to a change in clinical management for the target group of patients. The smaller the difference, the larger the required sample size. Statistical significance means that the observed difference, whatever its magnitude, cannot reasonably be considered as being due to chance. Statistical significance (denoted by the p-value) represents the strength of evidence against the null hypothesis [40]. The degree of clinical significance can be inferred only with the additional information of a confidence interval for the comparison between groups.

The third general approach aims to demonstrate equivalence between trial groups [39]. The same specifications are made as in the power-based approach, except that instead of specifying a particular target difference to be detected, the calculation is centered on the magnitude of difference beyond which the researchers would no longer accept that the treatments are 'equivalent'. The study is designed to have adequate power to produce a confidence interval for the difference between the groups, which does *not* include values greater than this limit.

There is no single answer for sample size determination; often the calculation proceeds around a 'circle of specifications' (involving, say, power, target difference and sample size) many times, starting and stopping at different points. For instance, it is not uncommon to commence with the 'textbook' approach of specifying power and target difference (along with alpha and the standard deviation) and calculating the sample size, then to reverse the argument by starting with how many subjects could be recruited and determining what differences could be detected with various probabilities! Furthermore, the ideal of the target being the *minimum* for clinical significance cannot always be met; rather, the aim in practice is to produce a convincing argument (among the researchers themselves, and also to funding bodies and regulatory agencies) that the sample size has an adequate chance of detecting differences that are (a) feasible, and (b) worthwhile detecting in clinical terms. A common failing is selecting a target difference that is too large, often derived from differences that have been observed or published previously rather than based on considered clinical judgment. Preliminary investigations (often termed 'elicitation exercises') into the levels of treatment effects that patients themselves consider worthwhile should be carried out much more commonly than is the case at present. Likewise, more evidence is required concerning the relationships between the responsiveness (sensitivity to change following treatment) of clinical and patient based outcome measures.

i) Pragmatic and explanatory trials

There is an important distinction between *pragmatic* and *explanatory* trials [41,42] and correspondingly, between *intention-to-treat* and *per-protocol* approaches to data analysis [20,37]. In pragmatic trials, data are analyzed by intention-to-treat, according to the group to which subjects were randomized, regardless of the extent of compliance with the intended treatment. In explanatory trials, data are analyzed accounting for compliance. This per-protocol approach may exclude serious non-compliers, analyze data according to treatment actually received, or allow for degree of compliance in a statistical model. At first sight, the explanatory approach appears more attractive. However, there are considerable limitations to the explanatory approach, particularly when the intention is to draw inferences from the trial to wider clinical practice.

The purpose of randomization is to produce groups that are, on average, comparable. A per-protocol analysis retains this property only in the unlikely situation when non-compliance is unrelated both to the patient's underlying state of health and the treatment received [20]. The intention-to-treat approach in pragmatic trials retains the full benefits of randomization and has the advantage that the comparison will more closely reflect the relative effectiveness of the treatments when applied in real clinical practice, where non-compliance obviously occurs [43]. In pragmatic trials, the interventions are designed to be as close as possible to treatment options in clinical practice (including 'cascades' of patient management choices) and entry criteria are usually relatively liberal. Pragmatic trials may involve a wide variety of outcome domains, including patient-completed questionnaires, and an economic evaluation of outcomes. Because of intention-to-treat data analysis, pragmatic trials will tend to yield lower estimates of treatment differences than explanatory trials. It may be of interest to gauge the effect of treatment given full compliance, so full data analysis may incorporate elements of intention-to-treat and per-protocol approaches [20].

The follow-up time for a trial should be at a fixed point (for logistical reasons, this is in practice often a short time window) relative to randomization rather than when treatment was actually received, since again this is the only way of ensuring a valid comparison. The planned timing of follow-up should allow for any likely delays in receiving treatment, e.g., due to surgical waiting lists.

In summary, it is established practice that unless there are strong reasons to the contrary the primary analyses (for both primary and secondary outcomes) of an RCT should be on an intention-to-treat basis [28,36]. Secondary analyses incorporating non-compliance and/or which treatment was actually received may be justified in addition to the primary analyses. Appreciable loss to follow-up in a trial (which is not the same as non-compliance with intended treatment, lack of efficacy, or the observation of adverse events) may present serious problems both in terms of generalizability of the findings to the wider population and, in the case of differential loss to follow-up across treatment groups, to the validity of the comparisons. Indeed, strictly speaking any missing outcome data means that not all of those allocated to the various randomization groups can be included in the analysis [28,44] and this might lead to the conclusion that the term 'intention-to-treat' should only be used if follow-up is complete. In practice complete follow-up occurs only rarely. Under current guidelines, intention-to-treat relates more to the broad strategy adopted by the researchers for data analysis [45]. Results should always be accompanied by a full and clear statement of how deviations from intended treatment and missing outcome measures have been handled in the analysis. The discussion should include how missing outcome data may have affected the conclusions [44]. Sensitivity analyses can be used to test the exclusion of, or assumptions about, missing values; practical examples of such analyses are becoming more common [46].

j) Data analysis

This section will not contain any technical details of statistical methods, which are available in standard texts [21,47] but rather will summarize concepts of data analysis. The emphasis here will be on RCTs, although many of the complex methods mentioned (e.g., multiple logistic regression analysis) are used in similar ways to analyze observational data. Appropriate techniques of data analysis will depend on the nature of the outcome variable. In practically all situations, hypothesis tests should be two-sided, rather than one-sided. One-sided tests are only appropriate if a difference in one direction is not just unlikely, but would not be of interest.

Regardless of the type and complexity of statistical techniques used in analysis, the general underlying principles behind hypothesis testing and estimation apply. In particular, the statistical significance of a hypothesis test should be interpreted critically. The actual p-value should be considered, rather than just whether or not it is below an arbitrary threshold such as 5% [28]; indeed, the p-value is better considered a measure of the strength of evidence against the null hypothesis, on a continuum or 'shades-of-gray' [40]. The direction and magnitude of the trial comparison should be presented with an appropriate confidence interval to indicate the possible clinical significance and precision of the comparison [28].

Data analysis for numerical outcome variables may use parametric or non-parametric methods. Simple parametric methods require that the data follow a normal distribution, while non-parametric methods do not have this requirement. Parametric methods of testing mean values include t-tests, confidence intervals for differences between group means, and analysis of variance. Regression techniques address more advanced issues such as stratification in randomization and allowance for baseline measures. Non-parametric methods include the Mann-Whitney test to compare two independent samples as in a parallel groups trial and the Wilcoxon matched-pairs signed-ranks test for paired data such as from a crossover trial [23]. Binary outcome variables can be analyzed using chi-square tests and confidence intervals for comparing proportions, and multiple logistic regression [48]. For time-to-event data (such as survival data), methods of data analysis include life tables, Kaplan-Meier survival curves, log rank tests, and Cox's proportional hazards regression [49].

How, then, should the analysis of data from an RCT proceed? An outline of the various stages of data analysis can be gleaned from the CONSORT statement [28,36]. The following discussion will concentrate on the underlying concepts of data analysis at a particular follow-up time relative to randomization, and considers initially the simplest case of just two trial groups. Multiple treatment groups will be covered briefly, but repeated measurements on outcomes and interim analyses involve considerably more complex methods of planning and analysis, for which expert help is essential [20,23,37,50].

The first stage of data analysis is to address the representativeness of randomized subjects compared to the target population of eligible patients. The number of eligible patients who were and were not randomized should be provided, along with reasons for the latter. The presentation of this information is facilitated by use of the ***CONSORT flow diagram*** [28,36]—indeed, its use is associated with improved quality of reporting of trials generally [51]. Descriptive statistics should be given of important characteristics of health care professionals approached for involvement in recruiting subjects to the trial, both for those taking part and those declining.

The second stage of data analysis is to compare the two groups at randomization (baseline) including demographic, prognostic, and outcome variables. A common error at this point is to rely on statistical testing for these comparisons [20,21,37]. If the randomization procedure has been performed correctly, then any statistically significant differences in baseline characteristics must be due to chance. Statistical testing of this kind is *not* a test of the comparability of trial groups; rather, it is a test of the allocation procedure [20, 21,37] It may be seriously misleading, particularly if lack of a statistically significant difference for a given characteristic is taken to imply comparability. Trials are not designed to detect potentially important differences in baseline characteristics that might be large enough to influence the comparison of the outcomes between the trial groups. The magnitude of this potentially influential difference for a baseline measure depends on the strength of its relationship with the outcome, and not on a p-value at randomization. Therefore, baseline comparability is best assessed by simply obtaining descriptive statistics for the groups and making a judgment as to whether any observed differences are likely to be influential or not. If differences are likely to be influential, they should be considered in the analyses. Notable exceptions to this are baseline measures of the outcome variables, which should be considered in the analysis regardless of the situation at baseline, since removing variance in the outcome measure that is purely attributable to differences between individuals at baseline has potentially marked benefits in terms of precision and power [20]. Investigators should consider stratifying the randomization on any strongly prognostic variable (for reasons of efficiency rather than bias). Since there are practical limitations to how many variables a trial can stratify for, a technique known as minimization

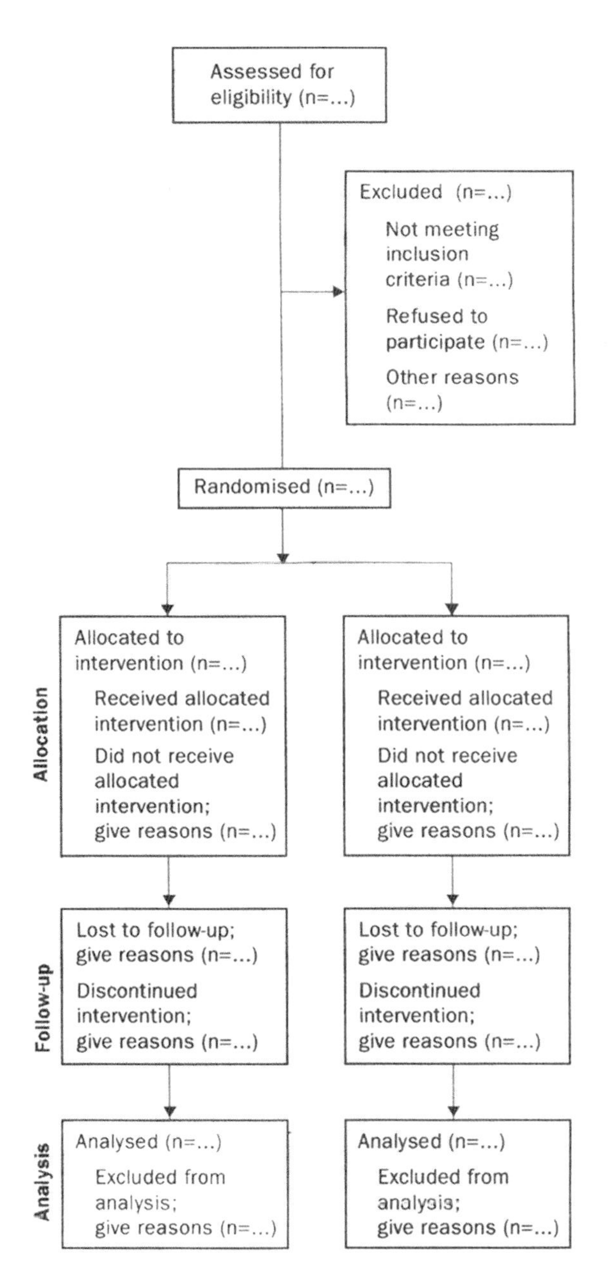

Flow diagram of the progress through the phases of a randomised trial

may also be considered [20,32]. Any variables stratified or minimized at randomization should be allowed for in the analysis [20].

The next stage of data analysis is to perform the primary analyses for the outcome variables. Primary outcomes should initially be analyzed by intention-to-treat comparisons of the groups as randomized, both using hypothesis tests for statistical significance and confidence intervals (CIs) for comparisons between the groups to assess clinical and statistical significance, usually adjusting for baseline measurements of the outcome variable. With a small number of primary outcomes, multiple testing is not a concern. However, when a large number of statistical tests are performed for secondary outcomes, corrections to the observed p-values should at least be considered. Similar issues of multiple testing for different outcomes are involved when there are more than two groups.

The most commonly used procedure for multiple testing is the Bonferroni correction [20,21,52]. The Bonferroni correction is fairly conservative in reducing the risk of a statistically significant effect occurring purely by chance, at the cost of reduced power for individual outcomes. This is particularly pertinent when, as is usually the case, the outcomes are positively associated with one another. While there are alternative procedures that improve this deficiency, none of them are entirely satisfactory [20]. It is emphasized that whatever strategy is adopted to deal with multiple testing, the major errors are to rely solely on p-values rather than present CIs as well, to over-simplify the presentation of p-values to just "NS" or "p<0.05" rather than to quote the actual p-values, and above all to report selectively the results of significance tests.

Another example of a "multiplicity" is where there are more than two treatment groups, e.g., when different doses of a drug are being investigated or when more than one 'active' procedure is being compared with placebo [20]. Similar issues to multiple testing of different outcomes are involved here, but there are a greater variety of commonly used procedures available to deal with the central concern of finding a difference purely by chance. Standard methods for dealing with this multiple comparisons problem include the procedures attributed to Tukey, Newman-Keuls and Dunnett [20, 23, 53].

More complex primary analyses adjust for baseline measurements and potentially important prognostic variables (including but not exclusively those that were unbalanced at randomization). They may also involve adjustments for center effects and the investigation of differential treatment effects across centers in multicenter trials [24]. The correct approach for continuous outcome variables is to use the (regression-based) technique known as the analysis of covariance [20,37]; the equivalent approach for binary outcomes is to use logistic regression. A commonly employed alternative for continuous outcome variables is to analyze simple change scores from baseline to follow-up (either in absolute or percentage terms), but for reasons of both bias and precision this is inferior to regression methods [20,37]. It is good practice to present both the (unadjusted) simple intention-to-treat results alongside those from the regression methods. In any case, the results from alternative analyses such as these should be compared in a sensitivity analysis of the conclusions [24].

Secondary analyses of trial data include per-protocol analyses with adjustments using regression methods for pertinent process measures such as degree of compliance with the allocated treatments. Secondary analyses also include planned subgroup analyses, such as different intervention effects across different age, ethnic, or disease severity groups. Subgroups should be analyzed by using appropriate interaction terms in regression models [28,37]. Using interaction terms rather than performing repeated, separate, subgroup-specific analyses considerably reduces the risk of false positive findings. [54]. Subgroup analyses should be carried out sparingly, specified in advance (preferably with a clinical rationale), and above all should not be reported selectively [28,54].

k) Reporting of randomized controlled trials

The CONSORT statement is specifically designed to provide standards for reporting RCTS [28, 36]. Adherence to these guidelines and the use of flow diagrams in particular is associated with improved quality in reporting of RCTs [51, 55]. Errors in presentation of statistical information are extensively covered in many textbooks [21, 47]. This section will emphasize the most important points on reporting of RCTs, to ensure an objective and comprehensive presentation of the trial itself, and also to facilitate any subsequent synthesis of research evidence including formal meta-analyses of RCTs. Meta-analyses are themselves the subject of separate reporting guidelines, the QUORUM statement [56]. Guidelines for reporting studies on diagnostic tests (the START document) will be published in 2001. However, such guidelines are not a panacea [31]; deficiencies in reporting are still common [55].

The CONSORT statement recommends clear statements about the objectives of the trial, intended study population, and planned comparisons. Subgroup or covariate analyses should be clearly specified and justified. The method of randomization should be stated, as should the unit of randomization; in most cases, this will be the individual subject but occasionally an aggregate group of subjects will be allocated jointly in a cluster randomized design [35]. Cluster randomized designs are also now the subject of separate reporting guidelines [57]. For all trials, specifications for the sample size calculation (primary outcomes, target differences, etc.) should be stated and justified. In addition, the precision actually obtained in a study must be presented. This requires confidence intervals as well as the observed p-values, at least for primary outcomes but preferably for all outcome variables. The principal confidence intervals should be for comparisons *between* the groups, rather than for differences in the outcomes *within* the trial groups [20,21]. Results should include a trial flow diagram, with numbers and reasons for the exclusion of eligible patients, randomization, and subsequent losses to follow-up [51]. Protocol deviations should be described and explained [37]. Finally, the discussion should include a brief summary of the trial's findings, possible explanations for the results, interpretation of the findings in light of the literature, limitations of the trial including internal and external validity, and the clinical and research implications of the study [28].

l) Conclusions

In conclusion, it is crucial that those intending to embark on research into incontinence plan the details of the study in advance. Many of the decisions to be made involve statistical issues; therefore it is vital that someone with relevant expertise is involved in the planning from the start. Statistics in general has been described as a combination of mathematics, logic and judgment [20], and this applies particularly to clinical trial design, conduct, analysis and reporting. Naturally, formally qualified biostatisticians are not the only professional group with the necessary expertise to address these issues, particularly since in the planning of studies the above three characteristics are probably stated in increasing order of importance. However, individuals with relevant statistical expertise are in a good position to contribute to research projects in these ways, if they are consulted sufficiently early in the process including at the piloting stage.

Furthermore, the benefits of such expertise will only fully be derived if the individuals are involved on an ongoing basis in the conduct of the trial. This is equally true of all the disciplines relevant to studies of health care technology and organization, including social scientists and health economists as well as statisticians and clinicians. Increasingly, the major funding bodies and international journals expect a sufficiently multi-disciplinary team to carry out and report on health services research. If for no other reason than because of their central position in influencing the purchasing and provision of health care, this is especially important for randomized controlled trials.

4. OUTCOME RESEARCH IN PATIENTS WITH LUTS, INCLUDING INCONTINENCE

INTRODUCTION

No single measure can fully express the outcome of an intervention. While every clinical trial must have a primary endpoint, complete collection and reporting of data is essential to progress in understanding and treating disease. It is good to know that a drug or procedure appears to be "safe and effective". It is better to know that treatment A is superior to treatment B. It is ideal to understand why one treatment is better than another— to understand why a treatment works for a particular patient and not for another. Understanding at this level requires correlation of outcomes with anatomic and physiologic variables. This degree of detail is often not obtained and is only rarely reported. Reports tend to concentrate on success or failure in achieving the primary endpoint (e.g., cure of stress incontinence); however, to understand outcomes, we need detailed data on improvement and deterioration in anatomy, symptoms, lower urinary tract function, complications of the intervention, and the effect on quality of life. Both subjective and objective measurements should be recorded and reported. Functional changes can occur without obvious symptoms and symptom improvement can occur without urodynamically demonstrable changes; therefore, it is necessary to correlate the subjective response with physiologic response if we are ever to fully understand therapies. Perceptions of the patient, doctor or therapist are frequently at variance and this must be reported. Patients' expectations may also influence the outcome of a study [58].

To obtain maximum information, it is important to chose and define the correct endpoints at the beginning of the study. Outcome variables should be chosen so that they will be relevant and may be incorporated into practice at the end of the study. We agree with recommendations from the ICS Standardization Committee [12]. For clarity, we have structured the recommendations as follows:

a) Baseline data:

b) Observations:

1. Patient's observation/Subjective measures

2. Clinician's observation/Objective measures

c) Tests

1. Quantification of symptoms—void diary and pad tests

2. Urodynamics

d) Follow-up

e) Quality of life measures

f) Socioeconomics

g) Toward a simple, inclusive outcome measure

a) Baseline data/demographics

Data collection in clinical research begins with complete demographic description of the subjects including age, race, sex, duration of symptoms, prior treatments, comorbidities, medications, etc. It is prudent to inquire about the use of naturopathic and alternative medicines since these can impact metabolism and clearance rates of certain conventional pharmaceutical agents. Obstetric and gynecologic history is important in women. Recommendations for minimum data collection are made in the proceedings of the NIH Terminology Workshop for Researchers in Female Pelvic Floor Disorders [59]. While few trials will be large enough to analyze the effect of these demographic factors on outcome, the potential use of meta-analysis makes a complete database valuable.

b) Observations

1. Subject's observation and subjective measures:

Validated patient completed symptom questionnaires and other validated instruments are recommended in trials for LUTS and incontinence. In addition to specific symptoms, the respondent's overall opinion of the condition should be included. Different methods to obtain this measure include: a question with a forced choice, a graded response, a statement with a Likert scale agree-disagree response, and a statement with a visual analog graded scale response. These global response instruments should have a symmetrical design with equivalent opportunity to express a negative as a positive outcome. Questionnaires should always be administered in private and by a third party. An ideal instrument would record all symptoms related to the lower urinary tract and relevant associated organ systems. At a minimum, this would comprise:

- Incontinence, stress induced
- Incontinence, urge induced
- Incontinence, other
- Frequency and nocturia
- Urgency
- Voiding/emptying symptoms
- Protection (e.g., pad use)
- Coping measures
- Pain
- Sexual function
- Bowel function

An ideal instrument would record both the objective severity of the symptom (e. g., how many times nocturia) and the impact or bother produced by the presence of the symptom (e. g., much greater for the individual who is unable to fall back to sleep easily). There is no general symptom measure with established methodological reliability. Therefore, researchers should clearly describe their instrument and procedure and provide reliability data or indicate their absence. As there is no one universally accepted, "ideal" instrument, trials are often conducted using multiple instruments to assess different domains. In the future, consideration may be given to use of the International Consultation on Incontinence Questionnaire (ICI-Q long form). Developed in response to the first Consultation, this is one instrument that meets these specifications. Unfortunately, clinical experience with this new instrument is lacking. Committee 6 provides a detailed discussion of available validated symptom scores.

RECOMMENDATIONS:

- **One or more validated symptom instruments should be chosen at the outset of a clinical trial to accurately define baseline symptoms and other areas in which the treatment may produce an effect.**
- **The same instruments should be administered after intervention throughout follow-up.**

2. CLINICIAN'S OBSERVATION AND OBJECTIVE MEASURES:

We have traditionally included functional, primarily urodynamic, data in the evaluation of lower urinary tract disorders. It is equally important to investigate the possible presence of anatomic changes in the lower urinary tract and its supporting structures. For example, in evaluating the results of stress incontinence surgery, there are few papers that report both anatomic and functional results adequately. Therefore, while one may get some idea about the effectiveness of a particular operation, it is impossible to determine if failure occurs because of technical factors (recurrent hypermobility) or due to an inherent limitation of the procedure (intrinsic sphincter dysfunction). Similarly, reports of biofeedback training for incontinence provide data about continence after intervention little information about muscular function is provided. Do patients fail because the intervention itself was unsuccessful (pelvic muscles remain weak) or because of an inherent limitation of the technique (incontinence persists despite successful muscular reeducation)? We can only make major progress in treating lower urinary tract dysfunction by merging a full understanding of the patient's symptoms with a detailed assessment of function and a complete description of anatomy. In parallel, a new concept for classification of objective observations in lower urinary tract disorders that recently has been suggested [60] visualizing all types of lower urinary tract dysfunction as being neurogenic—either primarily neurogenic because of disease/damage in the nervous system or secondarily neurogenic because of disease/damage in the lower urinary tract and/or their supporting structures. Only complete evaluation of both structure and function will allow us to ultimately devise an optimal classification of LUT disorders.

RECOMMENDATIONS:

- **Clinicians' observations of anatomy should be recorded using standardized, reproducible measurements.**
- **Pelvic muscle and voluntary sphincter function should be reported using a quantifiable scale.**
- **These measures should be repeated after intervention and correlated with primary clinical outcome measures.**

c) Tests

1. QUANTIFICATION OF SYMPTOMS—BLADDER DIARY AND PAD TESTS:

The diary (voiding diary, bladder diary, or frequency-volume chart) is a self-monitored record of selected lower urinary function that is kept for specific time periods. Variables include fluid intake, episodes of incontinence, pad use, voiding frequency (diurnal and nocturnal), total voided volume, mean voided volume, and the largest single void. Accuracy depends on the subject's ability to follow instructions. Reproducibility depends on the parameters used and improves with the number of days that self-recording is obtained. Diaries are reliable for assessing the number of incontinent episodes. In most instances, a single 24-hour diary is sufficient. Longer diaries (48-72 hours) are more reliable but have decreased subject compliance. The circumstances under which a diary is kept should approximate everyday life, and should be similar before and after intervention to allow for meaningful comparison. Reliability and validity data for specific diaries should be provided if available, or their absence indicated [61, 62, 63, 64]. The period of time the diary was used should be noted [65].

Urinary diaries are important in the evaluation of LUTS because they document functional bladder capacity, diagnose diurnal and nocturnal polyuria, and diagnose fluid restriction that may affect continence or other LUTS. Incontinence studies often use the number of incontinence episodes on the diary as the primary endpoint. While this may provide a clear endpoint, it does not provide the information necessary to interpret the data completely. Voided volumes are critical in this regard. Might urge incontinent patients fail to improve with anticholinergic medications because bladder capacity was normal at the outset? Is improvement in continence correlated with improvement in bladder capacity? If we are to understand our interventions completely, we need complete data.

Pad tests can be divided into short-term tests, generally performed under standardized conditions as office tests, and long-term tests, generally performed at home over 24 to 48 hours. Pad-weighing quantifies the amount of incontinence. 24-hour pad tests are reliable instruments for assessing the amount of urinary loss. Increasing the test duration to 48 or 72 hours increases reliability but decreases subject compliance. For short-term tests, the experimental conditions should be described. Standardized bladder volumes are recommended. The pad test quantifies incontinence in a way no other measure can replicate; therefore it can provide the key link in understanding outcome. A patient who experiences a decrease in the number of incontinence episodes from four to two per day may not be satisfied if the volume of urine loss is high. Similarly, cure of incontinence may not have a great impact on a patient with trivial volume of urine loss at baseline.

RECOMMENDATIONS:

- **Clinical trials of incontinence and LUTS should include bladder diaries as an essential baseline and outcome measure.**
- **The diary should include measured voided volume (for at least one day if a multi-day diary is employed).**
- **24-hour diaries are adequate for most studies.**
- **Clinical trials of incontinence and LUTS should include a pad test as an essential baseline and outcome measure.**

2. URODYNAMICS:

Detailed recommendations on the indications and conduct of urodynamic investigation are found in the report from committee 7. This discussion is limited to the role of urodynamics in clinical research. Urodynamic studies take on two major roles in research—describing subjects at entry and defining outcome. Most clinical trials do not enroll subjects based on specific urodynamic diagnoses but rather based on reported symptoms. This is appropriate because:

- Urodynamic tests add significant cost to clinical trials
- Urodynamic tests are not universally available
- No urodynamic test has 100% sensitivity or specificity

Subjects should not be stratified by urodynamic diagnosis. With the possible exception of a high detrusor leak point pressure in children with spina bifida, there are no studies that clearly define a predictive role for urodynamic testing in the management of LUTS and incontinence. One of our primary research goals should be to collect data to determine the predictive value of urodynamic testing prior to intervention.

We recommend the use of urodynamic studies to accurately characterize baseline lower urinary tract function and dysfunction. This information greatly facilitates understanding of the underlying disease and the actual effect of treatment, and even provides insight that can help improve urodynamic tests. How will we advance our understanding of the pathophysiology and treatment of urge incontinence if we do not perform cystometry during clinical trials?

How can we improve our selection of patients for surgical treatment of stress incontinence if we don't carefully study which patients succeed and which fail? Urodynamic tests are among the best tools currently available to understand the basic physiology and mechanisms of disease; these tests must be a fundamental part of our research efforts. Nevertheless, urodynamic testing is far from perfect in representing lower urinary tract function and dysfunction, and our research efforts should also be directed toward the development of new and better tools.

Interpretation of urodynamic signals remains an art, the art of detecting artifact. Direct interpretation of urodynamic data without careful and critical investigation of the accuracy and reproducibility of the measurements is inappropriate. Accurate urodynamic interpretation requires continuous observation and quality control of all signals with plausibility control. In addition to anatomical and physiological knowledge at least some basic knowledge of biomechanics is needed (e.g., muscle mechanics, fluid dynamics). The elementary physical-biomechanical properties of parameters and measurement should be understood. Procedures for performing urodynamic studies must be carefully standardized to ensure that consistent techniques are used for different subjects; this is particularly critical for different centers in a multicenter study.

The exact same technique must be used at baseline and follow-up. Studies with urodynamic endpoints require an evaluation of whether or not the study reproduces the symptom under investigation. Another source of potential error is investigator bias. In multicenter studies, this can be avoided by using a central reader for urodynamic tracings, after detailed annotation by the primary observer. In all studies the reader should be blinded.

RECOMMENDATIONS:

- **At this time, clinical studies should enroll subjects by carefully defined symptoms, not urodynamic findings.**
- **To determine the predictive value of urodynamic tests, urodynamics must be performed at baseline but subjects enrolled without prejudice of urodynamic test results.**
- **In the ideal clinical study, urodynamic tests are performed at baseline and exit to correlate symptom changes with physiologic changes.**
- **When these ideal conditions cannot be met, urodynamic tests should be performed on a subset of the larger group.**
- **In all trials, standardized urodynamic protocols (based on ICS recommendations) are defined at the outset. In multicenter trials, urodynamic tests are interpreted by a central reader to minimize bias.**

d) Follow-up

Minimal standards for evaluation of treatment outcomes in urinary incontinence have been presented by Blaivas et al. [16] in a report approved by the American Urological Association and the Urodynamics Society. Their recommendations are in agreement with the ICS, although they are more detailed and specific for certain patient groups and disorders. In addition to standard pre- and post intervention evaluation, they recommend evaluation of surgical, prosthetic, and implant therapies no less often than 1 to 3 months and 12 months after treatment, and thereafter at yearly intervals for as long as possible.

The method by which data were collected should be specified, e.g., prospective questionnaires or retrospective chart review. Individuals collecting data should be identified, e.g., independent research nurse, clinician. The interval between the time of evaluation and the last treatment should be specified. The exact type of data collected at each time point in follow-up will vary by individual studies and should be defined at the study's outset. Some general data are mandatory to collect at each post-treatment interval: the total number of patients treated, the number of subjects actually evaluated in the study, and the total number of subjects lost to follow up and the reasons why they were lost. Indications for retreatment and the time interval since the last treatment should be specified. Efficacy assessment should be done at a specific time interval after the last treatment. The protocol should further specify the criteria by which treatment success or failure is determined.

e) Quality of life measures

Health related quality of life (HRQOL) is a multidimensional construct that refers to an individual's perceptions of the effect of a health condition and its treatment on quality of life. Primary domains of HRQOL include physical, psychological and social functioning; overall life satisfaction and well-being; and perceptions of health status. Secondary domains include somatic sensations (symptoms), sleep disturbance, intimacy and sexual functioning, and personal productivity (e.g., household, occupational, volunteer, or community activities). It is important to know not only how successfully treatments eliminate incontinence, but also how a treatment affects a patient globally. Nonetheless, HRQOL can never be the sole outcome of clinical research. Our focus must always be on how successfully we have treated the target condition or symptom. If a treatment is effective but does not improve HRQOL due to some adverse effect, the treatment can be improved. The combination of HRQOL data and more traditional objective endpoints will allow us to understand the reasons behind our success and failures.

Three measurement approaches are commonly used to assess HRQOL: generic, condition-specific and dimension-specific. (These instruments are explained in the report from committee 6. Here only a few aspects of relevance to research are discussed.) Generic HRQOL instruments are designed to be used across groups by having established age and gender norms. Condition-specific instruments are designed to measure the impact of a particular condition. These instruments tend to be more responsive than generic instruments in detecting treatment effects. Symptom scales are considered condition-specific; generally, these scales should include measurement of the presence of a symptom as well as the "bothersome" or "troublesome" nature of it. The majority of generic and condition-specific instruments are multidimensional, i.e., they measure more than one aspect of HRQOL. Dimension-specific instruments, in contrast, are designed to assess a single component of HRQOL, such as emotional distress. The trend in assessing HRQOL outcomes has been toward the use of a multidimensional generic and/or condition-specific instrument, supplemented with dimension-specific instruments as needed.

The selection of an HRQOL instrument should be based on the purpose of the study. Descriptive epidemiological studies should consider both generic and condition-specific instruments. Intervention studies should include a condition-specific instrument. Dimension-specific instruments should be used when more detail about a specific subdomain of HRQOL is desired. Researchers should define HRQOL for their study, clearly describe their instrument(s) and data collection, and provide reliability data if available. Selected instruments should be reliable and sensitive. In adopting HRQOL instruments, results obtained in the study population should be compared with published norms. If a new instrument will be used in a study, adequate pretesting should be done to establish its clinimetric characteristics (e.g., reliability and sensitivity) and an established instrument should also be used to provide a comparison.

RECOMMENDATIONS:

- **Research in incontinence and LUTS should include both generic and condition-specific HRQOL instruments.**
- **Changes in HRQOL after therapy should be correlated with changes in individual symptoms, and with physiologic and anatomic outcome measures to learn how the particular therapy is working.**

f) Socioeconomic data as outcome measures [66]

A full discussion of the economic impact of urinary incontinence is detailed in the report of committee 14. We recommend that cost analyses be planned with clinical studies whenever possible. Costs are to some degree artificial, in that they are established by economic and political factors that are subject to change at any time. However, when basic units of work, time, and resources are carefully defined, cost analyses remain useful even if market forces change monetary costs in an unforeseen manner.

Economic measurements are divided into two broad categories: descriptive and comparative data. Descriptive data include the socioeconomic cost caused by the disease and its current treatment, and comparative data provide an economic evaluation of different treatment strategies and interventions.

Descriptive data: Cost of illness studies that are prevalence-based or incidence-based provide a baseline against which the economic consequences of a new intervention can be measured. They provide useful basic information for policy makers, as well as for researchers developing new treatments. Generally, such studies take a societal perspective and include direct costs (i.e., costs to the health care system or to patients) and indirect costs (e.g., loss of productivity due to disease or treatment, premature mortality).

Comparative data: Economic evaluations allow comparison of different courses of action in terms of their costs (inputs) and their consequences (outcomes). There are four types of evaluations:

- Cost Minimization Analysis (CMA) is appropriate when two interventions have an identical outcome and only costs need to be compared.
- Cost Effectiveness Analysis (CEA) is appropriate when two interventions for the same disease have similar outcomes, but to different degrees. Outcomes are measured by variables such as cure, function restored, symptom-free days, events avoided, or life-years saved. Costs and outcomes are compared and the additional cost to achieve an incremental unit of effectiveness is calculated.
- Cost Utility Analysis (CUA) is similar to cost effectiveness analysis, but outcome is expressed as a single measure incorporating survival and QoL, usually quality-adjusted life years (QALY). Cost utility analysis allows comparisons of treatments in different diseases.
- Cost Benefit Analysis (CBA) expresses the value of the outcome directly in monetary terms and allows comparison of interventions both inside and outside healthcare.

Costs: Costs of an intervention are a function of resource utilization (quantities) and cost (price). Data on utilization of relevant resources is usually collected directly within a trial, while costs are calculated outside the trial. Costs should be fully allocated including overhead and depreciation.

Economic evaluation: Socioeconomic decisions depend on knowing both the cost and outcome of therapies. It is not easy to define a single outcome measure that is acceptable and meaningful to patients, physicians, and health care purchasers. Ideally, a composite construct incorporating all the dimensions of disease would be most useful for economic evaluation.

RECOMMENDATIONS:

1. The type of economic evaluation should be chosen before starting a trial, based on the specific objectives to be addressed. Analysis is based on intention-to-treat, and dropouts must be handled in the same way as for the primary outcomes analysis of the trial.

2. Typical resource use to be collected in a study is:

a. Direct

- personnel (physician, nurse, technician) time;

- diagnostic tests, laboratory analyses;

- treatments (drugs, physiotherapy, etc.);

- treatment of side-effects;

- surgical interventions;

- days of hospitalization;

- miscellaneous (pads, laundry, etc);

b. Indirect

- days of absence from work.

3. Very few economic evaluations have been done in the field of urinary incontinence and more experience is needed to make firm recommendations. Researchers should consider both a condition-specific outcome measure for economic evaluation, and a quality of life instrument with utility properties to allow for comparison to other diseases.

g) Putting it Together: toward a simple, inclusive outcome measure

One group of researchers has proposed a simple scoring system to assess outcome of incontinence therapy combining the important non-invasive outcome measures—patient's perception, voiding diary, pad test [67]. Each item is scored "0" for cure, "1" for improvement, and "2" for failure. The total score (with range of 0 to 6) represents cured, improved (good, fair and poor) and failure (same or worse). This system has been used to assess the results of sling surgery and injection therapy

[68, 69]. This system has two important advantages, in that it is applicable to all types of incontinence and therapies, and it is inexpensive with no special equipment required. Consideration should be given to further investigation of this system in clinical trials.

Another instrument that has been developed and used in clinical trials is the SEAPI-QMM system [70]. The acronym SEAPI includes subjective and objective assessment of stress incontinence, emptying ability, anatomy, protection, and inhibition (urgency). The QMM includes a validated quality of life questionnaire, a mobility assessment and a mental status assessment. This is more cumbersome and expensive to use in its entirety but is more detailed; it may also be used without completing all domains.

III. CONSIDERATIONS FOR SPECIFIC PATIENT GROUPS

1. Men with LUTS, including Incontinence

We concur with recommendations in the ICS report on "Outcome Measures for Research in Adult Males with Symptoms of Lower Urinary Tract Dysfunction"[14]. The unique factors influencing research on lower urinary tract symptoms in adult men are the presence of the prostate and the possible presence of benign prostatic obstruction (BPO).

a) Prostate Size: If treatment could potentially change prostate volume, measurements of volume should be made before and after treatment. The method used to measure volume and its reliability and validity should be provided if available or their absence indicated. Timing of post-treatment testing depends on the treatment's mechanism of action. Correlation of outcome with change in prostate size should be reported. Consideration should be given to stratifying patients by prostate volume, as it is clear that response to medical therapy, at least, may be volume dependant.

b) Bladder outlet obstruction: As discussed in more detail by committee 7, routine urodynamic studies cannot be recommended prior to clinical trials on LUTS and incontinence. Urodynamic studies have not been demonstrated to predict response to treatment. However, detrusor pressure-uroflow studies (pQS) are highly desirable and should be included to document the presence and degree of change in bladder outlet obstruction whenever feasible. Results should be presented as stated in the ICS 1997 "Standardization Report on Pressure Flow Studies of Voiding, Urethral Resistance and Urethral Obstruction." Change in flow rates in response to treatment is sensitive, but the degree of change is meaningless unless pre-treatment detrusor voiding pressure is known. A slight decrease in outlet resistance might produce a pronounced increase in maximum urinary flow rate if outlet resistance is low before treatment. Conversely, a large decrease in outlet resistance might result in only a small increase in maximum urinary flow rate if outlet resistance was high before treatment and an element of obstruction persists. Reduction of residual urine volume after treatment indicates improvement of outlet conditions; such a reduction is likely to be more important in assessing treatment response than in establishing a diagnosis. Methods used for the assessment of bladder outlet obstruction should be stated and reliability and validity data should be provided if available, or their absence indicated. At this time there is not conclusive data demonstrating a differential response to treatment by degree of outlet obstruction and we do not recommend stratifying patients. This is an important area for future research.

Recommendations:

- **If treatment could change prostate volume, measurements of volume should be performed before and after treatment.**
- **Consider stratifying patients by prostate volume.**
- **Whenever feasible, detrusor pressure-uroflow studies should be performed before and after treatment to document the presence and degree of change in bladder outlet obstruction.**

2. Women with LUTS and incontinence

We concur with recommendations for outcome research in women by Blaivas et al. in 1997 [16,17]. We also refer to the ICS recommendations for outcome measures in women with lower urinary tract dysfunction [13] and the Proceedings of the NIH Terminology Workshop for Researchers in Female Pelvic Floor Disorders [59]. Unique factors influencing research on lower urinary tract symptoms in adult women include (1) ***hormonal effects*** on the lower urinary tract; (2) ***obstetric history*** and the influence of vaginal childbirth on the development of pelvic floor disorders; (3) assessment of ***pelvic organ prolapse*** and other measures on physical examination; (4) ***definitions of outcomes*** after treatment of lower urinary tract symptoms; and (5) ***sexual functioning.***

a) Hormonal effects

Our knowledge of hormonal influences on lower urinary tract function and symptoms is inadequate. Although estrogen has been advocated as a treatment for lower urinary tract symptoms, conclusive evidence of its benefit is lacking. A recent prospective study suggests that estrogen may actually be a risk factor for incontinence [71]. Evaluation of women in research studies should include assessment of menstrual and hormonal status. Information collected by history or questionnaire should include menopausal status (premenopausal; postmenopausal without hormone therapy; postmenopausal with hormone therapy); and hormone therapy if used (type, dose, and route of administration for estrogen and progestin).

b) Obstetric History

The unique influence of vaginal childbirth on the structure and function of the female pelvis remains incompletely understood. The need for basic clinical data on the study population and the specific aims of each study will determine the level of detail obtained for obstetric history. At a minimum in all studies, the number of vaginal deliveries should be ascertained. Other variables of potential interest include infant birthweight, length of second stage of labor, operative versus spontaneous vaginal delivery, use of midline or mediolateral episiotomy, and obstetric analgesia.

c) Pelvic Organ Prolapse

Studies of surgical treatment of incontinence (and other study types as appropriate) should include assessment for pelvic organ prolapse using the staging system approved by the ICS, the Pelvic Organ Prolapse Quantification (POP-Q) system [9] as described in the report of committee 8c. The POP-Q system includes measurement in centimeters of six vaginal sites relative to the hymen, plus three other measurements. The hymen marks the zero point of reference; positive numbers refer to prolapse beyond or distal to the hymen, and negative numbers refer to locations above or proximal to the hymen. Ordinal stages are defined by the most advanced site of prolapse affecting any of the six vaginal sites, as follows:

Stage 0: no prolapse.

Stage I: One or more of the vaginal sites or cervix is located at – 2 cm (2 cm above the hymen).

Stage II: One or more of the vaginal sites or cervix is located at – 1 cm, 0 cm, or + 1 cm (1 cm above or below the hymen, or at the hymen).

Stage III: One or more of the vaginal sites or cervix is located more than 1 cm beyond the hymen, but not to the maximal extent of protrusion.

Stage IV: Maximal extent of protrusion at one or more vaginal site or cervix.

Other measurements have not been standardized, such as assessment of urethral mobility (e.g., estimation on physical exam, cotton swab testing, perineal ultrasound, lateral cystogram), identification of paravaginal defects and perineal descent, pelvic muscle assessment, and pelvic imaging (e.g., defecating proctography, static or dynamic pelvic MRI). Detailed descriptions of their measurement should be included if they are used. Data should be presented as a continuum, not as a dichotomy of "normal" versus "abnormal" until those terms are clearly defined by evidence of clinical relevance.

Following recommendations made by the NIH Terminology Workshop for Researchers in Female Pelvic Floor Disorders, in general, prolapse is defined as descent of Stage I or greater at any site. An optimal anatomic outcome (cure) after intervention is defined as Stage 0, or no prolapse. A satisfactory anatomic outcome (improvement) after intervention is defined as Stage I. An unsatisfactory anatomic outcome (persistence or recurrence, failed treatment) after intervention is defined as Stage II or greater, or no change or worsening from pre-treatment stage.

d) Definitions of Outcomes for Lower Urinary Tract Symptoms in Women

The recommendations for outcomes from the NIH Terminology Workshop for Researchers in Female Pelvic Floor Disorders are detailed below. The recommendations emphasize that outcome after treatment for urinary incontinence should be defined in terms of stress incontinence symptoms, signs, and testing, but also in terms of associated symptoms and unwanted (side) effects resulting from an intervention, after return to baseline activities and medications. The suggested outcome definitions are detailed below. If these definitions are not adopted it is still imperative that researchers specify the outcome measures that will be used to define cure, failure, and improvement for each individual study protocol.

1. Stress Urinary Incontinence:

***Cure* of stress urinary incontinence is defined as:**

1. resolution of stress urinary incontinence symptoms;
2. resolution of the sign (negative full bladder cough stress test, performed under the same conditions as pre-treatment). In studies using urodynamics after intervention, absence of genuine stress incontinence should be documented.
3. no new symptoms or side effects. New symptoms or side effects should be specifically described and could include:

- new urinary symptoms such as urinary urgency, frequency, urge incontinence, with or without urodynamic changes of detrusor instability;

- change in sexual function;
- development or worsening of pelvic organ prolapse;
- adverse effect on bowel function;
- onset of urinary tract infections;
- surgical complications, such as foreign body reaction to grafts, or development of fistula or diverticula;
- osteitis or osteomyelitis;
- neuropathy; and
- others.

- **Failure of treatment of stress urinary incontinence is defined as any one of:**

1. persistent stress symptoms with the number of incontinent episodes unchanged, or worse, by voiding diary;
2. positive full bladder cough stress test (performed under the same conditions as pre-treatment) or genuine stress incontinence confirmed by urodynamic studies; and
3. presence or absence of new symptoms or side effects, as listed above.

- **Improvement of stress incontinence includes:**

1. persistent stress symptoms but with the number of incontinent episodes decreased by voiding diary;
2. positive full bladder cough stress test (performed under the same conditions as pre-treatment) or genuine stress incontinence confirmed by urodynamic studies; and
3. presence or absence of new symptoms or side effects, as listed above.

Since improvement has no standard definition, if improvement is used as an outcome, it must be specifically defined. In addition, when more than one characteristic is used to define an outcome (i.e., symptoms and sign), the characteristics will not be concordant in some situations. Possible categories to describe these situations include: (1) patient-observed treatment effect, with absence of stress symptoms and no side effects, but positive full bladder cough stress test; and (2) provider-observed treatment effect, with persistence of stress symptoms, no side effects, and negative full bladder cough stress test.

2. Urgency, Urge Incontinence, and Other Urinary Symptoms:

For outcomes related to urgency, urge incontinence and other urinary symptoms, *cure* is defined as the patient's statement (by history or questionnaire) that the symptom(s) is no longer present. *Failed* treatment is defined as the patient's statement that the symptom(s) is no better or worse, with objective data from a urinary diary. *Improvement* could include the patient's statement that the symptom(s) is less frequent or less bothersome, with evidence from a urinary diary.

Outcomes for detrusor overactivity should be defined separately for symptoms, as described above, and for urodynamic findings. Cure of detrusor overactivity is defined as the absence of involuntary phasic detrusor contractions on filling cystometry. Failure is defined as unimproved or worsened detrusor overactivity on urodynamics. Improvement has not been standardized and should be precisely defined for each study.

Although these recommendations advance the concept of global pelvic floor evaluation and emphasize the interrelatedness of pelvic organ function, there are limitations in compressing such broad outcome measures into only three categories. It is still critical to know whether a treatment corrects the intended problem. For example, if an operation reliably cures stress incontinence but causes dyspareunia, it may be more useful to report that there is a high cure rate plus a high complication rate. While appropriately emphasizing the significance of complications and adverse events, this system does not provide a means to fully express such complex outcomes. It also leaves a rather broad range of "improved" patients that must be further defined; when complete cures are relatively uncommon, this may diminish the impact of the outcome.

Sexual Function. Assessment of sexual function is an important part of measuring the impact of lower urinary tract symptoms on quality of life in women. Assessing change in sexual function should be a routine part of all studies of treatment for urinary symptoms. Some condition-specific quality of life instruments include sexual function, such as the Incontinence Impact Questionnaire[72]. A validated condition-specific instrument for assessing sexual function in women with urinary incontinence or pelvic organ prolapse has been recently published [73], and this or another valid instrument should be used in all surgical studies and whenever a higher level of detail regarding sexual function is appropriate.

Recommendations:

- **Data on hormonal status should be collected on women in all studies of incontinence and LUTS.**
- **At a minimum, data on vaginal parity should be collected on women in all studies. Additional obstetric history should be obtained as appropriate for individual studies.**
- **Studies of surgical treatment of incontinence (and other study types as appropriate) should include assessment for pelvic organ prolapse using the ICS staging system, the Pelvic Organ Prolapse Quantification (POP-Q) system.**

- **Outcomes (cure, failure, improvement) must be clearly symptoms and signs defined at the outset of all studies, based on changes in Complications and side effects may be included in the definition of outcomes but should also be reported separately.**
- **Assessment of sexual function should be included in all studies.**

3. Frail older and disabled people

We agree with recommendations for outcome research in frail older people as reported in the ICS Subcommittee on "Outcome Measures for Research of Lower Urinary Tract Dysfunction in Frail Older People" [15]. In addition, please refer to the full report of Committee 10c regarding conservative treatment in the elderly.

Frailty is defined as "a state of reduced physiological reserve associated with increased susceptibility to disability [74]." There remains a wide variation in functional capacity within this definition ranging from those requiring some assistance with activities of daily living to those suffering from dementia and severe physical handicaps. For this population there is little validated research showing long-term efficacy of treatment for urinary incontinence. Research in this population is difficult because of:

- heterogeneity of the population resulting in difficulty designing studies that account for comorbidity, drug use, intercurrent illness, and shorter life expectancy;
- lack of standardized terminology to define and measure cure and improvement;
- lack of validated research tools to measure baseline and outcome variables;
- lack of long-term follow up to gauge impact, durability, outcomes, and applicability of interventions;
- lack of information on the natural history of incontinence.

a) Considerations in study design

1. Baseline clinical data: Descriptive data regarding the patients' current care setting should be fully described (e.g., type of setting of the study such as home or nursing home; patient-staff ratio; usual continence care; direct and indirect costs of current care; patient, family and/or staff expectations; description of caregivers and their training; and system incentives or disincentives that may influence management options). Associated factors influencing incontinence or the potential response to treatment must also be accounted for (e.g., environmental factors contributing to incontinence such as toilet access, and associated comorbid conditions that influence incontinence or the effectiveness of intervention). Bowel status and concurrent medications are important in this population. Mobility is often impaired in these patients; impaired mobility impacts urinary control, therefore mobility should be assessed using validated instruments. Finally, the functional level and cognitive state of the patients should be characterized using standardized scales (Bartel Orcats ADL scales [75,76] and Mini-mental status Scale Examination [77], respectively).

There are age specific influences on lower urinary tract function but normative data are generally lacking in this frail population. In addition, the test-retest reliability and sensitivity to change of the more invasive measures of lower urinary tract function are poorly documented in the frail elderly. It is probably not appropriate to repeat invasive measures at follow-up in this frail population unless these measures are fundamental to the outcome of the intervention being studied.

The following information should be addressed and reported at the time of follow-up whenever possible:

- number and reason for dropouts and deaths (i.e. were they trial related)
- compliance issues (by patients, staff or caregivers), such as compliance to exercise programs, toileting protocols, or drug use)
- type of bladder training or toileting programs (if any)
- other intercurrent treatment including medication not directly related to bladder function that may influence outcome
- socioeconomic data including impact of the intervention on the patient
- changes in caregiver or staff status or numbers
- cost of the treatment
- cost-benefit data
- patient and/or caregiver satisfaction with the intervention
- risk benefit data

Because comorbidity and drug use contribute to the presence and severity of incontinence in this population, they should be stabilized before enrollment.

b) History and symptoms

Research in this group cannot be based solely on patients' subjective reporting of symptoms. In some cases, the patient's perspective of the problem may be less relevant than that of family members and caregivers. Patient-derived symptom response as an outcome measure should be supplemented by objective data from diaries, etc., and data derived from caregivers.

c) Outcome and other measures

It must be acknowledged that almost all measures used in the study of incontinence in the community dwelling population require separate validation for use with the frail elderly. In addition, establishing clear "clinically significant" outcomes and understanding the full socioeconomic costs of therapy are of particular importance in this population as the patients are often unable to participate in decision making.

d) Conclusion

Research methodology for studying incontinence in the frail and housebound elderly is fraught with pitfalls. This has compromised the usefulness of past research. There is a great need for basic research to validate practical and useful outcome measures that will allow meaningful results to be obtained. In addition, an understanding is required of the importance of defining clinical rather than statistical significance.

RECOMMENDATIONS:

- **This is a heterogeneous population requiring a detailed study design and careful description of baseline clinical data if results are to be interpretable**
- **There is a need for validation of all instruments and procedures used in incontinence research for the population of frail elderly patients**
- **"Clinically significant" outcome measures and relationships of outcome to socioeconomic costs are critically important to establishing the utility of treating urinary incontinence in this population.**

4. INCONTINENCE IN CHILDREN

In general, conducting clinical research in children is more difficult than in adults for a variety of reasons. However, the need for quality clinical research in children has been emphasized in an official report from the United States National Institutes of Health (NIH) from March 1998, published in response to statements from the 1996 U.S. Congress Appropriations committees calling for increased and improved funding of pediatric medical research. The document [78] sets forth the policy and guidelines on the inclusion of children in research involving human subjects that is supported or conducted by the NIH. The goal of this policy is to increase the participation of children in research so that adequate data will be developed to support the treatment modalities for disorders and conditions that affect adults and may also affect children. The document points out that, "The policy was developed because medical treatments applied to children are often based upon testing done only in adults, and scientifically evaluated treatments are less available to children due to barriers to their inclusion in research studies". The American Academy of Pediatrics has reported that only a small fraction of all drugs and biological products marketed in the U.S. have had clinical trials performed in pediatric patients and a majority of marketed drugs are not labeled for use in pediatric patients. Many drugs used in the treatment of both common childhood illnesses and more serious conditions carry little information in the labels about use in pediatric patients. It is the stated policy of NIH that children (i.e., individuals under the age of 21) must be included in all human subjects research, conducted or supported by the NIH, unless there are scientific and ethical reasons not to include them. Appropriate exceptions are listed in the document. The specific responsibilities of all involved parties—principle investigators, institutional review boards, involved institutions, peer review groups, and the NIH—are detailed. Finally, and perhaps most importantly, the document describes levels of risk and the corresponding nature of assent required for participation in research studies. All clinical investigators that work with children should be familiar with the contents of this NIH document.

Four overriding issues separate pediatric research from the general recommendations. First, physiology varies widely within the group referred to as "children", differs from adults, and changes with time. Because children are growing, any treatment, especially pharmacological and surgical therapy, may affect them profoundly in the long term. This is particularly true of the immature brain, nervous system and other incompletely developed systems. Second, compliance with therapy is more complicated as children may depend on caregivers to administer treatment in many studies. Third, reporting of symptoms and outcomes may be difficult. The child may be unable or unwilling to respond. Symptoms reported by a caregiver may not be interpreted in the same way as the child. Finally, the issue of informed consent becomes even more complex with children.

The pediatric population is not a homogenous group; neonates, infants, pre-pubescent children, and adolescents clearly differ physiologically and psychologically. The effect of illness and the treatment of that illness must be carefully studied in each age group. Studies should be robust enough to allow for evaluation of varying age groups when relevant. Urinary incontinence in children falls into four main categories: neuropathic (myelomeningocele and other less common neurogenic etiologies), pure nocturnal enuresis, detrusor overactivity, and dysfunctional voiding without neurologic disease. This issue of age groups is most crucial in children with myelomeningocele. These children may be on drug therapy from a very young age onward; the long-term safety of medications in children must be established in all age groups. Therapy for other causes of incontinence in children tends to start at a later age, by which time size is the main difference between children. We recommend that clinical studies have long-term (five years or more), open label extension arms to monitor safety, particularly focusing on normal growth and development and the effects on treatment of liver and central nervous system function. Most importantly for incontinence studies, normal maturation may significantly enhance or obscure response to an intervention.

Assessment of compliance with therapy is always difficult, and even more so with children. Compliance with voiding diaries, a significant issue in the adult population, may be even more problematic with children. Children may "act out" and refuse medications or other treatments. Children may be willing to comply with instructions from one parent or caregiver but not another. Personal problems of the caregiver may dramatically affect the child's compliance with a treatment protocol. We can only recommend that this potential problem be recognized and given even more attention than in trials with adults. Adequate support to the family member consenting to the trial may aid in compliance with treatment. Specific compliance issues should be identified whenever possible. If a treatment is not accepted by either the adult or the child (e.g., tablet size too large, taste of the medicine not acceptable, behavioral treatment schemes too rigid), then it cannot be effective in practice, no matter how theoretically beneficial it may be.

The NIH document details appropriate levels of consent required based on the risks inherent to a particular study. Depending on the age of the child, consent may be given by the parent in a purely surrogate role or the child may participate to some degree in the process. However, true informed consent of the subject is not possible in the vast majority of cases when children are involved. We recommend that an effort be made to include the child in the discussion of the trial with age specific language and illustrations when appropriate. It is important to include the primary care giver, when the consenting adult will not be administering the treatment. Such complex relationships exist where childcare is shared amongst more than one adult, or where an employee for the purposes of childcare exists, either inside or outside the home. As always, we recommend that that study designs ensure that children are always offered the standard of care when such exists. In fact, because so few treatments have ever been studied properly in children, there are many areas in which no treatment can properly be called "safe and effective".

Outcome measures are not as well developed in children as in adults. Validated, age-specific symptom and disease-specific quality of life instruments must be developed for the pediatric population. Early efforts in this area have been reported for dysfunctional voiding [79] and daytime incontinence [80] much more work remains to be done. Invasive urodynamics can rarely be used (except in the neurogenic population), as parents will not allow repeated instrumentation of the child. The reproducibility of urodynamic investigations in children is still under investigation.

RECOMMENDATIONS:

- **We support the NIH statement calling for increased clinical research in children. All investigators that work with children should be aware of the details of the document and particularly the issues surrounding informed consent.**
- **Long-term follow-up is of critical importance in the pediatric population in order to ascertain the effect of a treatment on normal growth and development**
- **Research is needed to develop standardized outcome measures including validated, age-specific symptom and disease-specific quality of life outcome measures.**

5. NEUROPATHIC LOWER URINARY TRACT DYSFUNCTION

Modern neurourologic care is generally successful in preventing late complications in neurogenic patients, maintaining renal function, and promoting independence in self-care. Lifelong urological follow-up is mandatory and there are many areas for further research to improve the lives of these patients. These recommendations add to those described before and focus on the specific characteristics of the neurogenic patient. Specific discussion of treatment in the neurogenic population is contained in reports from committees 10d and 11c. Reports from committees 2, 4, 7, and 15 are also relevant to this population. Statistical methods and research outcome are identical as described in the general recommendations. Emphasis is given to:

- classification of the neurogenic patient
- the specifics of history and evaluation, necessary for research studies
- the urodynamic evaluation, which is the key investigational tool in the evaluation of this specific, complex and difficult patient population

a) Classification

Classification of neurogenic voiding dysfunction has

three primary aims—to aid in discriminating or identifying an unknown underlying neurological disease process, to characterize the nature of the dysfunction so as to develop a treatment plan, and to assess the risk of secondary effects (e.g. on the upper tract) which may influence the necessity and aggressiveness of treatment. The latter two are clearly relevant to research in neurogenic incontinence and must be reflected in study design and patient description.

Despite this, it is difficult to find a good classification system of neurogenic voiding dysfunction as a base for research. The published systems are reviewed in detail by Wein [81]. Both the disease process and the site of the neurologic lesion(s) are relevant in the study of neurogenic voiding dysfunction, yet even this information is inadequate to predict the functional characteristics for an individual patient. There is no one that meets the broad needs of classification in this group. Typical or classic cases are often well described but it is especially difficult to handle patients with mixed and incomplete lesions. Thus, the classification systems necessarily oversimplify or become extremely cumbersome. Finally, it must be acknowledged that the complexity of neurologic diseases and variations in individual behavior almost always call for a customized approach to therapy, further complicating research in the neurogenic patient. All of these factors complicate study design as it becomes difficult to create workable inclusion and exclusion criteria.

b) History and evaluation

Study planning is best undertaken with the cooperation of urologist, neurologist, and other clinicians, who have specific interest and special training in the neuropathic patient. Baseline data collected by history in subjects with neuropathic lower urinary tract disorders should include:

- bladder volumes by diary or examination (functional, total capacity, post voiding residual urine);
- mechanism of bladder evacuation: normal or volitional, reflex evacuation, spontaneous involuntarily, Credé, sterile intermittent catheter (SIC), clean intermittent catheter (CIC), intermittent catheter by second person, suprapubic or urethral catheter;
- use of external appliances (e.g., diaper or pad use, condom catheter, urethral catheter, suprapubic tube);
- the typical time span of continence following last bladder evacuation.

Objective assessment of sacral nerve function should be determined. This includes:

- Perineal sensation (S 3-5)
- Bulbocavernous reflex (S 2-3)
- Bulboanal reflex (S 3-4)
- Cutaneous anal reflex (S 4-5)

Issues such a skin breakdown and fecal impaction frequently become relevant in this population compared to neurologically intact individuals.

c) Urodynamics

In contrast to the general recommendations, baseline urodynamics are required for research studies of the neurogenic incontinence. Because the nature of the lower urinary tract dysfunction cannot be accurately predicted based on the history and physical findings, urodynamic classification is mandatory. Neurogenic disorders commonly cause complex and generalized lower tract dysfunction, combining bladder and urethral sphincter abnormalities. In addition, data should be collected on symptoms and the underlying neurologic disease. While urodynamic classification alone is suboptimal, it is clearly preferable to classification by symptoms or disease alone (e.g., a study involving patients with hyperreflexic neurogenic bladder and coordinated sphincters will be more generalizable than one of urge incontinence in neurogenic patients or all multiple sclerosis patients).

Urodynamic studies in neurogenic disorders are qualitatively different compared to non-neurogenic disorders. For each subject, bladder function, sphincter function, and the coordination between the two must be fully described. In addition to data on stable or unstable filling, compliance is also of major importance. Elevated detrusor leak point pressure predicts upper urinary tract deterioration in children with myelomeningocele [82]and is important in all patients with non-compliant filling. Detailed analysis of voiding dynamics becomes more important (e.g., simultaneous Pves/Pabd during voiding, voiding time, shape of the Pd and Q curves) because of the possibilities of functional obstruction and impaired contractility, which are uncommon outside of the neuropathic population. Because the bladder and sphincter may be dyssynergic, assessment of sphincteric activity is essential. This may be accomplished by surface EMG of the pelvic floor, needle electrodes, fluoroscopy, ultrasound, or direct measurement of urethral pressure.

RECOMMENDATIONS:

- **Detailed urodynamic studies are required for classification of neurogenic lower urinary tract disorders in research studies because the nature of the lower tract dysfunction cannot be accurately predicted from clinical data. Videourodynamic studies are preferred but not mandatory.**
- **Change in detrusor leak point pressure should be reported as an outcome as appropriate, and can be considered a primary outcome in addition to symptom response.**

- **An area of high priority for research is the development of a classification system to define neurogenic disturbances. Relevant features would include the underlying diagnosis, the symptoms, and the nature of the urodynamic abnormality.**
- **It may sometimes be appropriate to group patients withurodynamically similar neurogenic bladder disorders of different etiologies in a clinical trial. However, great caution must be used if patients with progressive disease (e.g., multiple sclerosis) are grouped with patients having a stable deficit (e.g., traumatic spinal cord injury).**

IV. CONSIDERATIONS FOR SPECIFIC TYPES OF INCONTINENCE RESEARCH

1. BEHAVIORAL AND PHYSIOTHERAPY TRIALS

Non-pharmacologic, non-surgical treatments for incontinence comprise a wide variety of tools often grouped under the name of behavioral treatment. Because these treatments are generally very safe and applicable to most incontinent patients, there may be a tendency to use less stringent protocols. This must be discouraged.

The type of therapy must be defined with sufficient detail that other investigators can reproduce the study. The type of behavioral therapy should be clearly stated, including the duration of the total treatment period, duration of each treatment session, and number of treatment sessions. The time between qualification for study entry and start of therapy must be specified. Any devices used must be properly described. The background and training of the therapist should be defined. All instructions, training, and educational materials given the subjects should be reproduced or referenced. A complete description of all differences in the experience of the treatment and control groups should be provided.

As in other studies, the study population should be identifiable. When urodynamics are not used to describe the pathophysiology, other valid measures are employed. The usual clinical outcome measures suffice. In order to progress in our understanding of these treatments is important to correlate clinical outcome with physiologic changes. If the intervention is intended to increase the strength of pelvic floor muscle contraction, this should be measured and correlated with continence. Outcome measures in related organ systems (e.g., gastrointestinal and sexual functioning) should also be considered, as well as possible adverse outcomes.

It is important to distinguish between *specific* and *non-specific effects*, such as improvement related to the extra attention of the therapist, motivation, confidence gained, etc. The goal is to isolate what a particular therapy achieves on its own. However, in behavioral therapy, the non-specific effect is widely considered to be an essential, desirable and important part of the effect of the therapy. It therefore needs to be evaluated along with the specific effect. Carefully designed randomized controlled studies should allow separation of specific and non-specific effects. This is particularly important with techniques such as electrical stimulation and biofeedback where particular instrumentation or equipment may be credited with results that could be due to the efforts of the therapist.

It is often difficult to perform double-blind studies of behavioral technique. Clinicians and subjects often cannot be blinded. In quality assessment of studies, double blinding is often one of the criteria of methodological quality. It may not be reasonable to demand double-blinding in all behavioral studies, or, if double blinding is not accomplished, to consider such research less valuable. It is more realistic that we demand the 'most optimal and possible level of blinding'. This means that a relevant control group is established, that every effort is made to blind as many persons as possible, and that appropriate measures surrounding this issue are discussed in the manuscripts.

RECOMMENDATIONS:

- **Treatment protocols must be detailed to the degree that the work can easily be reproduced**
- **A structured examination of pelvic floor function should be included before and after treatments that are aimed at pelvic muscle training**
- **More work is needed to separate the specific and non-specific effects of treatment**

2. DEVICE TRIALS

The United States Food and Drug Administration (FDA) had established detailed guidelines for studies on intra-urethral and vaginal devices and urethral bulking agents in the treatment of urinary incontinence [83].Although devices and bulking agents differ considerably in risks to research subjects, they are grouped together for the purpose of FDA regulation. Requirements for the protection of human subjects are appropriate for the study of bulking agents, but are probably excessive for research on devices. Any researcher considering this area of investigation should be familiar with this FDA document, which outlines the entire conduct of studies from design through outcome measures. For the most part, these guidelines follow the general recommendations. Some specific issues invite comment.

1. Inclusion is limited to patients with "urinary incontinence due to ISD (intrinsic sphincter deficiency), as evidenced from urodynamic studies or radiographic assessment". While the concept of ISD is well understood, there is no consensus on its definition for clinical care or research.
2. Female subjects "must demonstrate an abdominal leak point pressure less than 65 cm H2O". There is no evidence to support this particular cutoff, and the clinical significance of this value is questionable given the wide variation in techniques for leak point pressure measurement.
3. The potential study population is markedly limited by exclusion of mixed incontinence, failure of a previous injection procedure for stress incontinence, neurogenic bladder, previous implantation of an artificial urinary sphincter, and patients taking medications affecting the bladder. These patients could potentially benefit from therapy, but cannot be included in research by this guideline.
4. The initial evaluation calls for urodynamic testing and a pad test but not a voiding diary. We recommend that voiding diaries be included in all incontinence studies.
5. Along with routine data collection, all studies must include urodynamic testing, cystoscopy, and pulmonary and liver function results at 12 month visits. Although this is because of issues specific to bulking agents, the requirements include all devices.
6. The Stamey grading scale (0-3) for stress urinary incontinence is recommended as the primary outcome measure. There is little evidence that this measure is as valid or reliable as other measures such as voiding diaries, pad tests, and leak point pressure measurements. While the Stamey grading scale is required by the FDA, researchers should use a variety of outcome measures as described in the general recommendations and in the specific recommendations for women.

One other important area of concern in device studies is patient recruitment procedures. We strongly support reporting according to the CONSORT guideline, including the flow diagram (Figure 1) for subject enrollment and follow-up. Subjects should be enrolled in a manner that minimizes selection bias. The protocol should detail the procedure by which consecutive patients meeting the inclusion criteria are selected. All situations in which a patient meets the inclusion/exclusion criteria but is not offered enrollment by the investigator should be documented. The number of patients who decline enrollment should be stated, along with the reasons. There should be a complete accounting of all patients in the study including the reasons for subject withdrawal; recommended loss to follow-up should not exceed 20% over the course of the study per the FDA.

RECOMMENDATIONS:

- **Researchers should be familiar with the FDA guidelines for research in devices. However, vaginal support devices, urethral stents, and urethral bulking agents are not intrinsically similar and these guidelines should be refined such that recommendations are appropriate to the risk involved in the treatment.**
- **Full reporting of studies following the CONSORT flow-chart (even for observational studies) will help to define the degree of selection bias inherent in this type of research**

3. PHARMOCOTHERAPY TRIALS

Drug trials are necessary so that new drugs can be clinically and scientifically evaluated for quality, efficacy and safety [47,84,85,86,87,88]. Since the 1960's administrative bodies such as the Food and Drug Administration have required that new pharmaceuticals undergo controlled investigations to establish efficacy. In order to comply with laws governing the release of new drugs to the general public, various phases of drug trials are undertaken. The specific stages and of study design have been discussed in detail in section IIB. Pharmacotherapy trials in incontinence have come closer to the ideals presented in the general recommendations than have other treatment modalities. Incontinence research has been greatly advanced in recent years with the introduction of new medications that have been carefully studied in several large RCTs. While the financial backing of the pharmaceutical industry has been largely responsible for this superior research, new conflicts and problems have arisen due to the changing economics of research. As stated in a joint editorial endorsed by members of the International Committee of Medical Journal Editors, ". . . published evidence of efficacy and safety rests on the assumption that clinical trials data have been gathered and are presented in an objective and dispassionate manner. . . We are concerned that the current intellectual environment in which some clinical research is conceived, study subjects are recruited, and the data analyzed and reported (or nor reported) may threaten this precious objectivity"[89]. Several of these issues are discussed below.

a) Payment for drug studies

Especially in the US, proceeds from clinical trials have become an increasingly important supplement to clinician income. Clinical research, previously limited to a few academic institutions, is now spread through all segments of the medical community. While this may improve the variety of patient representation in studies, it also makes safeguarding the rights of research subjects more difficult. Competition for revenue from research, aggressive advertising for research subjects, and dependence of clinicians on income from pharmaceutical companies are trends that bear close attention. Most quality peer-review scientific journals require a declaration of conflict of interest. It is preferable that researchers do not receive money directly from industry sponsors. An acceptable alternative is to have research funds paid into an appropriate research account and dispensed by an independent third party.

b) Clinical direction

In clinician-initiated, government-funded research, there has always been a lead investigator who is ultimately responsible for all aspects of the work. This paradigm may not be applicable to pharmaceutical research. The structure of the trial is determined by the company (perhaps with input from a group of consultants); there are typically a large number of sites, each of which enrolls relatively few subjects; and data analysis is performed centrally, often under the direction of the sponsoring company. Clinicians at each site cannot be intimately familiar with the entire process of the study. When results are reported, the paper may be written by an outside agency, and then passed to authors for editing and comments. This presents a real problem with favoritism and inevitably dilutes the force, impact, and responsibility of authorship. Standards of authorship defined by many journals should be followed and rely on the honor system for compliance. Academic leaders should work to establish standards for interactions between clinicians and industry.

A final issue of special relevance in trials of pharmaceutical agents (although germane to other treatment modalities) is the controversy regarding placebos in clinical trials. Regardless of whether a drug is effective or not, simply giving a drug to a patient may produce a beneficial response. To assess if a drug has an effect over and above the placebo response, it is usually tested against an inactive substance (placebo). In incontinence, the placebo effect may be quite large, anywhere from 30-50% in recent published studies. To account for this, investigators and regulators have generally demanded a placebo arm in most clinical trials of medication. On the other hand, the Helsinki Agreement (1989) states that "far from being useful, a placebo is unethical: in any medical study every patient including those in the control group, if any, should be assured of the best proven diagnostic and therapeutic method". Clinicians need to know how a new drug compares with established treatment. The FDA does not require placebo-controlled trials of drugs for approval. However, the sponsor will generally prefer to compare the drug with a placebo and not with a competitor, since it is usually easier to detect a difference between treatment and no treatment, compared to two active treatments. Researchers must carefully consider these issues in designing a relevant, ethical study. The report of committee 9 also addresses issues related to placebos.

RECOMMENDATIONS:

- **While considerable progress has been made in pharmaceutical research on urinary incontinence, few reports have followed the CONSORT document; this decreases the clarity and impact of the work. All randomized clinical trials should follow these reporting guidelines.**
- **Continuity in clinical direction from design through authorship is highly desirable. All authors should be able to accept responsibility for the published work and all potential conflicts of interest should be fully disclosed.**
- **Investigators must be sensitive to the conflicts regarding the use of placebos in clinical trials. While placebos are often desirable from a scientific standpoint, every consideration should be given to making sure that the interests of the subjects are kept at the forefront in designing safe, ethical research.**

4. SURGICAL STUDIES

Standards for surgical trials are detailed in recommendations from the ICS, the Society for Urodynamics and Female Urology (SUFU), and the American Urological Association (AUA) [12,13,14,15,16,17]. We support the adoption of these standards by clinical and basic science researchers, the peer review process, specialty and sub-specialty organizations, the health care industry, regulatory agencies and ultimately by clinicians. While discussion of surgical therapy for incontinence mainly applies to females with stress incontinence, most of these points are equally applicable to males undergoing surgery for post-prostatectomy incontinence and related problems.

Entry: The choice of surgical treatment involves significant selection bias on the part of both the patient and surgeon. If the study is not a randomized controlled trial, this bias should be acknowledged and the number of patients treated by other methods at the same institution during the same period should be reported. Of particular importance are those patients who would be eligible for surgery but who were not offered surgery or did not select an operation. Patients undergoing a different operation for incontinence other than the one under examination should be reported.

Baseline evaluation: All patients should undergo a comprehensive baseline evaluation as discussed in the general recommendations. Void diary and pad testing is of critical importance. In addition, we believe that urodynamic studies are valuable in patient selection and should be performed on all patients undergoing surgery. The issue is discussed in more detail in the report of committee 7.

Conduct of the study: The exact surgical procedure should be described in such detail that it could easily be reproduced in another study. Discussion should include measures taken to assure that all subjects were treated in the same fashion, and that surgical technique did not change or evolve during the study. It is important to avoid doing studies "on the learning curve". Any new technique, especially surgical ones, first should be allowed to find its intended form before it is compared to established techniques ("gold standards") or subjected to other comparisons.

Analysis: A concerted effort should be made to follow-up every patient. Follow-up should be considered to be to the date of the last exam or complete data collection. Accounting for patients "lost to follow-up" must be detailed.

Reporting: Reports of successful treatment should be limited to those subjects with a minimum of one year follow-up. However, unsuccessful treatments should be reported as rapidly as possible, to avoid exposing many more patients to inadequate treatment.

RECOMMENDATIONS:

- **There is a great need for randomized clinical trials in surgical treatment of urinary incontinence. Reports of observational studies should follow the CONSORT flow-chart, which will help to define the degree of selection bias inherent in this type of research**
- **We recommend urodynamic testing in all subjects involved in surgical research. However, evidence does not exist to support recommendations for minimal testing or the use of specific tests. Research into the predictive value of preoperative urodynamic studies would be most valuable.**
- **Reports of successful treatment should be limited to subjects with a minimum of one year follow-up.**

V. CONCLUSION

One of the key themes of this Second International Consultation on Incontinence has been examining and classifying data by levels of evidence. The goal of this section has been to aid researchers in their efforts to produce research of high quality. High quality research will win "high grades of evidence", lead to new recommendations in future Consultations, and drive our efforts to understand the etiology of incontinence, treat it effectively, and, prevent its occurrence. Ultimately, good research is credible. Credibility creates impact. Credible research draws others to follow and expand on the work while simultaneously guiding clinical care of patients. Unfortunately, much of the published work in the field has not been credible and has not effectively changed patient care. In most cases, this has been due to preventable deficiencies in planning and data collection.

We cannot be discouraged by the fact that much of the clinical research that has been carried out in lower urinary tract disorders has been of low quality. Instead, we should identify and promote what is good and tenable, and build on that knowledge. Continued multidisciplinary cooperation anchored in preclinical activities is an absolute precondition for successful clinical research in lower urinary tract dysfunction in the future.

In summary,

- All quality research, be it prospective or retrospective, clinical or preclinical, begins with detailed planning—establishing a clear and relevant hypothesis, developing a trial of appropriate magnitude to accept or reject the hypothesis, and defining methods of adequate sensitivity and specificity to produce credible data.
- Clinical research in incontinence must include a broad range of baseline and outcome measures including anatomic and physiologic variables, urodynamic testing, voiding diaries and pad tests, symptom assessment, and quality of life measures. Economic outcome assessment should be included whenever possible. In each area, data must be collected using structured, reproducible methodology. Symptom assessment and other instruments must be validated for the population being studied.
- The CONSORT statement should be adopted as criteria for publication of randomized clinical trials by researchers, reviewers, and editors.
- Baseline urodynamic assessment is required in the neurogenic population and recommended in surgical trials. However, baseline urodynamic studies are highly desirable in all types of incontinence research. There is a great need to critically examine the predictive value of urodynamic testing in order to refine our tools as well as the diagnosis and treatment of patients.
- The primary goal of clinical research is to improve the care of patients; the ultimate goal is to understand the nature of disease and how treatments actually work. We can make this progress by collecting comprehensive baseline and follow-up data, and correlating outcome to baseline characteristics and observed changes during treatment.

REFERENCES

1. Abrams P, Blaivas JG, Stanton SL and Andersen JT: The standardization of terminology of lower urinary tract function. Scand J Urol Nephrol suppl 114, 5-19, 1988.
2. Bates P, Bradley WE, Glen E, Melchior H, Rowan D, Sterling A, Hald T. First report on the standardization of terminology of lower urinary tract function. Urinary incontinence. Procedures related to the evaluation of urine storage: Cystometry, urethral closure pressure profile, units of measurements. Br J Urol 48:39-42, 1976, Eur Urol 2:274-276, 1976, Scand J Urol Nephrol 11:193-196, 1976, Urol Int 32:81-87, 1976.
3. Bates P, Glen E, Griffiths D, Melchior H, Rowan D, Sterling A, Zinner NR, Hald T. Second report on the standardization of terminology of lower urinary tract function. Procedures related to the evaluation of micturition: Flow rate, pressure measurement, symbols. Acta Urol Jpn 27:1563-1566, 1977, Br J Urol 49:207-210, 1977, Eur Urol 3:168-170, 1977, Scand J Urol Nephrol 11:197-199, 1977.
4. Bates P, Bradley WE, Glen E, Griffiths D, Melchior H, Rowan D, Sterling A, Hald T. Third report on the standardization of terminology of lower urinary tract function. Procedures related to the evaluation of micturition: Pressure flow relationships, residual urine. Br J Urol 52:348-359, 1980, Euro Urol 6:170-171, 1980, Acta Urol Jpn 27:1566-1568, 1980, Scand J Urol Nephrol 12:191-193, 1981.
5. Bates, P, Bradley WE, Glen E, Melchior H, Rowan D, Sterling A, Sundin T, Thomas D, Torrens M, Turner-Warwick R, Zinner NR, Hald T. Fourth report on the standardization of terminology of lower urinary tract function. Terminology related to neuromuscular dysfunction of lower urinary tract. Br J Urol 52:333-335, 1981, Urology 17:618-620, 1981, Scand J Urol Nephrol 15:169-171, 1981, Acta Urol Jpn 27:1568-1571, 1981.
6. Abrams P, Blaivas JG, Stanton SL, Andersen TJ, Fowler CJ, Gerstenberg T, Murray K. Sixth report on the standardization of terminology of lower urinary tract function. Procedures related to neurophysiological investigations: Electromyography, nerve conduction studies, reflex latencies, evoked potentials and sensory testing. World J Urol 4:2-5, 1986, Scand J Urol Nephrol 20:161-164, 1986.
7. Rowan D (Ch.), James ED, Kramer AEJL, Sterling AM and Suhel PF (ICS working party on urodynamic equipment). Urodynamic Equipment: technical aspects. J Med Eng Technol 11, 2, 57-64, 1987.
8. Andersen JT, Blaivas JG, Cardozo L and Thüroff, J. Lower Urinary Tract Rehabilitation Techniques : Seventh Report on the Standardization of Terminology of Lower Urinary Tract Function. Int Urogynecol J, 3:75-80, 1992.
9. Bump RC, Mattiasson A, Bø K, Brukaber LP, DeLancey JOL, Klarskov P, Shull BL and Smith ARB: The Standardization of Terminology of Female Pelvic Organ Prolapse and Pelvic Floor Dysfunction. Am J Obstet Gynecol, 175:10-17, 1996.
10. Thüroff J, Mattiasson A, Andersen JT, Hedlund H, Hinman F Jr, Hohenfellner M, Månsson W, Mundy AB, Rowland RG and Steven K. Standardization of Terminology and Assessment of Functional Characteristics of Intestinal Urinary Reservoirs. Neuroul Urodyn, 15:499-511, 1996, Br J Urol, 78:516-523, 1996, Scand J Urol Nephrol, 30:349-356,1996.
11. Griffiths D, Höfner K, van Mastrigt R, Rollema HJ, Spångberg A and Gleason D. Standardization of Terminology of Lower Urinary Tract Function:Pressure-Flow Studies of Voiding, Urethral Resistance, and Urethral Obstruction. Neurourol Urodyn 16:1-18, 1997.
12. Mattiasson A, Djurhuus JC, Fonda D, Lose G, Nordling J and Stöhrer M: Standardization of Outcome studies in patients with Lower Urinary Tract Dysfunction. A report on general principles from the Standardization Committee of the International Continence Society. Neurourol Urodyn 17:249-253, 1998.
13. Lose G, Fantl JA, Victor A, Walter S, Wells TJ, Wyman J and Mattiasson A: Outcome measures in adult women with symptoms of lower urinary tract dysfunction. Neurourol Urodyn 17:255-262, 1998.
14. Nordling J, Abrams P, Ameda JT, Donovan J, Griffiths D, Kobayashi S, Koyanagi T, Schäfer W, Yalla S and Mattiasson A: Outcome measures for research in treatment of adult males with symptoms of lower urinary tract dysfunction. Neurourol Urodyn 17:263-271, 1998.
15. Fonda D, Resnick NM, Colling J, Burgio K, Ouslander JG, Norton C, Ekelund P, Versi E and Mattiasson A: Outcome measures for research of lower urinary tract dysfunction in frail older people. Neurourol Urodyn 17:273-281, 1998.
16. Blaivas JG, Appell RA, Fantl JA, Leach G, McGuire EJ, Resnick NM, Raz S and Wein AJ: Standards of Efficacy of Treatment Outcomes in Urinary Incontinence: Recommendations of the Urodynamic Society. Neurourol Urodyn 16:145-147, 1997.
17. Blaivas JG, Appel RA, Fantl JA, Leach G, McGuire EJ, Resnick NM, Raz S and Wein AJ: Definition and Classification of Urinary Incontinence: Recommendations of the Urodynamic Society. Neurourol Urodyn 16:149-151, 1997.
18. Blaivas JG: Outcome measures for urinary incontinence. Urology Feb; 51 (2A Suppl):11-19, 1998.
19. Spilker B: Guide to clinical studies and developing protocols. Raven press New York, 1984.
20. Senn S. Statistical Issues in Drug Development. Chichester: Wiley, 1997.
21. Altman DG. Practical Statistics for Medical Research. London: Chapman & Hall, 1991.
22. Senn S. Cross-over Trials in Clinical Research. Chichester: Wiley;1993.
23. Armitage P, Berry G. Statistical Methods in Medical Research, 3rd edition. Oxford: Blackwell Science, 1994.
24. International Conference on Harmonisation web site. Statistical considerations in the design of clinical trials. Available at: http://www.ifpma.org/pdfifpma/e9.pdf. Accessibility verified May 29, 2001.
25. CONSORT web site. Statistical considerations in the design of clinical trials. Available at: http://www.consort-statement.org. Accessibility verified May 29, 2001.
26. Standards of Reporting Trials Group. A proposal for structured reporting of randomized controlled trials. JAMA 1994; 242: 1926-1931.
27. Altman DG. Better reporting of randomised controlled trials: the CONSORT statement. BMJ 1996;313:570-571.
28. Altman DG, Schulz KF, Moher D, Egger M, Avidoff F, Elbourne D, Gøtzsche PC, Lang T, for the CONSORT Group. The revised CONSORT statement for reporting randomised trials: explanation and elaboration. Annals of Internal Medicine 2001; 134: 663-694.
29. Egger M, Jüni P, Bartlett C, for the CONSORT Group. Value of flow diagrams in reports of randomized controlled trials. JAMA 2001;285:1996-1999.
30. Moher D, Jones A, Lepage L, for the CONSORT Group. Use of the CONSORT statement and quality of reports of randomized trials: a comparative before-and-after evaluation. JAMA 2001; 285:1992-1995.
31. Rennie D. CONSORT revised – improving the reporting of randomized trials. [Editorial] JAMA 2001;285:2006-2007.
32. Pocock SJ. Clinical Trials: a Practical Approach. Chichester: Wiley; 1983.

33. Black N. Why we need observational studies to evaluate the effectiveness of health care. Br Med J 312:1215-1218, 1996.

34. Peters TJ, Eachus JI. Achieving equal probability of selection under various random sampling strategies. Paediatric and Perinatal Epidemiology 1995;9:219-224.

35. Donner A, Klar N. Design and Analysis of Cluster Randomization Trials in Health Research. London: Arnold; 2000.

36. Moher D, Schulz KF, Altman D, for the CONSORT Group. The CONSORT statement: revised recommendations for improving the quality of reports of parallel-group randomized trials. JAMA 2001;285:1987-1991.

37. Matthews JNS. An Introduction to Randomized Controlled Clinical Trials. London: Arnold; 2000.

38. Campbell MJ, Julious SA, Altman DG. Estimating sample sizes for binary, ordered categorical, and continuous outcomes in two group comparisons. Br Med J 311:1145-1148, 1995.

39. Machin D, Campbell M, Fayers P, Pinol A. Sample Size Tables for Clinical Studies, 2nd edition. Oxford: Blackwell Science; 1997.

40. Sterne JAC, Davey Smith G. Sifting the evidence – what's wrong with significance tests? BMJ 2001;322:226-231.

41. Schwartz DS, Lellouch J. Explanatory and pragmatic attitudes in therapeutical trials. Journal of Chronic Diseases 20:637-648, 1967.

42. Newell DJ. Intention-to-treat analysis: implications for quantitative and qualitative research. Int J Epidemiology 21:837-841, 1992.

43. Peters TJ, Wildschut HIJ, Weiner CP. Epidemiologic considerations in screening. In: Wildschut HIJ, Weiner CP, Peters TJ, eds. When to Screeen in Obstetrics and Gynecology. London: WB Saunders, 1996:1-12.

44. Hollis S, Campbell F. What is meant by intention to treat analysis? Survey of published randomised controlled trials. BMJ 1999;319:670-674.

45. Lewis JA, Machin D. Intention to treat – who should use ITT? [Editorial] British Journal of Cancer 1993;68:647-650.

46. Richards SH, Bankhead C, Peters TJ, Austoker J, Hobbs FDR, Brown J, Tydeman C, Roberts L, Formby J, Redman V, Wilson S, Sharp DJ. A cluster randomised trial comparing the effectiveness and cost-effectiveness of two primary care interventions aimed at improving attendance for breast screening. Journal of Medical Screening 2001;8:91-98.

47. Bland M. An Introduction to Medical Statistics, 2nd edition. Oxford: Oxford University Press; 1995.

48. Collett D. Modelling Binary Data. London: Chapman & Hall; 1991.

49. Collett D. Modelling Survival Data in Medical Research. London: Chapman & Hall; 1994.

50. Matthews JNS, Altman DG, Campbell MJ, Royston P. Analysis of serial measurements in medical research. BMJ 300; 230-235, 1990

51. Egger M, Juni P, Bartlett C. Value of flow diagrams in reports of randomized controlled trials. JAMA 2001;285(15):1996-9.

52. Bland M. An Introduction to Medical Statistics, 2nd edition. Oxford: Oxford University Press 1995.

53. Zar JH. Biostatistical analysis, 2nd edition. New Jersey: Prentice-Hall, 1984.

54. Brookes ST, Whitley E, Peters TJ, Mulheran P, Egger M, Davey Smith G. Subgroup analyses in randomised controlled trials: quantifying the risks of false positives and negatives. Health Technology Assessment 2001;5(33).

55. Moher D, Jones A, Lepage L. Use of the CONSORT statement: revised recommendations for improving the quality of reports of parallel-group trials. Lancet 2001;357(9263):1191-4.

56. Moher D, Cook DJ, Eastwood S, Olkin I, Rennie D, Stroup DF, for the QUORUM Group. Improving the quality of reports of meta-analyses of randomised controlled trials: the QUORUM statement. Lancet 1999;354:1896-1900.

57. Elbourne DR, Campbell MK. Extending the CONSORT statement to cluster randomised trials: for discussion. Statistics in Medicine 2001;20:489-496.

58. Berry H, Bloom B, Mace BEW, Hamilton EDB. Expectation and patient preference-does it matter? JR Soc Med 73:34-38, 1980

59. Weber AM, Abrams P, Brubaker L, Cundiff G, Davis G, Dmochowski RR, Fischer J, Hull T, Nygaard I, Weidner AC. The standardization of terminology for researchers in female pelvic floor disorders. Int Urodynecol J Pelvic Floor Dusfunct 2001;12(3):178-86.

60. Mattiasson A: Characterisation of Lower Urinary Tract Disorders-A New View. Neurourol Urodyn 2001; 20(5):601-20.

61. Ryhammer AM, Laurberg S, Djurhuus JC, Hermann AP. No relationship between subjective assessment of urinary incontinence and pad test weight gain in a random population sample of menopausal women. J Urol 1998;159(3):800-3

62. Ryhammer AM, Djurhuus JC, Laurber S. Pad testing in incontinent women: a review. Int Urogynecol J Pelvic Floor Dysft 1999;10(2):111-5

63. Sandvik H, Seim A, Vanvik A, Hunscaar S, A severity index for epidemiological surveys of female urinary incontinence: comparison with 48 hour pad weighing tests. Neurourol Urodyn 2000;19(2):127-45

64. Groutz A, Blaivas JG, Chaikin DC, Resnick NM, Engleman K, Anzalone D, Bryzinski B, Wein AJ, Noninvasive outcome measures of urinary incontinence and lower urinary tract symptoms: a multi-center study of micturition diary and pad tests. J Urol 2000 Sep; 164(3 Pt 1):698-701

65. Nygaard I, Holcomb R, Reproducibility of the seven-day voiding diary in women with stress urinary incontinence. Int Urogynecol J Pelvic Floor Dysfunct 2000;11(1):15-7

66. Kobelt G. Economic considerations and outcome measurement in urge incontinence. Urology. 1997;50(6A Suppl):100-7; discussion 108-10.

67. Groutz A, Blaivas JG, Rosenthal JE. A Simplified urinary incontinence score for the evaluation of treatment outcomes. Neurourol Urodyn 2000;19(2):127-35

68. Groutz A, Blaivas JG, Hyman MJ, Chaikin DC. Pubovaginal sling surgery for simple stress urinary incontinence: analysis by an outcome score. J Urol 2001 May;165(5):1597-600.

69. Groutz A, Blaivas JG, Kesler SS, Weiss JP, Chaikin DC. Outcome results of transurethral collagen injection for female stress incontinence: assessment by urinary incontinence score. J Urol 2000 Dec;164(6):2006-9

70. Raz S and Erickson DR : SEAPI QMM Incontinence Classification System. Neurourol Urodyn 11:187-99, 1992

71. Grady D, Brown JS, Vittinghoff E, et. al.: Postmenopausal hormones and incontinence: the heart and estrogen/progestin replacement study. Obstet Gyecol 2001;97:116-20.

72. Shumaker SA, Wyman JF, Uebersac J, McClish DK, Fantl JA. Health-related quality of life measures for women with urinary incontinence: The urogenital distress inventory and the incontinence impact quetionnaire. Quality of Life Research 3:291-306, 1994.

73. Rogers RG, Kammerer-Doak D, Villarreal A, 2001, Coates K, Qualls C. A new instrument to measure sexual function in women with urinary incontinence or pelvic organ prolapse. Am J Obstet Gynecol 2001;184(4):552-8.

74. Buchner DM and Wagner EH, Preventing frail health, Clin Ceriatr Med 1992;8:1-17

75. Katz S, Ford A, Moskowitz R, et al. The index of ADL: A standardized measurement of biological and psychosocial function. JAMA 185; 914-919, 1963.

76. Mahoney FI, Barthel DW. Functional evaluation: The Barthel Index. Maryland State Med J 14; 61-65, 1965.

77. Folstein MF, Folstein S, McHugh PR. Mini Mental State: A practical method for grading the cognitive state of patients for the clinician. J Psych Res 12; 189-198, 1975.

78. Nih policy and guidelines on the inclusion of children as participants in research involving human subjects, Release Date: March 6, 1998, National Institutes of Health, at: http://grants.nih.gov/grants/ guide/notice-files/not98-024.html

79. Farhat W, Bagli DJ, Capolicchio G, O'Reilly S, Merguerian PA, Khoury A, and McLorie GA. The dysfunctional voiding scoring system: quantitative standardization of dysfunctional voiding symptoms in children. J Urol 2000;164:1011-15.

80. Sureshkumar P, Craig JC, Roy LP, Knight JF. A reproducible pediatric daytime urinary incontinence questionnaire. J Urol 2001;165:569-73.

81. Wein AJ. Pathophysiology and Categorization of Voiding Dysfunction. In Campbell's Urology, 7th edition, Walsh PC et al eds. WB Saunders, Philadelphia, 1998. 917-26

82. McGuire EJ, Woodside JR, Borden TA. Upper tract deterioration in patients with myelodysplasia and detrusor hypertonia: a follow up study. J Urol 129:823-6;1983

83. U.S. Food and Drug Administration – Center for Devices and Radiologic Health. Guidance Documents and Reports. Draft guidance for preclinical and clinical investigations of urethral bulking agents used in the treatment of urinary incontinence. Published November 29, 1995. http://www. fda.gov/cdrh/ ode/oderp850.html

84. Collier J and Dwight: Medicines and the NHS. Which Limited, 1997.

85. Collier J: Confusion over use of placebos in clinical trials. Editorial. Br Med J 311: 821-22, 1995.

86. Jones B, Jarvis P, Lewis J, Ebbutt A: Trials to assess equivalence: the importance of rigorous methods. Br Med J 313:36-39, 1996.

87. Herbison P: Letter to editor. Neurourol Urodyn 17: 513-14, 1998.

88. Henry D, Hill S: Comparing treatments. Br Med J 310:1279, 1995.

89. Davidoff F, DeAngelis CD, Drazen JM, Hoey J, Hojgaard L, Horton R, Kotzin S, Nicholls MG, Nylenna M, Overbeke AJPM, Cox HC, Van Der Weyden MB, Wilkes MS: Sponsorship, authorship, and accountability. JAMA 2001;286(10):1232-34.

2002

Organised by

International Consultation on Urological Diseases (ICUD)

NGO in official collaboration with WHO

*

International Continence Society (ICS)

In collaboration with

AUA

CAU

EAU

FIGO

SIU

UAA

and other medical associations

2nd International Consultation on Incontinence

Recommendations of the International Scientific Committee :

Evaluation and Treatment of Urinary Incontinence, Pelvic Organ Prolapse and Faecal Incontinence

◆◆◆

P. Abrams, K.E. Andersson, W. Artibani, L. Brubaker, L.Cardozo, D. Castro, J. Christiansen, J. Delancey, L. Denis, J. Donovan, D. Fonda, C. Fowler, J. Gosling, D. Griffiths, S. Herschorn, Y. Homma, T. Hu, S. Hunskaar, S. Khoury, H. Koelbl, A. Kondo, H. Madersbacher, M. Mitchell, J. Morrison, J. Mostwin, D. Newman, R. Nijman, O. Nishizawa, C. Payne, R. Shull, A. Smith. W. Steers, P. van Kerrebroeck, C. Norton, F. Richard, J. Thuroff, L. Wall, A. Wein, D. Wilson and U. Ulmsten
and *The Members of the Committees.*

INTRODUCTION

The 2nd International Consultation on Urinary Incontinence met from July 1-3, 2001 in Paris.

Organised by the International Continence Society (ICS) and the International Consultation on Urological Diseases (I.C.U.D.), NGO in official collaboration with the World Health Organisation (WHO), in order to ***develop recommendations*** for the diagnostic evaluation and treatment of ***urinary incontinence, faecal incontinence*** and ***pelvic organ prolapse.***

The recommendations are evidence based on a ***thorough review of the available literature*** and the ***global subjective opinion of recognised experts*** serving on focused subcommittees. The individual ***sub-committee reports*** were developed and ***peer reviewed*** by open presentation and comment. The Scientific Committee, consisting of the Chairmen of all the committees then ***refined the final recommendations.***

These recommendations published in ***2002*** will be ***periodically re-evaluated*** in the light of clinical experience and technological progress and research.

I. Definitions

The consultation agreed to use the new International Continence Society definitions (ICS) for lower urinary tract dysfunction (LUTD) including incontinence. These definitions will appear in the journal Neurourology and Urodynamics (issue 2, 2002;21:167-178) or can be viewed on the ICS website : www.icsoffice.org

The following ICS definitions are relevant:

1. Overactive Detrusor Function

Overactive detrusor function is characterised by involuntary detrusor contractions during the filling phase, which may be spontaneous or provoked.

The overactive detrusor is ***divided*** into ***idiopathic detrusor overactivity*** and ***neurogenic detrusor overactivity.***

Idiopathic Detrusor Overactivity is defined as overactivity when there is no defined cause.

Neurogenic Detrusor Overactivity is defined as overactivity due to a relevant neurological condition.

2. Urinary Incontinence

Urinary incontinence is ***involuntary loss of urine*** that is a social or hygienic problem.

Incontinence may be further defined according to the patient's symptoms:

- ***Urge Urinary Incontinence*** is the complaint of involuntary leakage accompanied by or immediately preceded by urgency.
- ***Stress Urinary Incontinence*** is the complaint of involuntary leakage on effort or exertion, or on sneezing or coughing.
- ***Nocturnal Enuresis*** is any involuntary loss of urine occuring during sleep.
- ***Post-micturition dribble*** and ***continuous urinary leakage*** denotes other symptomatic forms of incontinence.

The symptoms and signs of incontinence do not give a definite diagnosis and the ***cause*** of incontinence can only be absolutely determined by ***urodynamic studies*** (UDS). UDS allow the disease processes to be defined, for example ***Urodynamic stress incontinence*** is noted during filling cystometry, and is defined as the involuntary leakage of urine during increased abdominal pressure, in the absence of a detrusor contraction

CONTENT

II. Evaluation of Incontinence

The following was utilised to classify diagnostic tests and studies:

- ***A highly recommended test*** is a test that should be done on ***every patient.***
- ***A recommended test*** is a test of proven value in the evaluation of ***most patients*** and its use is strongly encouraged during initial evaluation.
- ***An optional test*** is a test of proven value in the evaluation of ***selected patients***; its use is left to the ***clinical judgement of the physician.***
- ***A not recommended test*** is a test of no proven value in the evaluation of most patients. However, such tests may be helpful in selected patients who do not fulfil the criteria for the standard (usual) patients.

This section primarily discusses the Evaluation ***of urinary incontinence*** with or without ***Pelvic Organ Prolapse*** (POP). The evaluation of ***Faecal Incontinence is*** summarized in the Algorithm VIII in this document.

I. HIGHLY RECOMMENDED TESTS DURING INITIAL EVALUATION

The ***main recommendations*** for this consultation have been abstracted from the ***extensive work*** of the 25 sub-committees of the ***2nd International Consultation on Incontinence (ICI)***. Each sub-committee has written a report that reviews and evaluates the published scientific work in each field of interest. Each report ends with detailed recommendations and suggestions for a programme of research.

The main recommendations should be read in conjunction with the management algorithms for children, men, women, pelvic organ prolapse, neurogenic patients, the frail older person and faecal incontinence.

The ***initial evaluation*** should be done on every patient presenting with incontinence to a health care professional.

1. History and General Assessment

Management of a disease such as incontinence requires caregivers to ***assess*** the sufferer as a «***whole individual***». Many factors may influence a particular individual's symptoms, some may cause incontinence, and other factors will determine the succcss of treatment. General assessment has a number of ***important components*** :

- ***Nature*** and ***duration*** of genitourinary and lower alimentary tract symptoms.
- ***Previous surgical procedures*** (in particular as they affect the genitourinary tract).
- ***Environmental issues***: these may include the social and cultural environment.
- ***Patient mobility***: individuals who have compromised mobility may need to be managed differently
- ***Mental status***: each individual needs to be assessed for their ability to understand proposed management plans and to enter into discussions when there are a range of treatment options. In some groups of patients formal testing of cognitive function is essential, eg. those thought to be suffering from dementia.
- ***Disease status:*** coexisting diseases may have a profound effect on incontinence sufferers, for example asthma patients with stress incontinence will suffer greatly during attacks. Diseases may also precipitate incontinence, particularly in frail older persons.
- ***Patient medication:*** it is always important to review every patient's medication and to make an assessment as to whether the treatment is in fact causing or worsening the patient's condition.
- ***Sexual function:*** at present little information exists on the impact of incontinence: this aspect of the patients life should be assessed where appropriate (depending on age).

- ***Bowel function:*** faecal incontinence is one of the subjects of this consultation and bowel function has considerable influence on urinary problems. Certain groups of urinary incontinent patients may have co-existing faecal incontinence, and/or constipation which may trouble them as much or even more than their urinary leakage.
- ***Assess patients goals or expectations of treatment***
- ***Assess patient's fitness*** for possible ***surgical procedures***

2. Assessment of Symptoms

A full history should be taken including:

- the ***frequency*** of incontinence
- the ***perceived quantity*** of leakage
- the ***perceived impact*** of leakage on every day life
- ***Pelvic organ prolapse*** (POP) symptoms

3. Physical Examination

There are a number of essential components in the examination of sufferers with incontinence and/or pelvic organ prolapse (POP).

- ***Abdominal examination*** after voiding in an effort to detect a palpable bladder.
- ***Perineal examination*** to assess sensation.
- ***Rectal examination*** to assess anal tone, pelvic floor function, the consistency of stool, and in the male, the prostate gland.
- ***External genitalia :*** including skin condition
- ***Vaginal examination*** to assess pelvic organ prolapse and with patient bearing down, pelvic floor function and oestrogen status.
- ***Stress test for urinary incontinence*** - patients with suspected stress incontinence should be asked to cough repeatedly and strain with a full bladder.

4. Urinalysis

As ***urinary infection*** is a readily detected and easily treatable cause of LUTS, urine testing is highly recommended. Testing may range from examination of urine in a ***clear glass container***, through ***dipstick*** testing, to ***urine microscopy.***

5. Tests before Further Investigation/ Treatment

a) Qualification of symptoms

The use of a simple frequency volume chart (example in Annex 1) is highly recommended to document the frequency of micturition, the volumes of urine voided, incontinence episodes and the use of incontinence pads.

b) Estimation of post void residual urine (PVR)

In patients with suspected voiding dysfunction, PVR is part of the initial assessment as the result is likely to influence management for example, in neurological patients.

PVR may be most accurately assessed by ultrasound. This will simultaneously provide information about bladder capacity and bladder wall changes, and can detect the presence of bladder stones, diverticula and a median prostate lobe.The invasive nature of any other means (i.e.catheterization) to determine residual urine, must be weighed against the benefits of the test.

Because of the marked intra-individual variability of residual urine volume, the test should be repeated to improve precision, if residual urine volume is significant at the first measurement.

II. RECOMMENDED DIAGNOSTIC TESTS

The tests below are recommended when the appropriate indication(s) is present. Some recommended tests become highly recommended in specific situations.

This section should also be read in conjunction with the relevant subcommittee reports.

1. Further Symptom and QoL Assessment

The use of a number of validated questionnaires is recommended for a more detailed assessment of the symptoms of incontinence and their impact on quality of life. The Consultation has developed a validated ***screening questionnaire for incontinence,*** the ***ICIQ-SF*** (short form). This is particularly suitable for epidemiological studies and for use in initial assessment of incontinent individuals (Annex 2).

The Consultation is developing a modular questionnaire including the assessment of symptoms and impact on quality of life for use in assessing the effectiveness of treatments for incontinence.

2. Detailed Physical Examination

Certain aspects of physical examination, when indicated, need to be more detailed.

a) Neurological examination:

concentrating on the ***sacral segments 2-4*** (the nerve supply of bladder and urethra, rectum and anal canal). Also examine ***lower limbs*** and ***observe gait.***

b) In Female patients

formal assessment is recommended when initial evaluation indicates the possibility of ***oestrogen deficiency, urethral diverticulum, urinary fistula or pelvic organ prolapse.***

c) Pelvic organ prolapse

should be assessed using the ***ICS classification*** (POPQ) recommended in order to properly document the extent of prolapse. In clinical work it's use would be optional.

3. Renal Function Assessment

Standard biochemical tests for renal function are recommended in patients with urinary incontinence ***and*** a high ***probability of renal impairment or prior to surgical interventions.***

4. Uroflowmetry and PVR

Uroflowmetry and the ***measurement of postvoid residual urine (PVR).*** These tests are recommended as a screening test for symptoms suggestive of voiding dysfunction, or suspicious physical signs.

5. Urodynamic Testing

a) Urodynamic evaluation is recommended :

- prior to ***invasive treatments***
- after ***treatment failure***
- as part of a ***long-term surveillance*** programme in neurogenic lower urinary tract dysfunction
- in ***"complicated incontinence".*** (For details please see relevant subcommittee reports).

b) The aims of Routine Urodynamic Evaluation are

- the detection of ***detrusor overactivity***
- the assessment of ***urethral competence*** during filling
- the determination of ***detrusor function*** during voiding
- the assessment of ***outlet function*** during voiding
- the measurement of ***residual urine***

c) It is recommended that Routine Urodynamic Evaluation should consist of

- ***filling cystometry*** (with provocation, and tailored to the individual patient's requirements) together with
- ***voiding cystometry***

6. Urinary Tract Imaging

Initial imaging may be by ***Ultrasound*** or ***plain X ray.***

a) Imaging of the lower urinary tract

is ***recommended*** in those with suspected lower tract or pelvic pathology.

b) Imaging of the upper urinary tract

is only ***recommended*** in ***specific situations.*** These include:

- neurogenic urinary incontinence e.g. myelodysplasia, spinal cord trauma,
- incontinence associated with significant post-void residual,
- co-existing loin/kidney pain,
- severe pelvic organ prolapse, not being treated
- suspected extra-urethral urinary incontinence,
- children with incontinence where indicated

7. Endoscopy

Endoscopy is ***recommended*** :

- when initial testing suggest ***other pathologies,*** e.g. microscopic haematuria raises the possibility of bladder tumour
- when ***pain or discomfort*** features in the patient's LUTS : these may suggest an intravesical lesion
- when appropriate in the evaluation of ***vesicovaginal fistula*** and extra-urethral urinary incontinence

III. OPTIONAL DIAGNOSTIC TESTS

1. Additional Urodynamic Testing

➡ If a more detailed estimate of ***urethral function*** is required then the following ***urethral function tests*** are optional :

- ***static*** and ***stress urethral pressure profilometry***
- abdominal ***leak point pressures***
- ***video-urodynamics*** and or ***electromyography***

➡ If ***initial urodynamics*** have ***failed*** to ***demonstrate*** the ***cause*** for the patient's incontinence then the following tests are optional:

- repeated provocative routine urodynamics
- ambulatory urodynamics

2. Pad Testing

Pad testing is an optional test for the routine evaluation of incontinence. Either a short test (20 min to 1 hr) or a ***24 hr test*** is suggested.

3. Neurophysiological Testing

The information gained by clinical examination and urodynamic testing may be enhanced by ***neurophysiological testing*** of ***striated muscle*** and ***nervous pathways.*** Appropriately trained personnel should perform these tests. The ***following neurophysiological tests*** are optional in patients with incontinence and suspected peripheral lesions.

- concentric needle EMG
- sacral reflex responses to electrical stimulation of penis/clitoris

4. Further Urinary Tract Imaging

a) Cysto-urethrography

in complicated or recurrent incontinence.

b) Ultrasound, CT or ***MRI*** imaging

of the lower urinary tract and pelvic floor are optional and should have a specific indication.

c) Simultaneous LUT imaging and urodynamics,

are an optional test in complicated or recurrent incontinence. The imaging modality may be ultrasound or Xray.

5. Imaging of the Central Nervous System, including Spine

Even if simple imaging, for example spinal X-rays in patients with suspected neurological disease, is normal then further imaging is still optional. The further methods include myelography, CT and MRI.

6. Endoscopy,

is an optional test in complicated or recurrent incontinence (e.g. after failed stress incontinence surgery in women, in post prostatectomy incontinence in men).

IV. TESTS NOT RECOMMENDED FOR THE INITIAL OR FURTHER EVALUATION OF INCONTINENCE

- ***Urinary tract imaging is*** not recommended unless there are specific indications (see above).
- ***Endoscopy of the urinary tract is not recommended unless there are specific indications (see above).***
- ***Gas cystometry*** is not recommended as part of the urodynamic evaluation of incontinence.

III. Management Recommendations

The management recommendations are derived from the detailed work in the subcommittee reports on management in children, men, women pelvic organ prolapse, the frail elderly, neurological patients and faecal incontinence. The management of incontinence is presented in ***algorithm form*** with ***accompanying notes.*** There are algorithms for

- I. Children,
- II. Men,
- III. Women,
- IV. Pelvic Organ Prolapse
- V. Neurogenic Incontinence
- VI. Frail and Disabled Older Men
- VII. Frail and Disabled Older Women
- VIII. Faecal Incontinence

These algorithms are divided into two for groups I, II, III, IV : the two parts, ***initial management*** and ***specialised management*** require a little further explanation.

The management algorithms are designed to be used for patients whose predominant problem is incontinence. However there are many other patients in whom the algorithms may be useful such as those patients with urgency and frequency suggestive of ***detrusor overactivity*** but without incontinence.

It should be noted that these algorithms, dated Paris 2002, represent the "***best opinion***" at that time. Our knowledge, developing from both a research base and because of evolving expert opinion, will inevitably ***change with time.*** The Consultation does not wish those using the algorithms to believe they are carved in tablets of stone: there will be changes both in the relatively short term and the long term.

➡ ***The algorithms for initial management***

are intended for use by all or any health care workers including health care assistants, nurses, physiotherapists, and family doctors as well as by specialists such as urologists and gynaecologists. The consultation has attempted to phrase the recommendations in the basic algorithms in such a way that they may be readily used by ***health care workers in all countries*** of the world in all continents, both in the developing and the developed world.

➡ ***The specialised algorithms***

are intended for use by specialists in the management of incontinence problems. The specialised algorithms, as well as the initial management algorithms are based on evidence where possible and on the expert opinion of the 1000 healthcare professionals who took part in the Consultation.

◆ **Essential components of basic assessment**

Each algorithm contains a core of recommendations relating to a number of essential components of basic assessment (see I to III Diagnostic Tests, above).

- General assessment
- Symptom assessment
- Assessment of quality of life impact
- Assessment of the desire for treatment
- Physical examination
- Urinalysis

◆ **Joint decision making**

The patient's desire for treatment. Today patient treatment is a matter for discussion and ***joint decision making*** between the patient and his or her health care advisors. This process of consultation includes the specific need to assess whether or not the sufferer of incontinence wishes to receive treatment and if so, what treatments he or she would favour. Implicit in this statement is the assumption that the health care worker will give an appropriate explanation of the patient's problem and the alternative lines of management, indications and risk. The assumption that patients almost always wish to have treatment is flawed and the need to consult the patient is paramount.

In each algorithm treatments are listed in the ***order in which they should be instituted.*** This order tends to list treatments in order of increasing invasiveness/complexity/cost.

In the ***initial management algorithms,*** treatment is ***empirically based,*** whilst, the ***specialized management*** algorithms rely on ***precise diagnosis*** from urodynamics and other testing.

I. CHILDREN

A. Initial management

1. Initial assessement should identify

➡ A group of children with ***complicated incontinence*** associated with:

- recurrent urinary infection
- voiding symptoms or evidence of poor bladder emptying
- urinary tract anomalies,
- previous pelvic surgery
- neuropathy

Complicated incontinence. Should have ***specialist management*** from the outset

➡ ***Two other main groups*** of children should be identified by initial assessment :

a) ***Nocturnal enuresis*** without other symptoms (mono-symptomatic).

b) ***Daytime symptoms*** of frequency, urgency, urge incontinence with or without night-time wetting

Children produce ***specific management problems*** for a variety of reasons: assessment requires ***help from their parents*** and carers; ***consent to treatment may be problematic***; and ***cooperation*** in both assessment and treatment ***may be difficult.***

In children, ***history*** and ***general assessment*** requires particular attention not only taking a full incontinence history but also in assessing bowel function, the child's social environment and the child's general and behavioral development: each should be formally assessed and recorded.

Physical examination should aim to detect a palpable bladder, any abnormality of the external genitalia, signs of incontinence and evidence of bony abnormalities in the gluteo-sacral area (eg. sacral dimple) or feet. If possible the child should be ***observed voiding.***

2. Treatment

Initial management should be instigated for those with «***uncomplicated***» nocturnal enuresis and or daytime symptoms.

➡ **a)** ***Mono-symptomatic nocturnal enuresis*** should be treated initially with the ***enuresis alarm***. Other recommended treatments are ***behavioral modification***, for example "star charts", and ***pharmacotherapy*** including anti-diuretic hormone analogues and antimuscarinic drugs.

➡ **b)** ***Daytime incontinence*** should be treated with bladder training (timed voiding) with or without antimuscarinic therapy.

Should initial treatment be unsuccessful in a and b

after a reasonable period of time (8-12 weeks), ***referral for a specialist's advice*** is highly recommended.

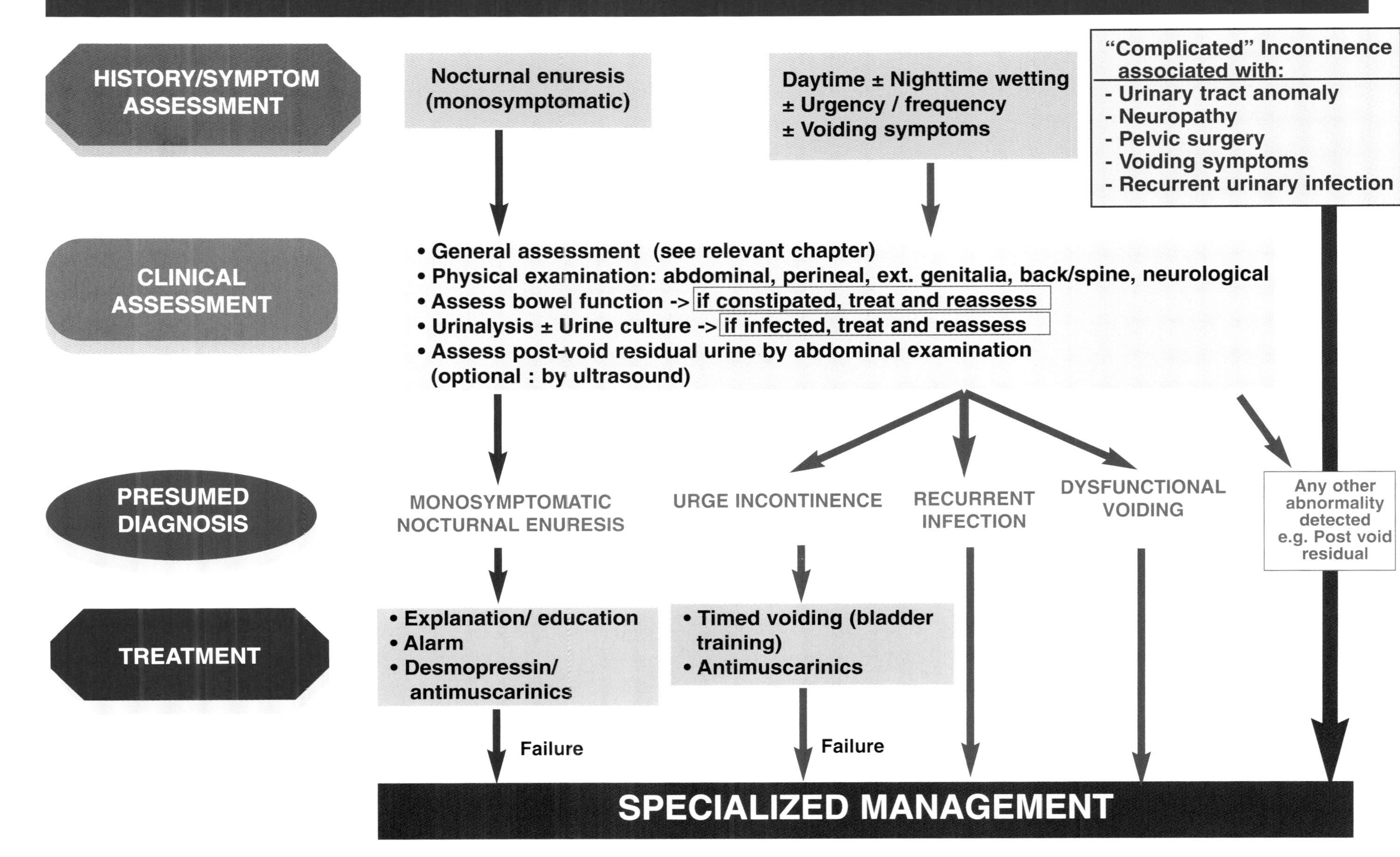
Initial Management of Urinary Incontinence in Children
HISTORY/SYMPTOM ASSESSMENT
Nocturnal enuresis (monosymptomatic)
Daytime ± Nighttime wetting
± Urgency / frequency
± Voiding symptoms
"Complicated" Incontinence associated with:
- Urinary tract anomaly
- Neuropathy
- Pelvic surgery
- Voiding symptoms
- Recurrent urinary infection
CLINICAL ASSESSMENT
• General assessment (see relevant chapter)
• Physical examination: abdominal, perineal, ext. genitalia, back/spine, neurological
• Assess bowel function -> if constipated, treat and reassess
• Urinalysis ± Urine culture -> if infected, treat and reassess
• Assess post-void residual urine by abdominal examination (optional : by ultrasound)
PRESUMED DIAGNOSIS
MONOSYMPTOMATIC NOCTURNAL ENURESIS
URGE INCONTINENCE
RECURRENT INFECTION
DYSFUNCTIONAL VOIDING
Any other abnormality detected e.g. Post void residual
TREATMENT
• Explanation/ education
• Alarm
• Desmopressin/ antimuscarinics
• Timed voiding (bladder training)
• Antimuscarinics
Failure
Failure
SPECIALIZED MANAGEMENT

I. CHILDREN

B. Specialized management

The ***group*** of children with "***complicated***" incontinence should have specialist management from the outset.

Three other groups of incontinent children are considered under ***specialist management:***

• those that have ***failed basic management***

• children whose incontinence is due to, or associated with, ***urinary tract anomalies***

• children without urinary tract anomalies, but with ***recurrent infection*** and, proven or suspected, ***voiding dysfunction***

1. Assessment

As part of further assessment, the measurement of urine flow (in children old enough), together with the ultrasound estimate of ***residual urine*** and the upper urinary tracts is ***highly recommended.***

Consideration should be given to the need for further ***renal imaging*** (nucleotide scanning, IVP) and /or ***lower urinary tract imaging*** and /or ***cysto-urethroscopy***. However, endoscopy is rarely indicated.

Urodynamic studies are ***highly recommended*** if ***invasive treatment*** is under consideration, for example, stress incontinence surgery if there is sphincteric incompetence, or bladder augmentation if there is detrusor overactivity.

Urodynamic studies are not recommended if the child has normal renal upper tract imaging and is to be treated by non invasive means, for example, bio-feedback (with or without electromyography) for dysfunctional voiding.

2. Treatment

The treatment of incontinence associated with ***urinary tract anomalies is complex*** and cannot be dealt with in an algorithm (please see children's subcommittee reports).

Children with bowel dysfunction should be treated with increased fibre, adequate fluid intake and adding bulking laxatives if necessary.

The treatment of stress and ***urge incontinence*** without voiding dysfunction is ***non-invasive*** and it is rare for invasive therapy to be considered: such children should only be dealt with by pediatric urologists with a special interest in incontinence.

When incontinence is associated with voiding dysfunction which results in significant post-void residuals (>30% of total bladder capacity) then initial treatment should be directed at achieving better bladder emptying by ***intermittent catheterisation*** : such therapy should be taught by those with special expertise in the care of children.

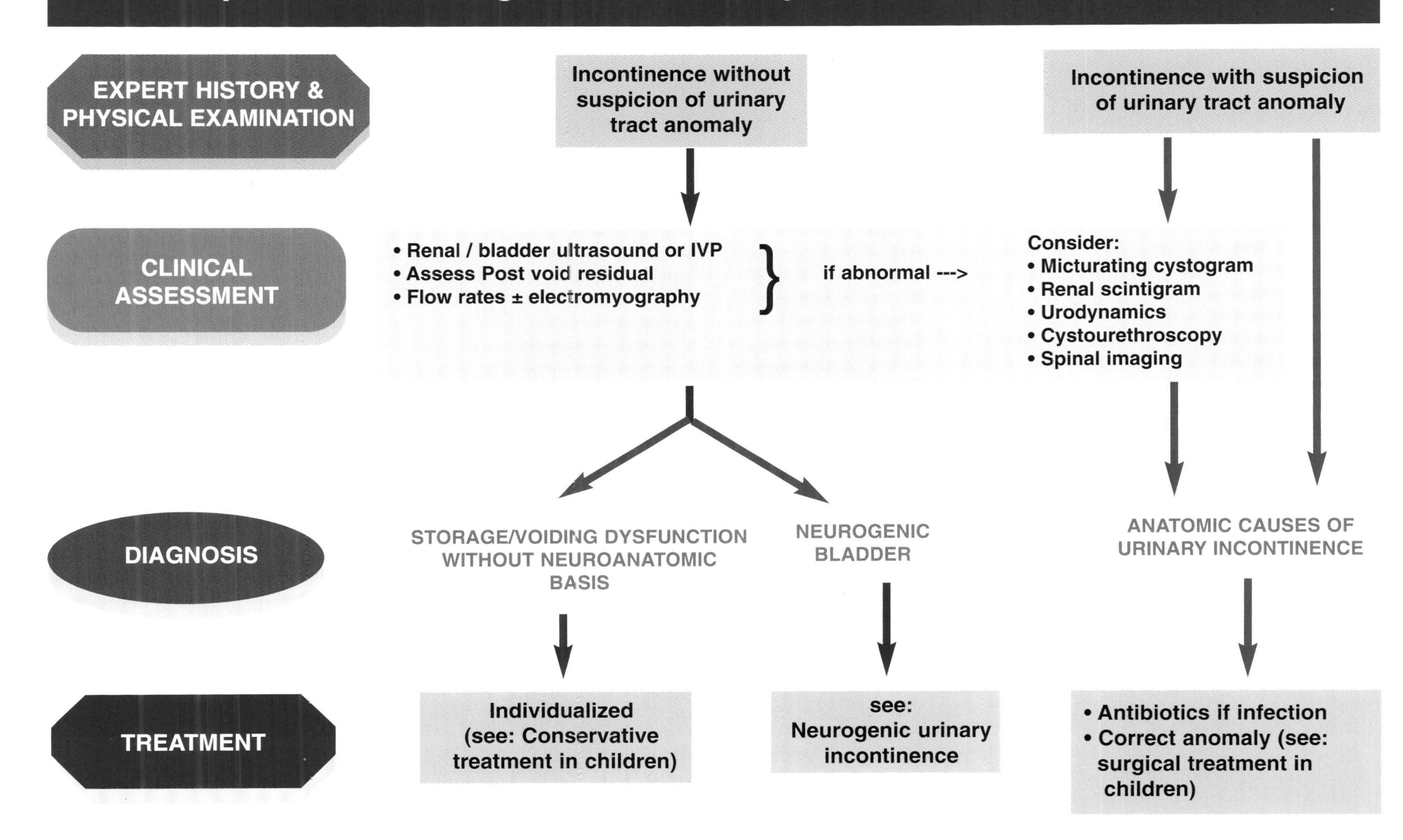

Specialized Management of Urinary Incontinence in Children
EXPERT HISTORY & PHYSICAL EXAMINATION
Incontinence without suspicion of urinary tract anomaly
Incontinence with suspicion of urinary tract anomaly
CLINICAL ASSESSMENT
• Renal / bladder ultrasound or IVP
• Assess Post void residual
• Flow rates ± electromyography
if abnormal --->
Consider:
• Micturating cystogram
• Renal scintigram
• Urodynamics
• Cystourethroscopy
• Spinal imaging
DIAGNOSIS
STORAGE/VOIDING DYSFUNCTION WITHOUT NEUROANATOMIC BASIS
NEUROGENIC BLADDER
ANATOMIC CAUSES OF URINARY INCONTINENCE
TREATMENT
Individualized (see: Conservative treatment in children)
see: Neurogenic urinary incontinence
• Antibiotics if infection
• Correct anomaly (see: surgical treatment in children)

II. MEN

A. INITIAL MANAGEMENT

1. Initial Assessement should identify :

Men with "complicated" incontinence associated with ***haematuria, pain, recurrent infection,*** or who are known to have, or who are thought to have ***poor bladder emptying*** are recommended for ***specialized management.*** Poor bladder emptying may be suspected from symptoms, physical examination or if imaging has been performed by X-ray or ultrasound after voiding.

Initial assessment aims to ***identify 3 groups of men*** suitable for ***initial management.***

a) Those with ***post-micturition dribble alone,***

b) Those with symptoms of ***urgency*** with or without urge incontinence, together with frequency and nocturia (overactive bladder) and

c) Those with ***post-prostatectomy incontinence***

2. Treatment

a) ***Post-micturition dribble*** requires ***no assessment*** and can usually be effectively treated by pelvic floor exercises and manual compression of the bulbous urethra at the end of micturition.

b) ***Urge incontinence*** and other overactive bladder symptoms should be treated by ***non-invasive*** means initially :

- pelvic floor exercises,
- bladder training and
- antimuscarinic drugs if detrusor overactivity is suspected as the cause for overactive bladder symptoms.
- alpha adrenergic antagonists (α-blockers), should be considered if it thought that there may also be bladder outlet obstruction

c) ***Post prostatectomy stress incontinence*** should also be treated initially by non- invasive means, by pelvic floor exercises.

Should initial treatment be unsuccessful

after a reasonable period of time (8-12 weeks), ***referral for a specialist's advice*** is highly recommended.

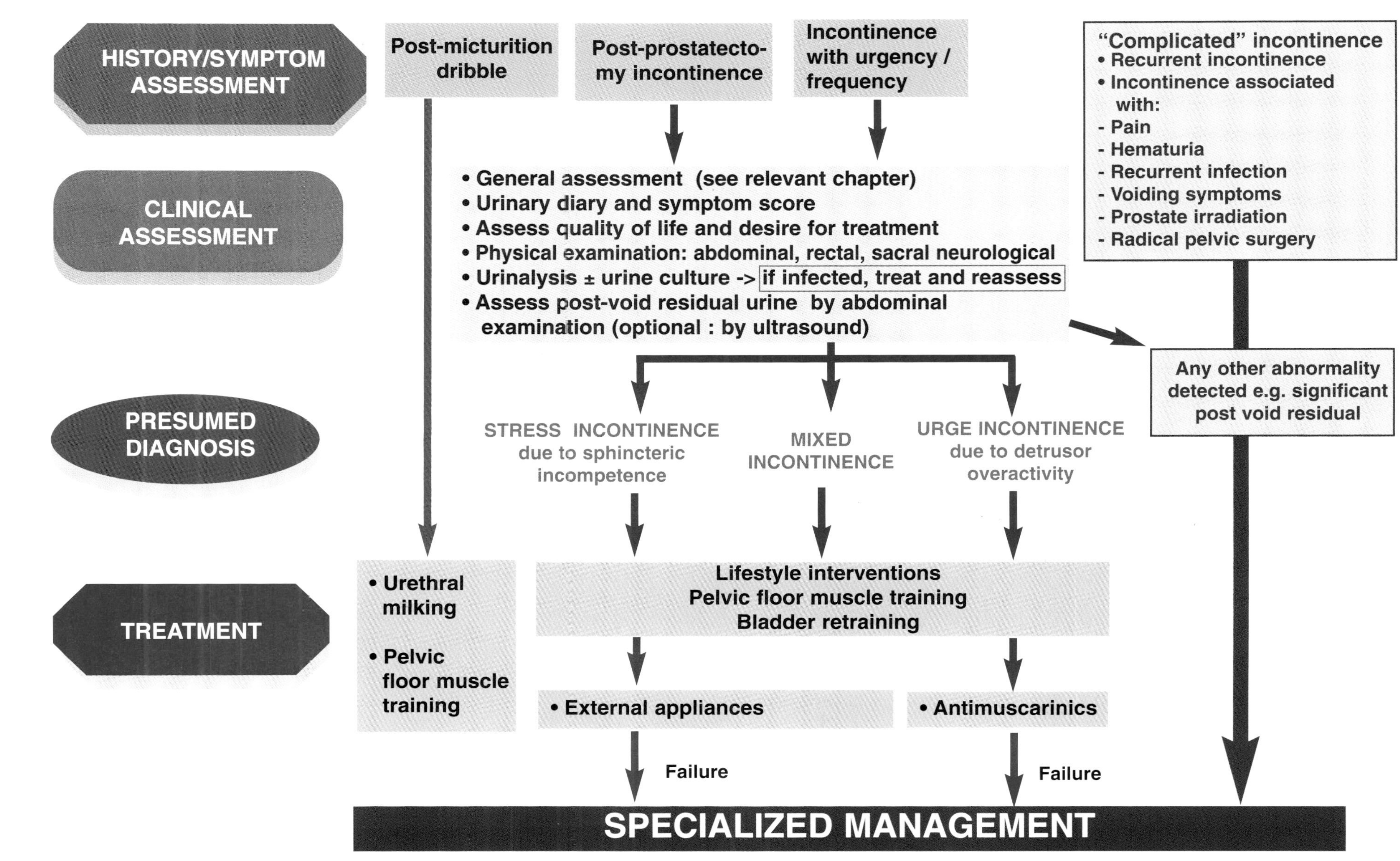
Initial Management of Urinary Incontinence in Men
HISTORY/SYMPTOM ASSESSMENT
CLINICAL ASSESSMENT
PRESUMED DIAGNOSIS
TREATMENT
Post-micturition dribble
Post-prostatectomy incontinence
Incontinence with urgency / frequency
"Complicated" incontinence
• Recurrent incontinence
• Incontinence associated with:
- Pain
- Hematuria
- Recurrent infection
- Voiding symptoms
- Prostate irradiation
- Radical pelvic surgery
• General assessment (see relevant chapter)
• Urinary diary and symptom score
• Assess quality of life and desire for treatment
• Physical examination: abdominal, rectal, sacral neurological
• Urinalysis ± urine culture -> if infected, treat and reassess
• Assess post-void residual urine by abdominal examination (optional : by ultrasound)
Any other abnormality detected e.g. significant post void residual
STRESS INCONTINENCE due to sphincteric incompetence
MIXED INCONTINENCE
URGE INCONTINENCE due to detrusor overactivity
• Urethral milking
• Pelvic floor muscle training
Lifestyle interventions
Pelvic floor muscle training
Bladder retraining
• External appliances
• Antimuscarinics
Failure
Failure
SPECIALIZED MANAGEMENT

II. MEN

B. SPECIALIZED MANAGEMENT

The specialist may first ***reinstitute initial management*** if it is felt that previous therapy had been inadequate,

1. Assessement

➡ ***Patients referred directly to specialized management*** are likely to require additional testing, cytology, cystourethoscopy and urinary tract imaging. If these tests prove normal then those individuals can be treated for incontinence by the initial or specialized management options as appropriate.

If symptoms suggestive of detrusor overactivity, or of sphincter incompetence persist, then ***urodynamic studies*** are highly recommended in order to arrive at a precise diagnosis.

2. Treatment

When basic management has failed

and if the patient's incontinence ***markedly disrupts*** his quality of life then ***invasive therapies*** should be considered.

➡ For ***sphincter incompetence*** the recommended option is the ***artificial urinary sphincter.***

➡ For the ***idiopathic detrusor overactivity,*** (overactive bladder) the recommended therapies are bladder augmentation, autoaugmentation, neuromodulation and urinary diversion.

➡ When ***incontinence*** has been shown to be associated with ***poor bladder emptying*** and detrusor underactivity, it is recommended that effective means are used to ensure bladder emptying, for example, intermittent catheterisation.

➡ If incontinence is associated with ***bladder outlet obstruction,*** then consideration should be given to surgical treatment to relieve obstruction. Alpha-blockers would be an optional treatment.

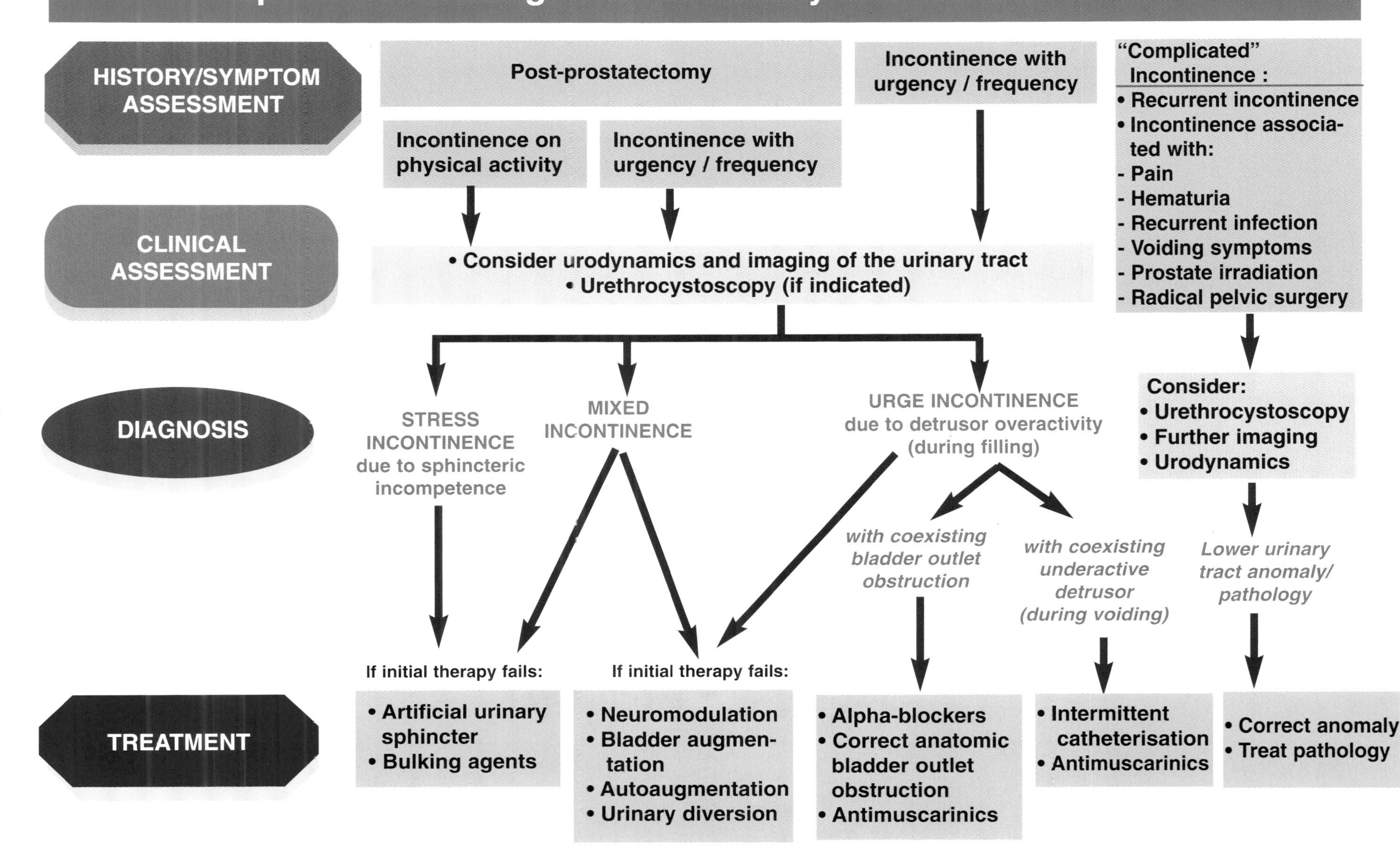

Specialized Management of Urinary Incontinence in Men
HISTORY/SYMPTOM ASSESSMENT
CLINICAL ASSESSMENT
DIAGNOSIS
TREATMENT
Post-prostatectomy
Incontinence on physical activity
Incontinence with urgency / frequency
Incontinence with urgency / frequency
"Complicated" Incontinence :
• Recurrent incontinence
• Incontinence associated with:
- Pain
- Hematuria
- Recurrent infection
- Voiding symptoms
- Prostate irradiation
- Radical pelvic surgery
• Consider urodynamics and imaging of the urinary tract
• Urethrocystoscopy (if indicated)
Consider:
• Urethrocystoscopy
• Further imaging
• Urodynamics
STRESS INCONTINENCE due to sphincteric incompetence
MIXED INCONTINENCE
URGE INCONTINENCE due to detrusor overactivity (during filling)
with coexisting bladder outlet obstruction
with coexisting underactive detrusor (during voiding)
Lower urinary tract anomaly/ pathology
If initial therapy fails:
• Artificial urinary sphincter
• Bulking agents
If initial therapy fails:
• Neuromodulation
• Bladder augmentation
• Autoaugmentation
• Urinary diversion
• Alpha-blockers
• Correct anatomic bladder outlet obstruction
• Antimuscarinics
• Intermittent catheterisation
• Antimuscarinics
• Correct anomaly
• Treat pathology

III. WOMEN

A. Initial management

1. Initial assessment should identify :

• ***"Complicated" incontinence group.***

In certain parts of the developing world, exceptionally severe incontinence results from childbirth injury and ***urinary fistula***. These devastating injuries affect millions of women in sub-Saharan Africa. These women form a special group of women with special needs who must be identified at initial assessment.

Others include those who also have ***pain*** or ***haematuria***, ***recurrent infections,*** suspected or proven ***voiding problems, significant pelvic organ prolapse*** or who have persistent incontinence or recurrent incontinence after ***previous surgery***, such as ***pelvic irradiation,*** radical ***pelvic surgery*** or ***previous surgery for incontinence.***

• ***Three other main groups*** of patients should be identified by initial assessment.

a) Women with stress incontinence on ***physical activity***

b) Women with ***urgency***, frequency and urge incontinence (overactive bladder)

c) Those women with ***mixed*** urge and stress incontinence

In women, ***abdominal, pelvic and perineal examinations*** should be a routine part of physical examination. Women should be asked to perform a "***stress test***" (cough and strain to detect leakage likely to be due to sphincter incompetence). Any pelvic organ prolapse or uro-genital atrophy, should be assessed. ***Vaginal or rectal examination*** allows the assessment of pelvic floor function, an essential step prior to the teaching of pelvic floor exercises. Vaginal examination is also an acceptable way to assess post-void residual urine if simple imaging methods are not available.

2. Treatment

➡ Initial treatment should include ***life style interventions*** in addition to therapies aimed at ***specific types of incontinence.*** Life style interventions include weight reduction, stopping smoking, and regulating food and fluid intake (including caffeine).

➡ ***Oestrogen deficiency*** and ***urinary infection*** should be treated at initial assessment and the patient reassessed after a suitable interval.

a) ***Presumed stress incontinence*** should be treated by pelvic floor exercise and/or by devices such as intra-vaginal supporting tampons, intra-urethral plugs and meatal occlusion devices.

b) ***Presumed urge incontinence*** should be treated by bladder retraining with or without antimuscarinic medication

c) Women with symptoms of ***both stress and urge leakage*** should have their ***predominant*** symptom ***treated initially.***

Initial treatment should be ***maintained for 8-12 weeks*** before reassessment and possible specialist referral.

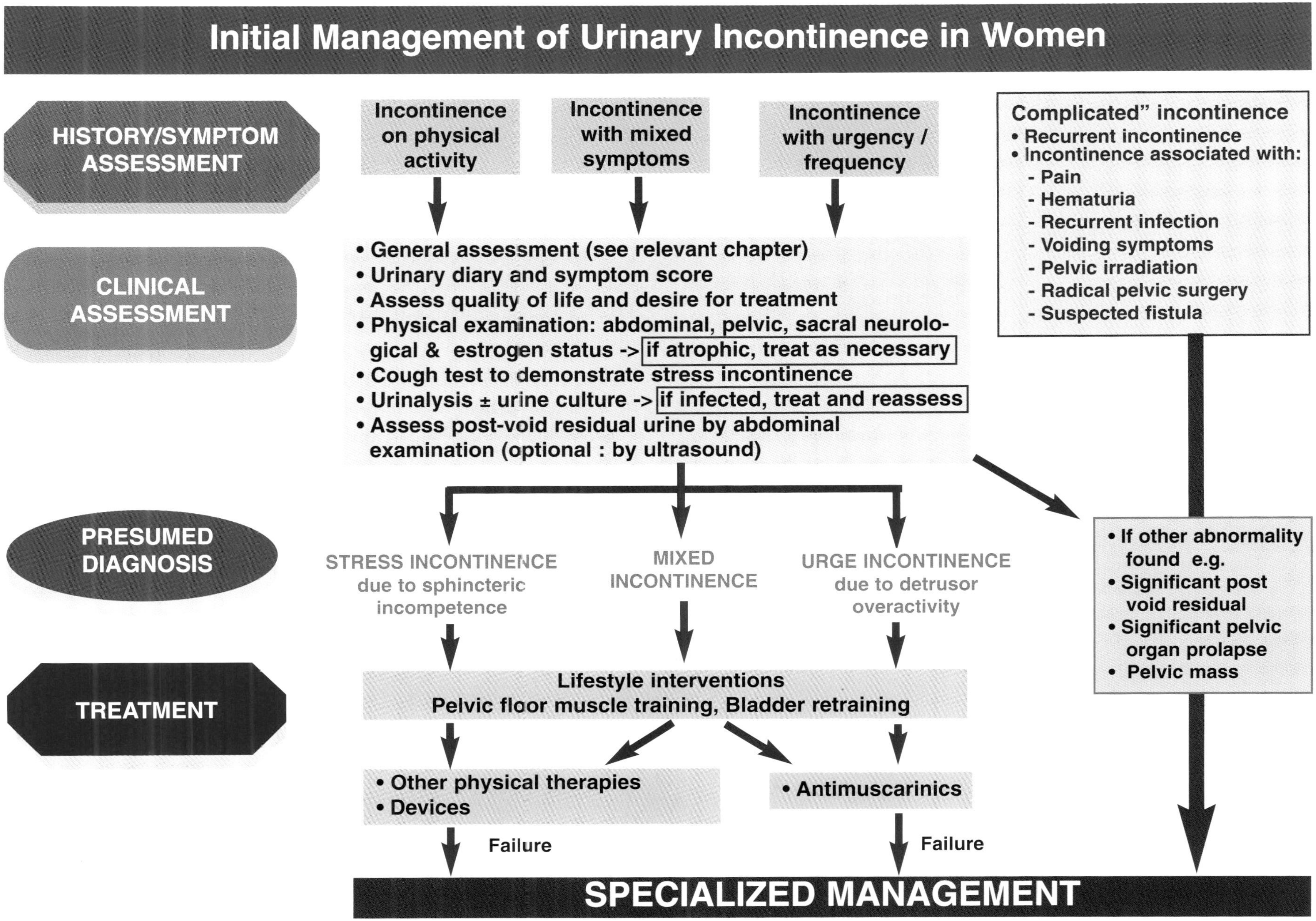

Initial Management of Urinary Incontinence in Women

HISTORY/SYMPTOM ASSESSMENT

Incontinence on physical activity

Incontinence with mixed symptoms

Incontinence with urgency / frequency

Complicated" incontinence
- Recurrent incontinence
- Incontinence associated with:
  - Pain
  - Hematuria
  - Recurrent infection
  - Voiding symptoms
  - Pelvic irradiation
  - Radical pelvic surgery
  - Suspected fistula

CLINICAL ASSESSMENT

- General assessment (see relevant chapter)
- Urinary diary and symptom score
- Assess quality of life and desire for treatment
- Physical examination: abdominal, pelvic, sacral neurological & estrogen status -> if atrophic, treat as necessary
- Cough test to demonstrate stress incontinence
- Urinalysis ± urine culture -> if infected, treat and reassess
- Assess post-void residual urine by abdominal examination (optional : by ultrasound)

PRESUMED DIAGNOSIS

STRESS INCONTINENCE due to sphincteric incompetence

MIXED INCONTINENCE

URGE INCONTINENCE due to detrusor overactivity

- If other abnormality found e.g.
- Significant post void residual
- Significant pelvic organ prolapse
- Pelvic mass

TREATMENT

Lifestyle interventions
Pelvic floor muscle training, Bladder retraining

- Other physical therapies
- Devices

- Antimuscarinics

Failure

Failure

SPECIALIZED MANAGEMENT

III. WOMEN

B. Specialized management

1. Assessement

Women who have *"**complicated" incontinence*** (see initial algorithm) may need to have ***additional tests*** such as cytology, cystourethroscopy or urinary tract imaging. ***If these tests are normal*** then they should be treated for incontinence by the initial or specialized management options as appropriate.

- ***Those women who have failed initial management*** and whose ***quality of life is impaired*** are likely to request further treatment. If initial management has been given an adequate trial then ***interventional therapy may be desirable.*** Prior to intervention ***urodynamic testing is highly recommended.*** Within the urodynamic investigation ***urethral function testing by*** *urethral pressure profile or leak point pressure* ***is optional.*** Systematic assessment for ***pelvic organ prolapse*** is highly recommended and it is suggested that the ICS method should be used in research studies. Urodynamics allow the precise diagnosis of the type of incontinence and therefore dictate the management plan.
- Women with ***co-existing pelvic organ prolapse*** should have their prolapse treated as appropriate
- Women in developing countries with ***birth/pregnancy injuries*** do not require urodynamic assessment and are best treated in specialist fistula units.

2. Treatment

- ***If genuine stress incontinence is confirmed*** then the treatment options that are recommended for patients with ***some degree of bladder-neck and urethral mobility*** include retropubic suspension procedures, and bladder neck/sub-urethral sling operations. Less invasive procedure may be offered to patients in specific circumstances, for example, needle suspensions in older, less fit, less energetic individuals. The correction of pelvic organ prolapse may be desirable at the same time.

For patients with ***intrinsic sphincter deficiency and limited bladder neck mobility,*** sling procedures, injectable bulking agents and the artificial urinary sphincter are recommended.

- ***Urge incontinence secondary to idiopathic detrusor overactivity*** (overactive bladder) may be treated by neuromodulation or bladder augmentation. Detrusor myectomy is an optional procedure (auto augmentation).
- Those patients with v***oiding dysfunction*** leading to ***significant post-void residual urine*** (>30% of total bladder capacity) may have bladder ***outlet obstruction*** or ***detrusor underactivity***. In women urethral dilatation is recommended to treat relative urethral narrowing. In most women with voiding dysfunction, the cause is detrusor underactivity, and intermittent catheterisation is recommended.
- Long -term low dose antibiotics are recommended if there are ***persistent infections.***

Specialized Management of Urinary Incontinence in Women

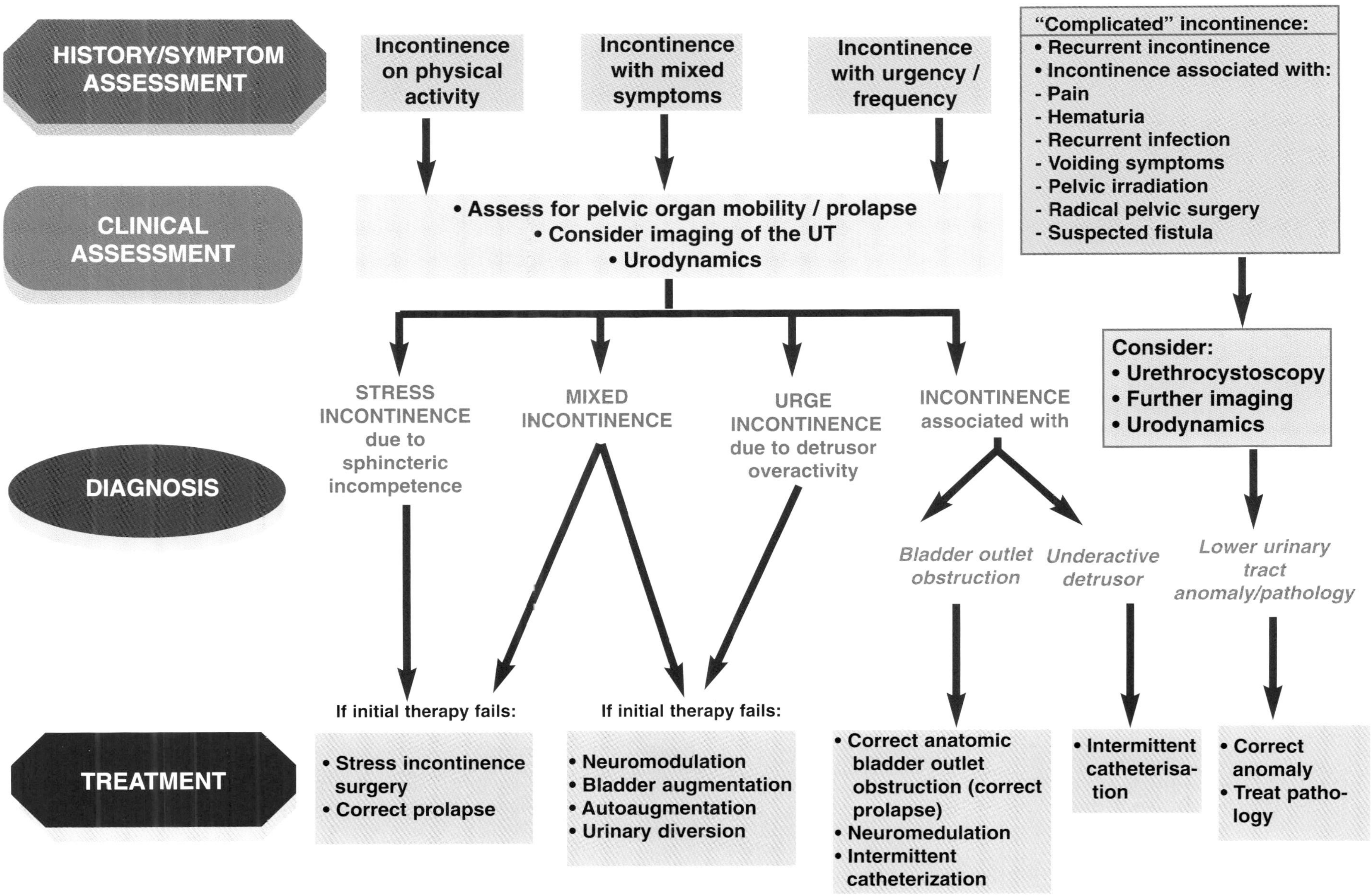

HISTORY/SYMPTOM ASSESSMENT

- Incontinence on physical activity
- Incontinence with mixed symptoms
- Incontinence with urgency / frequency

"Complicated" incontinence:
- Recurrent incontinence
- Incontinence associated with:
  - Pain
  - Hematuria
  - Recurrent infection
  - Voiding symptoms
  - Pelvic irradiation
  - Radical pelvic surgery
  - Suspected fistula

CLINICAL ASSESSMENT

- Assess for pelvic organ mobility / prolapse
- Consider imaging of the UT
- Urodynamics

Consider:
- Urethrocystoscopy
- Further imaging
- Urodynamics

DIAGNOSIS

- STRESS INCONTINENCE due to sphincteric incompetence
- MIXED INCONTINENCE
- URGE INCONTINENCE due to detrusor overactivity
- INCONTINENCE associated with
  - *Bladder outlet obstruction*
  - *Underactive detrusor*
- *Lower urinary tract anomaly/pathology*

TREATMENT

If initial therapy fails:
- Stress incontinence surgery
- Correct prolapse

If initial therapy fails:
- Neuromodulation
- Bladder augmentation
- Autoaugmentation
- Urinary diversion

Bladder outlet obstruction:
- Correct anatomic bladder outlet obstruction (correct prolapse)
- Neuromedulation
- Intermittent catheterization

Underactive detrusor:
- Intermittent catheterisa-tion

Lower urinary tract anomaly/pathology:
- Correct anomaly
- Treat patho-logy

IV. PELVIC ORGAN PROLAPSE

Introduction

Women may present with symptomatic pelvic organ prolapse (POP) with or without symptoms of urinary incontinence.

Evaluation for POP may be initiated by a carer or a health care worker.

1. Assessment

Symptom enquiry will reveal a range of symptoms with varying components of prolapse and incontinence symptoms.

- Need for prolapse replacement to improve urinary symptoms, or if replacement leads to symptoms, such as incontinence, this is significant.
- Need for prolapse replacement in order to micturate or defaecate is important.

Physical examination should define :

- the ***type*** and ***degree*** of prolapse : examining the women standing and straining is desirable
- ***Associated abnormalities*** such as ulcerations or sores of exposed vaginal/cervical. tissues, which may cause bleeding or copious discharge.
- ***Measurement of post void residual*** (PVR) is useful. If there is an anterior vaginal wall prolapse then the urethra may be distorted (kinked) leading to a significant PVR.

2. Treatment

In general it is considered wise to ***treat only symptomatic prolapse.***

Treatment of asymptomatic prolapse may result in new urinary, bowel or sexual dysfunction symptoms.

➡ ***Conservative treatment*** is safe and satisfactory for certain patients.

- Periodic re-evaluation may be preferred.
- ***Pessaries*** may be used with caution in the presence of sore/ulcers but there must be regular follow-up.

➡ ***Surgical treatments*** aim to restore the normal anatomy as far as is possible. Readers should refer to the chapter for full details of techniques

- ***Continence procedures*** may be needed in conjunction with ***prolapse procedures***, in these patients ***urodynamic*** studies are recommended prior to surgery, as they may be useful in selecting a specific procedure.

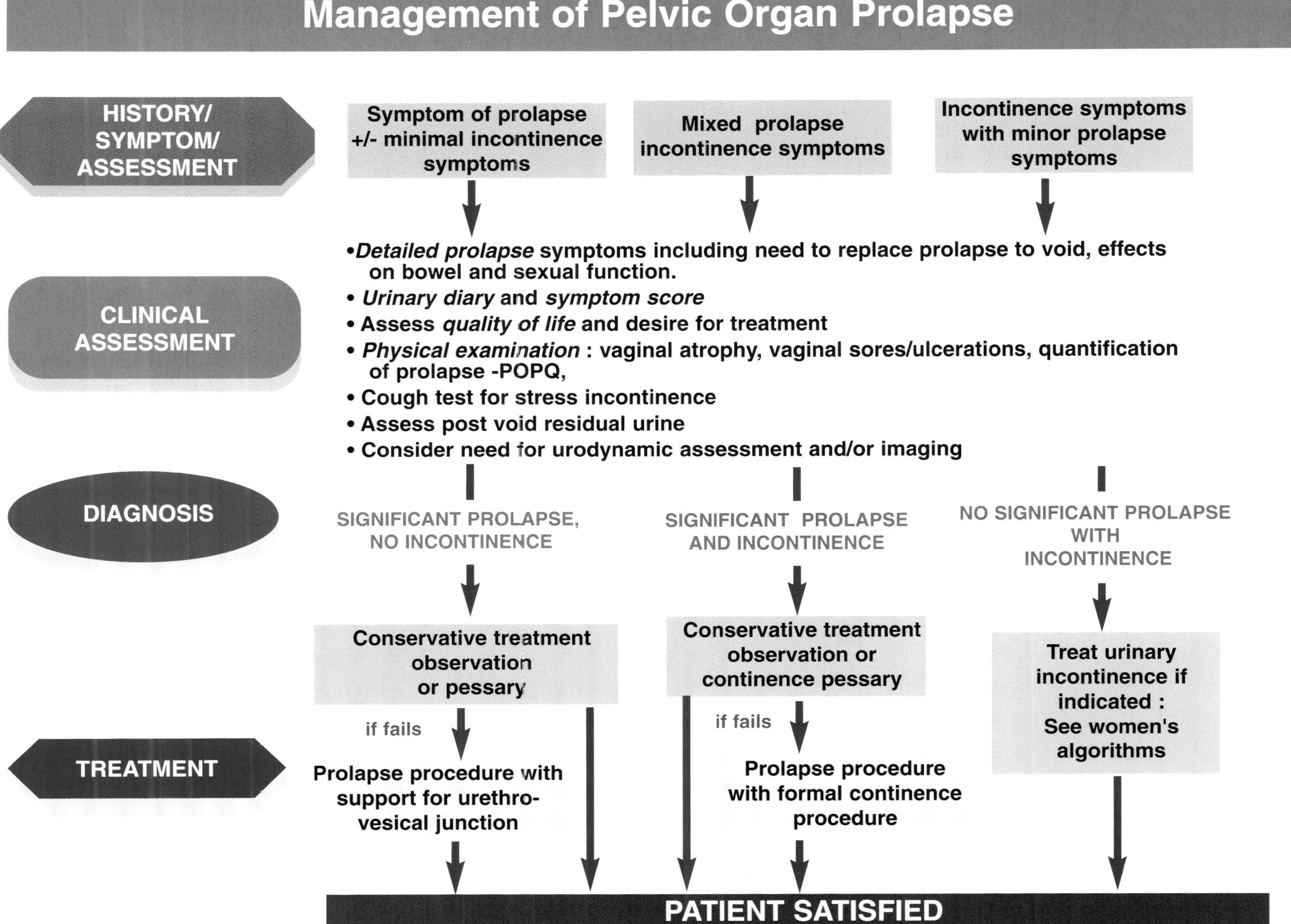
Management of Pelvic Organ Prolapse
HISTORY/ SYMPTOM/ ASSESSMENT
Symptom of prolapse +/- minimal incontinence symptoms
Mixed prolapse incontinence symptoms
Incontinence symptoms with minor prolapse symptoms
CLINICAL ASSESSMENT
•Detailed prolapse symptoms including need to replace prolapse to void, effects on bowel and sexual function.
• Urinary diary and symptom score
• Assess quality of life and desire for treatment
• Physical examination : vaginal atrophy, vaginal sores/ulcerations, quantification of prolapse -POPQ,
• Cough test for stress incontinence
• Assess post void residual urine
• Consider need for urodynamic assessment and/or imaging
DIAGNOSIS
SIGNIFICANT PROLAPSE, NO INCONTINENCE
SIGNIFICANT PROLAPSE AND INCONTINENCE
NO SIGNIFICANT PROLAPSE WITH INCONTINENCE
TREATMENT
Conservative treatment observation or pessary
if fails
Prolapse procedure with support for urethro-vesical junction
Conservative treatment observation or continence pessary
if fails
Prolapse procedure with formal continence procedure
Treat urinary incontinence if indicated : See women's algorithms
PATIENT SATISFIED

V. NEUROGENIC INCONTINENCE

A. INITIAL MANAGEMENT

1. Initial assessment

In assessing patients with incontinence due to neurogenic vesico-urethral dysfunction the management depends on an ***understanding of the likely mechanisms producing incontinence,*** which in turn depends on the ***site of the nervous system abnormality.*** Therefore, neurogenic incontinence patients can be divided as following:

Two groups of patients, one with peripheral nerve lesions (a) and the other with central lesions below the pons (b) should be managed by the specialist with a particular interest / training in neurological lower urinary tract dysfunction.

a) Peripheral lesions,

Including peripheral nerve lesions, for example the denervation that occurs after major pelvic surgery such as for cancer of the rectum or cervix. Also included are those lesions involving the lowest part of the spinal cord (conus/cauda equina lesions), eg. lumbar disc prolapse.

b) Central lesions below the pons

Suprasacral infrapontine spinal cord lesions, eg. traumatic spinal cord lesions, should be treated on a basis of urodynamic studies: the initial treatment should be maintained for 8-12 weeks, before reassessment and possible referral to the specialist.

c) Central lesions above the pons

suprapontine central lesions include for example cerebro-vascular accident, stroke, Parkinson´s Disease and multiple sclerosis

During initial assessment

- ***physical examination*** is important in helping to distinguish these 3 groups and a ***simple neurological examination*** should be a routine.
- An estimate of ***post-void residual PVR*** is highly recommended (preferably by ultrasound). If a significant PVR is found, then upper tract imaging is required.

2. Treatment

Initial treatment is suitable for the large group of patients with incontinence due to suprapontine conditions like strokes. At initial assessment, these patients need to be assessed for their degree of ***mobility*** and their ***ability to cooperate,*** as these two factors will determine which therapies are possible.

The treatments recommended are: behavioral (including timed voiding) and ***bladder-relaxant drugs*** for presumed detrusor overactivity. ***Appliances*** or catheters may be needed in patients who are immobile or cannot cooperate.

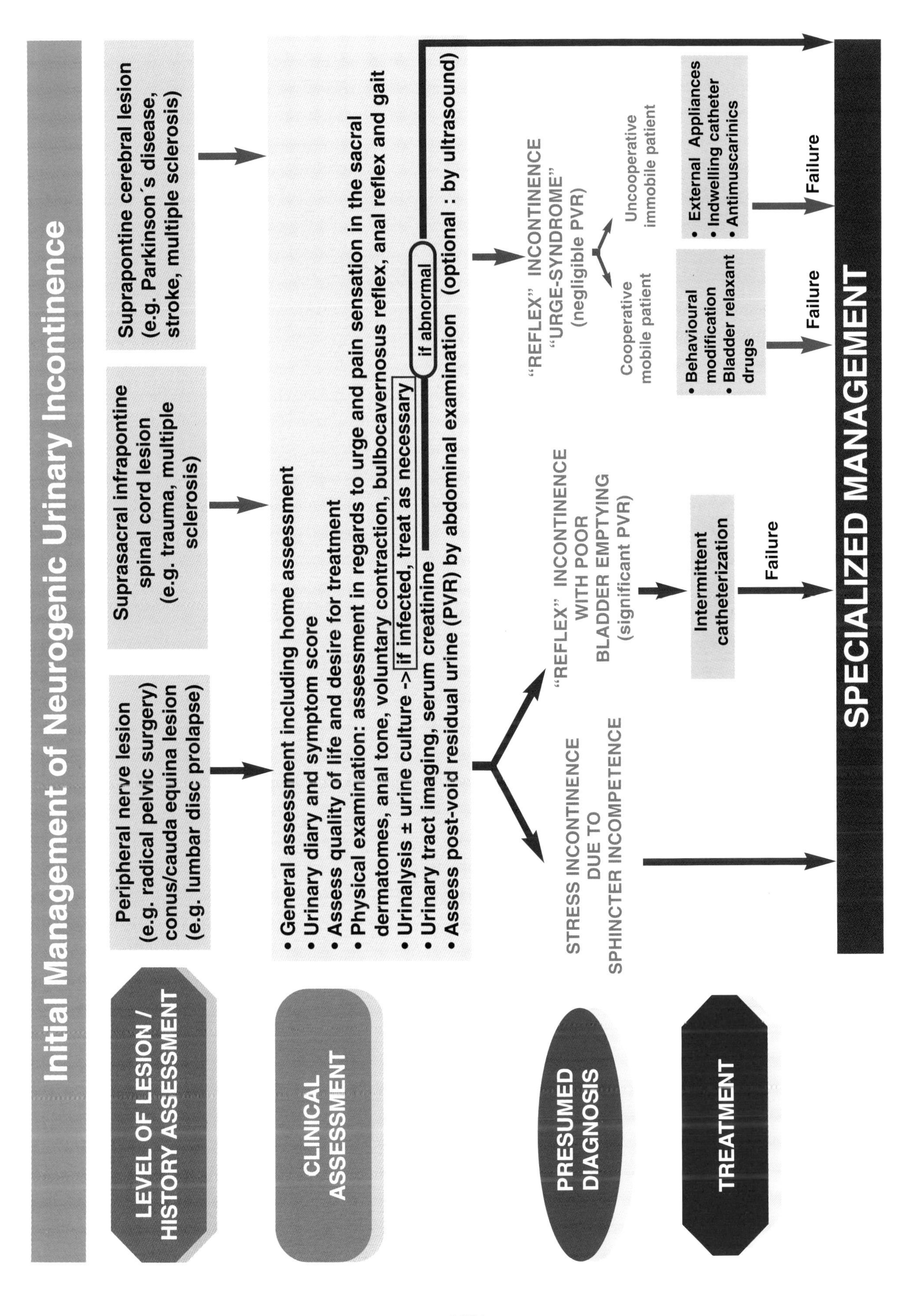

Initial Management of Neurogenic Urinary Incontinence
LEVEL OF LESION / HISTORY ASSESSMENT
Peripheral nerve lesion (e.g. radical pelvic surgery) conus/cauda equina lesion (e.g. lumbar disc prolapse)
Suprasacral infrapontine spinal cord lesion (e.g. trauma, multiple sclerosis)
Suprapontine cerebral lesion (e.g. Parkinson´s disease, stroke, multiple sclerosis)
CLINICAL ASSESSMENT
• General assessment including home assessment
• Urinary diary and symptom score
• Assess quality of life and desire for treatment
• Physical examination: assessment in regards to urge and pain sensation in the sacral dermatomes, anal tone, voluntary contraction, bulbocavernosus reflex, anal reflex and gait
• Urinalysis ± urine culture -> if infected, treat as necessary
• Urinary tract imaging, serum creatinine
• Assess post-void residual urine (PVR) by abdominal examination (optional : by ultrasound)
if abnormal
PRESUMED DIAGNOSIS
STRESS INCONTINENCE DUE TO SPHINCTER INCOMPETENCE
"REFLEX" INCONTINENCE WITH POOR BLADDER EMPTYING (significant PVR)
"REFLEX" INCONTINENCE "URGE-SYNDROME" (negligible PVR)
Cooperative mobile patient
Uncooperative immobile patient
TREATMENT
Intermittent catheterization
• Behavioural modification
• Bladder relaxant drugs
• External Appliances
• Indwelling catheter
• Antimuscarinics
Failure
Failure
Failure
SPECIALIZED MANAGEMENT

V. NEUROGENIC INCONTINENCE

B. Specialized management

1. Assessment

Most patients with ***peripheral or central lesions below the pons*** require specialized assessment and management.

Urodynamic studies are highly recommended in these patients to establish both bladder and urethral function. ***Upper urinary tract imaging*** is needed in most patients and more detailed renal imaging or ***renal function studies*** will be desirable in some.

Urodynamics will define the filling function, with detrusor overactivity and neurogenic stress incontinence secondary to denervation being the most common abnormalities. During voiding, sphincter overactivity and detrusor underactivity are both likely to lead to persistent failure to empty.

2. Treatment

Management is straightforward in concept although the therapeutic options are extensive. The algorithm details the recommended options.

For ***sphincter incompetence*** the recommended options are the artificial urinary sphincter, sling procedures (in women) and injectables in selected patients.

Combinations of abnormalities are common e.g. in meningomyelocele. Incontinence may be due to a combination of detrusor overactivity and neurogenic stress incontinence because of sphincter underactivity. Residual urine may be caused by detrusor underactivity as well as functional sphincter obstruction in the same patient. Each element of vesicourethral dysfunction needs to be dealt with. However, it must be remembered that ***preservation of upper tract function is of paramount importance.***

For detailed discussion please read the relevant chapters from the consultation.

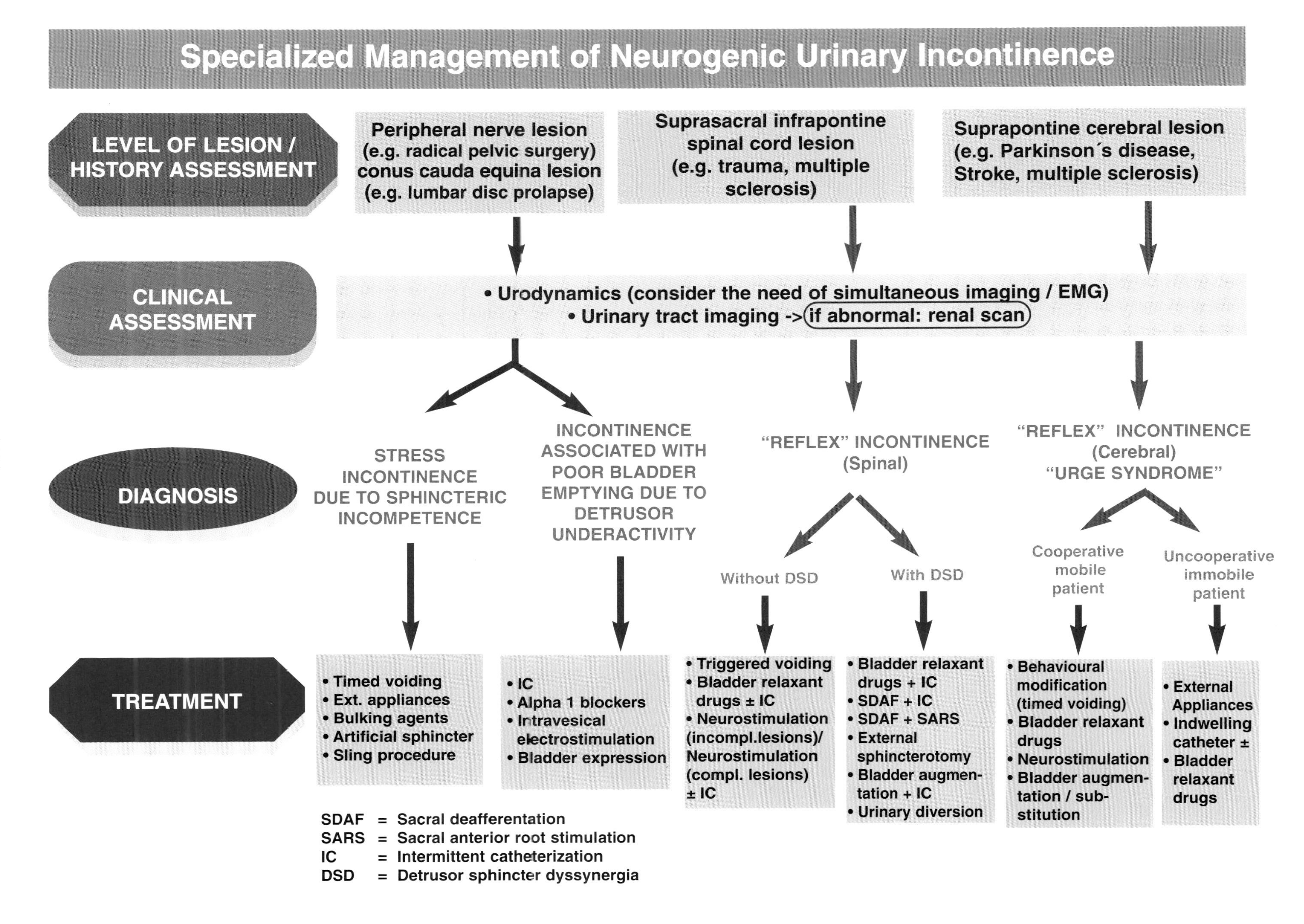
Specialized Management of Neurogenic Urinary Incontinence
LEVEL OF LESION / HISTORY ASSESSMENT
Peripheral nerve lesion (e.g. radical pelvic surgery) conus cauda equina lesion (e.g. lumbar disc prolapse)
Suprasacral infrapontine spinal cord lesion (e.g. trauma, multiple sclerosis)
Suprapontine cerebral lesion (e.g. Parkinson´s disease, Stroke, multiple sclerosis)
CLINICAL ASSESSMENT
• Urodynamics (consider the need of simultaneous imaging / EMG)
• Urinary tract imaging -> if abnormal: renal scan
DIAGNOSIS
STRESS INCONTINENCE DUE TO SPHINCTERIC INCOMPETENCE
INCONTINENCE ASSOCIATED WITH POOR BLADDER EMPTYING DUE TO DETRUSOR UNDERACTIVITY
"REFLEX" INCONTINENCE (Spinal)
"REFLEX" INCONTINENCE (Cerebral) "URGE SYNDROME"
Without DSD
With DSD
Cooperative mobile patient
Uncooperative immobile patient
TREATMENT
• Timed voiding • Ext. appliances • Bulking agents • Artificial sphincter • Sling procedure
• IC • Alpha 1 blockers • Intravesical electrostimulation • Bladder expression
• Triggered voiding • Bladder relaxant drugs ± IC • Neurostimulation (incompl.lesions)/ Neurostimulation (compl. lesions) ± IC
• Bladder relaxant drugs + IC • SDAF + IC • SDAF + SARS • External sphincterotomy • Bladder augmentation + IC • Urinary diversion
• Behavioural modification (timed voiding) • Bladder relaxant drugs • Neurostimulation • Bladder augmentation / substitution
• External Appliances • Indwelling catheter ± • Bladder relaxant drugs
SDAF = Sacral deafferentation
SARS = Sacral anterior root stimulation
IC = Intermittent catheterization
DSD = Detrusor sphincter dyssynergia

VI. Frail and/or Disabled Older Men

A. Initial Management

Frail older persons present different problems. Implicit in the terms "frail" is the realisation that such individuals may neither wish nor be fitter or younger enough to be considered for the full range of therapies likely to be offered to fitter or younger incontinent individual.

However, every person should be given the opportunity to achieve continence, irrespective of their frailty or disability. This can be ***"independent continence", "dependent continence"*** – dry with the assistance or reminder of a carer or "***social continence***" – dry with the use of appropriate aids and devices. Often dryness can be achieved by a combination of the above approaches.

1. Assessment

➡ During ***initial assessment*** the frail and/or disabled older person, besides a general continence assessment and a complete physical examination, needs to be assessed with specific inquiries into:

- Cognitive abilities
- Mobility and environment including access to toilet
- ADL (activities of daily living)
- Level of support available to the incontinent person
- Potentially reversible conditions that can cause or worsen incontinence in older people
- Medication, particularly diuretics or drugs that cause sedation or confusion

➡ The ***extent of investigation*** and ***management*** in frail and/or disabled older people should take into account

- Degree of bother to the patient and/or carer
- Patient motivation and level of cooperation
- Patient's comorbidities
- Prognosis and life expectancy

➡ ***Post-void residual urine*** (PVR) should be assessed, preferably by ultrasound, or by in/out catheter, since it influences the choice of management. There is no specific "cut off" for the different choices and the ranges listed below are provided as a broad guideline. It is often worthwhile to ***repeat the PVR*** since it can vary especially after reviewing drugs and treating constipation. A low PVR does not exclude outlet obstruction. Uroflowmetry may be helpful to rule out outlet obstruction but only if maximum flow is normal

2. Treatment

➡ ***Conservative and behavioural therapy*** includes pelvic floor muscle exercises, biofeedback, bladder training in the more fit or alert patient, assisted voiding for more disabled patients and prompted voiding for frailer and more cognitively impaired patients.

➡ ***Bladder relaxant drugs*** may be considered as an adjunct to these conservative treatments of detrusor overactivity, whilst ***α-blockers*** may be tried to assist bladder emptying. When they are being tried, it is important to dose titrate from a low dose, reviewing outcome and side effects regularly.

B. Specialised Management

If after initial assessment the frail older person is found to have incontinence with other significant factors (eg pain, haematuria) then consideration should be given to further assessment and investigation by a specialist.

Referral for specialised management may also be applicable for individuals who have not responded adequately to simple conservative measures provided they are motivated and if such intervention and/or management might improve their continence management and quality of life.

Age per se is not a contraindication to surgery for incontinence. However, in older people especially frail and/or disabled older people:

- ***Modifiable reversible conditions*** should be addressed prior to surgery
- Wherever possible, ***adequate trial of conservative treatment*** should be offered prior to surgery followed by reassessment of the need for surgery
- A ***urodynamic assessment*** should proceed surgery because clinical diagnosis may be inaccurate

Preoperative assessment plus perioperative care is essential to minimise postoperative geriatric complications such as delirium, infection, dehydration and falls.

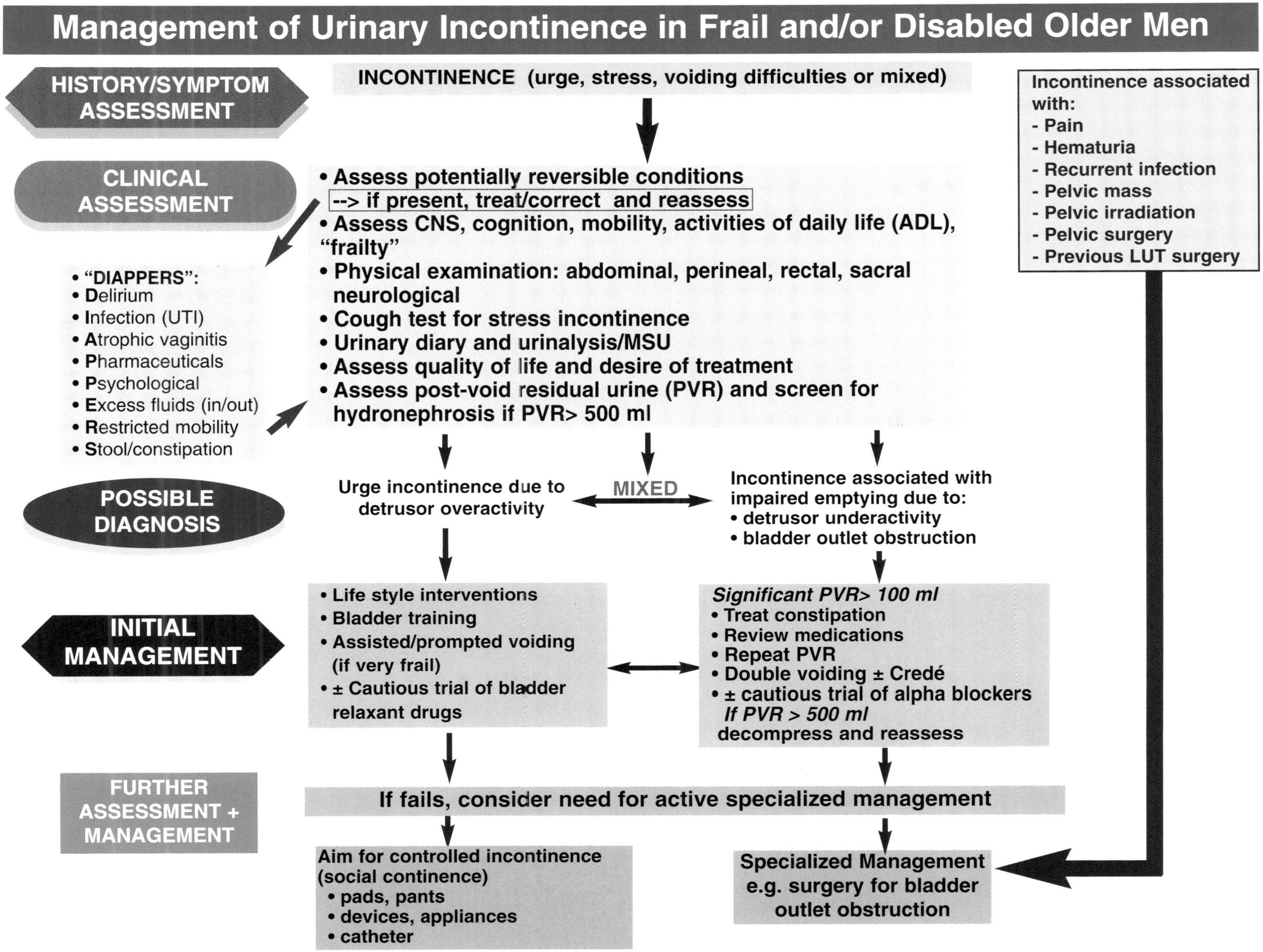

Management of Urinary Incontinence in Frail and/or Disabled Older Men

HISTORY/SYMPTOM ASSESSMENT

INCONTINENCE (urge, stress, voiding difficulties or mixed)

Incontinence associated with:
- Pain
- Hematuria
- Recurrent infection
- Pelvic mass
- Pelvic irradiation
- Pelvic surgery
- Previous LUT surgery

CLINICAL ASSESSMENT

- Assess potentially reversible conditions
  --> if present, treat/correct and reassess
- Assess CNS, cognition, mobility, activities of daily life (ADL), "frailty"
- Physical examination: abdominal, perineal, rectal, sacral neurological
- Cough test for stress incontinence
- Urinary diary and urinalysis/MSU
- Assess quality of life and desire of treatment
- Assess post-void residual urine (PVR) and screen for hydronephrosis if PVR> 500 ml

- "DIAPPERS":
- **D**elirium
- **I**nfection (UTI)
- **A**trophic vaginitis
- **P**harmaceuticals
- **P**sychological
- **E**xcess fluids (in/out)
- **R**estricted mobility
- **S**tool/constipation

POSSIBLE DIAGNOSIS

Urge incontinence due to detrusor overactivity

MIXED

Incontinence associated with impaired emptying due to:
- detrusor underactivity
- bladder outlet obstruction

INITIAL MANAGEMENT

- Life style interventions
- Bladder training
- Assisted/prompted voiding (if very frail)
- ± Cautious trial of bladder relaxant drugs

Significant PVR> 100 ml
- Treat constipation
- Review medications
- Repeat PVR
- Double voiding ± Credé
- ± cautious trial of alpha blockers

If PVR > 500 ml
decompress and reassess

FURTHER ASSESSMENT + MANAGEMENT

If fails, consider need for active specialized management

Aim for controlled incontinence (social continence)
- pads, pants
- devices, appliances
- catheter

Specialized Management e.g. surgery for bladder outlet obstruction

VII. Frail and/or Disabled Older Women

A. Initial Management

Frail older persons present different problems. Implicit in the terms "frail" is the realisation that such individuals may neither wish nor be fit enough to be considered for the full range of therapies likely to be offered to fitter or younger incontinent individual.

However, every person should be given the opportunity to achieve ***continence,*** irrespective of their frailty or disability. This can be ***"independent continence",*** ***"dependent continence"*** – dry with the assistance or reminder of a carer or "***social continence***" – dry with the use of appropriate aids and devices. Often dryness can be achieved by a combination of the above approaches.

1. Assessment

➡ During ***initial assessment*** the frail and/or disabled older person, besides a general continence assessment and a complete physical examination, needs to be assessed with specific inquiries into:

- Cognitive abilities
- Mobility and environment including access to toilet
- ADL (activities of daily living)
- Level of support available to the incontinent person
- Potentially reversible conditions that can cause or worsen incontinence in older people
- Medication, particularly diuretics or drugs that cause sedation or confusion

➡ ***The extent of investigation*** and ***management*** in frail and/or disabled older people should take into account:

- Degree of bother to the patient and/or carer
- Patient motivation and level of cooperation
- Patient's comorbidities
- Prognosis and life expectancy

It is highly recommended that ***post-void residual urine (PVR)*** is assessed preferably by ultrasound or by in/out catheter. Impaired bladder emptying may occur in older women because of pelvic organ prolapse, constipation, underactive detrusor, medications that impair bladder emptying, or postoperatively. The PVR therefore is a significant factor that should influence the choice of management. There is no specific "cut off" for the different choices and the ranges listed below are provided as a broad guideline.

Stress incontinence may coexist in older women with most other bladder conditions. It is appropriate to perform a cough stress test.

2. Treatment

It is sometimes worthwhile to ***repeat the PVR*** especially in the intermediate ranges listed or when medications could impact on it.

Conservative and behavioural therapy includes pelvic floor muscle exercises, biofeedback, bladder training in the more fit or alert patient, assisted voiding for more disabled patients and prompted voiding for frailer and more cognitively impaired patients.

Bladder relaxant drugs may be considered as an adjunct to these conservative treatments of detrusor overactivity. When they are being tried, it is important to dose titrate from a low dose, reviewing outcome and side effects regularly.

When PVR is high (eg greater than 500ml) the upper tracts should be screened to exclude hydronephrosis. However, treatment of coexisting conditions may reduce PVR, e.g treatment of constipation and stopping drugs with anticholinergic action.

In those patients where the various therapies fail, the patient can achieve ***"dependent continence"*** by assistance or prompting, and/or ***social continence*** with pads and/or appliances.

B . Specialised Management

If after initial assessment the frail older person is found to have incontinence with other significant factors (eg pain, haematuria) then consideration should be given to further assessment and investigation by a specialist.

Referral for specialised management may also be applicable for individuals who have not responded adequately to simple conservative measures provided they are motivated and if such intervention and/or management might improve their continence management and quality of life. Age per se is not a contraindication to surgery for incontinence. However, in older people especially frail and/or disabled older people:

- ***Modifiable reversible conditions*** should be addressed prior to surgery
- Wherever possible, ***adequate trial of conservative treatment*** should be offered prior to surgery followed by reassessment of the need for surgery
- A ***urodynamic assessment*** should proceed surgery because clinical diagnosis may be inaccurate

Preoperative assessment plus perioperative care is essential to minimise postoperative geriatric complications such as delirium, infection, dehydration and falls.

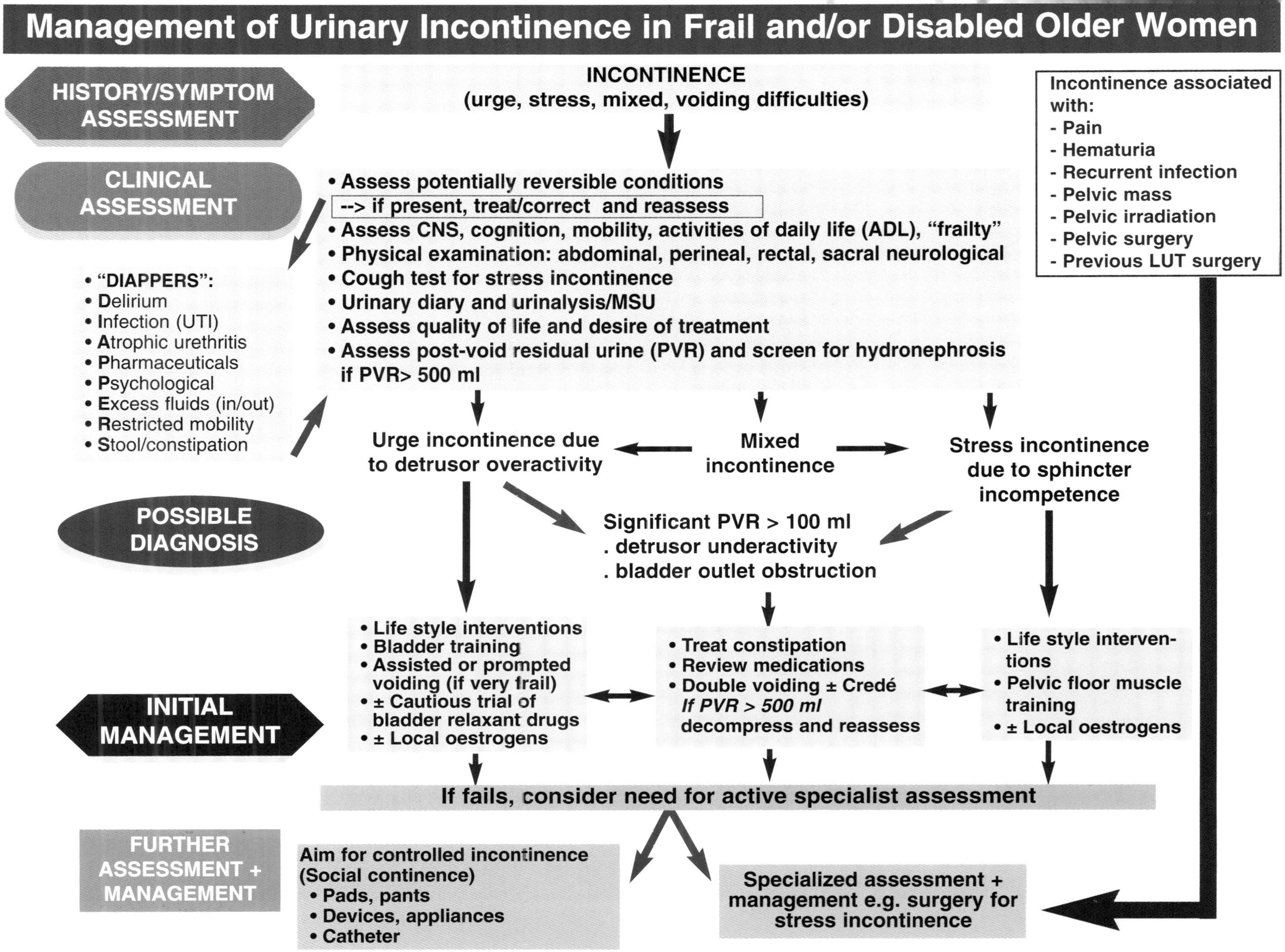

Management of Urinary Incontinence in Frail and/or Disabled Older Women

HISTORY/SYMPTOM ASSESSMENT

INCONTINENCE
(urge, stress, mixed, voiding difficulties)

Incontinence associated with:
- Pain
- Hematuria
- Recurrent infection
- Pelvic mass
- Pelvic irradiation
- Pelvic surgery
- Previous LUT surgery

CLINICAL ASSESSMENT

- Assess potentially reversible conditions
  --> if present, treat/correct and reassess
- Assess CNS, cognition, mobility, activities of daily life (ADL), "frailty"
- Physical examination: abdominal, perineal, rectal, sacral neurological
- Cough test for stress incontinence
- Urinary diary and urinalysis/MSU
- Assess quality of life and desire of treatment
- Assess post-void residual urine (PVR) and screen for hydronephrosis if PVR> 500 ml

- "DIAPPERS":
- **D**elirium
- **I**nfection (UTI)
- **A**trophic urethritis
- **P**harmaceuticals
- **P**sychological
- **E**xcess fluids (in/out)
- **R**estricted mobility
- **S**tool/constipation

POSSIBLE DIAGNOSIS

Urge incontinence due to detrusor overactivity

Mixed incontinence

Stress incontinence due to sphincter incompetence

Significant PVR > 100 ml
. detrusor underactivity
. bladder outlet obstruction

INITIAL MANAGEMENT

- Life style interventions
- Bladder training
- Assisted or prompted voiding (if very frail)
- ± Cautious trial of bladder relaxant drugs
- ± Local oestrogens

- Treat constipation
- Review medications
- Double voiding ± Credé
  If PVR > 500 ml decompress and reassess

- Life style interventions
- Pelvic floor muscle training
- ± Local oestrogens

If fails, consider need for active specialist assessment

FURTHER ASSESSMENT + MANAGEMENT

Aim for controlled incontinence
(Social continence)
- Pads, pants
- Devices, appliances
- Catheter

Specialized assessment + management e.g. surgery for stress incontinence

VIII. Management of faecal incontinence in adults

1. Initial assessment

Patients present with a ***variety of symptom complexes***.

Serious bowel pathology needs to be considered if the patient has a change in bowel habit or rectal bleeding.

History will include bowel symptoms, systemic disorders, local anorectal procedures, childbirth for women, medication, diet and effects of symptoms on lifestyle.

Examination will include anal inspection, abdominal palpation, a brief neurological examination, digital rectal examination and usually anoscopy and proctoscopy.

Two main symptoms are distinguished: urge faecal incontinence which is often a symptom of external anal sphincter dysfunction or intestinal hurry; and ***passive loss of stool*** may indicate internal anal sphincter dysfunction.

2. Initial management

➡ Once local or systemic pathology has been excluded, initial management includes

- patient information and education,
- diet and fluid advice, establishing a regular bowel habit with complete rectal evacuation and
- simple exercises to strengthen and enhance awareness of the anal sphincter.

➡ Anti-diarrhoeal medication can help if stools are loose.

➡ Initial management can often be performed in primary care. If this is failing to improve symptoms after 8-12 weeks, consideration should be given to referral for further investigations.

3. Investigations

A variety of anorectal investigations, including manometry, measurement of pudendal nerve terminal motor latencies, and anal ultrasound can help to define structural or functional abnormalities of anorectal function.

4. Specialised management

➡ ***Patients*** with a ***clearly disrupted external anal sphincter*** as seen on anal ultrasound often benefit from ***surgical sphincter repair,*** especially if the function of the remaining muscle is good.

➡ ***Those with sphincter disruption*** but ***poor function*** may achieve lesser results and should normally try ***conservative measures first.***

- "Biofeedback" therapy is usually a package of measures designed to enhance the patient's awareness of anorectal function, improve sphincter function and retrain the bowel habit.
- Electrical stimulation may help in selected cases.

➡ Products to manage ***severe faecal incontinence*** are ineffective in most cases. ***Severe faecal incontinence*** which ***fails to respond to management*** may lead to consideration of a novel surgical approach such as ***formation*** or ***implantation of a neosphincter***, ***sacral nerve stimulation,*** or ***formation of a colostomy.***

5. Special patient groups

The main chapter (refer) also gives algorithms for the management of ***third degree obstetric tears, soiling in children*** and faecal incontinence in ***older adults.***

Management of Faecal Incontinence

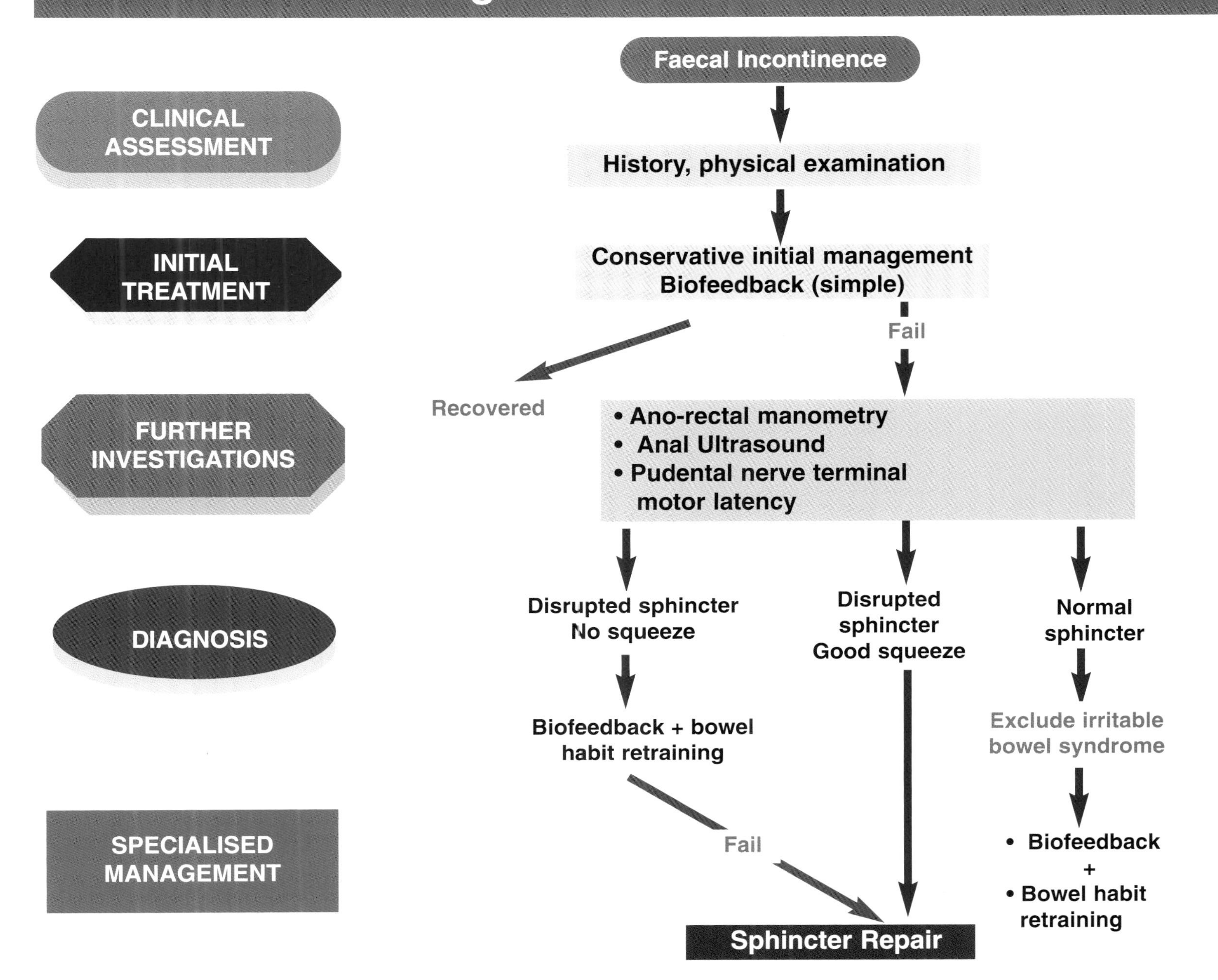

Faecal Incontinence
CLINICAL ASSESSMENT
History, physical examination
INITIAL TREATMENT
Conservative initial management
Biofeedback (simple)
Fail
Recovered
FURTHER INVESTIGATIONS
• Ano-rectal manometry
• Anal Ultrasound
• Pudental nerve terminal motor latency
DIAGNOSIS
Disrupted sphincter
No squeeze
Disrupted sphincter
Good squeeze
Normal sphincter
Biofeedback + bowel habit retraining
Exclude irritable bowel syndrome
Fail
SPECIALISED MANAGEMENT
Sphincter Repair
• Biofeedback
+
• Bowel habit retraining

IV. Recommendations for the Promotion, Education, and Organization for Continence Care

Progress has been made in the promotion of continence awareness, education of professionals and consumers, organization of the delivery of care and the delivery and public access to information on a worldwide basis. However, ***incontinence needs to be identified as a separate issue on the world health care agenda.*** All governments are encouraged to take an interest in and to support the development of continence services by actively planning policies and providing adequate funding. These should include a primary prevention strategy. For example, in developing countries with a high complication rate from childbirth, such prevention strategies could include ensuring that all births are attended by a qualified health care worker and also that there is access to secondary health care facilities for all in case of complications. The prevention strategy would include education in an attempt to prevent physically immature girls from becoming pregnant, as they have the highest incidence of complications.

The following are specific recommendations in three areas: promotion, education and organization

1. Promotion

Public awareness campaigns are essential in order to educate the public, break down taboos and to empower health-seeking behavior. The mass media, should wherever possible, be involved in raising public awareness.

Continence promotion should be ***health focused*** and ***use terminology***, which is understood by both the public and patient.

Public awareness campaigns could include ***increasing the visibility of the problem,*** advocate the need for research and evaluate the impact and efficacy of the program.

The Consultation supports the formation of a worldwide "Bladder Health" Day.

2. Education

The identification, assessment and management of incontinence must be a ***compulsory subject*** for all medical, nursing, and allied professional curricula and continuing education program. These programs should include basic principles of medical education that promotes change of knowledge, attitudes and behavior.

As professional education alone has not changed behavior, ***other tools are needed to augment*** or build on educational endeavors

3. Organization

The needs of service users (patients and carers) must be considered in planning continence services.

Continence services must be provided on a multi-disciplinary basis and proved a balance between community and specialist services.

Properly trained staff with the appropriate accreditation must deliver continence care.

Continence care should be based on ***agreed consensus recommendations.***

a) Delivery of Continence Services

The ***needs of service users*** (patients and carers) must be considered in planning continence services.

Continence services must be provided on a ***multi-disciplinary basis*** and provide a balance between community and specialist services.

National and regional ***service delivery models*** need to be developed and tested.

Properly ***trained professional staff*** with the appropriate supervision must deliver continence care.

Continence care should be based on ***agreed consensus recommendations***.

b) Worldwide Organization

Countries need to ***increase collaboration*** for use of scarce resources to further public awareness and education.

Organizations must undertake ***market research*** to better understand the needs of persons with incontinence; so as to ***set their own agenda and priorities*** rather than being led by the availability of funding.

Worldwide, countries are ***educating the public*** through self-help and support groups, telephone hotlines, Internet, brochures, and community outreach. These organizations, particularly the ***Continence Promotion Committee (CPC)*** of the ***International Continence Society (ICS)*** need to access marketing and public relation experts to broaden their efforts.

The CPC of ICS should be the ***central co-coordinating body*** to stimulate the collaboration of worldwide activity in the area of continence promotion.

V. Recommendations for Research

There are many goals of research—foremost to improve care of patients, but also to promote understanding of the disease process. We need a broad spectrum of information if we are to not only understand which treatments work but also how and why they work (or don't). The ultimate goal is to produce credible research. When research is inherently credible due to strong study design the impact is maximized. The clinical application of the research will be hastened and other investigators will be energized to use the information in their own quest for knowledge. Committee recommendations are reported as General recommendations for Incontinence Research, Recommendations for Specific Patient Groups, and Recommendations for Specific Types of Incontinence Therapy.

GENERAL RECOMMENDATIONS FOR CLINICAL RESEARCH IN INCONTINENCE

1. The first step of the planning phase involves reviewing previous and, if possible, ongoing work in the field. The work of the Cochrane Collaboration (www.cochrane.org) and its Cochrane Incontinence Group (www.otago.ac.nz/cure/) provide a tremendous asset to the potential investigator in defining the state of current knowledge and the key issues for further investigation.

2. Whenever possible, clinical research should be prospective, randomized, and multicenter. The randomized controlled trial (RCT) eliminates many of the biases that can corrupt research. While observational studies may be valuable in some areas, the bias that results from differential selection effects (both patient and clinician induced) cannot be eliminated, even by the use of advanced statistical methods. Multicenter trials involve a larger cross-section of the population and enhance the generalizability of the results.

3. Equivalence trials are underutilized. This design should be used to demonstrate that two treatments are similar in outcome or that there is no difference between treatment and controls. This can be of relevance when one treatment is significantly more cost-effective, offers a better quality of life, or is less toxic or time consuming for the patient when similar clinical outcome can be achieved. Failing to find a difference between two treatments is not the same as proving equivalence if this design is not used.

4. The study population should comprise a sample that is representative of the community overall—so that broad representativeness can be judged. This is as important for trials as for observational studies. Nevertheless, "the basic logic of clinical trials is comparative and not representative".

5. The Consolidated Standards of Reporting Trials (CONSORT) statement provides guidelines for reporting the design, detailed methods, and results of RCTs.

6. Specific outcome measures are discussed in detail by individual Committees. In almost all situations, the outcome set should include a dimension representing the viewpoint of the patient (such as a questionnaire relating to symptoms and impact on quality of life) as well as an appropriate clinical outcome measure.

7. Secondary outcomes and subgroup analysis are subject to the dangers of multiple hypothesis testing. Such measures should be defined at the outset of the trial and should be used sparingly. Analyses of such outcomes are often best viewed as exploratory, i.e., as hypothesis-generating exercises for which independent confirmation is essential.

8. Inclusion and exclusion criteria should provide a relevant population to address the study question, and together define the heterogeneity or homogeneity of the study population. Broadening the inclusion criteria can make a study more generalizable and facilitate recruitment. Making the entry criteria too broad, however, may dilute the effect being sought in the most suitable patients. If the study population is defined too narrowly with many exclusion criteria, applicability of the results may be limited and subject recruitment may be difficult. The committee feels that clinical incontinence research is in great need of more large-scale RCTs in almost all areas. Broad entry criteria to include as many patients as possible are desirable.

9. The *target difference* is arguably the most important quantity that must be specified in calculating sample size. The target difference is defined as the minimum difference needed for clinical significance, a difference that would lead to a change in clinical management for the target group of patients. This must be specified in the planning phase of the research.

10. It is established practice that unless there are strong reasons to the contrary the primary analyses (for both primary and secondary outcomes) of an RCT should be on an intention-to-treat basis. It may be of interest to gauge the effect of treatment given full com-

pliance, so secondary analyses incorporating non-compliance and/or which treatment was actually received may be justified in addition to the primary analyses.

11. The CONSORT statement is specifically designed to provide standards for reporting RCTs. Adherence to these guidelines and the use of flow diagrams in particular is associated with improved quality in reporting of RCTs. Meta-analyses are themselves the subject of separate reporting guidelines, the QUORUM statement. Guidelines for reporting studies on diagnostic tests (the START document) will be published in 2001.

12. Recommendations for minimum data collection in clinical research are published in the proceedings of the NIH Terminology Workshop for Researchers in Female Pelvic Floor Disorders and by the International Continence Society (ICS) Standardization committee. A broad demographic description of the patient population is desirable; while few trials will be large enough to analyze the effect of these demographic factors on outcome, the potential use of meta-analysis makes a complete database valuable.

13. One or more validated symptom instruments should be chosen at the outset of a clinical trial to accurately define baseline symptoms and other areas in which the treatment may produce an effect. An ideal instrument would record all symptoms related to the lower urinary tract and relevant associated organ systems—gastrointestinal and sexual function are particularly important. An ideal instrument would record both the objective severity of the symptom and the impact or bother produced by the presence of the symptom. In addition to specific symptoms, the respondent's overall opinion of the condition should be included. Research in incontinence and LUTS should include both generic and condition-specific HRQOL instruments.

14. Clinicians' observations of anatomy, particularly female pelvic support, should be recorded using standardized, reproducible measurements. Pelvic muscle and voluntary sphincter function should be reported using a quantifiable scale. These measures should be repeated after intervention and correlated with primary clinical outcome measures.

15. Clinical trials of incontinence and LUTS should include bladder diaries as an essential baseline and outcome measure. The diary should include measured voided volume (for at least one day if a multi-day diary is employed).

16. Clinical trials of incontinence and LUTS should include a pad test as an essential baseline and outcome measure.

17. Most clinical studies should enroll subjects by carefully defined symptoms, not urodynamic tests (UDS). Blinded baseline UDS are highly desirable in order to determine their predictive value. In the ideal clinical study, urodynamic tests are performed at baseline and exit to correlate symptom changes with physiologic changes. In multicenter trials, urodynamic tests should be interpreted by a central reader to minimize bias.

18. Follow-up of incontinence treatment is suggested at 1 to 3 months and 12 months after treatment, and thereafter at yearly intervals for as long as possible.

19. Socioeconomic data can be an important outcome measure and should be collected whenever possible.

RECOMMENDATIONS FOR SPECIFIC PATIENT GROUPS

1. In males, if treatment could change prostate volume, measurements of volume should be performed before and after treatment. It may be appropriate to stratify patients by prostate volume. Whenever feasible, detrusor pressure-uroflow studies should be performed before and after treatment to document the presence and degree of change in bladder outlet obstruction.

2. Significantly more research is needed in the frail elderly population. This is a heterogeneous population requiring a detailed study design and careful description of baseline clinical data if results are to be interpretable. There is a need for validation of all instruments and procedures used in incontinence research for the population of frail elderly patients. "Clinically significant" outcome measures and relationships of outcome to socioeconomic costs are critically important to establishing the utility of treating urinary incontinence in this population.

3. We support increased clinical research in children. All investigators that work with children should be aware of the details of the document and particularly the issues surrounding informed consent. Long-term follow-up is of critical importance in the pediatric population in order to ascertain the effect of a treatment on normal growth and development. Research is needed to develop standardized outcome measures including validated, age-specific symptom and disease-specific quality of life outcome measures.

4. Detailed urodynamic studies are required for classi-

fication of neurogenic lower urinary tract disorders in research studies because the nature of the lower tract dysfunction cannot be accurately predicted from clinical data. Change in detrusor leak point pressure should be reported as an outcome as appropriate, and can be considered a primary outcome in addition to symptom response.

RECOMMDATIONS FOR SPECIFIC TYPES OF INCONTINENCE RESEARCH

1. Treatment protocols in behavioral and physiotherapy trials must be detailed to the degree that the work can easily be reproduced. More work is needed to separate the specific and non-specific effects of treatment
2. The United States Food and Drug Administration (FDA) had established detailed guidelines for studies on intra-urethral and vaginal devices and urethral bulking agents in the treatment of urinary incontinence. However, these treatments are not intrinsically similar and the guidelines should be refined such that recommendations are appropriate to the risk involved in the treatment.
3. In pharmacotherapy trials, investigators must be sensitive to the conflicts regarding the use of placebos in clinical trials. While placebos are often desirable from a scientific standpoint, every consideration should be given to making sure that the interests of the subjects are kept at the forefront in designing safe, ethical research.
4. Continuity in clinical direction from design through authorship is highly desirable. All authors should be able to accept responsibility for the published work and all potential conflicts of interest should be fully disclosed.
5. There is a great need for randomized clinical trials in surgical treatment of urinary incontinence. We recommend urodynamic testing in all subjects involved in surgical research. However, evidence does not exist to support recommendations for minimal testing or the use of specific tests. Research into the predictive value of pre-operative urodynamic studies would be most valuable.
6. Reports of successful treatment should be limited to subjects with a minimum of one year follow-up.

SUMMARY

In summary,

- All quality research, be it prospective or retrospective, clinical or preclinical, begins with detailed planning—establishing a clear and relevant hypothesis, developing a trial of appropriate magnitude to accept or reject the hypothesis, and defining methods of adequate sensitivity and specificity to produce credible data.
- Clinical research in incontinence must include a broad range of baseline and outcome measures including anatomic and physiologic variables, urodynamic testing, voiding diaries and pad tests, symptom assessment, and quality of life measures. Economic outcome assessment should be included whenever possible. In each area, data must be collected using structured, reproducible methodology. Symptom assessment and other instruments must be validated for the population being studied.
- The CONSORT statement should be adopted as criteria for publication of randomized clinical trials by researchers, reviewers, and editors.
- Baseline urodynamic assessment is required in the neurogenic population and recommended in surgical trials. However, baseline urodynamic studies are highly desirable in all types of incontinence research. There is a great need to critically examine the predictive value of urodynamic testing in order to refine our tools as well as the diagnosis and treatment of patients.
- The primary goal of clinical research is to improve the care of patients; the ultimate goal is to understand the nature of disease and how treatments actually work. We can make this progress by collecting comprehensive baseline and follow-up data, and correlating outcome to baseline characteristics and observed changes during treatment.

Annex 1 : Bladder Charts and Diaries

Three types of Bladder Charts and Diaries can be used to collect data :-

Micturition Time Chart

- times of voiding and
- incontinence episodes

Frequency Volume Chart

- times of voiding with voided volumes measured,
- incontinence episodes and number of changes of incontinence pads or clothing.

Bladder Diaries

- the information above, but also
- assessments of urgency,
- degree of leakage (slight, moderate or large) and descriptions of factors leading to symptoms such as stress leakage, eg. running to catch a bus

It is important to assess the ***individual's fluid intake,*** remembering that fluid intake includes fluids drunk plus the water content of foods eaten. It is often necessary to explain to a patient with LUTS that it may be important to change the timing of a meal and the type of food eaten, particularly in the evenings, in order to avoid troublesome nocturia.

The micturition time and frequency volumes charts can be collected on a single sheet of paper (Fig. 1). In each chart/diary, the time the individual got out of bed in the morning and the time they went to bed at night should be clearly indicated.

Each chart/diary must be accompanied by clear instructions for the individual who will complete the chart/diary: the language used must be simple as in the suggestions given for patient instructions. There are a variety of designs of charts and diaries and examples of a detailed bladder diary are given. The number of days will vary from a single day up to one week.

INSTRUCTIONS FOR COMPLETING THE MICTURITION TIME CHART

This chart helps you and us to understand why you get trouble with your bladder. The diary is a very important part of the tests we do, so that we can try to improve your symptoms. On the chart you need to record :-

1. When you get out of bed in the morning, show this on the diary by writing ***'GOT OUT OF BED'.***
2. The ***time***, eg. 7.30am, ***when you pass your urine***. Do this every time you pass urine throughout the day and also at night if you have to get up to pass urine.
3. If you leak urine, show this by writing a 'W' (wet) on the diary at the time you leaked
4. When you go to bed at the end of the day show it on the diary - write ***'WENT TO BED'***.

INSTRUCTIONS FOR USING THE FREQUENCY VOLUME CHART

This chart helps you and us to understand why you get trouble with your bladder. The diary is a very important part of the tests we do, so that we can try to improve your symptoms. On the chart you need to record:-

1. When you get out of bed in the morning, show this on the chart by writing ***'GOT OUT OF BED'.***
2. The ***time,*** eg. 7.30am ***when you pass your urine***. Do this every time you pass urine throughout the day and also at night if you have to get up to pass urine.
3. Each time you pass urine, ***collect the urine*** in a measuring jug and ***record the amount*** (in mls or fluid ozs) next to the time you passed the urine, eg. 1.30pm - 320 mls.
4. ***If you leak urine,*** show this by writing 'W' (wet) on the diary at the time.
5. If you have a leak, please a***dd 'P'*** if you have to change a pad and ***'C'*** if you have to change your underclothes or even outer clothes. So, if you leak and need to change a pad, please write 'WP' at the time you leaked.
6. At the end of each day please write in the column on the right the ***number of pads you have used,*** or the ***number of times you have changed clothes.***
7. When you go to bed at the end of the day show it on the diary - write ***'Went to Bed'***

INSTRUCTIONS FOR USING THE BLADDER DIARY

This diary helps you and us to understand why you get trouble with your bladder. The diary is a very important part of the tests we do, so that we can try to improve your symptoms. On the chart you need to record :-

1. When you get out of bed in the morning, show this on the diary by writing ***'GOT OUT OF BED'.***
2. During the day please enter at the ***correct time the drinks you have during the day,*** eg. 8.00am - two cups of coffee (total 400 ml).
3. The ***time you pass your urine***, eg. 7.30am. Do this every time you pass urine throughout the day and night.
4. Each time you pass urine, collect the urine in a measuring jug and ***record the amount*** (in mls or fluid ozs) next to the time you passed the urine, eg. 1.30pm/320ml.
5. Each time you pass your urine, please write down ***how urgent was the need*** to pass urine:

'O' means it was not urgent.

+ means I had to go within 10 minutes.

++ means I had to stop what I was doing and go to the toilet.

6. ***If you leak urine,*** show this by writing an 'W' on the diary at the time you leaked.
7. If you have a leak, please add **'P'** if you have to change a pad and **'C'** if you have to change your underclothes or even outer clothes. So if you leak and need to change a pad, please write 'WP' at the time you leaked.
8. If you have a leakage please write in the column called 'Comments' whether you ***leaked a small amount*** or a ***large amount*** and ***what you were doing when you leaked,*** eg. 'leaked small amount when I sneezed three times'.
9. Each time you ***change a pad*** or ***change clothes,*** please write in the 'Comments' column.
10. When you go to bed at the end of the day show it on the diary - ***write 'Went to Bed'.***

Fig 1 : FREQUENCY / VOLUME CHART - STANDARD VERSION - 7 DAYS

Name: ______________________________

Date	**7:00 am Mid-day Midnight 6:00am**	**Pads used**

No. of drinks per day: ___________________

Fig. 2 : BLADDER DIARY Detailed version - one day

Name: ______________________ **Date:** ________________________

Urine passed Time/Amount	**Urgency?**	**Leakage?**	**Comments ?**	**Drinks - time, type and amount**
6:00 am 12:00 noon 6:00 pm 12:00 midnight				

Frequency - Volume chart - Standard Version - 7 days

Name: Pierre Smith

Date	7:00 am Mid-day Midnight 6:00am	Pads used
16th APRIL	UP 150 200 50 250 275 200 150 BED 2.30 5.30 7.30 7.30 9.30 WC 11.00 3.00 6.00 9.30 11.45 12 270 250	1
17th	UP 260 210 230 150 220 250 50 BED 275 200 7.30 10.00 1.00 3.30 7.30 9.30 11 11 1.30 4.00	0
18th	UP 300 150 200 275 100 150 175 125 BED 400 7.00 9.00 11.15 2.15 4.15 6.30 8.00 10.30 11 4.30	0
19th	UP 250 300 310 75 200 50 250 BED 260 220 200 7.30 10.30 2.15 3.00 W 5.50 9.00 10.15 10.30 12.00 2.30 5.00	0
20th	UP 150 250 275 175 200 250 100 100 BED 350 7.30 10.30 2.00 4.30 7.15 9.45 11.00 0.45 1 5.00	0
21st	UP 200 100 175 75 200 220 300 BED 200 350 300 8 9.00 WC 11.00 11.45 2.30 5.30 7.30 10 3.30 6.00	1
22nd	UP 150 220 150 290 300 110 150 BED 350 7.30 9.30 11.00 2.15 5.00 7.00 WC 9.30 11 (200) 4.30	1

No. of drinks per day: 7

BLADDER DIARY Detailed version - one day

Name: Maria Schmidt **Date:** 18th April 1998

	Urine passed Time	Amount	Urgency?	Leakage?	Comments?	Drinks - time, type and amount
	6:00 am					
GOT UP	7.15	200	0	–		800 – 2 cups coffee 400mls.
	7.30	100	+	–		
	11.30	275	++	W	Wet pants	11.00 can coke
	12:00 noon					
	12.30	150	+	–		12.30 1 glass water – 250mls
	3.00	220	0	–		3.30
	3.45	–	–	W	sneezed 3 times	cup tea – 200ml
	5.30	175	0	–		
	6:00 pm					6.30 glass water – 250mls.
	7.45	200	–	–		8.00 glass wine – 100 mls
	9.30	175	–	–		
BED	10.30	100	–	–		10.00 mug cocoa – 250ml
	12:00 midnight					
	3.30	250	–	–		

Annex 2 : ICIQ-SF

Initial number ☐☐ ☐☐ ☐☐☐

DAY ☐☐ MONTH ☐☐ YEAR ☐☐

Today's date

Many people leak urine some of the time. We are trying to find out how many people leak urine, and how much this bothers them. We would be grateful if you could answer the following questions, thinking about how you have been, on average, over the PAST FOUR WEEKS.

1 **Please write in your date of birth:** DAY ☐☐ MONTH ☐☐ YEAR ☐☐

2 **Are you** *(tick one)*: Female ☐ Male ☐

3 **How often do you leak urine?** *(Tick one box)*

never	☐	0
about once a week or less often	☐	1
two or three times a week	☐	2
about once a day	☐	3
several times a day	☐	4
all the time	☐	5

4 **We would like to know how much urine you think leaks.**
How much urine do you usually leak (whether you wear protection or not)? *(Tick one box)*

none	☐	0
a small amount	☐	2
a moderate amount	☐	4
a large amount	☐	6

5 **Overall, how much does leaking urine interfere with your everyday life?**
Please ring a number between 0 (not at all) and 10 (a great deal)

0 1 2 3 4 5 6 7 8 9 **10**

not at all — a great deal

ICIQ score: sum scores 3+4+5 ☐☐

6 **When does urine leak?** *(Please tick all that apply to you)*

never – urine does not leak	☐
leaks before you can get to the toilet	☐
leaks when you cough or sneeze	☐
leaks when you are asleep	☐
leaks when you are physically active/exercising	☐
leaks when you have finished urinating and are dressed	☐
leaks for no obvious reason	☐
leaks all the time	☐

Thank you very much for answering these questions.

INDEX

Indexer: Dr Laurence Errington
E-mail : laurence@errington-index.demon.co.uk

Abreviations: AI (or FI), anal (faecal) incontinence; BOO, bladder outlet obstruction; EMG, electromyography; LUT, lower urinary tract; QoL, quality of life; SEP, somatosensory evoked potentials; UI, urinary incontinence.

(Typesetter. Please retain indexer's name at top of printed index, subject to publisher's approval.)

A

B

D

E

F

G

H

I

J

M

N

Q

R

S

U

V

W

X

Y

Incontinence

2nd International Consultation on Incontinence Paris, July 1-3, 2001

2nd Edition 2002

ORDER FORM

Order from : **Plymbridge Distributors Ltd**
Estover Road, Plymouth PL6 7PY, United Kingdom
Customer Services : Tel. : +44 1752 202301 - Fax: +44 1752 202333
E-mail: cservs@plymbridge.com

ISBN	Author/Title (MRn°)	Quantity	Unit Price	total
1 898452 55 5	- Book "INCONTINENCE" 2nd Edition 2002		£ 100	
	- CD Rom "INCONTINENCE 2nd Edition 2002		£ 70	
	- BOOK + CD Rom		£ 120	

Mailing costs

	BOOK or Book + CD Rom	CD Rom alone
U.K	£ 5	£ 1.50
Europe	£ 14	£ 2

Sub total ________

Shipping ________

Total Enclosed ________

USA - BOOK or Book+ CD Rom
Surface £ 12 ❑ - Air £ 22 ❑ - DHL £26 ❑

USA - CD Rom alone
Surface £ 2 ❑ - Air £ 4 ❑ - DHL £ 13 ❑

REST OF THE WORLD
BOOKor Book + CD Rom £ 27 AIR ❑
CD Rom alone £ 4 AIR ❑

________ ***Cheque enclosed*** : Cheque must be drawn ***in sterling*** on a UK clearing Bank

________ ***Charge to*** : ❑ Visa ❑ MasterCard ❑ American Express

Card Number : ________________________ Exp Date : ____________

Name on the Card : ________________________ Issue Number: ____________

Signature : ____________________

Name : ____

Address (in full) : ____

____

____

Telephone N°: ____________________ Fax N°: ____________________

________________________________ Please print your name and

________________________________ address in **CAPITAL LETTERS**